General
&
Applied
Toxicology

ABRIDGED EDITION

General & Applied Toxicology

ABRIDGED EDITION

BRYAN
BALLANTYNE

■

TIMOTHY
MARRS

■

PAUL
TURNER

MACMILLAN

First published in 1993 in two volumes as
General and Applied Toxicology
by THE MACMILLAN PRESS LTD
London and Basingstoke

Hardcover ISBN: 0-333-49801-1 (two volumes)

Published in the United States and Canada by
STOCKTON PRESS, New York, 1993

Hardcover ISBN: 1-56159-107-6 (two volumes)

Abridged edition first published in the United Kingdom as
General and Applied Toxicology Abridged Edition
by MACMILLAN PRESS LTD, 1995
Brunel Road, Houndmills
Basingstoke, Hants RG21 2XS, England
Companies and representatives throughout the world.

Hardcover ISBN: 0-333-63166-8 (one volume)

Abridged edition published in the United States and Canada as
General and Applied Toxicology College Edition
by STOCKTON PRESS, 1995
49 West 24th Street, New York, N.Y. 10010, USA

Hardcover ISBN: 1-56159-167-X (one volume)

A catalogue record for this book is available from the British Library

10   9   8   7   6   5   4   3   2   1
04   03   02   01   00   99   98   97   96   95

Typeset by Input Typesetting Ltd, Wimbledon.
Printed in Great Britain by The Bath Press, Avon.

Contents

v

Preface

We were gratified by the reception and reviews given to *General and Applied Toxicology*, the parent edition of this volume. The stated objectives of the two-volume textbook were to give a comprehensive review of the scientific basis of toxicology and its applications, and to be used as a reference volume and a text for educational purposes. The first two objectives, according to remarks from colleagues, appear to have been achieved. However, because of reasons of cost and extensive coverage, the larger two-volume work was considered inappropriate to recommend for purchase by students. In view of this, and in response to comments by certain reviewers and requests by various academic departments, it was decided to revise the format of *General and Applied Toxicology*, and to issue the modified version as a soft covered text which we believe will find a better niche for educational purposes. Revisions have included omitting certain specialist chapters and including, in each chapter, a list of further reading. Contrary to the misconception of a few reviewers of *General and Applied Toxicology*, it was not intended to be a compendium of the toxicology of individual materials. This has been more than adequately covered by texts such as Volume 2 of *Patty's Industrial Hygiene and Toxicology*. Our text deals with principles.

The overall aim of this college version remains to present a comprehensive review of the scientific basis of toxicology and its applications. Coverage includes basic principles, definitions, laboratory aspects, interpretation, practical applications, and specialist considerations. Sections devoted to alternatives to whole animal testing and to ethical issues have been retained. We believe that this volume will be of use to those working for a first or higher degree in toxicology, and of value to those taking courses where toxicology is an important component.

During the preparation of this edition, we have received the utmost encouragement and guidance from Mrs. Rosemary Foster of Macmillan UK and Mr. Charles Regan of Stockton Press, USA.

Bryan Ballantyne
Danbury, Connecticut, USA

Timothy C. Marrs
London, UK

Paul Turner
London, UK

Contributors

G. E. Adams, PhD, DSc, FACR
Medical Research Council Radiobiology Unit, Chilton, Didcot, Oxford OX11 0RD, UK

Paul N. Adams, MB, BS, BDS, LRCP, MRCS, LDS (RCS), MFPM
Consultant in Pharmaceutical Medicine, 24 Greenhayes Avenue, Banstead, Surrey SM7 2JE, UK

John A. L. Amess, MB, FRCP, FRCPath
Department of Haematology, St Bartholomew's Hospital, West Smithfield, London EC1A 7BE, UK

Diana Anderson, BSc, MSc, PhD, DipEd, FIBiol, FRCPath, FIFST, FATS
BIBRA Toxicology International, Woodmansterne Road, Carshalton, Surrey SM5 4DS, UK

Janet Athis, BSc, PhD, MIBiol
Zeneca Central Toxicology Laboratory, Alderley Park, Macclesfield, Cheshire SK10 4TJ, UK

Ronald C. Backer, PhD, DABFT
Harrison and Associates Forensic Laboratories, 606 North Weatherford, Midland, Texas 79701, USA

Bryan Ballantyne, MD, DSc, PhD, FFOM, FACOM, FAACT, FATS, FRCPath, FIBiol
Applied Toxicology Group, Union Carbide Corporation, 39 Old Ridgebury Road, Danbury, Connecticut 06817, USA

Steven I. Baskin, PharmD, PhD, FCP, FACC, DABT
Biochemical Pharmacology Division, US Army Medical Research Institute of Chemical Defense, Aberdeen Proving Ground, Maryland 21010–5425, USA

D. Nicholas Bateman, BSc, MD, FRCP
The Wolfson Unit of Clinical Pharmacology, Claremont Place, University of Newcastle-upon-Tyne NE1 7RU, UK

Ian P. Bennett, MPhil
BIRAL, P.O. Box 2, Portishead, Bristol BS20 9JB, UK

Peter N. Bennett, MD, FRCP
School of Postgraduate Medicine, University of Bath, Wolfson Centre, Royal United Hospital, Bath BA1 3NG, UK

Sir Colin Berry, *KBE*, DSc, MD, PhD, FRCPath, FRCP, FFPM
Department of Morbid Anatomy, The Royal London Hospital, London E1 1BB, UK

C. Bouchard, PhD
Laboratoire de Cytologie, Universite Pierre et Marie Curie, Institut des Neurosciences, CNRS URA 1488, 75005 Paris, France

Joan M. Braganza, MB, MSc, FRCP
University Department of Medicine (Gastroenterology), Royal Infirmary, Manchester M13 9WL, UK

Lisa P. Brown, BSc, PhD
Consultant, 24 Highlands Heath, Bristol Gardens, Putney Heath, London SW15 3TR, UK

Heather D. Burleigh-Flayer, PhD
Bushy Run Research Center, 6702 Mellon Road, Export, Pennsylvania 15632, USA

John Caldwell, BPharm, PhD, DSc, CBiol, FIBiol
Department of Pharmacology and Toxicology, St. Mary's Hospital Medical School, London W2 1PG, UK

Mary Ellen Clinton, MD
Department of Neurology, School of Medicine, Vanderbilt University, Nashville, Tennessee 37212, USA

David M. Conning, MB, FRCPath, FIBiol, FIFST
The British Nutrition Foundation, High Holborn House, 52–54 High Holborn, London WC1V 6RQ, UK

P. F. D'Arcy, *OBE*, BPharm, PhD, DSc, FRPharmS, FRSC, FPSNI
Professor Emeritus, School of Pharmacy, The Queen's University of Belfast, Medical Biology Centre, 97 Lisburn Road, Belfast BT9 7BL, Northern Ireland, UK

Judith Deschamps, ALA, MI InfSc
Library, Department of the Environment, 2 Marsham Street, London SW1P 3EB, UK

Wolf-D Dettbarn, MD
Departments of Pharmacology and Neurology, School of Medicine, Vanderbilt University, 2100 Pierce Avenue, Nashville, Tennessee 37212, USA

G. E. Diggle, MB, BS, FFPM, Dip Pharm Med
Department of Health, Skipton House, 80 London Road, London SE1 6LW, UK

G. O. Evans, BSc, MSc
Drug Safety Evaluation, Welcome Research Laboratories, Beckenham, Kent BR3 3BS, UK

Andrew Forge, BSc, MSc, PhD
Institute of Laryngology and Otology, University College London Medical School, 330–332 Gray's Inn Road, London WC1X 8EE, UK

Shayne, C. Gad, PhD, DABT
Becton Dickinson, 21 Davis Drive, Research Triangle Park, North Carolina 27709, USA

Paul Grasso, BSc, MD, FRCPath, DCP, DTM&H
Robens Institute, University of Surrey, Surrey GU2 5XH, UK

P. Greaves, MB, FRCPath
Zeneca Pharmaceuticals, Safety of Medicines Department, Alderley Park, Macclesfield, Cheshire SK10 4TG, UK

Ernest S. Harpur, BSc, PhD, MRPharmS
Sterling Winthrop Pharmaceuticals Division, Sterling Winthrop Research Centre, Willowburn Avenue, Alnwick, Northumberland NE66 2JH, UK

Steven J. Hermansky, MS, Pharm D, PhD
Bushy Run Research Center, 6702 Mellon Road, Export, Pennsylvania 15632, USA

Paul M. Hext, BSc, PhD
Zeneca Central Toxicology Laboratory, Alderley Park, Macclesfield, Cheshire SK10 4TJ, UK

R. H. Hinton, BA, PhD, MRCPath
School of Biological Sciences, University of Surrey, Guildford, Surrey GU2 5XH, UK

H. P. A. Illing, PhD, FIBiol, FRSC
Health and Safety Executive, Magdelen House, Stanley Precinct, Bootle, Merseyside L20 3QZ, UK

Sam Kacew, PhD
Department of Pharmacology, University of Ottawa, 451 Smythe Road, Ottawa, Ontario KIH 8M5, Canada

James P. Kehrer, PhD
Division of Pharmacology and Toxicology, College of Pharmacy, University of Texas, Austin, Texas 78712, USA

A. B. G. Lansdown, BSc, PhD, FRCPath, CBiol, FIBiol
Department of Comparative Biology, Charing Cross and Westminster Medical School, London W6 8RP, UK

J. M. Lefauconnier, MD
INSERM U26, Hopital Fernand Widal, 200 rue du Faubourg St Denis, 75475 Paris, Cedex 10, France

Hon-Wing Leung, PhD, DABT, CIH
Applied Toxicology Group, Union Carbide Corporation, 39 Old Ridgebury Road, Danbury, Connecticut 06817, USA

Hilton C. Lewinsohn, MB, FFOM, FCCP, FACOEM, DIH
Center for Occupational and Environmental Health, P.O. Box 1050, 108 High Street, Exeter, New Hampshire 03833, USA

Edward A. Lock, MIBiol, PhD, FRCPath
Zeneca Central Toxicology Laboratory, Alderley Park, Macclesfield, Cheshire SK10 4TJ, UK

Edward U. Maduh, BPharm, MSc, PhD, RPh
Biochemical Pharmacology Division, US Army
Medical Research Institute of Chemical Defense,
Aberdeen Proving Ground, Maryland 21010–
5425, USA

Ronald D. Mann, MD, FRCP, FRCGP, FFPM,
FCP
Director of The Drug Safety Research Unit, Bur-
lesden Hall, Southampton SO3 8BA, UK

Timothy C. Marrs, MD, DSc, FRCPath, FIBiol,
DipTox RCPath
Department of Health, Skipton House, 80
London Road, London SE1 6LW, UK

A. David Martin, BSc, PhD
Pesticides Safety Directorate, Ministry of Agriculture, Fisheries and Food, Rothamsted, Har-
penden, Hertfordshire AL5 2SS, UK

Robert L. Maynard, BSc, MB, BCh, MRCPath,
FIBiol
Department of Health, Skipton House, 80
London Road, London SE1 6LW, UK

Patricia R. McElhatton, MSc, PhD, MIBiol,
CBiol
Department of Pharmacology and Toxicology,
UMDS, St. Thomas's Hospital, London SE1
7EH, UK

Douglas B. McGregor, PhD, FRCPath, FIBiol
Unit of Carcinogen Identification and Evaluation,
International Association for Research on
Cancer, 150 cours Albert-Thomas, 69372 Lyon,
Cedex, France

C. Meredith, MA, MSc, PhD
Immunotoxicology Department, BIBRA Toxi-
cology International, Woodmansterne Road,
Carshalton, Surrey SM5 4DS, UK

Klara Miller, MSc, PhD, FRCPath
BIBRA Toxicology International, Woodmansterne Road, Carshalton, Surrey SM5 4DS, UK

Karl E. Misulis, MD, PhD
Department of Neurology and Pharmacology,
School of Medicine, Vanderbilt University, Nash-
ville, Tennessee, USA

David J. Morgan, BA, ALA, MI InfSc
Library, Ministry of Agriculture, Fisheries and
Food, 3 Whitehall Place, London SW1A 2HH,
UK

James C. Norris, PhD
Bushy Run Research Center, 6702 Mellon Road,
Export, Pennsylvania 15632–8902

Frederick W. Oehme, DVM, PhD
Comparative Toxicology Laboratories, College of
Veterinary Medicine, Kansas State University,
Manhattan, Kansas 68506, USA

Alan J. Paine, BSc, PhD, MRCPath
Department of Toxicology, St. Bartholomew's
Hospital, London EC1A 7ED, UK

Dennis J. Paustenbach, PhD, CIH, DABT
McLaren/Hart ChemRisk, 1135 Atlantic Avenue,
Alameda, California 94501, USA

J. M. Ratcliffe, BSc, MSc, PhD
Department of Epidemiology, School of Public
Health, University of North Carolina, CB7400,
McGavaran-Greenberg Building, Chapel Hill,
North Carolina 275990–7400, USA

A. G. Renwick, BSc, PhD, DSc
Clinical Pharmacology Group, University of
Southampton, Southampton SO9 3TU, UK

Christopher Rhodes, BSc, PhD, FRSC, CChem,
FIBiol, DipTox RCPath
Zeneca Pharmaceuticals Group, Zeneca Inc.,
Wilmington, Delaware 19897, USA

Wilson K. Rumbeiha, BVM, PhD
Comparative Toxicology Laboratories, College of
Veterinary Medicine, Kansas State University,
Manhattan, Kansas 66506, USA

Michael D. Stonard, BSc, PhD
Zeneca Central Toxicology Laboratory, Alderley
Park, Macclesfield, Cheshire SK10 4TJ, UK

T. R. Stiles, MBA
Department of Quality Assurance, Huntingdon
Research Centre Ltd., Cambridgeshire PE18
6ES, UK

Frank M. Sullivan, BSc
Department of Pharmacology and Toxicology, UMDS, St. Thomas's Hospital, London SE1 7EH, UK

M. G. Thomas, BSc, CBiol, MIBiol
Senior Toxicologist, BP Oil, Product Stewardship Group, Oil Technology Centre, Chertsey Road, Sunbury-on-Thames, Middlesex TW16 7LN, UK

John A. Thomas, BS, MA, PhD, DipATS
Department of Pharmacology and Toxicology, Health Science Center, University of Texas, 7703 Floyd Curl Drive, San Antonio 78284–7722, USA

John A. Timbrell, BSc, PhD, MRCPath, FRSC, FIBiol
Toxicology Department, School of Pharmacy, University of London, London WC1N 1AX, UK

John A. Tomenson, BSc, Dip Stat Cantab, PhD
ICI Epidemiology Unit, Alderley Park, Macclesfield, Cheshire SK10 4TJ, UK

Paul Turner, CBE, MD, BSc, FRCP, FFPM
Department of Clinical Pharmacology, St. Bartholomew's Hospital, London EC1A 7BE, UK

D. J. Tweats, CBiol, BSc, PhD, FIBiol
Genetic and Reproductive Toxicology Department, Glaxo Group Research Ltd, Ware SG12 0DP, UK

Rochelle W. Tyl, PhD, DABT
Center for Life Sciences and Toxicology, Research Triangle Institute, Herman Building, 3040 Cornwallis Road, Research Triangle Park, North Carolina 27709–2194, USA

Tipton R. Tyler, MS, PhD, DABT
Applied Toxicology Group, Union Carbide Corporation, 39 Old Ridgebury Road, Danbury, Connecticut 06817, USA

D. W. Vere, MD, FRCP, FFPM
Department of Therapeutics, London Hospital Medical College, Turner Street, London E1 2AD, UK

David Walker, BVSc, MIBiol, FRCVS
APT Consultancy, Old Hawthorn Farm, Hawthorn Lane, Four Marks, Alton, Hampshire, UK

Robert Waller, BSc
Health Aspects of Environment and Food Division, Department of Health, Skipton House, 80 London Road, London SE1 6LW, UK

Gregory P. Wedin, PharmD, ABAT
Wedin Drug Inc., 1123 Hennepin Avenue North, Glencoe, Minnesota 55336, USA

Angela Wilson, PhD
Medical Research Council Radiobiology Unit, Chilton, Didcot, Oxford OX11 0RD, UK

PART ONE: INTRODUCTION AND BASIC CONCEPTS

1 Fundamentals of Toxicology

Bryan Ballantyne, Timothy C. Marrs and Paul Turner

INTRODUCTION

Toxicology, essentially concerned with addressing the potentially harmful effects of chemicals, is a recognized scientific and medical discipline encompassing a very large number of basic and applied issues. Although only generally accepted as a specific area of knowledge and investigation during this century, its principles and implications have been appreciated for aeons. Thus, the harmful lethal effects of certain substances—including plants, fruits, insect bites, animal venoms and minerals—have been known since prehistoric times. Indeed, the Greek, Roman and subsequent civilizations knowingly used certain substances and extracts for their lethality in hunting, protection, warfare, suicide and murder.

Current activity in toxicology is mainly, though not exclusively, concerned with determining the potential for adverse effects from chemicals, both natural and synthetic, in order to assess hazard and risk to humans and lower animal forms, and thus define appropriate precautionary, protective, restrictive and therapeutic measures. For example, substances used or of potential use in commerce, the home, the environment and medical practice may present variable types of harmful effects, whose nature is determined by the physicochemical characteristics of the material, its potential to interact with biological materials and the pattern of exposure. For man-made and man-used materials, a critical analysis may be necessary in order to determine the risk–benefit ratio for their employment in specific circumstances, and to determine what protective and precautionary measures are needed. Indeed, with drugs, pesticides, industrial chemicals, food additives and cosmetic preparations, mandatory toxicology testing and government regulations exist. Substances not occurring naturally are often referred to as xenobiotics.

HISTORY OF TOXICOLOGY

Except in a few countries, including the UK, where safety evaluation toxicology has been closely associated with pathology, toxicology as a discipline is a daughter science of pharmacology. Toxicology is therefore a young science. However, its origins are very old and it is likely that man undertook his first experiments in toxicology in a search for an acceptable diet when he moved out of the habitat in which he evolved. Of course many of these experiments must have had an unfortunate outcome. In Roman and Greek times poisons, generally of plant origin, were used for murder and suicide, while the potential danger of medicinal products and their adulterants has been recognized since Babylonian times. Poisoning for nefarious purposes has remained a problem ever since, and much of the earlier impetus to the development of toxicology was primarily forensic. Another motive for the development of toxicology has been the careful description of adverse reactions to medicinal products that began to appear in the eighteenth century. Thus, William Withering described digitalis toxicity in 1785, and about 1790 Hahnemann, the founder of homoeopathy, carried out toxicological studies on himself and his healthy friends with therapeutic agents of his time, including cinchona, aconite, belladonna, ipecacuanha and mercury. The introduction of anaesthesia was followed by formal enquiries into sudden deaths during chloroform anaesthesia in the closing years of the nineteenth century.

In World War I a variety of poisonous chemicals were used in the battlefields of northern France. This was the stimulus for much work on mechanisms of toxicity as well as medical countermeasures to poisoning. In fact, war or the prospect of war played as great a part in the development of toxicology as of many other sciences. Much of the basic work on organophosphates was stimulated by the discovery of these compounds in Germany in the 1930s. Although defence considerations stimulated this work, much of it, particularly that related to treatment, is applicable to organophosphate pesticides.

Occupational toxicology originated in the nineteenth century as a product of the industrial revolution, with early descriptions of occupational diseases induced by chemicals, such as cancer of the scrotum in chimney sweeps. Although in theory affected workers have always had some remedies at law, major advances in control of occupational disease of chemical origin came in the period after 1960 with the setting of threshold limit values (TLVs) and occupational exposure limits. Additionally, in western countries the increasing wealth of workers has enabled them to make use of existing legal remedies. These considerations have caused companies to take greater care of their workers and to devote greater resources to occupational hygiene.

Regulatory toxicology had its origins in the development of the chemical and pharmaceutical industries in the nineteenth and twentieth centuries. Regulatory toxicology now accounts for the vast majority of toxicological expenditure. However, none of the major national toxicology societies predates World War II. Toxicology has only come of age as a science in the last 30 years as concern for consumer and worker health and for the environment increased. The growth of the science has been fuelled by a succession of disasters such as Seveso, Bhopal and that of thalidomide, which have thrown up lacunae in knowledge of the toxic effects of substances, as well as the inadequacy of testing procedures. One of the earliest such disasters was the deaths of 107 people from poisoning by an elixir of sulphanilamide containing the solvent diethylene glycol in 1937 in the USA: this led to legislation forbidding the marketing of new drugs until cleared for safety by the US Food and Drug Administration (FDA).

Regulations have been elaborated at national, continental (EC and OECD) and international levels (WHO/FAO) for each major type of chemical, including human and veterinary drugs, pesticides, food additives and industrial chemicals. Because of a tendency for new tests to be required without old ones being abandoned, regulations have inclined to become ever more complex, with the result that the cost of animal toxicity testing has become a significant part of product development. New tests do not always imply added cost; thus, the advent of mutagenic-

ity tests *in vitro* may enable the avoidance of large numbers of very expensive and laborious long-term carcinogenicity bioassays. However, the complexity of toxicological regulations implies not only an effect on the profits of the companies developing the chemical or drug, but also a loss to the market of potentially useful substances. In some cases this has given rise to sufficient disquiet for legislative action to be taken. Examples of this are the 'orphan drug' procedure in the United States and the clinical trial exemption system in the UK. An interesting phenomenon has been that regulatory requirements have given rise to large departments within chemical and pharmaceutical enterprises, whose main role is to satisfy regulatory authorities as to the safety of the company's products. However, for reasons of size or economics, many companies have chosen not to develop their own toxicology facilities.

Organochlorine insecticides probably averted an epidemic of typhus at the end of World War II, but it was the persistence of these compounds in the environment that was probably the greatest stimulus to the evolution of environmental toxicology. A major landmark in the development of this branch of toxicology was the publication of *Silent Spring*, by Rachel Carson.

The emphasis in toxicology has moved from its origins in acute, particularly human, toxicology to long-term and non-target species toxicology. In parallel, stress has changed from study of natural, usually plant, compounds to that of the products of chemical synthesis. Additionally, a great amount of resources has gone into testing for carcinogenic potential in recent years, while there has been intensive study of *in vitro* alternatives to animals in toxicology studies.

A recent development has been the recognition that differing toxicology requirements may be a barrier to free trade. Within major trading blocks, such as the North American Free Trade Area and the EC, it has been necessary to elaborate common toxicological requirements for clearance of materials, while the General Agreement on Tariffs and Trade (GATT) may require the acceptance of Codex Alimentarium Commission (CAC) residue figures for pesticide residues and food additives for trade between the major blocks.

Clinical toxicology, the treatment of acute poisoning, was originally carried out by general physicians in general hospitals; in this respect it is an old branch of toxicology; indeed amyl nitrite, one of the earliest antidotes (for cyanide), was described in the 1880s. Much of the impetus for the development of clinical toxicology came from defence research establishments. Chelation therapy for heavy metal poisoning was discovered during a search for a method of treatment for organic arsenical poisoning during World War II, while oximes for organophosphate poisoning were developed during the 'cold war' in the 1950s and 1960s. As a distinct specialism clinical toxicology is quite new, having arisen out of the fact that clinicians may not have ready access to the information necessary to treat their poisoned patients successfully. Furthermore, clinical toxicologists need special skills and analytical expertise. In the USA in the 1950s the idea of specialist poisons information services arose. These services, which have access to information on the many thousands of possible chemicals which people may use to poison themselves, now exist in most developed countries. In some cases units exist not only to back up clinicians with information, but also to carry out hands-on treatment of poisoning.

Major, extensive and rapid developments in the scientific basis and practice of toxicology have been obvious since the early part of the 1950s. These developments have happened for a variety of reasons, principal among which are those listed in Table 1. Reflecting these developments has been a proliferation in the number of textbooks, monographs and journals devoted to general and

Table 1 Major driving forces for the recent expansion and development of the scientific basis and practice of toxicology

- Exponential increase in the number of synthetically produced industrial chemicals

- Major increase in the number and nature of new drugs, pharmaceutical preparations, tissue-implantable materials and medical devices

- Mandatory testing and regulation of chemicals used commercially, domestically and medically

- Enhanced public awareness of potential adverse effects from xenobiotics (non-naturally occurring) to man, animal and the environment

- Litigation, principally as a consequence of occupational-related illness, unrecognized or poorly documented product safety concerns (including drugs) and environmental harm

special aspects of toxicology; a proliferation of abstracting services related to toxicology information; the provision of courses at undergraduate and graduate levels dealing with general and specialized areas; and the establishment of a private industry devoted to toxicology testing and consultation. Along with these factors there has been an increase in the number of professional organizations and certification boards specifically devoted to toxicology. As a consequence of the markedly expanded scope of toxicology, the number of differing subdisciplines which have emerged and the need for varying professional activities, the practice of toxicology can be subdivided and described by areas of major involvement and specialization; the principal areas are shown in Table 2.

Historical aspects of toxicology have been reviewed in detail by Doull and Bruce (1991) and Decker (1987).

DEFINITION AND SCOPE OF TOXICOLOGY

The essence of toxicology is that it is a discipline concerned with studying the potential of chemicals, or mixtures of them, to produce harmful effects in living organisms and determining the implications of these effects. One overview definition covering the various facets of toxicology (Ballantyne, 1989), is:

> Toxicology is a study of the interaction between chemicals and biological systems in order to quantitatively determine the potential for chemical(s) to produce injury which results in adverse effects in living organisms, and to investigate the nature, incidence, mechanism of production, factors influencing their development, and reversibility of such adverse effects.

Within the scope of this definition, adverse effects are those which are detrimental to either the survival or the normal functioning of the individual. Inherent in this definition are the following key issues in toxicology:

(1) Chemicals, or their conversion products, require to come into close structural and/or func-

Table 2 Major subspecialities of toxicology

Speciality	Major functional components
Clinical	Causation, diagnosis and management of established poisoning in humans
Veterinary	Causation, diagnosis and management of established poisoning in domestic and wild animals
Forensic	Establishing the cause of death or intoxication in humans, by analytical procedures, and with particular reference to legal processes
Occupational	Assessing the potential of adverse effects from chemicals in the occupational environment, and the recommendation of appropriate protective and precautionary measures
Product	Assessing the potential for adverse effects from commercially produced chemicals and formulations, and recommendation on use patterns, and protective and precautionary procedures
Pharmacological	Assessing the toxicity of therapeutic agents
Aquatic	Assessing the toxicity on aquatic organisms of chemicals discharged into marine and fresh water
Toxinology	Assessing the toxicity of substances of plant and animal origin, and produced by pathogenic bacteria
Environmental	Assessing the effects of toxic pollutants, usually at low concentrations, released from commercial and domestic sites into their immediate environment and subsequently widely distributed by air and water currents and by diffusion through soil
Regulatory	Administrative function concerned with the development and interpretation of mandatory toxicology testing programmes, and with particular reference to controlling the use, distribution and availability of chemicals used commercially and therapeutically
Laboratory	Design and conduct of *in vivo* and *in vitro* toxicology testing programmes

tional contact with tissue(s) or organ(s) for which they have a potential to cause injury.

(2) When possible, the observed toxicity (or an end-point reflecting it) should be quantitatively related to the degree of exposure to the chemical (the exposure dose). Ideally, the influence of differing exposure doses on the magnitude and/or incidence of the toxic effect(s) should be investigated. Such dose–response relationships are of prime importance in confirming a causal relationship between chemical exposure and toxic effect, in assessing relevance of the observed toxicity to practical (in-use) exposure conditions, and to allow hazard evaluations and risk assessment.

(3) The primary aim of most toxicology studies is to determine the potential for harmful effects in the intact living organism, in many cases (and often by extrapolation) to man.

(4) Toxicological investigations should ideally allow the following characteristics of toxicity to be evaluated:

(a) The basic structural, functional or biochemical injury produced.

(b) Dose–response relationships.

(c) The mechanism(s) of toxicity: i.e. the fundamental chemical and biological inter-

actions and resultant aberrations that are responsible for the genesis and maintenance of the toxic response.

(d) Factors that may modify the toxic response; e.g. route of exposure, species, sex, formulation of test chemical and environmental conditions.

(e) Development of approaches for recognition of specific toxic responses.

(f) Is the toxic effect reversible, either spontaneously (healing) or by antidotal or other procedures (i.e. treatment)?

The word 'toxicity' is used to describe the nature of adverse effects produced and the conditions necessary for their induction; i.e. toxicity is the potential for a material to produce injury in biological systems. For pharmacologically active and therapeutic agents ('drugs') a description of the non-desired effects is most appropriately undertaken using the following specific terms.

Side-effects: undesirable effects which result from the normal pharmacological actions of the drug.
Overdosage: implies that toxicity will occur.
Intolerance: implies that the threshold dose to

produce a pharmacological effect is lowered; this may be a consequence of a genetic abnormality.

Idiosyncrasy: an abnormal reaction to a drug due to an inherent, frequently genetic, anomaly.

Secondary effects: those arising as an indirect consequence of the pharmacological action of a drug.

Adverse drug interactions: adverse effects produced by a combination of drugs, but not seen when the drugs are given separately at the same dose.

Toxicity (i.e. the potential to injure) requires to be clearly differentiated from the process of hazard evaluation, which examines the likelihood that a given material will exhibit its known toxicity under particular conditions of use.

DESCRIPTION AND TERMINOLOGY OF TOXIC EFFECTS

Precision in communication depends on a clear understanding of the definitions of technical and scientific terms in the context of their use. The following section discusses the derivation and meanings of frequently used expressions in toxicology.

A schematic representation of the basis for the general classification of toxic effects is given in Figure 1. Before toxicity can develop, a substance must come into contact with a body surface such as skin, eye or mucosa of the alimentary or respiratory tract; these are, respectively, the cutaneous, ocular, peroral and inhalation routes of exposure. Other routes of exposure, in experimental or therapeutic situations, are subcutaneous, intravenous, intramuscular and intraperitoneal.

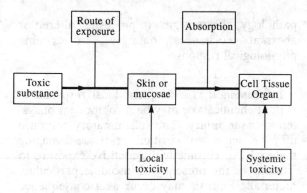

Figure 1 Basis for general classification of toxic effects

Harmful effects that occur at the sites where a substance comes into initial contact with the body are referred to as local effects. If substances are absorbed from the sites of contact, they or products of their bioconversion may produce toxic effects in cells, tissues or organs remote from the site of exposure; these remote responses are referred to as systemic effects. Many materials may produce both local and systemic toxicity. Also, since the nature and probability of toxicity depend on the number of exposures, this forms an additional general means for classifying toxic effect into those developing after a single (acute) exposure or multiple (repeated) exposures. Repeated exposure toxicity can cover a wide time-span; however, it is descriptively convenient to refer to short-term repeated (not more than 5 per cent of life-span), subchronic (5–20 per cent of life-span), and chronic (entire life-span or a greater portion of it). Examples of toxic effects classified according to site and to number of exposures are given in Table 3.

Additional descriptions of toxicity are by the time to development and the duration of induced effects. Thus, they may be described as temporary (reversible or transient) or permanent (persistent). Latent (delayed-onset) toxicity exists when there is a period free from signs following (usually) an acute exposure. Latent toxicity is of particular importance in clinical toxicology, since individuals exposed to chemicals of known latency in toxicity should be kept under review in order that any delayed adverse effects may be both promptly recognized and treated. Cumulative toxicity involves progressive injury produced by summation of incremental injury resulting from successive exposures. Examples of toxicity according to the time-scale for development and duration of effect are given in Table 4. Effects may also be classified, and described, according to the primary tissue or organ forming the target of toxicity—e.g. hepatotoxic, nephrotoxic, neurotoxic, genotoxic, ototoxic, immunotoxic, etc. A description of toxicity from a material requires inclusion of the following: whether effects are local, systemic or mixed; their nature and (if known) mechanism of toxicity; organs and tissues affected; and condition of exposure resulting in toxicity (including species, route and number or magnitude of exposure(s)).

Table 3 Examples of toxicity classified according to time-scale and site

Exposure	Site	Effect	Substance
Acute	Local	Skin corrosion Lung injury	Methylamine Hydrogen chloride
	Systemic	Kidney injury Haemolysis	Phenacetin Arsine
	Mixed	Lung injury and methaemoglobinaemia	Oxides of nitrogen
Short-term repeated	Local	Skin sensitization Lung sensitization Nasal septal ulceration	Ethylenediamine Toluene diisocyanate Chromates
	Systemic	Neurotoxic Liver injury	Acrylamide Arsenic
	Mixed	Respiratory irritation and neurobehavioural	Pyridine
Chronic	Local	Bronchitis Laryngeal carcinoma	Sulphur dioxide Nitrogen mustard
	Systemic	Leukaemia Angiosarcoma (liver)	Benzene Vinyl chloride
	Mixed	Emphysema and kidney injury Pneumonitis and neurotoxic	Cadmium Manganese

Table 4 Examples of toxicity classified according to time-scale for development or duration

Time-scale	Effect	Substance
Persistent	Testicular injury Scarring (skin/eye) Pleural mesothelia	Dibromochloropropane Corrosives Asbestos
Transient	Narcosis Sensory irritation	Organic solvents Acetaldehyde
Cumulative	Squamous metaplasia Liver fibrosis	Irritants (e.g. formaldehyde) Ethanol
Latent	Pulmonary oedema Peripheral neuropathy Pulmonary fibrosis	Phosgene Organophosphates (antiChE) Paraquat

NATURE OF TOXIC EFFECTS

The nature and magnitude of a toxic effect depend on many factors, among which are the physicochemical properties of the substance, its bioconversion, the conditions of exposure and the presence of bioprotective mechanisms. The latter factor includes physiological mechanisms such as adaptive enzyme induction, DNA repair mechanisms, phagocytosis, etc. Some of the frequently encountered types of morphological and biochemical injury constituting a toxic response are listed below. They may take the form of tissue pathology, aberrant growth processes, altered or aberrant biochemical pathways, or extreme physiological responses.

Inflammation is a frequent local response to irritant chemicals or may be a component of systemic tissue injury. The inflammatory response may be acute with irritant or tissue-damaging materials, or chronic with repetitive exposure to irritants or the presence of insoluble particulate materials. Fibrosis may occur as a consequence of the inflammatory process.

Necrosis, used to describe circumscribed death of tissues or cells, may result from a variety of pathological processes induced by chemical injury—e.g. corrosion, severe hypoxia, membrane damage, reactive metabolite binding, inhibition of protein synthesis and chromosome injury. With certain substances, differing patterns of zonal necrosis may be seen. In the liver, for example, galactosamine produces diffuse necrosis of the lobules (Mehendale, 1987), paracetamol (acetaminophen) mainly centrilobular necrosis, and certain organic arsenicals peripheral lobular necrosis (Ballantyne, 1978).

Enzyme inhibition by chemicals may inhibit biologically vital pathways, producing impairment of normal function. The induction of toxicity may be due to accumulation of substrate, or to deficiency of product or function. For example, organophosphate anticholinesterases produce toxicity by accumulation of acetylcholine at cholinergic synapses and neuromuscular junctions (Ellenhorn and Barceloux, 1988). Cyanide inhibits cytochrome oxidase and interferes with mitochondrial oxygen transport, producing cytotoxic hypoxia (Ballantyne, 1987).

Biochemical uncoupling agents interfere with the synthesis of high-energy phosphate molecules, but electron transport continues, resulting in excess liberation of energy as heat. Thus, uncoupling produces increased oxygen consumption and hyperthermia. Examples of uncoupling agents are dinitrophenol and pentachlorophenol (Williams, 1982; Kurt *et al.*, 1988).

Lethal synthesis occurs when foreign substances of close structural similarity to normal biological substrates become incorporated into biochemical pathways, and then metabolized to a toxic product. A classical example is fluoroacetate, which becomes incorporated in the Krebs cycle as fluoroacetyl coenzyme A, which combines with oxaloacetate to form fluorocitrate. The latter inhibits aconitase, blocking the tricarboxylic acid cycle and results, particularly, in cardiac and nervous system toxicity (Albert, 1979).

Lipid peroxidation in biological membranes by free radicals starts a chain of events causing cellular dysfunction and death. The complex series of events includes oxidation of fatty acids to lipid hydroperoxides which undergo degradation to various products, including toxic aldehydes. The generation of organic radicals during peroxidation results in a self-propagating reaction

(Horton and Fairhurst, 1987). Carbon tetrachloride, for example, is activated by a hepatic cytochrome *P*-450 dependent mono-oxygenase system to the trichloromethyl and trichloromethyl peroxy radicals; the former radical probably covalently binds with macromolecules, and the latter radical initiates the process of lipid peroxidation leading to hepatic centrilobular necrosis. The zonal necrosis is possibly related to high cytochrome *P*-450 activity in centrilobular hepatocytes (Albano *et al.*, 1982).

Covalent binding of electrophilic reactive metabolites to nucleophilic macromolecules may have a role in certain genotoxic, carcinogenic, teratogenic and immunosuppressive events. Important cellular defence mechanisms exist to moderate these reactions, and toxicity may not be initiated until these mechanisms are saturated.

Receptor interaction, at a cellular or macromolecular level, with specific chemical structures may modulate the normal biological effects mediated by the receptor; these may be excitatory or inhibitory. An important example is effects on Ca^{2+} channels (Braunwald, 1982).

Immune-mediated hypersensitivity reactions by antigenic materials are particularly important considerations for skin and lung, resulting, respectively, in allergic contact dermatitis and asthma (Cronin, 1980; Brooks, 1983).

Immunosuppression by xenobiotics may have important repercussions in increased susceptibility to infective agents and certain aspects of tumorigenesis.

Neoplasia, resulting from aberrations of tissue growth and control mechanisms of cell division, and leading to abnormal proliferation and growth, is a major consideration in repeated exposure to xenobiotics. The terms 'tumorigenesis' and 'oncogenesis' are general words used to describe the development of neoplasms; the word 'carcinogenesis' should be restricted specifically to malignant neoplasms. In experimental and epidemiological situations, oncogenesis may be exhibited as an increase in the total number of neoplasms, an increase in specific types of neoplasm, the occurrence of 'rare' or 'unique' neoplasms, or a decreased latency to detection of neoplasm.

Chemical carcinogenesis in many cases is a multistage process. The first, and critical, stage is a genotoxic event followed by other processes leading to the pathological, functional and clinical expression of neoplasia. One multistep model that has received most attention is the initiator–promoter scheme (Figure 2). The first stage, that of initiation, requires a brief exposure to a genotoxically active material which results in binding of the initiator or a reactive metabolite to cellular DNA; there is a low, or no, threshold for initiation. The second stage, that of promotion, permits the expression of the carcinogenic potential of the initiated cell. Promoting agents have the following characteristics:

- They need not be genotoxic.
- Repeated exposure is required after initiation.
- They show some evidence for reversibility.
- They may have a threshold for promoting activity.

Genotoxic initiators may also act in a promotional manner after initiation.

Substances causing or enhancing a carcinogenic process are respectively described as genotoxic and epigenetic carcinogens; the former are capable of causing DNA injury, and the latter exert oncogenic effects by mechanisms other than genotoxicity. Genotoxic materials acting directly with DNA are referred to as primary carcinogens; those requiring to be metabolically activated are procarcinogens, with the metabolically active electrophile being the ultimate carcinogen. Primary carcinogens include alkylene epoxides, sulphate esters and nitrosoureas; procarcinogens include polycyclic aromatic hydrocarbons, aromatic amines, azo dyes and nitrosamines.

Epigenetic carcinogens include the following differing functional classes: promoters, cocarcinogens, hormones, immunosuppressives and solid-state materials. Cocarcinogens, when applied just before or with genotoxic carcinogens, enhance the oncogenic effect. Various mechanisms may cause enhancement, including increased absorption, increased metabolic activation of procarcinogen, decreased detoxification or inhibition of DNA repair. One group of epigenetic carcinogens of current interest are the peroxisome proliferators, which induce liver tumours in experimental rodents. These materials produce hepatomegaly and hepatocyte peroxisome proliferation, and induce several liver enyzmes, including those of the peroxisomal fatty acid β-oxidation system. Phthalate esters are one class of compound producing peroxisomal proliferation and experimental hepatocarcinogenesis (Rao and Reddy, 1987). For the purposes of risk assessment, it is usually assumed that a threshold for oncogenesis does not exist with genotoxic carcinogens. In contrast, a threshold may exist with epigenetic carcinogens, but there is disagreement about the way in which data from studies with epigenetic carcinogens should be analysed for risk assessment purposes.

Genotoxic chemicals, which interact with DNA and possibly lead to heritable changes, may be conveniently classified as clastogenic or mutagenic. Clastogenic effects occur at the chromosomal level and are visible by light microscopy. They may involve simple breaks, rearrangement of segments or gross destruction of chromosomes. If severe, they may be incompatible with normal function, and cell death occurs. The relevance of chemically induced sublethal cytogenetic effects is not clearly understood, but could lead to dysfunction of the reproductive system and tissues with rapid cell turnover rates.

Mutagenic effects are focal molecular events in the DNA molecule, which involve either substitution of a base-pair, or deletion or addition of a base. Base-pair transformations ('point mutations') may occur by direct chemical transformation, incorporation of abnormal base analogues, or alkylation. Addition or deletion of a

Scheme	Initiator-promoter relations	Neoplasm
A	I	No
B	I P P P P P P P P	Yes
C	I P P P P P P P P P P	Yes
D	I P P P P P P P P P	Low/no
E	P P P P P P P P P P P P P P P P	No
F	P P P P P P P P P P P I	No
G	I I I I I I I I I I	Yes

Figure 2 Schematic representation of functional interrelationships between initiator and promoter in the two-stage mechanism of carcinogenesis. (A) An initiating dose of a genotoxic carcinogen is not by itself oncogenic. (B) If initiator dose is followed by multiple applications of an epigenetic promoter, neoplasia results (the classical initiator–promoter relationship). (C) If promotion is delayed after initiation, a neoplastic response occurs, indicating a persistent initiating process. (D) If promoter dosing is infrequent or doses are small, there may be no neoplasia or a low tumour incidence, indicating a threshold for the promoting effect. (E) Multiple applications of an epigenetic promoter alone do not result in neoplasia. (F) Initiation must precede promotion. (G) A genotoxic carcinogen may act as both initiator and promoter

base will result in a disturbance of the triplet code, and, hence, alteration of the codon sequence distal to the addition or deletion ('frameshift mutation'). Intracellular DNA repair enzymes are present, but if the repair mechanism is exceeded, then abnormal coding will be transcribed into RNA and expressed as altered protein structure and possibly function, depending on the molecular segmented affected. The relationship of chemically induced mutation to genetic abnormality is unclear. However, as noted above, it is now generally accepted that in genotoxic carcinogenesis the molecular DNA event of initiation is fundamental to multistage oncogenesis. There is now considerable evidence showing a good correlation (with some test systems) between carcinogenic and mutagenic potential. Thus, the use of certain mutagenicity test procedures has become widely accepted as a means of screening chemicals for their carcinogenic potential (Krisch-Volders, 1984; Brusick, 1988).

Developmental and reproductive toxicity are, respectively, concerned with adverse effects on the ability to conceive, and with adverse effects on the structural and functional integrity of the conceptus up to and around parturition.

Adverse effects on reproduction may result from a variety of differing effects on reproductive organs and their neural and endocrine control mechanisms (Barlow and Sullivan, 1982). Developmental toxicity deals with adverse effects on the conceptus from the stage of zygote formation, through the stages of implantation, germ layer differentiation, organ formation, and growth processes during intrauterine development and the neonatal period. The most extreme toxicity, death, may occur as preimplantation loss, embryo resorption, fetal death or abortion. Non-lethal fetotoxicity may be expressed as delayed maturation, including decreased body weight and retarded ossification. Structural malformations (morphological teratogenic effects) may be external, skeletal or visceral. The preferential susceptibility of the conceptus to chemical (and other environmental) insults in comparison with the adult state is related to: (1) small numbers of cells and rapid proliferation rates; (2) a large number of non-differentiated cells lacking defence capabilities; (3) requirements for precise spatial and temporal interactions of cells; (4) limited metabolic capacity; and (5) immaturity of the immuno-

surveillance system (Tyl, 1988). There is now increasing awareness that functional, in addition to structural, malformations of development may occur. Malformation from chemical exposure may result, among other mechanisms from (1) genotoxic injury; (2) interference with nucleic acid replication, transcription or translation; (3) essential nutrient deficiency; and (4) enzyme inhibition. The most sensitive period for induction of structural malformations is during organogenesis; functional teratogenic effects may be induced at later stages, particularly neurobehavioural malformations (Rodier, 1980).

Pharmacological effects may be induced by drugs and chemicals, and these may be significant as causes of temporary incapacitation or inconvenience in the occupational environment, as well as side-effects of medication. For example, narcosis from acute overexposure to an organic solvent may clearly be of relevance in safe workplace considerations; such a reversible narcosis needs to be differentiated from central nervous system injury resulting from long-term low-concentration solvent exposure (World Health Organization, 1985). Another important pharmacological effect, particularly from airborne materials in the workplace, is peripheral sensory irritation. Materials having such effects interact with sensory nerve receptors in skin or mucosae, producing local discomfort and related reflex effects. For example, with the eye there is pain or discomfort, excess lachrymation and blepharospasm. Although such effects are warning and protective in nature, they are also distracting and thus likely to predispose to accidents. For this reason peripheral sensory irritant effects are widely used in defining, along with other considerations, exposure guidelines for workplace environments (Ballantyne, 1984).

DOSAGE–RESPONSE RELATIONSHIPS

A fundamental concept in biology is that of variability. Individual members of the same species and strain differ to variable degrees with respect to their biochemical, cellular, tissue, organ and overall characteristics. Additionally, within a given individual there is a spectrum of variability in certain features—e.g. cell size and biochemical function within a particular cell series. The differences between individuals are usually a consequence of genetic factors. Since toxic effects are due to adverse effects on biological systems, or modifications of defence mechanisms, it is not unexpected that the majority of toxic responses will also show a variability between individuals of a given strain; also, because of genetic and biochemical variability, even larger discrepancies in response will be observed between species. It is axiomatic to the toxicologist that, within certain limits and under controlled conditions, there is a positive relationship between the amount of material to which given groups of animals are exposed and the toxic response, and that the response of a given animal may quantitatively differ from that of other animals in the same dosage group. As the amount of material given to a group of animals increases, so does the magnitude of the effect and/or the number who are affected. For example, a specific amount of a potentially lethal material given to a group of animals may not kill all of them; however, as the amount of material is increased so the proportion dying increases. This reflects the variability in the susceptibility of the population studied to the lethal toxicity of the test substance.

Likewise, if an irritant material is applied to the skin, as the amount is increased this is associated with (1) an increase in the number of the population affected and (2) an increase in the severity of the inflammation. For the two examples given above, death is an 'all-or-none' response (a quantal response), while inflammation may be considered from a dose–response viewpoint as having two elements—i.e. its presence or otherwise, and the degree of inflammation which represents a continuous (or graded) response. The above considerations, which reflect variability in biological systems, form the basis for the fundamental concept of dose–response relationships in both pharmacology and toxicology, there usually being a positive relationship between dose and response *in vivo* and in many *in vitro* test systems.

It follows from the above discussion that the amount of material to which an organism is exposed is one prime determinant of toxicity. The dose–response relationships for differing toxic effects produced by a given material in a particular species may vary. Thus, as discussed later, dose–response relationships have to be carefully interpreted in the context of the effect of interest

and the particular conditions under which the information was obtained.

The word 'dose' is most frequently used to denote the total amount of material to which an organism or test system is exposed; 'dosage' defines the amount of material given in relation to a recipient characteristic (e.g. weight). Dosage allows a more meaningful and comparative indicator of exposure. For example, 500 mg of a material given as a peroral dose to a 250 g rat or a 2000 g rabbit will result in respective dosages of 2 mg kg^{-1} and 0.25 mg kg^{-1}. It follows that comparative dosing should be expressed in dosage units. Dose in most reports usually implies the exposure dose—i.e. the total amount of material which is given to an organism by the particular route of exposure, or the amount incorporated into a test system. Another expression of dose is absorbed dose, which is the amount of material penetrating into the organism through the route of exposure. Absorbed dose may show a closer quantitative relationship with systemic toxicity than exposure dose, since it represents the amount of material directly available for metabolic interactions and systemic toxicity. A further expression of dose is target organ dose, which is the amount of material (parent or metabolite) received at the organ or tissue exhibiting a specific toxic effect. This should be expressed (if possible) in terms of the mechanistically causative molecule (parent chemical or reactive metabolite). Clearly target organ dose is a more precise quantitative indication of toxicity than exposure dose, since it is a measure of the amount of material at the site of toxicity, whereas exposure dose is total dose to the organism, and only a proportion of this (or metabolite) will ultimately gain access to the target site(s) for the toxic response. However, the estimation of target organ or tissue dose requires a detailed knowledge of the pharmacokinetics and metabolism of the material. For this reason, most information relates to the exposure dose.

The exposure dose is of practical importance, since it reflects the amount of material to which the organism is actually exposed and the likelihood of development of a particular toxic endpoint, and therefore is of particular use for hazard evaluation purposes. Absolute target organ doses allow a more detailed scientific evaluation of toxicity in relation to bioavailable chemical, and, when related to exposure dose, may be used for rational risk assessment procedures.

If a material is capable of inducing several differing types of toxicity, the dose (or dosage) of material required to cause the individual effects may differ, with the more sensitive toxic effect appearing at the lower dosages. The first distinct toxicity, at lower dosages, may not necessarily be the most seriously significant effect. For example, with epicutaneously applied materials, local inflammation may appear before more sinister systemic toxicity. Conversely, if the most significant toxicity occurs at lower dosages, then other toxicity at higher dosages may be overlooked.

Nature of the Dosage–Response Relationship

As discussed above, with a given population there is a quantitative variability in susceptibility to a chemical by individual members of that population. Thus, with a genetically homogeneous population of animals of the same species and strain, the proportion exhibiting a particular toxic effect will increase as the dosage increases. This is shown schematically in Figure 3 as a cumulative frequency distribution curve, where the number of animals responding (as a proportion of the total in the group) is plotted as a function of the dosage given (as a $\log_{10}$ function). In many instances there is a sigmoid curve, with a log-normal distribution and symmetrical about the mid-point. This is a typical dosage–response relationship, often loosely referred to as a dose–response relationship. There are several important elements to this curve that require consideration when interpreting its toxicological significance:

- The majority of those individuals responding do so symmetrically about the mid-point (i.e. the 50 per cent response value). The position of the major portion of the dosage–response curve around its mid-point is sometimes referred to as the potency.
- The mid-point of the curve (50 per cent response point) is a convenient description of the average response, and is referred to as the median effective dose for the effect being considered (ED_{50}). If mortality is the end-point, then this is specifically referred to as the median lethal dose (LD_{50}). The median

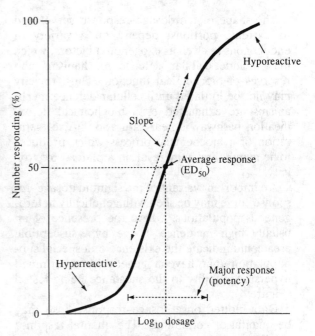

Figure 3 Typical sigmoid cumulative dosage–response curve for a toxic effect, which is symmetrical about the average (50 per cent response) point. The major response (potency) occurs around the average response. The slope of the curve is determined by the increase in response as a function of incremental increases in dosage. Hyperreactive and hyporeactive individuals are found at the extreme left and right sides of the curve, respectively

effective dosage is used for the following reasons: (1) it is at the mid-point of a log normally distributed curve; (2) the 95 per cent confidence limits are narrowest at this point.

- A small proportion of the population, at the left-hand side of the dosage–response curve, respond to low dosages; they constitute a hypersusceptible or hyperreactive group.
- Another small proportion of the population, at the right-hand side of the curve, do not respond until higher dosages are given; they constitute a hyposusceptible or hyporeactive group.
- The slope of the dose–response curve, particularly around the median value, gives an indication of the range of doses producing an effect. It indicates how greatly the response will be changed when the dosage is altered. A steep slope indicates that a majority of the population will respond over a narrow dosage range, and a flatter slope indicates that a much wider range of dosages is required to affect the majority of the population.

The shape of the dosage–response curve, and its extreme portions, depend on a variety of endogenous (as well as exogenous) factors, which may include cellular defence mechanisms and reserves of biochemical function. Thus, toxicity may not be initiated until cellular defence mechanisms are exhausted or a biochemical detoxification pathway is near saturation. Also, saturation of a biochemical process which produces toxic metabolites may result in a plateau for toxicity.

An important variant of the sigmoid dosage–response curve may be seen with genetically heterogeneous populations, where the presence of an usually high incidence in the hypersusceptible area could indicate the existence of a special subpopulation that have a genetically determined hypersusceptibility to the substance being tested (Figure 4).

Data plotted on a dosage–response basis may be quantal or continuous. The quantal response is 'all-or-none'—e.g. death. The graded, or variable, response is one involving a continual change in effect with increasing dosage—e.g. enzyme inhibition, degree of inflammation or physiological function such as heart rate. The dosage–response curve is often linearly transformed into a log–probit plot ($\log_{10}$ dose versus probit response) because it permits the examination of data over a wide range of dosages, and allows certain mathematical procedures (e.g. calculation of confidence limits and slope of response) (Figure 5). Quantal data can also be plotted as a frequency histogram or frequency distribution curve; this is done by plotting the percentage response at a given dose minus the percentage response at the immediate lower dose (i.e. response specific for the dosage). This procedure usually results in a gaussian distribution (Figure 6), reflecting the differential biological susceptibility of the test organism to the treatment. In such a normal frequency distribution curve the mean ± 1 standard deviation (SD) represents 68.3 per cent of the population; mean ± 2 SD represents 95.5 per cent and mean ± 3 SD is 99.7 per cent of the population.

It is important to stress that not only will the incidence of the effect of interest vary with dose, and determine the dosage–response relationship, but also the severity of magnitude of the effect will change with varying dosage. Thus, for any given dosage producing a particular response incidence, those responding may show a difference in the magnitude of the effect.

Absence of a clear dosage–response relationship in a controlled experiment may indicate a non-toxic or non-pharmacological action of the material. For example, an aminoalkyltrialkoxydisilane given by gavage to rats resulted in the following mortalities (expressed as (number dying)/(number dosed)): 16 g kg^{-1} (4/5), 8 g kg^{-1} (0/5), 4 g kg^{-1} (3/5) and 2 g kg^{-1} (0/5). Clearly there was no dosage–response relationship in this

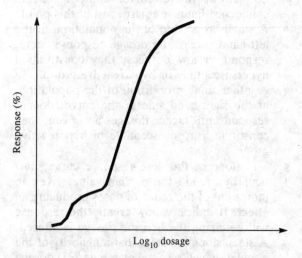

Figure 4 Variant of the sigmoid cumulative dosage–response curve due to enhanced hyperreactive response; this may represent a genetic variant in a proportion of the population causing enhanced sensitivity to the toxic effect

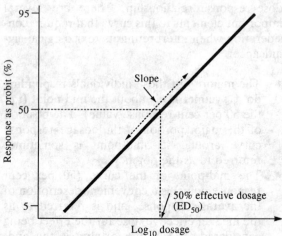

Figure 5 Linear transformation of dosage–response data by log–probit plot

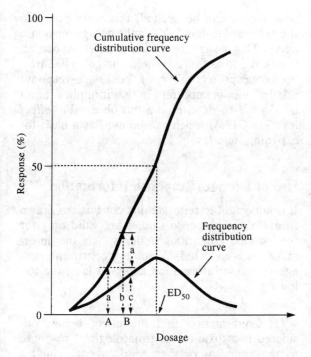

Figure 6 Relationship between cumulative frequency distribution curve and normal frequency distribution curve for quantal data. The cumulative frequency distribution curve shows the proportion responding for each dosage, and, hence, the expected total response for any given dosage. The frequency distribution curve shows the response specific for that dosage compared with lower dosages. For the frequency distribution curve, the response (c) at any dosage (e.g. B) is obtained by taking the total response at that dosage (b) and subtracting the response (a) at the immediate lower dosage (A)

study. Necropsy of dying rats showed that polymerization of the material had occurred in the stomach, producing a hard opalescent solid mass completely occluding the stomach. Thus, the cause of death was a consequence of mechanical obstruction and nutritional deprivation rather than intrinsic toxicity.

For drugs, one convenient indication of 'safety' often used is the ratio between the median effective dose causing death and that producing the desired therapeutic response (i.e. LD_{50}/ED_{50}); this is frequently referred to as the therapeutic index (TI_{50}). In general, the higher this ratio the greater the degree of safety with respect to lethality. However, very considerable caution is needed in applying this information. For example, if the slopes of the dosage–response curves for drug effectiveness and lethality are parallel, then the assumption of an equal therapeutic ratio over a

range of dosages and to a majority of the population is justified (Figure 7). If, however, the dosage–response curve for lethality is shallower than that for the therapeutic response (Figure 8), then there will be a decreasing therapeutic index at the lower dosages, and the hyperreactive groups may be at greater risk. One way which can be used to take into account differences in slopes is to calculate the ratio between that dosage causing a 1 per cent mortality (LD_1) and that producing near-maximum therapeutic efficacy (ED_{99}). This ratio, $(LD_1)/(ED_{99})$, is referred to as the margin of safety (Figure 8). A complete appraisal of safety-in-use, of course, also requires considerations on sublethal and long-term toxicity, and at therapeutic dosages the likelihood for side-effects and idiosyncratic reactions.

The slope of the dosage–response relationship, particularly around the mid-point, can be of value for more precisely assessing hazard or potential for overdose situations. Thus, for example, in considering lethality a steep slope indicates that a large proportion of the population will be at risk over a small range of doses. Likewise, with a material producing central nervous system depression, a steep slope implies that a small

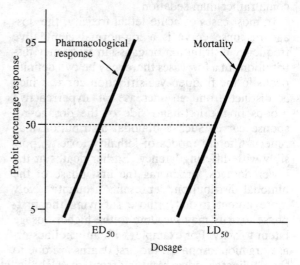

Figure 7 One simplistic method for assessing 'safety ratios' for drugs is by comparing the ratio between the therapeutically effective dose (e.g. ED_{50}) and that causing mortality (LD_{50}); this ratio of $(LD_{50})/(ED_{50})$ is referred to as the therapeutic index (TI_{50}). For parallel pharmacological effect and lethality dosage–response lines, the therapeutic index will be similar over a wide range of doses. However, non-parallel lines may give misleading conclusions if the TI_{50} is calculated (see Figure 8)

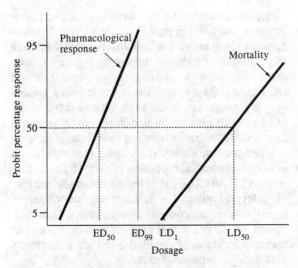

Figure 8 The TI_{50} may give a misleading index of drug safety if the dosage–response lines for pharmacological and lethal effects are not parallel. In the example shown in this figure, there may be a reasonable margin based on LD_{50} and ED_{50}. However, owing to the shallow slope of the mortality dosage–response line, the therapeutic index will be significantly lower at the 1 per cent and 5 per cent level, and thus the hyper-reactive group may be at greater risk. In this case a better index of safety will be the ratio of $(LD_1)/(ED_{99})$, which is referred to as the 'margin of safety'

incremental increase of dosage may result in coma rather than sedation.

In most cases of acute lethal toxicity, the dosage–response curve is a log-normal cumulative frequency distribution or gaussian frequency distribution. In a few cases there may be two definite peaks in the frequency distribution curve, which is distinct from an increase in hyperreactive groups in the left-hand side of the dosage–response curve. Such a bimodal distribution may reflect different modes of lethality toxicity, possibly with differing latency. Earlier deaths at the lower dosages, producing the first phase of the bimodal distribution, represents a quantitatively more potent toxicity; those surviving the first-phase toxicity may succumb to the higher-dosage latent toxicity. For example, with anticholinesterase organophosphates, the first deaths are due to the cholinergic crisis resulting from acetylcholinesterase inhibition, and late toxicity may result from delayed-onset peripheral neuropathy. In some cases log–probit plots will allow the determination of ED_{50} values for each subgroup in the bimodal distribution.

For many toxic effects, except genotoxic carcinogenesis, there is a dose below which no effect

or response can be elicited; this corresponds to the extreme left-hand side of the dosage–response curve. This dosage, below which no effect occurs, is referred to as the 'threshold dosage'. The threshold concept, a corollary of the dosage–response relationship, is important in that it implies that it is possible to determine a 'no observable effect level' (NOEL), which can be used as a basis for assigning 'safe levels' for exposure.

Use of Dosage–Response Information

It is important to reiterate that conclusions drawn from dosage–response studies are valid only for the specific conditions under which the information was collected. Within this constraint, dosage–response information allows at least the following:

(1) Confirmation that the effect being considered is a toxic (or pharmacological) response to the chemical or therapeutic agent. Thus, a positive dosage–response relationship is good evidence for a causal relationship between exposure and the development of toxicity or pharmacological effects.

(2) Quantitive dose–response information allows the determination of an average (median) response; gives the range of susceptibility in the population studied; and indicates where the dosage for hypersusceptible groups is expected.

(3) The slope of the dosage–response curve gives information on the range of effective dosages and the differential proportion of the population affected for incremental increases in dosage. With a shallow slope the range of effective doses is widespread; the proportion of the population additionally affected by incremental increases in dosage is small. In contrast, a steep slope implies that the effective dose for the majority of the population is over a narrow range, and there will be a significant increase in the proportion of the population affected for small incremental increases in dosage.

(4) The shape of the left-hand side of the dosage–response curve may indicate the existence of an unusually high hypersusceptible proportion of the population. This may, for example, indicate a genetically determined increased susceptibility to the chemical or pharmacologically active substance studied.

(5) The data may allow conclusions on 'threshold' or 'no-effect' dosages for the response.

(6) Quantitive comparison for a specific end-point may be made between different materials with respect to average and range of response, particularly if the information has been collected under similar conditions.

The above considerations are briefly illustrated in the following section.

Dosage–Response Considerations for Acute Lethal Toxicity

Death, a quantal response, is an end-point incorporated in many acute toxicity studies, and used for the calculation of LD_{50} values.

Acute lethal toxicity studies involve giving differing dosages of the test material to groups of laboratory animals of the same strain by a specific route of exposure, and under controlled experimental conditions—e.g. diet, caging, temperature, relative humidity, time of dosing. Mortalities at each dosage are recorded over a specified period of time, usually 14 days. By epicutaneous or respiratory exposure, the exposure time should be stated, since the degree of local injury and the potential for systemic toxicity are a function of this time. For routes other than inhalation, the exposure dosage is usually expressed as mass (or volume) of test material given per unit of body weight—e.g. ml kg^{-1} or mg kg^{-1}. For inhalation, the exposure dose is expressed as the amount of test material present per unit volume of exposure atmosphere—mg m^{-3} or ppm. Dose–response information collected for differing concentrations of an atmospherically dispersed material should be over similar periods of time in order to allow the most effective comparisons to be made. Alternatively, the effect of differing inhalation exposure doses can be achieved by exposing different groups to the same concentration of test substance for various exposure periods; this may allow the calculation of a median time to death (50 per cent response rate) for the population exposed to a specific atmospheric concentration of test material (Lt_{50}). By using both these approaches it is possible to reach conclusions on the differential sensitivity of a population to varying concentrations for a specified period of time, or to differing exposure periods for a given concentration.

Dosage–mortality data usually conform to the sigmoid cumulative frequency distribution curve (Figure 9A), which may be converted to a linear form using a log–probit plot (Figure 9B). Lethal toxicity is usually initially calculated and compared at a specific mortality level; most frequently used is that causing 50 per cent mortality in the population studied, since this represents the mid-point of the dosage range about which the majority of deaths occur and usually with a symmetrical distribution. This is the median lethal dose for 50 per cent of the population studied (LD_{50})—i.e. that dose, calculated from the dosage–mortality data, which causes death of half of the population dosed under the specific conditions of the test. This concept of the LD_{50} was introduced by Trevan (1927). By inhalation, the reference is the (lethal concentration)$_{50}$ (LC_{50}) for a specified period of time (i.e. *X*-h LC_{50}). However, as noted above, sometimes the Lt_{50} is a useful value.

Other values calculated may be the LD_5 and LD_{95}, which give statistical indications, respectively, of near-threshold and near-maximum lethal toxicity, and the range of doses over which a lethal response may occur.

Since the LD_{50}, for economical and ethical reasons, is usually conducted with only small numbers of animals, there is an uncertainty factor associated with the calculation of the LD_{50} (or

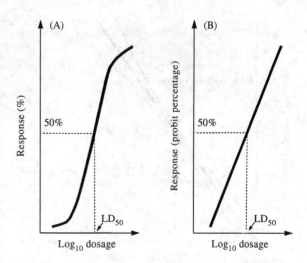

Figure 9 Dosage–mortality data plotted as a cumulative frequency distribution curve (percentage response versus $\log_{10}$ dosage) in A, and linearly transformed by log–probit plot in B

LC_{50}). This is estimated from the 95 per cent confidence limits—i.e. the dosage range for which there is only a 5 per cent chance that the LD_{50} (or other LD value) lies outside. Ninety-five per cent confidence limits are narrowest at the LD_{50} (Figure 10), which is another reason why this is an appropriate point for the comparison of acute lethal toxicity data.

The LD_{50}, by itself, is an insufficient index of lethal toxicity, particularly if comparisons are to be made between different materials. The whole of the dosage–response information should be examined, including the slope of the dosage–response line and 95 per cent confidence limits. For example, two materials with differing LD_{50} values but overlapping 95 per cent confidence limits are not regarded as being of significantly different lethal toxicity, since there is a statistical probability that the LD_{50} of one material will be within the 95 per cent confidence limits of the other. However, when there is no overlap of 95 per cent confidence limits, then the materials are considered to have significantly different lethal toxicity at the LD_{50} level (Figure 11). A particularly important consideration is that of the slope of the dosage–response curve (Figure 12). For example, if two materials have similar LD_{50} values with overlapping 95 per cent confidence limits and identical slopes on the dosage–response lines (and therefore statistically similar LD_{10} and LD_{90} values), they are lethally equitoxic over a wide

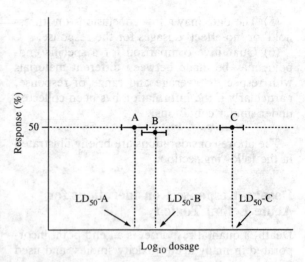

Figure 11 Comparison of the acute lethal toxicity of three compounds using LD_{50} data alone. Compounds A and B have overlapping 95 per cent confidence limits, and therefore have comparable acute lethal toxicity. Compound C, whose 95 per cent confidence limits are separate from those of A and B, is significantly less toxic (higher LD_{50} dosage) than either A or B, on the basis of LD_{50} values

dosage range (A and B, Figure 12). However, materials having similar LD_{50} values but differing slopes (and, hence, significantly different LD_{10} and LD_{90} values) may not be considered to be lethally equitoxic over a wide dosage range (A or B versus C, Figure 12). Thus, materials having a steep slope (A or B, Figure 12) may affect a much larger proportion of the population by incremental increases in dosages than is the case with materials having a shallow slope; thus, acute overdose may be a more serious problem affecting the majority of a population for materials with steeper slopes. In contrast, materials having a shallower slope (C, Figure 12) may present problems for the hyperreactive groups at the left-hand side of the dosage–response curve, and effects may occur at significantly lower dosages than for hyperreactive individuals associated with the steep slope group. It follows from the above that a proper interpretation of acute lethal toxicity information should include examination of LD_{50}, 95 per cent confidence limits, slope and extremes of the dosage–response curve.

It needs to be stressed that dosage–response information requires to be interpreted in terms of the conditions by which it was obtained; the following few examples are used to illustrate the care necessary.

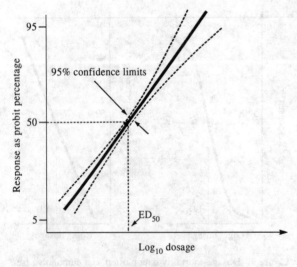

Figure 10 Dosage–mortality curve with 95 per cent confidence limits. The limits are closest at the ED_{50} and diverge as the extremes of the dosage response are reached

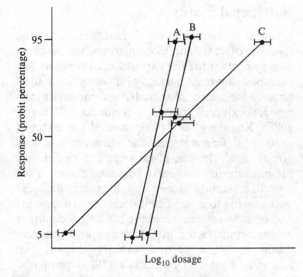

Figure 12 Influence of slopes of dosage–mortality data on the interpretation of LD_{50} data. All three materials (A, B and C) have overlapping 95 per cent confidence limits at the 50 per cent response level, and are therefore of comparable LD_{50}. Materials A and B have parallel dosage–response lines and overlapping confidence limits at 5 per cent and 95 per cent; therefore, these two materials are of comparable lethal toxicity over a wide range of doses. Material C with a shallower slope has significantly different LD_5 and LD_{95} values, and therefore over a wide range of doses has a lethal toxicity differing from that of materials A and B. With materials A and B, owing to the steep slope of the dosage–response line, a much larger proportion of the population will be affected by small incremental increases in dosage. With material C, there may be a greater hazard for the hyperreactive groups, since the LD_5 lies at a much lower dosage than for A and B

(1) The numerical precision of the LD_{50} lies only in the statistical procedures by which it is attained. If an experiment to determine LD_{50} is repeated at a later time, slightly different dosage–response data may be obtained because of biological and environmental variability, resulting in a different numerical value for the LD_{50}. Therefore, LD_{50} values should be regarded as representing an order of lethal toxicity under the specific circumstances by which the information was collected.

(2) An important consideration in interpreting the acute hazard from a chemical is the time to toxic effect. Thus, materials of similar LD_{50} but differing times to death may present different hazards. For example, with substances having similar LD_{50} and slope values, those having more rapid times to death can be considered as presenting a greater acute hazard. However, those substances with longer latency to effect may have a

potential to produce cumulative toxicity by repeated exposure. For example, the acute per-oral LD_{50} of 2,4-pentanedione in the rat is 0.58 g kg^{-1} and that of 2,2'-bis(4-aminophenoxyphenyl) propane (BAPP) is 0.31 g kg^{-1}, with respective times to death of 2–5 h and 13–14 days; on this basis, 2,4-pentanedione would be regarded as presenting a greater acute potential hazard than BAPP (Tyler and Ballantyne, 1988).

(3) A more complete interpretation of the significance of LD_{50} data may require consideration of the cause of death. If differing potentially lethal toxic effects are produced, it is important to know whether this can lead to a multimodal dosage–response curve, and thus to differing hazards by immediate or latent mortality or morbidity. Clearly latency is of importance in clinical toxicology for decisions on immediate medical management and observations and treatment for latent toxicity. For example, *tert*-butyl nitrite given by acute intraperitoneal injection to mice has a 30 min LD_{50} of 613 mg kg^{-1} and a 7 day LD_{50} of 187 mg kg^{-1}. The earlier deaths were probably related to cardiovascular collapse and methaemoglobin formation, whereas later deaths were due to liver injury (Maickel and McFadden, 1979).

(4) Acute LD_{50} data may not be a direct guide to defining lethal toxicity by multiple exposures. Thus, with a material producing significant cumulative toxicity, the acute lethal dose (and dosage) may be significantly higher than that producing death by multiple smaller exposures. For example, the 4 h LC_{50} for trimethoxysilane is 47 ppm (rat); however, in rats given 20 exposures, each of 7 h, over 4 weeks the LC_{50} was 5.5 ppm for that time period (Ballantyne *et al.*, 1988). Thus, the potentially lethal vapour concentration of trimethoxysilane for repeated exposure is significantly less than that for acute exposure.

Any investigation into lethal toxicity should attempt to allow the maximum amount of usable information to be obtained. For this reason, acute toxicity studies should be designed not only to determine lethal toxicity, but also to monitor for sublethal and target organ toxicity; this is made possible by incorporating into the protocol observations of clinical signs, body weight, haematology, clinical chemistry, urinalysis, gross and microscopic pathology, and such other specialized procedures as are considered appropriate for the material under test. In this way a significantly greater amount of relevant information can be obtained, and the most useful and meaningful information can be collected, to allow a comparative evaluation of acute toxicity and potential hazards and the potential for cumulative toxicity (Zbinden and Flury-Roversi, 1981).

Detailed discussions on dosage–response relationships and their toxicological and pharmacological relevance have been written by Tallarida and Jacob (1979), Timbrell (1982) and Sperling (1984).

FACTORS INFLUENCING TOXICITY

With both animal studies and human poisoning, the nature, severity, incidence and probable induction of toxicity depend on a large number of exogenous and endogenous factors. Some of the more important are as follows.

Species and Strain

Species and strain differences in susceptibility to chemical-induced toxicity may be due, to variable extents, to differences in rates of absorption, metabolic conversions, detoxification mechanisms and excretion. In some cases animal studies may give underestimates, and in other instances overestimates, for acute peroral toxicity to humans. For example, the acute peroral LD_{50} of ethylene glycol has been determined in several laboratory mammals to range from 4.7 to 7.5 g kg^{-1} (Sweet, 1985–1986a), and that for methanol to range from 5.63 to 7.50 g kg^{-1} (Sweet, 1985–1986b); both these chemicals are more toxic to humans with a minimal lethal dosage around 0.5–1.0 ml kg^{-1}.

Age

With some substances age may significantly affect toxicity, probably mainly owing to relative metabolizing and excretory capacities. In one extensive compilation of LD_{50} values for drugs to neonatal and adult mammals (Goldenthal, 1971), the ratio (LD_{50}-adult)/(LD_{50}-neonate) varied from <0.02 (for amidephrine) to 750 (for digitoxin).

Nutritional Status

Nutritional status may significantly influence the level of cofactors and biotransformation mechanisms important for the expression of toxicity. For example, diet may markedly influence the natural tumour incidence in animals, and modulate carcinogen-induced tumour incidence (Grasso, 1988). Khanna *et al.* (1988) studied the effect of protein deficiency on the neurobehavioural effects of acrylamide in rat pups exposed during the intrauterine and early postnatal stages. They found acrylamide more toxic in protein-deficient hosts, owing to a significant decrease in dopamine and benzodiazepine receptor binding. Feeding is an important factor in the design and interpretation of acute peroral toxicity studies. For example, Kast and Nishikawa (1981) compared the acute peroral toxicity of several antigastric ulcer drugs, and β-adrenoceptor agonists and blockers; the ratio (LD_{50} fed)/(LD_{50} fasted) for rats and mice ranged from 1.3 to 1.47, indicating a higher toxicity in the starved animals. The authors concluded that the greater acute toxicity in the starved animals was due to accelerated gastric emptying and intestinal absorption. The importance of dietary factors in toxicity has been reviewed by Angeli-Greaves and McLean (1981).

Time of Dosing

Diurnal and seasonal variations in toxicity may relate to similar variations in biochemical, physiological and hormonal profiles. Examples of temporal variations in biological activity include circadian dependence of metabolic adverse effects of cyclosporin (Malmary *et al.*, 1988), toxicity of methotrexate (Marks *et al.*, 1985) and seasonal variations in gentamicin nephrotoxicity (Pariat *et al.*, 1988).

Environmental Factors

A variety of environmental factors are known to influence the development of toxicity, including temperature, relative humidity and photoperiod. The influence of temperature may vary between differing chemicals and the effects investigated. For example, colchicine and digitalis are more toxic the higher the temperature (Lu, 1985); in contrast, studies on the behavioural toxicity of the anticholinesterase soman suggest that the lower the temperature the greater the susceptibility (Wheeler, 1987). The influence of temperature on toxicity is clearly an important consideration for materials used in arctic and tropical areas.

Exposure (Dosing) Characteristics

The nature, severity and likelihood of induction of toxicity are influenced by the magnitude, number, frequency and profiling of dosing. Thus, local or systemic toxicity produced by acute exposure may also occur by a cumulative process with repeated lower dosage exposures; also, additional toxicity may be seen with the repeated exposure situations. For example, acute exposure to formaldehyde vapour causes peripheral sensory irritant effects and (with sufficiently high concentration) injury and inflammatory change in the respiratory tract; short-term repeated vapour exposure may result in the development of respiratory sensitization; longer-term vapour exposure may cause squamous metaplasia and nasal tumours (Wartew, 1983). The relationships for cumulative toxicity by repetitive exposure compared with acute exposure toxicity may be complex, and the potential for repeated exposure cumulative toxicity from acutely subthreshold doses may not be quantitatively predictable. For example, the LC_{50} for a 4 h exposure to trimethoxysilane vapour is 47 ppm; by repeated exposure over a 4 week period (7 h/day, 5 days a week) the LC_{50} is 5.5 ppm (Ballantyne *et al.*, 1988). In contrast, acute exposure to benzene vapour for 26 h (95 ppm) or 96 h (21 ppm) produced severe bone marrow cytotoxicity, while a similar exposure dose given over a longer period of time (95 ppm for 2 h/day for 2 weeks) produced little toxicity (Toft *et al.*, 1982).

For repeated exposure toxicity, the precise profiling of doses may significantly influence toxicity. For example, with formaldehyde in a 4 week vapour inhalation study, it was determined that exposure of rats to 10 or 20 ppm by interrupted exposure over eight exposure periods produced more nasal mucosal cytotoxicity than did continuous exposures (Wilmer *et al.*, 1987). In a 4 week inhalation study with carbon tetrachloride, it was found that interruption of a daily 6 h exposure by 1–5 h periods of non-exposure caused more severe hepatotoxicity than with continuous exposures, but 5 min peak loads superimposed on a steady background only slightly aggravated the hepatotoxic effect of carbon tetrachloride vapour (Bogers *et al.*, 1977).

Formulation and Presentation

For chemicals given perorally or applied to the skin, toxicity may be modified by the presence of materials in formulations which facilitate or retard the absorption of the chemicals. With respiratory exposure to aerosols, particle size significantly determines the depth of penetration and deposition in the respiratory tract.

Miscellaneous

A variety of other factors may affect the nature and exhibition of toxicity, depending on the conditions of the study, for example, housing conditions, handling, dosing volume, etc. Variability in test conditions and procedures may result in significant interlaboratory variability in results of otherwise standard procedures (e.g. LD_{50} determination: Griffith, 1964; Hunter *et al.*, 1979).

BIOHANDLING AS A DETERMINANT OF SYSTEMIC TOXICITY

The induction of systemic toxicity results from a complex interrelationship between absorbed parent material and conversion products formed in tissues, their distribution in body fluids and tissues, binding and storage characteristics, and their excretion. Some of these factors are considered below (see also Figure 13).

Absorption

The absorption of a substance from the site of exposure may result from passive diffusion, facilitated diffusion, active transport or the formation of transport vesicles (pinocytosis and phagocytosis). The process of absorption may be facilitated or retarded by a variety of factors—e.g. elevated temperature increases percutaneous absorption by cutaneous vasodilation, and surface-active materials facilitate penetration. The integrity of the absorbing surface is important— e.g. the acute percutaneous LD_{50} for HCN (solution) is 6.89 mg kg^{-1} for rabbits with intact skin

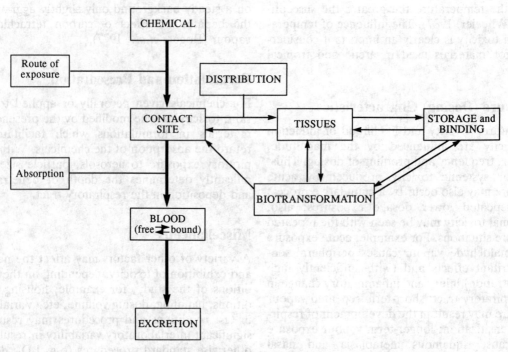

Figure 13   Possible fate of a chemical absorbed from the route of exposure

and 2.34 mg kg^{-1} if the skin is abraded (Ballantyne, 1987).

Biodistribution

After absorption, materials circulate either free or bound to plasma protein or blood cells; the degree of binding, and factors influencing the equilibrium with the free form, may influence availability for metabolism, storage and excretion. Within tissues there may be binding, storage, metabolic activation or detoxification; binding may produce a high tissue/plasma partition and be a source for slow titration into the circulation following the cessation of environmental exposure. Examples of storage sites include fat for lipophilic materials (e.g. chlorinated pesticides), and bone for fluoride, lead and strontium. The relationship between exposure dose and release rate may be complex: for example, volatile lipophilic materials are generally more rapidly desorbed than non-volatile lipophilic substances. Tissue permeability may be modified by tissue-specific barriers—e.g. the blood–brain barrier and the placenta. This may affect differential toxicity within classes of compounds—e.g. neurobehavioural effects produced by organomercuri-

als but to a lesser degree by inorganic mercury compounds (Lu, 1985).

Biotransformation

Metabolism of substances is conveniently classified under the following two major headings (Williams, 1959):

Phase I reactions   A functional group is introduced into the molecule by oxidation, reduction or hydrolysis.

Phase II reactions   There is conjugation of an absorbed material or its metabolite with an endogenous substrate.

For many materials there is an initial Phase I reaction to produce materials which are conjugated by Phase II processes. In other instances only a Phase II process may be utilized. Reactions of a Phase I type include oxidation, reduction and enzymic hydrolysis; Phase II reactions include conjugation with glucuronic acid, sulphate, glycine and glutathione, and acetylation and methylation. Phase I reactions, particularly, may result in the formation of toxic metabolites from relatively innocuous precursors—i.e. metabolic activation. Phase II conjugates are, in general, more water-soluble than parent compound or Phase I metabolites and, hence, usually more readily excreted. With toxic parent compounds, or toxic metabolites, there may be conversion to less toxic products—i.e. detoxification has occurred. Examples of metabolic activation and detoxification are given in Table 5. Many activation reactions are catalysed by a cytochrome *P*-450 dependent mono-oxygenase system, which is particularly active in liver. Clearly a major determinant of the likelihood of toxicity developing, and its severity, is the overall balance between absorption rate of a chemical, its metabolic activation and detoxification, and the excretion of toxic species.

Excretion

Substances may be excreted as parent compound, metabolites and/or Phase II conjugates. A major route of excretion is by the kidney, and in some cases the urinary elimination of parent compound, metabolite or conjugate may be used as a means for assessing absorbed dose. Some materials may be excreted in bile and thence in faeces; in such cases there may also be enterohepatic cycling. Certain volatile materials and metabolites may be eliminated in expired air. The excretion of materials in sweat, hair, nails and saliva is usually quantitatively insignificant, but these routes may be of importance for a forensic or industrial diagnosis of intoxication (Paschal *et al.*, 1989; Randall and Gibson, 1989). Materials excreted in milk may be transferred to the neonate.

General Considerations

The probability of adverse effects developing in response to chemical exposure depends particularly on the magnitude, duration, frequency and route of exposure. These will determine the amount of material to which an organism is exposed (the exposure dose) and, hence, to the amount of material which can be absorbed (the absorbed dose). The latter determines the amount of material available for distribution and toxic metabolite formation, and, hence, the likelihood of inducing a toxic effect. Opposing absorption and metabolite accumulation is elimination. Hence, for a given environmental exposure situation, the probability of inducing toxicity, and its magnitude, depend on the relationship between the rate of absorption, metabolism (activation and detoxification), and elimination of parent material and metabolites.

The amount of a material in contact with the absorbing surface is one of the principal determinants of absorbed dose. In general, the higher the concentration the greater the absorbed dose. However, if mechanisms other than simple diffusion across a concentration gradient are operating, a simple proportionate relationship between concentration and absorbed dose may not exist. In such instances, a rate-limiting factor could result in proportionately smaller increases in absorbed dose for incremental increases in concentration at the absorption site. Also, and in particular when there is absorption by active transport, there may be saturation of the absorption process and a ceiling value.

When there is repeated exposure, the relative amounts of biotransformation products, and the distribution and elimination of metabolites and

Table 5 Examples of metabolic transformations of chemicals

Biotransformation	Chemical	Conversion
Detoxification	Cyanide	Enzymic conversion to less toxic thiocyanate
	Benzoic acid	Conjugation with glycine to produce hippuric acid
	Bromobenzene	3,4-Epoxide reactive metabolite is enzymically hydrated to the 3,4-dihydrodiol or conjugated with glutathione
Activation	Carbon tetrachloride	Microsome enzyme metabolic activation to hepatotoxic trichloromethylperoxy radicals
	2-Acetylaminofluorene	*N*-hydroxylation to the more potent carcinogen *N*-hydroxyacetylaminofluorene
	Parathion	Oxidative desulphuration to the potent cholinesterase inhibitor paraoxon

parent compound, may be different from those following an acute exposure. For example, repeated exposure may induce and enhance mechanisms responsible for the biotransformation of the absorbed material. Thus they might alter the relative proportions of parent molecules and metabolites (activation and detoxification), and, hence, the probability for target organ toxicity. Also, if there is slow detoxification, storage and/or slow excretion, repeated exposures may lead to the accumulation of toxic species and, hence, a potential for cumulative toxicity.

ROUTES OF EXPOSURE

The primary tissue or system by which a material comes into contact with the body, and from where it may be absorbed in order to exert systemic toxicity, is the route of exposure. The frequent circumstances of environmental exposure are by ingestion (peroral), inhalation and skin or eye contact. Also, for investigational, therapeutic and certain forensic purposes, intramuscular, intravenous and subcutaneous injections may be routes of exposure.

The relationship between route and exposure, biotransformation and potential for toxicity, may be complex and also influenced by the magnitude and duration of dosing. Materials that undergo hepatic activation are likely to exhibit greater toxicity when given perorally than if absorbed across the lung or skin, owing to the high proportion of material passing directly via the portal vein following peroral dosing. In contrast, materials that undergo hepatic detoxification are likely to be less toxic perorally than when absorbed percutaneously or across the respiratory tract. However, in determining the relevance of route to biotransformation and toxicity, both the magnitude and time-scale for dosing should be considered. Thus, when a single large dose (bolus) of a metabolically activated material is given perorally, its rapid metabolism may result in the immediate development of a severe acute toxicity. However, if the same material is given perorally at much lower rates (e.g. by dietary inclusion), then there will be slow and sustained absorption, and in such circumstances the rate of generation of the toxic species may approach that resulting from continuous exposure by other routes. With materials that are detoxified by the liver, a slow continuous alimentary absorption will result in an anticipated low toxicity, compared with other routes of exposure. However, a peroral bolus may result in the detoxifying capacity of the liver being overwhelmed, and unmetabolized material may enter the circulation to initiate toxicity. A few comments on specific routes of exposure follow.

Peroral

If a materal is sufficiently irritant or corrosive, it will cause local inflammatory or corrosive effects on the upper alimentary tract. This may lead to, for example, fibrosis, dysphagia, and perforation with mediastinitis and/or peritonitis and the complications thereof. Additionally, carcinogenic materials may induce tumour formation in the alimentary tract. The gastrointestinal tract is an important route by which systemically toxic materials may be absorbed.

Percutaneous Absorption

Skin contact is an important route of exposure in the occupational and domestic environment. Local effects may include acute inflammation and corrosion, chronic inflammatory responses, immune-mediated reactions and neoplasia. The percutaneous absorption of materials can be a significant route for the absorption of systemically toxic materials (Billingham, 1977; Bronough and Maibach, 1985), and indeed is now a means for the systemic titration of pharmacologically active materials (Woodford and Barry, 1986). Factors influencing the percutaneous absorption of substances include skin site, integrity of skin, temperature, formulation and physicochemical characteristics, including charge, molecular weight, and hydrophilic and lipophilic characteristics (Billingham, 1977; Dugard, 1977; Stuttgen *et al.*, 1982; Kemppainen and Reifenrath, 1990).

Inhalation

The likelihood of toxicity from atmospherically dispersed materials depends on a number of factors, the most important of which include physical state and properties, concentration, and time and frequency of exposure. The water solubility of a gas or vapour influences the depth of penetration of a material into the respiratory tract. As water solubility decreases and lipid solubility increases, there is a more effective penetration towards the alveoli. Water-soluble molecules, such as formaldehyde, are more effectively scavenged by the upper respiratory tract.

The penetration and distribution of fibres and particulates in the respiratory tract are determined principally by their size. Thus, in general, particles having a mass medium aerodynamic diameter greater than 50 μm do not enter the respiratory tract; those >10 μm are deposited in the upper respiratory tract; those having a range of 10–2 μm are deposited in the trachea, bronchi and bronchioles; and only particles whose diameter is <1.2 μm reach the alveoli. Thus, larger insoluble particles are more likely to cause local reactions in the upper respiratory tract, and the potential for alveolar injury is greater with particles of smaller diameter. Fibres have aerodynamic characteristics such that those having diameters >3 μm are unlikely to penetrate the lung. In general, fibres having a diameter <3 μm and length not >200 μm will enter the lung. Fibres >10 μm may not be removed by normal clearance mechanisms. Several studies have indicated that fibres of diameter >1.5 μm and length <8 μm have maximum biological activity (Asher and McGrath, 1976; Stanton *et al.*, 1981). Dust may be a significant cause of lung disease (Conference, 1990).

The likelihood that inhaled substances will produce local effects in the respiratory tract depends on their physical and chemical characteristics (particularly solubility), reactivity with lining fluids, reactivity with tissue components and site of deposition. Depending on the nature of the material, conditions of exposure and biological reactivity, the types of response produced include acute inflammation and injury, chronic inflammation, immune-mediated hypersensitivity reactions and neoplasia. The degree to which inhaled gases, vapours and particulates are absorbed, and, hence, their potential to produce systemic toxicity, depend on molecular weight, solubility in tissue fluids, metabolism by lung tissue, diffusion rate and equilibrium state.

Eye

Local and systemic adverse effects may be produced by contamination with liquids, solids and atmospherically dispersed materials. Local effects include transient inflammation, permanent injury and hypersensitivity reactions. Penetration may lead to iritis, glaucoma and cataract. Systemically active amounts of material may be absorbed from periocular blood vessels and/or nasal mucosa following passage down the nasolachrymal duct (Shell, 1982; Ballantyne, 1983).

EXPOSURE TO MIXTURES OF CHEMICALS

Circumstances involving exposure to several xenobiotics can result in prior, coincidental or successive exposure to these chemicals, and the nature of the toxicity may vary considerably depending on the conditions of exposure. Thus, an evaluation of the hazards from exposure to multiple chemicals can be much more demanding than is the case for a single chemical. In assessing toxicity from mixtures it is important to consider: (1) chemical and/or physical interactions of the individual materials; (2) the effect that one chemical may have on the absorption, metabolism and pharmacokinetic characteristics of another; and (3) the possibility of interaction between parent compound and metabolites (Ballantyne, 1985). A convenient descriptive classification for effects produced by binary mixtures of chemicals is as follows.

Independent effects Substances qualitatively and quantitatively exert their own toxicity independent of each other.

Additive effects Materials with similar qualitative toxicity produce a response which is quantitatively equal to the sum of the effects produced by the individual constituents.

Antagonistic effects Materials oppose each other's toxicity, or one interferes with the toxicity of another; a particular example is that of antidotal action.

Potentiating effects One material, usually of low toxicity, enhances the expression of toxicity by another; the result is more severe injury than that produced by the toxic species alone.

Synergistic effects Two materials, given simultaneously, produce toxicity significantly greater than anticipated from that of either material; the effect differs from potentiation in that each substance contributes to toxicity, and the net effect is always greater than additive.

In assessing the toxicity of mixtures, the following need to be taken into consideration:

- Possible physical and chemical interactions — which may result in the formation of new substances or groupings, or influence bioavailability.
- Time relationships of the exposure for the various components.
- Route and conditions of exposure.
- Physical and physiological factors affecting absorption.
- Mutual influence of materials and metabolites on biotransformation, pharmacokinetic characteristics and target organ doses of toxic species.
- Relative affinities of the target sites.
- Potential for independent, additive, antagonistic and interactive processes between the various chemical species.

Mixtures may be complex and contain unreacted parent materials, major reaction and degradation products, and contaminants and trace additives. It is important to be aware that small quantities of high-toxicity materials may have equal, or greater, significance with respect to adverse health effects than major components. For example, serious consideration needs to be given to repeated exposure toxicity from small quantities of monomer residuals in polymeric materials — e.g. ethylene oxide, propylene oxide, vinyl chloride and formaldehyde (Ballantyne, 1989). The contribution to toxicity by trace materials is well illustrated by, for example, the presence of trialkyl phosphorothioate impurities in organophosphate anticholinesterases (Hollingshaus *et al.*, 1981) and the presence of 2,3,7,8-tetrachlorodibenzodioxin in chlorophenols (Kimbrough *et al.*, 1984).

Many instances of enhancement of toxicity by specific routes are known. Thus, on the skin the systemic toxicity of a material may be enhanced by other materials which facilitate percutaneous absorption. For example, the presence of a surface-active material may result in a carrier func-

tion, and the presence of a primary irritant may produce local erythema resulting in increased skin blood flow. If the viscosity of a material is increased, this may enhance local or systemic toxicity due to persistence on the skin.

The inhalation exposure dosage of chemicals may be modified by, for example, the presence of sensory irritants or HCN, which can alter the rate and depth of breathing. Some substances may cause anosmia, and, hence, remove an olfactory warning for other inhaled materials. Particulates may absorb other materials which, if inhaled, cause an increased local burden. When trace quantities of highly volatile and toxic materials are present in a substance, they may, depending on the condition of air movement, have a significant influence on toxicity and hazard. For example, if materials containing trace amounts of acrolein are handled in stagnant air conditions, then potentially toxic vapour concentrations of acrolein may develop; in contrast, when there is free airflow the acrolein vapour concentration may be low (Ballantyne *et al.*, 1989a). Thus, the degree of ventilation of an area may significantly influence the toxicity of the atmosphere resulting from vaporization of the individual constituents of a liquid mixture.

The endogenous determinants of overall toxicity resulting from exposure to a mixture of chemicals can be very complex. For example, toxicity may be altered by prior or simultaneous exposure, resulting in enhancement or suppression of metabolic activation or detoxification pathways. The potential for toxicity may depend on the equilibrium state, although this may be continually fluctuating. Modification of toxicity may also result from alteration of pharmacokinetic characteristics, variation in the biodistribution of absorbed materials and metabolites, modifying elimination of the toxic species, and competition for binding sites or receptors. All the above factors will influence the relative and absolute concentration of toxic species at target sites for toxicity. Detailed discussions on the toxicity and hazard evaluation of mixtures of substances have been presented in World Health Organization (1981), Murphy (1983), Ballantyne (1985) and National Research Council (1988).

DRUG TOXICITY

Adverse drug reactions can be classified in several ways. They may be divided into reactions due to overdosage, intolerance, side-effects, secondary effects, idiosyncrasy and hypersensitivity (see pp. 6–7). Some of these terms are difficult to define, however, and particular reactions are difficult to classify into one of them. Another system divides them into two types—Type A, which are the results of an exaggerated but otherwise normal pharmacological action of a drug, such as uncontrolled bleeding from an anticoagulant drug, and Type B, which are totally aberrant effects not expected from the known pharmacological actions of a drug, such as deafness from streptomycin. A third system divides them into three groups: dose-dependent, as in Type A above; dose-independent, which are of an allergic nature involving antigen–antibody reactions; and pseudoallergic reactions, where allergic reactions are mimicked by mediator release due to direct action of the drug or its metabolite on most cells.

Factors influencing dose-dependent drug toxicity include formulation, route of administration, pregnancy, age, genetic polymorphism of metabolism, environmental influences on metabolism, renal and hepatic excretion, disease, drug interactions and patient compliance.

In many countries evidence of adverse drug reactions is now sought in normal volunteers and patients in all phases of clinical trial leading up to licensing and marketing of a new product. Post-marketing surveillance (PMS) is then carried out to assess long-term safety in thousands of patients in order to detect low-frequency reactions which were not recognized in the relatively small number of patients studied in pre-marketing trials. There are a variety of post-marketing surveillance schemes, including voluntary reporting of possible cases of drug reaction, prospective cohort studies and case–control studies.

NATURE, DESIGN AND CONDUCT OF TOXICOLOGY STUDIES

Toxicology studies should permit, within the constraints of the time period studied, a quantitative determination of the potential for a chemical, or mixture of chemicals, to produce local and systemic adverse effects, and allow a determination of factors that may influence the nature, severity and possible reversibility of effects. Specific features that any toxicology testing programme should allow are as follows:

- The nature of the adverse effects—i.e. the fundamental pathological process.
- Relationship of the adverse effects to in-use and practical situations.
- Dose–response relationships (average, range, hyperreactive groups, no-effects and minimum-effects doses).
- Modifying factors.
- Effects of gross acute overexposure.
- Effects of repeated exposure (short- and long-term)
- Definition of allowable and non-allowable exposures.
- Definition of monitoring procedures.
- Guidance on protective and restrictive procedures.
- Guidance on first-aid and medical management.
- Definition of 'at-risk' populations (e.g. sex, pre-existing disease, genetically susceptible).

Information necessary for the above purposes can be obtained only from carefully designed and conducted studies. In many cases, it may not be economically possible to undertake a complete spectrum of toxicology studies, and in such circumstances it is necessary to consider carefully the most appropriate investigational approaches based on known physicochemical properties, existing and suspected toxicity and anticipated conditions of use. The relevance and credibility of a toxicology study can be no better than its design and conduct permit. For the purposes of hazard evaluation, there is a need to emphasize exposure conditions that may exist under practical conditions of use.

Toxicology testing programmes generally begin with single-exposure *in vivo* or *in vitro* studies and progress to evaluating the effects of long-term repeated exposures. Studies having specific end-points, such as teratology and reproductive effects, are conducted as the emerging toxicology profile and end-use exposure patterns dictate. Toxicology testing procedures can be conveniently subdivided into general and specific. General toxicology studies are those in which animals are exposed to a test material under appropriate conditions, and they are examined for all types of toxicity that the monitoring procedures permit. Specific toxicological studies are those in which exposed animals, or *in vitro* test systems, are monitored for a defined end-point.

General Toxicology Studies

These are usually conducted as a programme in the sequence of acute, short-term repeated, sub-chronic and chronic. Ideally, the protocol for general studies should include provision for some animals to be kept for a period after the end of dosing in order to determine if latency and reversibility, or otherwise, of toxic effects occurs. Acute studies give information on toxicity produced by a single exposure, including the effects of massive overexposure; they also give information of use for setting exposure conditions for short-term repeated exposure studies. The type of monitoring employed in general toxicology studies will depend on various considerations, including the chemistry of the test material, its known or suspected toxicity, degree of exposure and the rationale for conducting the test. In general, since multiple-exposure studies are most likely to produce the widest spectrum of toxicity, it is usual to employ the most extensive monitoring in these studies. The monitoring employed to detect functional toxicity in the living animal, and for the detection of toxic injury in dead animals, may include the following:

- Inspection, on a regular basis, for signs of toxic and/or pharmacological effects.
- Body weight before dosing and at appropriate intervals during the dosing and recovery phase.
- Food and water consumption.
- Haematology for assessment of peripheral blood and haematopoietic tissues.
- Clinical (serum) chemistry of various substances and of specific enzyme activities, and appropriate urinalysis.
- Gross and microscopic pathology with organ weight measurement.
- Special pathological or functional tests may be required on a case-by-case basis.

Specific Toxicology Studies

Many of these procedures are directed at determining a particular toxic effect for hazard evaluation purposes, but others are employed as 'screening' or 'short-term' tests to assess the potential of a substance to induce chronic effects or toxicity with a long latency. Some of the most frequently employed special toxicology methods are listed below:

Primary Irritation

These studies are designed to determine the potential of substances to cause local inflammatory effects, notably in skin and eye. In order to reduce the use of animals for eye irritancy testing, a variety of alternative procedures have been proposed, which include the use of enucleated eyes and various *in vitro* cell or tissue cultures, and the measurement of corneal thickness (Nardone and Bradlaw, 1983; Shopsis and Sathe, 1984; Ballantyne, 1986; Borenfreund and Borrero, 1984).

Peripheral Sensory Irritation

Methods to assess the potential to cause eye or respiratory tract discomfort with associated reflexes are particularly useful in occupational toxicology (Owens and Punte, 1963; Ballantyne *et al.*, 1977; Ballantyne, 1984).

Immune-mediated Hypersensitivity

Allergenic materials may produce hypersensitivity reactions by skin contact or inhalation, and several methods are available to determine the potential for chemicals to produce allergic contact dermatitis or asthmatic reactions (Goodwin *et al.*, 1981; Maurer *et al.*, 1984; Karol *et al.*, 1985).

Neurological and Behavioural Toxicity

To confirm the existence, nature, site and mechanism of toxic injury to the central and/or peripheral nervous system, a variety of approaches with varying degrees of sophistication are available. These include observational test batteries (Gad, 1982), light and electron microscopy (Spencer *et al.*, 1980), selective biochemical procedures (Abou-Donia *et al.*, 1987), and electrophysiological, pharmacological, tissue culture and metabolism techniques (Dewar, 1981; Mitchell, 1982).

Teratology

Most studies are currently directed at assessing the potential for chemicals to induce structural defects of development, and essentially involve administering the test material to the pregnant animal during the period of maximum organogenesis (Tuchmann-Duplessis, 1980; Beckman and Brent, 1984; Tyl, 1988). Recently there has been increasing interest in the development of test methods to assess for possible adverse functional effects resulting from exposure of the fetus both during gestation and in the early neonatal period (Zbinden, 1981; Vorhees, 1983).

Reproductive Toxicity

Reproductive studies are conducted to assess the potential for adverse structural and functional effects on gonads, fertility, gestation, fetuses, lactation and general reproductive performance. Exposure to the chemical may be over one or several generations. In view of the necessarily comparatively low doses used over these long-term studies, they may be not sufficiently sensitive to detect most potentially teratogenic materials. The basis for these tests has been reviewed (Mattison, 1983: Baeder *et al.*, 1985; Rao *et al.*, 1987.)

Metabolism and Pharmacokinetics

These studies may be of very considerable importance in the interpretation of conventional toxicology studies; in helping determine the mechanism of toxicity; in assessing the relationship between environmental exposure concentration and target organ toxicity; and in the design of additional studies to elucidate mechanisms of toxicity. Metabolic studies should yield information on the biotransformation of a material, the sites at which this occurs and the mechanism of biotransformation. Pharmacokinetic studies should allow a quantitative measurement of the rate of uptake, the absorbed dose, the biodistribution, tissue binding and storage, and the routes and rates of excretion of test material and metabolites (Oehme, 1980; Gibaldi and Perrier, 1982.

Genotoxicity

A number of tests, both *in vitro* and *in vivo*, are available to assess the mutagenic or clastogenic potential of chemicals. A positive genotoxic result is not necessarily a directly usable end-point *per se*, but may assist in defining a potential for adverse health effects or be used in screening for potential longer-term toxicity. Thus, materials with clear mutagenic activity may be suspected of being genotoxic carcinogens, and appropriate further studies may be required; clastogenic materials may be suspected of reproductive or haematological toxicity.

The most widely used *in vitro* mutagenicity test has probably been that described by Ames (1982), which utilizes histidine-dependent mutants of *Salmonella typhimurium*. The bacteria are incubated in a medium deficient in histidine; if the added test chemical is genotoxic, it causes a reverse mutation to the histidine-independent state, which permits bacterial growth.

Various mammalian cell culture preparations have been used to assess mutagenic potential. A commonly used test system is a forward gene mutation assay in Chinese hamster ovary (CHO) cells with a strain which is deficient in the enzyme hypoxanthine–guanine phosphoribosyl transferase (HGPRT), and which confers resistance to toxic purine analogues such as 6-thioguanine and permits growth of the cells in a medium containing such substrates. The presence of a mutant chemical will restore sensitivity to the presence of purine analogues, and this may be used to assess mutagenic potential quantitatively. Clastogenic potential can be assessed *in vitro* by exposing cultured cells and subsequently examining them by light microscopy for chromosome damage. It is usual to conduct *in vitro* genotoxicity studies in the presence and absence of a metabolic activation system in order to assess the possible influence of metabolism on the mutagenic potential of the test chemical. A homogenate of liver from animals given the polychlorinated biphenyl Arochlor, which induces a broad spectrum of hepatic cytochrome *P*-450 metabolizing enzymes, is frequently employed.

In vivo genotoxicity studies can be conducted in a variety of ways. For example, the specific locus test in mice involves exposure of non-mutant mice to the test substance and subsequently mating them to multiple-recessive stock. Mutant offspring have altered phenotypes such as hair or eye colour, ear length or hair structure. Clastogenic potential can be assessed *in vivo* by exposure to the test chemical, with subsequent examination of mitotically active tissue, such as bone marrow, for chromosome injury.

Combustion Toxicology

It has been estimated that 50–75 per cent of deaths occurring within a few hours of being exposed to a fire are the result of inhalation injuries and systemic toxicity (Ballantyne, 1981). The primary aim of combustion toxicology is to determine the adverse effects produced as a result of being exposed to heated or burning materials. Although considerable emphasis has been placed on acute effects, there is increasing concern about the long-term consequences of repeated exposure to the products of combustion in occupationally exposed individuals, such as firemen. The design and interpretation of appropriate studies may be difficult because of the large number of variables that may affect the nature, concentration and temporal characteristics of products of combustion. The major, though not exclusive, factors which influence the toxicity and hazard from a fire atmosphere include the nature of the materials available for heating or burning; the phase of the combustion process; temperature; air flow and oxygen availability; and potential for interaction between the combustion materials generated. All of these factors may require to be investigated and considered in evaluating the continually changing hazard from a fire. Principal lines of investigation and sources of information about toxicity and hazards from fire atmospheres are as follows:

(1) Physicochemical studies to determine the nature of the products of combustion generated under differing conditions of temperature and oxygen availability.

(2) Animal exposure studies.

(3) Clinical and forensic observations on fire casualties to determine the nature and cause of morbidity and mortality from exposure to a fire atmosphere.

Although investigations designed to investigate the nature and determinants for materials producing local respiratory or systemic toxicity are of clear importance, it is also necessary to be aware of the presence of materials which may produce sensory irritant or central nervous system depressant effects. Clearly, irritant effects on the eye or narcosis may impede escape from a potentially hazardous situation. Polymers, which constitute a major component of commercial and domestic buildings, provide good examples of the generation of toxic, irritant and neurobehavioural chemical species on combustion (Ballantyne, 1989).

Antidotal Studies

In addition to being aware of the likelihood for spontaneous reversibility of toxic injury (i.e. biochemical and morphological healing), it is of clear practical importance to investigate the induction of reversibility of toxicity by antidotal procedures (Marrs, 1988). Indications for such studies include high acute toxicity (including dose and time to onset of effects); serious (but potentially reversible) repeated-exposure toxicity; where there are indications that early treatment may reduce or abolish latent toxicity; suspicions of a potential for antidotal effectiveness based on considerations of mechanism of toxicity; and confirmation that antidotal treatment is effective for a new member of a chemical series for which a generic antidote has been established. Examples of chemicals for which specific antidotal treatment has been investigated include cyanides (Marrs, 1987), ethylene glycol (Baud *et al.*, 1988) and organophosphate anticholinesterases (Arena and Drew, 1986; Ellenhorn and Barceloux, 1988).

In addition to investigating specific antidotal therapy, it may also be necessary to confirm, or otherwise, whether standard methods of management and support are appropriate for particular substances or groups of materials. This investigation may include, for example, potential for aspiration hazards, influence of dilution (by giving fluid to drink), and potential for adverse interaction with drugs used to maintain cardiovascular or respiratory homoeostasis.

REVIEW OF TOXICOLOGY STUDIES

A critical review of toxicology studies requires detailed case-by-case considerations, but attention should be generally directed to the following:

- That the laboratory or institution reporting the studies has the necessary scientific and/or medical credibility, capabilities, experience and expertise in the areas being investigated.
- The objectives of the investigation should be precisely stated, and the study protocol should reflect this in detail.
- The work should be reported in a clear and

unambiguous manner, with all the necessary detail to allow the reader to undertake his or her own assessment of and conclusions about the study.

- There should have been adequate quality control procedures, and standards appropriate to good laboratory practices should have been followed.
- The material tested should be precisely specified, including stability, and the nature and amounts of any impurities, conversion products or additives.
- It should be confirmed that the methodologies which are used for exposure and to monitor the *in vivo* or *in vitro* studies are sufficiently specific and sensitive to allow the various objectives and end-points to be determined.
- Studies should be designed to allow a determination of the significance of the results and permit hazard and risk assessment procedures. For example, the number of test and control animals should be sufficient to allow for the detection of biological variability in response to exposure, to allow trends to be appreciated and to permit statistical analyses. There should be sufficient dose–response information to allow decisions on causal relationships, and the magnitude of doses which produce definite and threshold effects and those not producing toxicity.
- Monitoring should allow a determination of whether any injury produced is a direct consequence of toxicity or an effect which is secondary to toxicity at another site. A primary effect is one produced as a result of a direct toxic effect of a chemical, or metabolite(s), on a target organ or tissue. Secondary effects are those occurring, often at another non-target site, as a consequence of toxicity in the primary tissue or organ. For example, primary pulmonary injury produced by inhaled potent irritant materials may result in significant hypoxaemia and secondary hypoxic injury to other organs, including liver, kidney or brain. Ideally the study should be carefully assessed to allow a conclusion as to whether the toxicity induced is a consequence of the action of parent material or metabolite—e.g. comparison of routes involving, and not involving, first-pass effects.
- Detailed assessment is required to determine whether the numerical data have been appropriately and correctly evaluated. Thus, although there may be a statistically significant difference between a test group and the controls, this may not be of biological or toxicological significance. Conversely, changes or trends not of statistical significance, may be of biological and toxicological relevance. Quantitative information should be viewed against the study as a whole, normal biological variability, quantitative changes which imply pathological processes, and the magnitude of any changes as they may relate to an adverse effect.

The above considerations demand careful design of toxicological studies, taking into account all factors which are inherent in the defined and inferred objectives of the investigation.

To illustrate the care required in the interpretation of toxicology studies, a few examples are given below of different specific factors that need attention in particular studies:

- The acute peroral LD_{50} of undiluted diethylamine is <0.25 ml kg^{-1}, whereas with a 10 per cent aqueous solution, the acute peroral LD_{50} is 1.41 ml kg^{-1}, illustrating the influence of dilution of the test material on toxicity. A reciprocal relationship has been demonstrated with glutaraldehyde (Figure 14); in this case, acute peroral toxicity (as mg active material per kg) increases with dilution within the confines of the study.
- Materials with similar LD_{50} values may have differences in acute toxicity shown by other monitors of their toxicity. For example, 2,4-pentanedione has an acute peroral LD_{50} (rat) of 0.58 g kg^{-1}, similar to that of 2,2'-bis(4-aminophenoxyphenyl) propane (BAPP) at 0.31 g kg^{-1}; however, times to death were 2–5 h with 2,4-pentanedione and 3–4 days with BAPP, indicating a more serious acute potential hazard with 2,4-pentanedione.
- With inhalation studies, the method of generation of the test material in the atmosphere may be highly important, as indicated by the following three illustrative examples.
(1) For acute vapour inhalation studies, and in tests concerned with defining the effects of saturated vapour atmospheres, the vapour may be generated by static or dynamic

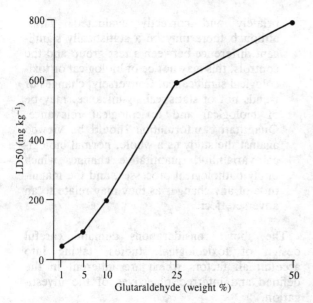

Figure 14 Influence of aqueous dilution on the acute peroral lethal toxicity (as LD_{50}) of glutaraldehyde to rats. As dilution increases, the LD_{50} becomes smaller (i.e. greater toxicity)

methods. Static methods involve placing a sample of the test material in the exposure chamber and allowing the atmosphere to equilibrate for an appropriate period of time; thus, all volatile components accumulate to vapour saturation in the chamber. Dynamically generated atmospheres are produced by passing air through the test material and transferring the atmosphere so generated into and through the chamber in a continuous manner; this results in components of the test material being present in the atmosphere in proportion to both their concentration in test material and their volatility. Thus, trace contaminants of highly volatile toxic materials will be present in much higher concentrations with static as opposed to dynamic conditions. For example, methoxydihydropyran (MDP) containing 0.03 per cent acrolein, when generated dynamically, did not produce mortalities with rats for a 4 h exposure period (MDP vapour, 7748 ppm; acrolein, trace). However, when the same material was used in a static exposure, there were mortalities due to the accumulation of acrolein vapour in the atmosphere (MDP 8044, ppm; acrolein, 240 ppm); acrolein has a 4 h LC_{50} of 8.3 ppm (Ballantyne *et al.*, 1989a).

(2) The relative humidity of the chamber atmosphere may influence inhalation toxicity with hydrolysable materials. For example, when tris(dimethylamino)silane (TDMAS) was generated as a vapour with moistened air, a 4 h LC_{50} of 734 ppm was determined (female rat), which accords stoichiometrically with toxicity due to dimethylamine formed by hydrolysis of TDMAS. However, when the vapour was generated under dry air conditions, a 4 h LC_{50} of 38 ppm was calculated from the exposure–mortality data, indicating a highly significantly greater intrinsic toxicity for the TDMAS molecule (Ballantyne *et al.*, 1989b).

(3) A marked difference in toxicity may be obtained for the same material generated in different modes. For example, short-term repeated exposure to vapour from 2-methacryloxypropyl trimethoxysilane does not produce any respiratory tract injury. However, when generated as an aqueous respirable aerosol, it produces laryngeal granulomas (Klonne *et al*, 1987).

- The use conditions of the test material may influence toxicity, with toxicity being modified by use pattern. Thus, the potential for cutting oil to induce cutaneous neoplasms is significantly enhanced after its industrial use, possibly owing to the generation of polycyclic aromatic hydrocarbons (Agarwal *et al.*, 1986).

HAZARD EVALUATION AND RISK ASSESSMENT

Toxicology is concerned with defining the potential for a material to produce adverse effects, while hazard evaluation is a process to determine whether any of the known potential adverse effects will develop under specific conditions of use. Thus, toxicology is but one of the many considerations to be taken into account in the hazard evaluation process. The following are some of the other factors that need to be considered in defining whether a defined use of a material will be hazardous, and are discussed in detail by Tyler and Ballantyne (1988):

- Physicochemical properties of the material.
- Use pattern.
- Characteristics of the handling procedure.

- Source of exposure and route of exposure, both normal and possible misuse.
- Control measures.
- Magnitude, duration and frequency of exposure.
- Physical nature of exposure conditions (e.g. solid, liquid, vapour, gas, aerosol, etc.).
- Variability in exposure conditions.
- Population exposed (e.g. number, sex, age, health status).
- Any experience and information derived from exposed human populations.

The general approach used to assess hazards is as follows:

(1) Search for all available health-related information on the substance and, if appropriate, substances of close chemical structure. This may include information on physicochemical properties, *in vivo* and *in vitro* toxicology, epidemiology, known occupational and domestic incidents, case reports, monitoring and use patterns.

(2) Detailed impartial review of information accessed, emphasizing those studies conducted by credible scientific standards and by relevant routes of exposure.

(3) Interpretation of the credible and relevant literature in order to define toxicity and, if possible, mechanism, dose–response relationships, and factors influencing toxicity (endogenous and exogenous).

(4) Conclusions regarding potential adverse effects from the substance under specific conditions of use.

(5) Determination of acceptable handling or use conditions, and acceptable exposure to the substance with respect to immediate and long-term conditions of use.

(6) Determination of the management of over-exposure situations.

The process and understanding of hazard evaluation, and its scientific basis, are now at a level where reliable interpretation and prediction can be made. A less reliable and scientifically limited evaluation process is that of risk assessment, which is currently an important developing component of regulatory and occupational toxicology. It is the objective of risk assessment processes to assess the probability that adverse health effects will develop from known, or suspected, toxic xenobiotics in the environment (e.g. drinking water or air) or workplace. Such quantitative risk assessments are most frequently conducted for worktime or lifetime exposure to low concentrations of xenobiotic. They are based on extrapolating dose–response relationships from animal studies, or occasionally human epidemiological data (1) to determine risk at known or anticipated range of occupational or environmental exposure doses, or (2) to assess 'risk-free' doses. The approaches that are currently most frequently employed are to assess risk from carcinogens, teratogens, reproductively active substances and genotoxic materials.

Currently, with most materials there is insufficient information on mechanisms of toxicity for particular materials to allow scientifically valid, appropriate mathematical models to be developed for a specific toxic effect. The current method of extrapolation makes many, often biologically unreasonable, assumptions, which include: (1) the existence (or otherwise) of thresholds for specific toxic end-points, (2) linearity of dose–response relationships, (3) comparability of metabolism and pharmacokinetic parameters between species, (4) the interaction between xenobiotics and biological systems at low concentrations, and (5) the statistical reliability and biological variability resulting from the relatively small numbers of animals that may technically and ethically be incorporated into animal studies. Thus, with current mathematical approaches of data extrapolation, quantitative risk assessments should be regarded as 'best guesses' for environmentally safe exposure dosages. The findings from quantitative risk assessment may result in risk management measures being undertaken (Hallenbeck and Cunningham, 1986). This involves the development and implementation of regulatory action, taking into account additional factors such as available control measures, cost–benefit analyses and 'acceptable' levels of risk, and taking note of various policy, social and political issues. To be encouraged is the developing science of 'Biological Risk Assessment', which allows a more rational risk analysis based upon incorporation of metabolism and pharmacokinetics, including interspecies differences, mechanisms of toxicity and influence of physiological variables (Clayson, 1987; National Research Council, 1987).

SPECIAL CONSIDERATIONS IN HUMAN HEALTH HAZARD EVALUATION

By the very nature of their design, laboratory studies are conducted under highly controlled conditions using healthy animals often of a particular weight range. The extrapolation of such information to a heterogeneous human population, with differing lifestyles and variable states of health, needs to be undertaken with considerable caution, taking into account all possible known and predictable variables.

The possible interactions of multiple exposures to a variety of chemicals or drugs has been discussed earlier in this chapter. Other illustrative examples are presented below.

Personal Habits

Many personal habits, including diet and the taking of medicinal products, may influence the response to a toxic chemical. Two factors that have received special attention are cigarette smoking and excessive alcohol consumption. Cigarette smoking may lead to increased body burdens of many of the combustion products found in smoke—in particular, carbon monoxide. Owing to the significantly increased carboxyhaemoglobin concentrations in smokers, they may be at greater risk in the occupational environment from carbon monoxide and materials that generate carbon monoxide such as methylene chloride. Other materials in cigarette smoke which may increase the exposure burden include hydrogen cyanide, hydrogen sulphide, acrolein and polycyclic aromatic hydrocarbons. In some instances there are clear indications of significantly enhanced toxicity—for example, synergism between cigarette smoking and asbestos (Hammond and Selikoff, 1973) or radon (Archer *et al.*, 1972). Heavy alcohol consumption may lead to chronic progressive liver injury and fibrosis, and thus increase susceptibility to hepatotoxic substances and impair detoxification pathways.

Co-existing Disease

Individuals with certain illnesses may be at greater risk from particular drugs or industrial chemicals. For example, those with established cardiovascular disease may be at increased risk from exposure to carbon monoxide or methaemoglobin-generating substances, since both may compromise available oxygen supply to the myocardium. Inhalation of irritant materials may aggravate chronic progressive pulmonary disease.

Genetically Susceptible Subpopulations

Individuals with genetically determined biochemical variants may be at greater risk from certain drugs and chemicals than those with normal biochemical characteristics. Some examples are given below.

- Individuals with hereditary methaemoglobinaemia may generate significant amounts of methaemoglobin at exposure doses of nitrites or aromatic amines which cause only minor methaemoglobin concentrations in the normal population.
- It is well known that slow acetylators are significantly more susceptible to the neurotoxic potential of isoniazid, whereas fast acetylators seem to be more likely to develop liver injury, since hepatotoxicity is caused by the metabolite acetylhydrazine (Breckenridge and Orme, 1987). Another aspect of acetylator status relates to the potential of arylamines to induce bladder cancer. Slow acetylators may be more susceptible to arylamine-induced bladder cancer (Cartwright *et al.*, 1987), possibly related to a higher urinary excretion of free arylamine (Derwan *et al.*, 1986).
- Individuals with glucose 6-phosphate dehydrogenase deficient erythrocytes may be at increased risk from haemolytic effects of oxidants because of the inability of the erythrocyte to generate sufficient NADPH and maintain an adequate concentration of reduced glutathione, resulting in haemolysis (Calabrese *et al.*, 1987). However, animal studies suggest that haemolytic effects occur only at exposure to otherwise toxic concentrations (Amoruso *et al.*, 1986).
- Exposure of persons with inherited uroporphyrinogen decarboxylase deficiency to dioxin can cause latent chronic hepatic porphyria to develop into porphyria cutanea tarda (Doss and Columbi, 1987).

Other genetically determined variants which have been implicated as increasing susceptibility to chemicals are α_1-antitrypsin deficiency (emphysema), aryl hydrocarbon hydroxylase deficiency (lung cancer), pseudocholinesterase variants (anticholinesterase toxicity) and thalassaemia (lead).

REFERENCES

Abou-Donia, M. B., Lapadula, D. M. and Carrington, C. D. (1987). Biochemical methods for the assessment of neurotoxicity. In Ballantyne, B. (Ed.), *Perspectives in Basic and Applied Toxicology*. John Wright, London, pp. 1–30

Agarwal, R., Gupta, K. P., Sushil, K. P. and Mehrotra, N. K. (1986). Assessment of some tumorigenic risks associated with fresh and used cutting oil. *Indian J. Exptl Biol.*, **24**, 508–510

Albano, E., Lott, K. A. K., Slater, T. F., *et al.* (1982). Spin-trapping studies on the free-radical products formed by metabolic activation of carbon tetrachloride in rat liver microsomal fractions. *Biochem. J.*, **204**, 593–603

Albert, A. L. (1979). *Selective Toxicity*. Chapman and Hall, London

Ames, B. N. (1982). The detection of environmental mutagens and potential carcinogens. *Cancer* **53**, 2034–2040

Amoruso, M. A., Ryer, J., Easton, D., *et al.* (1986). Estimation of risk of glucose-6-phosphate dehydrogenase-deficient red cells to ozone and nitrogen dioxide. *J. Occup. Med.*, **28**, 473–479

Angeli-Greaves, M. and McLean, A. E. M. (1981). Effect of diet on the toxicity of drugs. In Gorrod, A. W. (Ed.), *Drug Toxicity*. Taylor and Francis, London, pp. 91–100

Archer, V. E., Wagner, J. R. and Lurdin, F. E. Jr. (1972). Uranium mining and cigarette smoking effects in man. *J. Occup. Med.*, **15**, 204–211

Arena, J. M. and Drew, R. H. (1986). *Poisoning*. Charles C. Thomas, Springfield, Ill., pp. 146–188

Asher, I. M. and McGrath, P. V. (1976). *Symposium on Electron Microscopy of Microfibers*. Stock No. 017–012–002244–7. Superintendent of Documents, United States Government Printing Office, Washington, D.C.

Baeder, C., Wickramarante, G. A. S. and Hummler, H. (1985). Identification and assessment of the effects of chemicals on reproduction and development (reproductive toxicology). *Fd Chem. Toxicol.*, **23**, 377–388

Ballantyne, B. (1978). The comparative short-term mammalian toxicology of phenarsazine oxide and phenoxarsine oxide. *Toxicology*, **10**, 341–361

Ballantyne, B. (1981). Inhalation hazards of fire. In Ballantyne, B. and Schwabe, P. H. (Eds), *Respiratory Protection*. Chapman and Hall, London, pp. 351–372

Ballantyne, B. (1983). Acute systemic toxicity of cyanides by topical application to the eye. *J. Toxicol. Cut. Ocular Toxicol.*, **2**, 119–129

Ballantyne, B. (1984). Peripheral sensory irritation as a factor in the establishment of workplace exposure guidelines. In Oxford, R. R., Cowell, J. W., Jamieson, G. G. and Love, E. J. (Eds), *Occupational Health in the Chemical Industry*. Medichem, Calgary, Alberta, pp. 119–149

Ballantyne, B. (1985). Evaluation of hazards from mixtures of chemicals in the occupational environment. *J. Occup. Med.*, **27**, 85–94

Ballantyne, B. (1986). Applanation tonometry and corneal pachymetry for prediction of eye irritating potential. *Pharmacologist*, **28**, 173

Ballantyne, B. (1987). Toxicology of cyanides. In Ballantyne, B. and Marrs, T. C. (Eds), *Clinical Experimental Toxicology of Cyanides*. Butterworths, London, pp. 41–126

Ballantyne, B. (1989). Toxicology. In *Encyclopedia of Polymer Science and Engineering*, Vol. 16. Wiley, New York, pp. 879–930

Ballantyne, B., Dodd, D. E., Pritts, I. M., Nachreiner, D. S. and Fowler, E. M. (1989a). Acute vapor inhalation toxicity of acrolein and its influence as a trace contaminant in 2-methyoxy-dihydro-2H-pyran. *Human Toxicol.*, **8**, 229–235

Ballantyne, B., Dodd, D. E., Myers, R. C., *et al.* (1989b). The acute toxicity of tris(dimethylamino)silane. *Toxicol. Industr. Hlth*, **5**, 45–56

Ballantyne, B., Gazzard, M. F. and Swanston, D. W. (1977). Irritation testing by respiratory exposure. In Ballantyne, B. (Ed.), *Current Approaches in Toxicology*. John Wright, Bristol, pp. 129–138

Ballantyne, B., Myers, R. C., Dodd, D. E. and Fowler, E. H. (1988). The acute toxicity of trimethoxysilane (TMS). *Vet. Human Toxicol.*, **30**, 343–344

Barlow, S. M. and Sullivan, F. M. (1982). *Reproductive Hazards of Industrial Chemicals*. Academic Press, London

Baud, F. J., Galliot, M., Astier, A., *et al.* (1988). Treatment of ethylene glycol poisoning with 4-methylpyrolazone. *New Engl. J. Med.*, **319**, 97–100

Beckman, D. A. and Brent, R. L. (1984). Mechanisms of teratogenesis. *Ann. Rev. Pharmacol.*, **24**, 483–500

Billingham, D. J. (1977). Cutaneous absorption and systemic toxicity. In Drill, V. A. and Laza, P. (Eds), *Cutaneous Toxicity*. Academic Press, New York, pp. 53–62

Bogers, M., Appelman, L. M., Feron, V. J., *et al.* (1977). Effects of the exposures profile on the inhalation toxicity of carbon tetrachloride in male rats. *J. Appl. Toxicol.*, **7**, 185–191

Borenfreund, E. and Borrero, O. (1984). *In vitro* cytotoxicity assays. Potential alternatives to the Draize ocular allergy tests. *Cell Biol. Toxicol.*, **1**, 55–65

Braunwald, E. (1982). Mechanism of action of calcium-channel-blocking agents. *New Engl. J. Med.*, **307**, 1618–1627

Breckenridge, A. and Orme, M. L'E. (1987). Principles of clinical pharmacology and therapeutics. In Wetherall, D. J., Ledington, J. G. S. and Warrell, D. A. (Eds), *Oxford Textbook of Medicine*, 2nd edn, Vol. 1. Oxford University Press, Oxford, p. 77

Bronough, R. L. and Maibach, H. (1985). *Percutaneous Absorption*. Marcel Dekker, New York

Brusick, D. (1988). *Principles of Genetic Toxicology*. Plenum Press, New York

Brooks, S. M. (1983). Bronchial asthma of occupational origin. In Rom, W. N. (Ed.), *Environmental and Occupational Medicine*. Little, Brown, Boston, pp. 223–250

Calabrese, E. J., Moore, G. S. and Williams, P. (1987). The effect of methyl oleate ozonide, a possible ozone intermediate, on normal and G-6-PD deficient erythrocytes. *Bull. Environ. Contam. Toxicol.*, **29**, 498–504

Cartwright, R. A., Rodgers, M. J., Barham-Had, D., *et al.* (1987). Role of *N*-acetyltransferase phenotypes in bladder carcinogenesis: a pharmacogenetic epidemiological approach to bladder cancer. *Lancet*, **ii**, 842–846

Clayson, D. B. (1987). The need for biological risk assessment in reaching decisions about carcinogens. *Mutat. Res.*, **185**, 243–269

Conference (1990). Organic dust and lung disease. *Am. J. Industr. Med.*, **17**, 1–148

Cronin, E. (1980). *Contact Dermatitis*. Churchill Livingstone, Edinburgh

Decker, W. J. (1987). Introduction and history. In Maley, T. J. and Berndt, W. O. (Eds), *Handbook of Toxicology*. Hemisphere Publishing Corporation, Washington, D.C., pp. 1–19

Derwan, A., Jani, J. P., Shah, K. S., *et al.* (1986). Urinary excretion of benzidine in relation to acetylator status of occupationally exposed subjects. *Human Toxicol.*, **5**, 95–97

Dewar, A. J. (1981). Neurotoxicity testing. In Gorrod, J. W. (Ed.), *Testing for Toxicity*. Taylor and Francis, London, pp. 199–218

Doss, M. O. and Columbi, A. M. (1987). Chronic hepatic porphyria induced by chemicals: the example of dioxin. In Foa, V., Emmett, E. A., Maroni, M. and Columbus, A. (Eds), *Occupational and Environmental Chemical Hazards*. Ellis Horwood, Chichester, pp. 231–240

Doull, J. and Bruce, M. C. (1991). Origin and scope of toxicology. In Klaasen, C. D., Amdur, M. O. and Doull, J. (Eds), *Casarett and Doull's Toxicology: The Basic Science of Poisons*, 4th edn. Pergamon Press, New York, pp. 3–10

Dugard, P. H. (1977). Chapter 22. Skin permeability theory in relation to measurements of percutaneous absorption in toxicology. In Marzulli, F. N. and Maibach, H. I. (Eds), *Dermatotoxicology and Pharma-*

cology. Hemisphere Publishing Corporation, Washington, D.C., pp. 525–550

Ellenhorn, M. J. and Barceloux, D. G. (1988). *Medical Toxicology*. Elsevier, New York, pp. 1070–1103

Gad, S. C. (1982). A neuromuscular screen for use in industrial toxicology. *J. Toxicol. Environ. Hlth*, **9**, 691–704

Gibaldi, M. and Perrier, D. (1982). *Pharmacokinetics*. Marcel Dekker, New York

Goldenthal, E. I. (1971). A compilation of LD_{50} values in newborn and adult animals. *Toxicol. Appl. Pharmacol.*, **18**, 185–207

Goodwin, R. F. J., Crevel, W. R. W. and Johnson, A. W. (1981). A comparison of three guinea-pig sensitization procedures for the detection of 19 reported human contact sensitizers. *Contact Dermatitis*, **7**, 248–258

Grasso, P. (1988). Carcinogenicity tests in animals: some pitfalls that could be avoided. In Ballantyne, B. (Ed.), *Perspectives in Basic and Applied Toxicology*. John Wright, London, pp. 268–284

Griffith, J. F. (1964). Interlaboratory variations in the determination of acute oral LD_{50}. *Toxicol. Appl. Pharmacol.*, **6**, 726–730

Hallenbeck, W. H. and Cunningham, K. M. (1986). *Quantitative Risk Assessment for Occupational and Environmental Health*. Lewis Publishing, Chelsea, Michigan

Hammond, E. L. and Selikoff, J. J. (1973). Relation of cigarette smoking to risk of death of asbestos associated disease among insulation workers in the United States. In Bogorski, D., Timbrell, J. C., Wagner, J. C. and Davis, W. (Eds), *Biological Effects of Asbestos*. IARC Scientific Publications, No. 8, Lyon, pp. 312–317

Hollingshaus, J. G., Armstrong, D. and Toia, R. F. (1981). Delayed toxicity and delayed neurotoxicity of phosphorothiolate and phosphonothionate esters. *J. Toxicol. Environ. Hlth*, **8**, 619–627

Horton, A. A. and Fairhurst, S. (1987). Lipid peroxidation and mechanism of toxicity. *CRC Crit. Rev. Toxicol.*, **18**, 27–79

Hunter, W. J., Lingk, W. and Recht, P. (1979). Intercomparison study on the determination of single administration toxicity in rats. *J. Assoc. Off. Anal. Chem.*, **62**, 864–873

Karol, M. H., Stadler, J. and Magreni, C. (1985). Immunotoxicologic evaluation of the respiratory system: animal models for immediate and delayed-onset pulmonary hypersensitivity. *Fund. Appl. Toxicol.*, **5**, 459–472

Kast, A. and Nishikawa, J. (1981). The effect of fasting on oral acute toxicity of drugs in rats and mice. *Lab. Anim.*, **15**, 359–364

Kemppainen, B. W. and Reifenrath, W. G. (1990). *Methods for Skin Absorption*. CRC Press, Boca Raton, Florida

Khanna, V. K., Husain, R. and Seth, P. R. (1988).

Low protein diet modifies acrylamide neurotoxicity. *Toxicology*, **49**, 395–401

Kimbrough, R. D., Falk, H., Stehr, P., *et al.* (1984). Health implications of 2,3,7,8-tetrachlorodibenzo-dioxin (TCDD) contamination of industrial soil. *J. Toxicol. Environ. Hlth*, **14**, 47–93

Klonne, D. R., Garman, R. H., Snellings, W. M. and Ballantyne, B. (1987). The larynx as a potential target organ in aerosol studies in rats. In *Abstracts, 1987 International Symposium on Inhalation Toxicity*, Karger, Basel, p. 86

Krisch-Volders, M. (1984). *Mutagenicity, Carcinogenicity and Teratogenicity of Industrial Pollutants*. Plenum Press, New York

Kurt, T. L., Anderson, R., Petty, C., *et al.* (1988). Dinitrophenol in weight loss: the poison centre and public health safety. *Vet. Human Toxicol.*, **28**, 574–575

Lu, F. C. (1985). *Basic Toxicology*. Hemisphere Publishing Corporation, Washington, D.C.

Maickel, R. P. and McFadden, D. P. (1979). Acute toxicology of butyl nitriles and butyl alcohols. *Res. Commun. Chem. Pathol. Pharmacol.*, **26**, 75–83

Malmary, M.-F., Kabbaj, K. and Oustrin, J. (1988). Circadian dosing stage dependence in metabolic effects of cyclosporin in the rat. *Ann. Rev. Chronopharmacol.*, **5**, 35–38

Marks, V., English, J., Aherne, W. and Arendt, J. (1985). Chronopharmacology. *Clin. Biochem.*, **18**, 154–157

Marrs, T. C. (1987). The choice of cyanide antidotes. In Ballantyne, B. and Marrs, T. C. (Eds), *Clinical and Experimental Toxicology of Cyanides*. Butterworths, London, pp. 383–401

Marrs, T. C. (1988). Experimental approaches to the design and assessment of antidotal procedures. In Ballantyne, B. (Ed.), *Perspectives in Basic and Applied Toxicology*. John Wright, London, pp. 285–308

Mattison, D. R. (1983). *Reproductive Toxicology*. Alan R. Liss, New York

Maurer, T., Weirich, E. G. and Hess, R. (1984). Predictive contact allergenicity: influence of the animal strain used. *Toxicology*, **31**, 217–222

Mehendale, H. M. (1987). Hepatotoxicity. In Haley, T. J. and Berndt, W. O. (Eds), *Handbook of Toxicology*. Hemisphere Publishing Corporation, Washington, D.C., pp. 74–111

Mitchell, C. L. (1982). *Nervous System Toxicology*. Raven Press, New York

Murphy, S. D. (1983). General principles in the assessment of toxicity of chemical mixtures. *Environ. Hlth Perspect.*, **48**, 141–144

Nardone, R. M. and Bradlaw, J. A. (1983). Toxicity testing with *in vitro* systems. I. Ocular tissue culture. *J. Toxicol. Ocular Cut. Toxicol.*, **2**, 81–98

National Research Council (1987). *Pharmacokinetics in Risk Assessment*. National Academy Press, Washington, D.C.

National Research Council (1988). *Principles of Toxicological Interactions Associated with Multiple Chemical Exposures*. National Academy Press, Washington, D.C.

Oehme, F. W. (1980). Absorption, biotransformation, and excretion of environmental chemicals. *Clin. Toxicol.*, **17**, 147–158

Owens, E. J. and Punte, C. L. (1963). Human respiratory and ocular irritation studies utilizing *o*-chlorobenzylidene malononitrile aerosols. *Am. Industr. Hyg. Assoc. J.*, **24**, 262–264

Pariat, C., Courtois, P., Cambar, J., *et al.* (1988). Seasonal variations in gentamicin nephrotoxicity in rats. *Ann. Rev. Chronopharmacol.*, **5**, 461–463

Paschal, D. C., DiPietro, E. S., Phillips, D. L. and Gunter, E. W. (1989). Age dependence of metals in hair in selected U.S. population. *Environ. Res.*, **48**, 17–28

Randall, J. A. and Gibson, R. S. (1989). Hair chromium as an index of chromium exposure of tannery workers. *Br. J. Industr. Med.*, **46**, 171–175

Rao, M. S. and Reddy, J. K. (1987). Peroxisome proliferation and hepatocarcinogenesis. *Carcinogenesis*, **8**, 631–636

Rao, K. S., Schwetz, B. A. and Park, C. N. (1987). Reproductive risk assessment of chemicals. *Vet. Human Toxicol.*, **23**, 167–175

Rodier, P. M. (1980). Chronology of neuron development: animal studies and their clinical implications. *Childh. Neurol.*, **22**, 525–545

Shell, J. W. (1982). Pharmacokinetics of topically applied ophthalmic drugs. *Surv. Ophthalmol.*, **26**, 207–218

Shopsis, C. and Sathe, S. (1984). Uridine uptake inhibition as a cytotoxicity test: correlations with the Draize test. *Toxicology*, **29**, 195–206

Spencer, P. S., Bischoff, M. C. and Schaumburg, H. H. (1980). Neuropathological methods for the detection of neurotoxic diseases. In Spencer, P. S. and Schaumburg, H. H. (Eds), *Experimental and Clinical Neurotoxicology*. Williams and Wilkins, Baltimore, pp. 743–757

Sperling, F. (1984). Quantitation of toxicology—the dose-response relationship. In Sperling, F. (Ed.), *Toxicology: Principles and Practice*, Vol. 2. Wiley, New York, pp. 199–218

Stanton, M. F., Layard, M., Tegeris, A., *et al.* (1981). Relation of particle dimension to carcinogenicity in amphobile asbestosis and other fibrous minerals. *J. Natl Cancer Inst.*, **67**, 965–975

Stuttgen, G., Siebel, T. and Aggerbeck, B. (1982). Absorption of boric acid through human skin depending on the type of vehicle. *Arch. Dermatol. Res.*, **272**, 21–29

Sweet, D. V. (Ed.) (1985–1986a). *Registry of Toxic Effects of Chemical Substances*, Vol. 3. U.S. Department of Health and Human Services. Centers for Disease Control, NIOSH, p. 2360

Sweet, D. V. (Ed.) (1985–1986b). *Registry of Toxic*

Effects of Chemical Substances, Vol. 3. U.S. Department of Health and Human Services. Centers for Disease Control, NIOSH, p. 3060

Tallarida, R. J. and Jacob, L. S. (1979). *The Dose–Response Relation in Pharmacology*. Springer-Verlag, New York

Timbrell, J. A. (1982). *Principles of Biochemical Toxicology*. Taylor and Francis, London, Chapter 2

Toft, R., Olofsson, T., Tuneck, A., *et al.* (1982). Toxic effects on mouse bone marrow caused by inhalation of benzene. *Arch. Toxicol.*, **51**, 295–302

Trevan, J. W. (1927). The error of determination of toxicity. *Proc. Roy. Soc., B*, **101**, 483–514

Tuchmann-Duplessis, M. (1980). The experimental approach to teratogenicity. *Ecotoxicol. Environ. Safety*, **4**, 422–433

Tyl, R. W. (1988). Developmental toxicity in toxicologic research and testing. In Ballantyne, B. (Ed.), *Perspectives in Basic and Applied Toxicology*. Wright, London, pp. 206–241

Tyler, T. R. and Ballantyne, B. (1988). Practical assessment and communication of hazards in the workplace. In Ballantyne, B. (Ed.), *Perspectives in Basic and Applied Toxicology*. John Wright, London, pp. 330–378

Vorhees, C. V. (1983). Behavioural teratogenicity testing as a method of screening for hazards to human health: a methodological proposal. *Neurobehav. Toxicol. Teratol.*, **5**, 469–474

Wartew, G. A. (1983). The health hazards of formaldehyde. *J. Appl. Toxicol.*, **3**, 121–126

Wheeler, T. G. (1987). The behavioural effects of anticholinesterase insult following exposure to different environmental temperatures. *Aviat. Space Environ. Med.*, **58**, 54–59

Williams, P. L. (1982). Pentachlorophenol, an assessment of the occupational hazard. *Am. Industr. Hyg. Assoc. J.*, **43**, 799–810

Williams, R. T. (1959). *Detoxification Mechanisms*, 2nd edn. Chapman and Hall, London

Wilmer, J. W. G. M., Wouterson, R. A., Appleman, L. M., *et al.* (1987). Subacute (4-week) inhalation toxicity study of formaldehyde in male rats: 8-hour intermittent versus 8-hour continuous exposures. *J. Appl. Toxicol.*, **71**, 25–26

Woodford, R. and Barry, B. W. (1986). Penetration enhancers and the percutaneous absorption of drugs: an update. *J. Toxicol. Cut. Ocular Toxicol.*, **5**, 167–177

World Health Organization (1981). *Health Effects of Combined Exposures in the Workplace*. Technical Report Series No. 647, WHO, Geneva

World Health Organization (1985). *Chronic Effects of Solvents on the Central Nervous System and Diagnostic Criteria*. Environmental Health Criteria Series No. 5, WHO, Copenhagen

Zbinden, G. (1981). Experimental methods in behavioural teratology. *Arch. Toxicol.*, **48**, 69–88

Zbinden, G. and Flury-Roversi, M. (1981). Significance of the LD_{50} test for the toxicological evaluation of chemical substances. *Arch. Toxicol.*, **47**, 77–99

FURTHER READING

Albert, A. (1987). *Xenobiosis*. Chapman and Hall, London

Anderson, A. and Conning, D. M. (1994). *Experimental Toxicology. The Basic Issues*. Boca Raton, Florida

Calabrese, E. J. (1991). *Principles of Animal Extrapolation*. Lewis Publishers, Inc., Michigan

Calabrese, E. J. (1991). *Multiple Chemical Interactions* Lewis Publishers, Inc., Chelsea, Michigan

Hayes, A. W. (1994). *Principles and Methods of Toxicology*. 3rd edn. Raven Press, New York

Hodgson, E., Mailman, R. B. and Chambers, J. E. (1988). *Dictionary of Toxicology*. Van Nostrand Reinhold Company, New York [NB. Correct for current edition]

Ottoboni, M. A. (1991). *The Dose Makes the Poison*. 2nd edn. Van Nostrand Reinhold, New York

Sullivan, J. B. and Krieger, G. R. (Eds) (1992). *Hazardous Materials Toxicology*. Williams and Wilkins, Baltimore

For material specific toxicology, the following should be consulted:

Buhler, D. R. and Reed, D. J. (1987 and 1990). *Ethel Browning's Toxicity and Metabolism of Industrial Solvents*. 2nd edn, Vols. 1 and 2. Elsevier, Amsterdam

Clayton, C. D. and Clayton, F. E. (1993–1994). *Patty's Industrial Hygiene and Toxicology*. 4th edn, Vol. II, Parts A-F. John Wiley and Sons, Inc., New York

Hathaway, G. T., Proctor, N. H., Hughes, J. P. and Fischman, M. L. (1991). *Chemical Hazards of the Workplace*. Van Nostrand Reinhold, New York

Royal Society of Chemistry (1991). *The Agrochemicals Handbook*. 3rd edn. Royal Society of Chemistry, London

2 Principles of Testing for Acute Toxic Effects

Christopher Rhodes, Michael Thomas and Janet Athis

The scientist. He will spend thirty years in building up a mountain range of facts with the intent to prove a certain theory; then he is so happy in his achievement that as a rule he overlooks the main chief fact of all—*that his accumulation proves an entirely different thing*.
> Samuel L. Clemens (Mark Twain), 'The Bee', essay, 1917.

. . . animal studies are not helpful in the instant case because they involved different biological species. They are of so little probative force and so potentially misleading to be inadmissible.
> Ruling of a Federal Court Judge, USA.

INTRODUCTION

The collection of data on the acute toxic effects of substances has for many years been a focus for research in academic, industrial, contract and government research laboratories. It is common both to elective research and non-elective regulatory compliance work, involving a large number of substances from natural origin to chemicals synthesized by man and a wide range of species from both the plant and animal kingdoms. Investigation of acute toxicity has led to the identification of selective toxic action and the beneficial use of substances as pesticides in controlling the environment and as drugs for therapeutic use in domesticated animals and man (Albert, 1985). Natural agonists (Reuse, 1948) are selective molecules which contribute to the functioning of cells. Antagonists are inhibitors of natural agonists and are inevitably toxic at certain concentrations. This can be their most valuable property for use by man (Albert, 1985). However, most people perceive more inherent potential for harm from chemical antagonists synthesized by man than those produced in nature.

Several definitions of acute toxicity have been formulated: (1) 'the adverse change(s) occurring immediately or a short time following a single or short period of exposure to a substance or substances'; (2) 'adverse effects occurring within a short time of administration of a single dose of a substance or multiple doses given within 24 hours (in terms of human exposure it refers to life-threatening events following accidental overdosage, intentional, suicidal and homicidal attempts)'. An adverse effect (toxicity) can be defined as any effect that results in functional impairment and/or pathological and/or physiological and/or biochemical lesions that may affect the performance of the whole organism or that reduce the organ's ability to respond to an additional challenge (WHO Task Group, 1978; Vouk *et al.*, 1985). Pharmacodynamics, the study of the biochemical and physiological effects of chemicals and their mechanisms of action, is analogous to what can be considered as toxicodynamics.

Toxicity can be considered to be the capacity to cause injury; hazard the probability of injury occurring (Barnes, 1963; Oser, 1971); and safety the improbability of injury. Additionally, the amount of toxicant must reach a concentration sufficient to overcome the inherent reserve capacity within biological systems (threshold level) before it can elicit an adverse change (Hermann, 1971; Dinman, 1972; Farmer, 1974). The threshold assumption has as its premise a physiological reserve within the organism which requires depletion or significant alteration for a toxic response to occur. It is the consensus of various experts that acute toxic events exhibit threshold dose–response characteristics (Vouk *et al.*, 1985). For a toxic event to occur, the critical receptor in the organism has to come into contact with the toxicant. The concept of receptor–chemical interaction has been attributed to Langley (1905), which was the basis for chemotherapy as conceived by Ehrlich (1907). The drug–receptor theory of drug action (toxicant action), which has analogy in enzyme-substrate and ligand–protein theory, was further developed by Clarke (1933).

Hazard is a function of toxicity, exposure and

amount. Exposure (external dose) is a measure of the contact between the intoxicant and the outer or inner surface of the human body (e.g. skin, alveolar surface of lung or mucosal surface of gut). It is usually expressed in terms of concentrations of the intoxicant in the medium interfacing with the body surfaces. Once absorbed through body surfaces, the intoxicant gives rise to levels in various organs or tissues. Internal dose is measured in terms of concentrations in the tissues. Exposure and dose should include an indication of the time and frequency at which an individual is subjected to them. Acute exposure to toxins may result in death or sublethal responses, and the signs and symptoms may be overt or subtle. Consequences of acute exposure to toxins may be *non-specific*—reflecting a mass action effect; *specific*—inhibition of vital cellular receptors (antagonists) and enzymes (inhibitors), mimicking endogenous receptors (agonists); *reactive*—reflecting chemical modification of cellular chemistry which was described as 'lethal synthesis' by Peters (1963). Responses may occur as a consequence of biotransformation to reactive intermediates with subsequent modification of biochemical and physiological processes (McClean, 1971; Brown, 1980). The assessment of chemical toxicity and the demonstration of safety, including acute toxicity screening, has been an integral part of pharmaceutical and industrial research for many years. Smyth and Carpenter in 1944 described preliminary data on the oral, dermal and inhalation toxicity of a chemical. It is unfortunate that the terms 'acute lethality testing' and 'acute toxicity' have become synonymous (Zbinden and Flury-Roversi, 1981; Zbinden, 1986), as both regulatory bodies and industry expect more than lethality data to be generated from acute systemic toxicity studies. The study of acute toxic effects can be extremely broad. Objectives include the characterization of the acute biological effects of a chemical, defining clinical signs, describing a chemical's acute toxic syndrome so that intoxicated patients can be diagnosed and treated, and identifying target organs (OECD, 1981; Zbinden, 1984). Various regulatory guidelines combine, under the general heading of acute toxicity studies, evaluations of localized effects on skin and ocular tissues; these are dealt with in Chapters 24 and 30.

This chapter elaborates the principles of acute systemic toxicity assessment as it pertains to the evaluation of acute systemic effects in mammals leading to adverse changes in target organs which result in acute ill-health and death. Individual chapters which follow in this textbook cover parenteral, peroral, percutaneous, inhalation, ophthalmic and cutaneous toxicology. Comprehensive publications on acute toxicity assessment should be consulted for additional detail: Gad and Chengelis (1988), a text covering procedures in laboratory animals; Chan and Hayes (1989), a chapter on acute systemic and ocular irritation; Ellenhorn and Barceloux (1988), an encyclopaedic dissertation on the diagnosis and treatment of human poisoning. The reader's attention is also drawn to other books to which the present authors have referred: *Toxicology of Pesticides* (Hayes, 1975); *Acute Toxicity in Theory and Practice* (Brown, 1980); *Pesticides Studied in Man* (Hayes, 1982); *Animals and Alternatives in Toxicity Testing* (Balls *et al.*, 1983); *Goodman and Gilman's The Pharmacological Basis of Therapeutics* (Gilman *et al.*, 1985); *Casarett and Doull's Toxicology, The Basic Science of Poisons* (1986); *Alternatives to Animal Use in Research, Testing and Education* (US Congress, Office of Technology Assessment, 1986); *Handbook of Toxicology* (Haley and Berndt, 1987); *EPA Toxicology Handbook* (Government Institutes, 1988); *Principles and Methods of Toxicology* (Hayes, 1989).

DEVELOPMENT OF ACUTE TOXICITY ASSESSMENT

Classification

Many of the principles generally applied to acute (and chronic) toxicity evaluation were established in antiquity (this book, Chapter 1; Thompson, 1931; Guthrie, 1946; Mettler and Mettler, 1947; Leake, 1975; Decker, 1987). Primitive man undoubtedly observed previously healthy animals becoming ill and occasionally dying following their ingestion of or contact with various natural materials. The manuscripts of the ancient Egyptian societies (*Ebers Papyrus*, *c.* 1500 BC) and the Chinese-speaking peoples (*Yun Chi Ch i Ch ien*, *c.* 1023 BC) and the Sanskrit hymns and verses of the Indo-European Hindus (*Vedas*, *c.* 1500–1200 BC) are considered to be the earliest written records which contain references to poisonous substances and materials. The early Greek philosophers Hippocrates (*c.* 400 BC), Aristotle (*c.* 350 BC), and Theophrastus (*c.* 300 BC) describe the use of poisons; Pedanius Dioscorides (*c.* AD 50), a physician to Nero, introduced into his *De Materia Medica* the classification of poisons into plant, animal and mineral. Galen (*c.* AD 150); and the Persian physician Avicenna (*c.* AD 1000) further refined this classification, with the latter distinguishing oral from parenteral poisons—concepts which remain extant today.

Dose–Response and Animal Experimentation

Before the twentieth century the art of poisoning of man was the predecessor of acute toxicology testing in animals (Bruce and Doull, 1986; Decker, 1987). In early Greek and Roman times, the prevalence of assassination initiated efforts to discover antidotes. Zopyrus, physician to Mithridates VI, King of Pontus (*c.* 200 BC), adhering to the adage that 'the best model for man is man', is believed to have used prisoners to identify materials which acted as antidotes against ingested poisons. Eventually a guide to the treatment of accidental or intentional poisoning, *Poisons and Antidotes*, was published by the Judaic philosopher and physician, Moses Maimonides (*c.* AD 1198). During the Renaissance period many notorious poisoners, typified by the Borgias of Italy (*c.* AD 1500) and by Madame MonVoisin in France (*c.* AD 1680), further developed the poisoner's art of assassination. The Marquise de Brinvilliers (*c.* AD 1650) is claimed to have administered preparations of toxins to the sick and needy to evaluate potency, speed of onset, specificity, site of action, clinical signs and symptoms prior to their use in assassinations. A handbook of poisons, *De Venenis*, published in the fifteenth century by Peter of Albanos went to fourteen editions, so much was the interest in poisons. From such empirical observations, fundamental principles of toxicity assessment became apparent.

Paracelsus (Philippus Aureolus Theophrastus Bombastus von Hohenheim, *c.* AD 1500) is considered by many to have introduced the role of chemistry in medicine. Challenging the establishment views by ritualistically burning the books of Avicenna and Galen in front of his students, he emphasized in his teaching the concept of exper-

imentation. His insight into the relationship of dose and effect resulted in his often paraphrased quotation that 'the dose or amount of a chemical determines whether a substance is a remedy or a poison'. Orfila published his *Traité de Toxicologie*, in which he attempted a systematic correlation of chemically induced biological responses based on his observations of the effects of poisons on dogs (Orfila, 1817). Following in the steps of Joseph Plenck (1781), who published *Elementa Medicinae et Chirurgiae Forensis*, describing the role of chemistry in the detection of poisons, Orfila used chemical analysis of autopsy material for detecting and confirming accidental or intentional poisonings. The further advances in the application of experimentation to elucidate toxicity were made by the physiologists Claude Bernard (AD 1813–1878) and Magendie (AD 1783–1855). Bernard replaced Magendie's empirical method of experimentation with one of confirmation or refutation of a predefined hypothesis.

Anti-vivisection and Safety Evaluation

It was during this period that the views that animals were considered 'machines without consciousness' (Rene Descartes, AD 1644, *Discourse. The Principles of Philosophy*), were challenged as being morally wrong. Anti-vivisection lobbies arose against using animals in medical experimentation. In 1876 the UK introduced pivotal legislation inappropriately called 'The Cruelty to Animals Act', which required medical experimentation to be conducted only by licensed practitioners and under specified conditions. During the twentieth century legislation to protect the well-being of animals has been introduced by the governments of many countries (Figure 1). Recently, 110 years after the first legislation, the UK has introduced further legislation, The Animal (Scientific Procedures) Act (1986), and the United States has updated The Animal Welfare Act (1987). Some differences exist: for example, the UK act includes all vertebrate animals, whereas the USA act excludes certain classes of rodents (rats and mice) but includes others (guinea-pigs). It is probable that international harmonization of animal welfare legislation will follow the harmonization of study protocols (OECD, 1981) and all mammalian species will be the subject of equivalent animal

(A)

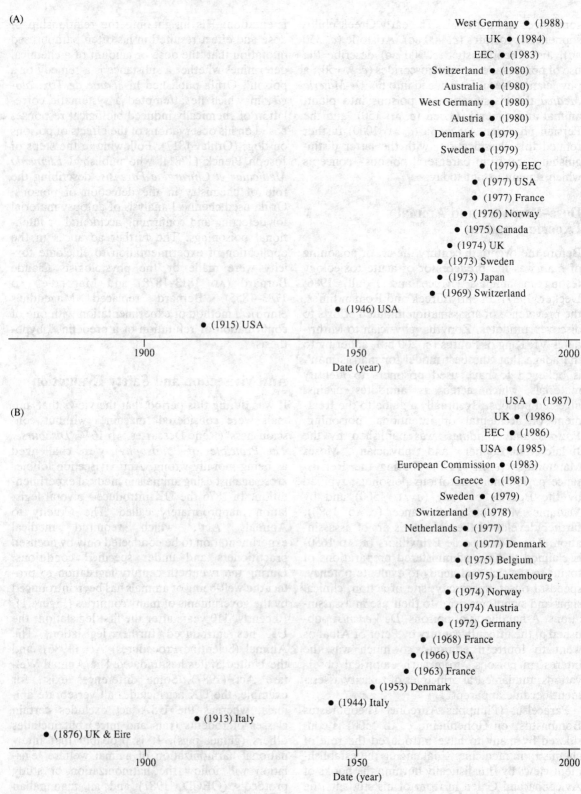

West Germany ● (1988)
UK ● (1984)
EEC ● (1983)
Switzerland ● (1980)
Australia ● (1980)
West Germany ● (1980)
Austria ● (1980)
Denmark ● (1979)
Sweden ● (1979)
● (1979) EEC
● (1977) USA
● (1977) France
● (1976) Norway
● (1975) Canada
● (1974) UK
● (1973) Sweden
● (1973) Japan
● (1969) Switzerland
● (1946) USA
● (1915) USA

1900   1950   2000
Date (year)

(B)

USA ● (1987)
UK ● (1986)
EEC ● (1986)
USA ● (1985)
European Commission ● (1983)
Greece ● (1981)
Sweden ● (1979)
Switzerland ● (1978)
Netherlands ● (1977)
● (1977) Denmark
● (1975) Belgium
● (1975) Luxembourg
● (1974) Norway
● (1974) Austria
● (1972) Germany
● (1968) France
● (1966) USA
● (1963) France
● (1953) Denmark
● (1944) Italy
● (1913) Italy
● (1876) UK & Eire

1900   1950   2000
Date (year)

Figure 1 Introduction of legislation related to the control of (A) chemical safety (B) experimentation on animals

welfare provisions to ensure their humane treatment, the minimizing of pain and discomfort, and the consideration of alternative approaches.

The increasing legislation for animal welfare has been paralleled by the increase in legislation for chemical safety (Figure 1), which in turn reflects the rapid development this century of the chemical industry. In 1901 a diphtheria epidemic in the USA resulted in the US Congress passing the Virus Act of 1902 regulating all biological products sold for the prevention of disease in man, with the purpose of achieving consistent potency and requiring batch-to-batch certification prior to release (Pendergast, 1984). In 1906 the US Congress passed the Pure Food and Drug Act, which led to the establishment of the Food and Drug Administration. In these early years the chief of the Bureau of Chemistry of the US Department of Agriculture did pioneering work on the tolerance of various additives to food, using human volunteers, the chemicals not having been previously evaluated in animals (Anderson, 1958). Quinine and digitalis were first tested in man before being given to animals (Baker and Davey, 1970). Since those early days, the use of surrogate species prior to exposure of man to chemicals has become the norm rather than the exception from both an ethical and a liability point of view.

International Hazard Labelling and Toxicity Ranking

Descriptions of lethality studies were published in the early 1900s (Sudmersen and Glenny, 1910). During the 1920s several experimentalists evaluated methods to describe the lethality of various biological materials such as insulin and digitalis extracts (Shackell, 1925; Trevan, 1927; Behrens, 1929). Trevan (1927) proposed an experimental design to define more accurately the lethal concentration or dose for biologically prepared therapeutic materials which were of a variable and inconsistent potency, and introduced the median lethal dose (LD_{50} and LC_{50}), terms consistent with the median effective dose (ED_{50}) used in pharmacology.

Deaths following the use of the antibiotic sulphanilamide which had been formulated in ethylene glycol (1937) led to the US Congress passing the Federal Food Drug and Cosmetic Act (1938) requiring the obligatory testing of drugs

for safety, using experimental animals. Advisory guidelines prepared by the staff of the US Food and Drug Administration (Lehman, 1959) have subsequently become standardized in International and National regulatory guidelines such as those prepared by the Organization for Economic Co-operation and Development (OECD).

The various legal acts and health and safety regulations of various countries place duties on persons who manufacture, import or supply chemical substances. Industry provides acute toxicity data as part of its extensive programme to establish the safety of products and to meet obligations under legislation for:

(I) the classification, packaging, labelling, requirements for transportation; (II) occupational control of safety and health; (III) the registration or re-registration of a new drug, food additive or pesticide for sale and use; (IV) new formulations of known products; (V) reassessment of a previously developed product's safety to maintain its continued sale and use.

The OECD identified 'information which should accompany chemicals when they are marketed, especially when traded internationally' as an important aspect of information exchange regarding chemicals when they reviewed international practices of labelling chemicals (OECD, 1984). In 1924 the International Convention for the Transport of Goods by Rail (CIM) dealt with the labelling of merchandise. A resolution on classification, labelling and international safety symbols for dangerous, harmful and toxic chemical substances was adopted by the International Labor Organization (1950). The recommendations of the United Nations Committee of Experts on the Transport of Dangerous Goods covering transport by land, sea and air were formulated into guidelines which are generally referred to as the 'Orange Book'. The UN Orange Book specifically refers to poisonous (toxic) dangerous goods with special recommendations which specify three packing groups primarily based on acute toxicity (Table 1). The International Air Transport Association (IATA) Restricted Articles Regulations (established in 1950) were adopted by 57 countries. The International Civil Aviation Organization (ICAO) and its 150 contracting states has adopted as of 1984 Annex 18 to the

Table 1 Acute systemic toxicity classification by country

Country, community	Title of category	Oral (LD$_{50}$) Solid (mg kg^{-1})	Liquid (mg kg^{-1})	Dermal (LD$_{50}$) Solid (mg kg^{-1})	Liquid (mg kg^{-1})	Inhalation (LC$_{50}$) Dust (mg l^{-1}h^{-1})	Gas/vapour (mg l^{-1}h^{-1})	Refs.
General								
Australia	Very toxic	≤5		≤40		0.5		1
	Toxic	>5-≤50		>40-≤200		>0.5-≤2		
	Harmful	>50-≤2000		>200-≤2000	>2-≤10	>2-≤10		
Canada	Very toxic	≤50		≤200		≤0.5ᵃ	gas≤2500ᵇ vapour≤1500ᵇ	2
	Toxic	>50-≤500		>200-≤1000		>0.5-≤2.5ᵃ	vapour 1500-≤2500ᵇ	
EEC/Norway	Very toxic	≤25		≤50		≤0.5ᵃ [≤0.25]ᶜ		3,4
	Toxic	>25-≤200		>50-≤400		>0.5-≤2ᵃ [>0.25-≤1]ᶜ		
	Harmful	>200-≤2000		>400-≤2000		>2-≤20ᵃ [>1-≤5]ᶜ		
Finland Poison	Class I	≤25		≤50		≤0.5		5
	Class II	≤200		≤400		≤2		
	Class III	≤2000		≤2000		≤20		
Japan	Toxic substance	≤30		≤100		≤200ᵈ		6,7
	Deleterious	>30-≤300		>100-≤1000		200-≤2000		
Sweden	Very toxic	≤25		≤50		≤0.5ᵃ		8
	Toxic	>25-≤200		>50-≤400		>0.5-≤2ᵃ		
	Harmful	>200-≤2000		400-≤2000		>2-≤20ᵃ		
	Less harmful	>2000		>2000			>20ᵃ	
Switzerland	Class 1	≤5						9
	Class 2	>5-≤50						
	Class 3	>50-≤500						
	Class 4	>500-≤2000						
	Class 5	2000-≤5000						
USA OSHA/ANSI	Highly toxic	≤50		≤200		≤2	gas ≤200ᵈ	10,11
	Toxic	>50-≤500		>200-≤1000		>2-≤20	gas 200-≤200ᵈ	
Transport								
United Nations	Group I	≤5		≤40		≤0.5ᵉ		12
	Group II	>5-≤50		>40-≤200		>0.5-≤2		
	Group III	>50-≤200	>50-≤500	200-≤2000		>2-≤10		
*Pesticides*ᵇ								
WHO Class Ia	Extremely hazardous	≤5	≤20	≤10	≤40			13
Class Ib	Highly hazardous	>5-≤50	>20-≤200	>10-≤100	>40-≤400			
Class II	Moderately hazardous	>50-≤500	>200-≤2000	>100-≤1000	>400-≤4000			
Class III	Slightly hazardous	≤500	≤2000	≤1000	≤4000			
EEC	Very toxic	≤5	≤25	≤10	≤50	≤0.5ᵃ		14,15,16
	Toxic	>5-≤50	>25-≤200	>10-≤100	>50-≤400	>0.5-≤2ᵃ		
	Harmful	>50-≤500	>200-≤2000	>100-≤1000	>400-≤4000	>2-≤20ᵃ		
USA (EPA)	Category I	≤50		≤200		≤0.2		17
	Category II	>50-≤500		>200-≤2000		>0.2-≤2		
	Category III	>500-≤5000		>2000-≤20,000		>2-≤20		
	Category IV	≤5000		≤20,000		≤20		

Notes to Table 1

[a] mg/l per 4 h.

[b] ppm/4 h.

[c] EEC inhalation criteria were originally based on the 1 h LC_{50}. They have since been changed to a 4 h LC_{50} without decreasing the exposure time (ref. 20). Adjusted inhalation limits are to be given in the proposed seventh amendment and these are shown in the □.

[d] ppm/h.

[e] UN list gives conversion rules to obtain the equivalent 1 h LC_{50} from the 4 h LC_{50}: exposures to dust and mists LC_{50} (4 h) $\times$ 4 = LC_{50} (1 h); exposures to vapours LC_{50} (4 h) $\times$ 2 = LC_{50} (1 h); UN list also gives criteria for assigning packing groups for liquids having toxic vapours using saturated vapour concentration and LC_{50}.

[f] UN transport list and EEC also give formulae for classification of formulations of pesticides; in addition, there is an Italian interpretation for the classification of pesticide formulations (ref. 18).

References in Table 1

1: Australian National Occupation Health and Safety Commission (1989).
2: Canadian Work Place Hazardous Materials Information System (1987).
3: Commission of the European Communities (1987).
4: Brandt, E. (1988).
5: Advisory Committee on Poisons (1987).
6: OECD (1984).
7: Wellenreuther, G. (1987).
8: Swedish Plastics and Chemicals Suppliers Association (1987).
9: Saxer, H.P. (1989).
10: US OSHA.
11: American National Standards Institute.
12: United Nations (1988).
13: World Health Organization (1985).
14: EEC (1978).
15: UK Statutory Instrument No. 1244 (1984).
16: Federal Republic of Germany (1988).
17: US Code of Federal Regulations (1988).
18: EEC Guidelines (1987).
19: EEC Guidelines (1988).
20: (1987) *Regulatory Toxicol. Pharmacol.*, **7**, 21–34.

Chicago convention 'The Safe Transport of Goods by Air' and the 'Technical Instructions for the Safe Transport of Goods by Air'. The World Health Organization (WHO) classifies pesticides into four toxicity groups, primarily on the basis of acute oral and dermal toxicity in the laboratory rat (Classification of Pesticides by Hazard, 1975).

A number of OECD countries have comprehensive regulations in addition to those summarized above for labelling based upon acute toxicity data. In Japan labelling requirements are specified under several laws, the primary ones being the Chemical Substances Control Law; the Drugs, Cosmetic and Medical Instruments Law; the Toxic and Deleterious Regulation Law; and the Agricultural Chemicals Regulation Law. In the Nordic countries hazardous product labelling is covered by the Act on Products Hazardous to Health and to the Environment (Sweden, 1973); Regulation Concerning Labelling, Sale, etc., of Chemical Substances and Products Which May Involve a Hazard to Health (Norway, 1982); Labelling of Dangerous Substances (Finland, 1978). In Europe the Dangerous Chemical Substances and Proposals Concerning Their Labelling, first published by the Council of Europe in 1962, with a final edition in 1978, was commonly referred to as the 'Yellow Book'. These regulations formed the basis for the European Communities (EC) Council Directive relating to Classification, Packaging and Labelling of Dangerous Substances (1967) and additional directives for solvents, paints and pesticides. In 1981 the 6th Amendment to the EEC Dangerous Substances Directive made it mandatory for every importer of a new substance to provide to the competent authorities of the Community a set of toxicological, ecotoxicological and physicochemical data before placing a new substance on the market.

Under the 6th Amendment Pre-Marketing Notification of New Chemicals Act, the EEC requires acute systemic toxicity assessment by at least two different routes of exposure (oral, dermal, inhalation being the most common) as well as assessment of eye and skin irritation. The Notification of New Substances Regulations (1982) identify the tests as those defined by Annex VI to the Council Directive 67/548/EEC (EEC, 1984), and these are based on those recommended by the Organization for Economic Co-operation and Development Guidelines for Testing of Chemicals (OECD, 1981a; b). The European Community's Classification, Packaging and Labelling Regulations apply to all substances which are hazardous to health and they stipulate that risk phrases (Table 2) as well as safety phrases (Table 3) have to appear on labels.

In the USA four federal agencies—the Food and Drug Administration (FDA), the Environmental Protection Agency (EPA), the Occupational Safety and Health Agency (OSHA) and the Consumer Product Safety Commission (CPSC)— administer numerous laws, the key ones being the Food, Drug and Cosmetics Act (FDCA) (1938), the Federal Insecticide, Fungicide and Pesticide Act (FIFPA) (1972), the Occupational Safety and Health Act (OSHA) (1970), the Toxic Substance Control Act (TSCA) (1976), the Consumer Product Safety Act (1972), the Federal Hazardous Substances Act (1960) and all their respective amendments. The latter act stipulates labelling requirements for hazardous substances (toxic, corrosive, irritant, strong sensitizer) for use in the household. Unlike the corresponding European regulation, TSCA does not have a mandatory requirement for a 'base set' of toxicological and ecotoxicological data prior to manufacture or marketing of a new substance, but its provisions under Section 8(e) of TSCA do require that adverse effects observed in toxicological studies and in man be notified to the EPA. The EPA under Section 4(a) of TSCA can require testing to be conducted to develop data with respect to health and environmental effects for which there is an insufficiency of data and experience. FDCA and FIFPA specify health and environmental testing requirements in animals for food additives, cosmetics, drugs and pesticides. The transport of

Table 2 European Community classification, packaging and labelling requirements related to acute toxic effects, risk phrases and label symbols

Symbol	Risk phrases	Code
St Andrew's Cross	Harmful	R20 by inhalation
		R21 by contact with skin
		R22 if swallowed
St Andrew's Cross	Irritation	R36 to eye
		R37 to respiratory system
		R38 to skin
		R41 risk of serious damage to eye
Skull and crossbones	Toxic	R23 by inhalation
		R24 in contact with skin
		R25 if swallowed
Skull and crossbones	Very toxic	R26 by inhalation
		R27 in contact with skin
		R28 if swallowed
Dripping test-tube over symbolized corroded hand and solid block	Corrosive	R34 causes burns
		R35 causes severe burns

Table 3 European Community classification, packaging and labelling regulations related to acute toxic effects, safety phrases

Route of exposure	Code	Safety phrase
Ingestion	S13	Keep away from food, drink, animal feedstuffs
	S20	When using, do not eat or drink
	S46	If swallowed, seek medical advice
Inhalation	S22	Do not breath dust
	S23	Do not breath gas/fumes/vapour/spray
	S38	In case of insufficient ventilation, wear suitable respiratory equipment
General	S44	If you feel unwell, seek medical attention
	S45	In case of accident, seek medical attention
Dermal	S24	Avoid contact with skin
	S25	Avoid contact with eyes
	S26	In case of contact with eyes rinse immediately with plenty of . . . .? . . .
	S27	Take off immediately all contaminated clothing
	S28	After contact with skin, wash immediately
	S36	Wear suitable protective clothing
	S37	Wear suitable gloves
	S39	Wear eye/face protection

hazardous materials in the US is subject to regulations covered by the Hazardous Materials Transportation Act administered by the Department of Transportation. It has provisions for labelling of toxic materials (Figure 2).

In Europe the Control of Substances Hazardous to Health (COSHH) and in the USA OSHA introduced statutory duties on employers to implement occupational hygiene measures appropriate to the type of hazard and the level of risk. Manufacturers of hazardous substances have two basic devices to impart the necessary information: (1) the material safety data sheet (MSDS) or bulletin (OSHA Hazard Communication standard); (2) the labels that they put on their containers. Acute systemic toxicity and irritancy tests define the appropriate symbols and phrases to be used in MSDS documents and on labels.

The data from acute systemic toxicity studies in laboratory animals are used to indicate the quantitative and qualitative differences between the toxicity of various substances but as yet there is not a complete harmonization between countries or regulations. The lay person needs to understand that the ingestion of no more than a taste of a *very toxic* material, a mouthful of *toxic* material or a pint of a *harmful* material would be expected to cause death. Ingestion of smaller amounts could well result not in death but in substantial ill-health effects, but it is important to recognize that the size of an adult would have a significant effect on the dose required to induce an effect when compared with a 10-year-old child or younger infant (Table 4).

Acute Poisoning in Man

The expanding use of synthetically and naturally produced chemicals has led to detrimental effects related to abuse of addictive substances, accidental, incidental and sometimes intentional poisoning of domesticated and wild animals, human adults and, most distressingly, children. The accidental release of chlorophenols at Seveso, of methyl isocyanate at Bhopal and of carbon dioxide from a lake in the Cameroons, and the use of chemicals in warfare, homicide and suicide; these typify for many the consequences of acute intoxication. In non-developed countries, accidents due to uncontrolled and incorrect use of synthetic chemicals have led to acute poisoning being a common cause of death and acute illness between 2 and 30 years of age. The American Association of Poisons Control Centers National Data Collection System estimated that 20 people per 1000 of the US population per annum in 1985 were reported as being exposed to poisonous substances, approximately 90 per cent of exposures occurring at home, 80 per cent being oral ingestion and 60 per cent being children under 5 years of age. In recent years there has been a decline in deaths arising from unintentional ingestion of toxins by children under the age of 5 (Ellenhorn and Barceloux, 1988). Approximately 90 per cent of reported exposures resulted in no signs of toxic

---

USA Department of Transportation regulation under the Hazardous Materials Transportation Act relating to poisons.

[29 Federal Regulations 18753, Dec. 29, 1964. Redesignated at 32 FR 5606, Apr. 5, 1967, and amended by Amdt. 173-94, 41 Fr 16081, Apr. 15, 1976.]

Class A Poisons

Class A poisons are defined not by testing, but rather by inclusion on a regulatory mandated list (Code of Federal Regulations 173, section 173.326), S 173.326 Poison A.

(a) For the purpose of Parts 170-189 of this subchapter extremely dangerous poison. Class A are poisonous gases or liquids of such nature that a very small amount of the gas or vapor of the liquid, mixed with air is dangerous to life. This class includes the following:
  1) Bromolactone.
  2) Cyanogen.
  3) Cyanogen chloride containing less than 0.9% water.
  4) Diphosgene.
  5) Ethyldichlorarsine.
  6) Hydrocyanic acid. (see class B poisons below)
  7) [Reserved].
  8) Methyldichlorarsine.
  9) [Reserved].
  10) Nitrogen peroxide (tetroxide).
  11) [Reserved].
  12) Phosgene (diphosgene).
  13) Nitrogen tetroxide-nitric oxide mixtures containing up to 33.2% weight nitric acid.
(b) Poisonous gases or liquids. Class A as defined in paragraph (a) of this section, except as provided in S 173.331, must not be offered for transportation by rail express.

Class B Poisons

By law those materials with oral LD_{50}s of 50 mg/kg or less in rats are classified as Class B poisons and must be labeled 'Poison'. Diluted solutions of hydrocyanic acid of not exceeding 5% strength are classed as poisonous articles in Class B.

Figure 2 United States Department of Transportation regulations

Table 4 Commonly stated amounts ingested by human adults and children – conversion to quantities

Amount	Quantity (ml)	Adult female (mg kg^{-1}) (50 kg; 120 lb)	Adult male (mg kg^{-1}) (100 kg; 240 lb)	Infant (mg kg^{-1}) (10 kg; 24 lb)
1 drop	0.05[a]	1	0.5	5
1 teaspoon	5	100	50	500
1 tablespoon	15	300	150	1 500
1 mouthful	40	800	400	4 000
1 cupful	200	4 000	2 000	20 000
1 glassful	200	4 000	2 000	20 000
1 mugful	340	6 800	3 400	34 000
1 pint	570	11 400	5 700	57 000

[a] The US Pharmacopeia official dropper delivers a drop of water with a weight between 45 and 55 mg.

effects, which if correct and representative, suggests that the incidence of acute toxicity is approximately 2 per 1000 of the population per annum.

Even from such traumatic situations of human poisoning, toxicologists need to look for data regarding human toxicology and dose–response relationships (Aldridge and Connors, 1985). Suicidal and homicidal sources of knowledge need analysis and comparison with experimental data from animal studies. Adverse effects of drugs in man provide opportunity for examining the process of hazard assessment by the retrospective analysis of clinical symptoms alongside experimental data from animals. Conventional toxicity testing using experiments with laboratory animals aims to detect and characterize the inherent potential for toxicity—this is hazard assessment, whereas risk assessment aims to extrapolate these data and predict the potential consequences for man at the exposure concentrations which are likely to prevail in a variety of circumstances. There is a need to extrapolate both qualitatively (*hazard assessment*) and quantitatively (*risk assessment*), using dose–response relationships obtained in animal studies to predict at what exposure level such responses may occur in man. Most toxicologists would agree that animal toxicity testing can reveal a chemical's potential toxicity for man, and that adverse consequences will not be seen in the majority of cases at exposure conditions which are without effect in animals (Gillette, 1984).

Pharmacology and clinical toxicology textbooks are a good source of information on the clinical signs and treatment of poisoning by drugs (Haddad and Winchester, 1983; Gilman *et al.*,

1985; Ellenhorn and Barceloux, 1988) and acute poisoning by commercial products (Gosselin *et al.*, 1984).

PRINCIPLES AND PROCEDURES

Acute Toxicity Studies

For most of the chemicals in widespread use, little toxicity information other than data from a set of short-term studies in the rat is published in the literature (Lorke, 1983). Although the most frequently performed test is an acute systemic toxicity assessment, the number of animals used in the protocol designs are far fewer than for chronic studies (Table 5), and form a relatively small proportion of the total number of animals used in experimental studies (Table 6). Reviews of studies completed against a broad spectrum of study types (pesticides, intermediates, dyes, pharmaceuticals, cutting oils, biocides, chlorinated solvents, surfactants, formulations) noted that a majority of these studies did not produce evidence of significant toxicity.

The use of laboratory animals has been an integral part of the screening for toxicity of chemicals (Paget, 1970). Some of these chemicals may damage one or more of the major organ systems with varying severity. Consequently there is a need to compare animal species to aid extrapolation of effects in man (Parke, 1983). In the past these lesions have been catalogued but the process of risk assessment now requires that toxicity should be understood (Weil, 1972). Defining the molecular basis of chemically induced lesions presents the best opportunity for achieving this

Table 5 Estimated number of animals used in typical (OECD) regulatory-style toxicity study protocols

Protocol	OECD Guideline number	Study type	Number of animals
Acute effects	401, 402, 403	Systemic effects	20–60[a,b]
	404	Irritancy	1–6
	405	Ocular irritancy	1–3
	406	Sensitization	10–30
Subchronic[b]	407, 410, 412	28 day subacute	80
	408, 411, 413	90 day subacute	160
Chronic and oncogenicity[b]	452	12 month rat	320
	451	18 month mouse	400
	451	24 month rat	400
Developmental and reproductive[b]	414	Rat	160
	414	Rabbit	96
	416	2nd generation rat parent	320
Genetic toxicity[b]	474	Micronucleus	20–60
	475	Cytogenetics	20–60
	478	Dominant lethal	1000
Toxicokinetics[b]	417	Metabolism (high, low, repeat)	24
		Distribution (high, low, repeat)	120
			3099

[a] Lower figure refers to limit test.
[b] Includes both sexes.

Table 6 Number of experiments conducted on living animals in the United Kingdom related to acute toxicity assessments[a]

	1980	1984	1985
Total number of experimental animals used	4 579 478	3 497 335	3 201 350
Acute toxicity[b] studies on:			
medicinal products (%)	6.48	6.06	6.42
other substances[c] (%)	5.21	4.24	4.73

[a] Home Office (1980, 1984, 1985, 1989). *Statistics on Experiments on Living Animals*. Great Britain Cmnd, 9574. HMSO London.
[b] Acute toxicity refers to studies for acute systemic effects, irritancy, allergenicity, pyrogens.
[c] Agricultural, industrial, household, cosmetic, food, environmental, chemical substances or products.

objective (Bridges *et al.*, 1983). However, before we are able to begin to understand toxicity, it is necessary to detect toxicity. Acute toxicity testing in whole organisms is a simple mechanism for achieving this. Traditionally, the emphasis in these types of studies was on determining the LD_{50}, time to death, the slope of the lethality curve, and the prominent clinical signs; however, non-lethal parameters of acute toxicity testing have been extensively reviewed by Sperling (1976) and Balazs (1976). Acute lethality testing designed to determine the amount of a chemical that causes death, with death as the only end-point, has come under extensive criticism (Sperling, 1976; Rowan, 1981; Zbinden and Flury-Roversi, 1981; British Toxicology Society, 1984; Zbinden, 1986; Society of Toxicology, 1989). Acute toxicity studies have achieved a level of notoriety in the public domain due to the efforts of animal welfare groups. A primary focus has been the 'LD$_{50}$ test'. Regrettably, a considerable amount of rhetoric has been used in the description of these tests, overshadowing more reasoned debate.

The primary goals of acute systemic toxicity studies depend principally on the circumstances in which the study data will be used (Gad and Chengelis, 1988). At the present time acute toxicity assessment involves the controlled exposure of various laboratory sentient animal species to a known chemical substance or preparation for a short period of time, following which the clinical signs are monitored for a period of time. While acute toxicity generally deals with the adverse effects of single doses, delayed effects may occur due to accumulation of the chemical in tissues or other mechanism, and it is important to identify any potential for these by repeated dose testing. Dosing periods distributed between the single dose and 10 per cent of life-span dosage are often called subacute. The OECD considered that this term was semantically incorrect and therefore, to distinguish such dosing periods from the classical subchronic, they may be described as 'short-term repeated dose studies'; this applies to 14-, 21- and 28-day studies. The terms 'para-acute' to describe dosing periods of a week or less and 'subacute' for single doses below acute dose levels have been recommended by Gad and Chengelis (1988), but these have not yet achieved popular usage. The main repeat-dose study protocols have usually employed durations of 14, 28 and 90 days, respectively. Other study durations have been used in toxicology, but the selection of these three durations is considered to represent a reasonable standardized approach. The term 'subchronic' has been used to embrace the toxic effects associated with repeated doses of a chemical over greater than a 10 per cent part of an average life-span of experimental animals.

Parameters Studied in Acute Systemic Toxicity Assessments

Establishing a dose–response relationship for exposures at which the probability of a known fraction of a population of a species under study will show lethality is not the only objective of acute systemic toxicity studies. In summary, acute studies establish the following:

- Dose ranges for subsequent studies.

- Potency, ranking from extreme to non-toxic.
- Identifying probable physiological systems/target organs being affected.
- Extent or degree of effect—e.g. subdued behaviour, coma, death.
- Minimal regulatory guideline requirements.

The following illustrates the additional data that can be obtained with appropriate protocol design:

Clinical signs: time of onset, duration and recovery
Morbidity: agonal changes; reflexes; pharmacological effects; dose–response curves (ED$_{50}$).
Lethality: dose–response (LD$_{50}$ with confidence limits); shape and slope of dose–response curve; estimation of median lethal dose (LD$_{50}$); estimation of minimum lethal dose (LD$_{01}$); estimation of certain lethal dose (LD$_{100}$).
Body weight: decreased body weight gain; body weight loss; reduced food consumption.
Target organ identification: necropsy and gross tissue examinations; histological examinations; blood clinical chemistry; haematology.
Physiological function: immunology; neuromuscular reflexes; behavioural screening; electrocardiogram; electroencephalogram.
Pharmacokinetic: therapeutic index; bioavailability (AUC, volume of distribution, half-life).
Pharmacodynamics: relationship between plasma and tissue levels and occurrence of clinical signs.

Identification of the probable physiological systems and target organs involved in acute systemic toxicity are important objectives when conducting these types of assessments (British Toxicology Society, 1984; ECETOC, 1985; Society of Toxicology, 1989). Often in the past, only a small selected amount of data from an acute toxicity study has been reported and recorded on informational databases. The data selected are often only the median lethal dose (LD$_{50}$), or median lethal concentration (LC$_{50}$).

Protocol Design

For valid conclusions to be reached, application of the scientific method requires the objective of the study to be defined, the use of homogeneous populations of experimental subjects, sensitive and selective indices of effects, and analysis of data by appropriate statistical approaches. While some protocols have been defined to meet various international regulations, for other regulations the exact protocols depend on the type of chemical substance and the country in which it will be registered for use (Zbinden and Flury-Roversi, 1981; Oliver *et al.*, 1985). There is a considerable amount of harmony in the requirements for acute oral, dermal, inhalation and parenteral toxicity. Often both sexes of two species, employing a route of exposure which is anticipated to be the most probable route of exposure for man, is necessary for regulatory purposes (Tables 7, 8). Laboratory mice and rats are the species typically selected. Additional species are required by some regulations and in these cases probe studies are often used to select an appropriate dose range and species. The use of parenteral and oral route comparisons was developed primarily in order to gain information about the bioavailability of the chemical without recourse to the development of a bioanalytical technique for determining the

chemical in biological matrixes such as urine and blood. It is questionable whether this estimate of bioavailability is appropriate, with the development of more appropriate pharmacokinetic methods of determining bioavailability. With certain materials the development of a bioanalytical technique may not be easily achieved and the use of a bioassay approach may be the only alternative. The use of a biological parameter other than lethality is clearly desirable in these instances. Zbinden and Flury-Roversi (1981) have documented several cases where lethality was of no biological relevance. The experimental design for acute systemic toxicity assessment has for many years been a modification of the Trevan approach of interval dose levels applied to groups of experimental animals such that an incidence of response can be achieved varying from zero incidence to 100 per cent response, and the median lethal dose can be derived (LD_{50}). The number of replicates and size of sample population will dictate whether the experimentally derived curve reflects the actual response. It is infrequent for control

Table 7 Summary of Regulatory Guidelines—dermal toxicity

	DOT	EEC	FDA	FHSA	FIFRA[a]	IRLG[a]	J MAFF	OECD	TSCA[a]
Species options and weight ranges:									
mouse	NR	≤20%	NR	NR	NR	NR	NR	NR	NR
rat	NR	≤±20% of mean	NS	NR	200–300 g	200–300 g	200–300 g	200–300 g	200–300 g
guinea-pig	NR	≤20%	NS	NR	350–450 g	350–450 g	350–450 g	350–450 g	350–450 g
rabbit	NS	≤20%	NS	2.3–3 kg	2–3 kg	2–3 kg	2–3 kg	2–3 kg	2–3 kg
Maximum dose level options:									
limit dose (mg/kg)	200	2000	NS	2000	≥200	≥2000	2000	2000	2000
Minimum number of groups	1	≥3	NS	1	≥3	≥3	≥3	≥3	≥3
Animals/group/sex	10	5	NS	10	5	5	5	5	5
Observation (days)	2	14	14	14	≥14	≥14	≥14	≥14	≥14
Data recording:									
body weights	NS	NS	NS	NS	Pre-test weekly at death	Pre-test weekly at death	Pre-test weekly at death	Pre-test weekly at death	Pre-test weekly at death
necropsy	NR	Required	NS	NR	Optional	Required	Optional	Optional	Optional
histopathology	NR	When indicated	NS	NR	NS	Optional	Optional	Optional	Optional
clinical chemistry	NS	NR	NS	NS	NS	NS	NS	NS	Optional

[a] Preferred species rabbit.
NS, not specific; NR, not required.
Based on Auletta (1988).

Table 8 Summary of Regulatory Guidelines—acute toxicity tests

	DOT	EEC	FDA[a]	FHSA	FIFRA	IRLG[b]	J MAFF[c]	OECD[d]	TSCA[d]
Species options:									
number required	1	2	4	1	1	1	2	2	2
species/weight									
mouse	NR	≤20%	NS	NR	NR	NR	NS	≤±20% of mean	≤±20% of mean
rat	200–300 g	≤20%	NS	200–300 g	≤±20% of mean	≤±20% of mean	NS	≤±20% of mean	≤±20% of mean
non-rodent	NR	≤20%	NS	NR	NR	NR	NS	NR	NR
Maximum limit dose (mg/kg)	50	5000	NS	5000	5000	≥5000	5000	5000	5000
Minimum number of groups	1	≥3	NS	1	≥3	≥3, prefer 4	≥5	≥3	≥3
Animals/group/sex	10	5	NS	10	5	5	5	5	5
Observations:									
days	2	14	≥7	14	14	14	14	14	14
body weights	NS	NS	NS	NS	Pre-test weekly at death	Weekly	Pre-test weekly at death	Pre-test weekly at death	Pre-test weekly at death
necropsy	NR	Required	Non-rodents[e]	NR	Optional	Required[e]	Optional	Optional	Required
histopathology	NR	When indicated	NS	NR	NS	Optional	Optional	Optional	Optional
clinical chemistry	NR	NS	NS	NR	NS	NS	NS	NS	Optional

[a] At least one to be a non-rodent.
[b] Rat.
[c] Rat plus one other species.
[d] Preferred species rat and mouse.
[e] For animals that die.
NR, Not required, NS, Not specified.
Based on Auletta (1988).

animals to be included in acute systemic studies but rather historical control data of survival clinical effect are used. Zbinden and colleagues refer to the positive control as the reference compound, and they have discussed some of the general criteria to be applied in the selection of reference compounds.

In systemic toxicity testing, experimental design should allow broad group classifications of extremely toxic, very toxic, toxic and practically non-toxic, and perhaps move away from the need to define the (LD_{50}). However, this point of view does beg the question, 'What data would be required to justify a nominated classification, if not the LD_{50}?' Lethality should not be the only dose-related systemic effect that would justify a classification, and more use would and could be made of the induced clinical signs (Tables 9, 10)— i.e. the use of qualitative judgements based on

semiquantitative rather than quantitative dose–response data (Rhodes *et al.*, 1988, 1989).

A wide variety of intrinsic and extrinsic factors can influence the outcome of a test (Morrison *et al.*, 1968; Balazs, 1976; DePass *et al.*, 1984; Auletta, 1988). Many investigations into the sources of variability in acute toxicity testing have been conducted and these have been recently reviewed by Elsberry (1986). In order to establish a dose–response relationship, the same species/ strain, sex and age should be divided randomly into equivalent-size groups, with the different groups treated at the same time of day with different dosages by the same route and observed for a set and consistent period of time. For a single exposure study a misdelivered dose would have a greater effect on the conclusions than for chronic exposure studies. Toxicity that is clearly the result of accidental events should not be considered in

Table 9 Physiological systems of mammalian organisms, potential target organs and clinical signs observed in acute systemic toxicity studies

Main body system	Organs	Examinations	Clinical signs
Integumentary	Skin, fur, claws	External observations	Piloerection, oedema, erythema, eruptions, colour, alopecia, irritation, necrosis
Musculature/skeletal	Muscles, tendons, bones, cartilage	Reflexes	Fasciculation, catalepsy, hyper/hypotonia
Nervous system	CNS—brain, spinal cord	Home-cage, external and in-hand passive observations, reflexes, provocation	Ataxia, convulsions (clonic and tonic), tremor, righting reflex, gait, prostration
	Peripheral—nerves and ganglia		
	Autonomic	Reflexes	Lachrymation, miosis, mydriasis, ptosis, exophthalmos, chromodacryorrhea
	Sensory, eye, ear, olfactory	External observations, reflexes	Anaesthesia, paraesthesia Corneal opacity, iritis, chemosis, conjunctivitis, nystagmus
Endocrine	Pancreas, adrenal, thymus, parathyroid, pituitary, pineal, testis, ovaries		
Cardiovascular	Heart[a], blood vessels, spleen	Palpitation, heart rate	Arrhythmia, bradycardia, tachycardia, vasodilation, vasoconstriction, hyperthermia, hypothermia
Respiratory	Lungs[a], nasal cavity, pharynx, larynx, bronchus	Breathing rate, external observation	Apnea, bradypnoea, dyspnoea, tachypnoea, cyanosis, nasal discharge, Cheyne–Stokes, Kussmaul, hypopnoea
Digestive system	Oral cavity, stomach, salivary glands, small/large intestine, rectum, colon, liver[a]	Excreta, external observation	Emesis, flatulence, constipation, diarrhoea, stained faeces, absence of faeces
Urinogenital	Kidney[a], bladder, ovary, testes, placenta, fetus, perineal region	External observation, excreta	Diuresis, rhinorrhea, anuria, polyuria
Lymphatic	Lymph nodes, thymus, spleen[a]		

[a] Typical organs occasionally removed at necropsy for additional histological evaluation if gross observation shows evidence of adverse change.

the final conclusion. All protocols should state the ceiling or limit dosage. Small differences in protocols are probably the major cause of the considerable laboratory-to-laboratory variations in results achieved (Lorke, 1983). There is some question concerning the utility of extensive pathological assessments as part of an acute study. Gross necropsies are the minimum requested by

Table 10   Clinical signs of systemic toxicity

Agonal
Signs of death

Alopecia
Deficiency of hair

Anaesthesia
Absence of or reduced response to external stimulus

Analgesia
Decrease in reaction to induced pain

Anuria
Absence of or reduction in urine excretion

Apnoea
Transient cessation of breathing following a forced
respiration

Arrhythmia
Abnormal cardiac rhythm

Asphyxia
Suspended animation due to lack of oxygen in blood,
suffocation

Ataxia
Incoordination of muscular action, loss of coordination
and unsteady gait

Blepharospasm
Rapid or spasmodic eyelid movement

Bradycardia
Decreased heart rate

Cardiac rhythm
Response of the heart muscle

Catalepsy
Animal tends to remain in position in which it is placed

Chemosis
Swelling/oedema of the conjunctival tissue

Cheyne–Stokes
Rhythmic waxing and waning of respiration

Chromodacryorrhoea
Red lachrymation/reddish conjunctival exudate/absence
of erythrocytes

Conjunctivitis
Inflammation of the mucus membranes of the eyelids
and junction with the cornea

Convulsion, asphyxial
Gasping and cyanosis accompanying clonic convulsions

Convulsion, clonic
Alternating contraction and relaxation of muscles,
observed as a cycling of the forelimbs

Convulsion, tonic
Persistent contraction of the muscles with rigid extension
of hindlimbs

Corneal opacity
Translucent and opaque to transmission of light

Corneal reflex
Touching of the cornea causing eyelid to close

Cyanosis
Bluish appearance of tail, mouth, footpads due to lack
of oxygenation of the blood

Diaphoresis
Production of perspiration

Diarrhoea
Frequent defaecation of fluid stools

Discharge
Excretion/secretion

Diuresis
Involuntary urination

Dyspnoea
Difficult or laboured breathing, gasping for air, slow
respiratory rate

Emaciation
Lean wasting muscle mass

Emesis
Vomiting and retching

Erythema
Redness of skin due to irritation and inflammation

Exophthalmos
Protrusion of the eyeball from the orbit

Exudates
Oozing secretion or discharge

Fasciculation
Rapid continuous contraction (twitching) involving
movements of skeletal muscle on the back, shoulders,
hindlimbs and digits

(continued)

Table 10 (continued)

Gait
Locomotory movement of the limbs during walking, normal carriage of body

Gasping
Strain for air or breath with open mouth, convulsive catching of breath often accompanied by a wheezing sound

Grip strength
Ability to retain hold with digits

Hyperactivity
Increased level of motor activity

Hyperpnoea
Deep and rapid breathing

Hypersensitivity
Excessive reaction to external stimuli such as light, noise or touch

Hypertonia
Increase in muscle tension

Hypo-activity
Low level of motor activity

Hypotonia
Generalized decrease in muscle tension and tone

Iritis
Inflammation of the iris

Jaundice
Yellow coloration of mucous membranes due to deposition of bile pigments

Kyphosis
Curvature of the vertebral column creating a hump back

Lachrymation
The secretion of tears

Lethargy
Inability to be aroused from stupor without relapse

Miosis
Constriction of the pupil irrespective of the presence or absence of light

Motor activity
Changes in frequency and nature of movements

Mydriasis
Excessive dilation of the pupil

Myotactic reflex
Ability to retract limb when extended over edge of a surface

Necrosis
Death of tissue

Nictitating membrane
Inner eyelid of many animals

Nystagmus
Involuntary rotational, horizontal or vertical movement of eyes

Oedema
Swelling of tissue filling with fluid

Opacity, cornea
As loss of transparency of the cornea

Opisthotonos
Tetanic spasm in which the head is pulled towards the dorsal position and the back is arched

Paralysis
Loss of motor function in all or part of the body

Piloerection
Raising of the hair/fur

Pinna reflex
Twitch of the outer ear elicited by light stroking of inside surface of ear

Polyuria
Increase above normal in the amount of urine excreted

Preyer's reflex
Involuntary movement of ears produced by noise

Prolapsus
Slipping forward or down of part of an organ, usually uterus or rectum

Prostration
Immobile, resting on ventral surface

Ptosis
Dropping of the upper eyelid associated with impaired conduction in the third cranial nerve and not reversed by stimulation

Pupillary reflex
Contraction of the pupil in response to light

Respiration irregular
Abnormal breathing rate

(continued overleaf)

Table 10 (continued)

Respiration laboured Breathing strained and difficult	*Stupor* Torpidity, dazed state
Righting reflex Ability to regain normal stance onto all four limbs	*Tachycardia* Increased heart rate
Salivation Excessive salivary secretion	*Tachypnoea* Rapid and unusually shallow respiration
Somnolence Drowsiness which can be aroused by external stimulation and with resumption of normal activities	*Torsion* Postural incoordination or rolling often associated with the vestibular system (ear canal)
Spasticity Uncontrolled involuntary movement of limbs	*Tremor* Trembling and quivering of the limbs or entire body
Startle reflex Response to external stimuli such as light, touch and noise	*Vasoconstriction* Blanching of skin or mucous membranes, body feels cold
Straub tail The carriage of the tail in an erect/vertical position (associated with interaction with opiate receptors)	*Vasodilation* Redness of skin and mucous membranes, body feels warm

most regulatory bodies. Protocols include necropsies on all animals found dead and those killed following the 2-week post-dosing observation period. Body weights are determined on day 1 (prior to dosing), day 7 and day 14, as required by most regulatory guidelines. Animals should not differ in age by more than 15 per cent: for example, the ratios of the LD_{50}s obtained in adult animals and those in neonates vary from 0.002 to 160 (Balazs, 1976).

Clinical Signs

Acute systemic studies are concerned with the detection of adverse changes to the body systems which are likely to be life-threatening following single exposure to chemicals. But they are also concerned with non-life-threatening responses that occur in other tissues which may lead to loss of function, ill-health and reduction in quality of life. The assessment of acute systemic toxicity is the assessment of the potential for severe health effects which result from the major systems of the body—cardiovascular, respiratory, central nervous system, excretory and locomotory—being compromised by adverse change. The aim of qualitative extrapolation of toxicity data from animals would be to predict potential signs of toxicity

in man and the symptoms that are likely to be described by someone who has been intoxicated—i.e. 'feeling drowsy', 'feeling nauseated'. Animals will not describe such symptoms: they have to be deduced from the clinical signs of toxicity and pharmacological responses expressed in the animal studies and observed and recorded by the toxicologist as cage-side observations. It should be remembered that when dealing with animals we are observing clinical signs: animals are not describing their symptoms. Clinical symptoms are the verbal descriptions of feelings provided by a human patient. The term 'clinical symptoms' is often misused when describing animal observations. Signs are overt and observable (Brown, 1984). Symptoms are apparent only to the subject of intoxication (e.g. headache) and can not be described or reported by animals (Balazs, 1970). Clinical signs can be reversible or irreversible. Reversible signs are those that dissipate as the chemical is cleared from the body. Irreversible signs are those that do not disappear and are accompanied by organic damage. Signs also represent pharmacological response which may be adverse. The reliability and accuracy of prediction from animal studies can be judged only when a chemical is assessed in both animals and man and any adverse reactions observed are compared (Griffin, 1985). Substantial gross macroscopic findings are rare in minimal acute studies and seldom suggestive of a specific effect. It is difficult to separate the chemical-associated effect from agonal and/or autolytic changes in animals found dead. It is difficult to come to a conclusion about the nature of a gross lesion without histological assessment. Confirmation of gross lesions is seldom done, because of the autolytic nature of many of the lesions. Pathological examinations in general and histological assessments in particular are most meaningful when the same organs are collected and examined from all animals regardless of the circumstances of death (Elsberry, 1986). The kidney and liver are most frequently the target organs of acute toxicity. The clinical laboratory package should be sufficient to detect possible damage to these organs. Serum parameters should include urea, glucose and total protein concentrations, and the activities of alanine aminotransferase, aspartate aminotransferase and alkaline phosphatase.

Liver

Liver structure and function are more often altered by acute exposures to chemicals as a consequence of the extensive role of the liver in biotransformation of absorbed exogenous substances. The most sensitive tests for hepatotoxicity are those that monitor elevation in the levels of serum transaminases (aspartate aminotransferase, ASP; alanine aminotransferase, ALT); gamma glutamyl transpeptidase (γ-GPT) and serum bile acids. Serum bile acid levels are specific for liver injury and reasonably sensitive, and are often observable by direct observation of yellowing of external surfaces (jaundice). Signs of hepatotoxicity are not often apparent from cage-side observation.

Kidney

As the kidneys receive one-quarter of the cardiac output and are the site of concentration and excretion of water-soluble exogenous materials, they are often a target for acute toxic response. Signs of renal intoxication, however, are rarely prominent in the acute phase. Polyuria and oliguria, proteinuria or haematuria and elevated serum creatinine or blood urea are often not seen until much of the kidney's capacity to filter, concentrate and reabsorb has been compromised.

Lung

Toxic pulmonary injury is most likely to occur in association with inhaled chemical agents, often by direct irritation—e.g. chlorine gas. However, severe acute toxicity to the lung has been observed following systemic absorption of certain compounds—i.e. methylfurans and some dipyridyl herbicides.

Nervous System

Functional and morphological disturbances of central, peripheral and autonomic systems often occur with acute intoxication—i.e. carbon disulphide, organophosphorus insecticides. The cerebral cortex, cerebellum, peripheral nerves, synapses and spinal cord are often the target for injury. Clinical signs of acute intoxication are often associated with the antagonism of CNS and PNS functions.

Haematopoietic System

While the haematopoietic system and the immune system may be target tissues following acute exposure, evidence of toxicity from clinical signs is limited. With regard to the blood, the most common acute lesion is induced haemolysis. Haematological assessment of blood, monitoring red and white cell counts, haematocrit, white cell differentials and blood coagulation factors such as clotting time are necessary to diagnose these tissues correctly as targets of acute toxicity.

External Organs

The skin can show evidence of irritation and eyes opacity of the cornea and/or lens following direct application, whole-body exposure or systemic exposure. To establish evident toxicity, more than a single exposure is often required. Direct contact of external tissues to toxicants often elicits immediate responses within a relatively short period of time following exposure.

Mortality

Mortality in each group is calculated on the basis of the number of animals that die (or are humanely killed because of morbidity) during the observation period, and is normally presented in percentage terms: (number dead/number dosed) $\times 100$. Delayed deaths (those occurring more than 24 h after dosing) are relatively rare and generally restricted to the 72 h period following dosing (Gad *et al.*, 1984; Bruce, 1985). The different laboratory practices of including or excluding animals killed because of morbidity may reflect some of the interlaboratory assessments of acute toxicity of equivalent chemicals.

In vivo Studies

Set Dose and Sequential Dosing Procedures

A small number of animals per dose are administered fixed dose levels approximating to current limits used for labelling. The top dose approximates to the limit dose specified by regulatory guidelines. The set-dose method works best if the doses are separated by constant multiples (Schutz and Fuchs, 1982; Lorke, 1983; British Toxicology Society, 1984). If there are no effects, the protocol defaults to a limit test. In a limit test, a single dose of the test article is given to one group of animals. Additional animals may be required to confirm the limit. Lorke's protocol design consists of 3 animals per dose at 10, 100 and 1000 mg kg^{-1}. Animals were observed for 14 days post dosing. Interestingly, 1 animal per group gave reliable results in 93 per cent of chemicals tested. Diechmann and LeBlanc estimated an LD$_{50}$ using 6 animals by analysing the responses of individual animals. The dose range was defined as 1.5× a multiplication factor. The approximate lethal dose was the highest dose that did not cause death. It has been suggested that to establish the acute toxicity of a chemical, one should move towards the maximum non-lethal dose, which, although inherently less accurate than the LD$_{50}$, better compares steep and flat dose–response curves (Tattersall, 1982).

A fixed dose design has been proposed for classification or labelling purposes (British Toxicology Society, 1984). Five rats per sex receive 50 mg kg^{-1}; if survival is less than 90 per cent, a second group of animals is given 5 mg kg^{-1}. If survival is again less than 90 per cent, the substance is classified as 'very toxic'. If survival is greater than 90 per cent, it is classified as 'toxic'. If survival is 90 per cent but there is evident toxicity after the 50 mg kg^{-1} dose, the substance is 'unclassified'. Evident toxicity refers to cage-side observations of clinical signs which are likely to be life-threatening. This protocol has been evaluated by several groups in the UK and is currently the subject of an international evaluation sponsored by the OECD. It would appear that this procedure will be accepted for regulatory purposes by the European Commission (EEC, 1989) and be introduced into Annex V of Directive 79/83/1/EEC as an alternative to the LD$_{50}$ for toxicity classification for labelling purposes.

Sequential Up-and-Down Dosing

The format for this type of procedure requires single animals to be exposed, with subsequent doses adjusted up or down by some constant factor depending on the outcome of the previous dose (Dixon and Wood, 1948; Brownlee *et al.*, 1953; Bruce, 1985). In Bruce's method, an individual animal is dosed; if an animal dies, the dose is decreased by a constant factor (suggested 1.3) and another animal is dosed at this level. If the animal does not respond, the dose is elevated by an equivalent constant factor until 5 animals have been dosed or the limit dose is reached. The data are analysed with the maximum likelihood methods (Bruce, 1985) or the use of the tables developed by Dixon (1965). In general, only 6–9 animals are required.

Rising-Dose Procedures

A single group of animals (usually 2) receives repeated exposure to the chemical throughout the study (often on alternate days), with the dose increasing at each administration by some constant factor such as doubling until toxicity, morbidity or lethality is observed in one or both animals or the limit dose is achieved. In one such rising-dose tolerance design, animals were exposed for 4 days to the initial dosage, followed by 3 days of recovery before the next 4-day dosing period at a raised dose level; the sequence was repeated for the three dosing cycles (Hazelett *et al.*, 1987).

Non-Rodent Acute Toxicity Studies

For non-rodents, rising-dose procedures are sufficient to support most regulatory submissions. Delayed effects, bioaccumulation due to incomplete clearance between administration, pharmacological accommodation, induction and inhibition of metabolism may all complicate the interpretation of this type of study. Under some international animal welfare regulations but not all, non-rodents can be re-used following a washout period.

The FDA and Canada require acute toxicity testing in at least one non-rodent species, although it has been suggested that is unnecessary to achieve lethal doses in non-rodent species. Animals often used are dog, monkey and ferret. Agricultural chemicals may have to be tested in domesticated farm animals. The rabbit is the species of choice for a variety of tests, such as dermal toxicity. The use of larger animals permits more extensive observation, such as complete physical examinations, palpations, behavioural checks, spinal reflex check, pupillary light responses, respiration rate, ECG recording and rectal temperature measurement. Blood samples can also be more easily collected to determine standard clinical chemistry and haematology profiles. The bioanalysis of plasma levels of parent compound and any significant metabolites would assist in interpretation but such analytical procedures are often unlikely to be available at the early evaluation stages of a chemical. Such rising multidose study designs can replace conventional 2-week studies conducted at a range of fixed dose levels. Gross necropsy examinations, measurement of major organ weights (both absolute and relative) and a battery of serum enzyme assays should all be part of the protocol.

Quality-Control Screen

Lethality screening is used in the quality control monitoring for the standardization of biologically derived materials for potency and the test for gross contamination or adulteration. Quality control tests for potency generally use a minimum number of groups of few animals dosed at the expected LD_{50}. Such quality assurance limit tests are almost exclusively conducted on mice. If mortality falls within the standardized range of expected responses, then the batch would be acceptable. Tests for contamination are often limit tests where only few animals are tested at a set limit dose (MLD, the minimum lethal dose, LD_{01}) with the anticipated outcome of 100 per cent survival. An occasional death may occur because the MLD is in the range of LD_{01}. There is cause for concern if the repeat response is again not 100 per cent survival, and the material should not be released until the cause of enhanced lethality is understood—i.e. possible infection in stock animals.

Rodenticide Testing

It should be remembered that the determination of the minimum dose to ensure lethality (LD_{100})

is still an objective in establishing the potency of rodenticides (FIFRA).

Other Species

EPA requires tests in aquatic non-vertebrates and vertebrates (fish, avian and feral species) for chemicals that may be released into the environment. These areas of acute toxicology assessment are more appropriately covered under 'ecotoxicology'.

Factors Affecting Acute Systemic Toxicity Studies

The various factors that influence the outcome of acute systemic toxicity studies are in many respects equivalent to those that modulate all biological studies. In assessing the extent of a toxic hazard, there are several important considerations related to route, severity, speed and duration of onset of effect (Table 11). As in any biological experiment in which a small sample is taken to estimate the population response, there are many factors that can act as variables.

(1) Interspecies differences relating to heterogeneity of populations, specific physiology, basal metabolic rate and size.

(2) Intraspecies variation regarding strain, sex, age.

(3) Environmental, including route of

Table 11 Factors affecting the assessment of acute toxic hazard

Factor	Type
Route of exposure	Ingestion, inhalation, dermal, parenteral
Severity of effect	Harmless, harmful, toxic, very toxic, extremely toxic, non-irritant, irritant, corrosive
Speed of onset	Immediate, delayed
Duration of effect	Acute, persistent, reversible, irreversible
Duration of exposure	Single short-duration (acute) Multiple short-duration (subacute) Multiple long-duration (subchronic) Continuous (chronic)

exposure, amount, physical form, formulation, exposure intervals, observation intervals.

(4) Statistical, including experimental bias, group size, size of population.

All the above factors contribute to the difficulties in achieving reproducible accurate and precise data. However, the route of exposure—the most common being gastrointestinal, inhalation, dermal, parenteral—has a major influence on the toxicity because of the effect of route of exposure on the rate and extent of absorption (bioavailability) of the chemical. The maximum plasma (tissue) level achieved, the time to maximum plasma levels and the duration of effect are affected by the clearance of the chemical from the system and the extent of distribution within the system. In turn, clearance can be modulated by the physiological changes induced by the chemical itself and the age and disease state of the organism under study.

Acute Inhalation Toxicity

Gases, vapours, smokes, dusts and aerosols, when inhaled, reach the absorptive surfaces of the lungs and the nasopharyngeal regions. This represents a major route of occupational and incidental exposure to toxins and a significant route of intentional exposure for drugs. In the lungs, inhaled intoxicants have ready access to the systemic circulation because of the extensive surface area and extensive vascularization. The close proximity of the gaseous phase to the vasculature allows toxicant exchange between inspired air and the blood and lymph. A number of factors affect the inhalation of aerosols—characteristics of the aerosols, architecture of the respiratory tract, breathing rate, tidal volume and residual capacity. The anatomy of nasal, buccal and pharyngeal regions, mucous distribution and the geometry of the air passages from nasal turbinates to the alveoli influence the extent and amount of toxicant entering the lungs. The respiratory rate (breaths min^{-1}) and tidal volume (ml) vary between species relative to their size—man has a breathing rate of 12–18 breaths min^{-1}, tidal volume of 750 ml; dog 20 breaths min^{-1} and 200 ml; guinea-pig 90 breaths min^{-1}, 2 ml; rat 160 breaths min^{-1}, 1.4 ml; mouse 180 breaths min^{-1}, 0.25 ml. The disposition of particles is not identical between species. Disposition in the respirat-

ory tract depends on the size of the particle or aerosol; those less than 1 μm in size reach the alveolar zone; those <5 μm are deposited in the trachea and bronchi; those of >5 μm diameter deposit in the nose and pharynx. It should be remembered that, unlike man, the rodent is an obligatory nose breather and the presence of a toxin may significantly change breathing rates.

Inhalation procedures are more complex and difficult to perform than are acute oral, dermal or parenteral procedures, requiring more sophisticated techniques of analysis, formulation preparation and exposure (Drew and Laskin, 1973). Acute inhalation toxicity is expressed as a function of concentration in the atmosphere and time of exposure, with 4 h being arbitrarily accepted as the maximum exposure for definition as acute. The practice of using many groups and numbers of animals to define an LC_{50} has been replaced by designs which determine the approximate lowest lethal concentration (Kennedy *et al.*, 1986). Exposure can be whole-body in an inhalation chamber or head-only, in which the animal is restrained with its head in an inhalation hood. There are limits to the amount of toxicants that can be presented as an atmosphere and commonsense should prevail for the concentration used for a limit test. Details of inhalation procedures are given in subsequent chapters.

Acute Dermal Toxicity

Contamination of the skin is considered by many to be the primary route of intentional, adventitious, incidental and accidental exposure to toxins. The several mechanisms of percutaneous diffusion of exogenous chemicals into and across the epidermis and into the vascular circulation are (1) diffusion through the cells of the stratum corneum, (2) diffusion between the cells of the stratum corneum, (3) diffusion down the skin appendages—hair follicles, and sweat and sebaceous glands. The rate and amount of transfer of toxin are influenced by the physical state of the toxicant, the physical state of the skin and the mode of presentation to the skin. Factors which are considered to make important contributions to the rate and extent of absorption and important during the design of acute dermal toxicity study are: (1) the nature of the vehicle; (2) the concentration of toxicant in the vehicle; (3) the state of hydration of the skin; (4) occluded or unoccluded exposure; (5) skin abrasion; (6) viscosity of the formulation; (7) ionization state of the toxicant—i.e. pK of toxicant and pH of formulation; (8) the ambient temperature. Fick's law of diffusion is considered to approximate percutaneous absorption kinetics of molecules:

$$F = \frac{Q_m}{At} = K_p\, C$$

where Q_m = amount of toxicant that penetrates the skin (mol); A = area of skin (cm^2); t = time (min); F = flux moles transferred / unit area in unit time (mol cm^{-2} min^{-1}); K_p = permeability constant (cm min^{-1}); and C = difference between external and internal concentration (mol cm^{-1}).

The general experimental design and principles are similar for dermal and oral acute toxicity studies. In acute dermal toxicity studies the rabbit has been the recommended species, presumably because of its preferred use in irritancy assessment. The rat, mouse or guinea-pig are adequate alternate species which are considerably easier to handle than the rabbit. The hair is removed in a manner which does not abrade the skin (abrasion increases the extent and rate of absorption of many chemicals) from an area of the dorsal surface (back, shoulder). The area is approximately 10 per cent of the body surface (rat 4 × 5 cm; rabbit 12 × 14 cm; guinea-pig 7 × 10 cm). There is a practical limit to the amount of a material that can be sensibly applied to the back of an animal, and most regulatory authorities accept a limit dose experiment at approximately 2000–5000 mg kg^{-1}.

Acute Parenteral Toxicity

Several parenteral routes of acute exposure are possible: intravenous, subcutaneous, intraperitoneal, intramuscular, intracerebral. Because of the toxicity which can be elicited by infectious organisms, it is essential that formulations for parenteral acute toxicity be sterile and procedures be aseptic. The intravenous route initially bypasses gut and liver first-pass effects but may demonstrate lung first-pass extraction. The principles and procedures for acute toxicity assessment by the parenteral route of administration are common with those described for oral administration.

STATISTICAL CONSIDERATIONS

Dose–Response/Effect Relationships

It is not the intention of this chapter to give a detailed appraisal of statistical approaches, and the reader should consult Gad and Chengelis (1988) and Chan and Hayes (1989) for in-depth analysis. One important way of expressing the severity of response is to establish the *dose effect*—the relationship between dose and the magnitude of a defined biological effect either in an individual or in a population sample (OECD, 1981)—or the *dose response*—the relationship between the dose and the proportion of a population sample showing a defined effect (Alarie, 1981; OECD, 1981a). For solids and liquids the dose is often expressed as mg or ml per kg body weight or as a concentration term expressed as parts per million (ppm) required to cause an effect or an increased incidence of effect. For gaseous or volatile materials concentration is expressed as mg l^{-1} h^{-1} or ppm h^{-1} to combine dose and length of exposure.

Paracelsus (1492–1541) in his work *The Third Principle* eloquently defined the dose–response concept, 'What is there that is not a poison? All things are poison and nothing [is] without poison. Solely the dose determines that a thing is not a poison' and the concept of a no-effect level or threshold dose, 'that while a thing may be a poison it may not cause poisoning' (Diechmann *et al.*, 1986). In an individual an effect may be graded from zero to a maximal value. Alternatively, a response may be either present or absent—i.e. a quantal response. Occasionally a response may have more than two possible outcomes and is referred to as a polychotomous response. Fundamental to acute toxicology is the relationship of response to log-normal distribution, which is commonly expressed in terms related to the principles of population statistics. Most often acute responses are expressed as percentage incidence occurring in an exposed population. Groups of experimental subjects are given various doses of a substance and observations are made, with the percentage responding plotted on the y-axis and the logarithm of the dose on the x-axis. The observed cumulative curve is often sigmoidal in shape.

In a population of subjects there is a range of sensitivity, and for a given population a frequency of response curve should be bell-shaped (if there were a sufficient number of studies), which when plotted as a cumulative frequency will show a sigmoidal relationship (Figure 3). The shape of the dose–response curve in the low-dose region often suggests that a safe level of exposure exists (Nordberg and Strangert, 1978). The general shape and relationship of this dose–response curve can be modelled by sampling over the range of response. How accurately and precisely this curve will model the true population response will depend upon the number of samples and the size of each sample chosen. Various mathematical transforms convert a sigmoidal curve into a straight line function. A log transform of a skewed distribution will often normalize the data (Figure 4).

Converting the percentile cumulative response into normal equivalent deviant ranges or probits will often transform a sigmoid response into a linear function (Gaddum, 1933; Finney, 1971).

This is expressed mathematically as:

$$dP = \frac{1}{\sigma\sqrt{2\pi}} \exp\left[\frac{-(x-\mu)^2}{2\sigma^2}\right]$$

where σ^2 = variance; μ = mean; and x = value at each dose, and dP = probability of response

then

$$P = \int_{-\infty}^{x} \frac{1}{\sigma\sqrt{2\pi}} \exp\left[\frac{-(x-\mu)^2}{2\sigma^2}\right] dx$$

A linear equation allows a more accurate statistical analysis and derivation of the median value, the slope and the confidence intervals (Figure 5). Caution must be exercised, as mathematically derived values may well suggest a level of exactitude and credibility which is not justified by the database being used. For many purposes these quantitative values are often no better than a qualitative judgement.

The concept of dose–response and the ranking of substances on the basis of the amount required to produce an effect is generally appreciated. What is not often appreciated is the reason for selecting the median effect dose or concentration (ED_{50}, LD_{50}, EC_{50}, LC_{50}). One could select a dose which would be insufficient to affect any animal in a group, or the dose required which is large enough to affect all the animals in a group. The former would be referred to as the minimum-

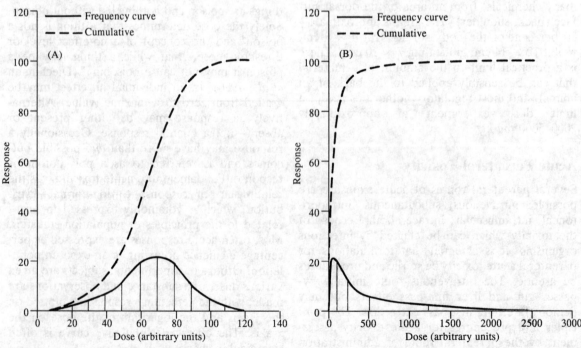

Figure 3 (A) Illustrative normal distribution response–frequency curve and cumulative response–frequency curve plotted against the dose. (B) Skewed distribution response–frequency curve and cumulative response–frequency curve plotted against dose

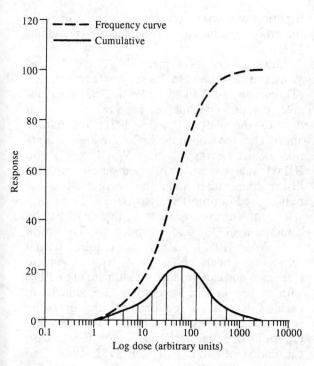

Figure 4 Plot of logarithmic transformation of skewed dose response

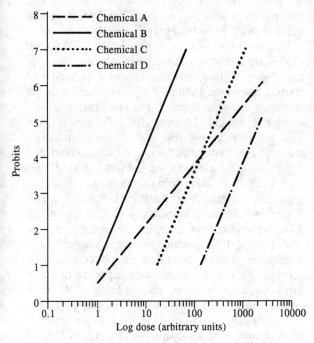

Figure 5 Comparison of probit lines for chemicals with equivalent LD_{50} and different slopes (A and C) and different LD_{50} and equivalent slopes (B,C,D)

effect dose level; the latter the certain-effect dose. Dependent upon the data required the minimum-effect dose level (ED_{01}) and the certain-effect dose level (ED_{100}) can be derived (Hermann, 1967; Farmer, 1974; Haley *et al.*, 1974). The estimated variance associated with these determinations will be greater than the variance for the median value, and often with small numbers of animals and dose groups, variances may be very large. For shallow slopes the ED_{01}, ED_{50}, ED_{100} may differ significantly; for steep response slopes they may be indistinguishable from each other (Figure 5). For another substance, the slope may be shallow with a large difference between the ED_{01}, ED_{50} and ED_{100}. Although the slopes vary between these two substances, as reflected by dissimilar minimum lethal effect level and certain-effect doses, their median-effect dose could be equivalent. The question remains whether it is better to rank substances on the basis of their minimum-effect dose, median-effect dose or maximum/certain-effect dose. The least variability for a derived value from a dose–response curve is the median-effect dose. Consequently this parameter has been selected as the reference point for comparing the relative toxicity of substances. Unfortunately, while the median-effect dose is often quoted, the confidence limits and the slopes are often not reported. All parameters are important in defining the response curve, although it is important to stress that it is questionable whether for lethality data these parameters need to be studied in a large number of animals.

Determination of the Median Lethal Dose (LD_{50}/LC_{50})

The LD_{50} value is the median lethal dose and is a statistically derived dose which, when administered in an acute toxicity test, is expected to cause death in 50 per cent of the treated animals in a given period. The LD_{50} is derived from a quantal dose–response curve where the specific response is death. When the route of exposure is inhalation, the term LC_{50} (median lethal concentration) is used. This is also used in aquatic toxicity testing. The LD_{50}/LC_{50} value is commonly misapplied when it is used to describe the acute toxicity of a chemical (Brown, 1984). The requirement to estimate the LD_{50} value with 95 per cent confidence limits has been the subject of criticism. Precise LD_{50} values are not required for the majority of its applications (Zbinden and Flury-Roversi, 1981; Chanter and Heywood, 1982; Oliver *et al.*, 1985). It is the statistical result of a single experiment, and is affected by many parameters, such as age, weight, health, food deprivation, route of administration, temperature, caging conditions, seasonal variation, genetic influence and strain of animal. A published source of LD_{50} values (Registry of Toxic Effects of Chemical Substances (RTECS)) was found to cite 62 sources for 87 LD_{50} measurements (Hodson, 1985). There is a lack of detail in the published sources of LD_{50} values with regard to experimental conditions, strain of animal and method of statistical analysis. It has been proposed that interlaboratory estimates could be better correlated if such information were published (Craver *et al.*, 1950).

The classic statistical methods for analysing lethality data have been extensively reviewed by Armitage and Allen (1959) and Morrison *et al.* (1968). If mortality at each dosage is plotted against dosages, a sigmoidal dose–response curve is obtained (Figure 3). The LD_{50} is simply the dose, either observed or calculated, that yields 50 per cent mortality. The LD_{50} is difficult to read off a sigmoidal curve and the small number of doses normally used make drawing an accurate lethal-dose curve difficult. The precision with which the curves are described will depend on the number of groups, the dose and the number of animals in each group.

In general, all methods of calculation and computation are more readily applied if the doses are evenly spaced and the group sizes are equal. The probit method, first developed by Bliss (1935, 1937) and later refined by Finney (1971, 1985) requires at least two groups of partial responses (i.e. mortality greater than 0 per cent but less than 100 per cent). The most common correction that will have either 0 per cent or 100 per cent lethality is to substitute 0.1 per cent for 0 per cent and 99.9 per cent for 100 per cent. The probit method is considered the standard and is required by certain regulatory authorities. The probit method uses the linear relationship resulting from plotting as ordinate values the transformed proportional response as probability units (probits) against the logarithmic transformation of the dose plotted as the abscissa value (Figure 5). Probits are based on a theoretical normal population distribution and converted into positive values by the arbitrary addition of the integer 5 (Gaddum, 1933).

Although graphical methods (Litchfield and Wilcoxon, 1949) and tables for easy computation (Thompson and Weil, 1952; Weil, 1952) are available, computer techniques are now more often used for the analysis (Davies, 1971). Alternative approaches have been the use of the logistic function Logits (Berkson, 1944; Waud, 1972) and RIDIT analysis, which is based on an empirical distribution rather than the theoretical distribution used in probit analysis (Bross, 1958).

The moving average method, first described by Thompson (1947) and amended by Thompson and Weil (1952), does not require partial responses, deals effectively with complete responses and can produce an estimate of an LD_{50} with as few as three groups of 3–5 animals in each. This method requires that the doses be separated by a constant geometric factor and that groups be of equal size. Tables allow for the easy calculation of the LD_{50} (Weil, 1952, 1983; Gad and Weil, 1982, 1986). An estimate of the LD_{50} and slope can be obtained from as few as three groups of 5 animals per group, provided that the data set has responses between 0 per cent and 100 per cent and two of these are less than and greater than 50 per cent, respectively.

The normit chi-squared, developed by Berkson (1955) does not require equally spaced doses or equal group sizes, but does require at least one partial response. Inclusion of complete response is better than for probit analysis, but the procedure is difficult (Waud, 1972). In general, the best pattern of response will definitely produce close to 100 per cent effect, a minimal effect and a partial effect close to the median effect. If this pattern is obtained, adding more groups does not generally change the results (Behrens, 1929). There is seldom a substantial difference in the LD_{50} determination if sexes are pooled (Schutz and Fuchs, 1982), which perhaps suggests that mixed-sex groups should be introduced as standard procedure. An alternative approach not generally used converts the median lethal molar concentration (T) into positive values similar to the pH scale, using $pT = -\log (T)$, values greater than unity demonstrating increasing orders of magnitude of toxicity (Luckey and Venugopal, 1977).

INTERSPECIES AND INTRASPECIES SIMILARITIES AND DIFFERENCES

Toxic effects depend on the concentration and duration of exposure of the toxicant to specific target sites (Gehring and Rao, 1981). Species differences in response are largely due to differences in pharmacokinetics and biotransformation. It has been claimed that reliable interspecies extrapolation is not justifiable (Garattini, 1986). It is also often stated that 'a species should be chosen which handles the compound in the same way as man' (Weil, 1972). Some have advocated the use of human cell cultures for investigating metabolic parameters prior to toxicity studies (Rodericks and Tardoff, 1983). The extent of absorption is remarkably consistent between different animal species for alarge variety of substances (Clark and Smith, 1984). The amount of the different metabolites reaching the systemic blood circulation and the well-perfused and poorly perfused tissues may differ markedly between species, owing to variations in the rate of biotransformation by the gastrointestinal system, lung, skin and liver. With large concentrations following acute exposure, often the rates of biotransformation are saturated and variability between species is reduced.

Distribution and elimination characteristics of substances tend to be more variable between species—in particular, elimination half-life and serum protein binding have shown marked differences between species (Tse, 1988). Consequently, interspecies variation in pharmacokinetic parameters such as absolute bioavailability, clearance and elimination half-life is often attributed to quantitative differences in disposition and quantitative rather than qualitative differences in biotransformation (Brodie, 1964). Others have indicated that extrapolation across species is appropriate for acute toxicity. For a series of chemicals in fish, mice and rats (Hodson, 1985), toxicity data extrapolated from one species predicted the response in another. When rat LD_{50}s (intraperitoneal route) were plotted against fish LD_{50}s (intraperitoneal route), a straight line with a correlation coefficient of 0.933 was obtained.

Allometric Scaling as an Aid to Species Extrapolation

The approximate 4000 different species of living mammals are clearly of very variable size and appearance, ranging from the tiny shrew (<10 g) through the rodent (5×10^2 g), rabbit (4×10^3 g), dog (10^4 g), man (10^5 g), elephant (3×10^7 g) to the largest mammal known to have lived, the blue whale (15×10^7 g)—a 10-million-fold difference in size. Mammals, including primates, have similar anatomy, physiology, biochemistry and cellular structure. Organ size and physiological function are correlated with body weight (Adolph, 1949; Dedrick, 1973; Boxenbaum, 1982). Allometric scaling has been used in various areas of the biological sciences. The general relationship which exists between various physiological parameters and the body weight is expressed as $X = aw^b$, where X is the physiological parameter, w is the body weight and a and b are constants. The relative weights of internal organs, pulse and breathing rates, consumption of oxygen, food and water intakes, microsomal enzyme activities, duration of pregnancy, latent periods of tumours, nerve and muscle cell dimensions, maturation time of bone marrow elements and duration of erythrocyte life can all be related to body weight and surface area (Pinkel, 1958).

Extrapolation of Acute Toxic Effects

The relationship between body weight and LD_{50} within a single species was established for groups of female mice of different weights (Lamanna and Hart, 1968). A straight line relationship existed between the logarithm of the body weight and the logarithm of the LD_{50}. The coefficients of regression differed for different chemicals, sexes and routes of administration. Using 278 chemicals and between 6 and 10 species of mammals, a linear relationship was demonstrated between log(body weight) of different mammalian species and log(oral LD_{50}) for individual chemicals (Krasovskii, 1975, 1976). Others have also found a linear relationship between the log(LD_{50})s of three anticholinesterase compounds (esterine, VX and paraoxon) and the log(body weight) of six species (mouse, hamster, rat, rabbit, dog and guinea-pig) for three routes of exposure—intravenous (iv), subcutaneous (sc) and intraperitoneal (ip), (Lebic *et al.*, 1984). The 'body weight' rule was used to calculate the acute median lethal concentration (LC_{50}) for the inhalation of nitrogen dioxide (NO_2) for a 70 kg man (Book, 1982). Extrapolation from the LC_{50} of NO_2 in 1 min (obtained in mouse, rat, guinea-pig, rabbit and dog), predicted 174 ppm as the LC_{50} for 1 min exposure to man. A published report of a fatality which occurred after acute exposure to 150 ppm NO_2 gives some credence to this extrapolation.

The familiar straight line relationship held for three non-steroidal anti-inflammatory drugs, when log (body surface area) or log (specific surface area)—i.e. surface area/body weight—was plotted against LD_{50} (Funaki, 1974). The relationship between log (LD_{50}) and log (body weight) was evaluated for seven chemicals, selected from substances most frequently reported as the intoxicants in human poisonings in the UK (OPCS, 1983; Onyon, 1986). The original literature-quoted LD_{50} values for paracetamol, aspirin, ethanol, amitriptyline, phenobarbitone, paraquat and sodium chlorate were critically evaluated and data of comparable standard were used to determine the range for each species (Table 12). Cases of human poisoning for these seven chemicals held by the UK National Poisons Information Service Database (Edwards *et al.*, 1984) were reviewed. Those cases with a complete follow-up were used to empirically determine the human LD_{50} and the minimum fatal dose. Only five chemicals had range of dose and known outcome adequate to allow the LD_{50} to be calculated (Table 13). These empirically derived human lethal doses were compared with those derived from standard linear regression statistics for log (LD_{50}) against log (body weight), log (body surface area) and log (basal metabolic rate) for the laboratory species for which values could be derived (Table 12). A reasonable prediction of the human lethal dose was obtained for paraquat (data on 12 mammalian species), phenobarbitone (6 mammalian species); the correct order of magnitude was obtained for ethanol (4 mammalian species) and aspirin (6 species); prediction was inadequate for paracetamol (3 species), amitriptyline (2 species); and prediction was not possible for sodium chlorate, which had only one literature LD_{50} value in the rat, of 1200 mg kg^{-1}. A prerequisite needed properly to define the straight line relationship appears to be a relatively large database including three or four animal species (Calabrese, 1986; Mordenti, 1986; Onyon, 1986; Yates and Kugler, 1986).

Physiologically Based Pharmacokinetic Scaling

Alternative approaches to extrapolation include physiologically based pharmacokinetic (PB-PK) models, which attempt to describe quantatitively the pharmacokinetic processes affecting the disposition of a chemical and its biotransformation from the time it is absorbed to the interaction with different and various body tissues (Gerlowski and Jain, 1983). Such models are used to quantify the magnitude and time-course of exposure to the chemical at the critical target tissue sites. They require data on anatomical and physiological parameters (Table 14) in the species under study and are designed to predict kinetic behaviour under a wide range of doses and routes of exposure. The application of such pharmacokinetic simulations to allow extrapolation of acute toxicity data obtained from animals and/or *in vitro* experiments on man is a future possibility which would enhance current allometric scaling approaches and integrate the subsequently obtained pharmacokinetic data on a substance with its acute and subacute data.

ALTERNATIVE APPROACHES

Alternative Approaches to Animal Experimentation

Current methodology for acute systemic toxicity assessment is undergoing evaluation and reform because of increasing societal demand for the development and use of *ex vivo*, *in vitro* and computer-aided quantitative structure–activity relationship (QSAR) models to replace, reduce and refine procedures (especially acute toxicity procedures) which employ animal experimentation. The development of 'alternatives' to detect and characterize changes to the underlying biochemical and physiological mechanisms involved in toxicological change without recourse to the use of studies in whole organisms seems unlikely. From our perspective the elimination of animal experimentation without losing the ability to detect, identify, characterize and understand toxicological events is a daunting and not to be

Table 12 Mean oral LD$_{50}$ information for different animal species

Species	Compound	Number of observations	Mean LD$_{50}$ (mg kg^{-1})	Range of LD$_{50}$s observed	Refs
Mouse	Paraquat	8	77	40–200	1–8
	Amitriptyline	8	202	27–310	1–8
	Phenobarbitone	5	266	200–350	1–5
	Paracetamol	14	777	250–1659	1–14
	Aspirin	14	1769	750–2875	1–14
	Ethanol	4	8213	7268–9488	1–4
Rat	Paraquat	19	134	40–200	1–10, 12–16, 21–25
	Phenobarbitone	6	349	162–660	1–3, 6, 9, 10
	Amitriptyline	5	403	257–530	1–5
	Aspirin	19	1683	920–3420	1–15, 17–21
	Paracetamol	8	3763	1944–4500	1–5, 7–9
	Ethanol	7	12 584	6162–17 775	1–4, 6–8
Guinea-pig	Paraquat	7	41	22–60	1–7
	Phenobarbitone	1	130	130	1
	Aspirin	5	1102	1075–1190	1–5
	Paracetamol	4	2968	2620–3500	1–4
	Ethanol	1	5560	5560	1
Rabbit	Paraquat	6	101	49–150	1–6
	Phenobarbitone	2	167.5	150–185	1, 2
	Aspirin	3	1303	1000–1800	1–3
	Ethanol	4	9149	6300–9905	1–4
Cat	Paraquat	7	40	30–70	1–7
	Phenobarbitone	1	175	175	1
Dog	Paraquat	3	45	20–75	1–3
	Phenobarbitone	1	150	150	1
	Aspirin	1	3000	3000	1

(1) Adolph (1949); (2) Alarie (1981); (3) Anderson (1981); (4) Anderson and Weber (1975); (5) Anon. (1972); (6) Axelson (1976); (7) Bainova *et al.* (1979); (8) Baker and Davey (1970); (9); (10) Barocelli *et al.* (1986); (11) Bartsch *et al.* (1976); (12) Baudot (1980); (13) Baumler (1977); (14) Bavin *et al.* (1952); (15) Behrendt and Cserepes (1985); (16) Beliles (1972); (17) Boissier *et al.* (1971); (18) Book (1982); (19) Boxenbaum (1982); (20) Boxenbaum (1980); (21) Boxill *et al.* (1958); (22) Boyd (1968); (23) Boyd (1959); (24) Boyd and Bereczky (1966); (25) Boyd (1970).

Table 13 Comparison of human LD$_{50}$ and lethality data with predicted human LD$_{50}$ values extrapolated from animal LD$_{50}$ data: regressions based upon log body weight (b.wt), log body surface area (BSA) and log basal metabolic rate (BMR)

Chemical	Empirically derived LD$_{50}$[a]	Predicted log b.wt	Predicted log BSA	Predicted log BMR
Paraquat	32–48	40–55	52	48
Phenobarbitone	95–143	121	125	185
Aspirin	3492	2019	2066	1698
Ethanol	3500–5000	7625	7851	9518
Paracetamol	42 857	22 518	24 303	13 910
Amitriptyline	64	2290	NP	NP
Sodium chlorate	508	NP	NP	NP

[a] Derived from reviewing human cases of poisoning; see text.

NP, Not possible to determine: insufficient data.

underestimated goal. Reduction in the use of animals for experimental purposes has been achieved. Between 1980 and 1988 the Swiss phar-maceutical companies Ciba-Geigy, Hoffman La Roche and Sandoz reported a reduction of 50 per cent in their use of animals in research (Pharma

Table 14 Physiological parameters in various animal species used in acute toxicity testing[a]

Parameter	Mouse	Ratio to mouse			
		Rat	Rabbit	Dog	Man
Weight (kg)	0.022	23	106	545	3182
Compartment volume (ml)					
plasma	1.0	20	70	500	3000
muscle	10.0	25	135	553	3500
kidney	0.34	11	44	176	824
liver	1.3	15	77	369	1038
gut	1.5	8	80	320	1400
heart	0.095	12	63	1263	3158
lungs	0.12	18	142	1000	
spleen	0.1	13	10	360	1600
marrow	0.6		78	200	2333
Plasma flow rate (ml min^{-1})					
plasma	4.38	19	119	117	838
muscle	0.5	45	310	276	840
kidney	0.8	16	100	113	875
liver	1.1	4	161	55	727
gut	0.9	16	123	91	778
heart	0.28	5.7	57	214	536
lungs	4.38	0.5	179	117	
spleen	0.05	19	180	270	4800
marrow	0.17		65	118	706

[a] Data from Gerlowski and Jain (1983); Clark and Smith (1984); Tse (1988).

Information, 1989). While the use of *in vitro*, *ex vivo* and computer-aided modelling can contribute to savings in resources, it should also be noted that alternative approaches can take considerably more time and resources than the use of *in vivo* studies in the laboratory-bred mouse and rat.

PB-PK modelling currently combines data from *in vivo*, *in vitro* and *ex vivo* studies to assist in the extrapolation of data generated in laboratory animals in its application to assessing safety to man. PB-PK modelling has been introduced into the regulatory environment for evaluation of chronic toxicity (Anderson *et al.*, 1987; EPA, 1987) but its use in acute toxicity is not yet apparent. Quantitative and semiquantitative approaches, many of them using sophisticated computerized treatments of biological data and chemical structure, have been applied with varying degrees of success to predict acute lethal toxicity (Tinker, 1982). They require extensive databases of known dose–effect or dose–response

relationships and are limited when the database contains only a few negative results.

QSAR prediction based upon associating structural elements or groups of molecules with toxicity (Enslein and Craig, 1978; Enslein *et al.*, 1983; Golberg, 1983) has been introduced on a commercial basis (TOPKAT, 1982), but it is still questionable whether such techniques are appropriate for general screening of new synthetic molecules, as opposed to their use in previously studied structurally similar series (ECETOC, 1986). The rapid increase in the development of QSAR may be attributed to the need to evaluate the potential toxicity of the large number of existing chemicals for which there are inadequate or no experimental data from studies in whole organisms. Prediction of biological activity from easily measurable physical and chemical properties of molecules is seen by many as an attractive alternative to whole-organism studies (Arcos, 1983; Moore, 1984).

Acute Systemic Toxicity Studied *In Vitro*

Considerable effort has gone into the development of *in vitro* and *ex vivo* procedures for the assessment of adverse effects of chemicals (King *et al.*, 1986; Purchase *et al.*, 1986). Bacteria, yeasts, Protista and preparations of higher organisms have been used for *in vitro* testing (Turner, 1983). The study of single cells rather than organs, tissue cultures or micromass preparations can provide usable information related to the problems of medical, veterinary or environmental safety (Pearson, 1986). The development of such tests is based on a series of assumptions, a principal one being that the manifestations of toxicity observed *in vitro* are relevant when extrapolated to conditions *in vivo*. The majority of us are aware that animals are complex biological entities, consisting of several organs and tissues, thousands of enzymes, tens of thousands of proteins and peptides, hundreds of thousands of different molecules and millions of cells. The diversity of animal species is built on an increasing level of organization from molecules through macromolecules, from cells to tissues, from organs to organisms. It is now well established that all animal cells have the same common features of a cell membrane enclosing subcellular organelles for cellular reproduction and energy generation as well as other more specialized cellular functions. A fundamental assumption in the *in vitro* assessment of systemic toxicity is that the disturbance of any part of the basic cellular system by toxins should lead to a common response such as general cytotoxicity (Benson *et al.*, 1986). Many different cell types have been used in cytotoxicity investigations and a large number of end-points for detecting cytotoxicity have been used: cell viability, cell morphology, cell proliferation, membrane damage, uptake or incorporation of precursors and metabolic activity. Hundreds of chemicals have now been studied in *in vitro* systems to determine their cytotoxicity to cells at various doses.

It is possible to perceive the development of a classification scheme for transforming the cytotoxicity ID_{50} values into categories of potential hazard statements comparable to those for LD_{50} values. For some industrial chemicals which are not to be manufactured in large amounts and are not for intentional exposure to man, the ability to label the potential hazard from a cytotoxicity index may well be all that is required. For example, potentially very toxic could be equivalent to a ID_{50} <10 μg ml^{-1}; potentially toxic >10 μg ml^{-1} or <100 μg ml^{-1}; potentially harmful >100 μg ml^{-1} but <1000 μg ml^{-1}; potentially non-toxic >1000 μg ml^{-1}. The use of molar units rather than concentration units may be more appropriate. Clearly with either there are many assumptions being made in this extrapolation of cytotoxicity in cells to the complex integrated organism. Many would not be able to recognize the limitation of a potential hazard label derived from a cytotoxicity test compared with a hazard label derived from an *in vivo* study using another animal as a surrogate for man.

What separates chemicals ranked by a cytotoxicity *in vitro* screen from those ranked by observing the response of a whole organism is the special functions of selected cells and tissues within the whole organism. It is these special cells and tissues which maintain homoeostasis, govern how much and at what rate a chemical is absorbed, transformed, distributed to the tissue and eventually excreted. The determination of the median lethal dose (LD_{50}) in a laboratory rat provides data which can rank chemicals with regard to their potential to cause lethality in other species but it may not necessarily predict the human toxic dose. Similarly, *in vitro* cytotoxicity ED_{50} data allow some ranking of the potential for chemicals to cause toxicity but cannot predict whether the effect will occur at all or at what dose the effect will be evident in the whole organism. The qualitative and quantitative pharmacokinetics and metabolic dissimilarities between species which compromise interspecies extrapolation clearly compromise extrapolation from cellular systems to man; intraspecies variation comprises extrapolation even when human tissues and cells are used. While possible routes of biotransformation are being predicted from chemical structures using computer-aided analysis (Wipke *et al.*, 1983), the prediction of internal dose (tissue level) will require very sophisticated modelling indeed.

Mechanism of Cell Injury

An understanding of the mechanism of cell injury offers a more rational basis for the design of reliable *in vitro* methods for toxicity screening than simple empiricism (Turner, 1983; Williams *et al.*, 1983; Purchase *et al.*, 1986). Elucidation of molecular change consequent on chemically induced injury is fundamental to developing an understanding of organ-selective toxicity. The study of isolated cells has the potential to aid in the identification of both the primary molecular mechanism and the cascade of consequent degenerative changes. Differentiation of the primary pathological and physiological events from secondary peripheral degenerative processes is required to elucidate the molecular mechanism of cell injury (Bach and Lock, 1982, 1985; Bach, 1988, 1989). Often very few cells are adversely affected compared with the total number of cells in an organ or tissue.

A wide range of cells isolated from humans have been used for examining pharmacological effects (Pearson and Chijioke, 1989). Studies of transport mechanisms of drugs across lipid membranes have been carried out as a model of absorption from the gut lumen (Taylor and Turner, 1981); the red blood cell/plasma concentration ratios were more reliable than organic solvent partition ratios in predicting distribution of drugs *in vivo*. The relationship between lipophilicity and membrane-stabilizing properties has led to understanding of the cardiac toxicity of a series of antidepressant and opiate drugs in overdose (Zaman *et al.*, 1984; Cassidy and Henry, 1986; Cassidy and Pearson, 1986; Henry and Cassidy, 1986). The effects of anti-inflammatory and antirheumatic drugs have been examined on isolated human peripheral blood mononuclear cell interactions (Lewis, 1989).

With our present knowledge of toxic mechanisms, pharmacokinetics and pharmacodynamics, *in vitro* cell cytotoxicity screens cannot replace studies *in vivo*. They may, as our knowledge develops and in combination with well-designed computer models, eventually predict a chemical's toxic potential to an organism. Their current application is limited to well-defined circumstances—e.g. pyrogenic evaluation using the *Limulus* amoebocyte lysate test. There are *in vitro* techniques other than cytotoxicity assays which can contribute to the *in vivo* assessment of systemic toxicity, such as the monitoring of the absorption of chemicals and the study of xenobiotic biotransformation (Gillette, 1986).

Gastrointestinal Absorption

The gastrointestinal (GI) barrier that separates the GI lumen and the splanchnic blood and lymph is a complex tissue. The permeability characteristics of the GI tract have been studied for many types of chemicals, including nutrients, drugs and industrial chemicals (Rozmann and Hanninen, 1986). The rate and extent (bioavailability) of absorption of a substance are determined by pharmacokinetic analysis of the concentration and amount of substance and metabolites in samples of blood, tissue, urine and other excreta taken during *in vivo* studies on animals or man following oral, dermal or inhalational exposure and comparing with parenteral exposure. *In vivo* bioavailability data often do not provide much information on the mechanism of absorption, whereas a variety of *in vitro* and *in situ* techniques permit direct assessment of the permeability characteristics in an isolated intestinal segment.

The *in vitro* method involves the isolation of a small segment of the GI tract, everting to place the mucosal surface to the outside and serosal surface to the inside, filling the lumen of the gut sac with physiological medium, tying each end of the segment and placing the intestinal sac in a flask of physiological saline, allowing the determination of the permeation rate of the substance from the bathing fluid into the lumen of the sac (Wilson and Wiseman, 1954). With the placement of a glass cannula at each end of the sac, serial sampling of the lumen content can be achieved

(Crane and Wilson, 1958). The limitation of this procedure is that the GI sac is without an intact blood circulation and the substance has to permeate the entire thickness of intestinal wall from mucosal to serosal surface through the epithelium, submucosa, muscularis and serosa. With a functional vasculature found *in vivo* a compound has only to traverse the epithelial layer between the mucosal surface and the villous blood capillaries (Perrier and Gibaldi, 1973). *In situ* methods in anaesthetized or surgically implanted animals are the only methods by which segments of the gut can be isolated and perfused with chemicals while maintaining the blood circulation intact (Doluisio *et al.*, 1969).

Skin Permeability (Percutaneous Absorption)

Skin contact is often the most significant route of exposure during manufacture, formulation or use of chemicals. Knowledge of the use of skin permeability of a chemical can make an invaluable contribution to the prediction of the risk of an adverse effect following exposure. The diffusion of chemicals through the skin is a passive process in which penetration of the stratum corneum is the rate-limiting step. The underlying epidermis and dermis are not considered to contribute significantly in determining the absorption rate of a chemical. Consequently, it is not necessary to keep the skin viable in order to determine the absorption rate, and this has led to the development of an *in vitro* technique for the determination of the percutaneous absorption of chemicals through excised skin from animal and human cadavers (Dugard, 1986; Scott *et al.*, 1986a). The technique is simple and employs a glass diffusion cell which consists of a donor chamber separated by a skin membrane from a receptor chamber. The chemical is applied to the epidermal surface and the lower chamber is filled with a receptor fluid. The receptor fluid is analysed periodically to determine the amount of chemical that has penetrated through the skin and an absorption rate is calculated. This technique is now used routinely to compare the percutaneous absorption of chemicals through human and animal skin (Dugard *et al.*, 1983; Scott *et al.*, 1986b). It is possible that *in vitro* permeability studies may eventually be used as preassessments prior to *in vivo* systemic toxicity studies. The *in vitro* technique is still developing, as is its use in predicting absorption through human skin for risk assessment purposes.

DATABASE FOR THE REVIEW OF ACUTE TOXICITY STUDIES

Assessment of the acute toxicity of substances is of primary importance in the overall evaluation of potential human health hazards. While a principal objective is the detection of adverse effects, it is often overlooked that an equally important objective is to establish the absence of adverse effects—i.e. the demonstration of safety. A second misconception is that the majority of industrial chemicals represent serious acute toxicity hazards. One purpose of acute toxicity tests is more often to confirm the absence of toxic responses. This view is supported by the relatively small proportion of marked effects in acute toxicity studies (Kobel and Gfeller, 1985; Rhodes *et al.*, 1986, 1989).

Many such studies are completed each year and elaborated computer-based systems are developed for the initiation of studies, and the capture of raw data, subsequent analysis and reporting. However, because of the relatively high throughput of studies, the data tend to be placed in archive in such a manner that they are not readily accessible for comparative assessment. In addressing this problem, systems for the handling of data from a wide range of toxicological studies have been developed (Clapp and McNamee, 1985). Retention of study data in a standardized format can be readily accessed, enabling comprehensive analysis. One such database comprises over 3000 acute systemic studies. Using standard classification systems to rank the responses, the following prevalence of toxic responses in each study type was obtained. In systemic toxicity studies 65 per cent of oral and 66 per cent of dermal studies were of low toxicity (>2000 mg kg^{-1}); 29 per cent and 24 per cent were in the harmful category, respectively; 5 per cent and 9 per cent were in the toxic category, respectively; and only 0.8 per cent and 0.9 per cent were in the very toxic category, respectively.

CONCLUSION

The detection and characterization of adverse changes following acute exposure to a chemical— i.e. the determination of the probable dose at which a chemical will be a poison rather than a remedy—is a large component in safety assessment. The principles for estimating this probable dose have for many years been based on the use of whole-animal experimental procedures. Advances in knowledge have established an increasing awareness and desire to minimize the use of whole-animal studies, establish humane approaches and introduce alternative *in vitro* approaches to meet these objectives. The authors, along with other scientists working in acute toxicology, recognize and welcome such advances, but we also advise that whole-animal experiments have intrinsic value for studying acute effects which should not be overlooked.

ACKNOWLEDGEMENTS

The authors wish to acknowledge the many academic, regulatory and industrial colleagues, especially ICI chemists, toxicologists, pharmacologists and biologists who over several years have contributed to discussions of ideas and approaches to acute toxicity assessment and to new developments. The opinions expressed are those of the authors alone and are not attributed to ICI PLC or ICI Americas Inc. The editorial and typing skills of Hilary M. Rhodes have contributed significantly to the production of this chapter.

REFERENCES

Adolph, E. F. (1949). Quantitative relations in the physiological constitutions of mammals. *Science*, **109**, 579–585

Alarie, E. F. (1949). Dose response analysis in physiological constitutions of mammals. *Environ. Hlth Perspect.*, **42**, 9–13

Alarie, Y. (1981). Dose response analysis in animal studies: Prediction of human responses. *Environ. Hlth Perspect.*, **42**, 9–13

Albert, A. (1985). *Selective Toxicity—the Physicochemical Basis of Therapy*, 7th edn. Chapman and Hall, London, New York

Aldridge, W. N. and Connors, T. A. (1985). Chemical accidents in toxicology. *Human Toxicol.*, **4**, 477–479

Andersen, M., Clewell, H., Gargas, F., Smith, F. and Reitz, R. (1987). Physiologically based pharmacokinetics and the risk assessment process for methylene chloride. *Toxicol. Appl. Pharmacol.*, **87**, 185–205

Anderson, M. E. (1981). Saturable metabolism and its relationship to toxicology. *CRC Crit. Rev. Toxicol.*, **11**, 105–150

Anderson, O. (1958). *The Health of a Nation: Harvey W. Wiley and the Fight for Pure Food*. University of Chicago Press, Chicago

Anderson, P. D. and Weber, L. J. (1975). Toxic response as a quantitative function of body size. *Toxicol. Appl. Pharmacol.*, **33**, 471–483

Anon. (1972). Paraquat poisoning. *Vet. Rec.*, **106**, 95

Arcos, J. C. (1983). Comparative requirements for pre-marketing and pre-manufacturing notifications in the EC countries and the USA. *J. Am. Coll. Toxicol.*, **2**, 131–135

Armitage, P. and Allen, I. (1959). Methods of estimating the LD_{50} in quantal response data. *J. Hyg.*, **48**, 398–422

Auletta, C. (1988). Acute systemic toxicity testing. In Gad, S. (Ed.), *Handbook of Product Safety Assessment*. Marcel Dekker, New York

Axelson, R. A. (1976). Analgesic induced renal papillary necrosis in the Gunn rat: The comparative nephrotoxicity of aspirin and phenacetin. *J. Pathol.*, **120**, 145–149

Bach, P. H. (1988). Towards the sensitive and selective diagnosis of chemically induced renal injury. *Xenobiotica*, **18**, 685–698

Bach, P. H. (1989). Morphological and biochemical changes in cultured cells exposed to toxic chemicals. In Payne, J. W. (Ed.), *In Vitro Techniques in Research: Recent Advances*, Vol. 7. Open University Press, Milton Keynes, pp. 91–108

Bach, P. H. and Lock, E. A. (1982). The use of renal tissue slices, perfusion and infusion techniques to assess renal function and malfunction. In Bach, P. H., Bonner, F. W., Bridges, J. W. and Lock, E. A. (Eds), *Nephrotoxicity: Assessment and Pathogenesis*. Wiley, Chichester, pp. 128–143

Bach, P. H. and Lock, E. A. (Eds) (1985). *Renal Heterogeneity and Target Cell Toxicity*. Wiley, Chichester

Bainova, A., Zaprianov, Z. and Kaloyanova-Simecnac, F. (1979). The effect of pesticides on the activity of monoamine oxidase (MOA) in rats. *Arch. Hig. Rada. Toksikol*, **30**, (S), 531–535

Baker, S. B. and Davey, D. G. (1970). The predictive value for man of toxicological tests of drugs in laboratory animals. *Br. Med. Bull.*, **26**, 208–211

Balazs, T. (1970). Measurements of acute toxicity. In Paget, G. (Ed.), *Methods in Toxicology*. F. A. Davies, Philadelphia, pp. 49–81

Balazs, T. (1976). Assessment of the value of systemic toxicity studies in experimental animals. In Mehlman, M., Shapiro, R. and Blumenthal, H. (Eds), *Advances in Modern Toxicology*, Vol. 1, Part 1, *New Concepts in Safety Evaluation*. Hemisphere Publishing Corporation, Washington, D.C., pp. 141–153

Balls, M., Riddell, R. J. and Worden, A. N. (Eds) (1983). *Animals and Alternatives in Toxicity Testing*. Academic Press, London

Barnes, J. M. (1963). Toxic hazards from drugs. *J. Pharm. Pharmacol.*, **15**, 75–91

Barocelli, E., Morini, G. and Silva, C. (1986). Antipyretic activity of new compounds 4-(3-oxo–1, 2-benziothiazolin–2-yl)phenylalkanoic acids, their esters, amides and 1,1-dioxide derivatives. *Pharmacol. Res. Commun.*, **18**, 171–185

Bartsch, W., Sponer, G., Dietmann, K. and Fuchs, G. (1976). Acute toxicity of various solvents in the mouse and rat. *Arzneimittel-Forsch.*, **26**, 1581–1583

Baudot, P. H. (1980). Comparative toxicology of bipyridium herbicides: Paraquat and Diquat. *Lyon Pharm.*, **31**, 7–17

Baumler, W. (1977). Application of herbicides and the effect on voles in forest plantations. *Anz. Schädlingskunde Pflanzenschutz*, **50**, 51–55

Bavin, E. M., Macrae, J., Seymour, D. E. and Waterhouse, P. D. (1952). The analgesic and antipyretic properties of some derivatives of salicylamide. *J. Pharm. Pharmacol.*, **4**, 872–878

Behrendt, W. A. and Cserepes, J. (1985). Acute toxicity and analgesic action of a combination of buclizine, codeine and paracetamol (Migraleve) in tablet and suppository form in rats. *Pharmatherapeutica.*, **4**, 322–331

Behrens, B. (1929). Evaluation of digitalis leaves in frog experiment. *Arch. Exp. Pathol. Pharmacol.*, **140**, 236–256

Beliles, R. P. (1972). The influence of pregnancy on the acute toxicity of various compounds in mice. *Toxicol. Appl. Pharmacol.*, **23**, 537–540

Benson, V., Clausen, J., Ekwall, V., Hesnten-Pettersen, A., Holme, J., Hogberg, J., Niemi, M. and Walum, E. (1986). Trends in Scandinavian cell toxicology. *Alternatives to Laboratory Animals*, **13**, 162–179

Berkson, J. (1944). Application of the logistic function to bio-assay. *J. Am. Stat. Assoc.*, **39**, 357–365

Berkson, J. (1955). Estimate of the integrated normal curve by minimum normit chi-square with particular reference to bioassay. *J. Am. Stat. Assoc.*, **50**, 529–549

Bliss, C. I. (1935). The calculation of the dosage mortality curve. *Anal. Appl. Biol.*, **22**, 134–167

Bliss, C. I. (1937). Some principles of bioassay. *Am. Sci.*, **45**, 449–466

Boissier, J. R., Drumont, C. and Ratouis, R. (1971). Etude pharmacologique d'un nouvel antidepresseur tricyclique. *Therapie*, **26**, 459–479

Book, S. (1982). Scaling toxicity from laboratory animals to people: An example with nitrogen dioxide. *J. Toxicol. Environ. Hlth*, **9**, 719–729

Boxenbaum, H. (1980). Interspecies variation in liver weight, hepatic blood flow and antipyrine intrinsic clearance: Extrapolation of data to benzodiazepine and phenytoin. *J. Pharmacokinet. Biopharmacol.*, **8** (2), 165–176

Boxenbaum, H. (1982). Interspecies scaling, allometry, physiological time and the ground plan of pharmacokinetics. *J. Pharmacokinet. Biopharmacol.*, **10**, 201–227

Boxill, G. C., Nash, C. B. and Wheeler, A. G. (1958). Comparative pharmacological and toxicological evaluation of *N*-acetyl-*p*-aminophenol, salicylamide and acetylsalicylic acid. *J. Am. Pharm. Assoc. Sci. Ed.*, **47**, 479–487

Boyd, E. M. (1959). The acute oral toxicity of acetylsalicylic acid. *Toxicol. Appl. Pharmacol.*, **1**, 229–239

Boyd, E. M. (1968). Analgesic abuse: Maximal tolerated dose of acetylsalicylic acid. *Canad. Med. Assoc. J.*, **99**, 790–798

Boyd, E. M. (1970). The oral 100-day LD_{50} index of Phenacetin in guinea-pigs. *Toxicol. Appl. Pharmacol.*, **16**, 232–238

Boyd, E. M. and Bereczky, G. M. (1966). Liver necrosis from paracetamol. *Brit. J. Pharmacol.*, **26**, 606–614

Brodie, B. B. (1964). Of mice, microsomes and men. *Pharmacologist*, **6**, 12–26

Bross, I. D. J. (1958). How to use RIDIT analysis. *Biometrics*, **14**, 18–38

Bridges, J. W., Benford, D. J. and Hubbard, S. A. (1983). Mechanisms of toxic injury. *Ann. N. Y. Acad. Sci.*, **407**, 42–63

British Toxicology Society (1984). A new approach to the classification of substances and preparations on the basis of their acute toxicology. *Human Toxicol.*, **3**, 85–92

Brown, V. K. (1980). *Acute Toxicity in Theory and Practice*. Monographs in Toxicology: Environmental and Safety Aspects, Bridges, J. W. and Grasso, P (Eds). Wiley, New York

Brown, V. K. (1984). The LD_{50} value—a frequently misapplied concept. *Alternatives to Laboratory Animals*, **12**, 75–79

Brownlee, K., Hodges, J. and Rosenblatt, M. (1953). The up-and-down method with small samples. *J. Am. Stat. Assoc.*, **48**, 262–277

Bruce, R. (1985). An up-and-down procedure for acute toxicity testing. *Fund. Appl. Toxicol.*, **5**, 151–157

Bruce, M. and Doull, J. (1986). Origin and scope of toxicology. In Klaassen, C. D., Amdur, M. and Doull, J. (Eds), *Casarett and Doull's Toxicology: The Basic Science of Poisons*, 3rd edn. Pergamon Press, New York, pp. 3–10

Calabrese, E. J. (1986). Animal extrapolation and the challenge of human heterogeneity. *J. Pharm. Sci.*, **75**, 1041–1067

Casarett and Doull's Toxicology (1986). *The Basic Science of Poisons*, 3rd edn. Klaasen, C. D., Amdur, M. O. and Doull, J. (Eds). Macmillan, New York

Cassidy, S. L. and Henry, J. A. (1986). Rapid *in vitro* techniques for the assessment of the membrane-stab-

ilizing activity of drugs. *Fd Chem. Toxicol.*, **6/7**, 807–809

Cassidy, S. L. and Pearson, R. M. (1986). Effects of trazodone and nadolol upon human sperm motility. *Br. J. Clin. Pharmacol.*, **22**, 119–121

Chan, P. K. and Hayes, A. W. (1989). Principles and methods of acute toxicity and eye irritancy. In Hayes, A. W. (Ed.), *Principles and Methods of Toxicology*, 2nd edn. Raven Press, New York, pp. 169–220

Chanter, D. O. and Heywood, R. (1982). The LD_{50} test: some considerations of precision. *Toxicol. Lett.*, **10**, 303–307

Clapp, M. J. L. and McNamee, J. A. (1985). On line capture of data from toxicity studies (ARTEMIS). *Med. Inform.*, **10**, No. 2, 115–121

Clark, B. and Smith, D. A. (1984). Pharmacokinetics and toxicity testing. *Crit. Rev. Toxicol.*, **12**, 343–385

Clarke, A. (1933). *The Mode of Action of Drugs on Cells*. Edward Arnold, London

Crane, R. K. and Wilson, T. H. (1958). *In vitro* method for the study of the rate of intestinal absorption of sugars. *J. Appl. Physiol.*, **12**, 145–146

Craver, B. N., Barrett, W. E. and Earl, A. E. (1950). Some requisites to making LD_{50} from different laboratories comparable. *Arch. Industr. Hyg. Occup. Med.*, **2**, 280–283

Davies, R. G. (1971). *Computer Programming in Quantitative Biology*. Academic Press, London, New York

Decker, W. J. (1987). Introduction and history. In Haley, J. and Berndt, W. (Eds), *Handbook of Toxicology*. Hemisphere Publishing Corporation, Washington, D.C., pp. 1–19

Dedrick, R. L. (1973). Animal scale-up. *J. Pharmacokinet. Biopharm.*, **1**, 435–461

DePass, L. R., Meyer, R. C., Weaver, E. V. and Weil, C. S. (1984). An assessment of the importance of number of dose levels, number of animals per dose level, sex and method of LD_{50} and slope calculations in acute toxicity studies. In Goldberg, A. M. (Ed.), *Alternative Methods in Toxicology*, Vol. 2: *Acute Toxicity Testing: Alternate Approaches*. Mary Ann Liebert, New York, pp. 139–154

Diechmann, W. B., Henscler, D., Holmstedt, B. and Keil, G. (1986). What is there that is not a poison? A study of the Third Defense by Paracelsus. *Arch. Toxicol.*, **58**, 207–213

Dinman, B. D. (1972). 'Non-concept' of 'no-threshold': Chemicals in the environment. *Science*, **175**, 495–497

Dixon, W. J. (1965). The up-and-down method for small samples. *J. Am. Stat. Assoc.*, **60**, 976–978

Dixon, W. J. and Wood, A. M. (1948). A method for obtaining and analyzing sensitivity data. *J. Am. Stat. Assoc.*, **43**, 109–126

Doluisio, J. T., Billups, N. F., Dittert, L. W., Sugitta, E. T. and Swintosky, J. V. (1969). Drug absorption.

1. An *in situ* rat gut technique yielding realistic absorption rates. *J. Pharm. Sci.*, **58**, 1196–1202

Drew, R. T. and Laskin, S. (1973). Environmental inhalation chambers. In Gray, W. I. (Ed.), *Methods of Animal Experimentation*, Vol. 4. Academic Press, London, New York, 1–41

Dugard, P. H. (1986). Absorption through the skin: Theory, *in vitro* techniques and their application. *Fd Chem. Toxicol.*, **24**, 749–753

Dugard, P. H., Scott, R. C., Ramsey, J. D., Mawdsley, S. J. and Rhodes, C. (1983). Percutaneous absorption of phthalate ester: *in vitro* experiments on human and rat epidermal membranes. *Human Toxicol.*, **3**, 561

ECETOC (1985). *Acute Toxicity Tests, LD₅₀ (LC50) Determination and Alternatives*. Oliver, G. J. A., Bomhard, E. M., Carmichael, N., Potokar, M. and Schutz, E. (Eds), Ecetoc Monograph No. 6. European Chemical Industry Ecology and Technology Center, Brussels

ECETOC (1986). *Structure activity relationships in toxicology and ecotoxicology: An assessment*. Choplin, F., Dugard, P., Hermens, J., Jaeckh, R., Marsmann, M. and Roberts, D. W. (Eds), Ecetoc Monograph No 8. European Chemical Industry Ecology and Toxicology Center, Brussels

Edwards, J. N., Wiseman, H. M. and Volans, G. N. (1984). Poisons information proceedings: The development of a computer database for case records. In Kostrewski, B. (Ed.), *Current Perspectives of Health Computing*, Cambridge University Press, Cambridge

EEC (1984). Annex V Commission Directive of 25th April 1984 adapting for the sixth time Council Directive 67/548/EEC (84/449/EEC). *Official Journal of the European Communities*, **27**, No. L 251, 1–223

EEC (1989). Annex 3. Commission statement on 'LD₅₀ and Classification schemes—the possibilities for change'. Brussels, 19–21 September 1989

Ehrlich, P. (1907). *Three Harber Lectures*. Royal Institute of Public Health, London; Lewis, London

Ellenhorn, M. J. and Barceloux, D. G. (1988). *Medical Toxicology Diagnosis and Treatment of Human Toxicology*. Elsevier, New York

Elsberry, D. (1986). Screening approaches for acute and subacute toxicity studies. In Lloyd, W. (Ed.), *Safety Evaluation of Drugs and Chemicals*. Hemisphere Publishing Corporation, Washington, D.C., pp. 145–151

Enslein, K. and Craig, P. N. (1978). A toxicity estimation model. *J. Environ. Pathol. Toxicol.*, **2**, 115–132 (supplement)

Enslein, K., Lander, T. R., Tomb, M. E. and Craig, E. N. (1983). A predictive model for estimating rat oral LD₅₀ values. In *Benchmark Papers in Toxicology*. Princeton Scientific Publishers, Princeton

EPA (1987). *Technical Analysis of New Methods and Data Regarding Dichloromethane Hazard Assessments*. Document EPA/600/8–87/029A. Environmental Protection Agency, Washington, D.C.

Farmer, J. (1974). Comparison of probit and logit models for estimation of LD₀₁. *Fed. Proc.*, **33**, 220

Finney, D. J. (1971). In *Probit Analysis*, 3rd edn. Cambridge University Press, Cambridge

Finney, D. J. (1985). The median lethal dose and its estimation. *Arch. Toxicol.*, **56**, 215–218

Funaki, H., (1974). Drug toxicity (LD₅₀) and 'dosis medicamentosa' for children in terms of body surface areas and body weight. *J. Kyoto Pref. Univ. Med.*, **83** (8), 467–477

Gad, S. and Chengelis, C. P. (1988). *Acute Toxicology Testing Perspectives and Horizons*. Telford Press, Caldwell, N.J.

Gad, S., Smith, A., Cramp, A., Gavigan, F. and Derelanko, M. (1984). Innovation designs and practices for acute systemic toxicity studies. *Drug Chem. Toxicol.*, **7**, 423–434

Gad, S. and Weil, C. (1982). Statistics for toxicologists. In Hayes, A. (Ed.), *Principles and Methods of Toxicology*. Raven Press, New York, pp. 273–320

Gad, S. and Weil, C. (1986). *Statistics and Experimental Design for Toxicologists*. Telford Press, Caldwell, N. J.

Gaddum, J. H. (1933). Reports on biological standards III. Methods of biological assay depending on a quantal response. *Med. Res. Cncl Spec. Rep.*, No. 813, London

Garratini, S. (1986). Toxic effects of chemicals: difficulties in extrapolating data from animals to Man. *CRC Crit. Rev. Toxicol.*, **16** (1), 1–29

Gehring, P. J. and RAO, K. S. (1981). Toxicology data extrapolation. In *Pattys Industrial Hygiene and Toxicology*, 3rd edn. Wiley, New York, pp. 567–594

Gerlowski, L. E. and Jain, R. K. (1983). Physiologically based pharmacokinetic modeling: principles and applications. *J. Pharm. Sci.*, **72**, 1103–1127

Gillette, J. R. (1984). Solvable and unsolvable problems in extrapolating toxicological data between animal species and strains. In *Drug Metabolism and Drug Toxicology (Workshop)*. Raven Press, New York, pp. 237–260

Gillette, J. R. (1986). On the role of pharmacokinetics in integrating results from *in vitro* and *in vivo* studies. *Fd Chem. Toxicol.*, **24**, 711–720

Gilman, A. G., Goodman, L. S., Rall, T. W. and Murad, F. (Eds) (1985). *Goodman and Gilman's The Pharmacological Basis of Therapeutics*, 7th edn. Macmillan, New York, Toronto, London

Golberg, L. (Ed.) (1983). *Structure-Activity Correlation as a Predictive Tool in Toxicology*. Hemisphere Publishing Corporation, Washington, D.C.

Gosselin, R. E., Smith, R. P. and Hodge, H. C. (Eds) (1984). *Clinical Toxicology of Commercial Products*, 5th edn. Williams and Wilkins, Baltimore

Government Institutes (1988). *EPA Toxicology Handbook*. Government Institutes, Rockville, Maryland

Griffin, J. P. (1985). Predictive values of animal toxicity studies. *Alternatives to Laboratory Animals*, **12**, 163–170

Guthrie, D. A. (1946). *A History of Medicine*. J. B. Lippincott, Philadelphia

Hadad, L. M. and Winchester, J. F. (Eds) (1983). *Clinical Management of Poisoning and Drug Overdose*. Saunders, Philadelphia

Haley, T. J. and Berndt, W. O. (1987). *Handbook of Toxicology*. Hemisphere Publishing Corporation, Washington, D.C.

Haley, T. J., Farmer, J. H., Dooley, K. L., Harmon, J. R. and Peoples, A. (1974). Determination of the LD_{01} and extrapolation of the LD_{001} for methylcarbamate pesticides. *Europ. J. Toxicol.*, **7**, 152–158

Hayes, W. J., Jr. (1975). *Toxicology of Pesticides*. Williams and Wilkins, Baltimore

Hayes, W. J., Jr. (1982). *Pesticides Studied in Man*. Williams and Wilkins, Baltimore

Hayes, A. W. (Ed.) (1989). *Principles and Methods of Toxicology*, 2nd edn. Raven Press, New York

Hazelett, J., Thompson, T., Mertz, B., Vuolo-Schuessler, L., Green, J., Tripp, S., Robertson, P. and Traina, V. (1987). Rising dose tolerance (RDT) study: A novel scenario for obtaining preclinical toxicology/drug metabolism data. *Toxicologist*, **7**, Abstract No. 846

Henry, J. A. and Cassidy, S. L. (1986). Membrane stabilising activity; a major cause of fatal poisoning. *Lancet*, **i**, 1414–1417

Hermann, E. R. (1967). Threshold prediction and characteristics of log-normal phenomena. *Environ. Res.*, **1**, 359–369

Hermann, E. R. (1971). Thresholds in biophysical systems. *Arch. Environ. Hlth*, **22**, 699–706

Hodson, P. V. (1985). A comparison of the acute toxicity of chemicals to fish, rats and mice. *J. Appl. Toxicol.*, **5** (4), 220–226

Kennedy, G. L., Jr., Ferenz, R. L. and Burgess, B. A. (1986). Estimation of acute oral toxicity in rats by determination of the approximate lethal dose rather than the LD_{50}. *J. Appl. Toxicol.*, **6**, 145–148

King, L. J., Wiebel, F. J. and Zucco, F. (Eds) (1986). Application of tissue culture in toxicology (Proceedings of the Third International Workshop, Urbino, Italy) *Xenobiotica*, **15** (Nos 8/9)

Kobel, W. and Gfeller, W. (1985). Distribution of eye irritation scores of industrial chemicals. *Fd Chem. Toxicol.*, **23**, No. 2, 311–312

Krasovskii, G. N. (1975). Species differences in sensitivity to toxic substances. In *Methods Used in the USSR for Establishing Biologically Safe Levels of Toxic Substances*. World Health Organization, Geneva, pp. 109–125

Krasovskii, G. N. (1976). Extrapolation of experimental data from animals to man. *Environ. Hlth Perspect.*, **13**, 51–58

Lamanna, C. and Hart, E. R. (1968). Relationship of lethal toxic dose to body weight of the mouse. *Toxicol. Appl. Pharmacol.*, **13**, 307–315

Leake, C. D. (1975). *An Historical Account of Pharmacology in the Twentieth Century*. Charles C. Thomas, Springfield, Ill.

Leblic, C., Coq, H. M. and Le Moan, G. (1984). Etude de la toxicité aigüe de L'Eserine, VX et le Paraoxon pour établir un modèle mathematique de l'être humain. (Proceedings of the 1st World Congress 'New Compd. Biol. Chem. Warfare: Toxicol. Eval.') Supplement. *Arch. Belg. Med. Soc.*, pp. 226–242

Lehman, A. J. (1959). Some relations of drug toxicity in experimental animals compared to man. In Staff of Division of Pharmacology of Food and Drug Administration, U.S. Department of Health, Education and Welfare (Eds), *Appraisal of Safety of Chemicals in Food and Drugs and Cosmetics*. Association of Food and Drug Officials of the United States

Lewis, G. P. (1989) The use of human cell cultures in the development of anti-rheumatic drugs. In Payne, E. J. (Ed.), *In vitro Techniques in Research: Recent Advances*. Open University Press, Milton Keynes

Litchfield, J. and Wilcoxon, F. (1949). A simplified method of evaluating dose-effect experiments. *J. Pharmacol. Exptl Therap.*, **96**, 99–113

Lorke, D. (1983). A new approach to acute toxicity testing. *Arch. Toxicol.*, **54**, 275–287

Luckey, T. D. and Venugopal, B. (1977). pT, a new classification system for toxic chemicals. *J. Toxicol. Environ. Hlth*, **2**, 633–638

McClean, A. E. M. (1971). Conversion by the liver of inactive molecules into toxic molecules. In Aldridge, W. N. (Ed.), *Mechanisms of Toxicity*. Macmillan, London

Mettler, C. C. and Mettler, F. A. (1947). *History of Medicine*. Blakiston, Philadelphia

Moore, J. A. (1984). Proposed design for a retrospective study of PMN hazard predictions. Memo to Science Advisory Board, 24 September. U.S. EPA

Mordenti, J. (1986). Pharmacokinetic scaling in mammals. *J. Pharm. Sci.*, **75**, 1028–1040

Morrison, J., Quilton, R. and Reinhert, H. (1968). The purpose and value of LD_{50} determinations. In Boyland, E. and Goulding, R. (Eds), *Modern Trends in Toxicology*, Vol. 1. Appleton-Century-Crofts, London, pp. 1–17

Nordberg, G. F. and Strangert, P. (1978). Fundamental aspects of dose response relationships and their extrapolation for non-carcinogenic effects of metals. *Environ. Hlth Perspect.* **22**, 97–102

OECD (1981a). *OECD Guidelines for the Testing of Chemicals*. Organisation for Economic Co-operation and Development, Paris

OECD (1981b). *OECD Guidelines for the Testing of Chemicals*. Section 4: Health Effects; 404 p. 2

OECD (1984). *Labelling of Chemicals: Overview of International Labelling Practices*. Organisation for Economic Co-operation and Development, Paris

OECD Test Guidelines (1981). Decision of the council concerning mutual acceptance of data in the assessment of chemicals. Annex 2. *OECD Principles of*

Good Laboratory Practices. Organisation for Economic Co-operation and Development, Paris

Oliver, G. J. A., Bomhard, E. M., Carmichael, N., Potokar, M. and Schultz, E. (1985). In *Acute Toxicity Tests, LD₅₀ (LC₅₀) Determination and Alternatives*. Monograph No. 6, ECETOC, Brussels

Onyon, L. J. (1986). *The Qualitative Extrapolation of Acute Toxicity Data from Animals to Man*. MSc Thesis. University of Surrey, Guildford

OPCS (1983). Office of Population Censuses and Surveys: *Mortality Statistics—Accidents and Violence*. OPCS, London

Orfila, M. J. B. (1817). *A General System of Toxicology, or a Treatise on Poisons*. Cox, London

Oser, B. L. (1971). Toxicity of pesticides to establish proof of safety. In White-Stevens, R. (Ed.), *Pesticides in the Environment*, Vol. 1, Part 2. Marcel Dekker, New York

Paget, G. E. (1970). *Methods in Toxicology*. Blackwell, Oxford

Parke, D. V. (1983). A more scientific approach to the safety evaluation of chemicals. In Turner, P. (Ed.), *Animals in Scientific Research: An Effective Substitute for Man?* Macmillan Press, London, pp. 7–28

Pearson, R. M. (1986). *In vitro* techniques: can they replace animal testing? *Human Reprod.*, 1, 559–560

Pearson, R. M. and Chijioke, P. C. (1989). In Payne, J. W. (Ed.), *In vitro* Technology in Research: Recent Advances. Open University Press, Milton Keynes

Pendergast, W. (1984). Biological drug regulations. In *The Seventy-fifth Anniversary Commemorative Volume of Food and Drug Law*. Edited and Published by the Food and Drug Law Institute, Washington, D.C., pp. 293–305

Perrier, D. and Gibaldi, M. (1973). Calculation of absorption rate constant for drugs with incomplete availability. *J. Pharm. Sci.*, 62, 1486–1490

Peters, R. (1963). *Biochemical Lesions and Lethal Synthesis*. Pergamon Press, Oxford

Pharma Information (1989). *Animal Experiments in the Research-based Pharmaceutical Industry—Answers to Some Important Questions*. Pharma Information, Basle

Pinkel, D. (1958). The use of body surface area as a criterion of drug dosage in cancer chemotherapy. *Cancer Res.*, 18, 853–856

Purchase, I. F. H., Conning, D., Balls, M., Rhodes, C., Davies, D. N. and Bridges, J. M. (Eds) (1986). International Conference on Practical *in vitro* Toxicology. *Fd Chem. Toxicol.*, 24, 447–818

Reuse, J. (1948). Action of antihistaminic compounds on the circulatory response of acetylcholine, the peripheral excitation of the vagus, and the actions of adrenaline and nicotine. *Br. J. Pharmacol.*, 3, 174

Rhodes, C., Jackson, S. J., Oliver, J. G. A., Pemberton, M. A. and Scott, R. C. (1986). *Toxicol. Lett.*, 31, Suppl. p. 221

Rhodes, C., Oliver, G. J. A., Pemberton, M. A. and Scott, R. C. (1989). Testing of chemicals for acute toxicity and irritancy: the contribution of *in vitro* techniques. In Payne, J. W. (Ed.) *In vitro Techniques in Research: Recent Advances*. Open University Press, Milton Keynes

Rhodes, C., Purchase, I. F. H., Pemberton, M. A. and Oliver, G. J. A. (1988). A balanced approach to the detection, characterization and mechanism of the toxicity of industrial chemicals. In *Proceedings of the Satellite Symposium on Toxicity Testing of Industrial Chemicals*, 4th International Congress of Toxicology, Tokyo

Rodericks, J. and Tardoff, R. G. (1983). Biological basis for risk assessment. In *Safety Evaluation and Regulation of Chemicals*, 1st Int. Conf., Boston, Mass. Karger, Basel, pp. 77–84

Rowan, A. (1981). The LD₅₀ Test: a critique and suggestions for alternatives. *Pharm. Technol.*, April, 65–92

Rozmann, K. and Hanninen, O. (Eds) (1986). *Gastrointestinal Toxicology*. Elsevier, Amsterdam, New York, Oxford

Russell, F. E., Sullivan, J. B., Egen, N. B., *et al.* (1985). Preparation of a new antivenin by affinity chromatography. *Am. J. Trop. Med. Hyg.*, 34, 141–150

Schutz, E. and Fuchs, H. (1982). A new approach to minimizing the number of animals in acute toxicity testing and optimizing the information of the test results. *Arch. Toxicol.*, 51, 197–220

Scott, R. C., Ramsey, J. D., Ward, R. J., Thompson, M. A. and Rhodes, C. (1986a). Percutaneous absorption: *In vitro* assessment. *Fd Chem. Toxicol.*, 24, 763–764

Scott, R. C., Ramsey, J. D., Ward, R. J., Thompson, M. A. and Rhodes, C. (1986b). *In vitro* absorption of 1-chloro-2,4-dinitrobenzene (DNCB) through human, hooded rat and mouse epidermis. *Br. J. Dermatol.*, 115, 47–48

Shackell, L. (1925). The relationship of dosage to effect. *J. Pharmacol. Expl Therap.*, 31, 275–288

Sidhu, K. S., Stewart, T. M. and Nelton, E. W. (1989). Information sources and support networks in toxicology. *J. Am. Coll. Toxicol.*, 8, 1011–1026

Smyth, J. F., Jr. and Carpenter, C. P. (1944). The place of the range finding test in the industrial laboratory. *J. Ind. Hyg. Toxicol.*, 26, 269

Society of Toxicology (1989). Comments on the LD₅₀ and acute eye and skin irritation tests. *Fund. Appl. Toxicol.*, 13, 621–623

Sperling, F. (1976). Nonlethal parameters as indices of acute toxicity: inadequacies of the acute LD₅₀. In Mehlman, M., Shapiro, R. and Blumenthal, H. (Eds), *Advances in Modern Toxicology*, Vol. 1, Part 1: *New Concepts in Safety Evaluation*. Hemisphere Publishing Corporation, Washington, D.C., pp. 177–191

Sudmersen, H. and Glenny, A. (1910). Variation in susceptibility of guinea-pigs to diphtheria toxin. *J. Hyg.*, 9, 399–408

Sullivan, J. B. and Russell, F. E. (1983). Isolation quantitation and subclassing of IgG antibody to Crotalidae venom by affinity chromatography and protein electrophoresis. *Toxicon*, Suppl. 3, 429–432

Tattersall, M. L. (1982). Statistics and the LD$_{50}$ study. In *New Toxicology for Old. Arch. Toxicol.*, Suppl. 5, 267–270

Taylor, E. A. and Turner, P. (1981). The distribution of propranolol, pindolol and atenolol between human erythrocytes and plasma. *Br. J. Clin. Pharmacol.*, **12**, 543–548

Thompson, C. J. S. (1931). *Poisons and Poisoners. With Historical Accounts of Some Famous Mysteries in Ancient and Modern Times.* Shaylor, London

Thompson, W. R. (1947). Use of moving averages and interpolation to estimate median effective dose. *Bacteriol. Rev.*, **11**, 115–145

Thompson, W. and Weil, C. (1952). On the construction of table for moving average interpolation. *Biometrics*, **8**, 51–54

Tinker, J. F. (1982). Qualitative structure–activity correlation: Results from several databases. Presented at *American Chemical Society National Meeting*, Kansas City, Missouri

TOPKAT (1982). *The HDI Predictive Service.* Health Designs, Rochester, N.Y.

Trevan, J. (1927). The error of determination of toxicity. *Proc. Roy. Soc. B*, **101**, 483–514

Tse, F. L. S. (1988). Non-clinical pharmacokinetics in drug discovery and development. In Welling, P. G. and Tse, F. L. S. (Eds), *Pharmacokinetics: Regulatory, Industrial, Academic Perspectives. Drugs and Pharmaceuticals Sciences.* Marcel Dekker, New York

Turner, P. (Ed.) (1983). *Animals in Scientific Research: An Effective Substitute for Man?* Macmillan Press, London

U.S. Congress, Office of Technology Assessment (1986). *Alternatives to Animals in Research, Testing and Education.* U.S. Government Printing Office, OTA-BA-273, Washington, D.C.

Vouk, V. B., Butler, G. C., Hoel, D. G. and Peakall, D. B. (Eds) (1985). *Methods for Estimating Risk of Chemical Injury: Human and Non-human Biota and Ecosystems.* SCOPE 26/SGOMSEC2. Wiley, Chichester, New York

Waud, D. (1972). Biological assays involving quantal responses. *J. Pharmacol. Exptl Therap.*, **183**, 577–607

Weil, C. (1983). Economical LD$_{50}$ and slope determination. *Drug Chem. Toxicol.*, **6**, 595–603

Weil, C. S. (1952). Table for convenient calculation of median effective dose (LD$_{50}$ or ED$_{50}$) and instructions in their use. *Biometrics*, **8**, 249–263

Weil, C. S. (1972). Guidelines to predict the (degree of) safety of a material(s) for man. *Toxicol. Appl. Pharmacol.*, **21**, 194–199

Westerfield, W. W. (1956). Biological response curves. *Science (Washington)*, **123**, 1017–1019

WHO Task Group on Environmental Health Criteria (1978). *Principle and Method for Evaluating the Toxicity of Chemicals*, Part 1, Vol. 6. World Health Organization, Geneva

Williams, G. M., Dunkel, V. C. and Ray, V. A. (Eds) (1983). Cellular systems for toxicity testing. *Ann. N. Y. Acad. Sci.*, **407**, 1–482

Wilson, T. H. and Wiseman, G. (1954). The use of sacs of everted small intestine for the study of the transference of substances from the mucosal to the serosal surface. *J. Physiol.*, **123**, 116–125

Wipke, W. T,. Ouchi, G. I. and Chow, T. J. (1983). In Goldberg, L. (Ed.), *Structure Activity Correlation as a Predictive Tool in Toxicology: Fundamental Methods and Applications.* Hemisphere Publishing Corporation, Washington, D.C.

Yates, F. E. and Kugler, P. N. (1986). Similarity principles and intrinsic geometries: Contrasting approaches to interspecies scaling. *J. Pharm. Sci.*, **75**, 1019–1027

Zaman, S., Lamb, J. M., Esberger, D. A. and Pearson, R. M. (1984). Inhibition of sperm motility by opiate drugs. *Br. J. Clin. Pharmacol.*, **18**, 320P

Zbinden, G. (1984). Acute testing, purpose. In Goldberg, A. (Ed.), *Acute Toxicity Testing: Alternative Approaches.* Mary Ann Liebert, New York, pp. 5–22

Zbinden, G. (1986). Invited Contribution: Acute toxicity testing, public responsibility and scientific challenges. *Cell. Biol. Toxicol.*, **2**, 325–335

Zbinden, G. and Flury-Roversi, M. (1981). Significance of the LD$_{50}$ test for the toxicological evaluation of chemical substances. *Arch. Toxicol.*, **47**, 77–99

FURTHER READING

Brown, V. K. (1980). *Acute Toxicity in Theory and Practice.* John Wiley and Sons, Chichester

Gad, S. C. and Chengelis, C. P. (1988). *Acute Toxicology Testing: Perspectives and Horizons.* Telford Press, Caldwell, New Jersey

Special report (1984). A new approach to the classification of substances and preparations on the basis of their acute toxicity. *Human Toxicology*, **3**, 85–92

van den Heuvel, M. J., Clark, D. G., Fielder, R. J., Koundakjian, P. P., Oliver, G. J. A., Pelling, D., Tomlinson, N. J. and Walker, A. P. (1990). The international validation of a fixed-dose procedure as an alternative to the classical LD$_{50}$ test. *Food and Chemical Toxicology*, **18**, 469–482

3 Biotransformation of Xenobiotics

John A. Timbrell

INTRODUCTION

For a xenobiotic to be absorbed into a biological system by passive diffusion generally requires it to be lipid-soluble and consequently not ideally suited for excretion. For example, very lipophilic substances such as the polychlorinated biphenyls are very poorly excreted and, hence, remain in an animal's body for many years.

After a xenobiotic has been absorbed into a biological system, it may undergo a biotransformation which leads to rapid excretion and therefore elimination of the compound from the animal. However, biotransformation may also change the biological activity of the substance. Thus, the metabolic fate of the compound can have an important bearing on its toxic potential, its disposition in the body and its excretion.

The products of metabolism are usually more water-soluble than the original compound. Indeed in animals, biotransformation seems directed at increasing water-solubility and, hence, excretion. For example, the analgesic drug paracetamol has a renal clearance value of 12 ml min^{-1}, whereas one of its major metabolites, the sulphate conjugate, is cleared at the rate of 170 ml min^{-1}.

Facilitating the excretion of a compound means that its biological half-life is reduced and, hence, its potential toxicity is kept to a minimum. Metabolism may also directly affect the biological activity of a foreign compound. For example, the drug succinylcholine causes muscle relaxation, but its action only lasts a few minutes because metabolism cleaves the molecule to yield inactive products (Figure 1). However, in some cases metabolism increases the toxicity of a compound. There are now many examples of this (see below) which have been documented but a relatively simple case is ethylene glycol. This is metabolized to oxalic acid, which is partly responsible for several of the toxic effects (Figure 2). Biotransformation is therefore an extremely important phase of disposition, as it may have a major effect on the biological activity of the

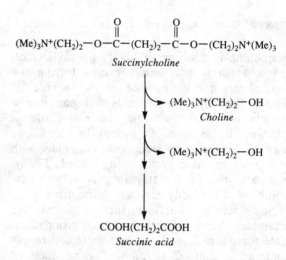

Figure 1 Metabolic hydrolysis of succinylcholine. From Timbrell (1982)

Figure 2 Metabolism of ethylene glycol. From Timbrell (1982)

compound, and by increasing polarity and so water-solubility, thereby increase excretion.

Rarely metabolism may actually decrease water-solubility and so reduce excretion. For example, acetylation decreases the solubility of some sulphonamides in urine and so may lead to crystallization of the metabolite in the kidney tubules, causing necrosis of the tissue.

Metabolism can be simply divided into two phases: phase 1 and phase 2. Phase 1 is the alteration of the original foreign molecule so as to add on a functional group which can then be conjugated in phase 2. This can best be understood be examining the example in Figure 3. The

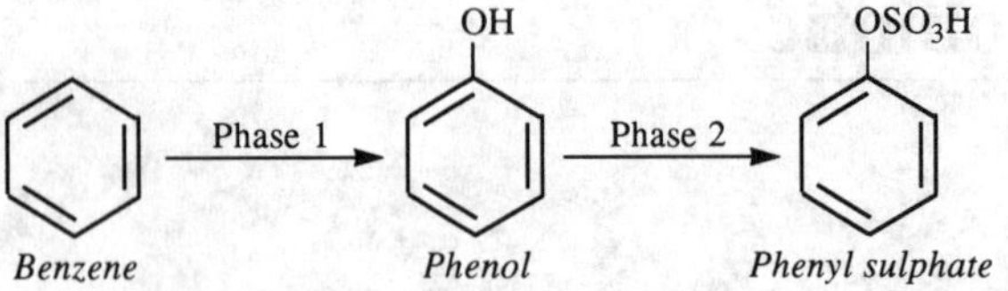

OH   OSO₃H

Benzene   Phenol   Phenyl sulphate

Figure 3 Benzene metabolism. From Timbrell (1982)

xenobiotic is benzene, a highly lipophilic molecule which is not readily excreted from the
animal except in the expired air, as it is volatile.
Phase 1 metabolism converts benzene into a
variety of metabolites, but the major one is
phenol. The insertion of a hydroxyl group allows
a phase 2 conjugation reaction to take place with
the polar sulphate group being added. Phenyl
sulphate, the final metabolite, is very water-
soluble and is readily excreted in the urine.

Some foreign molecules, such as phenol, for
example, already possess functional groups suitable for phase 2 reactions and therefore simply
undergo a phase 2 reaction. The products of
phase 2 biotransformations, such as glutathione
conjugates, may be further metabolized in what
are sometimes termed phase 3 reactions.

Biotransformation is almost always, although
not exclusively, catalysed by enzymes and these
are usually, but not always, found most abundantly in the liver in animals. The reason for this
location is that most foreign compounds enter the
body via the gastrointestinal tract and the portal
blood supply from this organ goes directly to the
liver (Figure 4). However, it is important to
remember that (1) the enzymes involved with the
metabolism of foreign compounds may be found
in many other tissues as well as the liver; (2) the
enzymes may be localized in one particular cell
type in an organ; (3) unlike the enzymes involved
in intermediary metabolism, those involved in the
biotransformation of xenobiotics are generally
non-specific and consequently are not always very
efficient; (4) enzymes normally involved in intermediary metabolism may catalyse the biotransformation of a xenobiotic if the chemical structure
happens to be suitable; (5) a xenobiotic may
undergo many different biotransformations and
the relative importance of each of these may be
affected by many factors.

The enzymes involved in biotransformation
also have a particular subcellular localization:
many are found in the endoplasmic reticulum,

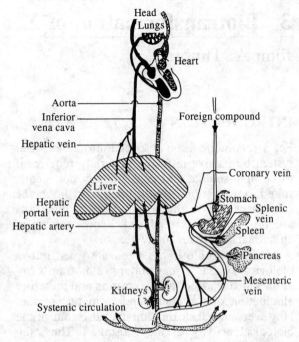

Figure 4 Blood supply of the liver. From Timbrell (1986)

some are located in the cytosol and a few are
found in other organelles such as the mitochondrion.

The various types of metabolic reactions are
shown in Table 1.

PHASE 1 REACTIONS

Oxidation Reactions

The majority of oxidation reactions which xenobiotics undergo are catalysed by one enzyme
system, the cytochrome *P*-450 monooxygenase
system. (Nebert and Gonzalez, 1985). However,
there are a number of other oxidative enzyme
systems whose importance in the biotransformation of xenobiotics is increasingly being recognized, and these will be discussed later in this
chapter. Cytochrome *P*-450 is a membrane-bound
enzyme system and is located in the smooth endoplasmic reticulum of the cell. After homogeniz-
ation and fractionation of the cell, the enzyme
system is isolated in the so-called microsomal
fraction. The liver has the highest concentration
of this enzyme, although it can be found in most
tissues. The reactions catalysed by cytochrome

Table 1 The major biotransformation reactions

Phase 1		Phase 2
Oxidation	Aromatic	Sulphation
	Aliphatic	
	Heterocyclic	Glucuronidation
	Alicyclic	
	of Nitrogen	Glutathione
	of Sulphur	conjugation
	N-hydroxylation	Acetylation
	Dealkylation	Amino acid
		conjugation
Reduction	Azo	Methylation
	Nitro	
Hydrolysis	Ester	
	Amide	
	Hydrazide	
	Carbamate	
Hydration		
Dehalogenation		

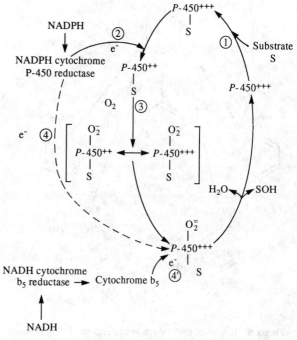

Figure 5 The cytochrome *P*-450 system. From Timbrell (1982)

P-450 also require NADPH and molecular oxygen, and the overall reaction is shown below:

$$SH + O_2 + NADPH + H^+ \rightarrow SOH + H_2O + NADP^+$$

where S is the substrate.

The sequence of metabolic reactions is shown in Figure 5 and involves four distinct steps: (1) addition of substrate to the enzyme; (2) donation of an electron; (3) addition of oxygen and rearrangement; (4) donation of a second electron and loss of water.

The cytochrome *P*-450 system is actually a collection of isoenzymes, all of which possess an iron atom in a porphyrin complex. These catalyse different types of oxidation reactions and under certain circumstances may catalyse other types of reaction such as reduction.

One important feature of cytochrome *P*-450 is its inducibility (Whitlock, 1989). Thus, treatment of an animal with certain substances may lead to an increase in the synthesis of one or more isoenzymes of cytochrome *P*-450, leading to an apparent increase in overall activity with respect to a particular substrate. There are now many known inducers of different isoenzymes of cytochrome *P*-450. Exposure of an animal to these substances clearly may have an effect on the metabolism of a compound and may influence its toxicity (see below).

The major types of oxidation reaction catalysed by the cytochrome *P*-450 system may be subdivided into: aromatic hydroxylation, aliphatic hydroxylation, alicyclic hydroxylation, heterocyclic hydroxylation, *N*-, *S*- and *O*-dealkylation, *N*-oxidation, *N*-hydroxylation, *S*-oxidation, desulphuration and deamination.

Aromatic hydroxylation, such as occurs with benzene (Figure 6), is a very common reaction for compounds containing an unsaturated ring. The initial products are phenols, but catechols, quinols and further hydroxylated products may be formed. One of the toxic effects of benzene is aplastic anaemia. This is believed to be due to an intermediate metabolite, possibly the hydroquinone, which may be formed in the bone marrow, the target site. Aromatic hydroxylation usually proceeds via an epoxide intermediate (Figure 7), which involves the addition of oxygen across the unsaturated double bond. The formation of this intermediate may have important toxicological implications (for example, the hepatotoxicity of bromobenzene discussed in detail later in the chapter). Epoxides are often chemically reactive and fairly unstable. They may give rise to

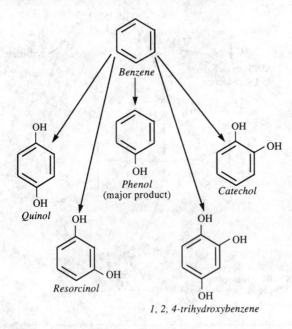

Figure 6   Routes of hydroxylation of benzene. From Timbrell (1982)

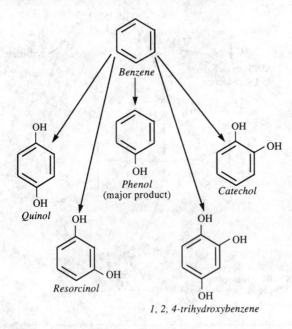

Figure 7   Oxidation of benzene to an epoxide

positively charged intermediates (electrophiles). The products formed *in vivo* will depend on the reactivity of the particular epoxide and they therefore may form a number of other metabolites, either phenols by chemical rearrangement or, following further metabolism, dihydrodiols, glutathione conjugates and catechols.

Destabilized epoxides, for example, will tend to form phenols by chemical rearrangement. The reactivity of metabolic intermediates may well determine the toxicity of the compound in question. However, extremely reactive intermediates are likely to react with many cellular constituents in the close proximity of their formation. Less reactive intermediates may travel to distant sites within or even outside the cell and react with more critical cellular targets (Monks and Lau, 1988) (see below). Also, aromatic hydroxylation is influenced by the substituents on the ring. Thus, a nitro or other electron-withdrawing group

will tend to direct hydroxylation to the *meta* and *para* positions, whereas an electron-donating group such as an amino group will be *ortho-* and *para*-directing.

Hydroxylation of unsaturated aliphatic compounds may also proceed with the formation of an epoxide across the unsaturated bond. For example, the toxic industrial intermediate vinyl chloride (Figure 8) undergoes such a biotransformation to yield chloroacetaldehyde. When the epoxide opens, there may be a shift in the chlorine atom to the adjacent carbon (Hathway, 1984).

Hydroxylation of a saturated aliphatic moiety such as that in propylbenzene may occur at one of three positions (Figure 9). Further metabolism will yield the aldehyde and then the acid from the 3-phenylpropan-1-ol. These further biotransformations may be catalysed by other enzymes than cytochrome *P*-450.

Alicyclic rings may also undergo hydroxylation catalysed by cytochrome *P*-450. For example, cyclohexane may be oxidized to cyclohexanol and then further to the *trans*-1,2-diol. Similarly, het-

Figure 8   Oxidation of vinyl chloride to an epoxide. From Timbrell (1982)

Figure 9   Hydroxylation of propylbenzene. From Timbrell (1982)

Figure 10 Dealkylation reactions. From Timbrell (1982)

Figure 11 Dealkylation of dimethylformamide via a stable hydroxymethyl intermediate. From Timbrell (1991)

2- Acetylaminofluorene ⟶ *N-Hydroxy-2-acetylaminofluorene*

Figure 12 *N*-Hydroxylation of acetylaminofluorene. From Timbrell (1982)

Figure 13 Oxidation of the pesticide aldicarb to sulphoxide and sulphone metabolites. From Timbrell (1982)

Parathion *Paraoxon*

Figure 14 Oxidative desulphuration of parathion. From Timbrell (1982)

erocyclic rings such as that in the drug hydralazine may be hydroxylated (see Figure 19 below). However, other enzymes may also be involved in this type of oxidation, such as the xanthine oxidases (see below).

Alkyl groups attached to N, O or S atoms are removed by dealkylation reactions which involve oxidation of the alkyl group. The intermediate hydroxyalkyl compound may be unstable and rearrange with loss of the respective aldehyde (Figure 10). Sometimes stable hydroxyalkyl products are produced, for example, when dimethylformamide undergoes metabolism (Figure 11). *S*-

Dealkylation may also involve a factor from the cytosol and so may not be a straightforward microsomal reaction. The chain length will have a bearing on whether dealkylation or oxidation of the alkyl group occurs. The longer the chain length the more likely is oxidation of the terminal carbon atom.

Nitrogen atoms in primary arylamines, arylamides and hydrazines may undergo hydroxylation which is catalysed by cytochrome *P*-450 (Figure 12). This reaction may result in a metabolic activation and so be responsible for toxicity (see below).

Nitrogen atoms in xenobiotics may also be oxidized by other oxidases (see below).

Sulphur atoms can also be oxidized by microsomal monooxygenases to yield *S*-oxides and sulphones such as in the pesticide aldicarb (Figure 13). Sulphur atoms may also be removed oxidatively and replaced by oxygen such as in the metabolism of the insecticide parathion (Figure 14).

(A) Halothane $\xrightarrow{O_2}$ ... $\longrightarrow$ ... $\longrightarrow$ *Trifluoroacetic acid*

(B) Halothane $\xrightarrow{e^-}$ ... $\xrightarrow{e^-}$ ...

1,1-Difluoro-2-chloroethylene

1,1,1-Trifluoro-2-chloroethane

Figure 15　Metabolism of the anaesthetic halothane showing both oxidative (A) and reductive (B) pathways. From Timbrell (1989)

Figure 16　Deamination of amphetamine

Trimethylamine　Trimethylamine-N-oxide

Figure 17　Oxidation of trimethylamine. From Timbrell (1982)

Similarly, halogen atoms may be removed via oxidative reactions, as shown for the metabolism of the anaesthetic halothane to trifluoroacetic acid (Figure 15).

Amine groups can also be removed oxidatively via a deamination reaction which may be catalysed by cytochrome *P*-450. For example, in the rabbit, amphetamine is metabolized in this way to phenylacetone (Figure 16). However, the initial attack is probably on the carbon atom to yield a carbinolamine, which can rearrange to the ketone with loss of ammonia as shown. Alternatively, the reaction may proceed via phenylacetoneoxime, which has been isolated as a metabolite and for which there are several possible routes of formation. The phenylacetoneoxime is hydrolysed to phenylacetone. *N*-Hydroxylation of amphetamine is also believed to take place and may also give rise to the observed metabolite, phenylacetone. The mechanism underlying the oxidative deamination of amphetamine has been a source of speculation and controversy but it illustrates

that there may be several routes of biotransformation to yield a particular metabolite (Gorrod and Raman, 1989).

Certain oxidation reactions are catalysed by enzymes other than the cytochrome *P*-450 monooxygenase system, such as the microsomal FAD-containing monooxygenase (Zeigler, 1984, 1985; Damani, 1988). This is responsible for the *N*-oxidation of tertiary amines such as dimethyl-aniline and trimethylamine (Figure 17). The enzyme requires NADPH and oxygen. The substrate specificity also includes secondary amines and sulphides, thioethers, thiols and thiocarbamates, and even organophosphates.

Alcohols, both aliphatic and aromatic, may be oxidized by alcohol dehydrogenase (Figure 18). This enzyme requires NADH and is cytosolic. The products from primary alcohols are aldehydes, whereas ketones are formed, more slowly, from secondary alcohols. The oxidation of an alcohol may result in a toxic metabolite being formed, such as that from allyl alcohol (Figure

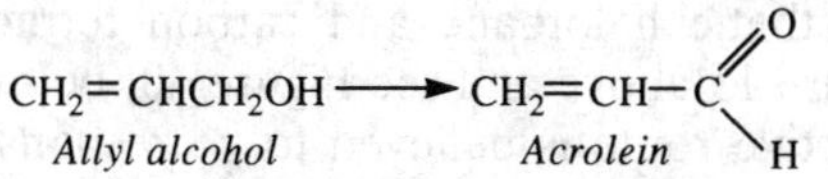

$$CH_2 = CHCH_2OH \longrightarrow CH_2 = CH - C \overset{O}{\underset{H}{\diagdown}}$$

Allyl alcohol   *Acrolein*

Figure 18 Oxidation of allyl alcohol. From Timbrell (1982)

18). A microsomal ethanol-metabolizing system has also been demonstrated.

Aldehydes may be further oxidized to acids by aldehyde dehydrogenase, another cytosolic enzyme which also requires NAD.

Other enzymes may also be involved in the oxidation of aldehydes, such as aldehyde oxidase and xanthine oxidase. These are also cytosolic enzymes which contain molybdenum and require flavoprotein cofactors (Beedham, 1988).

Xanthine oxidase also catalyses the oxidation of nitrogen heterocycles such as the purine hypoxanthine and also phthalazine to phthalazinone (Figure 19). Aldehyde oxidase will also catalyse the latter reaction. Some amines such as tyramine, found in certain foodstuffs such as cheese, are substrates for the monoamine oxidases. These are mitochondrial enzymes found in a variety of tissues, including the liver. The oxidative deamination of amines via the monoamine oxidases yields an aldehyde product (Figure 20). The action of monoamine oxidases may give rise to toxic products, however, such as the oxidation of allylamine to allyl aldehyde in heart tissue and the oxidation of the contaminant of certain 'home-made' drugs, 1-methyl-4-phenyl-1,2,3,6-tetrahydropyridine (MPTP), to a toxic metabolite

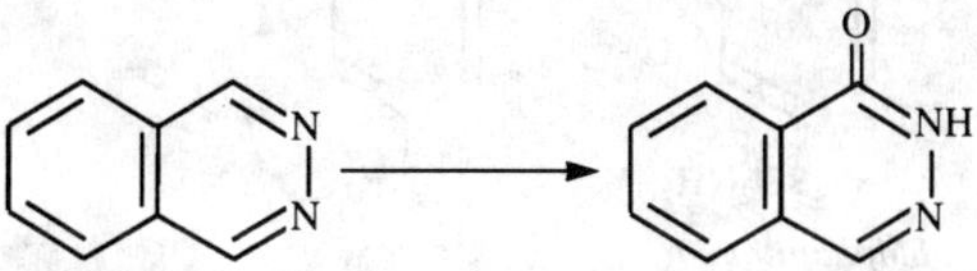

Phthalazine   *Phthalazinone*

Figure 19 Oxidation of the hydralazine metabolite phthalazine. From Timbrell (1982)

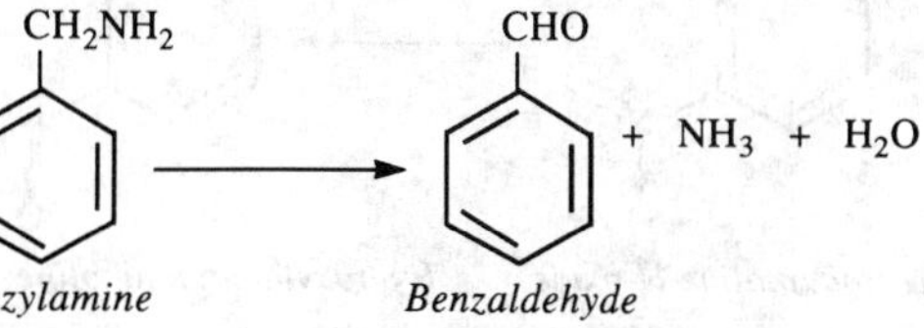

Benzylamine   *Benzaldehyde*

Figure 20 Oxidation of benzylamine by monoamine oxidase

responsible for degeneration of the substantia nigra in the brain.

Diamines such as putrescine are metabolized by the soluble enzyme diamine oxidase to dialdehyde products (Figure 21). Secondary and tertiary amines are less readily oxidized by these enzymes, dealkylation to the primary amine being preferred if it is possible.

Another group of enzymes which are involved in the oxidation of xenobiotics are the peroxidases (Larsson *et al.*, 1988). There are a number of these enzymes in mammalian tissues: prostaglandin synthase, found in kidney, lung, intestine and spleen; lactoperoxidase, found in mammary glands; myeloperoxidase, found in liver Kupffer cells and bone marrow cells, where it may be involved in the metabolic activation and therefore toxicity of benzene.

Uterine peroxidase has been suggested as being involved in the metabolic activation and toxicity of diethylstilboestrol.

The overall peroxidase-catalysed reaction may be summarized as follows:

peroxidase + H_2O_2 → compound I

compound I + RH_2 → compound II + $\cdot RH_2^+$

compound II + RH_2 → peroxidase + $\cdot RH_2^+$

Probably the most important is prostaglandin synthase. This is known to catalyse the oxidation of *p*-phenetidine, a metabolite of the drug phenacetin, a process which may be involved in the nephrotoxicity of the drug. The prostaglandin synthase-catalysed oxidation of this compound gives rise to free radicals which may be responsible for binding to DNA. Horseradish peroxidase will also catalyse the oxidation of this compound.

Reduction

Reduction may be catalysed by either microsomal or cytosolic reductases and by the gut bacteria, which also possess reductases. These are clearly important for substances taken orally, where contact with gut microflora is likely.

Reduction takes place under anaerobic conditions and utilizes NADH or NADPH. FAD

$$NH_2 - (CH_2)_4 - NH_2 \xrightarrow[\text{oxidase}]{\text{Diamine}} NH_2(CH_2)_3 - CHO$$

Figure 21 Oxidation of putrescine by diamine oxidase

may also be involved, possibly as a non-enzymic electron donor. The most commonly encountered types of reductive reaction are the reduction of nitro and azo groups. The reduction of azo groups such as those present in the drug Prontosil (Figure 22) is a two-step reaction involving first reduction to a substituted hydrazine, followed by a second reduction and cleavage to yield the amine.

Reduction of nitro groups is also an important route of biotransformation, such as for the compound nitrobenzene (Figure 23). Again this involves several steps, producing first a nitroso derivative, then a hydroxylamine and finally an amine. Reduction of nitro groups may be associated with toxicity. Nitrobenzene is haematotoxic in rats when given orally, causing methaemoglobinaemia and haemolysis, whereas given intraperitoneally or to rats without gut flora it is devoid of this toxicity. This is due to reduction of the compound in the gut to yield the nitroso and hydroxylamine metabolites which are responsible for toxicity to haemoglobin. Another example is nitroquinoline *N*-oxide, which is reduced to a hydroxylamine (Figure 24) which is believed to be carcinogenic.

Less common reduction reactions include reduction of aldehyde and keto groups, epoxides and double bonds.

Reductive dehalogenation, catalysed by the microsomal enzymes, may also occur in the metabolism of halogenated compounds such as the anaesthetic halothane and carbon tetrachloride (Figure 15 above and see Figure 40, below). The reductive route is believed to be responsible for the acute toxicity of halothane in rats when the oxygen tension is low. The reactive radical metabolites produced by the reductive pathway will covalently bind to liver protein and this may lead to toxicity. However, the oxidative pathway is probably more important in man under normal conditions of anaesthesia. This also gives rise to a reactive metabolite, trifluoroacetylchloride. Both the oxidative and reductive pathways involve cytochrome *P*-450. In the reductive mode the enzyme donates an electron to the substrate, which then loses a bromide ion, and a second electron is donated, which produces a radical species which may either react with protein or rearrange to other metabolic products.

Similarly, reductive dechlorination is also involved in the toxicity of carbon tetrachloride. Here, again, cytochrome *P*-450 donates an electron under reductive conditions and the products are chloride ion and the trichloromethyl radical (see Figure 40, below). This may then react further with oxygen to form the trichloromethylperoxy radical species, which is believed to cause the damage to lipids in cell membranes. Alternatively, the trichloromethyl radical may abstract a hydrogen atom from any of a variety of sources (such as glutathione) and the product will be chloroform.

Prontosil   *Sulphanilamide*

Figure 22   Reduction of the azo bond in Prontosil. From Timbrell (1982)

Nitrobenzene   *Aniline*

Figure 23   Reduction of nitrobenzene. From Timbrell (1982)

Nitroquinoline-N-oxide   *Hydroxylaminoquinoline-N-oxide*

Figure 24   Reduction of the carcinogen nitroquinoline *N*-oxide. From Timbrell (1982)

Hydrolysis

Esters and amides are hydrolysed by carboxyl-esterases and amidases, respectively, and there are a number of these enzymes occurring in a variety of tissues. They are usually found in the cytosol of cells, but microsomal esterases and amidases have also been described and some are also found in the plasma. Typical esterase and amidase reactions are shown in Figure 25. Esterases have been classified as type A, B or C on the basis of activity towards phosphate triesters. Thus, B-type esterases are all inhibited by paraoxon and have a serine residue at the active site which may be phosphorylated. However, there are a number of different enzymes within this group with different specificities. Esterases also have amidase activity and vice versa, and so these two activities may be part of the same overall activity. Hydrazides and carbamates may also be hydrolysed by amidases. Amidases have an important role in the toxicity of the drugs isoniazid and phenacetin, where hydrolysis is an important step in the metabolic activation (see Figure 44, below).

Hydration

Epoxides, which are three-membered rings containing an oxygen atom, may be reactive meta-bolic intermediates. They may undergo hydration catalysed by the enzyme epoxide hydrolase, which is located in the smooth endoplasmic reticulum, conveniently near to the cytochrome P-450 system which produces the epoxide. The reaction can normally be regarded as a detoxication reaction, as the dihydrodiol products are usually much less chemically reactive than the epoxide (Figure 26). The products are *trans* diols. However, there are examples where the diol is further metabolized to a more toxic metabolite. Both aromatic and aliphatic epoxides may be substrates for the enzyme.

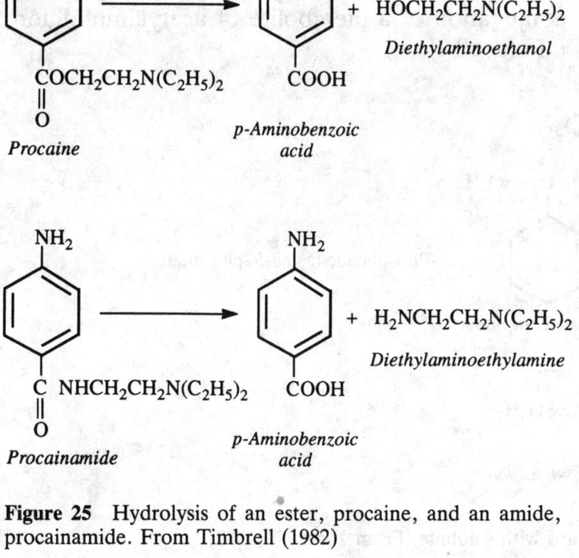

PHASE 2 REACTIONS

Phase 2 reactions, also known as conjugation reactions, involve the addition of a readily available, polar endogenous substance to the foreign molecule. This polar moiety is conjugated either to an existing group or to one added in a phase 1 reaction. The polar moiety renders the foreign molecule more water-soluble and so more readily cleared from the body and less likely to exert a toxic effect. The endogenous metabolites donated in phase 2 reactions include carbohydrate derivatives, amino acids, glutathione and sulphate. The mechanism involves formation of a high-energy intermediate: either the endogenous metabolite is activated as a high-energy derivative (type 1) or the substrate is activated (type 2).

Conjugation reactions are considered below.

Sulphation

The addition of the sulphate moiety to a hydroxyl group is a major route of conjugation for foreign compounds, and endogenous compounds, such as steroids, may also undergo sulphation. The reaction is catalysed by cytosolic sulphotransferase enzymes found particularly in the liver, gastrointestinal mucosa and kidney. The reaction also requires the coenzyme 3'-phosphoadenosine-

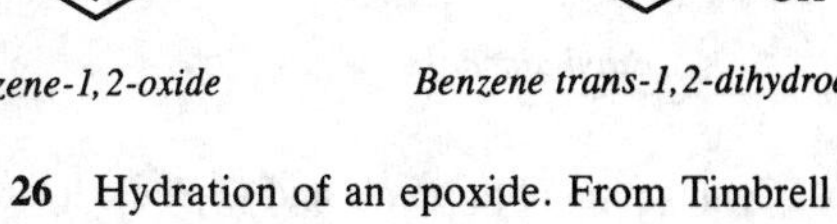

Figure 25 Hydrolysis of an ester, procaine, and an amide, procainamide. From Timbrell (1982)

Figure 26 Hydration of an epoxide. From Timbrell (1982)

5'-phosphosulphate (PAPS). This coenzyme is produced from inorganic sulphate ions and ATP in a two-stage reaction (Figure 27). Other anions may replace sulphate in the first reaction but the products are unstable. This may lead to toxicity by the depletion of ATP. The available inorganic sulphate in the body may also be depleted by large doses of compounds such as paracetamol which are conjugated with sulphate (see below).

There are a number of different sulphotransferases, classified by the particular type of substrate, and some of these exist in several forms. The product of sulphate conjugation is an ester which is very polar and water-soluble. Both aromatic and aliphatic hydroxyl groups may be conjugated with sulphate, as may *N*-hydroxy groups and amino groups (Figure 28).

Sulphate conjugation may be involved in the metabolic activation of compounds such as the carcinogen acetylaminofluorene (Mulder *et al.* 1988) (see below).

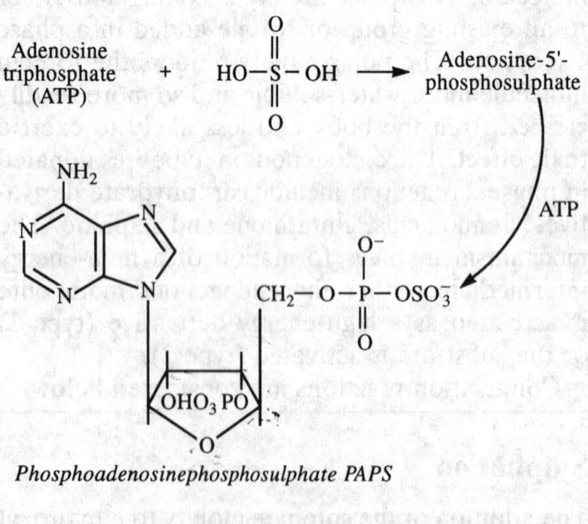

Glucuronidation

The addition of glucuronic acid, a polar and water-soluble carbohydrate molecule, to hydroxyl groups, carboxylic acid groups, amino groups and thiols is a major route of phase 2 metabolism. Uridine diphosphate glucuronic acid (UDPglucuronic acid) is the cofactor which donates glucuronic acid and, as with sulphation, the moiety added, glucuronic acid, is in a high-energy form as UDPglucuronic acid. UDPglucuronic acid is synthesized from glucose-1-phosphate in the cytosol in a two-step reaction (Figure 29).

The addition of the glucuronic acid to the xenobiotic molecule is catalysed by one of a number of glucuronosyl transferases which are microsomal enzymes. The enzymes are inducible in animals treated with compounds such as phenobarbitone.

The reaction involves nucleophilic attack by the recipient atom (oxygen, sulphur or nitrogen) at the C-1 carbon atom of the glucuronic acid. This displacement reaction involves an inversion of configuration resulting in the product being in the β configuration (Figure 30).

Other carbohydrates may also be involved in conjugation such as glucose, which is utilized by insects to form glucosides. Ribose and xylose may also be used in conjugation reactions.

As with sulphation, glucuronidation, although generally a detoxication reaction, may occasionally be involved in increasing toxicity, as with the conjugation of a metabolite of acetylaminofluorene (see below).

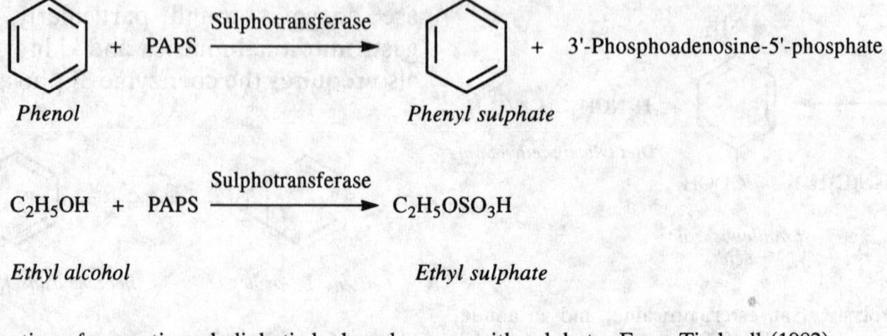

Phosphoadenosinephosphosulphate PAPS

Figure 27   Formation of the sulphate donor PAPS

Figure 28   Conjugation of aromatic and aliphatic hydroxyl groups with sulphate. From Timbrell (1982)

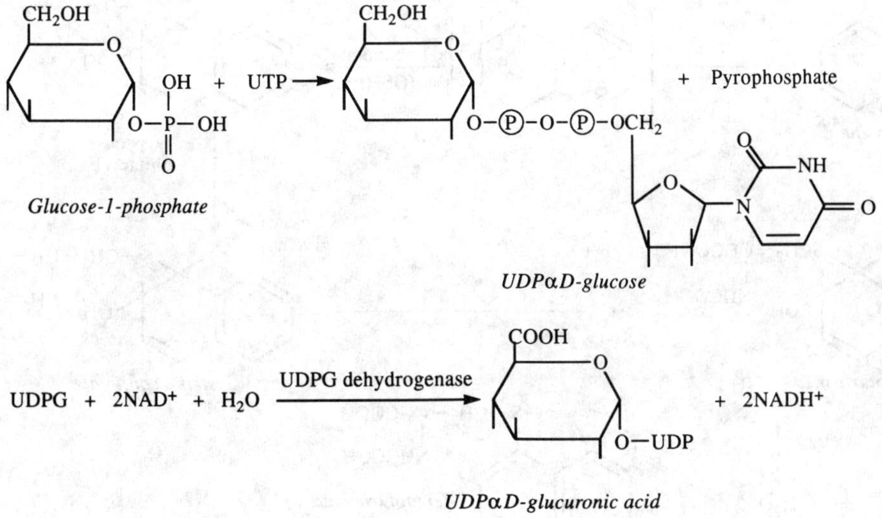

Figure 29 Formation of the glucuronic acid donor UPDG. From Timbrell (1982)

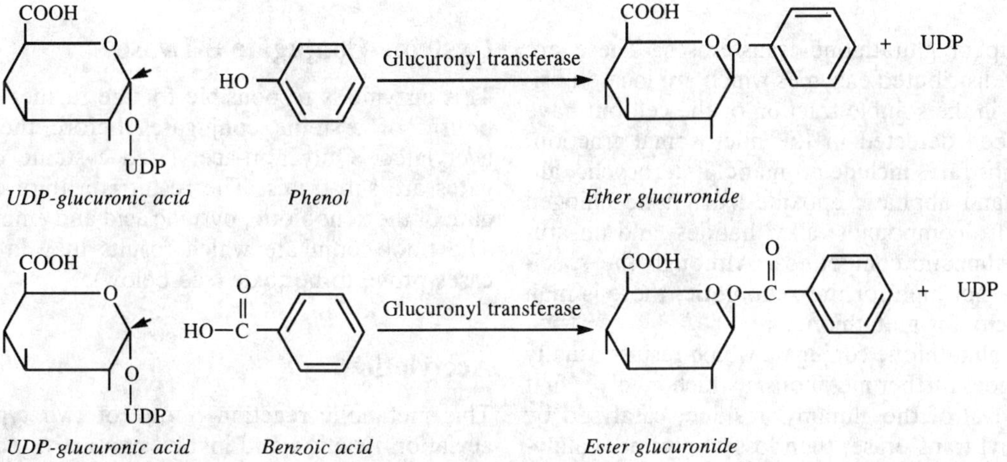

Figure 30 Formation of ether and ester glucuronide conjugates. From Timbrell (1982)

Glutathione Conjugation

This group of reactions involves the addition of glutathione to a molecule, usually with the subsequent removal of two amino acids to leave a cysteine conjugate. This is then acetylated to yield a mercapturic acid or *N*-acetylcysteine conjugate (Figure 31). Glutathione is a tripeptide (glu-cys-gly) found in many mammalian tissues, but especially the liver. It has a major protective role in the body, as it is a scavenger for reactive compounds of various types. The sulphydryl group attacks the reactive part of the foreign compound. This is a particularly important route of phase 2 metabolism from the toxicological point of view, as it is often involved in the removal of reactive intermediates. However, more recently this route has also been shown to be the cause of some toxic reactions (Van Bladeren *et al.*, 1988) (see below).

Normally the sulphydryl group of glutathione acts as a nucleophile and either displaces another atom or attacks an electrophilic site (Figure 31). Consequently, glutathione may react either chemically or in enzyme-catalysed reactions with a variety of compounds which are reactive/electrophilic metabolites produced in phase I reactions. The reactions may be catalysed by one of

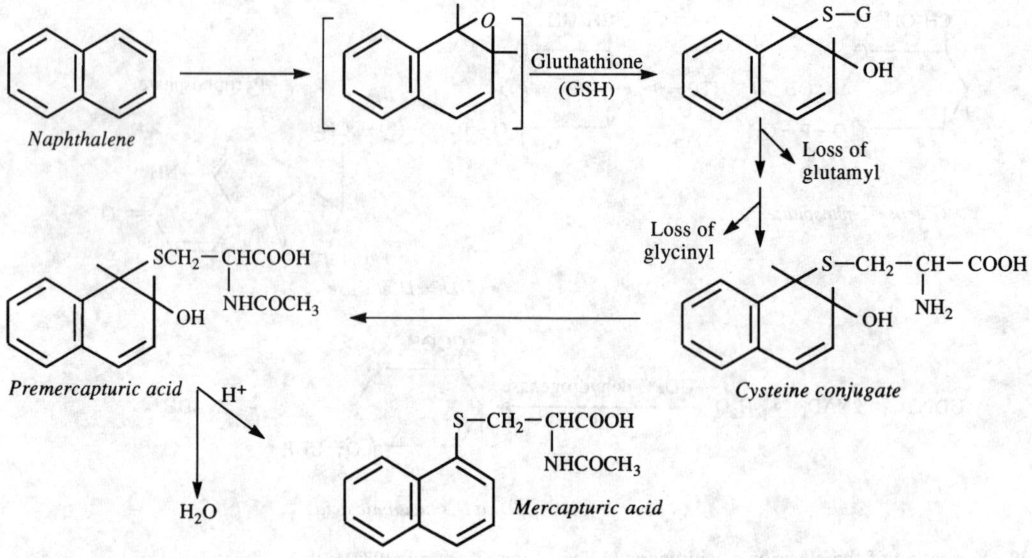

Figure 31   Metabolism of naphthalene to an *N*-acetylcysteine conjugate. From Timbrell (1982)

a group of glutathione transferases. These are widely distributed enzymes which are located primarily in the soluble fraction of the cell but have also been detected in the microsomal fraction. The substrates include aromatic, heterocyclic, alicyclic and aliphatic epoxides; aromatic halogen and nitro compounds; alkyl halides; and unsaturated aliphatic compounds. Although the specificity is not high for the xenobiotic, there is high specificity for glutathione.

The glutathione conjugate which results usually undergoes further metabolism which involves first a removal of the glutamyl residue, catalysed by glutamyl transferase, then loss of glycine, catalysed by cysteinyl glycinase, and finally the cysteine moiety is acetylated to give the *N*-acetylcysteine conjugate or mercapturic acid (Figure 31). The *N*-acetyltransferase which carries out this reaction is a microsomal enzyme found in liver and kidney but is not the same as the *N*-acetyltransferase which catalyses the acetylation of xenobiotic amine groups (see below). This further metabolism of conjugates such as illustrated for glutathione conjugates has been termed phase 3 metabolism.

Glutathione conjugates, or the cysteinyl–glycine conjugate which results from them, may be excreted directly into the bile and further metabolism may take place in the gastrointestinal tract.

Cysteine Conjugate β-Lyase

This enzyme is responsible for the further metabolism of cysteine conjugates before they are acetylated. Only non-acetylated cysteine conjugates are substrates. The result is a thiol conjugate of the xenobiotic, pyruvic acid and ammonia. The thiol conjugate which results may in some cases prove to be toxic (see below).

Acetylation

This metabolic reaction is one of two types of acylation reaction and involves an activated conjugating agent, acetyl coenzyme A (acetyl CoA). It is also notable in that the product may be less water-soluble than the parent compound. Acetylation is an important route of metabolism for aromatic amino compounds, sulphonamides, hydrazines and hydrazides (Figure 32). The enzymes involved are acetyltransferases and are found in the cytosol of cells in the liver, gastric mucosa and white blood cells. The enzymes utilize acetyl CoA as cofactor. The mechanism of the acetylation reaction involves first an acetylation of the enzyme, followed by addition of the substrate and then transfer of the acetyl group to the substrate. There are two enzymes (NAT 1 and NAT 2) in humans which differ markedly in activity and substrate specificity. In several species the possession of a particular mutant isoen-

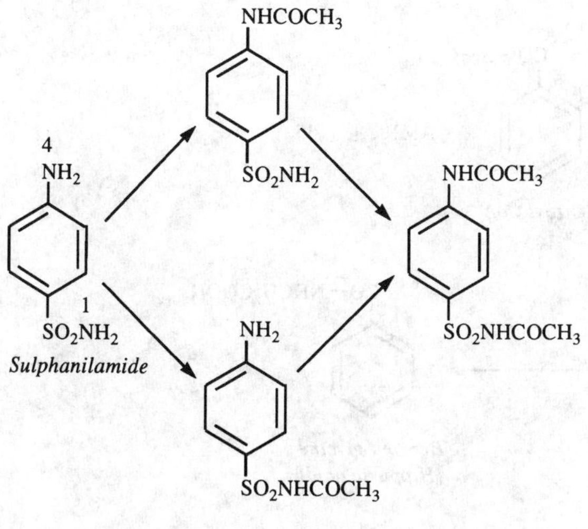

NHCOCH₃

4
NH₂

SO₂NH₂

NHCOCH₃

1
SO₂NH₂
Sulphanilamide

NH₂

SO₂NHCOCH₃

NHCOCH₃

SO₂NHCOCH₃

Figure 32 Acetylation of amino and sulphonamido groups. From Timbrell (1982)

zyme is genetically determined and gives rise to two distinct phenotypes known as 'rapid' and 'slow' acetylators. This has an important role in the toxicity of certain drugs such as hydralazine, isoniazid and procainamide, and these examples illustrate the importance of genetic factors in toxicology (Weber, 1987) (see below). As well as *N*-acetylation, a related reaction is *N,O*-trans-acetylation. This reaction applies to arylamines, which first undergo *N*-hydroxylation and then the hydroxylamine group is acetylated to yield an arylhydroxamic acid (see Figure 45, below). This may then transfer the acetyl group to another amine molecule or to the hydroxy group, to yield a highly reactive acyloxy arylamine which is capable of reacting, after a rearrangement, with proteins and nucleic acids (see below). The enzyme involved, an *N,O*-acyltransferase, is a cytosolic enzyme.

Amino Acid Conjugation

This is the second type of acylation reaction in which the xenobiotic itself is activated. Organic acids are the usual substrates for this reaction, with conjugation to an endogenous amino acid. The particular amino acid utilized depends on the species concerned and indeed species within a similar evolutionary group tend to utilize the same amino acid. Glycine is the most common amino acid used, but taurine, glutamine and ornithine are also utilized. The foreign carboxylic acid

group is first activated by reaction with Coenzyme A in a reaction which requires ATP and is catalysed by a mitochondrial ligase enzyme. The S-CoA derivative then reacts with the particular amino acid (Figure 33). This second reaction is catalysed by an acyltransferase enzyme which is found in the mitochondria. Two enzymes have been purified, each utilizing a different group of CoA derivatives.

Methylation

Hydroxyl, amino and thiol groups in both exogenous and endogenous compounds may be methylated by one of a series of methyltransferases (Figure 34). These enzymes are normally found in the cytosol, although a microsomal *O*-methyltransferase and an *S*-methyltransferase have been described. The cofactor required is *S*-adenosylmethionine, which is the methylation donor. As with acetylation, the methylation reaction tends to decrease rather than increase the water-solubility of the molecule. A number of metals such as mercury may also be methylated by microorganisms, a reaction which changes both the toxicity of mercury and its physicochemical characteristics and, hence, its environmental behaviour.

There are other minor reactions which a foreign molecule may undergo, but for information about these the interested reader should consult one of the texts or reviews given in the References. An important point, however, is that although a molecule is foreign to a living organism, it may still be a substrate for an enzyme involved in normal metabolic pathways, provided that its chemical structure is appropriate. For example, a foreign compound which is a halogenated fatty acid derivative may be metabolized by the β-oxidation pathway but might potentially interfere with that pathway. The possible involvement of enzymes of intermediary metabolism therefore widens the scope of potential metabolic reactions. Foreign compounds can be metabolized by a number of different enzymes simultaneously in the same animal and so there may be many different metabolic routes and metabolites. The balance between these routes can often determine the toxicity of the compound.

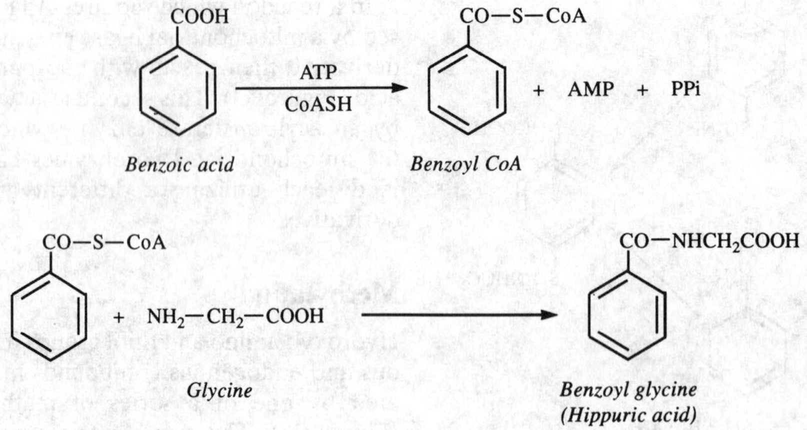

Figure 33 Conjugation of an aromatic acid with glycine. From Timbrell (1982)

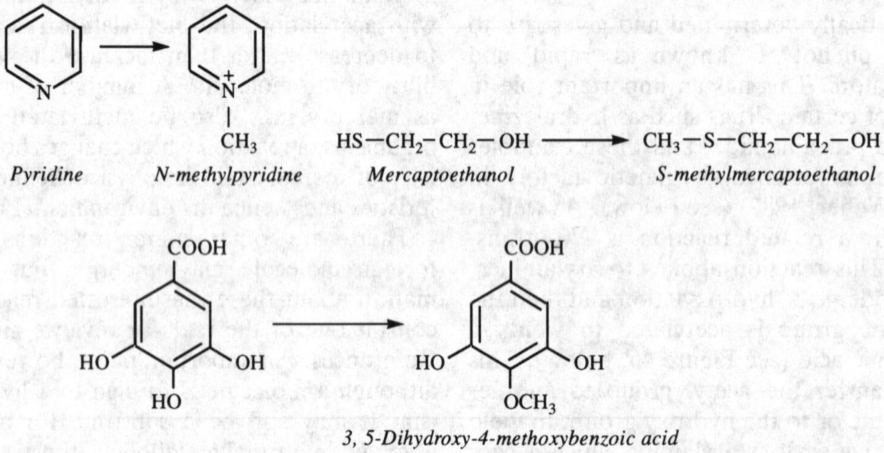

Figure 34 Methylation reactions. From Timbrell (1982)

FACTORS AFFECTING METABOLISM

Factors which affect metabolism may often affect the toxicity of a compound, either by changing the rate of removal of the parent compound or by altering the pattern of metabolites. Different species will often metabolize compounds differently, and so show differences in toxicity. Environmental factors such as dietary constituents and drugs taken by humans may influence the metabolism, and so alter the toxicity of a particular substance. In man genetic factors may play an important role in determining which

metabolic pathway is utilized and therefore whether a compound is toxic or not (Sitar, 1989; Weber, 1987).

The multiple forms of cytochrome *P*-450 may underlie the species differences in metabolism, the effects of age, sex, nutrition, strain and genetic differences. Different tissues may contain different isoenzymes and, hence, be differently susceptible to certain toxic compounds.

Species

Different species are utilized in the safety evaluation of chemicals, and in the environment widely different species may all be exposed to a chemical. These species may react very differently to xenobiotics. Indeed this difference in sensitivity is exploited in pesticides. Insecticides such as organophosphorus compounds and DDT are much more toxic to insects than to humans and other mammals. In the case of malathion this is due to a metabolic difference (Figure 35).

There are many species differences in metabolism which have been documented (Caldwell, 1980), but this section will mainly concentrate on those which are significant as far as toxicity is concerned.

Phase 1 reactions. These are quantitative differences between species in oxidation reactions but qualitative differences are perhaps less common. It is difficult to find a species pattern in these differences.

The aromatic hydroxylation of aniline has been shown to vary between various species (Table 2),

and those species such as the cat which produce more *o-* as opposed to *p*-aminophenol are more susceptible to the toxicity. The trend in this case is for carnivores to favour *ortho*-hydroxylation rather than *para*-hydroxylation. Another example of quantitative differences in metabolism between species is in the metabolism of ethylene glycol to oxalate (see Figure 2, above). The toxicity is partly due to the oxalic acid produced by the oxidative pathway and the toxicity correlates with the production of oxalate. Here again the cat is the species most susceptible to the toxicity, producing the most oxalate, followed by the rat, with the rabbit producing the least.

The *N*-hydroxylation of paracetamol (see below) also shows quantitative differences in metabolism between species, which accounts for species differences in hepatotoxicity. Thus, the rat is relatively resistant to the toxicity and metabolizes less via the toxic pathway, whereas the hamster is very susceptible. In contrast, the rat is well able to carry out *N*-hydroxylation of acetylaminofluorene (see Figure 12, above), a step which is necessary for the carcinogenicity of the compound (see Figure 45, below).

In the metabolism of the drug hexobarbitone there are striking differences between species, which correlate with the pharmacological effect (Table 3). The overall metabolic rate tends to decrease with the size of the species, and this would be expected to have some bearing on drug metabolism. In this example this is approximately true, apart from the rat and rabbit being transposed.

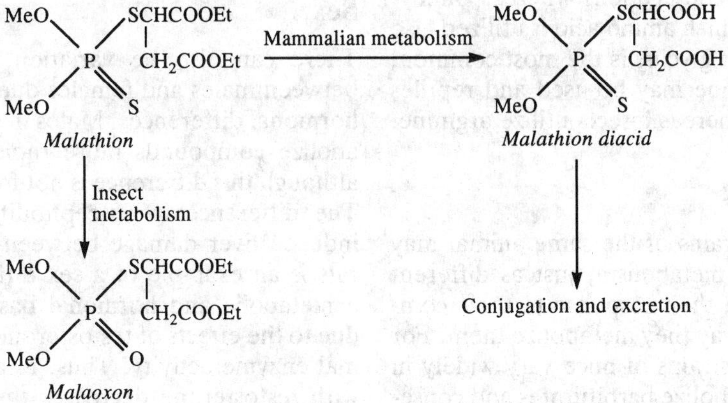

Table 2 Species differences in the hydroxylation of aniline

Species	% Dose excreted	
	o-Aminophenol	*p*-Aminophenol
Gerbil	3	48
Guinea-pig	4	46
Golden hamster	6	53
Chicken	11	44
Rat	19	48
Ferret	26	28
Dog	18	9
Cat	32	14

Data from Parke (1968).

Figure 35 Metabolism of malathion. From Timbrell (1982)

Table 3 Species differences in the metabolism and duration of action of hexobarbitone

Species	Duration of action (min)	Plasma half-life (min)	Relative enzyme activity ($\mu g\ g^{-1}\ h^{-1}$)	Plasma level on awakening ($\mu g\ ml^{-1}$)
Mouse	12	19	598	89
Rabbit	49	60	196	57
Rat	90	140	135	64
Dog[a]	315	260	36	19

[a] Dose in dogs: 50 mg kg^{-1}; other species 100 mg kg^{-1}.
Data from Quinn *et al.* (1958).

Another phase 1 reaction which shows a striking species difference which is a cause of selective toxicity is hydrolysis. Thus, the insecticide malathion is readily hydrolysed in mammals but in the insect the carboxylesterase enzyme is absent and oxidative metabolism is the major route (see Figure 35, above). This route leads to the production of malaoxon, which is toxic because it binds to the active site of cholinesterases.

A number of phase 2 reactions also show well-characterized species differences. For example, the metabolism of phenols in most mammals, and also birds, amphibians and reptiles but not fish, usually involves conjugation with either glucuronic acid or sulphate, depending on the species, but most species utilize a mixture of these two routes. The cat, however, cannot utilize glucuronic acid and the pig cannot usually conjugate with sulphate. There are also clear differences in the conjugation of organic acids. Carnivores favour glucuronic acid conjugation, herbivores favour amino acid conjugation, whereas omnivores utilize both. Which amino acid is utilized also varies, and although glycine is the most common, glutamine and taurine may be used and reptiles utilize ornithine, whereas insects utilize arginine.

Strain of Animal

Different inbred strains of the same animal may show variations in metabolism, just as different species may vary in their response to toxic compounds and in the way they metabolize them. For example, different strains of mice vary widely in their ability to metabolize barbiturates and consequently the magnitude of the pharmacological effect varies between these strains (Table 4). Vari-

Table 4 Strain differences in the duration of action of hexobarbitone in mice

Strain	Numbers of animals	Mean sleeping time (min) ± SD
A/NL	25	48 ± 4
BALB/cAnN	63	41 ± 2
C57L/HeN	29	33 ± 3
C3HfB/HeN	30	22 ± 3
SWR/HeN	38	18 ± 4
Swiss (non-inbred)	47	43 ± 15

Data from Jay (1955).

ations between human individuals may also be regarded similarly but will be considered separately in this chapter (see below).

Sex

There can also be variation in the responses between males and females due to metabolic and hormonal differences. Males in some species metabolize compounds more rapidly than females, although this difference is not found in all species. The difference in susceptibility to chloroform-induced liver damage between male and female rats is an example of a sex difference which has a metabolic and hormonal basis, thought to be due to the effects of testosterone on liver microsomal enzyme activity. Thus, treatment of females with testosterone decreases the LD_{50} and treatment of males with oestradiol increases the LD_{50} of chloroform. Similarly, there is a sex difference in the nephrotoxicity of chloroform in mice, with male mice being more susceptible. This difference can be removed by castration and restored by administration of androgens to the males. It may be that testosterone is increasing the microsomal enzyme-mediated metabolism of chloroform to toxic metabolites (Pohl, 1979).

Another example is the metabolism of ethylmorphine and hexobarbitone, which are clearly under hormonal control in the male rat. Castration of the animals significantly reduces the metabolism of both compounds. However, the normal rate of metabolism can be restored by the administration of androgens to the castrated animals.

Genetic Factors

Genetic variation in metabolism within the human population probably underlies much of the variability in response of that population to the toxic effects of foreign compounds. There are now many examples of toxic drug reactions which occur particularly in individuals who have a genetic defect or genetic difference in metabolism. Perhaps the best-known example of genetic variability in man is the acetylator phenotype (Weber, 1987). In this example the acetylation reaction (see above) shows genetic variations which are almost certainly due to the presence of different isoenzymes of the acetyltransferase. This difference in the isoenzymes results in a difference in activity of the enzyme and, hence, gives rise to rapid and slow acetylator phenotypes. The slow acetylator phenotype, which occurs to a variable extent in the population, depending on the racial origin (Table 5), is an important factor in a number of adverse drug reactions (Table 6). For example, the lupus syndrome induced by the drug hydralazine only occurs in slow acetylators. The metabolism of the drug is influenced by the acetylator phenotype, with more being metabolized by an oxidative pathway in the slow acetylators (Timbrell *et al.*, 1984). However, it is not yet known whether this is responsible for the toxic effect.

The acetylator phenotype is also believed to be a factor in isoniazid toxicity (see below) and bladder cancer, which occurs in workers exposed to aromatic amines. Thus, there is an increased incidence of the cancer in slow acetylators. This is postulated to be due to the decreased ability of

Table 5   Acetylator phenotype distribution in various ethnic groups

Ethnic group	Rapid acetylators (%)	Drug
Eskimos	95–100	INH
Japanese	88	INH
Latin Americans	70	INH
Black Americans	52	INH
White Americans	48	INH
Africans	43	SMZ
South Indians	39	INH
Britons	38	SMZ
Egyptians	18	INH

INH: isoniazid; SMZ: sulphamethazine.
Data from Lunde *et al.* (1977).

Table 6   Toxicities related to the acetylator phenotype

Xenobiotic	Adverse effect	Incidence
Isoniazid	Peripheral neuropathy	Higher in slow acetylators
Isoniazid	Hepatic damage	Higher in slow acetylators
Procainamide Hydralazine	Lupus erythematosus	Higher in slow acetylators
Phenelzine	Drowsiness/nausea	Higher in slow acetylators
Aromatic amines	Bladder cancer	Higher in slow acetylators

slow acetylators to detoxify the aromatic amines by acetylation (Cartwright *et al.*, 1982; Mommsen *et al.*, 1985).

A more recently discovered genetic factor in metabolism is the polymorphism in the hydroxylation of debrisoquine (Figure 36). This variation in oxidation has now been shown for a number of other drugs, such as phenytoin, sparteine and phenformin. Again there are two phenotypes, designated poor metabolizers and extensive metabolizers. Unlike the acetylator phenotype, how-

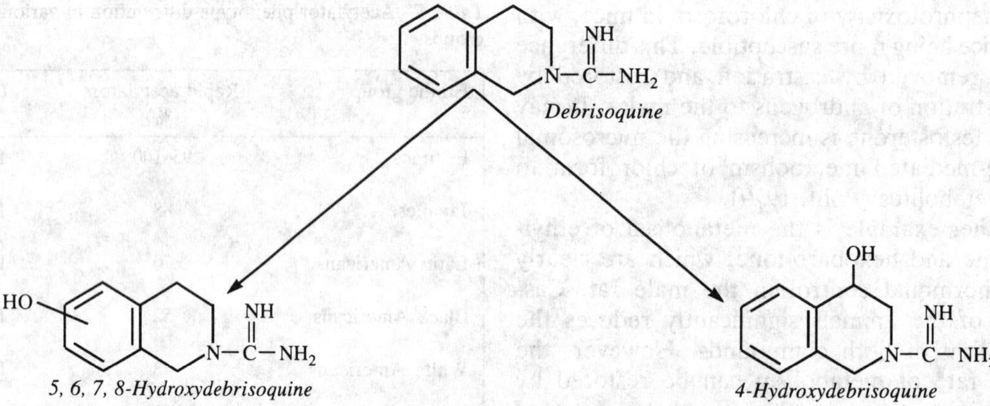

Figure 36   Metabolism of debrisoquine. From Timbrell (1982)

ever, the poor metabolizer phenotype is relatively uncommon, only occurring in about 7–9 per cent of the population. In some cases toxic reactions are associated with the poor metabolizer status. The difference between the poor metabolizers and extensive metabolizers is believed to be due to differences in the isozymes of cytochrome *P*-450 present in the particular subject. It has recently been shown (Gonzalez *et al.*, 1988) that human poor metabolizers have negligible amounts of the cytochrome *P*-450 isoenzyme *P*-450db1 in the liver microsomal fraction. There may also be other mutant alleles responsible for the poor metabolizer phenotype. It seems likely that there are several cytochrome *P*-450 isoenzymes for the oxidation of debrisoquine and similar substrates, with different affinities and capacities for a particular substrate. The extensive metabolizers may have all the isoenzymes, whereas the poor metabolizers may be deficient in the high-capacity isoenzyme. It also seems likely that not all of these isoenzymes are controlled by the polymorphism and that there may also be variations within one phenotype as well as between phenotypes (Tyndale *et al.*, 1989).

Environmental Factors

Exposure of animals to chemical substances via the environment, such as in the diet, air or water, may influence the metabolism and therefore the toxic response to the chemical of interest. Humans may be receiving medication with several drugs when exposure to an industrial chemical occurs, for instance. The intake of one drug may affect the metabolism of another. For example, overdoses of paracetamol are more likely to cause serious liver damage if the victim is also exposed to large amounts of alcohol or barbiturates. Both of these drugs influence drug metabolizing enzymes and thereby increase the metabolism and, in turn, the toxicity of paracetamol (see below).

The diet contains many substances, such as the naphthoflavones found in certain vegetables, which may influence the enzymes involved in drug metabolism. Cigarette smoking is also known to affect drug metabolism. One way in which a particular substance may influence the metabolism of another is by increasing the apparent activity of the drug metabolizing enzymes. This is known as induction. The induction of the microsomal monooxygenases, as well as a number of other enzymes, is now a well-known phenomenon and is caused by a large variety of compounds. It occurs in many species. However, these different inducers induce different isoenzymes of cytochrome *P*-450 and are therefore of importance for different types of substrates.

The first type of microsomal enzyme inducer to be described was the barbiturate phenobarbitone. When animals are exposed to repeated doses of this compound, there are a number of changes which can be observed. The liver of the animal exposed increases in weight, there is an increase in liver blood flow and the smooth endoplasmic reticulum proliferates. These changes are accompanied by an increase in the total amount of cytochrome *P*-450 in the liver. The activity of other enzymes found in the endoplasmic reticulum also increases. It is now known that enzymes in other organelles such as the peroxisomes may also be induced.

The effect of enzyme induction is that the metabolism of certain foreign compounds is increased. At the molecular level there is an increase in protein synthesis and underlying this an increase in mRNA synthesis. Since the initial discovery that phenobarbitone induced the enzymes responsible for its own metabolism, many other inducers have been discovered and studied, and some of these have been found to be different types of inducer. These different inducers induce different isoenzymes of cytochrome *P*-450 and do not necessarily cause all the changes observed with phenobarbitone induction, such as the increase in liver weight and blood flow. The inducers currently known can be separated into barbiturate-type inducers and the polycyclic aromatic hydrocarbon-type of inducer. These are the main types, but there are others which do not belong to one of these two groups, such as steroids, compounds such as the drug clofibrate and the acetone type of inducer. Each of these induces (a) different form(s) of the enzyme. These can in some cases be distinguished on the basis of spectral characteristics such as the absorption maximum for the carbon monoxide–cytochrome *P*-450 complex. There are also inducers which have a broader inducing ability, such as the compound Arochlor 1254, which may be both a barbiturate type of inducer and a polycyclic hydrocarbon type of inducer.

The isoenzymes induced by some of these compounds may represent only a small proportion of the total cytochrome *P*-450 present in the uninduced animal and therefore the induction may cause a big shift in the metabolic profile rather than a simple increase in the overall rate of metabolism. Thus, for the polycyclic hydrocarbon type of inducers the form of cytochrome *P*-450 induced normally only represents about 5 per cent of the total enzyme, whereas after induction the amount may be increased by a factor of 16. Furthermore, induction is not confined to the hepatic enzymes: those in other tissues may also be induced. The effect of different inducers on the metabolism of different compounds can be seen from the data in Table 7. Clearly, although all these compounds are inducers of cytochrome *P*-450, the effects on different substrates for the enzyme is different. These differential effects even extend to different isomers (Table 8). This

can be rationalized by the fact that there are many different isoenzymes and that these are induced by different compounds.

As well as influencing the metabolism of foreign compounds, enzyme induction may have effects on the metabolism of endogenous compounds and so disrupt normal physiological processes.

The mechanisms underlying induction are not all entirely clear but it is known to be a cellular response, which can be studied in isolated hepatocytes, for example. The synthesis of new protein is involved, as the induction process can be prevented by inhibitors of protein synthesis. Synthesis of RNA is required but not of DNA, and so it seems that the effect is at the level of transcription. For the polycyclic hydrocarbon type of inducer, studied with tetrachlorodibenzodioxin (dioxin), which is an exquisitely potent inducer, it seems that there is a cytosolic receptor which binds the inducer. The inducer–receptor complex is then transported to the nucleus and there causes mRNA coding for cytochrome *P*-450 to be synthesized. This then allows increased synthesis of the particular cytochrome *P*-450(s) for which the mRNA is coded. Presumably this involves derepression of the particular gene (Nebert and Gonzalez, 1985; Whitlock, 1989). However, to date no receptor for the barbiturate type of inducer has been found.

Consequences of Induction

Induction of drug metabolizing enzymes may lead to an alteration in the metabolism of a compound, which may then result in the toxicity being either increased or decreased. Prediction of which will occur is only possible with a knowledge of the metabolism and mechanism of toxicity of the compound in question. In some of the examples at the end of this chapter the effect of inducers will also be discussed.

Inhibition of Metabolism

Just as some of the enzymes involved in biotransformation may be induced, so these enzymes may also be inhibited, and this can have major consequences for toxicity (Netter, 1987). Such inhibitions are sometimes of major importance clinically with the interaction between drugs, and are probably more important than induction effects. Inhibition generally only requires a single dose of a compound rather than repeated doses

Table 7 Effects of different inducers on the metabolism of various substrates

Substrate	Inducer				
	Control	Pb	PCN	3MC	ARO
	(nmol product per min per nmol cytochrome *P*-450)				
Ethylmorphine	13.7 ± 0.8	16.8 ± 4.3	24.9 ± 3.5	6.4 ± 0.5	9.5 ± 1.2
Aminopyrine	9.9 ± 0.8	13.9 ± 1.7	9.7 ± 1.3	7.6 ± 1.8	13.7 ± 1.2
Benzphetamine	12.5 ± 1.2	45.7 ± 14.0	6.6 ± 0.7	5.7 ± 1.1	15.8 ± 2.7
Caffeine	0.5 ± 0.1	0.7 ± 0.1		0.5 ± 0.1	0.6 ± 0.1
Benzo[a]pyrene	0.1	0.1	0.1	0.3	

Pb, phenobarbitone; PCN, pregnenolone-16α-carbonitrile; 3MC, 3-methylcholanthrene; ARO, Arochlor 1254.
Data from Powis *et al.* (1977).

Table 8 The differential effect of cytochrome *P*-450 inducers on the hydroxylation of warfarin isomers

	Hydroxylated warfarin metabolites (nmol metabolite formed per nmol Cyt. *P*-450)			
	R-Isomer		*S*-Isomer	
	7-OH	8-OH	7-OH	8-OH
Control	0.22	0.04	0.04	0.01
Phenobarbitone	0.36	0.07	0.09	0.02
3-Methylcholanthrene	0.08	0.50	0.04	0.04

Data from Table 3.6 in Gibson and Skett (1986).

as does induction. The environmental impact of inhibition is, however, probably less than that of induction. Inhibition also may be relevant to the toxic effects of substances encountered in the workplace. For example, workers exposed to the solvent dimethylformamide seem more likely to suffer alcohol-induced flushes than those not exposed, possibly owing to the inhibition of alcohol metabolism.

There are many different types of inhibitor of the microsomal monooxygenase system. Thus, there are inhibitors which appear to bind as substrates and are competitive inhibitors, such as dichlorobiphenyl, which inhibits the *O*-demethylation of *p*-nitroanisole. There are those inhibitors which are metabolized to compounds which bind strongly to the active site of the enzyme, such as piperonyl butoxide, which probably acts by forming an inactive complex with cytochrome *P*-450, which becomes irreversibly inhibited. There

are indeed many compounds which form such inhibitory complexes with cytochrome *P*-450, including some commonly used drugs, such as triacetyloleandomycin. Some inhibitors destroy cytochrome *P*-450, such as carbon tetrachloride, cyclophosphamide, carbon disulphide and allyl-isopropylacetamide. Finally, there are those which interfere with the synthesis of the enzyme, such as cobalt chloride, which inhibits cytochrome *P*-450 *in vivo* by interfering with the synthesis of the haem portion of the enzyme.

Other enzymes which are also involved in biotransformation which also may be inhibited and which are toxicologically relevant are the esterases, which are inhibited by organophosphorus compounds. Inhibition of monoamine oxidases by drugs such as iproniazid is important clinically, because it results in the decreased metabolism of amines such as tyramine which may be ingested in the diet. These amines may thereby accumulate and can have profound physiological effects, which in some cases may be fatal.

Pathological State

The influence of disease states on metabolism and toxicity has not been well explored. Diseases of the liver might be expected to affect metabolism, but in practice different liver diseases can influence metabolism differently (Hoyumpa and Schenker, 1982). Indeed, some metabolic pathways are unaffected by liver damage. For example, the glucuronidation of paracetamol, morphine and oxazepam was not found to be affected by liver cirrhosis in human subjects. Conversely, the oxidation of a number of drugs such as barbiturates, antipyrine and methadone and the conjugation of salicylates with glycine were all depressed by cirrhosis. Disease states such as influenza are also known to affect drug metabolizing enzymes, possibly via the production of interferon in response to the infection.

Age

In general, animals at the extremes of age—neonates and geriatrics—are less able to metabolize foreign compounds than are adult animals between these extremes. However, the development of drug metabolizing ability is complex and depends on the particular substrate, and is influenced also by sex and species. For example, in the rat phase 1 metabolic activity may develop only after weaning for some demethylation reactions but the *p*-hydroxylation of aniline develops from birth. With phase 2 reactions, again, some are low at birth, such as glucuronidation, whereas acetylation and sulphation are at adult levels, even in the fetus in the guinea-pig.

In rats monooxygenase activity begins to decline when the animals reach 1 year of age.

These effects on drug metabolism may be translated into·differences in toxicity, but it is not always the young animal which is more susceptible. For example, paracetamol is less hepatotoxic in young mice than in adults. This may be due to the fact that the development of the cytochrome *P*-450 system required to activate paracetamol (see below) reaches maximum adult levels more slowly than hepatic glutathione levels (Hart and Timbrell, 1979).

Diet

Although there is a paucity of information in this area, it is clear that dietary deficiencies can affect the metabolism of foreign compounds by altering the enzymes involved (Gibson and Skett, 1986). Thus, a low-protein diet will generally decrease the activity of the monooxygenases and decrease the content of cytochrome *P*-450. For example, rats fed a low-protein (5 per cent) diet show 50 per cent of the *in vitro* microsomal enzyme activity of rats fed a normal diet (20 per cent protein). The effect occurs within 24 h and the enzyme activity is minimal after 4 days. *In vivo* findings are in agreement with these observations. The decrease in microsomal enzyme activity due to a low-protein diet may result in reduced toxicity. For example, carbon tetrachloride hepatotoxicity is less in protein-deficient rats when compared with normal animals. However, other changes may occur which have the opposite effect, and so paracetamol is more hepatotoxic in protein-deficient animals, possibly owing to decreased hepatic glutathione levels. As with protein deficiency, a dietary deficiency in lipid such as linoleic acid also tends to decrease levels of cytochrome *P*-450.

Changes in carbohydrate seem to have few effects on drug metabolism, although an increase in glucose intake seems to decrease hepatic cytochrome *P*-450 and inhibit barbiturate metabolism.

The effects of starvation seem to be variable, with some microsomal enzyme activities being increased and others decreased. Deficiencies in vitamins in general also reduce the activity of the monooxygenases, although there are exceptions to this.

Chiral Factors in Metabolism

The importance of chiral factors in metabolism and toxicity has been recognized only relatively recently. The presence of a chiral centre in a molecule, giving rise to isomers, may influence the routes of metabolism and toxicity of that compound. Alternatively, metabolism may yield a specific isomer as a product from a molecule without a chiral centre. For example, it has now been found that only the glutaminic acid derived from the *S*-(−) enantiomer of thalidomide is embryotoxic, not that formed from the *R*-(+) enantiomer.

Benzo[a]pyrene is metabolized stereoselectively by a particular cytochrome *P*-450 isenozyme, *P*-450c, to the (+)-7*R*,8*S* oxide, which, in turn, is metabolized by epoxide hydrolase to the (−)-7*R*,8*R* dihydrodiol. This metabolite is further metabolized to (+)-benzo[a]pyrene, 7*R*,8*S* dihydrodiol, 9*S*,10*R* epoxide, in which the hydroxyl group and epoxide are *trans* and which is more mutagenic than are other enantiomers. The (−)-7*R*,8*R* dihydrodiol of benzo[a]pyrene is ten times more tumorigenic than is the (+)-7*S*,8*S* enantiomer.

It was felt that in this case the configuration was more important for tumorigenicity than the chemical reactivity.

The hydroxylation of the drug bufuralol (Figure 37) in the 1 position only occurs with the (+) isomer, whereas for hydroxylation in the 4 and 6 position the (−) isomer is the substrate. Glucuronidation of the side-chain hydroxyl group is specific for the (+) isomer. A further complication in human subjects is that the 1-hydroxylation is under genetic control, being dependent on the debrisoquine hydroxylator status. The selectivity for the isomers for the hydroxylations is virtually abolished in poor metabolizers. As well as cytochrome *P*-450, other enzymes are specific for or form specific isomers. Thus, epoxide hydrolase forms *trans* dihydrodiols from cyclic epoxides. Glutathione transferases are also stereospecific enzymes.

TOXICATION VERSUS DETOXICATION

The biotransformation of foreign compounds is often regarded as detoxication because it usually converts compounds into more water-soluble, readily excreted substances. This tends to decrease the exposure of the animal to the compound and so tends to decrease the toxicity. However, in some cases the reverse occurs and a

metabolite is produced which is more toxic than the parent compound. There are many factors which affect this, such as the dose, availability of cofactors and the relative activity of the various drug metabolizing enzymes. There may also be several, competing pathways of metabolism— some leading to detoxication, others to toxicity. Factors which alter the balance between these competing pathways will alter the eventual toxicity. This balance between toxication and detoxication pathways (Figure 38) is very important in toxicology and underlies some of the factors which affect toxicity (Nelson and Harvison, 1987; Monks and Lau, 1988). Although in many cases the toxic metabolites are generated by the enzymes involved in phase I pathways, there are now a number of examples where phase II conjugation reactions are involved in toxication as opposed to detoxication processes.

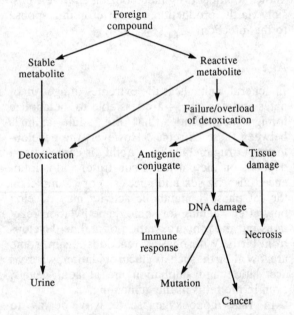

Figure 38 Some of the various consequences of biotransformation. From Timbrell (1989)

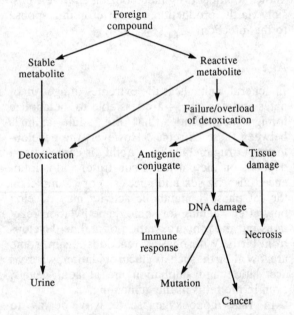

Figure 37   Stereo-selective hydroxylation of bufuralol. From Timbrell (1991)

Paracetamol

A prime example of the role of competing metabolic pathways in toxicity and the importance of endogenous cofactors is afforded by the drug paracetamol (acetaminophen) (Monks and Lau, 1988). This widely used drug is unfortunately sometimes taken in overdose. Such overdoses cause centrilobular hepatic necrosis in man and experimental animals, and a wealth of research has revealed that this toxicity is due in part to metabolism of the drug.

There are three pathways of metabolism for paracetamol (Figure 39), of which the two most important quantitatively are sulphate and glucuronic acid conjugation. The third, resulting in conjugation with glutathione, only represents a few per cent of the dose in humans. This latter pathway involves an initial reaction catalysed by cytochrome *P*-450, producing a reactive metabolite which is normally detoxified by conjugation with glutathione. The resulting glutathione conjugate is then further metabolized to a cysteine conjugate which is acetylated and excreted as a *N*-acetylcysteine conjugate or mercapturic acid.

Hepatotoxicity ensues when a sufficiently large dose of paracetamol is taken to deplete the liver of the majority of the glutathione (to 20 per cent or less in experimental animals). This means that the reactive metabolite is able to react with cellular macromolecules such as protein, covalently bind to these macromolecules and cause hepatic necrosis. The nature of the reactive metabolite has received much attention but seems to be a quinoneimine (*N*-acetyl-*p*-benzoquinoneimine; NAPQI). However, its precursor is not clear.

N-hydroxyparacetamol was postulated as the metabolite, produced by the microsomal monooxygenases, which yielded the quinoneimine after a chemical rearrangement involving dehydration. However, this metabolite has been synthesized, and studies with this compound and other indirect evidence have indicated that it is not likely to be the metabolite which is the precursor of the quinoneimine. Also, the 3,4-epoxide, another candidate for the precursor of the reactive intermediate, does not seem to be formed. 3-Hydroxyparacetamol is also formed but does not seem to be involved. In liver microsomal incubations both *in vitro* and *in vivo*, radiolabelled paracetamol binds covalently to protein, and the major adduct isolated from these protein conjugates is 3-cystein-*S*-yl-4-hydroxyaniline. However, the specific consequences of the covalent binding are as yet unclear.

It seems, however, that an electrophilic metabolite is involved in some way in the hepatotoxicity. It is clear that the NAPQI is a cytotoxic, reactive metabolite of paracetamol, produced via a cytochrome *P*-450 mediated oxidation, which will react with glutathione. It reacts with glutathione in two ways: (1) by forming a conjugate; (2) by oxidizing glutathione and being itself reduced back to paracetamol. NADPH can also reduce NAPQI back to paracetamol in a reaction which may involve glutathione reductase. Deacetylation of paracetamol can also occur, giving rise to *p*-aminophenol and subsequent metabolites. *p*-Aminophenol is a known nephrotoxin, and this might account for the nephrotoxicity seen after overdoses of paracetamol and occasionally reported with chronic dosage.

There are two main detoxication pathways for paracetamol: conjugation with (1) glucuronic acid and (2) sulphate. The oxidative pathway(s) leading to the mercapturic acid accounts for about 5 per cent in man. The deacetylation pathway is also presumably minor. However, this balance may be altered in a number of ways. Large doses of paracetamol may deplete animals of sulphate as well as glutathione. Metabolism may thereby

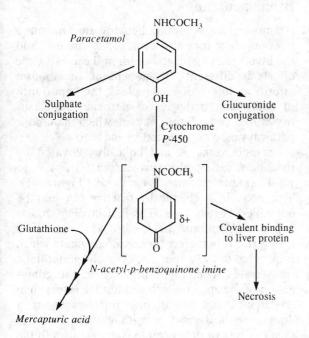

Figure 39 Metabolism of paracetamol. From Timbrell (1982)

be diverted through the oxidative pathway catalysed by cytochrome *P*-450 and more will be conjugated with glucuronic acid (Figure 39). Factors which affect the activity of the microsomal enzymes such as inducing agents will also alter this balance. For example, pretreatment of animals with phenobarbitone will increase the hepatotoxicity in some species (rats) by increasing the amount metabolized via the cytochrome *P*-450 pathway. However, this pretreatment will also increase the activity of glucuronyl transferase and in some species (hamsters) this effect will decrease the hepatotoxicity. In the hamster the oxidative pathway is quantitatively greater than in the rat, a factor which underlies the large difference in susceptibility to the hepatotoxicity between these two species.

Carbon Tetrachloride

Carbon tetrachloride is a potent hepatotoxin which has been extensively studied. The centrilobular hepatic necrosis, which is the major toxic effect it causes, is dependent upon metabolism via the cytochrome *P*-450 system. However, the enzyme system is acting as a reductase in this instance. Cytochrome *P*-450 donates an electron to the carbon tetrachloride molecule and thereby allows the homolytic cleavage of a carbon–chlorine bond (Figure 40). This yields the trichloromethyl radical and a chloride ion. The trichloromethyl radical may then react with oxygen to give the trichloromethylperoxy radical. Alternatively, the trichloromethyl radical can abstract a hydro-

gen atom from polyunsaturated lipids and thereby form a lipid radical and a stable product, chloroform. The lipid radical can then proceed to react with other cellular constituents and cause a cascade of disturbances within the cell, including peroxidation of lipids. Alternatively, the trichloromethyl radical can react covalently with lipids and proteins. The trichloromethylperoxy radical is believed to be the reactive metabolite responsible for lipid peroxidation.

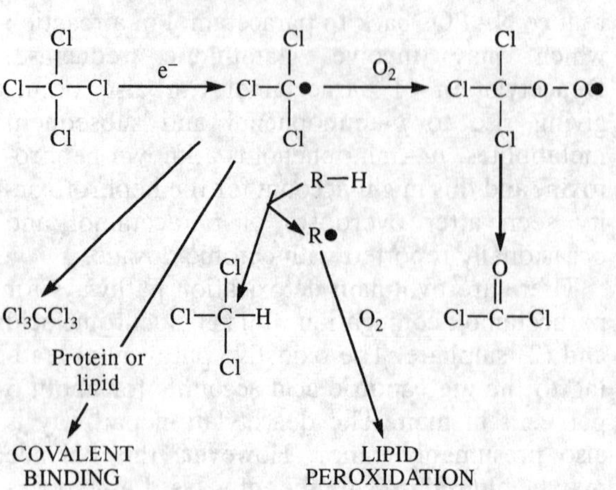

The oxygen concentration is important for the formation of the trichloromethylperoxy radical and the lipid peroxidation. As carbon tetrachloride is metabolically activated by cytochrome *P*-450 in the smooth endoplasmic reticulum, the reactive radicals formed are able to react with the enzyme itself and the lipids of the endoplasmic reticulum. The result is that cytochrome *P*-450 is destroyed by carbon tetrachloride. Consequently, if animals are given a small dose of carbon tetrachloride ($0.05 \, \text{ml kg}^{-1}$), a subsequent larger dose is less toxic than the same dose administered to a control animal (Glende, 1972). This is because the form of cytochrome *P*-450 which activates carbon tetrachloride is destroyed. Carbon tetrachloride is thus only hepatotoxic when it can be metabolically activated (Sesardic *et al.*, 1989).

Bromobenzene

Bromobenzene is another hepatotoxic compound but one which may also damage the kidneys, and the involvement of metabolism in these two toxic effects is different. Bromobenzene metabolism affords an interesting example of the importance of competing pathways of detoxication versus toxication and of the way in which metabolic pathways may be switched by inducers.

Bromobenzene is metabolically activated by oxidation, catalysed by cytochrome(s) *P*-450, to yield an intermediate 3,4-epoxide (Figure 41). This epoxide is chemically reactive but may be detoxified in two ways. The first involves conjugation with glutathione (Figure 41), eventually giving rise to a mercapturic acid conjugate which is excreted in the urine. The cytosolic glutathione transferases seem to be involved in the conjugation of the epoxide with glutathione rather than the microsomal glutathione transferases or a direct chemical reaction with glutathione. The second route of detoxication is metabolism to the dihydrodiol mediated by epoxide hydrolase. Just

Figure 40 Metabolism of carbon tetrachloride. From Timbrell (1986)

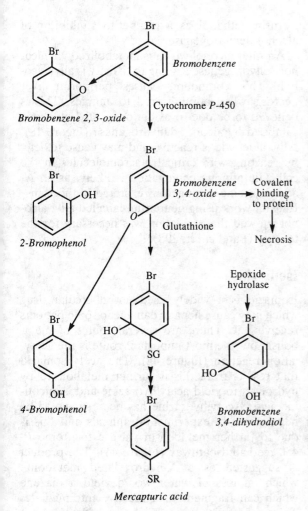

Figure 41 Some of the metabolic pathways for bromobenzene. From Timbrell (1982)

2,3-epoxide pathway, as indicated by an increased excretion of *o*-bromophenol, and decreases the toxicity (Table 9). Also, mice which have the cytochrome *P*-450 isoenzyme which catalyses the formation of the 3,4-epoxide show greater hepatic damage after doses of bromobenzene than do those who do not.

In vitro the 3,4-epoxide binds to microsomal protein and seems to prefer to bind to histidine residues, whereas the 2,3-epoxide binds to haemoglobin and prefers to bind to the cysteine residues. It is suggested that the 2,3-epoxide is more stable than the 3,4-epoxide and therefore reacts with a different target protein. However, the 3,4-epoxide was detected in both blood *in vivo* and hepatocyte incubation medium when animals or hepatocytes were exposed to bromobenzene. Clearly the reactive intermediate has sufficient stability to move within the hepatocyte and even leave the cell. There would seem to be an optimum reactivity for the epoxide in order for it to be toxic and react with critical sites on macromolecules. Reactive metabolites which are chemically too reactive will tend to interact with biological molecules indiscriminately and may never reach critical target molecules.

Further metabolism of the bromophenols may also occur, to give bromoquinols and bromocatechols. 2-Bromohydroquinone will deplete glutathione in both liver and kidney but only causes pathological damage in the kidney. It is believed that the diglutathione conjugate of bromohydroquinone (Figure 42) is the nephrotoxic agent (Monks and Lau, 1988).

as with paracetamol, a sufficiently large dose of bromobenzene will deplete the liver of glutathione and, hence, the reactive epoxide will bind to tissue macromolecules, a process which seems to underlie the liver necrosis.

There is also another oxidation pathway, however, also catalysed by cytochrome(s) *P*-450, which gives rise to another epoxide, the 2,3-epoxide, which is believed to be non-toxic. The evidence for this comes from the effect of inducers on the toxicity and metabolism, and illustrates switching of metabolic pathways. Pretreatment of animals with phenobarbitone increases metabolism via the 3,4-epoxide pathway and increases the toxicity. Conversely, pretreatment with 3-methylcholanthrene increases metabolism via the

Table 9 Effect of induction with 3-methylcholanthrene on the metabolism of bromobenzene in rats

Metabolites	% Total urinary metabolites	
	Control	3-MC Treated
4-Bromophenylmercapturic acid	72	31
4-Bromophenol	14	20
4-Bromocatechol	6	10
4-Bromophenyldihydrodiol	3	17
2-Bromophenol	4	21

Data from Zampaglione *et al.* (1973). Dose of bromobenzene 10 mmol kg^{-1}.

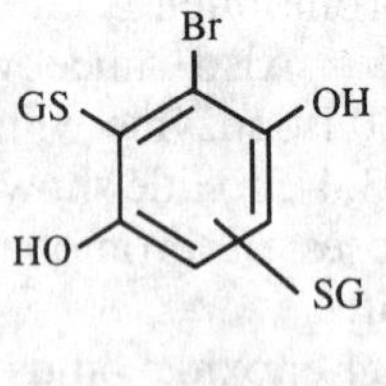

Figure 42   Diglutathione conjugate of bromobenzene

Methanol

Methanol is a widely used and readily available solvent which is often found in combination with ethanol. Consequently, it sometimes features in poisoning cases. The toxicity of methanol illustrates the role of metabolism in toxicity where a chemically reactive metabolite does not seem to be involved. Also, a species difference in detoxication is revealed. It also illustrates the importance of understanding the mechanism of toxicity in order to treat the poisoned patient in a rational way. Methanol is toxic mainly as a result of its metabolism to formic acid (Figure 43). This is a two-step reaction, with metabolism to formaldehyde being catalysed by either alcohol dehydrogenase or catalase. The second metabolic step to give formic acid is catalysed by either aldehyde dehydrogenase or formaldehyde dehydrogenase, an enzyme which requires glutathione.

The formic acid damages the optic nerve, seemingly by inhibiting the mitochondrial enzyme cytochrome oxidase and, hence, reducing the level of ATP available to the nerves. Humans and certain other primates are much more susceptible than are rodents to the toxicity of methanol. It seems that this is due at least in part to the accumulation of formic acid in the susceptible species compared with the non-susceptible species. Formic acid may be detoxified by the action of tetrahydrofolate, giving 10-formyl-tetrahydrofolate. This detoxication seems to be more efficient in rodents than in susceptible primates.

Because the metabolism is clearly important in the toxicity, treatment of the poisoning involves blocking the first step in the metabolic pathway

$$CH_3OH \longrightarrow HCHO \longrightarrow HCOOH$$
Methanol   Formaldehyde   Formic acid

Figure 43   Metabolism of methanol

by using ethanol as a competitive inhibitor of alcohol dehydrogenase.

Another alcohol which is metabolized via alcohol dehydrogenase leading to toxicity is allyl alcohol. This compound causes periportal liver necrosis when administered to animals. This is believed to be due to oxidation to allyl aldehyde catalysed by alcohol dehydrogenase (Figure 18). Allyl aldehyde is reactive and may cause toxicity by reacting with critical macromolecules in the cell. Glutathione conjugation is likely, as an *N*-acetylcysteine conjugate is excreted in the urine. Elegant work using deuterium-labelled allyl alcohol showed that oxidation was necessary for the toxicity (Patel *et al.*, 1983).

Isoniazid

Isoniazid is a widely used antitubercular drug which may cause hepatic damage in some patients receiving it. There are several routes of metabolism but the most important route is the acetylation reaction (Figure 44). The acetylisoniazid that results from this is further metabolized by hydrolysis to yield acetylhydrazine and isonicotinic acid. Acetylhydrazine has been shown to be hepatotoxic in experimental animals and this is due to further metabolism via a cytochrome *P*-450 mediated pathway (Figure 44). The product is suggested as a *N*-hydroxylated metabolite which on loss of water would yield a diazene which can fragment to a reactive intermediate. This may be either a radical or a carbonium ion which may react with proteins and cause hepatic necrosis. This pathway is induced by phenobarbitone, which also increases the covalent binding of the acetyl group to protein and the hepatotoxicity of acetylhydrazine. However, acetylhydrazine may also be further metabolized by a different route, a second acetylation step, which is a detoxication reaction. Both the primary acetylation step, giving acetylisoniazid, and this second step are influenced by the acetylator phenotype (see above).

Therefore, although rapid acetylators produce more acetylisoniazid and therefore more acetylhydrazine, this is then more extensively removed by acetylation to diacetylhydrazine in the rapid acetylator. When the plasma level of acetylhydrazine in human subjects after a dose of isoniazid was determined, it was found that the slow acetylator has a greater exposure to ace-

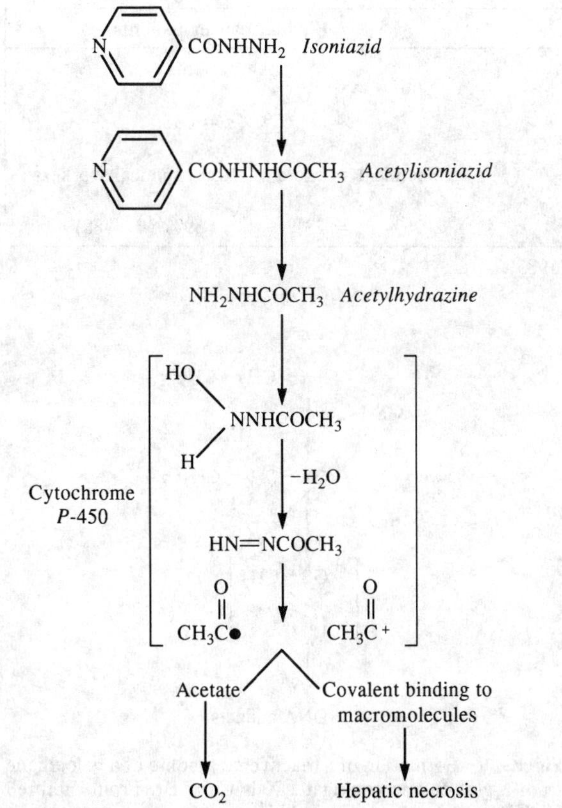

Figure 44 Part of the biotransformation of isoniazid. From Timbrell (1979)

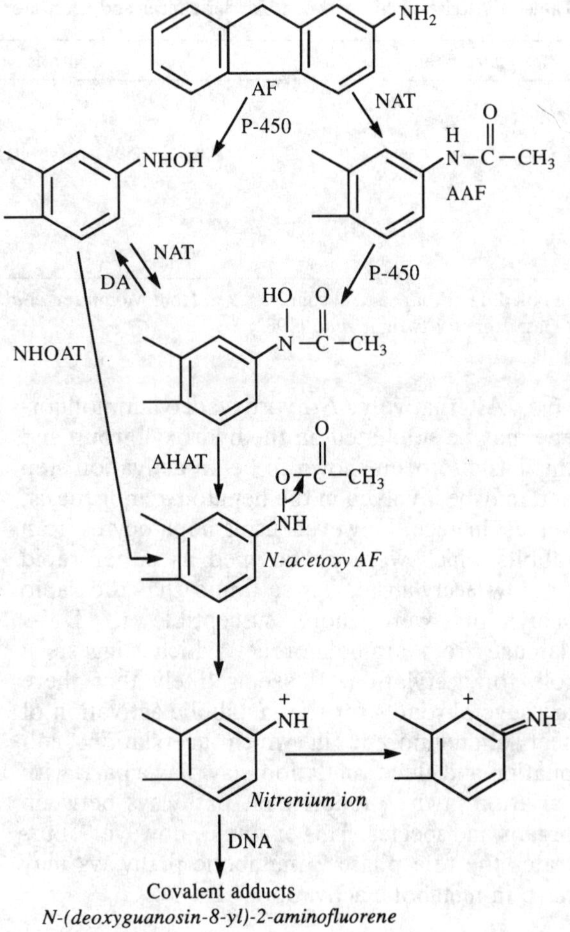

N-(deoxyguanosin-8-yl)-2-aminofluorene

Figure 45 Pathways of metabolic activation of aminofluorene

tylhydrazine. This example illustrates both the importance of competing detoxication and toxication routes of metabolism and also the influence which genetic factors may have on toxicity (Timbrell, 1979; 1991).

Aromatic Amines

Another example in which acetylation features is the carcinogenicity of aromatic amines. For some aromatic amines acetylation is a detoxication reaction. For example, 2-naphthylamine and benzidine both cause bladder cancer in man and it seems likely that the acetylation reaction reduces the carcinogenicity. Acetylated derivatives of benzidine are less reactive towards DNA and cause less damage to this macromolecule than does the parent compound. Several studies have shown that the slow acetylator is more at risk than is the fast acetylator from developing bladder cancer, and

this is especially so for those whose work may expose them to aromatic amines (Table 10).

However, acetylation may be an activation step, involved in the toxic pathway for some compounds such as aminofluorene, for example. There are several metabolic pathways involving acetylation and N-hydroxylation yielding *N*-acetoxy aminofluorene (Figure 45). The acetylation steps seem to involve similar but possibly distinct enzymes, either *N*-acetyltransferase (NAT), arylhydroxamic acid acetyl transferase (AHAT) or *N*-hydroxy-*O*-acetyl transferase (NHOAT). The *N*-acetoxy aminofluorene may rearrange to yield a reactive nitrenium ion which can react with DNA to give covalent adducts such as *N*-(deoxyguanosin-8-yl)-2-aminofluorene (Figure 45). This has been shown both *in vitro* and *in*

Table 10   Relationship between bladder cancer and acetylator phenotype in human subjects

Acetylator phenotype	Controls	Bladder cancer patients	
		All patients	
Slow	59% (n = 991)	65% (n = 681)[a]	
		Chemical workers	Non-chemical workers
Slow		96% (n = 23)	59% (n = 88)[b]

[a] Pooled data from several sources taken from Mommsen *et al.* (1985).
[b] Data from Cartwright *et al.* (1982).

vivo. Alternatively, *N*-hydroxyacetylaminofluorene may be sulphated on the hydroxyl group and this has also been shown to be an activation step and may be involved in the hepatocarcinogenesis, at least in mice. However, using hepatocytes from rabbits which were phenotyped as either rapid or slow acetylators, it was found that the rapid acetylators were more susceptible to DNA damage from aminofluorene, which suggests a role for acetylation. It seems likely that there are several routes for the metabolic activation of acetylaminofluorene in which acetylation, sulphation and glucuronidation may play a part, with variation in the predominant pathways between organs and species. This example, however, illustrates the role phase 2 metabolic pathways may have in metabolic activation.

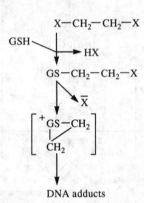

Figure 46   Formation of a reactive metabolite of a haloalkane from a glutathione conjugate. X is Cl or Br. From Timbrell (1991)

Haloalkanes

The toxicity of haloalkanes illustrates the role of glutathione conjugation in metabolic activation as opposed to detoxication. A number of haloalkanes with various structures are metabolically activated by conjugation with glutathione. For example, the compounds 1,2-dichloroethane and 1,2-dibromoethane are both conjugated with glutathione in a reaction catalysed by glutathione transferase (Figure 46). The resultant haloethyl glutathione conjugate can lose the halogen, to yield a charged episulphonium ion which can react with DNA. Incubation of 1,2-dibromoethane with DNA and glutathione transferase gives the adduct *S*-[2-(*N*[7]-guanyl)ethyl] glutathione. This interaction is believed to be responsible for the mutagenicity of these compounds.

Some haloalkanes are nephrotoxic and glutathione conjugation has been shown to mediate this toxic effect also. For example, hexachlorobu-

tadiene has been shown to be conjugated with glutathione, which is then further metabolized to a cysteine conjugate (Figure 47). This cysteine conjugate may then undergo further metabolism: either acetylation, deamination or cleavage by the action of the enzyme cysteine conjugate β-lyase. This gives rise to a thiol conjugate which has been shown to be nephrotoxic and is able to covalently bind to protein.

As well as enzymes commonly associated with drug metabolism, sometimes enzymes normally involved in intermediary metabolism may be responsible for metabolic activation. Thus, the metabolite of the drug valproic acid, 2-*n*-propyl-4-pentenoic acid, is believed to be involved in the hepatotoxicity. This metabolite, $\triangle^4$-VPA, is metabolized by the β-oxidation system, to give 3-oxo-$\triangle^4$-VPA. This is believed to be a reactive metabolite which inactivates the enzyme 3-ketoacyl-CoA thiolase, the terminal enzyme of the fatty acid oxidation system. This reactive metabolite may be

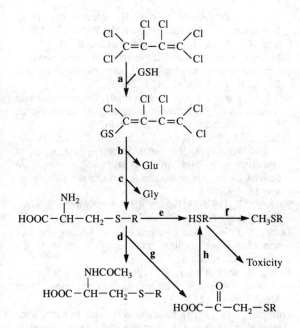

Figure 47 Metabolic activation of hexachlorobutadiene involving the action of β-lyase. The toxicity indicated is nephrotoxicity. R represents the 1,2,3,4,4-pentachlorobutadienyl moiety. GSH, glutathione. Glu, glutamate; Gly, glycine. The letters a–h represent the enzymes involved in the particular reactions: a, glutathione transferase; b, glutamyl transferase; c, dipeptidase; d, *N*-acetyltransferase; e, β-lyase; f thiol *S*-methyltransferase; g, deaminase; h, thiopyruvate lyase

involved in the hepatotoxicity of the drug (Baillie, 1992).

Thus, in conclusion it can be seen that biotransformation is often a crucial aspect of the toxicity of a compound and may in a variety of circumstances be the cause of toxicity rather than a process of detoxication.

REFERENCES

Anders, M. (ed.) (1985). *Bioactivation of Foreign Compounds*. Academic Press, New York

Baillie, T. A. (1992). Metabolic activation of valproic acid and drug-mediated hepatotoxicity. Role of the terminal olefin, 2-n-propyl-4-pentenoic acid. In Marnett, L. J. (Ed.), *Frontiers in Molecular Toxicology*. American Chemical Society. Washington DC

Beedham, C. (1988). Molybdenum hydroxylases. In Gorrod, J. W., Oelschlager, H. and Caldwell, J. (Eds), *Metabolism of Xenobiotics*. Taylor and Francis, London, pp. 51–58

Caldwell, J. (1980). Comparative aspects of detoxication in mammals. In Jakoby, W. B. (Ed.), *Enzy-*

matic Basis of Detoxication, Vol. 1. Academic Press, New York, pp. 85–111

Caldwell, J. and Jakoby, W. B. (1983). *Biological Basis of Detoxication*. Academic Press, New York

Cartwright, R. A., Glashan, R. W., Rogers, H. J., Ahmad, R. A., Barham-Hall, D., Higgins, E. and Kahn, M. A. (1982). Role of *N*-acetyltransferase phenotypes in bladder carcinogenesis: A pharmacogenetic approach to bladder cancer. *Lancet*, **ii**, 842–846

Damani, L. A. (1988). The flavin-containing monooxygenase as an amine oxidase. In Gorrod, J. W., Oelschlager, H. and Caldwell, J. (Eds), *Metabolism of Xenobiotics*. Taylor and Francis, London, pp. 59–70

Eling, T., Boyd, J., Reed, G., Mason, R. and Sivarajoh, K. (1983). Xenobiotic metabolism by prostaglandin endoperoxide synthetase. *Drug Metab. Rev.*, **14**, 1023–1053

Gibson, G G and Skett, P. (1986). *Introduction to Drug Metabolism*. Chapman and Hall, London

Glende, E. A. (1972). Carbon tetrachloride-induced protection against carbon tetrachloride toxicity. The role of the liver microsomal drug-metabolising system. *Biochem. Pharmacol.* **21**, 1679–1702

Gonzalez, F. J., Skoda, R. C., Kimura, S., Umeno, M., Zanger, U. M., Nebert, D. W., Gelboin, H. V., Hardwick, J. P. and Meyer, U. A. (1988). Characterisation of the common genetic defect in humans deficient in debrisoquine metabolism. *Nature*, **331**, 442–446

Gorrod, J. W., Oelschlager, H. and Caldwell, J. (Eds) (1988). *Metabolism of Xenobiotics*. Taylor and Francis, London

Gorrod, J. W. and Raman, A. (1989). Imines as intermediates in oxidative aralkylamine metabolism. *Drug Metab. Rev.*, **20**, 307–339

Hart, J. G. and Timbrell, J. A. (1979). The effect of age on paracetamol hepatotoxicity in mice. *Biochem. Pharmacol.*, **28**, 3015–3017

Hathway, D. E. (1984). *Molecular Aspects of Toxicology*. Royal Society of Chemistry, London

Hathway, D. E., Brown, S. S., Chasseaud, L. F. and Hutson, D. H. (Eds) (1970–1981) *Foreign Compound Metabolism in Mammals*, Vols 1–6. Chemical Society, London

Hawkins, D. R. (Ed.) (1988). *Biotransformations*, Vol. 1. Royal Society of Chemistry, London

Hoyumpa, A. M. and Schenker, S. (1982). Major drug interactions: effect of liver disease, alcohol and malnutrition. *Ann. Rev. Med.*, **33**, 113–50

Jakoby, W. B. (Ed.) (1980). *Enzymatic Basis of Detoxication*, Vols 1, 2. Academic Press, New York

Jakoby, W. B., Bend, J. R. and Caldwell, J. (Eds) (1982). *Metabolic Basis of Detoxication: Metabolism of Functional Groups*. Academic Press, New York

Jay, G. E. (1955). Variation in response of various mouse strains to hexobarbital (EVIPAL). *Proc. Soc. Exptl. Biol. Med.*, **90**, 378–380

Jenner, P. and Testa, B. (Eds) (1981). *Concepts in*

Drug Metabolism, Parts A, B. Marcel Dekker, New York

Ketterer, B. (1982). The role of non-enzymatic reactions of glutathione in xenobiotic metabolism. *Drug Metab. Rev.*, **13**, 161–187

Larsson, R., Boutin, J. and Moldeus, P. (1988). Peroxidase-catalysed metabolic activation of xenobiotics. In Gorrod, J. W., Oelschlager, H. and Caldwell, J. (Eds), *Metabolism of Xenobiotics*. Taylor and Francis, London, pp. 43–50.

Lunde, P. K. M., Frislide, K. and Hansteen, V. (1977). Disease and acetylation polymorphism. *Clin. Pharmacokin.*, **2**, 182–197

Mommsen, S., Barfod, N. M. and Aagaard, J. (1985). *N*-Acetyltransferase phenotypes in the urinary bladder carcinogenesis of a low risk population. *Carcinogenesis*, **6**, 199–201

Monks, T. J. and Lau, S. S. (1988). Reactive intermediates and their toxicological significance. *Toxicology*, **52**, 1–53

Mulder, G. J., Kroese, E. D. and Meerman, J. H. N. (1988). The generation of reactive intermediates from xenobiotics by sulphate conjugation and their role in drug toxicity. In Gorrod, J. W., Oelschlager, H. and Caldwell, J. (Eds), *Metabolism of Xenobiotics*. Taylor and Francis, London, pp. 243–250

Nebert, D. W. (1989). The Ah locus: Genetic differences in toxicity, cancer, mutations and birth defects. *CRC Crit. Rev. Toxicol.* **20**, 153–174

Nebert, D. W. and Gonzalez, E. J. (1985). Cytochrome P-450 gene expression and regulation. *Trends Pharmacol. Sci.* **6**, 160–164

Nelson, S. D. (1982). Metabolic activation and drug toxicity. *J. Med. Chem.*, **25**, 753–765

Nelson, S. D. and Harvison, P. J. (1987). Roles of cytochrome P-450 in chemically induced cytotoxicity. In Guengerich, F. P. (Ed.), *Mammalian Cytochromes P-450*. CRC Press, Boca Raton, Florida, pp. 19–80

Netter, K. J. (1987). Mechanisms of oxidative drug metabolism and inhibition. *Pharmacol. Therap.*, **33**, 1–9

Okey, A. B., Roberts, E. A., Harper, P. A. and Denison, M. S. (1986). Induction of drug metabolising enzymes; mechanisms and consequences. *Clin. Biochem.*, **19**, 132–141

Parke, D. V. (1968). *The Biochemistry of Foreign Compounds*. Pergamon Press, Oxford

Patel, J. M., Gordon, W. P., Nelson, S. D. and Leibman, K. C. (1983) Comparison of hepatic biotransformation and toxicity of allyl alcohol [1,1-^{2}H$_2$] allyl alcohol. *Drug Metab. Dispos.*, **11**, 164–166

Pohl, L. R. (1979). Biochemical toxicology of chloroform. *Rev. Biochem. Toxicol.*, **1**, 79–107

Powis, G., Talcott, R. E. and Schenkman, J. B. (1977). Kinetic and spectral evidence for multiple species of cytochrome P-450 in liver microsomes. In Ullrich, V., Roots, A., Hildebrandt, A., Estabrook, R. W.

and Conney, A. H. (Eds), *Microsomes and Drug Oxidations*, Pergamon Press, New York, 127–135

Quinn, G. P., Axelrod, J. and Brodie, B. B. (1958). Species, strain and sex differences in metabolism of hexobarbitone, amidopyrine, antipyrine and aniline. *Biochem. Pharmacol.*, **1**, 152–159

Reed, D. J. and Beatty, P. W. (1980). Biosynthesis and regulation of glutathione: toxicological implications. *Rev. Biochem. Toxicol.*, **2**, 213–241

Sesardic, D., Rich, K. J., Edwards, R. J., Davies, D. S. and Boobis, A. R. (1989). Selective destruction of cytochrome P-450d and associated monooxygenase activity by carbon tetrachloride in the rat. *Xenobiotica*, **19**, 795–811

Sitar, D. S. (1989). Human drug metabolism *in vivo*. *Pharmacol. Therap.* **43**, 363–375

Testa, B. (1989). Mechanisms of chiral recognition in xenobiotic metabolism and drug–receptor interactions. *Chirality*, **1**, 7–9

Testa, B. and Jenner, P. (1981). Inhibitors of cytochrome P-450s and their mechanism of action. *Drug Metab. Rev.*, **12**, 1–117

Timbrell, J. A. (1979). Studies on the role of acetylhydrazine in isoniazil hepatotoxicity. *Arch. Toxicol.* Suppl. 2, 1–8

Timbrell, J. A. (1982). *Principles of Biochemical Toxicology*. Taylor and Francis, London

Timbrell, J. A. (1986). The liver as a target organ. In Cohen, G. M. (Ed.), *Target Organ Toxicity*. CRC Press, Boca Raton, Florida

Timbrell, J. A. (1988). Acetylation and its toxicological significance. In Gorrod, J. W., Oelschlager, H. and Caldwell, J. (Eds), *Metabolism of Xenobiotics*. Taylor and Francis, London, pp. 259–266

Timbrell, J. A. (1989). *Introduction to Toxicology*. Taylor and Francis, London, pp. 145–173

Timbrell, J. A. (1991). *Principles of Biochemical Toxicology*, 2nd ed. Taylor and Francis, London

Timbrell, J. A., Facchini, V., Harland, S. J. and Mansilla-Tinoco, R. (1984). Hydralazine-induced lupus: Is there a toxic pathway? *Europ. J. Clin. Pharmacol.* **27**, 555–559

Tyndale, R. F., Inaba, T. and Kalow, W. (1989). Evidence in humans for variant allozymes of the non-deficient sparteine/debrisoquine monooxygenase (P450IID1) *in vitro*. *Drug Metab. Disp.*, **17**, 334–340

Van Bladeren, P. J., den Besten, C., Bruggeman, I. M., Mertens, J. J. W. M., van Ommen, B., Spenkelink, B., Rutten, A. L. M., Temmink, J. H. M. and Vos, R. M. E. (1988). Glutathione conjugation as a toxication reaction. In Gorrod, J. W., Oelschlager, H. and Caldwell, J. (Eds), *Metabolism of Xenobiotics*. Taylor and Francis, London, pp. 267–274

Weber, W. (1987). *The Acetylator Genes and Drug Response*. Oxford University Press, New York

Whitlock, J. P. (1989). The control of cytochrome P-450 gene expression by dioxin. *Trends Pharmacol. Sci.* **10**, 285–288

Williams, R. T. (1959). *Detoxication Mechanisms.* Chapman and Hall, London

Zampaglione, N., Jollow, D. J., Mitchell, J. R., Stripp, B., Hamrick, M. and Gillette, J. R. (1973). Role of detoxifying enzymes in bromobenzene-induced liver necrosis. *J. Pharmacol. Exp. Ther.*, **187**, 218–227

Zeigler, D. M. (1984). Metabolic oxygenation of organic nitrogen and sulphur compounds. In Mitchell, J. R. and Horning, M. G. (Eds), *Drug Metabolism and Drug Toxicity*. Raven Press, New York, pp. 33–53

Zeigler, D. M. (1985). Molecular basis for N-oxygenation of sec- and tert-amines. In Gorrod, J. W. and Damani, L. A. (Eds) *Biological Oxidation of Nitrogen in Organic Molecules*. Ellis Horwood, Chichester, pp. 43–52

FURTHER READING

Caldwell, J., Sangster, S. A. and Sutton, J. D. (1986). The role of metabolic activation in target organ toxicity. In Cohen, G. M. (Ed.), *Target Organ Toxicity, Vol. 1*. CRC Press, Boca Raton, Florida, pp. 37–54

Goldstein, J. A. and Faletto, M. B. (1993). Advances in mechanisms of activation and deactivation of environmental chemicals. *Environmental Health Perspectives*, **100**, 169–176

Haley, T. J. (1987). Absorption, distribution, biotransformation, conjugation, and excretion of xenobiotics. In Haley, T. J. and Berndt, W. O. (Eds), *Handbook of Toxicology*. Hemisphere Publishing Corporation, New York, pp. 20–43

Mulder, G. J. (1992). Glucuronidation and its role in regulation of biological activity of drugs. *Annual Review of Pharmacology and Toxicology*, **32**, 25–50

Sipes J. G. and Gandolfi, A. J. (1991). Biotransformation of toxicants. In Amdur, M. O., Doull, J. and Klaassen, C. D. (Eds), *Casarett and Doull's Toxicology. The Basic Science of Poisons*. 4th edn. Pergamon Press, New York, pp. 88–126

4 Toxicokinetics

A. G. Renwick

INTRODUCTION

In recent years there has been an increasing emphasis on the development of *in vitro* tests for specific organ toxicity in order to reduce the numbers of animals given toxic doses of chemicals. However, the logical interpretation of the results of such *in vitro* tests means a greater requirement for the definition of the *in vivo* concentrations of the chemical that could be present in the target organ, the time-course of exposure and the potential for accumulation during repeated dosing. Such information can only be obtained from the results of appropriate *in vivo* studies on the fate of the chemical within the body—that is, its *toxicokinetics*. Toxicokinetics are also of importance in extrapolating both *in vitro* and *in vivo* animal data to man. The basic techniques used in toxicokinetics, such as collecting timed blood and urine samples, can also be investigated in human volunteers, provided, of course, that it is ethical to administer the chemical to humans.

The outcome of *in vivo* toxicity studies is dependent on two main variables: (1) the delivery of the chemical to the site of action and (2) the activity of the chemical at the site of action.

The delivery of the chemical to the site of toxicity (Figure 1) depends on the processes of *absorption* from the site of administration into the general circulation and *distribution* via the blood to the site of action and all body tissues. The concentrations present at the site of action and the duration of exposure depend on the rate of *elimination* from the body, which may be by either *metabolism* or *excretion*. Studies on absorption, distribution, metabolism and excretion, which are often referred to simply as *ADME* studies, form an essential first step in the evaluation of the fate of the chemical in the body (Glocklin, 1982). Usually ADME studies involve following the fate of a radiolabelled dose of the chemical by measuring the total ^{14}C and radiolabelled metabolites in the excreta and also the tissue distribution by autoradiography at various

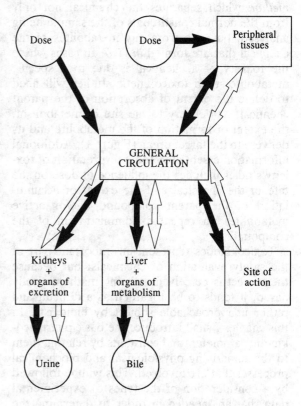

Figure 1 Delivery of chemicals to their site of action. This scheme assumes that the site of toxicity is not locally at the site of administration. Compounds absorbed from the gastro-intestinal tract are transported via the hepatic portal vein to the liver before they enter the general circulation. (Solid arrows refer to the parent compound; open arrows refer to metabolites). Compounds eliminated in the bile may re-enter the general circulation due to an entero-hepatic recirculation

times after dosing. Such studies clearly provide some information on the movement or kinetics of the chemical in the body but provide only a part of the total study of the toxicokinetics of the compound. The purpose of a radiolabelled compound is to provide information on the total balance of all compound-related products whether or not they have been identified and characterized. Thus, the strength of radiolabelled studies is the use of *non-specific detection methods* which allow the detection of all compound-related products. However, this strength is also a weakness in determining exposure of the body to the parent chemical itself or to specific identified metabolites.

Investigation of the kinetics of the parent molecule itself requires the use of a *specific detection method* which separates the chemical not only from the normal constituents of the sample being analysed, but also from any metabolites of the chemical that are formed *in vivo*. In cases where the toxicity of a chemical is due to a specific metabolite, then toxicokinetic studies will need to define the extent of absorption of the parent chemical, its delivery to the site of metabolism, the extent of formation of the metabolite and its delivery to the target organ (Figure 1). Additional information essential to the interpretation of toxicity studies includes the influence of dose on the fate of the chemical and the extent of accumulation of the parent compound and/or active metabolites on repeated administration of the compound.

Toxicokinetics represent an important part of the safety evaluation of chemicals, but because the subject is perceived as being mathematically based, it tends to be regarded as a difficult and rather unapproachable subject by biologists. In this chapter I shall introduce the basic pharmacokinetic parameters and constants by relating them to the underlying physiological and biochemical processes that are involved. This will be followed by a consideration of the types of experimental data that are needed in order to determine the various parameters. The chapter will conclude with a consideration of specific aspects related to the interpretation of high-dose, chronic animal studies.

PHARMACOKINETIC PARAMETERS AND CONSTANTS

Each of the basic processes involved in pharmacokinetics—i.e. absorption, distribution and elimination—may be described by parameters which define the *extent* to which the process occurs and the *rate* at which it occurs. These parameters are usually calculated from plasma concentration—time data.

Absorption

Absorption is the process of transfer of the chemical from the site of administration into the general circulation. Absorption from the gastrointestinal tract is studied most frequently because this is the common route of exposure of experimental animals via gavage dosing or by incorporation of the chemical into the diet. Oral administration is also the most common route by which humans are exposed to chemicals either as drugs or as intentional, incidental or accidental components of the diet. The process of absorption occurs whenever the compound is given by a route other than direct intravascular injection—for example, across the skin, via the airways, from subcutaneous sites and also from the peritoneal cavity.

Rate of Absorption

The rate of absorption depends on both the nature of the chemical and the site of administration.

Lipid-soluble chemicals can readily dissolve in membranes and therefore diffuse across cell walls. In contrast, ionized molecules do not readily enter the lipid membrane matrix in the ionized form and therefore only the un-ionized form freely diffuses across membranes (Figure 2). For strong acids and bases at pH 7.4, the un-ionized form on each side of the membrane is in

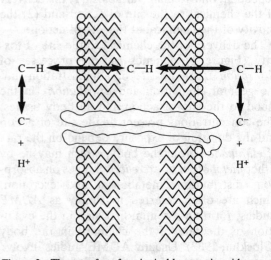

Figure 2 The transfer of an ionizable organic acid across a cell membrane. At equilibrium the concentration of the diffusible form (C-H) will be the same on each side of the membrane. The concentration of the ionized form (C⁻) will depend on the pK_a of the chemical and the pH of the solution

equilibrium with the ionized form, the concentrations of which may be orders of magnitude higher. Thus, only low concentrations of the un-ionized may be present, so that transfer of the chemical across membranes is very slow. For very strong acids and bases and also quaternary amines (which have a fixed positive charge), the absorption rate may be slower than the rate of transfer along the bowel by peristalsis, so that a fraction of the dose is lost in the faeces without ever being absorbed.

The rate of absorption also depends on the site of administration; for example, absorption across the skin is usually extremely slow, since it involves transfer across the stratum corneum—the main permeability barrier of the body. In contrast, absorption from the lungs tends to be rapid, since it involves transfer across a thin membrane which has a large surface area and a good blood supply.

Absorption from the gut is often complex, since chemicals are absorbed less effectively from the stomach than from the duodenum and jejunum because of the smaller surface area and lower pH. In consequence, there can be a delay before any appreciable absorption occurs, while the compound is in the stomach lumen. However, once the dose has left the stomach, it has a large surface area of well-perfused intestine which can allow very rapid absorption.

The kinetic parameter which describes the absorption rate is the absorption rate constant (k_a) or absorption half-life. These parameters assume that the rate of transfer of chemical into the plasma is proportional to the amount of chemical available to be absorbed—i.e. a first-order process (see later). This assumption is often a vast oversimplification and absorption may be zero-order or first-order and often involves a lag phase prior to significant absorption (Figure 3). In some cases absorption is complete and so rapid that the absorption rate constant cannot be calculated and the plasma concentration–time curve resembles an intravenous dose (Figure 3).

Extent of Absorption

There are a number of reasons why all of the dose of a chemical introduced into the gut lumen may not be able to pass into the general circulation (Table 1). The parameter which describes the extent of absorption is the *bioavailability (F)*, which is defined as the fraction of the dose which

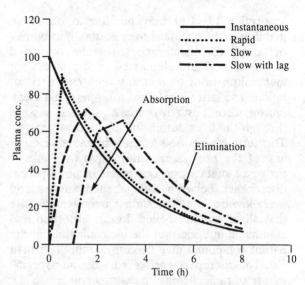

Figure 3 Plasma concentration–time curves of compounds, showing different rates of absorption from the site of administration

Table 1 Reasons for incomplete absorption from the site

Reason	Example
Incomplete dissolution	The formulation, e.g. tablet or suspension, is not completely dissolved during transit through the intestinal tract
Incomplete passage across absorptive epithelium	The compound is too polar to be absorbed completely before it is voided in the faeces (oral) or the unabsorbed dose is removed (transdermal). The rate of loss in exhaled air exceeds the rates of dissolution and absorption (inhaled gases)
Metabolism at the site of administration	The compound is metabolized or decomposes, owing to the pH or enzymes present in the gut lumen (oral). Inactivation by lung enzymes (inhalation)
Metabolism between site of administration and the general circulation	The compound is metabolized by the gut wall or liver prior to entering the general circulation

is transferred from the site of administration into the general circulation *as the parent compound*. Each of the processes in Table 1 can cause a decrease in the amount of parent chemical able to reach the general circulation. Incomplete absorption ($F < 1.0$) may be due to either an inability of the chemical to cross the lipid barrier of the epithelial membrane, so that the compound is unabsorbed and eliminated in the faeces, or metabolism prior to reaching the general circulation. The latter is referred to as *first-pass metabolism*, since it usually occurs on the first passage through the liver during the absorption process. This term is also used to describe metabolism at any of the presystemic sites listed in Table 1. First-pass metabolism can result in an apparent discrepancy between radiolabelled studies and toxicokinetic data. The former may demonstrate that all of a radiolabelled dose is absorbed and eliminated in urine, but the bioavailability of the parent compound may be considerably less than 1.0. The discrepancy arises from the non-specific nature of radiochemical measurements.

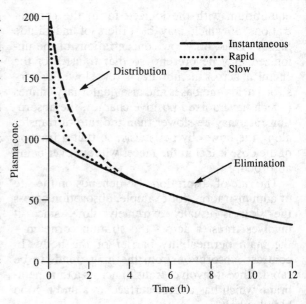

Figure 4 Plasma concentration–time curves following an intravenous bolus dose of chemicals, showing different rates of distribution from the blood into peripheral tissues

Distribution

Distribution is the process of transfer of the chemical from the general circulation into the body tissues. The process may be characterized as both rate and extent, and the corresponding parameters are the distribution rate constant(s) (α, k_{12} and k_{21}) and the apparent volume of distribution (V). Measurement of these parameters requires that the amount of compound which enters the general circulation be known, and therefore distribution parameters can be defined only when the chemical has been given by direct intravascular injection.

Rate of Distribution

Because distribution is usually rapid, the distribution rate constant is measured following the administration of a single rapid (bolus) intravenous dose (Figure 4). The rate of distribution into tissues may be slow for two possible reasons. First, if the chemical has a high affinity for and accumulates in a tissue or organ which is only slowly perfused—e.g. fat or muscle. For such a compound the rate at which the tissues and blood can reach equilibrium will be limited by the blood flow to the tissues. Second, the chemical may be polar, so that its rate of entry into the intracellular fluid of all tissues will be limited by its solubility in the lipid of the membrane.

Extent of Distribution

The tissues into which a chemical distributes can be identified by autoradiography but this technique cannot determine the overall extent to which a chemical has left the blood or plasma and entered the body tissues. In addition, autoradiography cannot differentiate between parent compound and metabolites. The apparent volume of distribution (V) is the parameter which relates the total amount of chemical in the body to the plasma concentration. It can be regarded as a dilution factor and represents the volume of plasma into which the chemical *appears* to have dissolved (see later).

Information on the concentration of a compound in a specific tissue can be determined only by analysis of that tissue. The data in Figure 5 show that cyclohexylamine rapidly enters the testes, which are the target for toxicity (Bopp *et al.*, 1986), and that concentrations in the testes are about four times higher than those in plasma. In contrast the hydroxylated metabolites (3- and 4-aminocyclohexanols) enter the testes less readily and did not show a high testes-to-plasma ratio even after chronic administration (Roberts *et al.*, 1989). These data illustrate that minor changes in molecular structure, such as the increase in polarity resulting from the hydroxyl-

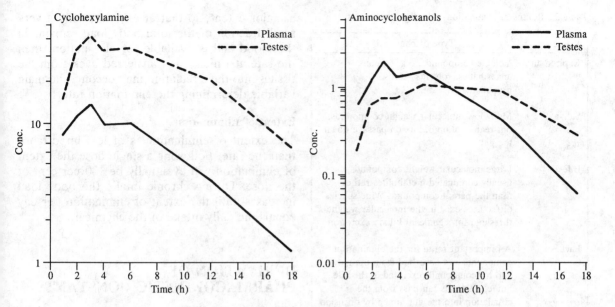

Figure 5 The concentrations of cyclohexylamine and its hydroxymetabolites (aminocyclohexanols) in the plasma (μg ml^{-1}) and testes (μg g^{-1}) of rats following a single oral dose. From Roberts and Renwick (1989)

ation of cyclohexylamine, can alter considerably the uptake into tissues.

Elimination

There are two principal mechanisms of elimination of foreign compounds from the body.

Metabolism eliminates the chemical from the body by converting it into a metabolite which is a different chemical species. The resulting metabolite may itself undergo further metabolism or it may be removed from the body by an excretory process. However, as far as the parent compound is concerned, it has been eliminated as soon as the initial metabolite has been formed. Thus, in the analysis of the kinetics of the parent compound it is essential that the assay methods separate the compound from all of its metabolites. The metabolism of foreign compounds has been the subject of numerous reviews and is discussed in detail in Chapter 3. Sometimes the initial metabolic step results in the generation of a toxic metabolite (Chapter 5), in which case the measurement of the concentration of parent compound provides information on the amount of substrate available for activation, but may not be the best estimate of body exposure to the toxic moiety. Under such circumstances toxicokinetics should concentrate on measurement of the toxic

moiety itself in plasma and tissues. When toxicity arises from the formation of an unstable reactive metabolite, exposure to the toxicant should be assessed by measuring the products formed from the unstable metabolite in either plasma, tissues or urine. For example, the extent of formation of the toxic quinoneimine metabolite of paracetamol can be assessed by measurement of the urinary excretion of the thio conjugates—i.e. the cysteine and mercapturic acid metabolites.

Excretion can occur via body fluids, faeces and expired air, the route of importance being determined by the nature of the compound (Table 2). When considering the toxicokinetics of a chemical, only the excretion of the chemical which is being measured is of importance. Confusion can arise when trying to relate studies with radiolabelled compounds to toxicokinetic data. For example, although all of the radioactivity may be eliminated in the urine, it is possible that this is all as metabolites and not as parent compound. Under such circumstances the renal clearance (see later) of the chemical itself will be negligible, and the kidneys will not be of importance in the elimination of the chemical *per se*.

The elimination of a chemical can be divided into both the rate and extent of elimination.

Table 2   Routes of elimination of foreign compounds

Route	Type of chemical
Expired air	Volatile compounds, e.g. gaseous anaesthetics, solvents, aerosol propellants
Saliva	Many low molecular weight compounds, but reabsorption occurs on passage down the gut
Bile	Large molecular weight compounds, usually conjugated metabolites rather than the parent compound. Wide species differences exist in the molecular weight threshold for significant biliary excretion
Faeces	An important route for the elimination of compounds not absorbed from the gut, and for compounds excreted in the bile. Some chemicals can pass from the circulation into the gut lumen by diffusion or active transport and thereby undergo elimination in the faeces
Urine	The major route of elimination for low molecular weight polar compounds. Lipid-soluble compounds are filtered at the glomerulus, but reabsorbed on passage down the renal tubule, and such compounds are eliminated by metabolism and their metabolites are removed in the urine and/or bile
Milk	Both water- and lipid-soluble compounds are present in milk. This route is usually of limited significance with respect to elimination from the mother but may be of critical importance with respect to exposure of the neonate
Hair	Quantitatively unimportant but the slow and directional growth of hair can allow an 'exposure history' to be determined based on the position of the chemical along the hair

Rate of Elimination

The rate of elimination is limited by two biological processes. First, the ability of the organs of elimination to extract the chemical from the circulation and remove it from the body by metabolism or excretion. Second, the extent to which the chemical remains in the circulation and is available for elimination rather than entering tissues. If the compound has entered the body tissues to a major extent, so that at any time only a very small fraction of the total body load remains in the blood and is available for elimination, then the rate at which it is transferred back from the tissues into the circulation may become the main variable determining the elimination rate.

Extent of Elimination

The extent of elimination is of less importance than the rate. Following a single dose the extent of elimination will eventually be 100 per cent of the dose. During chronic intake the body load increases until the extent of elimination per day equals the daily intake of the chemical.

DERIVATION OF PHARMACOKINETIC CONSTANTS

Most pharmacokinetic parameters are based on the measurement of the chemical in plasma samples collected at various times after dosing. In some cases the concentration in whole blood is used.

Basic Concepts

Before it is possible to describe the measurement of specific pharmacokinetic parameters, it is necessary to define certain basic concepts.

Order of Reaction

At low doses, most processes involved in toxicokinetics can be described as *first-order reactions*. That is, the rate of reaction is proportional to the amount of material present. Examples include passive diffusion, metabolism, protein binding and excretion, in which an increase in concentration will increase the amounts of chemical which cross a membrane, undergo metabolism, etc. The equation for such a reaction is:

$$\frac{dC}{dt} = kC$$

where dC/dt is the rate of change in concentration; k is the rate constant; and C is the concentration. The units of k are time^{-1}, and k can be regarded as the natural log of the proportion of the chemical that is changed within one unit of time. For example, if $k = 0.693$ h^{-1}, then the concentration will change by a factor of 2 (the anti-natural log of 0.693) each hour.

However, as the concentration of a chemical increases, a point may be reached at which no further increase in rate can occur; for example if a metabolizing enzyme is saturated. Under these conditions the rate of change in concentration is a fixed maximum amount and no further increase is possible. This is known as a *zero-order reaction*, which can be described by the equation

$$\frac{\mathrm{d}C}{\mathrm{d}t} = k$$

A straight line is obtained when the data for a zero-order reaction are plotted on a linear axis (Figure 6, left-hand panel). In contrast, for a first-order reaction the rate of change is proportional to the concentration, so that the slope decreases with decrease in concentration. Thus, first-order reactions can be described by exponential equations:

$$C_t = C_0 e^{-kt}$$

where C_t is the concentration at time t; C_0 is the initial concentration; and t is the time. Or, taking natural logs,

$$\ln C_t = \ln C_0 - kt$$

Therefore plotting the natural logarithm of the concentration ($\ln C_t$) against time (t) will give a straight line with an intercept of $\ln C_0$ and a slope of $-k$ (Figure 6, right-hand panel). If $\log_{10}$ is used, then the intercept is $\log_{10} C_0$ and the slope is $-k/2.303$. The zero-order decrease becomes non-linear when plotted on a logarithmic axis.

Half-lives

The rate constant (k) of a zero-order reaction can be described in terms of mass (or concentration) per unit time (e.g. $\mu g\ \min^{-1}$) and this value is a constant at all concentrations. In contrast, for first-order reactions the rate constant has units of time^{-1} (e.g. $\min^{-1}$), which are difficult to visualize. Therefore, the rate of a first-order reaction is normally described by a reciprocal of k, which therefore has units of time. A property of exponential decreases is that the time taken for the concentration to fall to 50 per cent of the initial value is a constant and independent of concentration. This parameter is the half-life ($t\frac{1}{2}$) of the decrease and is related to k by the equation

$$t_{\frac{1}{2}} = \frac{0.693}{k}$$

This can be seen graphically for the first-order reaction in Figure 6, where the concentrations

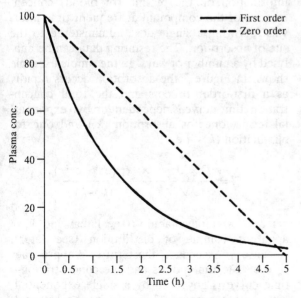
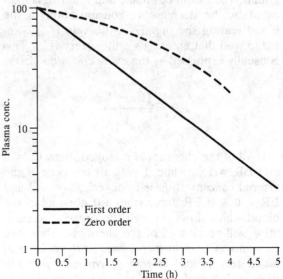

Figure 6 Graphical representations of first-order and zero-order decreases in concentrations plotted on linear (left) and logarithmic (right) axes

decrease by a factor of 2 between successive hourly intervals (i.e. 100, 50, 25, 12.5, 6.25, 3.125), so that the half-life in this case is 1 h. The half-life can be calculated from the slope of the decrease: for example, the initial concentration in Figure 6 is 100 and at 5 h the concentration is 3.125—i.e.

$$\ln 3.125 = \ln 100 - k \times 5$$

$$-k = \frac{\ln 3.125 - \ln 100}{5} = -0.693$$

$$k = 0.693 \text{ h}^{-1}$$

$$t_{\frac{1}{2}} = \frac{0.693}{0.693 \text{ h}^{-1}} = 1 \text{ h}$$

Real data are never calculated by taking two individual time-points, but are fitted by a least-squares regression programme to the ln concentration–time curve and the slope is used to calculate the half-life.

Clearance

A clearance process is one in which the chemical is removed permanently from the circulation— i.e. by metabolism or excretion. Thus, on passage through an organ of elimination the blood can be cleared, either totally or partially, of the compound. The extent of uptake and removal is indicated by the decrease in concentration in the blood leaving the organ via the vein (C_v) compared with that entering via the artery (C_a). This is usually expressed as the *extraction ratio* (ER):

$$\text{ER} = \frac{(C_a - C_v)}{C_a}$$

If all of the chemical is removed, then $C_v = 0$ and ER = 1.0, while if only 10 per cent of the arterial concentration is removed, $C_v = 0.9$ and ER = 0.1. If ER approaches 1.0, then all of the blood which flows through the organ of elimination will be cleared of the chemical. Thus, the clearance (CL), *which is defined as the volume of blood (or plasma) cleared of chemical per unit time*, will equal the blood (or plasma) flow through the organ (Q). If the extraction ratio is 0.1, then only one-tenth of the organ blood flow

will be cleared of the chemical—i.e.

$$\text{CL} = Q \cdot \text{ER}$$

The physiological significance of this is that if a compound has a very high extraction ratio, then changes in organ blood flow will not significantly affect the extraction efficiency of the organ, and consequently clearance will be dependent on and directly proportional to the organ blood flow. In contrast, if the extraction ratio is low, then uptake or extraction by the organ is dependent of the time available for uptake—i.e. the slower the organ flow (Q) the greater will be the extraction ratio (ER). Thus, a change in Q results in an opposite change in ER, so that CL remains relatively constant and independent of organ blood flow.

There are mathematical models which characterize the relationship between CL, Q and ER (see Wilkinson, 1976). In the context of the present chapter, the importance of this relationship is that if the doses of the chemical given to animals are sufficient to alter organ perfusion, then this could influence the clearance of the chemical if it has a high extraction ratio.

Absorption

Rate of Absorption

Measurement of the rate of absorption requires information on the plasma (or blood) concentrations of the compound at frequent time-intervals following a single dose administered to the site of absorption. The resulting data can be analysed by a number of ways. In the simple example shown in Figure 7 the absorption occurs rapidly as a first-order process and the total concentration–time curve is dependent on two exponential terms, one for absorption (k_a) and one for elimination (k)—i.e.

$$C_t = \frac{F \times \text{dose} \times k_a}{V} \frac{(e^{-kt} - e^{-k_a t})}{(k_a - k)}$$

where F = bioavailability (see later) and V = apparent volume of distribution (see later). Because k_a exceeds k, the term $e^{-k_a t}$ approaches zero at late time-points and the concentration–time curve is governed by a single exponential, e^{-kt}. This is shown in Figure 7 by the extrapolation line of the terminal data. If all the dose had

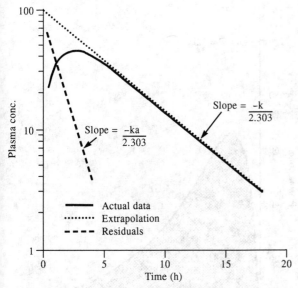

Figure 7 Plasma concentration–time curve following oral administration of a compound, showing simple first-order absorption

entered the circulation as a single bolus dose, then the concentration–time curve would have resembled this extrapolation line. The *difference* between the actual data obtained and the extrapolation line is due to the absorption of the chemical into the circulation. The differences or *residuals* between the actual data and the extrapolation line are then plotted (Figure 7) to derive the absorption rate constant.

The absorption and elimination of chemicals rarely show this simple pattern and more complex equations may be necessary. For example, if there is a lag time (t_{lag}) between dosing and measurable concentrations, then the time t in the equation above has to be replaced by $(t-t_{lag})$. In addition, if there is a clear distribution phase (see later), then a more complex equation may be required; in some cases the absorption rate can only be defined by comparison of oral and intravenous data. Readers are referred to Chapter 4 of Gibaldi and Perrier (1982) for further information. Characterization of the rate of absorption requires the collection of a number of blood samples (at least 3 or 4) during the absorption phase.

In some cases the rate of absorption does not resemble either a first- or zero-order input and the data cannot be fitted by any model. Under such circumstances the best estimate of absorption rate is the mean absorption time (MAT).

This is calculated using statistical moments analysis (see Gibaldi and Perrier, 1982, Chapter 11) from plasma concentration–time curve data after *both* oral and intravenous dosing.

$$MAT = MRT_{oral} - MRT_{iv}$$

where MRT = mean residence time (see later under 'dose-dependent kinetics').

In the brief description above, it is assumed that the compound is absorbed rapidly but eliminated slowly: for example, a lipid-soluble compound requiring metabolism. For highly polar molecules, absorption from the gut may be slow, while elimination from the blood, via the kidneys, may be rapid. However, the concentration–time curve still resembles that shown in Figure 7. The reason for this is that the exponential function which defines the later time-points is always that with the lower rate constant, whether it is k or k_a. Thus, for slowly absorbed/rapidly eliminated compounds the terminal slope is determined by k_a and the more rapid increase by k—a situation described as flip-flop kinetics.

Both the rate and extent of absorption from the gastrointestinal tract can be influenced by a number of variables, such as the nature and volume of the vehicle, the dose of compound (especially in relation to its solubility) and the presence of food in the gut lumen. Toxicokinetic studies should be performed under conditions which reflect the dosing regimen used in animal toxicity studies—e.g. gavage in corn oil, administration with diet, etc.

Extent of Absorption

The fraction of the dose absorbed (or bioavailability, F) can be determined only by reference to conditions in which it is known that all of the dose enters the general circulation *as the parent compound*—i.e. by reference to an intravenous dose given as a bolus or as a slow infusion. Because of the different shapes of the concentration–time curves following oral and intravenous doses (Figure 8), comparison of the concentrations at single time-points is meaningless.

The bioavailability can be calculated from the area under the plasma concentration–time curve (AUC) between administration and infinity following both routes of administration—i.e. if the doses are identical:

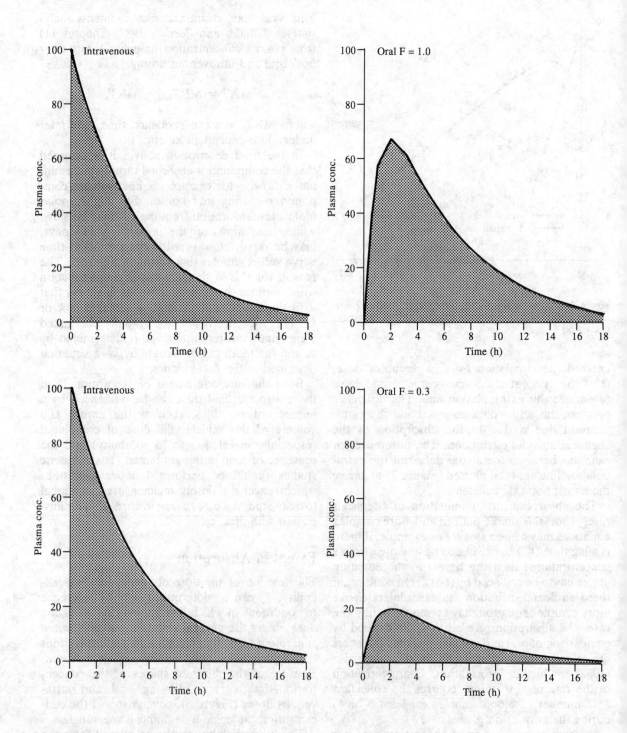

Figure 8 Comparison of area under the plasma concentration–time curves for a compound showing complete absorption (*F*=1.0; top panels) and a compound showing incomplete absorption (*F*=0.3; bottom panels). The reason for the incomplete bioavailability, e.g. first-pass metabolism or poor absorption from the gut lumen, cannot be determined without additional information

$$F = \frac{AUC_{oral}}{AUC_{iv}}$$

This is illustrated in Figure 8. In many cases acute toxicity may prevent the administration of a high iv dose, while a high oral dose may be essential to obtain measurable plasma concentrations. Under such circumstances different doses may be given by oral and intravenous routes and F is calculated as:

$$F = \frac{AUC_{oral} \times dose_{iv}}{AUC_{iv} \quad dose_{oral}}$$

The basis for this calculation is that plasma clearance (see later) is the same after each of the two separate doses (oral and intravenous). In clinical studies this is ensured by studying the same patient on two occasions. For animal toxicity studies it may be necessary to study different animals for each route, in which case the age and sex of the animals should be comparable. The AUC values must be calculated to infinity (see later), so that it is important that the concentration–time curves are followed for a sufficiently long time to allow accurate measurement of the terminal half-life.

Use of AUC data assumes that there is no saturation of elimination and that the intravenous dose with its possibly higher plasma concentrations does not produce cardiovascular, renal or metabolic effects which could alter the plasma clearance of the compound.

The bioavailability can also be calculated from urinary data. The percentage of the dose which is excreted in the urine *as the parent compound* is dependent on the amount of parent compound presented to the kidneys by the circulation—i.e. the percentage of the dose excreted in the urine to time t is proportional to the plasma AUC to time t. Thus, bioavailability (F) can be calculated as

$$F = \frac{\% \text{ oral dose in urine as the parent compound}}{\% \text{ intravenous dose in urine as the parent compound}}$$

where the percentage dose is measured until no more parent drug is excreted (i.e. $t = $ infinity).

Distribution

Rate of Distribution

The rate at which a compound distributes out of the blood into body tissues is usually rapid and can only be measured when the dose enters the circulation at a rate considerably greater than the rate of distribution. In effect, this means that usually the rate of distribution is measured following an intravenous bolus dose. The plasma concentration–time curve following a bolus dose depends on the rate and extent of distribution.

In the simplest case (Figure 4, bottom line) all distribution occurs between dosing and the collection of the first blood sample, so that distribution is essentially instantaneous. Thus, the concentration–time curve can be described by a single exponential term (k) dependent on elimination and the compound achieves instantaneous distribution within a single compartment (Figure 9).

However, normally a distinct distribution phase can be detected (Figure 4, top two lines), during which the chemical is undergoing *both* distribution and elimination. The tissues and blood eventually reach equilibrium and the concentration–time curve becomes a simple monoexponential decrease (Figure 4). For such compounds the body has to be regarded as comprising two compartments, with the chemical achieving instantaneous equilibrium in compartment 1 (the central compartment) but taking a finite time for equilibration between compartment 1 and compartment 2 (the peripheral compartment) (Figure 9). Thus, two exponential terms are necessary—

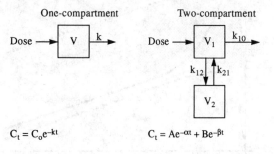

Figure 9 Simple one- and two-compartment models of distribution and elimination. More complex models involving three or more compartments with elimination from both central and peripheral compartments are sometimes necessary to provide a mathematical description of the plasma concentration–time curves. (The relationships between α, β, k_{10}, k_{12} and k_{21} are given in the text)

a rapid distribution rate (α) and the slower elimination rate (β). A more correct nomenclature for such multiple exponential rate constants is λ_1, λ_2, etc. and λ_z where these represent the rate constants for the fastest, next fastest and slowest rate, respectively. This nomenclature is receiving increasingly wide usage. The overall elimination rate (β or λ_z) or terminal half-life ($0.693/\beta$) is *not* equivalent to k_{10} but is a composite term involving k_{10}, k_{21} and k_{12}.

The concentration in the peripheral compartment is zero initially, and then rises during the distribution phase until equilibrium is reached, following which the concentrations decrease in parallel with those in the general circulation (Figure 10). The absolute concentration in the tissue will depend on the relative affinity of the blood and tissue for the compound. Tissues with different relative affinities may be part of compartment 2 and the only parameter that is shared is the rate of equilibration between blood and tissue (Figure 10). Thus, calculation of a mean concentration for compartment 2 is rarely of value. However, concentrations in compartment 2 can be predicted from a single post-equilibrium measurement and a knowledge of the terminal rate constant (β) in plasma.

The rate constants α and β and intercepts A and B can be calculated by the method of residuals (Figure 11). The 'micro'-rate constants k_{10}, k_{12} and k_{21} can be calculated as

$$k_{21} = \frac{A\beta + B\alpha}{A + B}$$

$$k_{10} = \frac{\alpha\beta}{k_{21}}$$

$$k_{12} = \alpha + \beta - k_{21} - k_{10}$$

It should be appreciated that such manipulations of derived data exaggerate any errors in the measurements. Accurate parameter estimates require that at least 3–4 blood samples are collected during each separate phase (e.g. α and β) and that the terminal phase is followed for as long as possible and for at least two half-lives. Some compounds may require three or more exponential terms (and compartments) to provide an adequate model.

Extent of Distribution

The shape of the concentration–time curve following a single bolus intravenous dose is dependent also on the extent to which the dose is

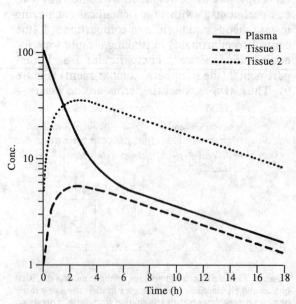

Figure 10 The concentration–time curve for a chemical in plasma (and tissues in the instantaneously equilibrating central compartment) and two tissues which are part of the slowly equilibrating peripheral compartment

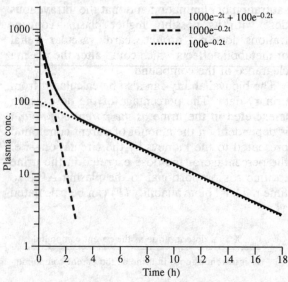

Figure 11 The use of the method of residuals to calculate distribution parameters. The terminal phase is given by $Be^{\beta t}$ (in this case $100e^{-0.2t}$) and the differences between the plasma concentrations and this line give the distribution phase $Ae^{-\alpha t}$ (in this case $1000e^{-2t}$)

retained in the central compartment or distributed to the tissues. This is illustrated in Figure 12. In the upper line ($C_t = 100e^{-2t} + 1000e^{-0.2t}$) only one-eleventh of the material is associated with the rapid phase of distribution to the tissues, so that the concentration–time curve almost resembles a monoexponential decrease; if the first sample had been taken at 1 h, the distribution phase could have been missed. In the lower line ($C_t = 1000e^{-2t} + 100e^{-0.2t}$) most of the dose undergoes the distribution phase, which is apparent until about 3 h after the dose.

The extent of distribution is characterized by the *apparent volume of distribution* (V), which can be calculated using a number of different methods. V is the parameter which relates the concentration in plasma (C) to the total body load (A_b) with which it is in equilibrium—i.e.

$$V = \frac{A_b}{C}$$

Thus, for a one-compartment system which shows instantaneous equilibrium:

$$V = \frac{\text{dose}}{C_0}$$

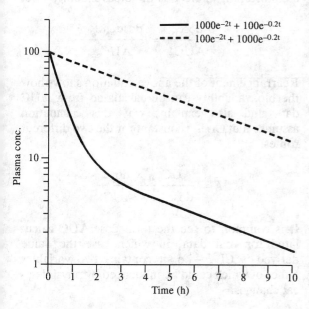

For a two-compartment system the situation is more complex.

Dose/$(A + B)$ gives the volume of the central compartment only, since the constant A is derived prior to distribution and the attainment of equilibrium. The volume of distribution can be calculated as dose/B, but this estimate does not take into account the volume of or amount of chemical in the central compartment. The apparent volume of distribution (V_β) is usually calculated as:

$$V_\beta = \frac{\text{dose}}{\text{AUC} \times \beta}$$

where AUC is the area under the plasma concentration–time curve.

It must be emphasized that the volume of distribution is not a real volume but is the volume of plasma (or blood if the concentration is measured in whole blood) in which the compound *appears* to have dissolved. If the concentration in plasma after equilibration with all the tissues is extremely low, then the apparent volume of distribution (A_b/C or dose/C_0) will be extremely high. For example, highly lipid-soluble compounds may have an apparent volume of distribution of 50 l per kg body weight—a physiological impossibility. Thus, all that the apparent volume of distribution really represents is the dilution factor between plasma concentration and body load. It provides an indication of the extent to which the compound has left plasma and entered the tissues, but it cannot provide information on uptake into specific tissues.

If a chemical enters a tissue but is eliminated without re-entering the general circulation, this is an elimination or clearance process and *does not contribute to the distribution parameters*.

Elimination

The overall rate of elimination (k or β) depends on two variables: the apparent volume of distribution and the clearance. This is illustrated in Figure 13 by analogy with the emptying of a container of water. In the case of a single compartment the rate at which the level falls in the container will be proportional to the flow through the tap (analogous to the clearance) but inversely proportional to the size of the container—i.e.

Figure 12 Plasma concentration–time curves for two compounds with the same rate constants (α and β) but with different proportions of the dose undergoing distribution

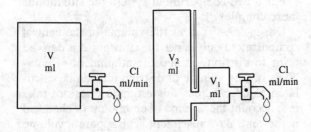

Figure 13   The relationship between volume, clearance and overall elimination. Rate of elimination ∝ CL/V

$$\text{rate} \propto \frac{CL}{V}$$

In the case of the 2-compartment system (Figure 13, right-hand side) the rate at which the level falls in V_1 is dependent on CL and the size of $(V_1 + V_2)$.

Clearance

The clearance (CL) of a chemical is perhaps the single most important pharmacokinetic parameter. It is defined as

$$CL = \frac{\text{rate of elimination of the chemical}}{\text{plasma concentration}} \quad \text{e.g.} \quad \frac{\mu g\ min^{-1}}{\mu g\ ml^{-1}}$$

For first-order reactions an increase in plasma concentration results in an increase in the rate of elimination, so that CL is constant. The units are volume time^{-1} (e.g. ml min^{-1}) and clearance represents the volume of plasma (or blood if concentrations are measured in whole blood) cleared of compound per unit time. The plasma clearance (CL) represents the sum of all individual clearance processes such as metabolism (CL_M), renal excretion (CL_R), biliary excretion (CL_B), etc.:

$$CL = CL_M + CL_R + CL_B + \ldots$$

Clearance is usually calculated from the area under the plasma concentration–time curve (AUC). The rate of elimination of the chemical from the body is the rate of change of body load (A_b)—i.e.

$$CL = \frac{dA_b}{dt} \times \frac{1}{C}$$

or

$$CL \times C dt = dA_b$$

If this equation is integrated between time equals zero and infinity, the term dA_B (the change in body load) becomes the dose administered, while $C dt$ (which is the area under the concentration–time curve for the time interval dt) becomes the AUC:

$$CL \times AUC = \text{dose}$$

or

$$CL = \frac{\text{dose}}{AUC}$$

For this equation to be valid both the dose and AUC needed to be defined properly.

Dose   The dose is that available to the organs of elimination. Thus, CL is calculated from the data following an *intravenous dose*, which can be given either as a bolus or as a slow infusion. If the dose is given orally, then the true dose available to the organs of elimination is $F \times$ dose administered, where F is the bioavailability—i.e.

$$CL = \frac{\text{dose}_{iv}}{AUC_{iv}} = \frac{\text{dose}_{oral} \times F}{AUC_{oral}}$$

Rearrangement of the above equation shows how the bioavailability can be calculated from AUC data and also explains why this calculation assumes that CL is a constant for the two different routes:

$$F = \frac{AUC_{oral} \times \text{dose}_{iv}}{\text{dose}_{oral} \times AUC_{iv}}$$

It is common to see the term dose/AUC calculated for oral data, in which case the value derived is CL/F—i.e. it contains two variables either of which could be influenced by physiological changes.

AUC   The AUC can be calculated by the trapezoidal rule between time zero and the last measured concentration, but needs to be extrapolated to infinity if the calculation of CL is to be valid. This is normally done by dividing the last measured concentration (C_{last}) by the terminal slope (β), which is derived from the terminal log-linear portion of the concentration–time curve. Thus, it is essential for the samples to be collected until a log-linear decrease is defined. The AUC can also be derived by fitting a suitable model to the data and calculating the AUC from the derived parameters, e.g. $AUC = C_0/k$ or $AUC = A/\alpha + B/\beta$.

The relationship between clearance, the terminal slope and the apparent volume of distribution can be derived from the simple definition of clearance—i.e.

$$CL = \frac{dA_b}{dt} \times \frac{1}{C}$$

For a first-order reaction, $dA_b/dt = kA_b$,

$$CL = \frac{kA_b}{C}$$

From the definition of apparent volume of distribution, $A_b = VC$,

$$CL = \frac{kVC}{C} = kV$$

or

$$k = \frac{CL}{V} \text{ and } t_{1/2} = \frac{0.693V}{CL}$$

This derivation has been included to emphasize (1) that the terminal elimination rate constant is a composite parameter which is dependent on two physiological variables (i.e. CL, which reflects the rate of extraction and removal from blood, and $1/V$, which reflects the amount of chemical remaining in the blood and available for clearance), and (2) that the interrelationship between CL, V and $t_{1/2}$ assumes that first-order kinetics apply (i.e. that the chemical does not show dose-dependent kinetics).

Renal clearance (CL_R) is the only specific clearance term that can be measured easily. CL_R may be defined as

$$CL_R = \frac{\text{rate of elimination in urine (as the parent compound)}}{\text{concentration in plasma}}$$

The rate of elimination in urine can be calculated by measuring the concentration of the chemical (C_u) in the volume of urine (V_u) produced in a known time interval (Δt). If the concentration in plasma at the mid-point of the urine collection is known, then CL_R can be calculated as:

$$CL_R = \frac{C_u \times V_u}{\Delta t} \times \frac{1}{C_{mid}}$$

where $C_u \times V_u$ is the total amount excreted (A_{ex}) over the time interval Δt.

The product $\Delta t \times C_{mid}$ is the AUC of the plasma concentration–time curve for the time interval Δt. Therefore, CL_R may be calculated also from plasma AUC data and the amount excreted unchanged (A_{ex}) over the same time interval—i.e.

$$CL_R = \frac{A_{ex\,(0-t)}}{AUC_{(0-t)}}$$

The terminal half-life can be calculated from serial timed urine collections:

$$CL_R = \frac{\text{rate of urinary excretion}}{C_{mid}}$$

$$\text{rate of urinary excretion} = C_{mid} \times CL_R$$

CL_R is a constant for a first-order reaction and therefore the rate of excretion at any time will be proportional to the plasma concentration. Therefore the decrease in excretion rate with time will mirror the decrease in plasma concentration. Thus, a graph of ln excretion rate against time will have a rate constant and half-life the same as that in plasma. Alternatively, the half-life can be calculated from the amount remaining to be excreted, using the sigma-minus method (see under trans-species comparisons). It is not possible to derive total plasma clearance (CL) or apparent volume of distribution (V) without taking blood samples.

Metabolic clearance (CL_M) cannot be measured readily, but since metabolism and renal excretion are the principal routes of total clearance (CL) in many cases, it can be assumed that

$$CL = CL_M + CL_R$$

$$CL_M = CL - CL_R$$

$$CL_M = \frac{dose}{AUC} - \frac{amount\ excreted\ unchanged}{AUC}$$

$$CL_M = \frac{(dose - amount\ excreted\ unchanged)}{AUC}$$

THE INTERPRETATION OF CHRONIC HIGH-DOSE ANIMAL FEEDING STUDIES

In many cases regulatory decisions are based on the use of chronic high-dose animal feeding studies to predict possible risk for man. However, such a protocol can lead to tissue accumulation and changes in clearance that would not be anticipated from single-dose studies.

Chronic Intake

During chronic intake the concentration of the chemical accumulates in the plasma and tissues as illustrated in Figure 14. Both of the hypothetical compounds shown in Figure 14 exhibit one-compartment kinetics with similar apparent volumes of distribution. Therefore the tenfold difference in the elimination rate constant arises from a tenfold difference in clearance. The compound in Figure 14 for which $k = 0.2\ h^{-1}$ shows negligible concentrations remaining at 24 h when the next dose is given. In contrast, the concentration of the other compound (where $k = 0.02\ h^{-1}$) at 24 h is 62 per cent of the value at $t = 0$, so that there is marked accumulation with successive doses. Eventually a steady state will be reached in which the rate of elimination per 24 h equals the rate of administration—i.e.

rate of input = rate of elimination

$$\frac{D \times F}{T} = CL \times C_{ss}$$

where D = dose administered; F = bioavailability; T = dose interval; CL = clearance; and C_{ss} = average plasma concentration at steady state.

The equation above is based on the definition of clearance (i.e. CL = rate of elimination/C) applied to the steady state condition when the rate of elimination exactly equals the rate of

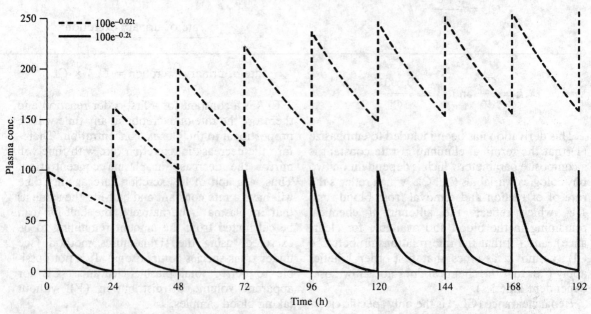

Figure 14 The accumulation of chemicals during chronic intake. In the examples shown above, the compounds are given as single intravenous bolus doses every 24 h. Both compounds exhibit monoexponential decreases (i.e. $C_t = C_0 e^{-kt}$)

administration. Thus, steady state data can be used to calculate the value of CL—i.e.

$$CL = \frac{D \times F}{T \times C_{ss}}$$

$T \times C_{ss}$ is the AUC for a dose interval at steady state, so that this equation can also be written as

$$CL = \frac{D \times F}{AUC_{0-T}}$$

This can be compared with the measurement of CL after a single dose, where

$$CL = \frac{D \times F}{AUC_{0-\infty}}$$

Thus, the AUC_{0-T} at steady state and the average steady state concentration (C_{ss}) can be calculated from the $AUC_{0-\infty}$ for a single dose:

$$AUC_{0-T} \text{ (steady state)} = AUC_{0-\infty} \text{ (single dose)}$$

$$C_{ss} = \frac{AUC_{0-\infty} \text{ (single dose)}}{T}$$

This is illustrated in Figure 15. Thus, if the dose interval is halved, then the value of C_{ss} will be doubled. *The AUC for a dose interval at steady state is the best estimate of exposure to the chemical and can be determined without fitting any specific model to the data.*

The increase to steady state for a compound which shows a simple monoexponential decline after an intravenous bolus dose is an inversion of the elimination phase—i.e. the percentage of steady state achieved after administration for 1, 2, 3, 4 and 5 half-lives is 50, 75, 87.5, 93.75, 96.875 per cent. Thus, it takes approximately 4–5 times the elimination (terminal) half-life to approach steady state. In contrast, for a compound which shows a more complex plasma concentration–time curve (Table 3) (for example, oral administration of a slowly absorbed compound such as saccharin), the percentage of steady state at time = t can be calculated from single-dose data as $AUC_{0-t}/AUC_{0-\infty} \times 100$. Thus, the time to steady state can be assessed without the fitting of any model (Figure 16).

For compounds which have a half-life of 6 h or less, 'steady state' will be reached within the first 24 h of regular dosing. However, there will be massive diurnal variations in concentration, as illustrated in Figure 14, where the half-life of one of the compounds is only 3.5 h (0.693/0.2 h^{-1}).

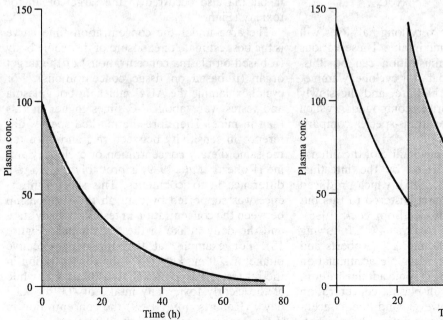

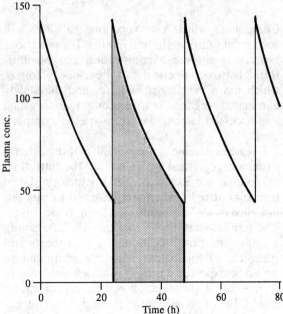

Figure 15 The relationship between $AUC_{0-\infty}$ for a single dose and AUC_{0-T} for a dose interval at steady state

Table 3 The use of single-dose data to predict the development of steady state

Time (t) (h)	C ($\mu g\ ml^{-1}$)	AUC_{0-t} ($\mu g\ ml^{-1}\ h^{-1}$)	% ss
0	0		
0.5	11.03	2.76	1.91
1	16.32	9.60	6.66
1.5	15.41	17.52	12.15
2	16.69	25.55	17.71
3	13.89	40.80	28.28
4	13.45	54.47	37.76
5	8.82	65.44	45.37
6	5.82	72.66	50.37
7	4.85	77.98	54.06
8	4.63	82.71	57.34
12	2.41	96.52	66.91
14	2.26	101.26	70.20
24	1.23	118.19	81.93
28	0.93	122.48	84.91
32	0.92	126.18	87.47
48	0.39	136.07	94.33
56	0.35	139.02	96.37
72	0.12	142.46	98.76
∞	–	144.25	100.00

The plasma concentration–time curve data are for a single dose of saccharin given orally to a human volunteer (data from Sweatman *et al.*, 1981).
C,   concentration.
AUC_{0-t}, area under concentration–time to the time of the plasma sample.
% ss,   percentage of steady state, $\dfrac{AUC_{0-t}}{AUC_{0-\infty}} \times 100$.

Compounds which have very long half-lives will accumulate during chronic intake. These various aspects of chronic administration can be illustrated by toxicokinetic data for cyclohexylamine, which has a very short half-life, and the slowly eliminated organo-chlorine compounds, which are discussed later under 'trans-species comparisons'.

Cyclohexylamine is a metabolite of the intense sweetener cyclamate formed by the intestinal microflora (see Renwick, 1986), which produced testicular atrophy when administered to rats but not mice in a 90 day study (see Bopp *et al.*, 1986). The terminal half-life in rats was 4.6 h following a single oral dose of 200 mg kg^{-1} (Roberts and Renwick, 1989), so that negligible accumulation would be expected during chronic administration. Wide diurnal variations in plasma concentration would be expected however and the concentration–time profile over 24 h during chronic dietary administration (Figure 17) was largely deter-

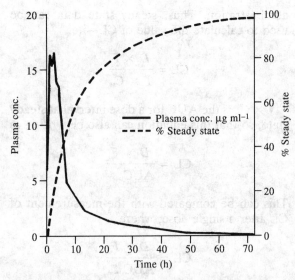

Figure 16 The relationship between single-dose kinetics and the development of steady state during chronic administration. The percentage of steady state at any time is the AUC to that time divided by the AUC to infinity times 100

mined by the nocturnal feeding habits of the rat. The concentration of cyclohexylamine in the testes increased rapidly following a single oral dose (Figure 5) and therefore the testes represent part of the rapidly equilibrating central compartment. Therefore the diurnal fluctuations detected in plasma also occurred in the target organ for toxicity (Figure 17).

The area under the concentration–time curve is the best estimate of exposure of the whole body (if based on plasma concentrations) or the target organ (if based on tissue concentrations). For cyclohexylamine the AUC values for both plasma and testes were about 2–3 times higher in rats than in mice. Therefore the marked species difference in sensitivity between rats and mice fed the same dietary concentration of cyclohexylamine (Roberts *et al.*, 1989) is probably related to a difference in toxicokinetics. This species difference was supported by data on the relationship between the concentration in testes at steady state and the daily intake in the test animals (Figure 18). For example, at the minimally effective intake of 200 mg kg^{-1} day^{-1} the concentration in the rat testes was approximately 30 μg g^{-1}, while at the clearly toxic daily intake of 400 mg kg^{-1} day^{-1} (Roberts *et al.*, 1989) the concentration in the testes was approximately 100 μg g^{-1}. In contrast an intake of 400 mg kg^{-1} day^{-1}, which is

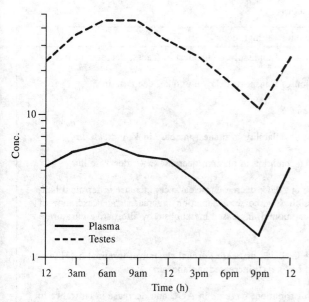

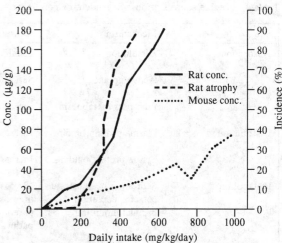

Figure 17 Concentration–time curves for cyclohexylamine in the plasma (μg ml^{-1}) and testes (μg g^{-1}) of rats given cyclohexylamine in the diet *ad libitum*. The animal room was dark between 9pm and 6am, during which time the animals consumed the diet. From Roberts and Renwick (1989)

Figure 18 The concentration of cyclohexylamine in the testes of rats and mice in relation to the daily intake. Concentrations were measured at 6am (from Roberts and Renwick, 1989) and the corresponding dose response for testicular atrophy in the rat was calculated (from Bopp *et al.*, 1986)

non-toxic in mice (Roberts *et al.*, 1989), produced concentrations of only about 25 μg g^{-1} in the mouse testes. The concentration–intake data in the rat showed clear evidence of non-linearity at intakes greater than about 200 mg kg^{-1} day^{-1}. This non-linearity was also detected in plasma and probably contributed to the steep dose–response relationship for testicular atrophy in the rat (Figure 18).

Dose-Dependent Kinetics

A non-linear relationship between dose and area under the plasma concentration–time curve is indicative of *dose-dependent* or *non-linear* kinetics. That is, the compound does not obey first-order kinetics at high doses. Non-linear kinetics can arise whenever an interaction between the chemical and a body constituent is saturated by the presence of excess chemical (Table 4).

Non-linear kinetics can be detected by studying a range of single doses but frequently is detected during chronic administration when the accumulation of the compound causes saturation. If saturation of elimination occurs during chronic administration, then the clearance will be reduced and the area under curve (AUC) for a dose inter-

val will be increased (see above). Thus, evidence of saturation of elimination is that the AUC for a dose interval at steady state exceeds the AUC to infinity of a single dose. In the example in Figure 18 the AUC for a dose interval at steady state was not measured and non-linearity was based on a single measurement taken at 6 am. Therefore the result in Figure 18 could have been obtained for reasons other than a decrease in clearance—for example, if high doses altered the pattern of food consumption or the rate of absorption of cyclohexylamine. In the case of cyclohexylamine, saturation of elimination had been demonstrated by single-dose studies, but it should be appreciated that the data in Figure 18 alone are indicative but not proof of saturation of elimination.

If the chemical causes induction of the enzymes which are responsible for its elimination, then the clearance will be increased during chronic administration. In consequence, the AUC for a dose interval will be reduced, compared with the AUC to infinity of a single dose.

It should be appreciated that age-related changes in physiological processes, such as renal blood flow, will occur during lifetime feeding studies. Therefore it is possible that concentrations at steady state may be age-dependent. The basic equation for mean steady state concentration (C_{ss}) still applies—i.e.

Table 4 Possible sources of dose-dependent or non-linear kinetics

Site	Mechanism	Consequences at high dose
Absorption	Dissolution	Elimination of undissolved chemical in faeces; decrease in F
	Active uptake	Saturation of transport; delayed uptake, decrease in F
	First-pass metabolism	Increase in F
Distribution	Plasma protein binding	Increased availability to tissues; increase in V; increase in $t_{1/2}$
	Tissue protein binding	Increased retention in plasma; decrease in V; decrease in $t_{1/2}$
Metabolism	Saturation by substrate cofactor depletion product inhibition	Increase in AUC; decrease in clearance; increase in terminal half-life possible (e.g. cofactor depletion); increased renal excretion of parent compound; increased metabolism by alternative unsaturated pathways
Excretion	Saturation of renal tubular secretion	Increase in AUC; decrease in renal clearance; terminal half-life not affected (see text); increased metabolism
Cardiac output	Decreased organ perfusion due to cardiovascular toxicity	Slower distribution; increase in AUC and decrease in clearance for compounds showing high renal or hepatic (metabolic) clearance, i.e. high extraction ratio

$$C_{ss} = \frac{\text{dose} \times F}{\text{CL} \times T}$$

Metabolic and physiological processes, such as renal blood flow, are immature in neonates (Blumer, 1990), so that clearances may be lower than in mature individuals. Thus, the neonatal phase of a two-generation protocol may result in excessively high plasma concentrations of compounds fed in the diet due both to a decreased clearance and to an enhanced intake due to the higher food intake in neonates per kg body weight. In ageing animals C_{ss} may increase, owing to an age-related decrease in clearance. In the case of N-acetylprocainamide the systemic clearance (dose$_{iv}$/AUC$_{iv}$) in 12-month-old rats was only 40 per cent of that in 3-month-old rats. However, the AUC$_{oral}$ showed a much less marked age-related change than the AUC$_{iv}$ because bioavailability was also decreased in 12-month-old rats (Yacobi *et al.*, 1982). This illustrates that the AUC$_{oral}$ is dependent on both the systemic clearance and the bioavailability which can vary independently.

If saturation of elimination is detected on giving increasing single doses, this is usually seen as slow elimination at high plasma concentrations, but the normal rate of elimination once

the concentration decreases and first-order kinetics apply (Figure 19). Under such circumstances the compound is said to obey Michaelis–Menten kinetics, that is:

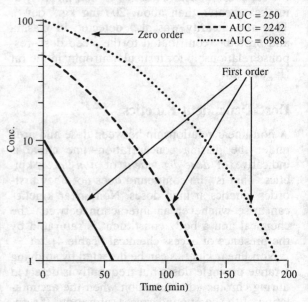

Figure 19 The plasma concentration–time curves for a compound showing saturation kinetics given at doses sufficient to give initial plasma concentrations of 10, 50 and 100 units. The compound is eliminated by a single saturable pathway

$$-\frac{dC}{dt} = \frac{V_{max}C}{K_m + C}$$

where dC/dt = rate of change of concentration; V_{max} = maximum rate of the enzyme-catalysed reaction (or transport); K_m = Michaelis constant of the enzyme; and C = concentration available to the enzyme.

At low concentrations $K_m \gg C$. Therefore $K_m + C$ approximates to K_m:

$$-\frac{dC}{dt} = \frac{V_{max}C}{K_m} = \text{constant} \times C = \text{first-order reaction}$$

At high concentrations $C \gg K_m$. Therefore $K_m + C$ approximates to C:

$$-\frac{dC}{dt} = \frac{V_{max}C}{C} = V_{max} = \text{zero-order reaction}$$

The true terminal half-life, which is measured when concentrations are very low, is not dose-dependent (see Figure 19). However, the measured half-life may indicate the possibility of saturation of elimination if the concentration–time curve is not followed for long enough—e.g. if measurements had been made for only 50 min after each dose in Figure 19.

The best indication of dose-dependent elimination is calculation of the clearance as dose/AUC to infinity. This is illustrated in Figure 19, which gives data for a compound showing a single exponential decrease at low concentrations and where K_m = 20 units and V_{max} = 1 unit per min. The initial plasma concentration is dependent only on the dose and the apparent volume of distribution (V) (C_0 = dose/V); therefore the three doses were in the ratio 1:5:10. However, the AUC values increased in the order 250:2242:6988—i.e. 1:9:28. Thus, the clearance (dose/AUC) decreased in the ratio 1:0.56:0.36, but the terminal half-life was 15 min for each dose.

A compound which shows non-linear pharmacokinetics similar to those depicted in Figure 19 is the solvent 1,4-dioxane (Dietz *et al.*, 1982), for which an increase in intravenous dose in rats from 3 mg kg^{-1} to 1000 mg kg^{-1} (333-fold) caused a 4439-fold increase in AUC. The disproportionate increase in AUC of dioxane at high doses was associated with a decrease in the urinary excretion of the metabolite β-hydroxyethoxyacetic acid and an increase in the elimination of the solvent itself in the expired air. However, during chronic daily administration of [^{14}C]-dioxane the body burden at steady state after allowing for differences in dose was only slightly higher after 1000 mg kg^{-1} day^{-1} compared with 10 mg kg^{-1} day^{-1}. This finding therefore suggests that the non-linear AUC difference between 1000 and 10 mg kg^{-1} as a single dose overestimated the difference at steady state. Studies on enzyme activities suggested that dioxane at high doses induces its own metabolism (Dietz *et al.*, 1982), so that an increase in V_{max} compensated for saturation of the enzyme.

Although the terminal half-life is not dose-dependent, non-linear kinetics can be demonstrated by the use of a time-based parameter derived from the AUC, i.e. the mean residence time, or MRT. The mean residence time is the ratio between the area under the first moment of the concentration–time curve (AUMC) and the area under the concentration–time curve (AUC):

$$\text{MRT} = \frac{\text{AUMC}}{\text{AUC}}$$

The AUMC is derived by the trapezoidal rule applied to a graph of $C \times t$, for each sample, against t for that sample and therefore does not require any fitting of the data to specific models. However, as for AUC, the AUMC data must be extrapolated to infinity for the above equation to be valid. Extrapolation from the last concentration–time point to infinity is achieved by the addition of

$$\frac{t_{last} \times C_{last}}{\beta} + \frac{C_{last}}{\beta^2}$$

where β is the terminal slope.

For the data in Figure 19 the AUMC values for the increasing doses were 5606, 77 427 and 354 639 (which have units of concentration $\times$ time^2), whereas the corresponding AUC values were 250, 2242 and 6988 (which have units of concentration $\times$ time). Thus, the MRT values, which are AUMC/AUC, have units of time and for the data in Figure 19 were 22.4, 35.3 and 50.7 min, thereby clearly demonstrating dose dependency. The MRT can be regarded as the mean time for which any one molecule of the chemical will be present in the body, and is analogous to but not identical with the half-life. The half-life $(t_{1/2})$ can be calculated as:

$$t_{1/2} = MRT \times 0.693$$

In the case of the lowest dose in Figure 19 the $t_{1/2}$ can be calculated as $22.4 \times 0.693 = 15$ min, which agrees with that derived from the terminal slope. Using the MRT to calculate the 'half-life' for the two higher doses is not logical, since the half-lives obtained will be composite values based on the whole concentration–time curve, which includes the slow, zero-order component (for which a half-life is not appropriate). However, such a calculation would demonstrate non-linear kinetics.

The statistical moment analysis can also be applied to an intravenous infusion (although a different correction is necessary—see Chapter 11 of Gibaldi and Perrier, 1982) and to oral administration to calculate the MAT (see earlier). In addition, it is possible to calculate a volume of distribution (V_{ss}) which is analogous to $V\beta$ (CL/β) by the equation

$$V_{ss} = CL \times MRT = \frac{dose}{AUC} \times \frac{AUMC}{AUC} \text{ (for a bolus dose)}$$

Dose-dependent kinetics can arise from the saturation of a number of protein–chemical interactions (Table 4). Therefore non-linear relationships can produce a range of different changes to the plasma concentration–time profile. A number of different approaches can be taken to demonstrate dose-dependent kinetics—e.g.:

(1) Dividing the plasma concentration for each time-point by the dose and plotting the resulting dose-adjusted data. For purely linear and first-order processes the adjusted data will be superimposable. A consistent dose-dependent deviation indicates that non-linearity is present but does not indicate the source.

(2) Fitting all doses to a common model and demonstrating systematic changes in parameter estimates.

(3) Measuring metabolite formation either in plasma or urine. A dose-dependent change in the ratio between the AUC for the parent compound and the AUC of the metabolite (or percentage in urine) would indicate saturation of metabolism.

(4) Measuring tissue-to-plasma ratio for a range of doses to detect saturation of protein binding in either tissue (if the unbound plasma protein concentration is measured) or possibly plasma (if total plasma concentration is measured).

Trans-Species Comparisons

The use of animal data to predict potential risks to humans or to establish safe exposure levels is based on the assumptions that both the toxicodynamics, or actions in the target organ, and the toxicokinetics in animals are relevant to humans. Despite basic similarities in their mammalian biology, there are wide differences between different animal species and between animals and humans in physiological processes, such as organ perfusion rates. There are also differences in biochemical processes such as foreign compound metabolism. In consequence, all extrapolations from animals to man must take into account differences in toxicokinetics. These differences are illustrated by data on chlorinated dibenzo-*p*-dioxins.

Chlorinated dibenzo-*p*-dioxins, such as 2,3,7,8-tetrachlorodibenzo-*p*-dioxin (TCDD), are among the most toxic chemicals known and produce acnegenic, carcinogenic, fetotoxic, immunosuppressive and teratogenic effects (HMSO, 1989). There are wide interspecies differences in acute toxicity of TCDD with the guinea-pig about 10–20 times more sensitive than the rat (Kociba *et al.*, 1976) or mouse (Beatty *et al.*, 1978; McConnell *et al.*, 1978), while the hamster appears to be the least sensitive species (Olson *et al.*, 1980b). The elimination half-life in guinea-pigs (30 ± 6 days; Gasiewicz and Neal, 1979) is similar to that in rats (Rose *et al.*, 1976) and only about twice that in hamsters (15 ± 3 days; Olsen *et al.*, 1980a). Differences in sensitivity to TCDD in different strains of rats cannot be related to differences in toxicokinetics (Pohjanvirta *et al.*, 1990). Thus, the species and strain differences in acute toxicity are not related to the ability to eliminate the compound.

Because of the slow elimination of [^{14}C]-TCDD, the elimination rate constant was calculated from the total amount of radioactivity recovered in urine and faeces each day using an adaptation of the *sigma-minus method* (Gibaldi and Perrier, 1982). This method is based on measurements of the excretion *of the parent compound* until no more can be detected in the urine (and/or faeces). For each collection time interval the amount remaining to be excreted is calculated as (the amount excreted as parent compound to infinity—the amount excreted up to that time); a plot of ln amount remaining to be excreted against the time at the end of the collection interval will have a slope of $-\beta$ (or $-\lambda_z$) and an intercept of ln total amount excreted unchanged. This method is applicable even in cases where excretion of the parent compound is not the major route of elimination because the amount of parent compound excreted at any time is proportional to the plasma concentration (*C*) and therefore the body load (*V* times *C*) of parent compound at that time. In the case of TCDD, the 'body burden' of TCDD remaining after each day was calculated as (dose administered − total ^{14}C recovered in excreta to that time). A plot of ln body burden against time was used to calculate the elimination half-life. This approach is particularly useful for calculating the elimination kinetics of compounds that are eliminated very slowly and also has the advantage of being non-invasive, and is illustrated in Table 5 and Figure 20. It should

be appreciated that in studies on slowly eliminated lipid-soluble compounds such as TCDD the radioactivity detected in the excreta may be present partly as metabolites (Neal *et al.*, 1982). Under such circumstances the sigma-minus method using excretion of total ^{14}C is only valid if the body burden is as parent compound and the metabolites, once formed, are eliminated rapidly—i.e. the rate limiting step is the initial metabolism of the parent compound.

The octachloro analogue of TCDD (OCDD) is 100–1000 times less potent than TCDD (Couture *et al.*, 1988) but it shows even slower elimination in rats with a half-life of 3–5 months, so that even greater accumulation is possible (Birnbaum and Couture, 1988). For compounds with such long half-lives, steady state will not have been reached at the end of a 7 week or 13 week study (Figure 21). In addition, if there is a minimum body burden or plasma concentration necessary for toxicity, this may have been reached only a short while before sacrifice. Clearly the interpretation of data from 'short-term' studies should take into account the half-life of the compound, since a 90 day study may be a steady state study for some

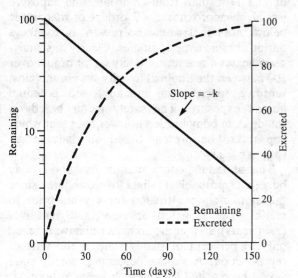

Figure 20 The calculation of the elimination rate constant from the cumulative elimination of the compound (see Table 5 for data). This analysis assumes that either the parent compound is excreted unchanged or the formation of excretable metabolites is the rate-limiting step

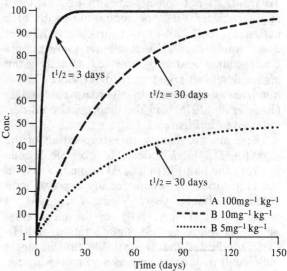

Figure 21 Accumulation of compounds during chronic administration. The compounds have similar apparent volumes of distribution but the clearance of A is 10 times greater than that of B, so that its half-life is 10 times less. Thus, daily intakes of 100 mg kg^{-1} of A and 10 mg kg^{-1} of B will give similar average steady state concentrations, while a dose of 5 mg kg^{-1} of B will give an average steady state concentrations one-half of that at a dose of 10 mg kg^{-1} day^{-1}

Table 5 Calculation of elimination rate constant by the sigma-minus method

Time (days)	% Dose excreted (as parent compound plus metabolites)				
	Urine	Faeces	Total	Cumulative total	Amount remaining
0	0.0	0.0	0.0	0.0	100.0
2	1.8	2.7	4.5	4.5	95.5
4	1.7	2.6	4.3	8.8	91.2
6	1.6	2.5	4.1	12.9	87.1
8	1.6	2.4	4.0	16.9	83.1
10	1.5	2.2	3.7	20.6	79.4
15	3.5	5.2	8.7	29.3	70.7
20	3.1	4.6	7.7	37.0	63.0
25	2.8	4.1	6.9	43.9	56.1
30	2.4	3.7	6.1	50.0	50.0
40	4.1	6.2	10.3	60.3	39.7
50	3.3	4.9	8.2	68.5	31.5
60	2.6	3.9	6.5	75.0	25.0
70	2.0	3.1	5.1	80.1	19.8
80	1.6	2.5	4.1	84.2	15.8
100	2.4	3.5	5.9	90.1	9.9
120	1.4	2.2	3.6	93.7	6.3
150	1.3	1.9	3.2	96.9	3.1

The data are for the excretion of a compound which is eliminated slowly by both urine and faeces with approximately 60 per cent of the dose excreted in faeces and 40 per cent in urine. The method assumes that the elimination of metabolites is formation rate limited and that there is no accumulation of metabolites.

Time = time at the end of the sequential collection intervals (e.g. 2 = 0–2; 30 = 25–30; and 150 = 120–150).

compounds but not for others (see Figure 21). Toxicologists not conversant with toxicokinetics might consider that, for compounds with such extremely long half-lives, animals given lower doses would eventually reach the same plasma concentration and body load as animals given higher doses but take longer to get there. This is *not* true as illustrated by the data for TCDD (Rose *et al.*, 1976) and the theoretical consideration given in Figure 21.

There are problems with extrapolation of the data for TCDD in rodents to possible human intakes. The half-life of TCDD in man, based on the elimination by occupationally exposed individuals, is about 7 years (Wolfe *et al.*, 1988); a recent report (Poiger, 1988) of the elimination of TCDD following self-administration of [³H]-TCDD indicated that the half-life (in this single individual) may be as long as 9 years. Using the value of 7 years it would take about 30–35 years of exposure for humans to reach steady state during constant intake. If the differences in half-life between animal species and humans are assumed to be due to differences in clearance, with no differences in the apparent volume of distribution, then it is possible to compare theoretical

steady state body burdens under differing rates of administration. These are summarized in Table 6 and indicate that the steady state body burden of TCDD in man from environmental exposure would be approximately 2 orders of magnitude below those that would be present in monkeys during chronic toxicity studies. Clearly this analysis indicates a reassuring safety factor of just over 100 between the minimal toxicity seen in the most sensitive species (the monkey) and potential human exposure. The safety factor based on steady state body burden is lower than that which appears to be present based on daily intake ($\mu g^{-1} kg^{-1} day^{-1}$).

The apparent safety margin based on body burden is probably a slight overestimate, since the monkeys were treated for 4 years prior to mating—i.e. a period of 'only' 1.46 half-lives (2.74 years), so that the animals will have reached only 64 per cent of steady state at the time of reproduction. A similar percentage steady state would be reached by a human being at approximately 10 years of age, whereas a woman giving birth at 25 years of age would have reached approximately 92 per cent of steady state. Thus, the apparent safety margin may have been over-

Table 6 Interspecies comparisons of theoretical steady state body burdens of TCDD at different rates of administration

Species	Half-life	Rate of administration	Steady state body burden
Rat	30 days	1.0 µg kg^{-1} day^{-1} [a] 0.1 µg kg^{-1} day^{-1} [a] 0.01 µg kg^{-1} day^{-1} [b]	approx. 20 µg kg^{-1} [a] approx. 2 µg kg^{-1} [a] 0.2 µg kg^{-1}
Guinea-pig	30 days	6 ng kg^{-1} day^{-1} [c]	0.12 µg kg^{-1}
Monkey	1000 days [d]	0.12 ng kg^{-1} day^{-1} [e]	0.08 µg kg^{-1}
Man	7 years [f]	0.0004 ng kg^{-1} day^{-1} [g]	0.0007 µg kg^{-1}

[a] Data from Gehring and Young (1978) at toxic doses during a 90 day study. Used as the basis for calculating the steady state body burdens in other species by correcting for half-life (assuming no species differences in the apparent volume of distribution).

$$\text{Body burden at steady state} = 20 \times \frac{\text{rate of administration (ng kg}^{-1}\text{ day}^{-1})}{1000} \times \frac{\text{half-life}}{30} \text{ (days)}$$

[b] Minimal effect level for carcinogenic effects (HMSO, 1989).
[c] Minimal effect level for immunotoxic effects (HMSO, 1989).
[d] Taken from HMSO (1989), p. 96.
[e] Minimal effect level for reproductive toxicity (HMSO, 1989).
[f] Taken from Wolfe *et al.* (1988).
[g] Daily intake from foods in West Germany (HMSO, 1989).

estimated by a factor of about 1.4. In contrast, if the limiting toxicity had been carcinogenicity in the rat, then steady state would have been approached in the animals after 4–5 months—i.e. after approximately 16 per cent of the animal's life. In contrast, the steady state for humans given in Table 6 would not have been approached until after 28–35 years—i.e. approximately 50 per cent of the life-span. Thus, the test animals would have been exposed to the steady state body burden for a considerably longer proportion of their life-span than would be possible in humans.

An interesting safety issue that is resolvable by toxicokinetic considerations concerns the intake of TCDD and related compounds by human infants via maternal milk. The concentrations of TCDD in human milk exceed those in meat, eggs and cow's milk (HMSO, 1989) and therefore higher plasma concentrations and body burdens might be anticipated. However, higher body loads would only occur if the intake of human milk extended for 4–5 times the half-life of the compound, which in the case of TCDD would mean 30–35 years! Exposure via human milk is of such limited duration, with respect to the half-life of TCDD, that even after 6 months' lactation the neonatal plasma concentrations would be only 5 per cent of the final steady state value. Thus, if

the daily intake in infants via maternal milk was as much as 20 times that in adults, then the infant would only just have reached the adult steady state plasma concentration after 6 months' suckling. Therefore, in reality, exposure via maternal milk would not pose an extra risk to the neonate, but would simply act as a 'loading dose', so that the adult steady state would be achieved more rapidly, and then subsequently maintained by the adult daily intake.

This detailed analysis of the case of TCDD illustrates the critical role that toxicokinetics can play in the design and interpretation of toxicity studies, especially when the compound has a very long half-life. In addition it should be appreciated that if as a result of the animal toxicity data it was decided that human intakes should be reduced immediately to negligible levels, it would take about 7 years before the existing body burdens decreased by 50 per cent, and about 30–40 years before they became negligible. In reality, comparison of the persistence of TCDD in mammalian organisms compared with the environment (DiDomenico and Zapponi, 1986) indicates that the latter would be rate-limiting in any attempted reduction of human body burden.

The body burden of TCDD in humans in Table 6 was calculated using a very simplistic analysis based on the body burdens of animals corrected for clearances (assuming that differences in half-lives are due to differences in clearance) and intakes; but it is probably realistic. Most TCDD accumulates in fat and to some extent the liver, and so it can be assumed that the body burden of a 70 kg human ($0.0007 \mu g\ kg^{-1} \times 70 = 0.049$ $\mu g\ kg^{-1}$ is concentrated in the 10 kg of fat, i.e. approximately $0.005 \mu g\ kg^{-1}$ of fat. This value is almost identical with that found in human body fat (approximately 6 ng kg^{-1}; HMSO, 1989, p.44).

The use of animal data to predict the body load of TCDD in humans in Table 6 is the simplest form of interspecies extrapolation. There are two principal methods by which more sophisticated extrapolations may be made—i.e. *allometry* and *physiologically based pharmacokinetic models*. The basis of both methods is that there are underlying basic similarities between mammalian species in the various processes involved in toxicokinetics. For example, (1) the intestine contains similar digestive enzymes and provides a large surface area for *absorption* via microvilli; (2) the compositions of blood and body tissues are similar across species with respect to fat and protein content, so that tissue *distribution* should be similar; (3) the perfusion of the organs of *elimination* and the basic metabolic and excretion processes within these organs are similar. Thus, reasonable estimates of human pharmacokinetic parameters should be derived from animal data after allowing for differences in body weight, cardiac output, etc. It should be emphasized that there are bound to be examples where clear species differences exist, especially with respect to specific pathways of metabolism, which render such extrapolations inappropriate.

Allometry is a mathematical extrapolation based on the body weight of the animal (Calder, 1981). Thus, the value of any parameter (P) is related to the mean body weight (W) of the species by an equation with two unknown variables:

$$P = aW^x$$

If the parameter estimate P is known in two or more species, then its value in a third species can be deduced from a simple regression equation of log P against log W. For example, the clearance values of the drug ceftizoxime in mice ($W = 23$ g), rats ($W = 180$ g), monkey ($W = 7500$ g) and dog ($W = 12\ 000$ g) are 84.4, 208.8, 2670 and

2340 ml h^{-1}, respectively (Mordenti, 1985). A regression of log clearance against log of body weight had a slope (x) of 0.573 and an intercept (log a) of 1.103 so that:

$$P = 12.69W^{0.573}$$

Using this equation, the clearance values calculated for mice, rats, monkeys, dogs and humans ($W = 70\ 000$ g) are 77, 249, 2108, 2760 and 7581 ml h^{-1}, respectively.

Interspecies comparisons of caffeine pharmacokinetics (Bonati *et al.*, 1985) showed that the apparent volume of distribution was linearly related to body weight (W) (i.e. $V = 0.79W^{1.00}$), while the plasma clearance (CL) showed a log-linear relationship (i.e. CL $= 6.26W^{0.739}$), the power term of which was similar to that for liver weight (L) (i.e. $L = 0.037W^{0.845}$).

Boxenbaum (1984) provides useful background information on the origins of allometry in pharmacokinetic scaling and extends this by the use of Dedrick plots in which plasma concentration—time curves in different species can be made superimposable if the concentration is corrected for dose (e.g. $\mu g\ ml^{-1}$ per mg kg^{-1}) and the time is corrected for body weight (e.g. min kg$^{-0.25}$). The basis for this latter correction is conversion to 'physiological time', which in effect relates body weight to the life-span of the animal. Thus, 100 min in the life of a 22 g mouse is physiologically equivalent to 751 min in the life of a 70 kg human. Although the approach of correcting pharmacokinetic data for the maximum potential life-span helped to linearize the relationship between intrinsic clearance of caffeine and body weight (Bonati *et al.*, 1985) the authors concluded that 'no practical use can yet be suggested for the resulting good fit'. Bachmann (1989) has applied allometry to the pharmacokinetics for a number of drugs in laboratory animals and man. For each drug there was a linear relationship between the log of the apparent volumes of distribution and the log of body weights, with correlation coefficients >0.95. The log of the clearance was not as closely related to the log of the body weight unless multiplied by the maximum life-span potential (MLP) for each species. This is shown in Figure 22, which also illustrates the principle of allometric analysis. Bachmann proposed that the clearance in a species could be calculated from the CL $\times$ MLP regression, since the term

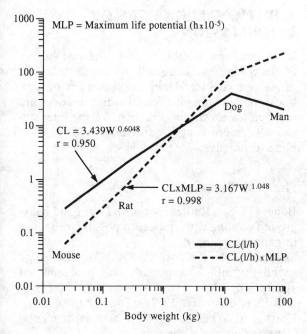

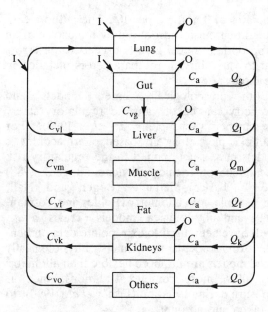

Figure 22 Interspecies scaling applied to the plasma clearance of phencyclidine. Data taken from Bachmann (1989)

Figure 23 A physiologically based pharmacokinetic model. The rate of delivery to an organ such as muscle (m) is given by the blood flow (Q_m) times the arterial concentration (C_a). The rate of removal from the organ is blood flow (Q_m) times the venous concentration (C_{vm}). Input functions (I) and output functions (O) can be first-order or Michaelis–Menten reactions. More complex models have been used, incorporating specific targets, such as bone marrow, or additional routes such as transdermal, in which case skin becomes a discrete compartment

CL × MLP divided by body weight (BW) was relatively constant across species. Thus, if the mean CL × MLP/BW was calculated for three animal species, this value could then be used to derive the clearance in a 70 kg human with a MLP of 9.9×10^5 h (113 years).

An alternative approach is that of *physiologically based pharmacokinetic modelling* (Gerlowski and Jain, 1983). The basis of the method is that each major organ system, plus any specialized sites, such as targets for toxicity, are taken as representing a physiological compartment. Each separate compartment has its own blood flow, tissue volume, uptake process, affinity for the compound (i.e. partition coefficient) and elimination process, as appropriate (Figure 23). Thus, the kinetics of the compound are described by a series of flow-related equations which can be solved following the incorporation of known physiological values and experimental estimates (e.g. partition coefficients). The value of this technique is that it allows an assessment of the impact of altered physiology (e.g. ageing and renal function) on the toxicokinetics and target organ exposure. More importantly, species differences can be predicted based on known differences in perfusion rates, etc. In cases where an important physiological value is not known for a species, this can be derived by allometry from species in which the values are known.

Simpler physiologically based models may be derived which are a compromise between physiological compartments and traditional rapidly and slowly equilibrating compartments. For example, Andersen *et al.* (1987) utilized a mixture of specific physiological compartments, liver, fat, lung and gut, with two general compartments 'richly perfused' and 'slowly perfused', in the analysis of the inhalation kinetics of dichloromethane.

The precision of a model similar to that used by Andersen *et al.* (1987) was investigated by Bois *et al.* (1990) for the saturable formation of the carcinogenic epoxide metabolite of tetrachloroethylene. The physiological model was coupled to a multistage model of carcinogenesis to predict cancer risk in humans exposed to 1 ng l^{-1} of tetrachloroethylene vapour. The median predicted incidence was 1.6 cancer per 10^6, and varying the parameter estimates within physiologically realistic bounds produced 5th and 95th percentile estimates of 0 and 6.8 per 10^6. The authors concluded that biases introduced by the choice of an inappropriate model greatly exceeded the errors due to variability in the parameters included in the model.

Both physiologically based models and allometry can be of value to regulatory safety assessments (Scheuplein *et al.*, 1990). For example, physiologically based pharmacokinetic models have been applied to the regulatory risk assessment of trichloroethylene (Bogen, 1988) and 1,1,1-trichloroethane (Bogen and Hall, 1989), while both allometry (Beliles and Totman, 1989) and physiological models (Travis *et al.*, 1990) have been used to extrapolate data on benzene from rodents to humans. Physiologically based models are far more flexible than allometry and allow more complex situations, such as exposure during lactation (Fisher *et al.*, 1990), to be taken into account.

The pharmacokinetics of TCDD in the rat have been fitted using a simple physiologically based model which allowed for enzyme induction (Leung *et al.*, 1990a). A similar model accurately predicted the influence of an inducing dose of TCDD on the concentration–time curve of the analogue 2-iodo-3,7,8-trichlorodibenzo-*p*-dioxin. Therefore autoinduction during high-dose animal toxicity studies on TCDD can be taken into account by these models in predicting the behaviour of TCDD at the lower environmental doses received by humans (Leung *et al.*, 1990b). A more complex physiological model has been developed for the fate of TCDD in man (Kissel and Robarge, 1988). A number of assumptions were made in the model, but trial simulations showed that the most important variables were adipose:blood partition coefficients and adipose perfusion. The model also estimated intake and body exposure on the basis of likely dietary sources, and accurately predicted the half-life and body burden in man. The model also showed that the half-life was dependent on the relative amount of faecal output compared with adipose tissue storage. The potential value of this approach was demonstrated by simulations which showed that faecal output of TCDD was significantly enhanced by the ingestion of 10 g per day of a non-absorbable oil, and that this reduced both the half-life and steady state concentration in adipose tissue by 60 per cent.

ADDITIONAL SOURCES OF INFORMATION

It has not been possible to cover the vast subject of toxicokinetics adequately within the confines of a single chapter. There are a number of textbooks and review articles to which readers are referred for further information, for the interpretation of more complex situations and for sampling techniques.

General Texts

Benet (1976)   Rather specialized but good background reading with respect to possible problems in geriatric animals.

Smyth and Hottendorf (1980)   Contains some useful examples, especially of problems of absorption.

Gibaldi and Perrier (1982)   The definitive text.

Curry and Whelpton (1983)   An experimental introduction to the subject.

Benet *et al.* (1984)   Based on a symposium, and therefore lacks the structure of Gibaldi and Perrier or Rowland and Tucker but contains some useful information.

Greenblatt and Shader (1985)   Introductory text (don't be put off by the title).

Clarke and Smith (1986)   Introductory text.

Rowland and Tucker (1986)   A more advanced text with useful chapters on interspecies scaling, dose- and time-dependent kinetics, and response modelling.

Review Articles

Gehring and Young (1978)   Contains interesting examples from the work of the pioneers in the application of pharmacokinetics to problems of animal toxicology.

Wilkinson (1984)   A clearly written article which deals with first-pass metabolism and dose-dependent kinetics and introduces physiological approaches.

O'Flaherty (1985)   A consideration of dose-dependent metabolism.

Wilkinson (1987)   A comprehensive review of the application of clearance concepts to the elimination of foreign components; not toxicology orientated, but an excellent source of references ($n = 525$).

Renwick (1989)   Similar to the present chapter

but with an expanded section on dose-dependent kinetics and metabolite kinetics, and worked examples.
Scheuplein *et al.* (1990) An interesting article on the value of toxicokinetic data to regulatory agencies such as the FDA.

Pharmacokinetic Data Fitting

Drug Metabolism Reviews (1984), Volume **15**, contains a series of valuable but mathematically complex articles by leading workers in the field of pharmacokinetics. Topics covered include compartmental models (Segre: pp. 7–53), physiological models (Rowland: pp. 55–74), models in health and disease (Balant: pp. 75–102), non-compartmental statistical moments (Nuesch: pp. 103–131), the weighting of data for regression analysis (Peck, Sheiner and Nichols: pp. 133–148), population pharmacokinetics (Sheiner: pp. 153–171) and population pharmacokinetics applied to destructively obtained experimental data (Lindstrom and Birkes: pp. 195–264). This last paper proposes the derivation of pharmacokinetic parameters from observations of the concentrations in the plasma and tissues of sacrificed animals, but the choice of an appropriately timed sampling protocol would be essential.

Sampling Techniques

Waynforth (1980) A textbook on surgical techniques in the rat.
Bakar and Niazi (1983) A simple and reliable method for chronic venous cannulation in the rat.
Cocchetto and Bjornsson (1983) Various methods of collecting rat body fluids – a useful review with 501 references.

REFERENCES

Andersen, M. E., Clewell, H. J., Gargas, M. L., Smith, F. A. and Reitz, R. H. (1987). Physiologically based pharmacokinetics and the risk assessment process for methylene chloride. *Toxicol. Appl. Pharmacol.*, **87**, 185–205

Bachmann, K. (1989) Predicting toxicokinetic parameters in humans from toxicokinetic data acquired from three small mammalian species. *J. Appl. Toxicol.*, **9**, 331–338

Bakar, S. L. and Niazi, S. (1983). Simple reliable method for chronic cannulation of the jugular vein for pharmacokinetic studies in rats. *J. Pharm. Sci.*, **72**, 1027–1029

Beatty, P. W., Vaughn, W. K. and Neal, R. A. (1978). Effect of alteration of rat hepatic mixed-function oxidase (MFO) activity on the toxicity of 2,3,7,8-tetrachlorodibenzo-*p*-dioxin (TCDD). *Toxicol. Appl. Pharmacol.*, **45**, 513–519

Beliles, R. P. and Totman, L. C. (1989). Pharmacokinetically based risk assessment of workplace exposure to benzene. *Regulatory Toxicol. Pharmacol.*, **9**, 186–195

Benet, L. Z. (1976) *The Effect of Disease States on Drug Pharmacokinetics*, American Pharmaceutical Association, Washington, D.C.

Benet, L. Z., Levy, G. and Ferraiolo, B. L. (1984). *Pharmacokinetics: A Modern View*, Plenum Press, London

Birnbaum, L. S. and Couture, L. A. (1988). Disposition of octachlorodibenzo-*p*-dioxin (OCDD) in male rats. *Toxicol. Appl. Pharmacol.*, **93**, 22–30

Blumer, J. L. (1990). The effect of physiological competence on toxicity: the response of neonates. In Volans, G. N., Sims, J., Sullivan, F. M. and Turner, P. (Eds), *Basic Science in Toxicology*. Taylor and Francis, London, pp. 375–389

Bogen, K. T. (1988). Pharmacokinetics for regulatory risk analysis: the case of trichloroethylene. *Regulatory Toxicol. Pharmacol.*, **8**, 447–466

Bogen, K. T. and Hall, L. C. (1989). Pharmacokinetics for regulatory risk analysis: the case of 1,1,1-trichloroethane (methylchloroform). *Regulatory Toxicol. Pharmacol.*, **10**, 26–50

Bois, F. Y., Zeise, L. and Tozer, T. N. (1990). Precision and sensitivity of pharmacokinetic models for cancer risk assessment: tetrachloroethylene in mice, rats and human. *Toxicol. Appl. Pharmacol.*, **102**, 300–315

Bonati, M., Latini, R., Tognoni, G., Young, J. F. and Garattini, S. (1985). Interspecies comparison of *in vivo* caffeine pharmacokinetics in man, monkey, rabbit, rat and mouse. *Drug Metab. Rev.*, **15**, 1355–1383

Bopp, B. A., Sonders, R. C. and Kesterson, J. W. (1986). Toxicological aspects of cyclamate and cyclohexylamine. *CRC Crit. Rev. Toxicol.*, **16**, 213–306

Boxenbaum, H. (1984). Interspecies pharmacokinetic scaling and the evolutionary-comparative paradigm. *Drug Metab. Rev.*, **15**, 1071–1121

Calder, W. M. (1981). Scaling of physiological process in homeothermic animal. *Ann. Rev. Physiol.*, **43**, 301–322

Clarke, B. and Smith, D. A. (1986) *An Introduction to Pharmacokinetics*. Blackwell, Oxford

Cocchetto, D. M. and Bjornsson, T. D. (1983). Methods for vascular access and collection of body fluids from the laboratory rat. *J. Pharm. Sci.*, **72**, 465–492

Couture, L. A., Elwell, M. R. and Birnbaum, L. S. (1988). Dioxin like effects in male rats following exposure to octachlorodibenzo-*p*-dioxin (OCDD) during a 13-week study. *Toxicol. Appl. Pharmacol.*, **93**, 31–46

Curry, S. H. and Whelpton, R. (1983). *Manual of Laboratory Pharmacokinetics*. Wiley, Chichester

DiDomenico, A. and Zapponi, G. A. (1986). 2,3,7,8-Tetrachlorodibenzo-*p*-dioxin (TCDD) in the environment: human health risk estimation and its application to the Seveso case as an example. *Regulatory Toxicol. Pharmacol.*, **6**, 248–260

Dietz, F. K., Stott, W. T. and Ramsey, J. C. (1982). Non-linear pharmacokinetics and their impact on toxicology: illustrated with dioxane. *Drug Metab. Rev.*, **13**, 963–981

Fisher, J. W., Whittaker, T. A., Taylor, D. H., Clewell, H. J. and Andersen, M. E. (1990). Physiologically based pharmacokinetic modeling of the lactating rat and nursing pup: a multiroute exposure model for trichloroethylene and its metabolite, trichloroacetic acid. *Toxicol. Appl. Pharmacol.*, **102**, 497–513

Gasiewicz, T. A. and Neal, R. A. (1979). 2,3,7,8-Tetrachlorodibenzo-*p*-dioxin tissue distribution, excretion, and effects on clinical chemistry parameters in guinea pigs. *Toxicol. Appl. Pharmacol.*, **51**, 329–339

Gehring, P. J. and Young, J. D. (1978). Application of pharmacokinetic principles in practice. In Plaa, G. L. and Duncan, W. A. M. (Eds), *Proceedings of the First International Congress on Toxicology*. Academic Press, London, pp. 119–141

Gerlowski, L. E. and Jain, R. K. (1983). Physiologically based pharmacokinetic modeling: principles and applications. *J. Pharm. Sci.*, **72**, 1103–1127

Gibaldi, M. and Perrier, D. (1982). *Pharmacokinetics*, 2nd edn. Marcel Dekker, New York

Glocklin, V. C. (1982). General considerations for studies of the metabolism of drugs and other chemicals. *Drug Metab. Rev.*, **13**, 929–939

Greenblatt, D. J. and Shader, R. I. (1985). *Pharmacokinetics in Clinical Practice*. Saunders, London

HMSO (1989). *Dioxins in the Environment*. Department of the Environment, Central Directorate of Environment Protection. Pollution Paper No. 27. Her Majesty's Stationery Office, London

Kissel, J. C. and Robarge, G. M. (1988). Assessing the elimination of 2,3,7,8-TCDD from humans with a physiologically based pharmacokinetic model. *Chemosphere*, **17**, 2017–2027

Kociba, R. J., Keeler, P. A., Park, C. N. and Gehring, P. J. (1976). 2,3,7,8-Tetrachlorodibenzo-*p*-dioxin (TCDD): results of a 13-week oral toxicity study in rats. *Toxicol. Appl. Pharmacol.*, **35**, 553–574

Leung, H.-W., Paustenbach, D. J., Murray, F. J. and Andersen, M. E. (1990a). A physiological pharmacokinetic description of the tissue distribution and enzyme-inducing properties of 2,3,7,8-tetrachlorodibenzo-*p*-dioxin in the rat. *Toxicol. Appl. Pharmacol.*, **103**, 399–410

Leung, H.-W., Poland, A., Paustenbach, D. J., Murray, F. J. and Andersen, M. E. (1990b). Pharmacokinetics of [^{125}I]–2-iodo-3,7,8-trichlorodibenzo-*p*-dioxin in mice: analysis with a physiological modeling approach. *Toxicol. Appl. Pharmacol.*, **103**, 411–419

McConnell, E. E., Moore, J. A., Haseman, J. K. and Harris, M. W. (1978). The comparative toxicity of chlorinated dibenzo-*p*-dioxins in mice and guinea pigs. *Toxicol. Appl. Pharmacol*, **44**, 335–356

Mordenti, J. (1985). Pharmacokinetic scale up: accurate prediction of human pharmacokinetic profiles from animal data. *J. Pharm. Sci.*, **74**, 1097–1099

Neal, R. A., Olson, J. R., Gasiewicz, T. A. and Geiger, L. E. (1982). The toxicokinetics of 2,3,7,8-tetrachlorodibenzo-*p*-dioxin in mammalian systems. *Drug Metab. Rev.*, **13**, 355–385

O'Flaherty, E. J. (1985). Differences in metabolism at different dose levels. In Clayson, D. B., Krewski, D. and Munro, I. (Eds). *Toxicological Risk Assessment*, Vol. 1. CRC Press, Boca Raton, Florida, pp. 53–90

Olson, J. R., Gasiewicz, T. A. and Neal, R. A.(1980a). Tissue distribution, excretion and metabolism of 2,3,7,8-tetrachlorodibenzo-*p*-dioxin (TCDD) in the golden Syrian hamster. *Toxicol. Appl. Pharmacol.*, **56**, 78–85

Olson, J. R., Holscher, M. A. and Neal, R. A. (1980b). Toxicity of 2,3,7,8-tetrachlorodibenzo-*p*-dioxin in the golden Syrian hamster. *Toxicol. Appl. Pharmacol.*, **55**, 67–78

Pohjanvirta, R., Vartiainen, T., Uusi-Rauva, A., Monkkonen, J. and Tuomisto, J. (1990). Tissue distribution, metabolism, and excretion of ^{14}C-TCDD in a TCDD-susceptible and a TCDD-resistant rat strain. *Pharmacol. Toxicol.*, **66**, 93–100

Poiger, H. (1988). Toxicokinetics of 2,3,7,8-TCDD in man: an update. Proceedings of *Dioxin '88, Umeå, Sweden*

Renwick, A. G. (1986). The metabolism of intense sweeteners. *Xenobiotica*, **16**, 1057–1071

Renwick, A. G. (1989). Pharmacokinetics in toxicology. In Hayes, A. W. (Ed.), *Principles and Methods of Toxicology*, 2nd edn. Raven Press, New York, pp. 835–878

Roberts, A. and Renwick, A. G. (1989). The pharmacokinetics and tissue concentrations of cyclohexylamine in rats and mice. *Toxicol. Appl. Pharmacol.*, **98**, 230–242

Roberts, A., Renwick, A. G., Ford, G., Creasy, D. M. and Gaunt, I. F. (1989). The metabolism and testicular toxicity of cyclohexylamine in rats and mice during chronic dietary administration. *Toxicol. Appl. Pharmacol.*, **98**, 216–229

Rose, J. Q., Ramsey, J. C., Wentzler, T. H., Hummel, R. A. and Gehring, P. J. (1976). The fate of 2,3,7,8,-tetrachlorodibenzo-*p*-dioxin following single and repeated oral doses to the rat. *Toxicol. Appl. Pharmacol.*, **36**, 209–226

Rowland, M. and Tucker, G. T. (1986). *Pharmacokinetics: Theory and Methodology*, Pergamon Press, Oxford

Scheuplein, R. J., Shoaf, S. E. and Brown, R. N. (1990). Role of pharmacokinetics in safety evaluation and regulatory considerations. *Ann. Rev. Pharmacol. Toxicol.*, **30**, 197–218

Smyth, R. D. and Hottendorf, G. H. (1980). Application of pharmacokinetics and biopharmaceutics in the design of toxicological studies. *Toxicol. Appl. Pharmacol.*, **53**, 179–195

Sweatman, T. W., Renwick, A. G. and Burgess, C. D. (1981). The pharmacokinetics of saccharin in man. *Xenobiotica*, **11**, 531–540

Travis, C. C., Quillen, J. L. and Arms, A. D. (1990). Pharmacokinetics of benzene. *Toxicol. Appl. Pharmacol.*, **102**, 400–420

Waynforth, H. B. (1980). *Experimental and Surgical Technique in the Rat*, Academic Press, London

Wilkinson, G. R. (1976). Pharmacokinetics in disease states modifying body perfusion. In Benet, L. Z. (Ed.), *The Effect of Disease States on Drug Pharmacokinetics*. American Pharmaceutical Association, Academy of Pharmaceutical Sciences, Washington, D. C., pp. 13–32

Wilkinson, G. R. (1984). Pharmacokinetic considerations in toxicology. In Mitchell, J. R. and Horning, M. G. (Eds) *Drug Metabolism and Drug Toxicity*. Raven Press, New York, pp. 213–235

Wilkinson, G. R. (1987). Clearance approaches in pharmacology. *Pharmacol. Rev.*, **39**, 1–47

Wolfe, W., Miner, J. and Peterson, M. (1988). Serum 2,3,7,8-tetrachloro-*p*-dioxin levels in air force health study participants—preliminary report. *J. Am. Med. Assoc.*, **259**, 3533–3535

Yacobi, A., Kamath, B. L. and Lai, C.-M. (1982). Pharmacokinetics in chronic animal toxicity studies. *Drug Metab. Rev.*, **13**, 1021–1051

FURTHER READING

Bryson, P. D. (1989). Pharmacokinetics and Toxicokinetics. In *Comprehensive Review in Toxicology*, Aspen Publishers, Rockville, Maryland, pp. 53–62

Grahame-Smith, D. G. and Aronson, J. K. (1992). The pharmacokinetic process. In *Oxford Textbook of Clinical Pharmacology and Drug Therapy*, Oxford University Press, pp. 13–40

Klaassen, C. D. (1991). Absorption, distribution and excretion of toxicants. In Amdur, M. O., Doull, J. and Klaassen, C. D. (Eds), *Casarett and Doull's Toxicology*, 4th edn. Pergamon Press, New York, pp. 50–87

Rescigno, A. and Thakur, A. K. (1991). *New Trends in Pharmacokinetics*. Plenum Press, New York

5 Physiologically-Based Pharmacokinetic Modelling

Hon-Wing Leung

INTRODUCTION

Pharmacokinetic (PK) models are used to make a rational prediction of the disposition of a chemical throughout the body (Gibaldi and Perrier, 1982). PK modelling has evolved over the past several decades. An early approach assumes that data on the internal environment of a chemical— e.g. tissue concentrations—cannot be obtained without employing invasive techniques. These PK models are developed to predict concentrations of chemicals in readily accessible media, such as blood and excreta. The plasma concentration, as an index of bioavailability, is assumed to mimic the biological effect in the entire system. Evidently this kind of approach cannot provide information on the concentration–time course of a chemical at the target site, which is not necessarily reflected by the blood concentration.

In recent years biologically based models which apply first principles such as material balance and incorporate physiological parameters are being developed, initially to describe the kinetics of therapeutic drugs (Himmelstein and Lutz, 1979), then to environmental chemicals (Menzel, 1987). These models include the exact physiology and anatomy of the animal species being described, as well as parameters such as blood flow, ventilation rates, metabolic constants, tissue solubilities and binding to macromolecules. These models are commonly known as physiologically based pharmacokinetic (PB-PK) models.

Classical Versus Physiological Pharmacokinetics

In early PK modelling the whole body is treated as a single compartment. More sophisticated models are created by the addition of peripheral compartments. In a multicompartment model the concentration–time course in the central compartment is typically curvilinear with a terminal linear portion. By the method of residuals or feathering, this kinetic behaviour is mathematically resolved into decaying exponential terms to account for the curvature of the data. The number of exponential terms corresponds to the number of compartments in the model, each representing an exchange between a peripheral tissue or organ with the central compartment. Obviously compartmentalization by such a rigid curve stripping process is a rather abstract mathematical construct and lacks physiological relevance.

In recent years physiological modelling has emerged as a pre-eminent approach to PK modelling (Clewell and Andersen, 1985; D'Souza and Boxenbaum, 1988). However, it must be emphasized that classical and physiological PK are not fundamentally incompatible; in fact, they share a common connection. The difference between them lies in the kinds of parameters on which the models are developed, and consequently they differ in their applications. In classical PK modelling no attempt is made to assign physiological correlates to model parameters. A compartment is simply considered as a kinetically homogeneous volume with transfer constants in and out of the compartment. In physiological PK a compartment is treated as individual organs or tissues arranged in precise anatomical configuration connected by the cardiovascular system. The transfer of chemicals between compartments is governed by actual blood flow rates and tissue solubilities (partition coefficients).

Because of a lack of biological constraints with conventional PK modelling, empirical data can be fitted by freely varying the model parameters. These best estimates of parameter values can then be statistically compared across experimental conditions, treatments or chemicals to establish whether apparent differences are significant. In contrast, in physiological PK modelling any major discrepancies between the physiological model prediction and experimental data will necessitate the reformulation of the model to account for the observed behaviour. Since classical models are constructed without conforming to anatomical reality, they cannot account for physiological or biochemical alterations such as body and organ weight changes (tissue growth or atrophy) or

Table 1   Physiologically based pharmacokinetic models for environmental toxicants

Chemical	Reference
Benzene	Medinsky *et al.* (1989); Travis *et al.* (1990)
2-Butoxyethanol	Johanson (1986)
Carbon tetrachloride	Paustenbach *et al.* (1988)
Chloroform	Corley *et al.* (1990)
1,2-Dichloroethane	D'Souza *et al.* (1988)
1,1-Dichloroethylene	D'Souza and Andersen (1988)
Dichloromethane	Andersen *et al.* (1987a)
Dieldrin	Lindstrom *et al.* (1974)
1,4-Dioxane	Leung and Paustenbach (1990)
2,2',4,4',5,5'-Hexabromobiphenyl	Tuey and Matthews (1980)
2-Iodo–3,7,8-trichlorodibenzo-*p*-dioxin	Leung *et al.* (1990b)
Kepone	Bungay *et al.* (1981)
Lead	Dalley *et al.* (1990)
Nickel	Menzel (1988)
Polychorinated biphenyls	Lutz *et al.* (1984)
Soman	Maxwell *et al.* (1988)
Styrene	Ramsey and Andersen (1984)
2,3,7,8-Tetrachlorodibenzofuran	King *et al.* (1983)
2,3,7,8-Tetrachlorodibenzo-*p*-dioxin	Leung *et al.* (1988, 1990a)
Tetrachloroethylene	Ward *et al.* (1988)
1,1,1-Trichloroethane	Reitz *et al.* (1988b); Dallas *et al.* (1989)
Trichloroethylene	Fisher *et al.* (1989, 1990)

enzyme induction and inhibition. While both classical and physiological models are capable of predicting tissue doses, albeit to somewhat different extents, classical models do not lend themselves to interspecies extrapolation of such dose–effect data.

THEORY AND PRINCIPLE OF PHYSIOLOGICAL MODELLING

The transfer of a chemical out of a single compartment follows Fick's law of simple diffusion, which states that the flux of a chemical is proportional to its concentration gradient. The differential rate equation describing this first-order process can be written as follows:

$$(\delta C/\delta t) = K \cdot \triangle C/V \qquad (1)$$

where C is the concentration of chemical in the compartment; K is the transfer constant; V is the volume of the compartment; and $\triangle C$ is the concentration gradient.

If the transfer is perfusion- or flow-limited, then the transfer constant is the rate of blood flow (Q) to the compartment. It follows, therefore:

$$(\delta C/\delta t) = Q(C_a - C_v)/V \qquad (2)$$

where C_a is the concentration of the chemical in the arterial blood entering the compartment and C_v is the concentration of the chemical in the venous blood leaving the compartment.

Since chemicals do not equilibrate freely in body fluids but, depending on their physicochemical properties, may be sequestered in tissue lipids, the concentration determined experimentally from a tissue sample is a composite of both the free and the sequestered form. Since transfer of a chemical in a tissue compartment is assumed to be flow-limited, the chemical concentration in the venous blood exiting from a tissue is equal to the concentration in the tissue fluid—i.e. the so-called free form. The partitioning of the chemical between the body fluid and tissue lipids is governed by tissue solubility or partition coefficient, P, as follows:

$$P = C/C_v$$

Substituting this into Equation (2), one obtains

$$(\delta C/\delta t) = Q(C_a - C/P)/V \qquad (3)$$

Equation (3) represents the fundamental relationship on which all PB-PK models are constructed. The expression for all non-metabolizing, non-eliminating and non-binding tissue compartments will have this same mathematical form. The expressions for blood and other eliminating tissues such as liver, kidney and lung are more complex, but are based on the same principles of flow, mass conservation and partitioning.

DEVELOPMENT OF PHYSIOLOGICAL PHARMACOKINETIC MODELS

The development of a PB-PK model is a highly integrative process. Figure 1 depicts the flow processes in the development of a PB-PK model. The first step involves defining the nature of the problem and reviewing the literature to assess the impact of mechanism on the choice of tissue dosimetrics. The actual model formulation is divided into four interwoven steps, as follows.

Selection of Appropriate Tissue Compartments

The most natural approach to the choice of tissue compartments in PB-PK modelling is to model a whole body by describing every organ and tissue. However, such detailed models, aside from the prohibitive labour and expenses to develop them, are not required in most circumstances. The selection should be governed by the degree of

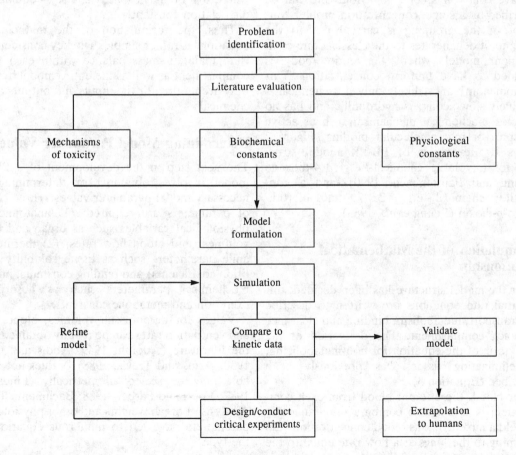

Figure 1 Flow chart of the development of a physiologically based pharmacokinetic model. Problem identification: the finding of a particular toxicity, in a particular organ, in a particular species. Literature evaluation: the integration of available information about the mechanism of toxicity, the pathways of chemical metabolism, the nature of the toxic chemical species, the tissue-binding characteristics and the physiological parameters of the target species. From these data a model is developed to estimate the appropriate measure of tissue exposure for a wide variety of exposure conditions. Reprinted with permission from National Academy Press, Washington, D.C.

detail necessary to provide a satisfactory depiction of the events. A knowledge of the chemical's mode and mechanism of action and its physico-chemical properties will help make such a judgement. For instance, if a substance is known to accumulate in, bind to, be metabolized by or be toxic to specific organs or tissues, these should form the integral compartments of the model that are described in detail. If a chemical is highly lipophilic, then the adipose tissues should be described as a separate compartment. Other 'non-target' organs and tissues may be lumped together with respect to similar kinds or properties—e.g. richly perfused tissues representing kidneys and other visceral organs, slowly perfused tissues representing skin and muscle. The tissues or organs in the same body group are considered to have common kinetic behaviour and can be described by a single concentration profile. Naturally, if the grouping is carried out to the extreme, it degenerates to the classical one-compartment model, where the entire body is assumed to have uniform concentration. This phenomenon is most likely only if a chemical is relatively slow-acting, is hydrophilic and has no complex biochemical mechanism such as active transport or macromolecular binding. Figure 2 shows two examples of PB-PK model structure for a volatile chemical—e.g. 1,4-dioxane (Leung and Paustenbach, 1990)—and a non-volatile chemical—e.g. 2,3,7,8-tetrachlorodibenzo-*p*-dioxin (Leung *et al.*, 1989).

Formulation of the Mathematical Relationship

After the model structure has been decided, differential rate equations are written to describe the transport, metabolism, binding and clearance for each compartment. The derivation of the basic form of the equation for non-metabolizing, non-eliminating tissues has previously been described (Equation 3).

For blood, the efferent blood from each compartment is assumed to combine simultaneously to yield a mixed venous blood concentration (C_b) returning to the lungs at a flow rate equal to the cardiac output (Q_b), as follows:

$$(\delta C_b/\delta t) = \Sigma(Q_i \cdot C_{vi})/Q_b$$

where i = name of tissue compartment.

For metabolizing tissues such as the liver, depending on the number and type of metabolic pathways, the basic differential equation is modified by the inclusion of terms describing a first-order metabolic process (K_f) or a saturable Michaelis–Menten type enzyme kinetics (K_m and V_{max}) or both:

$$V(\delta C/\delta t) = Q(C_a - C/P) - K_f(C/P) - (V_{max} \cdot C/P)/(K_m + C/P)$$

For tissues which exhibit specific binding, in addition to the amount partitioned by solubility, the total tissue concentration will also include the portion in bound form, as follows:

$$V\delta C/\delta t = Q(C_a - \{C/[(V \cdot C_v \cdot P) + (B \cdot C_v)/(K_b + C_v)]/V\}$$

where B = binding capacity and K_b = equilibrium dissociation constant.

Thus, the formulation of the mathematical equations is rather simple. The key consideration is to maintain mass balance within each tissue compartment as well as the entire model by carefully accounting for the inputs and outputs of the chemical.

Determining Model Parameter Values

The next step in the development of a PB-PK model involves obtaining or determining the necessary model parameter values. Three classes of parameters are required: (1) anatomic and physiological variables such as organ and tissue volumes, and blood flow rates; (2) thermodynamic parameters such as tissue solubility (partition coefficients) and binding constants; and (3) biochemical parameters such as absorption, excretion and metabolic constants.

Values for organ/tissue volumes, blood flows and ventilation rates can be readily obtained from the literature (Adolph, 1949; Addis and Gray, 1950; Arms and Travis, 1988). Values not available may be scaled allometrically (Lindstedt, 1987; Vocci and Farber, 1988; Bachmann, 1989). Analysis of organ weights and other physiological parameters have led to numerous equations of the type

$$X = \alpha W^\beta$$

where X = the parameter of interest; W = body weight; and α and β are numerical constants. In

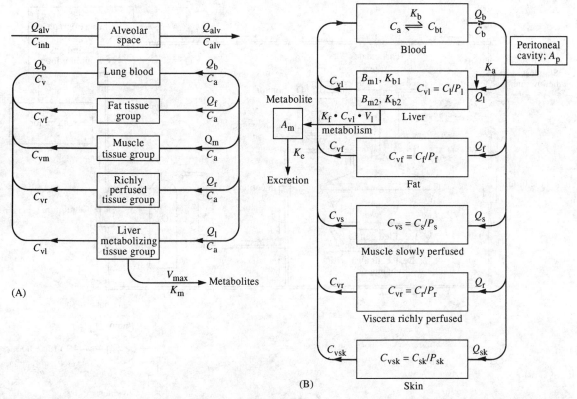

Figure 2 Two examples of physiologically-based pharmacokinetic model depicting the schematic of their model structures. Q_{alv} = alveolar ventilation rate; C_{alv} = alveolar concentration. (A) A volatile chemical: 1,4-dioxane. (B) A non-volatile chemical: 2,3,7,8-tetrachlorodibenzo-*p*-dioxin. C_b = concentration of free dioxin in blood; C_{bt} = concentration of total dioxin (free and bound) in blood; K_b = binding constant in blood; B_m = binding capacity to Ah receptor; B_{m2} = binding capacity to Ah receptor; K_{b1} = binding constant to Ah receptor; K_{b2} = binding constant to microsonial protein; K_a = absorption constant from GI tract to liver

general, organ size is directly proportional to body weight, and $\beta \approx 1$. For body surface area, flow rates, metabolic and clearance rates, they tend to vary to a fractional power of the body weight, and $\beta \approx \frac{2}{3}-\frac{3}{4}$. Like all procedures concocted to substitute for missing information, they only provide a best guess in the absence of data. When specific information becomes available, it should be used to adjust or to supplant the procedure (O'Flaherty, 1989).

Tissue:air partition coefficients for volatile chemicals can be determined by head space analysis with the vial equilibrium technique, using tissue preparations or homogenates (Fiserova-Bergerova and Diaz, 1986; Gargas *et al.*, 1989). As a rough approximation, a simple correlation approach which estimates tissue:air partition coefficients from water solubility and vapour pressure may be used (Paterson and Mackay, 1989). Tissue:blood partition coefficients are cal-

culated from the tissue:air partition coefficients by dividing by the corresponding blood:air partition coefficient:

$$P_i = P_{Ai}/P_{Ab}$$

where P_{Ai} = tissue:air partition coefficient and P_{Ab} = blood:air partition coefficient.

The metabolic constants V_{max} and K_m can also be estimated using a similar vial equilibrium technique with tissue homogenates *in vitro* (Sato and Nakajima, 1979), or with an *in vivo* technique by measuring gas uptake (Gargas *et al.*, 1986) or the exhalation rates of animals in an exposure chamber (Gargas and Andersen, 1989). Figure 3 shows the apparatus used for these experiments. In the gas uptake study, a closed recirculated exposure system is used to collect a series of uptake curves at a range of initial concentrations. The shapes of these curves are a function of P_i,

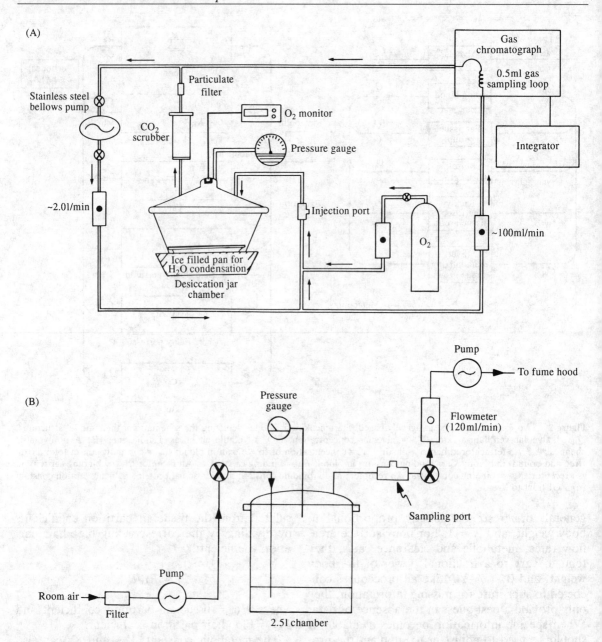

Figure 3 Schematic of the apparatus used to determine metabolic constants *in vivo*. (A) Gas uptake for highly volatile chemicals; (B) exhaled breath chamber for less volatile chemicals. Reprinted with permission from Academic Press, Orlando, Florida

V_{max} and K_m. Tissue partition coefficients are experimentally determined by the vial equilibration technique and incorporated into a PB-PK model which is then used to simulate the uptake process. An optimal fit of the family of uptake curves is then obtained by adjusting the biochemical constants for metabolism of the chemical. For materials of low vapour pressure which exhibit increasing blood and tissue solubilities, animals are first exposed by constant-concentration inhalation and then placed in exhaled breath chambers with fresh air flow. The chemical concentration in the chamber is serially analysed. The metabolic constants are estimated with the PB-

PK model by optimizing the fit of the elimination curves.

For non-volatile chemicals, tissue:blood partition coefficients may be estimated by using an *in vitro* equilibrium dialysis technique with tissue homogenates (Lin *et al.*, 1982), by single-pass perfusion of isolated organs *in situ* (Sultatos *et al.*, 1990), by bolus intravenous injection (Lam *et al.*, 1982) or by whole-body constant intravenous infusion *in vivo* (Chen and Gross, 1979). Metabolic constants for non-volatiles are determined with traditional enzyme assays by measuring the rate of disappearance of the substrate or the formation of product in tissue homogenates *in vitro* or in exposed animals.

In general, *in vivo* metabolic constants are quite difficult to determine empirically, and for ethical reasons it is nearly impossible to determine them for humans. In situations where only *in vivo* metabolic constants are available for the laboratory animal, V_{max} for humans may be scaled allometrically according to the fractional power rule. Alternatively, when *in vitro* data are available, the human *in vivo* V_{max} may be estimated proportionally, as has been demonstrated for methylene chloride (Reitz *et al.*, 1989). The Michaelis constant K_m generally is considered to be invariant among animal species.

Absorption rate constants are estimated from the rising portion of the blood concentration–time curve, and bioavailability is determined from the area under the blood curve following intravenous and other routes of administration.

Model Validation and Reformulation

Once the PB-PK model is configured and the requisite model parameters are collected, the model is subject to validation against kinetic, metabolic and toxicity information. This is accomplished by comparing the model predictions with experimental results. These exercises can suggest additional experiments to collect crucial data for verifying or improving model performance, as has been illustrated recently with methylene chloride (Reitz *et al.*, 1988b). When the model fails to accurately simulate known kinetic and toxicity behaviour despite modification of the model parameters consistent with physiological limits, the suggestion is that there may be additional mechanism(s) of action unaccounted for by the present model formulation. In such

an instance, the model structure will need to be reformulated to justify the discrepancies. Obviously there are multiple ways to restructure a PB-PK model if the objective is simply to improve the goodness of fit to the experimental results. However, model reformulation should be guided by plausible biological mechanisms, which can be verified experimentally. A model is validated when it is successful in simulating the empirical results. The more extensive the database a PB-PK model is validated against the more robust it is. A validated model can be used to make predictions of responses for a variety of exposure conditions, including ones which are difficult to perform experimentally. It also provides a means of predicting human kinetic behaviour when the biochemical constants and tissue-binding characteristics of the chemical have been determined in human tissues.

APPLICATIONS OF PB-PK MODELLING IN TOXICOLOGY

Risk Assessment

The most common application of PB-PK modelling in toxicology is dosimetric scaling in human health risk assessment. Because of ethical reasons, most toxicological data traditionally are derived from experimentations with laboratory animals. High exposure levels are also frequently employed to maximize the likelihood of observing effects. In order to assess the human health risk from exposure to a chemical from the animal toxicity data, it will be necessary to make extrapolations of the toxic response from: (1) the test species to human; (2) high to low exposure levels; and (3) the test route to another route of exposure.

Historically, exposure is expressed as the dose administered in proportion to body weight. This dosimetric method assumes that the response of the biological system is directly proportional to the initial concentration of the test material, which in turn correlates with the body volume. Interspecies dose adjustment is scaled according to an animal's body mass. A variation based on a similar concept of initial whole-body concentration is to scale according to body surface area (Freireich *et al.*, 1966). This latter scaling approach has lately become the method of choice for many risk assessment applications—e.g. the Environmental Protection Agency's Carcinogen Assessment Group. Despite its popularity, this form of dosimetric scaling is only marginally accurate for intraspecies extrapolation, and is rarely acceptable for interspecies extrapolation. The apparent unreliability of this approach is due to its failure to consider pharmacokinetic differences between species. The premise for this form of scaling assumes that the intensity of the toxic response correlates with the external exposure concentration or the amount of chemical administered. However, toxicity is not caused simply by the amount of chemical administered, but by the concentration of the chemical reaching the target tissues. Owing to the modifying effects of absorption, distribution, metabolism and excretion processes, target tissue dose is not always directly related to the amount of chemical administered. Another area where pharmacokinetics is important is extrapolation of biological response from high dose to low dose. At low exposure levels typically associated with environmental conditions, pharmacokinetic processes generally proceed at rates directly proportional to the chemical concentration. However, at the high doses used in toxicity studies, many pharmacokinetic processes, especially metabolism, have a finite capacity and may become saturated.

PB-PK modelling provides a means of estimating the tissue doses of chemicals and their metabolites over a wide range of exposure conditions in different animal species. It can provide a biologically based means of extrapolating from the animal results to predict effects in human populations. These techniques have been applied to the human cancer risk assessment of methylene chloride (Andersen *et al.*, 1987a), ethylene dichloride (D'Souza *et al.*, 1987), perchloroethylene (Chen and Blancato, 1987); trichloroethylene (Bogen, 1988), and 1,4-dioxane (Leung and Paustenbach, 1990). Figure 4 compares the interspecies scaling of doses, using the body volume correction and the PB-PK approach.

Another important application of PB-PK modelling in toxicological risk assessment is extrapolation from one route of exposure to another. Inter-route extrapolation is necessary because the bulk of toxicity testing has been conducted with the oral route, whereas environmental and occupational exposures typically occur by inhalation or skin contact. The general aspects of route-to-route extrapolation using PB-PK modelling has been described (Gillette, 1987). Specific examples include the dermal to inhalation extrapolation of organic chemical vapours (McDougal *et al.*, 1986, 1990), inhalation to oral extrapolation of trichloroethylene (Fisher, 1990) and methylene chloride (Angelo and Pritchard, 1987), and oral to dermal extrapolation of ethyl acrylate (Frederick, 1990).

Setting and Adjusting Exposure Standards

Occupational exposures to industrial chemicals traditionally have been evaluated by monitoring the airborne concentration of the chemicals. However, air monitoring does not represent the absorbed dose, since it ignores modifying processes such as bioavailability and metabolism. In addition, routes of exposure other than inhalation may contribute to the total body burden. In order accurately to determine the actual received dose, biological monitoring techniques can be used. Reference standards known as biological exposure indices (BEIs) defining the acceptable levels of chemical substances in biological media have been established. PB-PK models are well suited for setting BEIs, because they can readily be used to estimate chemical concentrations in a variety of body fluids or tissues corresponding to the airborne exposure concentrations. Leung and Paustenbach (1988) recently demonstrated that BEIs can be developed by exercising the PB-PK models at an exposure scenario corresponding to an 8 h inhalation at the Threshold Limit Value level. Table 2 gives the calculated BEIs for three common industrial chemicals.

Recently the PB-PK modelling approach has been advocated for setting occupational exposure limits (OELs) for work-shifts of longer duration than the standard 8 h per day, 5 days per week work schedule (Andersen *et al.*, 1987b). The rationale for adjusting OELs for unusual work-shifts is to ensure that workers are not placed at greater risk than those working a standard shift. Therefore, central to the development of a PB-PK model for adjusting OELs for non-conventional work-shifts is the quantification of the degree of risk associated with the standard work-shift such that the calculated OEL for the longer schedule poses no more than an equivalent risk. The selection of an appropriate risk index

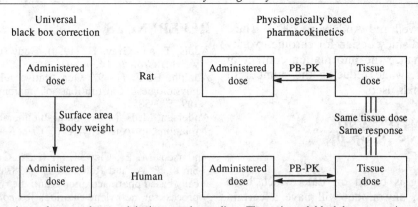

Figure 4 Comparison of approaches used in interspecies scaling. The universal black-box correction scales the external administered dose from animal to human on the basis of body size (body weight or body surface area). In the PB-PK approach, the equivalent human administered dose is estimated through a linkage of the internal tissue dose calculated by the respective animal and human PB-PK models.

Table 2 Tissue burdens in humans predicted by physiologically based pharmacokinetic modelling after an 8 h inhalation exposure to chemicals at the threshold limit value levels

	Styrene	Methylene chloride	1,4-Dioxane	Carbon tetrachloride
TLV (ppm)	50	50	25	5
Venous blood (mg l^{-1})	0.52	0.50	0.55	0.09
Fat (ppm)	9.88	3.53	0.28	1.85
Expired air (ppm)	17.27	26	0.083	1.7

depends on a chemical's mechanism of toxicity. For most systemic toxicants, the risk index is the integrated tissue dose—i.e. the concentration and time ($C \times t$) cross-product. An important advantage of PB-PK models is their ability to track the areas under the tissue or metabolism curves. Assuming that the area under the blood curve is the proper risk index associated with styrene exposure, Andersen *et al.* (1987b) determined that a 12 h exposure to 64 ppm was equivalent to an 8 h exposure to 100 ppm. In another example, blood carboxyhaemoglobin level was identified as the appropriate risk index for methylene chloride exposure. The OEL for non-standard work-shifts is determined by maintaining the end-of-shift blood carboxyhaemoglobin concentration at a level no greater than those observed after exposure to the 8 h time-weighted average OEL.

Refining Experimental Design in Toxicity Testing

Metabolism plays a salient role in regulating the toxicity of a multitude of chemicals. Almost all metabolic and many excretory processes utilize specific enzymes or binding proteins, which have limited capacity and may become saturated at high substrate concentrations. When these processes are saturated, internal dose parameters, such as area under the tissue curve or the amount of metabolite formed during inhalation exposure, are not linearly related to externally administered dose or inspired concentration (Andersen, 1981). PB-PK analysis of the dose-dependent processes provides an understanding of the relationship between external and internal dosimetrics under various exposure conditions. Recognition of these complex kinetic behaviours is essential to the proper design of toxicological experimentation. It is particularly relevant for dose selection in contemporary cancer bioassays, which emphasize the use of a maximum tolerated dose (MTD). The development of a comprehensive pharmacokinetic description to examine the influence of saturable processes on the delivery of a chemical to target tissues will aid in the correct selection of dosing regimen and test species. While some *in vivo* animal experimentation will always be necessary to test the accuracy of the predicted behaviour by the PB-PK model, this limited work requires fewer animals than conventional experimentation for assessing pharmacokinetic behaviour (Clewell and Andersen, 1985). Thus, a PB-PK guided study design for chronic toxicity testing will enhance the information content of the experiment, while reducing the number of laboratory animals used.

UNCERTAINTIES AND LIMITATIONS IN PB-PK MODELLING

Since modelling is based on data which have inherent errors, any model will have a certain degree of uncertainty associated with it. There are two important areas of uncertainties in the development of PB-PK models. The first concerns the selection of the proper model, and the second deals with the model parameters estimated. When a PB-PK model is used to make predictions, it should reflect these uncertainties in terms of confidence limits in the values predicted by the model, and the confidence regions around the estimated parameters.

As shown in Figure 1, the first step in PB-PK modelling is defining the problem to be solved. The next step is to postulate several plausible physiological mechanisms to describe the data set. The third step is to use the data to discriminate between candidate models. The selection of the best model and the estimation of model parameters can be guided by statistical analysis, often with the aid of computer programs (Blau and Neely, 1987). Since small changes in input data or in the goodness of fit to a set of experimental data may significantly affect the predicted output, and, in turn, the risk estimate when the PB-PK model is used to support quantitative risk assessment, the uncertainties associated with PB-PK model parameters should be carefully analysed. The systematic testing of the effects of the model parameters on the model predictions in PB-PK modelling is called sensitivity/variability analysis. This procedure of uncertainty evaluation in input parameters has recently been shown with PB-PK models for methylene chloride (Cohn, 1987; Portier and Kaplan, 1989), soman (Maxwell *et al.*, 1988), and tetrachloroethylene (Farrar *et al.*, 1989; Bois *et al.*, 1990). Finally, a PB-PK model is developed to provide insight to specific questions, and should never be used for extrapolation beyond its intended purpose. Furthermore, its use for prediction should come only after a thorough validation process.

REFERENCES

Addis, T. and Gray, H. (1950). Body size and organ weight. *Growth*, **14**, 49–80

Adolph, E. F. (1949). Quantitative relations in the physiological constitutions of mammals. *Science*, **109**, 579–585

Andersen, M. E. (1981). Saturable metabolism and its relationship to toxicity. *CRC Crit. Rev. Toxicol*, **9**, 105–150

Andersen, M. E., Clewell, H. J. III, Gargas, M. L., Smith, F. A. and Reitz, R. H. (1987a). Physiologically based pharmacokinetics and the risk assessment process for methylene chloride. *Toxicol. Appl. Pharmacol.*, **87**, 185–205

Andersen, M. E., MacNaughton, M. G., Clewell, H. J. III and Paustenbach, D. J. (1987b). Adjusting exposure limits for long and short exposure periods, using a physiological pharmacokinetic model. *Am. Industr. Hyg. Assoc. J.*, **48**, 335–343

Angelo, M. J. and Pritchard, A. B. (1987). Route-to-route extrapolation of dichloromethane exposure using a physiological pharmacokinetic model. In *Drinking Water and Health*, Vol. 8, *Pharmacokinetics in Risk Assessment*. National Academy Press, Washington, D.C., pp. 254–264

Arms, A. D. and Travis, C. C. (1988). *Reference Physiological Parameters in Pharmacokinetic Modelling*. U.S. EPA 600/6–88/004. Final report. (Available from NTIS, PB88–196019)

Bachmann, K. (1989). Predicting toxicokinetic parameters in humans from toxicokinetic data acquired from three small mammalian species. *J. Appl. Toxicol.*, **9**, 331–338

Blau, G. E. and Neely, W. B. (1987). Dealing with uncertainty in pharmacokinetic models using Simusolv. In *Drinking Water and Health*, Vol. 8, *Pharmacokinetics in Risk Assessment*. National Academy Press, Washington, D.C., pp. 185–207

Bogen, K. T. (1988). Pharmacokinetics for regulatory risk analysis: the case of trichloroethylene. *Regulatory Toxicol. Pharmacol.*, **8**, 447–466

Bois, F. Y., Zeise, L. and Tozer, T. N. (1990). Precision and sensitivity of pharmacokinetic models for cancer risk assessment: tetrachloroethylene in mice, rats, and humans. *Toxicol. Appl. Pharmacol.*, **102**, 300–315

Bungay, P. M., Dedrick, R. L. and Matthews, H. B. (1981). Enteric transport of chlordecone (Kepone) in the rat. *J. Pharmacokin. Biopharm.*, **9**, 309–341

Chen, C. W. and Blancato, J. N. (1987). Role of pharmacokinetic modelling in risk assessment: perchloroethylene as an example. In *Drinking Water and Health*, Vol. 8, *Pharmacokinetics in Risk Assessment*. National Academy Press, Washington, D.C., pp. 369–390

Chen, H. S. G., and Gross, J F. (1979). Estimation of tissue-to-plasma partition coefficients used in physiological pharmacokinetic models. *J. Pharmacokin. Biopharm.*, **7**, 117–125

Clewell, H. J. III and Andersen, M. E. (1985). Risk assessment extrapolations and physiological modelling. *Toxicol. Ind. Hlth.*, **1**, 111–122

Cohn, M. S. (1987). Sensitivity analysis in pharmacokinetic modeling. In *Drinking Water and Health*, Vol. 8, *Pharmacokinetics in Risk Assessment*, National Academy Press, Washington, D.C., pp. 265–272

Corley, R. A., Mendrala, A. L., Smith, F. A., Staats, D. A., Gargas, M. L., Conolly, R. B., Andersen, M. E. and Reitz, R. H. (1990). Development of a physiologically-based pharmacokinetic model for chloroform. *Toxicol. Appl. Pharmacol.*, **103**, 512–527

Dallas, C. E., Ramanathan, R., Muralidhara, S., Gallo, G. M. and Bruckner, J. V. (1989). The uptake and elimination of 1,1,1-trichloroethane during and following inhalation exposures in rats. *Toxicol. Appl. Pharmacol.*, **98**, 385–397

Dalley, J. W., Gupta, P. K., and Hung, C. T. (1990). A physiological pharmacokinetic model describing the disposition of lead in the absence and presence of L-ascorbic acid in rats. *Toxicol. Lett.*, **50**, 337–348

D'Souza, R. W. and Andersen, M. E. (1988). Physiologically based pharmacokinetic model for vinylidene chloride. *Toxicol. Appl. Pharmacol.*, **95**, 230–240

D'Souza, R. W. and Boxenbaum, H. (1988). Physiological pharmacokinetic models: some aspects of theory, practice and potential. *Toxicol. Industr. Hlth*, **4**, 151–171

D'Souza, R. W., Francis, W. R., Bruce, R. D. and Andersen, M. E. (1987). Physiologically based pharmacokinetic model for ethylene dichloride and its application in risk assessment. In *Drinking Water and Health*, Vol. 8, *Pharmacokinetics in Risk Assessment*. National Academy Press, Washington, D.C., pp. 286–301

D'Souza, R. W., Francis, W. R. and Andersen, M. E. (1988). Physiological model for tissue glutathione depletion and increased resynthesis after ethylene dichloride exposure. *J. Pharmacol. Exptl Therap.* **245**, 563–568

Farrar, D., Allen, B., Crump, K. and Shipp, A. (1989). Evaluation of uncertainty in input parameters to pharmacokinetic models and the resulting uncertainty in output. *Toxicol. Lett.*, **49**, 371–385

Fiserova-Bergerova, V. and Diaz, M. L. (1986). Determination and prediction of tissue-gas partition coefficients. *Int. Arch. Occup. Environ. Hlth*, **58**, 75–87

Fisher, J. W. (1990). Using inhalation kinetic data in the development of physiological models for oral absorption: a case study with trichloroethylene. *ILSI/EPA Workshop on Principles of Route-to-Route Extrapolation, Hilton Head, SC, March 19–21*

Fisher, J. W., Whittaker, T. A., Taylor, D. H., Clewell, H. J. III and Andersen, M. E. (1989). Physiologically based pharmacokinetic modelling of the pregnant rat: a multiroute model for trichloroethylene and its metabolite, trichloroacetic acid. *Toxicol. Appl. Pharmacol.*, **99**, 395–414

Fisher, J. W., Whittaker, T. A., Taylor, D. H., Clewell, H. J. III and Andersen, M. E. (1990). Physiologically based pharmacokinetic modelling of the lactating rat and nursing pup: a multiroute exposure model for trichloroethylene and its metabolite, trichloroacetic acid. *Toxicol. Appl. Pharmacol.*, **102**, 497–513

Frederick, C. B. (1990). Contact site carcinogenicity—estimation of an upper limit for risk of dermal carcinogenicity based on oral dosing site tumors. *ILSI/EPA Workshop on Principles of Route-to-Route Extrapolation, Hilton Head, SC, March 19–21*

Freireich, E. J., Gehan, E. A., Rall, D. P., Schmidt, L. H. and Skipper, H. E. (1966). Quantitative comparison of toxicity of anticancer agents in mouse, rat, hamster, dog, monkey and man. *Cancer Chemotherap. Rep.*, **50**, 219–244

Gargas, M. L. and Andersen, M. E. (1989). Determining kinetic constants of chlorinated ethane metabolism in the rat from rates of exhalation. *Toxicol. Appl. Pharmacol.*, **99**, 344–353

Gargas, M. L., Andersen, M. E. and Clewell, H. J. III (1986). A physiologically based simulation approach for determining metabolic constants from gas uptake data. *Toxicol. Appl. Pharmacol.*, **86**, 341–352

Gargas, M. L., Burgess, R. J., Voisard, D. E., Cason, G. H. and Andersen, M. E. (1989). Partition coefficients of low-molecular weight volatile chemicals in various liquids and tissues. *Toxicol. Appl. Pharmacol.*, **98**, 87–99

Gibaldi, M. and Perrier, D. (1982). *Pharmacokinetics*, 2nd edn. Marcel Dekker, New York

Gillette, J. R. (1987). Dose, species, and route extrapolation: general aspects. In *Drinking Water and Health*, Vol. 8, *Pharmacokinetics in Risk Assessment*. National Academy Press, Washington, D.C., pp. 96–158

Himmelstein, K. J. and Lutz, R. J. (1979). A review of the applications of physiologically based pharmacokinetic modeling. *J. Pharmacokin. Biopharm.*, **7**, 127–145

Johanson, G. (1986). Physiologically-based pharmacokinetic modeling of inhaled 2-butoxyethanol in man. *Toxicol. Lett.*, **34**, 23–31

King, F. G., Dedrick, R. L., Collins, J. M., Matthews, H. B. and Birnbaum, L. S. (1983). A physiological model for the pharmacokinetics of 2,3,7,8-tetrachlorodibenzofuran in several species. *Toxicol. Appl. Pharmacol.*, **67**, 390–400

Lam, G., Chen, M. L. and Chiou, W. L. (1982). Determination of tissue to blood partition coefficients in physiologically-based pharmacokinetic studies. *J. Pharm. Sci.*, **71**, 454–456

Leung, H. W. and Paustenbach, D. J. (1988). Application of pharmacokinetics to derive biological exposure indexes from threshold limit values. *Am. Industr. Hyg. Assoc. J.*, **49**, 445–450

Leung, H. W. and Paustenbach, D. J. (1990). Cancer

risk assessment of dioxane based upon a physiologically-based pharmacokinetic approach. *Toxicol. Lett.*, **51**, 147–162

Leung, H. W., *et al.* (1988). A physiologically based pharmacokinetic model for 2,3,7,8-tetrachlorodibenzo-*p*-dioxin in C57BL/6J and DBA/2J mice. *Toxicol. Lett.*, **42**, 15–28

Leung, H. W., *et al.* (1989). A physiologically-based pharmacokinetic model for 2,3,7,8-tetrachlorodibenzo-*p*-dioxin. *Chemosphere*, **18**, 659–664

Leung, H. W., *et al.* (1990a). A physiological pharmacokinetic description of the tissue distribution and enzyme inducing properties of 2,3,7,8-tetrachlorodibenzo-*p*-dioxin in the rat. *Toxicol. Appl. Pharmacol.*, **103**, 399–410

Leung, H. W., *et al.* (1990b). Pharmacokinetics of [^{125}I]-2-iodo-1,3,7,8-trichlorodibenzo-*p*-dioxin in mice: Analysis with a physiological modeling approach. *Toxicol. Appl. Pharmacol.*, **103**, 411–419

Lin. J. H., *et al.* (1982). *In vitro* and *in vivo* evaluation of the tissue-to-blood partition coefficient for physiological pharmacokinetic models. *J. Pharmacokin. Biopharm.*, **10**, 637–647

Lindstedt, S. L. (1987). Allometry: body size constraints in animal design. In: *Pharmacokinetics in Risk Assessment. Drinking Water and Health*, Vol. 8, National Academy Press, Washington, D.C., pp. 65–79

Lindstrom, F. T., *et al.* (1974). Distribution of HEOD (dieldrin) in mammals: I. preliminary model. *Arch. Environ. Contam. Toxicol.*, **2**, 9–42

Lutz, R. J., *et al.* (1984). Comparison of the pharmacokinetics of several polychlorinated biphenyls in the mouse, rat, dog, and monkey by means of a physiological pharmacokinetic model. *Drug Metab. Disp.*, **12**, 527–535

McDougal, J. N., *et al.* (1986). A physiological pharmacokinetic model for dermal absorption of vapors in the rat. *Toxicol. Appl. Pharmacol.*, **85**, 286–294

McDougal, J. N., *et al.* (1990). Dermal absorption of organic chemical vapors in rats and humans. *Fund. Appl. Toxicol.*, **14**, 299–308

Maxwell, D. M., *et al.* (1988). A pharmacodynamic model for soman in the rat. *Toxicol. Lett.*, **43**, 175–188

Medinsky, M. A., *et al.* (1989). A physiological model for simulation of benzene metabolism by rats and mice. *Toxicol. Appl. Pharmacol.*, **99**, 193–206

Menzel, D. B. (1987). Physiological pharmacokinetic modeling. *Environ. Sci. Technol.*, **21**, 944–950

Menzel, D. B. (1988). Planning and using PB-PK models: an integrated inhalation and distribution model for nickel. *Toxicol. Lett.*, **43**, 67–83

O'Flaherty, E. J. (1989). Interspecies conversion of kinetically equivalent doses. *Risk Anal.*, **9**, 587–598

Paterson, S. and Mackay, D. (1989). Correlation of tissue, blood and air partition coefficients of volatile organic chemicals. *Br. J. Industr. Med.*, **46**, 321–328

Paustenbach, D. J., *et al.* (1988). A physiologically based pharmacokinetic model for inhaled carbon tetrachloride. *Toxicol. Appl. Pharmacol.*, **96**, 191–211

Portier, C. J. and Kaplan, N. L. (1989). Variability of safe estimates when using complicated models of the carcinogenic process. *Fund. Appl. Toxicol.*, **13**, 533–544

Ramsey, J. C. and Andersen, M. E. (1984). A physiologically-based description of the inhalation pharmacokinetics of styrene in rats and humans. *Toxicol. Appl. Pharmacol.*, **73**, 159–175

Reitz, R. H., *et al.* (1988b). Incorporation of *in vitro* enzyme data into the physiologically-based pharmacokinetic (PB-PK) model for methylene chloride. *Toxicol. Lett.*, **43**, 97–116

Reitz, R. H., *et al.* (1989). *In vitro* metabolism of methylene chloride in human and animal tissues. *Toxicol. Appl. Pharmacol.*, **97**, 230–246

Sato, A. and Nakajima, T. (1979). A vial-equilibration method to evaluate the drug metabolizing enzyme activity for volatile hydrocarbons. *Toxicol. Appl. Pharmacol.*, **47**, 41–46

Sultatos, L. G., Kim, B. and Woods, L. (1990). Evaluation of estimations *in vitro* of tissue/blood distribution coefficients for organothiophosphate insecticides. *Toxicol. Appl. Pharmacol.*, **103**, 52–55

Travis, C. C., Qullen, J. L. and Arms, A. D. (1990). Pharmacokinetics of benzene. *Toxicol. Appl. Pharmacol.*, **102**, 400–420

Tuey, D. B. and Matthews, H. B. (1980). Distribution and excretion of 2,2′,4,4′,5,5′-hexabromobiphenyl in rats and man. *Toxicol. Appl. Pharmacol.*, **53**, 420–431

Vocci, F. and Farber, T. (1988). Extrapolation of animal toxicity data to man. *Regulatory Toxicol. Pharmacol.*, **8**, 389–398

Ward, R. C., *et al.* (1988). Pharmacokinetics of tetrachlorethylene. *Toxicol. Appl. Pharmacol.*, **93**, 108–117

FURTHER READING

Anderson, M. E. and Krishnan, K. (1994). Physiologically based pharmacokinetics and cancer risk assessment. *Envir. Hth. Perspec.*, **102**, Suppl., 103–108

Clewell, H. J. and Anderson, M. E. (1994). Physiologically-based pharmacokinetic modeling and bioactivation of xenobiotics. *Journal of Toxicology and Industrial Health*, **10**, 1–24

Droz, P. O. (1993). Pharmacokinetic modeling as a tool for biological modeling. *Int. Arch Occup. Envir. Hth.*, **65**, 553–559

Frantz, S. W., *et al.* (1994). The use of pharmacokinetics as an interpretive and predictive tool in chemical toxicology testing and risk assessment. *Reg. Toxicol. Pharmacol.*, **19**, 317–337

6 Biochemical Basis of Toxicity

John Caldwell

INTRODUCTION

In the past 30 or so years, the science of toxicology has progressively moved from being an activity based on the ability to observe and classify the harmful effects of chemicals in the animal body, relying principally on the tools of classical pathology to achieve these ends, to a discipline able to explain the effects of toxic compounds. This change has resulted from the widespread application of techniques and concepts from a wide range of basic sciences, triggered by the realization of the potential impact of exposure to a wide range of chemicals on human health. These changes were initially a reaction to the harmful effects of thalidomide, and the key molecules in the development of our understanding of toxic mechanisms (as opposed to a mechanistic understanding of chemical carcinogenicity) are paracetamol, bromobenzene and paraquat. Mechanistic explanations of toxic phenomena are critically important as they: (1) account for the origin of toxicity; (2) aid prevention of toxicity by chemical or biological means; and (3) provide a rational basis for the use of animal data to anticipate the consequences of human exposure to a particular chemical.

It is the purpose of this chapter to illustrate various mechanisms of toxicity, concentrating on those of general applicability rather than specialized areas such as reproductive and immunological toxicity, and to exemplify the use of such approaches to chemical safety evaluation.

MECHANISMS OF TOXICITY

The great majority of toxic compounds are chemically stable and produce their characteristic effects by interference with biochemical or physiological homeostatic mechanisms. This means that a full understanding of the pharmacology of toxic compounds is essential. In the case of drugs, it has been estimated that some 80 per cent of adverse reactions are the result of exaggerated pharmacological responses (Rawlins, 1981) and even if the compound under consideration has no specific actions appropriate for therapeutic application, it is still critical to have a proper knowledge of the compound's biochemical and molecular sites of action. Many adverse events are the consequence of disturbance of normal physiology and do not result in cell death.

Cytotoxicity, the causing of cell death, is often the consequence of exposure to a harmful chemical, but the number of cells which must be killed before the function of a tissue or organism is noticeably impaired is highly variable. Some cell types, notably the epithelia including the liver, have the ability to regenerate in response to insult while others, most notably neurons, cannot. Some organs, such as the liver, lung and kidney, have a substantial reserve capacity in excess of normal requirements and normal body function can be maintained in the presence of marked impairment.

Other chemicals can modify the regulation of cell division with harmful consequences. It has been understood for many years that non-lethal genetic alteration to somatic cells results in mutation (Williams and Weisburger, 1991), ultimately expressed as carcinogenesis. More recently, it has become clear that compounds not interacting directly with the genome can also produce cancer by so-called epigenetic mechanisms (Williams and Weisburger, 1991; see also Chapter 38). These may involve a proliferative response of epithelial cells to cytotoxicity, as is suggested to occur with high-dose carcinogens such as allyl isothiocyanate (see below) and chloroform, or a more direct action to enhance the rate of cell division seen with promoters such as phorbol esters and the peroxisome proliferators (Butterworth *et al.*, 1991). Increased cell replication, however caused, brings with it an increased chance of an unrepaired DNA lesion being fixed as a mutation. It has long been suspected that hyperplasia precedes neoplasia but the inevitability or otherwise of such a progression has never been established on pathological grounds alone.

There occurs a considerable extent of 'normal' damage to DNA by reactive oxygen species in the cell and it can be speculated that the non-genotoxic carcinogens act by enhancing the likelihood of this normal damage being fixed as a mutation, leading to cancer (Ames *et al.*, 1993).

Having established the fundamental differences between toxic chemicals which act (1) through physiological mechanisms, (2) through cytotoxicity, or (3) by causing proliferative lesions, we may now consider some basic mechanisms through which toxic chemicals may act.

RECEPTOR-MEDIATED EVENTS

Anything other than the most cursory description of receptor-mediated events is outside present consideration. However, it is important to appreciate that actions at the receptors for neurotransmitters and hormones, either as agonists or as antagonists of the physiological ligand, underlie numerous toxic responses. This is most clearly the case with neurotoxins, acting within and outside the central nervous system (CNS). In addition, it is now understood that a variety of toxic effects completely unrelated to any conceivable therapeutic or otherwise beneficial activity are mediated through receptor interactions. Interest has concentrated on the cytosolic receptors of the steroid hormone type and it is now clear that dioxin (TCDD) exerts most of, if not all, its toxic effects by binding to a specific receptor of the steroid hormone type (Lilienfeld and Gallo, 1989). More recently, a cytosolic binding protein has been identified for peroxisomal proliferators which has DNA-binding domains and which appears to activate gene transcription in the nucleus in a way analogous to the steroid hormones (Green, 1992).

DISTURBANCE OF EXCITABLE MEMBRANE FUNCTION

Excitable membranes are critical to the function of nerve and muscle, most notably in their ability to generate and propagate action potentials. This depends on the normal activity of ion channels and membrane ion pumps, which can be influenced by a variety of toxic compounds. The neur-

otoxicity of DDT is the result of interference with closing of sodium channels (Joy, 1982). The great majority of organic solvents are ethanol-like CNS depressants whose actions appear to be non-specific membrane effects (Rall, 1991).

DISTURBANCE OF NORMAL BIOCHEMICAL PROCESSES

The cells of the body maintain their function by a variety of closely coordinated synthetic and catabolic processes. The energy requirements of the body are met by the oxidation of carbohydrates and lipids, coupled to the synthesis of ATP by oxidative phosphorylation. The availability of oxygen to the tissues is obviously influenced by compounds affecting the transport of oxygen in the blood, e.g. those causing methaemoglobinaemia (Kiese, 1977), while the synthesis of ATP may be inhibited by uncoupling oxidative phosphorylation by compounds such as salicylate (Brenner and Simon, 1982). Under these circumstances, not only is there a loss of function owing to lack of ATP but there is also a marked rise in body temperature arising from excess heat production: this pyrexia can be fatal.

A number of compounds, notably quinones, are able to initiate redox cycling (Figure 1) with harmful consequences for the cell (Sies and Cadenas, 1983). These compounds are reduced by taking up an electron from NADPH to give a radical, which is then oxidized by molecular oxygen, returning the molecule to its original oxidized state and producing a series of reactive oxygen species from the primary product, superoxide anion radical $O_2^{\cdot-}$. These species include hydrogen peroxide, hydroxyl radical $OH^{\cdot}$, singlet oxygen $^1O_2$ and lipid peroxides. These are powerful oxidizing agents and can initiate a wide range of toxic responses including mutagenesis and carcinogenesis as a result of interactions with DNA, membrane damage by lipid peroxidation and biochemical disorders by enzyme inactivation. This underlies both the therapeutic and toxic actions of quinone drugs such as the anthracyclines, adriamycin and bleomycin, and the toxicity of agents such as paraquat and cephalosporin antibiotics (see below). The magnitude of any toxic response to such compounds is moderated by a variety of cellular defences such as glutathione peroxidase,

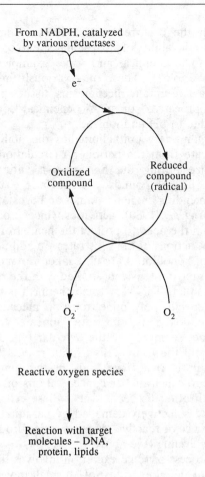

Figure 1 Formation of reactive oxygen species by redox cycling

catalase and superoxide dismutase and endogenous antioxidants, notably vitamins A, C and E.

ALTERED CALCIUM HOMEOSTASIS

Calcium ions have critical roles in cellular function and the intracellular levels and locations of calcium ions are tightly controlled by a variety of compartmentation processes and transport mechanisms. Various toxic chemicals can disrupt these with marked deleterious effects on the cell (Orrenius *et al.*, 1989). Increases in free intracellular calcium concentrations lead to changes to the cytoskeleton, blebbing and ultimately leakage of the plasma membrane, impaired mitochondrial function and activation of calcium-dependent degradative enzymes (proteases, phospholipases, endonucleases). Chemicals can raise intracellular calcium concentration in two ways, either by enhancing its influx (mainly caused by hormones and other chemicals acting via cytosolic receptors to enhance protein synthesis) or by impairing calcium transport. This latter mechanism is involved with the main chemicals inducing oxidative damage to the cell, e.g. free radicals, quinones and peroxides.

COVALENT BINDING TO CELLULAR MACROMOLECULES

It is now well understood that a great many toxic chemicals exert their effects by the covalent linkage of reactive metabolites to essential macromolecules of the cell (Brodie *et al.*, 1971). These include proteins, notably enzymes and membrane structural elements, lipids and nucleic acids (see below). The binding generally involves electrophilic metabolites binding to nucleophilic sites such as thiol, amino and hydroxy groups in the side chains of proteins and is essentially irreversible, depending solely on the turnover of the macromolecule in question for the repair of the lesion. In addition, other toxins may bind to protein so as to impair normal function without being converted first to reactive intermediates. This is best exemplified by the binding of metal ions to protein thiols, e.g. mercury ions in the kidney (Klaassen, 1991). Damage to lipids may take two forms, either covalent binding of reactive intermediates to free hydroxyl groups of lipids or the initiation of lipid peroxidation by free radicals derived from the compound *per se* or active oxygen species (superoxide, hydroxyl radical, etc.) produced by reactions such as redox cycling (see above).

GENOTOXICITY

Electrophilic compounds, generally formed by the oxidative metabolism of xenobiotics, are able to interact with various nucleophilic sites in DNA, principally O-6, N-7, N-2 and C-2 of guanine (Miller and Miller, 1985). Other compounds may interact with DNA by intercalation between the strands. In both cases, such interactions may alter gene expression: this is termed 'genotoxicity' and may cause the death of the cell but more frequently the result is a somatic mutation which can be the initiating event for a process ultimately leading to the development of cancer. Most compounds which are genotoxic in mammals are also mutagenic in bacteria, subject to the availability of an appropriate metabolic system for activation (Ashby and Tennant, 1988). It is important to appreciate that not all carcinogens are genotoxic and that proliferative lesions may also arise through mechanisms influencing cell division not operating at the genomic level. Such compounds are termed 'non-genotoxic' or 'epigenetic' carcinogens (see Chapter 38).

TISSUE SPECIFICITY OF TOXICITY

All the tissues and organs of the body are to a greater or lesser extent susceptible to toxicity but the effects of most toxic chemicals focus on one or more tissues or organs, the so-called *target organs of toxicity*. The examination of the reasons responsible for this specificity of action has proved extremely informative in developing a mechanistic understanding of the origin of the toxic response. In broad terms, the susceptibility of particular tissues and organs is a consequence of one or more of three factors:

- Tissue distribution of the chemical.
- Metabolic activation to toxic products within specific tissues.
- Biochemical differences between tissues exposed to the toxin.

Each of these may be illustrated by a considerable number of examples.

Role of Tissue Distribution

It is obviously the case that for a compound to exert a toxic effect it must be present at the site of action. The magnitude of any toxic effect will be dependent on the concentration of toxin to which the relevant target is exposed: this is the case for both reversible effects mediated by classical receptors and described by sigmoid dose–response curves (Ross, 1991) and for effects mediated through the formation of macromolecular adducts, where the concentration of adducts becomes the relevant index of exposure (Monro, 1992). There exists a substantial number of cases

in which the occurrence of toxicity is directly related to the ability of a particular site to concentrate a toxic chemical and some examples are listed in Table 1. These may variously involve specific active uptake mechanisms, tissue-specific binding processes, or physicochemical concentration due to pH and ionization.

The pulmonary epithelium has the ability to concentrate from the peripheral circulation and metabolize during the first pass a variety of endogenous compounds present in the circulation, including biogenic amines and prostanoids (Youdim *et al.*, 1980), activities which probably arise from the need to protect the heart from the stimulant actions of the substrates. In addition, a variety of xenobiotics are also taken up and this has been most intensively studied with the herbicide paraquat. This very toxic chemical is taken up by a specific polyamine transport mechanism, whose endogenous substrate appears to be putrescine, seemingly in the alveolar type I and II cells and the Clara cells (Smith *et al.*, 1989). The result is that these cells in the lung are exposed to much higher concentrations of paraquat than other tissues and it is these cell types which are selectively damaged by paraquat as a consequence of reactive oxygen species produced by redox cycling (see above).

The process of renal excretion involves the filtration, at the glomerulus, of all small molecules present in plasma followed by the progressive modification of the composition of the filtrate into urine by tubular reabsorption and secretion mechanisms. The aminoglycoside antibiotics, typified by gentamicin, are reabsorbed by the same mechanism as low molecular weight proteins and concentrated in the proximal tubular cell, bound to a number of organelles from which they are but slowly mobilized (Weinberg, 1988). The half-life for the loss of aminoglycosides from the renal cortex may be 100 times longer than the plasma elimination half-life. Some 10 per cent of

Table 1 Examples of chemicals whose toxicity is related to the ability of target organs to concentrate them

Compound	Tissue
Paraquat	Lung
Gentamicin, cephalosporins, sulphonamides	Kidney
Chloroquine	Eye
Kanamycin	Ear
Streptozotocin	Pancreas

all cases of acute renal failure have been attributed to the aminoglycosides (Bennett, 1983) and their nephrotoxicity is the result of a variety of biochemical abnormalities, most notably inhibition of phospholipases (Humes and O'Connor, 1988).

The cephalosporins are also concentrated within the renal cortex, being taken up by the same active transport process as *p*-aminohippurate (Wold, 1981). However, they are not transported out of the cell across the luminal membrane and so accumulate within the proximal tubular cell. The incidence and severity of the nephrotoxicity of cephalosporins correlate directly with their concentration within the renal cortex. A variety of mechanisms have been associated with nephrotoxicity and the most attractive of these involves redox cycling and the generation of reactive oxygen species (Kuo *et al.*, 1983).

In contrast, the nephrotoxicity of the sulphonamides is readily explicable on the basis of the physicochemical properties of their metabolites. Many of these are metabolized by *N*-acetylation, and the conjugates are readily excreted into the urine. However, they are poorly water soluble and can crystallize out in the lumen of the nephron, leading to nephrotoxicity by mechanical blockage of the tubules (Caldwell, 1982).

In recent years, there has been a great interest in the ability of a number of chemically inert and otherwise unremarkable molecules to give rise to a characteristic nephropathy and renal carcinoma in the male rat (EPA, 1991). This is associated with the accumulation of droplets of a specific protein, α_{2u}-globulin, in the kidneys and a list of compounds causing this notable renal toxicity, now generally referred to as 'α_{2u}-globulin nephropathy', is given in Table 2. None of these is geno-

Table 2 Compounds giving rise to α_{2u}-globulin nephropathy in male rats but not female rats or other species

1,4-Dichlorobenzene
Unleaded petrol
d-Limonene
Isophorone
Dimethyl methylphosphonate
Pentachloroethane
JP-4 jet fuel
JP-5 shale-derived jet fuel
Decalin (decahydronaphthalene)

Source: EPA (1991) and references therein.

toxic in a variety of short-term tests but it seems likely that they cause renal neoplasia after long-term, high-dose exposure as a result of the accumulation of hyaline protein droplets in the P2 segment of the renal tubule. The renal tumours are seen only in male rats and not in female rats or in mice of either sex.

α_{2u}-Globulin is a low molecular weight protein, approximately 18 000 daltons, whose synthesis under androgenic control is specific to the liver of male rats. Under normal conditions, it is filtered in the kidney, reabsorbed to the extent of about 50–60 per cent in the proximal tubule and degraded by lysosomal enzymes there. However, a range of simple hydrocarbons are able to bind to α_{2u}-globulin with remarkable consequences. The protein–hydrocarbon complex is filtered and reabsorbed by the kidney in the same way, but it is resistant to lysosomal breakdown and thus accumulates in the proximal tubular segment of the nephron. As more and more accumulates, the protein assumes the form of hyaline droplets, which are crystalline inclusion bodies. These lead to compensatory cell proliferation which in the long-term acts as a tumour promoter. This mechanism is now accepted to be a male rat-specific event with no significance for the safe human use of causative compounds (Flamm and Lehmann-McKeeman, 1991).

The pigment melanin is found in the skin and a variety of other tissues, notably the retina of the eye and the inner ear. Studies in animals of the tissue distribution of radiolabelled compounds, most notably by whole body autoradiography, have revealed that a significant number of compounds are concentrated in tissues rich in melanin (Ings, 1984). The role of melanin in this selective uptake may be most conveniently investigated by the comparison of tissue distribution in pigmented animals and albinos, which lack melanin. There appears to be two distinct modes of binding to melanin, differentiated on the basis of the half-life of the bound residue (Ings, 1984). When the half-life for depletion is up to 28 days, there occurs tight binding but the drug–melanin complex is reversible and seems not to have toxicological sequelae. There is a much smaller number of cases in which there occurs a much tighter, possibly covalent, linkage between the drug and melanin and here the turnover of the complex is essentially that of melanin itself, about three months. This pattern of melanin binding is generally associated with toxicity.

A number of compounds, most notably chloroquine and certain phenothiazines, produce a retinopathy which involves visual disturbance progressing to colour and night blindness. The effects of chloroquine are essentially irreversible because of the extremely long residence of the drug bound to melanin in the eye and the intensity of effects are directly related to the duration and size of dosage (Bernstein *et al.*, 1963; Burns, 1966). Although chlorpromazine only rarely causes retinopathy, certain other phenothiazines, notably thioridazine, have proved much more retinotoxic and one experimental member of this class caused blindness in volunteers (Boet, 1970). It is clear from tissue distribution and *in vitro* studies that this retinopathy is directly related to the very tight binding of the phenothiazine to melanin (Potts, 1962).

Kanamycin, neomycin and other aminoglycosides cause hearing disturbance, including tinnitus, loss of hearing acuity and frank deafness. This is 'nerve deafness' not involving mechanical damage to the ear and has been associated with binding to melanin in the stria vascularis of the inner ear, the site of toxicity (Denckner *et al.*, 1973).

Metabolic Activation

The great majority of toxic chemicals are unreactive and require metabolic activation to unveil their toxicity, in one of the following ways:

- The formation of chemically stable metabolites, which may have increased or changed activity relative to the parent compound.
- Formation of chemically reactive metabolites, most commonly electrophiles, able to interact with cellular constituents leading to toxicity.
- Formation as by-products of excess quantities of harmful endogenous compounds, notably active oxygen species.

The consequences for the cell of the formation of a reactive intermediate are governed by its inherent reactivity and by the balance of the activities of enzymes responsible for its formation and inactivation.

The reactivity of metabolites obviously covers a wide spectrum, from those which are essentially inert end-products whose fate will depend on their physicochemical properties, to those which are so reactive that they exist only in the active site of the enzymes catalyzing their formation. Such extremely reactive intermediates may act as suicide substrate inactivators of enzymes (Ortiz de Montellano *et al.*, 1981). We must next consider intermediates with lifetimes long enough to allow them to leave the immediate vicinity of the relevant enzyme and to which essential cellular organelles are exposed. The great majority of these are electrophiles which have been classified into 'hard' and 'soft' reactants (Ketterer, 1988). 'Hard' electrophiles react very well with nucleophilic sites such as the S atom of methionine in proteins and with nucleophilic N, O and C atoms in nucleic acid bases, but have poor reactivity with glutathione (GSH) and protein thiols. 'Soft' electrophiles, on the other hand, react well with thiols in glutathione and protein but not with other nucleophilic sites in biological macromolecules. Hard electrophiles are typically genotoxic intermediates such as the ultimate carcinogens *N*-sulphonyloxymethyl-4-aminoazobenzene and benzo[*a*]pyrene-7,8-diol-9,10-oxide (Djuric *et al.*, 1987; Coles *et al.*, 1988), while soft electrophiles are typified by *N*-acetyl-*p*-benzoquinoneimine (NAPQI), the cytotoxic (but not genotoxic) metabolite responsible for the hepatotoxicity of paracetamol. A numerical classification of 'hardness' and 'softness' is given by the second order rate constant for the reactivity of the electrophile with GSH: for NAPQI, the rate constant is 3×10^{-4} M s^{-1}, for the mutagenic but not carcinogenic epoxide of 1-nitropyrene it is 1.5 M s^{-1} while those for *N*-sulphonyloxymethyl-4-aminoazobenzene and benzo[*a*]pyrene-7,8-diol-9,10-oxide cannot be determined.

The cell possesses a number of enzymes which act to inactivate and detoxify reactive intermediates. Probably the most important of these in quantitative terms is GSH conjugation, in which the nucleophilic thiol of GSH (the tripeptide γ-glutamylcysteinylglycine) reacts with an electrophile, frequently under the catalysis of one or more of the glutathione *S*-transferases (GSTs). The reaction types involve attack on electrophilic centres (Caldwell, 1982), such as carbon atoms in strained oxirane rings, addition to α,β-unsaturated compounds and with carbonium ions. Electrophilic nitrogen atoms, including nitroso compounds and nitrate esters, and the electrophilic oxygen atoms in organic hydroperoxides are also attacked. The extent to which a particular reaction is catalyzed by the GSTs varies very widely and represents one discernible influence on the biological properties of their substrates. Thus, benzo[*a*]pyrene-7,8-diol-9,10-oxide is a good substrate for a number of hepatic GSTs and this together with the high concentration of GSH in the liver accounts for its lack of hepatocarcinogenicity in the rat (Ketterer, 1988). Aflatoxin B_1 2,3-oxide is a very poor substrate which is consistent with its hepatocarcinogenicity under normal circumstances (Ketterer, 1988): interestingly, induction with ethoxyquin of the GSTs, catalyzing its GSH conjugation, has a marked protective effect.

The cytochrome *P*-450-catalyzed oxidation of double bonds in alkenes and aromatic rings almost invariably produces an oxirane (arene oxide for aromatic rings, epoxide for alkenes) as the obligatory intermediate (Jerina *et al.*, 1970; Ortiz de Montellano, 1985). Arene oxides generally rearrange via the 'NIH Shift' to phenols but these and alkene oxides can exist free within the cell. Oxiranes are highly strained three-membered rings in which one or other of the carbon atoms can have marked electrophilic character depending on the substitution around the ring. Like other types of electrophiles, the reactivity of oxiranes covers a wide spectrum, from very stable cases like carbamazepine 10,11-oxide, which is a major urinary metabolite of this anticonvulsant (Faigle and Feldman, 1982), to the very reactive, like aflatoxin B_1 2,3-oxide as quoted above. As well as undergoing GSH conjugation, the oxirane ring is readily opened by water, generally catalyzed by an epoxide hydrolase (Ota and Hammock, 1980). Two distinct forms of this enzyme exist, one in the cytosol and one in the endoplasmic reticulum, the form involved in the metabolism of a particular substrate being determined by its structure. The activities of these enzymes represent a second major cellular defence mechanism against the toxic consequences of a reactive oxirane intermediate and in *in vitro* cytotoxicity and mutagenicity tests inhibition of epoxide hydrolases has been used to show the harmful consequences of an epoxide intermediate (Guest and Dent, 1980; Marshall and Caldwell, 1992).

Reactive metabolic intermediates are generally 'short range toxins' and their extreme reactivity (half-lives between 10 s and 1 min) strongly suggests that their toxicity involves reactions specific to particular tissues. However, although the liver is the major site of metabolism of xenobiotics in the body, it is relatively rarely a target organ for toxicity. It seems likely that in a number of cases reactive metabolites formed in the liver are in fact sufficiently stable to be transported to other organs where toxicity is expressed. In a small number of cases, it is apparent that metabolic activation is multiphasic, with a first step in the liver followed by further reactions in the target organ itself.

It must be remembered that not all toxic metabolites are reactive intermediates. On occasion, chemically stable products can be involved in toxicity, through their action at receptors, by physicochemical means, such as the renal toxicity of the sulphonamides (see above), or by retention in the body.

An example of activation by oxidation not involving an electrophile or a free radical is seen in the case of the solvent *n*-hexane (Bus, 1985). This is well known to produce a characteristic neuropathy, described as a 'dying back' of the axons of peripheral nerves, as well as testicular atrophy. These two toxic manifestations follow different time courses. The first clues that there might be a metabolic basis to this neuropathy was given by the fact that methyl *n*-butyl ketone (2-hexanone) gave pathologically similar effects and it was then demonstrated that *n*-hexane and 2-hexanone had a number of common metabolites. It is now clear that *n*-hexane is metabolized by sequential (ω-1)-hydroxylation at both ends of the chain (C-2 and C-5), so that 2,5-hexanedione is a common metabolite of both *n*-hexane and 2-hexanone. Various studies involving the feeding of a number of metabolites indicate that 2,5-hexanedione is the common neurotoxic metabolite of these solvents. Work with a range of related materials has shown that γ-diketones (1,4-diketones) or compounds metabolized to γ-diketones all give rise to axonopathies by binding to critical lysine residues in axonal proteins by Schiff's base formation leading to stable pyrrole derivatives.

Although most metabolic processes favour excretion from the body as a result of increases in polarity and water solubility, a small number of metabolites show increased lipophilicity relative to the parent compound and are retained in the body thereby. This is well established for a range of carboxylic acids and alcohols which are esterified with various lipids of the body (Caldwell and Marsh, 1983) and is also the case with certain end-products of the metabolism of glutathione conjugates. Glutathione conjugates undergo extensive metabolism by hydrolysis to the corresponding S-substituted cysteine, which may be N-acetylated to give a mercapturic acid, readily cleared in the urine of many species (Caldwell, 1982). However, the cysteine conjugates may also undergo other reactions of S-oxidation, transamination and the so-called 'thiomethyl shunt' (Caldwell *et al.*, 1989). This involves the cleavage of the cysteine conjugate by cysteine conjugate β-lyase to yield a thiol which is then methylated (Jakoby and Stevens, 1983). The thiomethyl conjugates so formed often undergo S-oxidation to give very lipophilic sulphones (Jakoby and Stevens, 1983). An example of the toxicological significance of this pathway is given by the metabolism of the polychlorinated biphenyl (PCB) 2,4,5,2′,4′,5′-hexachlorobiphenyl. This PCB is metabolized to a bisglutathionyl conjugate, which is progressively transformed as outlined to the very lipophilic 4,4′-bis(methylsulphonyl)-2,2′,5,5′-tetrachlorobiphenyl (Figure 2) (Brandt *et al.*, 1985). This accumulates in lung and kidney of mice and rats and was associated, in lung at least, with binding to a cytosolic protein. It is well known that PCBs accumulate in the tissues of various species exposed environmentally, the tissue residues generally being in the form of methylsulphones. Many of these methylsulphones are concentrated in the lung, which is of interest as the lung is a target organ for PCB toxicity in humans, as was shown in the Yusho incident in Japan, an epidemic of human PCB intoxication.

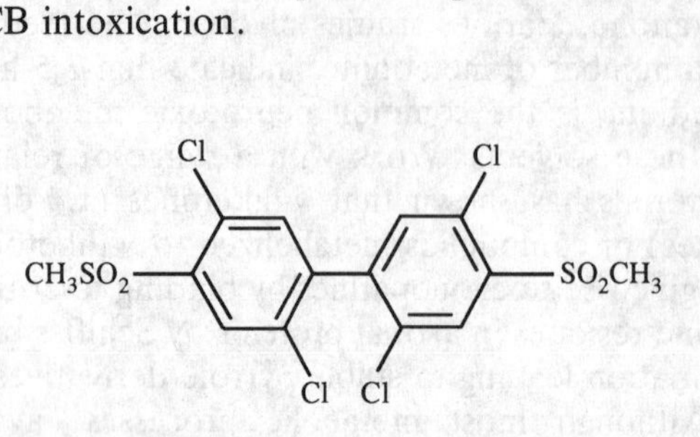

4,4′-Bis(methylsulphonyl)-2,2′,5,5′-tetrachlorobiphenyl

Figure 2 4,4′-Bis(methylsulphonyl)-2,2′,5,5′-tetrachlorobiphenyl, the lipophilic and pneumotoxic thioether metabolite of 2,4,5,2′,4′,5′-hexachlorobiphenyl

Metabolic Activation at the Site of Toxicity

The majority of examples where the toxicity of a compound is accounted for by metabolism within the site of toxicity are indeed seen in the liver. The liver necrosis caused by compounds such as paracetamol (acetaminophen) and carbon tetrachloride is the result of their metabolic activation in the liver. Paracetamol necrosis results from the cytochrome *P*-450 mediated formation of NAPQI in quantities sufficient to exceed the capacity of the glutathione conjugation mechanism to protect the hepatocyte (Prescott and Critchley, 1983). This knowledge has permitted the rational treatment of paracetamol overdose, many cases of which are fatal unless treated in time, by agents such as N-acetylcysteamine, which enhance the cell's protective pools of nucleophilic thiols (Prescott and Critchley, 1983).

The volatile general anaesthetic halothane is similarly activated by cytochrome *P*-450 to a very reactive trifluoracylating species whose toxicity is a consequence of the organism's immune response to the trifluoracylated proteins produced by the hepatocyte (Kenna, 1991). A single exposure to halothane has no harmful consequences, but can sensitize individuals so that subsequent doses can result in a fulminant hepatitis which has proved fatal (Stock and Strunin, 1985).

The metabolic activation of carbon tetrachloride, although also mediated by cytochrome *P*-450, by contrast involves one-electron chemistry. Its reductive dechlorination gives rise to chloride ion and the CCl_3· free radical which is cytotoxic as such and through initiation of lipid peroxidation (Anders and Pohl, 1985).

Tissue- or cell-specific activation of toxins also occurs outside the liver and one notable set of examples is seen in the lung. The lung is a highly heterogeneous organ, with over 40 cell types, and a number of indoles and furans are markedly pneumotoxic. These are selective for the Clara cells of the pulmonary epithelium which contain very large amounts of a number of cytochrome *P*-450 isozymes able to form reactive and cytotoxic epoxides from compounds such as the furan 4-ipomeanol (Boyd, 1977).

1-Methyl-4-phenyl-1,2,3,6-tetrahydropyridine (MPTP) is a neurotoxin first identified in illicitly synthesized samples of the opiate pethidine (meperidine). It causes selective destruction of dopaminergic neurons in the substantia nigra and produces a syndrome essentially indistinguishable from idiopathic Parkinsonism (Jenner and Marsden, 1987). MPTP is highly lipophilic and readily crosses the blood–brain barrier. Within the brain, it is oxidized in two steps by the 'B' form of monoamine oxidase (MAO-B; Singer *et al.*, 1987) to the pyridinium species MPP$^+$ (Figure 3), which inhibits mitochondrial respiration. This is a substrate for the dopamine uptake pump and is very toxic to nigral neurons in culture. MPP$^+$ destroys dopaminergic neurons when injected stereotactically into the substantia nigra, indicating it to be the ultimate neurotoxin of MPTP. The neurotoxicity of MPTP, which is irreversible, can be prevented by MAO-B inhibitors and dopamine uptake blockers, which prevent the formation of MPP$^+$ and its access to its site of action (Jenner, 1989).

Streptozotocin, a methylnitrosourea antitumour drug, is a widely used experimental tool for the induction of diabetes. It is also a pancreatic carcinogen which causes the selective destruction of the pancreatic islet cells, thereby preventing insulin release. Although the nitrosoureas are non-selective in their action, the glucose moiety apparently targets streptozotocin to the pancreas and releases the toxic and carcinogenic nitrosourea there (Srivastava *et al.*, 1982).

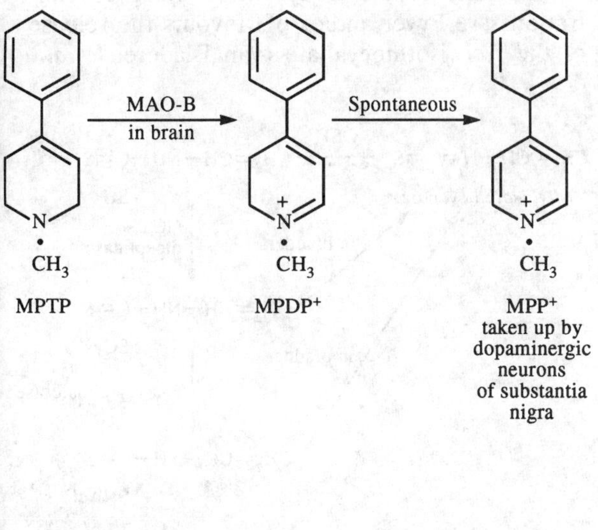

TRANSPORT OF REACTIVE INTERMEDIATES AROUND THE BODY FROM THEIR SITE OF FORMATION TO THEIR SITE OF ACTION

Extrahepatic Toxins Whose Metabolic Activation Occurs in the Liver

Although as has already been mentioned, reactive intermediates are generally thought of as 'short range toxins', it is now clear that a number of these are sufficiently stable to leave their site of formation and be transported to remote sites where they exert their toxicity. An early example of this is seen with the pyrrolizidine alkaloids present in various plants from the *Senecio, Heliotropium* and *Crotolaria* species which all too often contaminate human and animal foodstuffs (Culvenor, 1980). These alkaloids are typified by monocrotaline, which is highly toxic to liver and lung through its metabolite dehydromonocrotaline. *In vitro* studies show that only the liver has the ability to activate monocrotaline and its pneumotoxicity is due to the transport of the metabolite from the site of formation in the liver to the lung (Mattocks, 1972).

One of the earliest cases of the toxicity of a compound being directly related to its conversion to a reactive intermediate was bromobenzene, which is converted to bromobenzene 3,4-oxide. This binds covalently to hepatic macromolecules and this is presumed to underlie its hepatotoxicity (Brodie *et al.*, 1971). As well as having effects on the liver, bromobenzene is covalently bound and has toxic effects in a range of extrahepatic tissues. Despite its presumed high reactivity, the epoxide is able to escape from hepatocytes and is transported to the other tissues where part of its toxicity is expressed (Monks *et al.*, 1984). Bromobenzene 3,4-oxide can be detected in rat blood after administration of bromobenzene and although its half-life is very short (approximately 13.5 s), this is longer than the circulation time of the rat (5–10 s), which means that the hepatically-generated epoxide is available to the lung and other tissues (Lau *et al.*, 1984).

MPTP   MAO-B in brain → MPDP$^+$ Spontaneous → MPP$^+$ taken up by dopaminergic neurons of substantia nigra

Figure 3 Metabolic activation of MPTP by MAO-B in the brain

Metabolic Activation as a Consequence of Multiple Reactions in Multiple Tissues

This is typified by the nephrotoxicity of the halogenated solvent hexachlorobutadiene (Anders *et al.*, 1988) which is mediated through its glutathione conjugate and involves successive transformation in different organs, finishing in the kidney (Figure 4). The major site of formation of the glutathione conjugate, which occurs by displacement of a chlorine atom by the S- of glutathione, is the liver. The conjugate is then hydrolyzed by the liver, gut flora and kidney to the

corresponding *S*-substituted cysteine which is the proximate nephrotoxin. The cysteine conjugate is a substrate for the cysteine conjugate β-lyase of kidney which produces a reactive thiol which is the ultimate toxic metabolite. The tissue-specific expression of toxicity of hexachlorobutadiene thus involves metabolism first in the liver, giving a metabolite which is transported to the kidney, and then in the target organ, the kidney.

The urinary bladder is the target for the carcinogenicity of allyl isothiocyanate (AITC) and 2-naphthylamine. In both cases, the physicochemical conditions within the bladder result in the reversal of their metabolism, so that the urothelium is exposed to toxic compounds.

AITC, the pungent flavour principle of mustard and horseradish, has been shown to be a bladder carcinogen in male, but not female, rats (NTP, 1982). No effects were seen in the bladders of mice. The interpretation of the significance of the animal carcinogenicity data for the human safety of AITC is problematical in the absence of a clear-cut mechanism for tumorigenesis: the mutagenicity of AITC is far from clear (NTP, 1982), making a genotoxic mechanism unlikely. There is a strong possibility that a knowledge of the metabolism of AITC is relevant: AITC is detoxified by GSH conjugation in the liver and the glutathione conjugate is transformed to the corresponding mercapturic acid (*N*-acetylcysteine) (Ioannou *et al.*, 1984). This conjugation is reversible (Figure 5) so that AITC can be released at another site in the body where GSH concentrations are lower and/or pH favours the release of the free isothiocyanate (van Bladeren *et al.*,

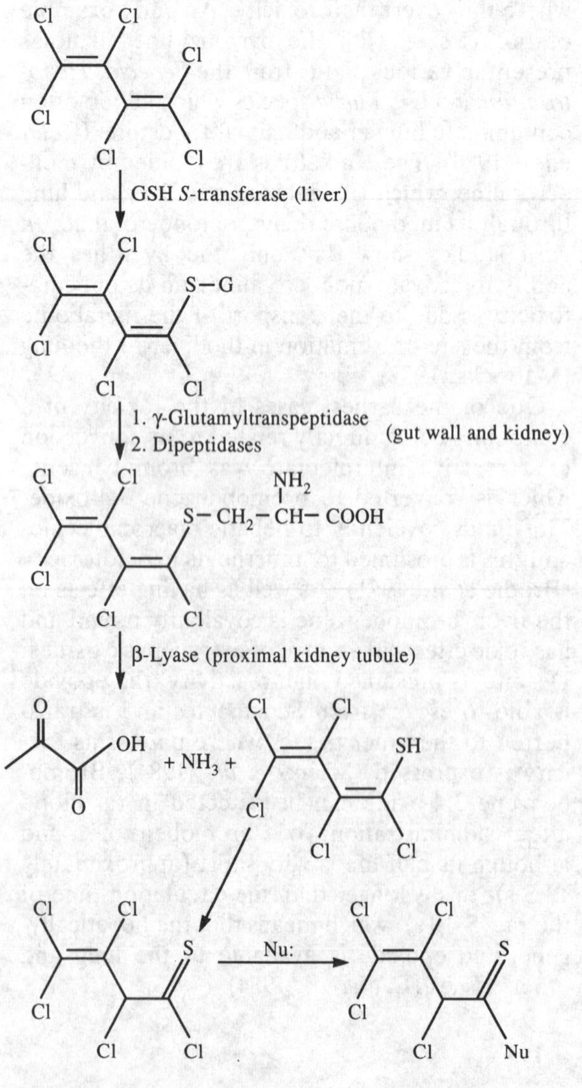

Figure 4 Metabolic activation of hexachlorobutadiene by the catabolism of its glutathione conjugate to a nephrotoxic electrophilic thiol

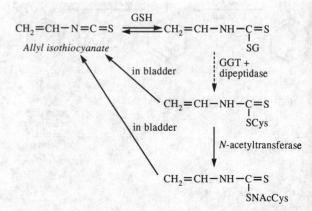

Figure 5 Reversible glutathione conjugation of allyl isothiocyanate, the basis for its toxicity to the urinary bladder

1987). It is reasonable to hypothesize that the tumours originate from chronic irritation of the bladder epithelium by AITC, a known strong irritant to skin and mucous membranes, liberated from its labile mercapturic acid conjugate under the conditions (temperature, basic pH, low or absent GSH levels, etc.) in the bladder. This prolonged irritation leads to hyperplasia and thence to neoplasia. The restriction of tumours to the male rat has been suggested to be related to the much lower urine flow in this sex (Ioannou *et al.*, 1984). Although knowledge of the metabolism of AITC is fragmentary, it is clear that there exist major differences between its fate in rats and mice (Ioannou *et al.*, 1984). AITC undergoes very extensive conjugation with glutathione in all species, but the subsequent fate of the glutathione conjugate is very variable. It is known that the further metabolism of the *S*-substituted cysteines produced by hydrolysis of glutathione conjugates shows very marked inter-species variability: while the major pathway in rats is almost invariably *N*-acetylation, yielding the mercapturic acid, in the mouse there occurs substantial transamination of the cysteine conjugate, giving thioglycollic and thioacetic acids (Caldwell *et al.*, 1989). In the case of isothiocyanate conjugates, these will cyclize to yield thiazolidin-2-thiones (Görler *et al.*, 1982). These may be expected to have very different reactivities from the mercapturic acid, which may account for the species specificity of tumour occurrence. The likely mechanism of tumorigenicity is thus a secondary mechanism, not involving genotoxicity, and which would be expected to show a dose-threshold. Comparison of human exposure from the diet, which is limited by sensory considerations (Fenwick *et al.*, 1982), with the doses required to evoke a small number of tumours in one sex of one animal species thus offers a sufficient margin of safety.

2-Naphthylamine is a genotoxic carcinogen which is activated by *N*-hydroxylation. Sulphation and/or acetylation of *N*-hydroxy-2-naphthylamine leads to nitrenium ions which give rise to DNA adducts and, ultimately, tumours in a variety of organs. In a detoxication reaction, *N*-hydroxy-2-naphthylamine is *N*-glucuronidated and this conjugate acts as a stable transport form which is excreted in the urine (Kadlubar *et al.*, 1977). The low pH (5–6) within the bladder of the average person eating a Western diet is low enough to break down the *N*-glucuronide, releasing the genotoxic *N*-hydroxy-2-naphthylamine in the lumen so as to allow it to attack the urothelium (Kadlubar *et al.*, 1977). This sequence of reactions is outlined in Figure 6.

CONCLUDING COMMENTS

The coverage of this chapter has hinted at the state of knowledge concerning various mechanisms of toxicity. The efforts of a number of disparate scientific disciplines, both chemical and biological, have combined to enable an understanding of the origin of a number of toxic reactions. There has been rapid progress in recent years and the applications of the techniques and concepts of molecular biology currently going on will enable this to continue.

It is important to appreciate that there remains a considerable problem in discerning cause and effect as far as toxicology is concerned which may be illustrated by the phenomenon of lipid peroxidation. This represents an important primary mechanism of cytotoxicity for a number of compounds, but it is also a general feature of dying cells. To delineate whether it is indeed a mechanism of toxicity or is simply the consequence of cell death caused some other way is problematical indeed and it is all too easy to be misled.

Molecular biology affords the opportunity to look for the first time at toxic mechanisms at the most fundamental level. This includes cytotoxicity, particularly now that programmed cell death, or apoptosis, is accessible to experiment. New insights are also possible into proliferative lesions, most importantly cancer, as knowledge develops of cellular regulatory processes. Basic mechanisms of reproductive toxicity are approachable for the first time with increased understanding of developmental biology.

The practical significance of a mechanistic basis of toxicity is that first and foremost it allows properly informed safety assessments to be made. The recognition of qualitative and/or quantitative differences in the occurrence of a toxic mechanism or a particular metabolic pathway between species and/or exposure situations provides a scientifically acceptable and objective basis for the extrapolation of data, most notably from animals to humans. This may be favourable, in that it may show that animal data overestimate human risk, as is the case with the peroxisome prolifera-

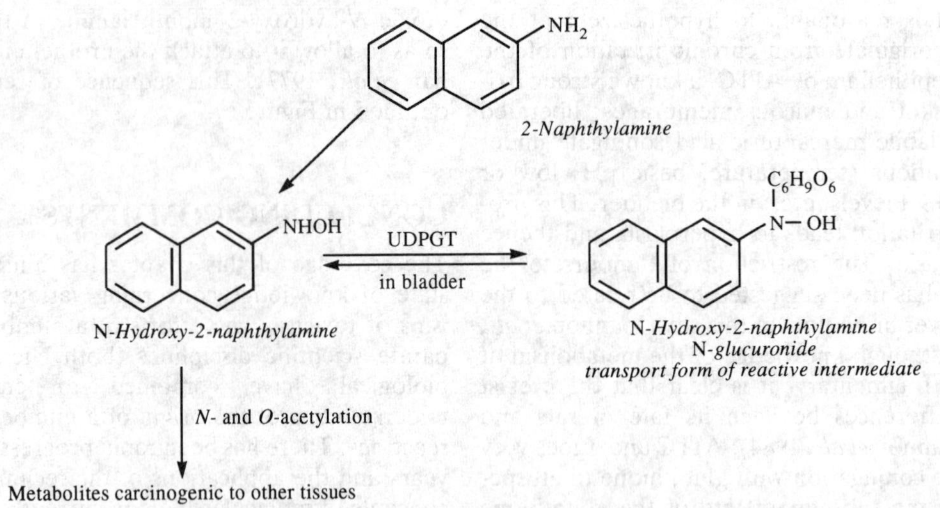

Figure 6   Metabolism of 2-naphthylamine, showing how the *N*-glucuronide of *N*-hydroxy-2-naphthylamine acts as a stable transport form for this reactive metabolite to the urinary bladder

tors and *d*-limonene (see above) but in other cases, like paracetamol, humans are seen to be at least as sensitive as test animals to a given compound.

Finally, it must be realized that the use of mechanistic approaches is not limited to their *post hoc* use to explain unwanted effects in toxicity tests. These approaches allow for the first time the design of improved tests whose end-points are far more relevant to the human situation and which allow the more economic and ethical deployment of test animals and other resources to support the safer and more effective use of chemicals in the human population.

REFERENCES

Ames, B. N., Shigenaga, M. K. and Gold, L. S. (1993). DNA lesions, inducible DNA repair and cell division: three key factors in mutagenesis and carcinogenesis. *Environ. Health Perspect.*

Anders, M. W. and Pohl, L. R. (1985). Halogenated alkanes. In Anders, M. W. (Ed.) *Bioactivation of Foreign Compounds*. Academic Press, New York, pp. 121–155

Anders, M. W., Lash, L., Dekant, W., Elfarra, A. A. and Dohn, D. R. (1988) Biosynthesis and biotransformation of glutathione S-conjugates into toxic metabolites. *CRC Crit. Rev. Toxicol.*, **18**, 311–341

Ashby, J. and Tennant, R. W. (1988). Chemical structure, *Salmonella* mutagenicity and extent of carcino-

genicity as indicators of genotoxic carcinogenesis. *Mutat. Res.*, **204**, 17–115

Bennett, W. M. (1983). Aminoglycoside nephrotoxicity. *Nephron*, **35**, 73–77

Bernstein, H. N., Zvaifler, N., Rubin, M. and Mansour, Sister A. M. (1963). The ocular deposition of chloroquine. *Invest. Ophthalmol.*, **2**, 381–392

Boet, D. J. (1970). Toxic effects of phenothiazines on the eye. *Doc. Ophthamol.*, **28**, 1–69

Boyd, M. R. (1977). Evidence for the Clara cell as a site of cytochrome P-450-dependent mixed function oxidase activity in lung. *Nature (Lond.)*, **269**, 713

Brandt, I., Lund, J., Bergman, Å., Klasson-Wheler, E., Poellinger, L. and Gustafsson, J.-Å (1985). Target cells for the polychlorinated biphenyl metabolite 4,4′-bis(methylsulfonyl)-2,2′,5,5′-tetrachlorobiphenyl in lung and kidney. *Drug Metab. Dispos.*, **13**, 490–496

Brenner, B. E. and Simon, R. R. (1982). Management of salicylate intoxication. *Drugs*, **24**, 335–340

Brodie, B. B., Reid, W. D., Cho, A. K., Sipes, I. G., Krishna, G. and Gillette, J. R. (1971). Possible mechanism of liver necrosis caused by aromatic organic compounds. *Proc. Natl Acad. Sci. USA*, **68**, 160

Burns, C. A. (1966). Ocular effects of indomethacin. Slit lamp and electroretinographic (ERG) study. *Invest. Ophthalmol.*, **5**, 325

Bus, J. S. (1985). Alkanes. In Anders, M. W. (Ed.), *Bioactivation of Foreign Compounds*. Academic Press, New York, pp. 111–120

Butterworth, B. E., Slaga, T., Farland, W. and McClain, M. (Eds) (1991). *Chemically Induced Cell Proliferation: Implications for Risk Assessment*. Wiley-Liss, New York

Caldwell, J. (1982). The conjugation reactions in

foreign compound metabolism: definition, consequences and species differences. *Drug Metab. Rev.*, **13**, 745–778

Caldwell, J. and Marsh, M. V. (1983). Interrelationships between xenobiotic metabolism and lipid biosynthesis. *Biochem. Pharmacol.*, **32**, 1667–1672

Caldwell, J., Weil, A. and Tanaka, Y. (1989). Species differences in xenobiotic conjugation. In Kato, R., Estabrook, R. W. and Cayen, M. N. (Eds), *Xenobiotic Metabolism and Disposition*. Taylor & Francis, London, pp. 217–224

Coles, B., Wilson, I., Wordman, P., Hinson, J. A., Nelson, S. D. and Ketterer, B. (1988). The spontaneous and enzymatic reaction of *N*-acetyl-*p*-benzoquinoneimine with glutathione: a stopped-flow kinetic study. *Arch. Biochem. Biophys.*, **264**, 253–260

Culvenor, C. C. J. (1980). Toxicology of pyrrolizidine alkaloids. In Smith, R. L. and Bababunmi, E. A. (Eds), *Toxicology in the Tropics*. Taylor & Francis, London, pp. 124–137

Denckner, L., Lindqvist, N. G. and Ullberg, S. (1973). Mechanism of drug-induced chronic otic lesions. *Experientia*, **29**, 1362

Djuric, Z., Coles, B., Fifer, E. K., Ketterer, B. and Beland, F. A. (1987). *In vivo* and *in vitro* formation of glutathione conjugates from the K-region epoxides of 1-nitropyrene. *Carcinogenesis*, **8**, 1781–1786

EPA (United States Environmental Protection Agency) (1991). *α2u-Globulin: Association with Chemically Induced Renal Toxicity and Neoplasia in the Male Rat*. EPA, Washington, DC

Faigle, J. W. and Feldman (1982). Carbamazepine biotransformation. In Woodbury, D. M., Penry, J. K. and Pippenger, C. E. (Eds), *Antiepileptic Drugs*, 2nd edn. Raven Press, New York, pp. 483–495

Fenwick, G. R., Heaney, R. K. and Mullin, W. J. (1982). Glucosinolates and their breakdown products in food and food plants. *CRC Crit. Rev. Food Sci. Nutr.*, **18**, 123–201

Flamm, W. G. and Lehmann-McKeeman, L. D. (1991). The human relevance of the renal tumor-inducing potential of *d*-limonene in male rats: implications for risk assessment. *Regulatory Toxicol. Pharmacol.*, **13**, 70–86

Görler, K., Krumbiegel, G. and Mennicke, W. H. (1982). The metabolism of benzyl isothiocyanate and its cysteine conjugate in guinea-pigs and rabbits. *Xenobiotica*, **12**, 535–542

Green, S. (1992). Receptor-mediated mechanisms of peroxisome proliferation. *Biochem. Pharmacol.*, **43**, 393–401

Guest, D. and Dent, J. G. (1980). Effects of epoxide hydratase inhibitors in forward and reverse bacterial mutagenesis assay systems. *Environ. Mutagen.*, **2**, 27–34

Humes, H. D. and O'Connor, R. P. (1988). Aminoglycoside nephrotoxicity. In Schrier, R. W. and Gottschalk, C. (Eds), *Diseases of the Kidney*. Vol. 2, 4th edn. Little, Brown, Boston, pp. 1229–1273

Ings, R. M. J. (1984). The melanin binding of drugs and its implications. *Drug Metab. Rev.*, **15**, 1183–1212

Ioannou, Y. M., Burka, L. T. and Matthews, H. B. (1984). Allyl isothiocyanate: comparative disposition in rats and mice. *Toxicol. Appl. Pharmacol.*, **75**, 173–181

Jakoby, W. B. and Stevens, J. (1983). Cysteine conjugate β-lyase and the thiomethyl shunt. *Biochem. Soc. Trans.*, **12**, 33–35

Jenner, P. (1989). MPTP-induced Parkinsonism: chemical basis of an age-related disease. In Volans, G. N., Sims, J., Sullivan, F. M. and Turner, P. (Eds), *Basic Science in Toxicology: Proceedings of the V International Congress of Toxicology*. Taylor & Francis, London, pp. 615–625

Jenner, P. and Marsden, C. D. (1987). MPTP-induced parkinsonism in primates and its use in the assessment of novel strategies for the treatment of Parkinson's disease. In Rose, F. C. (Ed.), *Parkinson's Disease: Clinical and Experimental Advances* Vol. 87, John Libbey, London, pp. 149–162

Jerina, D. M., Daly, J. W., Witkop, B., Zaltzman-Nirenberg, P. and Udenfriend, S. (1970). 1,2-Naphthalene oxide as an intermediate in the microsomal hydroxylation of naphthalene. *Biochemistry*, **9**, 147–156

Joy, R. M. (1982). Chlorinated hydrocarbon insecticides. In Ecobichon, D. J. and Joy, R. M. (Eds), *Pesticides and Neurological Disorders*. CRC Press, Boca Raton, Florida, pp. 91–150

Kadlubar, F. F., Miller, J. A. and Miller, E. C. (1977). Hepatic microsomal *N*-hydroxyarylamines in relation to urinary bladder carcinogenesis. *Cancer Res.*, **37**, 805–814

Kenna, J. G. (1991). The molecular basis of halothane-induced hepatitis. *Biochem. Soc. Trans.*, **19**, 191–195

Ketterer, B. (1988). Protective role of glutathione and glutathione transferases in mutagenesis and carcinogenesis. *Mutat. Res.*, **202**, 343–361

Kiese, M. (1977). *Methemoglobinemia, a Comprehensive Treatise*. CRC Press, Boca Raton, Florida

Klaassen, C. D. (1991). Heavy metals and heavy metal antagonists. In Gilman, A. G., Rall, T. W., Nies, A. S. and Taylor, P. (Eds), *Goodman and Gilman's The Pharmacological Basis of Therapeutics*, 8th edn. Pergamon Press, New York, pp. 1592–1614

Kuo, C. H., Maita, K., Sleight, S. D. and Hook, J. B. (1983). Lipid peroxidation: a possible mechanism of cephaloridine-induced nephrotoxicity. *Toxicol. Appl. Pharmacol.*, **67**, 78–88

Lau, S. S., Monks, T. J. and Gillette, J. R. (1984). Detection and half-life of bromobenzene-3,4-oxide in blood. *Xenobiotica*, **14**, 539–543

Lilienfield, D. E. and Gallo, M. A. (1989). 2,4-D, 2,4,5-T and 2,3,7,8-TCDD: an overview. *Epidemiol. Rev.*, **11**, 28–58

Marshall, A. D. and Caldwell, J. (1992). Influence of modulators of epoxide metabolism on the cytotoxicity of trans-anethole in freshly isolated rat hepatocytes. *Fd. Chem. Toxicol.*, **30**, 376–473

Mattocks, A. R. (1972). Toxicity and metabolism of *Senecio* alkaloids. In Harborne, J. (Ed.), *Phytochemical Ecology*. Academic Press, New York, pp. 179–200

Miller, E. C. and Miller, J. A. (1985). Some historical perspectives on the metabolism of xenobiotic chemicals to reactive electrophiles. In Anders, M. W. (Ed.), *Bioactivation of Foreign Compounds*. Academic Press, New York, pp. 3–28

Monks, T. J., Lau, S. S. and Gillette, J. R. (1984). Diffusion of reactive intermediates out of hepatocytes: studies with bromobenzene. *J. Pharm. Exp. Ther.*, **228**, 393–399

Monro, A. M. (1992). What is an appropriate measure of exposure when testing drugs for carcinogenicity in rodents. *Toxicol. Appl. Pharm.*, **112**, 171–181

NTP (National Toxicology Program) (1982). *NTP Technical Report on the Carcinogenesis Bioassay of Allyl Isothiocyanate*. DHHS Publication (NIH) 83–1790. Department of Health and Human Services. Washington, DC

Orrenius, S., McConkey, D. J. and Nicotera, P. (1989). The role of calcium in neurotoxicity. In Volans, G. N., Sims, J., Sullivan, F. M. and Turner, P. (Eds), *Basic Science in Toxicology*. Taylor & Francis, London, pp. 629–635

Ortiz de Montellano, P. R. (1985). Alkenes and alkynes. In Anders, M. W. (Ed.), *Bioactivation of Foreign Compounds*. Academic Press, New York, pp. 121–155

Ortiz de Montellano, P. R., Mico, B. A., Mathews, J. M., Kunze, K. L., Miwa, G. T. and Lu, A. Y. H. (1981). Selective inactivation of cytochrome P-450 isozymes by suicide substrates. *Arch. Biochem. Biophys.*, **210**, 717–728

Ota, K. and Hammock, B. D. (1980). Cytosolic and microsomal epoxide hydrolases. *Science (New York)*, **207**, 1479–1480

Potts, A. M. (1962). The concentration of phenothiazines in the eyes of experimental animals. *Invest. Ophthalmol.*, **1**, 522–530

Prescott, L. F. and Critchley, J. A. J. H. (1983). The treatment of acetaminophen poisoning. *Ann. Rev. Pharmacol.*, **23**, 87–101

Rall, T. W. (1991). Hypnotics and sedatives: ethanol. In Gilman, A. G., *et al.* (Eds), *Goodman and Gilman's The Pharmacological Basis of Therapeutics*, 8th edn. Pergamon Press, New York, pp. 345–382

Rawlins, M. D. (1981). Adverse reactions to drugs. *Br. Med. J.*, **282**, 974–976

Ross, E. M. (1991). Pharmacodynamics. In Gilman, A. G., Rall, T. W., Nies, A. S. and Taylor, P. (Eds), *Goodman and Gilman's The Pharmacological Basis of Therapeutics*, 8th edn. Pergamon Press, New York, pp. 33–48

Sies, H. and Cadenas, E. (1983). Biological basis of detoxicatiion of oxygen free radicals. In Caldwell, J.

and Jakoby, W. B. (Eds), *Biological Basis of Detoxication*. Academic Press, New York, pp. 181–211

Singer, T. P., Castagnoli, N. Jr, Ramsay, R. R. and Trevor, A. J. (1987). Biochemical events in the development of Parkinsonism induced by 1-methyl-4-phenyl-1,2,3,6-tetrahydropyridine. *J. Neurochem.*, **49**, 1–8

Smith, L. L., Lewis, C., Wyatt, I. and Cohen, G. M. (1989). The importance of epithelial uptake mechanisms in lung toxicity. In Volans, G. N., Sims, J., Sullivan, F. M. and Turner, P. (Eds), *Basic Science in Toxicology*. Taylor & Francis, London, pp. 233–241

Srivastava, L. M., Bora, P. S. and Bhatt, S. D. (1982). Diabetogenic action of streptozotocin. *Trends Pharmacol. Sci.* **3**, 376

Stock, J. G. L. and Strunin, L. (1985). Unexplained hepatitis following halothane. *Anesthesiology*, **63**, 424–439

Van Bladeren, P. J., Bruggeman, I. M., Jongen, W. M. F., Scheffer, A. G. and Temmink, J. H. M. (1987). The role of conjugating enzymes in toxic metabolite formation. In Benford, D. J., Bridges, J. W. and Gibson, G. G. (Eds), *Drug Metabolism — from Molecules to Man*. Taylor & Francis, London, pp. 151–170

Weinberg, J. M. (1988). The cellular basis of nephrotoxicity. In Schrier, R. W. and Gottschalk, C. (Eds), *Diseases of the Kidney*, Vol. 2, 4th edn. Little, Brown, Boston, pp. 1137–1195

Williams, G. M. and Weisburger, J. H. (1991). Chemical carcinogenesis. In Amdur, M. O., *et al.* (Eds), *Casarett and Doull's Toxicology*, 4th edn. Pergamon Press, New York, pp. 127–200

Wold, J. S. (1981). Cephalosporin nephrotoxicity. In Hook, J. B. (Ed.), *Toxicology of the Kidney*, Raven Press, New York, pp. 251–266

Youdim, M. B. H., Bakhle, Y. S. and Ben-Harari, R. R. (1980). Inactivation of monoamines by the lung. In *Metabolic Activities of the Lung*. Excerpta Medica, Amsterdam, pp. 105–122

FURTHER READING

Aust, S. D., Chignell, C. F., Bray, T. M., Kalyanaraman, B. and Mason, R. P. (1993). Free radicals in toxicology. *Toxicology and Applied Pharmacology*, **120**, 168–178

Calabrese, E. J. (1991). Comparative metabolism the principal cause of differential susceptibility to toxic and carcinogenic agents. In *Principles of Animal Extrapolation*. Lewis Publishers, Chelsea, Michigan. pp. 203–277

Kehrer, J. P. (1993). Free radicals as mediators of tissue injury and disease. *Critical Reviews in Toxicology*, **23**, 21–48

7 Alternatives to *in vivo* Studies in Toxicology

Shayne C. Gad

INTRODUCTION

The key assumptions underlying modern toxicology are (1) that other organisms can serve as accurate predictive models of toxicity in man; (2) that selection of an appropriate model to use is the key to accurate prediction in man; and (3) that understanding the strengths and weaknesses of any particular model is essential to understanding the relevance of specific findings to man. The nature of models and their selection in toxicological research and testing has only recently become the subject of critical scientific review. Usually in toxicology, when we refer to 'models', we really have meant test organisms, although, in fact, the manner in which parameters are measured (and which parameters are measured to characterize an end-point of interest) are also critical parts of the model (or, indeed, may actually constitute the 'model').

Although there have been accepted principles for test organism selection, these have not generally been the final basis for such selection. It is a fundamental hypothesis of both historical and modern toxicology that adverse effects caused by chemical entities in higher animals are generally the same as those induced by those entities in man. There are many who point to individual exceptions to this and conclude that the general principle is false. Yet, as our understanding of molecular biology advances and we learn more about the similarities of structure and function of higher organisms at the molecular level, the more it becomes clear that the mechanisms of chemical toxicity are largely identical in humans and animals. This increased understanding has caused some of the same people who question the general principle of predictive value to in turn suggest that our state of knowledge is such that mathematical models or simple cell culture systems could be used just as well as intact animals to predict toxicities in man. This last suggestion also missed the point that the final expressions of toxicity in man or animals are frequently the summation of extensive and complex interactions on cellular and biochemical levels. Zbinden has published extensively in this area, including a very advanced defence of the value of animal models (Zbinden, 1987). Lijinsky (1988) has reviewed the specific issues about the predictive value and importance of animals in carcinogenicity testing and research. Although it was once widely believed, and still is believed by many animal rights activists, that *in vitro* mutagenicity tests would entirely replace animal bioassays for carcinogenicity, this is clearly not the case on either scientific or regulatory grounds. Although there are differences in the responses of various species (including man) to carcinogens, the overall predictive value of such results, when tempered by judgement, is clear. At the same time, a well-reasoned use of *in vitro* or other alternative test model systems is essential to the development of a product safety assessment programme is both effective and efficient (Gad, 1990a).

The subject of intact animal models and their proper selection and use has been addressed elsewhere (Gad and Chengelis, 1992) and will not be further addressed here. However, alternative models which use other than intact higher organisms are seeing increasing use in toxicology for a number of reasons.

The first and most significant factor behind the interest in so-called *in vitro* systems has clearly been political—an unremitting campaign by a wide spectrum of individuals concerned with the welfare and humane treatment of laboratory animals (Singer, 1975). In 1959 Russell and Burch first proposed what have come to be called the 3 Rs of humane animal use in research—replacement, reduction and refinement. These have served as the conceptual basis for reconsideration of animal use in research.

Replacement means utilizing methods that do not use intact animals in place of those that do. For examples: veterinary students may use a canine cardiopulmonary-resuscitation simulator, Resusci-Dog, instead of living dogs; cell cultures may replace mice and rats that are fed new products to discover substances poisonous to humans.

In addition, using the preceding definition of animal, an invertebrate (e.g. a horseshoe crab) could replace a vertebrate (e.g. a rabbit) in a testing protocol.

Reduction refers to the use of fewer animals. For instance, changing practices allow toxicologists to estimate the lethal dose of a chemical with as few as one-tenth the number of animals used in traditional tests. In biomedical research, long-lived animals, such as primates, may be used in multiple sequential protocols, assuming that they are not deemed inhumane or scientifically conflicting. Designing experimental protocols with appropriate attention to statistical inference can lead to decreases or to increases in the numbers of animals used. Through co-ordination of efforts among investigators, several tissues may be simultaneously taken from a single animal. Reduction can also refer to the minimization of any unintentionally duplicative experiments, perhaps through improvements in information resources.

Refinement entails the modification of existing procedures so that animals are subjected to less pain and distress. Refinements may include administration of anaesthetics to animals undergoing otherwise painful procedures; administration of tranquillizers for distress; humane destruction prior to recovery from surgical anaesthesia; and careful scrutiny of behavioural indices of pain or distress, followed by cessation of the procedure or the use of appropriate analgesics. Refinements also include the enhanced use of non-invasive imaging technologies that allow earlier detection of tumours, organ deterioration or metabolic changes, and the subsequent early euthanasia of test animals.

Progress towards these first three Rs has been previously reviewed (Gad, 1990b). However, there is a fourth R—responsibility, which was not in Russell and Burch's initial proposal. To toxicologists this is the cardinal R. They may be personally committed to minimizing animal use and suffering, and to doing the best possible science of which they are capable, but at the end of it all, toxicologists must stand by their responsibility to be conservative in ensuring the safety of the people using or exposed to the drugs and chemicals produced by our society.

During the past decade, issues of animal use and care in toxicological research and testing have become one of the fundamental concerns of both science and the public. Are our results predictive of what may or may not be seen in man? Are we using too many animals, and are we using them in a manner that gets the answer we need with as little discomfort to the animals as possible? How do we balance the needs of man against the welfare of animals?

In 1984 the Society of Toxicology (SOT) held its first symposium and addressed scientific approaches to these issues. The last such symposium for SOT was in 1988. Each year that passes has brought new regulations, attempts at federal and state legislation in the USA and legislation in other countries, and demonstrations that directly affect the practice of toxicology. Increasing amounts of both money and scientific talent have been dedicated to progress in this area. At the same time, the public clearly supports animal use in research when they see a need and benefit. This is shown in Table 1.

During the same time-frame, interest and progress in the development of *in vitro* test systems for toxicity evaluations have also progressed. Early reviews by Hooisma (1982), Neubert (1982) and Williams *et al.* (1983) record the proceedings of conferences on the subject, but Rofe's 1971 review was the first found by this author. Although it is hoped that in the long term some of these (or other) *in vitro* methods will serve as definitive tests in place of those that use intact animals, at present it appears more likely that their use in most cases will be as screens. Goldberg and Frazier (1989) give a current overview of the general concepts and status of *in vitro* alternatives.

The entire product safety assessment process, in the broadest sense, is a multistage process in which none of the individual steps is overwhelm-

Table 1 Public opinon on animal use in research

A 1989 survey conducted for the American Medical Association (1989) sampled almost 1500 households and found that:

- Sixty-four per cent opposed organizations attempting to stop the use of animals in research testing.
- Seventy-seven per cent thought that animal research was necessary for progress in medicine.
- Other polls have given the same results in terms of medical research or general issues of animal research and testing, but a majority has been found to oppose animal testing of cosmetics as unwarranted (Cowley *et al.*, 1988).

ingly complex, but the integration of the whole process involves fitting together a large complex pattern of pieces. The single most important part of this product safety evaluation programme is, in fact, the initial overall process of defining and developing an adequate data package on the potential hazards associated with the product life-cycle (the manufacture, sale, use and disposal of a product and associated process materials). To do this, one must ask a series of questions in a highly interactive process, with many of the questions designed to identify and/or modify their successors. The first is—what information is needed?

Required here is an understanding of the way in which a product is to be made and used, and the potential health and safety risks associated with exposure of humans who will be associated with these processes. Such an understanding is the basis of a hazard and toxicity profile. Once such a profile has been established (as illustrated in Figure 1), the available literature is searched to determine what is already known.

Taking into consideration this literature information and the previously defined exposure profile, a tier approach (Figure 2) has traditionally been used to generate a list of tests or studies to be performed.* What goes into a tier system is determined by regulatory requirements imposed by government agencies as well as the philosophy of the parent organization, economics and available technology. How such tests are actually performed is determined on one of two bases. The first (and most common) is the menu approach: selecting a series of standard design tests as 'modules' of data. The second is an interactive/iterative approach, where strategies are developed and studies are designed, based on both needs and what has been learned to date about the product. This process has been previously examined in some detail. Our interest here, however, is in the specific portion of the process involved in generating data—the test systems.

TEST SYSTEMS: CHARACTERISTICS, DEVELOPMENT AND SELECTION

Any useful test system must be sufficiently sensitive to ensure that the incidence of false negatives is low. Clearly a high incidence of false negatives

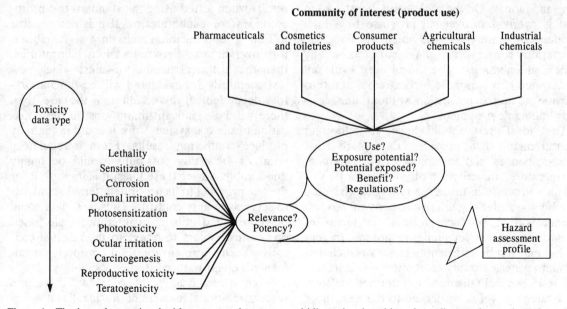

Figure 1 The hazards associated with a new product are a multidimensional problem depending on the product's intended use, its innate toxicity, its physicochemical properties, and the potential human and environmental exposure. This matrix diagrammatically illustrates the key questions involved in developing the final hazard assessment profile

* There is also the special case of pharmaceutical and pesticide products, where there are regulatory mandated minimum test batteries.

Tier testing

Testing tier	Mammalian toxicology	Genetic toxicology	Remarks
0	Literature review	Literature review	Upon initial identification of a problem, database of existing information and particulars of use of materials are established
1	Cytotoxicity screens Dermal sensitization Acute systemic toxicity Lethality screens	Ames test *In vitro* SCE *In vitro* cytogenetics Forward mutation/CHO	R&D material and low-volume chemicals with severely limited exposure
2	Subacute studies Metabolism Primary dermal irritation Eye irritation	*In vivo* SCE *In vivo* cytogenetics	Medium-volume materials and/or those with a significant chance of human exposure
3	Subchronic studies Reproduction Developmental toxicity Chronic studies Mechanistic studies	–	Any materials with a high volume or a potential for widespread or long-term human exposure or one that gives indications of specific long-term effects

Figure 2 The usual way of characterizing the toxicity of a compound or product is to develop information in a tier approach manner. More information is required (a higher tier level is attained) as the volume of production and potential for exposure increase. A common scheme is shown

is intolerable. In such a situation, large numbers of dangerous chemical agents would be carried through extensive additional testing only for it to be found that they possess undesirable toxicological properties after the expenditure of significant time and money. On the other hand, a test system that is overly sensitive will give rise to a high incidence of false positives, which will have the deleterious consequence of rejecting potentially beneficial chemicals. The 'ideal' test will fall somewhere between these two extremes and thus provide adequate protection without unnecessarily stifling development.

The 'ideal' test should have an end-point measurement that provides data such that dose–response relationships can be obtained. Furthermore, any criterion of effect must be sufficiently accurate in the sense that it can be used reliably to resolve the relative toxicity of two test chemicals that produce distinct (in terms of hazard to humans) yet similar responses. In general, it may not be sufficient to classify test chemicals into generic toxicity categories. For instance, if a test chemical falls into an 'intermediate' toxicity category, yet is borderline to the next more severe toxicity category, it should be treated with more concern than a second test chemical that falls at the less toxic extreme of the same category. Therefore, it is essential for a test system to be able to both place test chemicals in an

established toxicity category and rank materials relative to others in the category.

The end-point measurement of the 'ideal' test system must be objective. This is important, to ensure that a given test chemical will give similar results when tested using the standard test protocol in different laboratories. If it is not possible to obtain reproducible results in a given laboratory over time or between various laboratories, then the historical database against which new test chemicals are evaluated will be time/laboratory-dependent. If this condition is the case, then there will be significant limitations on the application of the test system since it could potentially produce conflicting results. From a regulatory point of view this possibility would be highly undesirable. Along these lines, it is important for the test protocol to incorporate internal standards to serve as quality controls. Thus, test data could be represented utilizing a reference scale based on the test system response to the internal controls. Such normalization, if properly documented, could reduce intertest variability.

From a practical point of view, there are several additional features of the 'ideal' test which should be satisfied. Alternatives to current *in vivo* test systems basically should be designed to evaluate the observed toxic response in a manner as closely predictive of the outcome of interest in man as possible. In addition, the test should be fast enough to ensure that the turnaround time for a given test chemical is reasonable for the intended purpose, very rapid for a screen, timely for a definitive test. Obviously the speed of the test and the ability to conduct tests on several chemicals simultaneously will determine the overall productivity. The test should be inexpensive, so that it is economically competitive with current testing practices. And finally, the technology should be easily transferred from one laboratory to another without excessive capital investment (relative to the value of the test performed) for test implementation.

It should be kept in mind that although some of these practical considerations may appear to present formidable limitations for any given test system at the present time, the possibility of future developments in testing technology could overcome these obstacles. In reality, these practical considerations are grounds for consideration of multiple new candidate tests on the basis of competitive performance. The most predictive test system in the universe of possibilities will never gain wide acceptance if it takes years to produce an answer or costs substantially more than other test systems that are only marginally less predictive.

The point is that these characteristics of the 'ideal' test system provide a general framework for evaluation of alternative test systems in general. No test system is likely to be 'ideal'. Therefore, it will be necessary to weigh the strengths and weaknesses of each proposed test system in order to reach a conclusion on how 'good' a particular test is.

In both theory and practice, *in vivo* and *in vitro* tests have potential advantages. Tables 2 and 3 summarize their advantages. How, then, might the proper tests by selected, especially in the case of the choice of staying with an existing test system or adopting a new one? The next section will present the basis for selection of specific tests.

Considerations in Adopting New Test Systems

Conducting toxicological investigations in two or more species of laboratory animals is generally accepted as being a prudent and responsible practice in developing a new chemical entity, especially one that is expected to receive widespread use and to have exposure potential over

Table 2 Rationale for using *in vivo* test systems

(1) Provides evaluation of actions/effects on intact animal and organ–tissue interactions.

(2) Either neat chemicals or complete formulated products (complex mixtures) can be evaluated.

(3) Either concentrated or diluted products can be tested.

(4) Yields data on the recovery and healing processes.

(5) Required statutory tests for agencies under such laws as the Federal Hazardous Substances Act (unless data are already available), Toxic Substances Control Act, Federal Insecticides, Fungicides and Rodenticides Act (FIFRA), Organization for Economic Cooperation (OECD) and Food and Drug Administration Laws.

(6) Quantitative and qualitative tests with scoring system generally capable of ranking materials as to relative hazards.

(7) Amenable to modifications to meet the requirements of special situations (much as multiple dosing or exposure schedules).

(8) Extensive available database and cross-reference capability for evaluation of relevance to human situation.

(9) The ease of performance and relative low capital costs in many cases.

(10) Tests are generally both conservative and broad in scope, providing for maximum protection by erring on the side of overprediction of hazard to man.

(11) Tests can be either single end-point (such as lethality, corrosion, etc.) or shot-gun (also called multiple end-point, including such test systems as a 13 week oral toxicity study).

human lifetimes. Adding a second or a third species to the testing regimen offers an extra measure of confidence to the toxicologist and the other professionals who will be responsible for evaluating the associated risks, benefits and exposure limitations or protective measures. Although undoubtedly broadening and deepening a compound's profile of toxicity, the practice of enlarging on the number of test species is an indiscriminate scientific generalization, as has been demonstrated in multiple points in the literature (Gad and Chengelis, 1988). Moreover, such a tactic is certain to generate the problem of species-specific toxicosis. This is defined as a toxic response or an inordinately low biological threshold for toxicity that is evident in one species or strain, while all other species examined are either unresponsive or strikingly less sensitive. Species-specific toxicosis usually implies that either different metabolic pathways for converting or excret-

Table 3 Limitations of *in vivo* testing systems which serve as a basis for seeking *in vitro* alternatives for toxicity tests

(1) Complications and potential confounding or masking findings of *in vivo* systems.
(2) *In vivo* systems may only assess short-term site of application or immediate structural alterations produced by agents. Specific *in vivo* tests may only be intended to evaluate acute local effects (i.e. this may be a purposeful test system limitation).
(3) Technician training and monitoring are critical (particularly in view of the subjective nature of evaluation).
(4) *In vivo* tests in animals do not perfectly predict results in humans if the objective is to exclude or identify severe-acting agents.
(5) Structural and biochemical differences between test animals and humans make extrapolation from one to the other difficult.
(6) Lack of standardization of *in vivo* systems.
(7) Variable correlation with human results.
(8) Large biological variability between experimental units (i.e. individual animals).
(9) Large, diverse and fragmented databases which are not readily comparable.

ing xenobiotics or anatomical differences are involved. The investigator confronting such findings must be prepared to address the all-important question, 'are humans likely to react positively or negatively to the test agent under similar circumstances?' Assuming that numerical odds prevail and that humans automatically fit into the predominant category would be scientifically irresponsible, whether on the side of being safe or at risk. Such a confounded situation can be an opportunity to advance more quickly into the heart of the search for predictive information. A species-specific toxicosis can frequently contribute towards a better understanding of the general case if the underlying biological mechanism either causing or enhancing toxicity is defined, and especially if it is discovered to uniquely reside in the sensitive species.

The design of our current tests appear to serve society reasonably well (i.e. significantly more times than not) in identifying hazards that would be unacceptable. However, the process can just as clearly be improved from the standpoint of both improving our protection of society and doing necessary testing in a manner that uses fewer animals in a more humane manner.

IN VITRO MODELS

In vitro models, at least as screening tests, have been with us in toxicology for some 20 years now. The last 5–10 years have brought a great upsurge in interest in such models. This increased interest is due to economic and animal welfare pressures and technological improvements.

Criteria against which an *in vitro* model should be evaluated for its suitability in replacing (partially or entirely) an accepted *in vivo* model are incorporated in the process detailed in Table 4, which presents the proposed steps for taking a new *in vitro* testing technology from being a research construct to a validated and accepted test system.

Table 4 Multistage scheme for the development, validation and transfer of *in vitro* test system technology in toxicology

STAGE I: STATEMENT OF TEST OBJECTIVE
(A) Identify existing test system and its strengths and weaknesses.
(B) Clearly state objectives for alternative test system.
(C) Identify potential alternative test system.
STAGE II: DEFINE DEVELOPMENTAL TEST DESIGN
(A) Identify relevant variables.
(B) Evaluate effects of variables on test system.
(C) Optimize test performance.
(D) Understand what the test does in a functional sense.
(1) Is it a simulation of an *in vivo* event?
(2) Is this simply a response to the presence of the agent?
(3) Is the measured response a functional step or link in the *in vivo* event of interest?
(4) Is this response an event or a property mechanistically linked to the *in vivo* event of interest or some intermediate stage?
(5) Is this an effect on some structure or function analogous to the *in vivo* structure or function?
STAGE III: EVALUATE PERFORMANCE OF OPTIMUM TEST
(A) Develop library of known positive- and negative-response materials of diverse structure and a range of response potencies (i.e. if the end-pont is irritation, then materials should range from non-irritating to severely irritating).
(B) Use optimum test design to evaluate the library of 'knowns' under 'blind' conditions.
(C) Compare correlation of test results with those of other test systems and with real case of interest— results in humans.

continued

Table 4 (continued)

> STAGE IV: TECHNOLOGY TRANSFER
> (A) Present and publish results through professional media (at society meetings, in peer-reviewed journals).
> (B) Provide hands-on training to personnel from other facilities and facilitate internal evaluations of test methods.
>
> STAGE V: VALIDATION
> (A) Arrange for test of coded samples in multiple laboratories (i.e. interlaboratory validation).
> (B) Compare, present and publish results.
>
> STAGE VI: CONTINUE TO REFINE AND EVALUATE TEST SYSTEM PERFORMANCE AND UTILIZATION
> (A) Continually strive for an understanding of why the test 'works' and its relevance to effects in man.
> (B) Remain sceptical. Why should any one of us be the one to make the big breakthrough? Clearly, there is some basic flaw in the design or conduct of the study which has given rise to these promising results. Doubt, check and question; let your most severe critic review the data; go to a national meeting and give a presentation; then go back home and doubt, check and question some more!

There are substantial potential advantages in using an *in vitro* system in toxicological testing which include isolation of test cells or organ fragments from homoeostatic and hormonal control, accurate dosing and quantification of results. It should be noted that, in addition to the potential advantages, *in vitro* systems *per se* also have a number of limitations which can contribute to their not being acceptable models. Findings from an *in vitro* system that either limit their use in predicting *in vivo* events or make them totally unsuitable for the task include wide differences in the doses needed to produce effects or differences in the effects elicited. Some reasons for such findings are detailed in Table 5.

Tissue culture has the immediate potential to be used in two very different ways by industry. First, it has been used to examine a particular aspect of the toxicity of a compound in relation to its toxicity *in vivo* (i.e. mechanistic or explanatory studies). Second, it has been used as a form of rapid screening to compare the toxicity of a group of compounds for a particular form of response. Indeed, the pharmaceutical industry has used *in vitro* test systems in these two ways for years in the search for new potential drug entities.

Table 5 Possible interpretations when *in vitro* data do not predict results of *in vivo* studies

> (1) Chemical is not absorbed at all or is poorly absorbed in *in vivo* studies.
> (2) Chemical is well absorbed but is subject to 'first-pass effect' in the liver.
> (3) Chemical is distributed so that less (or more) reaches the receptors than would be predicted on the basis of its absorption.
> (4) Chemical is rapidly metabolized to an active or inactive metabolite that has a different profile of activity and/or different duration of action from that of the parent drug.
> (5) Chemical is rapidly eliminated (e.g. through secretory mechanisms).
> (6) Species of the two test systems used are different.
> (7) Experimental conditions of the *in vitro* and *in vivo* experiments differed and may have led to different effects from those expected. These conditions include factors such as temperature or age, sex and strain of animal.
> (8) Effects elicited *in vitro* and *in vivo* by the particular test substance in question differ in their characteristics.
> (9) Tests used to measure responses may differ greatly for *in vitro* and *in vivo* studies, and the types of data obtained may not be comparable.
> (10) The *in vitro* study did not use adequate controls (e.g. pH, vehicle used, volume of test agent given, samples taken from sham-operated animals), resulting in 'artifacts' of method rather than results.
> (11) *In vitro* data cannot predict the volume of distribution in central or in peripheral compartments.
> (12) *In vitro* data cannot predict the rate constants for chemical movement between compartments.
> (13) *In vitro* data cannot predict the rate constants of chemical elimination.
> (14) *In vitro* data cannot predict whether linear or non-linear kinetics will occur with specific dose of a chemical *in vivo*.
> (15) Pharmacokinetic parameters (e.g. bioavailability, peak plasma concentration, half-life) cannot be predicted solely on the basis of *in vitro* studies.
> (16) *In vivo* effects of chemical are due to an alteration in the higher-order integration of an intact animal system, which cannot be reflected in a less complex system.

The theory and use of screens in toxicology have previously been reviewed (Gad, 1988a, b, 1989a, b). Mechanistic and explanatory studies are generally called for when a traditional test system gives a result that is either unclear or is one for which the relevance to the real-life human exposure is doubted. *In vitro* systems are particularly attractive for such cases because they can focus on very defined single aspects of a problem or pathogenic response, free of the confounding influence of the multiple responses of an intact higher-level organism. Note, however, that first one must know the nature (indeed the existence) of the questions to be addressed. It is then important to devise a suitable model system which is related to the mode of toxicity of the compound.

There is currently much controversy over the use of *in vitro* test systems—will they find acceptance as 'definitive test systems' or only be used as preliminary screens for such final tests? Or, in the end, not be used at all? Almost certainly, all three of these cases will be true to some extent. Depending on how the data generated are to be used, the division between the first two is ill-defined at best.

Before trying to definitively answer these questions in a global sense, each of the end-points for which *in vitro* systems are being considered should be overviewed and considered against the factors outlined to this point.

Lethality

Many of the end-points of interest in toxicology present a fundamental limitation to the development and use of an *in vitro* or non-mammalian system in place of established *in vivo* methods. While cytotoxicity is a component mechanism in many of these toxic responses, disruption or diminution of the integrated function of multiple cells and systems is just as important.

The evaluation of lethality (symbolized in the public mind by the LD_{50} test) would seem to offer a unique opportunity for the development and use of alternatives. Approaches to alternatives for lethality testing include no living materials at all (the SAR or computer model approaches), those that use no intact higher organisms (but rather cultured cells or bacteria) and those that use lower forms of animal life (invertebrates and fish, for example). Each of these approaches presents a different approach to the objective of predicting acute lethality in humans or, rarely, economic animals, and will be examined in turn.

There are systems that do not directly use any living organisms but, rather, seek to predict the lethality (in particular, the LD_{50}) of a chemical on the basis of what is known about structurally related chemicals. Such structure–activity relationship (SAR) systems have improved markedly over the last 10 years (Enslein *et al.*, 1983a; Lander *et al.*, 1984), but are still limited. Accurate predictions are usually possible only for those classes of structures where data have previously been generated on several members of the classes. For new structural classes, the value of such predictions is minimal. Accordingly, this approach is valuable when working with analogues in a series but not for novel structures. It is also a strong argument for getting as many data as possible into the published literature.

A more extensive and seemingly fruitful approach has been the use of various cultured cell systems. Kurack *et al.* (1986), for example, have developed and suggested a system based on cultured mammalian hepatocytes. The system does metabolize materials in a manner like mammalian target species, and has shown promise in a limited battery of chemicals. Such mammalian cell culture and bacterial screening systems have significant weaknesses for assessing the lethality of many classes of chemicals, since they lack any of the integrative functions of a larger organism. Thus, they would miss all agents that act by disrupting functions such as the organophosphate pesticides, most other neurologically mediated lethal agents, and agents that act by modifying hormonal or immune systems.

Clive *et al.* (1979) have reported on the correlation of the LC_{50}s of a variety of chemicals in mouse lymphoma cell cultures with their oral LD_{50}s in mice, as shown in Figure 3. No linear correlation is present, but highly cytotoxic substances (in this group) are significantly more toxic orally. Given the imprecision of some LD_{50} values, due to such factors as steepness of slope of the lethality curve, the lack of linear correlation should be no surprise. Most recently, Ekwall *et al.* (1989) have reported on the MEIC program system, which utilizes a battery of five cellular systems. For a group of ten chemicals, the system provided good correlation with, or predictive power of, rat LD_{50}s.

Recently Parce *et al.* (1989) reported on a biosensor technique in which cultured cells are confined to a flow chamber through which a sensor measures the rate of production of acidic metabolites. It is proposed to use this as a functional measure of cytotoxicity and as a screening

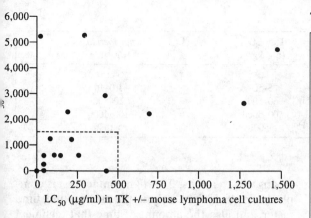

Figure 3 Graph showing a comparison of the lethalities of a group of eighteen drugs of diverse structure in *in vivo* (mouse) and *in vitro* (cultured mouse lymphoma cells) test systems. Correlation of these LD_{50}/LC_{50} values is very poor, though extreme high- and low-scale values seem to be more closely associated in the two systems

Table 6 Earthworm 48 h contact test—acute lethality

(1) Place filter paper of known size (9 cm, or 12 × 6.7 cm) in a Petri dish or standard scintillation vial.
(2) Dilute test article in acetone or some other volatile solvent.
(3) Slowly and evenly deposit known amounts of test article solution onto filter paper.
(4) Dry thoroughly with air or nitrogen gentle stream.
(5) Add 1.0 ml of distilled water to filter paper.
(6) Add worm (*L. rubellus*). Use 400–500 mg body weight range.
(7) Ten replicate vials per concentration.
(8) Store/incubate in the absence of light at 15–20°C for 48 h.
(9) Examine for lethality (swollen, lack of movement upon warming up to room temperature, lack of response to tactile stimulation).
(10) Express dose as $\mu g \, cm^{-2}$ and mortality as usual. Calculate LC_{50} using standard techniques.
(11) Always include negative and positive (benchmark) controls.

technique for a number of uses, including *in vivo* lethality.

Three lower species of intact animals have been proposed for use in screening or testing of the lethal effects of chemicals. First, some researchers have shown a good correlation between the lethality of chemicals to *Daphnia magnus* (the LC_{50} of the material dissolved in water) and the oral LD_{50} of the same chemicals in rats. This correlation is non-linear, but still suggests that more toxic materials could be at least initially identified and classified in some form of screening system based on *Daphnia*. A broader range of chemical structures will need to be evaluated, however, and some additional laboratories will need to confirm the finding. It must also be kept in mind that the metabolic systems and many of the other factors involved in species differences (as presented in Gad and Chengelis, 1988, 1992) contribute to a non-linear correlation and may also make the confidence in prediction of human effects in cases somewhat limited.

Earthworms have been one of the more common species used to test chemicals for potential hazardous impact on the environment. The 48 h contact test has proved to be a fast and resource-effective way of assessing acute toxicity of chemicals in earthworms and is outlined in Table 6. The standardized method, approved by the EEC, is discussed by Neuhauser *et al.* (1986). This test is for environmental impact assessment

where cross-laboratory comparisons are important. If, however, one wishes to adopt this technology for the purpose of screening new chemicals or releasing batches of antibiotics, then variants of this method may be acceptable, as internal consistency is more important than inter-laboratory comparisons. There are two important considerations. First, because of seasonal variation in the quality of earthworms obtained from suppliers, positive controls or comparator chemicals should be included on every assay run. Second, distilled water must be used, as worms are quite sensitive to contaminants that may occur in chlorinated water. The filter paper should completely cover the sides of the vessel, otherwise the worms will simply crawl up the sides to escape the adverse stimulus the chemical contact may provide.

Using these techniques, Roberts and Dorough (1984, 1985) and Neuhauser *et al.* (1986) have compared acute toxicity in a variety of organic chemicals in several earthworm species. While there are some obvious differences between worm species, in general the rank order of toxicity is about the same. *Lumbricus rubellus* tends to be the most sensitive species. All earthworms are very sensitive to carbofuran under the conditions of this test. Neuhauser *et al.* (1985a, b) have proposed a toxicity rating scheme based on acute lethality in the earthworms which is similar to the more familiar scheme based on acute

Table 7   Earthworm toxicity—toxicity rating

Rating	Designation	Rat LD_{50} (mg kg^{-1})	*Eisenia foetida* LC_{50} ($\mu g\ cm^{-2}$)
1	Supertoxic	<5	<1.0
2	Extremely toxic	5–50	1.0–10
3	Very toxic	50–500	10–100
4	Moderately toxic	500–5000	100–1000
5	Relatively non-toxic	>5000	>1000

From Neuhauser *et al.* (1985a and b).

lethality in rodents (Table 7). Roberts and Dorough (1985) and Neuhauser *et al.* (1986) have published extensive compilations of acute lethality in worms and compared these with acute lethality in rats and mice. A selection of these is shown in Table 8. Applying the rating scheme of Neuhauser, most chemicals receive about the same toxicity rating based on results in *Eisenia foetida* and mice. This may suggest that replacing the LD_{50} with the LC_{50} for rating toxicity (for transportation permits, for example) deserves serious consideration.

The main advantages of the 40 h contact test are the savings of time and money. The cost savings fall into three categories. First, earthworms are cheap. One hundred *L. rubellus* will cost about US $2.00. The one hundred mice they could replace in screens and quality control (QC) testing, for example, would cost $125.00–175.00 (£78–£110 at an exchange rate of $2.00 = £1.25). Second, earthworms require no vivarium space, and their use could reduce the number of rodents used, resulting in a net decrease in vivarium use. Third, adapting the 48 h contact test would require little capital investment, other than a dedicated under-the-counter refrigerator set at 15–20°C. Otherwise, the assay can be easily performed in a standard biochemistry laboratory. With regard to time savings, the standard lethality test with rodents requires 7–14 days of post-

dosing observations. The 48 h contact test is completed in 48 h. Not only is the turnaround time faster, but also the amount of time that technical personnel will have to spend observing animals and recording observations will be reduced. An incidental advantage of earthworms is that they are cold-blooded vertebrates, and thus are exempt from current animal welfare laws.

There are two main disadvantages to the use of earthworms in acute toxicity testing. First, there are a limited number of end-points. Other than death and a few behavioral abnormalities (Stenersen, 1979; Drewes *et al.*, 1984), the test does not yield much qualitative information. Second, there probably is some institutional bias. Because the test is basically low-technology (no tissue culture) and uses a non-mammalian model, it may be easy to dismiss the utility of the test.

Finally, the use of smaller species of fish as a surrogate for man has gained some supporters. Although, to date, the Medaka and rainbow trout have been proposed primarily as models for aquatic toxicity and carcinogenicity, there is no reason why they could not be used for screening water-soluble compounds for extreme acute toxicity.

Although the intact organisms would seem to be the most utilitarian on the face of it, they still will not totally replace mammalian systems, owing to the need to be concerned about those systems that are significantly different in the higher organisms. Still, it would appear that for those compounds for which human exposure is not intentional, testing in an intact lower organism system (or perhaps even in a cell culture system) should be sufficient to identify agents of significant concern. In these cases, lethality testing in intact mammals is probably unwarranted.

Table 8   Earthworm acute lethality—comparative values

Chemical	*Eisenia foetida* (LC_{50})	Mouse (LD_{50})
2,4-Dinitrophenol	0.6 (1)[a]	45 (2)
Carbaryl	14 (3)	438 (3)
Benzene	75 (3)	4 700 (4)
1,1,1-Trichloroethane	83 (3)	11 240 (5)
Dimethylphthalate	550 (4)	7 200 (5)

[a] ( ) = Toxicity rating as described in Table 7.

Ocular Irritation

Testing for potential to cause irritation or damage to the eyes remains the most active area for the development (and validation) of alternatives and the most sensitive area of animal testing in biomedical research. This has been true since the beginning of the 1980s. Table 9 presents an overview of the reasons for pursuing such alternatives. The major reason, of course, has been the pressure from public opinion.

Indeed, many of the *in vitro* tests now being evaluated for other end-points (such as skin irritation and lethality) are adaptations of test systems first developed for eye irritation uses. A detailed review of the underlying theory of each test system is beyond the scope of this chapter. Frazier *et al.* (1987) performed such a review, and

Table 10 presents an updated version of the list of test systems overviewed in that volume.

There are six major categories of approach to *in vitro* eye irritation tests. Because of the complex nature of the eye, the different cell types involved

Table 10 *In vitro* alternatives for eye irritation tests

I: MORPHOLOGY
(1) Enucleated superfused rabbit eye system (Burton *et al.*, 1981).
(2) Balb/c 3T3 cells/morphological assays (HTD) (Borenfreund and Puerner, 1984).

II: CELL TOXICITY
(1) Adhesion/cell proliferation
   (a) BHK cells/growth inhibition (Reinhardt *et al.*, 1985).
   (b) BHK cells/colony formation efficiency (Reinhardt *et al.*, 1985).
   (c) BHK cells/cell detachment (Reinhardt *et al.*, 1985).
   (d) SIRC cells/colony forming assay (North-Root *et al.*, 1982).
   (e) Balb/c 3T3 cells/total protein (Shopsis and Eng, 1985).
   (f) BCL/D1 cells/total protein (Balls and Horner, 1985).
   (g) Primary rabbit corneal cells/colony forming assay (Watanabe *et al.*, 1988).
(2) Membrane integrity
   (a) LS cells/dual dye staining (Scaife, 1982).
   (b) Thymocytes/dual fluorescent dye staining (Aeschbacher *et al.*, 1986).
   (c) LS cells/dual dye staining (Kemp *et al.*, 1983).
   (d) RCE-SIRC-P815-YAC-1/Cr release (Shadduck *et al.*, 1985).
   (e) L929 cells/cell viability (Simons, 1981).
   (f) Bovine red blood cell/haemolysis (Shadduck *et al.*, 1987).
   (g) Mouse L929 fibroblasts–erythrocin C staining (Frazier, 1988).
   (h) Rabbit corneal epithelial and endothelial cells/membrane leakage (Meyer and McCulley, 1988).
   (i) Agarose diffusion (Barnard, 1989).
(3) Cell metabolism
   (a) Rabbit corneal cell cultures/plasminogen activator (Chan, 1985).
   (b) LS cells/ATP assay (Kemp *et al.*, 1985).
   (c) Balb/c 3T3 cells/neutral red uptake (Borenfreund and Puerner, 1984).
   (d) Balb/c 3T3 cells/uridine uptake inhibition assay (Shopsis and Sathe, 1984).
   (e) HeLa cells/metabolic inhibition test (MIT–24) (Selling and Ekwall, 1985).
   (f) MDCK cells/dye diffusion (Tchao, 1988).

---

continued overleaf

Table 9 Rationales for seeking *in vitro* alternatives for eye irritancy tests

---

(1) Avoid whole-animal and organ *in vivo* evaluation.
(2) Strict Draize scale testing in the rabbit assesses only three eye structures (conjuctiva, cornea, iris) and traditional rabbit eye irritancy tests do not assess cataracts, pain, discomfort or clouding of the lens.
(3) *In vivo* tests assess only inflammation and immediate structural alterations produced by irritants (not sensitizers, photoirritants or photoallergens). Note, however, that the test was (and generally is) intended to evaluate any pain or discomfort.
(4) Technician training and monitoring are critical (particularly in view of the subjective nature of evaluation).
(5) Rabbit eye tests do not perfectly predict results in humans, if the objective is either the total exclusion of irritants or the identification of truly severe irritants on an absolute basis (that is, without false positives or negatives). Some (such as Reinhardt *et al.*, 1985) have claimed that these tests are too sensitive for such uses.
(6) There are structural and biochemical differences between rabbit and human eyes which make extrapolation from one to the other difficult. For example, Bowman's membrane is present and well developed in man (8–12 μm thick) but not in the rabbit, possibly giving the cornea greater protection.
(7) Lack of standardization.
(8) Variable correlation with human results.
(9) Large biological variability between experimental units.
(10) Large, diverse and fragmented databases which are not readily comparable.

Table 10 (continued)

III: CELL AND TISSUE PHYSIOLOGY
(1) Epidermal slice/electrical conductivity (Oliver and Pemberton, 1985).
(2) Rabbit ileum/contraction inhibition (Muir *et al.*, 1983).
(3) Bovine cornea/corneal opacity (Muir, 1984).
(4) Proptosed mouse eye/permeability test (Maurice and Singh, 1986).

IV: INFLAMMATION/IMMUNITY
(1) Chlorioallantoic membrane (CAM)
    (a) CAM (Leighton *et al.*, 1983).
    (b) HET–CAM (Luepke, 1985).
(2) Bovine corneal cup model/leukocyte chemotactic factors (Elgebaly *et al.*, 1985).
(3) Rat peritoneal cells/histamine release (Jacaruso *et al.*, 1985).
(4) Rat peritoneal mast cells/serotonin release (Chasin *et al.*, 1979).
(5) Rat vaginal explant/prostaglandin release (Dubin *et al.*, 1984).
(6) Bovine eye cup/histamine (Hm) and leukotriene C4 (LtC4) release (Benassi *et al.*, 1986).

V: RECOVERY/REPAIR
(1) Rabbit corneal epithelial cells–wound healing (Jumblatt and Neufeld, 1985).

VI: OTHER
(1) EYTEX assay (Gordon and Bergman, 1986; Soto *et al.*, 1988).
(2) Computer-based structure–activity (SAR) (Enslein, 1984, Enslein *et al.*, 1988).
(3) *Tetrahymena*/motility (Silverman, 1983).

and interactions between them, it is likely that a successful replacement for existing *in vivo* systems (such as the rabbit) would require some form of battery of such test systems. Many individual systems, however, might constitute effective screens in defined situations. The first five of these aim at assessing portions of the irritation response, including alterations in tissue morphology, toxicity to individual component cells or tissue physiology, inflammation or immune modulation, and alterations in repair and/or recovery processes. These methods have the limitation that they assume that one of the component parts can or will predict effects in the complete organ system. While each component may serve well to predict the effects of a set of chemical structures which determine part of the ocular irritation response, a valid assessment across a broad range of structures will require the use of a collection or battery of such tests.

The sixth category contains tests that have little or no empirical basis, such as computer-assisted structure–activity relationship models. These approaches can only be assessed in terms of how well or poorly they perform. Table 10 presents an overview of all six categories and some of the component tests within them, updated from the assessment by Frazier *et al.*, (1987) along with references for each test.

Given that there are now some 70 or more potential *in vitro* alternatives, the key points along the route to the eventual objective of replacing the *in vivo* test systems are thus: (1) How do we select the best candidates from this pool? (2) How do we want to use the resulting system (as a screen or test?)? (3) How do we select, develop and validate the system or systems that will actually be used?

There have been limited-scale validations of many of these tests. Most of the individual investigators have performed such 'validations' as part of their development of the test system, and in a number of cases trade associations have sponsored comparative and/or multilaboratory validations. At least for screening, several systems should be appropriate for use and, in fact, are used now by several commercial organizations. In terms of use within defined chemical structural classes, use of *in vitro* systems for testing of chemicals for non-human exposure should supplant traditional *in vivo* systems once validated on a broad scale by multiple laboratories. Broad use of single tests based on single end-points (such as cytotoxicity) is not likely to be successful, as demonstrated by such efforts as those of Kennah *et al.* (1989).

Dermal Irritation

Extensive progress has been made in devising alternative (*in vitro*) systems for evaluating the dermal irritation potential of chemicals since this author last reviewed the field (Gad and Chengelis, 1988). Table 11 overviews 20 proposed systems which now constitute five very different approaches.

The first approach (I) uses patches of excised human or animal skin maintained in some modification of a glass diffusion cell which maintains the moisture, temperature, oxygenation and elec-

Table 11 *In vitro* dermal irritation test systems

System	End-point	Validation data?[a]	References
I.			
Excised patch of perfused skin	Swelling	No	Dannenberg (1987)
Mouse skin organ culture	Inhibition of incorporation of [³H]-thymidine and [¹⁴C]-leucine labels	No	Kao *et al.* (1982)
Mouse skin organ culture	Leakage of LDH and GOT	Yes	Bartnik *et al.* (1989)
II.			
TESTSKIN—cultured surrogate skin patch	Morphological evaluation (?)	No	Bell *et al.* (1988)
Cultured surrogate skin patch	Cytotoxicity	No	Naughton *et al.* (1989)
III.			
Human epidermal keratinocytes (HEKs)	Release of labelled arachidonic acid	Yes	DeLeo *et al.* (1988)
Human polymorphonuclear cells	Migration and histamine release	Yes (surfactants)	Frosch and Czarnetzki (1987)
Fibroblasts	Acid		Lamont *et al.* (1989)
HEKs	Cytotoxicity	Yes	Gales *et al.* (1989)
HEKs	Cytotoxicity (MTT)	Yes	Swisher *et al.* (1988)
HEKs, dermal fibroblasts	Cytotoxicity	Yes	Babich *et al.* (1989)
HEKs	Inflammation mediator release	No	Boyce *et al.* (1988)
Cultured Chinese hamster ovary (CHO) cells	Increases in β-hexosaminidase levels in media	No	Lei *et al.* (1986)
Cultured C₃ H10T½ and HEK cells	Lipid metabolism inhibition	No	DeLeo *et al.* (1987)
Cultured cells—BHK21/C13 BHK21/C13 primary rat thymocytes	Cell detachment Growth inhibition Increased membrane permeability	Yes	Reinhardt *et al.* (1987)
Rat peritoneal mast cells	Inflammation mediator release	Yes (surfactants)	Prottey and Ferguson (1976)
IV.			
Hen's egg	Morphological evaluation		Reinhardt *et al.* (1987)
SKINTEX—protein mixture	Protein coagulation	Yes	Gordon *et al.* (1989)
V.			
Structure–activity relationship (SAR) model	NA	Yes	Enslein *et al.* (1987)
SAR model	NA	No	Firestone and Guy (1986)

[a] Evaluated by comparison of predictive accuracy for a range of compounds compared with animal test results. Not validated in the sense used in this chapter.

NA = not available.

trolyte balance of the skin section. In this approach, after the skin section has been allowed to equilibrate for some time, the material of concern is placed on the exterior surface and wetted (if not a liquid). Irritation is evaluated either by swelling of the skin (a crude and relatively insensitive method for mild and moderate irritants), by evaluation of inhibition of uptake of radiolabelled nutrients or by measurement of leakage of enzymes through damaged membranes.

The second set of approaches (II) utilizes a form of surrogate skin culture comprising a mix of skin cells which closely mirror key aspects of the architecture and function of the intact organ. These systems seemingly offer a real potential advantage but, to date, the 'damage markers' employed (or proposed) as predictors of dermal irritation have been limited to cytotoxicity.

The third set of approaches (III) is to use some form of cultured cell (either primary or transformed), with primary human epidermal keratinocytes (HEKs) preferred. The cell cultures are exposed to the material of interest, then either cytotoxicity, release of inflammation markers or decrease of some indicator of functionality (lipid metabolism, membrane permeability or cell detachment) is measured.

The fourth group (IV) contains two miscellaneous approaches—the use of a membrane from the hen's egg with a morphological evaluation of damage being the predictor end-point (Reinhardt *et al.*, 1987), and the SKINTEX system, which utilizes the coagulation of a mixture of soluble proteins to predict dermal response.

Finally, in group V there are two structure–activity relationship models which use mathematical extensions of past animal results correlated with structure to predict the effects of new structures.

Many of these test systems are in the process of evaluation of their performance against various small groups of compounds for which the dermal irritation potential is known. Evaluation by multiple laboratories of a wider range of structures will be essential before any of these systems can be generally utilized.

Irritation of Parenterally Administered Pharmaceuticals

Intramuscular (im) and intravenous (iv) injection of parenteral formulations of pharmaceuticals can produce a range of discomfort resulting in pain, irritation and/or damage to the muscular or vascular tissue. These are normally evaluated for prospective formulations before use in humans by evaluation in intact animal models—usually the rabbit (Gad and Chengelis, 1988).

Currently, a protocol utilizing a cultured rat skeletal muscle cell line (the L6) as a model is in an interlaboratory validation programme among more than ten pharmaceutical company laboratories. This methodology (Young *et al.*, 1986) measures creatine kinase levels in media after exposure of the cells to the formulation of interest, and predicts *in vivo* intramuscular damage based on this end-point. It is reported to give excellent rank-correlated results across a range of antibiotics (Williams *et al.*, 1987). The current multilaboratory evaluation covers a broader structural range of compounds.

Another proposed *in vitro* assay for muscle irritancy for injectable formulations is the red blood cell haemolysis assay (Brown *et al.*, 1989). Water-soluble formulations are gently mixed at a 1:2 ratio with freshly collected human blood for 5 s, then mixed with a 5 per cent w/v dextrose solution and centrifuged for 5 min. The percentage red blood cell survival is then determined by measuring differential absorbance at 540 nm, and this is compared with values for known irritants and non-irritants. Against a very small group of compounds (four), this is reported to be an accurate predictor of muscle irritation.

There is no current candidate alternative for the venous irritation test, but the *in vitro* alternative for pyrogenicity testing—the *Limulus* test—is one of the success stories for the alternatives movement. It has totally replaced the classical intact rabbit test in both research and product release testing. The test is based on the jelling or colour development of a pyrogenic preparation in the presence of the lysate of the amoebocytes of the horseshoe crab (*Limulus polyphemus*). It is simpler, more rapid and of greater sensitivity than the rabbit test it replaced (Cooper, 1975).

Sensitization and Photosensitization

There are actually several approaches available for the *in vitro* evaluation of materials for sensitizing potential. These use cultured cells from various sources and, as end-points, look at either biochemical factors (such as production of MIF—migration inhibition factor) or cellular events (such as cell migration or cell 'transformation').

Milner (1970) reported that lymphocytes from guinea-pigs sensitized to dinitrofluorobenzene (DNFB) would transform in culture, as measured by the incorporation of tritiated thymidine, when exposed to epidermal proteins conjugated with

DNFB. This work was later extended to guinea-pigs sensitized to *p*-phenylenediamine. He also reported (Milner, 1971) that his method was capable of detecting allergic contact hypersensitivity to DNFB in humans, using human lymphocytes from sensitized donors and human epidermal extracts conjugated with DNFB.

Miller and Levis (1973) reported the *in vitro* detection of allergic contact hypersensitivity to DNCB conjugated to leukocyte and erythrocyte cellular membranes. This indicated that the reaction was not specifically directed towards epidermal cell conjugates. Thulin and Zacharian (1972) extended others' earlier work on MIF-induced migration of human peripheral blood lymphocytes to a test for delayed contact hypersensitivity. Burka *et al.* reported in 1981 on an assay system based on isolated guinea-pig trachea. No further mention of this has been found in the literature. None of these approaches has yet been developed as an *in vitro* predictive test, but work is progressing. Milner published a review of the history and state of this field in 1983 which still provides an accurate and timely overview.

Any alternative (*in vitro* or *in vivo*) test for sensitization will need to be evaluated against a battery of 'known' sensitizing compounds. The Consumer Product Safety Commission in 1977 proposed such a battery, which is shown in Table 12. This has not yet been done for any of the proposed systems. Owing to the complexity of the system involved, it is unlikely that a suitable *in vitro* replacement system will be available soon.

Gad *et al.* (1986) have published comparative data on multiple animal and human test system data for some 72 materials. Such a database

Table 12 Requested reference compounds for skin sensitization studies (US Consumer Product Safety Commission)

Hydroxylamine sulphate	Penicillin G
Ethyl amino benzoate	*p*-Phenylenediamine
Iodochlorohydroxy quinoline (Clioquinol, Chinoform)	Epoxy systems (ethylenediamine, diethylenetriamine, diglycidyl ethers)
Nickel sulphate	Toluene-2,4-diisocyanate
Monomethyl methacrylate	Oil of Bergamot
Mercaptobenzothiazole	

should be considered for the development and evaluation of new test systems.

Phototoxicity and Photosensitization

The Daniel test for phototoxicity (also called photoirritant contact dermatitis) utilizes the yeast *Candida albicans* as a test species and has been in use for more than 20 years (Daniel, 1965). The measured end-point is simply cell death. The test is simple to perform and cheap, but does not reliably predict the phototoxicity of all classes of compounds (for example, sulphanilamide). Test systems utilizing bacteria have been suggested as alternatives over the last 10 years (Harter *et al.*, 1976; Ashwood-Smith *et al.*, 1980) for use in predicting the same end-point.

Most recently, ICI has conducted studies on an *in vitro* phototoxicity assay which involves using three cultured cell lines: the A431 human epidermal cell line (a derived epidermal carcinoma), normal human epidermal keratinocytes (a primary cell line derived from cosmetic surgery) and the 3T3 Swiss mouse fibroblast cell line. The protocol for this assay involves subculturing the particular cell type into microtitre tissue culture grade plates and incubating them over a period of 24 h. Following incubation, the cultures are exposed to the test compound at a concentration predetermined as non-toxic. After a 4 h exposure to the compound, the cell cultures are exposed to either UV A (320–400 nm) or UV A/B (280–400 nm) radiation for varying lengths of time. The degree of enhanced toxicity effected by either UV A or UV A/B radiation in the presence of the test compound relative to the control is assessed, using the MTT Assay. MTT, abbreviated from 3-(4,5-dimethylthiazol-2-yl)-2,5-diphenyl-tetrazolium bromide, undergoes a reduction reaction which is specific to mitochondrial dehydrogenases in viable cells. Work on validation of this test using 30 compounds of known phototoxic potential has shown a high degree of correlation between *in vitro* and *in vivo* results. Jackson and Goldner (1989) have described several other *in vitro* assay systems for this end-point.

The area of development of *in vitro* photosensitization assays has been a very active one, as the review of McAuliffe *et al.* (1986) illustrates. Such tests have focused on being able to predict the photosensitizing potential of a compound and variously employed cultured mammalian cell lines, red blood cells, micro-organisms and bio-chemical reactions. McAuliffe's group has developed and proposed a test that measures the incorporation of tritiated thymidine into human peripheral blood mononuclear cells as a predictive test (Morison *et al.*, 1982). They claim to have internally validated the test, using a battery of known photosensitizers.

Bockstahler *et al.* (1982) have developed and proposed another *in vitro* test system which uses the responses of two *in vitro* mammalian virus—host cell systems to the photosensitizing chemicals proflavine sulphate and 8-methoxypsoralen (8-MOP) in the presence of light as a predictive system. They found that infectious simian virus 40 (SV40) could be induced from SV40-transformed hamster cells by treatment with proflavine plus visible light or 8-MOP plus near-UV radiation. The same photosensitizing treatments inactivated the capacity of monkey cells to support the growth of herpes simplex virus. SV40 induction and inactivation of host cell capacity for herpes virus growth might be useful as screening systems for testing the photosensitizing potential of chemicals. Advantages (ease and speed of conduct) and disadvantages (use of potentially infective agent and the limited range of compounds evaluated to date) were found to be associated with both of these test systems.

Developmental Toxicity

The area of developmental toxicology actually is one of the earliest to have alternative models suggested for it, and has one of the most extensive and oldest literatures. This is, of course, partly owing to such models originally being used to elucidate the essential mechanisms and process of embryogenesis.

Because of the complicated and multiphasic nature of the developmental process, it has not been proposed that any of these systems be definitive tests, but rather that they serve as one form or another of a screen. As such, these test systems would either preclude or facilitate more effective full-scale evaluation in one or more of the traditional whole-animal test protocols.

The literature and field are much too extensive to review comprehensively here. There are a number of extensive review articles and books on the subject (Wilson, 1978; Clayton, 1981; Kochhar, 1981; Saxen, 1984; Homburger and Gold-berg, 1985; Faustman, 1988; Daston and D'Amato, 1989), which should be consulted by those with an in-depth interest.

The existing alternative test systems fall into six broad classes: (1) lower organisms; (2) cell culture systems; (3) organ culture systems; (4) submammalian embryos; (5) mammalian embryos; (6) others.

Table 13 provides an overview of the major representatives of these six groups, along with at least one basic reference to the actual techniques involved and the system components for each.

The comparative characteristics of these different classes of test systems are presented in Table 14. The key point is that these systems can be used for a wide range of purposes, only one of which is to screen compounds to determine the degree of concern for developmental toxicity.

The utility of these systems for screening is limited by the degree of dependability in predicting effects primarily in people and secondarily in the traditional whole-animal test systems. Determining the predictive performance of alternative test systems requires the evaluation of a number of compounds for which the 'true' (human) effect is known. In 1983 a consensus workshop generated a so-called 'gold standard' set of compounds of known activity (Smith *et al.*, 1983). The composition of this list has been open to a fair degree of controversy over the years (Flint, 1989; Johnson, 1989; Johnson *et al.*, 1989). However, an agreed-upon 'gold standard' set of compounds of known activity is an essential starting point for the validation of any single test system or battery of test systems because of the multitude of mechanisms for developmental toxicity. It is unlikely that any one system will be able to stand in place of segment II studies in two species, much less to accurately predict activity in humans. Their use as general screens or as test systems for compounds with little potential for extensive or intended human exposure will, however, probably be appropriate.

Target Organ Toxicity Models

This last model review section addresses perhaps the most exciting potential area for the use of *in vitro* models—as specific tools to evaluate and understand discrete target organ toxicities. Here the presumption is that there is reason to believe

Table 13 Alternative developmental toxicity test systems

Category	Test system	Model	References
I: Lower organisms	Sea urchins	Organism	Kotzin and Baker (1972)
	Drosophila	Intact and embryonic cells	Abrahamson and Lewis (1971)
	Trout	(Fish species)	MacCrimmon and Kwain (1969)
	Planaria	Regeneration	Best *et al.* (1981)
	Brine shrimp	Disruption of elongation; DNA and protein levels in *Artemia nauplii*	Kerster and Schaeffer (1983); Sleet and Brendel (1985)
	Animal virus	Growth of poxvirons in culture	Keller and Smith (1982)
	Slime mould	Dictyostelium discoidem	Durston *et al.* (1985)
	Medaka	(Fish species)	Cameron *et al.* (1985)
	'Artificial embryo'	*Hydra attenuata*	Johnson *et al.* (1982)
II: Cell culture	Protein synthesis of cultured cells	Pregnant mouse and chick lens epithelial cells	Clayton (1979)
	Avian neural crest	Differentiation of cells	Sieber-Blum (1985)
	Neuroblastoma	Differentiation of cells	Mummery *et al.* (1984)
	Lectin-mediated attachment	Tumour cells	Braun and Horowicz (1983)
III: Organ culture	Frog limb	Regeneration	Bazzoli *et al.* (1977)
	Mouse embryo limb bud	Inhibition of incorporation of precursor and of DNA synthesis	Kochhar and Aydelotte (1974)
	Metanephric kidney organ cultures	From 11 day mouse embryos	Saxen and Saksela (1971)
IV: Submammalian embryo	Chick embryo		Gebhardt (1972)
	Frog embryo	*Xenopus laevis*	Davis *et al.* (1981)
V: Mammalian embryo	Rat embryo culture	Whole postimplantation embryos	Brown and Fabro (1981); Cockroft and Steele (1989)
	Chernoff	Mouse embryo short test	Chernoff and Kavlock (1980)
	'Micromass cultures'	Rat embryo midbrain and limb	Flint and Orton (1984)
VI: Other	Structure–activity relationships (SAR)	Mathematical correlations of activity with structural features	Enslein *et al.* (1983b) Gombar *et al.* (1990)

(or at least suspect) that some specific target organ (nervous system, lungs, kidney, liver, heart, etc.) is or may be the most sensitive site of adverse action of a systemically absorbed agent. From this starting point, a system that is representative of the target organ's *in vivo* response would be useful in at least two contexts.

First, as with all the other end-points addressed in this chapter, a target organ predictive system could serve as a predictive system (in general, a screen) for effects in intact organisms, particularly man. As such, the ability to identify those

agents with a high potential to cause damage in a specific target organ at physiological concentrations would be extremely valuable.

The second use is largely specific to this set of *in vitro* models. This is to serve as tools to investigate, identify and/or verify the mechanisms of action for selective target organ toxicities. Such mechanistic understandings then allow for one to know whether such toxicities are relevant to man (or to conditions of exposure to man), to develop means either to predict such responses while they are still reversible or to develop the means to

Table 14 Developmental toxicity test system considerations

Possibility	*In vivo*	Organ culture	Cell culture	Lower organisms	Mammalian embryo culture	Submammalian embryos	Other
To study maternal and organ factors	Yes	No	No	No	No/Yes	No/Yes	NA
To study embryogenesis as a whole	Yes	No	No	No	Yes	Somewhat	NA
To eliminate maternal confounding factors (nutrition, etc.)	No	Yes	Yes	No	Yes	Yes	NA
To eliminate placental factors (barrier differences)	No	Yes	Yes	No	Yes	No	NA
To study single morphogenetic events	Difficult	Yes	No	Maybe	Yes	Yes	NA
To create controllable, reproducible conditions	Difficult	Yes	Yes	Yes	Yes	Yes	NA
For exact exposure and timing	Difficult	Yes	Yes	Yes	Yes	Yes	NA
For microsurgical manipulations	Difficult	Yes	No	Maybe	Yes	Yes	NA
For continuous registration of the effects	Difficult	Yes	Yes	No	Yes	Yes	NA
To collect large amounts of tissue for analysis	Yes	Difficult	Yes	No	Yes	No	NA
To use human embryonic tissue for testing	No	Yes	Yes	No	No	No	NA
Screening	Expensive	Yes	Yes	Yes	Yes	Yes	Yes

NA = not available.

intervene in such toxicosis (i.e. first aid or therapy), and finally to potentially modify molecules of interest to avoid unwanted effects while maintaining desired properties (particularly important in drug design).

In the context of these two uses, the concept of a library of *in vitro* models (Gad, 1989c) becomes particularly attractive. If one could accumulate a collection of 'validated', operative methodologies that could be brought into use as needed (and put away, as it were, while not being used), this would represent an extremely valuable competitive tool. The question becomes one of selecting which systems/tools to put into the library, and how to develop them to the point of common utility.

Additionally, one must consider what forms of markers are to be used to evaluate the effect of interest. Initially, such markers have been exclusively either morphological (in that there is a change in microscopic structure), observational (is the cell/preparation dead or alive or has some gross characteristic changed?), or functional (does the model still operate as it did before?). Recently it has become clear that more sensitive models do not just generate a single-end-point type of data, but rather a multiple set of measures which in aggregate provide a much more powerful set of answers.

There are several approaches to *in vitro* target organ models.

The first and oldest is that of the isolated organ preparation. Perfused and superfused tissues and organs have been used in physiology and pharmacology since the late nineteenth century. There is a vast range of these available, and a number of them have been widely used in toxicology (Mehendale, 1989, presents an excellent overview). Almost any end-point can be evaluated in most target organs (the CNS being a notable exception), and these are closest to the *in vivo* situation and therefore generally the easiest to extrapolate or conceptualize from. Those things that can be measured or evaluated in the intact organism can largely also be evaluated in an isolated tissue or organ preparation. However, the drawbacks or limitations of this approach are also compelling.

An intact animal generally produces one tissue preparation. Such a preparation is viable generally for a day or less before it degrades to the point of losing utility. As a result, such preparations are useful as screens only for agents that have rapidly reversible (generally pharmacological or biochemical) mechanisms of action. They are superb for evaluating mechanisms of action at the organ level for agents that act rapidly—but not generally for cellular effects or for agents that act over a course of more than a day.

The second approach is to use tissue or organ culture. Such cultures are attractive, owing to maintaining the ability for multiple cell types to interact in at least a near-physiological manner. They are generally not as complex as perfused organs, but are stable and useful over a longer period of time, increasing their utility as screens somewhat. They are truly a middle ground between the perfused organs and cultured cells. Only for relatively simple organs (such as the skin and bone marrow) are good models which perform in a manner representative of the *in vitro* organ available.

The third and most common approach is that of cultured cell models. These can be either primary or transformed (immortalized) cells, but the former have significant advantages in use as predictive target organ models. Such cell culture systems can be utilized to identify and evaluate interactions at the cellular, subcellular and molecular

level on an organ- and species-specific basis (Acosta *et al.*, 1985). The advantages of cell culture are that single organisms can generate multiple cultures for use, that these cultures are stable and useful for protracted periods of time, and that effects can be studied very precisely at the cellular and molecular levels. The disadvantages are that isolated cells cannot mimic the interactive architecture of the intact organ, and will respond over time in a manner that becomes decreasingly representative of what happens *in vivo*. An additional concern is that, with the exception of hepatocyte cultures, the influence of systemic metabolism is not factored in unless extra steps are taken. Stammati *et al.* (1981) and Tyson and Stacey (1989) present some excellent reviews of the use of cell culture in toxicology. Any such cellular systems would be more likely to be accurate and sensitive predictors of adverse effects if their function and integrity were evaluated while they were operational. For example, cultured nerve cells should be excited while being exposed and evaluated.

A wide range of target-organ-specific models have already been developed and used. Their incorporation into a library-type approach requires that they be evaluated for reproducibility of response, ease of use, and predictive characteristics under the intended conditions of use. These evaluations are probably at least somewhat specific to any individual situation. Tables 15–20 present overviews of representative systems for a range of target organs: respiratory, nervous system, renal, cardiovascular, hepatic, pancreatic, gastrointestinal and reticuloendothelial.

Table 15   Representative *in vitro* test systems for respiratory system toxicity

System	End-point	Evaluation	References
Isolated perfused rat and rabbit lungs (S)	Damage markers: exuadate of hormones	Correlation with results *in vivo*	Anderson and Eling (1976); Roth (1980); Mehendale (1989)
Alveolar macrophages (S)	Cytotoxicity: as a predictor of fibrogenicity	Correlation with *in vivo* fibrogenicity across a broad range of compounds	Reiser and Last (1979)
Lung organ culture (M,S)	Morphological: structure and macromolecular composition	Proposed from prior experience in pharmacology	Placke and Fisher (1987)
Hamster lung culture (M)	Morphological: structure and cell death	Correlation of *in vivo* effects of cigarette smoke	Stammati *et al.* (1981)

Letters in parentheses indicate primary employment of system: S = screening system; M = mechanistic tool.

Table 16   Representative *in vitro* test systems for neurotoxicity

System	End-point	Evaluation	References
Perfused rat phrenic nerve—hemidiaphragm (M)	Functional: release of ACh, conduction velocities, muscle response	Correlates with *in vivo* effects of trialkyltins	Bierkamper (1982)
Primary rat cerebral cells (S)	Observational: cell growth and differentiation	Cell diameter and outgrowth	Hooisma (1982)
Primary rat tissue culture (S)	Functional: receptor–ligand binding	Binding rates	Bondy (1982) Volpe *et al.* (1985)
Organotypic neural cultures (S)	Functional: electrophysiological and pharmacological properties	Correlation with *in vivo* results for a range of known active agents	Spencer *et al.* (1986) Kontur *et al.* (1987)
Isolated perfused brain (M)	Functional: biochemical and electrophysiological	Unknown	Mehendale (1989)
Cultured mouse otocyst (M)	Morphological	Unknown—a tool for potentially evaluating ototoxins	Harpur (1988)

Letters in parentheses indicate primary employment of system: S = screening system; M = mechanistic tool.

Table 17   Representative *in vitro* test systems for renal toxicity

System	End-point	Evaluation	References
Rat proximal tubular cells (S)	Functional: α-methylglucose uptake or organic ion transport	Correlation with effects of known nephrotoxin	Boogaard *et al.* (1989)
Rat cortical epithelial cells (S)	Functional: biochemical	Good correlation with *in vivo* for nephrotoxic metals and acetaminophen	Smith et al. (1986, 1987) Rylander *et al.* (1987)
Isolated perfused kidney (M)	Functional: biochemical and metabolic Morphological	Correlation with *in vivo* findings for some nephrotoxins	Mehendale (1989)
Renal slices (S,M)	Full range of functional (biochemical and metabolic)	Correlation with *in vivo* findings for a range of nephrotoxins. Still allows evaluation of a degree of cell-to-cell and nephron-to-nephron interactions	Smith *et al.* (1988)

Letters in parentheses indicate primary employment of system: S = screening system; M = mechanistic tool.

Table 18   Representative *in vitro* test systems for cardiovascular toxicity

System	End-point	Evaluation	References
Coronary artery smooth muscle cells (S)	Morphological evaluation—vacuole formation	Correlates with *in vivo* results	Ruben *et al.* (1984)
Isolated perfused rabbit or rat heart (M,S)	Functional: operational, electrophysiological, biochemical and metabolism	Long history of use in physiology and pharmacology	Mehendale (1989)
Isolated superfused atrial and heart preparations (S,M)	Functional: operational and biochemical	Correlation with *in vivo* findings for antioxidants	Gad *et al.* (1977 and 1979)

Letters in parentheses indicate primary employment of system: S = screening system; M = mechanistic tool.

Table 19 Representative *in vitro* test systems for hepatic toxicity

System	End-points	Evaluation	References
Primary hepatocytes (S,M)	Multiple: • Biotransformation • Genotoxicity • Peroxisome proliferation • Biliary dysfunction • Membrane damage • Ion regulation • Energy regulation • Protein synthesis	NA	See Tyson and Stacey (1989)[a]; Stammati *et al.* (1981)
Hamster hepatocytes (S)	Functional: biochemical	Correlates with *in vivo* effects of acetaminophen	Harman and Fischer (1983)
Rat liver slices (S)	Functional: alterations in ion content, leakage of damage markers, changes in biosynthetic capability Morphological: histopathological evaluation	Rank correlation with *in vivo* findings for a wide range of chemicals	Gandolfi *et al.* (1989)
Isolated perfused liver (M)	Functional: biochemical and metabolic	Correlation with *in vivo* findings for a wide range of chemicals	Mehendale (1989)

[a] Tyson and Stacey estimated in 1989 that there were 800 published studies of a toxicological nature on cultured hepatocytes.
Letters in parentheses indicate primary employment of system: S = screening system; M = mechanistic tool.
NA = not available.

Table 20 Representative *in vitro* test systems for other target organ toxicities

Organ	System	End-point	Evaluation	References
Pancreas	Isolated perfused intestines (M)	Functional: biochemical and metabolic	Correlation with *in vivo* findings for methylprednisolone	Mehendale (1989)
GI Tract	Isolated perfused intestines (M)	Functional: biochemical and metabolic	Limited	Mehendale (1989)
	Isolated superfused ileum (S)	Functional: pharmacological responses and biochemical	Correlation with *in vivo* findings for antioxidants and receptor-mediated agents	Gad *et al.* (1979)
Reticuloendothelial	Erythrocytes (S)	Observational: cytotoxicity Functional: inhibition of colony formation	Correlation with haemolytic effects	Stammati *et al.* (1981)
	Mouse bone marrow (M)		Correlates with *in vivo* benzene effects	Uyeki *et al.* (1977)
Testicular	Sertoli and germ cell cultures (S)	Observational: cytotoxicity Functional: steroid and hormone production	Correlation with *in vivo* effects for phytholate esters and glycol ethers	Garside (1988)

continued overleaf

Table 20 (continued)

Thyroid	Cultured thyroid cells (S,M)	Functional: biochemical and metabolic	Correlation with *in vivo* findings for a wide range of agents with thyroid-specific toxicity; evaluation against 'negative' compounds not significant	Brown (1988)

Letters in parentheses indicate primary employment of system: S = screening system; M = mechanistic tool.

These tables do not mention any of the new co-culture systems in which hepatocytes are 'joined up' in culture with a target cell type to produce a metabolically competent cellular system.

SUMMARY

The tools are currently at hand (or soon will be) to provide the practicing toxicologist with unique opportunities both for identifying potentially toxic compounds in a much more rapid and efficient manner than before and for teasing apart the mechanisms underlying such toxicities on a integrated basis (from the level of the molecule to that of the intact organism). The *in vitro* systems overviewed here, once 'validated' (that is, made reproducible and understood in how they function and fail, just as *in vivo* systems have come to be understood), will allow this to happen while reducing the need to have recourse to intact mammalian test systems. However, the intact animal models—and, indeed, man for pharmaceuticals— will still be an essential element in the safety assessment armamentarium for the foreseeable future.

REFERENCES

Abrahamson, S. and Lewis, E. B. (1971). The detection of mutations in *Drosophila melanogaster*. In Hollaender, A. (Ed.), *Chemical Mutagens. Principles and Methods of Their Detection*, Vol. 2. Plenum Press, New York, pp. 461–488

Acosta, D., Sorensen, E. M. B., Anuforo, D. C., Mitchell, D. B., Ramos, K., Santone, K. S. and Smith, M. A. (1985). An *in vitro* approach to the study of target organ toxicity of drugs and chemicals. *In Vitro Cell. Devel. Biol.*, **21**, 495–504

Aeschbacher, M., Reinhardt, C. A. and Zbinden, G. (1986). A rapid cell membrane permeability test using fluorescent dyes and flow cytometry. *Cell Biol. Toxicol.*, **2**, 247

American Medical Association (1989). Public support for animals in research. *Am. Med. News*, 9 June

Anderson, M. W. and Eling, T. E. (1976). Studies on the uptake, metabolism, and release of endogenous and exogenous chemicals by the use of the isolated perfused lung. *Environ. Hlth Perspect.*, **16**, 77–81

Ashwood-Smith, M. J., Poulton, G. A., Barker, M. and Midenberger, M. (1980). 5-Methoxypsoralen, an ingredient in several suntan preparations, has lethal mutagenic and clastogenic properties. *Nature*, **285**, 407–409

Babich, H., Martin-Alguacil, N., and Borenfreund, E. (1989). Comparisons of the cytotoxicities of dermatotoxicants to human keratinocytes and fibroblasts *in vitro*. In Goldberg, A. M. (Ed.), *In Vitro Toxicology: New Directions*. Mary Ann Liebert, New York, pp. 153–167

Balls, M. and Horner, S. A. (1985). The FRAME interlaboratory program on *in vitro* cytotoxicology. *Fd Chem. Toxic.*, **23**, 205–213

Barnard, N. D. (1989). A Draize alternative, *The Animal's Agenda*, **6**, 45

Bartnik, F. G., Pittermann, W. F., Mendorf, N., Tillmann, U., Kunstler, K. (1989). Skin organ culture for the study of skin irritancy. *Third International Congress of Toxicology*, Brighton, England

Bazzoli, A. S., Manson, J., Scott, W. J. and Wilson, J. G. (1977). The effects of thalidomide and two analogues on the regenerating forelimb of the newt. *J. Embryol. Exptl Morphol.*, **41**, 125–135

Bell, E., Parenteau, N. L., Haimes, H. B., Gay, R. J., Kemp, P. D., Fofonoff, T. W., Mason, V. S., Kagan, D. T. and Swiderek, M. (1988). Testskin: A hybrid organism covered by a living human skin equivalent designed for toxicity and other testing. In Goldberg, A. M. (Ed.), *Progress in In Vitro Toxicology*. Mary Ann Liebert, New York, pp. 15–25

Benassi, C. A., Angi, M. R., Salvalaoi, L. and Bettero, A. (1986). Histamine and leukotriene C4 release from isolated bovine sclerachoroid complex: a new *in vitro* ocular irritation test. *Chim. Agg.*, **16**, 631–634

Best, J. B., Morita, M., Ragin, J. and Best, J., Jr. (1981). Acute toxic responses of the freshwater planarian, *Dugesia dorothocephala*, to methylmercury. *Bull. Environ. Contam. Toxicol.*, **27**, 49–54

Bierkamper, G. G. (1982). *In vitro* assessment of neuromuscular toxicity. *Neurobehav. Toxicol. Teratol.*, **4**, 597–604

Bockstahler, L. E., Coohill, T. P., Lytle, C. D., Moore, S. P., Cantwell, J. M. and Schmidt, B. J. (1982). Tumor virus induction and host cell capacity inactivation: possible *in vitro* test for photosensitizing chemicals. *Journal of the National Cancer Institute*, **69**, 183–187

Bondy, S. C. (1982). Neurotransmitter binding interactions as a screen for neurotoxicity. In Prasad, K. N. and Vernadakis, A. (Eds), *Mechanisms of Actions of Neurotoxic Substances*. Raven Press, New York, pp. 25–50

Boogaard, P. J., Mulder, G. J. and Nagelkerke, J. F. (1989). Isolated proximal tubular cells from rat kidney as an *in vitro* model for studies on nephrotoxicity. *Toxicol. Appl. Pharmacol.*, **101**, 135–157

Borenfreund, E. and Puerner, J. A. (1984). A simple quantitative procedure using monolayer cultures for cytotoxicity assays (HTD/NR-NE). *J. Tissue Cult. Meth.*, **9**, 7–10

Boyce, S. T., Hansbrough, J. F. and Norris, D. A. (1988). Cellular responses of cultured human epidermal keratinocytes as models of toxicity to human skin. In Goldberg, A. M. (Ed.), *Progress in In Vitro Toxicology*. Mary Ann Liebert, New York, pp. 27–37

Braun, A. G. and Horowicz, P. B. (1983). Lectin-mediated attachment assay for teratogens. Results with 32 pesticides. *J. Toxicol. Environ. Hlth*, **11** (2), 275–286

Brown, C. G. (1988). Application of thyroid cell culture to the study of thyrotoxicity. In Atterwill, C. K. and Steele, C. E. (Eds), *In Vitro Methods in Toxicology*. Cambridge University Press, New York, pp. 165–188

Brown, N. A. and Fabro, S. (1981). Quantitation of rat embryonic development *in vitro*: A morphological scoring system. *Teratology*, **24**, 65–78

Brown, S., Templeton, L., Prater, D. A. and Potter, C. J. (1989). Use of an *in vitro* haemolysis test to predict tissue irritancy in an intramuscular formulation. *J. Parent. Sci. Technol.*, **43**, 117–120

Burka, J. F., Ali, M., McDonald, J. W. D. and Paterson, N. A. M. (1981). Immunological and non-immunological synthesis and release of prostaglandins and thromboxanes from isolated guinea pig trachea. *Prostaglandins*, **2**, 683–690

Burton, A. B. G., York, M. and Lawrence, R. S. (1981). The *in vitro* assessment of severe eye irritants, *Fd Cosmet. Toxicol.*, **19**, 471–480

Cameron, I. L., Lawrence, W. C. and Lum, J. R. (1985). Medaka eggs as a model system for screening potential teratogens. In *Prevention of Physical and Mental Congenital Defects*, Part C. pp. 239–243

Chan, K. Y. (1985). An *in vitro* alternative to the Draize test. In Goldberg, A. M. (Ed.), *In Vitro Toxicology. Alternative Methods in Toxicology*, Vol. 3. Mary Ann Liebert, New York, pp. 405–422

Chasin, M., Scott, C., Shaw, C. and Persico, F. (1979). A new assay for the measurement of mediator release from rat peritoneal in most cells. *Int. Arch. Allergy Appl. Immunol.*, **58**, 1–10

Chernoff, N. and Kavlock, R. J. (1980). A potential *in vivo* screen for the determination of teratogenic effects in mammals. *Teratology*, **21**: 33A–34A

Clayton, R. M. (1979). In Rowan, A. N. and Stratmann, C. J. (Eds), *Alternatives in Drug Research*. Macmillan Press, London, p. 153

Clayton, R. M. (1981). An *in vitro* system for teratogenicity testing. In Rowan, A. N. and Stratmann, C. J. (Eds), *The Use of Alternatives in Drug Research*. University Park Press, Baltimore, pp. 153–173

Clive, D., Johnson, K., Spector, J., Batson, A. and Brown, M. (1979). Validation and characterization of the L5178Y/TK mouse lymphoma mutagen assay system. *Mutation Res.*, **59**, 61–108

Cockroft, D. L. and Steele, C. E. (1989). Postimplantation embryo culture and its application to problems in teratology. In Atterwill, C. K. and Steele, C. E. (Eds), *In Vitro Methods in Toxicology*. Cambridge University Press, New York, pp. 365–389

Cooper, J. F. (1975). Principles and applications of the Limulus Test for pyrogen in parenteral drugs. *Bull. Parent. Drug Assoc.*, **3**, 122–130

Cowley, G., Hager, M., Drew, L., Namuth, T., Wright, L., Murr, A., Abbott, N. and Robins, K. (1988). The battle over animal rights. *Newsweek*, 26 December

Daniel, F. (1965). A simple microbiological method for demonstrating phototoxic compounds. *J. Invest. Dermatol.*, **44**, 259–263

Dannenberg, A. M., Moore, K. G., Schofield, B. H., Higuchi, K., Kajjki, A., Au, K., Pula, P. J. and Bassett, D. P. (1987). Two new *in vitro* methods for evaluating toxicity in skin (employing short-term organ culture). In Goldberg, A. M. (Ed.), *Alternative Methods in Toxicology*, Vol. 5. Mary Ann Liebert, New York, pp. 115–128

Daston, G. P. and D'Amato, R. A. (1989). *In vitro* techniques in teratology. In Mehlman, M. (Ed.), *Benchmarks: Alternative Methods in Toxicology*. Princeton Scientific, Princeton, N. J., pp. 79–109

Davis, K. R., Schultz, T. W. and Dumont, J. N. (1981). Toxic and teratogenic effects of selected aromatic amines on embryos of the amphibian *Xenopus laevis*. *Arch. Environ. Contam. Toxicol.*, **10**, 371–391

DeLeo, V., Hong, J., Scheide, S., Kong, B., DeSalva, S. and Bagley, D. (1988). Surfactant-induced cutaneous primary irritancy: An *in vitro* model-assay system development. In Goldberg, A. M. (Ed.), *Progress in In Vitro Toxicology*. Mary Ann Liebert, New York, pp. 39–43

DeLeo, V., Midlarsky, L., Harber, L. C., Kong, B.

M. and Salva, S. D. (1987). Surfactant-induced cutaneous primary irritancy: An *in vitro* model. In Goldberg, A. M. (Ed.), *Alternative Methods in Toxicology*, Vol. 5. Mary Ann Liebert, New York, pp. 129–138

Drewes, C., Vining, E. and Callahan, C. (1984). Noninvasive electrophysiological monitoring: a sensitive method for detecting sublethal neurotoxicity in earthworms. *Environ. Toxicol. Chem.*, 3, 559–607

Dubin, N. H., De Blasi, M. C., *et al.* (1984). Development of an *in vitro* test for cytotoxicity in vaginal tissue: effect of ethanol on prostanoid release. In Goldberg, A. M. (Ed.), *Acute Toxicity Testing: Alternative Approaches. Alternative Methods in Toxicology*, Vol. 2. Mary Ann Liebert, New York, pp. 127–138

Durston, A., Van de Wiel, F., Mummery, C. and de Loat, S. (1985). *Dictyostelium discoideum* as a test system for screening for teratogens. *Teratology*, 32, 21A

Ekwall, B., Bondesson, I., Castell, J. V., Gomez-Lechon, M. J., Hellberg, S., Hagberg, J., Jover, R., Ponsoda, X., Romert, L., Stenberg, K. and Watum, E. (1989). Cytotoxicity evaluation of the first ten MEIC chemicals: acute lethal toxicity in man predicted by cytotoxicity in five cellular assays and by oral LD50 tests in rodents. *Animal Technicians Laboratory Association*, 17, 83–100

Elgebaly, S. A., Nabawi, K., Herkbert, N., O'Rourke, J. and Kruetzer, D. L. (1985). Characterization of neutrophil and monocyte specific chemotactic factors derived from the cornea in response to injury. *Invest. Ophthalmol. Vis. Sci.*, 26, 320

Enslein, K. (1984). Estimation of toxicology end points by structure–activity relationships, *Pharmacol. Rev.*, 36, 131–134

Enslein, K., Blake, V. W., Tuzzeo, T. M., Borgstedt, H. H., Hart, J. B. and Salem, H. (1988). Estimation of rabbit eye irritation scores by structure-activity equations, *In Vitro Toxicol.*, 2, 1–14

Enslein, K., Borgstedt, H. H., Blake, B. W. and Hart, J. B. (1987). Prediction of rabbit skin irritation severity by structure–activity relationships. *In Vitro Toxicol.*, 1, 129–147

Enslein, K., Lander, T. R. and Strange, J. L. (1983b). Teratogenesis: A statistical structure-activity model. *Terat. Carcin. Mutagen*, 3, 289–309

Enslein, K., Lander, T. R., Tomb, M. E. and Craig, P. N. (1983a). *A Predictive Model for Estimating Rat Oral LD50 Values*. Princeton Scientific, Princeton, NJ

Faustman, E. M. (1988). Short-term tests for teratogens. *Mutation Res.*, 205, 355–384

Firestone, B. A. and Guy, R. H. (1986). Approaches to the prediction of dermal absorption and potential cutaneous toxicity. In Goldberg, A. M. (Ed.), *In Vitro Toxicology. Alternative Methods in Toxicology*, Vol. 3. Mary Ann Liebert, New York, pp. 516–536

Flint, O. P. (1989). Reply to Letter to the Editor. *Toxicol. Appl. Pharmacol.*, 99, 176–180

Flint, O. P. and Orton, T. C. (1984). An *in vitro* assay for teratogens with cultures of rat embryo midbrain and limb bud cells. *Toxicol. Appl. Pharmacol.* 76, 383–395

Frazier, A. M. (1988). Update: A critical evaluation of alternatives to acute ocular irritancy testing. In Goldberg, A. M. (Ed.), *Progress in In Vitro Toxicology*. Mary Ann Liebert, New York, pp. 67–75

Frazier, J. M., Gad, S. C., Goldberg, A. M. and McCulley, J. P. (1987). *A Critical Evaluation of Alternatives to Acute Ocular Irritation Testing*. Mary Ann Liebert, New York

Frosch, P. J. and Czarnetzki, B. M. (1987). Surfactants cause *in vitro* chemotaxis and chemokinesis of human neutrophils. *J. Invest. Dermatol.*, 88(3), Supplement, 52s

Gad, S. C. (1988a). Defining product safety information and testing requirements. In Gad, S. C. (Ed.), *Handbook of Product Safety Evaluation*. Marcel Dekker, New York, pp. 1–22

Gad, S. C. (1988b). An approach to the design and analysis of screening data in toxicology. *J. Am. Coll. Toxicol.*, 7(2), 127–138

Gad, S. C. (1989a). Principles of screening in toxicology: with special emphasis on applications to neurotoxicology. *J. Am. Coll. Toxicol.*, 8, 21–27

Gad, S. C. (1989b). Statistical analysis of screening studies in toxicology: with special emphasis on neurotoxicology. *J. Am. Coll. Toxicol.*, 8, 171–183

Gad, S. C. (1989c). A tier testing strategy incorporating *in vitro* testing methods for pharmaceutical safety assessment. *Humane Innovations and Alternatives in Animal Experimentation.*, 3, 75–79

Gad, S. C. (1990a). Industrial applications for *in vitro* toxicity testing methods: A tier testing strategy for product safety assessment. In Frazier, J. (Ed.), *In Vitro Toxicity Testing*. Marcel Dekker, New York

Gad, S. C. (1990b). Recent developments in replacing, reducing and refining animal use in toxicologic research and testing, *Fund. Appl. Toxicol.*, 15(1), 8–16

Gad, S. C. and Chengelis, C. P. (1988). *Acute Toxicology: Principles and Methods*. Telford Press, Caldwell, N.J.

Gad, S. C. and Chengelis, C. P. (1992). *Animal Models in Toxicology*. Marcel Dekker, New York

Gad, S. C., Dunn, B. J., Dobbs, D. W. and Walsh, R. D. (1986). Development and validation of an alternative dermal sensitization test: the Mouse Ear Swelling Test (MEST). *Toxicol. Appl. Pharmacol.*, 84, 93–114

Gad, S. C., Leslie, S. W. and Acosta, D. (1979). Inhibitory actions of butylated hydroxytoluene (BHT) on isolated rat ileal, atrial and perfused heart preparations. *Toxicol. Appl. Pharmacol.*, 48, 45–52

Gad, S. C., Leslie, S. W., Brown, R. G. and Smith, R. V. (1977). Inhibitory effects of dithiothreitol and sodium bisulfite on isolated rat ileum and atrium. *Life Sci.*, **20**, 657–664

Gales, Y. A., Gross, C. L., Karebs, R. C. and Smith, W. J. (1989). Flow cytometric analysis of toxicity by alkylating agents in human epidermal keratinocytes. In Goldberg, A. M. (Ed.), *In Vitro Toxicology: New Directions*. Mary Ann Liebert, New York, pp. 169–174

Gandolfi, A. J., Brendel, K., Tisher, R., Azri, S., Hanan, G., Waters, S. J., Hanzlick, R. P. and Thomas, C. M. (1989). Utilization of precision-cut liver slices to profile and rank-order potential hepatotoxins, *PMA — Drusafe East Spring Meeting*, 2 May

Garside, D. A. (1988). Use of *in vitro* techniques to investigate the action of testicular toxicants. In Atterwill, C. K and Steele, C. E. (Eds), *In Vitro Methods In Toxicology*. Cambridge University Press, New York, pp. 411–423

Gebhardt, D. O. E. (1972). The use of the chick embryo in applied teratology. In Woollam D. H. M. (Ed.), *Advances in Teratology*, Vol. 5. Academic Press, London, pp. 97–111

Goldberg, A. M. and Frazier, J. M. (1989). Alternatives to animals in toxicity testing. *Sci. Am.*, **261**, 24–30

Gombar, V. K., Borgstedt, H. H., Enslein, K., Hart, J. B. and Blake, B. W. (1990). A QSAR model of teratogenesis. *Quant. Struct.-Activ. Rel.*, **10**, 306–332

Gordon, V. C. and Bergman, H. C. (1986). *Eytex, an in vitro Method for Evaluation of Optical Irritancy*. National Testing Corporation Report, 26

Gordon, V. C., Kelly, C. P. and Bergman, H. C. (1989). SKINTEX, an *in vitro* method for determining dermal irritation. *International Congress of Toxicology*, Brighton, England

Harman, A. W. and Fischer, L. J. (1983). Hamster hepatocytes in culture as a model for acetaminophen toxicity: studies with inhibitors of drug metabolism. *Toxicol. Appl. Pharmacol.*, **71**, 330–341

Harpur, E. S. (1988). Ototoxicity. In Atterwill, C. K. and Steele, C. E. (Eds), *In Vitro Methods In Toxicology*. Cambridge University Press, New York, pp. 37–58

Harter, M. L., Felkner, I. C. and Song, P. S. (1976). Near-UV effects of 5,7-dimethoxycoumarin in *Bacillus subtilis*. *Photochem. Photobiol.*, **24**, 491–493

Homburger, F. and Goldberg, A. M. (1985). *In Vitro Embryotoxicity and Teratogenicity Tests*

Hooisma, J. (1982). Tissue Culture and Neurotoxicology. *Neurobehavioural Toxicology and Teratology*, **4**, 617–622

Jacaruso, R. B., Barlett, M. A., Carson, S. and Trombetta, L. D. (1985). Release of histamine from rat peritoneal cells *in vitro* as an index of irritational potential. *J. Toxicol. Cut. Ocular Toxicol.*, **4**, 39–48

Jackson, E. M. and Goldner, R. (1989). *Irritant Contact Dermatitis*, Marcel Dekker, New York

Johnson, E. M. (1989). Problems in validation of *in vitro* developmental toxicity assays. *Fund. Appl. Toxicol.*, **13**, 863–867

Johnson, E. M., Gorman, R. M., Gabel, B. E. C. and George, M. E. (1982). The *Hydra attenuata* system for detection of teratogenic hazards. *Terat. Carcin. Mutagen.*, **2**, 263–276

Johnson, E. M., Newman, L. M. and Fu, L. (1989). Letter to the Editor, *Toxicol. Appl. Pharmacol.*, **99**, 173–176

Jumblatt, M. M. and Neufeld, A. H. (1985). A tissue culture model of the human corneal epithelium. In Goldberg, A. M. (Ed.), *In Vitro Toxicology. Alternative Methods in Toxicology*, Vol. 3. Mary Ann Liebert, New York, pp. 391–404

Kao, J., Hall, J. and Holland, J. M. (1982). Quantitation of cutaneous toxicity: an *in vitro* approach using skin organ culture. *Toxicol. Appl. Parmacol.*, **68**, 206–217

Keller, S. J. and Smith, M. (1982). Animal virus screens for potential teratogens: poxvirus morphogenesis. *Terat. Carcin. Mutagen.*, **2**, 361–374

Kemp, R. V., Meredith, R. W. J., Gamble, S. and Frost, M. (1983). A rapid cell culture technique for assaying to toxicity of detergent based products *in vitro* as a possible screen for high irritants *in vivo*. *Cytobios*, **36**, 153–159

Kemp, R. V., Meredith, R. W. J. and Gamble, S. (1985). Toxicity of commercial products on cells in suspension: A possible screen for the Draize eye irritation test. *Fd Chem. Toxic.*, **23**, 267–270

Kennah, H. E., Albulescu, D., Hignet, S. and Barrow, C. S. (1989). A critical evaluation of predicting ocular irritancy potential from an *in vitro* cytotoxicity assay, *Fund. Appl. Toxicol.*, **12**, 281–290

Kerster, H. W. and Schaeffer, D. J. (1983). Brine shrimp (*Artemia salina*) Nauplia as a teratogen test system. *Ecotoxicol. Environ. Safety*, **7**, 342–349

Kochhar, D. M. (1981). Embryo explants and organ cultures in screening of chemicals for teratogenic effects. In Kimmel, C. A. and Buelbe-Saw, J. (Eds), *Developmental Toxicology*. Raven Press, New York, pp. 303–319

Kochhar, D. M. and Aydelotte, M. B. (1974). Susceptible stages and abnormal morphogenesis in the developing mouse limb, analyzed in organ culture after transplacental exposure to vitamin A (retinoic acid) *J. Embryol. Exptl. Morphol.*, **31**, 721–734

Kontur, P. J., Hoffmann, P. C. and Heller, A. (1987). Neurotoxic effects of methamphetamine assessed in three-dimensional reaggregate tissue cultures. *Dev. Brain Res.*, **31**, 7–14

Kotzin, B. L. and Baker, R. F. (1972). Selective inhibition of genetic transcription in sea urchin embryos. *J. Cell. Biol.*, **55**, 74–81

Kurack, G., Vossen, P., Deboyser, D., Goethals, F. and Roberfubid, M. (1986). An *in vitro* model for acute toxicity screening using hepatocytes freshly isolated from adult mammals. In Goldberg, A. M.

(Ed.), *In Vitro Toxicology*. Mary Ann Liebert, New York

Lamont, G. S., Bagley, D. M., Kong, B. M. and DeSalva, S. J. (1989). Developing an alternative to the Draize skin test: comparison of human skin cell responses to irritants *in vitro*. In Goldberg, A. M. (Ed.), *In Vitro Toxicology: New Directions*. Mary Ann Liebert, New York, pp. 175–181

Lander, T., Enslein, K., Craig, P. and Tomb, N. (1984). Validation of a structure-activity model of rat oral LD50. In Goldberg, A. M. (Ed.), *Acute Toxicity Testing: Alternative Approaches*. Mary Ann Liebert, New York, pp. 183–184

Lei, H., Carroll, K., Au, L. and Krag, S. S. (1986). An *in vitro* screen for potential inflammatory agents using cultured fibroblasts. In Goldberg, A. M. (Ed.), *In Vitro Toxicology. Alternative Methods in Toxicology*, Vol. 3. Mary Ann Liebert, New York, pp. 74–85

Leighton, J., Nassauer, J., Tchao, R. and Verdone, J. (1983). Development of a procedure using the chick egg as an alternative to the Draize test. In Goldberg, A. M. (Ed.), *Product Safety Evaluation. Alternative Methods in Toxicology*, Vol. 1, Mary Ann Liebert, Inc., New York, pp. 165–177

Lijinsky, W. (1988). Importance of animal experiments in carcinogenesis research. *Environ. Molec. Mutagen.*, **11**, 307–314

Luepke, N. P. (1985). Hen's egg chorioallantoic membrane test for irritation potential. *Fd Chem. Toxic.*, **23**, 287–291

McAuliffe, D. J., Hasan, T., Parrish, J. A. and Kochevar, I. E. (1986). Determination of photosensitivity by an *in vitro* assay as an alternative to animal testing. Goldberg, A. M. (Ed.), *In Vitro Toxicology*. Mary Ann Liebert, New York, pp. 30–41

MacCrimmon, H. R. and Kwain, W. H. (1969). Influences of light on early development and meristic characters in the rainbow trout (*Salmo gairdneri* Richardson). *Can. J. Zool.*, **47**, 631–637

Maurice, D. and Singh, T. (1986). A permeability test for acute corneal toxicity. *Toxicol. Lett.*, **31**, 125–130

Mehendale, H. M. (1989). Application of isolated organ techniques in toxicology. In Hayes, A. W. (Ed.), *Principles and Methods of Toxicology*. Raven Press, New York, pp. 699–740

Meyer, D. R. and McCulley, J. P. (1988). Acute and protracted injury to cornea epithelium as an indication of the biocompatibility of various pharmaceutical vehicles. In Goldberg, A. M. (Ed.), *Progress in In Vitro Toxicology*. Mary Ann Liebert, Inc., New York, pp. 215–235

Miller, A. E. Jr. and Levis, W. R. (1973). Studies on the contact sensitization of man with simple chemicals. I. Specific lymphocyte transformation in response to dinitrochlorobenzene sensitization. *J. Invest. Dermatol.*, **61**, 261–269

Milner, J. E. (1970). *In vitro* lymphocyte responses in contact hypersensitivity. *J. Invest. Dermatol.*, **55**, 34–38

Milner, J. E. (1971). *In vitro* lymphocyte responses in contact hypersensitivity II. *J. Invest. Dermatol.*, **56**, 349–352

Milner, J. E. (1983). *In vitro* tests for delayed skin hypersensitivity: lymphokine production in allergic contact dermatitis. Marzulli, F. N. and Maibach, H. D. (Eds), *Dermatotoxicology*. Hemisphere Publishing, New York, pp. 185–192

Morison, W. L., McAuliffe, D. J., Parrish, J. A. and Bloch, K. J. (1982). *In vitro* assay for phototoxic chemicals. *J. Invest. Dermatol.*, **78**, 460–463

Muir, C. K. (1984). A simple method to assess surfactant-induced bovine corneal opacity *in vitro*: Preliminary findings. *Toxicol. Lett.*, **23**, 199–203

Muir, C. K., Flower, C. and Van Abbe, N. J. (1983). A novel approach to the search for *in vitro* alternatives to *in vivo* eye irritancy testing. *Toxicol. Lett.*, **18**, 1–5

Mummery, C. L., van den Brink, C. E., van der Saag, P. T. and de Loat, S. W. (1984). A short-term screening test for teratogens using differentiating neuroblastoma cells *in vitro*. *Teratology*, **29**, 271–279

Naughton, G. K., Jacob, L. and Naughton, B. A. (1989). A physiological skin model for *in vitro* toxicity studies. In Goldberg, A. M. (Ed.), *Progress in In Vitro Toxicology*. Mary Ann Liebert, New York, pp. 183–189

Neubert, D. (1982). The use of culture techniques in studies on prenatal toxicity. *Pharmacol. Ther.*, **18**, 397–434

Neuhauser, E., Durkin, P., Malecki, M. and Antara, M. (1985a). Comparative toxicity of ten organic chemicals to four earthworm species. *Comp. Biochem. Physiol.*, **83C**, 197–200

Neuhauser, E., Loehr, C., Malecki, M., Milligan, D. and Durkin, P. (1985b). The toxicity of selected organic chemicals to the earthworm *Eisenia fetida*. *J. Environ. Qual.*, **14**, 383–388

Neuhauser, E., Loehr, C. and Malecki, M., (1986). Contact and artificial soil tests using earthworms to evaluate the impact of wastes in soil. In Petros, J., Lacy, W. and Conway, R. C. (Eds), *Hazardous and Industrial Solid Waste Testing: Fourth Symposium*, ASTM STP 886. American Society for Testing Materials, Philadelphia, pp. 192–202

North-Root, H., Yackovich, Demetrulias, F. J., Gucula, N. and Heinze, J. E. (1982). Evaluation of an *in vitro* cell toxicity test using rabbit corneal cells to predict the eye irritation potential of surfactants. *Toxicol. Lett.*, **14**, 207–212

Oliver, G. J. A. and Pemberton, N. A. (1985). An *in vitro* epidermal slice technique for identifying chemicals with potential for severe cutaneous effects. *Fd Chem. Toxicol.*, **23**, 229–232

Parce, J. W., Owicki, J. C., Kercso, D. M., Sigal, G. B., Wada, H. G., Muir, V. C., Bousse, L. J., Ross, K. L., Sikic, B. I. and McConnell, H. M. (1989).

Detection of cell-affecting agents with a silicon biosensor. *Science*, **246**, 243–247

Placke, M. E. and Fisher, G. L. (1987). Adult peripheral lung organ culture—A model for respiratory tract toxicology. *Toxicol. Appl. Pharmacol.*, **90**, 284–298

Prottey, C. and Ferguson, T. F. M. (1976). The effect of surfactants upon rat peritoneal mast cells *in vitro*. *Fd Chem. Toxicol.*, **14**, 425

Reinhardt, C. A., Aeschbacher, M., Bracker, M. and Spengler, J. (1987). Validation of three cell toxicity tests and the hen's egg test with guinea pig eye and human skin irritation data. In Goldberg, A. M. (Ed.), *In Vitro Toxicology—Approaches to Validation. Alternative Methods in Toxicology*, Vol. 5. Mary Ann Liebert, New York, pp. 463–470

Reinhardt, C. A., Pelli, D. A. and Zbinden, G. (1985). Interpretation of cell toxicity data for the estimation of potential irritation. *Fd Chem. Toxicol.*, **23**, 247–252

Reiser, K. M. and Last, J. A. (1979). Silicosis and fibrogenesis: fact and artifact. *Toxicology*, **13**, 51–72

Roberts, R. and Dorough, H. (1984). Relative toxicities of chemicals to the earthworm *Eisenia foetida*. *Environ. Toxicol.*, **3**, 67–78

Roberts, R. and Dorough, H. (1985). Hazards of chemicals to earthworms. *Environ. Toxicol. Chem.*, **4**, 307–323

Rofe, P. C., (1971). Tissue culture and toxicology. *Fd Cosmet. Toxicol.*, **9**, 685–696

Roth, J. A. (1980). Use of perfused lung in biochemical toxicology. *Rev. Biochem. Toxicol.*, **1**, 287–309

Ruben, Z., Fuller, G. C. and Knodle, S. G. (1984). Disobutamide-induced cytoplasmic vacuoles in cultured dog coronary artery muscle cells, *Arch. Toxicol.*, **55**, 206–212

Russell, W. M. S. and Burch, R. L. (1959). *The Principles of Humane Experimental Technique*. Methuen, London

Rylander, L. A., Phelps, J. S., Gandolfi, A. J. and Brendel, K. (1987). *In vitro* nephrotoxicity: response of isolated renal tubules to cadmium chloride and dichlorovinyl cysteine. *In Vitro Toxicol.*, **1**, 111–127

Saxen, L. (1984). Tests *in vitro* for teratogenicity. In J. W. Gorrod (Ed.), *Testing for Toxicity*. Taylor and Francis, London, pp. 185–197

Saxen, L. and Saksela, E. (1971). Transmission and spread of embrymic induction. II. Exclusion of an assimilatory transmission mechanism in kidney tubule induction. *Exptl Cell Res.*, **66**, 369–377

Scaife, M. C. (1982). An investigation of detergent action on *in vitro* and possible correlations with *in vivo* data. *Int. J. Cosmet. Sci.*, **4**, 179–193

Selling, J. and Ekwall, B. (1985). Screening for eye irritancy using cultured Hela cells. *Xenobiotica*, **15**, 713–717

Shadduck, J. A., Everitt, J. and Bay, P. (1985). Use of *in vitro* cytotoxicity to rank ocular irritation of six surfactants. Goldberg, A. M. (Ed.), *In Vitro Toxicology. Alternative Methods in Toxicology*, Vol. 3. Mary Ann Liebert, New York, pp. 641–649

Shadduck, J. A., Render, J., Everitt, J., Meccoli, R. A. and Essexsorlie, D. (1987). An approach to validation: comparison of six materials in three tests. Goldberg, A. M. (Ed.), *In vitro Toxicology—Approaches to Validation. Alternative Methods in Toxicology*, Vol. 5. Mary Ann Liebert, New York

Shopsis, C. and Eng, B. (1985). Uridine uptake and cell growth cytotoxicity tests: comparison, applications and mechanistic studies. *J. Cell. Biol.*, **101**, 87a

Shopsis, C. and Sathe, S. (1984). Uridine uptake inhibition as a cytotoxicity test: Correlation with the Draize test. *Toxicology*, **29**, 195–206

Sieber-Blum, M. F. (1985). Differentiation of avian neural crest cells *in vitro* (quail, chick, rodent). *Crisp Data Base* HD15311–04

Silverman, J. (1983). Preliminary findings on the use of protozoa (*Tetrahymena thermophila*) as models for ocular irritation testing in rabbits. *Lab. Anim. Sci.*, **33**, 56–59

Simons, P. J. (1981). An alternative to the Draize test. In Rowan, A. N. and Stratmann, C. J. (Eds), *The Use of Alternatives in Drug Research*. Macmillan Press, London

Singer, P. (1975). *Animal Liberation: A New Ethic for Our Treatment of Animals*. Random House, New York

Sleet, R. B. and Brendel, K. (1985). Homogenous populations of *Artemia nauplii* and their potential use for *in vitro* testing in developmental toxicology. *Terat. Carcin. Mutagen*, **5** (1), 41–54

Smith, M. A., Acosta, D. and Bruckner, J. V. (1986). Development of a primary culture system of rat kidney cortical cells to evaluate the nephrotoxicity of xenobiotics. *Fd Chem. Toxicol.*, **24**, 551–556

Smith, M. A., Acosta, D. and Bruckner, J. V. (1987). Cephaloridine toxicity in primary cultures of rat renal epithelial cells. *In Vitro Toxicol.*, **1**, 23–29

Smith, M. A., Hewitt, W. R. and Hook, J. (1988). *In Vitro* methods in renal toxicology. In Atterwill, C. K. and Steele, C. E. (Eds), *In Vitro Methods in Toxicology*. Cambridge University Press, New York, pp. 13–36

Smith, M. K., Kimmel, G. L., Kochhar, D. M., Shepard, T. H., Spielberg, S. P. and Wilson, J. C. (1983). A selection of candidate compounds for *in vitro* teratogenesis test validation. *Terat. Carcin. Mutagen*, **3**, 461–480

Soto, R. J., Servi, M. J. and Gordon, V. C. (1988). Evaluation of an alternative method of ocular irritation. In Goldberg, A. M. (Ed.), *Progress in In Vitro Toxicology*. Mary Ann Liebert, New York, pp. 289–296

Spencer, P. S., Crain, S. M., Bornstein, M. B., Peterson, E. R. and van de Water, T. (1986). Chemical neurotoxicity: detection and analysis in organotypic cultures of sensory and motor systems. *Fd Chem. Toxicol.*, **24**, 539–544

Stammati, A. P., Silano, V. and Zucco, F. (1981). Toxicology investigations with cell culture systems. *Toxicology*, **20**, 91–153

Stenersen, J. (1979). Action of pesticides on earthworms. Part I: Toxicity of cholinesterase-inhibiting insecticides to earthworms as evaluated by laboratory tests. *Pesticide Sci.*, **10**, 66–74

Swisher, D. A., Prevo, M. E. and Ledger, P. W. (1988). The MTT *in vitro* cytotoxicity test: correlation with cutaneous irritancy in two animal models. In Goldberg, A. M. (Ed.), *Progress in In Vitro Toxicology*. Mary Ann Liebert, New York, pp. 265–269

Tchao, R. (1988). Trans-epithelial permeability of fluorescein *in vitro* as an assay to determine eye irritants. In Goldberg, A. M. (Ed.), *Progress in In Vitro Toxicology*. Mary Ann Liebert, New York, pp. 271–284

Thulin, H. and Zacharian, H. (1972). The leukocyte migration test in chromium hypersensitivity. *J. Invest. Dermatol.*, **58**, 55–58

Tyson, C. A. and Stacey, N. H. (1989). *In vitro* screens from CNS, liver and kidney for systemic toxicity. In Mehlman, M. (Ed.), *Benchmarks: Alternative Methods in Toxicology*. Princeton Scientific, Princeton, N.J., pp. 111–136

Uyeki, E. M., Ashkar, A. E., Shoeman, D. W. and Bisel, J. U. (1977). Acute toxicity of benzene inhalation to hemopoietic precursor cells. *Toxicol. Appl. Pharmacol.*, **40**, 49–57

Volpe, L. S., Biagioni, T. M. and Marquis, J. K. (1985). *In vitro* modulation of bovine caudate muscarinic receptor number by organophosphates and carbamates. *Toxicol. Appl. Pharmacol.*, **78**, 226–234

Watanabe, M., Watanabe, K., Suzuki, K., Nikaido, O., Sugahara, T., Ishii, I. and Konishi, H. (1988). *In vitro* cytotoxicity test using primary cells derived from rabbit eye is useful as an alternative for Draize testing. In Goldberg, A. M. (Ed.), *Progress in In Vitro Toxicology*. Mary Ann Liebert, New York, pp. 285–290

Williams, G. M., Dunkel, V. C. and Ray, V. A. (Eds) (1983). *Cellular Systems for Toxicity Testing. Ann. N.Y. Acad. Sci.*, **407**

Williams, P. D., Masters, B. G., Evans, L. D., Laska, D. A. and Hattendorf, G. H. (1987). An *in vitro* model for assessing muscle irritation due to parenteral antibiotics. *Fund. Appl. Toxicol.*, **9**, 10–17

Wilson, J. G. (1978). Review of *in vitro* systems with potential for use in teratogenicity screening. *J.* **2**, 149–167

Young, M. F., Trombetta, L. D. and Sophia, J. V. (1986). Correlative *in vitro* and *in vivo* study of skeletal muscle irritancy. *Toxicologist*, **6**, 1225

Zbinden, G. (1987). *Predictive Value of Animal Studies in Toxicology*. Centre for Medicines Research, Carshalton, England

FURTHER READING

Anderson, D. (1993). The use of *in vitro* models in safety testing and research. In Anderson, R., Reiss, M., and Campbell, P. (Eds), *Ethical Issues in Biomedical Sciences*. Institute of Biology, London, pp. 47–68

Balls, M. (1993). How far advanced is the replacement of animal experimentation? *In Vitro Toxicology*, **6**, 149–161

Frazier, J. M. (1992). *In Vitro Toxicity Testing*. Marcel Dekker Inc., New York

Gad, S. C. (1994). *In Vitro Toxicology*. Raven Press, New York

Mayer, F. L., Whalen, E. A. and Rheins, L. A. (1994). A regulatory overview of alternatives to animal testing. *Journal of Toxicology, Cutaneous and Ocular Toxicology*, **13**, 3–22

McQueen, C. A. (1989). *In Vitro Toxicology: Model Systems and Methods*. Telford Press, Caldwell, New Jersey

Watson, R. R. (1992). *In Vitro Methods of Toxicology*. CRC Press, Boca Raton, Florida

8 Information Resources for Toxicology

J. Deschamps and D. Morgan

INTRODUCTION

The range and scale of toxicological information can be daunting. To take a historical perspective, for instance, we can go back approximately 4000 years to the earliest pharmacopoeias from Ancient Egypt, going on to the many Greek and Latin texts that deal with matters of toxicological interest. In the sixteenth century Paracelsus wrote a precursor of toxicology textbooks such as this. His work was the harbinger of an avalanche of toxicological literature, which has become all but overwhelming during the last hundred years.

As well as the plethora of information, there has been an inflation in costs. Some information is free—such as commercial chemical catalogues or government leaflets; other information is subsidized—such as the *Pesticide Manual* of the British Crop Protection Council. Most publications and databases have, however, increased their prices above the general rate of inflation, as have other information sources such as conferences. Since the time of first writing the growth in information sources and development of technology, particularly CD-ROM, has continued apace. References have been updated where information is readily available but some details will, inevitably, not be correct. No prices have been included for the sources listed in this chapter; a librarian/information officer would be able to advise.

There is no single, exhaustive source of toxicological data; several sources will be needed to obtain comprehensive information on a particular chemical. Printed sources are often quicker and easier to use, for instance, than computer databases; but interactive online searching can produce very precise results. Developments such as hypertext, electronic mail and non-text databases will produce exciting new options; new technology is leading to the blurring of functions between author, editor, publisher, database producer and librarian.

Toxicology is multidisciplinary and a variety of sources are needed to meet questions on anything from adverse drug reactions to complex environ-mental matters. Rather than categorize by toxicological topic, this short chapter will attempt to show the range of possible sources, with some specific but necessarily limited examples. The headings will be: 'Printed Sources'; 'Databases and Databanks'; and 'Research, Organizations and People'. By way of a conclusion, an attempt will be made to provide some guidance on data selection and quality criteria. The sources described have been divided into three major categories, but they are not mutually exclusive. Each has its own strengths and weaknesses, particularly regarding currency, quality, comprehensiveness and accessibility.

PRINTED SOURCES

The information explosion in scientific literature is unabated and toxicology has not escaped its effects. Two American authors have attempted to tackle the problem and have produced comprehensive volumes on toxicological information sources:

Wexler, P. (1988; 2nd edn), *Information Resources in Toxicology* (Amsterdam, New York: Elsevier Biomedical). ISBN 0444012141. This publication is well indexed and takes a broad view of the subject; it is probably the best book in this area.

Webster, J. K. (1987), *Toxic and Hazardous Materials, A Sourcebook and Guide to Information Sources* (Bibliographical Indexes in Science and Technology No. 2). (New York, London: Greenwood Press). ISBN 0313245754. This guide has chapters on twelve topics, such as acid rain and transportation of hazardous materials, each broken down into types of information source. Unfortunately, it is poorly in-dexed and the chapters are of uneven quality.

Both the above are written from an American perspective. Two slimmer British publications have been produced:

Fawell, J. K. and Newman, L. E. (1986), *Infor-

mation Sources in Toxicology (Publication 1060-M). (Medmenham: WRC).

Pantry, S. (1992; 3rd edn), *Health and Safety: A Guide to Sources Information* (CPI Information Reviews No. 6). (Edinburgh: Capital Planning Information). ISBN 0906011817.

Reference Works

Every library or information unit has a different set of textbooks and reference works. They remain the cheapest and simplest method of dealing with many requests. We can only attempt to list a few widely available works published since 1980; those also available as online databases are indicated.

American Conference of Governmental Industrial Hygienists, *Threshold Limit Values and Biological Exposure Indices* (Cincinnati OH: The Conference). Published annually.

Baselt, R. (1982), *Disposition of Toxic Drugs and Chemicals in Man* (Davis CA: Biomedical Publications). ISBN 093189008X.

Bismuth, C., and others (1987; 4th edn), *Toxicologie Clinique, Medicine, Sciences* (Paris: Flammarion).

Casarett, L. J., Doull, J., Klaasen, C. D. and Amdur, M. O. (1991; 4th edn), *Casarett and Doull's Toxicology; The Basic Science of Poisons* (New York: Macmillan). ISBN 0023646500.

Clayton, G. D. and Clayton, F. E. (Eds) (1985), *Patty's Industrial Hygiene and Toxicology* (Chichester, New York: Wiley). ISBN 0471831999. Newer editions of some volumes available.

Dreisbach, R. H. (1987; 12th edn), *Handbook of Poisoning: Prevention, Diagnosis and Treatment*, (Norwalk CT: Appleton and Lange). ISBN 0838536433.

Ellenhorn, M. J. and Barceloux, D. G. (1987), *Medical Toxicology: Diagnosis and Treatment of Human Poisoning* (New York: Elsevier). ISBN 0444011293.

Fawell, J. K. and Hunt, S. (1988), *Environmental Toxicology: Organic Pollutants* (Chichester: Ellis Horwood). ISBN 0745801943.

Garner, R. J. and Humphreys, D. S. (1988; 3rd edn), *Veterinary Toxicology* (London: Baillière Tindall). ISBN 0702012491.

Gilman, A. G., Goodman, L. S., Rall, T. W. and Murad, F. (1985; 7th edn), *Goodman and Gilman's The Pharmacological Basis of Thera-*

peutics (London: Collier Macmillan). ISBN 0080402968.

Glaister, J. C. (1986), *Principles of Toxicological Pathology* (London: Taylor and Francis). ISBN 0850663164.

Gosselin, R. E., Smith, R. P., Hodge, H. C. and Braddock, J. E. (1984; 5th edn) *Clinical Toxicology of Commercial Products* (London, Baltimore MD: Williams and Wilkins). ISBN 0683036327. Online through CIS (see 'Databases').

Haley, T. J. and Bernot, W. O. (Eds) (1988), *Toxicology* (London: Taylor and Francis). ISBN 0891168109.

Hamilton, A., Hardy, H. L. and Finkel, A. J. (1983; 4th edn), *Hamilton and Hardy's Industrial Toxicology* (Bristol, Boston MA: John Wright). ISBN 0723670277.

Hayes, W. A. (1989; 2nd edn), *Principles and Methods of Toxicology* (New York: Raven Press). ISBN 0881674397.

Hayes, W. J. (1982), *Pesticides Studied in Man* (Baltimore MD: Williams and Wilkins).

Hodgson, E. and Levi, P. E. (Eds) (1987), *Textbook of Modern Toxicology* (New York: Elsevier). ISBN 0444011315.

Lauwerys, R. (1982; 2nd edn), *Toxicologies Industrielles et Intoxications Professionelles* (Paris: Masson).

Manahan, E. E. (1989), *Toxicological Chemistry, A Guide to Toxic Substances in Chemistry* (Chelsea MI: Lewis Publishers). ISBN 0873711491.

Milman, H. A. and Weisburger, E. K. (Eds) (1985), *Handbook of Carcinogen Testing* (Park Ridge NJ: Noyes Publications). ISBN 0815510357.

Mitchell, J. R. and Horning, M. G. (Eds) (1984), *Drug Metabolism and Drug Toxicity* (New York: Raven Press). ISBN 0890049971.

Organisation for Economic Co-operation and Development, *OECD Guidelines for Testing of Chemicals* (Paris: OECD). ISBN 9264122214. Loose-leaf, updated irregularly.

Richardson, M. (1986), *Toxic Hazard Assessment of Chemicals* (Cambridge: Royal Society of Chemistry). ISBN 0851868975.

Richardson, M. (1992), *The Dictionary of Substances and their Effects* (Cambridge: Royal Society of Chemistry). ISBN 0851863310.

Royal Society of Chemistry (1991; 3rd edn), *Agrochemicals Handbook* (Cambridge: RSC).

ISBN 0851864163. Loose-leaf updating service available, also online via Dialog and DataStar.

Royal Society of Chemistry (1988), *European Directory of Agrochemical Products* (Cambridge: RSC). ISBN 0851867138.

Sax, N. I. (1986, 1988), *Hazardous Chemicals Information Annuals, Nos 1 and 2* (New York: Van Nostrand Reinhold). ISBN 0442281439, 0442281358.

Sax, N. I. and Lewis, R. J. (1988; 7th edn) *Dangerous Properties of Industrial Materials* (New York: Van Nostrand Reinhold). ISBN 0442280203.

Tatken, R. L. and Lewis, R. J. (Eds), *Registry of Toxic Effects of Chemical Substances (RTECS)* (Cincinnati OH: National Institute for Occupational Safety and Health). Published quarterly on microfiche, also CD-ROM and online.

Major Series

Much of the best summary information on toxicology is published in the form of series by the main organizations working in the field. In order to keep this section to reasonable length, only international and major UK or US series are listed. Addresses and more information are given in the section on 'Research, Organizations and People'.

Agency for Toxic Substances and Disease Registry: *ASTDR Toxicological Profiles* examine the state of knowledge for priority substances, often with useful tables and graphs; they are intended to help identify further research needs.

British Industrial Biological Research Association (BIBRA): Over a period of six years the Association has produced some 400 *Toxicity Profiles*. These briefly review available information and give a list of references. It is intended to update the profiles regularly.

Cold Spring Harbor Laboratory: *Banbury Reports* publish proceedings of conferences on toxicological and environmental subjects.

Commission of the European Communities (CEC): The *EUR* report series often includes titles of toxicological interest. In particular, it publishes the *Reports of the Scientific Committee on Cosmetology* and the *Reports of the Scientific Committee for Food*.

Environmental Protection Agency: A huge volume of reports is produced, mostly available on microfiche. The studies are indexed in *NTIS Government Reports Announcements*, and *EPA Publications: A Quarterly Guide*.

European Chemical Industry Ecology and Toxicology Centre: ECETOC issues three series: *Monographs, Technical Reports* and *Joint Assessments of Commodity Chemicals*.

Food and Agriculture Organization: *FAO Plant Production and Protection Papers* include the three annual volumes from the Joint FAO/WHO Expert Meetings on Pesticide Residues. JECFA (Joint FAO/WHO Expert Committee on Food Additives) reports are mostly published in the *Food and Nutrition Paper* series, including the JECFA *Specifications for Identity and Purity*, the *Food Additives Data System* (index to JECFA reports) and *Veterinary Residues Monographs*. The JECFA *Monographs on Toxicological Evaluation of Food Additives*, however, are now published by the Cambridge University Press. FAO also publishes the *Codex Alimentarius*.

Health and Safety Executive: The chief HSE series of interest is their *Toxicity Reviews*, though other series are of interest to those in the field of occupational health.

International Agency for Research on Cancer: *IARC Monographs* are definitive evaluations of carcinogenic hazards and are well supported by a *Supplement* series that acts as an index and gives additional summary data. The *Scientific Publications* series includes proceedings of conferences, an annual research register and other miscellaneous items; it is published for the Agency by Oxford University Press.

International Atomic Energy Agency (IAEA): *Safety* series includes relevant titles.

International Commission on Radiological Protection: *Annals of the ICRP* provide key data for radiation risk assessment.

International Programme on Chemical Safety (IPCS): The *Environmental Health Criteria* documents assess environmental and human health effects of exposure to chemicals, and biological or physical agents. A related *Health and Safety Guide* series give guidance on setting exposure limits for national chemical safety programmes.

International Register of Potentially Toxic Chemicals (IRPTC): The main series comprises the *Scientific Reviews of Soviet Literature on Toxicity and Hazards of Chemicals*. A computerized listing of *Chemicals Currently Being Tested for Toxic Effects* is issued periodically. IRPTC also publishes a number of monographs, in conjunction with Russia, such as *Long-term Effects of Chemicals on the Organism* and *Principles of Pesticide Toxicology*.

Monitoring and Assessment Research Centre (MARC): *MARC Technical Reports* give data and methods of approach for those involved in monitoring and assessment of environmental pollution. *General Reports* are synoptic reviews of environmental topics and *Research Memoranda* are short informal reports, sometimes including data and bibliographical information.

National Academy of Sciences: NAS provides many useful publications, including series on *Medical and Biologic Effects of Environmental Pollutants*, formerly *Biologic Effects of Atmospheric Pollutants*.

National Center for Toxicological Research: *Technical Report* series deals with drug and chemical toxicology studies.

National Institute for Occupational Safety and Health (NIOSH): At present 50 *Current Intelligence Bulletins* have been published on health hazards of materials and processes at work.

National Toxicology Program (NTP): A *Technical Report* series was begun by the National Cancer Institute to report results of their carcinogenicity bioassays and was taken up by the NTP, a consortium of US agencies. A status report is produced frequently by the Program, indexing studies under way as well as those published. The Program also issues an *Annual Review of Current DHHS, DOE and EPA Research Related to Toxicology*, an *Annual Plan* for each for each fiscal year, and an *Annual Summary Report on Carcinogens*.

World Health Organization (WHO): The *Technical Reports* series includes the summary reports of JECFA meetings; the *Food Additive* series is now published by Cambridge University Press (see FAO entry). The European office has produced a relevant *Environmental Health* series and another on *Health Aspects of Chemical Safety*.

Space constraints prevent any attempt at an exhaustive listing, although many commercial publishers produce useful series, such as the Karger series on *Concepts in Toxicology* and the Cambridge University Press series, *Cambridge Monographs on Cancer Research*.

Journals and Periodicals

A good way to stay up-to-date is to scan a selection of the many journals. Even newspapers can have a role as an alerting service to unexpected hazards. It is important, however, to avoid being swamped; use of abstracts or selective dissemination of information (SDI) should be considered. SDI will be discussed further under 'Databases and Databanks'. A quick review showed some 160 titles that could be considered as being in the core area of toxicology. A small selection of titles is given below; further titles can easily be traced from publications such as *Ulrich's International Periodicals Directory*.

Aquatic Toxicology
Archives of Environmental Contamination and Toxicology
Archives of Toxicology/Archiv für Toxicologie
Bulletin of Environmental Contamination and Toxicology
CRC—Critical Reviews in Toxicology
Clinical Toxicology
Developments in Toxicology and Environmental Science
Drug and Chemical Toxicology
Ecotoxicology and Environmental Safety
Environmental Toxicology and Chemistry
Food and Chemical Toxicology
Fundamental and Applied Toxicology
Human and Experimental Toxicology
IRPTC Bulletin
Journal de Toxicologie Clinique et Experimentale
Journal of the American College of Toxicology
Journal of Analytical Toxicology
Journal of Applied Toxicology
Journal of Biochemical Toxicology
Journal of Environmental Pathology, Toxicology and Oncology
Journal of Toxicology and Environmental Health
Journal of Toxicology, Clinical Toxicology
Journal of Toxicology, Cutaneous and Ocular Toxicology
Medical Toxicology
Molecular Toxicology
Neurotoxicology and Teratology
Pesticide and Toxic Chemical News
Pharmacology and Toxicology
Practical In Vitro Toxicology
Regulatory Toxicology and Pharmacology
Reproductive Toxicology

Reviews of Environmental Contamination and Toxicology
Toxic Substances Journal
Toxicity Assessment
Toxicity Review
Toxicologia
Toxicologic Pathology
Toxicological and Environmental Chemistry
Toxicologist
Toxicology
Toxicology Abstracts
Toxicology and Applied Pharmacology
Toxicology Forum
Toxicology and Industrial Health
Toxicology In Vitro
Toxicology Letters
Toxicon
Veterinary and Human Toxicology

Audiovisual Materials

Videocassettes and tape-slide programmes often include associated printed matter and a number are available on toxicological subjects. The National Library of Medicine produces an *Audiovisuals Catalog* and in the United Kingdom the Graves Medical Audiovisual Library has an extensive catalogue. The broadcasting media are sources of toxicological information and, sometimes, disinformation.

Other Printed Sources

A wide variety of additional publications can give relevant toxicological information. Legislation, standards and patents are all published sources but can vary considerably between different countries; some of the databases described later provide access to these. Another unusual form of publishing is the production of card sets, such as *TREMCARDS* for those transporting dangerous chemicals or the *IPCS International Chemical Safety Cards*.

A less well documented source of information is the 'grey literature'; care should be taken in its use, since it is often unreviewed and unedited. Material such as conference papers, translations, dissertations and manufacturers' leaflets is not always available through booksellers or indexed by secondary services. Even more difficult to obtain are internal reports produced by governments or commercial organizations. Such reports

are not always confidential but their existence is difficult to trace. In the United Kingdom Chadwyck-Healey produce a catalogue of non-HMSO publications and the British Library Supplementary Publications section holds many otherwise inaccessible items. A number of referral services are described later; these, too, can help trace grey literature.

DATABASES AND DATABANKS

'Databank' and 'database' are terms used rather loosely to cover a heterogeneous range of sources, and are sometimes even used to mean a library or information unit. Most of the cases cited below, however, are some form of text, mostly in electronic form. An unusual type of database covered by this definition is the bulletin board—e.g. Hazmat (US Federal Emergency Management Agency). Thus databases may sometimes be used for news or electronic mail but far more frequently they are used for literature searching. When starting a study of a compound or investigating a specific topic, electronic sources, such as computer databases or CD-ROM should be considered. Some databases, such as mini-Medline, are available on tape for loading on local computers but normally a remote host machine is used. Online searching of commercial databases can become expensive and CD-ROM is increasingly attractive; disk players are relatively cheap, will run with any IBM-compatible micro, avoid problems of line noise and allow unlimited use. In-house databases including minutes, letters and 'corporate intelligence' constitute another, increasingly popular, type of information resource. The great advantages of the electronic media are speed, the ability to refine searches and format the results, and non-text search options, such as chemical structure searching on Beilstein. Drawbacks include high costs, less browsing potential and lack of older material.

Databanks such as the Registry of Toxic Effects of Chemical Substances (RTECS) give summary data, statistics and structures, similar to a reference book. Databases such as Toxline are more like a library card catalogue, giving access to the literature. Electronic document delivery and full-text databases are being developed and have the potential to make information retrieval a seamless process.

In selecting which online host to use, the charge structure should be considered; some providers are moving away from the old system based mainly on the numbers of records printed. The same file can often be found as part of several different databases and at widely different cost. RTECS is part of Toxnet, CIS and the CCOHS systems listed below: it is also found in an old printed form, CD-ROM and on microfiche! The ubiquitous nature of RTECS data is a reminder that all sources should be treated with caution, particularly when data are sparse or duplicated. The frequency with which databases are updated also varies considerably between hosts, as does the quality of their manuals and search language. If frequent searches for new developments on a topic are required, then most systems allow SDI searches to be run regularly. Finally, users of electronic data should consider using a microcomputer to speed searches; with appropriate software this allows automatic dialing of hosts, auto-login, pre-prepared searches, and immediate downloading and reformatting.

An excellent guide to what is available online can be found in:

Farbey, R. (1987), *Medical Databases 1988* (London: Aslib). ISBN 0851422268. This listing gives summaries of database coverage, host systems and costs. A new edition appears every few years. Chemical databases, such as CAS, are not included, but the total still comes to over 120.

A brief selection of databases/databanks follows, with an indication of the media in which they are available, including non-electronic.

Aqualine: Produced by the UK Water Research Centre, this online bibliographical database covers water quality and pollution. The corresponding printed version is *Aqualine Abstracts*.
BIOSIS: BIOSIS offers 42 000 bibliographic records on life sciences, veterinary medicine and pharmacology; it is available online via BRS, DataStar, Dialog, ESA-IRS, STN and DIMDI. A subset is in Toxlit.
CAB Abstracts: Agricultural information, including toxicity and poisoning, is in this database from the Commonwealth Agricultural Bureaux. It is available in printed form or online via DIMDI, ESA-IRS or BRS.
Canadian Centre for Occupational Health and

Safety (CCOHS): This is a co-operative scheme with the International Occupational Safety and Health Information Centre of the International Labour Office (CIS-ILO). Two low-priced optical disks are available: one with NIOSHTIC, Canadian material and the database of CIS-ILO; the other with RTECS and the full text of 35 000 chemical safety information sheets.
Carcinogenic Potency Database: This printed source lists the standardized results of animal bioassays; it has been published in *Environmental Health Perspectives*, 1984, Vol. 58, pp. 1–319; 1986, Vol. 67, pp. 161–200; 1987, Vol. 74, pp. 237–329; 1989, Vol. 79, pp. 259–272.
CA Search (CAS) and CAS Online/DARC: CAS Online/DARC allows graphical structure and substructure searching, with subsequent text searching; it can be found through STN or DARC Telesystemes. Among the ordinary Chemical Abstracts files the Chemical Nomenclature file can be particularly useful before searching other databases to find synonyms and CAS numbers. CA is on Dialog, BRS, DataStar, Orbit, ESA-IRS and STN.
Chemical Carcinogenesis Research Information System (CCRIS): The US National Cancer Institute funds CCRIS, which is available on Toxnet (see below). A printed version of the Carcinogenicity Data Base is, however, available and covers some 1400 chemicals. Data are evaluated.
Chemical Exposure: This file is produced by the US Chemical Effects Center at Oak Ridge National Laboratory; it is available through Dialog. It concentrates on body burden data and is useful for target organ or tissue information, with 11 000 records on 600 chemicals.
Chemical Information Service (CIS): Originally developed under the auspices of the US EPA and NIOSH, CIS offers a collection of scientific and regulatory databases and data analysis programs. The various online services allow structure, substructure and full or partial name searching of 350 000 chemicals. Files include Merck Index, RTECS and CHRIS. Also specialist files such as Genetic Toxicity (GENETOX), Plant Toxicity (PHYTOTOX), Dermal Absorption (DERMAL) and Gastrointestinal Absorption (GIABS).
Computerized Clinical Information System (CCIS): Published by Micromedex, this database is available online, in microfiche or on CD-ROM. The files include full-text documents on pharma-

ceutical/commercial product toxicology (POISIN-DEX), industrial chemical toxicology and hazardous materials incidents response (TOMES) and pharmacology (DRUGDEX).

Chemicals Currently Being Tested for Toxic Effects (CCTTE): This is a project funded by IPCS and IRPTC. It comprises a registry of ongoing tests (not including carcinogenicity), together with a collection of critical reviews. An annual publication is produced from the database and is available from IRPTC in Geneva.

Environmental Health Information System: The CEC, UNEP, IARC and WHO Regional Office for Europe are in the process of setting up several statistical databanks and bibliographical databases. The Pan American Health Organization have similar schemes under the banner PAHO/PROECOS.

Excerpta Medica (EMBASE): Online database corresponding to 44 abstract journals and two literature indexes produced by Excerpta Medica, includes biomedicine, dermatology, environmental health and biological effects of chemical compounds. The file from 1973 to date contains about 4 400 000 records. Available in whole or part via BRS, DataStar, Dialog, DIMDI.

EXICHEM: This OECD database contains information on planned, ongoing and completed data gathering, testing, evaluation and risk management activities. The information is made available twice a year on diskettes.

Food Additives Data System: This is composed of printed volumes in the FAO *Food and Nutrition Paper Series*, providing an index to the evaluations published by the FAO/WHO Expert Committee for Food Additives between 1956 and 1987. The Papers issued so far are 30; 30/Rev 1; 30/Rev 1/Add 1; and 30/Rev 1/Add 2. Further updates are planned.

Food Science and Technology Abstracts: The International Food Information Service produces abstracts on all aspects of food science, including toxicology. The hosts include Dialog, DataStar, DIMDI and Orbit.

Genetic Activity Profiles: Short-term test activity profiles have been assembled by EPA/EHRT from references supplied by the Environmental Mutagen Information Center (EMIC), Oak Ridge, TN, USA. The agents were selected from those in IARC Monographs Supplement No. 6 on genetic and related effects. The database is available on floppy disk from EMIC; it gives

brief information and a graphic display for 330 substances. It is an interesting example of joint publication of a printed volume and computer software.

HAZDATA: Available from UK National Chemical Emergency Centre at Harwell, and designed to run on microcomputers, this database gives legislation details and chemical risk assessment information but also allows users to add their own data.

HSELINE: Produced by the UK Health and Safety Executive since 1977; this database includes bibliographical data on occupational health, toxic substances and environmental hazards. There are some 75 000 records, available via ESA-IRS Orbit and DataStar online or on CD-ROM from Silverplatter.

International Pharmaceutical Abstracts (IPA): This online database is produced by the American Society for Hospital Pharmacists and gives bibliographical information on drug toxicity. It is available through BRS, Dialog and ESA-IRS.

Martindale Online: Evaluated information on drugs and medicines (some 5000 compounds) is contained in this database, which corresponds to the printed *Martindale Pharmacopoeia*. This full-text database is searchable via DataStar.

NIOSHTIC: Database of US National Institute for Occupational Safety and Health Technical Information Centre; it includes 120 000 bibliographical records and is available online through Dialog and Orbit or on CD-ROM. Parts of the file are also in CCOHS.

Numerica: A number of programs and databases are available, such as Chemtest and Environmental Fate Database. Carcinogenicity Predictor analyses genetic toxicity data from any of 33 types of assay and can be used to produce graphical analysis of the prediction.

REPRORISK: Teratogen information on effects of drugs and environmental agents. Part of American Tomes Plus database, available on CD-ROM.

SEDBASE: Full-text database of evaluated information on drug toxicity, based on Mylers Side Effects of Drugs and EMBASE. Available on Dialog and DataStar.

Tomes Plus: American databases on toxicology, occupational health and environmental chemicals. Published by Micromedex on CD-ROM.

Toxic Release Inventory: 17 500 US manufacturing facilities are required to make an annual return to the EPA for some 300 chemicals. This database is made available to the public, an interesting attempt to give public access to information.

Toxline/Toxnet/Toxlit This huge database covers literature in all areas of toxicology. There are some 2.1 million entries but some are duplicates. Various hosts, such as DIMDI, Blaise and DataStar, offer versions of Toxline, and a CD-ROM copy became available in 1989. There have been 17 different contributors to Toxline and there is no consistent system of indexing; both free-text and CAS numbers should be used. The subfiles from CAS, IPA and BIOSIS have recently been split off, since their commercial providers require royalties, and are now searchable as Toxlit. Another spin-off has been Toxnet, which has the non-bibliographical files—e.g. Hazardous Substances Databank (formerly Toxic Substances Databank), Chemical Carcinogenesis Research Information System (CCRIS), RTECS, Directory of Biotechnology Information Resources (DBIR) and GENETOX.

RESEARCH, ORGANIZATIONS AND PEOPLE

Prior to publication of results useful information can still be obtained from research workers. Likewise, formal training and education will provide much unpublished information. Several international systems attempt to give details of current research: two in particular should be emphasized. The IPCS and IRPTC produce a *Computerised Listing of Chemicals Being Tested for Toxic Effect*; this register lists, by chemical name, research currently being done; it gives the name and address of the worker and reviews that have recently been completed. A second vital resource is the IARC *Directory of On-going Research in Cancer Epidemiology*; the 1989 volume is number 101 in the IARC scientific publications series.

Direct contact with an organization or individual is the most effective means of getting current and relevant information. Academic, government and trade directories or yearbooks help to target requests but are normally only national in coverage. A recent publication attempts to list contacts in nearly all Western countries:

Simeons, C. (1987), *Toxic Substances, Sources of Information*. Published by the author (21 Ludlow Avenue, Luton LU1 3RW, England). Concentrates on chemical hazards and transport of dangerous goods.

United Nations

Services offered by a variety of international organizations include not only published and semi-published literature but also access to corporate and individual expertise. Several bodies offering such services are part of the United Nations:

International Agency for Research on Cancer: IARC was established by the World Health Assembly in 1965. Its function is to promote and co-ordinate international research on the causes of cancer and its prevention. Staff carry out both epidemiological studies and laboratory work. IARC organizes many conferences and conducts a world-wide programme for education and training.

International Environmental Information System (INFOTERRA): This service covers the broad environmental subject area and operates on the referral principle—that is, it refers enquirers to sources of information or expertise, rather than providing substantive information direct to the user. However, factual information is often provided, especially to those in developing countries. There are two main components. First, there is an *International Directory*, which contains descriptions of some 6000 sources, such as government departments and research organizations; many of these sources are concerned with chemicals and related topics. Second, there is a network of national focal points in over 130 countries world-wide; each of these has links with, and knows about, information services and centres in its own country.

International Labour Organisation: This organization has been in existence since 1919. It aims to raise working and living standards world-wide. Its activities include development of international standards, research, and the collection and dissemination of information.

International Programme on Chemical Safety: The programme is a joint endeavour of UNEP, ILO and WHO. Its objectives are: to evaluate the effects of chemicals on human health and the environment; to develop guidelines on exposure limits for chemicals in air, food, water and the working environment; to develop methodology for toxicity testing, epidemiology and clinical studies, and risk assessment; to co-ordinate studies internationally and promote research; to develop information for coping with chemical accidents; to promote technical co-operation and training.

International Register of Potentially Toxic Chemicals: This service, together with other UNEP services, was largely designed to meet the needs of developing countries. Its main objective is to reduce the hazards associated with chemicals in the environment, and it supplies information to those responsible for human health and environmental protection. It thus covers not only chemical data but also regulations and standards. There is a central unit in Geneva and a network of national correspondents; it publishes *IRPTC Bulletin* twice a year. IRPTC has built up a network of data suppliers, such as NIOSH in the USA, and it collaborates with ECDIN, which holds its legal file online. Other computerized files include information on toxicity to animals and man, waste management and environmental fate.

World Health Organization: WHO was set up 40 years ago. It is the world's directing and co-ordinating authority on human health. It has numerous networks and other means of collecting and disseminating data, including seven periodicals. It publishes about 80 books each year, plus many working papers and drafts. Of particular interest is its environmental health and chemical safety subscription package, which should ensure delivery of all WHO publications in that area.

European Communities

In addition to the European Communities Information Offices in the member states, there are several major services, listed below. Attempts at a European research information service, ENREP, have not been successful.

Environmental Chemicals Data and Information Network (ECDIN): ECDIN may be regarded as the online equivalent of a chemical handbook. The files in the commercial version are accessible via DIMDI; they include basic identifiers and properties, occupational health and safety, toxicity, and environmental concen-

tration and fate. Although it contains some information on around 65 000 substances, many of the more specialized files are considerably smaller. Acute toxicity data, for example, are held for 18 000 substances and are mostly taken from RTECS; more extensive data in this field are held on about 1000–2000 compounds.

Eurotoxnet: This project will develop a computer database consisting of several interrelated files: cases of human poisoning; chemical substances; product information; analytical methods; bibliographical information; and addresses. Training will be offered at the Poison Centres in the United Kingdom, Italy and Belgium, and trainees will participate in the development of the system. It is hoped eventually to develop an expert system and provide extensive training in human toxicology and information technology. It will also link the national centres in the countries of the European Communities.

INVITTOX: This is an unusual information source, compiled by two pressure groups—ERGATT (European Research Group for Alternatives in Toxicity Testing) and FRAME (Federation for Replacement of Animals in Medical Experiments). It is a databank of research techniques and contacts. At present it offers a free enquiry service, funded by the CEC.

System for Information on Grey Literature in Europe (SIGLE): SIGLE is a European Communities-wide attempt to deal with gaps in the knowledge and supply of grey literature. The service has been available since 1984, and contains records dating from 1981 onwards; it is accessible via INKA or Blaise. Relevant subject areas include agriculture, biology and chemistry; UK input comes from the BL database called *British Reports, Translations and Theses.*

EXICHEM: This database, which contains details of research being carried out by member states on existing chemicals, is regularly updated both as a printed publication and on diskette. It is used as an aid to systematic investigation and to identify opportunities for co-operation in testing, reviewing and assessing substances.

Addresses

Agency for Toxic Substances and Disease Registry, Atlanta, GA 30333, USA
British Industrial Biological Research Associ-

ation, Woodmansterne Road, Carshalton, Surrey SM5 4DS, United Kingdom

British Library Document Supply Centre, Boston Spa, Wetherby, West Yorkshire LS23 7BJ, United Kingdom

Cold Spring Harbor Laboratory, Box 100, Cold Spring Harbor, NY 11724, USA

Commission of the European Communities, Office of Official Publications, 2 Rue Mercier, L–2985, Luxembourg (publications also via national agents)

ECDIN Group, Commission of the European Communities, Joint Research Centre, Ispra Establishment, I–21020 Ispra (Varesse), Italy

ECETOC, Avenue Louise 250, B–63 Brussels 1050, Belgium

Environmental Protection Agency, 401 Main Street SW, Washington DC 20406, United States

EUROTOXNET, Poisons Unit, Avonley Road, London SE14 5ER, United Kingdom

EXICHEM, Chemicals Division, Environment Directorate, 2 Rue Andre Pascal, 75775 Paris (Cedex 16), France

Food and Agriculture Organisation, Via della Terme di Caracalla, 00100 Rome, Italy (publications also via national agents)

Health and Safety Executive, Baynards House, 1 Chepstow Place, Westbourne Grove, London W2 4TF, United Kingdom

INFOTERRA/PAC, United Nations Environment Programme, PO Box 30552, Nairobi, Kenya

International Agency for Research on Cancer, 150 Cours Albert Thomas, F–69372 Lyon (Cedex 2), France

International Atomic Energy Agency, Wagramerstrasse 5, PO Box 100, A–1400 Vienna, Austria

International Commission on Radiological Protection, Clifton Avenue, Sutton, Surrey SM2 5PU, United Kingdom

International Labour Office, CH–1211 Geneva 22, Switzerland

International Programme on Chemical Safety, World Health Organization, CH–1211 Geneva 27, Switzerland

International Register of Potentially Toxic Chemicals, United Nations Environment Programme, Palais des Nations, CH–1211 Geneva 10, Switzerland

INVITTOX, 34 Stoney Street, Nottingham NG1 1NB, United Kingdom

Monitoring and Assessment Research Centre,

Octagon Building, 459A Fulham Road, London SW10 0QX, United Kingdom

National Academy of Sciences, 2101 Constitution Avenue, Washington, DC 20418, USA

National Center for Toxicological Research, Jefferson, AK 72079, USA

National Council on Radiation Protection and Measurements, 7910 Woodmont Avenue, Bethesda, MD 20814, USA

National Institute for Occupational Safety and Health, 5600 Fishers Lane, Rockville, MD 20857, USA

National Radiological Protection Board, Chilton, Didcot, Oxfordshire OX11 0RQ, United Kingdom

National Toxicology Program, Research Triangle Park, NC 27709, USA

Water Research Centre, Medmenham Laboratory, Henley Road, Medmenham, PO Box 16, Marlow, Buckinghamshire SL7 2HD, United Kingdom

World Health Organization, CH–1211 Geneva 27, Switzerland (publications also via national agents)

CONCLUSIONS

The tremendous increase in toxicological data in the past two decades has not been matched by better quality control or analysis. There are examples of information being misapplied or misunderstood. RTECS gives extreme cases and is not always accurate; it should not be used alone. The IARC listings of possible carcinogens have been used in some countries for framing legislation, but IARC base their classifications on some evidence of carcinogenicity in one or more published studies, not a full weight-of-evidence evaluation of all relevant data. The evaluations are intended as an input to, not a basis for, regulations. Likewise, doubtful extrapolations can be made from animal data to humans. Preambles and prefaces should be read with care and note taken of any caveats. A statement that a study has been undertaken in conformity with Good Laboratory Practice should be a favourable indication of quality. Guidance on the selection and evaluation of sources can be found in:

Richardson, M. L. (1986), *Toxic Hazard Assessment of Chemicals* (Cambridge: Royal

Society of Chemistry). ISBN 0851868975. Chapter 6, entitled 'Separating the wheat from the chaff', is particularly relevant.

A method sometimes suggested for quality control is use of Science Citation Index, or its online version, SciSearch, to look at the number of citations of a paper. Citations, however, can be biased in many ways: self-citation; in-house bias; citation copying (often perpetuating wrong references!); language/nationality bias; and even a tendency to cite papers written by those who will be the referees. Citation indexes are useful ways of following up somebody working in a field of interest but should not be used as a guide to the validity of a paper. Similarly, a long list of references at the end of a paper is no guarantee of quality.

The reputation of a journal is a nebulous thing but a look at the list of the editorial board, usually on the inside cover, can be revealing. Periodicals that do not have any refereeing system should certainly be treated with some caution. News items, letters, advertisements and other ephemeral types of information also need to be viewed differently but are useful alerting services.

The above are problems of validation and quality, but availability can be an even more difficult problem for someone seeking toxicological information. There is a growing tendency to cite items only submitted for publication or 'in press'; a considerable proportion of these never see the light of day and can cause immense frustrations for librarians and information staff. Publishers are normally helpful, but if the editorial office is in another country or on another continent, it can be expensive to trace publication details. A letter to the author of the original article may be the best method and may also help to discourage the practice. Unpublished material is probably also best tackled by a personal approach and can provide some useful contacts.

Having traced the bibliographical details, any library should be able to obtain the item. In Britain public libraries normally have a central reference collection for science and technology, while any branch will eventually get any book requested for a small fee. Some academic libraries provide a service for the local community and businesses. Behind them all stands the British Library, with the Science Reference and Information Service in London and the British Library Document Supply Centre at Boston Spa, which provides a loan and photocopy service. The British Library is a unique institution and is used world-wide, but most countries have some type of national library network. To get full use of the resources available, all organizations should employ qualified librarians or information scientists.

Other areas of difficulty arise from the complexity of chemical nomenclature; multiple publication of data; and sometimes even downright fraud in the presentation of results. A user of toxicological information should be aware of possible pitfalls and digest certain data with a unit of sodium chloride.

Databanks, such as IRPTC and ECDIN, are probably of the greatest value in providing an overview of a named chemical substance. They are strong on regulatory information and have good coverage of data taken from key works produced by international agencies. A limitation is that comprehensive data are available for only a comparatively small number of chemicals. Also, the extent to which data have been evaluated or validated is often unclear. IRPTC, in particular, gives access to a wide range of additional information through its network of National Correspondents.

Referral systems, such as INFOTERRA, do not themselves hold data but provide access to an extensive range of resources. Their weakness is an inbuilt communications delay, making them unsuitable for urgent requests. A strength is that they can provide publications and data which are not generally available, and access to specialist advice.

The same arguments apply to organizations as to referral services. The staff or organizations, even those with a remit to answer enquiries, often do not have the resources to do so or have to give priority to other work.

Bibliographical databases and research registers do not usually include data. Either the original documentation will have to be acquired or the researcher will have to be contacted in order to obtain the information needed. Coverage is not uniform; the quality and quantity of the coverage will vary considerably.

It is clear from the foregoing that there are a large number of ways in which to locate information on toxicology. Sometimes information will be diffuse and seeking it cumbersome. When, however, it is vital to exploit all possible options, the use of a wide range of resources, written and otherwise, will produce useful results.

ACKNOWLEDGEMENTS

This chapter has been seen by colleagues, whose help and advice is gratefully acknowledged. The views expressed are the authors' own and not necessarily those of the Departments for which they work.

PART TWO: TECHNIQUES IN TOXICOLOGY

9 The Design of Toxicological Studies

Alan J. Paine

INTRODUCTION

Toxicology is a unique form of science because it is more than a single discipline with one objective (Table 1). It is concerned with the assessment and subsequent management of potential chemical hazards to man, to other animals, and to the environment. In order to achieve this objective, the toxicologist needs a detailed knowledge not only of a chemical's primary and cumulative toxicity, but also of its 'no observed effect' level, as well as knowledge concerning its teratogenic, mutagenic and carcinogenic potential. Obviously these complex end-points cannot be determined from a single experiment, and when, as is often the case, precise toxicological mechanisms cannot be determined within an acceptable time-span, empirical procedures have been devised that permit pragmatic decisions to be made about probable safety. It is the objective of this chapter to provide a broad appreciation of these empirical procedures, as opposed to detailed methodologies, upon which assessments of risk are based in the real world of agricultural, industrial, medical and community practices.

Table 1 Definition and objectives of toxicology

Definition	The study of the adverse effects of chemicals on living organisms

Objectives
 (1) Hazard/risk assessment

   (A) Detect effects of chemicals as a cause of both acute and chronic illness = Fear what?

   (B) Exclude/minimize adverse effects:
     Balance economic benefits against the risk to protect the manufacturer, worker, consumer, environment and public = Avoid what?
                         Monitor what?

 (2) Aid the selection and development of therapeutic agents

 (3) Aid basic science = Knowledge of life processes

THE DOSE–RESPONSE RELATIONSHIP

The relationship between the degree of response and amount of chemical administered is the most fundamental and pervasive concept in toxicology. It also generates a vocabulary with which the student of toxicology needs to become familiar. The typical sigmoidal curve obtained by plotting response against administered dose is shown in Figure 1A. Figure 1B shows that lethality exhibits a normal Gaussian distribution. The data used to construct this histogram are the same as those used to generate the sigmoidal curve but the bars represent the percentage of animals that die at each dose minus the percentage that died at the lower dose. One can very clearly see that only a few animals responded at the lowest dose and only a small number responded at the highest dose. Larger numbers of animals responded to doses intermediate between these two extremes, and the maximum frequency of response occurred in the middle portion of the dose range. These curves can be transformed into a more manageable straight line (Figure 1C) by probit analysis (see Chapter 2), and the median lethal dose (LD_{50}) or for that matter the lethal dose for any percentage of the population (e.g. LD_{10}) can easily be determined.

The LD_{50} value in its simplest form is the dose of a compound that causes 50 per cent mortality in a population. A more precise definition is the statistically derived single dose that can be expected to cause death in 50 per cent of the animals under the specific conditions of the test. Thus, the LD_{50} value of a compound is not a mathematical constant but is a statistical term that describes the lethal response to a compound in a particular population under some discrete set of experimental conditions (e.g. age, general health and diet of the population). Although the numerical value of the LD_{50} has been used to classify and compare toxicity among chemicals, it must be remembered that lethality is only one of many indices in assessing toxicity (e.g. time to death).

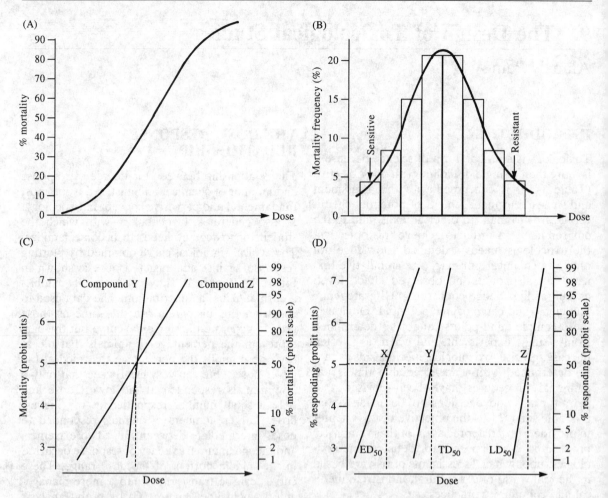

Figure 1 Typical dose–response curves. (A) shows the percentage mortality plotted against the log of the dose. (B) shows mortality frequency plotted against dose. (C) Comparison of the toxicities of two compounds X and Y. Although they have the same LD_{50}, the slope shows compound X to be more potent than compound Y. (D) Comparison of the dose–response curves for efficacy (X), toxicity (Y) and lethality (Z)

The slope of the log dose–response curve is perhaps more important in risk assessment than the numerical value of the LD_{50}, because more insight into the intrinsic toxic characteristics of a compound is available. For example, a steep slope may indicate rapid onset of action or faster absorption. A larger margin of safety may be predicted when a compound has a flat slope—i.e. a large increase in dose produces only a small increase in response. With the slope it is often possible to extrapolate the response to a low dose—for example, LD_1—or even to a no observable effect level (NOEL). Knowing the slope is especially important when comparing a series of compounds. For example, two compounds may have identical LD_{50} values but different slopes

indicating quite different toxicological characteristics (Figure 1C). Thus, LD_{50} is not equivalent to toxicity, as chemicals can induce irreversible damage to physiological, biochemical, immunological, neurological or anatomical systems, and, depending on the severity and extent of the disturbance, the animal may survive the toxic response. These non-lethal adverse effects are as undesirable as lethality and must be taken into account in the risk assessment of a chemical. Such non-lethal responses often follow a dose–response curve, and the term 'toxic dose' (TD) or more commonly 'effective dose' (ED) is used to describe these (Figure 1D). The term 'median effective dose' (ED_{50}) is often used in the standardization of biologically active compounds, such as drugs, and has a similar meaning to LD_{50} except that it is designed to examine non-lethal parameters such as pharmacological response or other non-lethal adverse effects. The ratio LD_{50}/ED_{50} defines the therapeutic index (TI) of a drug. The higher the index the greater the margin of safety with a drug, in that a large difference exists between the amount of a compound predicted to kill 50 per cent of the animals and the amount predicted to elicit a particular response in 50 per cent of the animals. The TI gives an even greater estimate of safety when the LD_1 or TD_1 is compared with the ED_{99}. What is being aimed for in the development of a pharmaceutical is a safety factor of 100–200-fold between the pharmacological and toxicological responses.

DURATION OF TOXICITY STUDIES

Essentially three types of study have become mandatory (see Chapter 42) in the course of safety evaluation of a chemical. These are as follows.

Acute studies demonstrate the adverse effects occurring within a short time, usually up to 14 days, following administration of a single dose of a substance or multiple doses given within 24 h.
Repeated-dose (subacute/subchronic) studies The definition of subchronic toxicity is confusing, as opinions differ as to the length of exposure that constitutes a subacute study. However, their purpose is the same—namely to demonstrate adverse effects occurring as a result of repeated daily doses of a chemical for part, not exceeding 10 per cent, of the life-span of an animal. Thus, 14, 21 and 28 day studies in rats are generally referred to as 'subacute' studies, while 90 day studies constitute 'subchronic' tests.
Chronic studies are those carried out over an animal's lifetime.

When these types of toxicity studies are translated into terms of human exposure, acute toxicity represents life-threatening crises of accidental catastrophes, overdoses or suicidal attempts. Subchronic/subacute toxicity represents frequent exposure to certain workplace and domestic chemicals, food additives, therapeutic agents or environmental pollutants at lower dose levels relative to accidental exposure. Chronic toxicity represents the daily ingestion of additives or agricultural residues in food.

ANIMAL HUSBANDRY AND OBSERVATIONS

The most important facet of any toxicological experiment is the condition of the test animals. Accordingly, all toxicity studies should be conducted in a controlled environment, which for rats means a temperature of $22\pm3°C$ with adequate ventilation (i.e. 10 changes of air per hour), relative humidity between 30 per cent and 70 per cent, and a 12 h light/dark cycle. The diet and quality of drinking water should be standardized and maintained throughout the experiment, and this should be carried out to Good Laboratory Practice standards (see Chapter 16) to ensure reproducibility/validity of data.

In brief, healthy young adult animals should be used, which means a body weight of 15–16 g for mice, 150–250 g for rats, 350–450 g for guinea-pigs and 2–3 kg for rabbits. Upon receipt the animals should be allowed to acclimatize to the conditions of the animal room for at least a week prior to dosing. During this period the animals should be individually and uniquely identified by tattooing or ear marking. Then all animals with health problems or body weights varying by more than 20 per cent of the mean body weight should be discarded and the remaining animals randomized, to ensure a homogeneous population, to the different dose groups.

For acute oral toxicity studies a minimum of 10 animals—5 male and 5 female—has been recommended in most regulatory guidelines. Therefore, rats and mice can be housed by sex and dose group according to current regulations concerning animal experimentation. Larger animals should be caged individually. For the determination of acute dermal and acute inhalation toxicities, 5 animals per dose level and sex are again sufficient, but these should be housed singly to prevent oral ingestion of the test substance by preening. Practical details of dosing by oral, dermal and inhalation routes are provided by Hayes (1982).

After dosing, observations should be made at frequent intervals in order to determine the onset of adverse effects, time to death or time to recovery. A mortality check should also be frequent enough to minimize unnecessary loss of animals due to autolysis or cannibalism. The observations should include any changes in the skin colour (e.g. cyanosis due to cardiac insufficiency), fur (e.g. piloerection due to disturbance of the autonomic nervous system), eyes (e.g. lachrymation indicating autonomic disturbances) and nostrils (e.g. discharge may indicate pulmonary oedema). Other pharmacotoxic signs such as tremor, convulsions, salivation, diarrhoea, lethargy, sleepiness, morbidity, etc., should be recorded in order to obtain the maximum amount of information from the experiment. Necropsies must be performed on animals that are moribund, found dead or killed at the end of the experiment. At necropsy changes in size, colour or texture of the major organs should be recorded and, if noted, tissues should be preserved in an appropriate fixative for histopathological examination. The procedures outlined in Table 2 attempt to summarize the considerable amount of work involved in toxicity tests.

TESTING FOR ACUTE TOXICITY

The objectives of an acute study are to define the intrinsic toxicity of a chemical, to assess the susceptible species, to identify the target organs of toxicity, to provide information for risk assessment after acute exposure to the chemical, and to provide information for the design and selection of dose levels for more prolonged studies. In the absence of data on the toxicity of a chemical, acute studies also help in formulating safety measures/monitoring procedures for all workers involved in the development and testing of a chemical. Accordingly, a battery of tests under different conditions and exposure routes should be conducted. In general, these tests should include determination of a chemical's oral (Chapter 16), cutaneous (Chapter 17) and inhalation (Chapter 18) toxicities, as well as skin and eye irritation studies (Chapters 20 and 24).

From a regulatory viewpoint, acute toxicity data are essential in the classification, labelling and transportation of a chemical (van den Heuvel *et al.*, 1987). From an academic standpoint, a carefully designed acute toxicity study can often produce information on the mechanism of toxicity and the structure–activity relationships within a particular class of chemicals. Therefore, acute toxicity tests should aim to record all lethal and non-lethal parameters.

Choice of Animal Species

In part the choice of species depends on the intended use of the chemical, but as humans will be intimately involved in its manufacture, distribution and use, acute toxicity tests, like all toxicity tests, should be conducted on an animal which will elicit compound-related responses similar to those which can be expected to occur in man. However, it should be appreciated that responses caused by a compound can vary greatly among species, owing almost entirely to differences in metabolism and pharmacokinetics (Tee *et al.*, 1987). Therefore, a sensible approach is to conduct acute oral toxicity studies in a variety of species of experimental animal under the assumption that if the toxicity of a compound is consistent in all the species tested, then there is a greater chance that such a response will occur in man. Although the response in different species is unlikely to be consistent, it is better to err on the safe side, with risk assessment being based on the most sensitive species unless there is justification, which usually comes from later studies (i.e. phase 1 studies for pharmaceuticals or occupational exposure data and/or human volunteer studies/or

Table 2 Consensus of basic procedure comprising acute, subchronic and chronic oral toxicity tests

	Acute oral	Subchronic oral	Chronic oral
Animals	Rats preferred	Rodent and non-rodent species	Rodent and non-rodent species
Sex	Males and females equally distributed per dose level		
Age and weight	Young adult weight variation within 20% of mean	Rodents 6 weeks; dogs 4–6 months old	

continued

Table 2 (continued)

	Acute oral	Subchronic oral	Chronic oral
No. per dose level	At least 10 animals (5 per sex)	At least 20 for rodents (10 per sex)	50 per sex group for rodents
Minimum no. of treatment groups	3 spaced appropriately to produce test groups with mortality rates between 10% and 90%	3 but not more than 10% mortality in high-dose group	3: low-dose should reflect expected human exposure. High-dose must produce an effect but not more than 10% mortality
Untreated control	Not necessary	Yes	Yes
Vehicle control	Yes, if suspending agent of unknown toxicity is used	Yes	Yes
Fasting	Rat overnight	Not appropriate	Not appropriate
Dosing	By gavage; single dose, same dose of vehicle. If necessary use divided doses over 24 h	Diet, gavage, drinking-water	Diet, gavage, drinking-water
Duration of study	At least 14 days	90 days	24 months in rats
Body weight determination	To be recorded before dosing, weekly thereafter and at death	Weekly and at termination	Weekly for first 13 weeks. Every 2 weeks thereafter and at termination
Food consumption	Weekly	Weekly	Weekly for first 13 weeks. Every 2 weeks thereafter and at termination
Necropsy	All animals	All test animals. Organ weights of liver, kidney, heart, lungs, brain, gonads, adrenals and spleen	
Histopathology	Examination of organs showing evidence of gross pathological change	All tissues high-dose and control groups. Liver, kidney, heart, lungs, target organs and any gross lesion in mid- and low-dose groups	All tissues all animals
Frequency of observation	Frequently during day of dosing. Once each morning and late afternoon thereafter	Daily	Daily
Observations to be made		Nature, onset, severity and duration of any effect observed. Ophthalmoscopy pretest and at termination on control and high-dose	
		Haematology/clinical chemistry: pretest monthly dosing mid-point termination	Pretest 3, 6, 12, 18, 24 months
		Urinalysis: dosing mid-point termination	Pretest 3, 6, 12, 18, 24 months

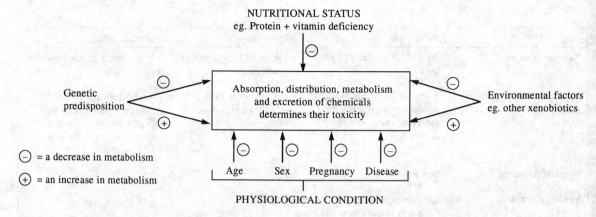

Figure 2 Factors affecting metabolism and toxicity

other chemicals), that such responses are less likely to occur in humans because of a dissimilarity in metabolism. Therefore, there is no absolute criterion for selecting a particular species, and most commonly rats, mice, rabbits and guinea-pigs are chosen for acute toxicity studies. However, toxicity within a particular species can vary with age, sex and health conditions, as well as genetic makeup (Figure 2). For example, immature animals may lack an effective xenobiotic metabolizing system. This may result in greater toxicity of the compound in an immature animal if an enzyme is responsible for detoxification or decrease toxicity if the enzyme system is responsible for activation (Table 3). Therefore, it is important to document all data on the animals' source, strain, sex, age, body weight and general health conditions.

Selection of Dose Levels

The purpose of an acute toxicity study is to establish the degree of toxicity of a new chemical entity, and the reader is reminded that formal determination of the LD_{50} value is not considered necessary nowadays and is more often measured in a semiquantitative limit test. In general, dose levels should be sufficient in number, at least three, to allow a clear demonstration of the dose–response relationship. In practice a pilot study will be needed to determine the order of toxicity. The British Toxicology Society's approach (van den Heuvel *et al.*, 1987) is to perform a preliminary 'sighting' study, using just three or four animals. Following administration, observations for effects are made. When toxicity

is not evident at the chosen dose level or where a severe toxic reaction requires, for animal welfare reasons, the removal of the animals from the study, the substance should be re-tested at the next higher or lower dose level (Table 4).

Principles of Acute Oral Tests

The test substance is dissolved in water, or corn oil/appropriate solvents if it is insoluble in aqueous media. If all attempts to dissolve the material fail, then appropriate suspending agents such as 0.5 per cent methyl cellulose or gum tragacanth in water can be used, provided that a homogeneous dosing preparation be produced. The dosing solution is administered by gastric intubation, and animals in the control groups should receive the same volume of vehicle, it being borne in mind that there are two methods of dosing the test material: (1) by varying the dosing volume, which means that animals are given different volumes of the same dosing solution; (2) by varying the concentration of the dosing solutions so that animals are given the same volume of vehicle.

The different methods of dosing can result in different toxicities for the same compound being obtained. For instance, when a large volume of corn oil is given orally, it will increase gastrointestinal mobility and have a laxative effect which may decrease the time the test substance is in the gut and available for absorption. Conversely, irritation of the gut will be decreased when the test substance is given in a diluted form. As the objective of an acute oral toxicity study is to determine systemic toxicity, which may include

Table 3   Consequences of metabolism

Process	Effect Pharmacological	Effect Toxicological	Example
Inactive compound activated by metabolism	Activation ———	——— Intoxication	Prontosil Fluoroacetate
Active compound changed into another active compound	Change in activity	———	Imipramine to desmethyl imipramine
		Detoxication or intoxication	Isoniazid — Peripheral neuropathy greater in slow acetylators — Hepatic damage greater in rapid acetylators
Active compound inactivated by metabolism	Inactivation	Detoxification	Barbiturates

Table 4   Investigation of acute oral toxicity using the BTS fixed-dose procedure criteria for classification for labelling purposes

Test dose (mg kg⁻¹)	Result	Action
5	Less than 90% survival	Classify as *very toxic*
	90% or more survival, but evident toxicity	Classify as *toxic*
	90% or more survival; no evident toxicity	Retest at 50 mg kg⁻¹
50	Less than 90% survival	Classify as *toxic*. Retest at 5 mg kg⁻¹ if not already tested at that dosage
	90% or more survival, but evident toxicity	Classify as *harmful*
	90% or more survival; no evident toxicity	Retest at 500 mg kg⁻¹
500	Less than 90% survival *or* evident toxicity and no deaths	Classify as *harmful*. Retest at 50 mg kg⁻¹ if not already tested at that dose
	No evident toxicity	*Unclassified*

Source: van den Heuvel *et al.* (1987).

gastrointestinal irritation, many toxicologists may choose constant concentration versus constant dose volume. However, most regulatory guidelines suggest a constant dose volume approach, with the dose volume being as small as possible and certainly not exceeding 10 ml kg⁻¹ body weight. Clearly the choice between constant concentration versus constant dose volume should be based on sound scientific judgement. If the dose is too large to be administered at a single time, it can be divided into equal doses with 3–4 h between them. Food should be withheld until the last dose, which should be given within 24 h of the first.

Principles of Acute Skin Tests

Skin exposure probably represents the most important route of exposure in the workplace, and, accordingly, knowledge of a chemical's dermal toxicity is prerequisite to its classification by regulatory authorities. The tests are commonly performed on rabbits and three types of dosing procedure are employed—namely unocclusive, semiocclusive and occlusive. In brief, the back or a band around the trunk of the animal is clipped free of hair, care being taken not to abrade the skin. The test substance should be applied uniformly to approximately 10 per cent of the body surface of the animal. Liquid test substances are generally applied undiluted. If the test substance is a solid, it is pulverized and moistened to a paste with physiological saline or appropriate solvent and spread evenly on the closely shaved skin. For the study to be meaningful, the effect of the vehicle on the dermal penetration of the test substance should be fully evaluated prior to the toxicity study. For occlusive or semiocclusive application, the application site is covered with an impervious material such as plastic sheet or with a porous gauze dressing, respectively. For unocclusive exposure, the test substance is applied to the skin as near to the head as possible, to prevent ingestion by preening of the application site. Alternatively, the correct amount of a liquid test substance may be applied underneath a plastic cuff with a long feeding needle, followed by gently rubbing the cuff to evenly distribute the test material.

The length of exposure ranges from 4 h to 24 h, depending on the guidelines followed, which, in general, agree that if no test-substance-related mortality is observed at 2 g kg^{-1}, testing at higher doses is not necessary. After 4–24 h exposure the site of application is inspected after gently removing the compound with cotton wool soaked in the appropriate solvent, and skin irritation can be assessed according to the scoring system described by Draize *et al*. (1944). However, the primary purpose of an acute dermal toxicity study is to provide information on the adverse, systemic effects of the test substance following percutaneous absorption.

Acute Inhalation Tests

Acute inhalation tests—technically difficult and specialized studies—may not be needed if inhalation exposure is not expected to occur because the physicochemical properties of the test substance are such that respirable particles cannot be generated even under the most favourable laboratory conditions. It is generally recognized that particles greater than 100 μm in diameter are unlikely to be inhaled, as they settle too rapidly. Those with diameters of 10–50 μm are likely to be retained in the nose and upper parts of the respiratory tract. Particles with diameters of less than 7 μm can reach the alveoli and are regarded as respirable. When inhalation studies are required, the exposure duration is usually 4–6 h and comprises either whole-body or head-only exposure. For details of the design of the different types of chambers as well as a discussion of the advantages/limitations of different methods of exposure, see Chapter 18 and Kennedy and Trochimowicz (1982). In brief, gases, followed by

volatile liquids, are the simplest atmospheres to generate and quantify. The quantity of a solid test substance in aerosols needs to be expressed in terms of both concentration and particle size.

Accordingly, the actual conduct of an inhalation experiment will differ for each type of material under study but the primary objective of an inhalation study is to derive a median lethal concentration (LC$_{50}$) following a single exposure, in much the same way as an LD$_{50}$ is derived from acute oral or dermal toxicity tests. The LC$_{50}$ value can then be used to derive short-term occupational exposure limits.

Interpretation of Data

It is accepted that all chemicals can produce toxicity under some experimental conditions—for example, if a sufficiently large dose is given. However, it would be misleading to conduct toxicity studies at unreasonably high dose levels just for the sake of demonstrating lethality/toxicity which may be irrelevant to compound itself. For example, extremely high oral doses of a practically non-toxic compound can cause blockage of the gastrointestinal tract and death (Chapter 1, pp. 14–15). However, such toxicity should not be related to the intrinsic characteristics of the test substance but rather to the fact that toxicity is a direct result of the physical blockage that was produced essentially by an inert substance. Accordingly, there must be a point where the toxicologist is confident to conclude that the test substance is practically non-toxic after acute exposure. For this reason an oral test limit of 5 g kg^{-1}, a cutaneous test limit of 2 g kg^{-1}, and an inhalation test limit of 50 mg m^{-3} are generally accepted. At these levels the investigator should conclude that administration of higher doses is not necessary.

REPEATED-DOSE (SUBACUTE AND SUBCHRONIC) TOXICITY STUDIES

Repeated-dose (subacute or subchronic) toxicity studies are designed to examine the adverse effects resulting from repeated exposure to a chemical at lower doses than used in acute studies. Primarily they demonstrate whether the accumulation of a compound, which may be virtually non-toxic in an acute study, disrupts vital body functions, rendering it toxic. Also, as repeated dose studies are conducted over longer periods of time, up to 10 per cent of the animal's life-span, than acute studies, they also demonstrate whether there is a latency period for the development of toxicity. Thus, although an animal may survive the acutely toxic action of a chemical, some irreversible damage to normal homoeostatic mechanisms may have occurred. A classical example of such an effect is the delayed neuropathy caused by many organophosphorous insecticides, which can manifest itself some weeks after the chemical has been eliminated from the body.

Such non-lethal adverse effects are obviously as undesirable as lethality itself, and so repeated-dose studies are considered to be essential for all new chemicals before their specific hazard can be assessed. Thus, unlike acute studies, the major end-point in a repeated-dose study is not mortality but some non-lethal parameter which can be defined by functional, biochemical, physiological or pathological effects (Table 5). Furthermore, the toxicological responses observed in a low-dose repeated-dose study may be quite different from those observed in a high-dose acute study. Certainly the pharmacokinetic profile of administering a small daily dose of a chemical in the diet will be very different from administering a large, single oral dose. For example, a single dose of a chemical may be detoxified and excreted harmlessly, while more prolonged exposure to the chemical may enhance its own metabolism,

leading to intoxication. Conversely, induction of the chemical's metabolism may lead to detoxification, depending on whether the parent compound or a metabolite is the toxic species (see Table 3, above). In view of the complicated changes in the disposition and metabolism of a chemical that can occur during prolonged exposure, a properly designed subchronic study will monitor a variety of clinical, haematological, biochemical and histopathological parameters (see Table 2, above) in order to detect a wide variety of effects. Such non-lethal adverse effects may be reversible, and therefore a reversibility phase is usually included in most subchronic studies. Obviously, irreversible changes will be weighted more heavily in reaching conclusions on the hazard a chemical may pose for humans.

Finally, the results of repeated-dose studies are generally extremely important in defining the no observable effect level and in selecting dose levels for chronic, reproductive (Chapter 39) and carcinogenicity (Chapters 37 and 38) studies.

Choice of Animal Species

Any common laboratory animal may be selected, but it is recommended that repeated-dose studies be conducted on at least two species, one being a rodent and the other a non-rodent. As with acute studies, the animal of choice should have a similar response to the test substance to that of humans. If this information is lacking, as is often the case, it is good practice to select the most sensitive species to evaluate the safety of a substance. Similarly, repeated-dose studies should always attempt to expose the animal by the route by which man is most likely to come into contact with the substance. In practice, dogs are the most commonly used non-rodent species, as, owing to their size, they have the advantage that blood samples can be collected during the study without it being necessary to kill the animal. The most common routes of administration employed in repeated-dose toxicity studies are oral, skin and respiratory. Thus, as repeated-dose studies are usually carried out over 10 per cent of the animal's life-span, oral and inhalation studies are usually carried out over 3 months in rodents and 1 year in dogs or monkeys, while repeated-dose skin studies are performed in a month or less.

Young and still-growing animals are preferred at the start of a subchronic study. Commonly rats

Table 5   Types of toxicity

> (1) Functional: based on clinical observations—e.g. behavioural toxicology, immunotoxicity
>
> (2) Biochemical: e.g. mechanism underlying dysfunction; absorption, distribution, metabolism and excretion of toxins
>
> (3) Structural: e.g. pathology based at the level of organs/tissues, including carcinogenesis
>
> (4) Environmental: e.g. Fear what? Monitor what? Ban what?
>
> (5) Newer aspects: e.g. irritancy, endocrine toxicology, genetic toxicology, reproductive toxicology, including fertility, teratology, postnatal development

and mice of 6–8 weeks of age are used, and, when dogs are chosen, these are 4–6 months old. Variation in responses due to sex differences may be important, and so each dose group should consist of equal numbers of male and female animals—usually 10–20 animals per sex per dose group for rodents and 6–8 per sex per dose group for dogs. The number of animals will need to be increased if interim kills are to be made and if the reversibility of effects is to be examined. In reversibility studies the animals are removed from the test compound at the end of the study and 2–4 weeks later are subjected to the same analyses as the animals comprising the main study.

Selection and Maintenance of Dose Levels

The primary purpose of a repeated-dose study is to define a no observable effect level as well as to determine which organs have the greatest susceptibility to the toxic effects of the chemical. Accordingly, ideal dose levels will be those that do not result in toxicity at the low dose, although this should be higher than the expected level of human exposure, only slight toxicity at the intermediate level and toxicity at the high dose, but not high enough to result in the death of more than 10 per cent of the group. In practice, this can only usually be achieved with a range-finding study of about 2 weeks duration prior to initiating the study. Toxicity in the pilot study is defined and based on the same measurements that will be employed in the main study.

In both repeated-dose and chronic toxicity studies the test substance is often incorporated into the diet or added to the drinking-water. The doses are commonly expressed in terms of concentration (parts per million; ppm) of the test substance in the diet or drinking-water or more usefully in terms of the test substance received by the animal [mg (kg body weight)$^{-1}$ day^{-1}]. In order to determine this, the exact amount of food or fluid consumed needs to be known. The approximate relationship of parts per million in the diet to mg (kg body weight)$^{-1}$ day^{-1} is shown in Table 6. However, food consumption varies from weaning to maturity, with younger animals consuming more food on a body weight basis. Therefore, in order to ensure constant dosing throughout the study, it will be necessary for the investigator to predict on a weekly basis changes

in body weight and food consumption, until they both stabilize, and adjust the concentration of the test substance in the diet according to the formulae shown in Table 7.

To avoid differences in food consumption due to changes in the calorific value of different batches of animal feed, the same batch of diet and, for that matter, the test substance should be used throughout the experiment. If different lots of test substance are used, its purity and chemical composition should not alter. Also, adequate mixing of the test substance with the diet should be ensured by monitoring its concentration at the top, middle and bottom of a batch of diet. In addition, samples of diet that have been kept at room temperature for the same duration as that for which the animals have been exposed to it should also be analysed to ensure the stability of the test material.

Finally, whenever food consumption appears excessive, account should be taken of the spillage of food. This can be very easily estimated if the animals are housed in cages with wire-grid bottoms and spilt food is collected on a sheet of absorbent paper. Obviously, faecal contributions to spilt food and food in the hopper are taken into account. In contrast, when a chemical is dosed via the drinking-water, spillage is more disastrous, because it cannot be recovered as easily as spilled feed. All oral dosing regimens are on a 7 day per week basis. A 5 days a week basis is usually sufficient for repeated-dose skin and inhalation studies.

Other methods of administration of the test substance include parenteral dosing, which is frequently used for pharmaceutical preparations, and subcutaneous or intramuscular implantation, which is commonly used for evaluating the toxicity of materials used in medical devices.

TESTING FOR CHRONIC TOXICITY

Nowadays the term 'chronic toxicity' encompasses investigations that include multigeneration reproduction studies and carcinogenicity tests. However, only classical chronic toxicity studies which are undertaken to define a safety factor between proposed use/exposure levels and toxicity will be described here. Chronic toxicity studies usually consist of three treatment groups plus a control group, and the xenobiotic is admin-

Table 6   Approximate relation of parts per million in the diet to mg per kg body weight per day

Animal	Weight (kg)	Food consumed per day (g) (liquids omitted)	Type of diet	Conversion factors	
				1 ppm in diet to mg (kg body weight)$^{-1}$ day^{-1}	1 mg (kg body weight)$^{-1}$ day^{-1} to 1 ppm in diet
Mouse	0.02	3	Dry laboratory chow diets	0.150	7
Chick	0.40	50		0.125	8
Rat (young)	0.10	10		0.100	10
Rat (old)	0.40	20		0.050	20
Guinea-pig	0.75	30		0.040	25
Rabbit	2.0	60		0.030	33
Dog	10.0	250		0.025	40
Cat	2	100	Moist, semi-solid diets	0.050	20
Monkey	5	250		0.050	20
Dog	10	750		0.075	13
Man	60	1 500		0.025	40
Pig or sheep	60	2 400	Relatively dry grain forage mixtures	0.040	25
Cow (maintenance)	500	7 500		0.015	65
Cow (fattening)	500	15 000		0.030	33
Horse	500	10 000		0.020	50

Source: WHO (1987).

Table 7   Formulae for dietary studies

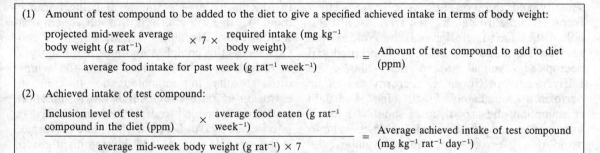

(1)   Amount of test compound to be added to the diet to give a specified achieved intake in terms of body weight:

$$\frac{\text{projected mid-week average body weight (g rat}^{-1}) \times 7 \times \text{required intake (mg kg}^{-1} \text{ body weight)}}{\text{average food intake for past week (g rat}^{-1} \text{ week}^{-1})} = \text{Amount of test compound to add to diet (ppm)}$$

(2)   Achieved intake of test compound:

$$\frac{\text{Inclusion level of test compound in the diet (ppm)} \times \text{average food eaten (g rat}^{-1} \text{ week}^{-1})}{\text{average mid-week body weight (g rat}^{-1}) \times 7} = \text{Average achieved intake of test compound (mg kg}^{-1} \text{ rat}^{-1} \text{ day}^{-1})$$

Source: Dr C. J. Powell, personal communication.

istered 7 days a week for 2 years to rats or for 18 months to mice. A second non-rodent species is usually utilized. Dose levels are usually selected after a 3 month range-finding study with enough doses to find a level which suppresses body weight gain slightly—i.e. by 10 per cent. This dose, defined as the maximum tolerated dose (MTD), is selected as the highest dose. The two other dose levels are usually ¼ MTD and ⅛ MTD. Alternatively, with a relatively non-toxic compound the dose may be chosen as not exceeding 100–200 times the anticipated human dose. Dose setting also requires careful consideration of the end-use of the chemical under study. For example, if the chemical is intended as a pharmaceutical which will only be used under medical supervision, then the dose levels may never be set at the MTD but rather will be related to the maximum therapeutic dose. Similarly, if the compound is expected to contaminate foodstuffs, the highest dose is likely to be 100 times the maximum detectable level in food.

Pharmacokinetic data (see Chapters 4 and 5) are also particularly pertinent in selecting the dose levels to be employed. For example, in its simplest form comparison of the day 1 and day 90 LD_{50} values, the so-called 'chronicity factor', will indicate something about the *in vivo* handling of the chemical. Thus, if the 90 day LD_{50} is much lower than the LD_{50} value derived from the acute study, it is probable that the compound is slowly metabolized and will accumulate within the animal during a chronic toxicity study. In such cases where the metabolism and/or excretion of a chemical becomes saturated, relatively minor pathways of metabolism may become of major significance to the toxic effects observed. Whatever dose levels are chosen, they are maintained in the same way as that described for repeated-dose studies.

INTERPRETATION OF THE RESULTS OF REPEATED-DOSE AND CHRONIC TOXICITY STUDIES

In life observations

Because all subacute, subchronic and chronic toxicity studies are expensive to perform, observations should be made frequently, and the onset, severity and duration of any observed effect recorded in plain English. Similarly, loss of valuable tissues due to autolysis must be avoided, and severely moribund animals should be killed and necropsied. Animals found dead should be refrigerated, not frozen, if necropsy cannot be performed immediately. Finally, food and fluid consumption and growth rates should be determined on a fixed schedule and double-checked to avoid dosing errors which may invalidate the study. Also, expression of the food consumed per unit weight gain is a useful way of assessing the effect of a treatment on eating habits and food utilization. Fluid consumption is a useful way of identifying an agent with a diuretic action.

Organ Weights

In terms of the total cost of a subchronic or chronic study, weighing the organs at necropsy is both cheap and may reveal a specific target organ response which could be confirmed by histopathological examination (see Chapter 10). The most easily dissected organs are the liver, lung, kidney, spleen and testes. However, considerable vari-

ation in the weight of other organs can occur— e.g. of heart due to entrapped blood, of adrenals due to adhering fat, of brain due to where the spinal cord is cut—but these variations can be avoided by careful dissection technique to a standardized protocol. Organ weights are best expressed as a percentage of the animal's body weight.

Histopathology

See Chapter 10 for details of appropriate techniques. Much emphasis is placed on histopathological changes which are supported by clinical chemistry.

Ophthalmoscopy

Ophthalmoscopy will reveal damage to the retina but examination may be difficult in rodents if they are bled, for haematology and clinical chemistry, from the retro-orbital sinus.

Haematology

Blood can easily be collected by venepuncture from large species and from the retro-orbital sinus in rodents under anaesthesia, it being borne in mind that this will interfere with subsequent ophthalmoscopy. Bleeding from the tail-tip of rodents avoids this complication but the tendency of investigators to 'milk' blood from the animal often results in anomalous results due to extrusion of extracellular fluids. At termination, rodents may be bled from the abdominal aorta or inferior vena cava. Bleeding should be performed at the same time of day and the treatment groups should be randomized to avoid spurious changes in blood constituents due to circadian rhythms, which can occur as a result of the time involved if the dose groups are bled in sequence.

The clinical characteristics of blood are determined after treatment with an anticoagulant, the choice of which depends on the analyses to be performed—e.g. chelating agents such as EDTA may interfere with clinical chemistry assays and, therefore, the anticoagulant chosen should be checked out. Blood used for clinical chemistry must not be haemolysed, as not only will this result in a lower haematocrit and erythrocyte count, but also red cell constituents such as LDH, aminotransferases, potassium and creatinine will be released into the plasma and may lead to falsely high values.

The classic haematological measurements are erythrocyte, leukocyte and differential leukocyte counts, haemoglobin concentration, haematocrit, platelet and reticulocyte counts. From these data the mean corpuscular haemoglobin (MCH), mean corpuscular haemoglobin concentration (MCHC) and mean corpuscular volume (MCV) can be calculated and blood dyscrasias identified which may necessitate evaluation of the bone marrow.

CLINICAL CHEMISTRY

Standardized techniques need to be applied within any one laboratory, and intra- and interlaboratory variance needs to be established before the values have any real meaning (see Chapter 11). Also, the introduction of automated equipment permits effortless analysis of nearly every biochemical parameter that can be measured, but before requesting a multitude of analyses the toxicologist should carefully think about selecting a battery of tests to identify specific target organ effects in the acute and subchronic studies and then focus on the area of concern in more depth in the chronic study.

URINALYSIS

Urinalysis is easy to perform but interpretation is fraught with difficulty due to the crude procedures often used in collection. Hair, room dust, bacteria, food and even the contents of the drinking-water bottle have been known to settle in urine collected in trays placed below cages. If there is a real concern and reason to consider urinalysis important, then the urine should be collected from sufficient animals in a manner that makes the analyses meaningful (e.g. use of metabolism cages), as the clinical chemistry of urine can provide useful toxicological information:

(1) If carefully collected over a specified period of time, the volume of urine may be useful for fluid balance assessments; e.g. diuresis, dehydration, etc.

(2) *Osmolality* Indicates the ability of the kidney to concentrate urine.

(3) *pH* Urine has a pH of 4.6–8.0 with a mean around 6.0, but its pH is meaningless unless urine is collected directly from the bladder, as dissolved CO_2 quickly dissipates after urination. Starvation and ketosis increase the acidity of urine.

(4) *Glucose* High levels of reducing sugars, which can be measured by simple dipstick methods, occur in diabetes.

(5) Coloration/turbidity increases when urine becomes supersaturated, and microscopy may show crystals indicating formation of kidney or bladder stones. Red coloration is indicative of haemoglobinuria, haematuria or hepatic porphyria.

CONCLUSION

The life of modern man has been greatly improved by the development of chemicals employed in all spheres of human activity. However, in doing so we must ensure that our own existence is not endangered by their uncontrolled use, about which we know so little but are beginning to learn more. What we do know is obtained from animal studies conducted under controlled conditions on a short-, intermediate- or long-term basis. All of these studies are looking for dose–response relationships so that we may extrapolate them to the human situation, which is often uncontrollable. Animal studies can tell us about no observable effect levels, which are used to derive acceptable daily intakes for environmental contaminants and other chemicals.

The toxicological studies described in this chapter are applicable to most xenobiotics and, when coupled with tests for reproductive toxicity, mutagenicity/genotoxicity, and carcinogenicity, will usually satisfy the regulatory requirements of most countries. Because of this overriding ambition, many toxicological experiments have become rather stereotyped. However, a toxicological experiment should not be different from an experiment in any other scientific discipline. Thus, its experimental design should be logical and, hence, there is no valid reason to adhere to a standard protocol if this is inappropriate for the specific test material. Regulatory guidelines are only a useful index of what is required and should not be used as a rigid checklist, because there are virtually no findings in experimental toxicology that can be simply extrapolated to man and his ecosystem without careful thought. When it is considered appropriate to modify an approach recommended by a particular regulatory agency, it is wise to discuss this with, and get agreement from, the agency in order to avoid subsequent administrative complications.

Furthermore, by performing experiments to a standardized protocol, toxicologists are missing real opportunities to unravel some of the most fascinating problems of biology by identifying chemical tools to probe life processes. There may often be too much emphasis on the generation of data with very little time available for scientific interpretation. It is this aspect of toxicological research that must be encouraged to survive or else the science will become as stereotyped as the studies conventionally performed for economic/ regulatory purposes. Therefore, consider abandoning a standard protocol if it is inappropriate, and feel free to increase the number of animals employed, particularly with regard to reversibility studies, because the best way of reducing the number of experiments performed on living animals is to conduct them properly. However, as noted above, studies carried out for regulatory agencies should be discussed with the agency before proceeding with extensive modifications.

It is essential to randomize the animals at the beginning of the study as well as during intermediate and terminal investigations. Always look for dose–response relationships and compare the data obtained with the controls as well as appropriate historical values for animals of the same age, sex and physiological condition. Above all, ensure that all observations are recorded in plain English. Remember that the primary purpose of a toxicological experiment is the same as that of any other scientific study—that is, that it can be repeated, blemishes and all!

REFERENCES

Draize, J. H., Woodward, G. and Calvery, H. O. (1944). Methods for the study of irritations and toxicity of substances applied topically to the skin and mucous membranes. *J. Pharmacol. Exptl Therap.*, **82**, 377–390

Hayes, A. W. (Ed.) (1982). *Principles and Methods of Toxicology*. Raven Press, New York

Kennedy, G. L. and Trochimowicz, H. J. (1982). Inhalation toxicology. In Hayes, A. W. (Ed.), *Principles and Methods of Toxicology*. Raven Press, New York, pp. 185–208

Tee, L. B. G., Davies, D. S., Seddon, C. E. and Boobis, A. R. (1987). Species differences in the hepatotoxicity of paracetamol are due to differences in the rate of conversion to its cytotoxic metabolite. *Biochem. Pharmacol.*, **36**, 1041–1052

van den Heuvel, M. J., Dayan, A. D. and Shillaker, R. O. (1987). Evaluation of the BTS approach to testing of substances and preparations for their acute toxicity. *Human Toxicol.*, **6**, 279–291

WHO (1987). *Principles for the Safety Assessment of Food Additives and Contaminants in Food*. Environmental Health Criteria No. 70. World Health Organization, Geneva

FURTHER READING

Ecobichon, D. J. (1992). *The Basis of Toxicity Testing*. CRC Press, Boca Raton, Florida

Svendsen, P. and Hau, J. (1994). *Handbook of Laboratory Animal Science, Vol. 2*. CRC Press, Boca Raton, Florida

World Health Organization (1978). *Principles and Methods for Evaluating the Toxicity of Chemicals. Environmental Health Criteria, No. 6*. World Health Organization, Geneva

10 Pathological Techniques in Toxicology

Peter Greaves

GENERAL APPROACHES

For over one hundred years microscopic evaluation of pathological alterations in human tissues has made major contributions to our understanding of diseases and remains a significant diagnostic tool in human medicine. Rather than diminish in importance in the face of novel imaging techniques, recent advances in immunology and biotechnology have served to reaffirm the central role of histopathology in the diagnosis of human diseases. This has occurred because the transfer of new technologies into the pathology laboratory has led to the development of new histological staining procedures. These new methods represent a logical extension to the use of special stains on tissue sections and have provided the pathologist with powerful new objective techniques which allow a more precise morphological and functional correlation of changes in tissues.

A similar spectrum of both classical histological and new technologies has also made important contributions in both experimental pathology and toxicology. Histopathological evaluation of tissue sections represents a major technique in experimental studies of human diseases. It also has a central role in conventional toxicology studies which are performed to assess the toxicity of many xenobiotics, including novel therapeutic agents and industrial chemicals.

The important place of histological assessment of tissues in regulatory toxicology has given rise to the development of an exacting professional discipline, that of the toxicological pathologist. The work of the toxicological pathologist requires rigorous training in comparative pathology and clinical pathology, as well as an understanding of the principles of toxicology and experimental method. It is also important to understand the kinetics and metabolism of administered xenobiotics, particularly therapeutic agents. Only in this way can pathological alterations be related to the degree of exposure of organs and tissues to administered agents and their metabolites (Zbinden, 1988). A thorough knowledge of pathological techniques applicable to experimental pathology and problem solving in toxicology is an important and integral component of the skills needed by the toxicological pathologist.

The aim of this chapter is to describe pathological techniques and technologies applicable to the morphological evaluation of alterations in tissue sections produced in laboratory animal species during the toxicity testing of chemicals. An attempt is also made to place the techniques in the context of the special problems of interpretation posed by changes induced by drugs and industrial chemicals in specific organs and organ systems.

Basic Techniques in Autopsy and Histology Practice

Fundamental to good histopathological evaluation of tissue sections is a detailed autopsy with careful observation of the organs for any abnormalities and appropriate selection of tissues. The autopsy is the responsibility of the pathologist. It is conducted or supervised by an experienced pathologist, usually with the help of trained prosectors.

Whereas in human autopsy practice and in experimental pathology studies, tissue sampling is usually directed towards particular lesions or organs of direct relevance to the problem under study, a more systematic approach is usually adopted in conventional toxicity studies. Most international regulatory guidelines require 30 or 40 tissues to be taken from all animals in most conventional toxicity studies, and these are usually defined by the standard protocols of laboratories performing regulatory work. It is important to remain acutely aware that even the most complete tissue list remains a selective process, and a careful inspection of the tissues for abnormalities at autopsy remains mandatory.

Less obvious is the fact that the selection of blocks and number of slides among different laboratories to achieve complete tissue lists may be quite different. For instance, some laboratories will take two blocks of tissue from the rat liver in carcinogenicity bioassays, others as many as four (Maronpot *et al.*, 1989). Thorough histological examination of the heart of the beagle dog requires at least five or six blocks to provide reasonable sampling of the four chambers, coronary arteries and areas sensitive to ischaemic damage, such as the papillary muscles of the left ventricle. However, this number of sections may appear unreasonable to many laboratories examining large numbers of dogs for toxicity studies. This highlights the difficulties of tissue selection and underlines the need for careful inspection of tissues at autopsy and modulation of the tissue sampling procedure to take account of the particular chemical under study.

For routine purposes, formalin or formol saline is employed by most laboratories for practically all organs except eyes and testes, where Bouin's, Zenker's or Davidson's fixative is used. Occasionally, Bouin's fluid is employed routinely for all tissues (Taradach and Greaves, 1984). Although fixation in Bouin's fluid produces excellent cytology, its cost-effectiveness leaves much to be desired when used routinely, and the simplicity of formalin is usually preferred. Microwave fixation has potential for the pathology laboratory engaged in toxicology (Boon and Kok, 1987), but it has not been exploited to any great extent in this context and initial results have not been entirely satisfactory. Haematoxylin and eosin remains the more widely used stain in most laboratories, supplemented where appropriate on a semiroutine basis with a Romanovsky stain for haemopoietic cells, periodic acid-Schiff (PAS) for hepatic glycogen, glomerular basement membrane and the acrosome on testicular germ cells, trichrome and elastic stains for the myocardium and blood vessels, and oil red O for neutral lipids.

Organ Weights

Some, but not all, regulatory guidelines indicate that some organs should be weighed during the course of the autopsy in conventional repeat-dose toxicity studies (Alder and Zbinden, 1988). The extent to which organs are weighed varies between laboratory, but organ weighing is a useful adjunct to macroscopic assessment. Therefore, the selection of organs for weighing is the primary responsibility of the study pathologist. Weighing helps to focus the histopathological

examination on key target organs such as the liver and kidney, the weights of which are quite frequently altered by administration of xenobiotics. Heart weight is a guide to potential cardiac alterations and is especially important in the assessment of cardiovascular drugs. Likewise, the lungs are weighed in inhalation studies, for this can provide a useful indication of the extent of oedema or accumulation of exudate. Brain weight is employed as a stable reference point in adult animals, for it is fairly independent of body weight changes. The weights of endocrine organs are useful guides to alterations in the endocrine status of laboratory animals. However, weighing a small and firmly attached organ such as the thyroid can severely disrupt its quality and orientation in the sections to offset any apparent advantage.

Testicular weights correlate with testicular toxicity, and weights can be compared with in-life measurement of testicular size (Heywood and James, 1978). Weighing the testis is a useful precaution at the early phase of development of a novel drug prior to any assessment of male fertility. By contrast, ovarian weight is highly variable, as a consequence of cyclical ovarian development, and is, therefore, a less sensitive indicator of treatment-induced changes in the female reproductive system.

Histopathological Evaluation of Conventional Toxicological Studies

Much has been written on methods in histopathological assessment. However, it requires, above all, a systematic and meticulous approach to the assessment of tissue sections correlating in-life observations, autopsy findings, organ weight and clinical pathology changes with histopathological alterations. Careful selection of diagnostic terminology is essential because many of the terms utilized in experimental pathology have been borrowed from human pathology, where they may be applied to quite specific clinical conditions not relevant to laboratory animal species. Lucid summary reports are also essential.

In conventional subacute and chronic toxicity studies as well as in carcinogenicity bioassays, a complete set of tissues from the top-dose and control animals is routinely examined. In addition, any target organs or tissues showing tumours or other macroscopic alterations at autopsy in animals from intermediate-dose groups are also assessed. This baseline approach is outlined in some of the regulatory guidelines. However, some pathologists avoid this selective approach and examine all tissues sampled from all animals. This approach is perhaps more costly from a histological processing point of view, but has the merit of completeness and forms a more satisfactory basis for the rapid reporting of all the salient histopathological findings in every dose group.

The error which develops from the increased awareness of a lesion by the pathologist only after examining a considerable number of animals has been aptly termed by Roe (1977) 'diagnostic drift'. It is important to have a good understanding of the nature of any lesion before grading is undertaken and for particular care to be given to selection of the 'cut-off' point for each grade (Greaves and Faccini, 1984). The appropriateness of blind slide reading as a means to avoid bias is another point of debate. However, blind slide reading as a routine process conflicts with the need to have relevant clinical, clinical pathology and macroscopic data to make an appropriate tissue diagnosis. For this reason, only doubtful lesions which persist after a careful and integrated non-blind review of these sections are those which should be evaluated in a properly designed blind review (Newberne and de la Iglesia, 1985).

Peer review of pathological findings and quality assurance audit of the processes in histopathological assessment have also become more important components of regulatory toxicology studies in recent years. It is generally accepted that a peer review or check of a percentage of the diagnoses in a particular study by a second pathologist provides a level of security for regulatory authorities. Some regulatory authorities have taken a clear stance on the audit of the processes which take place in the office of the toxicological pathologist. For instance, the UK regulatory authorities require a critical phase audit of this part of the study. This includes evaluation of the completeness, quality and labelling of glass slides given to the pathologist, review of the remarks made by the pathologist on missing or poor-quality slides, and verification that the pathologist has sufficient time to carry out the work required in the study protocol (Department of Health, 1988).

For over a decade the pathologist has been assisted in the evaluation of toxicity and carcino-genicity studies by computer recording, storage and collation of macroscopic findings and their corresponding histopathological diagnoses (Faccini and Naylor, 1979; Herrick *et al.*, 1983; Clapp and McNamee, 1985). This has been a particularly important contribution to the timely and accurate reporting of carcinogenicity studies where the number of observations in older animals render hand recording and tabulation a time-consuming process, prone to transcription error. This has had a significant impact in the development of novel drugs, as the carcinogenicity studies are usually performed towards the end of the development programme, where the results from these studies may be needed before the drug can be extensively employed for therapeutic purposes.

Histochemistry and Cytochemistry

Histochemistry is a tool which can be regarded as a system of chemical morphology which adds another dimension to the characterization of alterations in tissues. Changes to structures, cells or organelles can be assessed by the changes in their chemical structure or enzymatic activity. For instance the well-studied methods for alkaline phosphatase demonstrate activity at the cell membrane where active transport occurs and can be used to localize and detect changes in structures such as the surface of the intestinal epithelium and the brush border of proximal renal tubules (Faccini, 1982). The histochemical method for $5'$-nucleotidase is also an excellent marker for plasma membrane. Measures of peroxidase activity can be used to localize peroxisomes. Succinate dehydrogenase is used as an indicator for the Krebs' cycle and mitochondrial enzyme activity (reviewed by Chayen *et al.*, 1973). The enzyme gamma-glutamyl transpeptidase is regarded as the classical marker for neoplastic foci in the rodent liver. Glucose–6-phosphate dehydrogenase, the regulatory enzyme of the pentose phosphate shunt, which provides ribose for the synthesis of nucleic acids, is elevated in a number of malignant conditions in man (Ibrahim *et al.*, 1983) and can also be used as a marker for foci of hepatocellular alteration in rats (Greaves *et al.*, 1986).

It is important to note that the use of histochemical methods for the localization of tissue constituents or pathological alterations in this way is conceptually different from quantitative cytochemistry. This form of cytochemistry combines procedures for the production of insoluble chromophores by rigorous, controlled biochemical reactions with optical methods for their measurement (Chayen, 1984). To achieve enzyme measurement in this way, it is imperative to avoid techniques such as fixation, use of clearing agents and embedding media which produce loss of enzymatic activity. Therefore, supercooling of tissues and the use of colloid stabilizers are essential in order to facilitate chemical reactions and the precipitation of insoluble reaction products close to the sites of active groups where they are generated (Chayen, 1984). Coloured reaction products can then be visualized and measured by a spectrophotometer built around a microscope. This is coupled to a system to assess optically heterogeneous areas, using methods such as scanning and integrating microdensitometry.

Quantitative cytochemistry has advantages over biochemical measurements because it is nondisruptive, retains spatial relationships and relates activity measurement to histology. Moreover, it requires only small pieces of tissue. However, these advantages are offset by the fact that it is a labour-intensive technology. Quantitative cytochemical analysis has been undertaken to measure the effects of hormones in target tissues (Chayen, 1984), and in the characterization of the distribution of glycogen, glutathione and enzymatic activity within the liver lobule of rodents treated with xenobiotics (Irisarri and Mompon, 1983; Mompon *et al.*, 1987).

Immunocytochemistry

Immunocytochemistry of routinely fixed and processed tissues has been one of the major technological advances in the histopathological evaluation and diagnosis of human diseases, because it represents an independent, objective method of cell identification against which traditional subjective morphological criteria can be compared (Taylor and Kledzig, 1981). Immunocytochemistry has been particularly useful in the characterization of human neoplasms. However, unlike enzyme cytochemistry, it only demonstrates the presence of antigenic determinants and is unable to demonstrate activity of cellular systems. Although not widely employed in the histopathological evaluation of conventional toxicity and car-

cinogenicity studies, it represents a powerful tool for solving of certain problems in toxicology. Many of the commercially available monoclonal and polyclonal antisera cross-react well with the tissues of laboratory animals and can be used in the histopathological evaluation of toxicity studies, provided that appropriate controls are applied. Examples include polypeptide and protein hormones, metabolizing enzymes, structural proteins and cell markers such as S100 protein and intermediate filaments. Use of peroxidase-labelled or biotinated antibodies against bromodeoxyuridine (BrdUrd) represents an alternative to autoradiographic detection of cell proliferation using tritiated thymidine. Although haemopoietic cells retain species-specific surface markers, monoclonal antibodies to lymphocytic and monocytic surface membrane markers are available for rodents and dogs and can be used in the characterization of xenobiotic-induced alterations in the haemopoietic and lymphoid systems.

Lectin Histochemistry

A technique closely allied to immunocytochemistry is that of lectin histochemistry. The term 'lectin' is applied to proteins and glycoprotein extracted from invertebrates and lower vertebrates that have the capacity to bind sugar groups and glycoproteins in quite specific ways. For many years studies on red blood cells have been performed with the lectin concanavalin A, which possesses haemagglutination properties. More recently, lectins labelled with peroxidase or fluoroscein have been used to demonstrate specific sugar groups and glycoproteins histochemically in tissue sections (Nicholson, 1974; Spicer and Schulte, 1982). Lectin histochemistry has been used for the characterization of mucins, the demonstration of cell structures in normal tissues and changes in cell surface expression in malignant cells (Walker, 1985). In toxicology their primary use is in the characterization of changes induced by xenobiotics in structures which are well delineated by labelled lectins such as the biliary canaliculus, testicular germ cell acrosome, renal tubule, and bronchial and gastrointestinal epithelium (Geleff *et al.*, 1986; Masson *et al.*, 1986). Conventional formalin fixation and paraffin wax embedding is frequently adequate for the application of labelled lectin histochemistry, although alcoholic fixation or unfixed frozen sections may provide superior results.

Electron Microscopy

Although electron microscopy is widely used as a basic research tool, transmission electron microscopy also has a well-established role in the characterization of subcellular structural alterations in tissues which have been modified by the effects of xenobiotics. Despite the fact that electron microscopy only provides a static morphological assessment of cells, its ability to characterize changes in subcellular organelles can provide valuable information about any functional deficit. A common, almost routine application of electron microscopy in regulatory toxicology studies is the characterization of cytoplasmic alterations associated with liver weight changes and hepatocellular hypertrophy. Electron microscopy, in contrast to light microscopic examination, allows the characterization of changes such as proliferation of the smooth endoplasmic reticulum, peroxisomal or mitochondrial proliferation, and phospholipidosis. It is also important in the exclusion of subcellular degeneration in vital organs such as the heart when unexplained macroscopic or weight changes are seen without a light microscopic correlate.

A variety of methods for the selection, perfusion and immersion fixation of tissues have been proposed for the application of electron microscopy in toxicity studies. Optimum fixation is obtained by whole-body perfusion with an aldehyde fixative, but this may conflict with procedures necessary for other components of a toxicity study, such as routine histopathological examination, and biochemical, metabolism and kinetic studies. One compromise is perfusion fixation of freshly isolated samples of organs such as lung or liver. This provides superior tissue preparation to that obtained by immersion fixation (Roberts *et al.*, 1990).

Despite the technological advances in transmission electron microscopy, especially semiautomated tissue processing and staining, it remains a demanding and labour-intensive process. Furthermore, it is highly selective and only small samples of tissues can be examined. Therefore, any electron microscopic work performed within the context of a toxicity study should have precisely defined objectives so that appropriate samples are selected and examined. Electron microscopy is not a method for speculative study of tissues in toxicity studies and defining 'no effect dose levels'.

The use of larger, semithin (1–3 μm thick) plastic- or resin-embedded sections is a cost-effective compromise between electron microscopy and conventional light microscopy. Sometimes termed 'high-resolution light microscopy', light microscopic evaluation of semithin sections can provide a means of avoiding extensive use of the electron microscope, because it can locate cytoplasmic organelles in a way sometimes not possible in paraffin-embedded material.

Scanning electron microscopy is not considered a pivotal instrument in toxicological pathology. It has some applications, notably in the study of early chemical-induced changes on epithelial surfaces such as the gastrointestinal mucosa and the bladder epithelium. It also forms the basis for a robust technique for the examination of the middle ear in laboratory animals treated with ototoxic agents (Astbury and Read, 1982).

Immunocytochemistry can also be applied to electron microscopic study in order to define the subcellular distribution of antigenic sites. Ultrastructural autoradiography using tritium-labelled xenobiotics, especially when performed using quantitative methods such as the so-called hypothetical grain analysis, is valuable for the identification of sites of accumulation of drugs and chemicals within cells and may provide information on the possible modes of their cellular actions (Read *et al.*, 1985).

Morphometric Methods

Morphometry represents a powerful tool applicable to the light and electron microscopic evaluation of xenobiotic-induced cellular and tissue changes in animal toxicity studies. Morphometric study supports subjective histopathological descriptions or diagnoses by sharpening the distinction between normal and altered structures on a solid, quantitative basis. It also allows values of different variables to be compared and correlated (Pesce, 1987). Morphometry has been applied to the study of a variety of organ toxicities, notably in the liver, pulmonary tract and brain (Weibel, 1979; de la Iglesia and McGuire, 1981; de la Iglesia *et al.*, 1982; Barry and Crapo, 1985). Morphometric analysis requires application of good statistical methods in the choice of numbers of animals, of number of samples per animal and of the quantity of data points per sample, and in the final data analysis. In the measurement of the basic parameters such as volume density, surface density and numerical density, account should be taken of potential artefacts due to shrinkage of tissues following fixation and processing, as well as the problems posed by magnification factors (Barry and Crapo, 1985). Semiautomated digital image analysis has also been applied in the quantification of immunocytochemical staining in the toxicology laboratory (Levine *et al.*, 1987).

Application of Molecular Biology Technology

Recombinant DNA technology represents the most recent transfer of basic research technology into the pathology laboratory. Molecular probes have been used to examine the structure and expression of specific genes in both normal and neoplastic human tissues. Current applications in clinical and anatomical pathology include rapid microbiological diagnosis, study of oncogene expression, gene amplification and drug resistance of tumours, and molecular characterization of inherited diseases and their prenatal diagnosis (Fenoglio-Preiser and Willman, 1987).

These techniques have been widely applied to questions in experimental pathology, where they provide the pathologist with new opportunities for the study of mechanisms in pathological processess (DeLellis and Wolfe, 1987). They have been applied to the study of experimental tumorigenesis, particularly rodent models of hepatic carcinogenesis. Recent studies of activated oncogenes in hepatic neoplasms in B6C3F1 mice using DNA transfection techniques have suggested that they are finding a place in toxicology and human risk assessment. On the basis of patterns of oncogene activation shown by these methods, it may be possible to distinguish naturally occurring mouse hepatic neoplasms from those induced by administration of xenobiotics (Reynolds *et al.*, 1987).

METHODS APPLICABLE TO SPECIFIC ORGAN SYSTEMS

Skin and Subcutaneous Tissue

Careful visual inspection remains the principal component of the assessment of skin alterations or changes in the pelage of laboratory animals used in conventional toxicity studies. In studies in which compounds are administered systemically, any skin abnormalities detected during life or at autopsy should be examined histologically. In addition, sections taken from carefully selected standard sites should also be sampled for routine histopathological examination. Haematoxylin and eosin staining is sufficient for most purposes.

Drugs and chemicals given systemically may affect the skin in a number of ways. Pigmented skin or hair may lose its normal colour and albino skin may become coloured by administration of pigmented compounds or chemicals with pigmented metabolites. Agents with effects on sebaceous glands may alter the normal glossy pelage of laboratory animals. Compounds such as bleomycin, which adversely affect mitotic activity in squamous epithelium, lead to ulceration and inflammation in zones subjected to minor spontaneous trauma of everyday life, such as the feet and tail (Thompson *et al.*, 1972; Szczech and Tucker, 1985).

Studies conducted to study topical irritancy, contact sensitization or phototoxic activity usually employ rabbits or guinea-pigs. Here reliance is commonly placed on visual inspection and a semiquantitative assessment of the degree of erythema, swelling, erosion and ulceration of the treated skin without histopathological examination. A mouse ear model has been proposed for study of skin irritancy, on the basis that it can be more accurately quantified by the measurement of ear thickness (Patrick *et al.*, 1985). Although histopathological techniques are not routinely practised in the assessment of skin irritation and sensitization, histological examination can serve to define the nature of any induced changes. Semiquantitative histological examination has been shown to be a useful adjunct to naked eye assessment of the epidermis in experimental irritancy studies (Ingram and Grasso, 1975).

Immunohistochemical study of Ia antigen expression in antigen presenting cells of the epidermis has been used in studying delayed hypersensitivity reactions in the guinea-pig skin (Sobel and Colvin, 1986). The ultrastructural appearances of Langerhans' cells have also been shown to be modulated by topical application of sensitizing or irritating substances. Irritating agents cause their degeneration and vacuolation, whereas sensitization increases numbers of cytoplasmic Birkbeck granules and coated vesicles (Kolde and Knop, 1987).

Histological examination of injection site injury and the local damage around subcutaneously implanted biomaterials is an essential part of the assessment of their irritancy potential. It is important to evaluate not only the character and severity of the surrounding cellular reaction to these materials, but also the time-course of the inflammatory and healing process in comparison with known negative and positive control substances (Autian, 1972; Darby, 1987; Henderson *et al.*, 1987).

In carcinogenicity studies perfomed in rodents, tumours of the skin and subcutaneous tissues are usually adequately diagnosed by conventional microscopic techniques. In certain instances immunocytochemistry and electron microscopy are helpful in the characterization of soft-tissue tumours. Mesenchymal cells can be more accurately defined by the presence of immunoreactive myoglobin, lysozyme, alpha-1 antichymotrypsin, intermediate filaments and other cytoplasmic antigens, as well as by electron microscopic evaluation of subcellular structures such as myofilaments, cross-striations, basal lamina and lysosomes (Greaves and Barsoum, 1990).

Mammary Gland

In laboratory animals the mammary gland represents a sensitive indicator of the pituitary–gonadal axis. It is liable to develop neoplasms either spontaneously with advancing age or following prolonged hormonal derangement induced by administration of xenobiotics. For these reasons mammary glands are examined carefully in conventional toxicity studies, both during life and at autopsy, and this is followed by histological examination.

The basic structure of the mammary gland is similar in all laboratory animal species. It is composed of a system of alveolar buds or acini connected by a system of branching ducts which eventually converge on the nipple. Ducts and alveolar tissues are not static structures but respond to changes of the oestrous or menstrual cycles, pregnancy and lactation and to those xenobiotics which induce analogous hormonal alterations. Therefore, histological assessment of treatment-induced changes in these structures can provide useful information about the nature of associated hormonal derangements.

As laboratory rodents and beagle dogs possess several pairs of mammary glands, routine histological examination is usually conducted on a selected number of sites, frequently on one gland from each side plus any other showing macroscopic abnormality. Orientation remains a difficulty in small inactive glands but an attempt is made to take a section which includes the nipple, adjacent skin and underlying mammary ducts and acini.

Conventional haematoxylin and eosin stained sections are quite sufficient for mammary gland assessment, although myoepithelial cells which surround the ducts and acini may be difficult to visualize without special techniques. Immunocytochemical staining for cytokeratins and myosin is helpful in making this distinction (Warburton *et al.*, 1982; Dulbecco *et al.*, 1986). Myoepithelial and epithelial cells in the rat mammary gland have also been delineated on the basis of their activity in the histochemical reaction for ATPase. Myoepithelial cells show a reaction with Na^+/K^+-ATPase but epithelial cells only with Mg^{2+}-ATPase (Russo *et al.*, 1982).

Haemopoietic and Lymphatic Systems

In conventional toxicity studies blood, blood-forming organs and lymphoid tissues are routinely examined by light microscopy in conjunction with automated analysis of peripheral red and white blood cells. Weighing and careful histological examination of thymus, spleen and lymph nodes are widely considered to be important components in the examination of effects of xenobiotics on the immune system and form part of the first tier of procedures adopted in immunotoxicity testing batteries in the National Toxicology Program and at the Chemical Industry Institute of Toxicology (Dean *et al.*, 1986; Dean and Thurmond, 1987; Luster *et al.*, 1988).

Blood smears are commonly examined using classical Romanowsky stains, and conventional histological sections are taken from spleen, selected lymph nodes, thymus and decalcified bone marrow sections. The cellularity of bone marrow varies between different sites in laboratory animals. In rodents, bone marrow from the femur, sternum and vertebral bodies is considered to be the most representative (Cline and Maronpot, 1985; Wright, 1989). The cytology of bone marrow cells in decalcified, paraffin-embedded sections is not ideal, and Romanowsky-stained bone marrow smears provide better cytological detail. The technical problems posed by the need to decalcify bone have been surmounted in some toxicology laboratories by the use of 3 μm thick methyl methacrylate-embedded sections stained with modified Giemsa or gallamine blue–Giemsa supplemented by Gomori's stain for reticulin, a technique originally developed by Burkhardt and colleagues (1982) for human bone marrow biopsies.

Critical histological examination of lymph nodes requires good orientation of the tissue to provide the basis for a clear assessment of the relative sizes of cortex, paracortex and medulla and their three-dimensional orientation. A semiquantitative assessment based on a standard approach defined by the World Health Organization (WHO) represents a good method for characterization of functional alterations in the B- and T-cell zones of the lymphoid system (Cottier et al., 1972; van der Valk and Maijer, 1987).

Whereas the spleen functions as a blood storage organ and a site of extramedullary haemopoiesis, its discrete nature and small size in rodents make it a useful organ to weigh and subject to morphometric analysis of the periarteriolar lymphoid sheaths (T-cell zones) and germinal follicles (B-cell areas). Spleen weight does not appear to be a reliable indicator of haemopoietic cellularity in the dog.

Conventional histological stains are readily supplemented by a variety of antibodies for the immunohistochemical localization of monocytic cells and lymphoid subsets. While most reagents are monoclonal antibodies which require use of frozen tissue sections or smear preparations, many are commercially available for specific cells in the common laboratory animal species. For the mouse, these include antibodies to Thy-1 for T-lymphocytes and thymocytes, Lyt-1 for helper T-cells and Lyt–2 for cytotoxic/suppressor T-cells (Ahmed and Smith, 1983). An antibody to asialo

GM1 (ganglio-*n*-tetrosylceramide) has been employed as a marker for murine natural killer cells in the study of the toxicity of human recombinant interleukin–2 in the mouse (Anderson *et al.*, 1988). Mouse monoclonal antibodies W3/13, W3/25 and MRC OX8 have been employed immunocytochemically as pan-T-, helper T- and suppressor/cytotoxic T-lymphocytes, respectively, in the study of the effects of immune modulators in the laboratory rat, using both tissue sections and immunogold staining of peripheral blood smears (Evans *et al.*, 1988a). A mouse monoclonal antibody to Thy–1 can also be used to label canine T-lymphocytes (Evans *et al.*, 1988b). Antibodies to immunoglobulins or immunoglobulin light chains can be used in the characterization of B-lymphocytes, although, in contrast to many of the cell surface markers, they can be used in paraffin-wax-embedded sections.

Musculoskeletal System

An assessment of long bone growth is conveniently made by measurement of long bone length, the femur being frequently used for this purpose in laboratory animals. This measurement can also be conducted by radiographic means and is therefore an effective *in vivo* measure of bone growth in immature animals when treated by agents affecting bone (Robinson *et al.*, 1982).

Appropriate laboratory processing of bone is a prerequisite for its good histological assessment. Formalin is adequate for most purposes, followed by decalcification using acidic fluids and embedding in paraffin wax. Use of polarized light microscopy is helpful in the identification of bone types in decalcified sections, for it can demonstrate the patterns of collagen orientation. Undecalcified sections using methacrylate or similar hard embedding media, supplemented by stains such as von Kossa, Goldner trichrome or solochrome cyanine, are essential for the assessment of bone mineralization.

Choice of sampling site is particularly important in toxicity studies in laboratory animals. It should be an identical site in all animals within a particular study, for it has been shown that even modest differences in sampling site can influence histomorphological variables of bone (Anderson and Danylchuk, 1978). In long bones the focus of histological examination is usually directed to the metaphysis. Chondrocytes dividing in the metaphysis as columns of proliferating cells and maturing into hypertrophic cells are responsible for bone growth. Therefore, examination of this zone, particularly if morphometric analysis is also carried out, is an ideal place to evaluate bone formation and resorption in studies designed to evaluate xenobiotics which affect this process (Schenk *et al.*, 1986).

Use of vital fluorescent labels such as tetracycline, alizarin red S, calcein, procion or haematoporphyrin can be used to visualize sites of bone mineralization in tissue sections of bone from laboratory animals (Solheim, 1974).

Articular cartilage reacts to chemical insult only in a limited way (Mankin, 1974). However, like bone, it represents a stratified structure growing from the chondrosseous junction of the epiphysis which can be assessed histologically, using conventional processing and staining procedures. Special stains such as toluidine blue, safranine O, lectin histochemistry and immunocytochemistry or electron microscopy represent further tools for the study of chondrocytes, glycosaminoglycans and collagens in the matrix (Mankin, 1974; Brighton *et al.*, 1984; Gough *et al.*, 1985; Kirivanta *et al.*, 1987; Farnum and Wilsman, 1988).

Conventionally processed and stained sections of skeletal muscle are employed for most routine purposes, notably in the appraisal of intramuscular irritancy of locally injected drugs and embedded biomaterials. As at other sites of local damage, it is important to assess the extent and nature of local damage and the time-course of the repair process. The rabbit sacrospinalis muscle is the model of choice in the assessment of intramuscular preparations (Gray, 1981) but muscles in rat and dog are also used. Histological evaluation of muscle damage can be supplemented by histochemical methods for enzymes such as succinate dehydrogenase and acid phosphatase, which correlate with damage and repair activity (Salthouse and Willigan, 1972). Immunohistochemical stains for structural components such as myosin isoforms, collagens, fibronectin, myoglobin, laminin and desmin have also been used as adjuncts to assess alterations induced by xenobiotics in skeletal muscle (Helliwell, 1988).

Finally, it should be remembered that skeletal muscle fibres are heterogeneous in type and different types may respond differently to adverse stimuli. Though an oversimplification, two main types of fibres exist—the slow twitch or type I fibres and the fast twitch or type II fibres. These fibres are usually distinguished histochemically in frozen sections using their differences in myosin ATPase activity (Brooke and Kaiser, 1970; Pierobon-Bormioli *et al.*, 1980, 1981; Billeter *et al.*, 1981).

Pulmonary System

Nasal chambers are the structures which are first subjected to the effects of inhaled substances. Although they are not studied in great detail in conventional toxicity studies, it is vital that they be examined histologically when drugs and other chemicals are administered by inhalation. In rodents the small size of the bones of the nose and nasal sinuses makes a simple transverse blocking procedure following decalcification a cost-effective way to provide standardized histological sections (Young, 1981). For large animals, a more complex dissection is required for histological assessment of the nasal mucosa.

Careful inspection of the lungs in a good light after opening the thoracic cavity at autopsy provides important information about pathological alterations. Changes may be manifest by uneven collapse, enlargement or overinflation, patchy discoloration or stiffness of the lung parenchyma, as well as the presence of oedema or pleural effusions. Total weight or dry/wet weight ratios can be sensitive indicators of lung damage and oedema, although vascular congestion may be a confounding factor (Nemery *et al.*, 1987).

Various methods of lung fixation are available. Immersion fixation in neutral buffered formalin is widely employed for most routine purposes and has the advantage of retaining exudates and fluids within the air spaces and airways. Instillation of fixative via the trachea under constant pressure (25–30 cmH$_2$O) shows structural alterations well, although it has a tendency to dislodge exudates. Use of formalin vapour, perfusion fixation via the vasculature and freezing in liquid nitrogen are other methods which are employed (Tyler *et al.*, 1985; Nemery *et al.*, 1987).

Ultrastructural study has a place in the elucidation of selective structural damage to the pulmonary parenchyma, but the size of the lungs and the diversity of its cellular components create problems of fixation and sampling. The technical considerations of fixation for ultrastructural study of the lung in toxicology studies have been reviewed by Tyler and colleagues (1985). Extensive use of semithin sections is helpful for selection of samples, and a rigorous, tiered approach to random sampling is necessary for morphometric study (Barry and Crapo, 1985).

As in other tissues, immunocytochemical, cytochemical and autoradiological techniques are important in the study of the effects of xenobiotics on lung tissue. For instance, the pulmonary vascular leak syndrome of human recombinant interleukin-2 in mice has been studied by the use of the immunocytochemical method to demonstrate T-lymphocytes, macrophages, natural killer cells and lymphokine-activated killer cells (Anderson *et al.*, 1988). Mono-oxygenase enzymes and important structural components such as the collagens and laminin can also be studied in this way (Gil and Martinez-Hernandez, 1984; Linnoila and Petrusz, 1984). Mucin histochemistry is also helpful in the study of changes in the lining epithelium of the bronchi (Sturgess and Reid, 1973; Sturgess, 1985).

Cardiovascular System

Key to the pathological evaluation of the heart in toxicity studies is the careful visual inspection of the pericardium, myocardium, endocardium and valve cusps of each cardiac chamber. Cardiac weight in laboratory animals varies with body weight, body length, age and sex, and circulatory demand. For this reason, weighing the heart may be not only a useful guide to the toxic effects of xenobiotics on the myocardium, but also a measure of functional adaptation to cardiac workload. This is particularly true if individual ventricles are also weighed or ventricular wall thickness is measured, for this may provide information about any changes affecting predominantly the pulmonary or systemic circulation.

Careful sampling of representative sections of each cardiac chamber is also important for adequate histological assessment. These sections should include segments of the coronary arteries, valves and those zones sensitive to ischaemia, such as the endocardium and papillary muscles of the left ventricle. Issues relating to sampling have been reviewed by Piper (1981).

Conventional fixation, paraffin wax embedding, haematoxylin and eosin staining and connective tissue stains; fibrin and elastic stains are the cornerstones in the detection of myocardial and vascular alterations. Polarized light microscopy using formalin-fixed sections stained with picrosirius red is a powerful technique for the assessment of the distribution, size and orientation of collagen fibres within myocardial scar tissue (Pick *et al.*, 1989; Whittaker *et al.*, 1989).

Other histological techniques include the detection of early myocardial damage in formalin-fixed tissue, using demonstration of the loss of myosin, tropomyosin, ATPase, creatine kinase or lactate dehydrogenase from muscle fibres (Block *et al.*, 1983; Hayakawa *et al.*, 1984; Spinale *et al.*, 1989). Damaged muscle fibres stain red with the basic fuchsin–picric acid method or develop fluorescence in haematoxylin-stained sections (Al-Rufaie *et al.*, 1983).

Digestive System

The mouth is subjected to visual inspection in conventional toxicity studies and the tongue is commonly sectioned for histopathological examination of the oral mucosa. Major salivary glands are examined by conventional processing and staining techniques, although mucin histochemical stains are important in the study of alterations in mucin secretion in these glands. The mature dentition is not usually affected by xenobiotics, but some drugs such as anticancer agents have been shown to affect immature dentition (Stene and Koppang, 1976; Robinson and Harvey, 1989). For this reason, it may be necessary to examine the dentition histologically in animals treated with xenobiotics. This is performed using the techniques employed for bone.

Histological examination of the gastrointestinal tract itself is complicated by its great length and the fragility of the mucosa before fixation. Careful inspection without vigorous washing is essential to both locate lesions and avoid artefacts in histological sections which may mimic inflammation and ulceration. Although selective blocking is usually appropriate if preceded by careful macroscopic inspection; the so-called 'Swiss roll' techniques are valuable for a detailed histological survey of the gastrointestinal epithelium. These methods can be adjusted for use in laboratory rodents, larger animal species and man. They may be performed on fresh tissue or after fixation (Filipe and Branfoot, 1974; Greaves *et al.*, 1980; Moolenbeck and Ruitenberg, 1981).

Mucin histochemistry is an important tool for the study of xenobiotic-induced changes in the gastrointestinal mucosa. Both conventional mucin histochemistry and lectin histochemistry can be performed on formalin-fixed and paraffin-wax-embedded material. The techniques are applicable to study of the gastrointestinal mucosa from laboratory animals and man, although there are considerable interspecies differences in the distribution of glycoconjugates demonstrated by these methods (Sheahan and Jarvis, 1978; Tsiftis *et al.*, 1980; Greaves and Boiziau, 1984; Ishihara *et al.*, 1984). Argyrophil staining is useful in the characterization of enterochromaffin cells of the stomach and intestine because of their endogenous reducing activity. Argyrophil staining has been widely employed in the study of the effects of histamine H2 receptor blockers on enterochromaffin cells in the rodent gastrointestinal tract (Betton *et al.*, 1988; Hirth *et al.*, 1988; Streett *et al.*, 1988). Immunohistochemistry is also used for the characterization of these enterochromaffin cells in the mucosa, notably using antisera to histamine, histidine decarboxylase, neuron-specific enolase and chromogranin A (Betton *et al.*, 1988; Hirth *et al.*, 1988).

Monoclonal antibodies against lymphoid surface markers are used for the study of the mucosa-associated lymphoid system, or MALT, in laboratory animals (Bland and Warren, 1985; Ermak and Owen, 1986; Martin *et al.*, 1986). The so-called M-cells overlying Peyer's patches can only be adequately demonstrated at ultrastructural level or by their paucity of alkaline phosphatase activity (Owen and Bhalla, 1983). Mucosal mast cells in rats have been shown to be demonstrable in conventionally processed tissues by prolonged toluidine blue staining (Widgren and Enerbäck, 1983).

As the principal site of metabolism and detoxification of drugs and other xenobiotics, the liver is a frequent site of alterations in toxicity studies and is therefore the focus of careful histopathological assessment. In conventional studies the liver is usually weighed prior to fixation and selection of blocks for processing for light and electron microscopy as well as other techniques. The relatively large size of the liver presents problems of selection of tissue blocks, and considerable interlaboratory variation exists in the hepatic blocking schedule. For instance, blocks processed from the rat liver for routine histological examin-

ation in conventional toxicity studies may vary from 1 to 5+ (personal observations). In the National Toxicology Program (NTP) rat carcinogenicity studies the procedure involves the selection of two blocks taken from the widest parts of the left lobe and the right median lobe (Maronpot *et al.*, 1989). Selection of two blocks appears to be the generally accepted practice for routine rodent liver histopathological examination in many laboratories. Fine-needle aspiration of hepatic tissue from rodents, fixation in ethanol and staining with the Papanicolaou stain, in a manner similar to that used in human medicine, represents a method of sampling which can be used *in vivo* (Giampaolo *et al.*, 1989).

Electron microscopy, enzyme cytochemistry and latterly immunocytochemistry have well-accepted roles in the characterization of changes induced by xenobiotics in the liver of laboratory animals. It is frequently necessary to characterize the nature of cellular and subcellular changes such as proliferation of smooth endoplasmic reticulum, peroxisomes or mitochondria, and lysosomal alterations such as phospholipidosis, when treatment-induced changes in liver weight are recorded or when there is light microscopic evidence of hepatocyte hypertrophy.

As the liver possesses considerable functional heterogeneity within the lobule (Jungerman and Katz, 1982), cytochemical methods for reactions such as catalase, uricase, various dehydrogenases, alkaline phosphatase, 5'-nucleotidase and $NADH_2$ diaphorases as well as glutathione form a bridge for the pathologist between morphology and activity measured by classical biochemical techniques (Chayen, 1984; Mompon *et al.*, 1987). Although cytochrome P450 activity is difficult to measure directly by cytochemical techniques, immunocytochemistry can make a useful contribution here in the localization of immune-reactive metabolizing enzymes in tissue sections (Moody *et al.*, 1985; Foster *et al.*, 1986). A number of histochemical methods have been applied to the study of foci of cellular alteration in the rodent liver. These include the classical marker gamma-glutamyl transpeptidase, glucose-6-phosphate dehydrogenase and immunohistochemical demonstration of placental glutathione *S*-transferase (Farber, 1984; Greaves *et al.*, 1986; Tatematsu *et al.*, 1987). Immunocytochemical detection of oncogene proteins has also been used in the study of oncogene expression in the liver of carcinogen-treated rodents (Richmond *et al.*, 1988).

Another histochemical technique of potential importance is the direct Schiff's reaction, which can detect the presence of cellular aldehydes or free radicals produced *in vivo* when it is performed on cryostat sections (Rushmore *et al.*, 1987; Taper *et al.*, 1988).

Urinary tract

The kidney is particularly important in toxicology, because many xenobiotics or their metabolites are eliminated primarily through the urinary tract. In addition, the kidney is liable to be exposed quickly to peak concentrations of circulating xenobiotics by virtue of its high blood flow. Its ability to concentrate toxic solutes in renal tubular cells or in the tubular lumen is an additional risk factor.

Renal weight changes are a useful guide to renal toxicity but renal weight may also alter as a physiological response to changes in renal demand. Hence, it is essential that assessment of renal toxicity include careful visual inspection of the renal parenchyma at autopsy for appearances of toxicity such as swelling, pallor, congestion and haemorrhage, and this should be followed by histopathological examination. Inspection of the contents of the renal pelvis for crystals and mineral and cellular debris is also important at autopsy, for these substances may be lost in subsequent tissue handling and processing.

Conventional fixation and processing followed by haematoxylin and eosin staining supplemented by PAS is usually appropriate for most conventional toxicity studies. It is important that all parts of the nephron be examined microscopically, so histological sections should comprise both cortex and medulla and include the tip of the papilla.

A variety of techniques are available for more detailed study of xenobiotic-induced alterations in the nephron. Electron microscopy has an important and time-honoured place in the study of pathological alterations in both the glomerulus and the renal tubule, although perfusion fixation may be needed for good preservation of tubular cells for ultrastructural study. Light microscopy of plastic-embedded sections 1–3 μm thick is a useful compromise which provides excellent resolution of renal structures (Gregg *et al.*, 1990).

Various parts of the renal tubule show different enzyme activities which relate to the function of different segments (Guder and Ross, 1984). Histochemical demonstration of enzyme activities can therefore be used as markers for components of the nephron and for structural–functional studies. For instance, lysosomal enzyme activity is highest in the proximal tubule, reflecting the role of this segment in degradation of reabsorbed macromolecules. Therefore, enzyme cytochemical demonstration of acid phosphatase or other lysosomal enzymes outlines the proximal tubule. Demonstration of acid phosphatase at electron microscopic level using the cerium technique has been employed in the characterization of drug-induced alterations in proximal tubular lysosomes (Read *et al.*, 1988). Of special interest to the pathologist as cytochemical markers are brush border enzymes, alkaline phosphatase, 5′-nucleotidase and gamma-glutamyl transpeptidase. These are useful in the study of chemically induced tubular damage (Faccini, 1982). Measurement of enzyme activity in the urine is also a useful complementary, non-invasive technique for the assessment of tubular toxicity in man and laboratory animals, because cellular enzymes from damaged tubular cells spill into the urine in increased amounts (Kluwe, 1981; Zbinden *et al.*, 1988).

Immunocytochemistry can also be used to demonstrate the presence of brush border enzymes such as gamma-glutamyl transpeptidase (Yasuda and Yamashita, 1985). Immunocytochemical demonstration of Tamm–Horsfall proteins, localized at the surface membrane of the thick ascending loop of Henle, has also been used for the study of renal tubular changes induced by xenobiotics (Howie *et al.*, 1990).

In the study of drug-induced alterations to the juxtaglomerular apparatus, immunocytochemical staining using antisera to renin is superior to the classical, non-specific techniques for renin-containing granules such as the Bowie and Hartroft stains (Faraggiana *et al.*, 1982; Zaki *et al.*, 1982).

It is worth recording that labelled lectins can be used to localize different segments of the nephron histochemically, and this can often be performed on formalin-fixed, paraffin-wax-embedded material (Holthofer, 1983; Murata *et al.*, 1983; Schulte and Spicer, 1983). For instance, peanut lectin (*Phaseolus vulgaris*; PNA) and *Ricinus comminis* (RCA) stain the S1 and S2 segments of the rat proximal tubule, although the S2 segment remains poorly stained. The mouse proximal tubule brush border stains with *Lotus tetragonolobus* (LTA) (Schulte and Spicer, 1983).

Histological study of the bladder mucosa requires special care at fixation. The best orientation of the epithelium is obtained following inflation of the bladder with fixative at autopsy, for this removes folds which can give a misleading impression of the thickness of the epithelium. However, this procedure may dislodge exudates and other material from the bladder lumen, so care should be exercised in its application. Scanning electron microscopy is a useful special technique for the examination of chemically induced alterations to the superficial transitional epithelium.

Reproductive System

The effects of xenobiotics on the reproductive system are usually examined in special reproductive studies in which histopathological examination plays relatively little part. However, histopathological examination of the male and female reproductive tract is an important component of conventional toxicity studies. At an early stage in the development of a new medicine it represents the only assessment of potential treatment-related effects on the reproductive organs and germ cells, and therefore needs to be performed with some care. Special fixatives are routinely employed for light microscopic examination of the testes, because formalin is a particularly poor method of preservation of the germinal epithelium prior to embedding in paraffin wax. Immersion in Bouin's, Zenker's or Helly's fluid is commonly used, followed by paraffin wax embedding and staining with haematoxylin and eosin. PAS is used for the demonstration of the germ cell acrosome, for this enables the most precise staging of the germ cell cycle in all laboratory animal species as well as in humans (Clermont, 1972). More recently, the cycle of the seminiferous epithelium has been defined in formalin-fixed, plastic-embedded testis stained with toluidine blue (Russell and Frank, 1978; Ulvik *et al.*, 1982). This method provides excellent cytology of the germinal epithelium.

A number of quantitative and semiquantitative methods have been devised for the assessment of the effects of xenobiotics on testicular germ cells. These involve measurement of cross-sectional area of seminiferous tubules and germ cell–Sertoli cell ratios, and counting the number of spermatids per tubule.

The female reproductive system is usually examined histologically by conventional histological techniques but with close attention being paid to the cyclical alteration observed in the endometrium, vaginal mucosa and ovarian tissue. The ovary requires rigorous orientation if sections are to include cortex, medulla and hilar tissue. As ovarian function is closely linked to the endocrine system, it is important that in any histological assessment of the reproductive tract account be taken of endocrine organs. In the National Toxicology Program, alterations in reproductive organs induced by a variety of different chemicals were frequently associated with changes in the pituitary gland and adrenal cortex (Maronpot, 1987).

Endocrine System

The capacity of the mammalian organism to function as an integral and independent unit depends on the endocrine system operating in concert with the nervous system. Interrelationships between endocrine organs are complex, and over recent years it has become evident that there are close links between the hypothalamus, the pituitary gland and the rest of the endocrine and nervous systems. The nervous system releases substances which act as circulating hormones, and hormones released by endocrine cells also have local effects. Although endocrine cells are generally quite resistant to the direct toxic effects of xenobiotics, they are, by contrast, extremely sensitive to stimulation and inhibition by trophic or antitrophic substances, end organ feedback and systemic perturbations induced by administration of high doses of active chemicals. Furthermore, the close link between secretory function of endocrine tissue and its proliferative activity (Pawlikowski, 1982) concords with the frequent observation in toxicity studies that a common response to excessive stimulation is endocrine hyperplasia and neoplasia.

For these reasons histological examination of endocrine tissues is important in toxicity studies. Where technically possible, histological examination is preceded by weighing of the organs, although this may not be advisable for firmly bound organs such as the thyroid gland, for danger of disruption of histological sections. Total adrenal weight is not a good indicator of adenal medullary size, for it only represents 10–20 per cent of adrenal size (Neville, 1969).

A powerful tool of particular use in the examination of peptide-containing endocrine organs is immunocytochemistry. Antisera to many peptide hormones are widely available, and provided that appropriate dilutions and absorption controls are employed, they can be used in the examination of the endocrine tissues of most conventional laboratory animal species. They have superseded the tinctorial stains in the examination of the pituitary gland altered by drugs and hormones (El Etreby and Fath el Bab, 1977; El Etreby *et al.*, 1977; Zak *et al.*, 1985; Lloyd and Landefeld, 1986; Lloyd and Mailloux, 1987). Islet cell pathology is well demonstrated in both rats and dogs by immunocytochemical staining for insulin, somatostatin, glucagon and pancreatic polypeptide (Spencer *et al.*, 1986). C-Cells in the thyroid gland are clearly delineated in the thyroid by immunocytochemistry for calcitonin (DeLellis *et al.*, 1987). Immunohistochemical demonstration of the acidic protein chromogranin A is also a good general marker for many endocrine cells with secretory granules in different species (Hawkins *et al.*, 1989). Techniques of *in situ* hybridization for the detection of mRNA are also applicable to the identification of peptide-producing cells in the endocrine system (Bloch, 1985).

Immunostaining for non-polypeptide hormones such as steroids and catecholamines is less well developed, and conventional methods for histopathological assessment are still widely employed. Standard special stains for lipids using frozen sections and electron microscopy are applicable to the characterization of changes in the adrenal cortex. Immunocytochemical approaches have been used in the study of cytochromes *P*-450 in the adrenal cortex (Le Goascogne *et al.*, 1987).

The chromaffin reaction, which represents darkening on exposure to aqueous solutions of potassium dichromate as a result of oxidation and polymerization of catecholamines, also remains a useful stain in the study of catacholamine activity in the medulla (Tischler *et al.*, 1985). However, it may be less reliable than the use of formaldehyde vapour or glycoxylic acid treatment and fluorescence microscopy (Tischler and DeLellis, 1988). Neuron-specific enolase is consistently present in the rat and mouse adrenal medulla and can therefore be used as a histochemical marker for proliferative and neoplastic alteration in this tissue (Wright *et al.*, 1990). The examination of electron-dense granules in the medulla is also useful for the characterization of medullary cells (Rhodin, 1974).

Nervous System and Special Sense Organs

Careful histological examination of the nervous system frequently reveals subtle structural alterations which precede evidence of functional abnormality. However, it is clear that this sensitivity is dependent on identification of vulnerable zones and determination of the nature of the tissue alterations under study (Spencer *et al.*, 1980). To achieve this requires, therefore, careful selection of nervous tissues, and their appropriate fixation, processing and staining. This may be different from the techniques employed for other tissues.

Perfusion fixation of the brain is ideal for the exclusion of fixation artefact, although immersion fixation followed by conventional processing may be adequate for most routine purposes. However, it is essential to be aware of the artefacts which can develop in the immersion fixation of brain so that they are not confounded with treatment-induced alterations (reviewed by Garman, 1990).

It is important that the selection of blocks for histological examination be carefully performed to ensure that appropriate cerebral nuclei and fibre tracts are examined. In toxicity studies performed with pharmaceutical agents with effects on the central nervous system, appropriate cerebral nuclei and fibre tracts should be examined histologically. Guidelines for testing under the Toxic Substances Control Act (TOSCA) suggest that cross-sections of forebrain, centre of the cerebrum, midbrain, pons, medulla oblongata, cervical and lumbar spinal cord, Gasserian and dorsal root ganglia, dorsal and ventral root fibres, proximal sciatic, and sural and tibial nerves should be examined in a full neurotoxicological assessment (Environmental Protection Agency, 1985).

Standard sections can be obtained by the use of a metal mould with cross-channels for accurate slicing of the fixed brain and appropriate zones can be assessed by use of a stereotaxic atlas of neuroanatomy such as that of Paxinos and Watson (1986) for the laboratory rat.

In addition to haematoxylin and eosin, special stains for myelin, neuronal bodies, axons and glial cells are of additional help. Changes in peripheral nerve fibres are particularly well characterized in semithin plastic or epoxy-resin-embedded, toluidine blue-stained sections (Spencer *et al.*, 1980). Teased nerve fibre preparations are helpful in the demonstration of Wallerian degeneration, demyelination and regeneration (Griffin, 1990). Morphometric analysis of brain pathology, particularly neuronal loss, is also helpful in the characterization of neuronal toxicity (Robertson *et al.*, 1987).

Immunocytochemistry is important for the localization of neuropeptides, particularly in the hypothalamus. For instance, specific depletion of growth hormone releasing factor has been demonstrated by use of immunocytochemistry in the median eminence of rats treated with monosodium glutamate (Bloch *et al.*, 1984). Immunocytochemical localization of neurotransmitters can be combined with anterograde tracing with peanut lectin for the study of target fibre systems or neurons (Luiten *et al.*, 1988). Immunocytochemistry using antisera to glial fibrillary acid protein (GFA), S100 protein, neuron-specific enolase and cytoskeletal components may also provide valuable information in the identification of cell types and characterization of changes within them (Koestner, 1990). The topographical distribution of S100 and GFA proteins appears similar in most species but has been well studied in the rat (Ludwin *et al.*, 1976).

It also appears possible to localize cytochrome *P*-450 enzymes in neurons and glial cells of experimental animals by immunocytochemistry (Köhler *et al.*, 1988), and conventional quantitative enzyme cytochemistry is also applicable to neural tissues (Kuger, 1988). Electron microscopy also remains a valuable tool for problem solving in neuropathology, although it is technically demanding and labour-intensive (Jones, 1988).

Eyes are usually examined by conventional histological techniques after special fixation in a fluid such as Davidson's fluid to avoid as much artefact as possible in the lens and retina (Taradach and Greaves, 1984). The lens poses particular problems in histological processing but excellent results can be achieved with plastic embedding procedures (Heywood and Gopinath, 1988).

Likewise, the middle and inner ear can also be examined histologically after decalcification of the petrous bone and preparation of conventional sections. However, sectioning the cochlea to achieve the correct orientation requires considerable skill, and this method can only demonstrate small numbers of sensory cells in the organ. Engström and colleagues (1966) developed the surface preparation technique, which involves dissection of the cochlea and subdivision of the organ of Corti into short segments for examination by phase contrast microscopy. A modification of this technique using scanning electron microscopy is relatively simple to perform and can be used in the rat and other experimental animals (Astbury and Read, 1982; Liberman, 1990).

REFERENCES

Ahmed, A. and Smith, A. H. (1983). Surface markers, antigens and receptors on murine T and B cells. Part 2. *CRC Crit. Rev. Toxicol.*, **4**, 19–94

Alder, S. and Zbinden, G. (1988). *National and International Drug Safety Guidelines*. M. T. C. Verlag, Zollikon, Switzerland, pp. 20–182

Al-Rufaie, H. K., Florio, R. A. and Olsen, E. G. J. (1983). Comparison of the haematoxylin basic fuchsin picric acid method and the fluorescence of haematoxylin and eosin stained sections for the identification of early myocardial infarction. *J. Clin. Pathol.*, **36**, 646–649

Anderson, C. and Danylchuck, K. D. (1978). Bone remodeling rates of the beagle: A comparison between different sites on the same rib. *Am. J. Vet. Res.*, **39**, 1763–1765

Anderson, T. D., Hayes, T. J., Gately, M. K., Bontempo, J. M., Stern, L. L. and Truitt, G. A. (1988). Toxicity of human recombinant interleukin–2 in the mouse is mediated by interleukin-activated lymphocytes. Separation of efficacy and toxicity by selective lymphocyte subset depletion. *Lab. Invest.*, **59**, 598–612

Astbury, P. J. and Read, N. G. (1982). Improved morphological technique for screening potentially ototoxic compounds in laboratory animals. *Br. J. Audiol.*, **16**, 131–137

Autian, J. (1987). The new field of plastics toxicology—methods and results. *CRC Crit. Rev. Toxicol.*, **2**, 1–40

Barry, B. E. and Crapo, J. D. (1985). Application of morphometric methods to study diffuse and focal injury in the lung caused by toxic agents. *CRC Crit. Rev. Toxicol.*, **14**, 1–32

Betton, G. R., Dormer, C. S., Wells, T., Pert, P., Price, C. A. and Buckley, P. (1988). Gastric ECL-cell hyperplasia and carcinoids in rodents following chronic administration of H2-antagonists SK&F 93479 and oxmetidine and omeprazole. *Toxicol. Pathol.*, **16**, 288–298

Billeter, R., Heizmann, C. W., Howald, H. and Jenny, E. (1981). Analysis of myosin light and heavy chain types in single human skeletal muscle fibres. *Eur. J. Biochem.*, **116**, 389–395

Bland, P. W. and Warren, L. G. (1985). Immunohistologic analysis of the T-cell macrophage infiltrate in 1,2-dimethylhydrazine-induced colon tumors in the rat. *J. Natl Cancer Inst.*, **75**, 757–764

Bloch, B. (1985). L'hybridation *in situ*: méthodologie et applications à l'analyse des phénomènes d'expression génique dans les glands endocrines et le système nerveux. *Ann. Endocrinol.*, **46**, 253–261

Bloch, B., Ling, N., Benoit, R., Wehrenberg, W. B. and Guillemin, R. (1984). Specific depletion of immunoreactive growth hormone-releasing factor by monosodium glutamate in rat median eminence. *Nature*, **307**, 272–273

Block, M. I., Said, J. W., Siegel, R. J. and Fishbein, M. C. (1983). Myocardial myoglobin following coronary artery occlusion. An immunohistochemical study. *Am. J. Pathol.*, **111**, 374–379

Boon, M. E. and Kok, L. P. (1987). Microwave stabilization of unfixed tissue by microwave fixation. In *Microwave Cookbook of Pathology*. Coulomb Press Leyden, Leiden, pp. 71–77

Brighton, C. T., Kitajima, T. and Hunt, R. M. (1984). Zonal analysis of cytoplasmic components of articular cartilage chondrocytes. *Arth. Rheum.*, **27**, 1290–1299

Brooke, M. H. and Kaiser, K. K. (1970). Muscle fiber types: How many and what kind? *Arch. Neurol.*, **23**, 369–379

Burkhardt, R., Firsch, B. and Bartl, R. (1982). Bone biopsies in haematological disorders. *J. Clin. Pathol.*, **25**, 257–284

Chayen, J. (1984). Quantitative cytochemistry: a precise form of cellular biochemistry. *Biochem. Soc. Trans.*, **12**, 884–898

Chayen, J., Bitensky, L. and Butcher, R. G. (1973). *Practical Histochemistry*. Wiley, London

Clapp, M. J. L. and McNamee, J. A. (1985). The integration of modern computer technologies for effective toxicological data handling. *Med. Inform.*, **10**, 115–121

Clermont, Y. (1972). Kinetics of spermatogenesis in mammals: Seminiferous epithelium cycle and spermatogonial renewal. *Am. J. Anat.*, **112**, 35–45

Cline, J. M. and Maronpot, R. R. (1985). Variations in the histologic distribution of rat bone marrow cells with respect to age and anatomic site. *Toxicol. Pathol.*, **13**, 349–355

Cottier, H., Turk, J. A. and Sobin, L. (1972). A proposal for a standardized system of reporting human lymph node morphology in relation to immunological function. *Bull. Wld Hlth Org.*, **47**, 375–408

Darby, T. D. (1987). Safety evaluation of polymer materials. *Ann. Rev. Pharmacol. Toxicol.*, **27**, 157–167

Dean, J. H. and Thurmond, L. M. (1987). Immunotoxicology: An overview. *Toxicol. Pathol.*, **15**, 265–271

Dean, J. H., Lauer, L. D., House, R. V. and Thurmond, L. M. (1986). Immunomodulation: Assessing the immunoenhancing and immunosuppressive properties of xenobiotics. In *Toxicology in the Nineties*. 1985 Ciba-Geigy International Workshop. Mary Ann Liebert, New York, pp. 245–285

de la Iglesia, F. A. and McGuire, E. J. (1981). Quantitative stereology: Toxicologic pathology applications. *Toxicol., Pathol.*, **9**, 21–28

de la Iglesia, F. A., Sturgess, J. M. and Feuer, G. (1982). New approaches for the assessment of hepatotoxicity by means of quantitative functional-morphological interelationships. In Plaa, G. L. and Hewitt, W. R. (Eds), *Toxicology of the Liver*. Raven Press, New York, pp. 47–102

DeLellis, R. A. and Wolfe, H. J. (1987). New techniques in gene product analysis. *Arch. Pathol. Lab. Med.*, **111**, 620–627

DeLellis, R. A., Wolfe, H. J. and Morh, U. (1987). Medullary thyroid carcinoma in the Syrian golden hamster: An immunocytochemical study. *Exptl Pathol.*, **31**, 11–16

Department of Health (1988). The Quality Assurance Unit's role in the monitoring of specialist toxicology disciplines. The Department of Health GLP Monitoring Unit response to clarification sought by Quality Assurance Group, England

Dulbecco, R., Allen, W. R., Bologna, M. and Bowman, M. (1986). Marker evolution during the development of the rat mammary gland: Stem cells identified by markers and the role of myoepithelial cells. *Cancer Res.*, **46**, 2449–2456

El Etreby, M. F. and Fath el Bab, M. R. (1977). Effect of cyproterone acetate on cells of the pars distalis of the adenohypophysis in the beagle bitch. *Cell Tissue Res.*, **183**, 177–189

El Etreby, M. F., Schilk, B., Soulioti, G., Tüshaus, U., Wieman, H. and Günzel, P. (1977). Effect of 17ß-estradiol on cells of the pars distalis of the adenohypophysis in the beagle bitch: An immunocytochemical and morphometric study. *Endokrinologie*, **69**, 202–216

Engström, H., Ades, H. W. and Andersson, A. (1966). *Structure Patterns of the Organ of Corti*. Almqvist and Wiksell, Stockholm

Environmental Protection Agency (1985). Toxic Substances Control Act Guidelines, 40 DFR, part 798, subpart G, section 798.6400, Neuropathology. *Federal Register*, **50**, No. 188, 39461–39463

Ermak, T. H. and Owen, R. L. (1986). Differential

distribution of lymphocytes and accessory cells in mouse Peyer's patches. *Anat. Rec.*, **215**, 144–152

Evans, G. O., Flynn, R. M. and Lupton, J. D. (1988a). An immunogold labelling method for rat T lymphocytes. *Lab. Anim.*, **2**, 332–334

Evans, G. O., Flynn, R. M. and Lupton, J. D. (1988b). An immunogold labelling method for the enumeration of canine T-lymphocytes. *Vet. Quart.*, **10**, 273–276

Faccini, J. M. (1982). A perspective on the pathology and cytochemistry of renal lesions. In Bach, P. H., Bonner, F. W., Bridges, J. W. and Lock, E. D. (Eds), *Nephrotoxicity Assessment and Pathogenesis*. Wiley, Chichester, pp. 82–97

Faccini, J. M. and Naylor, D. (1979). Computer analysis and integration of animal pathology data. *Arch. Toxicol.*, Suppl. 2, 517–520

Faraggiana, T., Gresik, E., Tanaka, T., Inagami, T. and Lupo, A. (1982). Immunohistochemical localization of renin in the human kidney. *Histochem. Cytochem.*, **30**, 459–465

Farber, E. (1984). Chemical carcinogenesis: A current biological perspective. *Carcinogenesis*, **5**, 1–5

Farnum, C. E. and Wilsman, N. J. (1988). Lectin-binding histochemistry of intracellular glycoconjugates of the reserve cell zone of growth plate cartilage. *J. Orthop. Res.*, **6**, 166–179

Fenoglio-Preiser, C. and Willman, C. L. (1987). Molecular biology and the pathologist. General principles and applications. *Arch. Pathol. Lab. Med.*, **111**, 601–619

Filipe M. I. and Branfoot, A. C. (1974). Abnormal patterns of mucous secretion in apparently normal mucosa of the large intestine with carcinoma. *Cancer*, **34**, 282–290

Foster, J. R., Elcombe, C. R., Boobis, A. R., Davies, D. S., Sesardic, D., McQuade, J., Robson, R. T., Hayward, C. and Lock, E. A. (1986). Immunocytochemical localization of cytochrome P–450 in hepatic and extra-hepatic tissues of the rat with a monoclonal antibody against cytochrome P–450c. *Biochem. Pharmacol.*, **35**, 4543–4554

Garman, R. H. (1990). Artefacts in routinely immersion fixed nervous tissue. *Toxicol. Pathol.*, **18**, 149–153

Geleff, S., Böck, P. and Stockinger, L. (1986). Lectin binding affinities of the epithelium in the respiratory tract. A light microscopical study of ciliated epithelium in rat, guinea pig, and hamster. *Acta Histochem.*, **78**, 83–95

Giampaolo, C., Bray, K., Kowalski, B. and Rogers, A. E. (1989). Cytologic characteristics of neoplastic and regenerating hepatocytes in fine needle aspirates of rat liver. *Toxicol. Pathol.*, **17**, 743–753

Gil, J. and Martinez-Hernandez, A. (1984). The connective tissue of the rat lung: Electron immunocytochemical studies. *J. Histochem. Cytochem.*, **32**, 230–238

Gough, A. W., Barsoum, N. J., Renlund, R. C.,

Sturgess, J. M. and de la Iglesia, F. A. (1985). Fine structural changes during reparative phase of canine drug-induced arthropathy. *Vet. Pathol.*, **22**, 82–84

Gray, J. E. (1981). Appraisal of the intramuscular irritation test in the rabbit. *Fund. Appl. Toxicol.*, **1**, 290–292

Greaves, P. and Barsoum, N. J. (1990). Tumours of soft tissues. In Turusov, V. S. (Ed.), *Pathology of Laboratory Animals*, Vol. 1, *Tumours of the Rat*, 2nd edn. IARC, Lyon, pp. 597–623.

Greaves, P. and Boiziau, J.-L. (1984). Altered patterns of mucin secretion in gastric hyperplasia in mice. *Vet. Pathol.*, **21**, 224–228

Greaves, P. and Faccini, J. M. (1984). The pathological evaluation of toxicological studies. In *Rat Histopathology. A Glossary for Use in Toxicity and Carcinogenicity Studies*. Elsevier, Amsterdam, pp. 240–245

Greaves, P., Filipe, M. I. and Branfoot, A. C. (1980). Transitional mucosa and survival in human colorectal cancer. *Cancer*, **46**, 764–770

Greaves, P., Irisarri, E. and Monro, A. M. (1986). Hepatic foci of cellular and enzymatic alteration and nodules in rats treated with clofibrate or diethylnitrosamine followed by phenobarbital: Their rate of onset and their reversibility. *J. Natl Cancer Inst.*, **76**, 475–484

Gregg, N. J., Courtauld, E. A. and Bach, P. H. (1990). High resolution light microscopic morphological and microvascular changes in an acutely induced renal papillary necrosis. *Toxicol. Pathol.*, **18**, 47–55

Griffin, J. W. (1990). Basic pathology in the nervous system. *Toxicol. Pathol.*, **18**, 83–88

Guder, W. G. and Ross, B. D. (1984). Enzyme distribution along the nephron. *Kidney Int.*, **26**, 101–111

Hawkins, K. L., Lloyd, R. V. and Toy, K. A. (1989). Immunohistochemical localization of chromogranin A in normal tissues from laboratory animals. *Vet. Pathol.*, **26**, 488–498

Hayakawa, B. N., Jorgensen, A. O., Gotlieb, A. I., Zhao, M.-S. and Liew, C.-C. (1984). Immunofluorescent microscopy for the identification of human necrotic myocardium. *Arch. Pathol. Lab. Med.*, **198**, 284–286

Helliwell, T. R. (1988). Lectin binding and desmin staining during bupivicaine-induced necrosis and regeneration in rat skeletal muscle. *J. Pathol.*, **155**, 317–326

Henderson, J. D., Jr., Mullarky, R. H. and Ryan, D. E. (1987). Tissue biocompatibility and kevlar aramid fibres and polymethylmethacrylate composites in rabbits. *J. Biomed. Mater. Res.*, **21**, 59–64

Herrick, S. S., Davis, C., Donnelly, D. V., Lockhart, T., Marek, L. and Russell, H. (1983). Histopathology automated system. *Drug Inform. J.*, **17**, 287–295

Heywood, R. and Gopinath, C. (1988). Morphological assessment of visual dysfunction. *Toxicol. Pathol.*, **18**, 204–217

Heywood, R. and James, R. W. (1978). Assessment

of testicular toxicity in laboratory animals. *Environ. Hlth Perspect.*, **24**, 73–80

Hirth, R. S., Evans, L. D., Buroker, R. A. and Oleson, F. B. (1988). Gastric enterochromaffin-like cell hyperplasia and neoplasia in the rat: An indirect effect of the histamine H2-receptor antagonist, BL–6341. *Toxicol. Pathol.*, **16**, 273–287

Holthofer, H. (1983). Lectin binding sites in kidney. A comparative study of 14 animal species. *J. Histochem. Cytochem.*, **31**, 531–537

Howie, A. J., Gunson, B. K. and Sparke, J. (1990). Morphometric correlates of renal excretory function. *J. Pathol.*, **160**, 245–253

Ibrahim, K. S., Husain, O. A., Bitensky, L. and Chayen, J. (1983). A modified tetrazolium reaction for identifying malignant cells from gastric and colonic cancer. *J. Clin. Pathol.*, **36**, 133–136

Ingram, A. J. and Grasso, P. (1975). Patch testing in the rabbit using a modified patch test method. *Br. J. Dermatol.*, **92**, 131–142

Irisarri, E. and Mompon, P. (1983). Hepatic effects of fasting on 6 and 12 week old mice: A quantitative histochemical study. *J. Pathol.*, **140**, 176

Ishihara, K., Ohar, S., Azuumi, Y., Goso, K. and Hotto, K. (1984). Changes of gastric mucus glycoproteins with aspirin administration in rats. *Digestion*, **29**, 98–102

Jones, H. B. (1988). The role of ultrastructural investigations in neurotoxicology. *Toxicology*, **49**, 3–15

Jungerman, K. and Katz, N. (1982). Functional hepatocellular heterogeneity. *Hepatology*, **2**, 385–395

Kirivanta, I., Jurvelin, J., Tammi, M., Säämänen, A.-M. and Helminen, H. H. (1987). Weight bearing controls glycosaminoglycan concentration and articular cartilage thickness in the knee joints of young beagle dogs. *Arth. Rheum.*, **30**, 801–809

Kluwe, W. (1981). Renal function tests as indicators of kidney injury in subacute toxicity studies. *Toxicol. Appl. Pharmacol.*, **57**, 414–424

Koestner, A. (1990). Characterization of *N*-nitrosourea-induced tumors of the nervous system; their prospective value of studies of neurocarcinogenesis and brain tumor therapy. *Toxicol. Pathol.*, **18**, 186–192

Köhler, C., Eriksson, L. G., Hansson, T., Warner, M. and Ake-Gustafsson, J. (1988). Immunohistochemical localization of cytochrome P-450 in the rat brain. *Neurosci. Lett.*, **84**, 109–114

Kolde, G. and Knop, J. (1987). Different cellular reaction patterns of epidermal Langerhans cells after application of contact sensitizing, toxic and tolerogenic compounds. A comparative ultrastructural and morphometric time course analysis. *J. Invest. Dermatol.*, **89**, 19–23

Kuger, P. (1988). Quantitative enzyme histochemistry in the brain. *Histochemistry*, **90**, 99–107

Le Goascogne, C., Robel, P., Gouézou, M., Sananès, N., Baulieu, E.-E. and Waterman, M. (1987). Neurosteroids: Cytochrome P-450scc in rat brain. *Science*, **237**, 1212–1215

Levine, G. M., Brousseau, P., O'Shaughnessy, D. J. and Losos, G. J. (1987). Quantitative immunocytochemistry by digital image analysis. Application to toxicologic pathology. *Toxicol. Pathol.*, **15**, 303–307

Liberman, M. C. (1990). Quantitative assessment of inner ear pathology following ototoxic drugs or acoustic trauma. *Toxicol. Pathol.*, **18**, 138–148

Linnoila, I. and Petrusz, P. (1984). Immunohistochemical techniques and their application in the histology of the respiratory system. *Environ. Hlth Perspect.*, **56**, 131–148

Lloyd, R. V and Landefeld, T. D. (1986). Detection of prolactin messenger RNA in rat anterior pituitary *in situ* hybridization. *Am. J. Pathol.*, **125**, 35–44

Lloyd, R. V. and Mailloux, J. (1987). Effect of diethylstilbestrol and propylthiouracil on the rat pituitary. An immunohistochemical study. *J. Natl Cancer Inst.*, **79**, 865–873

Ludwin, S. K., Kosek, J. C. and Eng, L. F. (1976). The topographical distribution of S-100 and GFA proteins in adult rat brain: An immunohistochemical study using horseradish peroxidase-labelled antibodies. *J. Comp. Neurol.*, **165**, 197–208

Luiten, P. G. M., Wouterlood, F. G., Matsuyama, T., Strosberg, A. D., Buwalder, B. and Gaykema, R. P. A. (1988). Immunocytochemical applications in neuroanatomy. Demonstration of connections, transmitters and receptors. *Histochemistry*, **90**, 85–97.

Luster, M. I., Munson, A. E., Thomas, P. T., Holsapple, M. P., Fenters, J. D., White, K. L. Jr., Lauer, L. D., Germolec, D. R., Rosenthal, G. J. and Dean, J. H. (1988). Development of a testing battery to assess chemical induced immunotoxicity: National Toxicology Program's guidelines for immunotoxicity evaluation in mice. *Fund. Appl. Toxicol.*, **10**, 2–19

Mankin, H. J. (1974). The reaction of articular cartilage to injury and osteoarthritis. *New Engl. J. Med.*, **291**, 1285–1292

Maronpot, R. R. (1987). Ovarian toxicity and carcinogenicity in eight recent National Toxicology Program studies. *Environ. Hlth Perspect.*, **73**, 125–130

Maronpot, R. R., Harada, T., Murthy, A. S. K. and Boorman, G. A. (1989). Documenting foci of hepatocellular alteration in two-year carcinogenicity studies: Current practices of the National Toxicology Program. *Toxicol. Pathol.*, **17**, 675–683

Martin, M. S., Hammann, A. and Martin, F. (1986). Gut-associated lymphoid tissue and 1,2-dimethylhydrazine intestinal tumours in the rat: A histological and immunocytochemical study. *Int. J. Cancer*, **38**, 75–80

Masson, M. T., Villanove, F. and Greaves, P. (1986). Histological demonstration of wheat germ lectin binding sites in the liver of normal and ANIT treated rats. *Arch. Toxicol.*, **59**, 121–123

Mompon, P., Greaves, P. Irisarri, E., Monro, A. M.

and Bridges, J. W. (1987). A cytochemical study of the livers of rats treated with diethylnitrosamine/ phenobarbital, with benzidine/phenobarbital, with phenobarbital, or with clofibrate. *Toxicology*, **46**, 217–236

Moody, D. E., Taylor, L. A. and Smuckler, E. A. (1985). Immunofluorescent determination of the lobular distribution of a constitutive form of hepatic microsomal cytochrome P-450. *Hepatology*, **5**, 440–451

Moolenbeck, C. and Ruitenberg, E. J. (1981). The 'Swiss roll': A simple technique for histological studies of rodent intestine. *Lab. Anim.*, **15**, 57–59

Murata, F., Tsuyama, S., Suzuki, S., Hamada, H., Ozawa, M. and Muramatsu, T. (1983). Distribution of glycoconjugates in the kidney studied by use of labelled lectins. *J. Histochem. Cytochem.*, **31**, 139–144

Nemery, B., Dinsdale, D. and Verschoyle, R. D. (1987). Detecting and evaluating chemical-induced lung damage in experimental animals. *Bull. Eur. Physiopathol. Respir.*, **23**, 501–528

Neville, A. M. (1969). The adrenal medulla. In Symington, T. (Ed.), *Functional Pathology of the Human Adrenal Gland*, Part II. Livingstone, Edinburgh, pp. 219–234

Newberne, P. M. and de la Iglesia, F. A. (1985). Philosophy of blind slide reading in toxicological pathology. *Toxicol. Pathol.*, **13**, 255

Nicholson, G. L. (1974). The interactions of lectins with animal cell surfaces. *Int. Rev. Cytol.*, **39**, 89–190

Owen, R. L. and Bhalla, D. K. (1983). Cytochemical analysis of alkaline phosphatase and esterase activities and of lectin binding and anionic sites in rat and mouse Peyer's patch M cells. *Am. J. Anat.*, **168**, 199–212

Patrick, E., Maibach, H. I. and Burkalter, A. (1985). Mechanisms of chemically induced skin irritation. 1. Studies of time course, dose response and components of inflammation in the laboratory mouse. *Toxicol. Appl. Pharmacol.*, **81**, 476–490

Pawlikowski, M. (1982). The link between secretion and mitosis in the endocrine glands. *Life Sci.*, **30**, 315–320

Paxinos, G. and Watson, C. (1986). *The Rat Brain in Stereotaxic Coordinates*, 2nd edn. Academic Press, Sydney

Pesce, C. M. (1987). Biology of disease. Defining and interpreting diseases through morphometry. *Lab. Invest.*, **56**, 568–575

Pick, R., Jalil, J. E., Janicki, J. S. and Weber, K. T. (1989). The fibrillar nature and structure of isoproterenol-induced myocardial fibrosis in the rat. *Am. J. Pathol.*, **134**, 365–371

Pierobon-Bormioli, S., Sartore, S., Vitadello, M. and Schiaffino, S. (1980). 'Slow' myosins in vertebrate skeletal muscle. An immunofluorescence study. *J. Cell Biol.*, **85**, 672–681

Pierobon-Bormioli, S., Sartore, S., Vitadello, M. and Schiaffino, S. (1981). 'Fast' isomyosins and fibre types in mammalian skeletal muscle. *J. Histochem. Cytochem.*, **29**, 1179–1188

Piper, R. C. (1981). Morphologic evaluation of the heart in toxicology studies. In Balazs, T. (Ed.), *Cardiac Toxicology*. CRC Press, Boca Raton, Florida, pp. 111–136

Read, N. G., Astbury, P. J., Morgan, R. J. I., Parsons, D. N. and Port, C. J. (1988). Induction and exacerbation of hyaline droplet formation in the proximal tubular cells of the kidneys from male rats receiving a variety of pharmacological agents. *Toxicology*, **52**, 81–101

Read, N. G., Beesley, J. E., Blackett, N. M. and Trist, D. G. (1985). The accumulation of an aryloxylkylamidine (501C) and polymorphonuclear leucocytes: a quantitative electron microscopic study. *J. Pharm. Pharmacol.*, **37**, 96–99

Reynolds, S. H., Stowers, S. J., Patterson, R. M., Maronpot, R. R., Aaronson, S. A. and Anderson, M. W. (1987). Activated oncogenes in B6C3F1 mouse liver tumours: Implications for risk assessment. *Science*, **237**, 1309–1316

Rhodin, J. A. G. (1974). Adrenal (suprarenal) glands. In *Histology. A Text and Atlas*. Oxford University Press, New York, pp. 456–466

Richmond, R. S., Pereira, M. A., Carter, J. H., Carter, H. W. and Long, R. E. (1988). Quantitative and qualitative immunohistochemical detection of myc and src oncogene proteins in normal, nodule, and neoplastic rat liver. *J. Histochem. Cytochem.*, **36**, 179–184

Roberts, J. C., McCrossan, M. V. and Jones, H. B. (1990). The case for perfusion fixation of large tissue samples for ultrastructural pathology. *Ultrastruct. Pathol.*, **14**, 177–191

Robertson, D. G., Gray, R. H. and de la Iglesia, F. A. (1987). Quantitative assessment of trimethyltin induced pathology of the hippocampus. *Toxicol. Pathol.*, **15**, 7–17

Robinson, P. B., Harris, M., Harvey, W. and Papadogeargakis, N. (1982). Reduced bone growth on rats treated with anticonvulsant drugs: A type II pseudohypoparathyroidism? *Metab. Bone Dis. Rel. Res.*, **4**, 269–275

Robinson, P. B. and Harvey, W. (1989). Tooth root resorption induced in rats by diphenylhydantoin and parathyroidectomy. *Br. J. Exptl Pathol.*, **70**, 65–72

Roe, F. J. C. (1977). Quantitation and computerisation of histopathological data. Presentation at Ciba Symposium (unpublished)

Rushmore, T. H., Ghazarian, D. M., Subrahmanyan, V., Farber, E. and Ghoshal, A. K. (1987). Probable free radical effects on rat liver nuclei during early hepatocarcinogenesis with a choline-devoid low methionine diet. *Cancer Res.*, **47**, 6731–6740

Russell, L. D. and Frank, B. (1978). Characterization of rat spermiogenesis after plastic embedding. *Arch. Androl.*, **1**, 5–18

Russo, J., Tay, L. K. and Russo, I. H. (1982). Differentiation of the mammary gland and susceptibility to carcinogenesis. *Breast Cancer Res. Treat.*, **2**, 5–73

Salthouse, T. N. and Willigan, D. A. (1972). An enzyme histochemical approach to the evaluation of polymers for tissue compatibility. *J. Biomed. Res.*, **6**, 105–113

Schenk, R., Eggli, P. and Rosini, S. (1986). Quantitative morphometric evaluation of the inhibitory activity of new aminobisphosphonates on bone resorption in the rat. *Calcif. Tissue Int.*, **38**, 342–349

Schulte, B. A. and Spicer, S. S. (1983). Histochemical evaluation of mouse and rat kidneys with lectin-horseradish peroxidase conjugates. *Am. J. Anat.*, **168**, 345–362

Sheahan, D. G. and Jarvis, H. R. (1978). Comparative histochemistry of gastrointestinal mucosubstances. *Am. J. Anat.*, **146**, 103–132

Sobel, R. A. and Colvin, R. B. (1986). Responder strain-specific enhancement of endothelial and mononuclear cell Ia in delayed hypersensitivity reactions in (strain 2 × strain 13) F1 guinea pigs. *J. Immunol.*, **137**, 2132–2138

Solheim, T. (1974). Pluricolor fluorescent labeling of mineralizing tissue. *Scand. J. Dent. Res.*, **82**, 19–27

Spencer, A. J., Andreu, M. and Greaves, P. (1986). Neoplasia and hyperplasia of pancreatic endocrine tissue in the rat: An immunocytochemical study. *Vet. Pathol.*, **23**, 11–15

Spencer, P. S., Bischoff, M. C. and Schaumburg, H. H. (1980). Neuropathological methods for the detection of neurotoxic disease. In Spencer, P. S. and Schaumburg, H. H. (Eds), *Experimental and Clinical Neurotoxicology*. Williams and Wilkins, Baltimore, pp. 743–757

Spicer, S. S. and Schulte, B. A. (1982). Identification of cell surface constituents. *Lab. Invest.*, **47**, 2–4

Spinale, F. G., Schulte, B. A. and Crawford, F. A. (1989). Demonstration of early ischemic injury in porcine right ventricular myocardium. *Am. J. Pathol.*, **134**, 693–704

Stene, T. and Koppang, H. S. (1976). The effect of vincristine on dentinogenesis in the rat incisor. *Scand. J. Dent. Res.*, **84**, 342–344

Streett, C. S., Robertson, J. L. and Crissman, J. W. (1988). Morphologic stomach findings in rats and mice treated with the H2 receptor antagonists, ICI 125,211 and ICI 162,846. *Toxicol. Pathol.*, **16**, 299–304

Sturgess, J. and Reid, L. (1973). The effect of isoprenaline and pilocarpine on (a) bronchial mucus-secreting tissue and (b) pancreas, salivary glands, heart, thymus, liver and spleen. *Br. J. Exptl Pathol.*, **54**, 388–403

Sturgess, J. M. (1985). Mucociliary clearance and mucus secretion in the lung. In Witschi, H. P. and Brain, J. D. (Eds), *Toxicology of Inhaled Materials. General Principles of Inhalation Toxicology*. Springer-Verlag, Berlin, pp. 319–367

Szczech, G. M. and Tucker, W. E. Jr. (1985). Nail loss and foot-pad erosions in beagle dogs given BW 134U, a nucleoside analog. *Toxicol. Pathol.*, **13**, 181–184

Taper, H. S., Somer, M. P., Lans, M., de Gerlache, J. and Roberfroid, M. (1988). Histochemical detection of the in vivo produced cellular aldehydes by means of direct Schiff's reaction in CC14 intoxicated liver. *Arch. Toxicol.*, **61**, 406–410

Taradach, C. and Greaves, P. (1984). Spontaneous eye lesions in laboratory animals: Incidence in relation to age. *CRC Crit. Rev. Toxicol.*, **12**, 121–147

Tatematsu, M., Tsuda, H., Shirai, T., Masui, T. and Ito, N. (1987). Placental glutathione S-transferase (GST-P) as a new marker for hepatocarcinogenesis: *In vivo* short-term screening for hepatocarcinogenesis. *Toxicol. Pathol.*, **15**, 60–68

Taylor, C. R. and Kledzig, G. (1981). Immunohistochemical techniques in surgical pathology — A spectrum of 'new' special stains. *Human Pathol.*, **12**, 590–596

Thompson, G. R., Baker, J. R., Fleischman, R. W., Rosenkranz, H., Schaeppi, U. H., Cooney, D. A. and Davis, R. D. (1972). Preclinical toxicologic evaluation of bleomycin (NSC 125 006), a new antitumor antibiotic. *Toxicol. Appl. Pharmacol.*, **22**, 544–555

Tischler, A. S. and DeLellis, R. A. (1988). The rat adrenal medulla. 1. The normal adrenal. *J. Am. Coll. Toxicol.*, **7**, 1–19

Tischler, A. S., DeLellis, R. A., Perlman, R. L., Allen, J. M., Costopoulos, D., Lee, Y. C., Nunnemacher, G., Wolfe, H. J. and Bloom, S. R. (1985). Spontaneous proliferative lesions of the adrenal medulla in ageing Long-Evans rats. Comparison to PC12 cells, small granule-containing cells, and human adrenal medullary hyperplasia. *Lab. Invest.*, **53**, 486–498

Tsiftis, D., Jass, J. R., Filipe, M. I. and Wastell, C. (1980). Altered patterns of mucin secretion in precancerous lesions induced in the glandular part of the rat stomach by the carcinogen N-methyl-N'-nitro-N-nitrosoguanidine. *Invest. Cell. Pathol.*, **3**, 339–408

Tyler, W. S., Dungworth, D. L., Plopper, C. G., Hyde, D. M. and Tyler, N. K. (1985). Structural evaluation of the respiratory system. *Fund. Appl. Toxicol.*, **5**, 405–422

Ulvik, N. M., Dahl, E. and Hars, R. (1982). Classification of plastic-embedded rat seminiferous epithelium prior to electron microscopy. *Int. J. Androl.*, **5**, 27–36

van der Valk, P. and Maijer, C. J. L. M. (1987). Histology of reactive lymph nodes. *Am. J. Surg. Pathol.*, **11**, 866–882

Walker, R. (1985). The use of lectins in histopathology. *Histopathology*, **9**, 1121–1124

Warburton, M. J., Mitchell, D., Ormerod, E. J. and Rudland, P. (1982). Distribution of myoepithelial cells and basement membrane proteins in the resting, pregnant, lactating and involuting rat mammary gland. *J. Histochem. Cytochem.*, **30**, 667–676

Weibel, E. R. (1979). The lung and its gas exchange apparatus: an example of the use of stereology in studies of structure-function correlation. In Weibel, E. R. (Ed.), *Stereological Methods*, Vol. 1, *Practical Methods for Biological Morphometry*. Academic Press, New York, pp. 322–331

Whittaker, P., Boughner, D. R. and Kloner, R. A. (1989). Analysis of healing after myocardial infarction using polarized light microscopy. *Am. J. Pathol.*, **134**, 879–893

Widgren, U. and Enerbäck, L. (1983). Mucosal mast cells of the rat intestine: a re-evaluation of fixation and staining properties, with special reference to protein blocking and solubility of the granular glycosaminoglycans. *Histochem. J.*, **15**, 571–582

Wright, J. A. (1989). A comparison of rat femoral, sternebral and lumbar vertebral bone marrow fat content by subjective and image analysis of histological assessment. *J. Comp. Pathol.*, **100**, 419–426

Wright, J. A., Wadsworth, P. F. and Stewart, M. G. (1990). Neurone-specific enolase in rat and mouse phaeochromocytomas. *J. Comp. Pathol.*, **102**, 475–478

Yasuda, K. and Yamashita, S. (1985). Immunohistochemical study on gamma glutamyl transpeptidase in the rat kidney with monoclonal antibodies. *J. Histochem. Cytochem.*, **34**, 111

Young, J. T. (1981). Histopathologic examination of the rat nasal cavity. *Fund. Appl. Toxicol.*, **1**, 309–312

Zak, M., Kovaks, K., McComb, D. J. and Heitz, P. U. (1985). Aminoglutethimide stimulated corticotrophs. An immunocytologic, ultrastructural and immunoelectron microscopic study of the rat adenohypophysis. *Virchows Arch. Cell. Pathol.*, **49**, 93–106

Zaki, F. G., Keim, G. R., Takii, Y, and Inagami, T. (1982). Hyperplasia of the juxtaglomerular cells and renin localization in kidneys of normotensive animals given captopril. *Ann. Clin. Lab. Sci.*, **12**, 200–215

Zbinden, G. (1988). Biopharmaceutical studies, a key to better toxicology. *Xenobiotica*, **18**, Suppl. 1, 9–14

Zbinden, G., Fent, K. and Thouin, M. H. (1988). Nephrotoxicity screening in rats; general approach and establishment of test criteria. *Arch. Toxicol.*, **61**, 344–348

FURTHER READING

Glaister, J. (1986). *Principles of Toxicological Pathology*. Taylor and Francis, London

Haschek, W. M. and Rousseaux, C. G. (1991). *Handbook of Toxicologic Pathology*. Academic Press, San Diego, California

Newberne, J. W. (1994). The pathologist in litigation: a scientist's perspective. *Toxicological Pathology*, **22**, 222–225

11 Clinical Chemistry

M. D. Stonard and G. O. Evans

INTRODUCTION

The choice of tests which are employed in clinical chemistry is to some extent influenced by the guidelines for hazard assessment/safety evaluation of the various regulatory authorities (Table 1; Alder *et al.*, 1981—see Chapter 42 on Regulatory requirements). Other tests may be added on the basis of their diagnostic value or a particular known or suggested mechanism of action. For example, cholinesterases should be included where compound structures are similar to organophosphate or carbamate esters, which are known cholinesterase inhibitors.

In the early stages of the safety evaluation of development compounds, a variety of tests should be chosen to evaluate the broadest possible range of physiological and metabolic functions and to provide early indications of toxicity and possible target organs. At later stages, a tiered approach using more specialized targeted measurements may be required to characterize treatment-induced changes—e.g. urinary enzymes for monitoring nephrotoxicity (Kallner and Tryding, 1989). Few of the common biochemical parameters are independent of each other, and several measurements may be used to determine damage in a single organ—e.g. plasma enzymes in the assessment of hepatotoxicity. As the liver and kidneys are frequently the target organs in

toxicity studies, several of the traditional clinical chemistry measurements applied in the clinical situation can be used to detect damage to these organs. For the smaller laboratory animals, the number of analytes is governed partially by the restricted volume of plasma available for analysis.

Great emphasis is placed on the use of plasma enzymes as markers of organ damage, and therefore many enzymes have been investigated in toxicological studies (Table 2). The plasma activity of an enzyme depends on several factors, including the enzyme concentrations in different tissues, the intracellular location of the enzyme, the severity of tissue and cellular damage, the molecular size of the enzyme, and the rate of clearance of the enzyme from plasma.

The distribution of enzymes in different tissues varies between species, and therefore influences their diagnostic effectiveness in particular species (Clampitt and Hart, 1978; Keller, 1981; Lindena *et al.*, 1986). For example, plasma alkaline phosphatase (ALP) and lactate dehydrogenase (LDH) activities show greater variability in rats and monkeys when compared with man, and therefore have a poorer predictive or diagnostic value in these species. In young animals the osseous ALP isoenzyme is the dominant form in plasma, but in the adult rat the proportion of intestinal ALP in plasma is greater than in other species. Plasma γ-glutamyl transferase (GGT) activities are lower in most rodent species compared with the activity found in man, but the enzyme is a good marker of chemically induced cholestasis (Leonard *et al.*, 1984).

This general consideration of the diagnostic effectiveness of plasma enzyme measurements in different species also extends to other measurements, particularly hormones. For example, corticosterone is the primary glucocorticosteroid of rat adrenal tissue, and is therefore the plasma marker of choice in the rat. However, in canine plasma there are substantial quantities of both cortisol and corticosterone in comparison with human and guinea-pig plasma, where cortisol is the dominant glucocorticosteroid.

Table 1 Blood, plasma or serum tests suggested by regulatory authorities for toxicology studies

Acid/base balance (pH)	Glucose
Alanine aminotransferase	Hormones (miscellaneous)
Albumin	Inorganic phosphate
Alkaline phosphatase	Lactate dehydrogenase
Aspartate aminotransferase	Lipids (triglycerides, non-
Bilirubin (total)	esterified fatty acids)
Calcium	Potassium
Chloride	Protein
Cholesterol	Sodium
Cholinesterase	Total protein
Creatinine	Urea (or urea nitrogen)
Gamma-glutamyl	
transferase	

Table 2   Enzymes, their abbreviations and enzyme commission (E.C.) numbers

Abbreviation	Recommended name	EC number
ALT (GPT)	Alanine aminotransferase	2.6.1.2
AAP	Alanine aminopeptidase	3.4.1.2
ALP	Alkaline phosphatase	3.3.1.1
AMY	Amylase	3.2.1.1
AST (GOT)	Aspartate aminotransferase	2.6.1.1
CHE	Cholinesterase	3.1.1.8
CK (CPK)	Creatine kinase	2.7.3.2
GGT	γ-Glutamyl transferase	2.3.2.2
GLDH	Glutamate dehydrogenase	1.4.1.3
HBD	α-Hydroxybutyrate dehydrogenase	
ICDH	Isocitrate dehydrogenase	1.1.1.42
LDH	Lactate dehydrogenase	1.1.1.27
LAAP	Leucine arylamidase	3.4.11.2
LAP	Leucine aminopeptidase	3.4.11.1
LIP	Lipase	3.1.1.3
NAG	*N*-Acetylglucosaminidase	3.2.1.30
5′NT	5′-Nucleotidase	3.1.3.5
OCT	Ornithine carbamoyltransferase	2.1.3.3
SDH	Sorbitol dehydrogenase	1.1.1.14

Preanalytical Variables

It is necessary to distinguish between treatment-induced responses to a test material and normal biological variations, particularly where statistical differences are found for data in the absence of any other findings. When biological variation is considered, several preanalytical variables must be considered; they include species, genetic influences, sex, age, environmental conditions, chronobiochemical changes or cyclic biorhythms, diet and water intake, stress, exercise, and the route chosen for the administration of the test compound.

Clearly, there are major differences between species for reference clinical chemistry values in healthy laboratory animals (Mitruka and Rawnsley, 1977; Caisey and King, 1980; Loeb and Quimby, 1989), and these differences are not necessarily related to size or relative organ weight (Garattini, 1981). Genetic differences may occur in healthy animals—e.g. glomerular filtration rates vary between inbred strains of rats (Hackbarth *et al.*, 1981)—or the responses to a particular compound may vary between strains (Berdanier and Baltzell, 1986). Differences related to sex and age of laboratory animals are often observed (Nachbaur *et al.*, 1977; Nakamura *et al.*, 1983; Uchiyama *et al.*, 1985).

Several environmental factors which affect biological systems have been recognized including caging density, lighting, room temperature, relative humidity, cage bedding, cleaning procedures, etc. (Fouts, 1976). To some extent rodent accommodation is now designed to minimize the effects of such factors, but dogs may undergo periodic changes of housing, which may affect biochemical values (Kuhn and Hardegg, 1988). Parasitic or viral infections present in the animal stock may also affect some measurements—e.g. plasma proteins.

Cyclic variation of some analytes, particularly hormones, occurs in several laboratory animals (Jordan *et al.*, 1980; Orth *et al.*, 1988). Circadian rhythms may be altered by changing the light—dark cycles of the animals' accommodation, or they may be adapted by other experimental procedures—e.g. intravenous infusion effects of nutrients on blood glucose levels (Sitren and Stevenson, 1980). Other cyclic variations may be related to reproductive cycles or seasonal changes.

While in recent years attention has been drawn to the effects of differing diets in long-term carcinogenicity studies, diet or feeding regimens may also cause a marked effect on biochemical values, particularly in small rodents. Food restriction for 16–24 h in rats may produce changes in the composition of plasma enzymes, urea, creatinine and glucose (Jenkins and Robinson, 1975; Apostolou *et al.*, 1976; Kast and Nishikawa,

1981). Fasting may also lead to haemoconcentration effects.

The practice of fasting small laboratory animals overnight prior to blood collection may produce changes which differ from the findings for animals that have been fed. These differences may be due to (1) an alteration of the absorption or uptake of the test compound, (2) changes in the competitive binding of proteins with the test compound, (3) changes in metabolism rates or detoxification mechanisms or (4) modification of renal clearance. Treatment prior to sequential blood sampling in toxicology studies should be similar in respect to food and water intake. Fasting prior to blood collection also produces a transient reduction in body weight which distorts the growth curve.

Mineral imbalances in the diets may predispose some species to particular conditions—e.g. nephrocalcinosis with associated changes in plasma and urine biochemistry (Stonard *et al.*, 1984; Bertani *et al.*, 1989; Meyer *et al.*, 1989). Reduction of dietary protein may cause changes of plasma analytes (Schwartz *et al.*, 1973), and changes in the composition of dietary fat or the use of corn oil as a vehicle for test compounds may also produce effects on plasma chemistry measurements (Meijer *et al.*, 1987).

Biochemical changes occur in stress situations, and include changes of plasma corticosterone/cortisol, catecholamines and other analytes, although toxic effects may be variable in these situations (Vogel, 1987). Transport between breeding colonies and user laboratories or different environments (Bean-Knudsen and Wagner, 1987; Garnier *et al.*, 1990), caging arrangements (Riley, 1981) and restraint during experimental procedures (Pearl *et al.*, 1966; Gärtner *et al.*, 1980) appear to be stressful, with the potential to affect the levels of several analytes.

There are several general points to consider when collecting blood from laboratory animals, including the use of anticoagulants and the changes in blood composition which occur on standing.

When collecting blood, it is important to separate the plasma or serum as soon as possible; this reduces the effects of glycolysis which result in reduced glucose levels, and increased lactate, inorganic phosphate and potassium values. Sodium fluoride or fluoride/oxalate anticoagulants may be used to minimize the effects of glycolysis, but these anticoagulants interfere with other measurements, including enzymes and electrolytes.

Heparin or lithium heparinate are suitable anticoagulants for most plasma measurements. Inappropriate use of anticoagulants, and incorrect proportions of anticoagulant to blood volumes, may also cause errors. Samples collected with sequestrene (EDTA) or sodium citrate for haematological investigations are not suitable for several electrolyte and enzyme measurements.

For several enzyme measurements, it is preferable to use plasma rather than serum, owing to the relatively high erythrocytic concentrations of those enzymes, or other enzymes which may interfere with their measurements (Korsrud and Trick, 1973; Friedel and Mattenheimer, 1976).

Several other factors to be considered when collecting blood, particularly from smaller laboratory animals, include the sampling site, the choice of anaesthetic agent and the method for drawing the blood from the site of collection. In general, the collection of blood from dogs and most primates does not cause particular problems in terms of the sample volume required for clinical chemistry (Mitruka and Rawnsley, 1977; Fowler, 1982). However, the use of restraining procedures and sedatives for either large or small primates may affect biochemical values (Davy *et al.*, 1987).

For rodents, various sites and anaesthetic agents have been used, and the choice of blood collection procedure may markedly affect some biochemical measurements (Neptun *et al.*, 1985). For interim blood collections the retro-orbital plexus, tail or jugular veins may be used, whereas the major blood vessels (e.g. abdominal aorta) or cardiac puncture may be used at necropsy.

Anaesthetic agents used for rodents include halothane, ether, barbiturate, methoxyfluorane and carbon dioxide. Repeated anaesthesia may affect the analyte values, and blood collections repeated too frequently may cause anaemia. The collection of 0.5 ml of blood from a 20 g mouse represents more than a 20 per cent loss of blood volume for that animal. Combinations of different methods of blood collection within the same study for interim and terminal sampling points may confound interpretation of data and should be avoided if at all possible.

When collecting the blood with either a syringe or vacuum-container device, the choice of needle in relation to the proposed blood vessel site for collection is important (Conybeare *et al.*, 1988). Additionally, forcing blood from a syringe into the collection tube through a fine needle frequently increases the degree of haemolysis observed in the plasma samples.

Haemolysis and lipaemia may interfere with analyte determinations (Young, 1990), although the degree of interference may vary with a particular method (Powers *et al.*, 1986). Haemolysis may be compound-induced, but more frequently is due to problems in sample collection (Fowler, 1982); additional haematological data may be used to elucidate this situation. Interference due to haemolysis may affect the analytical results in several different ways. A change in plasma analyte concentration may occur because of a higher analyte concentration in erythrocytes—e.g. potassium.

Some enzymes occurring at relatively high concentrations in erythrocytes compared with plasma may interfere with the measurement of other enzymes—e.g. adenylate kinase interferes with creatine kinase (CK) measurements. Absorbance due to the presence of haemoglobin may affect absorbance measurements for a selected analyte, or haemoglobin may interfere with a chemical reaction—e.g. diazotization reactions for bilirubin (Chin *et al.*, 1979; Leard *et al.*, 1990). Some coloured compounds such as naphthoquinones may impart a pink or red colour to plasma which may be misinterpreted as haemolysis.

Turbidity caused by hyperlipaemic plasma may also interfere with the measurement of some analytes; this hyperlipaemia may be induced by the test material (Steinberg *et al.*, 1986) or may be caused by conditions such as severe ketosis. The turbidity due to lipaemia may be reduced by ultracentrifugation or precipitation techniques (Thompson and Kunze, 1984), but these procedures may disguise significant changes of analyte concentrations.

Analytical Procedures

The introduction of Good Laboratory Practice (GLP) requiring proven equipment maintenance, calibration and documentation, and, more importantly, the use of analytical equipment such as centrifugal analysers, has led to an overall improvement in analytical procedures when small volumes of plasma (3–50 µl per test) are used. Most laboratories use automated analytical methods for the common biochemical measurements, and adhere to quality control procedures within the laboratory; these laboratories may also participate in external quality assessment schemes. The level of precision or imprecision intra-assay is usually less than 5 per cent (expressed as a coefficient of variation) for most assays, but may be slightly higher for specialized assays—e.g. hormones or manual analytical methods.

Despite improvements in analytical procedures, large differences for reference (or control) ranges are observed between laboratories. Some of these differences are due to the use of methods and reagents formulated for the analysis of human samples, and these methods may not be suitable for all laboratory animal species. Dooley (1979) reported that substrate concentrations required for measurements of aspartate aminotransferase (AST) differed substantially between rat, dog, monkey and human sera. Other examples include the measurement of plasma creatinine using alkaline picrate reagent, in which the contribution of non-creatinine chromogens is greater in some laboratory species compared with humans (Evans, 1986b), and the differing affinities of various dyes for plasma albumin in different species (Evans and Parsons, 1988).

Xenobiotics may interfere with the analytical methods in several different ways. Direct interference with an assay may be chemical or physical, and the interference may be either negative or positive. Various guidelines have been proposed for testing for drug interference in clinical chemistry measurements (Kallner and Tryding, 1989), but seldom are the metabolites studied individually for possible interference with analytes. Additionally, the interference of a particular compound may vary with the analytical method (Evans, 1985). Comprehensive databases have been established for pharmaceuticals known to cause analytical interference with clinical chemistry methods (Young, 1990).

In general, the analytical variation is less than the biological variation, and the intra-animal variability differs for each analyte—e.g. Leissing *et al.* (1985) found in healthy dogs that intra-animal variability for sodium was less than 1 per cent, whereas it was more than 40 per cent for ALP. This intra-animal variation differs between species—e.g the analytical variation for glucose is small (with a coefficient of variation of <2 per cent for the method) but the biological variation observed in the marmoset was greater than in the dog, probably owing to stress during blood collection procedures (Fowler, 1982).

Although several analytes exhibit a normal (or Gaussian) distribution, other analytes show a skewed distributon to the right or are not continuous in nature. The distribution of analyte values may vary between and within long-term studies (Weil, 1982).

In rodent toxicology studies conducted for regulatory purposes, it is usual to compare differences between the treatment groups and a concurrent control group, while in studies using larger animals (i.e. primates, dogs, etc.), where group sizes of $n = 4$–6 per sex are common, the emphasis is both on differences, as already stated, and comparison with pretreatment values in the same animals. Where the number of animals within a study is small, it is advisable to take at least one baseline measurement and preferably more as a guide to intra-animal variations. It is sometimes necessary to compare the values obtained for a concurrent control group with the historical database, to ensure that differences between the concurrent control and treatment groups are not the consequence of an aberrant control group. Although historical reference ranges may be useful, there may be slight differences in the treatments (e.g. test vehicle) or animal populations studied. With samples taken from moribund animals in the absence of a concurrent control group, it is often difficult to distinguish between results expected due to toxicity and those results which would occur in moribund but untreated animals.

LIVER

Hepatic injury is well recognized as a toxicological problem, but the fact that the injuries are not a single entity is reflected by the choice of tests that may be used to detect hepatotoxicity. Xenobiotics may or may not produce functional and structural hepatic impairment. Drugs or metabolites may affect hepatic metabolizing enzymes or exhaust enzyme cofactors, resulting in either the inhibition of essential metabolic pathways or enhancement of alternative pathways with possible toxic byproducts (see Chapters 3 and 6).

Diagnostic tests for the evaluation of hepatic damage or dysfunction may be arbitrarily grouped as (1) plasma enzymes; (2) functional or clearance tests, including those tests which measure hepatic transport, uptake, conjugation and excretion; (3) tests to assess hepatic metabolism of proteins, lipids, carbohydrates and urate. The assessment of hepatic function and damage in animal species has been reviewed in the light of current practice in the UK (Woodman, 1988a).

Plasma Enzymes

Various factors affecting plasma enzyme measurements were discussed earlier in this chapter. In the early stages of tissue damage, cytoplasmic enzymes may leak from cells where membrane permeability has altered. As the severity of tissue damage progresses, enzymes normally present in subcellular organelles will be released into the circulation. Increased plasma enzyme activities may indicate loss of hepatocyte integrity with changes of parenchymal enzymes, or 'biliary' enzymes may indicate obstruction, proliferation, inflammation or neoplasia of the biliary system. Reduced plasma enzyme activities are also observed in some forms of liver injury—e.g. cholinesterase (see later discussion). In addition, some enzyme changes are the result of enzyme induction—e.g. increase of ALP that occurs with glucocorticosteroids (Dorner *et al.*, 1974; Eckersall, 1986).

Many of the enzymes listed in Table 2 have been used or tested as markers of hepatotoxicity. It should not be assumed that enzymes applied in human clinical practice show the same diagnostic value in various animal species (Woodman, 1981). The majority of plasma enzyme measurements for detecting hepatotoxicity are not specific to the liver and show a wide tissue distribution. Several of the enzymes commonly measured are affected by damage to extrahepatic tissue—e.g. AST and LDH following injury to cardiac or skeletal muscles.

Alanine aminotransferase (ALT, previously called GPT) is widely used as a sensitive marker of hepatotoxicity but does lack some specificity. In the dog the concentration of ALT found in the hepatic tissue is approximately 5 times that found in any other tissues, but tissue enzyme distribution studies show that this difference is much less in the guinea-pig, rat and rabbit (Clampitt and Hart, 1978; Lindena *et al.*, 1986). In some species plasma ALT activity is low and is less useful as a marker of hepatotoxicity (Davy *et al.*, 1984; Cowie and Evans, 1985). Plasma AST may also be elevated in hepatotoxicity where cellular and subcellular injury has occurred; the proportional activity of the two isoforms of the enzyme (mitochondrial and cytosolic) may indicate the extent of liver injury.

Several dehydrogenases have been used as screening tests for liver injury. The diagnostic value of LDH is limited, because it is widely distributed in the tissues and the tissue isoenzyme patterns vary between species. Sorbitol dehydrogenase is one of the more specific tests for hepatotoxicity, since it is confined mainly to the liver. Glutamate dehydrogenase (GDH), which is present in the liver at high concentrations, malate dehydrogenase (MDH) and isocitrate dehydrogenase (ICDH) activities also change following hepatic injury.

ALP is widely used as a marker of liver injury, particularly for cholestasis. However, the variable composition of plasma ALP alters its diagnostic value in different species. The dominant ALP isoenzyme in dog plasma is the hepatic form, but the osseous and intestinal isoenzymes are the dominant forms in rat plasma. The concentration of ALP in rat liver is very low, which limits its usefulness as an index of hepatic injury in this species. In the rat, the food intake affects the proportion of intestinal ALP in plasma (Pickering and Pickering, 1978a,b). In the majority of species, age-related changes are found due to the presence of osseous ALP. Various methods have been reported for separating the hepatic, intestinal and osseous ALP isoenzymes, including electrophoretic separations, heat lability, and inhibition studies with urea, levamisole and phenylalanine (Moss, 1982).

GGT is a useful marker of cholestasis, but its use as a marker of enzyme induction and of the presence of hepatic tumours is less predictive compared with data from human studies. The relative enzyme activity of GGT is highest in the kidney, of all the major organs. In the rat kidney the level of GGT is approximately 200 times higher than the level found in the liver: mouse, hamster and rat have lower GGT activity than that found in guinea-pig, rabbit and man. Although plasma GGT activity is lower in rodents

than in other species, it remains a good marker of cholestasis (Braun *et al.*, 1987).

Of the other plasma enzymes, ornithine carbamoyl transferase (OCT) is a sensitive liver-specific enzyme (Baumann and Berauer, 1985): arginase, 5-nucleotidase and leucine arylamidase (LAAP) may also be used. The half-life of arginase is shorter than that of ALT, and therefore plasma levels of arginase return to normal more rapidly; this point emphasizes the necessity to consider the relative half-lives for all of the enzymes used to test for hepatotoxicity. Whether through lack of technical simplicity, suitability for use with automated laboratory analysers or readily available reagents, some of the enzyme determinations mentioned are rarely used in regulatory toxicology studes—e.g. OCT.

Plasma Bilirubin

Increased plasma concentrations of total bilirubin (icterus) may follow excessive haem turnover by the reticuloendothelial system, alterations of hepatic clearance by microsomal conjugation, intrahepatic obstruction of the bile canaliculi, or extrahepatic obstruction of the bile duct. Where one of these conditions is truly severe, the measurement of conjugated (direct) and unconjugated (indirect) bilirubin may be helpful: extrahepatic obstruction is associated with increased concentrations of conjugated bilirubin, whereas plasma unconjugated bilirubin concentrations are increased in cases of haemolytic jaundice.

Plasma total bilirubin is lower (less than 8 μmol l^{-1}) in many laboratory animal species compared with the levels found in human plasma. Species such as the rat and the dog have a low renal threshold for bilirubin. The Gunn rat is unusual in that there is jaundice caused by a congenital defect in glucuronide formation, and this rat strain therefore serves as a useful model in elucidating bilirubin metabolism. The very low values found in rats (0.3–1.5 μmol l^{-1}) are below the limit of many photometric methods commonly used in the assay (Rosenthal *et al.*, 1981); this methodological problem is exacerbated when measurements of conjugated bilirubin are required.

When haemolytic jaundice occurs, the presence of plasma haemoglobin and other pigments may cause analytical interference at these low concentrations of plasma bilirubin. This has led to the suggestion that measurement of plasma total bilirubin is inappropriate in species such as the rat (Waner, 1990), although plasma bilirubin measurements still can be useful where cholestasis occurs. The binding of bilirubin by plasma proteins is complex in the presence of xenobiotics (Gautam *et al.*, 1984; Blanckaert *et al.*, 1986), and in the rat there are marked sex differences in hepatic conjugation of bilirubin (Muraca *et al.*, 1983).

Plasma Bile Acids

The development of various methods, including high-performance liquid chromatography, gas–liquid chromatography, radioimmunoassay and enzymatic methods, has encouraged several investigators to recommend this plasma measurement particularly as an indicator of cholestasis (Gopinath *et al.*, 1980; Woodman and Maile, 1981; Woodman, 1988a).

Total bile acids may be subdivided into primary (cholic and chenodeoxycholic) and secondary (deoxycholic and lithocholic) bile acids, with their taurine and glycine conjugates. The relative proportions of individual bile acids differ with species (Parraga and Kaneko, 1985). For example, the secondary bile acid, β-muricholate, is a prominent component of cholestasis in the rat (Greim *et al.*, 1972) but the reaction leading to its formation in man is absent (Hofmann, 1988). Simpler methods for total bile acids may not be appropriate for all species, and results must be interpreted in the light of these limitations. Secretion of bile acids alters after food intake, and the timing of blood samples in relation to food intake can be critical for the detection of changes. Hepatic uptake and the carrier-mediated transport system for bile acids differ from the mechanisms responsible for the transport of bilirubin and exogenous dyes (Alpert *et al.*, 1969; Schardsmidt *et al.*, 1975; Erlanger *et al.*, 1976).

Urine Bilirubin, Urobilinogen and Urobilin

Bilirubinuria can be a useful marker of hepatic necrosis or bile duct obstruction, but the low renal threshold in some animals reduces the usefulness of this test in borderline cases—e.g. increases of bilirubin may occur in the urine in the dog before changes of plasma total bilirubin (de Schepper and van der Stock, 1972).

Urobilinogen and stercobilinogen are formed from bile by the bacterial action of the intestinal flora, and enter the extrahepatic circulation to be excreted as urobilinogen. Urobilinogen may be increased following excessive breakdown of haemoglobin or hepatic dysfunction, including situations where there is a bypass via the enterohepatic circulation; urobilinogen is not elevated in cases of extrahepatic obstruction.

If exposed to strong light, urobilinogen is rapidly converted to urobilin. Both urobilinogen and urine bilirubin may be detected qualitatively by the use of test strips. Bile salts may also be elevated in some hepatobiliary conditions.

Exogenous Dyes

Several dye clearance and excretion tests have been used as indices of hepatic function. Bromsulphthalein (BSP or sulphbromophthalein) and indocyanine green (ICG) are the two commonly used cholephilic dyes (Jablonski and Owen, 1969). When administered intravenously, BSP binds principally to albumin and to a lesser extent to lipoprotein. In the hepatocytes the bound dye is removed from the circulation by conjugation with glutathione in the presence of glutathione transferase; the conjugated dye and a proportion of the free dye are excreted in the bile. These clearance measurements require additional blood collection procedures and accurately timed blood samples.

Approximately 50 per cent of liver functional mass has to be lost before the BSP clearance changes. Delayed dye clearance may be due to hepatic necrosis, cholestasis, reduced hepatic blood flow or renal dysfunction; obstruction of biliary excretion causes BSP retention. Several drugs may affect these dye clearance measurements, and one possible mechanism of interference is competitive binding of albumin with either BSP or the xenobiotic and/or its metabolite(s).

Marked differences are observed for BSP clearance determinations in various species. Both the rat and rabbit show greater ability to clear the dye than the dog—i.e. approximately 1 mg min^{-1} kg^{-1} in the first two species compared with 0.2 mg min^{-1} kg^{-1} in the dog. Therefore, it is essential to optimize BSP dosage and the timing of blood collections for each species studied (Klaassen and Plaa, 1967). The relationships of dosages and clearances for ICG between species is not identical with those determined with BSP (Klaassen and Plaa, 1969).

Plasma Proteins

Changes of plasma protein concentrations are not specific for hepatic necrosis, as discussed previously. Protein synthesis is altered by hepatocellular damage, with reduced hepatic synthesis of albumin, fibrinogen, alpha$_1$-antitrypsin, haptoglobin, transferrin, caeruloplasmin and other proteins.

Bile proteins have been detected in plasma of cholestatic rats following bile duct ligation (Hinton and Mullock, 1977), and increased concentrations of IgA and free IgA secretory component have been reported following chemically induced intrahepatic cholestasis (Wooley *et al.*, 1979). Changes of plasma proteins are more marked in chronic hepatotoxicity compared with acute or subchronic toxicity.

A reduction of plasma albumin is often accompanied by an increase in the γ-globulin fraction, and this is reflected by alterations of the albumin:globulin (A:G) ratio. Plasma protein electrophoresis using various matrices can provide more detailed information on changes of plasma protein. Flocculation or turbidity (thymol) tests based on the relative proportions of plasma proteins should be discarded in favour of more specific measurements of plasma proteins.

Impaired protein catabolism in diffuse liver disease can reduce the production of urea and, hence, is manifested as a reduced plasma urea concentration. Other related changes in severe liver damage include elevations in plasma ammonia and some amino acids such as taurine.

Plasma Lipids

Hepatic lipid content is altered by several xenobiotics, with accumulation of lipid in the parenchymal cells. Lipid accumulation in the liver often reflects changes in the rate of lipoprotein synthesis or a reduced ability to catabolize the non-esterified fatty acids which are formed when triglycerides are broken down. Several compounds of diverse structure have the ability in some rodent species to produce a hypolipidaemic response characterized by reductions in the circulating concentrations of triglycerides and/or cholesterol. These reductions in circulating lipids appear to reflect both structural and functional changes in the liver leading to differences in the metabolic handling of saturated fatty acids (Lock *et al.*, 1989). Fat accumulation in parenchymal cells does not necessarily lead to necrosis of hepatocytes, but some conditions involving fat accumulation may lead to the disruption of cellular integrity. Plasma lipid changes associated with hepatotoxicity may be detected by measuring plasma total cholesterol, triglycerides, ratio of esterified:free cholesterol, non-esterified fatty acids (Degen and van der Vies, 1985) and individual lipoprotein fractions.

KIDNEY

The primary functions of the kidney are in volume regulation, excretion of waste products, regulation of acid–base balance, regulation of electrolyte balance, and endocrine functions, including the renin–aldosterone axis, erythropoietin synthesis, 1,25-dihydroxycholecalciferol, and synthesis of prostaglandins and kinins. Nephrotoxic substances may impair some or all of these functions by a variety of toxic mechanisms (Commandeur and Vermeulen, 1990). It is important to recognize that renal function tests do not ensure identification of nephrotoxicity in all cases where structural alterations of the kidneys can be demonstrated by histopathology (Sharratt and Frazer, 1963). However, a combination of screening tests based on qualitative and quantitative measurements can be used to detect nephrotoxicity (Bovee, 1986; Fent *et al.*, 1988). Many xenobiotics are known to affect renal function, and these effects may vary between species because of the relative morphological differences of the kidneys (Mudge, 1982). The assessment of renal function and damage in animal species has been reviewed in the light of current practices in the UK (Stonard, 1990).

Glomerular Function

Glomerular function is commonly measured using creatinine and/or urea, as both of these endogenous substances are normally filtered from the plasma and reabsorbed or secreted to a minor extent. The degree of reabsorption or secretion differs from species to species. High values for plasma urea may occur in a variety of conditions other than renal failure—e.g. myocardial infarction, increased dietary nitrogen and gastrointestinal bleeding. Similarly, plasma creatinine concentration may also be affected by diet (Evans, 1987), although this is less well recognized. Although plasma creatinine is generally thought to be a better marker than urea of glomerular function, plasma creatinine measurements may be subject to analytical interference by endogenous non-creatinine chromogens or some xenobiotics—e.g. some cephalosporins (Evans, 1986b; Grotsch and Hajdu, 1987).

Determination of the glomerular filtration rate (GFR) by the measurement of endogenous creatinine involves the collection of timed urine samples, which may be difficult for small laboratory animals. More reliable measurements of GFR may be obtained by using exogenous inulin with or without radiolabel, [^{51}Cr]-EDTA, or iodothalamate. These determinations require additional infusion and accurately timed blood collection procedures, and may improve the accuracy of GFR determination but reduce the flexibility of study designs. These measurements may be affected by the use of particular anaesthetic agents for blood collection from small laboratory animals.

As glomerular filtration slows or ceases, plasma creatinine and/or urea will increase. The relationship between the loss of glomerular filtration capacity and plasma creatinine/urea is not linear. A significant amount of renal function capacity has to be lost before there is doubling of plasma creatinine or urea; conversely, plasma urea may remain within the normal range until renal function has been reduced by 50 per cent. The term 'BUN' should be used strictly for the determination of blood urea nitrogen (not plasma or serum urea). Non-creatinine chromogens lead to an underestimation of GFR. Glomerular function, plasma creatinine and urea, to a lesser extent, all show variation with age (Corman *et al.*, 1985; Goldstein, 1990).

Urinalysis

Urinalysis can be a useful non-invasive technique for monitoring nephrotoxicity, but it is important to give particular attention to the conditions for urine collection. Contamination of urine samples by diet and/or faeces may cause erroneous results for many parameters. Some assays may require the use of a preservative and/or cooling of the sample during collection. Simple observations of the urine appearance and colour may be useful, as the colour may be altered by the presence of exogenous and endogenous substances—e.g. blood, bilirubin, porphyrin and some drugs. Bromsulphthalein and phenolsulphthalein used for functional organ tests may impart colour to urine samples.

Several of the urinary measurements—e.g. glucose, pH, blood, ketones, urobilinogen, etc., can be made using one of several commercial test strips (or dipsticks). Certain pitfalls may be encountered as the test strips are designed for use in human clinical rather than laboratory animal practice; these pitfalls are primarily related to sensitivity and/or specificity—e.g. protein, osmolality (Evans and Parsons, 1986; Allchin and Evans, 1986c; Allchin *et al.*, 1987).

Urine volume and concentration may act as markers of nephrotoxicity. Many nephrotoxins will produce oliguria, whereas persistent polyuria may indicate an alteration of renal concentrating ability. Polyuria also may be a desired pharmacological response, such as that observed with diuretics. Osmolality, specific gravity or refractometry measurements can be used to monitor the renal concentrating ability, and additional information on renal tubular function may be obtained by using water deprivation or water loading techniques. The maximum osmolality that can be achieved varies with species, with both rat and dog giving values approximately twofold greater than in man (Schmidt-Nielsen and O'Dell, 1961). Additionally, the use of osmolar and/or free water clearance measurements can be used to differentiate between effects upon solute or water reabsorption (Bovee, 1986). Occasionally a urine specimen may appear to be extremely dilute, owing to the accidental addition of drinking-water by the animal in the metabolism cage.

Glycosuria may be detected conveniently by test strips using glucose oxidase methods, although these may be affected by several interferents, including ascorbate. Urinary glucose may reflect enhanced excretion because of elevated blood levels or be due to damage to the proximal tubules, where glucose is reabsorbed.

Changes of hydrogen ion concentration (pH) may reflect changes in tubular function or they may simply reflect dietary protein composition. High concentrations of xenobiotics or metabolites may also result in changes of urinary hydrogen ion concentration. Delays in analysing urine samples may cause hydrogen ion concentration values to be altered by ammonia produced by micro-organisms. Low pH may reflect catabolic states associated with severe toxicity.

Urine Cytology

Microscopic examination of urine sediment for the presence of erythrocytes, leucocytes, renal epithelial cells, bladder cells, spermatozoa, etc., may be used to detect renal tubular damage. The sediment may be examined unstained, although the use of stains helps to distinguish between renal epithelial cells and leucocytes (Prescott and Brodie, 1964; Hardy, 1970). The conditions used for collection, centrifugation and preparation of urine deposits are critical for semiquantitative analyses.

As the normal background of celluria differs from one species to another, and on the basis of a few published data on urine sediments in species other than man (Davies and Kennedy, 1967; Prescott, 1982), celluria appears to be of little benefit for monitoring chronic tubular injury and acute distal damage.

In acute proximal tubular damage, cells in urine may be a sensitive but unreliable indicator with four distinct phases. In the first phase there may be a delayed response, followed by a peak celluria in a second phase; there may be a recovery period despite continued exposure to the nephrotoxic substance in the third phase, which is followed by a final refractory phase where rechallenge is ineffective (Prescott and Ansari, 1969). Hyaline or granular casts associated with Tamm–Horsfall glycoprotein may be found in the tubular lumen and urine deposit.

The presence of blood in the urine may reflect non-specific systemic bleeding, renal or postrenal injury. Contamination of urine samples by blood from superficial injuries (e.g. skin abrasions) must always be considered as a possible explanation for blood in the urine. The presence of leucocytes in the urine may indicate bacterial infection.

Crystalluria may be due to the pH-dependent precipitation of urates or phosphates. Occasionally crystalluria may be due to the high urinary concentration of a xenobiotic or its metabolite(s).

Urine Protein

The measurement of urinary proteins can be used to assess glomerular integrity—i.e. the selective permeability of the glomerular membrane. This selectivity is altered by the action of various nephrotoxic agents, and this alteration may be monitored by continuing to measure urinary proteins. Tubular proteinuria may also occur with normal filtration of small-molecular-weight proteins but a failure of tubular reabsorption mechanism(s). Extrarenal proteinuria can occur as a result of inflammation, haemorrhage, or lower urinary tract infection.

Increased urinary protein levels are often the first signs of renal injury. Again test strips offer a simple method for the assessment of proteinuria, but they react mainly with albumin and are therefore not particularly useful in detecting the presence of other urinary proteins which may be found after renal tubular injury. Furthermore, the composition of the urinary proteins varies between species. The rat shows several qualitative and quantitative differences in protein excretion. The major protein in male rat urine is a low-molecular-weight protein, alpha$_{2u}$-globulin (Roy and Neuhaus, 1967), unlike other species, where albumin is the major urinary protein. Post puberty, male rats excrete more proteins than females and the amount of protein increases with age (Neuhaus and Flory, 1978; Alt *et al.*, 1980). The role of alpha$_{2u}$-globulin in light hydrocarbon nephropathy and hyaline droplet formation has received particular attention in recent years (Stonard *et al.*, 1985; Alden, 1986; Lock *et al.*, 1987).

Several methods for the quantitative measurement of urinary total protein are available (McElderry *et al.*, 1982; Dilena *et al.*, 1983), and there are several immunoassay techniques available for the measurement of specific proteins, although the choice of these methods is restricted by the lack of suitable purified proteins and specific antisera.

Primary tubular disorders may be distinguished from glomerular damage by the ratio of high- and low-molecular weight proteins in the urine. Techniques using various electrophoretic support media and buffers can provide additional information on the composition of urinary proteins (Allchin and Evans, 1986a; Stonard *et al.*, 1987; Boesken *et al.*, 1973).

The marked increase in urinary proteins which occurs in some nephrotic conditions may cause a marked reduction of plasma protein concentrations—e.g. albumin. One consequence of the reduction of plasma protein concentration will be alterations of the binding of xenobiotics to plasma proteins and of the concentrations of low-molecular-weight substances in the tubular fluid. For example, any substance 50 per cent bound to plasma protein has an effective filterable concentration of one-half of its total plasma concentration, and a fall in filterable plasma concentration will reduce the exposure of tubular cells to the xenobiotic or metabolite. Hypercholesterolaemia accompanies the hypoalbuminaemia found in nephrosis (March and Drablein, 1960).

Urine Enzymes

Urinary enzyme measurements provide useful information on the extent and site of renal injury, whereas plasma enzymes are poor markers of nephrotoxicity (Wright and Plummer, 1974; Stroo and Hook, 1977; Price, 1982; Guder and Ross, 1984; Stonard, 1987). However, of the many urinary enzyme measurements investigated, relatively few have proved to be of diagnostic value. In several acute studies with nephrotoxic substances, reasonable correlations between renal pathology and urinary enzyme excretion have been demonstrated (Cottrell *et al.*, 1976; Bhargava *et al.*, 1978). However, there are some examples where urinary enzymes do not appear to be as sensitive as other renal function indices (Stroo and Hook, 1977; Kluwe, 1981).

The enzymes which have received most attention are those localized in the proximal tubules. Those enzymes located on the brush border of the renal proximal tubules—e.g. ALP, GGT and alanine aminopeptidase—appear sometimes to act as earlier indicators of renal damage compared with other tests of renal toxicity (Wright *et al.*, 1972; Jung and Scholz, 1980; Salgo and Szabo, 1982). *N*-Acetyl-β-glucosaminidase

appears to be a useful enzyme marker of damage to the papilla of the kidney (Price, 1982). Several studies with papillotoxic agents have shown that increased urinary excretion of *N*-acetyl-β-glucosaminidase accompanies the increased volume and lower osmolality of the urine (Bach and Hardy, 1985; Stonard *et al.*, 1987).

The use of urinary enzymes to monitor glomerular damage is of limited value, as very few enzymes have been identified as specific markers of the glomeruli (Lovett *et al.*, 1982). The loss of plasma enzymes into the tubular fluid which accompanies glomerular damage makes it necessary to determine whether the increased enzymuria originates from damaged renal parenchymal tissues.

The presence of endogenous low-molecular-weight inhibitors in the urine may cause problems when urinary enzymes are being analysed, and these inhibitors require removal by dialysis, gel filtration or ultrafiltration (Werner *et al.*, 1969; Werner and Gabrielson, 1977). Several urinary enzymes are unstable and rapid analysis following collection is advisable. Contamination by faeces or diet can cause erroneous results, and the possible effect of the presence of a test substance or its metabolite(s) on an enzyme assay should always be considered. There is evidence of the effects of age, sex, urinary flow and biorhythms on urinary enzyme excretion (Grotsch *et al.*, 1985; Pariat *et al.*, 1990).

For some urinary enzymes which exist in isoenzymic forms—e.g. LDH and *N*-acetyl-β-glucosaminidase—the measurements of the isoenzymes can be more informative than the measurement of the total enzyme activity (Halman *et al.*, 1984).

Electrolyte Balance

Reduced fluid intake or excessive fluid loss by vomitus or diarrhoea will affect urine output. Although measurements of urinary cations—e.g. sodium and potassium—and anions may provide further evidence of renal dysfunction, this information may not help to identify the site of the lesion, as reabsorption of electrolytes can occur in various regions of the nephron.

Urinary electrolyte values are highly dependent on dietary intake. Plasma electrolyte measurements may be of some value, but are subject to many extrarenal influences. Urinary magnesium and calcium determinations may be important for some nephrotoxic substances—e.g. cisplatin (Magil *et al.*, 1986).

Perturbations of acid–base balance will often accompany severe electrolyte changes, but these measurements require controlled conditions, particularly for small laboratory animals. Measurements of renin, aldosterone and atrial natriuretic hormone are generally reserved for xenobiotics where the mode of action suggests that these assays will be useful for the understanding of the pathogenesis of renal changes.

The kidneys receive 20–25 per cent of the cardiac output, and it is sometimes important to measure the effective renal plasma flow (ERPF). This can be demonstrated by the active uptake and tubular secretion of the organic anion *p*-aminohippurate (PAH): the PAH transport is so efficient in many species that the PAH clearance indicates ERPF. A reduction of PAH clearance may be due to an alteration of renal blood flow by an effect on vasculature or a disruption of the active secretory process. Other organic cations, such as tetraethylammonium (TEA) and phenolsulphthalein (PSP), can also be used as indices of cationic tubular transport systems in the kidney (Plaa and Larson, 1965).

GASTROINTESTINAL TRACT

Nutritional status may influence the bioavailability and, hence, toxic effects on the gastrointestinal tract in several ways (George, 1984; Omaye, 1986; Aungst and Shen, 1986). Disturbances of gastrointestinal function are often accompanied by electrolyte imbalance due to fluid losses either by emesis (vomiting), volvulus (dilatation) or diarrhoea. Excessive salivation may also cause electrolyte perturbations. Prolonged or excessive losses of fluid via the gastrointestinal tract will affect packed cell volume (haematocrit) and plasma total protein, albumin, electrolytes, acid–base balance and osmolality values (Smith, 1986).

Electrolyte Balance

Hypo- or hypernatraemia may occur, depending on the proportional losses of electrolyte to water; these electrolyte changes are also reflected by plasma osmolality. In the presence of osmotically active solutes (e.g. mannitol) there may be significant differences between measured and calculated osmolality; similar differences may occur in the presence of hyperlipidaemia and hyperproteinaemia. These electrolyte measurements emphasize the need to separate plasma from erythrocytes as rapidly as possible in order to avoid changes in plasma potassium concentrations, although these changes are less in the dog than with other species.

Excessive losses of chloride-rich fluids (e.g. pancreatic secretion) may be monitored by plasma chloride measurements; changes in plasma chloride concentration which are not accompanied by a change in plasma sodium are usually associated with disturbances of acid–base balance where chloride concentration varies inversely to plasma bicarbonate.

Occult Blood

For compounds suspected of causing gastrointestinal bleeding or having ulcerogenic properties (e.g. non-steroidal anti-inflammatory compounds), the detection of faecal occult or frank blood may be of value. There are a number of available procedures for the detection of occult blood, and the majority of colorimetric qualitative tests are based on the pseudoperoxidase activity of haemoglobin. The sensitivity of these tests varies with the reagents used, and are subject to interferences from peroxidases and pseudoperoxidases present in food (Aldercreutz *et al.*, 1984; Johnson, 1989). Additionally, in animal studies it may be necessary to alter the sensitivity of a particular method in order to avoid false positive reactions associated with animal diets, particularly for carnivorous species (Dent, 1973). False positive reactions may also be caused by some cleaning fluids used in animal housing— e.g. hypochlorite solutions. Alternative methods for the detection of faecal occult blood include the use of radiolabelled erythrocytes (Walsh, 1982) or the detection of porphyrins by fluorescence (Boulay *et al.*, 1986), but these methods are not used widely.

Enzymes

Several enzyme measurements are available for assessing gastrointestinal function and toxicity, but these assays are not usually included in the majority of toxicology studies. Relatively simple assays are used for assessing pancreatic exocrine function (Boyd *et al.*, 1988), whereas the measurement of intestinal disaccharidases is more complex. Some of these enzyme measurements require the collection of gastric, pancreatic and other intestinal fluids, faeces or tissues.

Of the proteolytic enzymes, pepsin and trypsin can be measured by relatively simple techniques. Pepsinogen is the precursor of the proteolytic enzyme pepsin (EC 3.4.23.1), and is secreted by gastric parietal cells; it may be measured in plasma or gastric fluid by colorimetric, fluorimetric or radioimmunometric methods (Will *et al.*, 1984; Ford *et al.*, 1985; Tani *et al.*, 1987). Pepsinogen activities may be increased following peptic ulceration and by parasitic infections. Trypsin (EC 3.4.21.4) can be measured in faeces by gelatin digestion, chromogenic assays or immunoenzymometric methods (Fletcher *et al.*, 1986; Simpson and Doxey, 1988).

Measurement of intestinal disaccharidases may be useful, but these enzymes are subject to various factors, including age, nutritional status, hormonal influences due to glucocorticoids and thyroid hormones, diurnal variations, etc. (Henning, 1984). Duodenal or intestinal alkaline phosphatase is markedly reduced with some ulcerogens— e.g. cysteamine (Japundzic and Levi, 1987). Other enzyme changes occur in miscellaneous gastrointestinal conditions such as intestinal infarction or obstruction (Kazmlerczak *et al.*, 1988) and parasitic infections.

The two enzymes amylase and lipase have been widely used to detect pancreatitis, although there are wide variations in plasma amylase levels and the tissue distribution of amylase and its isoenzymes in different species (Rajasingham *et al.*, 1971; McGeachin and Akin, 1982). Pancreatic chymotrypsin activity can be measured in plasma following oral administration of *N*-benzoyl-1-tyrosyl-*p*-amino-benzoic acid.

Endocrine, Pancreatic Function and Carbohydrate Metabolism

For plasma glucose measurements, the use of an inhibitor (i.e. sodium fluoride) or rapid separation of the plasma is recommended to prevent glycolysis. Plasma glucose levels below 1.7 mmol l^{-1}, which would give rise to clinical signs of hypoglycaemia in man, do not appear to produce similar adverse effects in some other primates. With some rodent species it appears that the animals have to be fasted for much longer periods than other species to achieve similar reductions in plasma glucose. The ability of certain primates to store food in their buccal pouches often prevents the true measurement of 'fasting' glucose. Blood collection procedures may cause a marked elevation of plasma glucose where the animal is subject to stress, including restraint (Gärtner *et al.*, 1980).

The measurement of plasma and urinary glucose, and additional measurements of ketosis (i.e. urinary ketones), plasma 3-hydroxybutyrate, lipids and osmolality will all act as indicators of the severity of the disturbance to carbohydrate metabolism. The additional measurement of glycosylated haemoglobin may be useful when monitoring the effects of hypoglycaemic agents (Higgins *et al.*, 1982).

The molecular structures of the pancreatic hormones insulin and glucagon vary with animal species, and this prevents the universal application of immunoassays across different species, although there are degrees of cross-reactivity between some species (Berthet, 1963; Young, 1963).

Other Tests

Drug-induced pancreatitis may be accompanied by gross plasma lipid changes, and hypocalcaemia due to excessive loss of pancreatic secretion. Gross examination of faeces may show evidence of undigested fat in animals with severe pancreatic deficiency.

Other more specialized investigations for detecting gastrointestinal toxicity include measurement of intestinal permeability with polyethylene glycol polymers (Walsh, 1982), xylose absorption tests, and hydrogen or carbon isotopic pulmonary or 'breath' tests. Plasma gastrin measurements may be a useful adjunct to studies where antiulceration drugs are being investigated, but gastrin has a relatively short half-life (Koop *et al.*, 1982; Larsson *et al.*, 1986). Where gastrointestinal toxic effects are prolonged, marked reductions in the intake of essential nutrients such as vitamins (folate), amino acids, etc., may occur.

HEART

Enzymes

Enzymes are used as primary markers of cardiotoxicity, but timing and the methods of sample collection are particularly critical for the detection of cardiac damage; the importance of sample times has been shown in several studies where myocardial lesions have been induced by the administration of isoprenaline (Balazs and Bloom, 1982; Barrett *et al.*, 1988). Following cardiac damage, a large number of tissue enzymes are released into the plasma, but only a few of these enzymes are used commonly for the diagnosis of myocardial damage and congestive cardiac failure. These enzymes are CK, LDH, AST, and ALT to a lesser extent. None of these enzyme measurements is specific for cardiac tissue, and this has led to the use of isoenzymes, particularly for CK and LDH, to obtain additional information.

Creatine kinase (CK) is a dimeric molecule with subunits B and M; there are three cytosolic enzymes—the 'muscle' dimer MM, the brain dimer BB and the myocardial dimer MB (Lang, 1981). There are also mitochondrial isoenzymes and isoforms of CK. The tissue distribution of CK is not confined to the heart and the distribution pattern varies between species. Plasma CK activities may be markedly affected by skeletal muscle damage by either simple intramuscular injections or toxic myopathies.

LDH is a cytosolic tetrameric enzyme with five major isoenzymes in plasma consisting of H (heart) and M (muscle) subunits. The five isoenzymes are numbered according to decreasing anodic mobility during electrophoretic separation: LDH1 has four H subunits, LDH5 has four M subunits, and LDH2, LDH3 and LDH4 are hybrid combinations—containing HHHM, HHMM and HMMM, respectively (Markert and Whitt, 1975). The tissue distribution of LDH is widespread, and differences occur between the various species (Karlsson and Larsson, 1971). The broad normal ranges for plasma total LDH activity encountered in laboratory animals makes interpretation difficult; in the rat LDH5 is a major isoenzyme in plasma, and therefore a considerable increase of LDH1 is required before total plasma LDH values change significantly. Additional isoenzymes of LDH have been described, and some LDH isoenzymes may complex with some drugs—e.g. streptokinase (Poldlasek and McPherson, 1989).

The isoenzymes of CK and LDH may be separated by a variety of electrophoretic techniques or immunoinhibition methods, but the latter are limited by the specificity of the monoclonal antibodies currently available (Lang, 1981; Landt *et al.*, 1989). The plasma activities of the aminotransferases AST and ALT may also change following cardiac damage, although these enzymes are used more commonly as markers of hepatotoxicity.

Other plasma measurements which may be altered by cardiotoxic compounds include electrolytes, proteins other than enzymes, and lipids (Evans, 1991). Some of the preanalytical factors discussed previously may contribute to cardiotoxicity—e.g. obesity, nutritrional status, genetic variations, anaemia and thyroid function.

Electrolyte Balance

Disturbances of the intra- and extracellular equilibria of the cations sodium, potassium, calcium and magnesium may result in increased irritability of cardiac tissue and be associated with arrhythmias. As the balance of these cations is interrelated, an extreme change in the ionic balance of one cation may influence the concentrations of the other cations. The divalent cations—calcium and magnesium—are partially bound to plasma proteins particularly albumin, and it is necessary to consider the ionized and metabolically more important plasma fractions in relation to plasma proteins.

Cationic changes are accompanied invariably by disturbances of plasma anionic concentrations and acid–base balance. Where there are alterations of fluid balance such as occur with congestive cardiac failure, these may be reflected by changes in plasma osmolality and protein concentrations, particularly albumin. Following cardiotoxic changes, there may be alterations of the plasma protein pattern with increases in acute phase proteins—e.g. myoglobin, C-reactive protein and fibrinogen; these changes may be detected by electrophoretic techniques or selective methods for quantifying individual protein fractions.

The interpretation of changing values for plasma electrolytes may be complex where cardiac output is a consequence of the failure of other organ functions (e.g. the kidneys) and, conversely, where impaired cardiac damage affects renal function. This interrelationship of organ functions is seen with several anthracycline antitumour agents, which may cause cardiotoxic and nephrotoxic effects (Sinha, 1982). The procedures used for blood collection may affect the measurements of enzymes, cations and proteins used for the detection of cardiotoxicity.

Although haemoglobinuria, proteinuria and enzymuria may occur following myocardial infarction or damage to pulmonary arteries, urine tests are generally not helpful in the detection of cardiotoxicity.

Lipoproteins and Lipids

Various lipoproteins transport lipids in the plasma, and these lipoproteins are classified according to their physicochemical properties. The lipoproteins may be separated into chylomicra, very-low-density lipoproteins (VLDL), low-density lipoproteins (LDL), and high-density lipoproteins (HDL). The lipid and protein contents (apolipoproteins) also vary with the individual lipoprotein fractions. Adverse toxic and/or pharmacological effects on lipid metabolism can be monitored by measuring plasma cholesterol (total and free), triglycerides, non-esterified fatty acids, total lipids, phospholipids, lipoproteins (high- and low-density) and apolipoproteins. These measurements may be made using a variety of techniques, including chromogenic enzymatic assays, solvent extraction, electrophoresis, immunoassay, gas-liquid chromatography and ultracentrifugation. Initial information concerning alterations of plasma lipids may be obtained by measuring total cholesterol and triglycerides and by qualitative lipoprotein electrophoresis.

Plasma lipoproteins vary with age, sex, diet and the period of food withdrawal prior to sample collection. The proportion of chylomicra present in plasma is reduced after a period of fasting, but this selective food withdrawal may enhance the absorption of the test compound and, hence, its toxic or pharmacological effect.

Quantitative and qualitative differences of lipoproteins and lipids occur between species. These differences are observed for the rates of absorption, synthesis and metabolism (Beynon, 1988). Some of these differences are reflected by the plasma lipoprotein patterns; for example, the major plasma lipoprotein fraction in rats, dogs, mice, rabbits and guinea-pigs are the HDL fractions, whereas in old world monkeys the LDL fraction is the dominant fraction (Alexander and Day, 1973; Terpstra et al., 1981). These species differences lead to some additional methodological considerations when samples are analysed (Evans, 1986a). The testing of pharmaceutical agents such as hypolipidaemics in animal models, where atherosclerosis has been deliberately induced, may yield different responses from those obtained in healthy animals.

The effect of lipids on other plasma measurements has been briefly mentioned, and it is particularly relevant to the measurement of electrolytes. Sodium and potassium may be measured by the use of flame photometry or specific ion electrodes, and the differences observed between these two methods is accentuated in plasma samples with increased lipid content (Weisberg, 1989).

PLASMA PROTEINS

Perturbations of Plasma Proteins

Hypoproteinaemias are characterized by reductions in albumin and/or globulin fractions. In addition to reduced hepatic synthesis or increased renal excretion (discussed in previous sections on hepatotoxicity and nephrotoxicity), hypoproteinaemia may result from impaired nutritional status, some parasitic infections, haemorrhage, and impaired intestinal or pancreatic function. Severe hypoproteinaemia may be associated with oedema and ascites due to the osmotic influence of albumin, whereas hyperproteinaemia may be observed with dehydration. In some situations a compensatory increase in globulin fractions may occur where there are reductions of plasma albumin and total protein concentrations—e.g. plasma protein changes in rats treated with warfarin (Colvin and Lee Wang, 1974). Few protein changes are pathognomonic.

Albumin has an important colloidal osmotic effect and this protein fraction is also associated with binding of xenobiotics perhaps more frequently than other protein fractions; marked changes of drug-binding plasma proteins may clearly affect the apparent blood concentrations of test compounds, and hence toxicity. Other plasma proteins are involved in chelation of cations (e.g. caeruloplasmin, transferrin and metallothionein), binding of calcium and magnesium, antibody functions, clotting mechanisms, hormone metabolism, etc.

Protein measurements may be used to monitor inflammatory responses, although the timing of sample collection is again critical for the measurement of acute phase proteins (Betts *et al.*, 1964; Nakagawa *et al.*, 1984). Following inflammatory stimuli, several changes in the pattern of proteins synthesized by the liver occur, with elevations of the acute phase proteins and some reductions of other proteins. There are considerable variations of the acute phase response patterns found in different species, particularly for C-reactive protein, amyloid protein and alpha$_2$-macroglobulin (Kushner and Mackiewicz, 1987). Plasma amyloid protein is the major acute phase protein in the mouse, whereas alpha$_2$-macroglobulin is the major acute phase protein in the rat.

For rats and other small rodents, the site used for blood collection has a marked effect on the plasma protein values (Neptun *et al.*, 1985). Age and sex differences occur in the plasma protein values obtained for laboratory animals (House *et al.*, 1961; Reuter *et al.*, 1968; Coe and Ross, 1983; Wolford *et al.*, 1987).

Analytical Methods

Methods for assessing changes of plasma protein concentrations usually include measurement of total protein and albumin, and qualitative or quantitative separation of proteins by various electrophoretic techniques. Plasma protein values are slightly higher than corresponding serum values, owing to the presence of fibrinogen, although this protein fraction may precipitate during cold storage. Globulin values are usually determined as the difference between total protein and albumin concentrations, although the plasma globulin value will also include a contribution due to fibrinogen.

The bromocresol green dye-binding method for plasma albumin appears to be suitable for a majority of laboratory animal species, unlike some other albumin-binding dyes (Witiak and Whitehouse, 1969; Evans and Parsons, 1988). Simple electrophoretic techniques using cellulose acetate or agarose support media can be used to assess changes of albumin and globulin fractions, although the support media may affect the electrophoretic pattern (Allchin and Evans, 1986b).

Although albumin is usually the dominant electrophoretic band, there are marked species differences in the electrophoretic patterns. Using techniques such as two-dimensional immunoelectrophoresis, it is possible to demonstrate changes of plasma proteins which are not apparent using one-dimensional electrophoresis—e.g. in rats given hypolipidaemic agents (Hinton *et al.*, 1985).

Using cellulose acetate electrophoretic methods, it is possible to observe increases in plasma alpha- and beta-globulins following the injection of known irritants into rats (e.g. carrageenan). With quantitative immunolectrophoretic techniques applied in the same model of irritancy, it is possible to demonstrate changes which occur for over 20 individual proteins in acute phase response (Scherer *et al.*, 1977).

For compounds which act as immunomodulators (see Chapter 33), immunoglobulins may be measured by various immunological techniques. Immunoassay of individual proteins is dependent on obtaining specific antisera, although some antisera cross-react with several species (Hau *et al.*, 1990), and allow the use of such techniques as immunoturbidometry and single radial immunodiffusion.

CHOLINESTERASES

Cholinesterase enzymes are known targets for certain compounds, including organophosphate and carbamate esters, which are used as insecticides. Apart from the presence of the enzyme in the nervous system, where it serves to inactivate the neurotransmitter acetylcholine, cholinesterases are found in the blood.

Two principal types of cholinesterase enzyme have been identified in blood:

(1) Erythrocyte acetylcholinesterase (AChE; EC 3.1.1.7). This enzyme is bound to the stroma of erythrocytes and is characterized by preferential affinity for acetylcholine as substrate. It is also referred to as 'true' cholinesterase.

(2) Plasma or serum cholinesterase (ChE; EC 3.1.1.8). This enzyme exhibits heterogeneity (Ecobichon and Comeau, 1972; Unakami *et al.*,

1987) and shows less substrate specificity than AChE. It is also referred to as 'pseudo-' and 'non-specific' cholinesterase.

AChE in erythrocytes is identical in function to AChE found in the central nervous system, sympathetic ganglia and motor end plates. Its functional role in erythrocytes is unclear, but it has been suggested that it may have a protective role by acting as a 'sink' for part of the absorbed dose of anticholinesterase compounds (Wills, 1972). Even more conjectural is the physiological role of plasma ChE, which is also found in the liver (the major site of synthesis) and intestinal mucosa. Not all cholinesterase activity in brain can be accounted for by AChE. It has been estimated that some 15 per cent of the total activity may be attributable to pseudo/non-specific ChE in certain areas of white matter (Ecobichon and Joy, 1982). It is possible that the distribution and activities of AChE vary in different regions of the central nervous system, but this will not be reflected when total activity is measured in whole-brain homogenates.

Several methods have evolved for the measurement of cholinesterase activity (cf. review by Whittaker, 1986). The electrometric pH method (Michel, 1949) was for many years the method of choice in many laboratories, but has now been superseded by a superior colorimetric method (Ellman *et al.*, 1961) and its modifications for human and animal species (Voss and Sachsse, 1970; Pickering and Pickering, 1971). This method of Ellman *et al.* offers significant advantages in speed, sensitivity and reliability. The colorimetric method has been automated for both erythrocyte and plasma enzymes (Lewis *et al.*, 1981). The relative activity of erythrocyte to plasma ChE differs according to the nature of the alkyl substituent in the substrate.

There are significant pitfalls associated with the measurement of cholinesterases, especially when spontaneous reactivation of the inhibited enzyme occurs relatively rapidly. If the incubation time for the assay is significant in relation to the rate of reactivation, then the degree of inhibition may be underestimated. Also, further inhibition of cholinesterase may occur after blood sampling and is usually indicative of the presence of free inhibitor. Thus, if the rate of inhibition by free inhibitor exceeds the rate of reactivation, then the degree of inhibition may be overestimated.

Thus, for the generation of meaningful cholinesterase data, it is essential that the time which elapses between blood sampling and assay (including the incubation period) be reduced to a minimum.

In toxicology studies where organophosphates or carbamates are to be evaluated, it is usual (and essential) to measure cholinesterase activities in blood at various intervals during acute and chronic studies in more than one species: the dog and the rat are the preferred species. The more toxic the compound the more frequent should be the sampling. While concurrent control groups are used routinely in these studies, the study design for dog studies where the group sizes are smaller than for rodents, should incorporate two or more baseline measurements prior to treatment. This is essential, since several investigators have demonstrated that the variation in erythrocyte AChE and plasma ChE between individuals exceeds the variation between successive determinations in the same individual (Callaway *et al.*, 1951; Gage, 1967). The percentage difference from the mean baseline value which achieves statistical significance is, of course, dependent upon which enzyme is being assayed and upon the number of baseline measurements (Hayes, 1982). The interpretation of cholinesterase inhibition data is confounded by the various sources of variability (including analytical). Historically, the use of $\gg 20$ per cent inhibition of either enzyme activity has been used as the determinant of biological significance. The basis of this is a combination of analytical, inter- and intra-variability seen in the human population (Callaway *et al.*, 1951; Gage, 1967; Hackathorn *et al.*, 1983). Plasma ChE may be reduced for reasons other than inhibition by organophosphates and carbamates. These reasons have been tabulated (Whittaker, 1986), and include inherited, physiological, acquired and iatrogenic conditions.

The comparative sensitivity to man has been examined for a variety of organophosphates and carbamates in the preferred species—dog and rat. In all examples where cholinesterase inhibition was the critical effect, the dog was equally as sensitive or more sensitive than the rat (Appelman and Feron, 1986). These findings add substance to an earlier recommendation that cholinesterases should be measured in two species, one of which is the dog, because 'when plasma ChE or erythrocyte AChE provide the most sensitive index of cumulative effect, the response in the dog has approached very closely that in the human' (Lehman, 1959). However, it must be recognized that the mode of administration and differences in eating habits between the various species, including man, may influence the data regarding species sensitivity.

ENDOCRINE FUNCTION

Major toxic effects on the endocrine system appear to be relatively uncommon, on the basis of published literature. The extent to which this reflects the lack of relevant measurements or dismissal of any changes as non-specific or secondary to other effects is unclear. The susceptibility of the endocrine tissues to compound-induced lesions has been shown to be ranked in the following decreasing order of frequency: adrenal, testis, thyroid, ovary, pancreas, pituitary and parathyroid (Ribelin, 1984). Similar findings have been revealed by the Centre for Medicines Research (Table 3). Compounds affecting the adrenal and testis total approximately 70 per cent of all reports reviewed.

The release of peripheral hormones is controlled by the secretion of trophic hormones from the pituitary, which in turn are regulated by releasing hormones secreted by the hypothalamus (Table 4). The endocrine feedback axis is completed by circulating hormones modulating the output of releasing/trophic hormones from the hypothalamic–pituitary axis. Clearly, the

Table 3 Frequency of toxicity to endocrine glands[a]

Organ	Number of compounds with an effect	Weight change only	Species
Adrenals	44	27	Rat, dog, primate
Testes	24	10	Rat, dog
Thyroid	17	9	Rat, dog
Ovary	14	7	Rat, dog
Pituitary	11	6	Rat, dog, primate
Pancreas	4	0	Rat, dog, primate

[a] Data abstracted from the Toxicology database, Centre for Medicines Research (Woodman, 1988b).

measurements of circulating levels of one or more hormones together with other specific endocrine organ indicators of function are powerful tools in defining the level at which functional impairment occurs.

The majority of non-polypeptide hormones do not show species differences, and therefore several commercial test kits for human clinical use can be applied, although the circulating levels in some animal species present difficulties in analytical sensitivity. In contrast, the trophic hormones are polypeptides and require the use of species-specific reagents, which are often only available from relatively few sources. The majority of hormone assays utilize radioisotopes; however, several alternative approaches are now available—e.g. enzyme immunoassay, bioluminescence.

Adrenal Gland

The hormones of the adrenal cortex fall into three classes: (1) glucocorticoids, which influence the metabolism of carbohydrates, lipids and proteins, with the liver, muscles and adipose tissue as the major sites of action; (2) mineralocorticoids, which influence electrolyte transport by regulating renal sodium and potassium reabsorption and excretion, thereby affecting blood pressure homoeostasis; and (3) androgens and oestrogens.

The biosynthesis and secretion of these adrenal cortical hormones is under the direct control of a trophic hormone, adrenocorticotrophic hormone (ACTH) released by the pituitary. The secretion of ACTH is under a negative feedback control mechanism exercised by the circulating cortical hormones, of which cortisol is the most important in man and dog, and corticosterone in rat.

The circulating level of adrenal cortical hormone in rats depends on several factors, including age, season and strain (Wong *et al.*, 1983a; Kuhn *et al.*, 1983), sex and light (Critchlow *et al.*, 1963). It is also readily apparent that experimental (and pre-experimental) disturbance of animals has a pronounced effect upon the measurement of plasma cortisol (or corticosterone). It has been demonstrated that relatively innocuous stimuli, such as handling and change in environment, may induce significant increases in plasma corticosterone levels in rats (Barrett and Stockham, 1963; Jurcovicova *et al.*, 1984). Plasma corticosterone levels are high in young rats and decrease

Table 4 Hypothalamic–pituitary endocrine target axis, with examples of releasing and trophic hormones

Hypothalamus	Releasing hormones—e.g. corticotrophic releasing hormone (CRH), thyrotrophic releasing hormone (TRH), follicle stimulating releasing hormone (FRH), luteinizing hormone releasing hormone (LRH)
Pituitary	Trophic hormones—e.g. adrenocorticotropic hormone (ACTH), thyroid stimulating hormone (TSH), follicle stimulating hormone (FSH), luteinizing hormone (LH)
Endocrine target organ	Peripheral hormones—e.g. cortisol, corticosterone, aldosterone, thyroxine (T_4), triiodothyronine (T_3)
Peripheral circulation	Transport proteins Peripheral metabolism and excretion
End organ target	Receptor binding

dramatically during sexual development, reflecting a highly active adrenal gland during puberty.

The need for standardization in plasma corticosterone (and cortisol) measurements is illustrated by the circadian rhythm (D'Agostino *et al.*, 1982). In the dog a circadian rhythm is not apparent (Johnston and Mather, 1978); however, episodic secretion of cortisol and ACTH has been seen (Kemppainen and Sartin, 1984).

The need for standardization extends also to the mode of killing and blood sampling site, although the differences in corticosterone levels were less apparent than for some other hormones (Dohler *et al.*, 1978). Sequential termination and caging density may also affect plasma corticosterone measurements in laboratory animals (Dunn and Scheving, 1971).

The determination of plasma cortisol during periods of rest and following stimulation with ACTH can be used to diagnose whether adrenocortical function is perturbed (Garnier *et al.*, 1990). To further evaluate the functional status, direct assay of ACTH can be combined with administration of metyrapone, which is known to inhibit adrenal 11β-hydroxylase activity and cause a transient reduction in cortisol synthesis: this is normally sufficient to stimulate ACTH secretion from the pituitary, followed by a resultant increase in the secretion of 11-deoxycortisol (Orth *et al.*, 1988).

Toxic agents appear to interfere with the adrenal cortex by one of three direct mechanisms: (1) altering cholesterol synthesis; (2) altering conversion of cholesterol to △5-pregnenolone; and (3) altering 11β-hydroxylation. The plasma levels of unbound and metabolically active corticosteroids may also be measured indirectly by the effects on hepatic steroid metabolism or upon the plasma transport proteins.

Plasma volume and circulating electrolytes are the key regulators of mineralocorticoid secretion. The secretion of aldosterone is governed largely by the renin–angiotensin system and by plasma potassium and sodium concentrations. A circadian rhythm has been demonstrated for plasma aldosterone in the rat (Gomez-Sanchez *et al.*, 1976).

Thyroid Gland

The hormones of the thyroid gland arise from the iodination of tyrosine residues at positions 3 and 5 of the aromatic moiety to yield mono- and diiodotyrosines, which in combination give rise to triiodotyrosine (triiodothyronine, T_3) and tetraiodotyrosine (thyroxine, T_4). The requirement for iodine by the thyroid gland is met by dietary intake of iodide and uptake into the gland against a concentration gradient. Within the thyroid gland, the iodide is 'activated' by a peroxidase, and the receptors for this 'activated' iodine are the tyrosine residues in the protein, thyroglobulin (TBG). Most of the iodine within the gland is in a bound form as mono- and diiodotyrosines, with much smaller amounts as T_3 and T_4. Secretion and release of T_3 and T_4, the active hormones of the thyroid gland, are effected by proteolytic degradation of thyroglobulin.

The biosynthesis and secretion of these thyroid hormones is under the direct control of a trophic hormone, thyroid stimulating hormone (thyrotrophin, TSH), released by the pituitary. A reciprocal relationship exists between T_3 and T_4 production and TSH secretion, in which low circulating levels of thyroid hormones stimulate TSH release from the pituitary.

The problems of interspecies differences and relevance of findings to man are reflected well in the pituitary–thyroid axis—in particular, the binding and transport of these hormones by plasma proteins. Over 99.95 per cent of T_4 and more than 99.5 per cent of T_3 in blood are bound to carrier proteins (Robbins and Johnson, 1982). It is the unbound form of each hormone which is metabolically active, and for all species this generally amounts to less than 1 per cent. Several species are known to have plasma proteins which either bind with high affinity and low capacity or low affinity and high capacity. The low-affinity, high-capacity binding is provided mainly by albumin and/or a prealbumin in all species. However, differences exist between T_3 and T_4 binding to plasma proteins in different species (Woodman, 1988b). The low-affinity, high-capacity binding in the rat leads to a more rapid removal of thyroid hormones from the blood and conjugation by the liver such that metabolic half-lives in rat and man are widely different.

The two thyroid hormones differ in their physiological activity. Not only is T_3 almost twice as active as T_4, but also its onset of action is more rapid. Removal from the body involves hepatic uptake, conjugation with glucuronic acid and elimination of the conjugate in the bile.

Diurnal variations of plasma TSH, T_4 and T_3 have been observed in rats. Peak TSH levels occurred in the light period prior to peaks of T_3 and T_4 later (Jordan et al., 1980; Ottenweiller and Hedge, 1982). The circulating levels of both TSH and thyroid hormones in rats show a 24 h periodicity which is influenced by strain of rat and season of year but not age (Wong et al., 1983b); however, significant changes in 24 h mean serum levels of TSH and T_3 occur during pubertal development. Starvation of rats leads to reduced thyroid gland function, with thyroid concentrations of T_3 and T_4 increased, circulating levels of T_3 and T_4 decreased, and TSH secretion markedly depressed (Donati et al., 1966; Harris et al., 1978). Peripheral metabolism of T_4 is also decreased, which reflects both reduced deiodination and faecal excretion (Ingbar and Galton, 1975).

Sex-related differences in plasma concen-trations of canine TSH, T_3 and T_4 have been found, with TSH and T_4 levels higher in males and T_3 higher in females (Fukuda et al., 1975). Species differences in the levels of total and free T_3 and T_4 have been found in the serum of vertebrates—cattle, goats, guinea-pigs, horses, pigs, rats and sheep (Refetoff et al., 1970; Anderson et al., 1988).

Several commercial test kits which use the principle of radioimmunoassay (RIA) are available for the measurement of T_3 and T_4. Few require any modifications for the measurement of these hormones in laboratory animal species. In contrast, the measurement of TSH requires species-specific reagents because of the polypeptide nature of the hormone. Methods for its assay have been developed using a double-antibody RIA.

Testis

The weights of accessory glands, testes and epididymes are the primary indicators of a possible alteration in androgen status. Reductions in weight are indicative that androgen secretion is suboptimal or that testicular function has been compromised. The measurement of circulating hormones can often assist in the diagnosis of suspected reproductive toxicity. The testis can be functionally separated into the interstitial or Leydig cells and the seminiferous tubular compartments, which produce a complex fluid containing spermatozoa and a number of largely uncharacterized proteins.

The major function of the Leydig cells is the maintenance of spermatogenesis, which is partially mediated by the production of testosterone and dihydrotestosterone. Several radioimmunoassays have been described for testosterone and dihydrotestosterone, and the development of these sensitive assays has led to an assessment of Leydig cell function.

The endocrine control of testicular function is mainly exercised by the gonadotrophic hormones, luteinizing hormone (LH) and follicle-stimulating hormone (FSH), which are synthesized and released by the anterior pituitary gland. The principal target cells of the gonadotrophic hormones are the Leydig and Sertoli cells for LH and FSH, respectively. The homoeostatic control of the hypothalamo–pituitary–testicular (HPT) axis is complex, involving feedback modulation at several sites. Elevations of gonadotrophins are usually evidence of testicular injury. Leydig cell dysfunction usually leads to an increase in LH production, while increases in plasma FSH are usually indicative of damage to seminiferous tubules.

Apart from the technical aspects of performing these assays, there remain the questions of how and when to sample. LH is secreted in a pulsatile manner, and these pulses may cause plasma levels to vary by a factor of 2.5 or more from baseline values (Santen and Bardin, 1973). Collection procedures and storage procedures should be standardized to minimize any losses due to instability.

Seminiferous tubular function cannot be studied as easily, since many of its products are released into the tubular lumen which is contained within the 'blood–testis barrier'. This barrier has been shown to be capable of excluding from the tubular lumen many substances normally present in blood (Steinberger, 1981). It is clear that bloodborne components such as hormones and nutrients which can successfully permeate the blood–testis barrier can gain direct access to germ cells. Conversely, damage to this barrier caused by toxic substances or in disease would be expected to lead to release of extracellular and possible intracellular contents into blood, offering a possible screening mechanism of testicular dysfunction.

An androgenic binding protein (ABP) has been detected in the testis of rat, and appears to be identical with that in the epididymis. It is a heat-stable glycoprotein which is synthesized and released by Sertoli cells with a high affinity for testosterone and dihydrotestosterone (Gunsalus et al., 1981). The role of ABP is ill-defined at present. In the rat this protein has been isolated by affinity chromatography and a radioimmunoassay has been developed for its detection in tissues and body·fluids, especially blood (Gunsalus et al., 1978). The ability to measure an androgen binding protein of testicular origin in blood provides a novel method for the investigation of seminiferous tubular function (Gunsalus et al., 1978; Spitz et al., 1985).

The study of androgen-binding proteins in some species, including man, has been confounded by the existence of a closely related protein in serum. Testosterone–oestradiol binding globulin (TEBG) or sex hormone binding globulin (SHBG) is a glycoprotein of hepatic origin which has a greater affinity for androgens than for oestrogens. Further studies are needed to clarify the relationship between ABP and TEBG (Bardin et al., 1981; Cheng et al., 1985).

Several mammalian enzymes exist in testis-specific forms. The most widely studied of these is the testis-specific isoenzyme of LDH, referred to as LDH-X or LDH-C4. This isoenzyme possesses several properties which are distinct from the other isoenzymes of LDH. The synthesis of this unique gene product has been shown to occur at a precise stage of germ cell development. LDH-C4 is first detectable during the mid-pachytene stage of spermatocyte development, and continues throughout spermatid differentiation (Meistrich et al., 1977; Wheat et al., 1977). LDH-C4 is not normally detected in circulating blood but is present in seminal plasma under normal physiological conditions. Several studies of acute testicular toxicity in the rat have shown that elevations of plasma LDH-C4 can be detected (Haqqi and Adhami, 1982; Itoh and Ozasa, 1985; Reader et al., 1991).

The measurement of enzymes in seminal fluid and a variety of other fluids in animals as possible indicators of testicular damage is dependent upon a knowledge of the origin of these enzymes, since several accessory glands can contribute to the composition of semen. Some of these enzymes may in future be useful markers of testicular damage. In addition to LDH-C4, other enzymes are known to exhibit isoenzyme forms in which a testicular form has been demonstrated—e.g. phosphoglycerate kinase (Kramer, 1981; Vandeberg et al., 1981)—and some are known to be present in high activities in testicular tissue relative to other organs—e.g. branched-chain amino acid transferase (Mantamat et al., 1978).

SUMMARY

Clinical chemistry has a key role in toxicology studies, since it can provide advance warning of adverse effects that may be anticipated, e.g., by histopathology. By employing a combination of tests, it is possible to identify potential target organs and also to evaluate the functional status of major organs. As a general approach to the investigation of toxicity, a phased approach is recommended in which the first phase should include the traditional clinical chemistry tests, many of which have evolved from clinical practice. However, the timing of these tests is often governed by rigid protocols designed for regulatory submissions which therefore may not be appropriate to determine the period of maximal damage. The majority of these tests can be performed on automated equipment with a good throughput of samples per unit time, with high precision and with the use of relatively small volumes of body fluids. If confirmation is required of the first-phase results which may be indicative of toxicity in a single target organ, further studies should be targeted at this organ in order to characterize, where possible, the anatomical and subcellular localization of the lesion, the severity of the damage and functional impairment, and whether the changes observed are reversible or not. These further tests may be chosen on the basis of the known or suspected mechanism of action, using a more flexible study design with the sampling times geared to the evaluation of peak damage and/or dysfunction and recovery phase. The diagnostic effectiveness of the various analytes, enzymes and hormones, etc., has to be evaluated on a case-by-case basis for the relevant species. Some measurements (e.g. polypeptide hormone) require species-specific reagents, which may limit their application.

Several factors can contribute to biological variation, including husbandry practice, environmental control, genetic difference, diurnal rhythms, diet, etc. Thus, values generated in any given laboratory are unique to that laboratory. It cannot be emphasized too strongly that a concurrent control group must be a feature of the design of toxicology studies and therefore allows reference ranges from clinical chemistry parameters to be established. Equally important to the generation of meaningful data is the application of sound laboratory practices when collecting body fluids and the use of the same sampling site when making repeated measurements of the same analytes at intervals throughout a study. There are many examples of problems which can be overcome by reliance on the expertise and experience of the clinical chemist. These include a knowledge of the potential interferences (both endogenous and exogenous) which may lead to erroneous values, the lability of several analytes that require immediate analysis, and the need to adopt and

optimize assays to improve sensitivity in a particular species.

Finally, adherence to Good Laboratory Practice in the form of proven equipment maintenance, calibration and documentation is an absolute requirement in the clinical chemistry laboratory. A combination of internal quality control procedures with participation in an external quality assessment scheme permits the management and output of the laboratory to be monitored routinely and for unwanted trends and practices to be eliminated at the earliest opportunity.

REFERENCES

Alden, C. L. (1986). A review of unique male rat hydrocarbon nephropathy. *Toxicol. Pathol.*, **14**, 109–111

Alder, S., Janton, C. and Zbinden, G. (1981). *Preclinical Safety Requirements in 1980*. Swiss Federal Institute of Technology and University of Zurich

Aldercreutz, H., Partanen, P., Virkola, P., Liewendahl, K. and Turunen, M. J. (1984). Five guaiac-based tests for occult blood in faeces compared *in vitro* and *in vivo*. *Scand. J. Clin. Lab. Invest.*, **44**, 519–528

Alexander, C. and Day, C. E. (1973). Distribution of serum lipoproteins of selected vertebrates. *Comp. Biochem. Physiol.*, **46B**, 295–312

Allchin, J. P. and Evans, G. O. (1986a). A simple rapid method for the detection of rat urinary proteins by agarose electrophoresis and nigrosine staining. *Lab. Anim.*, **20**, 202–205

Allchin, J. P. and Evans, G. O. (1986b). Serum protein electrophoresis patterns of the marmoset, *Callithrix jacchus*. *J. Comp. Pathol.*, **96**, 349–352

Allchin, J. P. and Evans, G. O. (1986c). A comparison of three methods for determining the concentration of rat urine. *Comp. Biochem. Physiol.*, **85A**, 771–773

Allchin, J. P., Evans, G. O. and Parsons, C. E. (1987). Pitfalls in the measurement of canine urine concentration. *Vet. Rec.*, **120**, 256–257

Alpert, E., Mosher, M., Shankse, A. and Arias, I. M. (1969). Multiplicity of hepatic excretory mechanisms for organic anions. *J. Gen. Physiol.*, **53**, 238–247

Alt. J. M., Hackbarth, F., Deerberg, F. and Stolte, H. (1980). Proteinuria in rats in relation to age-dependent renal changes. *Lab. Anim.*, **14**, 95–101

Anderson, R. R., Nixon, D. A. and Akasha, M. A. (1988). Total and free thyroxine and triiodothyronine in blood serum of mammals. *Comp. Biochem. Physiol.*, **89A**, 401–404

Apostolou, A., Saidt, L. and Brown, W. R. (1976). Effect of overnight fasting of young rats on water consumption, body weight, blood sampling and blood composition. *Lab. Anim. Sci.*, **26**, 959–960

Appelman, L. M. and Feron, V. J. (1986). Significance

of the dog as 'second animal species' in toxicity testing for establishing the lowest 'no-toxic effect level'. *J. Appl. Toxicol.*, **6**, 271–279

Aungst, B. and Shen, D. D. (1986). Gastrointestinal absorption of toxic agents. In Rozman, K. and Hanninen, O. (Eds), *Gastrointestinal Toxicology*. Elsevier, Amsterdam, pp. 29–52

Bach, P. H. and Hardy, T. L. (1985). Relevance of animal models to analgesic-associated papillary necrosis in humans. *Kidney Int.*, **28**, 605–613

Balazs, T. and Bloom, S. (1982). Cardiotoxicity of adrenergic bronchodilator and vasodilating antihypertensive drugs. In Van Stee, E. W. (Ed.), *Cardiovascular Toxicology*, Raven Press, New York, pp. 199–200

Bardin, C. W., Musto, N., Gunsalus, G., Kotiten, N., Cheng, S. L., Larrea, F. and Becker, R. (1981). Extracellular androgen binding proteins. *Ann. Rev. Physiol.*, **43**, 189–198

Barrett, A. M. and Stockham, M. A. (1963). The effect of housing conditions and simple experimental procedures upon the corticosterone level in the plasma of rats. *J. Endocrinol.*, **26**, 97–105

Barrett, R. J., Harleman, H. and Joseph, E. C. (1988). The evaluation of HBDH and LDH isoenzymes in cardiac cell necrosis. *J. Appl. Toxicol.*, **8**, 233–238

Baumann, M. and Berauer, M. (1985). Comparative study on the sensitivity of several serum enzymes in detecting hepatic damage in rats. *Arch. Toxicol.*, Suppl. **8**, 370–372

Bean-Knudsen, D. E. and Wagner, J. E. (1987). Effect of shipping stress on clinicopathologic indicators in F344/N rats. *Am. J. Vet. Res.*, **48**, 306–308

Berdanier, C. D. and Baltzell, J. K. (1986). Comparative studies of the responses of two strains of rats to an essential fatty acid deficient diet. *Comp. Biochem. Physiol.*, **85A**, 725–727

Bertani, T., Zoja, C., Abbate, M., Rossini, M. and Remuzzi, G. (1989). Age-related nephropathy and proteinuria in rats with intact kidneys exposed to diets with different protein content. *Lab. Invest.*, **60**, 196–204

Berthet, J. (1963). Pancreatic hormones: glucagon. In von Euler, U. S. and Heller, H. (Eds), *Comparative Endocrinology*, Academic Press, London, pp. 410–423

Betts, A., Tanguay, R. and Freidell, G. H. (1964). Effect of necrosis on hemoglobin, serum protein profile and erythroagglutination reaction in golden hamsters. *Proc. Soc. Exp. Biol. Med.*, **116**, 66–69

Beynon, A. C. (1988). Animal models for cholesterol metabolism. In Beynon, A. C. and Solleveld, H. A. (Eds), *Biosciences*. Martinus Nijhoff, Dordrecht, pp. 279–288

Bhargava, A. S., Khater, A. R. and Gunzel, P. (1978). The correlation between lactate dehydrogenase activity in urine and serum and experimental renal damage in the rat. *Toxicol. Lett.*, **1**, 319–323

Blanckaert, N., Servaes, R. and Leroy, P. (1986).

Measurement of bilirubin–protein conjugates in serum and application to human and rat sera. *J. Lab. Clin. Med.*, **108**, 77–87

Boesken, W. H., Kopf, K. and Schollmeyer, P. (1973). Differentiation of proteinuric diseases by disc electrophoretic molecular weight analysis of urinary proteins. *Clin. Nephrol.*, **1**, 311–318

Boulay, J. P., Lipowitz, A. J., Klausner, J. S., Ellefson, M. L. and Schwartz, S. (1986). Evaluation of a fluorimetric method for the quantitative assay of fecal hemoglobin in the dog. *Am. J. Vet. Res.*, **47**, 1293–1295

Boyd, E. J. S., Rinderknecht, H. and Wormsley, K. G. (1988). Laboratory tests in the diagnosis of the chronic pancreatic diseases. Part 4. Tests involving the measurement of pancreatic enzymes in body fluid. *Int. J. Pancreatol.*, **3**, 1–16

Bovee, K. C. (1986). Renal function and laboratory evaluation. *Toxicol. Pathol.*, **14**, 26–36

Braun, J. P., Siest, G. and Rico, A. G. (1987). Uses of gamma-glutamyl transferase in experimental toxicology. *Adv. Vet. Sci. Comp. Med.*, **31**, 151–172

Caisey, J. D. and King, D. J. (1980). Clinical chemistry values for some common laboratory animals. *Clin. Chem.*, **26**, 1877–1879

Callaway, S., Davies, D. R. and Rutland, J. P. (1951). Blood cholinesterase levels and a range of personal variation in a healthy adult population. *Brit. Med. J.*, **2**, 812

Cheng, C. Y., Musto, N. A., Gunsalus, G. L., Frick, J. and Bardin, C. W. (1985). There are two forms of androgen binding protein in human testes. *J. Biol. Chem.*, **260**, 5631–5640

Chin, B. H., Tyler, T. R. and Kozbelt, S. J. (1979). The interfering effects of hemolyzed blood on rat serum chemistry. *Toxicol. Pathol.*, **7**, 19–22

Clampitt, R. B. and Hart, R. J. (1978). The tissue activities of some diagnostic enzymes in ten mammalian species. *J. Comp. Pathol.*, **88**, 607–621

Coe, J. E. and Ross, M. J. (1983). Hamster female protein. A divergent acute phase protein in male and female Syrian hamsters. *J. Exptl Med.*, **157**, 1421–1433

Colvin, H. W. and Lee Wang, W. (1974). Toxic effects of warfarin in rats fed different diets. *Toxicol. Appl. Pharmacol.*, **28**, 337–348

Commandeur, J. N. M. and Vermeulen, N. P. E. (1990). Molecular and biochemical mechanisms of chemically induced nephrotoxicity: a review. *Chem. Res. Toxicol.*, **3**, 171–194

Conybeare, G., Leslie, G. B., Angles, K. and Barrett, R. J. (1988). An improved technique for the collection of blood samples from rats and mice. *Lab. Anim.*, **22**, 177–182

Corman, B., Pratz, J. and Poujeol, P. (1985). Changes in the anatomy, glomerular filtration rate and solute excretion in aging rat kidney. *Am. J. Physiol.*, **248**, r282-r287

Cottrell, R. C., Agrelo, C. E., Gangolli, S. D. and

Grasso, P. (1976). Histochemical and biochemical studies of chemically induced acute kidney damage in the rat. *Fd Cosmet. Toxicol.*, **14**, 593–598

Cowie, J. R. and Evans, G. O. (1985). Plasma aminotransferase measurements in the marmoset (*Callithrix jacchus*). *Lab. Anim.*, **19**, 48–50

Critchlow, V., Liebelt, R. A., Bar-Sela, M., Mountcastle, W. and Lipscomb, H. S. (1963). Sex difference in resting pituitary-adrenal function in the rat. *Am. J. Physiol.*, **205**, 807–815

D'Agostino, J. B., Vaeth, G. F. and Henning, S. J. (1982). Diurnal rhythm of total and free concentration of serum corticosterone in the rat. *Acta Endocrinol.*, **100**, 85–90

Davies, D. J. and Kennedy, A. (1967). The excretion of renal cells following necrosis of the proximal convoluted tubule. *Br. J. Exp. Pathol.*, **48**, 45–50

Davy, C. W., Jackson, M. R. and Walker, J. M. (1984). Reference intervals for some clinical chemical parameters in the marmoset (*Callithrix jacchus*): effect of age and sex. *Lab. Anim.*, **18**, 135–142

Davy, C. W., Trennery, P. N., Edmunds, J. G., Altman, J. F. B. and Eichler, D. A. (1987). Local myotoxicity of ketamine hydrochloride in the marmoset. *Lab. Anim.*, **21**, 60–67

Degen, A. J. M. and van der Vies, J. (1985). Enzymatic microdetermination of free fatty acids in plasma of animals using paraoxon to prevent lipolysis. *Scand. J. Clin. Lab. Invest.*, **45**, 283–285

Dent, N. J. (1973). Occult blood detection in faeces of various animal species. *Lab. Pract.*, **22**, 674–676

de Schepper, J. and van der Stock, J. (1972). Increased urinary bilirubin excretion after elevated free plasma haemoglobin levels. 1. Variations in the calculated renal clearance of bilirubin in whole dogs. *Arch. Int. Physiol. Biochim.*, **80**, 279–281

Dilena, B. A., Penberthy, L. A. and Fraser, C. G. (1983). Six methods for determining urinary protein compared. *Clin. Chem.*, **29**, 553–557

Dohler, K.-D., Wong, C.-C., Gaudssuhn, D., von zur Muhlen, A., Gartner, K. and Dohler, U. (1978). Site of blood sampling in rats as a possible source of error in hormone determinations. *J. Endocrinol.*, **79**, 141–142

Donati, R. M., Warnecke, M. A. and Gallagher, N. I. (1966). The effect of acute starvation on thyroid function in rodents. *Experientia*, **22**, 270–272

Dooley, J. F. (1979). The role of clinical chemistry in chemical and drug safety evaluation by use of laboratory animals. *Clin. Chem.*, **25**, 345–347

Dorner, J. L., Hoffman, W. E. and Long, G. B. (1974). Corticosteroid induction of an isoenzyme of alkaline phosphatase in the dog. *Am. J. Vet. Res.*, **35**, 1457–1458

Dunn, J. and Scheving, L. (1971). Plasma corticosterone levels in rats killed sequentially at the 'trough' or 'peak' of the adrenocortical cycle. *J. Endocrinol.*, **49**, 347–348

Eckersall, P. D. (1986). Steroid induced alkaline phosphatase in the dog. *Israel J. Vet. Med.*, **42**, 253–259

Ecobichon, D. J. and Comeau, M. (1972). Pseudocholinesterases of mammalian plasma: physicochemical properties and organophosphate inhibition in eleven species. *Toxicol. Appl. Pharmacol.*, **24**, 92–100

Ecobichon, D. J. and Joy, R. M. (1982). *Pesticides and Neurological Disease*. CRC Press, Boca Raton, Florida

Ellman, G. L., Courtney, K. D., Andres, V. and Featherstone, R. M. (1961). A new and rapid colorimetric determination of acetylcholinesterase activity. *Biochem. Pharmacol.*, **7**, 88–95

Erlanger, S., Glasinovic, J. C., Poupon, R. and Dumont, M. (1976). In Taylor, W. (Ed.), *The Hepatobiliary System*. Plenum Press, New York, pp. 433–452

Evans. G. O. (1985). Changes of methodology and their potential effects on data banks for drug effects on clinical laboratory tests. *Ann. Clin. Biochem.*, **22**, 397–401

Evans, G. O. (1986a). The use of three esterase kits to measure plasma cholesterol concentration in the rat and three other species. *J. Comp. Pathol.*, **96**, 551–556

Evans, G. O. (1986b). The use of an enzymatic kit to measure plasma creatinine in the mouse and three other species. *Comp. Biochem. Physiol.*, **85B**, 193–195

Evans, G. O. (1987). Post-prandial changes in canine plasma creatinine. *J. Small Anim. Pract.*, **28**, 311–315

Evans, G. O. (1991). Biochemical assessment of cardiac function and damage in animal species. *J. Appl. Toxicol.*, **11**, 15–21

Evans, G. O. and Parsons, C. E. (1986). Potential errors in the measurement of total protein in male rat urine using test strips. *Lab. Anim.*, **20**, 27–31

Evans, G. O. and Parsons, C. E. (1988). A comparison of two dye binding methods for the determination of dog, rat and human plasma albumins. *J. Comp. Pathol.*, **98**, 453–460

Fent, K., Mayer, E. and Zbinden, G. (1988). Nephrotoxicity screening in rats: a validation study. *Arch. Toxicol.*, **61**, 349–358

Fletcher, T. S., Tsukamoto, H. and Largman, C. (1986). Immunoenzymometric determination of trypsin/alpha 1 protease inhibitor complex in plasma of rats with experimental pancreatitis. *Clin. Chem.*, **32**, 1738–1741

Ford, T. F., Grant, D. A. W., Austen, B. M. and Hermon-Taylor, J. (1985). Intramucosal activation of pepsinogens in the pathogenesis of acute gastric erosions and their prevention by the potent semisynthetic amphipathic inhibitor pepstatinyl-glycyl-lysyl-lysine. *Clin. Chim. Acta*, **145**, 37–47

Fouts, J. R. (1976). Overview of the field: environmental factors affecting chemical or drug effects in animals. *Fed. Proc.*, **35**, 1162–1165

Fowler, J. S. L. (1982). Animal clinical chemistry and haematology for the toxicologist. *Arch. Toxicol.*, Suppl. **5**, 152–159

Friedel, R. and Mattenheimer, H. (1976). Release of metabolic enzymes from platelets during blood clotting of man, dog, rabbit and rat. *Clin. Chim. Acta.*, **30**, 37–46

Fukuda, H., Greer, M. A., Roberts, L., Allen, C. F., Critchlow, V. and Wilson, M. (1975). Nyctohemeral and sex-related variations in plasma thyrotropin, thyroxine and triiodothyronine. *Endocrinology*, **97**, 1424–1431

Gage, J. C. (1967). The significance of blood cholinesterase activity measurements. *Res. Rev.*, **18**, 159–173

Garattini, S. (1981). Toxic effects of chemicals: difficulties in extrapolating data from animals to man. *CRC Crit. Rev. Toxicol.*, **16**, 1–29

Garnier, F., Benoit, E., Virat, M., Ochoa, R. and Delatour, P. (1990). Adrenal cortical response in clinically normal dogs before and after adaptation to a housing environment. *Lab. Anim.*, **24**, 40–43

Gärtner, K., Büttner, D., Döhler, K., Friedel, R., Lindena, J. and Trautschold, I. (1980). Stress response of rats to handling and experimental procedures. *Lab. Anim.*, **14**, 267–274

Gautam, A., Seligson, H., Gordon, E. R., Seligson, D. and Boyer, J. L. (1984). Irreversible binding of conjugated bilirubin to albumin in cholestatic rats. *J. Clin. Invest.*, **73**, 873–877

George, C. F. (1984). Food, drugs and bioavailability. *Br. Med. J.*, **289**, 1093–1094

Goldstein, R. S. (1990). In Volans, G. N., Sims, J., Sullivan, F. M. and Turner, P. (Eds), *Basic Science in Toxicology*, Taylor and Francis, London, pp. 412–421

Gomez-Sanchez, C., Holland, O. B., Higgins, J. R., Kem, D. C. and Kaplan, N. M. (1976). Circadian rhythms of serum renin activity and serum corticosterone, prolactin and aldosterone concentrations in the male rat on normal and low-sodium diets. *Endocrinology*, **99**, 567–572

Gopinath, C., Prentice, D. C., Street, A. E. and Crook, D. (1980). Serum bile acid concentration in some experimental lesions of rat. *Toxicology*, **15**, 113–127

Greim, H., Truzsch, D., Roboz, J., Dressler, K., Czygan, P., Hutterer, F., Schaffner, F. and Popper, H. (1972). Mechanism of cholestasis. 5. Bile acids in normal rat liver and in those after bile ligation. *Gastroenterology*, **63**, 837–845

Grotsch, H. and Hajdu, P. (1987). Interference by the new antibiotic Cefipirome and other cephalosporins in clinical laboratory test, with specific regard to the Jaffe reaction. *J. Clin. Chem. Clin. Biochem.*, **25**, 49–52

Grotsch, H., Hropot, M., Klaus, E., Malerczyk, V.

and Mattenheimer, H. (1985). Enzymuria of the rat: biorhythms and sex differences. *J. Clin. Chem. Clin. Biochem.*, **23**, 343–347

Guder, W. G. and Ross, B. D. (1984). Enzyme distribution along the nephron. *Kidney Int.*, **26**, 101–111

Gunsalus, G. L., Larrea, F., Musto, N. A., Becker, R. R., Mather, J. P. and Bardin, C. W. (1981). Androgen binding protein as a marker for Sertoli cell function. *J. Steroid Biochem.*, **15**, 99–106

Gunsalus, G. L., Musto, N. A. and Bardin, C. W. (1978). Immunoassay of androgen binding protein in blood; a new approach for study of the seminiferous tubule. *Science*, **200**, 65–66

Hackathorn, D. R., Brinkman, W. J., Hathaway, T. R., Talbot, T. D. and Thompson, L. R. (1983). Validation of whole blood method for cholinesterase monitoring. *Am. Industr. Hyg. Assoc. J.*, **44**, 547–551

Hackbarth, H., Baunack, E. and Winn, M. (1981). Strain differences in kidney function of inbred rats. 1. Glomerular filtration rate and renal plasma flow. *Lab. Anim.*, **15**, 125–128

Halman, J., Price, R. G. and Fowler, J. S. L. (1984). Urinary enzymes and isoenzymes of *N*-acetyl-β-glucosaminidase in the assessment of nephrotoxicity. In Goldberg, D. M. and Werner, M. (Eds), *Selected Topics in Clinical Enzymology*. Walter de Gruyter, Berlin, pp. 435–444

Hardy, T. L. (1970). Identification of cells exfoliated from the rat kidney in experimental nephrotoxicity. *Ann. Rheum. Dis.*, **29**, 64–66

Haqqi, T. M. and Adhami, U. M. (1982). Testicular damage and change in serum LDH isoenzyme patterns induced by multiple sub-lethal doses of apholate in albino rats. *Toxicol. Lett.*, **12**, 199–205

Harris, A. R. G., Fang, S. L., Azizi, F., Lipworth, L., Vagenakis, A. G. and Braverman, L. E. (1978). Effect of starvation on hypothalamic–pituitary–thyroid function in the rat. *Metabolism*, **27**, 1074–1083

Hau, J., Nilsson, M., Skovgaard-Jensen, H.-J., de Souza, A., Eriksen, E. and Wandall, L. T. (1990). Analysis of animal serum proteins against human analogous proteins. *Scand. J. Lab. Anim. Sci.*, **17**, 3–7

Hayes, W. J. (1982). *Pesticides Studied in Man*. Williams and Wilkins, Baltimore

Henning, S. J. (1984). Hormonal and dietary regulation of intestinal enzyme development. In Schiller, C. M. (Ed.), *Intestinal Toxicology*, Raven Press, New York, pp. 17–32

Higgins, P. J., Garlick, R. L. and Bunn, H. F. (1982). Glycosylated hemoglobin in human and animal red cells. *Diabetes*, **26**, 743–748

Hinton, R. H. and Mullock, B. M. (1977). Bile proteins in the serum of jaundiced rats. *Clin. Chim. Acta*, **78**, 159–162

Hinton, R. H., Price, S. C., Mitchell, F. E., Mann, A., Hall, D. E. and Bridges, J. W. (1985). Plasma protein changes in rats treated with hypolipidaemic drugs and with phthalate esters. *Human Toxicol.*, **4**, 261–271

Hofmann, A. F. (1988): Bile acids. In Arias, I. M., Jakoby, W. B., Popper, M., Schachter, D. and Shafritz, D. A. (Eds), *The Liver, Biology and Pathobiology*. Raven Press, New York, pp. 553–572

House, E. L., Pansky, B. and Jacobs, M. S. (1961). Age changes in blood of the golden hamster. *Am. J. Physiol.*, **200**, 1018–1022

Ingbar, D. H. and Galton, V. A. (1975). The effect of food deprivation on the peripheral metabolism of thyroxine in rats. *Endocrinology*, **96**, 1525–1532

Itoh, R. and Ozasa, H. (1985). Changes in serum lactate dehydrogenase isozyme X activity observed after cadmium administration. *Toxicol. Lett.*, **28**, 151–154

Jablonski, P. and Owen, J. A. (1969). The clinical chemistry of bromsulfophthalein and other cholephilic dyes. *Adv. Clin. Chem.*, **12**, 309–386

Japundzic, I. and Levi, E. (1987). Mechanism of action of cysteamine on duodenal alkaline phosphatase. *Biochem. Pharmacol.*, **36**, 2489–2495

Jenkins, F. P. and Robinson, J. A. (1975). Serum biochemical changes in rats deprived of food or water for 24 h. *Proc. Nutr. Soc.*, **34**, 37A

Johnson, D. A. (1989). Fecal occult blood testing. Problems, pitfalls and diagnostic concerns. *Postgrad. Med.*, **85**, 287–299

Johnston, S. D. and Mather, E. C. (1978). Canine plasma cortisol (hydroxycortisone) measured by radioimmunoassay; clinical absence of diurnal variation and results of ACTH stimulation and dexamethasone suppression tests. *Am. J. Vet. Res.*, **39**, 1766–1770

Jordan, D., Rousset, B., Perrin F., Fournier, M. and Orgiazzi, J. (1980). Evidence for circadian variations in serum thyrotropin, 3,5,3'-triiodothyronine, and thyroxine in the rat. *Endocrinology*, **107**, 1245–1248

Jung, K. and Scholz, D. (1980). An optimised assay of alanine aminopeptidase activity in urine. *Clin. Chem.*, **26**, 1251–1254

Jurcovicova, J., Vigas, M., Klir, P. and Jezova, D. (1984). Response of prolactin, growth hormone and corticosterone secretion to morphine administration or stress exposure in Wistar–AVN and Long–Evans rats. *Endocrinol. Experiment.*, **18**, 209–214

Kallner, A. and Tryding, N. (1989). I.F.C.C. Guidelines to the evaluation of drug effects in clinical chemistry. *Scand. J. Clin. Lab. Invest.*, **49**, Suppl. 195, 1–29

Karlsson, B. W. and Larsson, G. B. (1971). Lactic and malic dehydrogenases and their multiple molecular forms in the mongolian gerbil as compared with the rat, mouse and rabbit. *Comp. Biochem. Physiol.*, **40B**, 93–108

Kast, A. and Nishikawa, J. (1981). The effect of fasting on oral acute toxicity of drugs in rats and mice. *Lab. Anim.*, **15**, 359–364

Kazmlerczak, S. C., Lott, J. A. and Caldwell, J. H. (1988). Acute intestinal infarction or obstruction:

search for better laboratory tests in an animal model. *Clin. Chem.*, **34**, 281–288

Keller, P. (1981). Enzyme activities in the dog: tissue analyses, plasma values, and intracellular distribution. *Am. J. Vet. Res.*, **42**, 575–582

Kemppainen, R. J. and Sartin, J. L. (1984). Evidence for episodic but not circadian activity in plasma concentrations of adrenocorticotrophin, cortisol and thyroxine in dogs. *J. Endocrinol.*, **103**, 219–226

Klaassen, C. D. and Plaa, G. L. (1967). Species variation in metabolism, storage and excretion of sulfobromophthalein. *Am. J. Physiol.*, **213**, 1322–1326

Klaassen, C. D. and Plaa, G. L. (1969). Plasma disappearance and biliary excretion of indocyanine green in rats, rabbits and dogs. *Toxicol. Appl. Pharmacol.*, **15**, 374–384

Kluwe, W. M. (1981). Renal function tests as indicators of kidney injury in subacute toxicity studies. *Toxicol. Appl. Pharmacol.*, **57**, 414–424

Koop, H., Schwab, E., Arnold, R. and Creutzfeldt, W. (1982). Effect of food deprivation on gastric somatostatin and gastrin release. *Gastroenterology*, **82**, 871–876

Korsrud, G. O. and Trick, K. D. (1973). Activities of several enzymes in serum and heparinised plasma from rats. *Clin. Chim. Acta*, **48**, 311–315

Kramer, J. M. (1981). Immunofluorescent localization of PGK–1 and PGK–2 isozymes within specific cells of the mouse testis. *Dev. Biol.*, **87**, 30–36

Kuhn, E. R., Bellon, K., Huybrechts, L. and Heyns, W. (1983). Endocrine differences between the Wistar and Sprague–Dawley laboratory rat: influence of cold adaptation. *Horm. Metab. Res.*, **15**, 491–498

Kuhn, G. and Hardegg, W. (1988). Effects of indoor and outdoor maintenance of dogs upon food intake, body weight, and different blood parameters. *Z. Veruchstierkd.*, **31**, 205–214

Kushner, I. and Mackiewicz, A. (1987). Acute phase proteins as disease markers. *Disease Markers*, **5**, 1–11

Landt, Y., Vaidya, H. C., Porter, S. E., Dietzler, D. N. and Ladenson, J. H. (1989). Immunoaffinity purification of creatine kinase-MB from human, dog, and rabbit heart with use of a monoclonal antibody specific for CK-MB. *Clin. Chem.*, **35**, 985–989

Lang, H. (1981). *Creatine Kinase Isoenzymes*. Springer-Verlag, Berlin

Larsson, H., Carlsson, E., Mattsson, H., Lundell, L., Sundler, F., Sundler, G., Wallmark, B., Wanatabe, T. and Hakanson, R. (1986). Plasma gastrin and gastric enterochromaffin like cell activation and proliferation. *Gastroenterology*, **90**, 391–399

Leard, B. L., Alsaker, R. D., Porter, W. P. and Sobel, L. P. (1990). The effect of haemolysis on certain canine serum chemistry parameters. *Lab. Anim.*, **24**, 32–35

Lehman, A. J. (1959). *Appraisal of the Safety of*

Chemicals in Foods, Drugs and Cosmetics. Association of FDA Officials, Topeka

Leissing, N., Izzo, R. and Sargent, H. (1985). Variance estimates and individuality ratios of 25 serum constituents in beagles. *Clin. Chem.*, **31**, 83–86

Leonard, T. B., Neptun, D. A. and Popp, J. A. (1984). Serum gamma glutamyl transferase as a specific indicator of bile duct lesions in the rat liver. *Am. J. Pathol.*, **116**, 262–269

Lewis, P. J., Lowing R. K. and Gompertz, D. (1981). Automated discrete kinetic method for erythrocyte acetylcholinesterase and plasma cholinesterase. *Clin. Chem.*, **27**, 926–929

Lindena, J., Sommerfeld, U., Hopfel, C. and Trautschold, I. (1986). Catalytic enzyme activity concentration in tissues of man, dog, rabbit, guinea pig, rat, and mouse. *J. Clin. Chem. Clin. Biochem.*, **24**, 35–47

Lock, E. A., Charbonneau, M., Strasser, J., Swenberg, J. A. and Bus, J. S. (1987). 2,2,4-Trimethylpentane-induced nephropathy. II. The reversible binding of a TMP metabolite to a renal protein fraction containing alpha$_{2u}$ globulin. *Toxicol. Appl. Pharmacol.*, **91**, 182–192

Lock, E. A., Mitchell, A. M. and Elcombe, C. R. (1989). Biochemical mechanisms of induction of hepatic peroxisome proliferation. *Ann. Rev. Pharmacol. Toxicol.*, **29**, 145–163

Loeb, W. F. and Quimby, F. W. (1989). *The Clinical Chemistry of Laboratory Animals*. Pergamon Press, New York

Lovett, D. H., Ryan, J. L., Kashgarian, M. and Sterzel, R. B. (1982). Lysosomal enzymes in glomerular cells of the rat. *Am. J. Pathol.*, **107**, 161–166

McElderry, L., Tarbit, I. F. and Cassells-Smith, A. J. (1982). Six methods for urinary protein compared. *Clin. Chem.*, **28**, 356–360

McGeachin, R. L. and Akin, J. R. (1982). Amylase levels in the tissues and body fluids of several primate species. *Comp. Biochem. Physiol.*, **72A**, 267–269

Magil, A. B., Mavichak, V., Wong, N. L. M., Quamme, G. A., Dirks, J. H. and Sutton, R. A. L. (1986). Long-term morphological and biochemical observations in Cisplatin induced hypomagnesaemia in rats. *Nephron*, **43**, 223–230

Mantamat, E. E., Moreno, J. and Blanco, A. (1978). Branched-chain amino acid transferase in mouse testicular tissue. *J. Reprod. Fertil.*, **53**, 117–123

March, G. B. and Drablein, D. L. (1960). Experimental reconstruction of metabolic patterns of lipids nephrosis: key role of hepatic protein synthesis in hyperlipemia. *Metabolism*, **9**, 946–955

Markert, C. L. and Whitt, G. S. (1975). Evolution of a gene. *Science*, **189**, 102–114

Meijer, G. W., de Bruijne, J. J. and Beynen, A. C. (1987). Dietary cholesterol–fat type combinations and carbohydrate and lipid metabolism in rats and mice. *Int. J. Vit. Nutr. Res.*, **57**, 319–326

Meistrich, M. L., Trostle, P. K., Frapart, M. and

Erickson, R. P. (1977). Biosynthesis and localization of lactate dehydrogenase X in pachytene spermatocytes and spermatids of mouse testes. *Dev. Biol.*, **60**, 428–441

Meyer, O. A., Kristiansen, E. and Wurtzen, G. (1989). Effects of dietary protein and butylated hydroxytoluene on the kidneys of rats. *Lab. Anim.*, **23**, 175–179

Michel, H. O. (1949). An electrometric method for the determination of red blood cell and plasma cholinesterase activity. *J. Lab. Clin. Med.*, **34**, 1564–1568

Mitruka, B. M. and Rawnsley, H. M. (1977). *Clinical Biochemical and Hematological Reference Values in Normal Experimental Animals*. Masson, New York

Moss, D. W. (1982). Alkaline phosphatase isoenzymes. *Clin. Chem.*, **28**, 2007–2016

Mudge, G. H. (1982). Comparative pharmacology of the kidney; implications for drug-induced renal failure. In Bach, P. H., Bonner, F. W., Bridges, J. W. and Lock, E. A. (Eds), *Nephrotoxicity: Assessment and Pathogenesis*. Wiley, Chichester, pp. 504–518

Muraca, M., de Groote, J. and Fevery, J. (1983). Sex differences of hepatic conjugation of bilirubin determine its maximal biliary excretion in non-anaesthetised male and female rats. *Clin. Sci.*, **64**, 85–90

Nachbaur, J., Clarke, M. R., Provost, J. P. and Dancla, J. L. (1977). Variations of sodium, potassium, and chloride plasma levels in the rat with age and sex. *Lab. Anim. Sci.*, **27**, 972–975

Nakagawa, H., Watanabe, K. and Tsurufuji, S. (1984). Changes in serum and exudate levels of functional macroglobulins and anti-inflammatory effect of alpha-2-acute-phase-macroglobulin on carrageenin-induced inflammation in rats. *Biochem. Pharmacol.*, **33**, 1181–1186

Nakamura, M., Itoh, T., Miyata, K., Higashiyama, N., Takesue, H. and Nishiyama, S. (1983). Difference in urinary N-acetyl-β-D-glucosaminidase activity between male and female beagle dogs. *Renal Physiol. (Basel)*, **6**, 130–133

Neptun, D. A., Smith, C. N. and Irons, R. (1985). Effect of sampling site and collection method on variations in baseline clinical pathology parameters in Fischer 344 rats. *Fund. Appl. Toxicol.*, **5**, 1180–1185

Neuhaus, O. W. and Flory, W. (1978). Age dependent changes in the excretion of urinary proteins by the rat. *Nephron*, **22**, 570–576

Omaye, S. T. (1986). Effects of diet on toxicity testing. *Fed. Proc.*, **45**, 133–135

Orth, D. N., Peterson, M. E. and Drucker, W. D. (1988). Plasma immunoreactive propiomelanocortin peptides and cortisol in normal dogs and dogs with Cushing's syndrome: diurnal rhythm and responses to various stimuli. *Endocrinology*, **122**, 1250–1262

Ottenweiller, J. E. and Hedge, G. A. (1982). Diurnal variations of plasma thyrotropin, thyroxine and triiodothyronine in female rats are phase shifted after invasion of the photoperiod. *Endocrinology*, **111**, 509–514

Pariat, Cl., Ingrand, P., Cambar, J., de Lemos, E., Piriou, A. and Courtois, Ph. (1990). Seasonal effects on the daily variations of gentamicin-induced nephrotoxicity. *Arch. Toxicol.*, **64**, 205–209

Parraga, M. E. and Kaneko, J. J. (1985). Total serum bile acids and the bile acid profile as tests of liver function. *Vet. Res. Commun.*, **9**, 79–88

Pearl, W., Balazs, T. and Buyske, D. A. (1966). The effect of stress on serum transaminase activity in the rat. *Life Sci.*, **5**, 67–74

Pickering, C. E. and Pickering, R. G. (1971). Methods for the estimation of acetylcholinesterase activity in the plasma and brain of laboratory animals given carbamates or organophosphorus compounds. *Arch. Toxicol.*, **27**, 292–310

Pickering, C. E. and Pickering, R. G. (1978a). Studies of rat alkaline phosphatase. I. Development of methods for detecting isoenzymes. *Arch. Toxicol.*, **39**, 249–266

Pickering, R. G. and Pickering, C. E. (1978b). Studies of rat alkaline phosphatase. II. Some applications of the methods for detecting the isoenzymes of plasma alkaline phosphatase in rats. *Arch. Toxicol.*, **39**, 267–287

Plaa, G. L. and Larson, R. E. (1965). Relative nephrotoxic properties of chlorinated methane, ethane, and ethylene derivatives in mice. *Toxicol. Appl. Pharmacol.*, **7**, 37–44

Poldlasek, S. J. and McPherson, R. A. (1989). Streptokinase binds to lactate dehydrogenase subunit-M, which shares an epitope with plasminogen. *Clin. Chem.*, **35**, 69–73

Powers, D. M., Boyd, J. C., Glick, M. R. Kotschi, M. L., Letellier, G., Miller, W. G., Nealon, D. A. and Hartmann, A. E. (1986). *Interference Testing in Clinical Chemistry: Proposed Guidelines.* N.C.C.L.S. Document 6.13.EP7/P, Villanova, Pennsylvania

Prescott, L. F. (1982). Assessment of nephrotoxicity. *Br. J. Clin. Pharmacol.*, **13**, 303–311

Prescott, L. F. and Ansari, S. (1969). The effects of repeated administration of mercuric chloride on exfoliation of renal tubular cells and urinary glutamic-oxaloacetic transaminase activity in the rat. *Toxicol. Appl. Pharmacol.*, **14**, 97–107

Prescott, L. F. and Brodie, D. E. (1964). A simple differential stain for urinary sediment. *Lancet*, **ii**, 940

Price, R. G. (1982). Urinary enzymes, nephrotoxicity and renal disease. *Toxicology.*, **23**, 99–134

Rajasingham, R., Bell, J. L. and Baron, D. N. (1971). A comparative study of the isoenzymes of mammalian alpha amylase. *Enzyme*, **12**, 180–186

Reader, S. C. J., Shingles, C., Stonard, M. D. (1991). Acute testicular toxicity of 1,3-dinitrobenzene and ethylene glycol monomethyl ether in the rat: evaluation of biochemical effect markers and hormonal responses. *Fund. Appl. Toxicol.*, **16**, 61–70

Refetoff, S., Robin, N. I. and Fang, U. S. (1970). Parameters of thyroid function in serum of 16 selec-ted vertebrate species: a study of PBI, serum T_4, free T_4 and the pattern of T_4 and T_3 binding to serum protein. *Endocrinology*, **86**, 793–805

Reuter, A. M., Kennes, F., Leonard, A. and Sassen, A. (1968). Variations of the prealbumin in serum and urine of mice, according to strain and sex. *Comp. Biochem. Physiol.*, **25**, 921–928

Ribelin, W. E. (1984). The effects of drugs and chemicals upon the structure of the adrenal gland. *Fund. Appl. Toxicol.*, **4**, 105–119

Riley, V. (1981). Psychoneuroendocrine influences on immuno-competence and neoplasia. *Science*, **212**, 1100–1102

Robbins, J. and Johnson, M. L. (1982). Possible significance of multiple transport proteins for the thyroid hormones. In Albertini, A. and Ekins, R. P. (Eds), *Free Hormones in Blood*, Elsevier Biomedical, New York, pp. 53–64

Rosenthal, P., Blanckaert, N., Kabra, P. M. and Thaler, M. M. (1981). Liquid chromatographic determination of bilirubin and its conjugates in rat serum and human amniotic fluid. *Clin. Chem.*, **27**, 1704–1707

Roy, A. K. and Neuhaus, O. W. (1967). Androgenic control of a sex-dependent protein in the rat. *Nature*, **214**, 618–620

Salgo, L. and Szabo, A. (1982). Gamma-glutamyl transpeptidase activity in human urine. *Clin. Chim. Acta*, **126**, 9–16

Santen, R. J. and Bardin, C. W. (1973). Episodic LH secretion in man: pulse analysis, clinical interpretation, physiologic mechanisms. *J. Clin. Invest.*, **52**, 2617–2628

Schardsmidt, B. F., Waggoner, J. G. and Berk, P. D. (1975). Hepatic organic anion uptake in the rat. *J. Clin. Invest.*, **56**, 1280–1292

Scherer, R., Abd-el-Fattah, M. and Ruhenstroth-Bauer, G (1977). Some applications of quantitative two-dimensional immunoelectrophoresis in the study of the systemic acute-phase reaction of the rat. In Willoughby, D. A., Giroud, J. P. and Velo, G. P. (Eds), *Perspectives in Inflammation, Future Trends and Development.* MTP, Lancaster, pp. 437–444

Schmidt-Neilsen, B. and O'Dell, R. (1961). Structure and concentrating mechanism in the mammalian kidney. *Am. J. Physiol.*, **200**, 1119–1124

Schwartz, E., Tornaben, J. A. and Boxill, G. C. (1973). The effects of food restriction on hematology, clinical chemistry and pathology in the albino rat. *Toxicol. Appl. Pharmacol.*, **25**, 515–524

Sharratt, M. and Frazer, A. C. (1963). The sensitivity of function tests in detecting renal damage in the rat. *Toxicol. Appl. Pharmacol.*, **39**, 423–434

Simpson, J. W. and Doxey, D. L. (1988). Evaluation of faecal analysis as an aid to the detection of exocrine pancreatic insufficiency. *Br. Vet. J.*, **144**, 174–178

Sinha, B. K. (1982). Myocardial toxicity of anthracyclines and other antitumour agents. In van Stee, E. W.

(Ed.), *Cardiovascular Toxicology*, Raven Press, New York, pp. 181–198

Sitren, H. S. and Stevenson, N. R. (1980). Circadian fluctuations in liver and blood parameters in rats adapted to a nutrient solution by oral, intravenous and discontinuous intravenous feeding. *J. Nutr.*, **110**, 558–566

Smith, P. L. (1986). Gastrointestinal physiology. In Rozman, K. and Hanninen, O. (Eds), *Gastrointestinal Toxicology*. Elsevier, Amsterdam, pp. 1–23

Spitz, I. M., Gunsalus, G. L., Mather, J. P., Thau, R. and Bardin, C. W. (1985). The effects of the imidazole carboxylic acid derivative, tolmidamine, on testicular function. I. Early changes in androgen binding protein secretion in the rat. *J. Androl.*, **6**, 171–178

Steinberg, K. K., Freni-Titulaer, L. W. J., Rogers, T. N., Burse, V. W., Mueller, P. W., Stehr, P. A. and Miller, D. T. (1986). Effects of polychlorinated biphenyls and lipemia on serum analytes. *J. Toxicol. Environ. Hlth*, **19**, 369–381

Steinberger, E. (1981) Current status of studies concerned with evaluation of toxic effects of chemicals on the testes. *Environ. Hlth Perspect.*, **38**, 29–33

Stonard, M. D. (1987). Proteins, enzymes and cells in urine as indicators of the site of renal damage. In Bach, P. H. and Lock, E. A. (Eds), *Nephrotoxicity in the Experimental and Clinical Situation*. Martinus Nijhoff, Dordrecht, pp. 563–592

Stonard, M. D. (1990). Assessment of renal function and damage in animal species. *J. Appl. Toxicol.*, **10**, 267–274

Stonard, M. D., Foster, J. R., Phillips, P. G. N., Simpson, M. G. and Lock, E. A. (1985). Hyaline droplet formation in rat kidney induced by 2,2,4-trimethylpentane. In Bach, P. H. and Lock, E. A. (Eds) *Renal Heterogeneity and Target Cell Toxicity*. Wiley, London, pp. 485–488

Stonard, M. D., Gore, C. W., Oliver, J. A. and Smith, I. K. (1987). Urinary enzymes and protein patterns as indicators of injury to different regions of the kidney. *Fund. Appl. Toxicol.*, **9**, 339–351

Stonard, M. D., Samuels, D. M. and Lock, E. A. (1984). The pathogenesis of nephrocalcinosis induced by different diets in female rats, and the effect on renal function. *Fd Chem. Toxicol.*, **22**, 139–146

Stroo, W. E. and Hook, J. B. (1977). Enzymes of renal origin in urine as indicators of nephrotoxicity. *Toxicol. Appl. Pharmacol.*, **39**, 423–434

Tani, S., Ishikawa, A., Yamazaki, H. and Kudo, Y. (1987). Serum pepsinogen levels in normal and experimental peptic ulcer rats measured by radioimmunoassay. *Chem. Pharmacol. Bull.*, **35**, 1515–1522

Terpstra, A. H. M., Woodward, C. J. H. and Sanchez-Muniz, F. J. (1981). Improved techniques for the separation of serum lipoproteins by density gradient ultracentrifugation: visualization by prestaining and rapid separation of serum lipoproteins from small volumes of serum. *Anal. Biochem.*, **11**, 149–157

Thompson, M. B. and Kunze, D. J. (1984). Polyethylene glycol–6000 as a clearing agent for lipemic serum samples from dogs and the effect on 13 serum assays. *Am. J. Vet. Res.*, **45**, 2154–2157

Uchiyama, T., Tokoi, K. and Deki, T. (1985). Successive changes in the blood composition of the experimental normal beagle dogs accompanied with age. *Exptl Anim.*, **34**, 367–377

Unakami, S., Suzuki, S., Nakarishi, E., Ichonohe, K., Hirata, M. and Taninoto, Y. (1987). Comparative studies on multiple forms of serum cholinesterase in various species. *Exptl Anim.*, **36**, 199–204

Vandeberg, J. L., Yu Lee, C. and Goldberg, E. (1981). Immunohistochemical localization of phosphoglycerate kinase isozymes in mouse testes. *J. Exptl Zool.*, **217**, 435–441

Vogel, W. H. (1987). Stress—the neglected variable in experimental pharmacology and toxicology. *Trends Pharmacol. Sci.*, **8**, 35–38

Voss, G. and Sachsse, K. (1970). Red cell and plasma cholinesterase activities in microsamples of human and animal blood determined simultaneously by a modified acetylcholine/DTNB procedure. *Toxicol. Appl. Pharmacol.*, **16**, 764–772

Walsh, C. T. (1982). Methods in gastrointestinal toxicology. In Hayes, A. W. (Ed.), *Principles and Methods of Toxicology*. Raven Press, New York, pp. 475–486

Waner, T. (1990). Clinical chemistry in regulatory toxicology: the state of the art. In Kaneko, J. J. (Ed.). *Proceedings, IVth Congress, International Society for Animal Clinical Biochemistry*, University of California, pp. 61–68

Weil, C. S. (1982). Statistical analysis and normality of selected hematologic and clinical chemistry measurements used in toxicological studies. *Arch. Toxicol.*, Suppl. **5**, 237–253

Weisberg, L. S. (1989). Pseudohyponatremia: a reappraisal. *Am. J. Med.*, **86**, 315–318

Werner, M. and Gabrielson, D. (1977). Ultrafiltration for improved assay of urinary enzymes. *Clin. Chem.*, **23**, 700–704

Werner, M., Maruhn, D. and Atoba, M. (1969). Use of gel filtration in the assay of urinary enzymes. *J. Chromatog.*, **40**, 254–263

Wheat, T. E., Hintz, M., Goldberg, E. and Margoliash, E. (1977). Analyses of stage specific multiple forms of lactate dehydrogenase and of cytochrome c during spermatogenesis in the mouse. *Differentiation*, **9**, 37–41

Whittaker, M. (1986). *Cholinesterase*. Monographs in Human Genetics, Vol. II. Karger, Basel

Will, P. C., Allbee, W. E., Witt, C. G., Bertko, R. J. and Gaginella, T. S. (1984). Quantification of pepsin A activity in canine and rat gastric juice with the chromogenic substrate Azocoll. *Clin. Chem.*, **30**, 707–711

Wills, J. H. (1972). The measurement and significance of changes in the cholinesterase activities of erythrocytes and plasma in man and animals. *CRC Crit. Rev. Toxicol.*, **1**, 153–201

Witiak, D. T. and Whitehouse, M. W. (1969). Species differences in the albumin binding of 2,4,6-trinitrobenzaldehyde, chlorophenoxy-acetic acids, 2-(4′-hydroxybenzeneazo) benzoic acid and some other acidic drugs—the unique behaviour of plasma. *Biochem. Pharmacol.*, **18**, 971–977

Wolford, S. T., Schroer, R. A., Gallo, P. P., Gohs, F. X., Brodeck, M., Falk, H. B. and Ruhren, R. (1987). Age-related changes in serum chemistry and hematology values in normal Sprague–Dawley rats. *Fund. Appl. Toxicol.*, **8**, 80–88

Wong, C.-C., Dohler, K.-D., Atkinson, M. J., Geerlings, H., Hesch, R.-D. and von zur Muhlen, A. (1983a). Influence of age, strain and season on diurnal periodicity of thyroid stimulating hormone, thyroxine, tri-iodothyronine and parathyroid hormone in the serum of male laboratory rats. *Acta Endocrinol.*, **101**, 377–385

Wong, C.-C., Dohler, K.-D., Geerlings, H. and von zur Muhlen, A. (1983b). Influence of age, strain and season on circadian periodicity of pituitary, gonadal and adrenal hormones in the serum of male laboratory rats. *Hormone Res.*, **17**, 202–215

Woodman, D. D. (1981). Plasma enzymes in drug toxicity. In Gorrod, J. W. (Ed.), *Aspects of Drug Toxicity Testing Methods*. Taylor and Francis, London, pp. 145–156

Woodman, D. D. (1988a). Assessment of hepatic function and damage in animal species. *J. Appl. Toxicol.*, **8**, 249–254

Woodman, D. D. (1988b). The use of chemical biochemistry for assessment of endocrine system toxicology. In Keller, P. and Bogin, E. (Eds), *The Use of Clinical Biochemistry in Toxicologically Relevant Animal Models and Standardisation and Quality Control in Animal Biochemistry*. Hexagon-Roche, Basel, pp. 63–77

Woodman, D. D. and Maile, P. A. (1981). Bile acids as an index of cholestasis. *Clin. Chem.*, **27**, 846–848

Wooley, J., Mullock, B. M. and Hinton, R. H. (1979). Reflux of biliary components into blood in experimental intrahepatic cholestasis induced in rats by treatment with alpha naphthylisothiocyanate. *Clin. Chim. Acta*, **92**, 381–386

Wright, P. J., Leathwood, P. D. and Plummer, D. T. (1972). Enzymes in rat urine: alkaline phosphatase. *Enzymologia*, **42**, 317–327

Wright, P. J. and Plummer, D. T. (1974). The use of urinary enzyme measurements to detect renal damage caused by nephrotoxic compounds. *Biochem. Pharmacol.*, **23**, 65–73

Young, D. S. (1990). *Effects of Drugs on Clinical Laboratory Tests*. AACC Press, Washington, D.C.

Young, F. G. (1963). Pancreatic hormones: insulin. In von Euler, U. S. and Heller, H. (Eds), *Comparative Endocrinology*. Academic Press, London, pp. 371–402

FURTHER READING

Blick, K. E. and Liles, S. M. (1985). *Principles of Clinical Chemistry*. John Wiley and Sons, New York

Burtis, C. A. and Ashwood, E. R. (1994). *Clinical Chemistry*. W. B. Saunders Company, Philadelphia

Fernie, S., Wienshall, E., Malcolm, S., Bryce, F. and Arnold, D. L. (1994). Normative hematologic and serum biochemical values for adult rhesus monkeys (Macaca mulatta) in a controlled laboratory environment. *Journal of Toxicology and Environmental Health*, **42**, 53–72

12 Antidotal Studies

Timothy C. Marrs and D. Nicholas Bateman

INTRODUCTION

The Antidote

An antidote is defined in *Webster's New Collegiate Dictionary* as a remedy to counteract the effects of a poison. Remedies, in this sense, are usually visualized to be specific chemical entities, but sometimes this definition is broadened to include non-specific measures such as charcoal haemoperfusion, dialysis, and so on (Bateman and Chaplin, 1989). This chapter will not be dealing with these non-specific techniques.

Experimental studies on antidotes are carried out for the same reasons as on any other drug—namely, to demonstrate efficacy and to assess toxicity of the antidote in relation to its efficacy. Nevertheless, these therapeutic agents differ from many other drugs, both in the way they are used and in the manner in which their efficacy and toxicity can be appropriately assessed. Thus, antidotes are usually only used in life-threatening situations and are administered as a single dose, or for a short treatment course. This means that many of the toxicological data required for drugs used over longer periods in less serious diseases would be thought unnecessary by most toxicologists. Indeed, many antidotes, particularly older ones, have been introduced after minimal animal toxicity studies. Furthermore, randomized clinical trials, including a placebo group, are rarely possible in patients, because of ethical considerations. Although trials in humans can be designed, these often use a retrospective control group or a parallel group treated with an 'established antidote' and may therefore be less than satisfactory. Consequently, one is more than usually reliant on animal studies for the evaluation of efficacy.

The Poison

In a programme to develop a new antidote, some knowledge of the toxicology of the poison is required for two purposes: first, to identify an antidotal approach that is likely to be successful, and second, to enable the design and interpretation of an efficacy study.

The acute toxicity of a poisonous compound is traditionally quantified by the LD_{50}. Although the use of the LD_{50} test has been criticized on both humane and scientific grounds (e.g. British Toxicology Society, 1984; Society of Toxicology, 1989), most antidotal efficacy studies use experimental designs that require the use of this test (see below). When the LD_{50} is carried out, the slope of the log dose–probit mortality line should be recorded, because the slope is often changed by antidotal treatment (Natoff and Reiff, 1970); furthermore, the slope will be useful in the calculation of dosing schedules of the poison in studies in which the antidote is administered. Ideally, acute toxicity studies should be carried out in several species. Animals may show marked differences from humans in the quantitative or qualitative toxicity of a poison; such species differences will clearly influence the choice of a suitable model for animal experiments.

Where the object of the treatment is to ameliorate a non-lethal but crippling effect—for example, blindness in methanol poisoning—measurement of the ED_{50} (lowest dose giving the given effect in 50 per cent of the animals) for that effect will be needed. In such cases species sensitivity to the appropriate toxic effect will be an important consideration in the choice of species in efficacy studies.

The subacute or chronic toxicity of a poison is not usually of interest in the design of experiments to measure the effectiveness of antidotes. For poisons, in which late toxicity is an important toxicological effect in humans, delayed single-dose toxicity should be studied. Carbon monoxide is a good example of a poison with this pattern of toxicity (Garland and Pearce, 1967; Werner *et al.*, 1985). The ED_{50} may be a suitable measure of toxicity where the delayed effects are non-lethal.

It is reassuring for the toxicologist to know that the organ-specific toxicity of the poison is the same in an animal species as in man. Sometimes an indication of this may be gleaned from acute lethality studies. On most occasions the effects of sublethal doses of the poison will have to be studied, this usually being necessary, since death of some of the animals during LD_{50} studies makes interpretation of the histology, a useful indicator of organ-specific effects, difficult. Mechanistic studies on particular cell types within the target organ, while desirable and possibly helpful in the initial design of an antidotal approach, are in practice rarely necessary as a preliminary to the assessment of antidotes.

Elucidation of the metabolic pathways of the poison is most useful where conversion to a toxic metabolite is a prerequisite for toxicity. In such instances it is essential that the species used in experimental studies handle the poison in a similar manner to man. In the situation where the antidote and poison directly react together—for example, the chelating agents and metals—differences in metabolic handling of the toxin are likely to be less important. Knowledge of the pharmacokinetics of the poison in animals and man, while less useful in determining an antidotal mechanism, may be useful in designing animal efficacy studies and in the choice of an animal model.

INTRODUCTION OF NEW ANTIDOTES

The introduction of new antidotes has only rarely occurred by a chance finding of antidotal action—for example, as part of a screening programme. It has usually been based on an extensive substructure of knowledge of the mechanism of action of the poison. With the application of pharmacological, biochemical or chemical expertise, it has then been possible to find a way in which the poison could be detoxified or its toxic effects reversed. If one considers the introduction of antidotes at present available, it is clear that most antidotes have evolved from the discovery of an antidote that was less than optimal, a 'lead' compound (Burger, 1982). Analogous compounds were then studied, and usually the one with the best therapeutic index was eventually adopted as the standard treatment. Examples of this approach include the introduction of sodium nitrite, a component of the classical therapy for

cyanide, which arose from the discovery by Pedigo of the usefulness of amyl nitrite in cyanide poisoning (1888). Another example is the use of N-acetylcysteine for the treatment of paracetamol poisoning, which followed the earlier introduction of cysteamine. The discovery of the oxime organophosphorus antidotes, 2-PAM and later obidoxime, followed from discovery of the antidotal effect of hydroxylamine (Bismuth *et al.*, 1992), while the introduction of dicobalt edetate as a cyanide antidote by Paulet (1960) was an attempt to improve upon the experimentally effective but toxic inorganic cobalt salts. Thus, probably the single most challenging part of the process of bringing new antidotes into clinical practice is the discovery of 'lead' antidotes and this is usually dependent on an hypothesis for the mechanism of toxicity of a particular poison.

MECHANISM OF ANTIDOTAL ACTION

It is difficult to produce a classification of antidotes that is in all respects satisfactory, although a number of workers have attempted to do so (Marrs, 1987; Bismuth, 1987; Bateman and Chaplin, 1989; Marrs, 1992). To some extent this is because the mode of action of certain well-known antidotes is controversial, while others appear to act in more than one way.

It is possible to envisage a number of ways in which the toxic effects of poisons might be opposed (Table 1). Broadly, they can be divided into three main classes: (1) antidotes that remove the active poison from its site of action, usually by bringing about functional chemical detoxication of the poison; (2) antidotes that act at pharmacological receptors; and (3) antidotes that act by functional antagonism—that is, they reverse the secondary effects of a toxin. It should be noted, however, that antidotes may have actions in more than one of these classes.

Antidotes That Act Chemically

Antidotes That Act Directly on the Poison

The most simple and easily visualized mode of antidotal action is direct chemical reaction between an antidote and a poison to form a less toxic product which is more rapidly excreted.

Table 1 Mode of action of antidotes

Antidotes that act chemically
(1) Direct chemical detoxication
    (a) chelating agents (metals)
    (b) cobalt-containing cyanide antidotes
    (c) antibodies
        (i) monoclonal antibodies (soman)
        (ii) Fab fragments (digoxin)
(2) Enzymatic detoxication
    (a) cosubstrate
        sodium thiosulphate (cyanide)
    (b) exogenous enzymes
        (i) rhodanese
        (ii) acetylcholinesterase
    (c) prevention of formation of toxic metabolite
        ethanol (methanol, ethylene glycol)
(3) Antidote gives rise to a detoxifying substance
    methaemoglobin-formers (cyanide and sulphide)
(4) Antidote reacts with enzyme–poison complex
    oximes (organophosphates)
(5) Antidote acts on a toxic metabolite of poison
    reacts with toxic metabolite
        N-acetylcysteine and methionine (paracetamol)

Antidotes that act pharmacologically
(1) Antagonism at characterized pharmacological receptors
    (a) naloxone (opiates)
    (b) flumazanil (benzodiazepines)
    (c) prenalterol (β-blockers)
(2) Antagonism at other macromolecules
    oxygen (carbon monoxide)

Functional
(1) Diazepam as anticonvulsant (organophosphates)
(2) IV fluids in hypotension

There are numerous examples of such antidotes, including the chelating agents, used in poisoning with a variety of toxic metals, as well as the cobalt-containing cyanide antidotes and Fab fragments, used in digoxin poisoning. Studies *in vitro*, often unhelpful in antibody assessment, have been used in some of these examples to elucidate the chemistry of the reactions.

Chelating Agents
The term 'chelation' is often used with lack of precision. The word comes from the Greek for a claw and it has been argued that monothiol compounds should not be described as chelating agents, since they only have one reactive group. However, the term is often used to describe those drugs whose action is to complex metals. The beneficial effect is the result of the complex being less toxic than the free metal, with subsequent mobilization from critical sites of toxic action or elimination. In many instances all three processes contribute to antidotal efficacy.

One of the earliest chelating agents was dimercaprol (British Anti-Lewisite; BAL). Like many advances in toxicology, the introduction of this substance was stimulated by military considerations. Dimercaprol was intended for use in treating poisoning by the chemical warfare agent lewisite, an organic arsenic compound. The use of dithiol compounds had its origin in the suspicion, subsequently confirmed, that the toxicity of arsenic was due to its ability to combine with sulphydryl groups in biological molecules. Dimercaprol and some similar compounds were extensively studied by Stockenn and Thompson (1946), and dimercaprol was the first of the dithiol chelating agents to be used in clinical treatment. Recently two other related drugs have been introduced, dimercaptosuccinic acid (DMSA) and dimercaptopropanesulphonic acid (DMPS). These possess the same dithiol chelating grouping as dimercaprol but the molecules as a whole are more hydrophilic. Unlike dimercaprol, DMSA and DMPS can be used orally and have a better therapeutic index than the older drug.

As well as arsenic, the toxicity of many other metals is due, at least in part, to reaction with sulphydryl groups. It is, therefore, not surprising that the active part of some other chelators contains sulphydryl groups. Penicillamine, which is a monothiol chelator, has been used for some years for the treatment of Wilson's disease, a condition in which copper overload is responsible for hepatic and central nervous system toxicity. Therapy with penicillamine will mobilize a variety of other metals, including lead. Other chelating agents contain active groups other than thiols. Disodium calcium ethylenediamine tetraacetate and its analogues chelate lead and zinc and can be used in acute cadmium poisoning. Desferrioxamine is a compound of natural origin that binds iron and aluminium. A considerable amount of work has been carried out on reaction of the chelating agents (ligands) with metals, and it is possible to predict the efficacy of particular chelating agents in particular metal poisonings on the basis of the affinity constant of the metal and chelator (Ringbom, 1963; Pearson, 1968).

Despite their logical derivation, net affinity (conditional stability) constants of metal chelator complexes can be misleading. As discussed above, the beneficial action of the chelating agents is probably a combination of effects, detoxication by complexation, mobilization and elimination. In order to detoxify effectively, chelating agents must gain access to the tissue where the metal is exerting its action. In the case of mobilization, the process must occur in a toxicologically desirable direction (that is, away from the critical site of toxic action of the metal) if it is to be beneficial. Unfortunately, net affinity constants cannot predict the extent to which chelation occurs *in vivo*, or whether mobilization of the metal occurs in a beneficial way. Thus, Catsch and Harmuth-Hoehne (1975) found that penicillamine was a more effective mobilizing agent in mercury poisoning than diethylenetriamine pentacetate, while the corresponding affinity constants would suggest otherwise. In an attempt to refine studies *in vitro* Yokel and Kostenbauder (1987) hypothesized that hydrophobicity of the chelator–ligand complex was important in successful chelation therapy. They therefore studied chelating agents for use in aluminium poisoning *in vitro* in an octanol–aqueous system and *in vivo* in rabbits poisoned with this metal. They concluded that the ideal chelator should have a high affinity for the metal of interest, be sufficiently water-soluble to take by mouth, and be sufficiently lipid-soluble to distribute to sites of accumulation of the metal. If this is generally the case, partition studies would clearly improve the predictivity of *in vitro* studies of antidotes of this class. Nevertheless, the complete *in vitro* situation cannot adequately be approximated *in vivo*, even for chelating agents, a group of antidotes where *in vitro* studies should be the most promising.

Dicobalt Edetate and Hydroxocobalamin

It has been known for many years that transitional metals can form stable and often relatively non-toxic complexes with cyanide. Clinically, this property of the transitional metals has only been exploited in the cases of iron (see methaemoglobin below) and cobalt. Cobalt is a metal whose toxicity is well recognized and it was therefore generally considered that the toxicity of inorganic cobalt salts precluded clinical use. Muschett *et al.* (1952) showed that hydroxocobalamin (vitamin B12a) was an effective antidote in experimental cyanide poisoning of mice.

In clinical practice, hydroxocobalamin presents a number of problems. The molecular weight is high and it binds cyanide at the ratio of 1 mol hydroxocobalamin:1 mol cyanide. Although a concentrated preparation may soon be available (Rousselin and Garnier, 1985), very large volumes of the preparations currently available in the UK would be necessary. Paulet (1960) studied a number of cobalt derivatives in order to find a compound which had the antidotal effectiveness of hydroxocobalamin without its disadvantages and which lacked the toxicity of inorganic cobalt salts. The cobalt compounds studied were the chloride, acetate, gluconate and glutamate salts, and cobalt histidine and dicobalt edetate. The last two were effective and less toxic than the other compounds. On the basis of efficacy studies in dogs and acute lethality studies in mice, dicobalt edetate, in the formulation known as Kelocyanor, was widely adopted in Europe.

Fab Fragments and Monoclonal Antibodies

Antisera have long been used to treat poisoning with toxins of biological origin, such a botulinum toxin and toxins in snake venom: this approach can theoretically be adopted for other poisons. It is an attractive option for the many poisons where no chemically detoxifying antidote of sufficient efficacy and adequate lack of toxicity is available. Thus, monoclonal antibodies have reportedly been successful in experimental poisoning by the organophosphorus nerve agent soman (Lenz *et al.*, 1984), while monoclonal antibodies against paraquat have been produced (Johnston *et al.*, 1988). In the best-known example of immunotherapy for poisoning with a drug, the therapy of digoxin poisoning, whole antibodies are not used. Instead poisoning with this cardiac glycoside is treated with Fab antibody fragments (Stolshek *et al.*, 1988). These have the advantage that they can be eliminated by glomerular filtration (Cole and Smith, 1986) and are less immunogenic than whole antibodies. Immunotherapy can, in theory, be used to treat any poisoning where detoxicating antibodies can be made to the toxicant. However, in practice the size of the dose of poison makes the approach of limited practical value for many clinical poisonings. Biotechnology, making, as it does, large-scale manufacture of monoclonal antibodies easier, adds to the attraction of immunotherapy, making wider use likely in the future.

Antidotes That Act on the Poison via an Enzyme-Catalysed Reaction

The existence of enzymatic pathways of detoxication can be exploited in two main ways. Detoxifying cosubstrates can be used but will usually only be effective if the rate of reaction is cosubstrate-limited. Alternatively, the level of enzyme can be raised by injecting exogenous enzyme. A further way of influencing an enzymatic process is the exogenous supply of an alternative substrate, or use of an enzyme inhibitor.

Cosubstrates

Sodium thiosulphate is probably not the physiological sulphur donor for the enzyme rhodanese. Nevertheless, this cyanide antidote appears to act by increasing the supply of sulphur for the enzyme, which is normally rate-limited by sulphane sulphur availability. The rhodanese reaction accelerates the rate of cyanide transulphuration to thiocyanate, which is not very toxic. Sodium thiosulphate, when used alone, is not very effective, because, although it can increase the rate of cyanide transulphuration very considerably (Cristel *et al.*, 1977), the blood level of cyanide does not fall fast enough in the context of acute cyanide poisoning. A possible reason for this is that rhodanese is a mitochondrial enzyme, while sodium thiosulphate, administered intravenously, largely remains extracellular. Other sulphur compounds, including sodium ethane and propane thiosulphonates and tetrathionate, have been studied in the expectation or hope that they would enter mitochondria. In some animal studies they are superior to sodium thiosulphate, but they have not been used clinically. Cyanide detoxication by transulphuration has also been carried out experimentally using another endogenous enzyme: β-mercaptopyruvate sulphur transferase. In this case sodium β-mercaptopyruvate was the experimental antidote.

Exogenous Enzymes

Exogenous enzymes suffer from the disadvantage of being foreign proteins but have nevertheless been used experimentally as antidotes. Thus, in an attempt to place the rhodanese in the extracellular space, the use of intravenous bovine heart rhodanase accompanied by sulphur-containing cyanide antidotes has been studied in animals (Frankenberg, 1980). Another enzyme that has been studied is acetylcholinesterase in the treatment of anticholinesterase poisoning.

Alteration of Toxic Metabolite Formation

An enzymatic method of detoxication only applicable to indirectly acting poisons is to inhibit the formation of the toxic metabolite. Clinically, such an approach is adopted when ethanol is used to compete for the active site of the enzyme alcohol dehydrogenase and thus to inhibit the formation of formaldehyde and formic acid in methanol poisoning (Cooper and Kini, 1962). Ethylene glycol poisoning can be treated analogously. Additionally and in experimental studies, pyrazole or 4-methylpyrazole has been used to inhibit alcohol dehydrogenase in these poisonings (Clay *et al.* 1975).

Antidotes Giving Rise to a Detoxifying Substance

Methaemoglobin-forming Antidotes

A group of antidotes which do not themselves act by chemically binding the poison, but produce a substance that does, are the cyanide antidotes that induce a therapeutic methaemoglobinaemia. Methaemoglobin is a form of haemoglobin in which the ferrous iron has been oxidized to ferric iron. Methaemoglobin is unable to carry oxygen but it has a high avidity for cyanide and sulphide. The first of this group of antidotes introduced for use in cyanide poisoning was amyl nitrite. Although this is still sometimes used, the most widely available methaemoglobin-producer is sodium nitrite, and this is still used in the USA and elsewhere. The recently introduced 4-dimethylaminophenol (DMAP) is used in Germany, while hydroxylamine and 4-aminopropiophenone (PAPP) are primarily of military interest. Sodium nitrite and 4-dimethylaminophenol produce methaemoglobin in different ways, the former somewhat more slowly, but the aim in both cases is to produce methaemoglobinaemia of sufficient degree to bind substantial quantities of cyanide, without producing such a high level that there is appreciable danger of tissue anoxia. In fact, there appear to have been a number of instances where dangerously high levels of methaemoglobin have been produced, perhaps because of individual susceptibility, or overenthusiastic use of the antidotes. It is unfortunate that therapeutic monitoring of methaemoglobin during the treatment of cyanide poisoning is not usually possible, since common methods for measuring methaemoglobin do not separately measure cyanmethaemoglobin. Adverse outcomes seem to be more common with DMAP than with sodium nitrite, a fact which is surprising in view of the much longer time during which the latter has been used (van Heijst *et al.*, 1987; Marrs, 1989). It is also worth noting that some authorities doubt whether the main action of sodium nitrite is through its propensity to form methaemoglobin but is due possibly to a vasoactive effect (Way *et al.*, 1987).

Antidotes That React with an Enzyme–Poison Complex

Oximes

Hydroxylamine was studied as an antidote to poisoning with organophosphate anticholinesterases because it was, in certain respects, similar to the substrate of the enzyme, acetylcholine. It was superseded by the pyridinium oximes and organophosphate poisoning is now treated by an oxime together with atropine, an anticholinergic drug. The oxime that is in use in many countries is the monopyridinium oxime, pralidoxime chloride (2-PAM). The bispyridinium oxime, obidoxime, has certain advantages in the therapy of organophosphate chemical warfare nerve agents, but no major differences between the two in spectrum of activity has been demonstrated in the treatment of organophosphate pesticide poisoning. The major action of the oximes is the dephosphorylation and consequent reactivation of acetylcholinesterase. The major lacuna in their activity is acetylcholinesterase which has undergone 'ageing'. This process, which is the dealkylation of the alkylphosphorylated enzyme, renders it refractory to oxime reactivation (Bismuth *et al.*, 1992). It is probable that 'ageing' occurs to some extent with all organophosphate anticholinesterases and it is possible that it may cause a clinical problem in cases of organophosphate pesticide poisoning where treatment is initiated very late. It is, however, a very serious problem with the nerve agent soman, which complexes with acetylcholinesterases and whose complex ages with a half-life of a few minutes. Of the numerous oximes that have been studied, the only ones with much activity where 'ageing' has occurred are the Hagedorn oximes, such as H1–6. It is likely that the activity of this oxime, in situations where

appreciable 'ageing' has occurred, is attributable to effects other than acetylcholinesterase reactivtion. H1–6 has not been much studied for use in pesticide as opposed to nerve agent poisoning.

Antidotes That Act on a Toxic Metabolite of the Poison

In the case of poisons requiring metabolism before becoming toxic, any of the above antidotal methods could, in principle, be applied. In practice, however, poisoning with such materials is treated by bringing about direct reaction with the toxic metabolite.

Antidote Reacts with Toxic Metabolite

Paracetamol (acetaminophen) is toxic by virtue of its metabolic transformation to a reactive metabolite, *N*-acetyl-*p*-benzoquinoneimine (NABQI). Under normal conditions of use, paracetamol is harmless but in overdose NABQI causes cell damage and death leading to, among other things, hepatic necrosis. The lead antidote cysteamine, although effective in animal models, caused adverse reactions in man, especially nausea. Acetylcysteine probably acts by forming conjugates with NABQI. Methionine, an alternative sulphur donor, may also do so, but only after conversion in the liver to homocysteine (Prescott, 1983; Seddon *et al.*, 1987).

Antidotes That Act Pharmacologically

It is convenient to divide antidotes that act pharmacologically into those antidotes where antagonism occurs at characterized pharmacological receptors and those where antagonism occurs at other macromolecules. This division is somewhat artificial but is nevertheless useful.

Antidotes That Act at Characterized Pharmacological Receptors

Antidotes that act at characterized pharmacological receptors include naloxone, an antidote for opiates (Evans *et al.*, 1973), and flumazanil, which is effective in poisoning with benzodiazepines (Scollo-Lavgizzari, 1983). In severe poisoning with β-blockers, adrenergic agonists such as isoprenaline or the more specific and cardioselective prenalterol provide examples of receptor antagonism (Wallin and Hulting, 1983). Development of compounds within this class requires a knowledge of the pharmacological profile of a drug, and the particular pharmacological property responsible for toxicity.

Antidotes That Antagonize at Other Macromolecules

Carbon monoxide is poisonous by virtue of its tight binding to haemoglobin and other cellular components. Carbon monoxide can be displaced competitively from such sites by oxygen.

Related Antidotal Mechanisms

Antagonism of clinical poisoning does not necessarily take place at the same receptor as that at which the poison acts. Atropine is an anticholinergic drug and acts upon muscarinic cholinergic receptors. However, it is used as an antidote in poisoning with organophosphate and carbamate anticholinesterases, substances whose major action is not directly on the cholinergic receptor. The macromolecule with which the anticholinesterases bind is the enzyme acetylcholinesterase, and the poisoning follows on from the consequential accumulation of acetylcholine. It is this effect which is antagonized by atropine. Somewhat analogous is the use of physostigmine in atropine poisoning; this anticholinesterase promotes acetylcholine accumulation, which overcomes the effect of atropine.

Functional Antagonism

There are a number of antidotes which are used symptomatically in poisoning and as such are difficult to classify. In some cases, further study may show these to have antagonistic actions that belong to one of the above groups. An example is the use of diazepam to combat the convulsions and fasciculations produced by organophosphate poisoning (Sellström, 1992).

ASSESSMENT OF ANTIDOTAL EFFICACY

Antidotal efficacy can be assessed *in vitro*, in experimental animals and in human poisoning. However, the first and last of these approaches both have severe limitations. Studies *in vitro* cannot adequately simulate the situation *in vivo*, even for the most straightforward antidotes which directly react with and detoxify the poison.

Nevertheless, studies *in vitro* are useful preliminaries to animal studies, particularly in narrowing down the field of choice among a series of related antidotes (Marrs, 1992). Moreover, in mechanistic studies of the action of antidotes, an *in vitro* approach is often useful. The limitations inherent in poisons centre data are quite different. They are related to the uncontrolled nature of suicidal and accidental poisoning, and while the large multicentre trial is very useful, it is almost always used subsequent to animal studies.

Assessment of Antidotes in Experimental Animals

There are many ways in which studies of antidotal efficacy can be performed, and some of the factors to be considered in experimental design are listed in Table 2.

Animal Model

One of the main features requiring attention is the choice of species of experimental animal. However well conducted the study is in other respects, unless the behaviour of the poison and antidote are similar in the chosen species and in humans, the results will be valueless (see Calabrese, 1982; Marrs, 1987). Species suitability will be determined by similarity between the chosen species and humans in absorption, distribution, metabolism and excretion, and in the response to

Table 2   Variables in the design of efficacy studies

Animal model	(a)	Species, strain and sex
	(b)	Numbers and controls
Poison	(a)	Dose
	(b)	Route of administration
	(c)	Solvent and excipients
Antidote	(a)	Dose
	(b)	Route of administration
	(c)	Solvent and excipients
	(d)	Time of administration in relation to poison
End-point	(a)	Lethality
	(b)	Other
		(i) biochemical
		(ii) haematological
		(iii) electrophysiological
		(iv) histopathological
		(v) behavioural

the poison. The importance of these considerations depends on the mode of action of the poison: if it is a directly active one, such as cyanide, similarity in rate of endogenous detoxication would appear the most important consideration, while, for those substances which are toxic to humans only after a metabolic activation step, the occurrence of this conversion at a similar rate in the chosen species to that in man is probably the most important factor.

Major quantitative differences in lethality of chemicals between a given species and humans indicate that that species is often a poor choice. Such differences exist with respect to methanol (Clay *et al.*, 1975), ethylene glycol (Gessner *et al.*, 1961) and certain organophosphates (Crawford *et al.*, 1976). It must be further borne in mind that the choice of scarce, large or exotic animals will increase the cost of the experiment and thereby tend to reduce the numbers. All the foregoing considerations apply, of course, to the evaluation of any xenobiotic in animals. However, with antidotal studies the same considerations also apply with respect to the antidote, so that the species chosen must also be similar to the human in its handling of two substances, a fact which can greatly complicate the choice of animal model.

The species having been decided upon, the numbers of animals and controls must be determined. Two main types of experimental design have been adopted for the evaluation of antidotes.

In the first, 'LD$_{50}$ ratio', the LD$_{50}$ of the poison is measured with and without the administration of the antidote. This procedure has the advantage that the result is produced as a single figure, the protection ratio, but has the disadvantage that it is necessary to use a relatively large number of animals. Moreover, the slope of the treated and untreated log dose–probit mortality slopes may not be parallel (Natoff and Reiff, 1970), and this will impair the value of the single figure. The protection ratio design is usually employed when small laboratory animals are used, although there are exceptions, such as the use of sheep by Burrows and Way (1979), studying cyanide antidotes, and the use of monkeys by Dirnhuber *et al.* (1979) studying pyridostigmine prophylaxis in soman poisoning. The desire to use the protection ratio should not cause one to use an unsuitable species.

The other principal design is the comparison of survival in groups of animals given the same supralethal dose of poison, one group being treated with the antidote and the other being left untreated. The number of animals used is much less than with the protection ratio, but the information supplied is also less. This approach has been criticized on the grounds that antidotes capable of comparatively small increases in LD$_{50}$ of the poison can produce dramatic increases in survival (Way *et al.*, 1987); nevertheless, such experimental designs have frequently been used with large laboratory animals such as dogs. If this approach is adopted, it is essential to have an untreated but poisoned control group within the study. The reliance on literature LD$_{50}$, where animals nominally of the same strain may have been studied under different conditions and with different formulations of poison and antidote, is reprehensible and renders the study valueless.

Whichever type of design is adopted, consideration should be given to the inclusion of a treatment-only group.

Poison

The dose of poison used depends on the overall design of the study. Where a design of protection ratio type is used, dosing is, as with any LD$_{50}$ estimate, designed to bracket the lethal dose. Adjustment of the dose range upwards may be required in the antidote-treated group. Often sighting shots will be necessary preliminaries to the substantive experiment in both antidote-treated and untreated groups. Where survival is compared in two groups of animals, one poisoned and untreated and the other poisoned and treated with the antidote, the dose of poison chosen is usually a dose which will be supralethal in animals not treated with antidote, but against which there is a reasonable chance of survival with antidote. To obtain a reasonable idea of the maximum dose of toxicant against which an antidote will protect, it may be necessary to use several different doses of poison.

The poison should normally be given by the route by which it commonly gains access to man. In the case of a large number of poisons, this will be by mouth, so that gavage is appropriate in animal studies. Percutaneous and inhalation poisoning present problems, the former because the reproducibility of lethality figures tends to be poor, the latter because of the relative scarcity of inhalation facilities in laboratories. Intratracheal instillation has been used as a substitute, but it does not appear to be satisfactory, particularly with toxicants acting locally on the lung (Richards *et al.*, 1989).

Where poisoning by a pharmaceutical preparation is being studied, formulations are readily available for experimental purposes and are often used. The use of the formulation, rather than the pure active, ingredient, should also be considered with other formulated materials, such as pesticides.

Antidote

In the case of an antidote already in use in man, it may be appropriate to adjust dose to the size of the animal. In certain instances, however, the choice of dose is more complicated. For example, it would be unwise to ignore species differences in methaemoglobin generation when studying methaemoglobin-producing cyanide antidotes.

The antidote is usually assessed after administration by the route by which it will be used. Furthermore, while in the early stages of development an antidote will frequently be studied in its pure state, at some point it should be evaluated in the formulation in which it will be used clinically.

One of the most difficult points to resolve is the time relationship between administration of the poison and the antidote. This is a problem that is particularly important with rapidly acting poisons, and careful attention must be applied to this aspect of the design of the study if data are to be produced which can be extrapolated to clinical human poisonings. The use of prophylactic administration of antidotes is not valid, except where mechanistic studies are being carried out or when the antidote is intended for prophylactic use (Way *et al.*, 1987). However, when given after poisoning, there is still the problem of the precise time interval after the challenge at which the antidote should be administered. Usually the antidote is given at a fixed time after poisoning or at the onset of a well-defined clinical sign. Unfortunately, the time-interval has often been chosen so as to be unrealistic compared with the time between clinical poisoning and the normal clinical therapy. On the other hand, the use of clinical signs as a cue for antidote administration invites the possibility of observer bias. A possible solution is to use a fixed time-interval but one somewhat longer than those customarily employed. The temporal considerations discussed above tend to be much less important with poisons whose clinical effects have a slow onset, or in the treatment of chronic or delayed poisoning, than in acute poisoning.

End-point

Although the vast majority of antidote efficacy studies employ death or survival as the end-point, a possible alternative is change in time of survival. Efficacy of the antidote against a sublethal effect, often a behavioural one, has also been used. Biochemical end-points, such as reactivation of cholinesterase in organophosphate poisoning or mobilization of a metal in heavy metal poisoning, may be used, but these do not always correlate with clinical efficacy of the antidote.

Comparison of Antidotes

It is frequently necessary to evaluate a new antidote against an existing one. The aim should be to study both antidotes under reasonably realistic conditions. In this case the animal model chosen must be suitable for evaluation of the toxic effects of the poison and the antidotes, as well as be able clearly to show comparative efficacy. It may be appropriate to use control groups, these animals receiving antidotes alone; another group receiving the poison alone; and further groups receiving the poison together with each treatment. Alternatively, a full dose–response evaluation, which will yield a protection ratio for each antidote, can be carried out (see, e.g., Schwartz *et al.*, 1979; Although most of the variables discussed above in relation to assessment of single antidotes will also apply to an evaluation of two or more antidotes in the same study, it is usually more difficult to standardize experimental conditions in the latter.

The Assessments of Antidotes in Human Beings

Provided that certain ethical guidelines are followed (Royal College of Physicians of London, 1986) and given appropriate Ethical Committee approval, antidote studies may be carried out in human volunteers. Such studies would be performed for a number of different purposes.

It may be necessary to establish the pharmacokinetics of an antidote in man. Such studies may be carried out during clinical use, either as part of a controlled clinical trial, observationally during routine clinical use, or on healthy volunteers. Some compounds that are used as antidotes have already passed through such studies, since they are already used as therapeutic substances in other clinical situations. An example might be the use of a β-adrenergic antagonist in the management of theophylline poisoning.

A second area where it may be necessary to study effects of antidotes in volunteers is in the evaluation of adverse effects. Sometimes this may occur after the antidote has undergone clinical use, as is the case for studies that were carried out on acetylcysteine. In these experiments intradermal acetylcysteine was given to volunteers, and to patients who had undergone treatment for paracetamol poisoning and had suffered adverse reactions (Bateman *et al.*, 1984).

For antidotes that act as agonists or antagonists at pharmacological receptor sites, studies of the pharmacodynamic reaction in volunteers may be carried out prior to the administration of these drugs to patients. Thus, the opiate antagonist naloxone and the benzodiazepine antagonist flumazanil were studied in volunteers prior to being given to patients.

Clinical studies in patients may involve the use of single doses in intoxicated patients, with comparison with control groups to assess response. This technique was used when naloxone was introduced, and had been shown to be efficacious in opiate intoxication but without affecting benzodiazepine and barbiturate poisoning. In addition, clinical studies need to be done in patients to establish the appropriate dosing regimen, and this is particularly the case for pharmacological antagonists such as naloxone, where studies were carried out to clarify the most appropriate dosing format.

The greatest challenge to clinical toxicologists is the comparison of different antidotes in the same clinical condition.

REFERENCES

Bateman, D. N. and Chaplin, S. (1989). Antidotes to human toxins. In Turner, P. and Volans, G. N. (Eds), *Recent Advances in Clinical Pharmacology and Toxicology*. Churchill-Livingstone, Edinburgh, pp. 173–195

Bateman, D. N., Woodhouse, K. W. and Rawlins, M.

D. (1984). Adverse reactions to *N*-acetylcysteine. *Human Toxicol*, **3**, 393–398

Bismuth, C. (1987). Generalités. In Bismuth, C., Baud, F. J., Conso, F., Frejaville, J. P. and Garnier, R. (Eds), *Toxicologie Clinique*. Flammarion, Paris, pp. 2–24

Bismuth, C., Inns, R. H. and Marrs, T. C. (1992). The efficacy, toxicity and clinical use of oximes in anticholinesterase poisoning. In Ballantyne, B. and Marrs, T. C. (Eds). *Clinical & Experimental Toxicology of Organophosphates and Carbamates*. Butterworth-Heinemann, Oxford, pp. 555–577

British Toxicology Society, Working Party on Toxicity (1984). A new approach to the classification of substances and preparations on the basis of their acute toxicity. *Human Toxicol.*, **3**, 85–92

Burrows, G. E. and Way, J. L. (1979). Cyanide intoxication in sheep: enhancement of efficacy of sodium nitrite, sodium thiosulphate and cobaltous chloride. *Am. J. Vet. Res.*, **40**, 613–617

Burger, A. (1982). Drug design. In Hamner, C. E. (Ed.), *Drug Development*. CRC Press, Boca Raton, Florida, pp. 53–72

Calabrese, E. J. (1982). *The Principles of Animal Extrapolation*. Wiley, New York

Catsch, A. and Harmuth-Hoehne, A.-E. (1975). New developments in metal antidotal properties of chelating agents. *Biochem. Pharmacol.*, **24**, 1557–1562

Clay, K. L., Murphy, R. C. and Watkins, W. D. (1975). Experimental methanol toxicity in the primate: analysis of metabolic acidosis. *Toxicol. Appl. Pharmacol.*, **34**, 49–61

Cole, P. L. and Smith, T. W. (1986). Use of digoxin-specific Fab fragments in the treatment of digitalis intoxication. *Drug Intell. Clin. Pharmacol.*, **20**, 267–269

Cooper, J. R. and Kini, M. M. (1962). Biochemical aspects of methanol poisoning. *Biochem. Pharmacol.*, **11**, 405–416

Crawford, M. J., Hutson, D. H. and King, P. A. (1976). Metabolic demethylation of the insecticide dimethylvinphos in rats, in dogs and *in vitro*. *Xenobiotica*, **6**, 745–762

Cristel, D., Eyer, P., Hegemann, M., Kiese, M., Lörcher, W. and Weger, N. (1977). Pharmacokinetics of cyanide poisoning in dogs and the effect of 4-dimethylaminophenol or thiosulfate. *Arch. Toxicol.*, **38**, 177–189

Dirnhuber, P., French, M. C. and Green, B. (1979). The protection of primates against soman poisoning by pretreatment with pyridostigmine. *J. Pharm. Pharmacol.*, **31**, 295–299

Evans, L. J., Roscoe, P., Swainson, C. P. and Prescott, L. F. C. (1973). Treatment of drug overdose with naloxone, a specific narcotic antagonist. *Lancet*, **i**, 452

Frankenberg, L. (1980). Enzyme therapy in cyanide poisoning: effect of rhodanese and sulfur compounds. *Arch. Toxicol.*, **45**, 315–323

Garland, H. and Pearce, J. (1967). Neurological complications of carbon monoxide poisoning. *Quart. J. Med.*, **36**, 445–455

Gessner, P. K., Parke, D. V. and Williams, R. T. (1961). Studies in detoxification. *Biochem. J.*, **76**, 482–489

Johnston, S. C., Bowles, M., Winzor, D. J. and Pond, S. M. (1988). Comparison of paraquat-specific murine monoclonal antibodies produced by *in vitro* and *in vivo* immunization. *Fund. Appl. Toxicol.*, **11**, 261–267

Lenz, D. E., Brimfield, A. A. and Hunter, K. W. (1984). Studies using a monoclonal antibody against soman. *Fund. Appl. Toxicol.*, **4**, S156–S164

Marrs, T. C. (1987). Experimental approaches to the design and assessment of antidotal procedures. In Ballantyne, B. (Ed.), *Perspectives in Basic and Applied Toxicology*. John Wright, Bristol, pp. 285–308

Marrs, T. C. (1989). The antidotal treatment of acute cyanide poisoning. *Adv. Drug React. Acute Pois. Rev.* **4**, 179–200

Marrs, T. C. (1992). Principles in the development of antidotes to toxic materials. In O'Sullivan, J. B. and Krieger, G. B. (Eds), *Toxicology of Hazardous Matters*. Williams and Wilkins, Baltimore, pp. 46–60

Muschett, C. W., Kelley, K. L., Boxer, G. E. and Rickards, J. C. (1952). Antidotal efficacy of vitamin B12a (hydroxo-cobalamin) in experimental cyanide poisoning. *Proc. Soc. Exptl Biol. Med.*, **81**, 234–237

Natoff, I. L. and Reiff, B. (1970). Quantitative studies of the effect of antagonists on the acute toxicity of organophosphates in rats. *Br. J. Pharmacol.*, **40**, 124–134

Paulet, G. (1960). *L'intoxication cyanhydrique et son traitement*. Masson SA, Paris

Pedigo, L. G. (1888). Antagonism between amyl nitrite and prussic acid. *Trans. Med. Soc. Virginia*, **19**, 124–131

Pearson, R. G. (1968). Hard and soft acids and bases, HSAB. Part II. Underlying theories. *J. Chem. Educ.*, **45**, 643–648

Prescott, L. F. (1983). Paracetamol overdosage. Pharmacological considerations and clinical management. *Drugs*, **25**, 290–314

Richards, R. J., Atkins, J., Marrs, T. C., Brown, R. F. R. and Masek, L. (1989). The biochemical and pathological changes produced by the intratracheal instillation of certain components of zinc-hexachloro-ethane smoke. *Toxicol.*, **54**, 79–88

Ringbom, A. (1963). *Complexation in Analytical Chemistry*. Wiley/Interscience, New York

Rousselin, X. and Garnier, R. (1985). L'intoxication cyanhydrique: conduite à tenir en milieu de travail et aspect actuel du traitement de l'intoxication aigüe. *Doc. Méd. Trav.*, **23**, 1–8

Royal College of Physicians of London (1986). Research on healthy volunteers. *J. Roy. Coll. Phys. London*, **20**, 243–257

Schwartz, C., Morgan, R. L. and Way, J. L. (1979). Antagonism of cyanide intoxication with sodium pyruvate. *Toxicol. Appl. Pharmacol.*, **10**, 437–441

Scollo-Lavgizzari, G. (1983). First clinical investigation of the benzodiazepine antagonist TO 15–1788 in comatose patients. *Eur. Neurol.*, **22**, 7–11

Seddon, C. E., Boobis, A. R. and Davies, D. S. (1987). Comparative activation of paracetamol in the rat mouse and man. *Arch. Toxicol.*, Suppl II, 305–309

Sellström, Å. (1992). Anticonvulsants. In Ballantyne, B. and Marrs, T. C. (Eds), *Clinical & Experimental Toxicology of Organophosphates and Carbamates*. Butterworth-Heinemann, Oxford, pp. 578–586

Society of Toxicology (1989). SOT position paper comments on the LD_{50} and acute eye and skin irritation test. *Fund. Appl. Toxicol.*, **13**, 621–623

Stocken, L. A. and Thompson, R. H. S. (1946). British anti-lewisite 3, arsenic and thiol excretion in animals after treatment of lewisite burns. *Biochem. J.*, **40**, 548–554

Stolshek, B. S., Osterhout, S. K. and Dunham, G. (1988). The role of digoxin-specific antibodies in the treatment of digitalis poisoning. *Med. Toxicol.*, **3**, 167–171

van Heijst, A. N. P., Douze, J. M. C., van Kesteren, R. G., van Bergen, J. E. A. M. and van Dijk, A. (1987). Therapeutic problems in cyanide poisoning. *Clin. Pharmacol.*, **25**, 383–398

Wallin, G. J. and Hulting, J. (1983). Massive metaprolol poisoning treated with prenalterol. *Acta. Med. Scand.*, **324**, 253–255

Way, J. L., Leuing, P., Sylvester, D. M., Burrows, G., Way, J. L. and Tamulinas, C. (1987). Methaemoglobin formation in the treatment of acute cyanide intoxication. In Ballantyne, B. and Marrs, T. C. (Eds), *Clinical and Experimental Toxicology of Cyanides*. John Wright, Bristol, pp. 402–412

Werner, B., Back, W., Akerblom, H. and Barr, P. O. (1985). Two cases of acute carbon monoxide poisoning with delayed neurological sequelae after a 'free' interval. *J. Toxicol. Clin. Toxicol.*, **23**, 249–266

Yokel, R. A. and Kostenbauder, H. B. M. (1987). Assessment of aluminium chelators in an octanol/aqueous system and in the aluminium-loaded rabbit. *Toxicol. Appl. Pharmacol.*, **91**, 281–294

FURTHER READING

Jones, M. M. (1991). New developments in therapeutic chelating agents as antidotes for metal poisoning. *Critical Reviews in Toxicology*, **21**, 209–233

Meredith, T. J., Jacobsen, D., Haines, J. A. and Berger, J-C. (1993). *Naloxone, Flumazenil and Dantrolene as Antidotes*. Cambridge University Press

Parent-Massin, D. M., Sensebe, L., Leglise, M. C., Guern, G., Berthon, C., Riche, C. and Abgrall, J. F. (1993). Relevance of *in vitro* studies of drug-induced agranulocytosis. *Drug Safety*, **9**, 463–469

Scherrmann, J-M. (1994). Antibody treatment of toxin poisoning—recent advances. *Journal of Toxicology, Clinical Toxicology*, **32**, 363–376

13 Quality Assurance in Toxicology Studies

T. R. Stiles

BACKGROUND

As in any science, the value of a study or piece of work in toxicology has its foundations in the ability to reproduce the results of that study. In the conduct of preclinical safety evaluation studies certain laboratory principles entitled Good Laboratory Practice (GLP) were first introduced during 1979 in an attempt to assure the quality control, management, documentation and reproducibility of such work.

These first GLP regulations were promulgated by the United States Food and Drug Administration (FDA) following evidence that a number of toxicological studies being submitted to the FDA contained deficiencies and inaccuracies. An investigation was undertaken by the FDA in an attempt to quantify the problem and the deficiencies observed during these investigations were summarized in the preamble to the proposed Good Laboratory Practice Regulations as follows:

(1) Experiments were poorly conceived, carelessly executed, or inaccurately analysed or reported.

(2) Technical personnel were unaware of the importance of protocol adherence, accurate observations, accurate administration of test substance, and accurate record-keeping and record transcription.

(3) Management did not assure critical review of data or proper supervision of personnel.

(4) Studies were impaired by protocol designs that did not allow the evaluation of all available data.

(5) Assurance could not be given for the scientific qualifications and adequate training of personnel involved in the research study.

(6) There was a disregard for the need to observe proper laboratory procedures, animal care and data processing.

(7) Sponsors failed (in whole or in part) to monitor adequately the studies performed by contract testing laboratories.

(8) Firms failed to verify the accuracy and completeness of scientific data in reports of nonclinical laboratory studies in a systematic manner before submission to the FDA.

The problems were so severe at Industrial Bio-Test laboratories (IBT) and Biometric Testing Inc. that both laboratories were forced to stop undertaking preclinical studies. IBT had been one of the largest testing laboratories in the United States, with thousands of its toxicology studies serving to support the safety of drugs, pesticides and food additives. FDA and the United States Environmental Protection Agency (EPA) began reviewing all the compounds that relied on IBT and Biometric studies for support of safety. From the audits of the IBT studies, EPA found 594 of the 801 key studies, or 75 per cent, to be invalid. FDA's Bureau of Foods found 24 of 66 IBT studies, or 36 per cent, invalid. Criminal charges of fraud were brought against four IBT officials. Three of the officials were convicted.

The conclusion that studies affecting decisions relating to the safety of a product could be based upon invalid data was alarming to Congress, industry and the public. Faced with this evidence, Congress voted a special appropriation of 16 million dollars to support a Bioresearch Monitoring Program. From this programme came the first Draft GLP Standards in 1976.

CURRENT GLP STANDARDS

As time progresses, throughout the world more and more countries with pharmaceutical or agrochemical or chemical industries are introducing some form of GLP.

In the USA there are three Acts relating to GLP, one from FDA and two from EPA. They are:

(1) Food and Drug Administration, Title 21 Code of Federal Regulations Part 58, *Federal Register*, 22 December 1978 These

regulations have been amended on a number of occasions, the most recent of which was published in the *Federal Register* on 4 September 1987.

(2) Environmental Protection Agency, Federal Insecticide, Fungicide and Rodenticide Act (FIFRA) Title 40 Code of Federal Regulations Part 160, *Federal Register*, 17 August 1989 These were first published on 29 November 1983.

(3) Environmental Protection Agency, Toxic Substances Control Act (TSCA) Title 40 Code of Federal Regulations Part 792, *Federal Register*, 17 August 1989 These were first published on 29 November 1983.

Japan has four ministries which have issued GLP Regulations: those of the Ministry of Health and Welfare and the Ministry of Labour are combined within one document:

Japan Ministry of Health and Welfare Notification No. Yakuhatsu 313, Pharmaceutical Affairs Bureau, 31 March 1982, and subsequent amendment, Notification No. Yakuhatsu 870, Pharmaceutical Affairs Bureau, 05 October 1988;
Japan Ministry of Agriculture, Forestry and Fisheries, 59 NohSan, Notification No. 3850, Agricultural Production Bureau, 10 August 1984;
Japan Ministry of International Trade and Industry, Directive 31 March 1984 (Kanpogyo No. 39 Environmental Agency, Kikyoku No. 85 MITI)

In the European Community (EC) numerous directives have been issued. All directives are addressed to the current twelve member countries and are required to be implemented by national legislation in each member nation.
The following is a list of current EC Directives applicable to GLP:

Directive 79/831/EEC. The first European Community Directive requiring testing to be undertaken in accordance with GLP was 79/831/EEC, the so-called Sixth Amendment, on notification of new industrial chemicals. It did not specify the GLP Principles, although EC countries had been implementing the Principles of Good Laboratory Practice, published by the Organization for Economic Cooperation and Development (OECD) in 1981. Many European laboratories implemented GLP, therefore, before the

first, more explicit, European directive was adopted by the end of 1986: Directive 87/18/EEC. This directive, the first one dealing with GLP, states that the OECD Principles of Good Laboratory Practice will apply whenever, in EC regulations, the application of GLP is required for the safety testing of chemicals and preparations. This Directive also requires the member countries to take the necessary enforcement measures and appoint responsible monitoring authorities.

Apart from creating obligations to member countries, the directive also restricts their rights: it is no longer acceptable to refuse the results of safety testing on GLP grounds if the OECD GLP has been applied. This provision is not limited to a specific geographical area and applies therefore equally to data originating from EC member countries and non-member countries.

Directive 88/320/EEC. The second GLP Directive, 88/320/EEC, was adopted on 30 June 1988 and should have been implemented nationally before 1 January 1989. It elaborates on the obligation of Directive 87/18/EEC for national authorities to monitor compliance with the OECD Principles of Good Laboratory Practice. The national authorities should follow the OECD guidance for compliance monitoring, and in a recent update of this directive the full texts of the relevant OECD guidance documents have been attached.

New in this directive is the requirement for national monitoring units to submit, once a year, a report on inspection activities to the Commission, with a summary of the findings. These reports will be circulated to other member countries.

Member countries are obliged to accept the results of GLP compliance monitoring activities in other countries. Directive 88/320/EEC provides, however, a procedure for solving problems—e.g. when a GLP or regulatory agency in one country has questions on the compliance monitoring procedures in another country or when there is a specific concern on GLP compliance for a specific study.

For completeness, two other EC directives should be mentioned. The first one is Directive 89/569/EEC, mandating the Commission to agree to the adoption of the 1989 OECD decision on GLP (C(89)87(Final)) on behalf of the EC member countries. The second is Directive 90/19/

EEC, giving a full translation of OECD inspection guidance, instead of just a reference to these OECD documents which was already included in Directive 88/320/EEC.

To date the following EC countries have implemented functioning GLP programmes: Belgium, Denmark, France, Germany, The Netherlands, Italy and the UK.

Within the UK the following GLP Principles have been issued through the Department of Health. Compliance with these principles is monitored by the United Kingdom Department of Health (DH) GLP Monitoring Authority:

Good Laboratory Practice, The United Kingdom Compliance Programme, Department of Health 1989. The principles were first published in 1986.

Within the UK for a facility to claim it is operating in compliance with GLP a 'Certificate of Compliance' is required which is issued by the Department of Health GLP Monitoring Authority. Such Certificates are only issued following a satisfactory inspection performed by that Authority.

To assist in the application and understanding of Good Laboratory Practice, the UK GLP Monitoring Authority has produced the following advisory leaflets which cover specific areas of GLP:

No. 1 1989 *The Application of GLP Principles to Computer Systems*
No. 2 1990 *The Application of GLP Principles to Field Studies*
No. 3 1991 *Good Laboratory Practice and the Role of Quality Assurance*
No. 4 1992 *Good Laboratory Practice and the Role of the Study Director*

These advisory leaflets and the UK Compliance Programme can be obtained from: The Director, Department of Health, UK GLP Monitoring Authority, Room 501A, Skipton House, 80 London Road, Elephant and Castle, London SE1 6LW.

Besides the US, Japan and the EC, the OECD has played a major role in introducing GLP. This organization, which consists of Australia, Austria, Belgium, Canada, Denmark, Finland, France, Germany, Greece, Iceland, Ireland, Italy, Japan, Luxembourg, the Netherlands, New Zealand, Norway, Portugal, Spain, Sweden, Switzerland, Turkey, UK, USA, produced its own GLP principles which were accepted by all member countries in 1982:

Good Laboratory Practice in the Testing of Chemicals, Paris, 1982, ISBN 92-64-12367-9 It is these principles which now form the foundation of the International Principles of Good Laboratory Practice.

Other countries have published GLP guidelines but in practice these have been based upon OECD and are therefore very similar and unnoteworthy. The other Quality Standards which might be applicable to a toxicology study are the British Standards Institute BS 5750 *Quality Systems* and its International equivalent ISO 9000 series. These standards contain a number of the same elements but in practice the GLP principles have been written specifically for the conduct of toxicology studies and are therefore more appropriate.

SCOPE OF GLP

As GLP principles are continuing to be developed and being adopted by more countries, their scope and applications grow. Rather than attempting to identify the requirements of each country, it is more accurate to state that any study undertaken to assess the safety of a test substance and submitted in support of a safety assessment should be undertaken in compliance with GLP. This will include all kinds of toxicity studies from *in vitro* mutagenicity studies to acute, subchronic, and long-term toxicity/carcinogenicity studies.

While it should now be possible to identify which studies should be conducted in compliance with GLP, one further factor should be remembered when implementing GLP within a facility: that dual standards within a laboratory can be detrimental to the overall quality of work within that laboratory. Within the UK a facility is inspected for GLP compliance in addition to individual studies being inspected, and therefore, where possible, it is advised that GLP be applied to a whole facility and all the work it performs rather than to individual studies.

GLP PRINCIPLES

It would be very easy to write a book on GLP principles and their application, as the interpretations and applications to different possible situations are numerous. This chapter will identify the essential elements of GLP as they apply to toxicology studies. These elements themselves provide the environments within which good-quality work can be undertaken.

Personnel

Personnel involved in a toxicology study should:

- Have sufficient education, training and experience or combination thereof to enable them to undertake assigned functions.
- Have a record of training and experience and a job description. The training record should indicate in which procedures the individual has attained competence. Such records and job description should not only be prepared for those individuals directly involved in the study, but also include staff from support areas.
- Take the necessary personal and health precautions to avoid contamination of test system and test article.
- Wear, and change as often as necessary, clothing appropriate for the duties performed — to prevent microbiological/radiological, or other contamination of test systems and test article.

Management

The responsibilities of 'Management' in terms of GLP are as defined in the various GLP standards and regulations. These include, but are not limited to, the following. Management of the testing facility has responsibility for ensuring that the work performed within the testing facility is carried out in accordance with the principles of Good Laboratory Practice. As a minimum, management should:

- Designate a Study Director for each study.

- Replace the Study Director promptly if it becomes necessary to do so during the study, and record the action.
- Ensure that personnel employed on the study have sufficient training and experience to perform their duties, and that each individual clearly understands the functions he/she is to perform.
- Ensure that there are sufficient personnel for the proper conduct of studies and that their health, insofar as it may affect the integrity of studies, is monitored.
- Maintain a record of the qualifications, training and experience, together with a job description, for each professional and technical person involved in the study.
- Ensure that the laboratory facilities, equipment and experimental data handling procedure are of an adequate standard.
- Authorize all written Standard Operating Procedures (SOPs). These SOPs should be adequate to ensure high quality and accuracy of data generated during the conduct of the study.
- Assure that test and control articles or mixtures have been appropriately tested for identity, strength, purity, stability and uniformity as applicable.
- Ensure that a study protocol has been prepared for each study which is then approved by the sponsor prior to the start of the study. This document should also be authorized by management.
- Establish arrangements for a quality assurance programme and ensure that any problems reported during the monitoring of the study are communicated to the Study Director, and that corrective actions are taken and documented.
- Identify an archivist to take responsibility for the archive.

Study Director

For each study, management should appoint a Study Director. The Study Director is the individual responsible for ensuring that the study is conducted in compliance with GLP, as well as being responsible for the interpretation, analysis, documentation and reporting of results. The Study Director is the single point of control on a study.

As a minimum the general responsibilities of a

Study Director on any given study are to: ensure that all aspects of the study are conducted in compliance with GLP and that a study protocol is prepared which will include all the information required by GLP.

Also he must agree the final protocol with management and the sponsor; approve the study protocol; document and approve all/any changes to the study protocol prior to effecting such changes; and ensure prompt distribution of the protocol prior to animal arrival/study start to all relevant individuals.

In relation to the conduct of the study, he should ensure that the study is conducted in compliance with the study protocol and all relevant SOPs; document and approve prior to the event any planned deviations to departmental SOPs; ensure that all experimental data, including observations of responses of the test system, are accurately recorded and verified; and promptly notify the study sponsor, Quality Assurance Unit (QAU), and management of any unscheduled event which could compromise the integrity/outcome of the study, and ensure that such events are fully and completely documented.

When the report is prepared, he is responsible for the preparation of a final report which accurately records all the results generated during the course of the study and contains all the various information required by GLP. He must prepare a GLP compliance statement for inclusion in the final report indicating the compliance of the reported study and accepting responsibility for the validity of the data generated during the course of the study. Additionally, he must approve the final study report. So that the study can be investigated retroactively, he must ensure that all raw data, specimens, slides, study protocol and other documentation, including the final report, are retained and transferred to archives as soon as practicable on completion of the study. It should be noted, however, that once archived, these data become the responsibility of the retention management.

On submission of data and specimens to archives, the Study Director should ensure preparation of an inventory which details the type and amount of specimens and documentation sent for retention. This inventory should accompany the data to the archive, as it will be used to account for the data sent.

The Study Director is not required to observe every data collection event, but should assure that data are collected as specified by the protocol and the SOPs and that data collection includes the accurate recording of unanticipated responses of the test system. The Study Director should also review data periodically, to promote the accurate recording of data and to assure that data are technically correct. Systems must be in place to ensure that the Study Director is promptly notified of unforeseen circumstances that may have an effect on the integrity of the study.

Quality Assurance

There must exist, within a testing facility, an organizational group known as the Quality Assurance Unit, separate from and independent of the personnel directly engaged in the control and conduct of a study, which shall give assurance to the highest level of management that such work is conducted and reported to a high standard of quality and in accordance with existing GLP regulatory requirements.

Operating Principles

The test facility should have a documented quality assurance programme to ensure that studies performed are in compliance with the principles of Good Laboratory Practice. The object is to ensure that the study plan and SOPs are followed by periodic inspections of the test facility and/or by auditing the study in progress.

Documentation

A copy of all studies should be maintained, documenting type, data, test article, test system, Study Director, sponsor and study status. In addition, copies of protocols and amendments should be kept. Written records of inspections undertaken by QAU and any action taken by the Study Director and management to correct adverse findings should be kept and the final report reviewed, to confirm that the methods, procedures and observations are accurately described, and that the reported results accurately reflect the raw data of the study. It should be possible to ascertain that the study plan and SOPs are available to personnel conducting the study. The QAU should advise management if the facilities, equipment, personnel, methods, practices, records and controls are not considered to be in conformance with current GLP Regulations.

The QAU is a mechanism used to monitor ongoing studies to determine that the protocols and written SOPs have been followed. Thus, the QAU within a testing facility is charged with the responsibility for assuring the regulatory agency, the facility management and the Study Director that the facilities, equipment, personnel, methods, practices, procedures, records and controls are designed and function in conformance with GLP and the protocol for individual nonclinical laboratory studies.

The Quality Assurance Unit is required periodically to inspect each phase of a study to assure its compliance. Such inspections should be documented in a manner which details the problems noted and the actions taken to resolve those problems.

Laboratory Areas

GLP requires that a separate area should be provided, as necessary, for the various operations and activities, to prevent possible contamination or mix-ups occurring on a study and that testing facilities are of a suitable size and construction for the purpose intended. If a testing facility is too small to handle its planned volume of work, there may be an inclination to mix incompatible functions. Examples might include the simultaneous conduct of studies with incompatible species in the same room, setting up a small office in the corner of an animal housing area, or housing an excessive number of animals in a room. The facility should be constructed of materials which facilitate cleaning. Heating, ventilation and air conditioning systems should be of adequate capacity to produce environmental conditions which comply with employee and animal health and safety standards, and should be designed to prevent cross-contamination.

In principle, a facility should be designed and constructed to ensure the adequacy of the facility for conducting toxicity studies and to ensure the quality and integrity of study data.

Animal Care Facilities

Facilities should be adequate for separation of species or test systems, isolation of individual projects, quarantine of animals and routine or specialized housing of animals.

Separate areas must be provided, as appropriate, for the diagnosis, treatment and control of laboratory animal diseases. These areas should provide effective isolation for the housing of animals either known or suspected of being diseased, or of being carriers of disease, from other animals.

Facilities must be available for the collection and disposal of all animal waste and refuse or for safe sanitary storage of waste before removal from the testing facility. Disposal facilities shall be so provided and operated as to minimize vermin infestation, odours, disease hazards and environmental contamination.

There should also be storage areas, as needed, for feed, bedding, supplies and equipment. Storage areas for feed and bedding should be separated from areas housing the test systems and should be protected against infestation or contamination. Perishable supplies shall be preserved by appropriate means.

Equipment

Equipment used in the generation, measurement or assessment of data, and equipment used for facility environmental control, must be appropriate in design and of adequate capacity to function according to the protocol and be suitably located for operation, inspection, cleaning and maintenance.

Written records should be maintained of all inspection, maintenance, testing, calibrating and/or standardizing operations. These records should contain the date on which maintenance was performed, the type of maintenance undertaken (inspection, routine maintenance, non-routine maintenance), and the actual work undertaken. Equipment used for the generation, measurement or assessment of data should also be adequately tested, calibrated and/or standardized before use.

Standard Operating Procedures

A testing facility must have SOPs in writing, setting forth the methods and procedures that management is satisfied are adequate to ensure the quality and integrity of the data generated in the course of a study. When the Study Director, pathologist or other principal scientist recognizes a need for a variation in the SOP on a given study, this is acceptable, provided that the modification is agreed by the Study Director and is documented in the raw data of the study. Significant changes in established SOPs should be properly authorized in writing by management. This may require the revision/reissue of the SOP. Within each laboratory area, staff should have immediately available to them the SOPs relating to their tasks. Published literature such as operating manuals and text books may be used as supplementary information to the SOP. A historical file of SOPs, and all revisions thereof, including the dates of such revisions, should be maintained in archives. SOPs should be periodically reviewed to maintain their accuracy.

Standard Operating Procedures should be available for, but not be limited to, the following categories of laboratory activities. The details given under each heading are to be considered as illustrative examples.

Test Substances (Including Control and Reference Substances)

The integrity and identification of the test substances is of great importance.

(1) Documentation of receipt, identification, characterization, handling, formulation and storage of substances, including expiry date, where appropriate.
(2) Testing of homogeneity and stability of test substance mixtures with carriers.
(3) Administration of test substance.

Test System

(1) Procedures for receipt, transfer, proper placement, identification and care of animals or other test system.
(2) Test system, observations and examinations.
(3) Laboratory tests and analyses.
(4) Handling of animals found moribund or dead during the study.
(5) Experimental work using micro-organisms.
(6) Autopsy procedures.
(7) Collection and identification of specimens.
(8) Histopathology and other post-mortem studies.
(9) Field studies.

Equipment

(1) Use of equipment.
(2) Maintenance, cleaning, calibration and/or standardization.
(3) Identification and instructions for use of computer hardware and software.

Documentation

(1) Data collection, handling, storage and retrieval.
(2) Preparation of reports.

SOPs should be treated as 'controlled documents'; their distribution should be monitored to enable, when appropriate, SOPs to be reissued and old or out-of-date SOPs to be withdrawn.

Protocol

For each study an approved protocol should be written which indicates the work to be undertaken and the methodologies involved in the conduct of that study. Such a protocol should be distributed and available to all staff engaged in the authorized amendment by the Study Director and these changes should be maintained with each copy of the protocol. The protocol should be prepared and distributed prior to the arrival of the test system.

The following is a guide to the items to be included in a study protocol.

General

Study number: it is usual for a study to have a unique number by which it is identified. This number should appear on all data, records or specimens as a means of study identification.
Name and address of the testing facility: the postal address of the testing facility. The address of any company or individual to which certain tests or analyses may be subcontracted should also be identified.
Descriptive title: this should include the type of study, i.e. toxicity, metabolism, etc; the compound name or code number; species of the animal; and, if appropriate, route of administration and duration of study in weeks.
Name and address of sponsor.
Name of sponsor's monitoring scientist.

Background to Study

Statement of purpose of study.

Justification for test system selection. A number of possible justifications could include:

- Because this species/strain metabolizes the test compound in the same way as man.
- Because previous studies with this test compound have been undertaken in this species/strain/substrain and the present work is required for comparison to be done in the same species.
- To meet the requirements/recommendations of the governmental regulatory agencies.
- Because the sponsor instructed you to use this species/strain/substrain without giving further reasons—i.e. the statement 'at sponsor request'.
- Because the sponsor has substantial amounts of background data or experience with this species/strain/substrain.
- To compare findings with those obtained with other species/strains.
- Because of intended use of test compound (this applies, for example, with veterinary compounds when the target animal might be the species of choice).

Reference to test guideline: this is a requirement of OECD GLPs. If no test guideline is applicable, then a statement to that effect is preferred to omission of this category.

Name of Study Director: self-explanatory; however, it is pointed out that you cannot have two Study Directors for the same study.

Proposed Study Dates

These dates must be included in the protocol.

Delivery of animals: if animals were ordered specifically for the study, then the date of arrival at the test facility should be entered into the protocol. If, however, the animals are selected from stock, it is the date on which the animals were allocated to the study from stock that should be placed in the protocol.

First day of dosing: fairly straightforward except when a staggered start is to be operated, in which case all dates for the first day of dosing for each group or sex should be given (time relative to first dose or day of pregnancy is acceptable).

Interim sacrifice(s): the dates on which all interim sacrifices are to be made should be given in the protocol (times relative to first dose are acceptable).

Final sacrifice/completion of laboratory work: the date on which the final sacrifice is due to commence or the date of anticipated completion of laboratory work should be indicated in the protocol.

Test System

Species: dog, mouse, rat, rabbit, etc. Scientifically, primates are not a species but an order; the correct description of a species would be, for example, Cynomolgus monkey (*Macaca fascicularis*).

Strain: Beagle would be the strain of dog, New Zealand White the strain of rabbits, Large White the strain of pig, etc. In the case of the rat, Wistar and Sprague–Dawley are technically the strains and CFHB and CFY the substrains.

Supplier: the name and address of the animal supplier. In the case of primates and avian species, whether home-bred or wild-caught should be stated.

Body weight range: the body weight range of animals used should be stated as well as the time-point to which this range applies—i.e. on receipt, at first dose.

Age: this should be at the time of commencement of pre-dose period; however, provided that sufficient information is given to enable the calculation of this figure, then that is sufficient.

Test Control and Substances

Name/code number: the test substance name and/or code numbers plus alternative names should be given.

Identity: chemical name or structure.

Strength: concentration of solution, if applicable.

Purity: for radiochemicals, reference should be made to radiochemical purity and to specific activity.

Stability: the period over which the test material can be used.

Batch number(s): purity and batch number of the test material.

Test Substance Mixtures

Method and frequency of preparation: a brief description of methods in dose preparation and the frequency of preparation should be given.

Frequency of dispensing should be provided, if appropriate.

Tests to determine homogeneity, stability and concentration: the protocol should state that tests to identify these parameters are being made and identify the organization which is peforming them, if not your own.

Description of dosing vehicle: details of any suspending/dispersing agents should be given.

Test System Treatment and Maintenance

Location of study: inclusion of building by name or number.

Environmental conditions: temperature and humidity ranges and light/dark cycles.

Number of groups: the number of treatment and control groups on the study.

Number of each sex per group.

Method of animal identification: tattoo, earmark, etc.; the numbers used should be recorded in the protocol.

Route of administration: for all administrations it should be stated whether by capsules, dietary, gastric intubation, etc (oral is not sufficient).

Reason for choice of route: the reason for choice to some extent will be covered in the statement of purpose, but a justification should still be given—e.g. because that is the route by which the test compound will be administered to man.

Dosage levels: this should include appropriate units and any control substances used as well as test compound.

Method, frequency and duration of dosing: the method of dosing should include brief details of the procedure to be followed. The frequency should be interpreted as number of times per day, number of days per week, number of weeks' administration. Duration is interpreted as the number of days or weeks the test system is exposed to the test compound. *Note*: Any periods of recovery/withdrawal from treatment should be specified.

Description of experimental design: the protocol as a whole should define the design of the study.

Methods for the control of bias: this section should be used to identify the method used to ensure a random or bias-free allocation of animals to treatment groups or location within the animal unit.

Description and identification of diet: this should include the name of suppliers, and commercial name and form of diet—i.e. powder, pellet, gran-

ules, etc. Any supplementary items of diet should also be identified—i.e. fruit, bread, blackcurrant juice, etc. Further descriptions or identification is not necessary.

Expected level of contaminant expected to be present in the diet and capable of affecting the study: the Study Director should be aware of any possible contaminant that could be present in the diet being used that could have an effect upon the test material or test system. All such possible contaminants should be identified in the protocol.

Reference to determine absorption: if this is to be done by the testing facility, the methods used should be stated in the protocol.

Observations

Type, frequency and methods of specified tests, analyses, observations, examinations and measurements: self-explanatory and including body weights, food and water consumption, clinical signs, ophthalmoscopy, clinical pathology, gross pathological examination, organ weights, histopathological examination, etc.

Records to be maintained: it should suffice that a statement in the protocol indicates that all records will be maintained of all test measurements and analyses as listed in the protocol.

Proposed statistical methods: an outline of the methods to be used should be included, with a comment that further examination using different statistical methods may be performed, dependent on the results generated.

Archiving: location of archiving of all raw data samples and specimens associated with the study should be given.

GLP statement: the protocol should give an indication as to where the study is to be conducted in compliance with GLP.

Dates and signatures of protocol approval: the signature page should be numbered as part of the protocol. The protocol approval page should be signed and dated by the Study Director, management and the sponsor.

CONDUCT OF STUDY

The study should be conducted as defined in the study protocol and appropriate SOPs. All data generated during the conduct of a study, except those that are generated by automated data collection systems, must be recorded directly, promptly and legibly in ink. All data entries should be dated on the date of entry and signed or initialled by the person entering the data. Any change in entries, made so as not to obscure the original entry, must indicate the reason for such change, and should be dated and signed or identified at the time of the change. In automated data collection systems, the individual responsible for direct data input should be identified at the time of data input. Any change in automated data entries must be made so as not to obscure the original entry, must indicate the reason for change and should be dated, and the responsible individual should be identified.

STUDY REPORT

For each study as defined by the protocol a final report should be produced. As a minimum, this report should contain the following information:

- Name and address of the facility performing the study and the dates on which the study was initiated and completed.
- Objectives and procedures stated in the approved protocol, including any changes in the original protocol.
- Statistical methods employed for analysing the data.
- The test and control articles identified by name, Chemical Abstracts number or code number, strength, purity, and composition or other appropriate characteristics.
- Stability of the test and control articles under the conditions of administration.
- Description of methods used.
- A description of the test system used. Where applicable, the final report shall include the number of animals used, sex, body weight range, source of supply, species, strain and substrain, age and procedures used for identification.
- A description of the dosage, dosage regimen, route of administration and duration.
- A description of all circumstances that may have affected the quality or integrity of the data.
- The name of the Study Director, the names of other scientists or professionals, and the names of all supervisory personnel involved in the study.

- A description of the transformations, calculations or operations performed on the data, a summary and analysis of the data, and a statement of the conclusions drawn from the analysis.
- The signed and dated reports of each of the individual scientists or other professionals involved in the study.
- The locations where all specimens, raw data and the Final Report are to be stored.

The Final Report should also contain the following signed and dated statements:

Study Director: the Study Director should prepare a statement indicating that the study was conducted in compliance or not, as the case may be, with GLP. The statement should also indicate with which GLP Standards compliance is claimed.

Quality Assurance: the Quality Assurance Unit should prepare a statement to indicate that they have audited this final report and found it to be a true, complete and accurate reflection of the data generated on the study. The dates on which study inspection were conducted and the dates on which management were informed should also be reported.

ARCHIVES

All raw data, documentation, protocols, final reports and specimens generated as a result of a study must be retained.

Such materials should be placed in an archive for orderly storage and expedient retrieval of all raw data, documentation, protocols, specimens, and interim and final reports. Conditions of storage should minimize deterioration of the documents or specimens in accordance with the requirements for the time-period of their retention and the nature of the documents or specimens.

Once accepted into the archive, the responsibility for the retention of the study raw data, specimens and samples becomes that of management. It is management's responsibility to appoint an individual(s) to this function.

The facility should have adequate and suitable space for the secure storage of all data and specimens for completed studies.

Access to the archives should be restricted to authorized personnel.

Data and specimens should be retained in such a way as to preclude, as far as is practical, the risk of degradation of items retained.

Records should be maintained of when, by whom, and for what reasons, data or samples were accessed or retrieved.

In addition to raw data, the final study report should be held in the archive.

Systems should be in a place which ensure the prompt and accurate retrieval of all stored material.

APPLICATION OF GLP TO COMPUTER SYSTEMS: SYSTEMS DEVELOPMENT

When GLP was first promulgated, few companies had on-line data capture systems. As time has passed, more and more computer systems have been developed and introduced within organizations. With this increase in computerization has come a growing interest from GLP monitoring bodies in the way such systems have been designed, developed, introduced, operated and controlled in order that compliance with GLP is maintained throughout an organization.

The Department of Health GLP Monitoring Unit published, in December 1988, a document entitled *The Application of GLP Principles to Computer Systems*. As the title suggests, this document identifies and applies those elements of GLP which relate to computer systems.

The FDA, in the absence of any official regulatory intent, organized a meeting to which were invited 66 individuals from industry, government and academia on 11 October 1987, at the Red Apple Conference Center in Arkansas. The purpose of the meeting was to prepare a reference book which would present current concepts and procedures in the computer automation of toxicology laboratories and would describe effective means for ensuring the quality of computerized data systems. The book from this consensus meeting, titled *Computerised Data Systems for Nonclinical Safety Assessment, Current Concepts and Quality Assurance*, was published in September 1988.

The direction of both the DH and FDA documents is to ensure as far as possible that computers involved in the capture and/or manipulation of data used in support of safety assessment are developed, tested, introduced and operated in such a way as to ensure data integrity.

There are many aspects of GLP which apply to computer systems. Here attention is concentrated on the development phase of a computer system and its compliance with GLP.

Introduction

As with any project, the planning phase is critical to its success. During the early phase of systems development the risk of failure is high but the cost of failure is low. As the system is developed, the reverse applies, the risk is reduced but the cost increases (see Figure 1). This just emphasizes the importance of logically planned system development.

The sequence of events now listed outlines an approach which should help to achieve the successful development of the system (see Figure 2). This approach can be defined as simply Good Computing Practice—an approach which many organizations may have already adopted. For a system to comply with GLP, the areas which are mostly critical and essential for compliance are system validation (acceptance testing) and the operation and use of the system. Should the system not have been developed 'in-house', then clearly little control can be placed on the development of that system. However, the key GLP requirements for system validation (acceptance testing) and the operation and use of the system can still be applied.

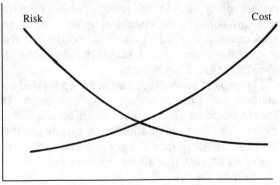

Design development implementation use

Figure 1 Systems development risk/cost ratio

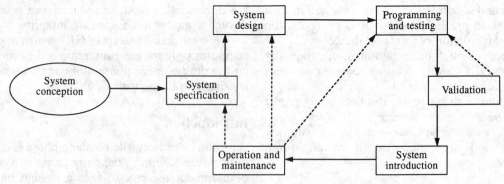

Figure 2　System development life-cycle

System Conception

It is at this stage that an 'idea' is developed. The user will document broad descriptions of the areas the system will cover, its objectives and benefits. A feasibility study and preliminary analysis of the needs of the proposed system may be conducted to establish the project scope, cost and time estimations, as well as potential impact upon existing systems. On completion of this phase it is recommended that a report be prepared which will outline the concepts and estimated costs, timings and manpower required for the project. Approval to continue to the next phase should be obtained.

System Specification

Once approval to continue has been given, a project team should be established. This team should contain representatives from the systems programmers, users, plus, as appropriate to the system being developed, other personnel with relevant skills. If the system is to be used in an area covered by GLP, then it is appropriate for a Quality Assurance representative to be a member of the project team.

The project team leader must be appointed to manage the project and the project team. It should be remembered that the successful completion and implementation of a system in the main will depend upon the project manager. It is therefore critical that this individual be capable of fulfilling the role.

During this phase, detailed information concerning the proposed system is obtained. Each system function is analysed to assure that it is fully understood. Functional requirements are determined through analysis of existing and proposed systems. In particular, the specific functions that the system is intended to perform must be analysed and documented.

Identifying the actual requirements for the final system is one of the most difficult tasks associated with software development. It requires the ability to understand both the process or activity being computerized and the needs of the individuals who will be using or supporting the system.

It is critical during this phase that the systems programmers clearly understand the user requirement. Failure to communicate requirements clearly will ensure that the user does not get the system.

The needs of the system having been analysed and identified, these should be clearly documented in the system specification. This document specifies the requirements of the system, and may include raw data definitions, information flows, descriptions of processing functions, performance requirements, system availability requirements, security considerations and error handling. The system specification conveys the user's needs and ideas to all involved in the project. It is from the detail contained within the specification that the system will be designed.

It should be remembered that it is easier to correct the specification now than after the system has been designed and built. Time spent earlier will save money later.

Before proceeding to the next phase, the system specification should be reviewed and approved by personnel involved in the project. This will help to assure that the document is complete, and that the requirements are compatible and in accord with the user's needs. Management should also approve the specification, thus ensuring commitment to the project.

System Design

System design is the process of defining the data structures, components, modules, interfaces and test approach for the software system identified in the system specification document. System design translates the requirements from the specification into detailed guidelines to be followed during the programming and testing phase.

This phase will typically identify in detail the system overview, screen designs, report layouts, data descriptions, system configuration, system security, file design, module specification and system validation plan. At this stage it is also necessary to consider how the system will be released into operational use and the possible effect/interaction with existing systems.

Programming and Testing

During the programming and testing phase, the system development team codes the system modules according to the information generated in the detailed design documentation.

Tests are executed on an iterative basis until each module performs according to its module specification and until the testing requirements for that module have been satisfied. Problems encountered during these tests may be documented by programmers in appropriate test or error logs.

Concurrent with the programming and testing phase, system documentation, such as software maintenance manuals, hardware maintenance manuals, user manuals, vendor manuals, back-up procedures, change control procedures and security, may be prepared.

With a large system it may be appropriate to develop the system in modular form. Before proceeding to validation, the modules should be combined and tested as a whole to ensure that the system operates.

System Validation

At the end of the programming and testing phase, as far as the development staff are concerned, the system operates as designed and could be used. However, for use in a GLP environment it is necessary to test/validate a system and to document and prove its successful operation.

Systems validation is a series of tests undertaken to assure the correct operation of the system. While attention is focused on software, the validation process must consider the total environment in which the system is used.

If a validation test fails, the action taken will depend upon the cause and impact of the failure. In some cases a decision may be taken to implement the system with a cosmetic error such as a misspelled title on a report. Where correction is necessary, the extent of validation necessary following change is a professional subjective assessment made within and approved by the project team. In most cases the system will be released for production use after certain specified tests have been repeated. This decision must be clearly recorded.

The systems validation phase would include a review of all necessary documentation. The executed validation plan, including test or error logs, the user manuals and any other updated documentation, should be approved. Results of the system validation should be archived with other records of the system.

System Introduction

The validation procedures having successfully been undertaken, the system is now ready for introduction and integration into production. However, before the cross-over from the old system, be it manual or computerized, it is first necessary to ensure that the environment is ready and prepared for the system. This procedure will include distribution of SOPs and user guides as well as other approved documents. Users should be trained according to their specific needs and responsibilities.

Operation and Maintenance

The system and its environment are dynamic and therefore require constant management to ensure continued operation in compliance with specification. The system development life-cycle does not end with system introduction. The operation and maintenance phase of the life-cycle covers the system as it continues to evolve. During this phase, services to support the user are put in place, including a continuation of user training and the authorization of new users.

System performance should be regularly assessed during this phase to provide an ongoing evaluation of software and/or hardware performance and to identify necessary changes. Procedures should be followed for the implementation of system changes as well as reporting of 'bugs' and their resolution (change control procedures). Ideally, these procedures should uniquely identify each 'bug' report or enhancement request so that it can be linked to the proper programme version when it is implemented.

Change control covers changes to hardware, application and system software, and documentation. Procedures may include controls which assure that the proposed modification is reviewed and approved or rejected by both users and those responsible for support of the system. Such controls assure that with each modification or revision, the documentation (user and system) accurately reflects the functions and operations of the system. Procedures for determining the degree of testing are necessary to assure the proper functioning of the system following any modification. Specific changes made to the system must be documented.

Modification to software or changes to hardware may require part or all of the system development life-cycle to be repeated.

CONCLUSION

The purpose of GLP is to assure the quality and integrity of the data submitted in support of the safety of regulated products. To this end, most of the requirements of GLP would have been considered familiar and reasonable by any conscientious scientist. Protocols and SOPs, adequate facilities and equipment, full identification of test substance, proper animal care, equipment maintenance, accurate recording of observations, and accurate reporting of results are basic necessities for the conduct of a high-quality, valid toxicity study, or any scientific study.

FURTHER READING

Dent, N. J. (1994). European compliance issues: good research practices. *Journal of the American College of Toxicology*, **13**, 78–85

Dybkaer, R. (1994). Quality assurance, accreditation, and certification: needs and possibilities. *Clinical Chemistry*, **40**, 1416–1420

Horri, I. (1994). Data management for toxicological studies. *Environmental Health Perspectives*, **102**, Supplement, 71–75

Turnheim, D. (1993). Benefits of good laboratory practice as a tool to improve testing. *Human and Experimental Toxicology*, **12**, 528–532

14 Evaluation of Toxicity in Human Subjects

Peter N. Bennett

INTRODUCTION

Humans experience toxic effects from exposure to substances in the environment, from food additives, from drugs or from substance abuse. Sometimes that toxicity is recognized but the individual deems the risk to be sufficiently small to be worth taking—e.g. continuing to smoke tobacco; sometimes it is unrecognized or, if recognized, then it is unquantified. This chapter considers how toxicity in humans is recognized and how the risk to the individual is assessed. While many substances may be harmful to us, the responses that humans show, and the means we have developed to recognize them and assess the hazard they pose, have been best developed in relation to medicinal drugs. Much of the information cited here will therefore relate to drug therapy, although it is relevant to human toxicity in general.

A Historical Perspective

In the early years of this century the number of drugs in use was far less than it is now. The USA Food and Drug Administration (FDA) was concerned primarily with the safety of food, as the name suggests, and this was reflected by the legislation under which it operated. Public awareness that drugs have the capacity to harm as well as to heal evolved largely from specific incidents which aroused concern, and which were followed by governmental action. A brief account is therefore given of the reasons why certain laws and regulations were required for public protection; these were necessarily accompanied by the development of scientific methods designed to evaluate hazard and minimize risk from drugs and other substances.

Sulphanilamide-Massengill

The introduction of the sulphonamides in 1935 was a major therapeutic advance against common bacterial infections. Sulphanilamide was marketed in 1937 in the USA as tablets and capsules, but there was a demand for a liquid form which could be taken more easily—for example, by children. The issue was addressed by the S. E. Massengill Company of Tennessee. Because sulphanilamide is insoluble in the usual vehicles, several industrial solvents were tried and diethylene glycol (a constituent of antifreezes) was found to be suitable; with the addition of flavouring and water, an elixir was made. The mixture was checked for appearance, fragrance and flavour, but no animal tests and no special clinical trials were conducted. About 1100 l were marketed, and this was compatible with the prevailing law in the USA. Later the same year came the first news of deaths in patients who had received the sulphanilamide elixir, and despite vigorous attempts by the Company and the FDA to recall it, about 93 people died, mainly children.

The marketing of Sulphanilamide-Massengill was compatible with existing USA law, except that use of the word 'elixir' implied an alcoholic solution, whereas it was a solution in diethylene glycol. The Report of the Secretary of Agriculture (Report, 1937) pointed out that 'A few simple and inexpensive animal tests would have quickly demonstrated the toxic properties of both diethylene glycol and the elixir'. The USA Congress then moved quickly and enacted more comprehensive legislation, including the provision that no new drug and no modification of an existing drug be licensed until the entire formulation had been submitted to the FDA. Later this legislation had the effect of limiting the exposure of US citizens to thalidomide before its teratogenic and other adverse effects were discovered.

Thalidomide

By the 1950s there were many new drugs; penicillin was available, as were thiazide diuretics, adrenal steroids and ganglion blockers for hypertension. Each was hailed for the therapeutic advance it signified but, unrecognized, the capacity of scientific medicine to invent new medicines was outstripping its ability safely to introduce these agents to clinical use, and there was a price to pay. Thalidomide was marketed in

1956 in West Germany and 2 years later in the UK as what seemed to be a safe and effective hypnotic and sedative. Commencing about 1957, paediatric clinics noticed an unaccountable increase in cases of phocomelia, a congenital deformity principally of the long bones with substantially normal or rudimentary hands and feet, giving the extremities the appearance of the flippers of a seal (for photographs, see Taussig, 1962; Ward, 1962). A case–control study showed a strong association between maternal use of thalidomide and phocomelia. Accounts of the thalidomide incident are given by Woollam (1962) and Mellin and Katzenstein (1962).

The impact of this disaster on the public was profound, for the worst had happened: a nonessential drug had produced devastating congenital deformities. Furthermore, the legislation of the time did not, in general, provide for routine testing of new drugs in pregnant animals. Governments around the world enacted laws and created regulations that demanded far more stringent animal and human testing. In the UK these are covered by the Medicines Act 1968. The administrative systems so established are the basis of the national drug regulatory agencies in operation today.

Practolol

Practolol, a beta₁-selective adrenergic receptor antagonist, was introduced in the UK in 1970 and developed to the highest prevailing scientific standard, which included review by the UK drug regulatory authorities. Some 200 000 patient-years of experience had been gained with patients taking practolol before case reports of adverse reactions in skin (Rowland and Stevenson, 1972; Felix and Ive, 1974) and the eye and other tissues (Wright, 1975) appeared in the literature. Soon the whole oculomucocutaneous syndrome was defined, and its association with practolol. The lesson from practolol was that, despite extensive testing in animals, toxicity can occur through an idiosyncratic reaction in a small number of persons. Their identification gave impetus to the development of methods for evaluation of toxicity from drugs after they have become generally available—i.e. post marketing surveillance (see Chapter 43).

Benoxaprofen

Benoxaprofen, a nonsteroidal anti-inflammatory drug, was introduced to drug regulatory agencies for licensing from about 1979 onwards. Its mode of action suggested that benoxaprofen might cause less gastric bleeding than others of this class, and preliminary data supported this view. Soon reports began to appear associating benoxaprofen with photosensitivity, oncholysis and deaths from cholestatic jaundice (Goudie *et al.*, 1982; Halsey and Cardoe, 1982; Hindson *et al.*, 1982; Taggart and Alderdice, 1982), and it was withdrawn from marketing in 1982. Those who were most at risk were the elderly, and it became evident that the reason for their special sensitivity was that the action of benoxaprofen is terminated by renal excretion, which is often impaired in this age group. The experience of benoxaprofen draws attention to groups of persons who are at risk from drugs used in doses that are safe for the rest of the population; such groups may be readily identifiable, as are the young and the old, or identification may require special testing, as with those who are genetically deficient in their ability to carry out certain metabolic reactions necessary to inactivate drugs—e.g. glucose–6-phosphate dehydrogenase deficiency, slow oxidizers.

The examples above illustrate the growth of awareness about toxicity in humans. While the instances cited refer to medicinal drugs, they could also apply to toxicity from other sources—e.g. additives to pharmaceutical formulations (Young *et al.*, 1987); chemicals in the environment, including ionizing radiation; and herbal preparations. It is evident that legislation and regulation were *reactive* to specific incidents, as is generally the case. The challenges of modern scientific toxicology, however, are to be *proactive*—i.e. to forewarn and therefore to avoid hazard, failing which, to identify it rapidly and quantify it in as low a frequency as is possible. That is what much of this chapter will discuss.

TYPES AND SOURCES OF TOXICITY

Toxic effects of substances present in different ways, which therefore demand different approaches to their evaluation. They are commonly classed as follows.

Dose- and Time-related Effects

Injury is related to the degree of exposure—i.e. there is a dose–response relation—and the reaction can be expected in any member of the population who receives a sufficiently large dose. The notion of dose includes both the amount of substance in question and the time over which exposure takes place—i.e. a time–response relation applies. It thus encompasses, e.g., acute hepatic necrosis after an overdose of paracetamol, and hepatic fibrosis after repeated dosing with methotrexate.

Special forms of such effects include the following.

Carcinogenesis, the generation of neoplastic change—e.g. asbestos causing mesothelioma.
Teratogenesis, the causation of anatomical abnormalities in the fetus—e.g. isotretinoin, the anti-acne agent.
Mutagenesis, the production of abnormality in the genetic material of the organism such that there is a permanent alteration of its hereditary constitution; the latter may be manifest in a later generation. There is strong evidence that ethylene oxide, a gas used for sterilization of rubber and plastic equipment, is mutagenic.

Idiosyncratic Effects

Injury occurs only in individuals who are susceptible because of particular attributes. These are broadly of two types.

Immunological

Any of the standard allergic mechanisms may be involved, namely:

Type I Immediate-type, involving IgE antibodies and the release of pharmacologically active substances from mast cells and leukocytes—e.g. anaphylactic reaction to benzylpenicillin.
Type II Autoallergy, where the combination of the foreign compound with protein provokes the formation of antibodies which combine with antigen to activate complement and cell damage results—e.g. haemolysis with α-methyldopa, or drug-induced agranulocytosis.
Type III Complex-mediated hypersensitivity, where antibody reacts with soluble antigen to form complexes that activate complement or attach to mast cells, causing the release of inflammatory mediators; vasculitis, glomerulonephritis and serum sickness are examples of this type.
Type IV Cell-mediated (delayed) hypersensitivity, where receptors specific to the allergen develop on T-lymphocytes and any subsequent challenge causes a tissue reaction—e.g. contact dermatitis with industrial chemicals.

Genetic

The risk of toxicity usually arises from enzyme deficiency. Examples include:

Hepatic porphyrias, where deficient conversion of porphyrins to haem exposes affected individuals to risk from drugs which have the common property of increasing the activity of delta-amino-laevulinic acid synthase.
Glucose-6-phosphate dehydrogenase (G-6-PD) deficiency, where haemolysis occurs in affected persons who take oxidant substances.
Defective carbon oxidation, where affected individuals exhibit adverse responses to standard doses of drugs whose inactivation involves oxidation of their carbon centres—e.g. debrisoquine (hypotension), bufuralol, timolol (increased beta-blockade), nortriptyline (postural hypotension), nifedipine (prolonged cardiovascular action).
Acetylator status Slow acetylators respond adversely to standard doses of hydralazine and procainamide (antinuclear antibodies in plasma, and some proceed to systemic lupus erythematosus), and dapsone (haemolytic anaemia); fast acetylators appear to be at greater risk from isoniazid (acute hepatocellular necrosis from an active metabolite).

Other Factors

Susceptibility to toxic effects may arise for other reasons.

Extremes of age Neonates who received chloramphenicol developed the grey syndrome (cardiovascular collapse) because of immaturity in their capacity to form the glucuronic acid conjugate which inactivates the drug (Burns *et al.*, 1959; Craft *et al.*, 1974). There is increasing definition of adverse drug reactions among children in hospital (Choonara and Harris, 1984) and in the community (Woods *et al.*, 1987).

Multiple drug therapy and differences in pharmacokinetics and pharmacodynamics are factors that predispose the elderly to adverse reactions to drugs—e.g. to digoxin, diuretics and psychotropics (Nolan and O'Malley, 1989).

Disease of the liver and kidney predisposes to accumulation of, and toxic effects from, substances which are normally cleared by these organs. Patients with hepatic cirrhosis, for example, are extremely sensitive to the effects of opioids, partly because drugs of this class are ordinarily inactivated by hepatic metabolism.

ATTRIBUTION OF CAUSE

A central issue in attempting to evaluate toxicity of substances in humans is the degree of certainty with which the occurrence of an event can be attributed to an agent. The following relationship was proposed in an attempt to rationalize the difficulty in respect of injury due to drugs (Karch and Lasagne, 1976).

Definite
- The time sequence from taking the drug is reasonable.
- The event corresponds to what is known of the drug.
- The event ceases on stopping the drug.
- The event returns on restarting the drug.

Probable
- The time sequence is reasonable.
- The event corresponds to what is known of the drug.
- The event ceases on stopping the drug.
- The event is not reasonably explained by the patient's disease.

Possible
- The time sequence is reasonable.
- The event corresponds to what is known of the drug.
- The event could have been the result of the patient's disease or other therapy.

Conditional
- The time sequence is reasonable.
- The event does not correspond with what is known about the drug.

- The event could not reasonably be explained by the patient's disease.

Doubtful Not meeting the above criteria.

Evaluation of Toxicity

Evaluating toxicity in humans relies substantially on assembling and then examining data according to criteria such as the above. The evidence comes broadly as two types.

Experimental Studies

In experimental studies clinical trials of new drugs are conducted on relatively small numbers of subjects, principally with the aim of establishing therapeutic efficacy and its relation to toxicity. Entry to these is strictly controlled by predetermined inclusion and exclusion criteria, as is allocation of treatment; only the commoner toxic effects are likely to be uncovered by such studies. They comprise: preclinical studies of animals and tissue culture; clinical trials of Phase I, Phase II and Phase III (see later, pp. 307–308).

Observational Studies

In observational studies the groups to be compared have to be compiled from subjects who are being treated in routine medical care, or who are not—i.e. the controls. These are referred to as Phase IV or postmarketing surveillance studies; they are designed mainly to identify and quantify adverse and toxic reactions, often of low frequency, and eventually involve large numbers of subjects. They comprise: case reports, cohort studies and case–control studies.

Specific systems that have been created to undertake postmarketing surveillance will be described, and include: voluntary reporting, prescription event monitoring, medical record linkage and hospital-based monitoring systems.

Some impression of the practical difficulty of detecting adverse reactions to drugs is given in Table 1, which lists the numbers of patients who must be monitored to detect adverse events, with no background incidence and with a 95 per cent chance of detecting reactions, of differing frequency.

Table 1 Numbers of patients required to detect adverse reactions

Expected incident of adverse reaction	Number of patients required for:		
	1 event	2 events	3 events
1 in 100	300	480	650
1 in 200	600	960	1300
1 in 1000	3000	4800	6500
1 in 2000	6000	9600	13 000
1 in 10 000	30 000	48 000	65 000

From: *Safety Requirements for the First Use of New Drugs and Diagnostic Agents in Man.* CIOMS, Geneva, (1983) with permission.

EVALUATION BY EXPERIMENTAL STUDIES

Preclinical Studies in Animals and Tissue Culture

A brief account is given here, for animal testing forms part of the process whereby toxicity is evaluated in humans. Studies on animals are required by law for drug regulatory purposes. In part these provide pharmacodynamic and pharmacokinetic data, but their prime purpose is to give an indication of whether injury may be caused by a drug that is intended for humans. Animal experiments should therefore reflect the proposed clinical use. Where a drug is to be given in single doses, animal studies of 14 days are common; where humans may be exposed to the drug for 30 days or more, animal studies extend for 180 days or more.

Special studies are required for drugs that may cause chromosome damage. These may involve tissue culture of peripheral blood lymphocytes, bone marrow cells or epithelial fibroblasts. Gross abnormalities are readily distinguished in the metaphase stage, when chromosomes are at their most condensed. More refined techniques can detect, for example, rearrangements of material within a chromosome (sister chromosome exchanges). Extensive studies on pregnant animals are carried out to establish effects on fertility and the risk of teratogenesis. While the predictive value of such tests remains an issue, they have been mandatory for new drugs since the thalidomide disaster. Testing is designed to investigate all stages of the reproductive process from damage to male and female gametes, to embryogenesis, fetal effects, uterine growth and development, parturition, postnatal effects such as suckling, later effects such as behaviour, and second-generation effects.

Carcinogenicity studies are undertaken whenever suspicion arises from the chemical structure of a substance or of its metabolites, or chromosome studies, or from histology after repeated dose administration. Substances may be found to be carcinogenic in animals, however, without real suspicion of similar effects in humans (e.g. the diuretic drug spironolactone), raising again the issue of predicting human toxicity from animal data. In a very real sense, therefore, humans are their own best experimental animals and, once safety screening in animals is complete, the ultimate evaluation of toxicity must lie in observing, recording and analysing the effects of substances on human beings.

Clinical Trials of Drugs

All new chemicals that are intended for therapeutic use undergo a process during which their therapeutic efficacy is evaluated in relation to the adverse effects they cause—i.e. the establishment of the risk:benefit ratio that determines their value in relation to other drugs and their place in therapy. The process involves formal clinical studies in which (apart from those of the earliest phase) equivalent groups of patients are randomly allocated to receive test substances, including placebo where necessary, in order to answer precisely framed questions—i.e. the randomized, controlled trial. Details of the design, statistical validity and conduct of these studies are beyond the remit of this chapter, but an outline of the individual Phases is given in so far as these relate to evaluating toxicity.

Phase I establishes the clinical pharmacology of a drug in healthy volunteers; in it the absorption, distribution, metabolism, excretion (pharmacokinetics) and biological effects (pharmacodynamics) of the drug are determined, and, where practicable, its safety, tolerance and efficacy. In broad terms this is likely to involve about 100 volunteers, and clearly this number affords little opportunity, and there is indeed little intent, to study toxicity.

Phase II sees the investigation of the pharmaco-kinetics and, more particularly, the pharmacody-namics of the drug in patients (i.e. the clinical effects on the target disease) and addresses the issue of the therapeutic dose range. This may involve up to 500 patients.

Phase III is the phase of formal randomized con-trolled therapeutic trials where efficacy, safety and comparison with other drugs are the issues. The activity may encompass 1000–3000 patients within the structured and systematized monitor-ing of the clinical trial, including the search for toxicity developing during the period of obser-vation (usually weeks or months). Clinical trials are, by their nature, unlikely to uncover toxicity after long-term use (e.g. vascular disease from hormonal contraception) or toxicity in vulnerable groups (e.g. pregnant women, and patients with renal or hepatic disease, as these are normally excluded from the studies).

Ethical Aspects

A common feature of the type of study referred to in the above Phases is that experiments are conducted on healthy volunteers or patients. Over recent years there has been increasing awareness of the ethical aspects of such activity. These encompass, for example, the scientific val-idity of the research and the reasons for under-taking it, the competence of the investigators, the quality of the information given to the experi-mental subject and the form (written or oral) in which it is given, and the provision of adequate recompense in the event of harm resulting from participating in the study.

The basic provisions to guide investigators are set out in the Declaration of Helsinki of 1964 and its subsequent amendments (World Medical Association, 1989). Various institutions provide more detailed advice. In the UK the Royal Col-lege of Physicians of London has published recommendations on research involving healthy volunteers (Report of the Royal College of Phys-icians of London, 1986) and on patients (Report of the Royal College of Physicians of London, 1990a). The protocols which describe the conduct of clinical trials should be reviewed by indepen-dent research ethics committees (called Insti-tutional Review Boards in the USA) which have the power to accept, amend or reject studies. Their function has been described in respect of the UK (Report of the Royal College of Phys-

icians of London, 1990b) and the USA (Night-ingale, 1991). Within the European Community, the protection of trial subjects, provision for ethics review, informed consent and other aspects of experiments on human subjects are compre-hensively defined in the document *Good Clinical Practice for Trials on Medicinal Products in the European Community* (111/3976/88), the back-ground to which has been reviewed (Sauer, 1991).

EVALUATION BY OBSERVATIONAL STUDIES

Phase IV or postmarketing surveillance studies take place when the drug is being used in the patient community at large. It is then subject to influences that include a variety of reactions to colourings and preservatives (Pollock *et al.*, 1989), interaction with other drugs, use in the presence of other diseases and incorrect com-pliance with the dosage regimen. Postmarketing surveillance of individual drugs may encompass up to or over 10 000 patients, and the systems used provide the most effective means of identify-ing and quantifying toxicity, including the recog-nition of low-frequency adverse effects.

The evaluation of toxicity in this complex phase is effected by differing epidemiological approaches and surveillance systems. Often the first evidence of an adverse event is a *case report* to a medical journal; *voluntary reporting schemes* such as the UK 'Yellow Card' system are a form of systematized case-reporting. Suspicions raised by voluntary reports may need to be verified and, epidemiologically, there are two main approaches, the *cohort* and the *case–control* study. *Prescription event monitoring* is a type of cohort study. Other forms of surveillance such as *medical record linkage* can be adapted to perform either cohort or case–control studies, depending on the nature of the scientific question. Among these related elements, it is convenient first to consider case reports, cohort studies and case–control studies, and then the formal systems for surveillance.

Case Reports

Case reports can provide the hypotheses that stimulate formal surveillance studies, and experi-ence records that these are often the first evidence of toxicity from a drug or other substance. Venning (1983a, b), in an assessment of how serious new adverse reactions to drugs were detected, found that the first alert for 13 of 18 reactions came from case reports by individual physicians. Clearly there is a problem for the reporting physician in distinguishing between coincidence and cause, but, where documentation of the event is good, such reports appear to have a high degree of sensitivity, for Venning (1982) also found that 35 of 47 (75 per cent) reports were validated within 18 years; where documentation was less complete, only 7 of 19 reactions were authenticated at the time of publication. Edwards *et al.* (1990) have suggested diagnostic criteria for case reports to reduce the frequency of spurious associations in cases reported to the World Health Organization (WHO) Collaborating Centre.

Case reports tend to reveal the idiosyncratic type of reaction, which, by definition, is of low frequency. Evidence shows that the initial report soon prompts the appearance of others as the association becomes recognized, as was the case with practolol. Delays introduced while a series of cases is assembled, and by the publication process, mean that alerting by case report may be less rapid than by, for example, voluntary reporting systems.

Cohort Studies

In an *observational* cohort study a group of patients who are taking a drug is identified and also a comparable group who are not (the controls). In a prospective study both are then monitored to determine the outcome; less commonly the groups are analysed retrospectively. These studies are expensive to conduct, as large numbers of subjects must be followed for months or years. Observational cohort studies may be either randomized or non-randomized.

A randomized cohort study requires that within a monitored population of patients each individual is given an equal chance of receiving the active drug or the placebo. This approach was adopted in the World Health Organization trial of the lipid-lowering drug clofibrate for the prevention of ischaemic heart disease (Committee of Principal Investigators, 1978). Unexpectedly, patients who took clofibrate were found to have a 47 per cent excess risk of death, which returned to normal when the drug was discontinued (Committee of Principal Investigators, 1984); there remains a strong suggestion that the drug caused the extra deaths.

In a non-randomized study a group of patients who are being treated with the drug are compared with a group who are not taking it, as they have no need of it. An example is the Royal College of General Practitioners study of oral contraceptives. This began in 1968, recruited 46 000 women and 1400 general practitioners, and quantified the risk of arterial disease (Layde *et al.*, 1983) and mortality (Layde *et al.*, 1981). A similar enquiry into the histamine H_2 receptor antagonist cimetidine encompassed nearly 20 000 patients and controls, and confirmed the safety of this drug in normal clinical practice (Colin-Jones *et al.*, 1985a, b). This type of surveillance does, however, depend on the identification and recording of reactions in the general practitioner's notes and may underreport information that is sensitive — e.g. concerning sexual function.

Observational cohort studies are thus suitable for identifying and quantifying the commoner, but not the idiosyncratic, type of drug toxicity. *Experimental* cohort studies are the randomized controlled trials conducted mainly in Phases II and III of clinical assessment (above).

Case–Control Studies

The researcher assembles a group of patients with the condition in question (e.g. a form of cancer) and a control group who do not have the disease but are similar in relevant respects, such as age, gender, habits and location. In an investigation of drug toxicity, the drug histories of both groups are compared, and a causal link may be established if there is an excess of drug takers in the disease group. Thus, the analysis is retrospective.

A case–control study of a suggested environmental hazard illustrates well the use of this technique (Gardner *et al.*, 1990a, b). In 1984 a report pointed to a possible raised incidence of cancer, mainly childhood leukaemia and lymphoma, in and around the English village of Seascale, near the Sellafield nuclear plant (Independent Advisory Group, 1984). It was necessary to identify as completely as possible the cases of leukaemia and lymphoma that occurred in the area from 1950 to 1985. The diversity of sources used to compile these cases helps to illustrate the rigour and scope of the effort required. They comprised (1) case records from a former local childhood cancer survey; (2) pathology records from the district general hospital; (3) registered death entries, both locally and at medical referral centres; (4) death certificates for the locality, and more widely for those mentioning leukaemia; (5) death entries for the locality at the Office of Population Censuses and Surveys; (6) registrations with the regional and a national cancer registry; (7) circular letters to general practitioners; and (8) pre-school illness notifications.

The searches identified 52 cases of leukaemia, 23 of non-Hodgkin's lymphoma and 22 of Hodgkin's disease; these were compared with 1001 controls from the same locality or area, matched for age and gender, and obtained from registers of live births at the Office of Population Censuses and Surveys. The principal finding was an important one in environmental toxicology: the relative risk of leukaemia was higher in children whose fathers worked at the nuclear installation and who had high radiation dose recordings before the child's conception.

Voluntary Reporting Schemes

Schemes that provide for voluntary or spontaneous reporting of adverse reactions to drugs have been established in many countries, usually as independent agencies that advise the drug regulatory authorities. With the impetus delivered by the thalidomide incident, the UK initiated a reporting scheme in 1964, the 'Yellow Card' system. A supply of reply-paid letter-cards is made available to doctors, dentists, coroners and drug manufacturers, who are invited to report details of all suspected reactions, however minor, that could conceivably be related to a new drug. Such drugs are signified by an inverted black triangle opposite their listing in the British National Formulary. In addition, reports are requested for any serious reaction (disabling, incapacitating, life-threatening, fatal) in an established drug. General medical practitioners supply about 70 per cent of the reports and hospital doctors most of the remainder. The number received rose from 4000 in 1965 to over 20 000 in 1991. These are retained in the Adverse Reactions Register which now has in excess of 210 000 reports. Reactions that involve the skin and appendages, and the nervous, gastrointestinal and cardiovascular systems comprise 83 per cent of the entries.

Over 20 other countries now operate voluntary reporting schemes and all supply their information to the WHO Adverse Reaction Collaborating Centre, in Uppsala in Sweden. This enormous database can reinforce or refute signals of adverse reactions from individual contributors.

Authentication of Reports

The individual reports of adverse reactions are at best internal early warnings. Licensing authorities must live with pressures that require them to prevent continued exposure of patients to an identified hazard, while simultaneously not curtailing the use of a valuable drug. There is therefore a need to validate or refute reports in short order. In the UK the Committee on Safety of Medicines (CSM) operates a team of some 200 medically qualified field workers who interview reporting physicians. The genuineness of a report is examined by a searching enquiry for, e.g., evidence that the patient actually took the suspect drug, alternative explanations for the adverse reaction, the possible contribution of other drugs taken by the patient, or evidence of the effects of past exposure to the suspect or to similar drugs.

Limitations of Voluntary Reporting Schemes

Voluntary reporting systems cannot accurately define the incidence of adverse reactions and this is their important limitation. The reason is that, once a reaction has been proposed, there remains uncertainty both about the number of patients who have experienced it (the numerator) and about the number of patients exposed to the drug (the denominator). There is no doubt that all voluntary schemes are compromised by under-reporting, and surveys in the UK suggest that rarely are more than 10 per cent of serious reactions reported (Rawlins, 1988a). Cumulated reports suggest that reporting is probably particularly low where the adverse reaction has a long latency—e.g. tardive dyskinesia with chronic neuroleptic treatment—or occurs only on withdrawal of the drug—e.g. long-term use of benzodiazepine anxiolytics.

Some indication of the number of patients who receive a drug may be obtained in the UK from sampling the Prescriptions Pricing Authority (PPA), which processes all National Health Service prescriptions to remunerate the dispensing pharmacists, from Intercontinental Medical Statistics (IMS), an independent organization, or from sales figures. This information, together with the number of reports, does therefore give some clue to the lower limit of the risk of toxicity from a drug. National registers—e.g. for death, cancer, congenital abnormalities (see pp. 380–381)—may also be consulted to relate disease trends to drug use.

Rawlins (1988a) identified important independent determinants of the number of yellow cards received by the CSM as:

The inherent toxicity of the drug—i.e. those with a low therapeutic ratio (maximum tolerated dose: minimum effective dose) tend to generate significant numbers of severe reactions.
Usage, as indicated from data collected by the PPA or IMS (see above).
Marketing life The incidence is highest in the first 2 years, partly because doctors alter their prescribing habits once the profile of toxicity is recognized and partly because there is less reporting as reactions become known.
Publicity Prior to the communications to the medical literature of the skin (Felix and Ive, 1974) and ocular (Wright, 1975) effects of practolol, the UK CSM had received only 6 accounts of adverse reactions that were later related to the drug, yet such was the publicity that subsequently surrounded the issue that within 18 months the number had risen to 1038 reports.

Achievements of Voluntary Reporting Schemes

Despite these innate constraints on their application, voluntary reporting schemes have yet proved useful; their achievements have been defined by Rawlins and colleagues, and the following account refers extensively to their published experience (Rawlins, 1988b; Rawlins *et al.*, 1989).

Early Warning of Drug Toxicity
Voluntary reporting schemes begin to operate as soon as a drug is marketed, and indeed they were introduced as 'early warning' systems. They can be swiftly successful, as witness the single report of suspected mercurial poisoning that prompted the withdrawal of a proprietary preparation as treatment for nappy-rash, or the 7 reports of anaphylaxis with a desensitizing vaccine which caused a batch of the vaccine to be withdrawn

(Inman and Weber, 1986). More commonly the reasons for ascribing an adverse effect to a compound relate to the number of reports and the known pharmacology and toxicology of the substance; the case becomes stronger if the event is serious and exceptional. Acute dystonias and acute anaphylaxis are almost always due to drugs; some conditions attract attention because their setting is unusual—e.g. gynaecomastia in otherwise healthy males. Attribution becomes more difficult when a drug is linked with a disease that may be caused by any one of several agents, but the association may be strengthened if an uncommon condition (e.g. peripheral neuritis, fibrosing alveolitis) is supported by a collection of reports. An adverse event that is an exaggeration of the pharmacological or therapeutic action (e.g. lowering of blood pressure) can be more difficult to identify but the time relationship may help, as in first-dose hypotension with angiotensin-converting enzyme inhibitors.

Voluntary reporting schemes are much less likely correctly to identify adverse events that are common in the treated population—e.g. dysrhythmias in patients receiving antidysrhythmic drugs; these are best brought to light by an appropriately designed therapeutic trial, as was suggested by the CAST study of flecainide and encainide (Echt *et al.*, 1991).

Voluntary reporting from various countries has alerted drug relatory authorities to toxic reactions to drugs, as Table 2 demonstrates. The rising number of adverse reactions identified with successive decades attests to the increasingly comprehensive coverage obtainable by this system.

Characterization of Iatrogenic Syndromes
'Yellow Card' reports provide data on the patient (gender, age, indication for treatment), the drug (dose, duration of treatment) and the adverse reaction (clinical and pathological characteristics, time relation to drug administration, outcome). There are enough characteristics, therefore, to delineate specific drug-related syndromes, where a sufficient number of reports give concurring findings. Some examples appear in Table 3. Hypotheses generated from spontaneous reports may be supported from case reports in the medical literature, but usually after a delay due to the time involved in publication.

The reports provide, in addition, a means of

Table 2 Some early warnings of new adverse reactions identified through spontaneous reporting schemes

Year	Drug	Reaction	Country
1965	Ibufenac	Hepatotoxicity	UK
1975	Metoclopramide	Extrapyramidal reactions	UK, Argentina
1976	Aprindine	Agranulocytosis	Holland
1976	Glafenine	Anaphylaxis	Holland
1977	Clozapine	Granulocytopenia	Finland
1980	Tienilic acid	Hepatotoxicity	USA
1981	Bromocriptine	Pulmonary toxicity	Finland
1981	Mebhydrolin	Granulocytopenia	Austria, Japan, UK
1981	Mianserin	Blood dyscrasias	UK, New Zealand
1982	Amiodarone	Hepatotoxicity, pulmonary toxicity	UK
1983	Zomiperac	Anaphylaxis	USA
1983	Zimelidine	Guillain–Barré	Sweden, UK
1984	Captopril	Cough	New Zealand
1986	Nifedipine	Gum hyperplasia	Holland, Israel, UK
1987	Pivmecillinam	Oesophageal injury	Sweden, UK
1988	Nefopam	Urinary retention	UK

From Rawlins *et al.* (1989), with permission.

Table 3 Some examples of the clinical delineation of iatrogenic syndromes through spontaneous reporting schemes

Year	Drug	Reaction	Country
1970	Oral contraceptives	Thromboembolism	Sweden, Denmark, UK
1974	Bismuth subgallate	Encephalopathy	Australia
1977	Nitrofurantoin	Eosinophilic lung lesions	Sweden, Finland, UK, Holland
1978	Halothane	Hepatotoxicity	UK
1978	Emepronium bromide	Oesophageal injury	Finland, UK
1979	Phenylpropanolamine	Childhood psychosis	Sweden
1985	Enalapril	Hypotension, renal failure	UK
1985	Metoclopramide	Dyskinesia	UK
1986	Desensitizing vaccines	Anaphylaxis, bronchospasm	UK
1987	Ketoconazole	Hepatotoxicity	UK
1987	Pivmecillinam	Oesophageal injury	Sweden, UK
1989	Mianserin	Blood dyscrasias in the elderly	UK

From Rawlins *et al.* (1989), with permission.

examining the influence of certain variables on toxicity—for example, dose.

In the 1960s an excess incidence of certain forms of thromboembolic disease was noted among users of the oral contraceptive pill; evidence suggested a higher risk with mestranol than with ethinyloestradiol (Inman, 1970). When the reports were analysed by oestrogen dose level, however, the excess risk of thromboembolism with higher doses became clear (Inman *et al.*, 1970). This finding led to introduction of the low-dose oral contraceptives now in use. Other spontaneous reports drew attention to the danger of hypotension with the first dose of prazosin (Committee on Safety of Medicines, 1975) and enalapril (Committee on Safety of Medicines, 1986a).

Voluntary reporting has also provided evidence of susceptibility to toxicity by age or gender. Thus, the elderly were shown to be vulnerable to disorders of haematopoiesis (including agranulocytosis) with mianserin (Committee on Safety of Medicines, 1983) and co-trimoxazole (Committee on Safety of Medicines, 1985). Reports involving the dopamine-receptor antagonist drug metoclopramide showed that extrapyramidal reactions (dystonia–dyskinesia) were significantly more common in young adults and especially girls and women aged 12–19 years, whereas parkinsonian reactions occurred more often in the elderly (Bateman *et al.*, 1985). Similarly, extrapyramidal reactions with prochlorperazine and haloperidol were reported more commonly in the young, although in this case no gender effect was discerned (Bateman *et al.*, 1986). The statistical logic for testing the effect of single factors in drug monitoring was defined by Finney (1986), and was developed to investigate the influence of two or more factors simultaneously by using generalized linear models (Simpson *et al.*, 1987)

Comparisons of Toxicity between Drugs

Voluntary reports of adverse reactions may sometimes be used to compare the relative toxicities of drugs within the same therapeutic class. One approach is to use the number of reports for each drug by major organ system to create histograms and so to compile individual drug 'profiles' (Inman and Weber, 1986; Speirs, 1986). Such profiles drew attention to the special liability of protriptyline to cause photosensitive skin reactions compared with four other tricyclic antidepressants. Profile analysis can provide alerting signals to toxicity where there is difficulty in identifying the incidence of adverse reactions to a drug, or its volume of use.

An alternative approach is to relate the number of reports about individual drugs in a class to their number of prescriptions for comparable marketing periods. Use of this technique drew attention to the greater toxicity of zimelidine and nomifensine compared with other antidepressants (Committee on Safety of Medicines, 1986b). The greater risk of lactic acidosis with phenformin than with metformin, another biguanide, was also highlighted by this methodology (Bergman *et al.*, 1978).

Data on comparative toxicity between drugs derived from voluntary reporting must be regarded with caution because of the statistical problems of confounding and bias (Sachs and Bortnichak, 1986). Rawlins (1988a) drew attention to a larger number of 'Yellow Card' reports of acute airways obstruction provoked by atenolol (a relatively cardioselective beta-adrenoceptor antagonist) compared with propranolol (nonselective). To conclude that atenolol is more likely to cause bronchospasm is erroneous; almost certainly doctors prescibed atenolol more often for asthmatics or chronic bronchitics in the mistaken belief that its pharmacological properties made it the better choice, and thus it became overrepresented as a cause of bronchospasm.

Conclusions

Voluntary reporting schemes are the first line in postmarketing surveillance to detect and evaluate toxicity from drugs. They provide an internal alerting signal, which may eventually produce evidence that is strong enough to warrant regulatory action. Such systems are limited by being unable to provide accurate estimates of the incidence of adverse events, but they can reveal rare hazards that are not found by formal clinical trials. Through the growth of information technology and international co-operation in data collection—i.e. the World Health Organization's International Collaborative Programme on Drug Monitoring—voluntary reporting is likely to provide monitoring for ever larger numbers of patients.

Prescription Event Monitoring

Prescription event monitoring (PEM) is operated by the Drug Safety Research Unit (DSRU) of Southampton University, UK. It makes use of fact that within the National Health Service all prescriptions written by general medical practitioners are processed by a single authority, the Prescriptions Pricing Authority (PPA), to enable pharmacists to be remunerated for the drugs they dispense. Pricing clerks, who inspect each prescription, may thus identify prescriptions for selected drugs together with the names of the doctor and patient, photocopies of which are sent to DSRU.

Event data are collected by DSRU by means of a simple questionnaire sent to the prescribing doctor to complete from the patient's notes. An event is defined as 'any new diagnosis, any reason for a referral to a consultant or admission to hospital (e.g. operation, accident or pregnancy), any unexpected deterioration (or improvement) in a concurrent illness, any suspected drug reaction, or any other complaint which was considered of sufficient importance to enter in the patient's notes'. As an example, 'a broken leg is an event. If more fractures were associated with this drug they could have been due to hypotension, CNS effects or metabolic disease' (Inman *et al.*, 1986a). Thus, the system monitors *events*, without a judgement about causality being made at the time of reporting. The scheme is strongly supported by doctors; only 1 in 200 of general practitioners does not take part, and response rates range from 55 per cent to 75 per cent.

When a decision is taken to investigate a drug, an initial target of 20 000 patients who received it is usually set; this may be difficult if a new drug is slow to achieve a place in the market. DSRU attempts to undertake a PEM study on any new chemical entity that shows likelihood of being widely used in general medical practice. Priority is given to the first few members of an entirely new class of drug (e.g. ACE inhibitors) or to any drug with a known problem.

Inman *et al.* (1986b) described the use of PEM to compare toxicity associated with the non-steroidal anti-inflammatory drugs (NSAIDs) benoxaprofen, fenbufen, zomiperac, piroxicam and indomethacin (as Osmosin, a controlled-release formulation), as particular hazard is attached to the use of drugs of this class. The study highlighted excess photosensitivity with benoxaprofen, and headache and gastrointestinal events with indomethacin. Interestingly, a deficiency of cases of myocardial infarction was detected with zomiperac and indomethacin, and a similar though less marked effect was noted for piroxicam and benoxaprofen. A cardioprotective effect of NSAIDs other than aspirin (Julian *et al.*, 1988) seems feasible in view of their common mode of action on prostaglandin synthesis. This example illustrates how PEM can generate hypotheses about drug effects.

The system has also been used to test hypotheses, as in the case of erythromycin estolate. Data obtained by voluntary reporting to the CSM suggested a much higher incidence of jaundice with the estolate than with other forms of this drug. In a PEM study 12 000 forms relating to patients were dispatched, 76 per cent were returned, of which 16 recorded 'jaundice' as an event; in only 3 of these could the antibiotic have been considered as a possible cause of the jaundice and in each case the stearate, rather than the estolate, form of the drug had been used. The results indicated that jaundice was not commoner with the estolate, and in any case was a rare event (incidence $\ll 1{:}1000$) (Inman and Rawson, 1983).

Conclusions

The different findings with the 'Yellow Card' system (which may have been due to selective reporting) emphasize the complementary nature of the two schemes. PEM records any adverse event in selected drugs with a 3–12 month delay and provides a good estimate of the incidence of adverse reactions, but not of rare ($<1{:}1000$) events. Voluntary reporting involves a continuous

review of all suspected adverse reactions in all drugs being used, with a potentially faster response time; it does not supply a reliable estimate of their incidence but is better at detecting rare events.

Medical Record Linkage

Every member of the population creates certain vital records during the course of his or her life; these include birth, marriage and death certificates, and medical records of immunization, admission to hospital and prescriptions for drugs. These are deposited in many different places. The concept of record linkage is that all the important records about a single person may be brought together in an accessible form. The term is not recent, having been coined by Dunn in 1946 (Dunn, 1946), but its development has been slow. The opportunity is best in countries which have evolved highly structured national health services, as in Scandinavia and the UK, but medical report linkage operates on the largest scale in North America, utilizing the databases of co-operative or state-sponsored health care schemes.

North America

For many people health care is delivered by private co-operative schemes or by programmes supported by individual states. Those who provide the care (e.g. doctors, pharmacists) are remunerated through computerized billing which permits the identification of the patient, the drugs used, the date of the service and the disease; these data are used for clinical and epidemiological research. For example, where a cohort study is planned, all patients exposed to a certain drug or with a certain disease may be enrolled. Control groups for any specified cohort can be matched for age, gender, diagnosis and drug. The time relationship between use of a drug and a subsequent illness can be examined, as can the consequences of re-exposure of a patient to the same drug.

The patient population to which such schemes have access tends to be large (millions) and diversified, but the eligibility requirements of the Medicaid programme, for example, ensure an overrepresentation of young children, women of childbearing age and the elderly, and a deficit of employed males; this skewedness limits applicability of the findings to the general population. On the other hand, large paediatric databases may provide out-patient information for an age group in which formal studies of exposure to drugs are few, and are mostly limited to hospital studies. Drugs taken by pregnant women and monitored to term give the opportunity to relate birth defects to fetal exposure to drugs.

Groups that are involved in this area include those in Seattle (Jick *et al.*, 1984, 1987; Jick, 1985) and Saskatchewan (Guess *et al.*, 1988). Others utilize the databases of state-supported systems such as Medicare (Avorn *et al.*, 1986) and Medicaid. Using the Tennessee Medicaid data, Ray *et al.* (1987) demonstrated a strong association between use of central nervous system depressants (antipsychotics, antidepressants, hypnotics) and hospitalization with hip fracture, a finding that is interesting for its similarity (in its implications) to the Oxford Record Linkage Study's observation (see below) of an association between use of minor tranquillizers and admission to hospital with road accidents (Skegg *et al.*, 1979). Ray *et al.* (1989) also made the contrasting finding of a strong negative association between risk of hip fracture and long-term thiazide diuretic use, a finding which may be explained by the calcium-retaining effect of this class of drug.

Some record linkage studies have attracted criticism on methodological grounds. Shapiro (1989a) reviewed the general epidemiological criteria that should be satisfied to establish causality: that exposure and outcome be adequately defined, that the time of exposure and its relationship to outcome be relevant to the hypothesis at issue, that bias and confounding be controlled, and that dose–response and duration–response relationships be demonstrable where these might be anticipated. He observed that few of the elements were satisfied in a selected series of record linkage studies. The subsequent exchanges between some of their authors (Faich and Stadel, 1989; Strom and Carson, 1989) and himself (Shapiro, 1989b) are worth reading as a critique of this form of record linkage.

Apart from the systems in the USA, record linkage has developed in countries with highly organized national health services. Such schemes seem more likely to be representative of the population as a whole.

Finland

Finland (population 5 million) maintains nationwide computerized health surveillance registries in congenital malformations, cancer, hospital discharges, entitlement to free drugs and adverse drug reactions. These are notified to a central databank as a routine part of maintaining patients' medical records.

Over many years the Finnish authorities have used the Malformation Register to respond rapidly to case reports of potential teratogenic effects in pregnancy—e.g. of imipramine (Indanpaan-Heikkila and Saxen, 1973), diazepam (Saxen and Saxen, 1975) and short-term hyperthermia in the Finnish sauna (Saxen *et al.*, 1982). The use of the Finnish Malformation Register was reviewed by Saxen (1983).

Availability of the Finnish Adverse Drug Reactions Register enables an assessment to be made of the risk of blood disorders, notably agranulocytosis and neutropenia, associated with drug use. These identified apparent excess risk with the antidepressant drug clozapine (Indanpaan-Heikkila *et al.*, 1977) and the immunomodulator drug levamisole (Teerenhovi *et al.*, 1978). The incidence of drug-induced agranulocytosis appears higher in Finland than in other countries and is a cause of controversy.

United Kingdom

The Oxford Record Linkage Study began in 1962 (Acheson, 1967) with the linkage of birth, death, hospital admissions and obstetric records for about 350 000 people, and it has since expanded to include other records in a population of over 2 million. The system has been used to study the recurrence of various conditions and the outcome of illnesses, and to seek associations between different conditions (Baldwin and Acheson, 1987).

In the mid-1970s record linkage was extended to study adverse reactions to drugs, with the computerization of data from patients of selected general practices; these included basic biographic data (gender, date of birth), prescriptions dispensed (photocopies obtained from the PPA) and records of morbidity and mortality (mainly from the Oxford Record Linkage Study). The system demonstrated an excess risk of bronchopneumonia among users of the laxative liquid paraffin (Skegg, 1986), so reinforcing clinical evidence of adverse effects of this drug on the lung (liquid paraffin has since been withdrawn from the UK market). Record linkage also demonstrated an association between use of minor tranquillizers and admission to hospital with road accidents (Skegg *et al.*, 1979).

A record linkage system specifically designed for drug surveillance was established on Tayside in Scotland (Crombie *et al.*, 1984); it has provided largely reassuring data on long-term use of the histamine H_2 receptor antagonist cimetidine (Beardon *et al.*, 1988a,b) and of gastrointestinal events in patients taking NSAIDs (Beardon *et al.*, 1989).

Hospital-based Monitoring Systems

In addition to the community-based schemes outlined above, specialized monitoring is conducted in hospitals.

The Boston Collaborative Drug Surveillance Program

In 1966 a scheme was started in which specially trained nurses monitored acute adverse drug reactions in medical in-patients (Slone *et al.*, 1966); over subsequent years data were collected from surgical, psychiatric and paediatric patients, using similar methodology. Their combined activities constitute the Boston Collaborative Drug Surveillance Program (BCDSP), which now involves continuously monitored samples from patients in teaching hospitals throughout the USA and beyond. The scheme has thus assembled a substantial body of information about short-term toxicity to drugs used in hospital; Lawson (1986) lists 32 drugs which have been the subject of detailed reports from the BCDSP. An interesting reassuring product of this work was the finding, among 26 462 consecutive admissions, of 24 drug-related deaths, with only 6 deaths thought to have been preventable (Porter and Jick, 1977a); this reinforces the general impression that serious adverse reactions to drugs are uncommon events. Indeed one of the advantages of comprehensive and uniform data collected from a large number of patients is that low-frequency events can be detected; thus, Porter and Jick (1977b) were able to identify 119 episodes of drug-attributed anaphylaxis, convulsions, deafness and extrapyramidal reactions in 38 812 patients who had received over 250 000 course of drug therapy.

The Aberdeen–Dundee System

The in-patient Scottish Morbidity Return is used to obtain details of the patient and the diagnosis, and this information is linked with a standardized prescription sheet giving the drugs that were administered, to form a patient–drug file (Crooks *et al.*, 1965). The scheme covers some 4300 beds and about 70 000 discharges per year. In general, the system has been used to investigate suspected adverse reactions to drugs, for it has the capacity rapidly to identify patients who have received a suspect drug; follow-up by inspection of case records or by interview then becomes possible. Specific enquiries using the system include a possible association between spironolactone and the development of breast cancer, and between cimetidine and gastric cancer; these and other aspects of the system are described by Moir (1986)

INFORMATION SOURCES IN THE EVALUATION OF TOXICITY

The world scientific literature contains a wealth of information relating drugs and other chemicals to biological effects, and chemical structure to activity and toxicity, in both animals and man. This general body of knowledge is consulted whenever toxicity to a substance is evaluated, and literature surveys become ever easier with the advance of information search systems.

In addition, most countries maintain, to a varying degree, national systems of records for monitoring trends in disease and mortality among their citizens. In the UK the National Health Service Central Register (NHSCR) holds the names of almost everyone in the country; its records include the facts of birth and death, which can be linked with data on death certificates. The rise and fall in mortality due to asthma in young persons in England and Wales was charted by Inman and Adelstein (1969) and correlated with the sales of pressurized aerosol inhalers. Their conclusion that deaths were due to misuse of the aerosols led to more stringent advice being given to asthmatics on how often to use these devices.

Cancer cases are registered regionally and nationally, and are linked with the NHSCR, so that prospective studies are possible, as with the mortality returns.

The Office of Population Censuses and Surveys (OPCS) maintains records of general biographical data. A routine 10 per cent sample of all (non-psychiatric) patients discharged from or dying in hospital is analysed as the Hospital In-patient Enquiry and publishes its findings annually.

Data on babies with congenital malformations are collected from each health district and forwarded to the OPCS. Trends on each of 66 categories of malformation are analysed continuously so that changes may be monitored—e.g. in the incidence of specific categories, or within a district as compared with the national data.

CONCLUDING COMMENTS

The identification of drug-induced illness was analysed by Jick (1977) as follows.

If a drug commonly induces an otherwise rare illness, then the effect is likely to be discovered by clinical observation during the experimental (clinical trial) phases of its development unless it occurs in patients who are specifically excluded (e.g. pregnant women), when detection will occur later.

If a drug rarely induces an otherwise common illness, the effect is likely to remain undiscovered.

If a drug rarely induces an otherwise rare illness, the effect is likely to remain undiscovered until it is marketed, when it should be detected by clinical observation (case reports) and post-marketing surveillance, and confirmed by case–control studies.

If a drug commonly induces an otherwise common illness, the effect is unlikely to be discovered by clinical observation, but a very common effect may be revealed by formal therapeutic trials and case–control studies.

In this chapter the evaluation of toxicity in humans has been taken largely from the perspective of pharmaceuticals, because the legal, regulatory and monitoring systems for detecting and quantifying adverse reactions are best-developed in this area. At present there seems to be no pressing general need for more extensive legislative or regulatory action; within the EEC, the adoption of common guidelines for Good Clinical Practice provides for uniform standards of experimental evaluation. The various observational systems that have been developed for postmarketing surveillance are complementary, each with strengths and weaknesses, but with passage of time and the growth of information technology, their databases will become ever larger, and their capacity to detect toxicity will become ever more sensitive.

Evaluation of toxicity becomes easier when susceptible groups within the population can be identified. It was only comparatively recently that the special sensitivity of the elderly to adverse drug reactions was widely appreciated. Once their special risk is known, certain groups—e.g. those at the extremes of age, the diseased, the pregnant—are readily recognized. But some members of the population are susceptible to substances because of particular metabolic or immunological characteristics, and these are not distinguished by obvious physical factors. Challenges for the future may lie in identifying these individuals—e.g. by screening for enzyme deficiencies or for the presence of antibodies in plasma—and in developing strategies to avoid their exposure to substances to which they are susceptible.

REFERENCES

Acheson, E. D. (1967). *Medical Record Linkage*. Oxford University Press, London

Avorn, J., Everitt, D. E. and Weiss, S. (1986). Increased antidepressant use in patients prescribed betablockers. *J. Am. Med. Assoc.*, **255**, 357–360

Baldwin, J. A. and Acheson, E. D. (Eds) (1987). *A Textbook of Medical Record Linkage*. Oxford University Press, Oxford

Bateman, D. N., Rawlins, M. D. and Simpson, J. M. (1985). Extrapyramidal reactions with metoclopramide. *Br. Med. J.*, **291**, 930–932

Bateman, D. N., Rawlins, M. D. and Simpson, J. M. (1986). Extrapyramidal reactions to prochlorperazine and haloperidol in the United Kingdom. *Quart. J. Med.*, **59**, 549–556

Beardon, P. H. G., Brown, S. V. and McDevitt, D. G. (1988a). Post-marketing surveillance: A follow-up study of morbidity associated with cimetidine using record linkage. *Pharm. Med.*, **3**, 185–193

Beardon, P. H. G., Brown, S. V. and McDevitt, D. G. (1988b). Four-year mortality among cimetidine takers in Tayside: Results of a controlled study using record linkage. *Pharm. Med.*, **3**, 333–339

Beardon, P. H. G., Brown, S. V. and McDevitt, D. G. (1989). Gastrointestinal events in patients prescribed non-steroidal anti-inflammatory drugs: A controlled study using record linkage. *Quart. J. Med.*, **71**, 497–505

Bergman, U., Boman, G. and Wilholm, B.-E. (1978).

Epidemiology of adverse drug reactions to phenformin and metformin. *Br. Med. J.*, **2**, 464–466

Burns, L. E., Hodgman, J. E. and Cass, A. B. (1959). Fatal circulatory collapse in premature infants receiving chloramphenicol. *New Engl. J. Med.*, **261**, 1318–1321

Choonara, I. A. and Harris, F. (1984). Adverse drug reactions in medical patients. *Arch. Dis. Childhd*, **59**, 578–580

Colin-Jones, D. G., Langman, M. J. S., Lawson, D. H. and Vessey, M. P. (1985a). Post-marketing surveillance of the safety of cimetidine: twelve-month morbidity report. *Quart. J. Med.*, **54**, 253–268

Colin-Jones, D. G., Langman, M. J. S., Lawson, D. H. and Vessey, M. P. (1985b). Post-marketing surveillance of the safety of cimetidine: mortality during second, third and fourth years of follow up. *Br. Med. J.*, **291**, 1084–1088

Committee of Principal Investigators (1978). A cooperative trial in the primary prevention of ischaemic heart disease using clofibrate. *Br. Med. J.*, **40**, 1069–1118

Committee of Principal Investigators (1984). WHO cooperative trial on primary prevention of ischaemic heart disease with clofibrate to lower serum cholesterol: final mortality follow-up. *Lancet*, **2**, 600–604

Committee on Safety of Medicines (1975). *Prazosin and Loss of Consciousness*. Adverse Reactions Series, No. 12

Committee on Safety of Medicines (1983). *Mianserin (Bolvidon, Norval)*. Current Problems, No. 10

Committee on Safety of Medicines (1985). *Deaths Associated with Co-trimoxazole, Ampicillin and Trimethoprim*. Current Problems, No. 15

Committee of Safety of Medicines (1986a). *Adverse Reactions to Enalapril (Innovace)*. Current Problems, No. 17

Committee on Safety of Medicines (1986b). CSM update: Withdrawal of nomifensine. *Br. Med. J.*, **293**, 41

Craft, A. W., Brocklebank, J. T., Hey, E. N. and Jackson, R. H. (1974). The 'grey toddler'. Chloramphenicol toxicity. *Arch. Dis. Childhd*, **49**, 235–237

Crombie, I. K., Brown, S. V. and Hamley, J. G. (1984). Postmarketing drug surveillance by record linkage in Tayside. *J. Epidemiol. Comm. Hlth*, **38**, 226–231

Crooks, J., Clark, C. G., Caie, H. B. and Mawson, W. B. (1965). Prescribing and administration of drugs in hospital. *Lancet*, **1**, 373–378

Dunn, H. L. (1946). Record Linkage. *Am. J. Publ. Hlth*, **36**, 1412–1416

Echt, D. S., Liebson, P. R., Mitchell, L. B., Peters, R. W., Obias-Manno, D., Barker, A. H., Arensberg, D., Baker, A., Friedman, L., Greene, H. L., Huther, M. L., Richardson, D. L. and the CAST Investigators (1991). Mortality and morbidity in patients receiving encainide, flecainide, or placebo. *New Engl. J. Med.*, **324**, 781–787

Edwards, I. R., Lindquist, M., Wilholm, B.-E. and Napke, E. (1990). *Lancet*, **336**, 156–158

Faich, G. A. and Stadel, B. V. (1989). The future of automated record linkage for postmarketing surveillance: A response to Shapiro. *Clin. Pharmacol. Therap.*, **46**, 387–389

Felix, R. and Ive, F. A. (1974). Skin reactions to practolol. *Br. Med. J.*, **2**, 333

Finney, D. J. (1986). Statistical logic in the monitoring of reactions to therapeutic drugs. In Inman, W. H. W. (Ed.), *Monitoring for Drug Safety*, 2nd edn. MTP, Lancaster, pp. 423–442

Gardner, M. J., Hall, A. J., Snee, M. P., Downes, S., Powell, C. A. and Terrell, J. D. (1990a). Methods and basic data of case–control study of leukaemia and lymphoma among young people near Sellafield nuclear plant in West Cumbria. *Br. Med. J.*, **300**, 429–434

Gardner, M. J., Snee, M. P., Hall, A. J., Powell, C. A., Downes, S. and Terrell, J. D. (1990b). Results of case–control study of leukaemia and lymphoma among young people near Sellafield nuclear plant in West Cumbria. *Br. Med. J.*, **300**, 423–429

Goudie, B. M., Birnie, G. F., Watkinson, G., Mac-Sween, R. N., Kisssen, L. H. and Cunningham, N. E. (1982). Jaundice associated with the use of benoxaprofen. *Lancet*, **1**, 595

Guess, H. A., West, R., Strand, L. M., Helston, D., Lydick, E. G., Bergman, U. and Wolski, K. (1988). Fatal upper gastrointestinal haemorrhage or perforation among users of nonsteroidal anti-inflammatory drugs in Saskatchewan, Canada 1983. *J. Clin. Epidemiol.*, **41**, 35–43

Halsey, J. P. and Cardoe, N. (1982). Benoxaprofen: side-effect profile in 300 patients. *Br. Med. J.*, **284**, 1365–1368

Hindson, C., Daymond, T., Diffey, B. and Lawlor, F. (1982). Side effects of benoxaprofen. *Br. Med. J.*, **284**, 1368–1369

Idanpaan-Heikkila, J., Alhava, E., Olkinuora, M. and Palva, I. P. (1977). Agranulocytosis during treatment with clozapine. *Eur. J. Clin. Pharmacol.*, **11**, 193–198

Idanpaan-Heikkila, J. and Saxen, L. (1973). Possible teratogenicity of imipramine/chloropyramine. *Lancet*, **2**, 282–284

Independent Advisory Group (1984). *Investigation of the Possible Increased Incidence of Cancer in West Cumbria [Black Report]*. HMSO, London

Inman, W. H. W. (1970). Role of drug-reaction monitoring in the investigation of thrombosis and 'The Pill'. *Br. Med. Bull.*, **26**, 248–256

Inman, W. H. W. and Adelstein, A. M. (1969). Rise and fall of asthma mortality in England and Wales in relation to use of pressurised aerosols. *Lancet*, **2**, 279–285

Inman, W. H. W. and Rawson, N. S. B. (1983). Erythromycin estolate and jaundice. *Br. Med. J.*, **286**, 1954–1955

Inman, W. H. W., Rawson, N. S. B. and Wilton, L. V. (1986a). Prescription-event monitoring. In Inman, W. H. W. (Ed.), *Monitoring for Drug Safety*, 2nd edn. MTP, Lancaster, p. 217

Inman, W. H. W., Rawson, N. S. B. and Wilton, L. V. (1986b). Prescription-event monitoring. In Inman, W. H. W. (Ed.), *Monitoring for Drug Safety*, 2nd edn. MTP, Lancaster, pp. 218–223

Inman, W. H. W., Vessey, M. P., Westerholm, B. and Engelund, A. (1970). Thromboembolic disease and the steroid content of oral contraceptives. A report to the Committee on Safety of Drugs. *Br. Med. J.*, **2**, 203–209

Inman, W. H. W. and Weber, J. C. P. (1986). Post-marketing surveillance in the general population. 1. The United Kingdom. In Inman, W. H. W. (Ed.), *Monitoring for Drug Safety*, 2nd edn. MTP, Lancaster, pp. 23–25

Jick, H. (1977). The discovery of drug-induced illness. *New Engl. J. Med.*, **296**, 481–485

Jick, H. (1985). Use of automated data bases to study drug effects after marketing. *Pharmacotherapy*, **5**, 278–279

Jick, H., Madsen, S., Nudelman, P. M., Perera, D. R. and Stergachis, A. (1984). Post-marketing follow-up at Group Health Cooperative of Puget Sound. *Pharmacotherapy*, **4**, 99–100

Jick, S. S., Perera, D. R., Walker, A. M. and Jick, H. (1987). Nonsteroidal anti-inflammatory drugs and hospital admissions for perforated peptic ulcer. *Lancet*, **2**, 380–382

Julian, D. G., Pentecost, B. L. and Chamberlain, D. A. (1988). A milestone for myocardial infarction. *Br. Med. J.*, **297**, 497–498

Karch, F. E. and Lasagne, L. (1976). Evaluating adverse drug reactions. *Adverse Drug Reaction Bull.*, **59**, 204–207

Lawson, D. H. (1986). Intensive monitoring studies in hospitals. 1. The Boston Collaborative Drug Surveillance Program. In Inman, W. H. W. (Ed.), *Monitoring for Drug Safety*, 2nd edn. MTP, Lancaster, pp. 255–276

Layde, P. M., Beral, V. and Kay, C. R. (1981). Further analyses of mortality in oral contraceptive users. *Lancet*, **1**, 541–546

Layde, P. M., Ory, H. W., Beral, V. and Kay, C. R. (1983). Incidence of arterial disease among oral contraceptive users. *J. Roy. Coll. Gen. Pract.*, **33**, 75–82

Mellin, G. W. and Katzenstein, M. (1962). The saga of thalidomide. *New Engl. J. Med.*, **267**, 1184–1193, 1238–1244

Moir, D. C. (1986). Intensive monitoring in hospitals 11: the Aberdeen–Dundee system. In Inman, W. H. W. (Ed.), *Monitoring for Drug Safety*, 2nd edn. MTP, Lancaster, pp. 277–289

Nightingale, S. L. (1991). An established position: The USA Experience. In Bennett, P. N. (Ed.), *Ethical Responsibilities in European Drug Research*. University of Bath Press, Bath, pp. 29–38

Nolan, L. and O'Malley, K. (1989). Adverse drug reactions in the elderly. *Br. J. Hosp. Med.*, **41**, 446–457

Pollock, I., Young, E., Stoneham, M., Slater, N., Wilkinson, J. D. and Warner, J. O. (1989). Survey of colourings and preservatives in drugs. *Br. Med. J.*, **299**, 649–651

Porter, J. and Jick, H. (1977a). Drug related deaths among medical in patients. *J. Am. Med. Assoc.*, **237**, 879–881

Porter, J. and Jick, H. (1977b). Drug induced anaphylaxis, convulsions, deafness and extrapyramidal symptoms. *Lancet*, **1**, 587–588

Rawlins, M. D. (1988a). Spontaneous reporting of adverse drug reactions. 1. The data. *Br. J. Clin. Pharmacol.*, **26**, 1–5

Rawlins, M. D. (1988b). Spontaneous reporting of adverse drug reactions. 11. Uses. *Br. J. Clin. Pharmacol.*, **26**, 7–11

Rawlins, M. D., Breckenridge, A. M. and Wood, S. M. (1989). National adverse drug reaction reporting—a silver jubilee. *Adverse Drug Reaction Bull.*, **138**, 516–519

Ray, W. A., Griffin, M. R., Downie, W. and Melton, L. J. (1989). Long-term use of thiazide diuretics and risk of hip fracture. *Lancet*, **1**, 687–690

Ray, W. A., Griffin, M. R., Schaffner, W., Baugh, D. J. and Melton, L. J. (1987). Psychotropic drug use and risk of hip fracture. *New Engl. J. Med.*, **316**, 363–369

Report (1937). Deaths due to elixir of Sulfanilamide-Massengill. *J. Am. Med. Assoc.*, **109**, 1985–1989

Report of the Royal College of Physicians of London (1986). Research on healthy volunteers. *J. Roy. Coll. Physicians*, **20**, 243–257

Report of the Royal College of Physicians of London (1990a). *Research Involving Patients*. Royal College of Physicians, London

Report of the Royal College of Physicians of London (1990b). *Guidelines on the Practice of Ethics Committees in Medical Research involving human subjects*, 2nd edn. Royal College of Physicians, London

Rowland, M. G. M. and Stevenson, C. J. (1972). Exfoliative dermatitis and practolol. *Lancet*, **2**, 1130

Sachs, R. M. and Bortnichak, E. A. (1986). An evaluation of spontaneous adverse drug reaction monitoring systems. *Am. J. Med.*, **81** (Suppl. 5b), 49–55

Sauer, F. (1991). Ethical aspects of EEC pharmaceutical legislation. In Bennett, P. N. (Ed.), *Ethical Responsibilities in European Drug Research*. University of Bath Press, Bath, pp. 29–38

Saxen, L. (1983). Twenty years of study of the etiology of congenital malformations in Finland. In Kalter, H. (Ed.), *Issues and Reviews in Teratology*, Vol. 1, Plenum Publishing Corp., New York, pp. 73–110

Saxen, L., Holmberg, P. C., Nurminen, M. and Kuosma, E. (1982). Sauna and congenital defects. *Teratology*, **25**, 309–313

Saxen, I. and Saxen, L. (1975). Association between maternal intake of diazepam and oral clefts. *Lancet*, **2**, 498

Shapiro, S. (1989a). The role of automated record linkage in postmarketing surveillance of drug safety: A critique. *Clin. Pharmacol. Therap.*, **46**, 371–386

Shapiro, S. (1989b). Automated record linkage: A response to the commentary and letters to the editor. *Clin. Pharmacol. Therap.*, **46**, 395–398

Simpson, J. M., Bateman, D. N. and Rawlins, M. D. (1987). Using the adverse reactions register to study the effects of age and sex on adverse drug reactions. *Stat. Med.*, **6**, 863–867

Skegg, D. C. G. (1986). Medical record linkage. In Inman, W. H. W. (Ed.), *Monitoring for Drug Safety*, 2nd edn. MTP, Lancaster, pp. 291–301

Skegg, D. C. G., Richards, S. M. and Doll, R. (1979). Minor tranquillizers and road accidents. *Brit. Med. J.*, **1**, 917–919

Slone, D., Jick, H., Borda, I., Chalmers, T. C., Feinlieb, M., Muench, H., Lipworth, L., Bellotti, C. and Gilman, B. (1966). Drug surveillance using nurse monitors. *Lancet*, **2**, 901–903

Speirs, C. J. (1986). Prescription-related adverse reaction profiles and their use in risk-benefit analysis. In D'Arcy, P. D. and Griffin, J. P. (Eds), *Iatrogenic Diseases*. Oxford University Press, Oxford, pp. 93–101

Strom, B. L. and Carson, J. L. (1989). Automated data bases for pharmacoepidemiology research. *Clin. Pharmacol. Therap.*, **46**, 390–394

Taggart, H. McA. and Alderdice, J. M. (1982). Fatal cholestatic jaundice in elderly patients taking benoxaprofen. *Br. Med. J.*, **284**, 1372

Taussig, H. B. (1962). A study of the German outbreak of phocomelia. *J. Am. Med. Assoc.*, **180**, 1106–1114

Teerenhovi, L., Heinonen, E., Grohn, P., Klefstrom, P., Mehtonen, M. and Tilikainen, A. (1978). High frequency of agranulocytosis in breast-cancer patients treated with levamisole. *Lancet*, **2**, 151–152

Venning, G. R. (1982). Validity of anecdotal reports of suspected adverse drug reactions: the problem of false alarms. *Br. Med. J.*, **284**, 249–252

Venning, G. R. (1983a). Identification of adverse reactions to new drugs 1: What have been important

adverse reactions since thalidomide? *Br. Med. J.*, **286**, 199–202

Venning, G. R. (1983b). Identification of adverse reactions to new drugs 11: How were 18 important adverse reactions discovered and with what delays? *Br. Med. J.*, **286**, 289–292

Ward, S. P. (1962). Thalidomide and congenital abnormalities. *Br. Med. J.*, **2**, 646–647

Woods, C. G., Rylance, M. E., Cullen, R. E. and Rylance, G. W. (1987). Adverse reactions to drugs in children. *Br. Med. J.*, **294**, 869–870

Woollam, D. H. M. (1962). Thalidomide disaster considered as an experiment in mammalian teratology. *Br. Med. J.*, **2**, 236–237

World Medical Association (1989). World Medical Association Declaration of Helsinki: Recommendations guiding physicians in biomedical research involving human subjects. *41st World Medical Assembly, Hong Kong, September 1989*

Wright, P. (1975). Untoward effects associated with practolol administration: oculomucocutaneous syndrome. *Br. Med. J.*, **1**, 595–598

Young, E., Patel, S., Stoneham, M., Rona, R. and Wilkinson, J. D. (1987). The prevalence of reaction to food additives in a survey population. *J. Roy. Coll. Physicians Lond.*, **21**, 241–247

FURTHER READING

Bulger, R. E., Heitman, E. and Reiser, S. J. (Eds) (1993). Research with human subjects. Part VI. In *The Ethical Dimensions of the Biological Sciences*, Cambridge University Press, pp. 143–172

Royal College of Physicians (1990). *Guidelines on the Practice of Ethics Committees in Medical Research Involving Human Subjects*, 2nd edn. Royal College of Physicians, London

van Gelderen, C. E. M., Savelkoul, T. J. F. and Sangster, B. (1990). Studies in humans. II. Human volunteer studies. *Food and Chemical Toxicology*, **28**, 775–778

Wilks, M. F. and Wollen, B. H. (1994). Human volunteer studies with non-pharmaceutical chemicals: metabolism and pharmacokinetic studies. *Human and Experimental Toxicology*, **13**, 383–392

PART THREE: TOXICITY BY ROUTES

15 Parenteral Toxicity

D. Walker

INTRODUCTION

'Parenteral' is defined, for the purposes of this book, as the administration of a test substance by any route other than peroral, percutaneous and inhalational (including intranasal and intratracheal). In toxicity studies this is usually by injection but infusion and implantation are also used, either of which may or may not require surgical interference. The standard routes of injection in toxicology are intravenous, subcutaneous, intramuscular and intraperitoneal. Less frequently employed routes include intracutaneous, intra-arterial, intracerebral, intrapleural and intrathecal. Parenteral routes are commonly used to determine acute toxicity, especially of novel pharmaceutical products, whatever their intended clinical mode of administration. Such routes are not as popular as oral dosing for repeat-dose experiments, particularly life-span studies. Indications for, and disadvantages of, various routes of injection are discussed subsequently, but it is pertinent here to consider the relative merits in toxicology of oral and parenteral routes as a whole.

Ingestion is the most common, the most convenient and the safest method of drug administration in the human subject. It is also the usual route of exposure to food additives and contaminants. Therefore, it is not surprising that it is the route most favoured in animal toxicology, particularly for long-term studies. Dietary inclusion is a convenient, economical method of dosing, more practical and less stressful than repeated injections in small rodents. Nevertheless it has limitations such as chemical instability of the test substance in the diet, depression of palatability, erratic or incomplete absorption, inability of the rodent to vomit, and physiological alterations which tend to confound estimations of 'no-effect' levels. These include changes brought about in intestinal flora, laxation bulk or high osmotic load, caecal enlargement and retarded growth caused by high intake of non-digestible substances.

Parenteral injections provide the advantage of more rapid and predictable absorption. They are preferable when gastrointestinal absorption is poor, and are essential for polypeptide drugs and other compounds which are digested by intestinal enzymes or otherwise degraded and destroyed. On the other hand, parenteral formulations may necessarily include preservatives and other ingredients not required for oral drugs, and these may introduce toxicological complications. Also, careful attention to technique is necessary to avoid artefacts. Parenteral injections should be aseptic, and even so the direct introduction of exogenous substances into tissue is often irritant or necrogenic. Finally, no parenteral routes are very practical for the daily dosing of small rodents in life-span carcinogenicity studies.

The contents of this chapter have been arranged in the following sequence of sections:

Indications Although the intended clinical route determines, more than any other factor, that selected for prior toxicology, there are also indications for parenteral administration in toxicity studies on oral drugs, pesticides and industrial chemicals. Objectives include estimation of absorption, determination of mechanism, and investigation of pathogenesis. The indications for the parenteral route described in this section are intended to illustrate the experimental benefits of facility and expediency which accrue from this approach.

Techniques Injection technique is an art which by itself may determine the success or failure of an experiment. Animals are not usually co-operative subjects and, if overrestrained or underconditioned, readily become stressed. At the stage of experimental design the toxicologist should contemplate carefully the practicality of route, site and frequency of injection with respect to the chosen species model. Some practical aspects of conventional injection technique are described in this section, together with a consideration of infusion methods and a discussion on the possible introduction to toxicology of new routes reflecting novel systems of drug delivery.

Artefacts and alterations There are well-known artefacts in toxicology resulting from errors in technique or imprudent selection of route. These include with intravenous injection too rapid or perivascular injection, and intramuscularly myodegeneration and subcutaneous sarcoma. Also, the introduction of exogenous substances into tissues may exert more subtle alterations which are primarily local effects and yet have a profound influence on systemic toxicity. These may not always be anticipated, appreciated or even discovered, and it is the intention in this section to alert the unwary toxicologist to their potentially complicating properties.

Vehicles and additives Solvents and excipients often constitute a large proportion of the total volume of parenteral drug products. They are usually regarded as pharmacologically inert and conventionally in toxicity studies this is affirmed by an absence of findings in control groups. However, the vehicle is an important determinant of bioavailability, and in large or repeated doses it may result in local or systemic toxicity *per se*. The attempt in this section is not to present a toxicological review of drug formulations but to remind the reader that sometimes findings may be ascribed to a constituent other than the active principle.

Quality control tests Biological quality control tests for pyrogenicity, abnormal toxicity and local reactivity are performed usually, and often statutorily, on batch samples of finished pharmaceutical and medical products. They are included in this chapter because the specified routes of administration are almost invariably parenteral. In this section the common prescribed methods are described and subjected to critical appraisal. The descriptions have a historical flavour, and one subsection is devoted to an *in vitro* technique which is currently poised to replace the rabbit pyrogen test, perhaps the best example in toxicology of a well-validated alternative to animal use.

The theme of this chapter is an illustration of the various aspects of parenteral toxicity by a collation of published examples and personal experiences. There has been no intention to provide a comprehensive review, and it may well be that some readers will recall examples of their own more apposite than those selected. To them the apology of omission or oversight is offered in advance.

INDICATIONS

The indications for parenteral toxicity are important because the selection of route in animal studies has not always been prudent or even applicable and a correct choice is essential to achieve experimental objectives. The indications for parenteral administration in animal toxicology are a simulation of the intended route in man and veterinary species, an estimation of absorption, a determination of intrinsic toxicity, an investigation of gastrointestinal target pathogenesis, and a facilitation of certain bioassays for carcinogenicity.

Intended Route

For potential medical pharmaceutical products the dose route in the animal model should be the same as that proposed clinically for the human patient. This concept is invariable in guidelines issued by regulatory authorities concerned with the assessment and registration of new drugs. There are two main indications for parenteral therapy in man: (1) inadequate absorption of the active ingredient by the gastrointestinal tract after ingestion and (2) a clinical requirement to confine or concentrate the desired pharmacological effect in a target organ or tissue. Examples of both reasons are listed (Table 1). Veterinary medicine adds a third, that of facility, because it is often easier to inject large animals than to dose them by mouth. Also, the oral route is contraindicated for antibiotics in several animals, such as ruminants and rabbits, because digestion in these species depends considerably on a normal gastrointestinal flora.

Patients are also exposed by parenteral routes to inserted or surgically implanted medical devices which may incorporate plasticizers to impart flexibility or clarity. Low levels of phthalate esters have been detected in the tissues of patients exposed to medical devices (Jaeger and Rubin, 1970). It follows that plasticizers and/or finished products should be tested by parenteral route toxicology. A good example of this was the

Table 1   Indications for parenteral therapeutic routes

Reason	Example
Inadequate absorption after oral dosing	
Large polar molecules excreted unchanged in the faeces	Aminoglycoside antibiotics (e.g. streptomycin)
Digestion by pancreatic or intestinal proteolytic enzymes	Polypeptide hormones (e.g. insulin)
Gastrointestinal inactivation and/or hepatic conjugation	Catecholamines (e.g. adrenaline)
Gastrointestinal irritation and/or emesis	Chemotherapeutic alkaloids (e.g. emetine)
Need to target pharmacological effect	
Prompt bactericidal action in life-threatening infections	Certain antibiotics (e.g. benzylpenicillin)
Rapid depression of the central nervous system	Barbiturate anaesthetics (e.g. thiopentone sodium)
Infiltration anaesthesia, nerve block and intrathecal injection	Local anaesthetics (e.g. lignocaine)
Reversal of disturbed body fluid volume or composition	Plasma volume expanders (e.g. dextran-saline)
Intra-arterial administration for local tumour delivery	Cytotoxic drugs (e.g. vincristine)

demonstration of antifertility and mutagenicity in a dominant-lethal study on di-2-ethylhexyl phthalate injected subcutaneously in mice (Agarwal *et al.*, 1985). The oral route would have been not only inappropriate but also misleading, because the compound is hydrolysed in the intestine. Medical devices may also incorporate heavy metals such as nickel, which is oxytocic and allergenic and increases coronary artery resistance. Potential sources of repeated nickel exposure include prostheses, indwelling intravenous needles and heater tanks for dialysis fluids (Sunderman, 1983).

Estimation of Absorption

Pharmacokinetics is an integral part of toxicology and few candidate drugs escape a parenteral study in animals, whatever their intended clinical route. Frequently acute toxicity manifests itself best by a parenteral route, and intravenous injection is the most convenient procedure for determining half-life. Medical regulatory authorities invariably include, in their guidelines on testing for acute toxicity, a requirement to use at least one route which ensures systemic absorption, e.g. intravenous, intramuscular, subcutaneous. Availability has been expressed as the ratio in areas under the blood concentration–time curves between oral and intravenous routes after equivalent doses (Rowland, 1972). When the areas are equal, the drug is fully available. If the area ratio is less than unity, the drug is incompletely available because of poor absorption, metabolism on entry to the systemic circulation, or a combination of both. Similarly, good gastrointestinal absorption is indicated by comparable LD_{50}

values obtained in the same species by gavage and intraperitoneal injection, e.g. the cholinergic rodenticide phosacetim (Dubois *et al.*, 1967). Conversely, a higher parenteral LD_{50} value indicates poor availability from the injection site, e.g. subcutaneous trimethoprim (Honda *et al.*, 1973). Even intramuscular administration may occasionally provide absorption inferior to oral dosing, although this is the exception to the rule, e.g. aqueous chloramphenicol suspension in dogs (Watson, 1972).

It is well acknowledged that the absorption of drugs from diet mixtures is determined with difficulty and that comparable intravenous doses provide helpful information on first-pass gut–hepatic metabolism and biliary excretion. In the absence of a parenteral dose, the presence of drugs or metabolites in the faeces following biliary excretion might be misinterpreted as incomplete absorption after oral administration (Smyth *et al.*, 1979). Parenteral dosing is also expedient in another context with respect to absorption after ingestion. That is the situation when good absorption from the gastrointestinal tract has been established in man but not in any of the commonly used laboratory animals. Then it is more practical and economic to inject the compound into a rat than to continue searching for a species which absorbs it like man.

Tin compounds as a group illustrate well the close relation between absorption and toxicity (Winship, 1988). Only about 5 per cent of inorganic tin salts are absorbed from the gastrointestinal tract and as a result their toxicities are low. On the other hand, many of the organotin compounds are toxic, especially trimethyltin and triethyltin, which are well absorbed after ingestion.

Most of the other alkyl and aryl tin compounds are poorly absorbed from the gastrointestinal tract and are consequently less toxic by oral dosing than by parenteral administration.

Significant differences in toxicity, reflecting availability, have been demonstrated in repeat-dose studies between oral and parenteral routes, even for readily absorbed compounds. Dietary inclusion often results in a rather flat blood level curve, but intravenous or intraperitoneal injections cause high peaks followed by exponential declines. This difference was examined for lithium administered to rats over 22 weeks (Plenge *et al.*, 1981). Both functional and structural evidence of nephrotoxicity were more pronounced in the dietary group than in rats receiving daily intraperitoneal injections. It was postulated that regenerative processes were allowed to operate during the periods of very low serum lithium levels between injections, which were continuously exceeded in the dietary inclusion group. These findings were correlated with therapeutic schedules, plasma lithium levels and diuresis in manic-melancholic patients to propose that their twice-daily dose should be reduced in frequency and increased in amount.

Intrinsic Toxicity

The true toxic potential of a compound can only be assessed when it is administered in a form which is readily available for absorption and distribution to its target sites. Occupational exposure to many highly toxic industrial chemicals and pesticides is usually via oral, inhalational and percutaneous routes. Consequently, parenteral administration might be considered inappropriate to toxicological evaluations of these substances. However, these occupational routes often minimize or preclude absorption, especially when the toxic compound is formulated in an inert fluid vehicle or powder carrier. Therefore, to determine intrinsic toxicity, an essential requirement despite low risk, a parenteral route of administration may be necessary. Also, for an expensive novel compound, low-volume injections are more economical than large doses given by less absorptive routes.

Pyrethrins (pyrethrum) and their synthetic analogues (pyrethroids) have come to be regarded as one of the safest chemical classes of insecticides. Allergy to natural pyrethrum has long been known, and contact facial paraesthesia is an established occupational hazard of workers handling some of the cyanopyrethroids. Otherwise, scientifically validated cases of human systemic toxicity following peroral, inhalational or percutaneous exposure to pyrethroids are rare. Nevertheless they are extremely toxic in laboratory animals by intravenous injection. When the earliest analogues were synthesized, their acute toxicities were compared by oral and intravenous routes in rats (Verschoyle and Barnes, 1972). The intravenous LD_{50} results, and those of natural pyrethrins, were usually well below 10 mg kg^{-1} but corresponding oral values were several hundred times higher. Moreover, the intravenous effects were rapid and signs of toxicity following sublethal doses were short-lived in survivors. It was inferred that these compounds acted *per se* without metabolic activation to more toxic molecules.

Subsequently it was shown that many pyrethroids are highly potent neurotoxins but that they are rapidly metabolized to less toxic compounds by hydrolysis of a central ester bond or by oxidative attack at several sites (Gray and Soderlund, 1985). It was confirmed that intrinsic toxicity was well demonstrated by intravenous administration, which minimized metabolism, and that the oral, and even intraperitoneal, routes hindered interpretation of pyrethroid toxicity by involving complex pharmacokinetic and pharmacodynamic factors. Furthermore, it was shown that an even more target-direct parenteral route, intracerebral, could elucidate structure–activity relations. Thus, structural features which permitted rapid metabolism (e.g. *trans* substitution, possession of a primary alcohol moiety) also conferred low intrinsic neurotoxicity and those which provided metabolic stability (e.g. *cis* substitution, possession of an (*S*)-α-cyano substituent) were more toxic.

Parenteral dosing has similarly been used to confirm the predicted property of environmental contaminants to cause toxic changes by providing doses exceeding those to which workers might be exposed or which would be impractical in animal models by the inhalational route. An example of this was the exposure of Fischer–344 rats in an inhalation chamber 20 h a day, 5½ days a week, for 9 months to diluted diesel exhaust providing a maximum concentration of particulates at 1.5 mg m^{-3} (Chen and Vostal, 1981). This did not increase lung or liver microsomal activity of aryl hydrocarbon hydroxylase, which is known to be induced by polyaromatic hydrocarbons. The total mass of hydrocarbons deposited in the lung during the inhalation exposure was estimated and an equivalent dose (2 mg kg^{-1}) of extractable hydrocarbons was injected intraperitoneally daily for 4 days. Again this failed to induce the enzyme but similarly administered doses 10–50 times higher did. Ambient concentrations were estimated at levels approximately 100 times lower than those to which the rats were exposed. Thus, hazard was demonstrated and risk was determined negligible.

Gastroenteric Target Pathogenesis

Perhaps the most common clinical symptoms of drug toxicity in human patients, even at therapeutic dose levels, are nausea and vomiting. Occasionally these may be accompanied by pathological changes such as gastric and intestinal erosion or ulceration. Nausea following ingestion of a medicine may indicate local mucosal irritation but frequently it is the result of a central effect after absorption or a combination of both mechanisms. It is well recognized in, and a considerable cause of discomfort to, cancer patients receiving intravenous cytotoxic drugs. Common culprits include cisplatin, dacarbazine, cyclophosphamide, doxorubicin, fluorouracil, etc. Necrosis and desquamation of intestinal epithelium have been demonstrated in laboratory animals following parenteral administration of nitrogen mustards, and their emetic property in patients has been attributed to stimulation of the central nervous system. Cyclophosphamide causes nausea and vomiting with equal frequency following intravenous injection or ingestion. Intravenous fluorouracil therapy may cause oral or colostomic stomatitis, proctitis and possible enteric injury at any level. These gastrointestinal effects of cytotoxic drugs have been summarized (Calabresi and Parks, 1975).

Another pharmaceutical class, the non-steroidal anti-inflammatory drugs, is notorious for its property of inducing gastric ulceration and emesis. The nausea caused by salicylates involves receptors in both the gastric mucosa and the brain medulla, the former stimulated by direct irritation. In man centrally induced nausea and emesis appear at plasma salicylate concentrations of about 0.27 mg ml^{-1} but the same effects may occur at much lower levels as a result of local irritation (Woodbury and Fingle, 1975).

It is most likely that many novel candidate oral drugs in these or other classes will possess similar undesirable properties, and this poses a double problem for the toxicologist—their detection and pathogenesis. Detection is hindered by the inability of the rat to vomit and by its gastric differences from man, anatomical and chemical. The investigation of pathogenesis must necessarily involve a parenteral route, if only to negate a purely local mechanism. Gastric ulceration caused by aspirin after oral dosing is well documented in man and rat, and yet, despite prolonged and prolific use of the drug, the pathogenesis of its lesion is still incompletely understood. However, the parenteral route has made significant contributions. These include the demonstration that both aspirin and sodium salicylate, its hydrolysis product, cause gastric mucosal injury in rats by intravenous injection but only in the presence of luminal acid. Also, pretreatment with exogenous prostaglandin, either by intraluminal instillation or by subcutaneous injection, has a protective effect which is complete against aspirin and incomplete against sodium salicylate (Rowe *et al.*, 1987).

Another example of gastrointestinal lesions evoked by either oral or parenteral routes has been provided from the acute toxicology of the trichothecene toxin T-2 (Fairhurst *et al.*, 1987). LD$_{50}$ values in rats, mice and guinea-pigs by intravenous, intragastric, subcutaneous, intraperitoneal and intratracheal routes ranged between 1 mg kg^{-1} and 14 mg kg^{-1}. Oral sublethal doses caused pigeons to vomit and produced lymphocytolysis and mucosal ulceration in the gastrointestinal tract of rats. The latter recalled similar descriptions in various species after parenteral dosing, and so it was inferred that these changes in the gut were not due to the luminal presence of T-2. A possible explanation offered was biliary excretion of an active metabolite.

Carcinogenesis

Regulatory authorities require evidence of lifespan carcinogenicity studies in experimental animals, by the intended clinical routes, for new drugs which are to be given to man continuously or intermittently for prolonged periods or which have chemical structures suggestive of a carcinogenic potential. Most of these are formulated for ingestion, which minimizes practical difficulties of animal dosing. However, parenteral products in these categories create an experimental problem, because of the relatively small size of rodents, the animals in which the majority of carcinogenicity studies are now conducted. This limits the availability of injection sites and repetitive dosing is likely to lead to local intolerance. Fortunately, the intravenous route is required infrequently. For instance, it is unnecessary to test for carcinogenicity cytotoxic drugs which may be given repetitively by this route. Also, the intraperitoneal route, not favoured in man, is inappropriate, although it has been used in animals for carcinogenicity studies on poorly absorbed materials. The subcutaneous route is more popular but may provide sarcomas which do not represent true carcinogenic potential (see below). The intramuscular route is compromised by the limited availability of sites and the probability of local reaction following repetitive injections (see below). This might be avoided by a restriction of dosing to twice weekly or the use of a larger species such as the dog, but the latter is not a serious alternative. Remote tumours in the dog have been induced by parenteral injections but routine use of dogs as a model for carcinogenesis is precluded by a prolonged latent period of up to 10 years and the prohibitive cost which this would incur (Bonser, 1969).

Although parenteral routes are not easily incorporated in routine or standard protocols for carcinogenicity, they have been invaluable in the investigation of mechanisms. This applies particularly to the polycyclic hydrocarbons, which require relatively few administrations to exert their effects and are characterized by short periods of latency. For example, in the Syrian hamster a genetic influence was discovered by the difference in mean latency from 9 to 15–16 weeks between various inbred strains simply by single subcutaneous injections of 9,10-dimethyl-1,2-benzanthracene (Homburger, 1972). Also, in the same species and by the same route an inverse relationship was demonstrated between mean induction time of nasal or laryngeal tumours and dose of diethylnitrosamine after only 12 weekly injections (Montesano and Saffioti, 1968).

Another popular experimental application of the parenteral route is the expediency of localizing carcinogens to their target tissues with the objectives of confining tumours to the organ under study, increasing yields and foreshortening latent periods. Thus, via surgical intervention in rats, local adenocarcinomas have been induced by direct implantation of 7,12-dimethylbenzanthracene crystals in the pancreas (Dissin et al., 1975), and squamous cell carcinomas have been produced in the lung by intrapulmonary injection of 3-methylcholanthrene in beeswax pellets (Hirano et al., 1974).

A similar target approach via parenteral methods was used to investigate the effects of asbestos and so circumvent the technical demands of inhalation toxicology. Mesotheliomas were first induced in the rat by direct intrapleural application of dusts (Wagner, 1962). Then it was discovered, almost fortuitously, that two subcutaneous injections in mice of 10 mg asbestos suspended in 0.4 ml saline, one in each flank and repeated twice at intervals of 5 weeks, produced extensive inflammatory and proliferative changes in the pleural and peritoneal serosae within 2 years (Roe et al., 1967). These were much more conspicuous than local inflammatory and neoplastic reactions at the administration sites, which the experiment was designed to investigate. Thus, the unexpected transport of fibres from subcutis to serosa facilitated further the study of asbestos pathogenesis. Other workers in this field reverted to direct implantation of the rat visceral pleura with asbestos carried on fibrous glass pledgets and, after numerous experiments by this technique, inferred that its carcinogenicity was primarily related to structure shape rather than physicochemical properties (Stanton and Wrench, 1972).

Parenteral carcinogenicity testing would be incomplete without a mention of the once-fashionable, now almost obsolete, neonatal mouse test. A small dose of the test substance was injected into subcutaneous tissues or into the peritoneal cavity, once within 24 h of birth, and the mice were allowed to live for about a year. Sometimes supplementary injections were administered over the first week or two. The appeal of this assay was the small quantity of compound required, the restricted dosing and a reduction in the adult study duration. There was a common belief that newborn animals were more responsive to carcinogens than adults, but a review of 30 studies, mostly on genotoxic agents, did not confirm this unequivocally (Toth, 1968). Despite some enthusiasm for the method and its application to food additives, with the attribution of hepatocarcinogenicity to safrole (Epstein *et al.*, 1970), doubts about its value and validity grew. An increased incidence of liver cell tumours in mice parenterally exposed at birth was regarded as unreliable evidence of carcinogenic potential (Roe, 1975). Finally, it was concluded that the range of neoplasms produced was restricted, that induction of common tumours was not a good indication of carcinogenicity and that the neonate might react differently to the adult because of its immunological and enzymatic immaturity (Grasso and Grant, 1977). Now it would appear that the neonatal mouse test has fallen into disuse.

TECHNIQUES

The common parenteral routes in toxicology are intravenous, subcutaneous, intraperitoneal and intramuscular. It is not intended here to describe in detail the numerous techniques for these routes in the various species of animal used in toxicity studies, because there is a plethora of relevant scientific publications. Moreover, most techniques have been collated in several standard texts on laboratory animals, to which the interested reader is referred. These include the rabbit (Bivin and Timmons, 1974), the rat (Kraus, 1980) and most species, with good illustrations (Green, 1979) and useful tabular summaries of injection sites, needle sizes and suggested maximum volumes (Flecknell, 1987). These texts describe techniques applicable to all scientific procedures or to anaesthetization. The following remarks apply specifically to toxicology.

Injection Technique

Intravenous

Numerous veins have been suggested for intravenous injections in the various laboratory species but some of them, in small rodents, necessitate sedation or anaesthesia and surgical exposure. As such they are unsuitable for routine toxicology, where the important criteria of technique are simplicity, often repeatability, and always avoidance of undue stress. In conscious animals the author's

preferred veins for repeated injections are: lateral caudal in mice and rats, marginal ear in rabbits and guinea-pigs, cephalic in dogs, saphenous in marmosets and alar in chickens. Injection may be facilitated in rodents by warming the animal or its tail to promote vasodilation and by simple restraint systems, all of which are well described in publications on animal technology. Successful intravenous injections rely on simple preparations such as clipping or shaving fur, good illumination, slight magnification, sharp needles and swabbing with surgical spirit, which not only provides asepsis but also renders veins more conspicuous. A series of injections into a frequently used vein should follow a cycle of distal to proximal. In this way it is possible to deliver large volumes (over 40 ml) into the same vein of pyrogen test rabbits twice a week almost indefinitely. The administration of large volumes to fractious or frightened animals may be facilitated by a break in the needle, connecting the cut ends with flexible polythene tubing (Nicholls, 1970). The speed of intravenous injection has a profound effect on acute toxicity (see below).

Subcutaneous

Injections into the subcutaneous tissues are considerably easier, even in small rodents. The advised site in all toxicology species is the dorsal neck or back. The technique is to pick up a tent of loose skin and to inject into it, but care is necessary to avoid passing the needle through the two layers. The injected area is usually massaged and large volumes can be divided to multiple sites. It should be noted that absorption may vary with site, because different LD_{50} values have been reported for dorsal and ventral subcutaneous injections in mice (Balazs, 1970).

Intraperitoneal

The intraperitoneal route is sometimes regarded as hazardous because there is a risk of penetrating viscera such as liver, intestines or urinary bladder. In practice, with the subject firmly restrained in dorsal recumbency and the use of a small needle carefully inserted, such errors are infrequent. The risk may be reduced further by prior starvation but great care is necessary injecting viscous or oily fluids, which require heavy pressure on the plunger of the syringe. Probably of more concern to the toxicologist is the extreme sensitivity of the peritoneum, which may react to some compounds by acute shock or severe local reaction, so confounding systemic toxicity. The intraperitoneal route is preferred to intravenous injection in neonatal rats, since their veins are so small. It is a hazardous technique, although an unconventional dorsal approach claims safety (Hornick, 1986).

Intramuscular

The usual sites for intramuscular injection are the same for virtually all laboratory animals used in toxicology. They are the posterior thigh muscles and the quadriceps. The former, usually providing the larger muscle mass, is favoured more frequently but is disadvantageous, because there is a risk of hitting the sciatic nerve or delivering the injected material into a fascial plane. These pitfalls may be avoided by careful consideration of anatomy or by injecting into the quadriceps, although this approach seems to be more painful. Intramuscular injections may penetrate blood vessels but the risk of this is difficult to estimate. The simple precaution of withdrawing the plunger of the syringe before depressing it is not always reliable when fine needles enter small blood vessels. Local reaction to intramuscular injection merits much attention in veterinary medicine (see below).

Other Routes

Less frequently used routes of injection utilized in toxicology include intrapleural, intra-arterial, intrathecal, intracerebral and intracerebroventricular. These are not common in standard protocols and are more frequently employed in studies on mechanisms. Anaesthesia and surgical exposure are usually necessary. Actual techniques are often described in the methods sections of papers on relevant toxicity studies.

Infusion Systems

One prime objective of clinical pharmacology is the maintenance of a fairly constant blood concentration of the drug within an established therapeutic range. Blood levels below this are ineffectual and those above it may be toxic. This objective is not difficult to achieve with drugs which have a prolonged half-life but compounds which are rapidly excreted may thwart it. Necessarily drugs have to be administered by inconvenient regimens with short intervals between doses, and this may result in unacceptably high

peaks in blood levels. The problem is exaggerated in some animal models in which the half-life of certain drugs may be more than an order of magnitude less than that in man (Nau, 1983).

Attempts to avoid excessive fluctuations in blood level have been the main thrust in the emergence, over the last decade or more, of a whole new industry developing novel delivery, particularly rate-controlled, systems (Urquhart, 1982). Examples of their application in human therapy include insulin for diabetic ketoacidosis, cisplatin for solid tumours, nitroglycerine for angina and scopolamine for motion sickness. Even veterinary medicine has been influenced, with slow or pulsed release of anthelmintics and trace elements from glass bullets or corrosive devices residing in the ruminant stomach. The rate-controlled methods are mainly conventional infusion systems and implanted devices. It is reasonable to expect that drugs intended for these systems should be tested for toxicity in similar animal models, but such methods at present are not common in routine toxicology. Presumably cost and impracticability are deterrents. Nevertheless they offer attractive features, not the least of which is the means by which steady states of rapidly excreted compounds may be achieved.

The basic components of an intravenous infusion system in laboratory animals are a flexible indwelling securely anchored cannula, an extension line usually burrowed subcutaneously to a convenient point of exit, an electrically operated infusion pump, and a mechanical contrivance to permit movement and prevent self-mutilation. Clinical microprocessor-controlled pumps may be used despite their large size, because they will deliver as little as 0.1 ml h^{-1}. Like injection techniques and choice of veins, infusion systems in laboratory animals are the subject of many publications, although few of them apply to toxicology. Most suffer to varying extents from the disadvantages of anaesthesia, surgical exposure and postoperative complications of leakage and stress. Favoured veins in the rat are the jugular, femoral and caudal. At least one non-surgical method has been described in this species, providing continuous infusion for a week via the lateral caudal vein (Rhodes and Patterson, 1979).

Presumably the impracticality of conventional infusion systems in laboratory animals will always preclude their routine use in toxicology, but they have permitted valuable insights into mechanisms, particularly of cytotoxic drugs, because they provide the means by which protracted delivery may be compared with bolus injection. Some comparative studies with this objective have shown little difference in host toxicity between the two methods, e.g. for doxorubicin, cytosine arabinoside and neocarzinostatin in a rat model of acute myelogenous leukaemia (Ensminger *et al.*, 1979). In others toxicity was reduced by continuous infusion, e.g. the pulmonary fibrogenesis of bleomycin, the cardiac toxicity of doxorubicin and the myelosuppression of fluorouracil (Carlson and Sikic, 1983). Similarly, infusion LD_{50} values of alkylating agents were lowered by bolus injections, e.g. mechlorethamine, phenylalanine mustard and carmustine (Valeriote and Vietti, 1985). However, it should not be assumed that infusion is invariably less toxic. A 24 h infusion of fenoldopam mesylate administered at a rate of 0.005 mg kg^{-1} min^{-1} (total 7.2 mg kg^{-1}) caused medial necrosis in the splanchnic arteries of rats but daily intravenous injections of 20 mg kg^{-1} for 12 days had no effect (Yuhas *et al.*, 1985). Presumably these differences are functions of variable rates of enzyme induction and detoxification.

Intravenous infusion systems have also proved their worth in the toxicology of addictive drugs by providing the means for self-administration through lever-activation. By this method cocaine was found to be considerably more toxic to rats than heroin (Bozarth and Wise, 1985).

Osmotic Minipumps

An attractive alternative to intravenous infusion is the subcutaneous implantation of self-powered miniature diffusion cells (Pinedo *et al.*, 1976) or osmotic minipumps (Ray and Theeuwes, 1987). Some of these devices are small enough to implant into mice. The necessary surgery is simple and the duration of anaesthesia is brief.

A range of Alzet miniature osmotic pumps is commercially available. The smallest, which is suitable for mice, measures 17 mm × 6 mm, has a reservoir capacity of 0.1 ml and pumps at a rate of 0.001 ml h^{-1} for 3 days. Larger versions, for dogs, will deliver either 0.005 ml h^{-1} for 2 weeks or 0.0025 ml h^{-1} for 1 month. Each pump consists of a collapsible impermeable reservoir surrounded by concentrated sodium chloride invested by a semipermeable membrane (Figure

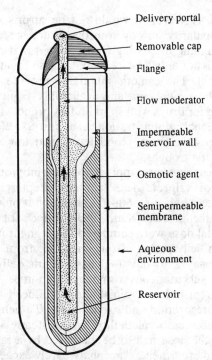

Figure 1 The Alzet osmotic minipump (cross-section). Reproduced by permission of Charles River UK Ltd

1). The reservoir is filled with the test substance by injection and capped with the flow moderator, and then the pump is implanted. The osmotic agent imbibes tissue water which gradually compresses the reservoir and displaces its contents through the delivery portal. Rate and duration of delivery are preset at manufacture. Duration may be extended by serial implantation. Osmotic minipumps are usually implanted subcutaneously or intraperitoneally, but can be fitted with simple catheters for delivery to remote target sites, e.g. intravenous, intracerebroventricular, into solid organs, etc. They are produced in sterile packs and manufactured from tissue-compatible components. The wall of the elastomeric reservoir is inert to most aqueous drug formulations, dilute acids, bases and alcohols, but is incompatible with natural oils.

Osmotic minipumps are advantageous over infusion systems by virtue of their simplicity of insertion, particularly an absence of any cumbersome external connections, so that the test animal is unrestricted and less stressed. Nevertheless their use in toxicology is not widespread. Probable reasons for this include cost, necessity for serial implantation and incompatibility with oily vehicles. However, it would not be surprising if their popularity improved in the future, because it is becoming increasingly appreciated that drug toxicity is not only dose-related, but also regimen-dependent. The osmotic minipump provides the means by which constant availability could be achieved for drugs with short half-lives and whose conventional administration results in a cycle of high, possibly toxic, blood levels and low sub-therapeutic troughs.

This concept was applied to the embryotoxicology of valproic acid, an antiepileptic drug which has a half-life of 8–16 h in man but only 48 min in the mouse (Nau, 1983). Effects of the same total dose were compared in pregnant mice between daily subcutaneous injections from gestational day 7 to day 14 and constant delivery from a subcutaneous osmotic minipump. The intermittent bolus administration produced high rates of resorption and exencephaly. To achieve comparable embryolethality by the steady state system, the dose had to be increased by a factor of 10 and even then exencephaly barely exceeded control values. Similar results were obtained in pregnant rats with sodium salicylate (Gabrielsson *et al.*, 1985). Unlike valproic acid, this drug is pharmacokinetically similar in man and rodent. Its fetal adverse effects following daily intravenous injections were reduced by constant delivery into the jugular vein via an indwelling catheter from a subcutaneous osmotic minipump. The difference was more evident at the lower analgesic dose of 75 mg kg^{-1} day^{-1} than at the higher antirheumatic level of 150 mg kg^{-1} day^{-1}.

These examples may illustrate the most apposite application of osmotic minipumps to toxicology, because conventional bolus dosing at a brief time of embryo susceptibility could exaggerate teratological properties. However, other applications have been described. The pulmonary fibrogenic effect of bleomycin injected into tumour-bearing mice was significantly reduced by continuous infusion of the same total dose from an osmotic minipump (Sikic *et al.*, 1978). Conversely, lung damage in rats injected subcutaneously with paraquat was increased by a similar dose delivered from an osmotic minipump (Dey *et al.*, 1982). Obviously the effect of dosing regimens on toxicity is drug-specific and the contrivance of steady state availability may increase or decrease it. The future contribution to toxicology of rate-control systems such as osmotic mini-

pumps and transdermal devices is difficult to predict. Suffice it to say that any means of improving species bioequivalence which circumvents differences in metabolism, absorption and excretion must improve the model.

ARTEFACTS AND ALTERATIONS

Many sequelae of parenteral injections are the effects of technique or local perturbation which either modify systemic toxicity of the test substance or completely misrepresent it. Obviously the toxicologist must be fully aware of such potential artefacts and alterations. The common examples are intravenous rapid injection, subcutaneous sarcoma, intramuscular reaction and intraperitoneal sensitivity. There are also other more subtle changes which are not always anticipated or even considered in the determination and description of toxic effects.

Intravenous

One of the therapeutic, and consequently toxicological, reasons for intravenous injection is the introduction into the bloodstream of hypertonic, irritant or even vesicant solutions, because the endothelium is relatively refractory and the drug is rapidly and greatly diluted. It follows that careful technique is necessary to avoid partial perivascular injection with its possible consequences of local inflammatory reaction in and around the sensitive venous adventitia. This might not influence acute toxicity but it could end prematurely the experimental life of affected animals in repeat-dose studies or pyrogen testing laboratories. Lesions at the caudal vein site of administration were found in over 50 per cent of 1422 rats injected daily for 4 weeks with a variety of test articles (Kast and Tsunenari, 1983). They included periphlebitis, phlebitis, cushion-like swellings of the intima and thrombosis with hair penetration of the caudal vein wall.

The physicochemical properties of intravenously administered substances are important considerations. Oily vehicles are contraindicated and drugs which either precipitate blood constituents or haemolyse erythrocytes should not be injected by this route. Nevertheless emulsions of vegetable oil, lecithin and water or saline have been given intravenously to the dog. Other considerations include total volume, osmolarity and acidity (Balazs, 1970). Overwhelming volumes should be avoided and hypotonicity may increase toxicity, but a wide range of pH is permissible for slowly administered solutions. Concentrated solutions of compounds with low aqueous solubility may precipitate in the blood. The effect of this on toxicity was described for the pyrethroid cismethrin in rats (Gray and Soderlund, 1985). Its intravenous injection in a concentrated form reduced acute toxicity and delayed its onset. This was attributed to initial precipitation in the pulmonary capillaries and subsequent slow release into the bloodstream before final distribution to target nervous tissue.

Pulmonary embolism of hair and skin fragments is another pathological artefact of intravenous injection which has been recognized in experimental mice, rats, rabbits and dogs. Pulmonary thromboarteritis and/or giant cell granulomas with hair or skin particles were discovered in over 25 per cent of 1422 rats after daily injections in the caudal vein for a month (Kast and Tsunenari, 1983). Pathologists should note that this incidence was derived from the examination of single left lobe sections, so that the true percentage of affected rats was probably higher. Findings were similar in rabbits injected through an ear vein but the incidence was lower.

Regimen-dependence and differences in toxicity between bolus dosing and continuous infusion have been discussed above. One determinant of these differences is the actual delivery speed of administration and the effect this has on activating detoxification or compensatory mechanisms. It is well recognized that the rapidity with which many compounds are injected intravenously profoundly influences their acute toxicities. This is one reason why the intravenous median lethal dose is almost as much a function of technique as it is of a compound's inherent toxicity. Despite this, it is surprising how few reports on acute toxicity are qualified by any mention of injection speed, let alone its measurement. In general, intravenous administration should be slow but this is subject to wide interpretation. Slow has been defined as not more than 0.02 ml s^{-1} with concomitant advice for a limit on total volume of 0.1–0.5 ml for rodents and 2 ml for larger laboratory animals (Balazs, 1970). However, it should be considered that, for some drugs, a slow infusion might equilibrate with the

rate of detoxification and so nullify a toxic response. Moreover, there are exceptional indications for rapid injection. One such was the requirement to simulate the clinical accident of injecting local anaesthetics intravenously. For this a dog model was used (Liu *et al.*, 1983). It was demonstrated that the toxicities of lignocaine (lidocaine), etidocaine, bupivacaine and tetracaine for the canine central nervous system were directly proportional to their human anaesthetic potencies.

There are probably numerous examples of too-rapid intravenous injection in toxicology, mostly unpublished. Pyrogen test technicians are very familiar with the lethal consequences in rabbits of injecting adrenaline, potassium salts and other products too fast. The author was once requested to investigate the death of a racehorse after the reputedly rapid intravenous injection of a veterinary multivitamin preparation (Walker, 1981). Injection of the diluted product into the caudal vein of mice at a volume rate of 12.5 ml kg^{-1} had no effect when the speed of delivery was timed at 0.025 ml s^{-1}. When this was increased to 0.167 ml s^{-1}, the same dose approximated the LD_{50}.

Similarly, with infusions it might be expected that acute toxicity would relate positively to the time rate of delivery. Probably for many drugs this holds but sometimes results are confusing, if not anomalous. Thus, in mice perfused via a caudal vein with phytic acid at a total constant dose of 0.28 mg g^{-1} convulsive deaths occurred when the delivery rate was approximately 0.03 mg g^{-1} min^{-1} but not when it was reduced to <0.02 mg g^{-1} min^{-1} or increased to >0.05 mg g^{-1} min^{-1} (Gersonde and Weiner, 1982). The observed toxicity was consistent with the ability of phytic acid to bind calcium, and the seemingly anomalous result was tentatively ascribed to the rapidity with which hypocalcaemia elicited the compensatory response of parathyroid hormone secretion.

By a completely different mechanism, mechanical rather than pharmacological, the delivery rate of an intra-arterial infusion may determine its toxicity, particularly its topographical distribution. The cerebral distribution of ^{14}C-labelled iodoantipyrine was investigated in rhesus monkeys infused via the cervical segment of the internal carotid artery (Blacklock *et al.*, 1986). After a slow infusion of 0.4 ml min^{-1} isotope deposition in the ipsilateral hemisphere was markedly heterogeneous, but a fast rate of 4 ml min^{-1}, and retrograde needle direction to promote mixing, produced uniform distribution. The authors attributed the heterogeneous deposition to drug streaming within the internal carotid artery and its branches. They suggested that this might be the cause of focal cerebral and retinal toxicity sometimes observed in patients treated for brain tumours by slow intra-arterial chemotherapeutic infusion.

Subcutaneous

Clinically the subcutaneous route is used for non-irritant drugs. It provides a reasonably even slow rate of absorption which may be retarded further by various techniques such as the combination of zinc and protamine with insulin or the incorporation of vasoconstrictor agents in formulations of local anaesthetics. In toxicology it is the route of choice for drugs which are intended for subcutaneous administration and is also used for oral compounds which are poorly absorbed from the gastrointestinal tract of the animal model. The subcutaneous tissues of rats and other animals readily react to the introduction of an irritant with the formation of a sterile abscess, particularly when the formulation is designed to provide a depot. This type of abscess is the result of necrotic tissue attracting a purulent exudate. It may occur even after intraperitoneal injection when an irritant such as oxytetracycline leaks into the subcutis from the needle as it is advanced through the body wall (Porter *et al.*, 1985). Subcutaneous infection is not so common, even though aseptic technique is sometimes disregarded in toxicology. Nevertheless it has been recorded as, for example, in dogs which received a daily subcutaneous injection of suspended cortisone acetate for three or four weeks (Thompson *et al.*, 1971).

The most notorious artefact of subcutaneous injections in toxicology is the sarcoma of carcinogenicity studies, particularly those conducted in the rat. The subcutaneous method came into fashion 50 years ago to demonstrate the carcinogenicity of substances whose chemical structure suggested this property but failed to exhibit it when applied topically like the coal-tar derivatives. Then it became used to screen drugs, food additives and other chemicals for carcinogenicity. Eventually it was realized that numerous substances which induced subcutaneous sarcomas in rodents, after repeated injections of high doses, were not intrinsically carcinogenic. The method fell into disrepute and is now used less frequently and with more caution in its interpretation.

The unravelling of this phenomenon and the postulation of a pathogenesis constituted a comprehensive review which cited numerous subcutaneous studies (Grasso and Golberg, 1966). Most of the following remarks are excerpts from this thorough publication. The authors defined three physical categories of materials which had been shown to induce subcutaneous sarcoma: water-soluble compounds, substances which dissolved initially and then came out of solution at the injection site, and implanted solids. The water-soluble compounds included hypertonic solutions of various sugars and saline, food colours and aldehydes, although some positive results from earlier studies were not confirmed by later work. The tumorigenic water-soluble substances exhibited three common factors: neoplasms were restricted to local sarcomas, they resulted from the frequent administration of high doses and they had latent periods of about 40 weeks. Examples of materials which came out of solution to accumulate at the injection site as foreign bodies were carboxymethylcellulose and iron-dextran. Examples of implanted solids included many plastics and other materials, which appeared to produce sarcomas irrespective of their chemical composition. Their tumorigenic property seemed to depend more on physical characteristics such as shape and size.

Pathogenetic studies on the reaction of implanted solids were particularly enlightening. The gradual development of a thick connective tissue capsule invariably preceded tumour formation by several months. This was an essential step in tumorigenesis, because sarcomas did not appear if the capsule failed to develop or if it was surgically excised. Moreover, once the capsule had fully formed, removal of the implant did not prevent the malignant outcome. It was suggested that a similar mechanism operated in the induction of sarcomas by repeated injections of fluid. It was postulated that frequent repetitive trauma of young fibroblasts at the injection site impeded normal repair and eventually disrupted the homoeostatic forces controlling these cells so that their autonomous proliferation ensued.

The problem was, and still is, a distinction between the consequence of this 'indirect' mechanism and the effects of 'true' carcinogens which act directly on intracellular receptors at the injection site. Interpretation is facilitated when true carcinogens induce remote tumours. When local tumours alone develop, it is necessary either to confirm carcinogenicity by demonstrating dose-dependence or to refute it by establishing the nature of an indirect mechanism as described above.

The authors of this review concluded that malignant transformation of subcutaneous fibroblasts could be induced by implanted or repeatedly injected materials either by virtue of their carcinogenic properties or through non-specific physical or physicochemical factors. They further inferred that the neoplastic outcome of physicochemical insults which derange normal fibrosis did not constitute a carcinogenic property. These conclusions were soon affirmed in a WHO publication which recommended that the routine testing of food additives and contaminants by subcutaneous injection should be considered inappropriate unless this was necessary to circumvent poor gastrointestinal absorption (World Health Organization, 1967). This recommendation would seem to be equally appropriate to the testing of drugs, and indeed a subsequent WHO publication addressed the potential invalidity of pharmaceutical studies which resulted in local sarcomas alone (World Health Organization, 1969). The conclusions of the review authors have stood the test of time, now over 20 years, and remain basically unchanged (Grasso, personal communication).

Intramuscular

After intramuscular injection drugs in aqueous solution are soon available but absorption from oils and repository suspensions is protracted. Isotonic and slightly hypertonic solutions are better tolerated than hypotonic formulations, and even irritant compounds, precluded from the subcutaneous route, may be injected into muscle. The intramuscular route is well used in human patients but is more favoured by veterinary practice because of its practicality in large animals. It has been claimed that actual site of intramuscular deposition is an important determinant of bioavailability but, although differences between muscles have been demonstrated for a few drugs in some species, this is not invariable. For example, gentamicin is equally absorbed from the longissimus dorsi and biceps femoris muscles of dogs (Wilson *et al.*, 1989). In toxicology, intramuscular administration is indicated for the study of novel drugs intended by this route, but the relatively small mass of muscle available in rats and rabbits limits the frequency of injection, even of non-irritant drugs. This is one reason why it has not been widely adopted for carcinogenicity studies, although it should be noted that rhabdomyosarcomas have been induced in rats by this route following single injections of cobalt salts and repeated doses of triphenylmethane food dyes (Magee, 1970).

Those well-recognized artefacts of intramuscular injection, accidental intravascular injection and trauma of the sciatic nerve, have already been mentioned in the section on technique (see above). Both occur in clinical, especially veterinary, medicine. The high risk of injecting the sciatic nerve by overpenetrating the posterior thigh muscles has been emphasized in the cat (Baxter and Evans, 1973) and in the weanling pig (Van Alstine and Dietrich, 1988), with consequent advice to prefer the quadriceps and neck sites, respectively.

There is a similar danger of nerve damage in most laboratory species used for toxicology. The author gave rats single injections of licensed tetracycline into the posterior thigh muscles at a high dose rate of 50 mg kg^{-1} (Walker, 1973). Paralysis was almost immediate, characterized by flexion of the lateral digits, and subsequently improved but was still evident a week later, when histopathology of the injection sites revealed necrotic foci surrounded by inflammatory cells and regenerating muscle fibres. This reaction is typical of myonecrogenic drugs, irrespective of damage to the sciatic nerve. The rabbit, with its relatively large dorsal mass of lumbar muscle, is preferable for local toxicology. This model was used to predict human tolerance to different esters of clindamycin by single injections of 50 mg in 1 ml (Gray *et al.*, 1974). Within 24 h the normal range of serum creatine phosphokinase (62 ± 19 iu l^{-1}) was markedly elevated by clindamycin 2-phosphate (to 1500 iu l^{-1}) and clindamycin hydrochloride (to 4100 iu l^{-1}). The authors inferred that an activity of >3000 iu l^{-1} in the rabbit test would be too irritant in the human and that values <2000 iu l^{-1} would be clinically tolerable. They emphasized the sensitivity of this assay by advice to handle the animals carefully.

Allusion has been made to the prominence of the intramuscular route in veterinary therapeutics. This merits special attention not only because it so often results in muscle damage, but also because there is a related aspect of drug residues in food animals, a matter of considerable current concern to consumer and legislator. Consequently, the rest of this subsection is apportioned entirely to the clinical toxicology of local intramuscular reaction caused by veterinary pharmaceutical products.

A myonecrogenic property is common in licensed veterinary parenteral antibiotics and has been well documented, especially by Danish workers. It has been shown that most preparations of penicillin, streptomycin and their combinations are relatively innocuous after intramuscular injection of pigs and cattle, but tetracycline, oxytetracycline, erythromycin and tylosin cause severe local reaction: necrosis occurs within 6 days and scarring at 3 weeks (Rasmussen and Høgh, 1971). These findings were confirmed in a subsequent histopathological study which revealed, on the sixth day, fibrovascular proliferation and myoregeneration after penicillin and streptomycin but necrosis surrounded by demarcating reaction after the other antibiotics (Svendsen, 1972). In the porcine sites there were foreign-body giant cells and, when the vehicle was oily, cyst formations in the demarcating zones. After 3 weeks the more severe reactions had become thick layers of scar tissue surrounding residual foci of necrosis. Subsequent studies provided similar findings in the hen (Blom and Rasmussen, 1976) and added sulphonamides, trimethoprim and their potentiating combinations to the list of myonecrogenic products (Rasmussen and Svendsen, 1976).

Local reaction is not confined to antibiotics and chemotherapeutic agents. It has also been ascribed to vaccines, vitamins, metallic salts and other compounds. Iron in various formulations is commonly injected into the ham muscle of piglets a few days old to prevent anaemia, although modern recommendations are for alternative sites. The local reaction to some of these preparations is, within 24 h, acute inflammation, hyaline myodegeneration and siderophagocytosis, but there are claims that careful attention to injection technique, particularly direction of delivery

towards the popliteal lymph node, is mitigating (Schmitz *et al.*, 1976). Acute myodegeneration and fatal hyperkalaemia may also occur in vitamin E-deficient piglets injected by the intraperitoneal route with iron-dextrose, but this is an entirely different pathogenesis, possibly peroxidation (Patterson *et al.*, 1971).

Another metal commonly used in veterinary medicine which forms irritant salts is copper. The sheep is particularly susceptible to its deficiency and toxicity. The pharmaceutical search for suitable parenteral compounds to prevent swayback in lambs provided a choice between soluble but systemically toxic salts and safer but less efficacious complexes (Suttle, 1981). An example of the latter was the copper salt of methionine, which causes undesirable reactions in sheep and cattle. The pathogenesis of these lesions was investigated by the author (Walker, 1975). Single 0.02 ml injections were administered into the posterior thigh muscles of rats providing a dose rate of 2 mg kg^{-1} (Cu), about twice the ovine recommendation. Within 3 days the reaction was a central blue focus of unabsorbed copper methionine surrounded by necrotic tissue. On the fourth day this changed strikingly to liquefaction, which progressed for 2 weeks as necrotic tissue became copious sterile pus. Then the abscess resolved, to leave a small dry residual nodule of large vacuolated histiocytes and foreign material. Eventually this disappeared completely and the absence of scar tissue was remarkable by contrast with the effects of antibiotics described above.

Intraperitoneal

Although the peritoneal cavity provides a large surface area through which drugs may be readily absorbed, it is not a common parenteral route in human medicine. Reasons for this include its sensitivity to irritants, a danger of infection and a proclivity to form adhesions. Even so, it is a valuable route for dialysis in the treatment of drug overdosage and for total parenteral nutrition when intravenous feeding is compromised by catheter sepsis or venous thrombosis. A rabbit model has been used to evaluate intraperitoneal nutrition (Stone *et al.*, 1986). In toxicology the intraperitoneal route is used more frequently than intended clinical administration might dictate, probably because it may achieve absorption comparable to intravenous injection and is technically simpler. It has not been widely adopted for carcinogenicity studies, because it does not correspond with the usual exposures to drugs, food additives and pesticides. However, it has found application in the study of genotoxic carcinogens and in the determination of promoting activity. It has been shown, for example, that the antioxidant butylated hydroxytoluene enhances the formation of lung tumours in mice after a single dose of ethyl carbamate irrespective of route, intraperitoneal or oral (Witschi, 1981).

The accidental risk of penetrating viscera by the intraperitoneal route has been mentioned above in the section on techniques. This error in rats was investigated by injecting viscous oily iodinated radiopaque media into the left caudal quadrant of the peritoneal cavity (Lewis *et al.*, 1966). Radiographs revealed that some of the contrast media was not injected into the peritoneal cavity in 20 per cent of animals. Misdirected material was discovered mainly in the gastrointestinal tract, but also in retroperitoneal, subcutaneous and intravesical sites. Insoluble materials injected into the peritoneal cavity rapidly elicit focal granulomatous plaques on visceral and parietal surfaces. Foreign-body granulomas so caused by single injections in young rodents may persist for life. However, the artefact of most concern to the toxicologist is acute peritonitis.

The typical inflammatory reaction of the rat peritoneum to the introduction of an irritant was observed by the author, determining the acute toxicity of copper methionine by this route (Walker, 1976). Within hours of a single injection peritoneal fluid was increased, and in survivors a week later adhesions of the liver lobules were invariably present. Acute peritonitis may be so severe that it contributes to lethality. This occurred following the intraperitoneal injection of sterigmatocystin in rats (Purchase and van der Watt, 1969). Then the investigator is presented with a dilemma of interpretation; should the lethal contribution be regarded as an integral feature of toxicity or should it be disregarded as an artefact of administration? The dilemma may be resolved by injecting another group intravenously to accord a gratuitous effect to the intraperitoneal route.

This was strikingly illustrated by the injection of copper acetate in chicks (McCormick and Fleet, 1988). Mortality following a single dose of 1.84 mg kg^{-1} (Cu) was 46 per cent by intraperi-

toneal injection but only 4 per cent by intravenous administration, even though the accumulation of copper at 24 h in total hepatic tissue and cytosol was comparable for both routes. Copious peritoneal fluid, equivalent to 41 per cent of total plasma volume, was observed 1–3 h after intraperitoneal injections but not after intravenous administrations. The peritoneal fluid was assumed to be plasma, because it was clear, was amber-coloured and lacked red blood cells. The authors were impressed by the extent and rapidity with which this fluid formed, postulated its pathogenesis by increased permeability of peritoneal capillaries, and inferred that death was caused by haemoconcentration, not by hepatotoxicity.

Another difference between these routes was demonstrated by the administration of lead acetate to mice (Maintani *et al.*, 1986). Following a single dose of 30 mg kg^{-1} (Pb), the intraperitoneal injection induced twice as much metallothionein in the liver as did the intravenous administration despite a lower hepatic concentration of the metal. This difference prompted the authors to suggest a role of leucocytic endogenous mediator or interleukin 1, produced by peritoneal leucocytes, for metallothionein induction.

The intrapleural route has often been used in toxicology to circumvent inhalation exposure but, like the peritoneum, the pleura is highly sensitive. This was shown in anaesthetized rats by the intrapleural instillation, via a surgical incision, of 2 μm inert polystyrene microspheres suspended in sterile phosphate buffered saline (Valdez and Lehnert, 1988). Lavage of the intrapleural space, 24 h after instillation, revealed a threefold increase in the population of free cells, particularly polymorphonuclear leucocytes but also mononuclear phagocytes. Even the saline vehicle alone caused a 40 per cent increase in the number of pleural cells.

VEHICLES AND ADDITIVES

Basically a parenteral drug is a sterile solution, suspension or emulsion of an active constituent in a carrier described as a vehicle or excipient. The formulation may also include other ingredients such as suspending or emulsifying agents, preservatives, antioxidants, buffers and chelating compounds. Usually these additives are incorporated in such small amounts that they have no toxic effects either experimentally or clinically. Therefore, there is no attempt here to list them or to review their inherent toxicities. Vehicles, on the other hand, often constitute a considerable proportion of the formulation, are vital determinants of bioavailability and, consequently, merit more attention. It is assumed that their pharmacological activity is minimal, and this is usually confirmed by negative findings in control groups conventionally dosed with the vehicle alone. However, the examples cited in this section should alert toxicologists to the potential influences which vehicles may exert on systemic or local toxicity.

Ideally the vehicle should be compatible with the active constituent and should possess no toxic effects at the recommended clinical dose. Also, novel drugs should be tested for toxicity in the vehicle proposed for the final product. Sometimes initial studies may suggest a change in formulation. If this involves vehicle substitution, then bioavailability and toxicity studies must be repeated, because such a change can have profound effects on the release pattern of the active constituent. For example, when a lyophilized water-soluble glycinate salt of chloramphenicol became available in veterinary medicine to replace the customary solution of propylene glycol, it was found that both the duration and magnitude of plasma antibiotic concentrations were significantly increased in dogs after intramuscular injection (Bergt and Stowe, 1975).

Excipient Solvents

The term 'excipient' is usually defined as any more or less inert substance included in a formulation in order to confer a suitable consistency or form to the product. It also has a wider application to embrace substances with slight pharmacological activity, and probably this is more apposite in toxicology. Even water, the essential or true excipient of aqueous solutions, influences toxicity by its effect on osmolarity. The intravenous injection of rats with distilled water, at a volume rate of 1 ml kg^{-1}, induces hypotensive bradycardia, and its LD_{50} value in mice is 44 ml kg^{-1} compared with 68 ml kg^{-1} for isotonic saline (Balazs, 1970). Thus, the intravenous injection of 1 ml hypotonic solution might kill a mouse simply because of its excipient action. Moreover, such overwhelming volumes should be avoided, even

by intravenous infusion, because excessive hydration may alter renal clearance.

Aqueous excipients also have local effects, albeit more detectable biochemically than morphologically. Thus, single 1 ml injections of normal saline and sterile water into the dorsal muscles of rabbits raised, within 24 h, serum creatine phosphokinase activities from a normal level of 62 ± 19 iu l^{-1} to 223 iu l^{-1} and 537 iu l^{-1}, respectively (Gray *et al.*, 1974). Among the non-aqueous solvents, vegetable oils and polyethylene glycol are probably the most pharmacologically inert. Mineral oils, because of their intolerable effects at the injection site, have now been abandoned as vehicles except as inflammatory adjuvants for experimental vaccines. Vegetable oils are common vehicles for intramuscular injections, and polyethylene glycols are used for the subcutaneous and intravenous routes. The solubility of water-insoluble components often increases exponentially with increasing concentrations of solvent in water. Thus, to reduce dose, the concentration of a non-aqueous solvent may be kept up to 40 per cent. However, the dose of such a solvent should not exceed 20 per cent of its LD_{50} value (Balazs, 1970). Compatibility of solutions incorporating non-aqueous solvents with plasma should be investigated *in vitro* before definitive formulation.

Glycerol formal is another common organic solvent for experimental drugs and provides a good example of the variable influence which a vehicle may confer on toxicity according to its application and route of administration. In general, it is regarded as rather inert, and this was illustrated by its negligible effect in dose volumes of up to 0.2 ml kg^{-1} on the acute intravenous toxicities of various pyrethrins and pyrethroids in rats (Verschoyle and Barnes, 1972). Moreover, by the intraperitoneal route, it increased the LD_{50} value of cismethrin above that determined by oral dosing, a contrary expectation for pyrethroids (Gray and Soderlund, 1985). On the other hand, glycerol formal administered intramuscularly to the pregnant rat was embryotoxic and teratogenic in positive relation to dose from 0.25 ml kg^{-1} to 1.0 ml kg^{-1} per day (Aliverti *et al.*, 1978). This prompted the authors to recommend more teratology on solvents proposed for toxicity studies.

Another undesirable property of glycerol formal, which it shares with other vehicles such as propylene glycol, is local irritancy. Propylene glycol is completely miscible with water and dissolves in many oils. It used to be a common vehicle for veterinary antibiotics such as chloramphenicol and oxytetracycline. The well-known painful response by animals to intramuscular injections of these formulations was attributed, at least in part, to the propylene glycol base (Bergt and Stowe, 1975). Glycerol formal, which contributes 75 per cent of the vehicle for certain potentiated sulphonamides, has been similarly implicated. Both of these solvents cause intramuscular necrosis. This was demonstrated in pigs 6 days after injections with 5 ml doses of 33 per cent glycerol formal and 40 per cent propylene glycol (Rasmussen and Svendsen, 1976). Loss of creatine phosphokinase from the intramuscular site of rabbits injected with propylene glycol or glycerol formal has been proposed as a predictive tool for local toxicity (Svendsen *et al.*, 1978).

Oily Vehicles

Parenteral drugs with a poor aqueous solubility are commonly formulated in vegetable oils as solutions, suspensions or emulsions. Oil is slowly absorbed from an intramuscular or subcutaneous injection site, and the duration of pharmacological action of drugs dissolved or emulsified in oily vehicles is prolonged by comparison with that of aqueous formulations. When a drug, dissolved entirely in an oily solvent, is injected into muscle, it is partitioned between the oil and the surrounding aqueous tissue phase and then absorption occurs mainly via the latter, followed by diffusion through capillaries. The absorption rate of the oily solvent itself, such as methyl oleate, is much slower than that of the drug dissolved in it (Tanaka *et al.*, 1974).

It has been assumed that the fate of injected oil was a local metabolic degradation, phagocytosis and absorption into the blood. It is now known that some of it is absorbed into the lymphatic system, although this may be a minor pathway. The first human case history of lymphadenopathy following repeated oil-based injections was a 17-year-old male who presented with an enlarged left inguinal lymph node (Ahmed and Greenwood, 1973). The lymphadenopathy was a foreign body giant cell reaction to cystic spaces which contained neutral fat and it was attributed to therapy for diabetes insipidus by regular self-administered injections of pitressin tannate in arachis oil into the left thigh.

Then a comprehensive study was performed in dogs, rabbits and rats on the fate of vegetable oils after intramuscular injection (Svendsen and Aaes-Jørgensen, 1979). The vehicles tested were sesame oil, containing mainly long-chain saturated and unsaturated fatty acids such as oleic and linoleic, and a commercial product, composed only of short-chain fatty acids, particularly caprylic and capric. In different experiments administration was single or repeated, sometimes ^{14}C-labelled, and detection of oil was by histology, including frozen sections, liquid scintillation counting and autoradiography. Pulmonary oil microembolism occurred in dogs injected with either vehicle intramuscularly once a week for 6 months at a volume dose rate of 0.45 ml kg^{-1}. The iliac lymph nodes in the sesame group were enlarged and cystic, owing to the presence of oil. Pulmonary microembolism was also detected in rabbits and rats injected three times a week for 2 and 5 weeks, respectively. The authors concluded that both vehicles caused pulmonary microembolism by a lymphogenic pathway despite different absorption characteristics. However, the doses were considerably higher than those recommended clinically for most depot preparations and were administered more frequently.

Quite apart from its own fate, the oil used as a drug vehicle may exert secondary or remote effects which the unwary toxicologist could miss. In a 74 week study on progesterone, beagles were injected subcutaneously and aseptically daily in different dorsal sites with the hormone dissolved in 90 per cent ethyl oleate, 7 per cent ethanol and 3 per cent benzyl alcohol (Capel-Edwards *et al.*, 1973). The vehicle volume dose rate was 0.07 ml kg^{-1} up to week 36 and 0.2 ml kg^{-1} thereafter. Reactions at the injection sites occurred in all dogs, including controls injected with the vehicle alone, especially after the increase in dose volume at 37 weeks. They included sterile abscesses which ulcerated and healed. The ensuing haematological changes included neutrophil leucocytosis, increased erythrocyte sedimentation rate, mild anaemia, haemosiderosis and thrombocytosis. These were interpreted as representing a low-grade chronic inflammatory condition and, since they occurred in control as well as progesterone-treated animals, were regarded as secondary effects of the subcutaneous reaction caused by the oily vehicle.

Other Ingredients

Examples of some common non-vehicular ingredients of parenteral drug formulations are as follows: the preservatives chlorocresol, benzoic acid, sorbic acid, phenol, benzethonium chloride and the esters of parahydroxybenzoic acid; the antioxidants sodium metabisulphite and formaldehyde sulphoxylates; the chelating agents citric acid and disodium ethylenediamine tetraacetic acid. Many of these compounds are toxic but they rarely increase pharmaceutical toxicity, because of their low inclusion rates. Moreover, dilution may decrease toxicity. For example, the intraperitoneal LD_{50} values determined in the rat for sodium metabisulphite, an antioxidant added to solutions for peritoneal dialysis, were 498 ml kg^{-1}, 650 ml kg^{-1} and 740 ml kg^{-1} for 25 per cent, 5 per cent and 1.25 per cent solutions, respectively (Wilkins *et al.*, 1968). However, the toxicologist should not disregard minor ingredients of novel formulations and should always consider their potential roles in unexpected circumstances. For instance, the consumption of a single meal containing only 1 per cent benzoic acid may be fatal to the cat (Clarke, 1975) Also, it should be noted that autoclaving parenteral solutions may alter the relative proportions of constituents.

The author encountered one case of preservative toxicity, albeit in a statutory quality control test without clinical repercussions (Walker, 1979). The test, on allergen extracts, required no deaths in five mice, each weighing approximately 20 g, within 24 h of 1 ml intraperitoneal injections of the final product. Infrequently, but expensively, batches failed and phenol, incorporated in the product at a 0.4 per cent concentration, was thought to be responsible. An intraperitoneal LD_1 for phenol was determined as 190 mg kg^{-1}. This suggested that one in every 100 mice might die from phenol toxicity *per se*; i.e. one in 20 batches of extract would fail irrespective of any allergen toxicity. As a result the test dose was reduced.

QUALITY CONTROL TESTS

Biological quality control tests are conducted routinely, and usually statutorily, on batch samples of finished pharmaceutical and biological products and on medical devices or extracts prepared from them. They are also performed on drugs and materials undergoing development, but less frequently. The statutory obligations are compliance with pharmacopoeial methods or other official standards. These tests are designed to provide a broad screen for the detection of microbiological, endotoxic or chemical contamination and misformulation which might result in overdosage. Their objectives are variously described as verifications of freedom from 'unexpected or unacceptable biological reactivity' and 'abnormal or undue toxicity'. Collectively and historically, they have probably been of considerable benefit in the protection of patients from contaminated parenteral injections and tissue implantations, but conceivably their future role may diminish as chemical analyses and microbiological assays become increasingly sophisticated as a result of good manufacturing practice. For each type of test there are numerous variations on a theme, which include differences between national pharmacopoeias and modifications of these official methods by the quality control departments of the manufacturers. Most biological quality control tests may be distinguished from other more or less standard toxicological protocols by their dependence on numerical pass–fail criteria, of either magnitude (e.g. temperature response in pyrogen tests) or frequency (e.g. lethality in safety tests). Usually, but not invariably, their interpretation does not require toxicological or pathological expertise. Nevertheless they are included in this chapter because almost invariably their methods involve parenteral routes.

The most commonly conducted biological quality control tests are for pyrogenicity of parenteral products in rabbits, abnormal toxicity of pharmaceuticals in mice, safety of biologicals in guineapigs, muscle implantation of medical devices in rabbits and intracutaneous reactivity of rubber or plastic extracts in rabbits. These tests are described and evaluated below. There are other tests in this broad category which, because of their relatively infrequent use, are not appraised here. These include blood pressure response to depressor substances in cats and anaphylaxis of potential allergens in guinea-pigs. Few regulatory authorities now seem to require the traditional methods of antigenicity testing (Ronneberger, 1977).

The Pyrogen Test

The rabbit pyrogen test has been used extensively now for nearly 50 years, principally to detect bacterial endotoxins in finished pharmaceutical parenteral products. In fact, the method is probably the oldest and most frequently used protocol in animal toxicology. Even so, its demise is being hastened by the increasing adoption of an alternative *in vitro* technique. Most pyrogens are bacterial endotoxins, lipopolysaccharide components of Gram-negative bacteria. They are potent ubiquitous substances, resistant to steam sterilization, and readily contaminate parenteral solutions from inadequately treated water and raw materials. A positive response in the rabbit test may be obtained with tap-water. The necessity for high-quality water to carry parenteral drugs was recognized by the detection of pyrogens in rabbits and the attribution of a microbiological origin to them (Seibert, 1923). This led to the design and adoption of the rabbit pyrogen test in a standard protocol which was first officially recognized in the US Pharmacopeia in 1942.

The suitability of the rabbit model was thoroughly investigated by a direct comparison of the response between man and animal following the intravenous injection in both species of purified endotoxins in various doses. The endotoxins were prepared from *Salmonella typhosa, Escherichia coli* and *Pseudomonas* (Greisman and Hornick, 1969). Human volunteers were inmates of a house of correction. The experimental design included a recognition of differences between the species such as circadian influence in man and emotional lability in the rabbit. It was found that, on a unit body weight basis, rabbit and man were similarly sensitive to threshold pyrogenic quantities of endotoxin. This work, preceded and succeeded by thousands of pyrogen tests on numerous products, validated the rabbit model.

The objective of the rabbit pyrogen test is the measurement of temperature rise following intravenous aseptic injection of sterile test substance. Official methods are well described in current editions of pharmacopoeias (e.g. British Pharmacopoeia, 1988; European Pharmacopoeia, 1986;

United States Pharmacopeia, 1990). Dose rates for licensed products are prescribed in the pharmacopoeial monographs and those for developmental compounds are usually determined by the clinical intention or an increase on this below the level of acute intravenous toxicity. Other protocols include extraction procedures for medical devices (e.g. British Standard 5736/5, 1982) and limitations on the reuse of rabbits previously exposed to antigenic materials or cytotoxic drugs (Personeous, 1969).

All methods require the initial use of three rabbits preconditioned to the technique. Minimum weights are stipulated but neither sex nor breed is specified. Injections are administered in a marginal ear vein at volume rates of between 0.5 ml kg^{-1} and 10 ml kg^{-1}. Temperatures are recorded by rectal thermocouple or thermister probe thermometers at intervals for up to 90 min before injection (to derive the baseline: initial or control) and for 3 h afterwards (to determine the maximum). The difference between the maximum and the initial (BP) or control (USP) temperature is the response. Differences between the British and American methods comprise rabbit conditioning before definitive use, rabbit qualification according to previous use, rabbit eligibility with respect to baseline temperature, pass–fail criteria of summed or individual response, and retest requirements following an inconclusive result. The prolonged perpetuation of these differences has little to commend it, since the specifications were set arbitrarily and each method has been used extensively to test numerous identical products. Fortunately, both methods address the biological vagaries of the rabbit model. Thus, environmental conditions are specified to allay excitement, conditioning is obligatory, and reuse, which improves the reliability of response (Weary and Wallin, 1973), is neither discouraged nor permitted so frequently that it might influence sensitivity (Webb, 1969). Also, immature rabbits, which are significantly more resistant than mature animals to endotoxic pyrogens (Greisman and Hornick, 1969), are precluded from use.

The rabbit pyrogen test has been managed traditionally in some laboratories by quality control chemists or microbiologists, not toxicologists, and this may be one reason why some of its limitations and contraindications are not always recognized. Several substances and even whole drug classes thwart the test objective by their inherent pharmacological, toxicological or antigenic properties. Examples compiled from relevant publications (Personeus, 1969; Cooper *et al.*, 1971) and the author's own experiences are listed (Table 2).

The LAL Test

Injection fever, a hazard of parenteral administration first recognized in the latter part of the nineteenth century, is now part of medical history. The occurrence in patients of febrile reactions to injections has been eliminated by a combination of decontaminating parenteral water, batch pyrogen testing of finished products and aseptic administration technique. The contribution of the rabbit test is difficult to assess but it has probably been considerable. Now, however, its replacement by an *in vitro* technique seems imminent.

The search for an alternative method was prompted by the high cost of the rabbit test in labour and time; its shortcomings, which have been tabulated; its non-quantitative nature; and perhaps latterly a modern inclination to avoid the use of live laboratory animals. However, the precipitant factor for this search was the inapplicability of the rabbit test to short-lived radiopharmaceuticals. This led directly to the first successful application of an *in vitro* alternative (Cooper *et al.*, 1971). It was based on the discovery by previous workers that a lysate of circulating amoebocytes from the horseshoe crab, *Limulus polyphemus*, reacted in aqueous media with picogram quantities of endotoxin to form a gel. Limulus amoebocyte lysate (LAL) became commercially available and its use to test a variety of parenteral products was soon investigated. Excel-

lent correlation was obtained with results by the rabbit test after due allowance was made for the greater sensitivity of the LAL method (Eibert, 1972).

In 1973 the US Food and Drug Administration declared LAL a biological product, subject to licensing requirements, which could be used voluntarily by pharmaceutical manufacturers for the in-process testing of drugs but which was not suitable to replace the rabbit test. This provided the means of gaining experience in the use of LAL and establishing a database. Its production was improved considerably, and modern yields of LAL now consistently exceed 100 times the original endotoxin sensitivity. More extensive correlations with the rabbit test were recorded (Mascoli and Weary, 1979) and in 1980 recognition by the US Pharmacopeia was a significant benchmark. In 1987 a guideline was published on the validation of LAL testing on end-products for human and veterinary drugs, biological products and medical devices (United States Food and Drug Administration, 1987). These set forth acceptable conditions for its use in lieu of the rabbit test. At about the same time official methods were prepared in America and Europe which are now published under the heading of 'Bacterial Endotoxins' (European Pharmacopoeia, 1987; United States Pharmacopeia, 1990).

The LAL test was not described in the 1988 British Pharmacopoeia, although its use was suggested for radiopharmaceuticals intended for administration into cerebrospinal fluid (British Pharmacopoeia, 1988). However, an edited version of the European method appeared in the 1989 Addendum (British Pharmacopoeia Addendum, 1989). The introduction to this stated: 'It is expected that this *in vitro* test will find progressive

Table 2 Pharmacological and iatrogenic interference with the rabbit pyrogen test

Drug class	Example	Complicating effect on pyrogen test
Antipyretic analgesics	Certain steroids	Reversal of pyrogenic response
Hypnotics and anaesthetics	Phenothiazines	Hypothermia decreasing normal temperature
Antigenic agents	Plasma proteins	Potential anaphylactic reaction on reuse
Cytotoxic drugs	Mitozantrone	Progressive nephropathy with reuse
Acutely toxic substances	Potassium salts	Death by too-rapid injection
Miscellaneous	Amphotericin B	Hyperthermia increasing normal temperature

application in appropriate monographs of both the British and European Pharmacopoeias in place of the *in vivo* test for pyrogens.'

Thus, it seems that we are about to witness a considerable substitution of the long-established rabbit test by an *in vitro* technique which must be one of the best-validated alternatives of all those introduced to toxicology during the last two decades. The regulatory authorities have been prudent to insist on a prolonged delay before its official adoption, and even now it is not certain that the LAL test will replace the rabbit method completely. It will not, for example, detect pyrogenicity attributable to chemical contamination, particulate matter and live Gram-positive bacteria, although these exclusions may be largely overcome by good manufacturing practice. Other limitations of the LAL test have been identified (Assal, 1989) and it seems likely that a minority of substances will require the rabbit method for some time yet.

Abnormal Toxicity Tests

The abnormal toxicity or safety test is, by modern toxicological standards, a relatively crude assay, simple and cheap to conduct but completely nonspecific in its objective. A typical method for general pharmaceuticals is the intravenous injection of five mice and their subsequent observation for one or two days. If no mouse dies, the batch is released. Traditionally for biological products two guinea-pigs also are injected, by the intraperitoneal route. Extracts prepared from medical devices are tested in two groups of mice: test or sample (extract) and control or blank (extractant). For each of the above three product categories there are slight, but incongruous, differences in the national method specifications (Table 3). The quantity of test substance to be injected is specified by the individual monograph, except that the dose for a biological product may be the label recommendation subject to a maximum volume, as tabulated. Body weights, when stipulated, are very approximately 20 g for mice and 300 g for guinea-pigs. The delivery rate for intravenous injections in mice, unless otherwise prescribed, is 0.02–0.03 ml s^{-1}. In most specifications there is a provision for retest when results are inconclusive, and usually the American versions require more animals than the initial number tested.

National variations in the methods probably have minimal influence on the outcome, but there is little merit in their perpetuation and they frustrate laboratories routinely testing to international specifications. The value of the abnormal toxicity test is difficult to assess but almost certainly it has detected contamination or misformulation. However, in this author's experience, failures are extremely rare and usually attributable to faulty technique or intentional overconcentration of active ingredient or preservative to validate the method. The test does not seem to have attracted much scientific appraisal. Good injection technique is essential to avoid spurious results, and the importance of animal acclimatization or conditioning has been emphasized by its effect on body weight which, in some specifications, must not decrease over the test duration (Prasad *et al.*, 1978).

Local Reaction Tests

Intracutaneous tests in rabbits on polar and nonpolar extracts of medical devices and plastics are the local equivalents of the systemic toxicity or systemic injection methods in mice. Specified methods of extraction and extractants (Table 3, footnote) are identical. Two rabbits are used for each type of extractant and intracutaneous injections of 0.2 ml are administered in the clipped dorsal skin. The effects of the injections are compared after 24 h, 48 h and 72 h between the test or sample extract on one side of the spinal column and the control or blank extractant on the other. The British method (British Standard 5736/4, 1981) specifies ten test and five control injection sites per rabbit; the American method (United States Pharmacopeia, 1990), five for each. In both methods the local effects of erythema and oedema are accorded standard numerical ratings and the mean difference between test and control sides determines the outcome.

Implantation tests in rabbits are also required for medical devices and plastics, but in this case to evaluate the local effects of direct contact between solid samples and muscle tissue. The British specification (British Standard 5736/2, 1981) is for medical devices intended for long-term implantation, such as hip prostheses, and for short-term use within the body or in contact with mucosal surfaces, such as urinary catheters. The American specification (United States Phar-

Table 3 Summary of British, European and American tests for abnormal toxicity or safety

Reference[a]	Title of test	Number and species	Dose and route[b]	Test duration	Pass criteria
General pharmaceuticals					
BP 1988, A184	Abnormal Toxicity Method A	5 mice	0.5 ml iv	24 h	No deaths
EP 1986, V.2.1.5	Abnormal Toxicity General	5 mice	0.5 ml iv	24 h	No deaths
BP(Vet.) 1985, A121	Abnormal Toxicity Method A	5 mice	ns iv	24 h	No deaths
USP 1990, 1500	Safety (non-biologics)	5 mice	0.5 ml iv	48 h	Neither deaths (0/5) nor toxicity ($\leqslant$1/5)
Biological products					
BP 1988, A185	Abnormal Toxicity Method B	5 mice	$\leqslant$ 1 ml ip	7 days	Neither deaths nor
		2 guinea-pigs	$\leqslant$ 5 ml ip	7 days	signs of ill-health
EP 1986, V.2.1.5	Abnormal Toxicity Human Use Immunosera and Vaccines	5 mice	$\leqslant$ 1 ml ip	7 days	Neither deaths nor
		2 guinea-pigs	$\leqslant$ 5 ml ip	7 days	signs of ill-health
EP 1986, V.2.1.5	Abnormal Toxicity Veterinary Use Immunosera and Vaccines	5 mice	0.5 ml sc	7 days	Neither deaths nor
		2 guinea-pigs	$\geqslant$ 2 ml ip	7 days	significant local or systemic reaction
BP(Vet.) 1985, A121	Abnormal Toxicity Method B	5 mice	0.5 ml ip	7 days	Neither deaths nor
		2 guinea-pigs	5 ml ip	7 days	signs of ill-health
BP(Vet.) 1985, 159	Safety (non-avian vaccines)	$\geqslant$2 target	cr $\times$ 2	$\geqslant$7 days	No abnormal reaction
USP 1990, 1500	Safety (biologics)	$\geqslant$2 mice	0.5 ml ip	7 days	No loss of weight,
		$\geqslant$2 guinea-pigs	5 ml ip	7 days	unexpected response or deaths
Extracts of solids					
BS 5736/3, 1981	Systemic Toxicity (medical devices)	6 mice $\times$ 2 groups	50 ml kg^{-1} iv/ip[c]	3–14 days	No pathological or clinical differences between extract and extractant groups
USP 1990, 1499	Systemic Injection (elastomeric plastics)	5 mice $\times$ 2 groups	50 ml kg^{-1} iv/ip[c]	72 h	No reaction to sample significantly greater than that to blank

[a] BP = British Pharmacopoeia (1988); EP = European Pharmacopoeia (1986); USP = United States Pharmacopeia (1990); BP(Vet) = British Pharmacopoeia (Veterinary) (1985); BS 5736/3 = British Standard 5736 Part 3 (1981).

[b] iv = intravenous; ip = intraperitoneal; sc = subcutaneous; ns = not specified (refer to monograph); cr = clinical recommendation (label).

[c] Route of injection in the tests for medical devices (British) depends on the extractant (and therefore the extract): iv for polar (saline), ip for non-polar (sesame or cottonseed oil). Additional extractants are specified for plastics (American): alcohol in saline iv and polyethylene glycol 400 ip.

macopeia, 1990) is for plastics and other polymers intended for fabricating containers or their accessories, and for use in medical devices, implants and other materials. The American method stipulates the aseptic implantation of four sterile smooth sample strips, each measuring 10 mm $\times$ 1 mm, at intervals on one side of the spinal column and two similar negative control strips on the opposite side. Implantation is via wide-bore hypodermic needles into the paravertebral muscles of two healthy adult rabbits. The animals are killed after a minimum period of 72 h and, following a delay for bleeding to cease, the implantation sites are dissected. The material passes the test if, in each rabbit, the reaction to not more than one of the four sample strips is significantly greater than that to the control material. The British method is similar but specifies not fewer than three rabbits, additional implantation of positive control strips (such as tin-stabilized polyvinylchloride), a duration of 7 days, and histology of the sites if any macroscopic reaction to the test material is negative. It also advocates a less objective assessment of the results. The anaesthetic suggested is pentobarbitone (pentobarbital) but the neuroleptic–analgesic combination of fluanisone and fentanyl citrate is preferable because it is safer in rabbits and reversible.

In the author's experience one problem of the implantation test is a tendency for the strips to migrate from their implantation sites, even to subcutaneous positions, and this often prolongs the search for them. Nevertheless it is an effective detection system for toxic ingredients of solid materials which leach in contact with tissue fluid. It is important to recognize the microscopic effects of the standard negative control strips (additive-free polyethylene). These are typical of skeletal muscle in contact for a week with a foreign body and comprise mild mononuclear cell infiltration, multinucleated giant cell formation, fibroplasia, slight dystrophic calcification, muscle fibre atrophy and centripetal migration of sarcolemmal nuclei. Also, traumatic haemorrhage is common. Positive reactions are similar but more pronounced and additionally include focal necrosis and exudation, particularly of heterophils. It is a useful test, not only for finished products, but also to identify unacceptable changes in formulation or manufacturing process such as the introduction of chlorinating cycles to remove bloom on latex catheters (Walker, 1982).

REFERENCES

Agarwal, D. K., Lawrence, W. H. and Autian, J. (1985). Antifertility and mutagenic effects in mice from parenteral administration of di-2-ethylhexyl phthalate. *J. Toxicol. Environ. Hlth*, **16**, 71–84

Ahmed, A. and Greenwood, N. (1973). Lymphadenopathy following repeated oil-based injections. *J. Pathol.*, **111**, 207–208

Aliverti, V., Bonanomi, L. and Mariani, L. (1978). Teratogenic evaluation of glycerol formal in the rat. *Proc. 20th Cong. Europ. Soc. Toxicol., Berlin*, Abstract No. 84

Assal, A. N. (1989). Comments on pyrogen testing methods. *Anim. Tech.*, **40**, 129–131

Balazs, T. (1970). Measurement of acute toxicity. In Paget, G. E. (Ed.), *Methods in Toxicology*. Blackwell, Oxford, pp. 49–81

Baxter, J. S. and Evans, J. M. (1973). Intramuscular injection in the cat. *J. Small Anim. Pract.*, **14**, 297–302

Bergt, G. and Stowe, C. M. (1975). Comparison of bioavailability of two chloramphenicol preparations on dogs after intramuscular injection. *Am. J. Vet. Res.*, **36**, 1481–1482

Bivin, W. S. and Timmons, E. H. (1974). Basic biomethodology. In Weisbroth, S. H., Flatt, R. E. and Kraus, A. L. (Eds), *The Biology of the Laboratory Rabbit*. Academic Press, New York, pp. 76–77

Blacklock, J. B., Wright, D. C., Dedrick, R. L., Blasberg, R. G., Lutz, R. J., Doppman, J. L. and Oldfield, E. H. (1986). Drug-streaming during intra-arterial chemotherapy. *J. Neurosurg.*, **64**, 284–291

Blom, L. and Rasmussen, F. (1976). Tissue damage at the injection site after intramuscular injection of drugs in hens. *Br. Poult. Sci.*, **17**, 1–4

Bonser, G. M. (1969). How valuable the dog in the routine testing of suspected carcinogens? *J. Natl Cancer Inst.*, **43**, 271–274

Bozarth, M. A. and Wise, R. A. (1985). Toxicity associated with long-term intravenous heroin and cocaine self-administration in the rat. *J. Am. Med. Assoc.*, **254**, 81–83

British Pharmacopoeia (1988). Vol. II. HMSO, London, 1074, A183-A185

British Pharmacopoeia Addendum (1989). HMSO, London, A132

British Pharmacopoeia (Veterinary) (1985). HMSO, London, 159, A120-A121

British Standard 5736/2 (1981), 5736/3 (1981), 5736/4 (1981), 5736/5 (1982). British Standards Institution, London

Calabresi, P. and Parks, R. E. (1975). Alkylating agents, antimetabolites, hormones, and other antiproliferative agents. In Goodman, L. S. and Gilman, A. (Eds), *The Pharmacological Basis of Therapeutics*, 5th edn. Macmillan, New York, pp. 1248–1307

Capel-Edwards, K., Hall, D. E., Fellowes, K. P., Vallance, D. K., Davies, M. J., Lamb, D. and Robertson, W. B. (1973). Long-term administration of progesterone to the female beagle dog. *Toxicol. Appl. Pharmacol.*, **24**, 474–488

Carlson, R. W. and Sikic, B. I. (1983). Continuous infusion or bolus injection in cancer chemotherapy. *Ann. Intern. Med.*, **99**, 823–833

Chen, K.-C. and Vostal, J. J. (1981). Aryl hydrocarbon hydroxylase activity induced by injected diesel particulate extract vs inhalation of diluted diesel exhaust. *J. Appl. Toxicol.*, **1**, 127–131

Clarke, E. G. C. (1975). *Poisoning in Veterinary Practice*. Association of the British Pharmaceutical Industry, London, p. 10

Cooper, J. F., Levin, J. and Wagner, H. N. (1971). Quantitative comparison of *in vitro* and *in vivo* methods for the detection of endotoxin. *J. Lab. Clin. Med.*, **78**, 138–148

Dey, M. S., Breeze, R. A., Dey, R. A., Kreiger, R. I., Naser, L. J. and Renzi, B. E. (1982). Disposition and toxicity of paraquat delivered subcutaneously by injection and osmotic pump in the rat. *Toxicologist.*, **2**, 96

Dissin, J., Mills, L. R., Mains, D. L., Black, O. and Webster, P. D. (1975). Experimental induction of pancreatic adenocarcinoma in rats. *J. Natl Cancer Inst.*, **55**, 857–864

Dubois, K. P., Kinoshita, F. and Jackson, P. (1967). Acute toxicity and mechanism of action of a cholinergic rodenticide. *Arch. Int. Pharmacodyn.*, **169**, 108–116

Eibert, J. (1972). Pyrogen testing: horseshoe crabs vs rabbits. *Bull. Parent. Drug Assoc.*, **26**, 253–260

Ensminger, W. D., Greenberger, J. S., Egan, E. M., Muse, M. B. and Moloney, W. C. (1979). Technique for preclinical evaluation of continuous infusion chemotherapy with the use of WF rat acute myelogenous leukaemia. *J. Natl Cancer Inst.*, **62**, 1265–1268

Epstein, S. S., Fujii, K., Andrea, J. and Mantel, N. (1970). Carcinogenicity testing of selected food additives by parenteral administration to infant Swiss mice. *Toxicol. Appl. Pharmacol.*, **16**, 321–334

European Pharmacopoeia (1986). 2nd edn. Maisonneuve, Sainte-Ruffine, V.2.1.4.-V.2.1.5

European Pharmacopoeia (1987). 2nd edn. Maisonneuve, Sainte-Ruffine, V.2.1.9

Fairhurst, S., Marrs, T. C., Parker, H. C., Scawin, J. W. and Swanston, D. W. (1987). Acute toxicity of T2 toxin in rats, mice, guinea-pigs and pigeons. *Toxicology.*, **43**, 31–49

Flecknell, P. A. (1987). Non-surgical experimental procedures. In Tuffery, A. A. (Ed.), *Laboratory Animals: An Introduction for New Experimenters*. Wiley, Chichester, pp. 225–246

Gabrielsson, J., Paalzow, L., Larsson, S. and Blomquist, I. (1985). Constant rate of infusion—improvement of tests for teratogenicity and embryotoxicity. *Life Sci.*, **37**, 2275–2282

Gersonde, K. and Weiner, M. (1982). The influence of infusion rate on the acute intravenous toxicity of phytic acid, a calcium-binding agent. *Toxicology*, **22**, 279–286

Grasso, P. and Goldberg, L. (1966). Subcutaneous sarcoma as an index of carcinogenic potency, *Fd Cosmet. Toxicol.*, **4**, 297–320

Grasso, P. and Grant, D. (1977). Short-term toxicity tests for carcinogenicity: A brief review. In Ballantyne, B. (Ed.), *Current Approaches in Toxicology*. John Wright, Bristol, pp. 219–220

Gray, A. J. and Soderlund, D. M. (1985). Mammalian toxicology of pyrethroids. In Hutson, D. H. and Roberts, T. R. (Eds), *Insecticides*. Wiley, Chichester, pp. 193–248

Gray, J. E., Weaver, R. N., Moran, J. and Feenstra, E. S. (1974). The parenteral toxicity of clindamycin 2-phosphate in laboratory animals. *Toxicol. Appl. Pharmacol.*, **27**, 308–321

Green, C. J. (1979). *Animal Anaesthesia*. Laboratory Animals, London, pp. 135–205

Greisman, S. E. and Hornick, R. B. (1969). Comparative pyrogenic reactivity of rabbit and man to bacterial endotoxin. *Proc. Soc. Exp. Biol.*, **131**, 1154–1158

Hirano, T., Stanton, M. and Layard, M. (1974). Measurement of epidermoid carcinoma development induced in the lungs of rats by 3-methylcholanthrene-containing beeswax pellets. *J. Natl Cancer Inst.*, **53**, 1209–1219

Homburger, F. (1972). Chemical carcinogenesis in Syrian hamsters. In Homburger, F. (Ed.), *Progress in Experimental Tumor Research. Pathology of the Syrian Hamster*. Karger, Basel, pp. 165–166

Honda, K., Matuyama, D., Mitarai, H., Nakamura, T., Ota, E. and Tejima, Y. (1973). Toxicological studies on sulphamethoxazole–trimethoprim combination—acute and subacute toxicities. *Chemotherapy*, **21**, 175–186

Hornick, P. (1986). A new method of giving repetitive intraperitoneal injections to neonatal rats. *Lab. Anim.*, **20**, 14–15

Jaeger, R. J. and Rubin, R. J. (1970). Plasticizers from plastic devices: extraction, metabolism and accumulation in biological systems. *Science*, **170**, 460–461

Kast, A. and Tsunenari, Y. (1983). Hair embolism in lungs of rat and rabbit caused by intravenous injection. *Lab. Anim.*, **17**, 203–207

Kraus, A. L. (1980). Research methodology. In Baker, H. J., Lindsey, J. R. and Weisbroth, S. H. (Eds), *The Laboratory Rat. Research Applications*. Academic Press, New York, pp. 20–22

Lewis, R. E., Kunz, A. L., and Bell, R. E. (1966). Error of intraperitoneal injections in rats. *Lab. Anim. Care.*, **16**, 505–509

Liu, P. L., Feldman, H. S., Giasi, R., Patterson, M. K. and Covino, B. G. (1983). Comparative CNS toxicity of lidocaine, etidocaine, bupivacaine and tetracaine in awake dogs following rapid intravenous administration. *Anesth. Analg.*, **62**, 375–379

McCormick, C. C. and Fleet, J. C. (1988). The toxicity of parenteral copper in the chick: dependence on route of administration. *J. Nutr.*, **118**, 1398–1402

Magee, P. N. (1970). Tests for carcinogenic potential. In Paget, G. E. (Ed.), *Methods in Toxicology*. Blackwell, Oxford, p. 173

Maintani, T., Watahiki, A. and Suzuki, K. T. (1986). Induction of metallothionein after lead administration by three injection routes in mice. *Toxicol. Appl. Pharmacol.*, **83**, 211–217

Mascoli, C. C. and Weary, M. E. (1979). Limulus amebocyte lysate (LAL) test for detecting pyrogens in parenteral injectable products and medical devices: advantages to manufacturers and regulatory officials. *J. Parent. Drug Assoc.*, **33**, 81

Montesano, R. and Saffiotti, U. (1968). Carcinogenic response of the respiratory tract of Syrian golden hamsters to different doses of diethylnitrosamine. *Cancer Res.*, **28**, 2197–2210

Nau, H. (1983). The role of delivery systems in toxicology and drug development. *Pharm. Int.*, **4**, 228–231

Nicholls, P. J. (1970). Trouble-free intravenous injection of rabbits. *J. Inst. Anim. Tech.*, **21**, 12

Patterson, D. S. P., Allen, W. M., Berrett, S., Sweasy, D. and Done, J. T. (1971). The toxicity of parenteral iron preparations in the rabbit and pig with a comparison of the clinical and biochemical responses to iron-dextrose in 2 days old and 8 days old piglets. *Zbl. Vetmed. A.*, **18**, 453–464

Personeus, G. R. (1969). Pyrogen testing of biologicals and small volume parenterals. *Bull. Parent. Drug Assoc.*, **23**, 201–207

Pinedo, H. M., Zaharko, D. S. and Dedrick, R. L. (1976). Device for constant sc infusion of methotrexate: plasma results in mice. *Cancer Treat. Rep.*, **60**, 889–893

Plenge, P., Mellerup, E. T. and Norgaard, T. (1981). Functional and structural rat kidney changes caused by peroral or parenteral lithium treatment. *Acta Psychiat. Scand.*, **63**, 303–313

Porter, W. P., Bitar, Y. M., Strandberg, J. D. and Charache, P. C. (1985). A comparison of subcutaneous and intraperitoneal oxytetracycline injection methods for control of infectious disease in the rat. *Lab. Anim.*, **19**, 3–6

Prasad, S., Gatmaitan, B. R. and Oconnell, R. C. (1978). Effect of a conditioning method on general safety test in guinea-pigs. *Lab. Anim. Sci.*, **28**, 591–593

Purchase, I. F. H. and van der Watt, J. J. (1969). Acute toxicity of sterigmatocystin to rats. *Fd Cosmet. Toxicol.*, **7**, 135–139

Rasmussen, F. and Høgh, P. (1971). Irritating effect and concentrations at the injection site after intramuscular injection of antibiotic preparations in cows and pigs. *Nord. Vet.-Med.*, **23**, 593–605

Rasmussen, F. and Svendsen, O. (1976). Tissue damage and concentration at the injection site after intramuscular injection of chemotherapeutics and vehicles in pigs. *Res. Vet. Sci.*, **20**, 55–60

Ray, N. and Theeuwes, F. (1987) Implantable osmotically powered drug delivery systems. In Johnson and Lloyd-Jones (Eds), *Drug Delivery Systems*. Ellis Horwood, Chichester, pp. 120–138

Rhodes, M. L. and Patterson, C. E. (1979). Chronic intravenous infusion in the rat: a nonsurgical approach. *Lab. Anim. Sci.*, **29**, 82–84

Roe, F. J. C. (1975). Neonatal induction of hepatic and other tumours. In Butler, W. H. and Newberne, P. M. (Eds), *Mouse Hepatic Neoplasia*. Elsevier, Amsterdam, pp. 133–142

Roe, F. J. C., Carter, R. L., Walters, M. A. and Harington, J. S. (1967). The pathological effects of subcutaneous injections of asbestos fibres in mice: migration of fibres to submesothelial tissues and induction of mesotheliomata. *Int. J. Cancer.*, **2**, 628–638

Ronneberger, H. (1977). Antigenicity testing of parenteral drugs in animal models. In Duncan, W. A.

M. and Leonard, B. J. (Eds), *Clinical Toxicology*. Excerpta Medica, Amsterdam, pp. 141–142

Rowe, P. H., Starlinger, M. J., Kasdon, E., Hollands, M. J. and Silen, W. (1987). Parenteral aspirin and sodium salicylate are equally injurious to the rat gastric mucosa. *Gastroenterology.*, **93**, 863–871

Rowland, M. (1972). Influence of route of administration on drug availability. *J. Pharm. Sci.*, **61**, 70–74

Schmitz, H., Schaub, E. and Müller, A. (1976). Intramuscular iron therapy. *Schweiz. Archiv Tierheilk.*, **118**, 441–479

Seibert, F. B. (1923). Fever-producing substance found in some distilled waters. *Am. J. Physiol.*, **67**, 90

Sikic, B. I., Collins, J. M., Mimnaugh, E. G. and Gram, T. E. (1978). Improved therapeutic index of bleomycin when administered by continuous infusion in mice. *Cancer Treat. Rep.*, **62**, 2011–2017

Smyth, R. D., Gaver, R. C., Dandekar, K. A., Van Harken, D. R. and Hottendorf, G. H. (1979). Evaluation of the availability of drugs incorporated in rat laboratory diet. *Toxicol. Appl. Pharmacol.*, **50**, 493–499

Stanton, M. F. and Wrench, C. (1972). Mechanisms of mesothelioma induction with asbestos and fibrous glass. *J. Natl Cancer Inst.*, **48**, 797–821

Stone, M. M., Mulvihill, S. J., Lewin, K. J. and Fonkalsrud, E. W. (1986). Long-term total intraperitoneal nutrition in a rabbit model. *J. Pediatr. Surg.*, **21**, 267–270

Sunderman, F. W. (1983). Potential toxicity from nickel contamination of intravenous fluids. *Ann. Clin. Lab. Sci.*, **13**, 1–4

Suttle, N. F. (1981). Comparison between parenterally administered copper complexes of their ability to alleviate hypocupraemia in sheep and cattle. *Vet. Rec.*, **109**, 304–307

Svendsen, O. (1972). Histologic changes after intramuscular injections with antibiotic preparations. *Nord. Vet.-Med.*, **24**, 181–185

Svendsen, O. and Aaes-Jørgensen, T. (1979). Studies on the fate of vegetable oil after intramuscular injection into experimental animals. *Acta Pharmacol. Toxicol.*, **45**, 352–378

Svendsen, O., Rasmussen, F., Nielsen, P. and Steiness, E. (1978). The loss of creatine phosphokinase (CPK) from the intramuscular injection site of rabbits as a predictive tool for local toxicity. *Proc. 20th Congr. Europ. Soc. Toxicol., Berlin*, Abstract No. 56

Tanaka, T., Kobayashi, H., Okumura, K., Muranishi, S. and Sezaki, H. (1974). Intramuscular absorption of drugs from oily solutions in the rat. *Chem. Pharm. Bull.*, **22**, 1275–1284

Thompson, S. W., Sparano, B. M. and Diener, R. M. (1971). Vacuoles in the hepatocytes of cortisone-treated dogs. *Am. J. Pathol.*, **63**, 135–145

Toth, B. (1968). A critical review of experiments in chemical carcinogenesis using newborn animals. *Cancer Res.*, **28**, 727–738

United States Food and Drug Administration (1987).

Guideline on Validation of the Limulus Amebocyte Lysate Test as an End-product Endotoxin Test for Human and Animal Parenteral Drugs, Biological Products, and Medical Devices. US Food and Drug Administration, Rockville

United States Pharmacopeia XXII (1990). US Pharmacopeial Convention, Rockville, pp. 1493–1500, 1515

Urquhart, J. (1982). Rate-controlled drug dosage. *Drugs*, **23**, 207–226

Valdez, Y. E. and Lehnert, B. E. (1988). A procedure for instilling agents into the pleural space compartment of the rat without co-administration into the lung compartment. *Anim. Tech.*, **39**, 1–8

Valeriote, F. and Vietti, T. (1985). Comparison of cytotoxicity of single dose and infusion of alkylating agents. *Cancer Drug Delivery*, **2**, 11–18

Van Alstine, W. G. and Dietrich, J. A. (1988). Porcine sciatic nerve damage after intramuscular injection. *Comp. Fd Anim.*, **10**, 1329–1332

Verschoyle, R. D. and Barnes, J. M. (1972). Toxicity of natural and synthetic pyrethrins to rats. *Pest. Biochem. Physiol.*, **2**, 308–311

Wagner, J. C. (1962). Experimental production of mesothelial tumours of the pleura by implantation of dusts in laboratory animals. *Nature*, **196**, 180–181

Walker, D. (1979). Acute toxicity: how and why? *Proc. Symp. Assoc. Vet. Ind., London*, pp. 7–16

Walker, D. (1981). An alternative to the LD$_{50}$: the study of acute sublethal effects. *Proc. Symp. Dutch Soc. Toxicol., Utrecht*, pp. 60–73

Watson, A. D. J. (1972). Chloramphenicol plasma levels in the dog: a comparison of oral, subcutaneous, and intramuscular administration. *J. Small Anim. Pract.*, **13**, 147–151

Weary, M. E. and Wallin, R. F. (1973). The rabbit pyrogen test. *Lab. Anim. Sci.*, **23**, 677–681

Webb, F. W. (1969). The importance of uniformity in biological control. In Brown, A. M. (Ed.), *Uniformity*. Carworth Europe, Huntingdon, pp. 11–32

Wilkins, J. W., Greene, J. A. and Weller, J. M. (1968). Toxicity of intraperitoneal bisulfite. *Clin. Pharmacol. Therap.*, **9**, 328–332

Wilson, R. C., Duran, S. H., Horton, C. R. and Wright, L. C. (1989). Bioavailability of gentamicin in dogs after intramuscular or subcutaneous injections. *Am. J. Vet. Res.*, **50**, 1748–1750

Winship, K. A. (1988). Toxicity of tin and its compounds. *Adverse Drug React. Acute Poisoning Rev.*, **7**, 19–38

Witschi, H. P. (1981). Enhancement of tumor formation in mouse lung by dietary butylated hydroxytoluene. *Toxicology.*, **21**, 95–104

Woodbury, D. M. and Fingle, E. (1975). Analgesic–antipyretics, anti-inflammatory agents, and drugs employed in the therapy of gout. In Goodman, L. S. and Gilman, A. (Eds), *The Pharmacological Basis of Therapeutics*, 5th edn. Macmillan, New York, p. 328

World Health Organization (1967). Procedures for investigating intentional and unintentional food additives. *Wld Hlth Org. Tech. Rep. Ser.*, 348

World Health Organization (1969). Principles for the testing and evaluation of drugs for carcinogenicity. *Wld Hlth Org. Tech. Rep. Ser.*, 426

Yuhas, E. M., Morgan, D. G., Arena, E., Kupp, R. P., Saunders, L. Z. and Lewis, H. B. (1985). Arterial medial necrosis and haemorrhage induced in rats by intravenous infusion of fenoldopam mesylate, a dopaminergic vasodilator. *Am. J. Pathol.*, **119**, 83–91

FURTHER READING

Perkin, C. J. and Stejskal, R. (1994). Intravenous infusion in dogs and primates. *Journal of the American College of Toxicology*, **13**, 40–47

16   Peroral Toxicity

Tipton R. Tyler

INTRODUCTION

In assessing the toxic properties of any substance, careful consideration must be given to the manner in which it is introduced into the animal. A rapid review of the toxicological literature will quickly reveal that the peroral route is certainly the most common method of administration encountered. There are a number of reasons for this, not the least of which is the ease of dose administration and quantitative determination. It is a route by which a large number of substances gain entrance into the animal body. Thus, many pharmaceutical preparations are designed to be administered orally. Environmental contaminants which enter drinking-water supplies will be inadvertently ingested. It is virtually impossible to avoid ingestion of traces of chemical residues used on field crops, used in animal husbandry and used in food processing or in food packaging. In addition, it is often important to gain toxicological information on substances which could be accidentally swallowed or swallowed in suicidal or homicidal incidents.

At times the peroral route of administration is used to study the toxic effects of a material when the primary concern is by some other mode of exposure, i.e. inhalation or skin exposure. Often this is done because it is far easier to obtain a quantitative estimate of dose when delivered perorally. Route-to-route extrapolation requires an in-depth knowledge of a number of biological, chemical and physical processes, including an understanding of the anatomy, physiology, and pharmacodynamics and pharmacokinetics of the test substance. It should be remembered that one of the precepts of toxicology is that, whenever technically feasible, test substances should be studied by the route of administration which is appropriate to the problem under investigation. This is particularly important in the field of risk assessment, where route-to-route extrapolations add to the uncertainty already inherent in the imprecise approximations and assumptions used to obtain the risk estimates.

This chapter will review techniques used in peroral administration studies, discuss variables in the design of peroral studies which may influence the expression of toxicological responses, and point out some specific characteristics of peroral administration which must be carefully considered when attempting route-to-route extrapolation. Initially, however, it is important to review some anatomical features and physiological processes which can affect toxicological responses of perorally administered chemical substances.

ANATOMICAL CONSIDERATIONS

Anatomical features which can affect the toxic manifestations of ingested substances both between various animal species and within the same species include:

- The structure of the gastrointestinal (GI) tract, particularly the upper portion of the tract, which is often involved when dosing animals by gavage or intubation.
- The type of cellular lining in various parts of the GI tract.
- The location and nature of glands which empty secretions into the tract.
- The blood supply and drainage patterns from various parts of the tract.
- The innervation of the tract.

Morphology

The arrangement of the pharynx, epiglottis and oesophagus determine the ease with which substances can be administered to animals by gavage or intubation. In rats and mice these structures are relatively straight and unobstructed by folds of tissue. Grasping these animals by folds of skin on the dorsal aspect of the head and neck with gentle extension of the neck allows for easy passage of an animal feeding needle into the oesophagus and stomach (Figure 1). Accomplished technicians can dose several animals a minute by this

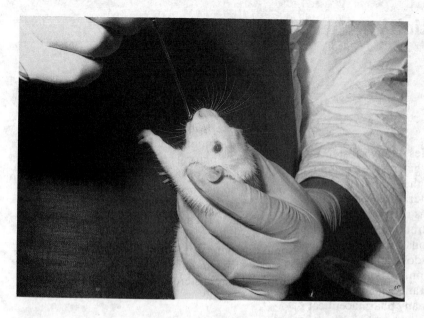

Figure 1   Typical procedure used in gavage dosing of a rat

method with amazingly few errors; errors in which the material inadvertently gains entrance to the trachea (lunging the animal). The structure in guinea-pigs and rabbits, on the other hand, is complicated by folds of tissue which impede the direct entrance of rigid feeding needles and often flexible tubing is employed in dosing rather than the stainless steel needles. This procedure usually requires more time. In general, technical considerations, including animal size, require the use of flexible intubation for dogs, monkeys and other larger mammals.

The gastrointestinal tract is exposed to a wide variety of chemical and physical conditions, some of which are quite hostile or incompatible with life. Organisms, therefore, have developed resistant cellular linings of this tube to protect the surrounding visceral elements from the GI tract contents. The mouth and oesophagus of rodents are lined with keratinized stratified squamous epithelium, while that of primates and man is of the non-keratinized type (Ham and Cormack, 1979). This type of cellular lining is designed primarily for protection against mechanical abrasion and chemical corrosion rather than for absorptive function. The cells undergo continual renewal, with mitotic division taking place in the deepest 2–3 layers, the older cells being displaced towards the lumen.

All rodents have two distinct areas of the

stomach—the non-glandular stomach, or forestomach, and the glandular stomach (Figure 2). The forestomach is developed to the greatest degree in ruminant species (consisting of the rumen and abomasom) and to different degrees in various rodent species, and is not present in man or primates. The function of this organ is generally believed to be for the storage of food, although in ruminants and some other species (Bauchop and Martucci, 1968; Dellow *et al.*, 1983; Grajal *et al.*, 1989) it acts as a fermentation vessel from which the animal derives a major portion of its energy needs. The cellular lining of the forestomach is a continuation of the oesophageal keratinized squamous epithelium. There are relatively few glands scattered in the submucosa of the oesophagus and forestomach; those which are present secrete mucus, primarily for the purpose of lubrication to assist in the passage of food.

In rodents the true or glandular stomach is separated from the forestomach by an elevated border, the dividing or limiting ridge. This distinct structure assists in maintaining some degree of separation of the stomach contents between either the forestomach or the true or glandular stomach. In contrast to the forestomach, the mucosal lining of the true stomach is thicker and characterized by a columnar lining which forms numerous tubular glands or gastric pits lined by

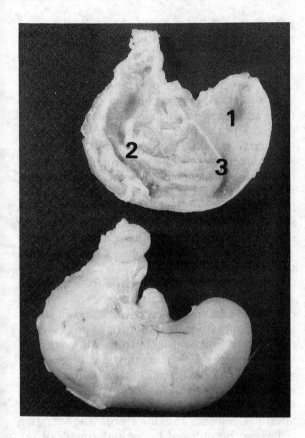

Figure 2 Intact and longitudinal section of rat stomach: 1, non-glandular stomach, or forestomach; 2, glandular stomach; 3, limiting ridge

three types of secreting cells: neck cells, which secrete mucus which acts to protect the lining from the hostile, acidic environment; parietal cells, which secrete hydrochloric acid; and chief cells, which secrete digestive proenzymes, including pepsinogen.

The flow of gastric contents from the stomach to the duodenum is controlled by the pyloric sphincter. This structure normally remains closed, limiting the flow of stomach contents to the small intestine. The sphincter is controlled by both hormones and nervous impulses, and is influenced by factors such as the degree of distension of the duodenum, the degree of irritation to the duodenal mucosa, the acidity of the duodenal chyme, the degree of osmolality of the chyme and the presence of products of digestion, particularly those of meat and to a lesser extent fat (Guyton, 1981).

The epithelium of the small intestine is designed to perform efficient absorptive functions, but, in addition, performs some secretory functions. The walls of the small intestine are highly convoluted in nature. The mucosal lining is arranged in tiny projections known as intestinal villi. The epithelial cells lining the luminal surface and forming the intestinal villi are characterized by possessing numerous microvilli. The entire structure, therefore, possesses a tremendous surface area through which absorption can occur. The columnar cells lining the small intestine are in a process of continual renewal; it is estimated that the entire intestinal epithelium is renewed every third day (Ham and Cormack, 1979).

In addition to the epithelial cells lining the tract, glandular structures are also present. The ducts of the exocrine glands, the liver and pancreas empty into the small intestine in the very upper portion of the duodenum. Brunner's glands, composed of goblet cells, are also found in great number, primarily in the submucosa of the proximal portion of the duodenum. These glands secrete mucus into the lumen which acts both as a protective coating of the lining and to serve in a lubricating role. Various digestive enzymes are secreted from the crypts of Lieberkühn. The primary function of the large intestine is to absorb water. The epithelial lining differs from that of the small intestine in that no villi are present. The secretory cells of the crypts of Lieberkühn are primarily goblet cells which secrete mucus for lubricating and protective purposes. As the chyme passes through the large intestine, therefore, the liquid aqueous phase is absorbed and the solid material becomes more concentrated, the flow of semisolid faecal material from the tract being controlled by the external and internal anal sphincters. In some species the caecum is well developed and serves as a vessel in which digestion occurs through fermentation.

Circulation

The circulatory pattern of the gastrointestinal tract must be considered when extrapolating toxicological data obtained from peroral studies to other routes of exposure. Arterial blood is supplied by a number of arteries. However, the veins draining the tract, from the lower oesophagus to the very distal portion of the rectum, flow into the portal vein. All portal vein blood empties into the sinusoids of the liver; thus, all material absorbed from the lower portion of the oesophagus to the rectum is delivered to the liver prior to entering the general systemic circulation. During this 'first pass' the liver, being the major organ for the metabolism of most xenobiotic substances and many other endogenous chemicals, may modify, through metabolic processes, a significant portion of an absorbed nutrient or toxicant. Thus, a major portion of an absorbed chemical can be metabolized prior to being delivered to the potential target organ through systemic circulation. This can lead to either enhancement of toxicity in the case of metabolic activation, or moderation of the toxicity in the case of detoxification, over what might occur by another route of administration where the liver is not the first organ encountered—i.e. pulmonary or dermal exposure. Expressions of toxic responses moderated by the hepatic portal pattern of blood circulation are often referred to as 'first pass effects'.

In contrast to the venous drainage of the major portion of the gastrointestinal tract, the drainage of the buccal cavity, the mouth and the tongue, is into the jugular vein and, hence, directly enter the general systemic circulation, bypassing the hepatic–portal loop. This is the reason that certain drugs which are rapidly metabolized by liver enzymes are administered by buccal absorption, i.e. nitroglycerin. An analogous pattern exists at the juncture of the rectum and anus. Here there is an anastomosis of veins of the hepatic portal system and the systemic system (Johnson, 1981). This pattern of circulation allows a portion of a pharmaceutical rectal suppository preparation to be absorbed directly into the systemic circulatory system.

Innervation

Movement of contents through the gastrointestinal tract is controlled by peristaltic contractions of the smooth muscle fibres within the structural portion of the walls of the tube. The contractions of these muscle fibres are mediated by the autonomic nervous system and, to some extent, by hormonal secretions. The gastrointestinal tract has an intrinsic nervous system that extends from the oesophagus to the anus. This intrinsic system is under the control of both parasympathetic and sympathetic signals from the brain. With the exception of the very proximal and distal portion of the tract, parasympathetic innervation arises from the vagus nerve. The sympathetic innervation arises from the spinal cord between segments T-8 and L-3, the preganglionic fibres passing to various ganglia, and the postganglionic fibres accompanying the blood vessels to the various parts of the tract. In general, stimulation of the parasympathetic system increases strength and frequency of mixing and propulsive contractions of the smooth muscles of the gastrointestinal tract wall, thereby leading to an increased movement of contents through the tract. Sympathetic stimulation, on the other hand, has an opposite effect, and strong sympathetic stimulation can completely block the movement of the contents through the tract.

Afferent nerve fibres also arise in the gut wall and are stimulated by such processes as irritation of the mucosa and distension of the wall of the tract. Signals from these fibres are processed in the medulla and contribute to overall control of the movement of contents through the tract. In addition, in some species these afferent fibres send signals to the vomiting centre in the medulla, leading to emesis or the expulsion of gastric and intestinal contents (Smith, 1986). The vomiting reflex can be initiated by various stimuli of the gastrointestinal tract, i.e. irritation or distension of various segments of the tract, and also by direct action of agents on an area known as the chemoreceptor trigger zone of the vomiting centre in the medulla itself, i.e. chemical emetics such as ipecac (Venho, 1986). Not all mammalian species are capable of vomiting; in general, rodents and rabbits are believed to be incapable of expressing the vomiting reflex, while dogs, cats, monkeys and man certainly exhibit the reflex when stimulated. The fact that an animal may exhibit the reflex can cause problems in administering certain test substances by the peroral route.

PHYSIOLOGICAL CONSIDERATIONS

Physiological factors which affect the absorption of both nutrients and environmental chemical substances include:

- The concentration of the substance in the GI tract contents.

- The pH of the GI tract contents.
- The ionic concentration of the GI tract contents.
- The rate of passage of the contents through the tract.
- The surface area available for absorption.
- The blood supply to the serosal side of the GI tract wall.

Factors Affecting pH and Volume

The pH of the milieu is particularly important in the case of ionic materials, as they are absorbed almost entirely in the non-charged state, i.e. as free acids or free bases. Crouthamel *et al.* (1971) demonstrated that the un-ionized forms of the drugs sulfaethidole and barbitone (barbital) were absorbed 3–5 times faster from either the stomach or the intestine of the rat than the ionized forms. Shanker *et al.* (1957) demonstrated that acids having a pK_a value greater than 2 were, in general, well absorbed from the stomach of rats when introduced in a 0.1 M HCl solution. Strong acids such as sulphonic acids, phenolsulphophthalein and 5-sulphosalicylic acid were not absorbed under these conditions, nor were organic bases having a pK_a greater than 2.5. On the other hand, the absorption of acids was distinctly depressed when they were introduced into the rat stomach in 0.15 M sodium bicarbonate solution, while a marked increase in the absorption of bases was noted under these conditions.

The pH and volume of GI tract contents are controlled by a number of hormonal and neurological mechanisms, and vary in accordance with the feeding cycle. In the postprandial state the stomach secretes HCl at only a fraction of the maximal rate. The empty stomach, therefore, contains a relatively small volume of acidified fluid. HCl is secreted by the parietal cells of the glandular stomach, secretion primarily under control of the hormone gastrin and the parasympathetic mediator acetylcholine. Other mediators of HCl secretion include histamine and perhaps an intestinal-derived hormone, enterooxyntin (Johnson, 1985). Gastric secretion is stimulated by the anticipation of feeding, and by tasting, smelling, chewing and swallowing food. These stimuli to gastric secretion are mediated through the nervous system, and, in particular, by impulses delivered by the vagus nerve. In addition to the neurological stimulation of the secretory pathways, the secretion of gastrin and subsequently HCl is stimulated by distension of the stomach and the presence of specific molecular species such as amino acids and peptides.

The ingestion of food increases the pH of the acidic fluid in the empty stomach by dilution, thus permitting the release of gastrin and the release of HCl from the parietal cells. As the digestion process continues, the release of HCl eventually overwhelms the buffering capacity of the chyme. Gastrin secretion is inhibited at pH values below 3 and blocked at pH values of 2 and less. Therefore, by a classic feedback mechanism, further gastrin release and consequently HCl secretion is prevented.

Secretions from the cells of the intestinal lining tend to neutralize chyme flowing from the stomach. The secretion of fluid and bicarbonate by the mucosal cells of the duodenum is controlled by the quantity of acid which flows through the cardiac valve (Johnson, 1985). These secretions, both enzymes and bicarbonate, are produced from the acinar cells. It is the pancreatic secretions, however, which account for the major portion of neutralization of acid coming from the stomach. Pancreatic secretions not only are under control of the acid environment, but also respond to nervous stimuli arising primarily from the vagus nerve. Pancreatic secretions are also under hormonal control, being stimulated by release of secretin and cholecystokinin. Secretin appears to control the release of the alkaline component of the pancreatic and intestinal secretions, water and bicarbonate, while cholecystokinin stimulates the release of the enzymatic component, i.e. pepsin, amylases and lipases.

Factors Affecting Movement of Contents

Mixing and movement of the contents down the intestinal tract occur by the rhythmic contractions, peristalsis, of the stomach and intestine. The contractions are produced by the layers of smooth muscle which comprise the outer layer of the gastrointestinal tract walls. In the stomach nervous impulses arise primarily from the vagus nerve, bringing about strong contractions of the smooth muscle layers. In the small intestine the contractions are controlled by activities of the smooth muscle cells themselves as well as being initiated by nervous impulses (Weisbrodt, 1985). Humoral substances, endogenous and exogenous chemicals, and physical distension affect the motility of the GI tract. Adrenaline (epinephrine) inhibits, while serotonin stimulates contractions. Gastrin, cholecystokinin and other hormones (i.e. motilin) stimulate contractions, whereas secretin has an inhibitory action.

Under normal conditions the contractions of the stomach result in mixing ingested food with the gastric secretions. The peristaltic activity within the small intestine occurs in relatively short segments, primarily leading to mixing action allowing for maximum contact with the vast surface area of the intestinal lining. The small and the large intestine are capable of undergoing co-ordinated contractions which can cause the movement of the chyme through the entire tract in a relatively short period of time. In addition, there appear to be other mechanisms which promote the rapid movement of certain materials throughout the upper gastrointestinal tract. Frederick and co-workers (1992), for instance, have demonstrated that in rats up to 15 per cent of a gavage dose of ethyl acrylate administered in corn oil can be recovered from the duodenum and 3 per cent from the ileum within 1–2 min after administration.

The effect of the rate of passage of GI tract contents can be complex. Upon first consideration, the longer a solute remains in contact with an absorptive surface, the greater the likelihood of absorption. Thus, physiological states or conditions which impede transport through the intestinal tract would be expected to increase the amount of material absorbed. There are conditions, however, where prolonged retention in parts of the tract may lead to decreased absorption and a reduction in the toxicity of an environmental chemical or the efficacy of a pharmaceutical preparation. Thus, retention of acid-labile penicillin or erythromycin in the stomach can lead to drug degradation and a lowering of the efficacy of these antibiotics (Welling, 1984).

Factors Affecting Circulation

An increase in blood flow to the GI tract accompanies the postprandial increase in GI tract secretions and motility. The increase in blood flow is relatively greater to the gastric and intestinal mucosa and pancreas than to the GI tract musculature. This increase in blood flow is mediated by hormones secreted from the intestinal mucosa: glucagon and cholecystokinin act to increase the blood flow to the intestine and pancreas, and gastrin to the gastric mucosa. Presumably the blood flow to the GI tract tissue results from vasodilatation caused by the indirect release of local vasodilator metabolites along with direct stimulatory action of cholecystokinin and acetylcholine released by vagal discharge.

ABSORPTION MECHANISMS

There are five different means by which nutrients and exogenous materials can pass from the mucosal side of the GI tract across to the serosal side:

- Passive diffusion through a lipid membrane.
- Diffusion through pores.
- Active energy-dependent transport.
- Absorption through lymphatics.
- Absorption of macromolecules by pinocytosis.

Effects of pH and Volume

A number of barriers are present to impede the simple diffusion of molecules across the membranes of the epithelial cells lining the tract. First, the molecules must traverse the unstirred layers of fluid lying immediately adjacent to the membrane, then cross the mucous layer coating the membrane and finally cross the bilipid membrane itself into the cell. Once within the cytoplasm of the cell, the molecule must pass through the cytoplasm and then through the basement membrane and the capillary or lymphatic wall membranes. The bilipid structure of the cell membranes greatly favours the absorption of hydrophobic species over hydrophilic species. This, then, accounts for the greater absorption rate of un-ionized species over ionized species, as demonstrated by Crouthamel et al. (1971) and Schanker et al. (1957). The fact that ionized forms are absorbed to a slight degree may be the result of microenvironments of lower pH in the unstirred layers immediately adjacent to the membrane, or to the acidity of the membrane itself. The process of diffusion is driven by the concentration gradient across the membrane, and thus the fluid volume in the tract can have a major influence on the rate at which ingested material may appear in the bloodstream. Presumably, the greater the volume of fluid present, the more dilute the various solutes. Herein lies the basis for the often given advice in poisoning cases of diluting the offending material by 'giving two glasses of water'. As it turns out, this is not always appropriate advice. For instance, dilution of glutaraldehyde in water actually increases its peroral toxicity, the LD_{50} of the material being reduced from 733 mg kg^{-1} (expressed as contained glutaraldehyde) in the rat when administered as a 50 per cent solution to 123 mg kg^{-1} as a 1 per cent solution (Tyler and Ballantyne, 1988). As discussed above, ingestion of food is a powerful stimulant for both the secretion of gastric and intestinal secretions and the release of acid in the stomach. Therefore, it would be expected that the effects, particularly acute effects, of an orally administered toxicant may be greatly influenced by the prandial state of the animal.

The transport of an absorbed molecule into the bloodstream is driven by a large concentration gradient between the luminal side and the serosal side of the intestine. Because of rapid blood flow and concomitant rapid removal of solutes, concentration gradients are invariably favourable for movement from the gut into the circulatory system. The major impediment to absorption of nutrients and exogenous chemicals, then, is the initial movement across the mucosal cell membrane.

It is believed that a major portion of the water present in the GI tract is reabsorbed through pores which are present in the apical junctions of the epithelial cell lining. These pores are large enough to allow penetration of small molecules, particularly small ionized species. The net direction of flow of water is either from the tract into the serosal fluid, as is generally the case when the contents are either iso-osmotic or hypotonic, or into the tract, as might occur when the gastrointestinal contents are hyperosmotic or in certain pathological states. Vogel *et al.* (1975) studied the effect of water flow on the toxicity of atropine, an azoniaspiro compound, phenobarbitone (phenobarbital) and nicotine by infusing solutions of these substances into the duodenum of rats. Mannitol was concomitantly infused to adjust the osmotic concentration of the contents and thus the flow of water from the serosal side to the mucosal side of the GI tract. Toxic effects were increased by a factor of 2–4, with a decrease in osmotic concentration from triple-isotonicity to isotonicity for three of the four materials, the only exception being with the azoniaspiro compound. No explanation for this latter discrepancy was given.

The depression of absorption of solutes resulting from the flow of water from the serosa into the lumen of the intestine has been termed solvent drag. As demonstrated by the work of Vogel *et al.*, this process can play an important role in the rate of absorption from the intestine and, hence, toxicity of certain compounds, primarily small water-soluble ions.

Active Transport

The active transport or energy-dependent transport mechanisms of absorption are primarily reserved for nutrients—i.e. amino acids, sugars, essential vitamins and minerals, etc. There are examples where specific exogenous substances can also be absorbed from the gastrointestinal tract by these same transport systems. For instance, pyrimidines and amino acids are absorbed by active transport systems. 5-Fluorouracil and 5-bromouracil, which are actively transported across the rat intestinal epithelium by the process which transports natural pyrimidines (Schanker and Jeffrey, 1961), and penicillamine and levodopa utilize an active transport mechanism for natural amino acids. Some toxic metals, such as lead and aluminium, are also absorbed by processes designed for the transport of essential metals. Chlorothiazide has been demonstrated to be absorbed by a non-saturable active absorption process (Welling, 1984).

Lymphatics

Absorption by way of the lymphatics is limited to non-polar materials and occurs by mechanisms analogous to that by which fatty acids are absorbed. Bile salts play an important role in dispersing triglycerides and other fat-soluble molecules and are critical in the formation of micelles which allow dissolution of the fatty materials within the chyme. The fact that rats do not possess a gall bladder may lead to differences in their ability to absorb materials efficiently by way of the lymphatics. Fatty acids, derived from the hydrolysis of triglycerides by various lipases, migrate to the brush border of the mucosal cells, and readily diffuse through the mucosal membrane into the cytosol of the cell. Once in the cell, the fatty acids are reincorporated into triglycerides within the endoplasmic reticulum and packaged into chylomicrons, a conglomerate of triglycerides, cholesterol and phospholipids encased in a protein coat. The highly non-polar nature of the interior of the chylomicron provides an ideal environment to entrain other lipid-soluble molecules. The protein coat provides a hydrophilic exterior to the conglomerate which is extruded from the cell into the serosal fluid and into the central lacteals of the villi. The chylomicrons are pumped through the lymphatic system and empty into the systemic circulatory system at the entrance of the thoracic duct in the veins of the neck.

In this manner, fatty lipophilic materials avoid entering the hepatic portal circulatory system and possibly first pass effects of metabolism by liver enzymes. Sieber (1976) has shown that p,p'-dichlorodiphenyltrichloroethene (p,p'-DDT) and some structurally related analogues are absorbed through the lymphatics. The extent of lymphatic absorption, however, is limited, presumably because of the relatively slow rate of movement of lymph through the lymphatics as compared with movement of blood through the general circulatory system. The extent of absorption may also vary greatly, depending on the vehicle in which a test substance is administered. Thus, Sieber recovered only 15 per cent of a dose of p,p'-DDT in the lymph when administered in ethanol, compared with 34 per cent when administered in corn oil.

p-Aminosalicylic acid (PAS) and tetracycline have also been demonstrated to be absorbed by way of the lymphatics; however, both of these drugs are also rapidly distributed throughout the extracellular fluid, including lymph, when administered by the intravenous route (DeMarco and Levine, 1969). This finding suggests that care is required in interpretation of data in which accountability of a substance in lymph is used to determine absorption through lymphatics after peroral dosing. Other materials which have been shown to be absorbed by way of the lymphatics include 3-methylcholanthrene, polychlorinated biphenyls and benzpyrene.

Macromolecules

The direct absorption of macromolecules from the gastrointestinal tract is well established and has grave toxicological implications in some instances—i.e. the absorption of *Botulinum* toxins, which are proteins of molecular weight ranging from 200 000 to 400 000 daltons. Macromolecules are believed to be absorbed by pinocytosis. Intestinal mucosa in the area of the Peyer's patches, which are lymphoid follicle aggregates, are believed to be particularly active in this respect (Aungst and Shen, 1986). Once taken into the mucosal cells, the macromolecules are transported to the general circulation by way of the lymphatics. The process is age-dependent, the ability to absorb large molecules decreasing with age. Thus, the newborn are able to obtain immunity to disease states through the absorption of immunoglobulins in the colostrum of milk.

PRACTICAL IMPLICATIONS

Procedures Used for Peroral Dosing

In general, the procedures used in administering test substances to animals can be grouped into one of two categories: those procedures in which the material is administered as a bolus and those in which it is administered more or less on a continuous basis.

In the first category the most common means of administration, at least in rodents, is by gavage. In this procedure, described previously, the material is fed through an animal feeding needle directly into the animal's stomach. A similar procedure using a flexible tube is often used for dogs, monkeys and farm animals. In these larger species gelatin capsules filled with the test substance are also commonly used; in this case, however, the test substance is generally in a solid form. Gavage administration of test materials can be accomplished quite rapidly and automated systems have been adapted from equipment designed for cutaneous application in which animals are weighed, the weights are down-loaded to a computer and the dosing volume for each individual animal, based on body weight, is automatically calculated. The animal handler then inserts the feeding needle into the animal's stomach and the dosing volume is automatically dispensed (Wilson *et al.*, 1991).

The gavage procedure is fairly labour-intensive and can represent a major cost factor in large studies. To appreciate this, consider that in a 2-year study usually 50 animals of each species and each sex are used in each dosage group. In addition, 30 or more additional animals of each sex are included in each dosage group for satellite studies, interim sacrifices or recovery groups. Thus, in a two-species study with three dosage groups and two control groups (vehicle control and naïve control) more than 1500 animals may have to be dosed every day, 5–7 days a week for 24 or more months.

Alternatively, studies are carried out in which the test material is incorporated into the feed or dissolved in the animal's drinking water. When incorporated into feed, care must be taken to produce a uniform dispersion of the material. Differences in density and/or particle size can lead to the non-homogeneous mixing or the settling out of the test substance in the fines. Animals may refuse to eat feed in cases where the test chemical imparts unacceptable taste. Rodents often waste material, tossing the feed out of the feed cups and thus making it impossible to determine accurately feed consumption and, therefore, impossible to obtain an accurate estimate of dose.

Although dispersion is not a problem with soluble test materials administered in drinking water, stability often is. As an example, the decompositon rate of vinyl acetate in water was found to be approximately 8.5 per cent per day at room temperature and 5 per cent per day at 5°C (Lijensky and Reuber, 1983). A chronic drinking-water study was conducted with the ester in rats using a procedure in which solutions were prepared on a weekly basis. It was estimated that the animals received at least half the nominal dose. The effect of the decomposition products was not considered in the evaluation of the results of the study. In a subsequent chronic study with the material, drinking water was prepared daily, a labour-intensive procedure, to reduce the influence of the hydrolysis products, and was overformulated by 5 per cent to compensate for the daily rate of hydrolysis (Shaw *et al.*, 1988).

In addition to instability, volatile materials may evaporate from the water into room air. Evaporation will occur at the tip of the drinking water tube and can lead to an overestimate of the actual dose to the animal. As with feeding studies, animals will refuse to drink and/or waste water containing chemicals which impart an unpalatable taste.

Under ideal conditions, the choice of dosing procedures should be dictated by the type of exposure anticipated in normal use or as encountered in the environment. If, in its end use, a material will be administered in bolus form, as is the case with many drugs which are designed to be administered by capsule, then certainly administration by gavage is appropriate. On the other hand, when data from a study will be used to estimate the risk from chronic exposure to a contaminant in food or water, a feeding or drinking water study would be more appropriate. A material entering the gastrointestinal tract as a bolus, contrasted with the more uniform pattern when ingested in feed or water, will affect both the rate of absorption and peak plasma concentrations in both the hepatic portal and the systemic circulatory systems. In the case of bolus administration, hepatic metabolic enzyme systems may become saturated, allowing higher concentrations of unmetabolized chemical to enter the systemic circulation, possibly influencing toxic response.

More often than not, the physical and/or chemical properties of a test substance dictate the manner in which it will be administered. Chemicals that are insoluble in water cannot be administered in drinking water. Volatile chemicals are not suited for feeding studies. Reactive materials will not maintain the degree of purity required for testing when formulated in feed or water. Under these conditions gavage administration is sometimes the only rational alternative available.

The chemical intermediate 2-ethylhexanol (2-EH) is a case in point. This chemical was nominated for chronic testing under the provisions of the Toxic Substances Control Act (EPA, 1990). The concern arose from possible exposure to the chemical in the environment due to its high production volume. In the 'Rule' the oral route of exposure was specified for the chronic testing. The material is an industrial chemical intermediate, and, considering its noxious nature, it would be highly unlikely that repeated exposure would occur as a result of swallowing bolus doses. Therefore, a means of more uniform administration was sought. Although this alcohol has a relatively low vapour pressure, 0.05 mmHg at

20°C, it was found to evaporate rapidly when formulated in feed. The maximum solubility in water was found to be approximately 0.06 per cent. A short-term repeated (11 day) exposure study was conducted with water saturated with 2-EH, the maximum dosage achieved being about 160 mg kg^{-1} day^{-1}. At this dose no toxic effects were noted in either rats or mice. This procedure of dosing, therefore, proved to be unacceptable for a guideline study which requires demonstration of toxicity.

Interest was expressed in conducting a feeding experiment with microencapsulated 2-EH. Microencapsulation is a process whereby the test material is uniformly coated with a degradable but impervious material (Melnick *et al.*, 1987a). Microencapsulation has been used in feeding studies to prevent evaporation of volatile materials and to mask objectionable tastes (Aida *et al.*, 1989; Melnick *et al.*, 1987b; Yuan *et al.*, 1991). Microcapsules of 2-EH were prepared, using food-grade modified corn starch as the coating medium. Again, a short-term repeated study was conducted with this material in rats and mice. By use of this technique, 2-EH was shown to remain stable in the feed. In rats dosages of up to 2700 mg kg^{-1} day^{-1} were achieved and produced toxic effects, as expected. In contrast, dosages of greater than 5000 mg kg^{-1} day^{-1} were attained in mice, this being in the range of the single-dose LD$_{50}$ of between 3.2 and 6.4 mg kg^{-1} for this species. Even at this dose no appreciable toxicity was noted, which suggests that microencapsulated 2-EH may not be appropriate for chronic feeding studies in mice. After conducting several more short-term repeated studies using various dosing vehicles, the only feasible procedure for conducting the chronic study was by gavage using an aqueous emulsifier for the dosing vehicle.

Dosing Vehicles

It is often necessary when conducting studies by gavage to dilute the test substance in a dosing vehicle. Usually an aqueous vehicle is preferred, but often materials are insoluble in water and a more non-polar medium is required. For such materials corn oil is generally the vehicle of choice. Administering test substances in corn oil can have a profound influence on the toxicity observed. Kim and co-workers (1990) found that

carbon tetrachloride at single doses of 10 mg kg^{-1} and 25 mg kg^{-1} in corn oil caused less severe hepatic injury than when given at these same dosages either undiluted or as an aqueous emulsion to rats. Although clearly affecting the severity of the injury, the formulations appeared to have little effect on the time-course of hepatic injury as evaluated by serum enzyme activities and histopathological examination. In contrast, the hepatotoxicity of chloroform in mice was shown to be enhanced by formulation in corn oil over that when administered as an aqueous emulsion (Bull *et al.*, 1986). Both the corn oil and aqueous emulsion formulations produced significantly decreased body weights and increased liver weights when given to B6C3F1 mice at dosages of from 60 mg kg^{-1} day^{-1} to 270 mg kg^{-1} day^{-1} for 90 days. The effect in corn oil, however, was greatly enhanced over that when administered as the emulsion. Further, the mice receiving the corn oil formulation demonstrated clear pathological changes in liver, whereas similar lesions were not seen in animals administered corn oil without chloroform or in animals receiving chloroform at similar dosages in the emulsion.

Jorgenson *et al.* (1985) have postulated that differences in carcinogenic response in female mice obtained in two bioassays with chloroform may be explained by the formulation. These workers could not confirm a previous finding that chloroform induced hepatocellular carcinomas in female B6C3F1 mice (Reuber, 1979). In the NCI study an 80 per cent incidence of hepatocellular carcinomas was observed when the chlorinated hydrocarbon was administered in corn oil at a dosage of 238 mg kg^{-1} day^{-1}, 7 days a week for 78 weeks. Jorgenson and co-workers found only a 2 per cent incidence of hepatocellular carcinoma when they administered the chemical in drinking water at a dosage of 263 mg kg^{-1} day^{-1}. These authors suggested that either the dosing regimen, bolus versus the more gradual dosing via drinking water, or the dosing vehicle may have accounted for the discrepancies in the two bioassays.

Other examples of the effect of vehicle on absorption and subsequent toxicity include 1,1-dichloroethylene, which, when given to fasted rats in corn oil or mineral oil, has been shown to enhance hepatic injury compared with when given as an aqueous emulsion (Chieco *et al.*, 1981). The dosing vehicle had little effect on subsequent liver injury when 1,1-dichloroethylene was given by gavage to fed animals. Administering corn oil formulations of methylene chloride, dichloroethane, trichloroethylene and chloroform decreased the rate and extent of uptake, as measured by area under the blood concentration–time curve and peak plasma concentrations, compared with that when administered in aqueous solution (Withey *et al.*, 1983). Thus, with the exception of carbon tetrachloride, corn oil formulations of chlorinated hydrocarbons appear to enhance the toxic response to the liver. Perhaps the anomalous behaviour of carbon tetrachloride results from a different mechanism of hepatic toxicity, that believed to occur through the formation of free radicals, a mechanism which, perhaps, is enhanced by more rapid uptake and corresponding higher peak plasma concentrations.

Ingestion of significant quantities of corn oil will clearly increase the flow of lymph. As described previously, this can lead to an increase in quantity of lipophilic material (i.e. *p,p'*-DDT and analogues) absorbed through the lymphatics (Sieber, 1976). This mechanism may also account for the enhancement of maximum plasma levels and bioavailability, and an increase in the duration of the absorption time of the refractory antibiotic griseofulvin when administered as a corn oil emulsion compared with administration as an aqueous suspension (Bates and Carrigan, 1975).

Prandial State

The presence of food or, for that matter, even the anticipation of the presence of food, can have a profound effect on the physiological state of the gastrointestinal tract. The manner in which the ionic milieu, the pH and the fluid volume affect the absorption, and subsequently the toxicity of drugs and chemicals can be complex. Common advice has suggested that 'gastric absorption is favoured by an empty stomach in which the drug, in undiluted gastric juice, will have good access to the mucosal wall' and that 'only when a drug is irritating to the gastric mucosa is it rational to administer it with or after a meal' (Goldstein *et al.*, 1974). This advice clearly is not universal for all drugs, and does not reflect the effect of prandial state on the known toxicity of many chemicals. Welling (1977) reviewed the effect of food and diet on the gastrointestinal absorption,

grouping a series of drugs into four different categories:

- drugs whose absorption may be reduced by food;
- drugs whose absorption may be delayed by food;
- drugs whose absorption may be unaffected by food;
- drugs whose absorption may be increased by food.

The first category was represented by members of the penicillin family, tetracycline, aspirin and several other materials. The second group contained many of the sulpha and cephalosporin drugs. Drugs which appeared to be unaffected by the prandial state included theophylline and prednisone, while those which were enhanced by the presence of food in the gastrointestinal tract included griseofulvin, nitrofurantoin, propoxyphene and a few others. No generalizations could be made as to what structural or other features contributed to either a depression or an enhancement of absorption in the presence or absence of food. In a later paper, however, Welling (1984) discussed the effects of stomach emptying time, which could enhance the absorption of drugs, particularly basic drugs, by increasing the percentage dissolved prior to passing into the small intestine and by prolonging the time in which the drug comes in contact with the absorptive surface, the mucosal wall. In addition, food interactions can affect the absorption of specific molecules—for instance, absorption of penicillamine and tetracyclines is impeded by chelation with heavy metals and complex formation with proteins.

In addition to the effect of dosing vehicle, the effect of prandial state on the absorption of chlorinated hydrocarbons has been studied. Chieco *et al.* (1981) demonstated that the hepatotoxicity of 1,1-dichloroethylene was diminished in fasted animals when administered in aqueous suspension. The metabolism of vinylidene chloride was shown to be diminished in fasted rats (McKenna *et al.*, 1978). A 50 per cent increase in the amount of parent compound was eliminated in exhaled air of fasted rats compared with fed rats receiving a single 50 mg kg^{-1} oral dose of ^{14}C labelled chemical. In addition, fasting also resulted in an increased concentration of covalently bound metabolites in the liver and, in contrast to the experience with 1,1-dichloroethylene, led to an enhancement of hepatotoxicity. The increased covalent binding and hepatotoxicity may have resulted from depleted concentrations of glutathione in the livers of the fasted animals.

The acute peroral toxicity of epoxidized soybean oil and polypropylene glycol were both shown to be widely divergent, depending on whether or not rats were fed or fasted when dosed (Tyler and Ballantyne, 1988). The LD_{50} values obtained under the two prandial states are shown in Table 1. In this case feeding has opposite effects on the toxicity of these two dissimilar materials. The reasons for this discrepant behaviour are not understood at this time. In contrast to the effects of prandial state with these chemicals, Bates and Carrigan (1975) found no effect on the absorption, maximum plasma concentrations or bioavailability when griseofulvin was given orally in corn oil emulsion to either fed or fasted rats.

Results obtained in studies where animals have been fasted for prolonged periods of time, over 20 h, may reflect functional changes in the intestinal mucosa (Doluisio *et al.*, 1969). Although fasting for up to 20 h had little effect on intestinal absorption of salicylic acid, barbital, haloperidol or chlorpromazine in a surgical preparation, significant decrements in the absorption rate were noted when trials were conducted with rats fasted for over 20 h. Krasavage and Terhaar (1981) investigated the effect of prandial state on a series of glycol ethers (Table 2). These chemicals, monoethers of ethylene glycol, are solvents which are soluble in water as well as in less polar solvents. The ethylene glycol monoethers are, in general, more toxic than the diethylene glycol monoethers. However, prandial state also appears to play a moderating role in the toxic activity of these solvents, animals dosed in the fed state universally demonstrating resistance to the toxic effects of the chemicals. The mechanism of toxicity of monobutyl and monopropyl ethers in rodents differs from that of the lower homologues,

Table 1 Effect of feeding and fasting on the acute oral LD_{50} in rats

Epoxidized soybean oil	Fasted	64
	Fed	19
Polypropylene glycol	Fasted	0.8
	Fed	4

the methyl and ethyl ethylene glycol ethers, with the toxic effects of the former being produced primarily through effects on red blood cells leading to haemolysis. The moderating effect of feeding appears to have less influence on this toxic activity than it has on the toxic effects of the other glycol ethers. In addition, the moderating effects of feeding appear to be accentuated in rats compared with mice.

Effects of Direct Contact

Severely irritating and corrosive materials can produce toxic effects by direct action on the oesophagus and stomach. Such effects are commonly encountered in accidental swallowing, but occasionally these effects can complicate the interpretation of animal studies when administering test materials by gavage. In humans, particularly in the case of accidental poisonings in children caused by swallowing caustic materials, severe injury and fatalities may result from oesophageal perforation and resulting local and systemic complications. More commonly oesophageal burns occur, leading later to the development of strictures and possible infection. The development of strictures appears to be directly correlated to the severity of the burn. Thus, third-degree burns, defined by ulcerations, white plaques and sloughing of the mucosa in a circumferential pattern, lead to a high incidence of stricture formation requiring surgical correction (Anderson *et al.*, 1990). In cases where caustics happen to reach the stomach with minimal injury, regurgitation may result in further injury to the oesophagus and exacerbate an already critical condition. This, together with aspiration hazards, is the basis of the first-aid advice not to induce vomiting in cases of swallowing caustic or severely irritating chemicals.

In studies where irritating materials are given to animals by gavage, little opportunity exists for irritation or corrosive injury to the oesophagus, since the test material is injected through an animal feeding needle or a tube directly into the stomach. Rodents are believed to lack the vomiting response and therefore regurgitation of materials back into the oesophagus is not ordinarily encountered. However, in practical situations oesophageal perforation or tears can occur in a dosage-related manner, suggesting that materials do come into contact with the oeso-

Table 2 Effect of prandial state on acute toxicity (LD_{50}) of a series of glycol ethers

	Rats (mmol kg^{-1})		Mice (mmol kg^{-1})	
	Fasted	Fed	Fasted	Fed
Ethylene glycol monomethyl ether	29.7	51.7	51.7	59.4
Ethylene glycol monoethyl ether	39.2	90	27.2	59.4
Ethylene glycol monopropyl ether	29.7	59.4	17.1	29.7
Ethylene glycol monobutyl ether	14.8	14.8	12.9	17
Diethylene glycol monomethyl ether	59.4	103	59.4	68.2
Diethylene glycol monoethyl ether	78.4	119	45	45
Diethylene glycol monopropyl ether	45	64.8	25.8	38.5
Diethylene glycol monobutyl ether	45	59.4	14.8	34.1
Ethylene glycol mono-2-ethyl hexyl ether	45	29.6	42	22.4

Unpublished data obtained from the Eastman Kodak Company, Rochester, New York.

phageal tissue, particularly in the area of the gastro-oesophageal junction. Such dose-related injury has been seen in rats repeatedly administered diethylene glycol monobutyl ether by gavage (Hobson *et al.*, 1987) and when isopropanol was administered to rats by gavage in a repeated-dose reproductive probe study (Table 3). Presumably, the oesophageal injury was exacerbated by repeated direct exposure to the irritating properties of these materials through

Table 3 Treatment-related oesophageal injury produced by gavage of isopropanol to rats

Dose[a] (mg kg^{-1})	% of dead with oesophageal injury
0	0
0.1	0
0.5	0
1.0	57
1.75	8
2.5	25

[a] Given as an aqueous solution at a dosage volume of 5 ml kg^{-1}.

some sort of regurgitating process in the area of the gastro-oesophageal junction.

A second type of direct irritation to the rodent gastrointestinal tract occurs in the forestomach. A number of chemicals have been shown to produce severe irritation to the forestomach tissue when given by gavage: butylated hydroxyanisole; propionic acid; ethyl acrylate; diglycidyl resorcinol ether; epichlorohydrin; methyl acrylamidoglycolate methyl ether; and aristolochic acid. Ethyl acrylate, for instance, has been shown to cause forestomach tumours in rats and mice when administered in corn oil by gavage (NTP, 1986). In that study there was no increase in the incidence of tumours in any other organ or tissue. In addition, a 27-month bioassay in rats and mice by inhalation was without a carcinogenic response (Miller *et al.*, 1985); a lifetime mouse skin painting study did not result in the induction of skin tumours at the site of contact (DePass *et al.*, 1984); a 2-year drinking water study in rats did not result in forestomach tumours or an increase in any other tumour type; and a study in which dogs, which do not possess a forestomach, were administered ethyl acrylate by capsule for a 2-

year period did not induce a carcinogenic response (Borzelleca *et al.*, 1964).

The relationship between the irritant response and forestomach tumours is not clear; however, Ghanayem and co-workers (1991) have shown that administration of ethyl acrylate in corn oil to rats for 13 weeks results in severe epithelial hyperplasia of the forestomach without involvement of the glandular stomach or the liver. There was a significant decrease in the incidence and severity of forestomach mucosal hyperplasia in animals treated in a similar manner for 13 weeks and sacrificed 8 weeks later. An even greater decline in the severity of the response was noted in animals allowed a 19-month recovery period, with no tumours developing in the forestomach of these animals. In a following study these workers demonstrated that repeated oral gavage administration of ethyl acrylate in corn oil to rats for either 6 months or 12 months produced extensive mucosal cell proliferation in the forestomach (Ghanayem *et al.*, 1992). In those animals dosed for 6 months there was a significant time-dependent regression in cell proliferation at 2 and 15 months after cessation of dosing, with no evidence of neoplasia. In those rats dosed for 12 months, on the other hand, papillomas were observed in 2 of 5 animals at 2 months, and squamous cell carcinomas or papillomas were seen in 4 of 13 animals at 9 months after dosing had been discontinued. These data suggest that local effects of irritation produced by gavage administration can have a profound influence on the toxicity of a material and that the length of time over which the irritation takes place is a critical factor in eliciting the toxic response, particularly as related to neoplastic events associated with chronic irritation.

CONSIDERATIONS IN HAZARD EVALUATION AND RISK ASSESSMENT

From the foregoing discussion it is abundantly clear that, once ingested, there are numerous factors which affect the manner in which chemical toxicants pass through and are absorbed from the gastrointestinal tract. It is equally clear that differences exist between animal species with regard to both anatomical structure and physiological function. In addition, hepatic portal circulation and potential absorption through the central lacteals of the intestinal villi, with subsequent lymphatic absorption, provide unique differences in the uptake and disposition of toxicants from the gastrointestinal tract as compared with uptake by other typical routes of exposure to environmental chemicals (i.e. the skin and respiratory tract) or by intravenous administration of pharmaceutical preparations or social poisons. A clear understanding of, and accountability for, these factors and differences is essential when attempting to extrapolate hazards and risks from studies which have been conducted by oral administration in laboratory animals to exposure in humans, either by ingestion or by other routes.

Anatomical and Physiological Considerations

As pointed out above, one of the more obvious distinguishing anatomical differences between the gastrointestinal tract of humans and that of rodents is the presence of a food storage compartment in the stomach, the forestomach. The epithelial lining of this structure is very similar to that of the human oesophagus; however, the residence time of food in the oesophagus is transient, whereas that in the forestomach may be prolonged. Other, less obvious, differences exist between common laboratory animals and man which can influence passage and absorption and subsequently the toxicity of environmental chemicals and drugs. Table 4, for instance, demonstrates the proportional differences between

Table 4 Comparison of lengths of intestinal segments between man and rats[a]

Segment	Human length (cm)	Human % of total	Rats length (cm)	Rats % of total
Small intestine	500	–	125	–
duodenum	25	5	10	8
jejunum	190	38	110	88
ileum	285	57	5	4
Large intestine	170	–	24	–
caecum	7	4	6	25
colon	108	64	10	42
rectum	55[b]	32	8	33

[a] Adapted from DeSesso and Mavis (1989).
[b] Includes both sigmoid colon and rectum.

lengths of various segments of the intestinal tract of humans and of rats. In the rat the jejunum accounts for approximately 88 per cent of the ileum and 4 per cent of the length of the small intestine, while the corresponding proportions in humans are 38 per cent and 57 per cent, respectively. In addition to differences in the length of various segments of the small intestine, there are differences in the mucosal structure—i.e. the intestinal villi of rats are about twice as long as those of man or other non-rodents (DeSesso and Mavis, 1989).

In addition to species differences in the structure of the gastrointestinal tract, differences also exist in physiological function. For most mammalian species, both rodent and non-rodent, the anterior portion of the stomach is generally less acidic than the posterior portion, ranging in pH from about 4.3 in the pig to 6.9 in the hamster, a species with a prominent limiting ridge (Calabrese, 1983). Posterior gastric pH ranges from about 2.2 in the pig to 4.2 in the cat. The rabbit, on the other hand, is an exception to this pattern, producing notably acidic gastric fluid and demonstrating little difference in the pH between the two portions of the stomach, fluid in both the anterior and posterior parts falling in a pH range of around 1.9. The distribution and kinds of microflora may also differ between animal species. Although the gastric contents of most contain few micro-organisms, the forestomach and upper small intestine of the rat support a considerable population of microflora.

First-pass Effect Considerations

The hepatic portal circulatory pattern, which is unique to the gastrointestinal tract, requires special consideration when attempting quantitatively or qualitatively to extrapolate effects encountered by oral administration to other routes of exposure. As has been pointed out previously, all material absorbed from the distal portion of the oesophagus to the distal rectum is transported by way of the portal vein to the liver. The liver, being a primary organ of metabolism, can have a major influence on the concentrations of parent toxicant and metabolites which enter the general circulatory system. The bioavailability of the anti-inflammatory drug diclofenac sodium, for instance, can be reduced by values ranging from 50 per cent to 60 per cent when given orally

(Peris-Ribera *et al.*, 1991). Propranolol and lignocaine (lidocaine) are two other drugs which have been shown to be rapidly metabolized by the liver and exhibit differences in plasma time–concentration patterns when administered orally compared with methods in which they directly enter the systemic circulation.

Considerations of Bolus versus Continuous Dosing

Bolus administration can also affect the concentration–time pattern of ingested chemicals and therefore affect potential toxic responses. Table 5 demonstrates the effect of bolus dosing versus continuous dosing on the developmental toxicity of ethylene glycol in mice. Acute toxic responses may be elicited by high peak concentrations and thus toxicity is accentuated by gavage dosing, and diminished when given in feed or water. High portal vein concentrations of chemicals which have poor affinity for active sites on metabolic enzymes (high Michaelis constants) can saturate these enzymes, resulting in breakthrough of the chemical into the systemic circulation. Cumulative toxicity, on the other hand, may be uninfluenced or diminished by bolus doses. Dosing chemicals in corn oil vehicle may increase the amount absorbed by way of the lymphatics, reducing the effect of hepatic portal circulation, since corn oil will stimulate the flow of lymph. Careful consideration must be given to these variables when, as so often is the case, oral toxicity data are the only data available, and extrapolation is attempted to predict what air concentration of a chemical will produce similar toxic effects when exposure is by inhalation.

Localized Effect Considerations

The forestomach has been shown to be the site of both neoplastic and non-neoplastic lesions, possibly associated with an irritant response and

Table 5 Effect of bolus compared with continuous dosing of ethylene glycol on developmental effects in mice

Procedure	Minimum effect level	NOEL
Gavage[a]	500	150
Drinking-water[b]	≈2000	≈1000

[a] Tyl *et al.* (1989).
[b] NTP (1984).

associated cellular hyperplasia. It is important to note the difference in anatomical structure and function between rodents and humans. Thus, it is difficult to evaluate the significance of a chemically induced tumorigenic response in this structure, particularly when the chemical produces no similar carcinogenic response in other organs or tissues and does not exhibit genotoxic activity. In addition, irritation, hyperplasia and eventual tumour formation appear to be more related to the concentration of test substance in the dosing solution than to total dose administered (Davis *et al.*, 1986; Clayson *et al.*, 1990). Although consideration has been given to the use of the forestomach as a model for the human oesophagus, attempts to demonstrate similar reactivities for the oesophageal and forestomach mucosa in various species have been unsuccessful (Wester and Kroes, 1988). Taken as a whole, critical evaluation is required in determining appropriate classification of chemicals which produce a carcinogenic response in the forestomach of rodents alone, and without evidence of genotoxic activity.

Consideration of Gastrointestinal Parameters in Modelling

Current efforts in attempts to extrapolate toxicity data between species and routes of administration centre around the use of physiologically based pharmacokinetic models. These models, which are based on realistic anatomical and physiological concepts, account for major differences encountered in route-to-route extrapolations, such as the hepatic portal circulation, and species-to-species extrapolations, such as proportional differences in organ perfusion. On the other hand, the effect of dosing vehicle, differences in epithelial cell type, effects of prandial state and local effects of chemical insult prove harder to account for in these models. Staats and co-workers (1991) attempted to explain differences in the gastrointestinal absorption of trichloroethylene when administered to rats by gavage in either water or corn oil. A physiologically based pharmacokinetic model which incorporated a two-compartment gastrointestinal tract simulated blood concentration–time-course data more accurately than did a model incorporating a one-compartment description. Curiously, although the physiologically based pharmacokinetic approach is usually based on specific anatomical and physio-

logical considerations, in this case the selection of the compartments was arbitrary. Although the authors suggested that the compartments might represent the stomach and small intestine, respectively, no terms specific for these two distinct portions of the tract were incorporated into their model to account for physiological differences or transport.

Frederick *et al.* (1992), on the other hand, have developed a physiologically based pharmacokinetic model which includes a description of the interaction of ethyl acrylate on the tissues of the entire gastrointestinal tract. The model was designed to describe the effects resulting from tissue contact as measured by glutathione depletion, this being an important factor in understanding the mechanism of toxicity of this chemical. This model incorporated both portions of the rodent stomach, the forestomach and the glandular stomach, the duodenum and the remainder of the small intestine, and the caecum, large intestine and colon.

Both of these models demonstrate the complexity and difficulties involved in addressing anatomical, physiological and mechanistic details in attempts to extrapolate toxicological information obtained in peroral studies in one species to health risks by other routes of exposure in other species.

SUMMARY

From the above discussion it is clear that numerous factors affect the passage of drugs and chemicals through and absorption from the gastrointestinal tract. These factors involve both anatomical features, which can differ between species, and physiological features, the function of which can be influenced by conditions under which a material is administered. Any attempt to extrapolate toxic effects of chemicals obtained after oral dosing of animals must take into consideration:

(1) Anatomical differences between the species of comparison including such factors as the presence of a forestomach; pH differences between various segments of the gastrointestinal tract; the presence or absence of microflora in various parts of the gastrointestinal tract; other factors which may be specific to the chemical under study—i.e. length of intestinal segments,

presence or absence of a gall bladder, prevalence of Peyer's patches, etc.

(2) Physiological differences between routes of administration, including hepatic portal circulation; lymphatic absorption; possible pharmacological effects of the chemical on the function of the gastrointestinal tract—i.e. possible effects on gastric motility or blood circulation.

(3) The influence of conditions under which a material was administered: the prandial state of the animal; mode of dosing—more or less continuous, as opposed to bolus dosing; possible effects of dosing vehicle on absorption and metabolism; direct effects of the chemical at the site of contact.

All such factors will influence the extrapolation of results obtained from animal testing, particularly as they apply to extrapolation between rodents and humans and between the peroral route of administration and other common routes of exposure, including inhalation and skin absorption.

REFERENCES

Aida, Y., Ando, M., Takada, K., Momma, J., Yoshimoto, H., Nakaji, Y., Kurokawa, Y. and Tobe, M. (1989). Practical application of microcapsulation for toxicity studies using bromodichloromethane as a model compound. *J. Am. Coll. Toxicol.* **8**, 1177–1187

Anderson, K. D., Rouse, T. M. and Randolph, J. G. (1990). A controlled trial of corticosteroids in children with corrosive injury on the esophagus. *New Engl. J. Med.*, **323**, 637–640

Aungst, B. and Shen, D. D. (1986). Gastrointestinal absorption of toxic agents. In Rozman, K. and Hanninen, O. (Eds), *Gastrointestinal Toxicology*, Elsevier, New York, pp. 35–36

Bates, T. and Carrigan, P. (1975). Apparent absorption kinetics of micronized griseofulvin after its oral administration on single- and multiple-dose regimens to rats as a corn oil-in-water emulsion and aqueous suspension. *J. Pharm. Sci.*, **64**, 1475–1481

Bauchop, T. and Martucci, R. W. (1968). Rumen-like digestion of the Langur monkey. *Science* **161**, 698–700

Borzelleca, J. F., Larson, P. S., Hennigar, G. R. Jr, Huf, E. G., Crawford, E. M. and Smith, R. B. Jr (1964). Studies on the chronic oral toxicity of monomeric ethyl acrylate and methyl methacrylate. *Toxicol. Appl. Pharmacol.*, **6**, 29–36

Bull, R. J., Brown, J. M., Meierhenry, E. A., Jorgen-son, T. A., Robinson, M. and Stober, J. A. (1986). Enhancement of the hepatotoxicity of chloroform in B6C3F1 mice by corn oil: implications for chloroform carcinogenesis. *Environ. Hlth Perspect.*, **69**, 49–58

Calabrese, E. J. (1983). Absorption—interspecies differences. In *Principles of Animal Extrapolation*. Wiley, New York, pp. 45–47

Chieco, P., Moslen, M. T. and Reynolds, E. S. (1981). Effect of administrative vehicle on oral 1,1-dichloro-ethylene toxicity. *Toxicol. Appl. Pharmacol.*, **57**, 146–155

Clayson, D. B., Iverson, F., Nera, E. A. and Lok, E. (1990). The significance of induced forestomach tumors. *Ann. Rev. Pharmacol. Toxicol.*, **30**, 441–463

Crouthamel, W. G., Tan, G. H., Dittert, L. W. and Doluisio, J. T. (1971). Drug absorption. IV. Influence of pH on absorption kinetics of weakly acidic drugs. *J. Pharm. Sci.*, **60**, 1160–1163

Davis, R. A., Siglin, J. C., Becci, P. J. and Friedman, M. A. (1986). Concentration dependence and reversibility of gastric lesions induced by repeated gavage of acrylic monomers. *Toxicologist*, **6**, 188

Dellow, D. W., Nolan, J. V. and Hume, I. D. (1983). Studies on the nutrition of macropodine marsupials. V. Microbial fermentation in the forestomach of *Thyogale thetis* and *Macropus eugenii*. *Aust. J. Zool.*, **31**, 433–443

DeMarco, T. J. and Levine, R. R. (1969). Role of the lymphatics in the intestinal absorption and distribution of drugs. *J. Pharmacol Exptl Ther.*, **169**, 142–151

DePass, L. R., Fowler, E. H., Meckley, D. R. and Weil, C. S. (1984). Dermal oncogenicity bioassays of acrylic acid, ethyl acrylate and butyl acrylate. *J. Toxicol. Environ. Hlth*, **14**, 115–120

DeSesso, J. M. and Mavis, R. D. (1989). *Identification of Critical Biological Parameters Affecting Gastrointestinal Absorption. The MITRE Corporation, Report No. MTR–89W00223.* McLean, Virginia

Doluisio, J. T., Tan, G. H., Billups, N. F. and Diamond, L. (1969). Drug absorption. II. Effect of fasting on intestinal drug absorption. *J. Pharm. Sci.*, **58**, 1200–1201

EPA (1990). Part 799: Identification of specific chemical substance and mixture testing requirements—2-ethylhexanol. *Code of Federal Regulations* Part 40, 605–606

Frederick, C. B., Potter, D. W., Chang-Mateu, M. I. and Andersen, M. E. (1992). A physiologically-based pharmacokinetic and pharmacodynamic model for the oral dosing of rats with ethyl acrylate and its implications for risk assessment. *Toxicol. Appl. Pharmacol*, **114**, 246–260

Ghanayem, B. I., Matthews, H. B. and Marenpot, R. R. (1991). Sustainability of forestomach hyperplasia in rats treated with ethyl acrylate for 13 weeks and regression after cessation of dosing. *Toxicol. Pathol.* **19**, 273–279

Ghanayem, B. I., Sanchez, I. M. and Elwell, M. R. (1992). Sustainability of ethyl acrylate (EA) induced forestomach (FS) cell proliferation (CP) for 12, but not 6 months, leads to carcinogenesis after cessation of dosing in male F344 rats. *Toxicologist*, **12**, 268

Goldstein, A., Aronow, L. and Kalman, S. M. (1974). *Principles of Drug Action: The Basis of Pharmacology*, 2nd edn. Wiley, New York, pp. 129–217

Grajal, A., Strahl, S. D., Parra, R., Dominguez, M. G. and Neher, A. (1989). Foregut fermentation in the hoatzin, a neotropical leaf-eating bird. *Science*, **245**, 1236–1238

Guyton, A. C. (1981). Chapters 63–66. *Textbook of Medical Physiology*, 6th edn. Saunders, Philadelphia, pp. 784–834

Ham, A. W. and Cormack, D. H. (1979). The digestive System. In *Histology*, 8th edn. Lippincott, Philadelphia, pp. 645–693

Hobson, D. W., Wyman, J. F., Lee, L. H., Bruner, R. H. and Uddin, D. E. (1987). *The Subchronic Toxicity of Diethylene Glycol Monobutyl Ether Administered Orally to Rats*. Naval Medical Research and Development Command, NMRI 87–48. NTIS, Springfield, Virginia

Johnson, F. R. (1981). The Digestive System. In Romanes, G. J. (Ed.), *Cunningham's Textbook of Anatomy*, 12th edn. Oxford University Press, New York, pp. 411–489

Johnson, L. R. (1985). Gastric secretion & pancreatic secretion. In Johnson, L. R. (Ed.), *Gastrointestinal Physiology*, Mosby, St. Louis, pp. 63–93

Jorgenson, T. A., Meierhenry, E. F., Rushbrook, C. J., Bull, R. J. and Robinson, M. (1985). Carcinogenicity of chloroform in drinking water to male Osporne–Mendel rats and female B6C3F1 mice. *Fund. Appl. Toxicol.*, **5**, 760–769

Kim, H. J., Odend'hal, S. and Bruckner, J. V. (1990). Effect of dosing vehicles on the acute hepatotoxicity of carbon tetrachloride in rats. *Toxicol. Appl. Pharmacol.*, **102**, 34–49

Krasavage, W. J. and Terhaar, C. J. (1981) *Comparative Toxicity of Nine Glycol Ethers: I. Acute Oral LD50*. Eastman Kodak Company, Health Safety and Human Factors Laboratory. Rochester, New York

Lijensky, W. and Reuber, M. D. (1983). Chronic toxicity studies of vinyl acetate in Fischer rats. *Toxicol. Appl. Pharmacol.*, **68**, 43–53

McKenna, M. J., Zempel, J. A., Madrid, E. O., Braun, W. H. and Gehring, P. J. (1978). Metabolism and pharmacokinetic profile of vinylidene chloride in rats following oral administration. *Toxicol. Appl. Pharmacol.*, **45**, 821–835

Melnick, R. L., Jameson, C. W., Goehl, T. J. and Kuhn, G. O. (1987a). Applications of microencapsulation for toxicology studies, I. Principles and stabilization of trichloroethylene in gelatin–sorbitol microcapsules. *Fund. Appl. Toxicol.*, **8**, 425–431

Melnick, R. L., Jameson, C. W., Goehl, T. J., Maronpot, R. R., Collins, B. J., Greenwell, A., Harring-ton, F. W., Wilson, R. E., Tomaszewski, K. E. and Agarwal, D. K. (1987b). Application of Microencapsulation for toxicology studies. II. Toxicity of micro-encapsulated trichloroethylene in Fischer 344 rats. *Fund. Appl. Toxicol.*, **8**, 432–442

Miller, R. R., Young, J. T., Kociba, R. J., Keyes, D. G., Bodner, K. M., Calhoun, L. L. and Ayres, J. A. (1985). Chronic toxicity and oncogenicity bioassay of inhaled ethyl acrylate in Fischer 344 rats and B6C3F1 mice. *Drug Chem. Toxicol.*, **8**, 1–42

NTP (1984). *Ethylene Glycol: Fertility Assessment in CD-1 Mice When Administered in Drinking Water*. Report No. NTP–82–FACB–015. National Institute of Environmental Health Sciences, Research Triangle Park, North Carolina

NTP (1986). *Carcinogenesis Studies of Ethyl Acrylate in F344/N Rats and B6C3F1 Mice (Gavage Studies)*. NIH Publication No. 87–2515. NTP Public Information Office, National Toxicology Program, Research Triangle Park, North Carolina

Peris-Ribera, J.-E., Torres-Molina, F., Garcia-Carbonell, M. C., Aristorena, J. C. and Pla-Delfina, J. M. (1991). Pharmacokinetics and bioavailability of diclofenac in the rat. *J. Pharmacokin. Biopharm.*, **19**, 647–664

Reuber, M. D. (1979). Carcinogenicity of chloroform. *Environ. Hlth Perspect.*, **31**, 171–182

Schanker, L. S. and Jeffrey, J. J. (1961). Active transport of foreign pyrimidines across the intestinal epiphelium. *Nature* **190**, 727–728

Schanker, L. S., Shore, P. A., Brodie, B. B. and Hogben, C. A. (1957). Absorption of drugs from the stomach I. The rat. *J. Pharmacol. Exptl Ther.*, **120**, 528–539

Shaw, D. C., Zubaidy, A. J., Clary, J. J., Rickard, R. W., Tyler, T. R., Vinegar, M. B. and Carpanini, F. (1988). Chronic oral toxicity and carcinogenicity study of vinyl acetate administered in drinking water. *Toxicologist* **8**(1), 162

Sieber, S. M. (1976). The lymphatic absorption of p,p'-DDT and some structurally-related compounds in the rat. *Pharmacol.* **14**, 443–454

Smith, P. L. (1986). Gastrointestinal physiology. In Rozman, K. and Hanninen, O. (Eds), *Gastrointestinal Toxicology*. Elsevier, New York, pp. 1–28

Staats, D. A., Fisher, J. W. and Connolly, R. B. (1991). Gastrointestinal absorption of xenobiotics in physiologically based pharmacokinetic models: A two-compartment description. *Drug Metab. Disp.*, **19**, 144–148

Tyl, R. W., Fisher, L. C., Kubena, M. F., Losco, P. E. and Vrbanic, M. A. (1989). Determination of a developmental toxicity 'no observable effect level' for ethylene glycol (EC) by gavage in CD-1 mice. *Terato.*, **39**, 487

Tyler, T. R. and Ballantyne, B. (1988). Practical assessment and communication of chemical hazards in the workplace. In Ballantyne, B. (Ed.), *Perspec-*

tives in Basic and Applied Toxicology. John Wright, London, pp. 330–378

Venho, V. M. K. (1986). Toxicants in the gastrointestinal tract: Drugs. In Rozman, K. and Hanninen, O. (Eds), *Gastrointestinal Toxicology*. Elsevier, New York, pp. 367–368

Vogel, G., Becker, U. and Ulbrich, M. (1975) The relevance of the osmolarity of the intestinal fluid to the effectiveness and toxicity of drugs given by the intraduodenal route—solvent drag influence on the intestinal absorption of drugs. *Arzneim.-Forsch*, **25**, 1037–1039

Weisbrodt, N. W. (1985). Motility of the small intestine. In Johnson, L. R. (Ed.), *Gastrointestinal Physiology*, 3rd edn. Mosby, Princeton

Welling, P. G. (1977). Influence of food and diet on gastrointestinal drug absorption: A review. *J. Pharmacokin. Biopharm.*, **5**, 291–334

Welling, P. G. (1984). Interactions affecting drug absorptions. *Clin. Pharmacokin.*, **9**, 404–434

Wester, P. W. and Kroes, R. (1988). Forestomach carcinogens: Pathology and relevance to man. *Toxicol. Pathol.*, **16**, 165–171

Wilson, R. E., Fisher, L. C. and Van Miller, J. P. (1991). Dosing developmental cutaneous toxicity studies using an automated dual delivery system. *Toxicologist*, **11**, 342

Withey, J. R., Collins, B. T. and Collins, P. G. (1983). Effect of vehicle on the pharmacokinetics and uptake of four halogenated hydrocarbons from the gastrointestinal tract of the rat. *J. Appl. Toxicol.*, **3**, 249–253

Yuan, J., Jameson, C. W. Goehl, T. J. and Collins, B. J. (1991). Molecular encapsulator: A novel vehicle for toxicology studies. *Toxicol. Meth.*, **1**, 231–241

FURTHER READING

Koster, A. S., Richter, E., Lauterbach, F. and Hartmann, F. (1989). *Intestinal Metabolism of Xenobiotics*. Gustav Fisher Verlag, Stuttgart

Rozman, K. and Hannanen, O. (1986). *Gastrointestinal Toxicology*. Elsevier, Amsterdam

17 Percutaneous Toxicity

Hon-Wing Leung and Dennis J. Paustenbach

INTRODUCTION

The skin is an important portal of entry for many chemical substances. An understanding of the percutaneous absorption of chemicals is essential in the evaluation of the potential of a chemical to cause systemic toxicity following skin exposure. While the percutaneous absorption of many industrial chemicals in liquid state and those dissolved in a liquid vehicle have been evaluated, only a handful of chemicals in other physical states, e.g. gas or vapour, and those associated with other environmental matrices, e.g. contaminated soil or water, have been studied. Since the behaviour of chemicals in such physical forms can be quite different from that of neat chemicals (matrix effect) and the law of simple diffusion may not be applicable, the estimation of skin uptake of chemicals from various matrices must be carefully conducted.

Most laboratory studies on percutaneous absorption have traditionally been performed with chemicals at high concentrations. These experimental data, therefore, may not be applicable for the low concentrations usually encountered in the environment. Recent developments in various mathematical models may provide a means to overcome this constraint and allows the estimation of skin uptake over a wide range of exposure conditions. In addition, these models also enable the testing of the various factors influencing the skin uptake of chemicals from matrices, thus yielding crucial information on the matrix effect.

CHARACTERISTICS OF THE SKIN AFFECTING PERCUTANEOUS ABSORPTION

The barrier function of the skin is believed to reside almost entirely in the stratum corneum (Scheuplein and Blank, 1985). Although hair follicles and sweat ducts may facilitate the passage of chemicals, their total area is relatively small in humans, and for most chemicals absorption through the general skin surface is the preferred route (Dugard, 1983). In short, for humans, hairy skin seems to be no more permeable than non-hairy skin. However, in the case of some molecules that penetrate the bulk of the stratum corneum slowly, such as electrolytes and polar molecules, the route through follicles and ducts may predominate (Scheuplein, 1980). In humans the capacity of these 'shunts' to facilitate transfer is limited by the small fraction of skin area that consists of shafts and pores (Blank, 1964; Scheuplein, 1965, 1967). However, for mouse skin, hair appears to contribute significantly to overall percutaneous absorption (Kao et al., 1988). These observations suggest that some correction factor should be applied when extrapolating from animal data to predict the human response.

FACTORS AFFECTING PERCUTANEOUS ABSORPTION

The concentration of the applied chemical and the surface area of contact are the two most important factors affecting absorption of a chemical through the skin. The greatest potential for absorption occurs when a high concentration of a chemical is spread over a large surface area of the body (Wester and Noonan, 1980). However, the relationship between the concentration of an applied chemical and the efficiency of its absorption is not necessarily linear. The rate of percutaneous absorption can either decrease or increase with increasing dose, depending on the type of chemical (Wester and Noonan, 1980). Usually, percutaneous uptake will increase if the skin has been damaged by the chemical.

The solvent used to deliver a chemical to the skin (vehicle) will usually have an effect on the efficiency of absorption. The ability of a chemical to penetrate the skin is dependent on two consecutive physical events: the chemical must first diffuse out of the vehicle to the skin surface, and then penetrate the skin en route to the site of action (Ostrenga *et al.*, 1971). If the membrane diffusion constant for the chemical and the thickness and solvent properties of the membrane are unchanged by the nature of the external vehicle, then the rate of absorption is proportional to the chemical potential of the vehicle. When the chemical potential and chemical concentration are linearly related, Fick's laws of diffusion should hold for the vehicle (Dugard, 1983).

The site of application of a chemical can be an important factor affecting the rate of percutaneous absorption. The palm allows about the same penetration as the forearm; the abdomen and the dorsum of the hand have twice the penetration of the forearm; the scalp, the angle of the jaw, the postauricular area and the forehead have fourfold greater penetration; and the scrotum allows almost total absorption (Maibach *et al.*, 1971).

The condition of the skin, such as loss of barrier function of the stratum corneum through disease or damage, will also affect percutaneous absorption. Absorption can be almost 100 per cent if all the barrier function is removed. Some solvents such as dimethyl sulphoxide actually dissolve lipids, thus destroying the barrier function and carrying the chemical rapidly into the bloodstream. Damage due to occupations such as bricklaying, or covering of the applied dose, as with bandaging or putting on clothing after a cutaneous application, will increase absorption. Occlusion changes the hydration and temperature of the skin and prevents loss through wiping or evaporation of an applied dose (McLaughlin, 1984).

The frequency of application is another factor which will often affect the degree of percutaneous absorption. Absorption of a single application of a high concentration of a chemical will often be greater than where the equivalent concentration is applied in equally divided doses (Wester *et al.*, 1977). This is possibly because the initial treatment may have altered the barrier function of the stratum corneum, resulting in an increased absorption for subsequent applications (Wester *et al.*, 1980). Thus, the effects of repeated application will depend on the ability of the individual chemical to cause damage to the stratum corneum.

The skin contains many of the enzymes that are contained in the liver; thus, metabolism by the skin could affect absorption. The metabolizing potential of skin has been estimated to be about 2 per cent of that of the liver with most of the enzyme activity localized in the epidermal layer (Pannatier *et al.*, 1978). The more slowly a chemical is absorbed through the skin, the greater the opportunity for some metabolism to occur. For most chemicals, metabolism by the skin is too small to be worthy of consideration.

RATE AND BIOAVAILABILITY OF PERCUTANEOUS ABSORPTION

Percutaneous absorption is defined as the transport of externally applied chemicals through the cutaneous structures and the extracellular medium to the bloodstream. One of the most interesting phenomena about the percutaneous absorption of organic solvents is that the chemicals often appear in the blood and exhaled air long after skin exposure has ended (Wester and Maibach, 1987). This phenomenon is due to three consecutive processes: (1) a penetration phase — i.e. the passage of a chemical through the superficial skin structures, the stratum corneum and the epidermis, to the extracellular medium; (2) a resorption phase during which a rapid diffusion occurs from the extracellular fluid to the blood via the cutaneous circulation; and (3) lipid-rich tissues such as adipose slowly release the absorbed chemical after cessation of exposure. The skin behaves as a rate-limiting barrier which only allows penetration of chemicals at a relatively slow rate. The skin structure which is largely responsible for this barrier function is the stratum corneum (Marzulli and Tregear, 1961). The living cells of the epidermis are relatively more permeable than are those the stratum corneum and do not govern the rate-limiting step under most circumstances.

The simplest way to model the rate of skin absorption is to assume that Fick's first law of diffusion at steady state is applicable:

$$J = \delta Q / \delta t = K_p \cdot \nabla C = D \cdot k \cdot \nabla C / e$$

where J = flux; $\delta Q / \delta t$ = rate of chemical absorbed; K_p = permeability constant; ∇C = concentration gradient; D = diffusion constant in the stratum corneum; k = stratum corneum–vehicle partition coefficient of the chemical; e = thickness of the stratum corneum. The concentration gradient is equal to the difference between the concentration above and that below the membrane. Since the concentration below is usually negligible relative to the concentration above, the concentration gradient can be approximated to equal the applied chemical concentration.

The above equation describes the kinetics of the penetration process through the skin at steady state. It must be emphasized that it is an oversimplification and is an approximation for most *in vivo* exposure situations, where true steady-state conditions are rarely attained. None the less, this equation includes the most important factors which account for the percutaneous absorption of chemicals. The two factors which strongly influence the transfer rate are the partition coefficient and the diffusion coefficient of the stratum corneum. Since it is rather difficult to measure skin–vehicle partition coeffficients, these two constants are sometimes multiplied together to give a permeability constant. From the equation, it can be seen that the absorption intensity is proportional to the concentration of the chemical and the application area. Thus, for the same quantity of chemical, the systemic effect will be greater in proportion when the skin is occluded (Wepierre and Marty, 1979). Table 1 shows the absorption rate of 34 chemicals through the human skin.

The diffusion constant represents the rate of migration of a chemical through the stratum corneum. As the stratum corneum has a non-negligible thickness, there is a period of transient diffusion during which the rate of transfer through the skin rises to reach a steady state (Figure 1). The steady state is maintained thereafter indefinitely, provided that the system remains constant. The common method of analysing kinetic profiles such as the one depicted in Figure 1 is to determine the lag time (T_L) by extrapolating the linear portion of the curve to the x axis. The diffusion coefficient is then given by $D = e^2/6T_L$.

Depending on the type of chemicals, the lag time sometimes can be as long as several hours or even days. From an exposure assessment standpoint, if the exposure time is shorter than the lag time, it is unlikely that there will be significant systemic absorption and accumulation (Flynn, 1990). The partition coefficient in the diffusion equation illustrates the importance of solubility characteristics for a chemical to penetrate

Table 1 Steady-state skin penetration rates in humans. Adapted from Kasting *et al.* (1987)

Chemical	log K_{ow}[a]	J[b] (mg cm^{-2} h^{-1})
Paracetamol (acetaminophen)	0.47	4.6
Benzoic acid	1.95	720
Benzyl alcohol	1.02	1060
Caffeine	−0.02	1.5
Clonidine HCl	−2.60	1.4
Dextromethorphan	4.13	10
Diazepam	2.80	4.7
Ethacrynic acid	3.95	740
5-Fluorouracil	−0.92	3.2
Frusemide (furosemide)	1.46	0.21
Griseofulvin	2.18	0.24
Hydralazine HCl	−1.53	20
Hydrocortisone	1.61	0.42
Ibuprofen	3.51	430
Indolyl-3-acetic acid	1.41	11
Indomethacin	3.08	0.25
Isosorbide dinitrate	1.22	4.8
Ketoprofen	3.00	12
Methyl salicylate	2.46	1350
Minoxidil	1.24	0.81
Morphine sulphate	−1.76	0.19
Naproxen	3.18	4.8
Nicotinic acid	−0.20	2.2
Nifedipine	2.12	0.07
Oestradiol	2.69	11
Pentazocine	2.19	0.68
Piroxicam	0.05	0.7
Propranolol HCl	−0.45	6.6
Salicylamide	0.89	53
Salicylic acid	2.24	1900
Sulindac	4.53	0.03
Terbutaline sulphate	−1.90	0.04
Testosterone	3.31	35
Triamcinolone acetonide	2.53	0.18

[a] Octanol-water partition coefficient
[b] J = flux

the skin (Anderson *et al.*, 1988; Surber *et al.*, 1990). Examination of the data presented in Table 1 reveals that there is a direct correlation between the *n*-octanol–water partition coefficient (K_{ow}) of the chemicals and their skin penetration rate. The stratum corneum typically mimics the characteristics of a lipophilic structure (Elias *et al.*, 1981; Raykar *et al.*, 1988).

Lipophilic chemicals tend to accumulate in the stratum corneum and a high concentration of the chemical is achieved at the point of contact. Assuming that the chemical is at least slightly soluble in water, penetration at this level will be rather rapid, owing to migration into the inter-

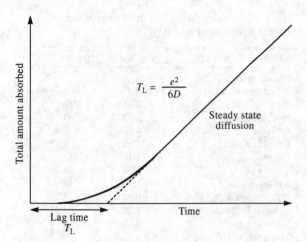

$$T_L = \frac{e^2}{6D}$$

Steady state diffusion

Total amount absorbed

Lag time
T_L

Time

Figure 1 Typical time-course of penetration for chemical diffusion through intact human skin. T_L = lag time; e = thickness of the membrane; D = diffusion constant

cellular spaces (Scheuplein, 1965). With purely lipophilic chemicals, however, penetration may not extend beyond the stratum corneum. For these chemicals the stratum corneum behaves as a storage site, and the chemicals can be released over a long period of time. This phenomenon, known as the 'reservoir effect' (Vickers, 1963), may explain why sometimes a single exposure to certain chemicals in the skin can lead to prolonged effects (Rougier *et al.*, 1985). Accordingly, the stratum corneum is an effective barrier for hydrophilic substances, which therefore have very low skin absorption rates.

In Vivo Studies

Historically, percutaneous absorption of a chemical through the skin has most often been studied in humans. More recently, studies have also been performed with laboratory animals. In addition, some studies have used athymic rodents grafted with human skin (Klain *et al.*, 1985).

The rate of absorption and the percentage of a chemical absorbed through the skin (bioavailability) *in vivo* are usually determined by measuring the total radioactivity in blood or excreta following a topical application of a radiolabelled compound. The amount of radioactivity retained in the body or excreted through expiration or sweat can be determined by measuring the amount of radioactivity excreted following an intravenous injection. Three indirect methods for

estimating the bioavailability of a chemical following topical administration can be used:

(1) If an intravenous dose is assumed to have maximum bioavailability (i.e 100 per cent), the extent of absorption following a cutaneous dose can be estimated by comparing the total quantity in the body compartment after giving equivalent doses by both the intravenous and cutaneous routes (Andersen and Keller, 1984). The total dose can be represented as the concentration–time integral carried out to infinite time—i.e. the area under the plasma concentration–time curve (AUC_∞).

bioavailability = AUC_∞ (cutaneous)/AUC_∞ (intravenous)

The radioactivity in the blood or excreta consists of a mixture of the parent compound and any metabolites. Since a radiolabel does not distinguish between the parent chemical and its metabolite(s), the bioavailability determined with this methodology actually represents the composite absorption of the parent chemical and its metabolite(s). Specific chemical assays are necessary to quantify the absolute bioavailability of chemicals which undergo metabolism as they are absorbed through the skin.

(2) This method calculates the extent of absorption by monitoring the cumulative amount of the chemical in all routes of excretion (urine, faeces, exhaled air, etc.) over infinite time following topical administration. Thus:

bioavailability = total amount in excreta/applied dose

In reality, the duration of excreta collection is only for a finite time, since collection of excreta over an extremely prolonged period is impractical. For certain chemicals, especially those which have low whole-body clearance, there may be a considerable portion of the absorbed dose remaining in the body at the cessation of the collection period. Thus, the total amount recovered in the excreta does not represent the total dose absorbed. This residual amount and any material excreted in routes not assayed can be estimated by determining the amount excreted following an intravenous administration (Wester and Maibach, 1985) and through use of standard pharmacokinetic models. Thus:

bioavailability = total excreted (cutaneous)/total
excreted (intravenous)

(3) The last method, which is the most expedient but also the least reliable, consists of quantifying the amount of a chemical recovered from the skin surface after topical administration:

bioavailability = (applied dose − dose remaining
on skin)/applied dose

The limitation of this surface recovery method is that it is prone to inaccuracies. Losses of the chemical from the skin may occur as a result of evaporation, and total recovery from the skin is difficult to ascertain with high confidence.

Several human *in vivo* studies have been reported (Stewart and Dodd, 1964; Feldmann and Maibach, 1969, 1974). Owing to the potential toxicity of many chemicals, *in vivo* human percutaneous absorption studies have been largely supplanted by experiments with laboratory animals. Unfortunately, there are a number of difficulties associated with the extrapolation of animal data to humans—e.g. animal species variation, different sites of application, differences between shaved versus unshaved skin and difference in skin metabolism (or lack of).

Some rules of thumb are available for extrapolating animal data to estimate skin uptake in humans. In general, the penetration of chemicals through the human skin is similar to that of the pig, miniature swine or squirrel monkey, and much slower than that of the rat and rabbit (Bartek *et al.*, 1972; Bartek and LaBudde, 1975). Table 2 illustrates the quantitative differences among the most frequently used test animals for four different pesticides.

Table 2 *In vivo* percutaneous absorption of pesticides in several animals and humans. Adapted from Bartek and LaBudde (1975) and Feldmann and Maibach (1974)

Pesticide	% Dose absorbed			
	Rabbit	Pig	Squirrel monkey	Human
DDT[a]	46.3	43.4	1.5	10.4
Lindane	51.2	37.6	16	9.3
Parathion	97.5	14.5	30.3	9.7
Malathion	64.6	15.5	19.3	8.2

[a] *p,p'*-Dichlorodiphenyltrichloroethane

In Vitro Studies

Starting in the 1980s, *in vitro* studies using human skin were conducted more frequently for estimating percutaneous absorption (Dugard *et al.*, 1984). In these studies a piece of excised human skin is attached to a diffusion apparatus which has a top chamber to hold the applied dose of a chemical, an O-ring to hold the skin in place, and a temperature-controlled bottom chamber containing saline or other solvents (plus a sampling port to withdraw fractions for analysis). Although human forearm skin is optimal, it is difficult to obtain, so it is common practice to use abdominal skin. It is generally believed that properly conducted *in vitro* tests using human skin, for most classes of chemicals, can be a reasonably good predictor of the absorption rate in humans (Bronaugh *et al.*, 1982). However, owing to the fragile nature of the technique, these studies must be carefully interpreted.

Mathematical Models

Models Based on Chemical Thermodynamics

Berner and Cooper (1987) envisioned that there exist two parallel pathways of diffusion for the cutaneous transport of chemical substances. The flux of polar molecules at constant concentration is independent of the partition coefficient in the stratum corneum (for simplicity, the *n*-octanol–water partition coefficient (K_{ow}) is commonly used as a substitute). This pathway is referred to as the polar or aqueous pathway. With lipophilic substances the flux becomes a function of the partition coefficient, and this pathway is referred to as the non-polar or lipophilic pathway. On the basis of this concept, Fiserova-Bergerova *et al.* (1990) proposed a mathematical model to evaluate the percutaneous absorption potential of industrial chemicals. The flux of a chemical across the skin can be related to its physicochemical properties, as shown in the following empirical equation:

$$J = (C/15)(0.038 + 0.153 K_{ow}) e^{-0.016\,MW}$$

where J = flux of the chemical across the skin; C = saturated aqueous solution concentration of the chemical; K_{ow} = octanol–water partition coefficient; and MW = molecular weight of the chemical.

Critical fluxes are determined by comparing the skin uptake rate under specified exposure conditions with the inhalation uptake rate during exposure to the time-weighted average ambient occupational exposure limits of steady-state conditions. The specified exposure condition for the critical flux can be calculated assuming exposure of 2 per cent of the body surface area (equivalent to the stretched palms and fingers) to a saturated aqueous solution of the chemical (Fiserova-Bergerova *et al.*, 1990). If the flux of a chemical exceeds the critical flux by 30 per cent, the chemical should be classified as possessing cutaneous absorption potential. If the flux of a chemical exceeds three times the critical flux, the chemical should be classified as possessing cutaneous toxicity potential. Based on this scheme, an evaluation of the chemicals listed in the threshold limit value (TLV) booklet (ACGIH, 1987) revealed that a percutaneous absorption potential is predicted for 48 chemicals and a significant percutaneous toxicity potential is indicated for 77 chemicals (Table 3).

McKone (1990) described a mathematical model for predicting the uptake fraction of various industrial chemicals on soil. The model is used to estimate the amount of chemical that crosses the stratum corneum into the underlying tissue layer only. To differentiate this absorptive process from bioavailability which also includes transport into blood, it is referred to as an uptake fraction. The approach is based on the concept of fugacity (Kissel and Robarge, 1988; Kissel and McAvoy, 1989). Fugacity, which is directly related to concentration, measures the tendency of a chemical substance to move from one phase to another. Because the skin has a fat content of about 10 per cent and soil has an organic carbon content of only about 1–4 per cent, a chemical in a soil matrix placed on the skin will ultimately move from the soil to the underlying adipose layers of the skin surface. However, the rate at which this process occurs is crucial for determining whether appreciable uptake occurs during the period of time between deposition on the skin and removal by evaporation, washing or other processes. It is the mass-transfer coefficients of the soil–skin layer and the soil–air layer that define the rate at which these competing processes occur.

McKone's model (1990) predicts that the uptake fraction of a chemical in soil is particularly sensitive to the values of the octanol–water partition coefficient (K_{ow}), the air–water partition coefficient (K_h) and the mass of soil deposited on the skin (I_s). When K_h is very small (<0.001), i.e. there is little vapour loss, the only loss mechanisms are mass transfer and wash-off. Under this condition, the uptake fraction is inversely porportional to K_{ow} and I_s. When $I_s = 10$ mg cm^{-2} and $K_{ow} \leqslant 10^4$, the uptake is almost complete over a period of 12 h (Figure 2). When $K_h > 0.001$, there is competition between vapour loss and diffusion as removal mechanisms for contaminants bound to soil particles, and vapour loss becomes more important in controlling uptake fraction. Under such conditions, the model predicts that the uptake fraction decreases strongly when K_{ow} is large, but is less sensitive to soil loading when K_{ow} is small (Figure 3).

McKone's model (1990) is intended for first-order estimates of percutaneous uptake of chemicals from a soil matrix. The uptake fraction varies with the duration of exposure, soil deposition rate and chemical properties of the deposited compound. Results based on this model reveal that the efficiency of contaminant uptake can depend strongly on the amount or depth of soil on the skin surface. When the amount of soil on the skin is <1 mg cm^{-2}, a rather high uptake fraction, approaching unity in some cases, is predicted. With 20 mg cm^{-2} of soil, the model predicts an uptake of 0.5 per cent, which is comparable to the 1 per cent measured in the uptake studies with soil-bound dioxin in rats (Poiger and Schlatter, 1980; Shu *et al.*, 1988). Because of the diverse variations of the uptake fraction with soil loading, it is recommended that the results obtained from experiments with a single soil loading should not be applied to all human soil-exposure scenarios. Recently McKone's model has been extended to evaluate the joint time- and loading-dependencies of six aromatic hydrocarbons (Burnmaster and Maxwell, 1991).

Describing the transport of chemicals from soil through the human skin is not a simple process, but its behaviour is predictable and a few generalizations can be made if the controlling factors are quantified and accounted for. First, for compounds with a $K_{ow} \leqslant 10^6$ and a $K_h < 0.001$, it is not unreasonable to assume 100 per cent uptake in 12 h. Second, for compounds with a $K_h \geqslant 0.01$, the uptake fraction is unlikely ever to exceed 40 per cent in 12 h and will be well below this when

Table 3 Industrial chemicals with ambient occupational exposure limits that have percutaneous absorption potential or percutaneous toxicity potential. Adapted from Fiserova-Bergerova *et al.* (1990)

Percutaneous absorption potential		Percutaneous toxicity potential	
Acetone	Isoamyl alcohol	Acetic acid	Formaldehyde
n-Amyl acetate	Isopropanol	Acetonitrile	Formamide
Atrazine	Methoxychlor	Acetylsalicylic acid	Formic acid
1,3-Butadiene	Methyl acetate	Allyl alcohol	Furfural
n-Butyl acetate	Methyl *n*-amyl ketone	2-Aminopyridine	Glycerin
p-tert-Butyltoluene	Methyl chloroform	Aniline	Hexylene glycol
Cumene	Methyl ethyl ketone	Benzene	Hydrazine
Cyclohexanone	Methyl isoamyl ketone	Biphenyl	Isobutyl alcohol
o-Dichlorobenzene	Methyl isobutyl ketone	*n*-Butanol	Isopropylamine
1,1-Dichloroethane	Methyl propyl ketone	*sec*-Butanol	Lindane
1,2-Dichloroethylene	Metribuzin	*n*-Butyl acrylate	Mesityl oxide
Diethyl ketone	Naphthalene	*n*-Butylamine	Methanol
Diuron	Nitromethane	Carbon disulphide	2-Methoxyethanol
Enflurane	Pentaerythritol	Carbon tetrachloride	4-Methoxyphenol
Ethanol	*n*-Propyl acetate	Chloroform	Methylamine
Ethyl acetate	Propylene dichloride	Chloropicrine	*n*-Methyl aniline
Ethyl benzene	Strychnine	*o*-, *m*-, *p*-Cresol	Methyl *n*-butyl ketone
Ethyl ether	Styrene	Cyclohexanol	Methyl chloride
Ethyl formate	Toluene	Dichloroethyl ether	Methylene chloride
Halothane	1,2,4-Trichlorobenzene	Dicyclopentadiene	Methyl iodide
n-Heptane	Trichloroethylene	Dieldrin	Morpholine
Hexachloroethane	Trimethyl benzene	Diethanolamine	*p*-Nitroaniline
n-Hexane	*o*-, *m*-, *p*-Xylene	2-Diethylaminoethanol	*p*-Nitrotoluene
		Diethylene triamine	Pentachlorophenol
		Diisopropylamine	*p*-Phenylene diamine
		N,N-Dimethyl aniline	Phenyl ether
		Dimethyl phthalate	Phenyl mercaptan
		Dioxane	Propoxur
		Dimethylacetamide	*n*-Propyl alcohol
		Dimethyl formamide	Fenchlorphos (Ronnel)
		Diphenylamine	1,1,2,2-Tetrachloroethane
		Ethanolamine	Thioglycolic acid
		2-Ethoxyethanol	*o*-, *p*-Toluidine
		Ethylamine	Tributyl phosphate
		Ethyl butyl ketone	Trichloroacetic acid
		Ethylene glycol	1,1,2-Trichloroethane
		Ethyl mercaptan	Triethylamine

$K_{ow} > 10$. Third, for compounds with a $K_h \geq 0.1$, we can expect ≤ 3 per cent uptake in 12 h. In most occupational settings, contaminated soil will rarely be in contact with the skin for more than 4 h before it is washed off. Consequently, this should be accounted for when conducting a risk assessment.

Pharmacokinetic Models

Guy *et al.* (1982) presented a four-compartment pharmacokinetic model to describe the percutaneous absorption of chemicals. In this model (Figure 4) movement of a chemical through the various compartments representing the skin struc-

tures is described by first-order rate constants. K_1 describes the chemical diffusion from the skin surface through the stratum corneum; K_2 relates to diffusion through the viable epidermis; and K_3 measures the back-diffusion of chemical from the viable epidermis to the stratum corneum. The ratio K_3/K_2, therefore, may be regarded as the relative affinity or the partition coefficient of the chemical for the stratum corneum compared with the viable epidermis. The larger the value of K_3, the higher the affinity for the stratum corneum and therefore the larger the reservoir effect. Finally, K_4 measures the clearance of the chemical from the capillary blood. This pharmacokin-

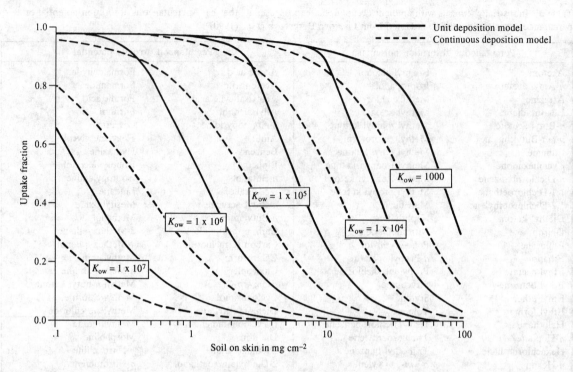

Figure 2   Based on the unit and continuous deposition models and for the range of octanol–water partition coefficients (K_{ow}) listed, this graph shows the uptake fraction of various chemicals during 12 h plotted against soil deposition per unit area of exposed skin with the dimensionless Henry's law constant $K_n \ll 0.001$

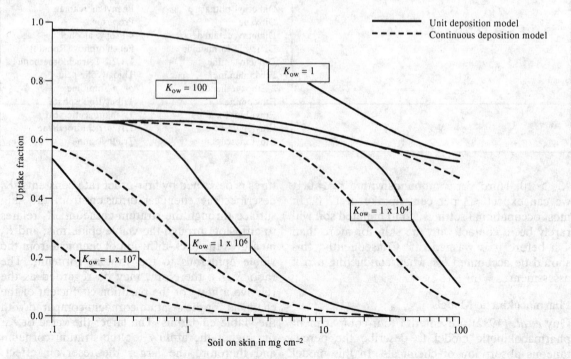

Figure 3   Based on the unit and continuous deposition models and for the range of octanol–water partition coefficients (K_{ow}) listed, this graph shows the uptake fraction of various chemicals during 12 h plotted against soil deposition per unit area of exposed skin with the dimensionless Henry's law constant $K_n = 0.001$

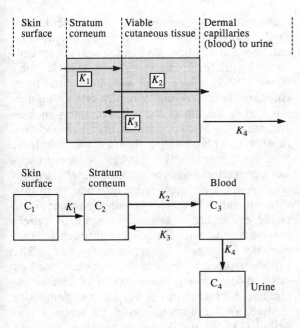

Figure 4 Schematic representation of the four-compartment pharmacokinetic model to describe the percutaneous absorption of chemicals. C_1, C_2, C_3 and C_4 are concentrations of chemical in respective compartments

etic model has been used to predict the skin absorption of a variety of steroid compounds and has been found to provide good agreement with actual experimental data (Guy *et al.*, 1982, 1983). This model has also been used to predict the disposition of a chemical in the skin and plasma as a function of its physicochemical properties (Guy and Hadgraft, 1984). Furthermore, if the model is configured with an input rate constant to the skin surface, it can be used to assess vehicle effects.

Zatz (1985) developed a multicompartmented membrane model that treated the barrier membrane as a series of spaces filled with immiscible liquids and assumed that transport from one space to another is a first-order process (Figure 5). The donor compartment contains the chemical

in solution. The living portion of the epidermis as well as the portion of the dermis separating the stratum corneum (SC) from the capillaries are combined into the AQ compartment. The sink compartment, which represents the circulation, collects all chemical that reaches it. The advantage of this model is that it is possible to study conditions under which the simple form of Fick's law does not apply, i.e. non-steady-state conditions. Two general types of experimental conditions were studied. The first, referred to as the 'infinite dose' situation, requires that the amount of chemical lost by penetration be too small to alter the donor concentration. The second, referred to as the 'finite dose' situation, describes the condition in which the donor concentration decreases during the experiment. The model parameters used in these two experimental conditions are shown in Table 4.

In the infinite dose system the concentration profile is essentially linear once steady state has been reached. The steady-state flux, J, is proportional to K, K_I/K_{-I} and V. Increasing the number of compartments, N, which is analogous to increasing the membrane thickness, has the effect of decreasing the steady-state flux. In the

Table 4 Parameter values used in the multicompartmented membrane model. Adapted from Zatz (1985)

Parameter	Infinite dose	Finite dose
Number of stratum corneum compartments	5	5
Volume of compartment, V	0.0002	0.0002
Donor concentration	10	10
Donor volume	100	0.002
K	0.4	0.4
K_I	45	45
K_{-I}	1	1
K_A	2	2
K_{-A}	2	2
K_S	2	2

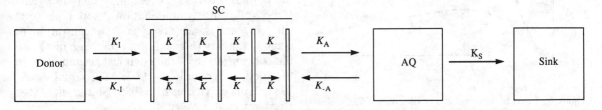

Figure 5 Schematic representation of a multicompartmented membrane model. Standard values for model parameters are given in Table 4

finite dose system the chemical solution is applied as a thin film. Because of the deposition of a limited amount of the chemical on the skin surface, the donor concentration may decrease as penetration proceeds. All other model parameters being the same, penetration is reduced under finite dose conditions (Figure 6). This is because the chemical concentration in the donor is continuously reduced, which results in a decrease in the gradient across the membrane. While J is directly proportional to K, K_I/K_{-I} and V under the infinite dose condition, changing K_I/K_{-I} or V has a smaller impact on J than changing K or N under the finite dose condition. This may be due to a significant loss of material from the donor, which is a source of the chemical. Because the donor and the first stratum corneum compartment are linked reversibly, there is a tendency towards a pseudoequilibrium distribution in which the actual transmembrane gradient is not as large as would be anticipated from the K_I/K_{-I} ratio. These modelling results indicate that the mechanism by which fluxes are affected must be considered when extrapolating to non-steady-state conditions for various chemical formulations.

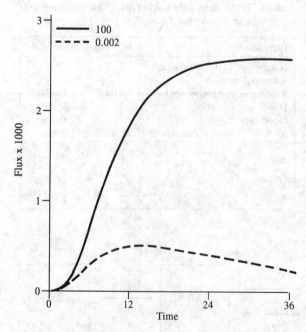

Figure 6 Effect of donor volume on penetration flux as simulated by the multicompartmented membrane model. The donor volumes of 100 ml cm^{-2} and 0.002 ml cm^{-2} represent the infinite dose and finite dose conditions, respectively

A physiologically based pharmacokinetic model was recently developed to describe the percutaneous absorption of volatile organic contaminants in dilute aqueous solutions (Shatkin and Brown, 1991). The model contained three body compartments: stratum corneum, viable epidermis and blood. Physiological parameters such as volume of the body compartments and blood flow rates were obtained directly from the literature. Partition coefficients between compartments were estimated from the octanol–water partition coefficients. Chemicals were assumed to diffuse through fully hydrated stratum corneum and viable epidermis in a dissolved state by purely passive means, with the passage through stratum corneum being the rate-limiting step. The exposure scenario modelled was either hand or full-body immersion into a vessel of solute-contaminated water of a known volume. Sensitivity analyses of the various model parameters suggested that the uptake of chemicals in aqueous solutions was most markedly influenced by epidermal blood flow rates, followed by epidermal thickness and the fat content in the stratum corneum. In general, thicker and fattier skin would provide better barriers to percutaneous penetration of chemicals. The model also predicted that the daily dose of some volatile organic contaminants in tap-water absorbed during a 20 min bath may be similar in magnitude to either ingested or indoor inhalation dose of that chemical (Shatkin and Brown, 1991).

FACTORS USED IN EXPOSURE CALCULATIONS

The typical media of concern for assessing cutaneous contact to environmental chemicals are fly-ash, sediment, house dust and soil. There are a number of parameters which can influence the degree of cutaneous bioavailability of chemicals in complex matrices. These may include ageing (time following contamination), soil type (e.g. silt, clay and sand), type and concentration of cocontaminants (e.g. oil and other organics) and the concentration of the chemical contaminant in the media (Scheuplein, 1967; McConnell *et al.*, 1984; Paustenbach *et al.*, 1986; Shu *et al.*, 1988; Brewster *et al.*, 1989).

The bioavailability of a chemical in soil will be very much affected by its physicochemical properties. Chemicals of large molecular weight will often bind to the soil and be less water-soluble, while smaller molecules will frequently be water-soluble, less tightly bound and relatively bioavailable (McKone, 1990). The cutaneous bioavailability of various chemicals in soils (Poiger and Schlatter, 1980; McConnell *et al.*, 1984; Umbreit *et al.*, 1986; Brewster *et al.*, 1989; Shu *et al.*, 1988; Skrowronski *et al.*, 1988; Goon *et al.*, 1990, 1991) and in fly-ash (Van den Berg *et al.*, 1984) have been determined. These studies showed that differing media and chemicals can yield dramatically different cutaneous bioavailabilities.

To calculate the cutaneous exposure to a chemical, one needs to know, in addition to the percutaneous absorption rate and bioavailability, the area of exposed skin, the concentration of the chemical, and the duration and frequency of the exposure (Paustenbach, 1989; Sheehan *et al.*, 1991).

One scenario is that of a thin film of chemical on the skin. For this finite mass scenario:

$$\text{percutaneous absorption} = C{\cdot}A{\cdot}f{\cdot}x{\cdot}r{\cdot}t$$

where C = concentration of the chemical; A = skin surface area; f = frequency of exposure; x = thickness of the film layer; r = percutaneous absorption rate; and t = duration of exposure.

Another scenario is where there is an excess amount of a chemical on the skin. In this case, the thickness of the chemical layer is not calculated and steady-state kinetics is assumed:

$$\text{percutaneous absorption} = C{\cdot}A{\cdot}f{\cdot}K_p{\cdot}t$$

where K_p = permeability constant.

Skin Surface Area

An important factor in assessing percutaneous toxicity is the surface area of the skin that is exposed. The 'rule of nines' may be used for estimating the surface area of certain regions of the total body (Snyder, 1975): head and neck, 9 per cent; upper limbs, each, 9 per cent; lower limbs, each 18 per cent; front or back of trunk, 18 per cent. The USEPA (1989) has estimated the exposed skin surface area (arms, hands, legs and feet) of 2897 cm² for children 0–2 years old, 3400 cm² for children 2–6 years old and 2940 cm² for adults (adult is assumed to wear pants, open-

necked, short-sleeved shirt, shoes, with no hat or gloves). Table 5 gives the skin surface areas commonly used when conducting exposure assessments of workers (Snyder, 1975).

Percutaneous Absorption of Chemicals in an Aqueous Matrix

The percutaneous uptake of heptachlor and chlordane from water in humans was studied (Scow *et al.*, 1979). The water flux (J) through the skin was taken to be 0.2–0.5 mg cm⁻² h⁻¹, while the flux of the chemical was estimated by multiplying the water flux by the weight fraction of the chemical in water. At a concentration of 1 ppb, the flux of the chemical was 0.2×10^{-9} mg cm⁻² h⁻¹. Using a representative body surface area of 18 000 cm², if one swam for 4 h per day in water containing 1 ppb chlordane, the amount of chlordane absorbed was estimated to be as much as 0.013–0.036 µg. Beech (1980) estimated the amount of chloroform absorbed over a 3 h period by a 6-year-old boy swimming in water containing 0.0005 mg chloroform per cm³. The

Table 5 Representative surface areas of the human body (adult male). Adapted from Snyder (1975)

Body portion	Area (cm²)
Whole body	18 000
Head and neck	1620
head	1260
back of head	320
neck	360
back of neck	90
Torso	6480
back	2520
chest	2520
sides	1440
Upper limbs	3240
upper arms (elbow–shoulder)	1440
lower arms (elbow–wrist)	1080
hands	720
hands (1 side)	360
upper arms (back of)	360
lower arms (back of)	270
Lower limbs	6480
thighs	3240
lower legs (knee–ankle)	2160
feet	1080
soles of feet	540
thighs (back of)	810
lower legs (back of)	540
Perineum	180

average 6-year-old is assumed to have a surface area of 8800 cm². The permeability constant (K_p) for chloroform in aqueous solution was 0.125 cm h⁻¹. The flux through the skin was calculated to be:

$$0.125 \text{ cm h}^{-1} \times 0.0005 \text{ mg cm}^{-3} = 0.000\ 062\ 5 \text{ mg cm}^{-2}.\text{h}^{-1}$$

The percutaneous absorption is then:

$$0.000\ 062\ 5 \text{ mg cm}^{-2}\ \text{h}^{-1} \times 8800 \text{ cm}^2 \times 3 \text{ h} = 1.65 \text{ mg chloroform}$$

Byard (1989) evaluated the percutaneous absorption of 1,1,1-trichloroethane (TCA) from daily hygiene activities such as bathing and showering. He calculated a cutaneous vapour, cutaneous water and inhalation dose of 0.0072 µg kg⁻¹ day⁻¹ for a 10 min shower exposure to 50 l of water containing 1 ppb TCA. Using a half-life for volatilization of 10 min, the TCA release would be about 24 µg, since percutaneous uptake and volatilization are competing processes, and much of the water does not make direct cutaneous contact. In addition, he estimated that 0.0475 µg kg⁻¹ of TCA was absorbed from skin contact during a 20 min bath.

Showering appears to be an event where an individual can be exposed to elevated concentrations of volatile compounds in the air within a confined space and the entire body skin area is exposed to contaminants in the water. Recent work suggests that the uptake of chloroform from a single, 10 min shower was about 0.46 µg kg⁻¹ day⁻¹, with 0.24 µg kg⁻¹ day⁻¹ from inhalation and 0.22 µg kg⁻¹ day⁻¹ from cutaneous exposure (Travis and Hester, 1990). Comparisons have been made of the concentration of chloroform in exhaled breath after a normal shower with municipal tap-water and those after an inhalation-only exposure to chloroform. The resulting concentrations were 6–21 µg kg⁻¹ day⁻¹ for the shower exposure and 2.4–10 µg kg⁻¹ day⁻¹ for inhalation-only exposure (Jo *et al.*, 1990). The concentration in exhaled breath after showering was approximately twice as high as that after inhalation-only exposure, indicating that the contribution to the absorbed dose due to percutaneous absorption was about equivalent to inhalation absorption.

Morgan *et al.* (1991) measured the percutaneous absorption of a range of volatile organic chemicals (VOC) in aqueous solutions. Rats were exposed to 2 ml of ⅓, ⅔ or saturated aqueous VOC solutions for 24 h in a surgically attached cutaneous exposure cell. Absorption of VOC was rapid, along with about 0.18 ml of water (Table 6). VOC in blood rapidly attained a peak level and then declined to near-control levels by 24 h. This kinetic pattern was due to a decreasing exposure concentration along with rapid distribution and elimination of VOC. These results indicate that significant amounts of VOC can be absorbed through the skin following cutaneous exposure to low levels of these chemicals in aqueous solutions.

Percutaneous Absorption of Liquid Solvents

While the percutaneous absorption of chemical solutes usually proceeds by simple diffusion, the skin uptake of non-aqueous liquids, including liquid solvents, is not governed by Fick's law. Consequently, the uptake of a pure liquid through the skin needs to be determined by direct *in vivo* skin contact techniques. Stewart and Dodd (1964) conducted a series of human experiments in which the skin of the hands was exposed to carbon tetrachloride, trichloroethylene, tetrachloroethylene, methylene chloride or 1,1,1-trichloroethane. Table 7 gives the percutaneous absorption rates of some common industrial liquid solvents in humans.

Paustenbach (1988) estimated the amount of 2-methoxyethanol absorbed by a worker wearing a heavily contaminated glove on one hand for about 30 min:

$$\text{percutaneous uptake} = A{\cdot}J{\cdot}t/W = 8 \text{ mg kg}^{-1} \text{ day}^{-1}$$

where: $A = 400 \text{ cm}^2$; $J = 2.8 \text{ mg cm}^{-2} \text{ h}^{-1}$; $t = 0.5 \text{ h day}^{-1}$; $W = 70 \text{ kg}$. For comparison purposes, the amount of 2-methoxyethanol taken up via inhalation by the same worker who is exposed for 8 h day⁻¹ (10 m³ of air inhaled) at the TLV of 16 mg m⁻³ (assuming an 80 per cent uptake efficiency) was also estimated:

$$\text{inhalation uptake} = (16)(10)(0.8)/70 = 1.8 \text{ mg kg}^{-1} \text{ day}^{-1}$$

These calculations indicate that the uptake of 2-methoxyethanol following 30 min of skin

Table 6 Volumes of aqueous chemical solutions absorbed after 24 hr cutaneous exposure. Adapted from Morgan *et al.* (1991)

Chemical	Volume of chemical solution absorbed (ml)[a]			
	Neat	Saturated	⅔ Saturated	⅓ Saturated
Bromochloromethane	1.3	0.30	0.22	0.20
Dibromomethane	0.82	0.29	0.23	0.14
1,2-Dichloroethane	1.08	0.29	0.24	0.32
Chloroform	1.48	0.37	0.32	0.22
Benzene	0.62	0.21	0.26	0.14
Trichloroethylene	0.93	0.50	0.44	0.31
Carbon tetrachloride	0.54	0.39	0.22	0.36
1,1,1-Trichloroethane	0.59	0.25	0.27	0.19
Toluene	0.56	0.27	0.31	0.68
m-Xylene	0.65	0.38	0.51	0.56
Styrene	0.31	0.20	0.26	0.19
Ethyl benzene	0.24	0.20	0.18	0.17
Tetrachloroethylene	0.55	0.24	0.30	0.18
n-Hexane	0.98	0.33	0.14	0.21
Water	0.18			

[a] Calculated by subtracting the volume remaining from the initial 2 ml volume.

Table 7 Percutaneous absorption rates of some common industrial liquid solvents in humans. Adapted from Tsuruta (1990)

Liquid solvent	Percutaneous absorption rate (mg cm^{-2} h^{-1})
Aniline	0.2–0.7
Benzene	0.24–0.4
2-Butoxyethanol	0.05–0.68
Carbon disulphide	9.7
Ethylbenzene	22–33
Methanol	11.5
Methyl *n*-butyl ketone	0.25–0.48
Nitrobenzene	2
Styrene	9–15
Toluene	14–23
Xylene (mixed)	4.5–9.6
m-Xylene	0.12–0.15

exposure (one hand) is about 4.5 times greater than the uptake from inhalation for 8 h at the TLV. From this example, it is clear that the cutaneous route of entry can significantly contribute to the total absorbed dose.

Percutaneous Absorption of Chemicals in Gaseous Matrix

The absorption of several chemicals in the gaseous phase through the human skin has been studied. Recently, McDougal *et al.* (1990) developed a chamber system to measure the whole-body percutaneous vapour absorption in rats. The flux of a chemical across the skin and the permeability constant were determined on the basis of the concentrations of the chemical in the blood during exposures by using a physiologically based pharmacokinetic model. Table 8 shows the permeability constants measured in these studies. In most cases the absorption of vapours through the skin amounted to less than 10–30 per cent of the total dose received from a mixed percutaneous and inhalation exposure. The permeability constant for this set of chemical vapours appeared to be directly proportional to lipophilicity, but was independent of the exposure concentration. While there was a good agreement between the rat and the human in the relative ranking of the permeability constants among the chemicals studied, for individual chemicals the rat skin appeared, in general, to be 2–4 times more permeable than the human skin. This is consistent with the data of Bartek and LaBudde (1975), which showed that the skin absorption of chemicals in rats and rabbits is 5–10 times higher than in humans. Figure 7 shows the dependence of absorption rates of aniline vapours through the respiratory tract and skin on the air concentration. The rate of aniline absorption via inhalation appeared to be linearly proportional to the vapour concentration, while that via skin exposure became non-linear as the aniline vapour concentration increased.

Table 8 Percutaneous absorption of chemical vapours. Adapted from McDougal *et al.* (1990), Riihimaki and Pfaffli (1978) and Johanson and Boman (1991)

Chemical	Skin uptake in a mixed exposure (%)	Permeability constant (cm h^{-1})	
		Rat	Human
Styrene	9.4	1.75	0.35–1.42
m-Xylene	3.9	0.72	0.24–0.26
Toluene	3.7	0.72	0.18
Perchloroethylene	3.5	0.67	0.17
Benzene	0.8	0.15	0.08
Halothane	0.2	0.05	
Hexane	0.1	0.03	
Isoflurane	0.1	0.03	
Methylene chloride		0.28	
Dibromomethane		1.32	
Bromochloromethane		0.79	
Phenol			15.74–17.59
Nitrobenzene			11.1–25.00
2-Butoxyethanol			2.1–28.8
1,1,1-Trichloroethane			0.01

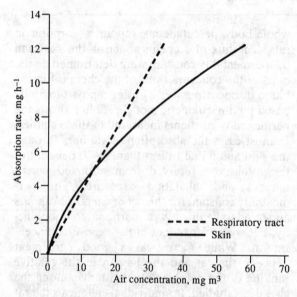

Figure 7 Absorption rate of aniline vapours through the respiratory tract and skin as dependent on the air concentration

In most workplaces, the airborne concentration of chemicals is too low for the uptake of vapours through the skin to be significant. However, respirators are often worn when in environments where the airborne concentrations of solvents can be as much as 10- or 1000-fold higher than the TLV. Assuming that a person wears an airline respirator for 30 min in a room containing 50 ppm (250 mg m^{-3}) nitrobenzene (50 times the current

TLV), the amount of nitrobenzene absorbed through the skin can be calculated as follows:

$$uptake = C_a \cdot A \cdot t \cdot K_p \cdot i / W$$

where K_p = cutaneous permeability constant of vapour and i = inhibition factor for clothing.

On the basis of a controlled study of nitrobenzene vapour absorption by persons who wore respirators, a cutaneous permeability constant of 11 cm h^{-1} and 25 cm h^{-1} at air concentrations of 5 mg m^{-3} and 20 mg m^{-3}, respectively, has been estimated (Piotrowski, 1977). For the purposes of this assessment, all but the skin on the feet was considered exposed. The head and arms were assumed not to be covered with clothing (surface area = 5000 cm^2), while the rest of the body (surface area = 13 000 cm^2) was covered with clothing. The available data (Piotrowski, 1977) suggest that clothing reduces the percutaneous uptake rate of vapours by about 20 per cent, i.e. the inhibition factor. On the basis of this information, the amount of nitrobenzene vapour absorbed through the skin would be:

$$uptake = (250 \text{ mg m}^{-3})(25 \text{ cm h}^{-1})(0.5 \text{ h})(5000 +$$
$$(13\,000)(0.8) \text{ cm}^2)(10^{-4} \text{ m}^3 \text{ cm}^{-3})/70 \text{ kg}$$
$$= 70.2 \text{ mg kg}^{-1}$$

From this example, it is clear that if one enters an environment which contains high concentrations of airborne contaminants, even if a supplied-air respirator is worn to control inhalation exposure, percutaneous uptake of the chemical vapour may be significant.

Wipe Samples

Wipe samples are frequently collected to assess the cleanliness of the environment. Hospitals were among the first to rely on this method. Recently, wipe samples have frequently been collected within buildings to evaluate the potential for indoor air hazards. For example, following numerous fires involving transformers containing polychlorinated biphenyls (PCBs), wipe samples of walls, floors and furniture were collected to determine the degree of contamination by PCBs or the toxic byproducts such as dioxins and furans. These samples were then used quantitatively to predict the possible degree of human exposure and uptake of these chemicals.

In general, wipe samples have been used simply for industrial hygiene and housekeeping practices. Criteria that have been established were often intended only as an indicator of acceptable cleanliness. However, these data can be used to estimate uptake through the skin if the degree of skin contact with the contaminated surfaces is measured. For example, if one knows the number of times a valve handle, a door knob or a drum is handled, the surface area of the palm of the hand and the percutaneous uptake rate of the contaminant, then dose can be estimated. One of the most thorough evaluations which relied upon wipe sample data and time–motion studies was conducted by the National Institute of Occupational Safety and Health (NIOSH) when they attempted to estimate the amount of dioxin absorbed by chemical operators in a 2,4,5-T manufacturing plant (Marlow *et al.*, 1990). Similar analyses have been conducted for offices where PCB fires occurred (Kim, 1983).

GENERALIZATIONS

Although cutaneous exposure to chemicals due to splashes and incidental contact, as well as contamination of gloves and clothes, has been commonplace in industrial settings, for decades the human health hazard has rarely been quantified. This has been in part due to a lack of knowledge about the percutaneous absorption rate and the degree of exposure. The other reason is that for many years many industrial hygienists and occupational physicians assumed that personal protective clothing and gloves probably prevented contact with liquid chemicals and dusts. Today there is good evidence that many liquids and vapours do penetrate most barriers at a low but measurable rate. While a fair amount of information is now available about the uptake of neat chemical liquids through the human skin, there is a paucity of data about the effects of media on percutaneous absorption. Human exposures at hazardous waste sites or in contaminated buildings rarely involve substances in neat physical form. Instead, workers can be exposed to contaminated soils and dusts transported indoors through open windows or tracking, or to soot due to fires involving highly toxic materials (such as in PCBs or plastics). Adults doing gardening or yard work, and children playing in fields, may be exposed to soils contaminated by the deposition of particulate emissions from cars, smelters, foundries, incinerators or other industrial processes. Exposure to organic solvents in water during showering or swimming represents another source of potential exposure.

As a result of the emerging interest in exposure and health risk assessments, relatively reliable techniques for estimating the percutaneous absorption of chemicals are now available. In those instances where precise estimates are needed, chemical- and media-specific tests can be performed using either human skin *in vitro* or animal skin *in vivo*. If animal data are generated, the clear differences between the animal and human skin must be accounted for. While specific experimental data on the effects of matrix on percutaneous absorption will be most valuable, the development of mathematical models provides a useful tool to allow toxicologists and industrial hygienists to predict these complex processes. Unlike empirical studies, a mathematical model can readily be used not only to simulate a wide range of exposure conditions, including those at non-steady state, but also to evaluate the influence of various biological or physicochemical factors, such as contact area, membrane thickness, molecular size, lipophilicity or volatility, on percutaneous absorption. These uptake rates, coupled with reasonable estimates of human exposure, should give occupational health professionals the kind of tool needed to identify those hazards worthy of attention.

A review of the present data suggests the following conclusions:

(1) The bioavailability of chemicals bound to media, such as soil and fly-ash, can range from 0.01 per cent to nearly 100 per cent. Consequently, it is important that media effects be accounted for;

(2) The rate of percutaneous absorption in the workplace can be appreciable for those chemicals with a high K_{ow}. For example, studies of nitrobenzene, phenol, dimethyl formamide, dimethyl acetamide, carbon tetrachloride and several glycol ethers suggest that even if relatively good hygienic practices are in place, the dose due to percutaneous absorption can often be as much as one-half of that due to inhalation. Although for many chemicals such an increase in the daily uptake may pose no significant hazard, for those chemicals where the margin of safety between the TLV and toxic effects is small, such an incremental contribution to dose should not be overlooked;

(3) The percutaneous absorption of chemical vapours is particularly worthy of consideration when the atmospheric concentration of the chemical is 10–1000-fold higher than the TLV, even when the worker is wearing protective clothing and using adequate respiratory protection.

REFERENCES

ACGIH (1987). *Threshold Limit Values and Biological Exposure Limits for 1987–1988*. American Conference of Governmental Industrial Hygienists, Cincinnati

Andersen, M. E. and Keller, W. C. (1984). Toxicokinetic principles in relation to percutaneous absorption and cutaneous toxicity. In Drill, V. A. and Lazar, P. (Eds), *Cutaneous Toxicity*. Raven Press, New York, pp. 9–27

Anderson, B. D., Higuchi, W. I. and Raykar, P. V. (1988). Heterogeneity effects on permeability: Partition coefficient relationships in human stratum corneum. *Pharmacol. Res.*, **5**, 566–573

Bartek, M. J. and LaBudde J. A. (1975). Percutaneous absorption *in vitro*. In Maibach, H. I. (Ed.), *Animal Models in Dermatology*. Churchill Livingstone, New York, p. 103

Bartek, M. J., LaBudde, J. A., and Maibach, H. I. (1972). Skin permeability *in vivo*: comparison in rat, rabbit, pig and man. *J. Invest. Dermatol.*, **58**, 114–123

Beech, J. A. (1980). Estimated worst-case trihalomethane body burden of a child using a swimming pool. *Med. Hypothesis*, **6**, 303–307

Berner, B. and Cooper, E. R. (1987). Models of skin permeability. In Kydonieu, A. F. and Berner, B. (Eds), *Transdermal Delivery of Drugs*, Vol. II. CRC Press, Boca Raton, Florida, pp. 107–130

Blank, I. H. (1964). Penetration of low-molecular weight alcohols into skin. I. The effect of concentration of alcohol and type of vehicle. *J. Invest. Dermatol.*, **43**, 415–420

Brewster, D. W., Banks, Y. B., Clark, A. M. and Birbaum, L. S. (1989). Comparative dermal absorption of 2,3,7,8-tetrachlorodibenzo-*p*-dioxin and three polychlorinated dibenzofurans. *Toxicol. Appl. Pharmacol.*, **97**, 156–166

Bronaugh, R. L., Stewart, R. F., Congdon, E. R. and Giles, A. L. Jr. (1982). Methods for *in vitro* percutaneous absorption studies. I. Comparison with *in vivo* results. *Toxicol. Appl. Pharmacol.*, **62**, 474–480

Burnmaster, D. E. and Maxwell, N. I. (1991). Time- and loading-dependence in the McKone model for dermal uptake of organic chemicals from a soil matrix. *Risk Anal.*, **11**, 491–497

Byard, J. (1989). Hazard assessment of 1,1,1-trichloroethane in groundwater. In Paustenbach, D. J. (Ed.), *The Risk Assessment of Environmental and Human Health Hazards: A Textbook of Case Studies*. Wiley, New York, pp. 331–344

CDHS (1986). *The Development of Applied Action Levels for Soil Contact: A Scenario for the Exposure of Humans to Soil in a Residential Setting*. California Department of Health Services, Sacramento

Driver, J. H., Konz, J. J. and Whitmyre, G. K. (1989). Soil adherence to human skin. *Bull. Environ. Contam. Toxicol.*, **17**, 1831–1850

Dugard, P. H. (1983). Skin permeability theory in relation to measurements of percutaneous absorption in toxicology. In Marzulli, F. N. and Maibach, H. I. (Eds), *Dermatotoxicology*. Hemisphere Publishing Corporation, Washington, D.C., p. 102

Dugard, P. H., Walker, M., Mawdsleit, S. J. and Scott, R. C. (1984). Absorption of some glycol ethers through human skin *in vitro*. *Environ. Hlth Perspect.*, **57**, 193–198

Dutkiewicz, T. and Piotrowski, J. (1961). Experimental investigations on the quantitative estimation of aniline absorption in man. *Pure Appl. Chem.*, **3**, 319–323

Dutkiewicz, T. and Tyras, H. (1967). A study of the skin absorption of ethylbenzene in man. *Br. J. Industr. Med.*, **24**, 330–332

Elias, P. M., Cooper, E. R., Korc, A. and Brown, B. E. (1981). Percutaneous transport in relation to stratum corneum structure and lipid composition. *J. Invest. Dermatol.*, **76**, 297–301

Feldmann, R. J. and Maibach, H. I. (1969). Percutaneous penetration of steroids in man. *J. Invest. Dermatol.*, **52**, 89–94

Feldmann, R. J. and Maibach, H. I. (1974). Percutaneous penetration of some pesticides and herbicides in man. *Toxicol. Appl. Pharmacol.*, **28**, 126–132

Fiserova-Bergerova, V., Pierce, J. T. and Droz, P. O. (1990). Dermal absorption potential of industrial chemicals: criteria for skin notation. *Am. J. Industr. Med.*, **17**, 617–635

Flynn, G. L. (1990). Physicochemical determinants of skin absorption. Paper presented at the *ILSI-EPA Workshop on Principles of Route-to-Route Extrapolation*, Hilton Head, South Carolina

Goon, D., Hatoum, N. S., Jernigan, J. D., Schmitt, S. L. and Garvin, P. J. (1990). Pharmacokinetics and oral bioavailability of soil-adsorbed benzo(a)pyrene in rats. *Toxicologist*, **10**, 872

Goon, D., Hatoum, N. S., Klan, M. J., Jernigan, J. D. and Farmer, R. G. (1991). Oral bioavailability of aged soil-adsorbed benzo(a)pyrene in rats. *Toxicologist*, **11**, 1356

Guy, R. H. and Hadgraft, J. (1984). Prediction of drug disposition kinetics in skin and plasma following topical application. *J. Pharm. Sci.*, **73**, 883–887

Guy, R. H., Hadgraft, J. and Maibach, H. I. (1982). A pharmacokinetic model for percutaneous absorption. *Int. J. Pharm.*, **11**, 119–129

Guy, R. H., Hadgraft, J. and Maibach, H. I. (1983). Percutaneous absorption: Multidose pharmacokinetics. *Int. J. Pharm.*, **17**, 23–28

Hanke, J., Dutkiewicz, T. and Piotrowski, J. (1961). The absorption of benzene through human skin. *Med. Pr.*, **12**, 413–426

Jo, W. K., Weisel, C. P. and Lioy, P. J. (1990). Routes of chloroform exposure and body burden from showering with chlorinated tap water. *Risk Anal.*, **10**, 575–580

Johanson, G. and Boman, A. (1991). Percutaneous absorption of 2-butoxyethanol vapour in human subjects. *Br. J. Industr. Med.*, **48**, 788–792

Kao, J., Hall, J. and Helman, G. (1988). *In vitro* percutaneous absorption in mouse skin: influence of skin appendages. *Toxicol. Appl. Pharmacol.*, **94**, 93–103

Kasting, G. B., Smith, R. L. and Cooper, E. R. (1987). Effect of lipid solubility and molecular size on percutaneous absorption. In Shroot, B. and Schaefer, H. (Eds), *Pharmacology and the Skin*, Vol. 1: *Skin Pharmacokinetics*. Karger, Basel, pp. 138–153

Kim, N. (1983). *An Evaluation of the Human Health Risks of PCB Soot Following a Transformer Fire*. New York State Department of Health, Albany

Kimbrough, R. D., Falk, H., Stehr, P. and Fries, G. (1984). Health implications of 2,3,7,8-tetrachlorodibenzo-*p*-dioxin (TCDD) contamination of residential soil. *J. Toxicol. Environ. Hlth*, **14**, 47–93

Kissel, J. C. and McAvoy, D. R. (1989). Reevaluation of the dermal bioavailability of 2,3,7,8-TCDD in soil. *Haz. Waste Haz. Matls*, **6**, 231–248

Kissel, J. C. and Robarge, G. M. (1988). Assessing the elimination of 2,3,7,8-TCDD from humans with a physiologically-based pharmacokinetic model. *Chemosphere*, **17**, 2017–2027

Klain, G. J., Reifenrath, W. G. and Black, K. E. (1985). Distribution and metabolism of topically applied ethanolamine. *Fund. Appl. Toxicol.*, **5**, S127-S133

Lepow, M. L., Bruckman, L., Gillette, M., Markowitz, S., Robino, R. and Kapish, J. (1975). Investigations into sources of lead in the environment of urban children. *Environ. Res.*, **10**, 415–426

McConnell, E. G., Lucier, R., Rumbaugh, P., Albro, D., Harvan, J., Hass, M. and Harris, M. W. (1984). Dioxin in soil: bioavailability after ingestion by rats and guinea pigs. *Science*, **223**, 1077–1079

McDougal, J. N., Jepson, G. W., Clewell, H. J. III, Gargas, M. L. and Andersen, M. E. (1990). Dermal absorption of organic chemical vapours in rats and humans. *Fund. Appl. Toxicol.*, **14**, 299–308

McDougal, J. N., Jepson, G. W., Clewell, H. J. III, MacNaughton, M. G. and Andersen, M. E. (1986). A physiological pharmacokinetic model for dermal absorption of vapors in the rat. *Toxicol. Appl. Pharmacol.*, **85**, 286–294

McKone, J. E. (1990). Dermal uptake of organic chemicals from a soil matrix. *Risk Anal.*, **10**, 407–419

McLaughlin, T. (1984). *Review of Dermal Absorption*. Exposure Assessment Group, US Environmental Protection Agency, Washington, D.C. EPA Report 600/8–84/033

Maibach, H. I., Feldmann, R. J., Milby, T. H. and Serat, W. F. (1971). Regional variation in percutaneous penetration in man. *Arch. Environ. Hlth*, **23**, 208–211

Marlow, D., Sweeney, M. H. and Fingerhut, M. (1990). Estimating the amount of TCDD absorbed by workers who manufactured 2,4,5-T. Presented at the *10th Annual International Dioxin Meeting*, Bayreuth, Germany

Marzulli, F. N. and Tregear, R. T. (1961). Identification of a barrier layer in the skin. *J. Physiol.*, **157**, 52–53

Maxfield, M. E., Barnes, R. R., Azar, A. and Trochimowicz, H. T. (1975). Urinary excretion of metabolite following experimental human exposures to DMF or to DMAC. *J. Occup. Med.*, **17**, 506–511

Michaud, J. and Paustenbach, D. J. (1992). Selecting an appropriate clean-up level for buildings where PCB fires occurred. *Toxicologist*, **12**, abstract 105

Morgan, D. L., Cooper, S. W., Carlock, D. L., Sykora, J. J., Sutton, B., Mattie, D. R. and McDougal, J. N. (1991). Dermal absorption of neat and aqueous volatile organic chemicals in the Fischer 344 rat. *Environ. Res.*, **55**, 51–63

Ostrenga, J., Steinmetz, C. and Poulsen, B. (1971). Significance of vehicle composition. I. Relationship between topical vehicle composition, skin penetrability, and clinical efficacy. *J. Pharm. Sci.*, **60**, 1175–1183

Pannatier, A., Jenner, B., Testa, B. and Etter, J. C. (1978). The skin as a drug-metabolizing organ. *Drug Metab. Rev.*, **8**, 319–343

Paustenbach, D. J. (1988). Assessment of the developmental risks resulting from occupational exposure to select glycol ethers within the semiconductor industry. *J. Toxicol. Environ. Hlth*, **23**, 29–75

Paustenbach, D. J. (1989). A survey of environmental risk assessment. In Paustenbach, D. J. (Ed.), *The Risk Assessment of Environmental and Human Health Hazards: A Textbook of Case Studies*. Wiley, New York, pp. 27–124

Paustenbach, D. J. and Leung, H. W. (1992). Techniques for assessing the health risks of dermal contact with chemicals in the environment. In Wang, R. G., Knaak, J. B. and Maibach, H. I. (Eds), *Health Risk Assessment through Dermal and Inhalation Exposure and Absorption of Toxicants*. CRC Press, Boca Raton, Florida

Paustenbach, D. J., Shu, H. P. and Murray, F. J. (1986). A critical examination of assumptions used in risk assessment of dioxin contaminated soil. *Regulatory Toxicol. Pharmacol.*, **6**, 284–307

Piotrowski, J. (1977). *Exposure Tests for Organic Compounds in Industrial Toxicology*. Publication No. 77–144, National Institute for Occupational Safety and Health, Cincinnati

Poiger, H. and Schlatter, C. H. (1980). Influence of solvents and absorbents on dermal and intestinal absorption of TCDD. *Fd Cosmet. Toxicol.*, **18**, 477–481

Que Hee, S. S., Peace, B., Scott, C. S., Boyle, J. R., Bornschein, R. L. and Hammond, P. B. (1980). Evolution of efficient methods to sample lead sources, such as house dust and hand dust, in the homes of children. *Environ. Res.*, **38**, 77–95

Raykar, P. V., Fung, M. and Anderson, B. D. (1988). The role of protein and lipid domains in the uptake of solutes by human stratum corneum. *Pharm. Res.*, **5**, 140–150

Riihimaki, V. and Pfaffli, P. (1978). Percutaneous absorption of solvent vapors in man. *Scand. J. Work Environ. Hlth*, **4**, 73–85

Roels, H. A., Buchet, J. P., Lauwerys, R. R., Bruax, P., Claeys-Thoreau, F., Fontaine, A. and Verduyn, G. (1980). Exposure to lead by the oral and pulmonary routes of children living in the vicinity of a primary lead smelter. *Environ. Res.*, **22**, 81–94

Rougier, A. D., Dupuis, D., Lotte, C. and Roguet, R. (1985). The measurement of the stratum corneum reservoir. A predictive method for *in vivo* percutaneous absorption studies: influence of application time. *J. Invest. Dermatol.*, **84**, 66–68

Scheuplein, R. J. (1965). Mechanism of percutaneous absorption. I: Routes of penetration and the influence of solubility. *J. Invest. Dermatol.*, **45**, 334–343

Scheuplein, R. J. (1967). Mechanism of percutaneous absorption. II. Transient diffusion and the relative importance of various routes of skin penetration. *J. Invest. Dermatol.*, **48**, 79–88

Scheuplein, R. J. (1980). Percutaneous absorption: Theoretical aspects. In Mauvais-Jarvis, C., Vickers, C. F. H. and Wepierre, J. (Eds), *Percutaneous Absorption of Steroids*. Academic Press, New York, p. 9

Scheuplein, R. J. and Blank, I. H. (1985). Permeability of the skin. *Physiol. Rev.*, **51**, 702–747

Scow, K., Wechsler, A. E., Stevens, J., Wood, M. and Callahan, M. (1979). *Identification and Evaluation of Waterborne Routes of Exposure from Other Than Food and Drinking Water*. US Environmental Protection Agency. Washington D.C. EPA–440/4–79–016

Shatkin, J. A. and Brown, H. S. (1991). Pharmacokinetics of the dermal route of exposure to volatile organic chemicals in water: a computer simulation model. *Environ. Res.*, **56**, 90–108

Sheehan, P., Meyer, D. M., Sauer, M. M. and Paustenbach, D. J. (1991). Assessment of the human health risks posed by exposure to chromium contaminated soils at residential sites. *J. Toxicol. Environ. Hlth*, **32**, 161–201

Shu, H. P., Teitelbaum, P., Webb, A. S., Marple, L., Brunck, B., Dei Rossi, D., Murray, F. J. and Paustenbach, D. J. (1988). Bioavailability of soil-bound TCDD: dermal bioavailability in the rat. *Fund. Appl. Toxicol.*, **10**, 648–654

Skrowronski, G. A., Turkall, R. M. and Abdel-Rahman, M. S. (1988). Soil absorption alters bioavailability of benzene in dermally exposed male rats. *Am. Industr. Hyg. Assoc. J.*, **49**, 506–511

Snyder, W. S. (1975). *Report of the Task Group on Reference Man*. International Commission of Radiological Protection Publication No. 23. Pergamon Press, New York

Stewart, R. D. and Dodd, H. C. (1964). Absorption of carbon tetrachloride, trichloroethylene, tetracloroethylene, methylene chloride, and 1,1,1-trichloroethane through the human skin. *Am. Industr. Assoc. J.*, **25**, 439–446

Surber, C., Wilhelm, K. P., Maibach, H. I., Hall, L. L. and Guy, R. L. (1990). Partitioning of chemicals into human stratum corneum: implications for risk assessment following dermal exposure. *Fund. Appl. Toxicol.*, **15**, 99–107

Travis, C. C. and Hester, S. T. (1990). Background exposure to chemicals: What is the risk? *Risk Anal.*, **10**, 463–466

Tsuruta, H. (1990). Dermal absorption. In Fiserova-Bergerova, V. and Ogata, M. (Eds), *Biological Monitoring of Exposure to Industrial Chemicals*. American Conference of Governmental Industrial Hygienists, Cincinnati, pp. 131–136

Umbreit, T. H., Dhun, P. and Gallo, M. A. (1986).

Acute toxicity of TCDD-contaminated soil from an industrial site. *Science*, **232**, 497–499

USEPA (1989a). *Exposure Factors Handbook*. Office of Remedial Response. US Environmental Protection Agency, Washington, D.C. Publication 540/1-88/001

Van den Berg, M., Olie, K. and Hutzinger, O. (1984). Uptake and selective retention in rats of orally administered chlorinated dioxins and dibenzofurans from fly-ash and fly-ash extract. *Chemosphere*, **12**, 537–544

Vickers, C. F. H. (1963). Existence of reservoir in the stratum corneum. *Arch. Dermatol.*, **88**, 20–23

Wepierre, J. and Marty, J. P. (1979). Percutaneous absorption of drugs. *Trends Pharmacol. Sci.*, inaugural issue, 23–26

Wester, R. C. and Maibach, H. I. (1985). *In vivo* methods for percutaneous absorption measurements. In Bronaugh, R. L. and Maibach, H. I. (Eds), *Percutaneous Absorption. Mechanisms, Methodology, Drug Delivery*. Dermatology Series, Vol. 6. Marcel Dekker, New York, pp. 245–266

Wester, R. C. and Maibach, H. I. (1987). Percutaneous absorption of organic solvents. In *Occupational and Industrial Dermatology*, 2nd edn. Yearbook Medical, Chicago, pp. 213–226

Wester, R. C. and Noonan, P. K. (1980). Relevance of animal models for percutaneous absorption. *Int. J. Pharm.*, **7** 99–110

Wester, R. C., Noonan, P. K. and Maibach, H. I. (1977).

Frequency of application on percutaneous absorption of hydrocortisone. *Arch. Dermatol.*, **113**, 620–622

Wester, R. C., Noonan, P. K. and Maibach, H. I. (1980). Percutaneous absorption of hydrocortisone increases with long-term administration. *Arch. Dermatol.*, **116**, 186–188

Wieczorek, H. (1985). Evaluation of low exposure to styrene. II. Dermal absorption of styrene vapours in humans under experimental conditions. *Int. Arch. Occup. Environ. Hlth*, **57**, 71–75

Zatz, J. L. (1985). Computer simulation using multi-compartmented membrane models. In Bronaugh, R. L. and Maibach, H. I. (Eds), *Percutaneous Absorption, Mechanisms, Methodology, Drug Delivery*. Dermatology Series, Vol. 6. Marcel Dekker, New York, pp. 165–181

FURTHER READING

Bronaugh, R. L. and Maibach, H. I. (1985). *Percutaneous Absorption*. Marcel Dekker, Inc., New York

Grandjean, P. (1990). *Skin Penetration*. Taylor and Francis, London

Kemppainen, B. W. and Reifenrath, W. G. (1990). *Methods for Skin Absorption*. CRC Press, Boca Raton, Florida

Shroot, B. and Schaefer, H. (1987). *Skin Pharmacokinetics*. S. Karger Ag, Basel

18   Inhalation Toxicology

Paul M. Hext and Ian P. Bennett

INTRODUCTION

Inhalation represents one of the major routes by which the body can be exposed by accident or design to foreign materials. Once having entered the respiratory tract, inhaled materials may be readily absorbed or may react directly with the tissues present. In investigating the fate or effects of inhaled materials a number of problems are encountered which are unique to this route of exposure. In the first instance it is necessary to ensure that the material under investigation can reach the target site or sites within the respiratory tract at concentrations appropriate to the needs of the study. The experimentalist must therefore have an understanding of the anatomy of the respiratory tract, mechanisms of deposition, particularly in the case of aerosols, and species differences with respect to these points, since in most cases studies are performed in species other than man. Second, in conducting inhalation studies the exposure and generation systems must be appropriate to the requirements of the study. The latter is particularly important in the case of studies performed for regulatory purposes, where very high atmospheric concentrations are advocated if the material under test has a low toxic potential. Atmospheres, once generated, must also be monitored or analysed at regular intervals to demonstrate stability and, if an aerosol, that the particle size characteristics are acceptable. The foregoing indicates that inhalation toxicity studies involve a considerable technological input which may vary extensively according to the physical and chemical characteristics of the material being investigated. The inhalation toxicologist must therefore understand a number of disciplines, such as aerosol physics, that are not normally encountered in general toxicology.

The aim of this chapter is to provide the reader with a review of the basic principles and practices involved in conducting inhalation studies. It is not possible here to cover in detail the theoretical backgrounds to technology and study design, or the structure of the respiratory tract, its functions and responses to exposure, all of which are essential for a full understanding of the science of inhalation toxicology. These topics are extensively covered in textbooks dedicated to this topic and the reader should refer to these if a greater depth of knowledge is required (see References and Bibliography).

DOSIMETRY

The most important parameter in the majority of toxicity tests is the dose administered to the experimental animal or system. In all modes of administration apart from inhalation, it is easy to determine the dose, since this is usually administered on an easily controlled weight per kilogram body weight basis. In inhalation studies it is clearly more difficult to assess the dose received by the animal, since this is dependent on several factors, the major ones being: (1) atmospheric concentration, (2) duration of exposure, (3) pulmonary physiological characteristics of the test species during the exposure period(s) and (4) deposition/absorption patterns of the test material. It is readily apparent that the dose must be a product of concentration (C) and time (T) for any given exposure, provided that (3) and (4) remain constant. This $C \cdot T$ product is commonly used to relate exposure to the magnitude of a toxic response and is frequently referred to as 'Haber's law', following from the work of Haber (1924), who investigated the comparative lethalities of potential war gases. In many cases, particularly those involving relatively short-duration exposures to materials such as phosgene which have a predominantly direct action on the pulmonary system, the observed toxicity follows Haber's law. However, with increasing interest in relationships between concentration and exposure time, and in mechanisms of toxicity, it is becoming increasingly apparent that many materials do not follow Haber's law. This is frequently seen with those exhibiting systemic toxicity. Such toxicity depends upon the combined processes of uptake by the respiratory tract, tissue distribution, metabolism in potential target organs and elimination. Since many of these processes may be highly efficient at low concentrations but saturable at higher concentrations, a basis for non-linear relationships between concentration, time and toxic phenomena becomes quite apparent. A more detailed appraisal of the toxicokinetics of inhaled materials is beyond the scope of this chapter but is addressed in more detail in the general texts referred to in the References and Bibliography.

The respiratory parameters of an animal will dictate the volume of air inhaled and, hence, the quantity of test material entering the respiratory system. While it is possible, and is frequent practice, to refer to standard respiratory parameters for different species, such as minute volume, in order to calculate inhaled dose with time, it is quite common for toxic materials to influence considerably the breathing patterns of test animals. The most common examples of this are irritant vapours, which can reduce the respiratory rate by up to 80 per cent. This phenomenon results from a reflexive pause during the breathing cycle due to stimulation by the inhaled material of the trigeminal nerve endings situated in the nasal passages. The duration of the pause and, hence, the reduction in the respiratory rate is concentration-related, permitting concentration–response relationships to be plotted. This has been investigated extensively by Alarie (1981), and forms the basis of a test screen for comparing quantitatively the irritancy of different materials and assessing appropriate exposure limits for human exposure when respiratory irritancy is the predominant cause for concern (see Chapter 20).

While irritancy resulting from the above reflex reaction is one cause of altered respiratory parameters during exposure, there are many others. These include other types of reflex response, such as bronchoconstriction, the narcotic effects of many solvents, the development of toxic signs as the exposure progresses, or simply a voluntary reduction in respiratory rate by the test animal due to the unpleasant nature of the inhaled atmosphere. The extent to which these affect breathing patterns and, hence, inhaled dose can only be assessed by actual measurements during the exposure. Such measurements are being incorporated increasingly into routine toxicity

tests in order to estimate more accurately the inhaled dose. Methodology is relatively simple and has been adapted to small experimental animals from the standard plethysmographic techniques used on human subjects. From these parameters it is possible to assess the quantities of test atmosphere breathed in by the animal. It must be remembered that these techniques do not give the quantity of the inhaled material that is absorbed by, or deposited in, the respiratory tract.

In the case of aerosols, the particle size dictates the quantities and regional deposition of the particles. An approximation of dose can therefore be obtained by reference to plots of deposition efficiency as a function of particle size. Figure 1 is an example, based on the studies of Raabe *et al.* (1977, 1988), of such a plot, and shows the total and regional deposition curves for various particle sizes in the rat. Factors governing such deposition are considered later in this chapter. For more accurate assessment or determination of dose for both particulate and vapour atmospheres, chemical analysis of tissues or exposure to radioisotopically labelled materials may be required in conjunction with measurement of respiratory physiology parameters.

PHYSICAL CHARACTERISTICS AND REGIONAL ABSORPTION/ DEPOSITION

The fate of an inhaled material depends upon both its physical and chemical characteristics and

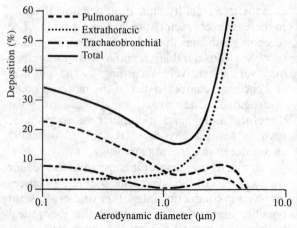

Figure 1 Deposition pattern of particles in the respiratory tract of the rat. From Raabe *et al.* (1977, 1988)

the physical and biological characteristics of the respiratory tract. Although suggesting complexity, all atmospheres to which man or animals may be exposed may be divided initially according to the physical form of the test material and then aspects of the respiratory tract addressed individually to these groups. Thus, atmospheres are divided into those which are vapours or gases and those which are aerosols. The latter term refers to both liquids and solids suspended in the air and encompasses other terms often used for solid aerosols, such as 'particulates' and 'dusts'.

Gases and Vapours

An initial assumption that is made frequently regarding a vapour or gas is that, owing to its physical form, it will penetrate and be absorbed uniformly throughout the respiratory tract. This assumption is incorrect generally. The chemical characteristics and concentration of the material and conditions or characteristics of the respiratory tract all influence the sites to which the atmosphere may penetrate and the proportion absorbed. When an atmosphere is inhaled, it encounters saturated humidity and comes into contact with the tissue lining the various regions of the respiratory tract. Many gases or vapours — for example, ammonia, formaldehyde and sulphur dioxide — are extremely soluble in water and therefore will be absorbed rapidly in the upper respiratory tract. At lower concentrations, which indeed may be as high as hundreds or thousands of parts per million (ppm), there may be a total absorption in these regions with none of the atmosphere penetrating to the lower respiratory tract. Therefore any direct toxic effects of this class of material will be confined generally to these regions, particularly the nasal passsages, where the pattern and type of lesion are characteristic of exposure to this class of material (Buckley *et al.*, 1984). With increasing concentration a gradient will develop such that the material may penetrate eventually to the alveolar regions with subsequent progression throughout the tract of any material-induced toxicity. With materials which have low solubility in water the humidity in the respiratory system has little effect on upper respiratory tract absorption and these materials penetrate readily to the pulmonary regions, even at relatively low concentrations, where they may

exert toxicity. Well-known examples of this class are ozone and nitrogen dioxide.

The site of deposition of vapours according to their solubility in water is only a general rule. Other factors may have a considerable influence on where vapours may deposit or become absorbed. In mixed atmospheres, where both a vapour and particulate are present, the vapour may adsorb onto the particle and the deposition pattern then is governed by the influence of particle deposition, which is addressed later in this section.

The metabolizing capacity of different areas of the respiratory tract may influence also the regional uptake of vapours. For example, the nasal passages are known now to be rich in cytochrome *P*-450 monooxygenase enzymes (Hadley and Dahl, 1982, 1983), by virtue of which they have a considerable capacity to metabolize inhaled materials. If the metabolite proves to be toxic, then the observed tissue effects may be site-specific. This accounts for the ability of some compounds — e.g. 3-trifluoromethylpyridine (Lock and Hext, 1988) and methyl bromide (Hurtt *et al.*, 1987) — to induce upper respiratory tract lesions that are specific to the olfactory epithelium. Another result of the metabolic capacity of these regions is that not only may the inhaled vapour be absorbed totally in this region, but also the compound that enters the blood stream may be the metabolite rather than the parent compound. The bronchiolar regions also have cells (Clara cells) that are capable of metabolizing inhaled xenobiotics with the potential of cell- or site-specific toxicity (Hook *et al.*, 1990). It is therefore apparent from this brief outline of vapour or gas absorption that there are many factors governing the site at which this occurs and the quantity absorbed.

Aerosols

An aerosol can be considered as a suspension of particles in a gas, air being the gas in the majority of cases applicable to inhalation toxicity. When such an atmosphere is inhaled, the particles may deposit anywhere within the respiratory tract, the actual deposition site being dictated by their size. Before the relationship between size, deposition mechanism and site can be understood, it is necessary to realize that it is not the physical size of the particle that is important here but the aerodynamic size, which will vary according to a number of potential variables, the most important of which is the density. Shape—for instance, a fibre—will also have an influence but this is usually less than might be expected.

The aerodynamic diameter of a particle is determined by use of specialized instrumentation and is defined as the diameter of a sphere of unit density having the same settling velocity as the particle in question. Instrumentation used for assessing aerodynamic size and particle size distribution in atmospheres will be covered later. More detailed treatises on the physical aspects of aerosols may be found in Hidy (1984), Hinds (1982) and Vincent (1989), as well as in those texts referred to in the introduction.

Deposition of particles within the respiratory tract is governed by five principal mechanisms—namely inertial impaction, gravitational sedimentation, Brownian diffusion, interception and electrostatic precipitation.

Impaction

Impaction occurs where the airstream undergoes a directional change (Figure 2A). The momentum of the particle is such that it is unable to change course and deposits on the wall of the airway. Particles of aerodynamic size of greater than 0.5 μm may deposit by this mechanism. This mechanism can operate only where there is a combination of both velocity and directional change, and is confined predominantly to the upper respiratory tract and higher branching points in the trachaeo-bronchial system of man but can operate down to the alveolar duct region of smaller experimental animals. Factors influencing deposition by this mechanism include the physical size and density of a particle and breathing pattern.

Gravitational Sedimentation

All particles are subjected to gravity, and when this force exceeds other forces to which the particle is subjected, such as velocity and buoyancy, the particle will deposit on the wall of the respiratory tract (Figure 2B). This mechanism predominates in the lower regions of the respiratory tract, where velocities are low. Factors influencing deposition by this mechanism are those mentioned above for impaction, with the addition of residence time within the respiratory tract.

Brownian Diffusion

Very fine particles, i.e. those less than approximately 0.5 μm, are subject to bombardment by gas molecules and thus acquire random movement in air, termed Brownian movement. Within the respiratory tract particles moving in such a manner may contact the wall of the airway and deposit (Figure 2C). Deposition by this mechanism is favoured by air velocities being low or absent, and therefore predominates in the bronchiolar and alveolar regions.

Interception

Where there is a change in direction of the airflow, irregularly shaped particles such as fibres or fume aggregates may make partial contact with the wall of the airway and become deposited (Figure 2D).

Electrostatic Charge

Aerosols generated for inhalation experiments frequently carry substantial electrostatic charge as a result of the methods of generation employed. Such charges can enhance the fraction and site of deposition of the inhaled aerosol by both particle–particle charge interaction and particle–respiratory tract charge interaction.

Regional Deposition of Particles

When conducting inhalation studies with aerosols, it is important to understand the relationship between particle size and regional deposition. Particles of aerodynamic size exceeding 10 μm

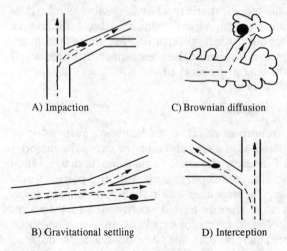

A) Impaction   C) Brownian diffusion

B) Gravitational settling   D) Interception

Figure 2 Diagrammatic representations of the mechanisms influencing the deposition of particles in the respiratory tract

will be deposited primarily in the nose. Many particles smaller than this will deposit in this region but they are also capable of penetrating to other regions. In man it is considered that particles of less than 7 μm are capable of penetrating to the alveoli, although the deposition efficiency in this region increases somewhat as the particle size is reduced further. Most inhalation studies, however, are conducted in experimental animals and allowance may need to be made for differences in particle deposition patterns compared with man. A comparison of respiratory tract deposition in different species can be found in the review paper of Schlesinger (1985). The rat, for example, the most commonly used species for toxicity testing, is an obligate nose-breather and has a complex nasal turbinate structure which will filter out many of the relatively fine particles which would be expected normally to penetrate to the alveoli. Thus, whereas 7 μm is considered to represent the upper size limit for particles that can reach the alveolar regions in man, this is more likely to be in the region of 3–4 μm in the rat, as shown in Figure 1.

EXPOSURE SYSTEMS

Exposure systems for short- or long-term inhalation studies fall into three main categories: whole-body, nose/head-only and masks. Systems using masks are only suitable for larger experimental species and will not be dealt with here. The remaining two categories can be divided further into those operating in the dynamic or static modes. In dynamic systems the test atmosphere passes through the exposure chamber and is renewed continuously. This ensures atmospheric stability and no reduction in oxygen concentration as a result of the respiration of the test animals. It is the mode in which the great majority of inhalation studies are conducted and is the only mode in which reasonable numbers of test animals can be exposed to materials for appreciable periods of time. Static systems are sealed and generally depend upon the air within the chamber to maintain any exposed animals. The exposure time is therefore relatively short, although some systems, in order to extend the exposure time, are designed to replace the consumed oxygen and remove exhaled carbon dioxide. The atmospheric concentration generally will

not remain stable in these systems. If the atmosphere is generated continuously, then it will increase in concentration, whereas if generated only at the initiation of a study, it will decrease, owing to absorption by the test animal and also adsorption onto the walls of the exposure system. The advantage of static systems is that they are relatively simple to operate and will consume only a fraction of the material required to generate a dynamic atmosphere at equivalent concentrations. Thus, they are used predominantly in research studies, particularly if the test material is isotopically labelled, or for other specialized applications, such as assessing the toxicity of products evolved during the combustion of materials.

Dynamic systems, of whatever size or design, must involve a considerable amount of ancillary equipment to maintain appropriate conditions of airflow, temperature and relative humidity. There is a wide range of designs currently in use, some being commercially available, whereas others have been designed and built by individual laboratories. Figure 3A shows the general design for a chamber of approximately 250 l capacity in which small experimental species may be exposed whole-body to experimental atmospheres and Figure 3B shows a typical nose-only exposure chamber. The latter mode of exposure is used frequently for exposure to particulates, since it reduces to an absolute minimum the deposition of test atmosphere on the pelt of the test animal. This is an important factor to take into account when exposure is to aerosols which may exert systemic toxicity, since with whole-body exposure the quantities depositing in the fur and subsequently ingested during grooming can exceed considerably the quantity depositing in the respiratory tract (Langard and Nordhagen, 1980; Iwasaki *et al.*, 1988).

The main criteria for the design and operation of any dynamic system are:

- The concentration of the test atmosphere must be reasonably uniform throughout the chamber and should increase and decrease at a rate close to theoretical at the start or end of the exposure. Silver (1946) showed that the time taken for a chamber to reach a point of equilibrium was proportional to the flow rate of atmosphere passing through the chamber and the chamber volume. From this, the con-

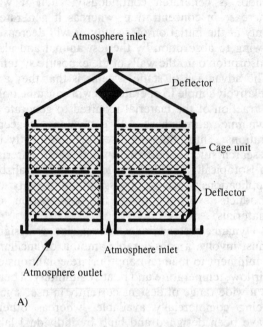

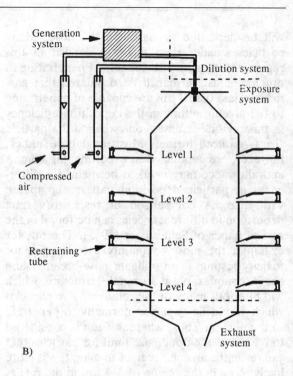

Figure 3 Typical designs for short-term whole-body (A) and nose-only (B) exposure systems

centration–time relationship during the 'run-up' and 'run-down' phase could be expressed by the equation

$$t_x = k \cdot \frac{V}{F}$$

where t_x = time required to reach x per cent of the equilibrium concentration;
k = a constant of value determined by the value of x;
V = chamber volume; and
F = chamber flow rate.

The t_{99} value is quoted frequently for exposure chambers, representing the time required to reach 99 per cent of the equilibrium concentration and providing an estimate of chamber efficiency. Thus, at maximum efficiency, the theoretical value of k at t_{99} is 4.605, and the closer to this that the results of evaluation of actual chamber performance fall, the greater the efficiency and the better the design of the chamber.

• Flow rates must be controlled in such a way that they are not excessive, which might cause streaming effects within the chamber, but must be adequate to maintain normal oxygen levels, temperature and humidity in relation to the number of animals being exposed. A minimum of 12 air changes per hour is advocated frequently and is appropriate in most cases. However, the chamber design and housing density also need to be taken into account and some designs, such as that of Doe and Tinston (1981), function effectively at lower air change rates.

• Chamber materials should not affect the chemical or physical nature of the test atmosphere.

In addition, it is desirable, and frequently a regulatory necessity, to monitor and record air flow, temperature and humidity within the chamber.

The above criteria apply equally to those chambers already illustrated (Figure 3) which are designed predominantly for short-term studies (days to months) and to those built on a larger scale to accommodate large numbers of experimental animals for durations of up to several years. The latter can vary from a relatively simple design of 2 m³ capacity (similar to Figure 3A) to the more complex design described by Doe and Tinston (1981), where the cages are suspended on carriers which rotate within the chamber. More detailed considerations of theoretical and practical design and operation of inhalation chambers may be found in Drew (1978), Leong (1981) and MacFarland (1983).

ATMOSPHERE GENERATION

Atmosphere generation systems fall into two classes: those concerned with particulate atmospheres, such as aerosols of solids or liquids, and those concerned with non-particulate atmospheres, such as gases or vapours. In all cases there should be sufficient control over the generation system to provide reasonably stable atmospheres. Gases and vapours should normally be controlled to within 5–10 per cent of target concentration with little difficulty whereas particulates, which present invariably the greater difficulties of control, may vary acceptably to within 20 per cent of target.

Gases and Vapours

Gases and vapours may be generated in several ways, including direct dilution of a gas with clean air, and vaporization of a liquid either by the addition of heat or by increasing the surface area of the liquid. The latter is achieved frequently either by atomization or by passing the liquid over glass beads (as described by Miller *et al.*, 1980) or similar apparatus designed to increase the surface area of the liquid.

Particulates

The generation of particulate atmospheres is more complicated, owing to the physical characteristics of the material and of the generated aerosol. The latter, for inhalation studies, must be capable generally of penetrating to all regions of the respiratory tract. Aerosol generation systems must therefore be capable of producing particles of a suitable size. It is convenient to consider liquid and solid aerosol generation systems separately.

Aerosol Generation from Liquids

There are two commonly used processes by which an aerosol can be generated under laboratory-controlled conditions: condensation from saturated vapours or dispersion of solutions or suspensions by aerosolization or nebulization. Condensation generators produce only relatively low concentration aerosols, but can be used to produce aerosols containing a very narrow range of particle sizes. Aerosols of materials with only moderate volatility at ambient temperature and pressure may be generated as condensation aerosols. This involves heating the test material and passing air over or through it, to carry away the vapour phase created by the raised temperature. The air then passes through a flue, where it is cooled to room temperature. This causes the vapour phase to become supersaturated and to condense onto any nuclei present in the air stream. The nuclei grow until the vapour phase of the test material reaches a new point of saturation. An aerosol produced in this way is usually monodisperse—i.e. all the particles have a very similar size. The mass concentration of the aerosol will be limited by the change in saturated vapour concentration caused by the increase in temperature. Only aerosols of essentially pure materials should be generated in this way, as the removal of the vapour phase from above the heated material may cause a fractional distillation from mixtures of chemicals with different vapour pressures.

Atomization and Nebulization

Atomizers and nebulizers are two methods of liquid atomization which use compressed air as a motive force. The former are very simple devices which use a high-velocity air jet to disrupt a stream of the test liquid as it leaves a narrow orifice. There are many designs based on this principle. An example of a commercially available atomizer that may be used to produce test atmospheres is the Schlick atomizer (Figure 4A; Gustav Schlick GmbH, Germany), which is made from stainless steel and is therefore suitable for use with a wide range of liquids, including organic solvents. This atomizer is representative of the most common type of atomizer, where the air jet forms an annulus around the inner liquid jet as shown. The Schlick is designed as an industrial device used, for example, in spray drying, spray painting or glue spreading, but it is suited equally to generation of atmospheres in inhalation toxicity. The extended inner jet prevents volatile materials evaporating within the jet throat, which

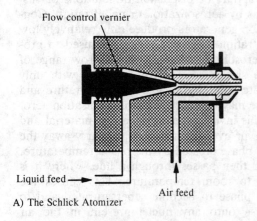

A) The Schlick Atomizer

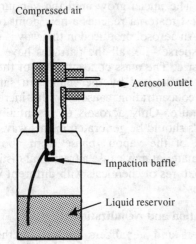

B) The Wright Nebulizer

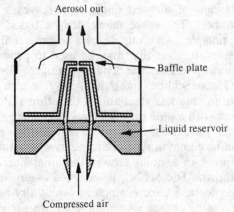

C) The Acorn Nebulizer

Figure 4   Commonly used liquid aerosol generation systems

could result in precipitated solute blocking the jet and causing either stoppages or irregular operation.

Atomizers produce a broad-spectrum aerosol containing a wide range of particle sizes. However, although the mean diameter of the aerosol can vary substantially, atomizers generate aerosols with large mean diameters and as such their use may be limited to inhalation toxicology, so more suitable devices such as the nebulizer have been developed.

Nebulizers are more sophisticated than atomizers. The main difference between the two types of aerosol generator is the inclusion of some form of size selection device in the nebulizer. This is usually a baffle placed in the path of the air–liquid mixture. The Wright nebulizer (Wright, 1958; Figure 4B) is an example and is constructed generally from polyacrylic resin. This does, however, preclude the use of this device with materials containing many organic solvents. Several other nebulizers have been designed to provide aerosol therapy via the respiratory tract and are equally applicable to inhalation toxicology. One example, the Acorn nebulizer (Medic-aid, Chichester, Sussex, UK), is shown diagrammatically in Figure 4C. The performance of this and a number of similar devices has been characterized extensively by Clay *et al.* (1983), Bretz *et al.* (1984) and Newman *et al.* (1985). Such devices are usually very compact. Since they are generally injection-moulded from polyacrylic resins or similar materials, they may similarly be unsuitable for materials which contain organic solvents. However, they do offer the most consistent output between different generators, owing to their closely controlled method of manufacture.

Aerosol Generation from Solids

There are two main forms of dry particle dispersion system: those that disperse from a compressed sample of the test material and those that disperse from the free-flowing material. Both types are in common use.

One widely used dust generation system is the Wright Dust Feed Mechanism (Wright, 1950; Figure 5A), which is available in a number of different commercial forms. The material to be generated is first packed and compressed into a hard cake and during aerosol production a thin layer is scraped off into the air stream. The scra-

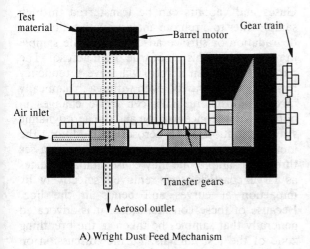

A) Wright Dust Feed Mechanism

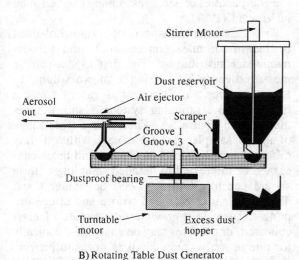

B) Rotating Table Dust Generator

Figure 5   Commonly used solid aerosol generators

per is driven into the cake by a series of gears powered by a constant-speed motor. The gears can be adjusted to achieve a range of scraper advancement speeds, and, hence, dust generation rates. Systems based on compressing material into a hard cake are not suitable for materials which are near to their melting point at room temperature. If such materials were used, the pressure could cause the melting point of the material to be exceeded, resulting in fusion into a solid or wax.

The other major group of dust generation systems disperse material directly from the freely flowing bulk sample without any compaction into a cake. The Rotating Table Dust Generator (RTDG) was described by Mark *et al.* (1985) and

represents an inexpensive system of this type. The device is shown in Figure 5B. The bulk material is placed into a hopper and a stirrer blade is passed down the centre. The hopper exhaust is positioned over a groove in the rotating table. Several concentric grooves of different depths may be cut into each table to extend the range of concentrations available without changing the table. Dust from the hopper fills the groove as it rotates beneath the hopper exhaust. After the dust has been levelled, it is transferred beneath the inlet of an air ejector which lifts it from the groove. The air velocity and turbulence within the air ejector dissociate the test material into individual particles. The concentration of the test aerosol can be adjusted and controlled by altering the rate at which the table rotates, by using a different groove or by adjusting the air flow through the air ejector. Other systems using free-flowing powders include those based on air jet mills (Bernstein *et al.*, 1984) and fluidized beds (Carpenter and Yerkes, 1980).

The atmosphere generation systems described above are provided as examples of the wide range of systems, based on an equally wide range of principles, that can be used to generate atmospheres suitable for use in determining the inhalation toxicity of a material. Although many generators will produce atmospheres from a range of different materials, there are also many specialized generation systems that have been developed to create a specific atmosphere from one material or, at the most, a narrow class of materials. For more detail of the principles and practices of atmosphere generation the reader is referred to books in the general reference list which describe these more fully.

ATMOSPHERE ANALYSIS

An atmosphere having been generated, it is necessary to confirm that the atmosphere is chemically and physically suitable to provide a valid assessment of the inhalation toxicity of the test material. This is a two-stage process: the first stage involves the collection of a representative sample of the atmosphere, generally from the breathing zone of the test animals; the second is concerned with a determination of the physical and chemical nature of the atmosphere. The frequency of sampling for analysis is dependent on a number of factors, including the stability of the test atmosphere, the method of sampling or analysis and the concentration of test material. All these factors need to be considered for each new material, but as a general rule sampling should be performed at least hourly during exposure. Instruments are now available to give continuous qualitative, semiquantitative or quantitative assessments of both particulate and non-particulate atmospheres. These help both to assess continuously the stability of test atmospheres and to reduce the frequency of sampling.

Vapours and Gases

When vapours and gases are considered, the first stage represents few problems generally. However, the possible reactivity of the atmosphere with components of the sampling system and the volume taken for analysis must be considered in every case. The latter is important, since the flow rate through and atmosphere distribution within the inhalation chamber must be unaffected by the volume removed for sampling. In general, the sampling rate should not represent greater than 5–10 per cent of the total chamber flow rate.

Atmospheres of vapours or gases can be considered as homogeneous mixtures and, as such, would be unaffected by the physical nature of the sampling process. In this instance the process becomes a matter of collecting sufficient material to allow a meaningful chemical analysis. The amount needed can vary enormously, depending on the type of analysis to be peformed. Gas Chromatography (GC), High Performance Liquid Chromatography (HPLC), Gas Chromatography/Mass Spectrometry (GCMS) and Infra-red Gas Analysis (IRGA) are all commonly used to measure non-particulate atmosphere concentrations, as are 'wet' chemistry and spectrophotometry. Many of these methods may be automated in order to take and analyse samples repeatedly from a range of inhalation and exposure chambers. The results may be collated with a microcomputer as well as being used to trigger alarms should the measured concentration fall outside a pre-set range.

Particulates

Particulate atmospheres are more complicated to analyse than are non-particulate atmospheres.

Gases and vapours can be transferred through sample lines to a remote analyser with little or no degradation or surface adsorption of the sample in many cases. This is not true of an aerosol. The particles within an aerosol will have a tendency to settle out by gravity, even within a dynamically mixed atmosphere. This can cause changes in both the mass concentration and the aerodynamic size distribution of an aerosol. In addition, the inertial forces acting on an aerosol as it passes through a sample line may cause similar changes as larger particles are removed selectively by impaction at curves and bends in the line. Because of these considerations, it is advocated generally that samples be taken in the breathing zone of the test animals. Further discussion on the complexities of aerosol sampling can be found in Vincent (1989).

Two fundamental aspects of an aerosol must be measured: mass concentration and aerodynamic size distribution. The first aspect can be measured easily by drawing a known volume of test atmosphere, at a known flow rate, through a filter. A basic sampling system is shown schematically in Figure 6A. There are a wide range of aerosol samplers available, each with a slightly different sampling inlet efficiency, and those concerned or interested in detailed sampling criteria should consult Vincent (1989) or similar texts. The filter mass is weighed before and after sampling to provide a gravimetric estimate of mass collected, or the filter may be analysed chemically for one or more components in order to provide a more detailed description of the chemical nature of the aerosol. The atmospheric concentration of the particulate is calculated simply from the mass collected divided by the volume of air sampled.

The aerodynamic size distribution of an aerosol is determined generally by use of a cascade impactor (see Figure 6B). In such a device the aerosol is accelerated repeatedly through a series of increasingly finer jets that play upon a flat collection surface. As the particles are accelerated, they achieve sufficient momentum to prevent them following the change in direction of the air flow and they are deposited by impaction onto the collection plate. In this way particles with increasingly smaller aerodynamic diameters are collected on to the successive stages. The impactor is designed such that under defined operating conditions the particle size of material

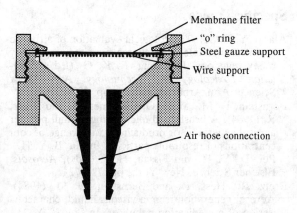

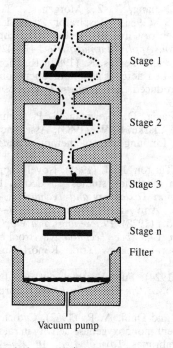

A) A typical open-faced total gravimetric sampler

B) A typical cascade impactor

Figure 6 Typical designs of (A) a sampler for measuring the total particulate present in an aerosol and (B) a cascade impactor for determination of the particle size distribution of an aerosol

Table 1 Tabulation of cascade impactor data for plotting of particle size distribution

Aerodynamic diameter cut-off (µm)	Weight on stage (mg)	% of total	Cumulative % (less than previous cut-off)
9.8	0.305	6.1	
6.0	0.425	8.5	93.9
3.5	0.32	6.4	85.4
1.55	1.15	23.0	79.0
0.93	0.60	12.0	56.0
0.52	0.75	15.0	44.0
Filter	1.45	29.0	29.0
Total	5.000	100.0	

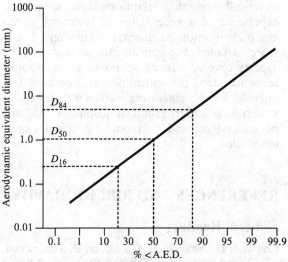

Figure 7 Logarithmic-probability plot of data (Table 1) derived from atmosphere sampling using a six-stage cascade impactor. Plotting cumulative percentage of deposited material against aerodynamic cut-off for each stage allows graphical derivation of mass mean aerodynamic diameter (D_{50}) and geometric standard deviations (GSD)

collecting on each stage is known; hence, the quantity of material depositing on each stage can be assigned a specific 'cut-point'. This information is then converted to cumulative percentage, as shown in Table 1, and then linearized by plotting 'cut-point' particle size against cumulative percentage on log-probability paper, as shown in Figure 7. From such a plot the particle size distribution is demonstrated graphically and the mean aerodynamic diameter (D_{50}) can be found. The distribution of particle size can be expressed as the Geometric Standard Deviation (GSD), which is calculated from the particle sizes at the 16 per cent or 84 per cent points (these represent one standard deviation from the mean) according to the following equations:

$$\text{GSD} = \frac{D_{84}}{D_{50}} \text{ or } \frac{D_{50}}{D_{16}} \text{ or } \sqrt{\frac{D_{84}}{D_{16}}}$$

In recent years a range of direct reading instruments based on some indirect measurement of aerodynamic diameter via, for example, light scattering or radio-opacity, have become available. These are becoming increasingly used for continuous monitoring of aerosols to assess real-time variability and to provide a means of quality control when calibrated against an 'absolute' system such as gravimetry or cascade impaction.

CONCLUSION

This chapter provides a basic introduction to the principles and practice of inhalation toxicology. It should be apparent that this discipline is very technically oriented, requiring knowledge and experience of a wide range of technical equipment in addition to general toxicology. While more detailed theoretical information on the aspects covered can be found in the textbooks recommended, the difficulties encountered frequently when generating different classes of materials as experimental atmospheres can only be understood and overcome by actual experimentation.

REFERENCES AND BIBLIOGRAPHY

General Reading

Crapo, J. D., Smolko, E. D., Miller, F. J., Graham, J. A. and Hayes, A. W. (Eds) (1989). *Extrapolation of Dosimetric Relationships for Inhaled Particles and Gases*. Academic Press, San Diego

Fiserova-Bergorova, V. (Ed.) (1983). *Modelling of Inhalation Exposure to Vapours: Uptake, Distribution and Elimination*, Vols 1, 2. CRC Press, Boca Raton, Florida

McClellan, R. O. and Henderson, R. F. (Eds) (1989). *Concepts in Inhalation Toxicology*. Hemisphere Publishing Corporation, New York

Mohr, U. (Ed.) (1989). *Inhalation Toxicology, the Design and Interpretation of Inhalation Studies and Their Use in Risk Assessment*. Springer-Verlag, New York

Phalen, R. F. (1984). *Inhalation Studies: Foundations and Techniques*. CRC Press, Boca Raton, Florida

Salem, H. (Ed.) (1987). *Inhalation Toxicology*. Marcel Dekker, New York

Witschi, H. P. and Brain, J. D. (Eds) (1985). *Toxicology of Inhaled Materials*. Springer-Verlag, Berlin

Specific Topics

Alarie, Y. (1981). Toxicological evaluation of airborne chemical irritants and allergens using respiratory reflex reactions. In Leong, B. K. G. (Ed.), *Inhalation Toxicology and Technology*. Ann Arbor Science, Ann Arbor, Michigan, pp. 207–231

Bernstein, D. M., Moss, O., Fleissner, H. and Bretz, R. (1984). A brush feed micronising jet mill powder aerosol generator for producing a wide range of concentrations of respirable particles. In Liu, B. Y. H.., Pui, D. Y. H. and Fissan, H. J. (Eds), *Aerosols*. Elsevier Science, New York, pp. 721–724

Bretz, R., Hess, R. and Bernstein, D. M. (1984). Aerosol generation from a viscous liquid: characterisation of a medication nebuliser. In Liu, B. Y. H., Pui, D. Y. H. and Fissan, H. J. (Eds), *Aerosols*. Elsevier Science, New York, pp. 717–720

Buckley, L. A., Jiang, X. Z., Morgan, K. T. and Barrow, C. S. (1984). Respiratory tract lesions induced by sensory irritants at the RD_{50} concentration. *Toxicol. Appl. Pharmacol.*, **74**, 417–429

Carpenter, R. L. and Yerkes, K. (1980). Relationship between fluid bed aerosol generator operation and the aerosol produced. *Am. Industr. Hyg. Assoc. J.*, **41**, 888–894

Clay, M. M., Pavia, D., Newman, S. P., Lennard-Jones, T. and Clarke, S. W. (1983). Assessment of jet nebulisers for lung aerosol therapy. *Lancet*, **ii**, 592–594

Doe, J. E. and Tinston, D. J. (1981). Novel chambers for long term inhalation studies. In Leong, K. J. (Ed.), *Inhalation Toxicology and Technology*. Ann Arbor Science, Ann Arbor, Michigan, pp. 77–88

Drew, R. T. (Ed.) (1978). *Proceedings of a Workshop on Inhalation Chamber Technology*. Brookhaven National Laboratory, New York. Report Number BNL 51318

Haber, F. R. (1924). Funf Vorträge aus den Jahren 1920–1923 (No. 3: *Die Chemie in Kreize*). Springer, Berlin

Hadley, W. H. and Dahl, A. R. (1982). Cytochrome P-450 dependent monooxygenase activity in rat nasal epithelial membranes. *Toxicol. Lett.*, **10**, 417–422

Hadley, W. H. and Dahl, A. R. (1983). Cytochrome P-450 dependent monooxygenase activity in nasal membranes of six species. *Drug Metab. Disp.* **11**, 275–276

Hidy, G. M. (1984). *Aerosols—An Industrial and Environmental Science*. Academic Press, Orlando, Florida

Hinds, W. C. (1982). *Aerosol Technology—Properties, Behaviour and Measurement of Airborn Particles*. Wiley, New York

Hook, G. E. R., Gilmore, L. B., Gupta, R. P., Patton, S. E., Jetten, A. M. and Nettesheim, P. (1990). The function of pulmonary Clara cells. In Thomasson, D. G. and Nettesheim, P. (Eds), *Biology, Toxicology and Carcinogenicity of Respiratory Epi-*

thelium. Hemisphere Publishing Corporation, New York, pp. 38–59

Hurtt, M. E., Morgan, K. T. and Working, P. K. (1987). Histopathology of acute toxic responses in selected tissues from rats exposed to methyl bromide. *Fund. Appl. Toxicol.* **9**, 352–365

Iwasaki, M., Yoshida, M., Ikeda, T. and Tsuda, S. (1988). Comparison of whole-body versus snout-only exposure in inhalation toxicity of fenthion. *Japan. J. Vet. Sci.*, **50**, 23–30

Langard, S. and Nordhagen, A. L. (1980). Small animal inhalation chambers and the significance of dust ingestion from the contaminated coat when exposing rats to zinc chromate. *Acta Pharmacol. Toxicol.*, **46**, 43–46

Leong, B. K. J. (Ed.) (1981). *Inhalation Toxicology and Technology*. Ann Arbor Science, Ann Arbor, Michigan.

Lock, E. A. and Hext, P. M. (1988). Selective toxicity of 3-trifluoromethylpyridine (3-FMP) to rat olfactory epithelium. *Toxicologist*, **8**, 6P

MacFarland, H. N. (1983). Designs and operational characteristics of inhalation exposure equipment – a review. *Fund. Appl. Toxicol.*, **3**, 603–613

Mark, D., Vincent, J. H., Gibson, H. and Witherspoon, W. A. (1985). Application of closely graded powders of fused alumina as tests dusts for aerosol studies. *J. Aerosol Sci.*, **16**, 125–131

Miller, R. R., Letts, R. L., Potts. W. J. and McKenna, M. J. (1980). Improved methodology for generating controlled test atmospheres. *Am. J. Industr. Hyg. Assoc. J.*, **41**, 844–846

Newman, S. P., Pellow, P., Clay, M., and Clarke, S. W. (1985). Evaluation of jet nebulisers for use with gentamycin solutions. *Thorax*, **40**, 671–676

Raabe, O. G., Yeh, H., Newton, G. J., Phalen, R. F. and Velasquez, D. J. (1977). Deposition of inhaled monodisperse aerosols in small rodents. In Walton W. H. (Ed.), *Inhaled Particles IV*. Pergamon Press, Oxford, pp. 3–21

Raabe, O. G., Al-Bayati, M. A., Teague, S. V. and Rasolt, A. (1988). Regional deposition of inhaled monodisperse coarse and fine aerosol particles in small laboratory rodents. In Dodgson, J., McCallum, R. I., Bailey, M. R. and Fisher, D. R. (Eds), *Inhaled Particles VI*. Pergamon Press, Oxford, pp. 53–63

Schlesinger, R. B. (1985). Comparative deposition of inhaled aerosols in experimental animals and humans: a review. *J. Toxicol. Environ. Hlth*, **15**, 197–214

Silver, S. D. (1946). Constant flow gassing chambers: principles influencing design and operation. *J. Lab. Clin. Med.*, **31**, 1153–1161

Vincent, J. H. (1989). *Aerosol Sampling—Science and Practice*. Wiley, Chichester

Wright, B. M. (1950). A new dust feed mechanism. *J. Sci. Instrum.*, **27**, 12–15

Wright B. M. (1958). A new nebuliser. *Lancet*, **ii**, 24–25

FURTHER READING

Barrow, C. S. (1986). *Toxicology of the Nasal Passages*. Hemisphere Publishing Corporation, Washington D.C.

McClellan, R. O. and Henderson, R. F. (1989). *Concepts in Inhalation Toxicology*. Hemisphere Publishing Corporation, New York

Medinsky, M. A., Kimbell, J. S., Morris, J. B., Gerde, P. and Overton, J. M. (1993). Advances in biologically based models for respiratory tract uptake of inhaled volatiles. *Fundamental and Applied Toxicology*, **20**, 265–272

Warheil, D. B. (1993). *Fiber Toxicology*. Academic Press, San Diego

Wischi, H. P. and Brain, J. D. (1985). *Toxicology of Inhaled Materials*, Springer-Verlag, Berlin

PART FOUR: TARGET ORGAN TOXICITY

19 Neurotoxicology

J. M. Lefauconnier and C. Bouchaud

INTRODUCTION

Cellular Elements of Nervous Tissue

There are two cell populations in nervous tissue: neurons and glial cells. Some discussion of their organization is necessary, as neurotoxins have a predilection to injure some cell constituents. Neurons are cells specialized in generation, reception and transfer of information. They interact with other neurons, with muscle cells and with sensory and glandular cells. Information is transmitted by release of neurotransmitter from the presynaptic axon terminal, the transmitter substance crossing the synaptic cleft and binding to the receptors of the post-synaptic membrane of the following cell.

The neuron has a very characteristic appearance in histological sections, with a perikaryon or soma (cytoplasm around the nucleus) rich in granular endoplasmic reticulum (Nissl substance), which is the site of protein synthesis. Several short dendrites leave the soma in addition to the axon, which can be very long. The axon has no granular endoplasmic reticulum, and its cytoskeleton has neurofilaments and microtubules which are the rails for bidirectional transport of molecules and cellular organelles. At its synaptic ending, the axon may endocytose neurotoxins, viruses as well as neurotransmitters, and allow them to enter the nerve cell, to join the perikaryon by retrograde transport.

The glial cells include the macroglia (astrocytes and oligodendrocytes) and microglia. The macroglia is of the same embryological origin as the neuron, while the microglia is of mesenchymal origin, as are endothelial cells. The axon is very often in close relation with oligodendroglial cells in the central nervous system (CNS) or with Schwann cells in the peripheral nervous sytem (PNS). These cells are responsible for myelination. Astrocytes are star-shaped cells, the processes of which are often in close relation with endothelial cells and also meningeal cells which cover the central nervous system. A trophic and an axonal guiding role has been attributed to them. It also seems that they transmit chemical factors which give rise to the blood–brain barrier (BBB) in endothelial cells. The microglia is a type of resident macrophagocytic cell that can become active as a result of damage.

The Blood–Brain Barrier

This barrier between the blood and the central nervous system plays an essential role in the selection of molecules that enter the nervous system. It is formed by the non-fenestrated endothelial cells of brain microvessels which differ from other endothelial cells in several ways. These non-fenestrated endothelial cells are bound to other endothelial cells by tight junctions which prevent the entry of proteins and other water-soluble substances of low molecular weight. Vesicular transfer, which exists in other endothelial cells, is very low. The endothelial cells of capillaries are surrounded by a basal lamina which also encloses pericytes. Formation of the blood–brain barrier (BBB) occurs during development by astrocytic induction (for review, see Risau and Wolburg, 1990).

There are some areas of the CNS without a blood–brain barrier—namely the choroid plexus, neurohypophysis, eminentia media, pineal gland, area postrema and subfornical organ. The capillaries of these areas have a fenestrated endothelium, but there are tight junctions between the ependymal cells.

In brain, fluid compartments, containing CSF, communicate with the brain extracellular space, the CSF being secreted mainly by the choroid plexus. The CSF fills the ventricles, which are lined with ependymal cells (a variety of macroglia), and the subarachnoid space, which separates the pia mater from the arachnoid. The meningeal barrier is situated in a layer of specialized cells at the border of the arachnoid membrane with the dura mater (Nabeshima *et al.*, 1975).

Sensory and autonomous ganglia are not protected by the BBB, their neurons thus being particularly exposed to neurotoxins. However, the peripheral nerve has a barrier isolating it from the environment: the perineurium forming a connective tissue sheath. The inner layers of perineurial cells are connected by tight junctions (Rechthand and Rapoport, 1987). In addition, a blood–nerve barrier is provided by capillary and endothelial cells which are bound by tight junctions.

Neurotoxins and Cell Permeability

The target of a neurotoxin can be either on the cell surface (the plasma membrane) or inside the cell. As in other tissues, the permeability is proportional to the lipid/water partition coefficient, and lipophilic substances are able passively to diffuse through the lipid bilayer, an essential structure of biological membranes. Lipophilic substances which pass via a vascular route can reach the parenchyma of the nervous system and act upon neurons and glial cells.

A lipid abnormality can cause an alteration in the function of membranes and a greater sensitivity to toxic alterations. Since brain, spinal cord and peripheral nerves are the organs with the highest lipid concentration after adipose tissue, it is evident that lipid solubility of toxic molecules plays a fundamental role in neurotoxicology. However, one protein, P-glycoprotein, which is present at the BBB, is able to eject lipophilic substances from endothelial cells (Cordon-Cardo et al., 1989).

For hydrophilic molecules an effective transmembrane transport can exist only if there are selective carriers or channels (for ions) in the plasma membrane. Hydrophilic toxic molecules can be transported by these carriers or have an action on them, or bind to protein receptors or to ionic channels. The interaction with a receptor can trigger an intracellular response.

CELLULAR AND MOLECULAR TARGETS FOR NEUROTOXINS

A substance is neurotoxic when it causes a pathological modification of the function of the nervous system by interaction with one or more type of constituent cell (neurons, glial cells, endothelial cells). Neurotoxins may have a variety of origins; they may be biological, or inorganic or organic chemicals. In extreme instances neurotoxins can cause cellular death, and when this cellular death involves the neurons, the intoxication can have serious consequences, as there is no renewal of neurons after birth. Finally, neurotoxins can affect the evolution of several types of glial cells: microglial cells which can multiply and clear the organism of debris and astrocytes which can divide and heal damaged regions.

Neurotoxins can be classified according to their targets or according to their functions. Some neurotoxins are active on the CNS regions or on the PNS. Others are ototoxic and/or vestibulotoxic or oculotoxic, and are discussed in Chapter 31. Some act on specific cellular functions. This specificity has been called 'selective cell vulnerability'. Finally, some will act on the developing nervous system. In addition, the type of effect of toxic substances can vary according to the dose.

Neuronal Lesions

The neurotoxins described here will be either those which produce specifically neuronal lesions or those which affect all cells (for example, carbon monoxide) but give a symptomatology which is mainly neuronal, although the histopathological changes can also affect the glial cells. Neurons seem to be very sensitive to neurotoxins, possibly because neuronal dysfunction results in specific signs.

Action on Nucleic Acids

Nearly all deoxyribonucleic acid (DNA) is found in the nucleus, where transcription to messenger ribonucleic acid (mRNA) occurs. mRNA then moves to the cytoplasm, where it associates with transfer RNA (tRNA) and ribosomal RNA (rRNA) for protein synthesis. After birth, neurons do not multiply and DNA synthesis stops. On the other hand, glial and endothelial cells continue to divide. Glial cells can occupy considerable areas—for example, after cellular death caused by neurotoxins.

A large number of drugs can interfere with cell division and have been used in cancer treatment. These drugs, in general, are not neurotoxic, as they are excluded from the CNS by the BBB. However, some of them—for example, methotrexate—can show neurotoxicity (due to astrocytic alterations) when administered intrathecally in the treatment of meningeal leukaemia or parenchymal tumours or when administered after irradiation has impaired the BBB. Clinical manifestations are either meningeal irritation, paraparesis or encephalopathy leading in severe cases to coma and death. The neuropathological manifestations are periventricular necrosis, fibrinoid degeneration and small vessel thrombosis (Weiss *et al.*, 1974). In addition, some drugs that are excluded from the nervous system by the BBB can reach it via unprotected regions, such as sensory ganglia or cells of the circumventricular organs. Doxorubicin (adriamycin) is such a drug, and, while it has not been shown to be harmful in humans, is neurotoxic in animals (Cavanagh, 1986). It induces clear nuclear areas in rat spinal ganglion cells, probably due to a decrease in the size of chromatin areas. There is also a loss of Nissl substance and thus of protein synthesis (Cho *et al.*, 1980). Cisplatin produces similar results.

In the nucleus, actinomycin D can prevent the transcription of DNA into RNA by binding to DNA and inhibiting the action of RNA polymerase. Similarly, amanitine, an alkaloid derived from the toxic mushroom *Amanita phalloides*, inhibits RNA polymerase. These substances cannot cross the BBB *in vivo*.

Action on Protein Synthesis

Protein synthesis is carried out in ribosomes, localized in polysomes or in granular endoplasmic reticulum which constitutes the Nissl substance. Methyl mercury acts on protein synthesis and leads to the disappearance of Nissl substance. Autoradiography has shown that methyl mercury inhibits the incorporation of $[^{14}C]$-leucine into neurons of the CNS (Yoshino *et al.*, 1966). However, the lesions are more extensive in the sensory ganglia which have no BBB.

Action on Energy Metabolism

Sugars and fatty acids are oxidized to H_2O and CO_2 in the mitochondria. Recovery of the available energy is very efficient, but requires the presence of molecular oxygen. The supply of oxygen can be impaired by certain poisons—for example, carbon monoxide (Ginsberg, 1980). Carbon monoxide binds to metals to form metal carbonyls. It binds reversibly to the iron of haemoglobin, myoglobin and cytochromes, and competes with oxygen on the haemoglobin molecule. It seems that it can also modify the affinity of the remaining sites for their substrate, so that oxygen is

delivered to the tissues less easily than under normal conditions.

Carbon monoxide intoxication occurs mainly in attempted suicide and rapidly leads to loss of consciousness. A notable feature is that, when the patient does not die, he or she usually regains consciousness and becomes neurologically normal: but, at a variable time after the intoxication (2–5 weeks), there is often an abrupt deterioration with confusion and cortical dysfunction which may lead to death.

Neuropathological studies show the same modifications as in hypoxic and ischaemic lesions with other causes. When death occurs a few hours after intoxication, there is congestion of brain and meningeal vessels and sometimes small haemorrhages. In patients dying later, there is often brain oedema and lesions of the cortex, and in one-half of the cases parenchymal necrosis. There are often lesions of the hippocampus and less often of the cerebellum and globus pallidus. Changes in the white matter lesions are also seen with myelinopathy and astrocytosis.

It seems that the toxicity of carbon monoxide depends not only on its competition with oxygen for the binding sites on haemoglobin, but also on an impairment of cerebral perfusion and on oligaemia. These effects have been demonstrated in experimental studies in animals (Ginsberg, 1980).

Energy metabolism can also be modified at the level of enzymes or coenzymes. This can be important for axonal transport which uses proteins (dyneine and kinesine) which require ATP. Some glycolytic enzymes (glyceraldehyde-3-phosphate dehydrogenase, phosphofructokinase) can be inhibited by neurotoxins. This is true for 2,5-hexanedione (2,5-HD), carbon disulphide and acrylamide (Spencer *et al.*, 1979), but this process may not be the cause of their neurotoxicity. In addition, some intoxications result in symptoms similar to those of beri-beri, a disease due to a thiamine deficiency (Cavanagh, 1988). Signs and symptoms of this type are seen in arsenic poisoning. Arsenic binds to lipoic acid, which has a role, like thiamine, in pyruvate decarboxylation. Some drugs (nitrofurans and nitroimidazoles) also cause a neuropathy which is similar to that observed in thiamine deficiency; however, it is not responsive to thiamine therapy. Thallium, which binds to mitochondrial membranes, can also have such an effect. The ATPases are very important enzymes in brain cells, as they are necessary for the formation of action potentials. ATPases have been shown to be inhibited by a rather large number of neurotoxins, but the assays have generally been made *in vitro* and it is difficult to extrapolate to the *in vivo* situation, because the presence of the BBB can greatly modify the concentration of the neurotoxin *in vivo*. Maier and Costa (1990) assayed brain ATPase in animals intoxicated with a single dose of substances known to have an effect on ATPase *in vitro*. They used chlordecone, an organochlorine pesticide, organotins (triethyltin and tributyltin), mercuric chloride and methyl mercury. There was no difference in ATPase activity in treated animals, despite the appearance of neurotoxic symptoms not exhibited by control animals. The metals assayed in brain showed that the concentration was too low to inhibit ATPase. These experiments thus show that although ATPase is easily inhibited *in vitro*, this is not true *in vivo*, at least after only one injection.

Action on the Metabolism of Amino Acids

This action occurs mainly through interaction with vitamin B_6 constituents: pyridoxine, pyridoxal, pyridoxamine. When phosphorylated, those substances become important coenzymes in amino acid metabolism. One drug has particularly marked neurotoxicity of this type—namely isoniazid: (INH; Holtz and Palm, 1964), the hydrazide of isonicotinic acid, a widely used antituberculosis drug. INH affects coenzyme synthesis by inhibiting pyridoxal phosphokinase, the enzyme which phosphorylates pyridoxal to pyridoxal phosphate. As INH is a hydrazine, it can also chelate pyridoxal phosphate which can then inhibit pyridoxal phosphokinase more strongly than INH alone. The chelation of pyridoxal phosphate by INH acts on enzyme systems using pyridoxal phosphate as coenzyme, including transamination and decarboxylation. In humans, peripheral neuropathy is the most frequent manifestation of neurotoxicity, and neuropathy is also observed in some experimental studies—for example, in the rat. The neuropathy includes axonal degeneration which is most marked in the distal part of the nerve and is associated with signs of sensory and motor neuropathy. Regeneration rapidly follows degeneration, and the neuropathy can be prevented by the administration of pyridoxine. In humans, convulsions are also sometimes observed

with isoniazid. They are probably due to a decreased GABA concentration resulting from inhibition of glutamate decarboxylase. Convulsions are usually caused by treatment at higher doses than those which cause peripheral neuropathy. It is interesting that excessive ingestion of pyridoxine can also cause a sensory axonal neuropathy.

Another type of neurotoxicity involving amino acids is that observed in hepatic encephalopathy: it is discussed below (p. 413).

Action on Synapses

Excitable cells have numerous synaptic contacts. At these junctions neurotransmitters are released and bind to specific receptors. Neurotransmitters are destroyed by enzymatic processes in the synaptic cleft; moreover, transmitters can be inactivated by endocytosis triggered in the presynaptic membrane. Neurotoxicity can act at the pre- and postsynaptic membrane by the action of false neurotransmitters or of excitatory amino acids. An example of a target for neurotoxins is given below (pp. 411–412).

Action on the Cytoskeleton and Axonal Transport

The cytoskeleton is a major constituent of the neuronal cytoplasm. There are three types of 'neurofibrils': the microtubules (diameter, 24 nm), the neurofilaments (diameter, 10 nm) and the very fine (6 nm) actin-like microfilaments.

Intoxication with aluminium results in the abnormal accumulation of neurofilaments in the perinuclear region of neuronal cell processes causing the other cell organelles to be displaced peripherally. In humans it has been shown that dialysis encephalopathy, which is a progressive dementia observed in patients undergoing renal dialysis, is probably due to aluminium intoxication, as the plasma and the brain aluminium concentrations in these patients are considerably increased. Discontinuation of the use of aluminium-containing dialysate has caused a marked decrease in the incidence of this disease. Aluminium has a high affinity for transferrin, an iron-transporting protein. It has been suggested that aluminium, bound to this protein, could enter brain by transcytosis, thanks to the presence of an endothelial cell receptor. Morris *et al.* (1989) showed that the accumulation of aluminium in the brain of a patient with dialysis encephalopathy corresponded to the regions of high transferrin receptor density.

Colchicine and Vinca alkaloids (vincristine, vinblastine) produce changes similar to those produced by aluminium, accompanied by the depolymerization of microtubules. Vinca alkaloids and colchicine do not act either on brain or on nerve, which are protected by barriers, but on sensory ganglia (Weiss *et al.*, 1974). The toxic action of Vinca alkaloids in other tissues consists of inhibition of the mitotic spindle: hence their utilization as anticancer agents. This activity cannot occur in the nervous system, as neurons do not divide, but these agents dissociate the microtubules, an essential element of the axonal cytoskeleton (rails allowing anterograde and retrograde transport). Some degree of sensory neuropathy is observed in nearly all patients treated with Vinca alkaloids, and their neurotoxicity limits their therapeutic use.

The axon is the highly specialized part of the neuron. It is responsible for generating and propagating bioelectric currents and is also a duct for bidirectional transport.

Proximal Axonopathies

Proximal axonopathies affect the initial segment of the axon where action potentials arise. A toxin that particularly damages this part of the axon is iminodipropionitrile (IDPN), which causes a lesion of slow axonal transport (Griffin *et al.*, 1985), with proximal axonal swelling and distal axonal atrophy. This intoxication also induces a proliferation of astrocytic subpial processes and the formation of myelin vacuoles with secondary demyelination.

Distal Axonopathies

Distal axonopathies have been observed in the CNS and in the PNS, and central–peripheral distal axonopathy (Spencer and Schaumburg, 1976) is the name given to a group of toxic metabolic diseases of obscure pathogenesis in which there is symmetrical axonal degeneration, beginning distally in long central and peripheral nervous system processes and spreading proximally along these and other shorter processes with time. The reduction in the amount of cytoskeletal transport elements outweighs the modest retardation in transport and results in proximal axonal atrophy.

This was first observed in neuropathies due to organophosphorus compounds. In these neuropathies, organophosphorus compounds phosphorylate a membrane-bound protein with esterase catalytic activity, the neuropathy target esterase (NTE) (Johnson, 1990). This protein can be inhibited by two groups of compounds: one is non-neurotoxic and can protect the NTE; the other undergoes a second reaction which has been called aging (Clothier and Johnson, 1980). This modifies the structure of the protein or its environment and leads to neurotoxicity.

It has also been shown that the link between distal axonopathies produced by carbon disulphide (CS_2), acrylamide and 2,5-hexanedione (2,5-HD) is the accumulation of 10 nm neurofilaments prior to distal axonal degeneration (Spencer and Schaumburg, 1976). This accumulation of filaments is observed in portions of the axon proximal to nodes of Ranvier and leads to massive axonal swelling. The propensity for change in the distal part of the axon in systemic intoxication can be explained by the toxin inactivating material required for the maintenance of axonal integrity, the neuronal soma being unable to meet the axonal demand for the replacement of this material.

Subacute Myelo-opticoneuropathy

An epidemic of SMON (subacute myelo-opticoneuropathy) occurred in Japan over a long period. Extensive clinical and scientific investigation of this disease showed that it was due to clioquinol, a drug used for the treatment of a wide variety of abdominal disorders. Clioquinol caused abdominal symptoms (different from those it was used to treat) and shortly afterwards neurological symptoms: bilateral ascending paraesthesia of the lower extremities and weakness of the lower limbs. There were also increased reflexes in the lower extremities and bladder disturbance while bilateral visual impairment was frequent. Neuropathological studies showed a central distal axonopathy and degenerative changes affecting the visual pathways. (Rose and Gawel, 1984).

Lesions in Schwann Cells and Oligodendrocytes

Lesions in Schwann cells and oligodendrocytes are very different from those observed in the neuron and mainly affect the myelin sheath. Oligodendrocytes and Schwann cells form a segmented chain of myelin which envelops axons in intimately apposed concentric layers in both the CNS and PNS.

Diphtheria toxin inhibits the synthesis of the proteolipid of myelin and of the basic protein in the Schwann cell. Myelin destruction is not affected. The result is a marked slowing of conduction in affected axons.

Myelin-associated vacuolation is a change induced by many toxic compounds acting on oligodendrocytes. The location of the vacuoles varies, depending on the time-course and severity of the intoxication of the cell. If myelin-associated fluid accumulation reflects effects in the metabolism of oligodendrocytes, then its presence may be taken as a sensitive indicator of oligodendrocyte dysfunction. An example is what is seen in some isoniazid intoxications. We have already seen that isoniazid produces peripheral neuropathy in humans. Experimental animal studies have investigated both peripheral neuropathy (in rats) which can be prevented by pyridoxine, and CNS manifestations (in chicks and dogs) which cannot be prevented by pyridoxine (Blakemore, 1980). Chicks show tremor, ataxia and convulsions. Pathological changes are largely restricted to the white matter of the CNS, the lesions appearing as intense vacuolation which can be seen to be associated with the myelin sheath. Shortly afterwards, myelin sheaths are lost and a marked astrocytosis appears. In the dog the most prominent pathological change is vacuolation of the white matter, the most common location of these vacuoles being within the myelin sheath arising from the separation of the intraperiod line. Vacuolation also arises from swelling of the cytoplasm of the internal oligodendrocyte tongue, distension of the periaxonal space and focal swelling of the axon.

Changes in oligodendrocytes are most common at high doses. These cells show cytoplasmic swelling or nuclear pyknosis with loss of ribosomes, concentration of microtubules and sometimes mitochondrial swelling or the presence of small vacuoles and/or osmiophilic bodies. Astrocytic hypertrophy is the other prominent change in the CNS of dogs with isoniazid intoxication and either accompanies the white matter vacuolation or is found with a focal distribution in the cortical grey matter. The lesions observed in Cuprizone (bis-

cyclohexanone oxaldihydrazone) intoxication in mice are very similar.

Other substances cause impairment only in the myelin sheath, as, for example, triethyltin (Watanabe, 1980). In the 1950s a very serious drug intoxication occurred in France due to contamination of diethyltin diiodide (Stalinon) by triethyltin (TET). TET is very neurotoxic: patients had increased intracranial pressure of sudden onset and many died. The neuropathological examination showed severe and widespread oedema in the white matter. Subacute experimental studies with TET in rats showed weakness of the hindlimbs followed by paralysis and later tremor and convulsions. If TET dosing was interrupted, the rats recovered and histological examination showed that the predominant change was a diffuse spongiosis of the white matter due to numerous vacuoles. In advanced lesions, histological techniques revealed normally stained myelin forming a spongy array. Neuropathy was also manifested by the separation of the lamellae of the myelin sheaths at the intraperiod line. In TET animals, there was an increase in the water content of the brain and spinal cord associated with an increase in sodium and chloride. Cerebral oedema was not associated with modification of the extracellular space or of the permeability of the BBB to large molecules. Hexachlorophene neurotoxicity is somewhat similar. It has occasionally been observed in humans mainly after dermal application or after use as an anthelminthic agent. It was observed with greater frequency in premature infants who had been bathed in water which contained hexachlorophene (Towfighi, 1980). In experimental studies, the neuropathological findings in orally dosed animals consist of a diffuse intramyelinic oedema in the CNS and vacuolation of myelin in the PNS of rats of all ages.

Acetyl ethyl tetramethyl tetralin (Spencer *et al.*, 1980) is used in scent and does not cause toxicity in humans. However, it is neurotoxic in animals, colouring nervous tissue blue and bringing about vacuolation of myelin. The neuropathology is rather similar to that of TET and hexachlorophene but, in addition to the oedematous vacuoles in the myelin sheath, there is an accumulation of granular inclusions in the neuronal perikarya and in the cytoplasm of glial cells. This poisoning is also characterized by the action of phagocytes of haematological origin on the damaged myelin. Remyelination occurs during the intoxication, which probably means that Schwann cells are not prevented from functioning.

Lesions in Astrocytes

There are many toxins that lead to neuronal dysfunction but very few that lead to astrocyte dysfunction. An exception is methionine sulphoximine (MSO), which has been used as an astrocyte toxin. It is an inhibitor of glutamine synthetase, which is immunologically localized only to the astrocytes. The administration of MSO causes an absence of enzyme activity a few hours after administration and afterwards seizures, if the animal is intoxicated with a high dose. Neuropathological studies carried out in animals which had not suffered seizures showed development of Alzheimer II-like glia in which astrocytic nuclei were deformed, watery and often surrounded by a clear halo. This change was present mainly in the deeper neocortical layers and was accompanied by an accumulation of glycogen granules which was observed in the superficial layers.

Glutamine synthetase is a key enzyme in the glutamate/glutamine pathways, and a possibility raised by Yamamoto *et al.* (1989) is that its inhibition leads to an impairment of glutamate metabolism. Glutamate in excess can lead to seizures and this substance is ultimately metabolized via the tricarboxylic cycle, resulting in the accumulation of glycogen; there is also an increase in ammonia.

Another neurotoxin that has an effect on astrocytes is ouabain, but its neurotoxic effect can only occur after intracerebral injection, as it does not cross the BBB.

Changes in Endothelial Cells

Endothelial cells have a very important role in neurotoxicity because of their tight junctions which almost completely exclude hydrophilic substances that do not have carriers. They can also metabolically alter some lipophilic substances. The endothelium of cerebral microvessels seems to be particularly weak in the thalamus, where microhaemorrhages are frequently observed—for example, in seizures due to convulsants. The other lesions of endothelial cells will be described below.

EXAMPLE OF A TARGET FOR NEUROTOXINS: THE SPINAL CORD MOTOR NEURON

The motor neuron controls muscle function, by providing synaptic contact between the axon terminal and striated muscle cells, in the form of the motor endplate or neuromuscular junction. In vertebrates the neurotransmitter is acetylcholine and the synapse is said to be cholinergic. Stimulation of motoneurons causes the liberation of acetylcholine contained in synaptic vesicles by a calcium-dependent process.

Acetylcholine acts on the nicotinic receptor situated on the membrane of the muscle cell. It is destroyed in the synaptic cleft by an enzyme, acetylcholinesterase, synthesized in the endoplasmic reticulum of the perikaryon of the neuron.

The different sites of action of neurotoxins in the spinal cord motoneuron are as follows:

- The plasma membrane: tetanus toxin specifically binds to the neuronal surface and is used in immunochemistry for distinguishing neurons from non-neuronal cells. Its specific receptor is probably, as with cholera toxin, a ganglioside in the plasma membrane. It modulates the activity of the motoneuron by inhibiting gamma-aminobutyric acid (GABA) and glycine release. This leads to rigidity and muscle spasms.
- The endoplasmic reticulum of the perikaryon: organophosphorus compounds and carbamates inhibit acetylcholinesterase activity.
- The axon: a disturbance of transport by IDPN leads to axonal swelling due to neurofilament accumulation in the insertion cone of the axon.
- The level of the nodes of Ranvier, where impulse conduction takes place; blocking of sodium channels by tetrodotoxin may lead to paralysis.
- The synaptic ending: blocking of the liberation of acetylcholine by botulinum toxin prevents the exocytosis of the transmitter or, the reverse, continuous liberation of acetylcholine by the venom of the black widow spider.
- The neuromuscular synaptic cleft: lack of breakdown of the liberated acetylcholine due to the inhibition of acetylcholinesterase by organophosphorus compounds leads to fasciculation followed by paralysis.

- The acetylcholine postsynaptic receptors: where the binding by a snake venom bungarotoxin leads to paralysis.
- Schwann cells: these form the myelin sheath around the axon, of which the attack by diphtheria toxin causes demyelinization leading to paralysis.

EFFECT OF NEUROTOXINS ON THE BLOOD–BRAIN BARRIER

Introduction

The BBB is formed by endothelial cells of brain cerebral capillaries which are linked by tight junctions and have a very small vesicular transfer capability. The two plasma membranes of the endothelial cells are not symmetrical and do not have exactly the same carriers. The luminal membrane, on the blood side, has several carriers which are mainly for glucose, ketone bodies and amino acids. There are several carriers for amino acids, one for basic amino acids, one for neutral amino acids transported by the L system, which is sodium-independent, and one for acidic amino acids which are transported by a low-activity system. At the abluminal membrane there are transport systems which are similar to those of the luminal membrane for glucose and for ketone bodies, but they are different for the amino acids. Besides the system for basic amino acids and the L system for neutral amino acids, there are additionally two sodium-dependent systems for neutral amino acids, the A and ASC systems, and a very active sodium-dependent system for glutamic acid. In addition there is Na^+/K^+-ATPase, which creates the sodium gradient.

The BBB can be studied in animals *in vivo* and the unidirectional transfer constant can be determined, but as the BBB is formed by the endothelium of brain microvessels which can be isolated, *in vitro* studies can also be performed; this has the great advantage of giving information on the processes of transport at the abluminal membrane.

The BBB is important in toxicology for the following reasons.

(1) It plays an essential role in preventing a direct passage of substances from blood to brain. Substances in general can enter the brain according to their partition coefficient. Entry is rapid for lipophilic substances, except for those which are excluded by the P-glycoprotein (Cordon-Cardo *et al.*, 1989). The degree of entry is very low for hydrophilic substances and for protein-bound substances, with the exception of substances bound to proteins which have a receptor on the endothelial cell membrane and thus can enter brain: such a protein is transferrin. Hydrophilic substances can also enter into the few areas without a barrier, such as the circumventricular organs. In these areas there are fenestrated capillaries.

(2) However, thanks to the presence of carriers in its membranes, the BBB allows entry of all the metabolites necessary for brain function. Toxic substances can have an action on these carriers and modify the entry of metabolites into the brain.

(3) Brain endothelial cells contain enzymes which can metabolize some lipophilic toxic substances (Ghersi-Egea *et al.*, 1988).

(4) Lesions of the endothelial cells can cause impairment of permeability and sometimes brain oedema.

Toxic Alterations to Blood–Brain Transport

These modifications can affect the carriers or the concentration of transported substances.

Mercury

Mercury is a toxic substance which can be in elemental, inorganic or organic form. It can enter the animal or human body via inhalation, by ingestion or through the skin. Mercury vapour is readily oxidized to the mercuric ion in blood or tissue, while with organic mercury cleavage is very low for methyl mercury but higher for ethyl and higher alkyl mercuries. Most patients intoxicated by inorganic mercury are victims of occupational exposure. The critical organ for inorganic mercury is the kidney, but mercury also affects the nervous system, the most characteristic neurological feature being tremor. The nervous system is the principal target of organic mercury, which was responsible for two very serious intoxications. One in Japan, named 'Minamata disease', was caused by eating fish exposed to mercury; the other, in Iraq, was caused by seed grain treated with a methyl mercury fungicide. The main clinical symptoms were sensory and visual disturbance and cerebellar ataxia; tremor was less frequent than in inorganic mercury intoxication. Neuropathology showed cerebral atrophy, predominantly in the occipital lobe, and atrophy of the cerebellar folia with disintegration of granule cells. Among the intoxicated persons were pregnant women. Methyl mercury has been shown to be particularly damaging to the developing nervous system and in this case resulted in encephalopathy in fetuses at doses which did not cause lesions in the mothers.

After a single injection, inorganic mercury is detected in the cerebellar grey matter, the area postrema, the hypothalamus and areas near the ventricles. Organic mercury is believed to enter brain more easily because of its high lipid solubility, but its high uptake may also be due to formation of a complex between mercury and cysteine in blood. This complex may enter the brain by the amino acid carrier for methionine, as the structure of the complex is similar to that of methionine, which is transported by the L system carrier, present in the luminal membrane of the endothelial cell (Aschner and Clarkson, 1988). When methyl mercury is given orally, its uptake is rather slow. Distribution is relatively uniform, and in dogs predominates in the calcarine cortex and cerebellum. The mercury content in brains of patients with Minamata disease was studied a long time after death in 1979 by electron microscopical X-ray analysis (Shirabe *et al.*, 1979). This showed the mercury to be present in the cytoplasm of the neurons bound to selenium and sulphur.

Methyl mercury has a considerable facility for entering cells and dissolving in membranes. Since both inorganic and organic mercury bind to SH groups it may well be irrelevant for toxicity which form enters the cell provided there is a minimal quantity present. In the damaged CNS the largest neurons tend to survive, seeming to be able to tolerate a much larger amount of mercury than small cells (Cavanagh, 1977). Small neurons have a smaller total number of ribosomes than large neurons and it seems that cell death occurs when a critical proportion of the ribosomes of the cell is damaged by mercury.

Yoshino *et al.* (1966) observed that in animals intoxicated by methyl mercury a plateau in the brain mercury concentration occurred as early as 1 day after the ip injection and before the onset of neurological symptoms, which appeared several days later. For this reason they studied rat brain metabolism both at the neurologically unaffected stage and at the affected stage. The only abnormality noticed in the latent stage was an inhibition of the incorporation of [U-^{14}C]-leucine into brain cortical proteins. This appeared before the development of neurological signs and symptoms at a time when oxygen consumption, aerobic and anaerobic glycolysis, and sulphydryl enzyme activities were still unchanged.

However, as brain protein synthesis is regulated by amino acid availability, the inhibition of leucine incorporation could be due to a decrease in amino acid blood–brain transport. Steinwall and Olsson (1969) have shown, using a semiquantitative technique, that blood–brain transport of [^{75}Se]-selenomethionine is decreased in animals receiving mercuric chloride. Pardridge (1976) studied the problem in animals not previously intoxicated, using a quantitative technique with mercury present only in the injection solution. Mercury did not increase the blood–brain transport of sucrose but considerably decreased the transport of cycloleucine and tryptophan. Amino acid transport has also been studied on isolated microvessels (Tayarani *et al.*, 1987). They found that amino acid uptake was normal at mercury doses lower than 10^{-5} M. But at this concentration, similar to that observed in Minamata patients, the uptake of all amino acids was decreased.

Aluminium has also been reported to affect the permeability of the BBB (Banks and Kastin, 1985).

Hepatic Encephalopathies

Hepatic encephalopathies have been observed mainly in alchoholic patients, often those with portacaval shunts. These patients have a high level of neutral amino acids in the CSF. Studies of the blood–brain transport of amino acids in rats fitted with a portacaval anastomosis showed a large increase in the transport of neutral L amino acids, while there was no increase in the transport of basic amino acids (James *et al.*, 1979). It has been suggested that this increase could be due to brain increase in glutamine (ammonia + glutamate). The efflux of glutamine from brain could be explained by exchange with the neutral amino acids (Jeppsson *et al.*, 1985).

Enzymes in the Endothelial Cell

The endothelial cells of cerebral microvessels contain a number of enzymes which are not present in other endothelial cells and which can affect neurotoxicity. For example, monoamine oxidase (MAO), known to have a role in monoamine detoxification, has been shown to influence the toxicology of MPTP (1-methyl-4-phenyl-1,2,4,6-tetrahydropyridine). Parkinsonism usually occurs in old people, but it has been observed in the USA in the very young. They were found to be using a new synthetic heroin contaminated with MPTP (Langston, 1985). Administration of MPTP destroys dopaminergic neurons and causes a Parkinsonian-like syndrome in humans and other primates, but not in rats. It was believed that MPTP neurotoxicity was due to enzymatic oxidation to give 1-methyl-4-phenyldihydropyridine (MPDP$^+$), which is further oxidized to MPP$^+$ (1-methyl-4-phenylpyridinium ion). MPP$^+$ given systemically is itself not neurotoxic, because it is a polar water-soluble substance and thus unable to cross the BBB. What is surprising is the different susceptibility to MPTP among species. It is not neurotoxic to rats when injected systemically, but is neurotoxic when injected directly in the substantia nigra. Kalaria *et al.* (1987) suspected that the resistance of rats to systemic MPTP could be due to metabolism of MPTP in endothelial cells at the BBB, transforming it into MPP$^+$. This would prevent it reaching the dopaminergic cells, since it is very hydrophilic, in contrast to MPTP. MAO-B activity was effectively very high in rat cerebral endothelial cells, while it was very low in human cerebral endothelial cells.

The cerebral endothelium contains other enzymes such as acetylcholinesterase, butyrylcholinesterase, gamma-glutamyl transpeptidase or ATPases which may have a role in neurotoxicity, but at the moment they have not been often studied in relation to toxicological problems.

Other enzymes in cerebral microvessels can metabolize lipophilic molecules. NADPH, cytochrome *P*-450 reductase, epoxide hydrolase, UDP glycuronosyl transferase, and NADH reductase have been measured by Ghersi-Egea *et al.* (1988). Their inducibility was different from that in liver.

Modification of the Permeability of the Blood–Brain Barrier

The permeability of the BBB can be physiologically modified, by action of adrenergic neurotransmitters (Palmer, 1986). Some drugs, such as antidepressants, have been shown to increase the permeability of the BBB to water, probably by a β-adrenergic mechanism. In addition, the permeability of the BBB can be modified in what is called cerebral vasogenic oedema. Cerebral oedema has been divided into vasogenic oedema, due to an increase in permeability of the BBB, and cytotoxic oedema, due to intra-cellular swelling (Klatzo, 1967). We shall give two examples of vasogenic oedema: convulsions due to organophosphorus compounds and lead intoxication in immature animals.

Modifications Due to Seizures

Convulsive seizures, produced by a large number of epileptogenic agents, can be the cause of BBB lesions. This is the case with cholinesterase inhibitors such as carbamates, including pyridostigmine and physostigmine, which are reversible short-term inhibitors, and the relatively irreversible organophosphorus compounds (OPs) which generally have actions of longer durations. Toxicologically, these substances are important, as they are used in agriculture as insecticides and can also have military applications, as chemical warfare agents. Organophosphorus compounds belong to the family of phosphates (paraoxon, parathion, diisopropylphosphorofluoridate (DFP), tabun) or of methylphosphonates (sarin, soman). The phosphonates are remarkably toxic, causing death after percutaneous administration. Most of them inhibit acetylcholinesterases and non-specific cholinesterases equally but some of them act only on one enzymatic type, those inhibiting the acetylcholinesterases being the most dangerous. Attempts have been made to localize cholinesterases using organophosphorus inhibitors labelled with tritium.

The inhibition of cholinesterases by organophosphorus compounds, leads to a hypercholinergic state, as, when the inhibitor dose is high enough, acetylcholine, the transmitter at cholinergic synapses, is no longer hydrolysed. This can result in neuronal death and astrocytic oedema in several cerebral structures but mainly in the hippocampus. These lesions are illustrated in Figures 1 and 2.

Seizures, with onset at doses near the LD_{50}, are accompanied by a reversible lesion of the BBB. This lesion can be demonstrated in animals by extravasation of a dye, Evans blue, which binds *in vivo* to plasma proteins after iv injection. Leakage of the stained proteins is bilateral and limited to some cerebral areas—for example, the septum and thalamus. It lasts only a few hours and corresponds to cerebral signs of hyperactivity, such as seizures and hyperoxia. OPs cause an astrocytic oedema not only during the convulsive period, but also during the following days (Carpentier *et al.*, 1990), the origin of the oedema being vasogenic. In addition, neuronal death occurs 48–72 h after administration of the toxicant. These neuronal lesions occur mainly in the hippocampus, where there are no BBB lesions. There is thus no relation between the increase in vascular permeability and the observed neuronal death. The

opening of the BBB is therefore due not to the inhibition of cholinesterases but to the convulsions. Prior anticonvulsant treatment does not prevent the inhibition of cholinesterases but prevents the opening of the BBB. Recent research shows that populations of non-cholinergic receptors, in particular GABA and dopamine receptors, are modified by OPs and that for cholinergic receptors the number of muscarinic receptors decreases (down regulation: Bouchaud *et al.*, 1990). Organophosphorus compounds thus have a complex action. The antidote to organophosphorus intoxication is a combination of an anticonvulsant (diazepam), an anticholinergic substance (atropine for muscarinic receptors, D-tubocurarine for nicotinic receptors) and a reactivator of inhibited acetylcholinesterases.

Modifications in Young Animals

Lead has long been known and utilized by man. It is absorbed by ingestion or inhalation, and transported by blood mainly in the erythrocytes. If lead salts are dissolved in saline and administered by the intra-arterial injection method of Takasato *et al.* (1984), which avoids mixture with plasma, transport into the CNS is rapid and seems to be effected by passive transport. From plasma, transport is much slower, as lead binds to albumin and cysteine. However, lead transport is much more rapid than that of calcium, with which it does not seem to interfere. It is possible that transport is linked to the potential difference across the luminal plasma membrane of the endothelium. Lead uptake into brain by this system is reduced by active transport back into the capillary lumen by the Ca^{2+}-ATP-dependent pump (Deane and Bradbury, 1990).

In the nervous system, lead intoxication can give rise to either encephalopathy or peripheral neuropathy. Encephalopathy has been rarely observed in adults, and then mostly in those drinking 'moonshine'. But encephalopathy has often been observed in children between 1 and 3 years old, an age when they may eat pigment-based paints containing lead. Lead encephalopathy in children generally follows chronic lead poisoning. Typically there is intestinal colic and loss of orientation, followed by stupor, coma and seizures. There is papilloedema, and neurological findings often include blindness. The diagnosis can be made by assay of lead in blood and by the finding of inhibition of aminolaevulinate dehy-

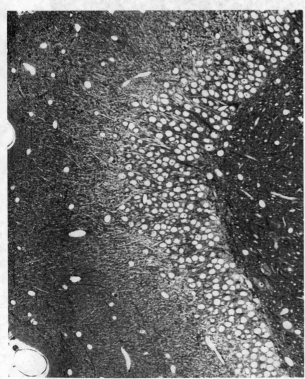

Figure 1 Encephalopathy observed 1 h after soman intoxication (soman is an organophosphorus compound, inhibiting the cholinesterases and inducing seizures). CA_3 area of the hippocampus. Astrocytic oedema is evident. Toluidine blue; ×700. Courtesy P. Carpentier.

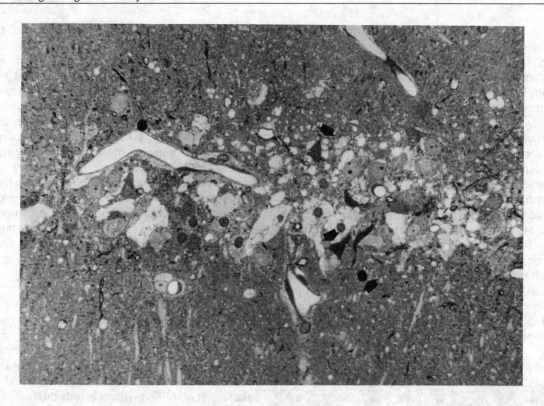

Figure 2 Encephalopathy observed 24 h after soman intoxication. CA$_1$ area of the hippocampus. In addition to the oedema there are many 'dark' neurons. Toluidine blue; ×1750. Courtesy P. Carpentier.

dratase or an accumulation of its substrate. There is also accumulation of zinc protoporphyrin in red cells.

Neuropathology normally shows brain swelling, sometimes with collapsed ventricles. The abnormalities are mainly related to the blood vessels. There is an amorphous acidophilic periodic acid–Schiff (PAS)-positive exudate around blood vessels in the brain, spinal cord and meninges, and mineralized concretions are visible within the vessel wall. In a few cases there are extravasated erythrocytes, while swelling of capillary endothelial cells is often observed and some capillaries are necrotic. These changes are seen throughout the nervous system and in the meninges but are more conspicuous in the cerebrum and the cerebellum. There are foci of astrocytic proliferation, and the white matter and astrocytes appear oedematous, while in some cases there is a variable number of necrotic neurons, especially in the cerebellum. Almost all these alterations are those of vasogenic cerebral oedema, but there is also a slight cytotoxic oedema component. Chelation

therapy and supportive measures have reduced mortality from childhood lead encephalopathy to less than 5 per cent. However, morbidity, such as mental retardation, seizures or convulsions, remains high.

A problem that has arisen in the last 15 years is the question of whether elevated lead levels found in a rather high number of children can be responsible for alterations in psychological and classroom performances. This problem was examined by Needleman and Gatsonis (1990), who reviewed the studies on the neuropsychological function in many children in which lead was assayed in blood or teeth. They concluded that lead at low doses was associated with a deficit in psychometric intelligence.

Experimental Animal Disease

In all animal studies, the susceptibility to encephalopathy has been found to be higher for young animals than for adult animals. This has been particularly studied in the rat since the description by Pentschew and Garro (1966) of lead encephalopathy in young rats, who had ingested lead via their mother's milk and developed haemorrhagic encephalopathy mainly in the cerebellum and spinal cord. The encephalopathy was associated with capillary vasculopathy. Dilated capillaries were lined with necrotic endothelial cells and later with a hypertrophic endothelium. There was also brain oedema, which developed after the haemorrhage. This encephalopathy regressed if the young rat did not die during the haemorrhagic period, the brain lesions disappearing in spite of the persistence of a high brain lead level (Lefauconnier *et al.*, 1983).

The characteristics of the BBB change during development and it is possible that lead, for a reason at present unknown, interferes with this development and leads to encephalopathy. Gebhart and Goldstein (1988) have studied bovine adrenal endothelial cells and rat brain astrocytes in culture. They have shown that rat brain astrocytes are more sensitive than endothelial cells to the cytotoxic effect of lead acetate. In coculture the two cell types demonstrated a distinctive cellular organization and the astrocytes were less sensitive to the cytotoxic effect of lead than when they were cultured alone. The problem is different in lead encephalopathy, but the endothelial cells are perhaps a little further from the astrocytes in young animals than in adults, and when these cells are in closer contact, the pathological changes perhaps decrease.

EFFECT OF NEUROTOXINS ON MEMBRANE RECEPTORS AND CARRIERS

Venoms and Toxins of Biological Origin

Biological toxins are characterized by great specificity. They interact with various constituents of the neuron and can disturb its various functions, particularly protein synthesis, axonal transport and synaptic transmission. Numerous neurotoxins bind to receptors on the neuronal or the muscular plasma membrane and so can be used as markers for the localization of receptors. They are thus pharmacological agents which allow the molecular approach of the identification of receptors and investigation of their physiology.

Biological neurotoxins originate from vertebrate or invertebrate organisms, from animal venoms, plants, bacteria or fungi. They act in a manner which is now well-known, especially in the case of toxins of animal origin. Many have a spectacular action on the neuromuscular junction and the regional pathology they bring about is particularly well-understood in the case of the motor neuron which innervates muscle fibres.

Bacterial toxins have actions on the plasma membrane of the neuron and in particular on its presynaptic portion. The two best-known are:

(1) Tetanus toxin from the bacterium *Clostridium tetani* which produces the muscular spasms characteristic of tetanus after contamination of wounds. It binds to the neuronal plasma membrane; this binding to a specific receptor is used in immunochemistry to identify nerve cells, the receptor being absent on glial cells. After intramuscular injection *in vivo*, the toxin is taken up by the presynaptic endings and is transported by the retrograde axoplasmic flux in the perikaryon of motor neurons. The result of poisoning with tetanus toxin is the loss of control of motor neurons, probably by glycinergic systems.

(2) Botulinum toxin from *Clostridium botulinum*, a species of bacteria which contaminate improperly preserved food. The first signs are cranial nerve pathology, then a bilateral motor deficit and often a respiratory muscle paralysis. Botulinus toxin has a well-known action as an inhibitor of acetylcholine, the transmitter at the neuromuscular junction. Electrophysiological techniques have shown that the toxin blocks the liberation of acetylcholine by making the liberation system less sensitive to excitatory Ca^{2+} ions of the presynaptic transmitter flux. Ricin, from the seeds of castor oil plant, is 100 times less active.

Venom neurotoxins disturb neuromuscular transmission either at the presynaptic level or at the postsynaptic level. Their molecular action is even better known. Some toxins bind to K^+ channels and can be classified into a number of subclasses (Castle *et al.*, 1989). This is the case with apamine (from bee venom), with nojiutoxin (from scorpion venom) and with dendrotoxin (from Mamba snake venom). Several toxins extracted from animals or plants bind to the Na^+ channels in the membrane of excitable cells (neurons and muscle cells) and block synaptic transmission. This is the case with saxitoxin and tetrodotoxin. The latter is highly toxic and is found in the organs of fugu (a Japanese fish). This excellent fish is particularly appreciated by the Japanese; it must be prepared by competent cooks, who remove the organs containing the neurotoxin. Saxitoxin is synthesized by various sea dinoflagellates which can be ingested without any harm by shellfish. These contaminated shellfish are very toxic for humans. Tetrodotoxin and saxitoxin are very dangerous neurotoxins. It is now known that they prevent the diffusion of Na^+ ions through the transmembrane channels. They constitute valuable tools for molecular biology, owing to their selectivity: they allowed the quantification of the sodium channels on excitable cells, the purification of their constitutive protein and the sequencing of the amino acids.

Endogenous and Exogenous Neuroexcitatory Amino Acids

The excitotoxic amino acids are either synthesized in brain (endogenous amino acids) or are transported to brain from the environment (exogenous amino acids). They cause depolarization by acting on excitatory neurotransmitter receptors: NMDA (*N*-methyl-D-aspartic acid), AMPA (5-methyl-4-isoxazole propionic acid), kainate, L AP4 (L-2-amino-4-phosphonobutanoic acid), situated on the soma or the dendrites of the neuron. This depolarization is accompanied by increased membrane permeability to cations, the action of the amino acids ceasing when they are taken up by the membrane. As neurotoxic amino acids act on receptors on the soma or dendrites of the neuron and do not act on the axon, they have been used experimentally as axon-sparing agents.

Endogenous amino acids play a very important role as excitatory neurotransmitters. It has been shown that there is good correspondence between excitatory properties and neurotoxicity because excessive concentrations of an amino acid can cause continuous depolarization and an increase in membrane permeability. This needs energy to restore ionic equilibrium and can also be associated with a large increase in intracellular calcium. Both can be the cause of cellular death (Olney, 1986). Endogenous amino acids can act as neurotoxic substances, because the process of uptake does not work efficiently; in epilepsy a small deficit in the process of uptake can cause an extra-

cellular accumulation of the amino acids which provoke convulsions. This neurotoxicity has also been shown recently to be a complication of pathologies which are not neurotoxic, such as brain ischaemia, brain hypoxia, and hypoglycaemia. Brain cell degeneration observed in adult-onset olivopontocerebellar degeneration (Plaitakis *et al.*, 1982), Huntington's chorea (Beal *et al.*, 1986) and Alzheimer's disease (Maragos *et al.*, 1987) may involve similar processes. These amino acids are:

- L-Glutamic acid, which has been used for a long time as a flavour enhancer; its toxicity was not known. In young animals it causes serious retinal lesions and damage to the arcuate nucleus of the hypothalamus. In adults 'the Chinese restaurant syndrome' seems to be due to monosodium glutamate.
- L-Aspartic acid. This amino acid bound to phenylalanine constitutes aspartame. It has been authorized by regulatory authorities as a sweetener, because of its low toxicity in animal experiments.

Exogenous amino acids can also be neurotoxic in the same way as endogenous amino acids; in fact they can even be more toxic, as they are not taken up by the membranes. The role of the uptake process has been shown, for example, for D- and L-homocysteic acid. The L-amino acid has an uptake process and is much less toxic than the D-amino acid. Whereas endogenous amino acids are synthesized in brain and can thus easily interact with receptors, exogenous amino acids are generally of dietary origin and are transported in the blood. They must then cross the BBB, which has either a very low carrier-mediated uptake for some acidic amino acids or a very small uptake as a function of their partition coefficient. This is the case for kainic acid, which is an excitotoxic amino acid and causes convulsions when administered systemically. Its blood–brain transport measured *in vivo* is very low, while measurements on isolated microvessels do not show any transport. It is thus an extracellular amino acid. A very toxic amino acid can exert a certain neurotoxicity, even if its partition coefficient is very low. In addition, these amino acids can act on circumventricular organs which have no BBB. Some exogenous amino acids are as follows:

- Kainic acid is a very potent excitotoxic amino acid. It comes from seaweed, which has been used for hundreds of years in the Orient as a home remedy for intestinal worms, but at doses below those causing neurotoxic effects.
- Ibotenic acid is found in some mushrooms and has been used for its fly-killing properties. It is thought to be responsible for the neurotoxicity of the amanita mushrooms.
- Alanosine is an experimental antibiotic and antileukaemic agent. It is several times more potent than glutamic acid as a neurotoxic agent and slightly less potent than homocysteic acid in immature animals, where it necrotizes neurons in the same regions of brain and retina that are affected by glutamic acid.

Lathyrism is a well-known disease in which there is spastic paraparesis due to pyramidal tract involvement, probably induced by excessive consumption of the vegetable *Lathyrus sativus* in periods of famine. β-*N*-Oxalylamino-L-alanine, an amino acid, has been found to be present in *Lathyrus sativus* and to induce corticospinal dysfunction similar to that seen in animals consuming a fortified diet of this vegetable (Spencer *et al.*, 1986). This amino acid is a potent agonist of the excitatory transmitter glutamate and is probably causally related to lathyrism in man. A disease that occurred in the Chamorro people of the island of Guam is also possibly due to such a mechanism (transmitter antagonism). After World War II, a disease consisting of, in various degrees, amyotrophic lateral sclerosis, Parkinsonism and dementia, called hereditary paralysis, was frequently observed in these people. During the war they had a high consumption of sago palm seeds (*Cycas cincinalis*) and the frequency of the disease decreased when they changed to American food. Laboratory investigation of the seeds revealed the presence of several subsances, including an unusual non-protein amino acid: β-*N*-methylamino-L-alanine. Spencer *et al.* (1987) studied the effects of this amino acid on monkeys, which developed a disease similar to that observed in man. He speculated that the diseases of the Chamorros were not hereditary, as had been thought, but were elicited by different doses of the cycad toxin. People who had left the island when they were about 20 years old and perfectly healthy to live in the USA, and had not eaten cycad seeds, subsequently developed the disease about 30 years after their arrival in the USA.

Another disease which may occur as a possible consequence of neurotoxicity but not only of a neurotoxic amino acid is Parkinson's disease. This involves abnormally reduced activity of dopaminergic neurons. No cause for this disease is known but it has already been observed in the pathology of the Chamorro people. Moreover, it has also been shown (see above) that MPTP could give a symptomatology similar to that of this disease.

An interesting hypothesis has been put forward by Calne *et al.* (1986): Alzheimer's disease, Parkinson's disease and motor neuron disease are due to environmental damage to specific regions of the CNS which remains subclinical for several decades but makes those affected especially prone to the consequences of age-related neuronal attrition. In support of this hypothesis, Calne *et al.* (1985) reported that four members of a family had been injected with a drug that contained MPTP. Two who had received a high dose had Parkinsonian symptomatology. Two who received a lower dose had absolutely no neurological sign. They all underwent a PET (positron emission tomography) examination and even the two with no symptomatology had an image very similar to that of Parkinsonism.

'False Neurotransmitters'

It has been shown in animals that certain chemical substances can produce degeneration of either catecholaminergic or serotoninergic neurons, characterized by a transmitter of the monoamine group (catecholaminergic and serotoninergic neurons). This selective lesioning makes these neurotoxins tools of choice for the production of experimental lesions in these systems.

It is now considered that these substances are 'false neurotransmitters' which enter neurons by the same uptake route as true transmitters, to which they are very similar. As soon as they enter the neuron they are probably degraded into diverse cytotoxic molecules, perhaps by autoxidation with a production of superoxide ion, H_2O_2, or hydroxyl radicals.

The first neurotoxic substance of the monoaminergic system to be discovered was an analogue of dopamine, 6-hydroxydopamine (6-OHDA), which has effects on the sympathetic nervous system (it causes chemical sympathectomy) and on the CNS. This substance also causes denervation of the noradrenaline and dopamine system (Baumgarten *et al.*, 1972).

Two serotoninergic substances have high toxicity: these include 5,6- and 5,7-dihydroxytryptamine (5,6- and 5,7-DHT), which lead to the death of serotoninergic neurons in the CNS by a mechanism probably similar to that of 6-OHDA (Figure 3).

In general, chemical sympathectomy is obtained in laboratory animals after iv injection of a dose of 6-OHDA, which does not seem to have a cytotoxic action on non-catecholaminergic neurons.

However, in the CNS these three neurotoxins behave like dopamine and serotonin and cannot cross the endothelium of cerebral microvessels. In order to produce the lesions, the toxin must be put in direct contact with neurons thought to be catecholaminergic or serotoninergic by intraventricular, intracisternal or intraparenchymatous administration.

Animal experiments have shown that some substances cause selective neuronal death, allowing identification of neuronal projections. A good example is 3-acetylpyridine (3-AP). It is a highly toxic substance for some cerebral neurons (inferior olive, hypoglossal nucleus). After intraperitoneal injection 3-AP causes the death of neurons in the inferior olive of the rat. The inferior olive is a structure which innervates the cerebellar cortex (Desclin, 1974) and the climbing fibres degenerate, resulting in a cortex without olivary afferents. This permits analysis of the significance of the climbing fibres in the normal cerebellum.

CONCLUSION

When the neurotoxic dose is sufficiently high to cause cellular death, a phagocytic process begins. In brain, the destruction is carried out by specialized cells of mesenchymal origin (microglia). These cells evolve in brain very early in development and remain latent in the cerebral parenchyma. It seems that they are activated by dead elements in their proximity and are perhaps able to change their place in the cerebral parenchyma. They are thus resident cells which become phagocytic.

When neurotoxins cause a lesion in the cerebral microvessels, this is accompanied by micro-

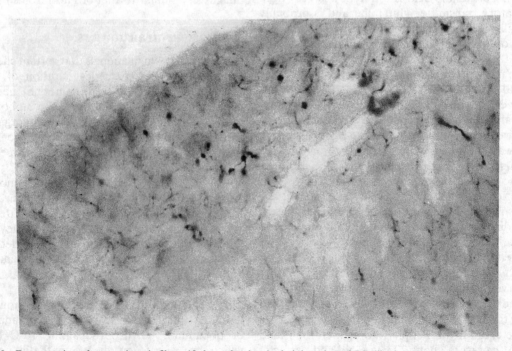

Figure 3   Degeneration of serotoninergic fibres 10 days after local administration of 5,7-dihydoxytryptamine. Nucleus tractus solitarius. ×500. Courtesy M. Arluison.

haemorrhages, especially in sensory areas such as the thalamus. If the haemorrhage is of sufficient intensity, this may permit circulating monocytes to cross the endothelial barrier, become fixed in the perivascular area and be transformed to active macrophages.

Since we first wrote this chapter it has become rather clear that oxygen radicals play a role in several neuropathological affections and also in neurotoxicological mechanisms. For a review on this subject refer to Lebel and Bondy (1991) and Halliwell (1992).

This review was supported in part by DRET (direction de recherches et études techniques) grant 91–156.

REFERENCES

Aschner, M. and Clarkson, T. W. (1988). Uptake of methylmercury in the rat brain: effects of amino acids. *Brain Res.*, **462**, 31–39

Banks, W. A. and Kastin, A. J. (1985). Aluminum alters the permeability of the blood–brain barrier to some non-peptides. *Neuropharmacology*, **24**, 407–412

Baumgarten, H. G., Haylett, D. G. and Jenkinson, D. H. (1972). Evidence for degeneration of indoleamine containing nerve terminals in rat brain, induced by 5,6-dihydroxy tryptamine. *Z. Zellforsch.*, **125**, 553–559

Beal, M. F., Kowall, N. W., Ellison, D. W., Mazurek, M. F., Swartz, K. J. and Martin, J. B. (1986). Replication of the neurochemical characteristics of Huntington disease by quinolinic acid. *Nature*, **321**, 168–171

Blakemore, W. F. (1980). Isoniazid. In Spencer, P. S. and Schaumburg, H. H. (eds), *Experimental and Clinical Neurotoxicology*. Williams and Wilkins, Baltimore, London, pp. 476–489

Bouchaud, C., Mailly, P., Chollat-Namy, A., Delamanche, I. S. and Vergé, D. (1990). Quantitative autoradiographic analysis of neuroreceptors in rat brain after acute or chronic soman intoxication. *Third International Meeting on Cholinesterases*, La Grande Motte. p. 117

Calne, D. B., Langston, J. W., Martin, W. R. W., Jon Stoessl, A., Ruth, T. J., Adam, M. J., Pate, B. D. and Schulzer, M. (1985). Positron emission tomography after MPTP: observations relating to the cause of Parkinson's disease. *Nature*, **317**, 246–248

Calne, D. B., McGeer, E., Eisen, A. and Spencer, P. (1986). Alzeimer's disease, Parkinson's disease, and motoneuron disease: abiotrophic interaction between ageing and environment? *Lancet*, **II**, 1067–1070

Carpentier, P., Delamanche, I. S., Blanchet, G. and

Bouchaud, C. (1990). Seizure-related opening of the blood–brain barrier induced by soman: possible correlation with the acute neuropathology observed in poisoned rats. *Neurotoxicology*, **11**, 501–516

Castle, N. A., Haylett, D. G. and Jenkinson, D. H. (1989). Toxins in the characterization of potassium channels. *TINS*, **12**, 59–65

Cavanagh, J. B. (1977). Metabolic mechanisms of neurotoxicity caused by mercury. In Roizin, L., Shiraki, H. and Grčević, N. (Eds), *Neurotoxicology*. Raven Press, New York pp. 283–288

Cavanagh, J. B. (1986). Sensorimotor neuropathy and cisplatin and adriamycin toxicity. *J. Neurol. Neurosurg. Psychiat.*, **49**, 964–965

Cavanagh, J. B. (1988). Lesion localisation: implications for the study of functional effects and mechanisms of action. *Toxicology*, **49**, 131–136

Cho, E-S., Spencer, P. S. and Jortner, B. S. (1980). Doxorubicin. In Spencer, P. S. and Schaumburg, H. H. (Eds), *Experimental and Clinical Neurotoxicology*. Williams and Wilkins, Baltimore, London, pp. 430–439

Clothier, B. and Johnson, M. K. (1980). Reactivation and aging of neurotoxic esterase inhibited by a variety of organophosphorus esters. *Biochem. J.*, **185**, 739–747

Cordon-Cardo, C., O'Brien, J. P., Casals, D., Rittman-Grauer, L., Biedler, J. L., Melamed, M. R. and Bertino, J. R. (1989). Multidrug-resistance gene (P-glycoprotein) is expressed by endothelial cells at blood–brain barrier sites. *Proc. Natl Acad. Sci. USA*, **86**, 695–698

Deane, R. and Bradbury, M. W. B. (1990). Transport of lead–203 at the blood–brain barrier during short cerebrovascular perfusion with saline in the rat. *J. Neurochem.*, **54**, 905–914

Desclin, J. C. (1974). Histological evidence supporting the inferior olive as the major source of cerebellar climbing fibres in the rat. *Brain Res.*, **77**, 365–384

Gebhart, A. M. and Goldstein, G. W. (1988). Use of an *in vitro* system to study the effects of lead on astrocyte-endothelial cell interactions: a model for studying toxic injury to the blood–brain barrier. *Toxicol. Appl. Pharmacol.*, **94**, 191–206

Ghersi-Egea, J-F., Minn, A. and Siest, G. (1988). A new aspect of the protective functions of the blood–brain barrier: activities of four drug-metabolizing enzymes in isolated rat brain microvessels. *Life Sci.*, **42**, 2515–2523

Ginsberg, M. D. (1980). Carbon monoxide. In Spencer, P. S. and Schaumburg, H. H. (Eds), *Experimental and Clinical Neurotoxicology*. Williams and Wilkins, Baltimore, London, pp. 374–394

Griffin, J. W., Parhad, I., Gold, B., Price, D. L., Hoffman, P. N. and Fahnestock, K. (1985). Axonal transport of neurofilament proteins in IDPN neurotoxicity. *Neurotoxicology*, **6**, 43–54

Halliwell, B. (1992). Reactive oxygen species and the

central nervous system. *J. Neurochem.*, **59**, 1609–1623

Holtz, P. and Palm, D. (1964). Pharmacological aspects of vitamin B_6. *Pharmacol. Rev.*, **16**, 113–178

James, J. H., Jeppsson, B., Ziparo, V. and Fischer, J. E. (1979). Hyperammonaemia, plasma aminoacid imbalance, and blood–brain aminoacid transport: a unified theory of portal-systemic encephalopathy. *Lancet*, **II**, 772–775

Jeppsson, B., James, J. H., Edwards, L. L. and Fischer, J. E. (1985). Relationship of brain glutamine and brain neutral amino acid concentrations after portacaval anastomosis in rats. *Eur. J. Clin. Invest.*, **15**, 179–187

Johnson, M. K. (1990). Contemporary issues in toxicology. Organophosphates and delayed neuropathy—Is NTE alive and well? *Toxicol. Appl. Pharmacol.*, **102**, 385–399

Kalaria, R. N., Mitchell, M. J. and Harik, S. I. (1987). Correlation of 1-methyl-4-phenyl-1,2,3,6-tetrahydropyridine neurotoxicity with blood–brain barrier monoamine oxidase activity. *Proc. Natl Acad. Sci. USA*, **84**, 3521–3525

Klatzo, I. (1967). Neuropathological aspects of brain edema: Presidential address. *J. Neuropathol. Exptl Neurol.*, **26**, 1–14

Langston, J. W. (1985). MPTP and Parkinson's disease. *TINS*, **8**, 79–83

Lebel, C. P. and Bondy, S. C. (1991). Oxygen radicals: common mediators of neurotoxicity. *Neurotox. Teratol.*, **13**, 341–346

Lefauconnier, J. M., Hauw, J. J. and Bernard, G. (1983). Regressive or lethal lead encephalopathy in the suckling rat. *J. Neuropathol. Exptl Neurol.*, **42**, 177–190

Maier, W. E. and Costa, L. G. (1990). Na^+/K^+-ATPase in rat brain and erythrocytes as a possible target and marker, respectively, for neurotoxicity: studies with chlordecone, organotins and mercury compounds. *Toxicol. Lett.*, **51**, 175–188

Maragos, W. F., Greenamyre, J. T., Penney, J. B. and Young, A. B. (1987). Glutamate dysfunction in Alzheimer's disease: an hypothesis. *TINS*, **10**, 65–68

Morris, C. M., Candy, J. M., Oakley, A. E., Taylor, G. A., Mountfort, S., Bishop, H., Ward, M. K., Bloxham, C. A. and Edwardson, J. A. (1989). Comparison of the regional distribution of transferrin receptors and aluminium in the forebrain of chronic renal dialysis patients. *J. Neurol. Sci.*, **94**, 295–306

Nabeshima, S., Reese, T., Landis, D. M. and Brightman, M. W. (1975). Junctions in the meninges and marginal glia. *J. Comp. Neurol.*, **164**, 127–170

Needleman, H. L. and Gatsonis, C. A. (1990). Low-level lead exposure and the IQ of children. *J. Am. Med. Assoc.*, **263**, 673–678

Olney, J. W. (1986). Excitotoxic amino acids. *NIPS*, **1**, 19–23

Palmer, G. C. (1986). Neurochemical coupled actions of transmitters in the microvasculature of the brain. *Neurosci. Biobehav. Rev.*, **10**, 79–101

Pardridge, W. M. (1976). Inorganic mercury: selective effects on blood–brain barrier transport systems. *J. Neurochem.*, **27**, 333–335

Pentschew, A. and Garro, F. (1966). Lead encephalomyelopathy of the suckling rat and its implications on the porphyrinopathic nervous diseases. *Acta Neuropathol.*, **6**, 266–278

Plaitakis, A., Berl, S. and Yahr, M. D. (1982). Abnormal glutamate metabolism in an adult-onset degenerative neurological disorder. *Science*, **216**, 193–196

Rechthand, E. and Rapoport, S. I. (1987). Regulation of the microenvironment of peripheral nerve: role of the blood–nerve barrier. *Prog. Neurobiol.*, **28**, 303–343

Risau, W. and Wolburg, H. (1990). Development of the blood–brain barrier. *TINS*, **13**, 174–178

Rose, E. C. and Gawel, M. (1984). Clioquinol neurotoxicity: an overview. *Acta Neurol. Scand.*, **70** (Suppl. 100), 137–145

Shirabe, T., Eto. K. and Takeuchi, T. (1979). Identification of mercury in the brain of Minamata disease victims by electron microscopic X-ray analysis. *Neurotoxicology*, **1**, 349–356

Spencer, P. S., Foster, G. V., Sterman, A. B. and Horoupian, D. (1980). Acetyl ethyl tetramethyl tetralin. In Spencer, P. S. and Schaumburg, H. H. (Eds), *Experimental and Clinical Neurotoxicology*. Williams and Wilkins, Baltimore, London, pp. 296–308

Spencer, P. S., Ludolph, A., Dwivedi, M. P., Roy, D. N., Hugon, J. and Schaumburg, H. H. (1986). Lathyrism: evidence for role of the neuroexcitatory amino acid BOAA. *Lancet*, **II**, 1066–1067

Spencer, P. S., Nunn, P. B., Hugon, J., Ludolph, A. C., Ross, S. M., Roy, D. N. and Robertson, R. C. (1987). Guam amyotrophic lateral sclerosis-parkinsonism-dementia linked to a plant excitant neurotoxin. *Science*, **237**, 517–522

Spencer, P. S., Sabri, M. I., Schaumburg, H. H. and Moore, C. L. (1979). Does a defect of energy metabolism in the nerve fiber underlie axonal degeneration in polyneuropathies? *Ann. Neurol.*, **5**, 501–507

Spencer, P. S. and Schaumburg, H. H. (1976). Central-peripheral distal axonopathy—The pathology of dying-back polyneuropathies. In Zimmerman, H. M. (Ed.), *Progress in Neuropathology*. Grune and Stratton, New York, pp. 253–295

Steinwall, O. and Olsson, Y. (1969). Impairment of the blood–brain barrier in mercury poisoning. *Acta Neurol. Scand.*, **45**, 351–361

Takasato, Y., Rapoport, S. I. and Smith, Q. R. (1984). An *in situ* brain perfusion technique to study cerebrovascular transport in the rat. *Am. J. Physiol*, **247**, H484–H493

Tayarani, I., Lefauconnier, J. M. and Bourre, J. M. (1987). The effect of mercurials on amino acid transport and rubidium uptake by isolated rat brain microvessels. *Neurotoxicology*, **8**, 543–552

Towfighi, J. (1980). Hexachlorophene. In Spencer, P. S. and Schaumburg, H. H. (Eds), *Experimental and Clinical Neurotoxicology*. Williams and Wilkins, Baltimore, London, pp. 440–445

Watanabe, I. (1980). Organotins (triethyltin). In Spencer, P. S. and Schaumburg, H. H. (Eds), *Experimental and Clinical Neurotoxicology*. Williams and Wilkins, Baltimore, London, pp. 545–557

Weiss, H. D., Walker, M. D. and Wiernik, P. H. (1974). Neurotoxicity of commonly used antineoplastic agents. *New Engl J. Med.*, **1**, 75–81; **2**, 127–133

Yamamoto, T., Iwasaki, Y., Sato, Y., Yamamoto, H. and Konno, H. (1989). Astrocytic pathology of methionine sulfoximine-induced encephalopathy. *Acta Neuropathol.*, **77**, 357–368

Yoshino, Y., Mozai, T. and Nakao, K. (1966). Biochemical changes in the brain in rats poisoned with an alkylmercury compound, with special reference to the inhibition of protein synthesis in brain cortex slices. *J. Neurochem.*, **13**, 1223–1230

FURTHER READING

Arlien-Søborg, P. (1992). *Solvent Neurotoxicity*, CRC Press, Boca Raton, Florida

Chang, L. W. (1994). *Principles of Neurotoxicology*. Marcel Dekker, Inc., New York

LoPachin, R. M. and Aschner, M. (1993). Glial-neuronal interactions: relevance to neurotoxic mechanisms. *Toxicology and Applied Pharmacology*, **118**, 141–158

Tilson, H. and Mitchell, C. (1992). *Neurotoxicology*. Raven Press, New York

Weiss, B. and O'Donoghue, J. L. (1994). *Neurobehavioural Toxicity: Analysis and Interpretation*. Raven Press, New York

20   Peripheral Sensory Irritation

Bryan Ballantyne

INTRODUCTION

The majority of investigations into, and causes of, adverse affects from occupational exposure to chemicals relate to toxicological phenomena. However, certain reversible pharmacological or physiological effects may be a cause of discomfort, distraction, or inattention. These include nauseating smells and induction of narcosis, which may lead to uncomfortable working conditions and/or be a contributory factor to accidents, and hence have been used in part to assign occupational exposure limits such as Threshold Limit Values (ACGIH, 1991–92: Amoore and Hautala, 1983). Another common source of discomfort and distraction is that of peripheral sensory irritation (PSI) which involves the interaction of materials with sensory receptors in exposed body surfaces, producing discomfort or pain at the site of contact together with related reflexes. Effects on the eye and respiratory tract are those usually experienced, have the greatest practical significance, and may be a factor in assigning occupational exposure limits.

NATURE OF PERIPHERAL SENSORY IRRITATION

The word irritation, sometimes used loosely in toxicological discussions, is used to describe two differing basic processes. Unqualified, an irritant response usually refers to an inflammatory response following local contact with the causative material. In contrast, PSI is a pharmacological effect involving the interaction of chemicals with sensory receptors in skin or mucosae at the site of contamination, causing local sensation (discomfort or pain) with associated local reflexes and, in some cases, systemic reflexes (Figure 1). These effects disappear on removal of the stimulus. Most substances causing a PSI effect will, usually at higher concentrations, also produce inflammation. Thus, PSI may be a warning (pro-

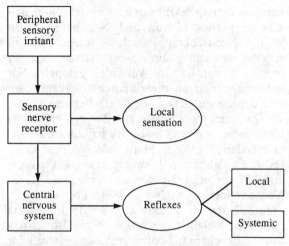

Figure 1   Schematic representation of effects produced by peripheral sensory irritants

tective) indication of exposure to a potentially harmful material.

The major characteristics of peripheral sensory irritants are that:

(1) they act locally; i.e. at the site of contamination of skin or mucosae;

(2) they stimulate sensory nerve receptors and produce local discomfort with locally mediated reflexes; and

(3) there may be associated systemic reflexes, usually automatic in type.

In general it is considered that peripheral sensory (PS) irritants interact non-specifically with sensory nerve receptors. The phrase 'common chemical sense' has been used to differentiate this sensory function from other chemically-induced sensations, such as taste or smell (Keele, 1962). Chemicals inducing PSI are of widely differing structure, and there are generally no identifiable specific morphological receptors. However, in skin PSI materials show some selectivity in that they excite polymodal nociceptors and warm thermoreceptors (Foster and Ramage, 1981). The sensitivity of the receptors is divorced from their mechano- and thermoreceptive functions (Green and Tregear, 1964).

A wide variety of chemical structures are capable of causing PSI effects. For example, with aldehydes, the degree of irritation increases with α, β unsaturation (Moncrief, 1944), and molecules having C=C and carbonyl groupings, particularly in the presence of a halogen, confer irritant properites (Dixon and Needham, 1946). With a given chemical nucleus, introduction of specific chemical groupings may change sensory irritant potential to variable extents. For example, based on measurement of respiratory rate depression (RD_{50}, see later) 3-chlorostyrene was 2.6 times more potent and β-nitrostyrene 364 times more potent as a sensory irritant than styrene (Alarie, 1973a). Many homologous series show a relationship between molecular weight and PSI potential (Neilson and Vinggaard, 1988: Neilson and Yamagiwa, 1989). For example, Figure 2 shows increasing PSI with increasing molecular weight for a series of N-(3'-hydroxy-4'-methoxyphenyl)-2-chloroamides. A similar relationship has been shown for a series of n-alkylamines (Table 1). However, for some series there may be little influence on PSI potential by changing molecular weight, as for example a series of N-phenyl-2-chloroamides (Table 2).

A characteristic effect of many sensory irritant materials is the development of tachyphylaxis, i.e. a progressive decrease in sensory irritant

Table 1 Depression of respiratory rate produced by alkylamines in male Ssc:CF-1 mice by nasal breathing (RD_{50}) and breathing through a tracheal cannula (tRD_{50}). For the higher member of the series, sensory irritant potential increases with molecular weight

Amine	RD_{50} (ppm)	tRD_{50} (ppm)
Diethylamine	184	549
Triethylamine	186	691
Dibutylamine	81	101
Cyclohexylamine	27	78

Source: after Nielsen and Yamagiwa (1989).

response with sequential applications of test material. Cross-tachyphylaxis between differing sensory irritants can occur, suggesting a similar mode of action for certain different PSI materials and stimulation of the same sensory receptor (Foster and Ramage, 1981). Using a depression of respiratory rate model, Chang and Barrow (1986) showed that formaldehyde pretreatment of rats induced significant cross-tolerance to the sensory irritant effects of chlorine, i.e. a shift to the right of the concentration–response curves. Babiuk *et al.* (1985) showed that formaldehyde pre-exposure of rats resulted in cross-tolerance with acetaldehyde (RD_{50} increased three- to fivefold) and acrolein (RD_{50} increased fivefold), but no cross-tolerance was evident to sensory irritation by propionaldehyde, butyraldehyde, crotonaldehyde, cyclohexane carboxaldehyde, 3-cyclohexene-1-carboxaldehyde, as benzaldehyde. These data indicate that cross-tolerance is not a generalized phenomenon.

If tolerance and cross-tolerance do occur then this is clearly of practical significance because repeated exposure to a particular chemical, or pre-exposure to another, may result in reduced sensory warning on subsequent exposures and a correspondingly lesser degree of protection. As differing mechanisms of neural stimulation probably occur between differing chemical groups to produce a PSI response, the mechanism of tolerance is not known. Also, it has been proposed that chemically-induced histopathological changes in the nasal epithelium may be a cause for tolerance and cross-tolerance in some instances. Tolerance and cross-tolerance in the PSI response have been reviewed by Bos *et al.* (1992).

Experimental studies indicate that sensory irritant materials interact with membrane-associated

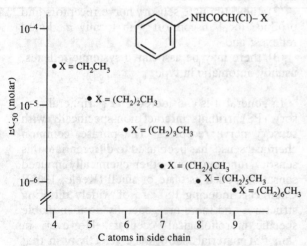

Figure 2 Influence of molecular weight on sensory irritant potential in the guinea pig blepharospasm test for a homologous series of N-(3'-hydroxy-4'-methoxyphenyl)-2-chloroamides. Source: Ballantyne (unpublished data).

Table 2   Peripheral sensory irritation for a series of *N*-phenyl-2-chloroamides as revealed by guinea pig blepharospasm (EC_{50}). Over a wide range, molecular weight has only a small effect on sensory irritant potential

$$NHCOCH_2 - X$$

N-Phenyl-2-chloro-	X	EC_{50} (molar)	95% Confidence limits
-propionamide	$-CH_3$	8.70×10^{-5}	$(6.61–11.43) \times 10^{-5}$
-butyramide	$-CH_2CH_3$	4.30×10^{-5}	$(3.52–5.37) \times 10^{-5}$
-valeramide	$-(CH_2)_2CH_3$	3.54×10^{-5}	$(2.72–4.60) \times 10^{-5}$
-hexanamide	$-(CH_2)_3CH_3$	2.87×10^{-5}	$(2.18–3.77) \times 10^{-5}$
-heptanamide	$-(CH_2)_4CH_3$	2.68×10^{-5}	$(2.05–3.50) \times 10^{-5}$
-octanamide	$-(CH_2)_5CH_3$	1.15×10^{-5}	$(0.87–1.50) \times 10^{-5}$
-nonanamide	$-(CH_2)_6CH_3$	1.07×10^{-5}	$(0.82–1.40) \times 10^{-5}$
-decanamide	$-(CH_2)_7CH_3$	1.25×10^{-5}	$(0.92–1.65) \times 10^{-5}$

Source: Ballantyne (unpublished data).

binding sites, and that binding affinity is a major factor in determining the potency of the PSI response (Green *et al.*, 1979). In some cases these effects may be in association with -SH or $-NH_2$ groups of membrane proteins or enzymes, and/or amide nitrogen of the peptide bond (Dixon and Needham, 1946; Silver *et al.*, 1967; Alarie, 1973a; Schauenstein *et al.*, 1977; Douglas, 1981). However, differing mechanisms may operate for different chemical groups. For example, the PSI potential of saturated aliphatic aldehydes diminishes with their dehydration constant, which may determine their degree of cross-linking with receptor proteins. In contrast, unsaturated aliphatic aldehydes such as acrolein and crotonaldehyde do not hydrate to any degree, but they undergo addition reactions with -SH, $-NH_2$, and other groups (Schauenstein *et al.*, 1977; Steinhagen and Barrow, 1984). For higher molecular weight less reactive aldehydes, the sensory irritant effects may result from physiological mechanisms involving thermodynamic and solubility properties of the molecule in a lipid bilayer containing receptor protein (Luo *et al.*, 1983; Neilson and Alarie, 1982).

Although PSI effects may be induced in the skin, the two most important practical sites are the eye and respiratory tract, as effects in these tissues are detrimental to the performance of coordinated tasks and because sensory irritant effects in the skin occur only at exposure concentrations much higher than those causing respiratory and ocular effects.

Eye

On the eye, PSI materials produce local itching, discomfort or pain (depending on exposure concentration) together with excess lachrymation and blepharospasm as local reflexes. These local sensory and reflex effects will clearly result in a warning of exposure to an irritant substance and a disturbance of vision; depending on the degree of stimulation there may be partial or complete visual incapacitation. Systemic autonomic reflexes may develop, including increases in systolic and diastolic blood pressure and bradycardia. Following cessation of the PSI stimulation, sensory and reflex effects diminish; an example of diastolic blood pressure changes is shown in Figure 3.

An additional consequence of sensory irritation of the eye is a transient increase in intraocular pressure (Figure 3). This is most likely to occur following splash contamination of the eye with a sensory irritant in solution (Ballantyne *et al.*, 1976; Ballantyne, 1983), but has been demonstrated following vapour exposure (Ballantyne *et al.*, 1976; Ballantyne, 1977). The basic cause of the increased intraocular pressure is unknown in most cases, but there appears to be an association between the magnitude and duration of increased intraocular pressure and inflammatory potential as evidenced by conjunctival hyperaemia. Changes in local blood flow, mostly congestion at the episceral venous plexus, may be a causal factor. However, following contamination of one eye with a PSI material, there is an increase in

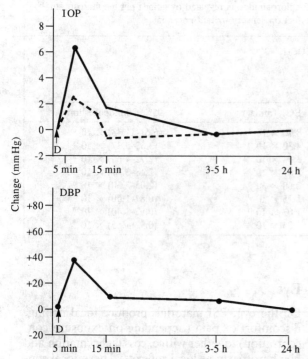

Figure 3 Effect of a potent sensory irritant stimulus on the eye in humans. At D, a human volunteer subject had 0.05 per cent dibenz[*b,f*]-1,4-oxazepine (in polyethylene glycol 300) applied to one eye. There were transient increases in diastolic blood pressure (DBP) and intraocular pressure (IOP) in the contaminated eye (—) and (to a lesser extent) in the contralateral eye (- - -)

intraocular pressure both in the contaminated eye and, to a lesser degree, in the contralateral eye (Figure 3). This indicates the probable existence of a systemic, as well as local, cause for the increase of intraocular pressure (Ballantyne *et al.*, 1977a). Thus, in addition to local changes in blood flow, the following may be factors in the production of transient ocular hypertension: (1) squeezing of the eyeballs during blepharospasm, (2) reflex contraction of the extraocular muscles, and (3) increase in central venous pressure resulting from the pain and stress of potent sensory irritation (Collins *et al.*, 1967; Miller, 1967; Rengstorff, 1975; Ballantyne, 1977a). The transient increase of intraocular pressure that occurs with non-injurious concentrations of a PSI material is unlikely to be detrimental, except possibly for susceptible individuals in whom there may be precipitation or exacerbation of glaucoma (Ballantyne *et al.*, 1973a; Rengstorff, 1975).

Respiratory System

Persons inhaling PSI materials will experience discomfort or pain in the nose, nasopharynx, throat, and possibly chest; local reflexes include coughing, sneezing, and increased secretions, increase or decrease in breathing rate, and decreased tidal volume. As with sensory irritation of the eye there may be transient hypertension with bradycardia. The clinical presentation varies somewhat depending principally on the chemical nature of the material, its solubility, and the principal site of receptor activation (Table 3).

A feature characteristic of materials producing PSI is that they stimulate afferent cholinergic fibres in the nasal mucosa, leading to a reduction in the rate of breathing and a reduction in tidal volume (Cauna *et al.*, 1969; James and Daly, 1969; Ulrich *et al.*, 1972). A variety of sensory receptors are present in the lower respiratory tract, whose morphology and probable physiological functions have been reviewed in detail elsewhere (Crofton and Douglas, 1981; Widdicombe, 1981). With respect to sensitivity to inhaled irritant materials, the most important appear to be the J-receptors and airways irritant receptors. Stimulation of the J-receptors produces apnoea, rapid shallow breathing and systemic hypertension with bradycardia. Stimulation of the airways irritant receptors causes hyperpnoea and bronchoconstriction (Douglas, 1981).

The overall effect of stimulation of the lower respiratory tract receptors is, in most species, an increase in breathing rate and tidal volume. This is a characteristic response to PSI materials which are also capable of causing primary irritation or an allergic response in animals sensitized to the antigen. With many materials, PSI effects are produced by trigeminal nerve stimulation at concentrations significantly lower than those causing

Table 3 Effects produced by peripheral sensory irritant materials on the respiratory tract irritant receptors

Site	Effect
Nasal mucosa	Decreased breathing rate Decreased tidal volume
Lung	Increased breathing rate[a] Decreased tidal volume Bronchospasm

[a] A few species have decreased breathing rate (e.g. mouse).

features characteristic of lower respiratory tract receptor stimulation. Therefore, if there is a biologically-effective respiratory challenge with a peripheral sensory irritant material, the trigeminal reflex will usually predominate. This regional difference in sensitivity of response forms the basis for techniques, discussed below, concerned with assessing the margin of warning for respiratory tract injury provided by the PSI response.

SIGNIFICANCE OF SENSORY IRRITATION

The biological and practical significance of PSI responses is as follows.

Biological Warning

The local sensations produced by PSI materials give a warning of the presence of such materials in the immediate environment. Such biological warning effects will cause those so exposed to seek a source of uncontaminated air. Because PSI materials may also cause local tissue injury at higher concentrations, a determination of the exposure conditions leading to sensory irritation may be an important factor in determining, or qualifying, occupational exposure limits (Ballantyne, 1981).

Biological Protection

The local reflexes resulting from PSI are important as protective mechanisms limiting further exposure. For example, lacrimation removes material from the surface of the eye, and blepharospasm restricts further access of material. With the respiratory tract, decreased breathing rate, decreased tidal volume and cough, all limit inhalation of irritant material.

Harassment and Incapacitation

In the context of an occupational environment, both the sensory and the reflex effects may be distracting and harassing, producing variable degrees of incapacitation. For example, intermittent blepharospasm with excess lacrimation results in an impairment of vision and harassment, which are detrimental to efficient working.

Equally important is the fact that the affected individual is likely to be at an increased risk from accidents and physical injury. Peripheral sensory effects may, therefore, be an important cause of impairment of safe and efficient working conditions.

Injury Without Warning

While the biological importance of a positive peripheral sensory irritant response is clear, the absence of such a response with materials capable of causing tissue injury is also important to know. Such an absence of warning on contact is clearly conducive to injury. Examples of substances which may injure the eye without giving a sensory warning include methyl bromide and dimethyl sulphate (Grant, 1986). In some circumstances, a potent peripheral sensory irritant material has been used as an additive to give warning of the presence of a dangerous material devoid of sensory irritant effects; for example, the inclusion of chloropicrin in methyl bromide used for fumigation.

In relation to hazard evaluation, recent studies have indicated that certain potent peripheral sensory irritant materials can partially inhibit the phagocytic capacity of pulmonary macrophages (Hogg *et al.*, 1983).

The above considerations are clearly relevant to the development of sensory irritant effects in the following illustrative examples.

(1) *Occupational exposure*. Some atmospherically dispersed materials in the workplace may produce PSI effects, causing partial physical incapacitation, discomfort, and/or difficult working conditions. This is a factor frequently taken into account in establishing occupational exposure limits (discussed later in this chapter).

(2) *Riot control agents*. By the very nature of their intended use, riot control agents ('tear gases') produce marked PSI effects resulting in harassment, hindering the conduct of unlawful activity, and causing the malefactors to leave the area. This use of PSI materials requires a detailed knowledge of their acute and long-term toxicology, and the ratio between those concentrations producing harassing effects and those which are threshold for the induction of adverse effects.

(3) *Products of combustion*. Some materials

produced during combustion processes may, in addition to being toxic, also produce PSI effects. Moderately low concentrations of such materials may produce harassing or incapacitating effects which can impede escape from the areas of a fire. Such materials include sulphur dioxide, hydrogen chloride, and toluene diisocyanate.

QUANTITATIVE ASPECTS OF THE SENSORY IRRITANT RESPONSE

As with many toxicological phenomena, there is a positive relationship between the proportion of a population responding to a PSI stimulus and the concentration of the material to which the population is exposed. A plot of proportionate response against exposure concentration yields a sigmoid curve typical of many biological responses (Figure 4). This indicates that while there is a response by a major proportion of the population over a well-defined range around the median, a small proportion of the population (at the left-hand side of the curve) are hyper-reactive to sensory irritant stimulation, and also a small portion (at the right-hand side) are hyporeactive. The concentration–response data are usually converted to linear configuration by log-probit plot. As with other acute phenomena, it is possible to calculate a 50 per cent response level, with 95 per cent confidence limits, to allow comparison of the potency of different materials with respect to peripheral sensory irritation under defined conditions. However, and as discussed in detail later, to obtain the best possible practical estimate of comparative sensory irritant potency it is necessary to consider a variety of other factors, including the slope of the concentration–response regression line.

A variety of expressions, discussed below, are used numerically to express the peripheral sensory irritant response.

For effects that can be objectively evaluated it is common to refer to the effective concentration, i.e. a concentration which produces the specific effect under consideration. In such circumstances, and when adequate concentration–response data exist, it is usual to express sensory irritancy potency as the EC_{50}, i.e. the concentration, calculated from the concentration–response data, which effectively causes a sensory irritant response in 50 per cent of the population under the specific conditions of the observations. Examples of effects which involve the determination of an effective concentration include blepharospasm and change in breathing rate.

When measurements on specific effects are made in laboratory models for particular PSI effects, then specific expressions may be used to refer to the effect produced. For example, calculation of the effective concentration to produce a 50 per cent depression of breathing rate is usually referred to as the respiratory depression 50 or RD_{50}.

For subjective evaluations in humans, such as the degree of discomfort produced by a sensory irritant, it may be possible to determine a threshold for the induction of discomfort, i.e. where the effects are so slight as to pass unnoted. This is clearly of value in defining the concentration at which it is anticipated that peripheral sensory effects will appear. In such circumstances, the threshold for a 50 per cent response under the conditions of the observations can be calculated, ie. the TC_{50}.

Above the TC_{50} it is possible to study the onset, duration, and nature of subjective PSI effects as a function of exposure concentration (or dosage) of irritant. At sufficiently high suprathreshold concentrations it is possible to investigate effects that may be so marked and intolerable (incapacitating) as to interfere with the performance of

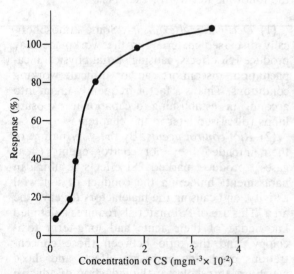

Figure 4 Concentration–response for threshold sensation induced by an aerosol of *o*-chlorobenzylidene malononitrile to the human eye

voluntary and coordinated activities. In these cases a concentration causing incapacitation in 50 per cent of the exposed population may be calculated, i.e. the IC_{50}. Also, it may be useful to compare differing IC levels, as exemplified below.

The relationship between exposure concentration and time to produce defined levels of incapacitation is shown in the left-hand curve of Figure 5. By comparing the three curves for IC_{16}, IC_{50} and IC_{84}, it can be seen that for any given exposure concentration the proportion of the population responding increases with time. This indicates a variable latency between individuals for the same concentration of PSI material. Also, the curves show that, within certain limits, any given degree of incapacitation or harassment (as expressed in this case by IC_{16}, IC_{50} and IC_{84}) can be produced by a variety of reciprocally related exposure times and concentrations. A description of the effectiveness of PSI therefore requires information on concentration, exposure time, latency (tolerance) time, and proportionate response.

The reciprocal relationship between time and concentration also has implications for exposure dosage. Figure 5 (right curves) shows that for any given level of incapacitation (i.e. fixed proportion of the population responding) exposure dosages are greater for the high concentration-short duration conditions than for the low concentration-long duration exposures. Thus, increasing the exposure concentration shortens the effective response time but results in a greater exposure dose to produce an equipotent harassing effect.

FACTORS INFLUENCING THE SENSORY RESPONSE

A variety of factors, both endogenous and environmental, may influence the conditions required to induce sensory irritation and the latency and duration of the effects. Some of the more important of these are briefly discussed below.

Concentration of Irritant

The concentration of peripheral sensory irritant is a determinant of the following:

(1) The proportion of the population responding (e.g. Figure 5)
(2) The latency to onset of effects; in general, the higher the concentration the shorter the time to onset of effects (Figures 5 and 6).
(3) For a brief (pulsed) exposure, the duration of the sensory irritant effect; in general, the higher the concentration the longer the duration (Figure 6).
(4) The higher the concentration the more marked the effect. For example, with increasing concentration an intermittent blepharospasm will become sustained, and threshold sensation becomes progressively more severe until incapacitating pain is experienced.

Particle Size

For PSI materials in particulate form, size is an important determinant of both the site and severity of irritant effects. For example, small particles of a respirable size rapidly produce ocular and respiratory effects, whereas large particles produce predominantly ocular irritation with prolonged recovery times. Such a differential effect has been shown, for example, by Owens and Punte (1963) for particles of approximately 1 and 60 μm MMAD.

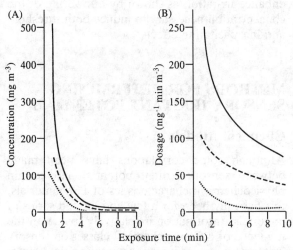

Figure 5 Relationship between concentration and times (left) and exposure dosage and time (right) to produce different levels of incapacitation. [A] incapacitating concentration (C) and [B] incapacitating dose (Ct) are plotted as a function of the time required to produce intolerable effects in 16 (.....), 50 (- - -) and 84 (——) per cent of the population studied. Source: after McNamara *et al.* (1968)

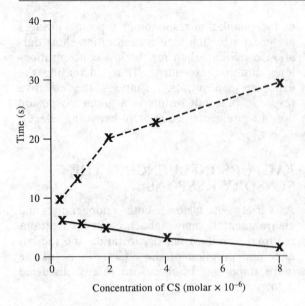

Figure 6 Influence of the concentration of *o*-chlorobenzylidene malononitrile, dissolved in polyethylene glycol 300, on the time to onset (——) and duration (- - -) of human eye discomfort. Source: Ballantyne and Swanston (1973a)

Personality

There are significant personality factors in tolerance to pain, and a similar variability exists between individuals with respect to the discomfort produced by peripheral sensory irritants. Under a given set of conditions, some will tolerate the discomfort more readily than others. This is clearly a practical factor when considering the variability of response to sensory irritation in an occupational environment.

Motivation and Distraction

Increased motivation and distracting influences generally raise the threshold for induction of PSI effects, and enhance tolerability for suprathreshold levels of sensory irritancy. Thus, in an occupational environment the concentration at which sensory discomfort is appreciated may be significantly higher than that causing threshold effects in humans under carefully controlled laboratory situations. It follows that the values derived for PSI materials in experimental situations probably represent the most sensitive index for the effect, and thus provide the most reliable estimates on which to base occupational exposure guidelines.

Tolerance

Individuals may develop tolerance if exposure to a peripheral sensory irritant is gradual and to low concentrations, i.e. the individual adapts by a decrease in the apparent feeling of discomfort and harassment (Beswick *et al.*, 1972). The phenomenon of tolerance is clearly of importance in the workplace, because an adaptation to a warning of potentially harmful chemicals may result in a decrease of safe working conditions. This is a factor which needs to be kept in mind when deciding on an appropriate safety margin in assigning workplace exposure guidelines based on peripheral sensory irritation.

Temperature and Humidity

It has been determined that increased environmental temperature and humidity may decrease endurance to peripheral sensory irritation (Punte *et al.*, 1963).

Vehicle

When sensory irritants in solution make contact with body surfaces, then any vehicle used to dissolve the active material may modify its sensory irritant potential. Surface active materials, for example, may facilitate penetration and thus enhance irritation as shown by a lowering of the concentration necessary to induce both threshold and incapacitating effects.

METHODS FOR DETERMINING SENSORY IRRITANT POTENTIAL

Chemical Models

Although some correlations have been made between sensory irritant potential and certain physicochemical characteristics of PSI materials, this has only been for a few and limited series of materials. Information is relatively sparse on the influence of differing chemical classes on sensory irritancy, as are comparisons between the physicochemical properties of irritant versus non-irritant species.

In an attempt to predict materials likely to be peripheral sensory irritants, a variety of artificial membranes have been used to simulate reactivity with biological membranes. These have included monolayers and bilayers of lecithin, with monitoring of phase transitions to measure interaction. Techniques used to investigate transitions include differential scanning calorimetry, electron spin resonance, and X-ray diffraction. The use of these artificial membranes has not generally been promising as a reliable biological screening method for sensory irritant potential.

Biological Models

A variety of biological models, of varying degrees of sensitivity and of sophistication, are available for assessing the qualitative and quantitative potential of substances to cause PSI. Some of the more commonly used are briefly reviewed below.

Isolated Intestinal Segment

This is a non-specific method based on the use of isolated segments of intestine which are suspended in an incubating bath and supported to allow contraction of the segment to be mechanically measured. Sensory irritant is added to the bath at varying concentrations and a determination made of those concentrations causing contraction of the segment.

Frog Flexor Reflex

This also is a general and non-specific method, which involves a determination of the minimum concentration of irritant required to cause withdrawal of the hindlimb of decerebrate frogs from test solutions. This approach has found use as a reliable screening test for materials having peripheral sensory irritant potential (Feniak, 1966).

The procedure involves sequentially immersing the hindlimb in increasing concentrations of the irritant in solution. After each immersion, the leg is washed with saline and a 5-min period allowed to elapse before immersion of the limb in the next concentration. The time between immersion and its reflex withdrawal after each concentration is recorded (T). Log molar concentration is plotted against T and extrapolated to infinite time by fitting a template of a standard curve. By this means the minimum irritating concentration (T_m) can be estimated. The mean minimum irritating concentration ($\bar{T}$), obtained from a minimum of six animals, is used for comparative purposes. The frog flexor reflex test is simple, economic, and easy to conduct. However, it is insensitive compared with other biological models (Table 4). It may also show poor reproducibility and tachyphylaxis can develop. In spite of these restrictions, the frog flexor reflex correlates well with the simple guinea pig blepharospasm test (Table 5), but is less well correlated with the depression of respiration test in mice (Table 6).

Neurophysiological Preparations

These are neural pathway-specific methods involving the recording of action potentials in afferent nerves from tissue preparations to which PSI materials are applied. Afferent nerve activity measurement has been undertaken for the following:

(1) Recording ciliary nerve activity in response to stimulation of the cornea. This is usually conducted by using an excised cat eye mounted in a warm chamber, with the cornea exposed; the attached long ciliary nerve is laid over recording electrodes (Green and Tregear, 1964). Sensory discharge can be produced by light tactile stimuli to the cornea or cooling its surface; the respective thresholds are 0.1–1.0 g and 5–20°C (Green and Tregear, 1964).

(2) Nasopalatine, ethmoidal, or sphenoidal nerve recording with stimulation of the nasal mucosa. The rat has been successfully used for such studies (Kulle and Cooper, 1975). For example, Tsubone and Kawahl (1991) used the ethmoidal nerve to record afferent activity during exposure of rats to various irritant gases. They found that formaldehyde and acrolein stimulate the nasal sensory system at concentrations of <1 ppm, with stimulation being much weaker for acetaldehyde. The concentrations, in ppm, producing a 50 per cent increase in nerve activity were 1.8 (formaldehyde), 1.2 (acrolein) and 908 (acetaldehyde).

(3) Laryngeal nerve recording in response to stimulation of the laryngeal mucosa with peripheral sensory irritants. The preparation consists of an anaesthetized and tracheotomized cat, with recording of afferent nerve activity from the recurrent laryngeal nerve. Unlike the corneal preparation, the larynx is a more complex and slowly adapting one (Dirnhuber *et al.*, 1965).

(4) For skin, a convenient biological model is by topical application of test material to the hindlimb with recordings taken from the saphenous nerve (Foster and Ramage, 1981).

Table 4 Comparison of sensory irritant potential by frog flexor reflex, guinea pig blepharospasm and respiratory rate depression in mice

Compound	Frog flexor reflex T_m (molar)	Guinea pig blepharospasm EC_{50} (molar)	Respiratory rate depression in mice RD_{50} (molar)
o-chlorobenzylidene malononitrile	9.78×10^{-6}	2.16×10^{-5}	6.00×10^{-8}
2-chloroacetophenone	1.10×10^{-4}	9.00×10^{-5}	3.40×10^{-7}
N-(4′-hydroxy-3′-methoxyphenyl)-2-chlorooctanamide	2.14×10^{-6}	7.70×10^{-7}	3.82×10^{-8}

Source: Ballantyne (unpublished data).

Table 5 Comparison of peripheral sensory irritant potency measured by the frog flexor reflex and guinea pig blepharospasm methods

Compound	Frog flexor T_m (molar)	Blepharospasm EC_{50} (molar)
N-(4′-hydroxy-3′-methoxyphenyl)-2-chlorodecanamide	1.64×10^{-6}	3.58×10^{-7}
N-(3′-hydroxy-4′-methoxyphenyl)-2-chloroheptaneamide	1.89×10^{-6}	2.83×10^{-6}
N-(3′-hydroxy-4′-methoxyphenyl)-2-chlorononanamide	1.97×10^{-6}	$9.5 \ \times 10^{-7}$
N-nonanoylvanillylamide	2.00×10^{-6}	$3.3 \ \times 10^{-7}$
N-(4′-hydroxy-3′-methoxyphenyl)-2-chlorononanamide	2.10×10^{-6}	3.17×10^{-7}
N-(4′-hydroxy-3′-methoxyphenyl)-2-chlorooctanamide	2.14×10^{-6}	7.69×10^{-7}
N-(3′-hydroxy-4′-methoxyphenyl)-2-chlorooctanamide	3.32×10^{-6}	2.03×10^{-6}
N-(4′-hydroxy-3′-methoxyphenyl)-2-chloroheptanamide	5.23×10^{-6}	1.90×10^{-6}
o-chlorobenzylidene malononitrile	9.78×10^{-6}	2.16×10^{-5}
Dibenz[*b*,*f*]-1:4-oxazepine	2.09×10^{-5}	3.48×10^{-5}
4-Methyldibenzoxazepine	2.20×10^{-5}	9.30×10^{-5}
3-Methyldibenzoxazepine	4.16×10^{-5}	5.40×10^{-5}
β,β-Diacetyl-3-chlorostyrene	9.43×10^{-5}	1.30×10^{-4}
2-Chloroacetophenone	1.10×10^{-4}	9.00×10^{-5}
Phenanthridine	1.77×10^{-3}	4.11×10^{-3}

Correlation coefficient $(r) = 0.99$ $(p < 0.001)$.
Source: Ballantyne (unpublished data).

Blepharospasm Test

The induction of blepharospasm in conscious animals in response to topically applied solutions or to materials dispersed in the atmosphere is a technique frequently used to assess the potential of a substance to cause sensory irritant effects on the eye. It is a simple and reliable method for this purpose. For solutions, the test involves applying increasing concentrations of the substance to the surface of the cornea, and recording the proportion of the population which develops blepharospasm following the initial blink reflex.

In this way a concentration–response relationship can be obtained and the EC_{50} for blepharospasm calculated. It is important that if the substance has to be dissolved or diluted, then an appropriate inert solvent is required.

For materials in the atmosphere, a similar approach is undertaken in which sequential exposure to increasing concentrations of the test substance is carried out.

There is a species variation in sensitivity to substances applied to the eye (Table 7). In general, the guinea pig is the most suitable test spe-

Table 6 Comparison of peripheral sensory irritant potency measured by the frog flexor reflex and mouse respiratory rate depression

Compound	Frog flexor T_m (molar)	Respiratory depression RD_{50} (molar)
o-Chlorobenzylidene malononitrile	9.78×10^{-6}	6.00×10^{-8}
Dibenz[*b*,*f*]-1,4-oxazepine	2.09×10^{-5}	2.30×10^{-7}
2-Chloroacetophenone	1.10×10^{-4}	3.40×10^{-7}
N-(4'-hydroxy-3'-methoxyphenyl)-2-chlorooctanamide	2.14×10^{-6}	3.82×10^{-8}
N-(4'-hydroxy-3'-methoxyphenyl)-2-chlorononanamide	2.10×10^{-6}	1.43×10^{-7}
N-(4'-hydroxy-3'-methoxyphenyl)-2-chlorodecanamide	1.64×10^{-6}	2.16×10^{-7}

Correlation coefficient (r) = 0.76 (p = 0.079).
Source: Ballantyne (unpublished data).

Table 7 Comparison of blepharospasm-inducing effects of solutions of *o*-chlorobenzylidene malononitrile (CS) and dibenz[*b*,*f*]-1,4-oxazepine (CR) applied to the eye of various species[a,b]

Material	Blepharospasm EC_{50} (molar)			Sensation TC_{50} (molar) Man
	Guinea pig	Rabbit	Man	
CS	$2.2(1.9–2.4) \times 10^{-5}$	$5.9(3.8–10.0) \times 10^{-5}$	$3.2(2.1–6.1) \times 10^{-6}$	$7.3(4.2–11.2) \times 10^{-7}$
CR	$3.5(2.8–4.3) \times 10^{-5}$	$7.9(5.1–12.5) \times 10^{-5}$	$8.6(6.8–12.5) \times 10^{-7}$	$4.9(3.8–6.5) \times 10^{-7}$

[a] Solvent was polyethylene glycol 300.
[b] Results as 50% response with 95% confidence limits.
Source: Ballantyne and Swanston (1973a,b).

cies because of its size, cost and sensitivity to peripheral sensory irritant materials. It is reproducible, free from tachyphylaxis, and differentiates between irritants of close chemical structure. It does not correlate well with the depression of breathing rate test (Table 8).

Depression of Breathing Rate

Inhalation of PSI materials by conscious animals causes a decrease in breathing rate, which is reflexly induced by stimulation of cholinergic trigeminal sensory receptors in the nasal mucosa. The depression in breathing rate results from an expiratory pause (Alarie, 1981a). The technique involves the use of a head-only exposure to differ-

Table 8 Comparison of peripheral sensory irritant potential measured by guinea pig blepharospasm and mouse plethysmography

Compound	Plethysmography RD_{50} (molar)	Blepharospasm EC_{50} (molar)
N-undec-10-enonyl-4-hydroxy-3-methoxybenzylamine	2.04×10^{-8}	1.55×10^{-7}
cis-*N*-(4-cyclohexylmethyl)cyclohexylacetamide	2.95×10^{-8}	8.83×10^{-7}
N-(4'-hydroxy-3'-methoxyphenyl)-2-chloroheptanamide	3.82×10^{-8}	7.69×10^{-7}
2-Chloro-3,4-dimethyoxy-ω-nitrostyrene	7.10×10^{-8}	9.26×10^{-6}
N-(4'-hydroxy-3'-methoxyphenyl)2-chlorononanamide	1.43×10^{-7}	3.17×10^{-7}
N-(4'-hydroxy-3'-methoxyphenyl)-2-chlorodecanamide	2.16×10^{-7}	3.58×10^{-7}
Dibenz[*b*,*f*]-1,4-oxazepine	2.30×10^{-7}	3.48×10^{-5}
N-phenyl-2-chlorooctanamide	3.08×10^{-7}	1.15×10^{-5}
2-Chloroacetophenone	3.40×10^{-7}	9.00×10^{-5}

Correlation coefficient (r) = 0.68 (p = 0.06).
Source: Ballantyne (unpublished data).

ing concentrations of test substance in the atmosphere, and breathing rate is measured with a body plethysmograph. Using a minimum of four animals, the mean peak proportionate depression of breathing rate (R) for a given concentration (C) can be calculated. Up to a limiting value, there is a relationship between increasing concentration of inspired PSI material and depression of respiratory rate (Figure 7). As C and C/R are linearly related, a least squares regression between C/R and C can be undertaken. By this approach, a concentration causing a 50 per cent depression of breathing rate can be calculated for the population studied; this is usually referred to as the RD_{50}:

$$RD_{50} = (1/KR_s)/(1/50 - 1/R_s)$$

where $R_s = 1/slope$, and $K = slope/intercept$.

The mouse is the usual species used in this test, although strain differences in sensitivity occur. It has been shown that there is a factor of about 10 between the least and most sensitive strains of mouse (Alarie *et al.*, 1980). Swiss–Webster mice are most frequently used, although it has been shown that there are no differences between B6C3F1 and Swiss–Webster mice (Steinhagen and Barrow, 1984). The rat is an inappropriate species (Babuik *et al.*, 1985). Methods for studying peripheral sensory irritancy by respiratory exposure have been published elsewhere (Alarie, 1973a,b, 1981b; Ballantyne *et al.*, 1977b). Lists of RD_{50} values are available (Alarie, 1981b,c; Bos *et al.*, 1992).

As discussed previously, for any given substance there is usually a marked difference in the concentration causing a typical sensory irritant response by stimulation of sensory receptors in the nasal mucosa and that concentration necessary to stimulate pulmonary receptors. In most instances, in the intact conscious animal, the nasal trigeminal response will dominate. It follows that determination of the difference between concentrations causing nasal and pulmonary irritation may be used as an index of the margin of warning for potential injury provided by the peripheral sensory irritant response. A considerable amount of valuable work has been conducted in this area using intact mice to determine the peripheral sensory irritant response from trigeminal nerve stimulation, and that from tracheal cannulated mice to measure the pulmonary receptor response (Alarie, 1981a). The mouse, unlike other species, undergoes a decrease in breathing rate in response to pulmonary receptor stimulation. The expression tRD_{50}/RD_{50}, which is the ratio of the concentration causing a decrease in breathing in cannulated mice versus that for intact mice, may be used as a guide to the margin of safety produced by nasal sensory irritant warning. An example for alkylamines is shown in Table 1. Methods are available to allow measurement of lung injury and comparison with sensory irritation. These include measurement of changes in respiratory function including resistance (Matijak-Schaper *et al.*, 1983) and detection of pulmonary oedema by a sensitive method based on injection of ^{51}Cr-ethylenediaminetetraacetic acid followed by lung lavage (Valentini *et al.*, 1983).

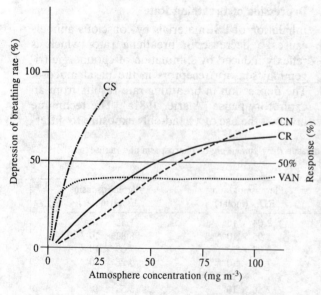

Figure 7 Relationship between depression of breathing rate in conscious mice and airborne exposure concentration for several peripheral sensory irritant materials. CS=*o*-chlorobenzylidene malononitrile; CN=2-chloroacetophenone; CR=dibenz[*b,f*]-1,4-oxazepine; VAN=*N*-nonanoyl vanillylamide

Studies in Human Subjects

The various animal studies discussed above allow the detection of materials causing peripheral sensory irritant effects based on the reflex changes induced. They do not, however, allow for the assessment of subjective discomfort or pain, which is an important component for the evaluation of PSI in humans. In view of this, and because of the difference in sensitivity between animals models and humans to certain PSI materials, it is desirable to conduct tests for assessing irritant potential in human volunteer subjects. Such tests should, of course, only be conducted providing that there is adequate information on the toxicology of the material to ensure that the procedure carries no risk to the volunteers. Such studies allow not only a quantitative assessment of sensory irritant potential at threshold and suprathreshold levels, but permit a determination of variability and the influence of environmental factors on the response.

Eye Irritation

As with the animal models, it is possible to determine the concentration of irritant which causes blepharospasm in human subjects. In addition, it is also possible to determine the degree of local discomfort produced at various concentrations, and define a threshold for sensation and an indication of concentrations causing marked discomfort. PSI of the eye may be relatively easily assessed for solutions by the direct application of carefully measured droplets (Ballantyne and Swanston, 1973a,b). For vapours or gases, tests may be conducted in a chamber with the subject wearing half-face respiratory protective equipment, or using a chamber specially equipped with eye ports (Bender *et al.*, 1983). Table 7 shows some examples of EC_{50} values for blepharospasm in animals and humans, and TC_{50} for sensation in humans. These examples show that the human eye is more sensitive to the blepharospasm-inducing effect of the materials tested than either the rabbit or guinea pig eye. Also, with humans the most sensitive indication of the peripheral sensory irritant effect on the eye is sensory discomfort.

Kjaergaard *et al.* (1990) demonstrated that photographic measurement of changes in conjunctival redness was a reproducible and sensitive method for assessing sensory irritation of the eye, in which comparisons are made before and after irritant provocation. This non-invasive objective method may be useful particularly in studies of irritation resulting from environmental pollution, and has been successfully used to study exposure to formaldehyde, *n*-decane, tobacco dust and

birch pollen (Bach *et al.*, 1988; Kjaergaard and Pederson, 1989; Kjaergaard *et al.*, 1989, 1990).

Inhalation

For respiratory tract irritation it is usual to determine the concentration causing discomfort; for example, chest pain, cough, or nasal irritation. Exposures may be conducted in chambers of a size sufficient to house the volunteers comfortably, and equipped with facilities for sampling the atmosphere in the breathing zone. In some instances a wind tunnel may offer a convenient exposure environment to control and alter concentrations of the test material. In order to avoid complications due to ocular stimulation, either comfortable airtight goggles may be worn or the irritant delivered by mask.

Skin

To determine the degree of discomfort produced by applying a PSI material to the skin, various concentrations of the substance can be used and the discomfort produced subjectively assessed. In choosing the site, it is important to remember that there are anatomical regional variations in the sensitivity of skin to peripheral sensory irritation (Ballantyne *et al.*, 1973a,b).

Because the epidermis presents a barrier for the access of peripheral sensory irritant substances to subepidermal sensory nerve receptors, a method which has been used to overcome this and obtain a comparative evaluation of substances is the blister base technique. This involves the creation of a blister on the forearm by covering the area with tape having perforations at regular intervals, to which is applied a paste of 0.2 per cent cantharidin in kaolin. The tape and paste are removed after six hours and the blisters allowed to develop overnight.

Total Body Exposure

In occupational situations with unprotected subjects PSI materials may access the skin, eye, and respiratory tract, and produce effects in one or all of these tissues. For such situations, controlled studies of PSI materials on human subjects are most meaningful by whole body exposure. In this way it can be determined if any particular tissue is more susceptible, and obtain information on relative warning effects on these tissues. For example, Lundquist *et al.* (1992) studied the effect on human volunteer subjects of dimethylamine vapour which was increased in concentration from 0 to 12 ppm over a one-hour period (average concentration 10 ppm). A moderate to strong olfactory response with distinct subjective nasal and ocular irritation was noted; some, but not all, subjects showed adaptation. Nasal irritation appeared to be a slightly more sensitive index, but there was a significant correlation between ocular and nasal effects ($r = 0.87$, $p < 0.001$). It is of interest to note that in a mouse plethysmography study they found the threshold for depression of breathing rate to be 32 ppm.

INTERPRETATION OF PERIPHERAL SENSORY IRRITATION DATA

Ideally, information derived from the use of animal models should give an indication of the concentration range over which sensory irritant effects may be expected to occur in humans. However, most animal models are less sensitive to peripheral sensory irritants than is the human. In general, studies with animal models can detect those materials having a potential to produce peripheral sensory irritant effects, but they usually do not rank different substances in their order of potency for humans. Also, they may not accurately predict the concentration range over which effects may be anticipated in humans. An example of the difference in the assessment of the relative potency of materials is provided by a comparison of three potent peripheral sensory irritant materials; 2-chlorobenzylidene malononitrile (CS), dibenz[b,f]-1:4-oxazepine (CR) and 2-chloroacetophenone (CN). Table 9 shows that by the frog flexor reflex, guinea pig blepharospasm

and mouse plethysmography methods, the order of PSI potency is CS>CR>CN. However, studies on human subjects show that the TC_{50} and IC_{50} by respiratory exposure give an order of potency CR>CS>CN.

In comparing the relative potency of different sensory irritant materials, and when adequate concentration–response data are available, it is important to review the EC_{50} and 95 per cent confidence limits to determine if there are significant differences in potency at the 50 per cent response level. However, and as with any analysis of dose–response information, it is of the utmost importance to take into consideration the slope of the regression line. For example, if two materials have significantly different EC_{50} values and the slopes of the dose–response regression lines are essentially parallel, then it can be confidently stated that the two materials are not significantly different over a wide range of concentrations with respect to peripheral sensory irritant potency under the conditions of the study. In contrast, if the slopes are not similar this may have important influences on the differential interpretation of the practical relevance of the data. For example, the two materials shown in Figure 8 have identical EC_{50} values and 95 per cent confidence limits, indicating no difference in PSI potency at the 50 per cent response level. However, because of differences in the slopes of the regression lines there are significant differences between the two materials for sensory irritant potency at the high response (EC_{95}) and low response (EC_5) regions; this has important implications for the interpretation of these data. For the material having the steeper slope, once a concentration is reached which causes sensory irritation in a minor pro-

Table 9 Comparison of the sensory irritant potential of 2-chloroacetophenone (CN), o-chlorobenzylidene malononitrile (CS) and dibenz[b,f]-1,4-oxazepine (CR) using animal models and observations in humans

Compound	Animal models			Human studies	
	GPB[a] EC_{50} (molar)	FFR[b] T_m (molar)	MP[c] RD_{50} (μg l^{-1})	TC_{50}[d] (μg l^{-1})	IC_{50}[e] (μg l^{-1})
CN	9.00×10^{-5}	1.10×10^{-4}	52.5	0.4	20.0
CS	2.16×10^{-5}	9.78×10^{-6}	11.5	2.3×10^{-3}	3.6
CR	3.48×10^{-5}	2.09×10^{-5}	46.0	2.0×10^{-3}	0.7

[a] Guinea pig blepharospasm (Ballantyne, unpublished data).
[b] Frog flexor reflex (Ballantyne, unpublished data).
[c] Mouse plethysmography (Ballantyne *et al.*, 1977b).
[d] Threshold concentration for respiratory effects (Ballantyne, 1977).
[e] Incapacitating concentration for respiratory effects (Ballantyne, 1977).

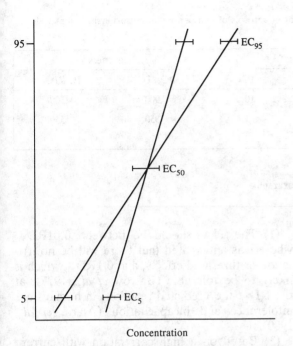

Figure 8 Comparison of two sensory irritants having similar EC_{50} values but differing concentration–response line slopes. This has implications for hyper-reactive individuals with the shallow slope, and safety margins for materials with steep slopes (see text)

portion of the exposed population, then only a small incremental increase is necessary to cause an effect in the majority of the population. Thus, in such circumstances, it may be necessary to add a wide margin below this restricted concentration range to ensure adequate protection. In contrast, with the material having a shallow slope, the concentration range over which the majority of the population will be affected is much greater. However, because of the shallow slope there will clearly be an interest in protecting the small proportion of the population who are hypersensitive.

It follows from the above discussion that when the PSI potential of different substances are being compared it is necessary to consider both the 50 per cent response level (with 95 per cent confidence limits) and the slope of the concentration–response regression line. The fact that slopes may differ for various substances has two implications. First, it may not be possible to calculate a true statistical potency ratio. Second, the relative potency of two materials can vary for differing levels of sensory irritation. Although it may not be possible to calculate a true potency ratio, it can be useful to determine the comparative

potency of materials at different levels of irritancy (Ballantyne, 1977); this may be defined as follows:

$$\text{Comparative Potency} = \frac{\text{Concentration of A}\atop\text{causing a defined response}}{\text{Concentration of B}\atop\text{causing the same response}}$$

Also, during considerations of the relevance of incapacitating effects of PSI it is useful to compare the threshold levels (TC_{50}) and incapacitating levels (IC_{50}) to determine if the difference between these values is sufficient to enable threshold effects to give adequate warning of a potentially incapacitating exposure. A useful expression is the ratio IC_{50}/TC_{50} (effectiveness ratio). A high value for the effectiveness ratio indicates that threshold irritation will give a good warning of potentially incapacitating effects. However, if the ratio is small, then a small incremental increase in concentration will convert a threshold effect into a incapacitating effect. For example, using the data shown in Table 9, the effectiveness ratios (IC_{50}/TC_{50}) for CS and CR are respectively 900 and 350 at the 50 per cent level (Table 10). This indicates that although there is a significant margin between the threshold and incapacitating concentrations for both materials, the proportionate increase in atmospheric concentrations to convert a threshold effect to an incapacitating effect does not have to be as great with CR as with CS. Another feature of importance in comparing threshold and incapacitating effects is also shown in Table 10, namely, that the comparative potency of two materials may differ at the threshold level from that at the incapacitating level, because of differences in the concentration–response lines. For example, the comparative potency data at the IC_{50} and IC_{75} levels of incapacitation show that CR is five and nine times, respectively, more potent than CS.

SENSORY IRRITATION AS A FACTOR IN OCCUPATIONAL EXPOSURE LIMITS

Occupational exposure limits (OELs), such as the Threshold Limit Values (TLVs) developed by the American Conference of Governmental Indus-

Table 10 Comparison of the respiratory tract potency in humans of aerosols of two peripheral sensory irritant materials at differing levels of irritant effect

Material	Level of irritancy (mg m^{-3})[a]			Effectiveness ratio	
	TC_{50}	IC_{50}	IC_{75}	IC_{50}/TC_{50}	IC_{75}/TC_{50}
CS	4.0×10^{-3}	3.6	10.0	900	2500
CR	2.0×10^{-3}	0.7	1.1	350	550
CS/CR[b]	2.0	5.1	9.1		

[a] For a 1-min exposure.
[b] Potency ratio.
CS = o-chlorobenzylidene malononitrile; CR = dibenz[b,f]-1,4-oxazepine.
Source: Ballantyne (1977).

trial Hygienists (ACGIH, 1991–92), are derived by a detailed consideration of all available and credible information from laboratory studies and observations on exposed humans. The OEL will usually be assigned on the basis of the most sensitive indicator(s) of toxicity, i.e. the adverse effects produced by the lowest acute or repeated exposure concentration. As PSI materials produce distraction and/or incapacitating effects, which may predispose to accidents, many OELs are assigned on the basis of sensory irritation. This is particularly useful when sensory irritation effects occur at concentrations lower than those causing toxicity by acute or repeated exposure, and thus give a warning of potential overexposure.

For some materials, information on sensory irritation in humans is available, allowing a reasonable estimate for threshold and incapacitating effects and thus permitting reliable OELs to be assigned. Where data are sufficient, attention should be paid to threshold and incapacitating concentrations, slopes of the dose–response relationship, and effectiveness ratios. Also, consideration should be given to development of tolerance.

In the absence of reliable human data, or else to support and confirm human data, PSI studies in animals have been widely used to predict OELs to prevent sensory irritation. Most widely used have been RD_{50} values obtained from plethysmography studies in mice. Those with a belief that RD_{50} values can be used for assigning OELs have supported their case by comparing RD_{50} data for known irritants with ACGIH TLV values (Barrow *et al.*, 1977; Alarie *et al.*, 1980; Ceaurriz *et al.*, 1981; Steinhagen and Barrow, 1984; Nielsen and Yamagiwa, 1989). Examples of OEL predictive models are as follows:

(1) The TLV should be between $0.01RD_{50}$, where it is anticipated that there will be no irritation or threshold effects, and $0.1RD_{50}$, which is likely to be tolerable (Barrow *et al.*, 1977); at the RD_{50}, the predicted reactions in humans are intolerance and incapacitation (Alarie *et al.*, 1980).

(2) Based on a high correlation with current TLVs, $0.03RD_{50}$ has been recommended for establishing a TLV for a PSI material (Alarie, 1981b,c).

Bos *et al.* (1992) have questioned the suitability of the RD_{50} test as a means for assigning OELs. Their doubts are based on interlaboratory variations, the finding that severe toxicity may be seen below the RD_{50} with some compounds, and the fact that the rationale for deriving an OEL from RD_{50} data is based on empirical findings. They recommend the following with regard to application of the sensory irritation test:

(1) Because of the interspecies variations, two species (i.e. rat and mouse) should be used, with the results from the more sensitive species being chosen.

(2) Time–response and log concentration–response curves should be provided.

(3) Exposure should be prolonged until a plateau response is obtained.

(4) Verification should be obtained that no pulmonary irritation is occurring.

(5) For every compound, it should be verified whether the observed response is the result of irritation or toxicity.

REFERENCES

ACGIH (1991–92). *Threshold Limit Values for Chemical Substances and Physical Agents and Biological Exposure Indices*. American Conference of Governmental Industrial Hygienists. Cincinnati, OH

Alarie, Y. (1973a). Sensory irritation of the upper airways by airborne chemicals. *Toxicol. Appl. Pharmac.*, **24**, 279–297

Alarie, Y. (1973b). Sensory irritation by airborne chemicals. *CRC Crit. Rev. Toxicol.*, **3**, 299–363

Alarie, Y. (1981a). Toxicological evaluation of airborne chemical irritation and allergens using respiratory reflex reactions. In Leong, B. K. J. (Ed.), *Proceedings of the Inhalation Toxicology and Technology Symposium*. Ann Arbor, Michigan, pp. 207–331

Alarie, Y. (1981b). Bioassay for evaluating the potency of airborne irritants and predicting acceptable levels of exposure in man. *Fd Cosmet. Toxicol.*, **19**, 623–626

Alarie, Y. (1981c). Dose-response analysis in animal studies: prediction of human responses. *Envir. Hlth Perspec.*, **42**, 9–13

Alarie, Y., Kane, L. and Barrow, C. (1980). Sensory irritation: the use of an animal model to establish acceptable exposure to airborne irritants. In Reeves, A. L. (Ed.), *Toxicology: Principles and Practice*, Vol. 1. Wiley, New York, pp. 48–92

Amoore, J. E. and Hautala, L. (1983). Odor as an aid to chemical safety. *J. Appl. Toxicol.*, **3**, 275–289

Babiuk, C., Steinhagen, W. H. and Barrow, C. S. (1985). Sensory irritation response to inhaled aldehydes after formaldehyde pretreatment. *Toxicol. Appl. Pharmac.*, **79**, 143–149

Bach, B., Molhave, L. and Pederson, O. F. (1988). *Human Reactions to Formaldehyde Vapor*. Institute of Environmental and Occupational Medicine, Aarhus

Ballantyne, B. (1977). Biomedical and health aspects of the use of chemicals in civil disturbances. In Scott, R. B. and Frazer, J. (Eds), *Medical Annual*. Wright, Bristol, pp. 7–41

Ballantyne, B. (1981). Toxic effects of inhaled materials. In Ballantyne, B. and Schwabe, P. H. (Eds), *Respiratory Protection: Principles and Applications*. Chapman and Hall, London, pp. 93–134

Ballantyne, B. (1983). Local ophthalmic effects of dipropylene glycol monomethyl ether. *J. Toxicol. Cut. Ocular Toxicol.*, **2**, 125–138

Ballantyne, B. and Swanston, D. W. (1973a). The irritant potential of dilute solutions of orthochlorobenzylidene malononitrile (CS). *Acta Pharmac. Toxicol.*, **32**, 266–277

Ballantyne, B. and Swanston, D. W. (1973b). The irritant effects of dilute solutions of dibenzoxazepine (CR) on the eye and tongue. *Acta Pharmac. Toxicol.*, **35**, 412–423

Ballantyne, B., Beswick, F. W. and Price Thomas, D. (1973a). The presentation and management of individuals contaminated by solutions of dibenzoxazepine. *Med. Sci. Law*, **13**, 265–268

Ballantyne, B., Gall, D. and Robson, D. C. (1973b). Effects on man of drenching with dilute solutions of *o*-chlorobenzylidene malononitrile (CS) and dibenz[*b*,*f*]-1:4-oxazepine (CR). *Med. Sci. Law*, **16**, 159–170

Ballantyne, B., Gazzard, M. F. and Swanston, D. W. (1976). The ophthalmic toxicology of dichloromethane. *Toxicology*, **6**, 173–187

Ballantyne, B., Gazzard, M. F. and Swanston, D. W. (1977a). Applanation tonometry in ophthalmic toxicology. In Ballantyne, B. (Ed.) *Current Approaches in Toxicology*. Wright, Bristol, pp. 158–192

Ballantyne, B., Gazzard, M. F. and Swanston, D. W. (1977b). Irritancy testing by respiratory exposure. In Ballantyne, B. (Ed.) *Current Approaches in Toxicology*. Wright, Bristol, pp. 129–138

Barrow, C. S., Alarie, Y., Warrick, J. and Stock, M. (1977). Comparison of the sensory irritant response in mice to chlorine and hydrogen chloride. *Arch. Environ. Health*, **3**, 68–76

Bender, J. R., Mullin, L. S., Graepel, G. J. and Wilson, W. E. (1983). Eye irritation response of humans to formaldehyde. *Am. Industr. Hyg. Assoc. J.*, **44**, 463–465

Beswick, F. W., Holland, P. and Kemp, K. H. (1972). Acute effects of exposure to orthochlorobenzylidene malononitrile (CS) and the development of tolerance. *Br. J. Industr. Med.*, **29**, 298–306

Bos, P. M. J., Zwart, A., Reuzel, P. G. J. and Bragt, P. C. (1992). Evaluation of the sensory irritation test for assessment of occupational health risk. *Crit. Rev. Toxicol.*, **21**, 423–450

Cauna, N., Hinderer, K. H. and Wentges, R. T. (1969). Sensory receptor organs in human nasal respiratory mucosa. *Amer. J. Anat.*, **14**, 295–300

Ceaurriz, J. C. de, Micillino, J. C., Bonnet, P. and Guenier, J. P. (1981). Sensory irritation caused by various industrial airborne chemicals. *Toxicol. Lett.*, **9**, 137–143

Chang, J. C. F. and Barrow, C. S. (1986). Sensory irritation tolerance of F-344 rats exposed to chlorine or formaldehyde gas. *Toxicol. Appl. Pharmac.*, **76**, 319–327

Collins, C. C., Bach-y-Rita, P. and Loeb, D. R. (1967). Intraocular pressure variation with oculorotatory muscle tension. *Am. J. Physiol.*, **213**, 1039–1043

Crofton, J. and Douglas, A. (1981). *Respiratory Diseases*, 3rd edn. Blackwell Scientific Publications, Oxford

Dirnhuber, P., Gree, D. M. and Tregear, R. T. (1965). Excitation of sensory neurones in the cat larynx by ω-chloroacetophenone and *n*-nonanoylvanillylamide. *J. Physiol. (Lond.)*, **178**, 41–42

Dixon, M. and Needham, D. M. (1946). Biochemical research on chemical warfare agents. *Nature*, **158**, 432–438

Douglas, R. (1981). Inhalation of irritant gases and

aerosols. In Widdicombe, J. (Ed.), *Respiratory Pharmacology*. Pergamon Press, Oxford, pp. 297–333

Feniak, G. (1966). The common chemical sense of the frog. *Suffield Technical Paper No. 310* (March). Suffield Experimental Station, Canada

Foster, R. W. and Ramage, A. G. (1981). The action of some chemical irritants on somatosensory receptors of the cat. *Neuropharmacology*, **20**, 191–198

Grant, W. M. (1986). *Toxicology of the Eye*, 3rd edn. Charles C. Thomas, Springfield, Illinois

Green, D. M. and Tregear, R. T. (1964). The action of sensory irritants on the cat's cornea. *J. Physiol. (Lond.)*, **175**, 37–38

Green, D. M., Balfour, D. J. K. and Muir, A. (1979). Effect of methyl substitution on the irritancy of dibenz[b,f]-1:4-oxazepine (CR). *Toxicology*, **12**, 151–153

Hogg, S. I., Curtis, C. G., Russell, N. J., Upshall, D. G. and Powell, G. M. (1983). The effects of sensory irritants on phagocytosis by pulmonary macrophages. *Environ. Res.*, **30**, 492–497

James, J. E. A. and Daly, M. de B. (1969). Nasal reflexes. *Proc. R. Soc. Med.*, **62**, 1287–1293

Keele, C. A. (1962). The common chemical sense and its receptors. *Arch. Int. Pharmacodyn. Ther.*, **139**, 547–557

Kjaergaard, S. and Pederson, O. F. (1989). Dust exposure, eye redness, eye cytology and mucous membrane irritation in a tobacco industry. *Int. Arch. Occup. Environ. Health*, **61**, 519–525

Kjaergaard, S., *et al.* (1989). Human exposure to indoor pollutants: n-decane. *Environ. Int.*, **15**, 473–482

Kjaergaard, S., *et al.* (1990). Assessment of changes in eye redness by a photographic method and the relation to sensory eye irritation. *Int. Arch. Environ. Health*, **62**, 133–137

Kulle, T. J. and Cooper, G. P. (1975). Effects of formaldehyde and ozone on the trigeminal nasal sensory system. *Arch. Environ. Health*, **30**, 237–243

Lundquist, G. R., Yamagiwa, M., Pederson, O. F. and Nielsen, G. D. (1992). Inhalation of diethylamine. *Amer. Industr. Hyg. Assoc. J.*, **53**, 181–185

Luo, J. E., Nielsen, G. D. and Alarie, Y. (1983). Formaldehyde: an exception in the series of saturated aldehydes, aliphatic alcohols and alkylbenzenes. *Toxicologist*, **3**, 74

McNamara, B. P., Vocci, F. J. and Owens, J. E. (1968). The toxicology of CN. *Edgewood Arsenal Technical Report Series No. 4207*. Aberdeen Proving Ground, Maryland

Matijak-Schaper, M., Wong, K-L. and Alarie, Y. (1983). A method to rapidly evaluate the acute pulmonary effects of aerosols in unanesthetized guinea-pigs. *Toxicol. Appl. Pharmac.*, **69**, 451–460

Miller, D. (1967). Pressure of the lid on the eye. *Arch. Ophthalmol.*, **78**; 328–330

Moncrief, R. H. (1944). *The Chemical Senses*. Leonard Hill Ltd, London

Nielsen, G. D. and Alarie, Y. (1982). Sensory irritation, pulmonary irritation and respiratory stimulation by airborne benzene and alkylbenzenes. *Toxicol. Appl. Pharmacol.*, **65**, 459–477

Nielson, G. D. and Vinggaard, A. M. (1988). Sensory irritation and pulmonary irritation of C3-C7 n-alkylamines. *Pharmacol. Toxicol.*, **63**, 293–304

Nielson, G. D. and Yamagiwa, M. (1989). Structure activity of airway irritative aliphatic amines. *Chem. Biol. Interact.*, **71**, 223–244

Owens, E. J. and Punte, C. L. (1963). Human respiratory and ocular irritation studies using orthochlorobenzylidene malononitrile aerosol. *Am. Industr. Assoc. J.*, **24**, 262–264

Punte, C. L., Owens, E. J. and Gutentag, E. J. (1963). Exposure to ortho-chlorobenzylidene malononitrile. *Arch. Environ. Health*, **6**, 366–374

Rengstorff, R. H. (1975). The effect of external ocular irritation on intraocular pressure. *Amer. J. Optom. Physiol. Optics*, **52**, 587–590

Schauenstein, E., Esterbaauer, M. and Zollne, H. (1977). *Aldehydes in Biological Systems*. Pion Ltd, London

Silver, R. F., Kerr, A. K., Frandson, P. D., Kelley, S. J. and Holmes, H. L. (1967). Synthesis and chemical reactions of some conjugated heteroenoid compounds. *Can. J. Chem.*, **45**, 1001–1006

Steinhagen, W. H. and Barrow, C. S. (1984). Sensory irritation structure-activity study of inhaled aldehydes in B6C3F1 and Swiss-Webster mice. *Toxicol. Appl. Pharmac.*, **72**, 495–503

Tsubone, H. and Kawahl, M. (1991). Stimulation of the trigeminal afferent nerve of the nose by formaldehyde, acrolein and acetaldehyde gas. *Inhal. Toxicol.*, **3**, 211–222

Ulrich, C. E., Haddock, M. P. and Alarie, Y. (1972). Airborne chemical irritants. *Arch. Environ. Health*, **24**, 37–42

Valentini, J. E., Wang, K-L. and Alarie, Y. (1983). Single tracer technique to evaluate pulmonary edema and its application to detect the effect of hexamethylene diisocyanate trimer aerosol exposures. *Toxicol. Appl. Pharmacol.*, **69**, 461–470

Widdicombe, J. G. (1981). Physiological response to inhaled materials. In Ballantyne, B. (Ed.), *Respiratory Protection: Principles and Applications*. Chapman and Hall, London, pp. 47–64

FURTHER READING

Cometto-Muniz, J. E. and Cain, W. S. (1994). Sensory reactions of nasal pungency and odor to volatile organic compounds: the alkylbenzenes. *American Industrial Hygiene Association Journal*, **55**, 811–817

Schaper, M. (1993). Development of a database for sensory irritants and its use in establishing occupational exposure limits. *American Industrial Hygiene Association Journal*, **54**, 488–544

21 Responses of the Kidney to Toxic Compounds

Edward A. Lock

INTRODUCTION

The mammalian kidney is an extremely complex organ, both anatomically and functionally, and plays an important role in the control and regulation of homoeostasis. In this regard it has a key role in the regulation of extracellular fluid volume and electrolyte composition. The kidney is also the site of synthesis of hormones and certain vasoactive prostaglandins and kinins that influence systemic metabolic function. For example, renin, the stimulus for the formation of angiotensin, and aldosterone are formed in the kidney. 25-Hydroxyvitamin D_3 undergoes hydroxylation specifically in the kidney to 1,25-dihydroxyvitamin D_3, which plays a key role in promoting bone resorption and calcium absorption from the gut. Erythropoietin, an important stimulus for erythrocyte formation in the bone marrow, is also synthesized in the kidney.

A toxic insult to the kidney may affect some or all of these functions but, in general, it is markers of excretory function such as blood urea nitrogen, or creatinine, and the presence of glucose, protein or electrolytes in urine which are commonly monitored as indicators of renal dysfunction.

RENAL STRUCTURE AND FUNCTION

The kidney can be divided into two major anatomical areas—the cortex and the medulla. The cortex forms the major part of the kidney and receives most of the blood supply and, hence, nutrients. Thus, when a foreign chemical enters the bloodstream, a high percentage will be delivered to the cortex and, hence, have a greater chance of altering cortical function than medullary. Some chemicals, however, will be delivered to the medulla and, because of the anatomy of the vasa rectae and loops of Henle, can become trapped by the countercurrent system in this region of the nephron. Thus, a foreign chemical can achieve relatively high concentrations in the medulla although the blood flow is relatively poor.

The functional anatomy of the kidney is based on the nephron structure which has three separate elements, the vasculature, the glomerulus, and the tubular component (Figure 1). All nephrons have their major vascular components and glomeruli in the cortex. The proximal convoluted tubules (pars convoluta) are located in the cortex, with the straight portions of the proximal tubules (pars recta) extending into the outer stripe of the outer medulla (Figure 2). Those nephrons whose glomeruli are close to the cortical surface (cortical nephrons) send their loops of Henle down into

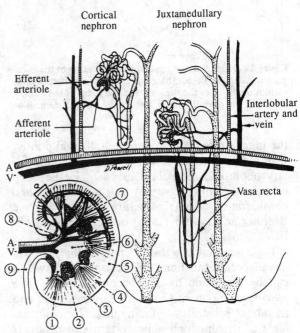

Figure 1 A sagittal section of a human kidney is illustrated diagrammatically (lower left). Numbers (1)–(9) indicate the following: (1) minor calix: (2) fat in sinus: (3) renal column of Bertin: (4) medullary ray: (5) cortex: (6) pelvis: (7) interlobar artery: (8) major calix: and (9) ureter. The letter A indicates the renal artery, and the letter V indicates the renal vein. Insert (a) from the upper pole is enlarged to illustrate the relationships between the juxtamedullary and the cortical nephrons and the renal vasculature. From Tisher (1976). With permission

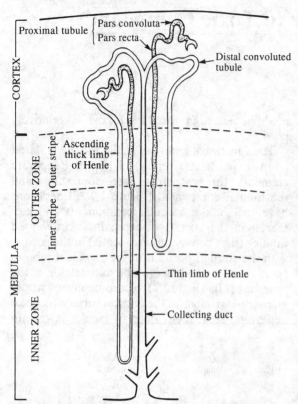

Figure 2 Diagram of the structural organization of the mammalian kidney to demonstrate the relationships between the various segments of the nephron and the zones of the kidney, especially the medulla. From Tisher (1976). With permission

the inner stripe of the inner medulla, while those with glomeruli close to the medulla (juxtamedullary nephrons) send their loops of Henle deep into the medulla (Figure 2). For a more detailed consideration of renal structure and function see Brenner and Rector (1986) or Seldin and Giebisch (1985).

Each anatomically distinct part of the nephron has a specific function or functions, all of which can be perturbed by a nephrotoxic insult. The vascular component serves to deliver oxygen and metabolic substrates to the nephron for maintenance of its function, while certain end products of metabolism and other materials are delivered to the tubule for excretion. The blood supply also enables reabsorbed materials and those synthesized in the kidney to be returned to the systemic circulation.

The glomerulus contains a very specialized capillary network which is relatively porous and acts as a selective filter of components from

plasma. On the basis of molecular weight and net charge, certain materials and chemicals will be filtered into the tubular lumen, while others will be retained in the circulation. (See Dworkin and Brenner, 1985, and Maunsbach *et al.*, 1980, for more detailed information.) The tubular part of the nephron selectively reabsorbs the majority, about 98 per cent, of the salts and water in the filtrate. In a normal healthy kidney there is almost complete reabsorption of filtered glucose and amino acids and selective elimination of end or waste products of metabolism. The proximal tubule is also able to actively secrete certain chemicals into the urine; the excretion of some organic compounds and the elimination of hydrogen and potassium ions occur primarily via this route. (See Greger *et al.*, 1981, Moller and Sheikh, 1983, and Weiner, 1985, for more detailed information.)

Depending on the size of a toxic insult, chemicals may produce changes in renal function which are mild and reversible or which are permanent, and if severe enough they will cause death. For example, nephrotoxicity may be expresssed as a minor perturbation in tubular reabsorption such as a mild or transient glucosuria or proteinuria, as a decreased concentrating ability (for example, polyuria) or, following a more severe insult, as acute renal failure associated with anuria and elevations in creatinine and blood urea nitrogen.

SUSCEPTIBILITY OF THE KIDNEY TO TOXIC INSULT

The two kidneys comprise about 1 per cent of the body weight, but receive about 25 per cent of the cardiac output, and about one-third of the plasma water that reaches the kidney is filtered. Maintenance of renal function requires delivery of large quantities of oxygen and metabolic substrates to the kidney. Thus, the kidney, especially the pars recta of the proximal tubule, is particularly susceptible to agents that produce cellular anoxia— for instance, a decrease in blood pressure or blood volume, as in shock or haemorrhage (Glaumann and Trump, 1975; Venkatchalam *et al.*, 1978). Similarly, dehydration, due to either increased heat output or decreased water intake, or a chemical which causes a decrease in plasma volume (Lock, 1979) can lead to a marked alteration in renal function.

Potentially toxic chemicals present in the bloodstream will be delivered to the kidneys in large quantities, especially to the cortex, which receives about 80 per cent of the total renal blood flow. This, together with the ability of the kidney to concentrate tubular fluid, may enhance the toxic effect on the proximal tubular cells, by generating a high concentration of the chemical in the tubular lumen. In addition, if a chemical which has been filtered at the glomerulus and concentrated within the tubule is then reabsorbed, by a passive or active mechanism, it will pass through the cells of the nephron at relatively high concentrations and potentially lead to intracellular toxicity. Finally, many organic chemicals undergo active transport from the blood into proximal tubular cells and then diffuse into the tubular lumen. Thus, the proximal tubular cells can be exposed to higher concentrations than those present in plasma. This active transport occurs in all three segments of the proximal tubule, although considerable variation exists from segment to segment depending on the species (Roch-Ramel and Weiner, 1980; Greger *et al.*, 1981; Weiner, 1985).

The renal medulla receives a much lower blood flow and therefore receives relatively less potential toxic chemical via the bloodstream. However, as the chemical passes down the nephron into the medulla the countercurrent mechanisms may lead to a chemical becoming concentrated in this region and the papilla to a concentration many times greater than that in the plasma (Duggin and Mudge, 1976; Mudge, 1982).

Once a chemical has become concentrated in a renal cell, it may act directly or require further metabolism to produce a toxic response. A direct-acting chemical presumably acts by interfering with important metabolic events—for instance, inhibition of mitochondrial function or of key enzymes involved in energy metabolism. Alternatively, the chemical may be converted to a reactive species that may bind covalently to critical sites in proteins or initiate lipid peroxidation leading to cellular damage. In the latter case the chemical could have already undergone metabolism in another organ and the stable metabolite have entered the kidney where further metabolism to generate a reactive species occurs.

Most of the common enzymes involved in the metabolism of foreign compounds, such as cytochrome(s) *P*-450 and glutathione-*S*-transferases, are present in renal tissue, although the specific activities of these enzymes are usually lower than that found in the liver (Anders, 1980). However, the nephron has a very marked cellular heterogeneity and there are major differences in the relative amounts of certain enzymes in the different regions of the nephron (Figure 3) (Guder and Ross, 1984). Thus, any measurement of enzyme activities in whole kidney as opposed to renal cortex or medulla or isolated glomeruli or proximal tubular cells can grossly underestimate the metabolic capabilities of these regions of the kidney. As a foreign chemical passes down the nephron, it may undergo metabolism by a number of different enzymes. For example, paracetamol, on entering a proximal tubular cell, may undergo oxidation by cytochromes *P*-450, whereas once it has entered the medulla, it can undergo co-oxidation via the endoperoxidase synthetase pathway (Mohandas *et al.*, 1981). Frequently the intrarenal location of injury represents the site of accumulation of either the chemical or its metabolite, or the location of the enzymes which are responsible for activating it.

The kidney is also under the influence of the sympathetic nervous system (Gottschalk *et al.*, 1985), and chemicals which have a direct action on renal sympathetic nerves can alter renal vascular resistance or renin secretion and influence renal function *per se*.

MEASUREMENT OF THE EFFECT OF CHEMICALS ON RENAL FUNCTION

A number of non-invasive techniques are available to assess whether a chemical has had a marked effect on the kidney in both experimental animals and man. A battery of simple tests has evolved which can be applied to urine to give an indication of renal injury. These measurements can be conducted on a temporal basis during feeding studies in experimental animals, or in man exposed to a potentially harmful compound in the workplace, or during drug therapy. The various advantages and disadvantages of these techniques will not be discussed in detail in this chapter. Readers are referred to the following review articles and papers therein: Stonard, 1987; Dawnay and Cattell, 1987; Lauwerys and Bernard, 1989; Stonard, 1990.

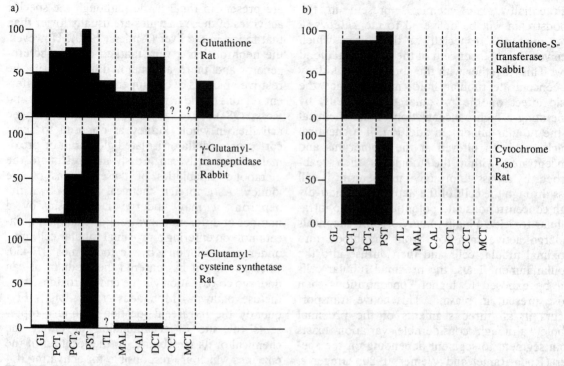

Figure 3 Distribution of glutathione, glutathione-related enzymes and enzymes related to drug metabolism along the nephron. Glutathione, γ-glutamyl transpeptidase (E.C. 2.3.2.1), glutamyl cysteine synthetase (E.C. 6.3.2.2), glutathione-S-transferase (E.C. 2.5.1.18) and cytochrome P-450 were measured from microdissected rat and rabbit nephron. Activities were related to tubular dry weight or protein (P-450). The abbreviations of nephron segments used are: GL, glomerulus; PCT_1, early proximal convoluted tubule; PCT_2, late proximal convoluted tubule; PST, proximal straight tubule; TL, loop of Henle, thin limbs; MAL, medullary thick ascending limb; CAL, cortical ascending limb; DCT, distal convoluted tubule; CCT, cortical collecting tubule; MCT, medullary collecting tubule. Modified from Guder and Ross (1984) with permission.

The standard battery of measurements includes urine volume and osmolality, urinary pH and the excretion of the electrolytes Na^+ and K^+. The presence of glucose or excess protein in urine and changes in urinary sediment would all indicate abnormalities in renal function. The increased excretion of specific enzymes of renal origin in urine can indicate abnormality of function. Certain enzymes that increase in the urine can be of postrenal origin—for instance, the bladder—and as such are not indicative of renal damage. However measurement of N-acetyl-β-D-glucosaminidase, which is primarily of renal origin, has been successfully used as an early indicator of renal transplant rejection in man (Yuen *et al.*, 1987) and for the detection of chemically induced renal injury in experimental animals as well as man (Price, 1982; Stonard, 1987).

Once an indication of renal dysfunction has been suggested by this simple battery of assays, it may be necessary to examine in more detail this effect on renal function and to quantify this response. More specific information indicating whether the insult has occurred to the proximal tubule and/or the glomerulus can be gained by characterizing the proteins excreted in urine on a molecular weight basis, low-molecular-weight proteinuria being indicative of a tubular site of injury, while excretion of high-molecular-weight protein (>80 000) is indicative of glomerular injury (Stonard, 1987). High-resolution ¹H NMR spectroscopy has also been used to provide an initial biochemical screen for detecting abnormal patterns of metabolites in urine (Bales *et al.*, 1984). Studies in experimental animals have indicated that this technique can provide valuable information regarding the probable site of toxic action of a chemical to the nephron. Proximal tubular toxins produce marked glycosuria, aminoaciduria and lactic aciduria, whereas papillary toxins cause early increases in trimethylamine N-oxide and dimethylamine (Figure 4) (Gartland *et*

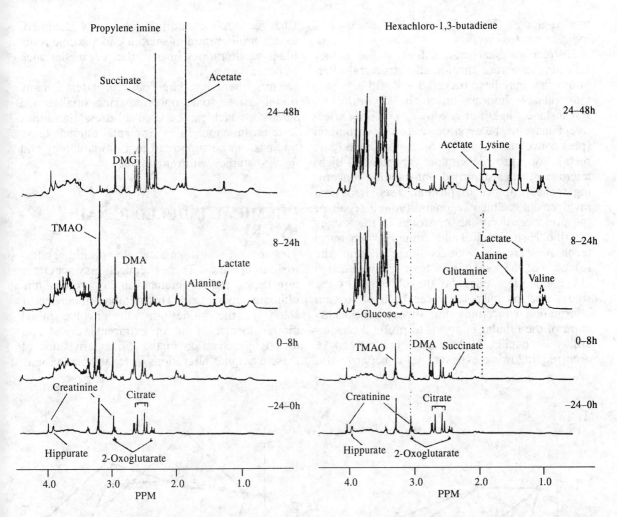

Figure 4 400 MHz ^{1}H NMR spectra of urine from rats before and after dosing with 200 mg kg^{-1} hexachloro-1,3-butadiene or 20 μl kg^{-1} propylene imine. DMA, dimethylamine; TMAO, trimethylamine *N*-oxide; DMG, *N-N*-dimethylglycine. From Gartland *et al.* (1989). With permission

al., 1989). Small blood samples can be taken at varous times after treatment and the concentration of plasma creatinine or blood urea nitrogen can be monitored to give some indication of altered renal excretory function. Further information on renal function can be obtained by measuring (1) renal clearance of insulin to determine glomerular filtration and (2) renal clearance and excretion of *p*-aminohippuric acid to determine renal plasma flow, from which renal blood flow can be estimated. Alternatively, radiolabelled microspheres or an electromagnetic flowmeter may be used to specifically measure renal blood flow in experimental animals.

These techniques will enable the detection of abnormal renal function *in vivo;* however, it can be difficult to ascertain whether this malfunction is a direct effect of the chemical or is secondary to altered renal haemodynamics. The toxic effect of chemicals may be evaluated *in vitro* by adding the chemical or its metabolite directly to renal cortical slices or isolated proximal tubular cells/tubules. Alterations in transport of the organic cations tetraethylammonium (TEA) and *N*-methylnicotinamide (NMN) or the organic anion *p*-aminohippurate (PAH) across the basolateral membrane have been used as indices of nephrotoxicity (Kacew, 1987). Leakage of lactate dehydrogenase, loss of intracellular ATP and altered transport of the non-metabolized sugar α-methyl-glucose (Figure 5) have also been used to indicate cytotoxicity.

Histopathological examination of the kidney following exposure can identify structural alterations that may have occurred and will also provide valuable information on the area affected. For instance, light microscopy can identify selective damage to the nephron caused by chromium (pars convoluta), hexachloro-1,3-butadiene (pars recta) or propyleneimine (papilla). Light microscopy can also provide information concerning the appearance of protein casts, lysosomal involvement, cellular regeneration and repair or the presence of crystals or stones in the kidney or urine. Histochemical and immunocytochemical techniques are also valuable in evaluating the response of the kidney to a toxic insult (Bach *et al.*, 1987). Depending on the objective of the study, electron microscopy can be used to gain information concerning the subcellular localization of the tubular injury or to probe the glomerulus or papilla for changes that may have occurred following exposure to a nephrotoxin.

Changes in mitochondria can be easily identified, as can proliferation of smooth endoplasmic reticulum or alterations in the other organelles such as peroxisomes.

Thus, there is a large battery of tests, many non-invasive, some only requiring small blood samples, which can be used to assess alterations in renal function. In experimental animals these findings can be supported by histopathology and *in vitro* studies with renal tissue.

CHEMICAL INDUCED RENAL INJURY

This section will discuss certain specific nephrotoxic compounds. These chemicals may act either directly or require metabolism to produce the ultimate nephrotoxin. This metabolism may occur solely in the kidney or may involve initial biotransformation in an extrarenal organ followed by activation in the kidney. In some of these examples alterations in renal function may

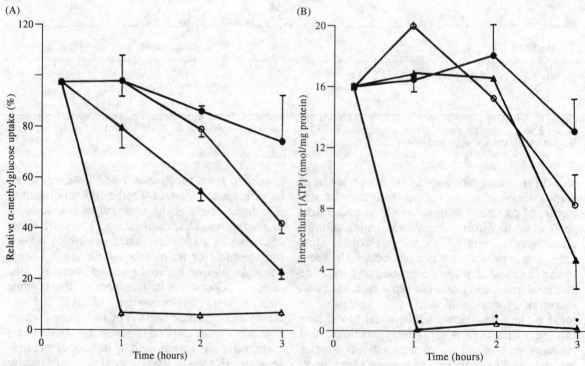

Figure 5 The effect of mercuric chloride on the integrity of isolated rat renal proximal tubular cells *in vitro*. (A) α-methylglucose transport; (B) intracellular ATP concentrations. Control (●), mercuric chloride, 10 μM (○), 100 μM (▲), 1 mM (△). From Boogaard *et al.* (1989). With permission

be secondary to changes in blood pressure or blood volume, or to hormonal or neural effects. It is not the intention of this section to discuss all known chemicals which have been reported to cause renal injury. Instead the focus will be on areas where there is some understanding of the mechanisms of nephrotoxicity.

Heavy Metals

Several heavy metals are nephrotoxic, since the kidney concentrates them prior to excretion and they are potent inhibitors of a large number of metabolic processes. However, several mechanisms exist which protect the kidney against heavy metals—for example, the presence of metallothionein and other high-affinity metal-binding proteins, and the compartmentalization of the metals into lysosomes. Relatively little is known about the precise biochemical mechanisms of metal transport into proximal renal tubular cells. Specific metal transport systems on the brush border membrane have not been identified. Metals enter proximal tubular cells by endocytosis following the binding of the metal itself or a metalloprotein complex such as Cd–metallothionein to the brush border membrane (Foulkes, 1988). This endocytotic process is followed by the intracellular release of the metal from the membrane or the protein–metal complex via lysosomal degradation. The distribution of the released metal will then depend on the presence of various high-affinity binding sites or sinks within the cell (Cain, 1987; Fowler *et al.*, 1987; Fowler, 1989).

Low doses of a number of heavy metals produce a similar response—for example, leakage of glucose and amino acids into urine and diuresis. If the dose of metal is increased, then renal tubular necrosis occurs which can lead to renal shutdown, a marked elevation in blood urea and ultimately the death of the animal. The histological pattern of injury is one of necrotic proximal tubules with dilatation of the tubular lumen which contains proteinaceous casts. This necrosis is thought to be due to a combination of ischaemia secondary to vasoconstriction and a direct cytotoxic action of the heavy metal, since renal ischaemia produced by temporary clamping of the aorta or sustained hypotension causes renal tubular necrosis which is mainly localized to the pars recta region (Glaumann and Trump, 1975; Kreisberg *et al.*, 1976; Ven-

katchalam *et al.*, 1978). The fall in blood pressure is thought to trigger the release of renin, which activates angiotensin, a potent vasoconstrictor. The site of renal necrosis produced by ischaemia is the same as that seen with several heavy metals, which suggests a vascular component in the acute renal failure. However, chronic salt loading of rats, which depletes intrarenal renin prior to administration of a heavy metal, can protect against the functional impairment without affecting the extent of necrosis (DiBona *et al.*, 1971; Flamenbaum *et al.*, 1973), which indicates a role for the direct action of heavy metals on the tubular epithelium. There is also frequently a good correlation between the renal localization of a heavy metal and the site of morphological damage. On the basis of the above it seems plausible to conclude that the nephrotoxicity of heavy metals occurs by two distinct mechanisms: (1) acute renal failure mediated through the release of renin, which can be prevented by depletion of intrarenal renin, and (2) proximal tubular necrosis, which seems to be due to accumulation of the metal in the proximal tubular cells.

Inorganic Mercury

Extensive data are available on the nephrotoxicity of mercuric chloride ($HgCl_2$), primarily because of its use as a model compound to produce acute renal failure in experimental animals. Functional impairment probably results from both vasoconstriction and a direct cytotoxic effect of the metal. Small nephrotoxic doses of $HgCl_2$ produce a selective necrosis histologically located in the pars recta of the proximal tubule (Rhodin and Crowson, 1962; Gritzka and Trump, 1968). The location of the lesion in this region is consistent with the localization of the metal (Taugner *et al.*, 1966). However, as the dose of $HgCl_2$ is increased, the injury extends into the pars convoluta (Rhodin and Crowson, 1962). The basic biochemical mechanism whereby $HgCl_2$ produces renal cellular damage is unclear. $HgCl_2$ will readily react with thiol groups in proteins and enzymes (Webb, 1966) in the latter case, causing inhibition of cellular function. It has, however, been difficult to identify *in vivo* those proteins most sensitive to mercury (Vallee and Ulmer, 1972). The earliest pathological changes following $HgCl_2$ are loss of brush border membranes, dispersion of ribosomes and the clumping of smooth membranes in the cytoplasm (Ganote *et al.*, 1975;

McDowell *et al.*, 1976). These changes are followed by the appearance of vacuoles in the cytoplasm and clumping of nuclear chromatin. Rupture of the plasma membrane and mitochondrial changes are late changes associated with the onset of renal necrosis. Histochemical studies have shown that enzyme activities associated with the brush border membranes—e.g. alkaline phosphatase and 5'-nucleotidase—were decreased as early as 15 min following $HgCl_2$ administration (Zalme *et al.*, 1976). Kempson *et al.* (1977) found a threefold increase in the urinary excretion of alkaline phosphatase, within 3 h of $HgCl_2$ administration. Thus, the changes following $HgCl_2$ are first associated with the brush border membranes and apical vacuole and only later with mitochondria and other structures within the cell. Procedures for the isolation of brush border membrane vesicles from the kidney have been devised and can be used to study transport of substrates (Boumendil-Podevin and Podevin, 1983). These have been used to examine the effect of a number of heavy metals including $HgCl_2$ on membrane function (Berndt and Ansari, 1990). $HgCl_2$ inhibited glucose transport by brush border vesicles at a time when no effect was seen on basolateral membrane vesicle function, which supports the suggested selective action of metals on membrane function.

Organomercurials

The rate of decomposition of organomercurials to form Hg^{2+} appears to reflect the relative nephrotoxicity of these chemicals, the ranking order (from least to most toxic) being $MeHg^+ < EtHg^+ < PhHg^+ < MeoEtHg < Hg^{2+}$ (Magos, 1982). The alkyl mercurials, which decompose quite slowly, can produce renal injury, although their primary action is on the nervous system. For example, the victims of the ethyl mercury epidemics in Iraq showed polyuria or oliguria with urinary casts and excretion of albumin (Jalili and Abbasi, 1961). However, in the large epidemics following methyl mercury exposure the kidneys of even the most severely affected people were spared (Bakir *et al.*, 1973). Nevertheless, chronic administration of methyl mercury will produce renal damage in rats (Fowler, 1972; Magos and Butler, 1972; Klein *et al.*, 1973; Mitsumori *et al.*, 1984) and mice (Mitsumori *et al.*, 1990). Fowler (1972) showed that chronic administration of methyl mercury to rats produced ultrastructural damage to the pars recta of the

proximal tubule which included proliferation of smooth endoplasmic reticulum, degeneration of mitochondria and cellular necrosis. These lesions are also seen following inorganic mercury exposure to rats (Rhodin and Crowson, 1962; Gritzka and Trump, 1968), which supports the view that it is the release of inorganic mercury that is responsible for the renal injury. Chronic administration of methyl mercury in the diet for 2 years to mice caused nephropathy and a high incidence of renal tumours in male mice (Mitsumori *et al.*, 1990).

Mercury-induced Glomerulonephritis

Mercury has been reported to produce an immunologically-mediated glomerulonephritis in both man and experimental animals (Druet *et al.*, 1987a, b). The cause of this glomerulonephritis is not well understood and different mechanisms may operate depending upon species and strain. Administration of $HgCl_2$ 1 mg kg^{-1} three times a week to the Brown Norway strain of rat produces an autoimmune response with an increase of circulating IgE, IgG and antiglomerular basement membrane antibodies; these latter antibodies can be found deposited along the glomerular capillary wall and this deposition is associated with the occurrence of marked proteinuria and the nephrotic syndrome. This autoimmune disease in the Brown Norway rat is not dose-dependent, since lower doses induce the same response, nor does the route of administration (oral, topical or parenteral) influence the response. Also important is the fact that several mercurials ($HgCl_2$, methyl mercury or various pharmaceuticals containing mercury) all induce this response to various degrees. The autoimmune response is under genetic control, the Brown Norway rat being the only strain out of 22 tested which responded. However, glomerular lesions have also been induced with $HgCl_2$ in various other strains of rats, the immune response being different from that seen in the Brown Norway rat. In these strains it was characterized as an immune-complex-type glomerulonephritis with the presence of antinuclear antibodies. It therefore seems that the mechanism responsible for the autoimmune glomerulonephritis can be different, depending on the strain of rat tested. Mercuric chloride will also produce an autoimmune response in rabbits and mice (Roman-Franco *et al.*, 1978; Albini *et al.*, 1982).

Cadmium

Damage to proximal renal tubules is a characteristic feature of long-term, but not acute, cadmium exposure in both humans and experimental animals (Buchet *et al.*, 1980, Lauwerys *et al.*, 1980; Goyer, 1989, and references therein). Acute doses of Cd^{2+} accumulate predominantly in the liver, whereas following chronic exposure in the diet it is the kidney which ultimately accumulates the highest concentration of Cd^{2+}. Cd^{2+} or Cd^{2+}–protein complexes accumulated by hepatic parenchymal cells induce the synthesis of metallothionein, a low-molecular-weight cysteine-rich protein (Kagi *et al.*, 1984), which binds cadmium very avidly. This Cd^{2+}–metallothionein complex is then thought to be very gradually released from the liver and taken up by endocytosis into renal proximal tubular cells, where free Cd^{2+} can be generated due to lysosomal degradation of the complex. The kidney is able to accumulate large concentrations of Cd^{2+}–metallothionein without obvious damage until a critical concentration of between 100 and 200 μg Cd^{2+} g^{-1} renal cortex is attained at which renal injury is initiated (Friberg, 1984). Proximal tubular cells can synthesize metallothionein in response to a rise in intracellular Cd^{2+} concentration and the onset of renal injury may reflect a saturation of all the available binding sites in the cell (both constitutive and induced). The toxic species which precipitates the renal damage is almost certainly free (non-metallothionein-bound) cadmium. It is known that Cd^{2+} *per se* is a very potent inhibitor of enzymes and biochemical pathways (Vallee and Ulmer, 1972; Webb, 1977), whereas Cd^{2+}–metallothionein is not.

Administration of Cd–metallothionein to rats produces a very marked nephrotoxicity at much lower doses than does Cd^{2+} itself. In this acute model considerably more Cd^{2+} is delivered to the kidney than in the low-level chronic situation such that the defence mechanism(s), e.g. metallothionein, may not be adequately induced to afford protection; see Cain (1987) and references therein.

Other Metals

Two other metals which are nephrotoxic should be mentioned—chromium and lead. Acute necrosis of the proximal convoluted tubule has been reported in man following exposure to hexavalent chromium (Cr^{6+}) (Franchini *et al.*, 1978; Jao *et al.*, 1983). Various studies have confirmed these findings in rodents. The primary site of action of Cr^{6+} is on the convoluted portion of the proximal tubule (Evan and Dail, 1974; Berndt, 1975), which is different from that seen with mercury. These morphological findings are supported by functional studies where, for example, glucose reabsorption, a function of the convoluted part of the proximal tubule, is severely affected, which leads to marked glucosuria (Berndt, 1975). As with the other metals, the earliest morphological change following Cr^{6+} administration is to the brush border membrane (Evan and Dail, 1974; Kirschbaum *et al.*, 1981), although how the metal is transported into renal cells is not understood.

Lead is probably the most abundant nephrotoxic metal and because of industrial exposure there are considerable clinical data. Lead-induced nephrotoxicity is characterized morphologically by the presence of lead intranuclear inclusion bodies, karyomegaly, cytomegaly and ultrastructural changes in mitochondria, primarily in the pars recta of the proximal tubule. These changes are accompanied in severe cases by functional changes in glucose, amino acid and phosphate reabsorption (Goyer, 1982). Chronic exposure of experimental animals to lead salts produces a similar spectrum of renal changes to those seen in man (Goyer and Rhyne, 1973). The majority of lead present in blood is located in the red cell; only the lead bound to proteins or ligands which are filterable at the glomerulus is available for uptake into renal cells. As with the other metals, lead may enter renal tubular cells via endocytosis and then be released, presumably from secondary lysosomes. In addition, there is some evidence from *in vitro* studies that lead can enter renal cells by passive diffusion (Vander *et al.*, 1979). Once inside the cell, any free metal will initially bind to certain high-affinity lead-binding proteins which are present in the kidney in high concentrations. These proteins are thought to carry lead into the nucleus, where *de novo* synthesis of a unique acidic protein results in metal precipitation to form the classical lead intranuclear inclusion bodies (Fowler, 1989).

Entry of lead into the nucleus raises the issue of carcinogenesis. Lifetime exposure to high doses in rats and mice produces an increased incidence of renal adenoma and adenocarcinoma

(Choie and Richter, 1980). However, no renal tumours were induced in hamsters or rabbits and the renal tumour incidence in man occupationally exposed to lead is not increased (Goyer, 1982). Mitochondria are extremely sensitive to lead and, following chronic *in vivo* administration, mitochondrial swelling, which is associated with decreased respiratory control, has been reported (Goyer and Krall, 1969; Fowler *et al.*, 1980). Certain enzymes involved in haem biosynthesis are also very sensitive to lead—in particular, δ-aminoaevulinic acid dehydratase. Inhibition of this enzyme *in vivo* results in urinary excretion of δ-aminolaevulinic acid dehydratase. Inhibition of this enzyme *in vivo* results in urinary excretion of δ-aminolaevulinic acid and forms the basis of biological monitoring for lead.

Antineoplastic Agents: Cisplatin

The platinum antitumour drugs—for example, cisplatin (*cis*-dichlorodiammine platinum II)—are widely used for the treatment of a range of cancers (Loehrer and Einhorn, 1984; Rosenberg, 1985) but nephrotoxicity is frequently a side-effect which limits the dosage (Borch, 1987). Clinical manifestation of renal functional impairment includes elevation in blood urea and creatinine, some proteinuria and enzymuria and, in severe cases, the presence of cells and casts in the urine. Electrolyte disturbances are also common, particularly hypomagnesaemia, which may be related to impaired renal tubular absorption (Goldstein and Mayor, 1983; Litterst and Weiss, 1987). Histopathology of the human kidney showed focal tubular necrosis primarily to the distal tubule and collecting ducts, with some dilatation of the convoluted tubules and the presence of casts (Gonzalez-Vitale *et al.*, 1977; Dentino *et al.*, 1978). In experimental animals cisplatin produces marked impairment of renal function (Goldstein *et al.*, 1981; Safirstein *et al.*, 1981); however, the onset of this renal lesion is delayed. Following a single dose to the rat, histopathological alterations were minimal over the first 2 days but by day 3 changes to brush border membranes occurred selectively in the pars recta of the proximal tubule. By day 5 the predominant pattern of injury was widespread necrosis to the pars recta of the proximal tubule, which by day 7 had started to show extensive regeneration (Dobyan *et al.*, 1980). No histopathological changes were seen in

the distal tubule, in contrast to the findings in man.

The mechanisms underlying cisplatin nephrotoxicity and the basis of the delayed onset of toxicity are not fully understood. The platinum moiety *per se* may not be responsible for the nephrotoxicity, as the *trans* isomer of cisplatin is not nephrotoxic (Daley-Yates and McBrien, 1985). Platinum complexes are characterized by their slow rates of ligand substitution in comparison with other metal complexes. When cisplatin is dissolved in water, the more labile chloride ligands are displaced in a stepwise fashion (Figure 6) to form aquated complexes. In plasma at a chloride concentration of 110 mM, cisplatin would be expected to exist predominantly as the neutral dichloro complex. In contrast, the aquated species would be expected to dominate at the lower chloride concentration of the cytosol. An important property of the aquated platinum complexes is that the water ligands are far more reactive than the chloride ligands and are readily replaced by a variety of biological nucleophiles. Cisplatin itself as well as the aquated species will readily react with thiol groups in proteins (enzymes) and with glutathione, cysteine and methionine. Thus, a metabolite of cisplatin rather than the platinum moiety itself may mediate the nephrotoxicity of the drug.

Selenium (Baldew *et al.*, 1989) and a number of thiol ligands such as glutathione, diethyldithi-

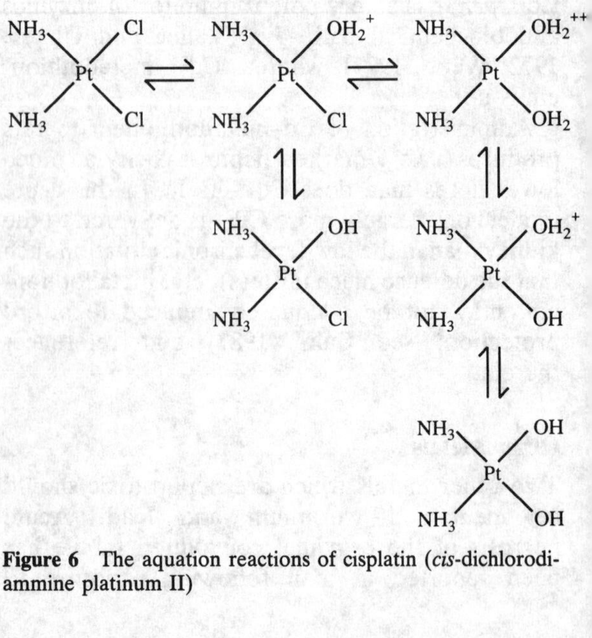

Figure 6 The aquation reactions of cisplatin (*cis*-dichlorodiammine platinum II)

ocarbamate (Borch and Markman, 1989), 4-methylthiobenzoic acid (Boogaard *et al.*, 1991a) and metallothionein (Boogaard *et al.*, 1991b) have been shown to afford some protection against the nephrotoxicity produced by cisplatin. Similarly, administration of cisplatin in hypertonic saline reduced the nephrotoxicity and lowered kidney platinum concentrations in both rat (Litterst, 1981) and man (Borch and Markman, 1989). Thus, the data suggest that the retention of platinum or an aquated platinum complex in renal tubular cells and its reactivity with cellular nucleophiles may account for the nephrotoxicity.

Immunosuppressive Agents: Cyclosporin A

Cyclosporin A is a highly lipophilic, cyclic undecapeptide of fungal origin with potent immunosuppressive activity. It is widely used in renal and bone marrow transplantation. The major clinical problem associated with cyclosporin A usage is nephrotoxicity, which is manifested as a decrease in glomerular filtration rate (GFR). This effect is in part due to altered renal haemodynamics; several studies in experimental animals (Murray *et al.*, 1985; Barros *et al.*, 1987; Whiting and Thomson, 1989) and man (Myers *et al.*, 1984; Curtis *et al.*, 1986) have shown that cyclosporin A causes an increase in renal vascular resistance and a reduction in renal blood flow. Cyclosporin A causes both acute and chronic toxicity, and these may occur by different mechanisms. The mechanisms underlying the altered renal function are unclear but studies have focused on factors that control renal haemodynamics; eicosanoids, the renin–angiotensin system, and the renal sympathetic nervous system (see Whiting and Thomson, 1989, for a review). For example, cyclosporin A increases the level of the vasoconstrictor eicosanoid thromboxane A_2 in rat urine (Kawaguchi *et al.*, 1985; Perico *et al.*, 1986) and administration of thromboxane synthetase inhibitors can ameliorate the nephrotoxicity (Smeesters *et al.*, 1988, Grieve *et al.*, 1990). This treatment does not, however, normalize GFR, which suggests that other factors are also involved. Administration of angiotensin converting enzyme inhibitors such as captopril (Barros *et al.*, 1987) to cyclosporin-treated rats also improved renal function, although evidence for the involvement of angiotensin II in the pathogenesis is not well established. The acute haemodynamic effects of cyclosporin A can also be abolished by the con-comitant infusion of phenoxybenzamine or by renal denervation, which suggests that the increase in renal vascular resistance may be mediated in part by circulating catecholamines and/or the renal sympathetic nervous system (Murray *et al.*, 1985).

Morphological studies of experimental acute cyclosporin A nephrotoxicity have shown early sublethal cellular changes confined to the pars recta of the proximal tubule. However, whether these degenerative changes are a direct result of the chemical or are secondary to the ischaemia is currently unclear (Myers, 1986; Mihatsch *et al.*, 1989).

In vitro studies in which cyclosporin A has been added to renal cells have indicated that the chemical can have a direct action on cellular systems. Cyclosporin A will prevent the uptake of glucose by LLC-PK$_1$ cells (Scoble *et al.*, 1979), which suggests that the glycosuria seen *in vivo* (Grieve *et al.*, 1990) could be due to a direct effect of the chemical. Cyclosporin A has recently been shown to inhibit renal cortical synthesis of DNA, RNA and protein (Buss *et al.*, 1989). Changes in mitochondrial morphology and function following cyclosporin A have also been observed; however, conflicting findings have been reported (Backman *et al.*, 1986; Pfaller *et al.*, 1986; Aupetit *et al.*, 1988; Brokenness and Pfeiffer, 1989) and the precise location of the alteration remains unclear. However, recent studies have shown that cyclosporin A is a potent inhibitor of the mitochondrial matrix enzyme peptidyl-prolyl *cis–trans* isomerase and thereby inhibits mitochondrial membrane transport (Griffiths and Halestrap, 1991). Inhibition of renal mitochondrial peptidyl-prolyl *cis–trans* isomerase may be relevant to the mechanism of nephrotoxicity.

Acute cyclosporin A nephrotoxicity is related to the concentration of the circulating drug. Although it is still unclear as to whether the unchanged drug or a metabolite is responsible for the toxicity, most information supports the view that it is the parent compound (see Burke *et al.*, 1989). There is good evidence that alteration of the hepatic metabolism of cyclosporin A in both man and experimental animals can affect the extent of renal functional impairment. For example, inducers (e.g. phenobarbitone, phenobarbital) or inhibitors (e.g. ketoconazole) of cyclosporin A metabolism will either lower or raise the cyclosporin A circulating blood level and thereby reduce or potentiate the nephrotoxicity (Burke *et al.*, 1989).

Chronic cyclosporin A nephrotoxicity is characterized by an irreversible and potentially progressive nephropathy (Hall *et al.*, 1985; Mihatsch *et al.*, 1989). The haemodynamic consequences are a persistent renal vascular resistance associated with a marked decline in GFR and renal blood flow and systemic hypertension. Morphologically the nephropathy is characterized by a diffuse interstitial fibrosis or striped fibrosis with glomerular and arteriolar thrombi (Mihatsch *et al.*, 1989). Thus cyclosporin A produces marked changes in the renal vasculature and has a direct effect on the proximal tubule, which leads to an alteration in those factors regulating vascular tone.

Therapeutic Agents

Aminoglycosides

Nephrotoxicity related to aminoglycosides is still a major limitation in their clinical use. Kahlmeter and Dahlager (1984) reviewed over 10 000 patients in clinical trials with aminoglycosides and found a frequency of nephrotoxicity resulting from gentamicin and tobramycin of about 14 per cent and from netilmicin and amikacin of 9 per cent. Similarly, Hall *et al.* (1983) reviewed cases of hospital-acquired acute renal failure and showed that 11 per cent of over 2000 cases were attributable to aminoglycosides.

The aminoglycosides consist of two or more amino sugars which are cationic at physiological pH joined by a glycosidic linkage to a hexose nucleus (Figure 7). The clinically relevant aminoglycosides are gentamicin, tobramycin, netilmicin, amikacin, streptomycin and neomycin C. These antibiotics are primarily excreted by glomerular filtration. A small amount of the cationic drug binds to anionic phospholipids (primarily phosphoinositides) located on the brush border membrane of the proximal tubule (Feldman *et al.*, 1982) and the bound aminoglycoside then enters the renal tubular cell by endocytosis and is stored in secondary lysosomes. This process leads to the accumulation of the antibiotic in proximal tubular cells (Silverblatt and Kuehn, 1979; Vandewalle *et al.*, 1981), where it can persist for days. Some aminoglycoside may be absorbed from the basolateral membrane, but

this represents only a minor contribution to the cellular aminoglycoside concentration (Kaloyanides and Pastoriza-Munoz, 1980). Location of the drug in the pars convoluta and pars recta of the proximal tubule is in agreement with the histopathological location of necrosis in this region of the cortex. Ultrastructural examination of the renal cortex showed marked hypertrophy of the lysosomes in the proximal tubule and the presence of concentric lamellar material (myeloid bodies) within these organelles (Kosek *et al.*, 1974; De Broe *et al.*, 1984).

The earliest functional changes are alterations in renal concentrating ability, proteinuria and enzymuria and in acid–base balance (see review by Kaloyanides and Pastoriza-Munoz, 1980; Appel, 1982; Kaloyanides, 1984; Davey and Harpur, 1987; Walker and Duggin, 1988). In addition to renal tubular necrosis, functional and ultrastructural changes occur in the glomerulus, where these polycationic antibiotics may alter the anionic charge of the glomerular endothelium (Appel, 1982; Cojocel *et al.*, 1983).

The biochemical events leading to renal tubular necrosis are believed to be initiated by the binding of the cationic aminoglycoside to negatively charged phospholipid bilayers. This impairs the degradation of phosphatidylinositol by binding to phosphatidylinositol-4,5-bisphosphate and preventing its metabolism to the triphosphate (Kaloyanides and Ramsammy, 1989). The binding of the aminoglycosides also alters the activation and redistribution of the protein kinase C complex. Impairment of phosphoinositide metabolism probably results in altered Ca^{2+} membrane transport, which can lead to cellular injury and slow repair to damaged cell membranes. Calcium has been shown to inhibit the binding of gentamicin to renal membranes, and calcium loading can protect against the renal injury produced by this drug (Humes *et al.*, 1984). Administration of an anionic polypeptide such as poly-L-aspartic acid with gentamicin will protect against the nephrotoxicity (Gilbert *et al.*, 1989; Ramsammy *et al.*, 1989). It is believed that poly-L-aspartic acid binds gentamicin, thereby displacing it from negatively charged membrane lipids and relieving the inhibition of phospholipid metabolism. Gentamicin inhibits oxidative phosphorylation in renal cortical mitochondria *in vitro* (Simmons *et al.*, 1980). This is probably due to altered mitochondrial calcium transport, which can influence mito-

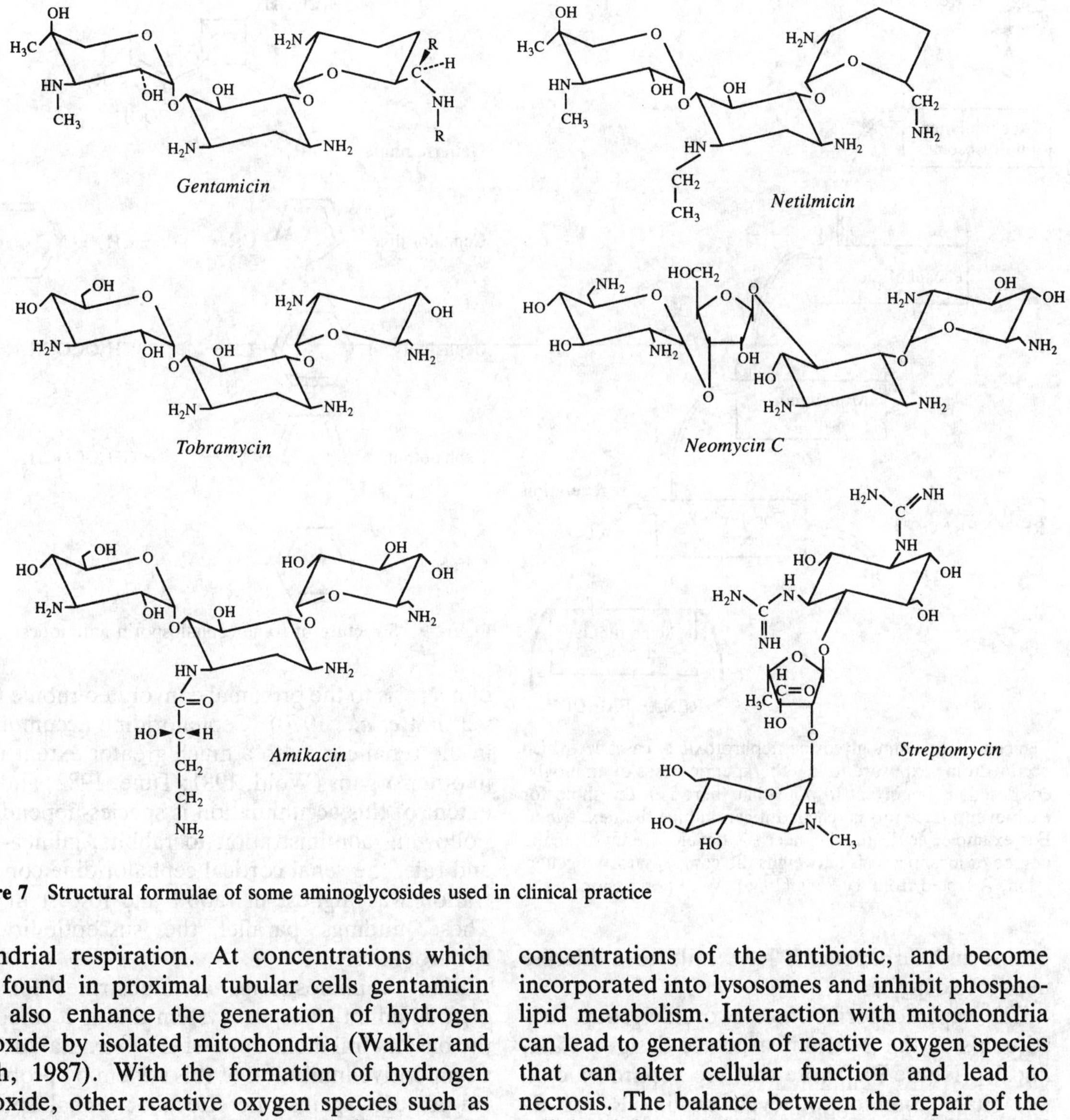

Figure 7 Structural formulae of some aminoglycosides used in clinical practice

chondrial respiration. At concentrations which are found in proximal tubular cells gentamicin will also enhance the generation of hydrogen peroxide by isolated mitochondria (Walker and Shah, 1987). With the formation of hydrogen peroxide, other reactive oxygen species such as superoxide anion and hydroxyl radicals can be produced. Hydroxyl radical scavengers and iron chelators (desferrioxamine) have been shown to protect against the acute renal injury produced by gentamicin (Walker and Duggin, 1988), implicating a role for free radicals in aminoglycoside nephrotoxicity.

Thus the following cascade of events is thought to occur (Tulkens, 1986; Figure 8). The drug is filtered at the glomerulus and enters the tubular lumen, where it binds to apical cell membrane phosphoinositols. These complexes undergo endocytosis, thereby developing high intracellular concentrations of the antibiotic, and become incorporated into lysosomes and inhibit phospholipid metabolism. Interaction with mitochondria can lead to generation of reactive oxygen species that can alter cellular function and lead to necrosis. The balance between the repair of the cellular injury and the extent and duration of the necrosis determines the extent of the renal failure.

β-Lactam Antibiotics

The β-lactam antibiotics include the penicillins, cephalosporins, carbapenems and several structurally related compounds. With the exception of guanylureidopenicillin, none of the penicillins are directly nephrotoxic. However, at least two cephalosporins (cephaloridine and cephaloglycin) and a carbapenem (imipenem) have proved to be highly nephrotoxic, while several other cephalos-

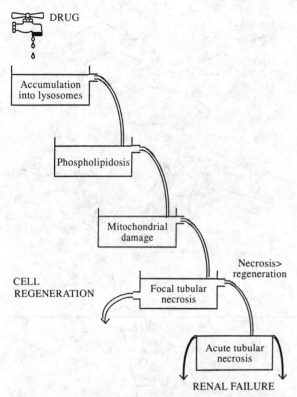

Figure 8   The aminoglycoside nephrotoxicity cascade, which occurs during exposure to low therapeutic doses of aminoglycosides. It is important to note that there is a threshold for each event; once this is reached it can induce the next event. For example, acute tubular necrosis develops only after the degree of focal necrosis outweighs the compensatory regeneration. Adapted from Tulkens (1986). With permission

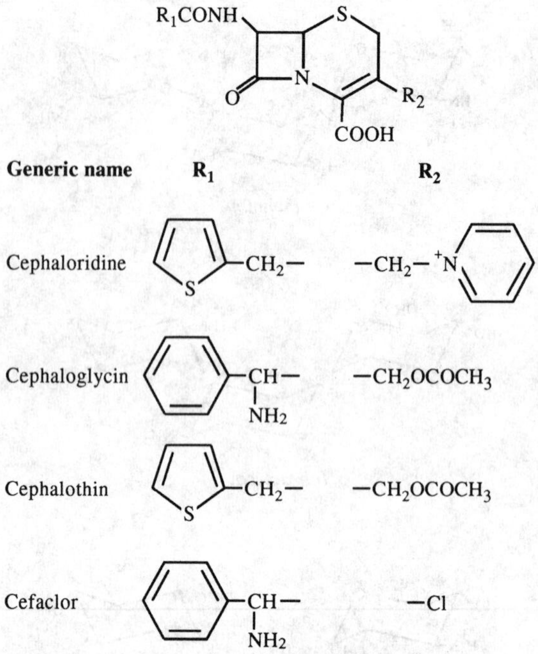

Figure 9   Structure of some cephalosporin antibiotics

porins and carbapenems have mild to moderate nephrotoxicity.

The cephalosporins have two side-group substituents on the β-lactam structure designated R_1 and R_2 (Figure 9). Those that are nephrotoxic do not share common or even similar R_1 or R_2 groups, although no cephalosporin with $R_2 = H$ is nephrotoxic. One common feature of the nephrotoxic cephalosporins is a comparatively unstable bond between the β-lactam ring and the R_2 substituent which favours release of the R_2 group. The acylating potential of the leaving group is an important factor in determining nephrotoxicity (Tune, 1986).

Cephaloridine causes renal tubular injury in both experimental animals and man which is characterized by a decreased GFR, glycosuria, enzymuria and proteinuria. These changes are frequently accompanied by histological evidence

of necrosis to the proximal convoluted tubule (Silverblatt *et al.*, 1970). Cephaloridine accumulates in the renal cortex to a much greater extent than in other organs (Wold, 1981; Tune, 1982) and the extent of this accumulation is species-dependent. Following administration to rabbits, guinea-pigs and rats, the renal cortical cephaloridine concentration was highest in rabbit and lowest in rat. These findings parallel the susceptibility to nephrotoxicity.

Many cephalosporins are substrates for the organic anion transport system that is located on the basolateral membrane of the proximal tubule. Competitive inhibition of this system by probenecid protects against the effects of cephalosporins (Tune and Hsu, 1990). Not only transport into a renal cell but also its rate of efflux into the tubular fluid is an important factor in determining the toxicity. With different β-lactams the renal concentration can vary by several orders of magnitude and it is the area under the concentration–time curve (AUC) in the tubular cell that is important with regard to toxicity. For example, β-lactams that are rapidly and efficiently transported across the basolateral membrane and then rapidly transported from the cell into the tubular lumen have comparatively low AUCs—e.g. cephalothin and cefaclor. Lower rates of secretion can be caused either by restricted movement from the cell into the tubular lumen giving very high AUCs (e.g. cephaloridine) or by little or no secretory transport into the cell, resulting in very low intracellular antibiotic concentrations (e.g. ceftazidime). As a consequence of these widely different intracellular AUCs, cephaloridine is very toxic and ceftazidime non-toxic to the kidney (Tune and Hsu, 1990).

The nephrotoxic β-lactams share two important properties, one or both of which are lacking in the non-toxic β-lactams (Tune, 1986). The first, as discussed above, is the ability to concentrate within cells in the proximal tubule and the second is their acylating potential. For example, the nephrotoxic β-lactam cephaloglycin covalently binds to proteins within renal tubular cells to a far greater extent than do the non-toxic β-lactams such as cephalothin (Browning and Tune, 1983). Consistent with this is the finding that cephaloridine depletes glutathione levels in the renal cortex (Kuo *et al.*, 1983). Prior treatment with agents that deplete glutathione will potentiate the nephrotoxicity of cephaloridine, which suggests that glutathione plays a protective role by scavenging the acylating moiety (Kuo and Hook, 1982). It has been postulated that cephaloridine can generate superoxide anion via a redox cycle, catalysed by NADPH-cytochrome *P*-450 reductase (Kuo *et al.*, 1983; Goldstein *et al.*, 1986). The superoxide anion formed ultimately leads to lipid peroxidation (Cojocel *et al.*, 1985) and the consequent oxidation of reduced glutathione in the renal cortex (Kuo *et al.*, 1983). In support of the lipid peroxidation hypothesis are the findings that animals fed diets deficient in vitamin E or selenium are more susceptible to the nephrotoxicity of cephaloridine. The lipid peroxidative injury mechanism has been shown to be limited mainly to cephaloridine.

Several lines of study suggest that the toxic cephalosporins and imipenem produce their tubular injury by an action on mitochondria. (1) Respiration is reduced in mitochondria isolated from animals dosed with the nephrotoxic β-lactams. (2) The mitochondrial respiratory toxicity is an early event occurring 0.5–1 h after administration of a single dose; (3) it is associated with a marked depletion of cortical ATP by 1.5 h; and (4) it precedes the first indications of ultrastructural damage by 5 h. The resulting lesion resembles that produced by ischaemic injury to the kidney

(Tune, 1986). Recent studies indicate that the nephrotoxic β-lactams selectively acylate and inactivate the transport systems that carry anionic substrates into the mitochondrial matrix (Tune *et al.*, 1988, 1989; Tune and Hsu, 1990).

Paracetamol

Paracetamol (*N*-acetyl-*p*-aminophenol; acetaminophen) is a widely used analgesic and antipyretic drug. It is the major active metabolite of phenacetin, which has been used in analgesic mixtures and implicated in the aetiology of analgesic nephropathy (Duggin, 1980; Bach and Bridges, 1985; Gregg *et al.*, 1989). Large doses of analgesic mixtures containing aspirin and phenacetin given over a prolonged period of time produce medullary interstitial nephritis, papillary damage and chronic renal failure in man (Kincaid-Smith, 1978).

Paracetamol is capable of producing analgesic nephropathy in rats but only when fed at large doses for long periods of time (Molland, 1978). Paracetamol and its conjugates have been shown to concentrate within cells of the inner medulla rather than plasma or renal cortical cells (Duggin and Mudge, 1976). Dehydration of animals leads to a greater concentration of these chemicals in the medulla, which is consistent with the finding of enhanced toxicity during dehydration. Thus, trapping of paracetamol or its metabolites in the countercurrent concentrating mechanism in the medulla may play a role in the medullary toxicity. The NADPH-independent prostaglandin endoperoxidase synthetase (PES) system containing a fatty acid cyclooxygenase and prostaglandin hydroperoxidase is located predominantly in the inner medulla (Spry *et al.*, 1986). This enzyme complex is able to metabolize paracetamol to generate a reactive metabolite that covalently binds to protein (Boyd and Eling, 1981; Mohandas *et al.*, 1981; Moldeus *et al.*, 1982). Glutathione, antioxidants and inhibitors of PES will reduce the covalent binding of paracetamol to rabbit medullary tissue (Mohandas *et al.*, 1981; Moldeus *et al.*, 1982). The conversion of paracetamol to its reactive intermediate by PES probably involves a one-electron oxidation and hydrogen abstraction to form the phenoxy radical of paracetamol, which may undergo a further one-electron oxidation to *N*-acetyl-*p*-benzoquinoneimine (NAPQI). NAPQI can either react with glutathione to form a glutathione conjugate or redox cycle and generate oxidized glutathione (Moldeus *et al.*, 1982) (Figure 10). This redox cycling could cause a marked depletion of glutathione in the inner renal medulla, since these cells already have a low level of reduced glutathione (Mohandas *et al.*, 1984). The concentration of reduced glutathione is critical in preventing the covalent binding of reactive paracetamol metabolites to renal proteins. When the levels of glutathione are reduced, the reactive metabolite of paracetamol will react with cysteine residues in proteins to

form 3-cystein-*S*-yl-4'-hydroxyaniline adducts (Hoffman *et al.*, 1985). Thus, the available evidence suggests that paracetamol toxicity to the inner renal medulla is probably due to its ability to concentrate in that part of the kidney, and undergo activation via the PES system to NAPQI, which subsequently binds to critical protein thiol groups and ultimately results in cell death.

Compound analgesics containing aspirin and phenacetin have a synergistic effect on the devel-

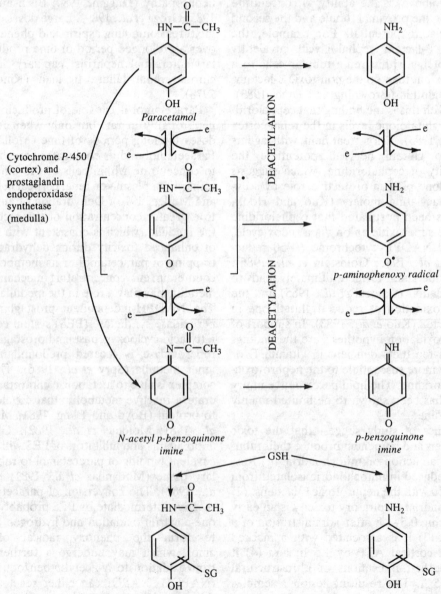

Figure 10   Proposed pathways of activation of paracetamol

opment of chronic medullary necrosis (Molland, 1978). Aspirin is only a modest inhibitor of the cyclooxygenase component of the PES system; however, it is readily deacetylated to salicylate, which is effective at depleting renal glutathione levels (Duggin, 1980). Thus, the presence of other analgesics may potentiate the medullary toxicity of paracetamol.

Following acute overdose of paracetamol, renal cortical necrosis has been reported to occur in patients, in addition to hepatic damage (Boyer and Rouff, 1971). The histological pattern of damage seen with paracetamol resembles that seen with other chemicals that damage the cortex, and includes loss of brush border membranes, mitochondrial changes, sloughing of cells into the tubular lumen and disruption of the basement membrane (Kleinman *et al.*, 1980).

In the liver paracetamol undergoes metabolism primarily via conjugation to form the non-toxic glucuronide or sulphate conjugates. However, a small amount undergoes metabolism via cytochrome *P*-450 to form NAPQI, which can covalently bind to critical thiol groups in proteins. Normally this reactive metabolite is conjugated with reduced glutathione to render it non-toxic; however, following large doses of paracetamol the concentration of reduced glutathione in liver cells can be depleted and then toxicity may ensue (Hinson, 1980; Monks and Lau, 1988). Metabolism of paracetamol to a reactive intermediate is also thought to be required for the induction of renal tubular necrosis (McMurtry *et al.*, 1978). Two different mechanisms for the generation of a reactive metabolite within the renal cortex have been proposed. The first is analogous to that reported for the liver, namely that NAPQI is generated via a pathway mediated by cytochrome *P*-450 mediated (Figure 10) in cells in the proximal convoluted tubule. Evidence for this mechanism includes the demonstration of NADPH-dependent covalent binding of paracetamol to renal cortical microsomes (McMurtry *et al.*, 1978; Mohandas *et al.*, 1981). The second proposed mechanism involves the deacetylation of paracetamol to *p*-aminophenol. *p*-Aminophenol then undergoes one-electron reduction and hydrogen abstraction to form the 4-aminophenoxy radical, which in turn may undergo further oxidation to form *p*-benzoquinoneimine (Figure 10). Evidence to support this mechanism of activation includes identification of *p*-aminophenol as a urinary

metabolite of paracetamol (Newton *et al.*, 1982), and the demonstration of NADPH-independent covalent binding of [^{14}C]-ring-labelled but not [^{14}C]-acetyl-labelled paracetamol to renal homogenates (Newton *et al.*, 1983b). *p*-Aminophenol is about five times more potent as a nephrotoxin than paracetamol, a single dose producing a marked renal tubular necrosis (Davis *et al.*, 1983; Newton *et al.*, 1983a).

Thus, there are at least three separate biochemical pathways for the generation of a radical intermediate from paracetamol. The first is mediated by PES, the second by cytochrome *P*-450 and the third by deacetylation.

Halogenated Hydrocarbons

Chloroform

Chloroform is both hepatotoxic and nephrotoxic in most mammalian species, including man (Pohl, 1979; Davidson *et al.*, 1982). The magnitude of chloroform-induced nephrotoxicity varies with species, and in mice there are unique sex and strain differences. Male ICR mice are susceptible to chloroform-induced renal injury, while female mice are resistant (Smith *et al.*, 1983, 1984). The renal lesions induced in male mice by acute doses of chloroform include swelling of the tubular epithelium, increased renal weight, marked necrosis of the proximal tubular epithelium and the presence of tubular casts (Hewitt, 1956). Changes in renal function include glucosuria, proteinuria, an elevation of blood urea nitrogen and a decreased secretion of organic anions and cations (Plaa and Larson, 1965; Kluwe and Hook, 1978; Rush *et al.*, 1984).

The mechanism of chloroform-induced nephrotoxicity has recently been shown to be similar to that established in the liver—namely generation of phosgene (see Smith, 1986, for a review). Studies with renal cortical slices from rats (Paul and Rubinstein, 1963), and rabbits (Bailie *et al.*, 1984) and renal microsomes from male but not female mice (Smith and Hook, 1984) have demonstrated that [^{14}C]-chloroform is metabolized to [^{14}C]O$_2$, a known degradation product of phosgene. Furthermore, studies in male mouse renal homogenates showed that phosgene can be trapped by two molecules of glutathione to form diglutathione dithiocarbonate, which undergoes further metabolism to 2-oxothiazolidine-4-carboxylic acid

(OTZ) (Branchflower *et al.*, 1984; Pohl *et al.*, 1984). Administration of chloroform to male mice causes renal glutathione depletion (Branchflower *et al.*, 1984), which suggests that phosgene is also formed *in vivo*. Deuterated chloroform is less nephrotoxic than chloroform *in vivo* and in renal slices, which suggests that metabolism is required for toxicity (Ahmadizadeh *et al.*, 1981). The metabolism of chloroform requires NADPH and oxygen and can be inhibited by carbon monoxide and metyrapone (Smith and Hook, 1984). Thus, in the kidney chloroform can undergo oxidative dechlorination catalysed by cytochrome *P*-450 (Bailie *et al.*, 1984) to give phosgene. This can covalently bind to nucleophiles (glutathione or cellular macromolecules) at or near the site of generation and cause cellular injury.

The marked sex and strain differences in chloroform-induced nephrotoxicity in the mouse (for references see Lock, 1987a) appear to be related to the rate of metabolism via cytochrome *P*-450 (Pohl *et al.*, 1984). The concentration of cytochrome *P*-450 is about fivefold greater in the kidneys of male as compared with female mice (Smith *et al.*, 1984). Castration of male mice converted their pattern of cytochrome *P*-450 expression to that seen in females (Henderson *et al.*, 1990) and reduced their susceptibility to chloroform (Smith *et al.*, 1984). Similarly, testosterone pretreatment of female mice resulted in a suppression of the female cytochrome *P*-450 profile and induction of the male pattern (Henderson *et al.*, 1990), thus rendering them susceptible to the nephrotoxic effects of chloroform (Smith *et al.*, 1984). These findings plus those of Clemens *et al.* (1979) suggest that the androgen-induced renal susceptibility to chloroform is mediated via the androgen receptor, which may control the expression of cytochrome *P*-450 genes.

In other species the primary target organ for chloroform is the liver, with nephrotoxicity being either absent or only mild (Kluwe, 1981). This suggests that perhaps the cytochrome *P*-450 which can metabolize chloroform to phosgene is either absent or present in low concentrations in the kidney of these species. Following chronic low level exposure to chloroform an increased incidence of renal tumours has been reported in male rats and, in one study, in male mice (see Davidson *et al.*, 1982). Whether the mechanism of carcinogenicity is the same as that which pro-

duces the acute nephrotoxicity in male mice or is entirely separate is not clear.

Haloalkenes

Hexachloro-1,3-butadiene (HCBD) is a by-product formed during the manufacture of chlorinated solvents. The kidney appears to be the primary target for HCBD toxicity in rats, mice and other mammalian species (Lock, 1988). In the rat HCBD produces a well-defined lesion in the pars recta of the proximal tubule, the earliest morphological changes occurring in the mitochondria (Ishmael *et al.*, 1982). The morphological changes are associated with renal functional impairment such as glucosuria, proteinuria and loss of concentrating ability (Lock, 1988).

Treatment with inducers or inhibitors of hepatic and/or renal cytochrome *P*-450 prior to HCBD administration had little or no effect on the nephrotoxicity (Lock and Ishmael, 1981; Hook *et al.*, 1982). These studies indicated that activation of HCBD by cytochrome *P*-450 was not responsible for the nephrotoxicity. HCBD administration to male rats causes a depletion of hepatic but not renal non-protein sulphydryl content (reduced glutathione). Studies *in vitro* with rat liver microsomes and cytosol indicated that HCBD underwent direct conjugation with glutathione to form *S*-(1,2,3,4,4-pentachloro-1,3-butadienyl)glutathione (PCBD-GSH) (Wolf *et al.*, 1984). Administration of PCBD-GSH, or its further metabolites the cysteine conjugate (PCBD-CYS) or mercapturate (PCBD-NAC), or bile from an HCBD-treated rat, all produced necrosis to the pars recta of the proximal tubule, identical with that seen with HCBD (Nash *et al.*, 1984; Ishmael and Lock, 1986). These data suggest that HCBD undergoes conjugation with glutathione in the liver, and is then eliminated in bile. In the bile and gastrointestinal tract it can undergo further metabolism to the PCBD-CYS. Following enterohepatic circulation, it may be delivered unchanged to the kidney or may be N-acetylated in the liver prior to renal uptake (Figure 11). Metabolism of PCBD-GSH may also occur in the brush border of proximal tubular cells to afford PCBD-CYS, prior to renal cell uptake.

The susceptibility of the proximal tubule to glutathione-derived conjugates of HCBD appears to be related to their ability to accumulate in that part of the nephron. PCBD-NAC appears to

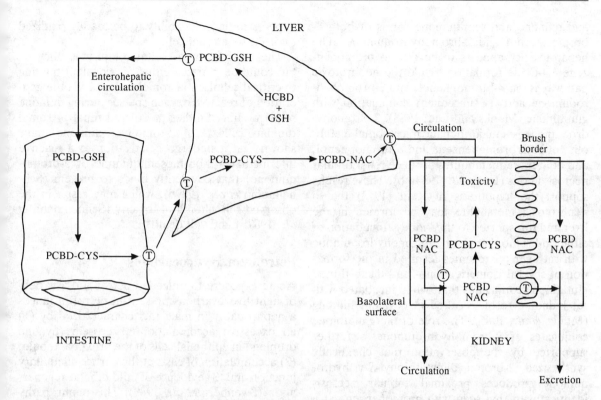

Figure 11 Inter-organ co-operativity and metabolism of hexachloro-1,3-butadiene (HCBD). For a more detailed scheme with supporting evidence see Lock (1987b) and Stevens and Jones (1989). T represents a transport process

enter proximal tubular cells via the organic anion transport system (Lock *et al.*, 1986) and treatment of rats with probenecid (an inhibitor of organic anion transport) completely prevents the accumulation and nephrotoxicity of HCBD or PCBD-NAC (Lock and Ishmael, 1985). Once accumulated within the cell, PCBD-NAC undergoes deacetylation to PCBD-CYS and then becomes covalently bound to renal macromolecules (Figure 11). The enzyme responsible for the activation of PCBD-CYS, and indeed other haloalkene cysteine conjugates, is cysteine conjugate β-lyase. Metabolism of cysteine conjugates by this enzyme results in the formation of pyruvate, ammonia and an electrophilic mercaptan moiety (see reviews by Anders *et al.*, 1988; Lock, 1988; Dekant *et al.*, 1989, 1990) which will readily react with thiols (glutathione), intracellular proteins and nucleic acids (Anders *et al.*, 1988; Dekant *et al.*, 1989, 1990). These latter events are believed to account for the cytotoxicity and carcinogenicity of HCBD. The critical proteins with which the reactive moiety interacts have not been identified, but PCBD-CYS impairs mitochondrial function

in vitro (Jones *et al.*, 1986; Schnellmann *et al.*, 1987a, 1989a), which leads to changes in mitochondrial membrane potential and intracellular calcium levels. Morphological evidence suggests that the mitochondria are early markers of renal damage (Ishmael *et al.*, 1982). The localization of cysteine conjugate β-lyase in the mitochondrion (as well as the cytosol) (Stevens, 1985; Lash *et al.*, 1986) may explain these findings.

Several other halogenated compounds (tri- and perchloroethylene, tetrafluoroethylene, chlorotrifluoroethylene and dichloroacetylene) have been shown to undergo metabolism via conjugation with glutathione, followed by cysteine conjugate β-lyase mediated activation of the cysteine conjugate to produce renal toxicity (Odum and Green, 1984; Green and Odum, 1985; Dekant *et al.*, 1986, 1989).

Bromobenzene

Bromobenzene is both nephrotoxic and hepatotoxic. The metabolism of bromobenzene is complex, with multiple reactive metabolites being formed, including two epoxides, phenol oxide(s) and quinone and semiquinone forms of both 4-bromocatechol and 2-bromohydroquinone. The hepatotoxicity appears to be due to bromobenzene-3,4-oxide formation, while the nephrotoxic pathway is via *o*-bromophenol, and 2-bromohydroquinone and its subsequent conjugation with glutathione (Monks and Lau, 1988). 2-Bromohydroquinone is a major hepatic microsomal metabolite of both bromobenzene and *o*-bromophenol, and both these metabolites produce renal tubular necrosis in rats (Lau *et al.*, 1984a,b). These results support the hypothesis of Reid (1973) that a nephrotoxic metabolite may be formed in the liver and transported to the kidney. Incubation of either *o*-bromophenol or 2-bromohydroquinone with rat liver microsomes resulted in the formation of several isomeric mono- and disubstituted glutathione conjugates that, when incubated with rat kidney cytosol, resulted in covalent binding (Monks *et al.*, 1985). The role of the glutathione conjugates of 2-bromohydroquinone is further supported by the observation that chemically synthesized 2-bromo-(diglutathionyl-*S*-yl)hydroquinone produces proximal tubular necrosis identical with that seen with bromobenzene at a dose which is only 0.3 per cent of that of the parent compound (Monks *et al.*, 1985).

The glutathione conjugates of 2-bromohydroquinone require further metabolism to their cysteine conjugates to exert their toxicity, since metabolism via γ-glutamyltransferase and the subsequent transport into renal cells is critical to the development of the toxicity (Monks *et al.*, 1988; Monks and Lau, 1990a). However, in contrast to HCBD, metabolism via cysteine conjugate β-lyase does not appear to be involved, as inhibition of this enzyme with aminooxyacetic acid gave only minor protection against 2-bromo-(diglutathionyl-*S*-yl)hydroquinone nephrotoxicity (Monks *et al.*, 1988). Thus, the mechanism of transport and intracellular bioactivation of 2-bromo-(diglutathionyl-*S*-yl)hydroquinone appears to be different from that seen with the haloalkene glutathione conjugates. Conversion of the glutathione conjugate of 2-bromohydroquinone to the cysteine conjugate results in the formation of a compound that is more readily oxidized than either 2-bromohydroquinone itself or the glutathione and mercapturate conjugates (Monks and Lau, 1990b). Thus, the nephrotoxicity of 2-bromo-(dicysteinyl-*S*-yl)hydroquinone

appears to lie in its ability to be readily oxidized once inside a renal cell.

The mechanism of cellular injury is unclear, but could be initiated either via covalent binding to critical cellular macromolecules or via the generation of reactive oxygen species during quinone redox cycling. Studies in isolated renal proximal tubular cells with bromohydroquinone have shown that it undergoes activation to a reactive intermediate (2-bromosemiquinone or 2-bromoquinone) that covalently binds to protein (Schnellmann *et al.*, 1989b), which may result in the observed mitochondrial toxicity (Schnellmann *et al.*, 1987b) and cell death.

Petroleum Hydrocarbons

Acute exposure to unleaded petrol and a variety of light hydrocarbons present in petrol produces a nephropathy in male rats characterized by (1) an excessive accumulation of protein (hyaline droplets) in epithelial cells of the proximal tubule, (2) accumulation of casts at the cortico-medullary junction and (3) evidence of mild tubular regeneration (Swenberg *et al.*, 1989). This nephropathy only occurs in male rats; female rats and mice of either sex to not show any renal pathology. A number of chemicals present in unleaded petrol when tested alone have been shown to produce the nephropathy (Halder *et al.*, 1985) and, in particular, 2,2,4-trimethylpentane and decalin have been used as model compounds. Certain other industrial chemicals (1,4-dichlorobenzene, isophorone), natural products (D-limonene) and pharmaceuticals (levamisole) also produce this male-rat-specific nephropathy. Chronic exposure of male rats to unleaded petrol, 1,4-dichlorobenzene, isophorone or D-limonene ultimately leads to the induction of a low incidence of renal adenomas and carcinomas (Swenberg *et al.*, 1989).

Studies on the mechanism of pathogenesis have shown that the protein which accumulates in the proximal tubular cells is α_{2u}-globulin, a low-molecular-weight protein (18 700 daltons) that is synthesized in the liver of adult rats and is freely filtered at the glomerulus (see Swenberg *et al.*, 1989, for references). Female rats excrete less than 1 per cent of the α_{2u}-globulin that male rats excrete (Vandoren *et al.*, 1983). The chemical itself or a metabolite has been shown to bind reversibly to α_{2u}-globulin (Lock *et al.*, 1987; Charbonneau *et al.*, 1989; Lehman-McKeeman *et al.*,

1989) and this chemical–protein complex is then thought to be taken up by the proximal tubular cells (primarily in the S_2 segment) by endocytosis. These complexes appear to be quite resistant to, or impair, lysosomal degradation, which leads to their accumulation as polyangular droplets (Figure 12). Lysosomal overload is thought to lead to individual cellular necrosis which is followed by repair and regeneration (Short *et al.*, 1987, 1989). It has been suggested that a sustained increase in renal cell proliferation can promote initiated cells to form preneoplastic foci and lead to renal neoplasia (Swenberg *et al.*, 1989). The development of the renal toxicity and increased cell proliferation is dependent on the presence of α_{2u}-globulin. The NCI Black–Reiter strain of male rat cannot synthesize α_{2u}-globulin and is refractory to the nephrotoxicity (Ridder *et al.*, 1990). Similarly, other species that do not synthesize the protein do not develop the toxicity. Man does not synthesize α_{2u}-globulin and, by inference, would not be expected to be at risk. However, it is not known whether these hydrocarbons or their metabolites can bind to other low-molecular-weight proteins and, if so, whether the same biochemical events as those observed with α_{2u}-globulin could occur.

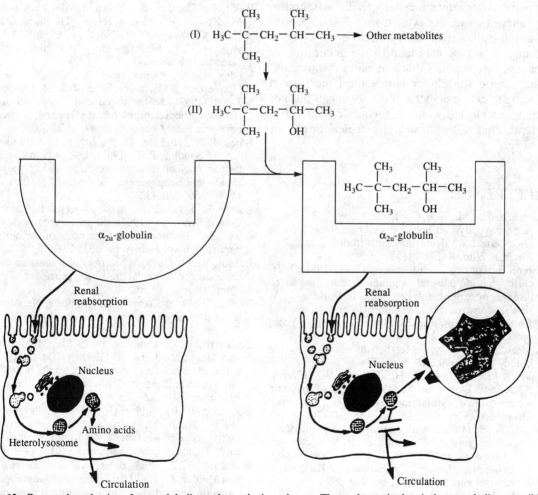

Figure 12   Proposed mechanisms for α_{2u}-globulin nephropathy in male rats. The nephrotoxic chemical or metabolite reversibly binds to α_{2u}-globulin, altering the structure of the protein and decreasing its lysosomal catabolism in S_2 segment renal epithelial cells. This results in α_{2u}-globulin accumulation, lysosomal overload and cytotoxicity. Sustained increases in compensatory cell proliferation associated with chronic exposure result in greater 'fixation' of spontaneous DNA damage and promotion of such initiated cells to renal tumours. From Swenberg *et al* (1989). With permission

SUMMARY

Chemically induced injury to the kidney can occur as a result of the direct effect of a chemical or a metabolite on renal cells or indirectly by altering renal haemodynamics, or by a combination of both. The site along the nephron which is damaged is frequently the site of cellular accumulation of the chemical or a metabolite. Nephrotoxic chemicals may enter renal tubular cells by endocytosis either as the chemical *per se* or a chemical–protein complex. Alternatively, some chemicals are actively transported into renal cells on endogenous transport systems. Once concentrated inside cells, the chemical may be released from its intracellular binding site and cause cytotoxicity. Alternatively, renal specific metabolism by enzymes such as cytochrome *P*-450, prostaglandin endoperoxidase synthetase or cysteine conjugate β-lyase may lead to the generation of reactive electrophiles that can cause cytotoxicity. The precise subcellular biochemical mechanism leading to cytotoxicity for most chemicals has not been established, but mitochondria are frequently, but not exclusively, a critical target for toxicity.

REFERENCES

Ahmadizadeh, M., Kuo, C.-H. and Hook, J. B. (1981). Nephrotoxicity and hepatotoxicity of chloroform in mice: effect of deuterium substitution. *J.Toxicol. Environ. Hlth*, **8**, 104–111

Albini, B., Glurich, I. and Andres, G. A. (1982). Mercuric chloride-induced immunologically mediated diseases in experimental animals. In Porter, G. A. (Ed.), *Nephrotoxic Mechanisms of Drugs and Environmental Toxins*. Plenum, New York, pp. 413–423

Anders, M. W. (1980). Metabolism of drugs by the kidney. *Kidney Int.*, **18**, 636–647

Anders, M. W, Lash, L. H., Dekant, W., Elfarra, A. A. and Dohn, D. R. (1988). Biosynthesis and metabolism of glutathione-S-conjugates to toxic forms. *CRC Crit. Rev. Toxicol.*, **18**, 311–341

Appel, G. B. (1982). Aminoglycoside nephrotoxicity: physiologic studies of the sites of nephron damage. In Whelton, A. and Neu, H. C. (Eds), *The Aminoglycosides: Microbiology, Clinical use and Toxicology*. Marcel Dekker, New York, pp. 269–282

Aupetit, B., Ghazi, A., Blanchouin, N., Toury, R., Shechter, E. and Legrand, J. C. (1988). Impact on energy metabolism of quantitative and functional cyclosporine-induced damage of kidney mitochondria. *Biochim. Biophys. Acta*, **936**, 325–331

Bach, P. H. and Bridges, J. W. (1985). Chemically-induced renal papillary necrosis and upper urothelial carcinoma. *CRC Crit. Rev. Toxicol.*, **15**, 217–439

Bach P. H., Gregg, N. J. and Wachsmuth, E. D. (1987). The application of histochemistry at the light microscope level to the study of nephrotoxicity. In Bach, P. H. and Lock, E. A. (Eds), *Nephrotoxicity in the Experimental and Clinical Situation*, Vol. 1. Martinus Nijhoff, Lancaster, pp. 19–84

Backman, L., Appelkvist, E. L., Brunk, U. and Dallner, G. (1986). Influence of cyclosporin A treatment on intracellular membranes of hepatocytes. *Exptl Mol. Pathol.*, **45**, 31–43

Bailie, M. B., Smith, J. H., Newton, J. F. and Hook, J. B. (1984). Mechanism of chloroform nephrotoxicity: IV, Phenobarbital potentiation of *in vitro* chloroform metabolism and toxicity in rabbit kidneys. *Toxicol. Appl. Pharmacol.*, **74**, 285–292

Bakir, F., Damluji, S. F., Amin-Zaki, L. Murtadha, M., Khalidi, A., Al-Rawi, N. Y., Tikriti, S., Dhahir, H. I., Clarkson, T. W., Smith, J. C. and Doherty, R.A. (1973). Methylmercury poisoning in Iraq. *Science*, **181**, 203–241

Baldew, G. S., Hamer, C. J. A., Van den Los, G., Vermeulen, N. P. E., de Goeji, J. J. M. and McVie, J. G. (1989). Selenium-induced protection against *cis*-diamminedichloroplatinum (II) nephrotoxicity in mice and rats. *Cancer Res.*, **49**, 3020–3023

Bales, J. R., Higham, D. P., Howe, I., Nicholson, J. K. and Sandler, P. J. (1984). Use of high resolution proton nuclear magnetic resource spectroscopy for rapid multi-component analysis of urine. *Clin. Chem.*, **30**, 426–432

Barros, E. J. G., Boim, M. A., Ajzen, H., Ramos, L. O. and Schor, N. (1987). Glomerular haemodynamics and hormonal participation on cyclosporin nephrotoxicity. *Kidney Int.*, **32**, 19–25

Berndt, W. O. (1975). The effect of potassium dichromate on renal tubular transport processes. *Toxicol. Appl. Pharmacol.*, **32**, 40–52

Berndt, W. O. and Ansari, R. A. (1990). Nephrotoxicity of metals: effects on plasma membrane function. *Toxicol. Lett.*, **53**, 87–92

Boogaard, P. J., Lempers, E. L. M., Mulder, G. J. and Meerman, J. H. N. (1991a). 4-Methylthiobenzoic acid reduces cisplatin nephrotoxicity in rats without compromising anti-tumour activity. *Biochem. Pharmacol.* **41**, 369–375

Boogaard, P. J., Mulder, G. J. and Nagelkerke, J. F. (1989). Isolated proximal tubular cells from rat kidney as an *in vitro* model for studies of nephrotoxicity. *Toxicol. Appl. Pharmacol.*, **101**, 144–157

Boogaard, P. J., Slikkerveer, A., Nagelkerke, J. F. and Mulder, G. J. (1991b). The role of metallothionein in the reduction of cisplatin-induced nephrotoxicity by Bi^{3+}-pretreatment in the rat *in vivo* and *in vitro*. Are the antioxidant properties of metallothionein more relevant than platinum binding? *Biochem. Pharmacol.*, **41**, 369–375

Borch, R. F. (1987). The platinum anti-tumour drugs. In Powis, G. and Prough, R. A. (Eds), *Metabolism and Actions of Anti-Cancer Drugs*. Taylor and Francis, London, pp. 163–193

Borch, R. F. and Markman, M. (1989). Biochemical modulation of cisplatin toxicity. *Pharmacol. Ther.*, **41**, 371–380

Boumendil-Podevin, E. F. and Podevin, R. A. (1983). Isolation of brush border and basolateral membranes from rabbit kidney cortex–vesicle integrity and membrane sidedness of the basolateral fraction. *Biochim. Biophys. Acta*, **735**, 86–93

Boyd, J. A. and Eling, T. E. (1981). Prostaglandin endoperoxide synthetase-dependent co-oxidation of acetaminophen to intermediates which covalently bind *in vitro* to rabbit renal medullary microsomes. *J. Pharmacol. Exptl Ther.*, **219**, 659–664

Boyer, T. D. and Rouff, S. L. (1971). Acetaminophen-induced hepatic necrosis and renal failure. *J. Am. Med. Assoc.*, **218**, 440–441

Branchflower, R. V., Nunn, D. S., Highet, R. J., Smith, J. H., Hook, J. B. and Pohl, L. R. (1984). Nephrotoxicity of chloroform: metabolism to phosgene by the mouse kidney. *Toxicol. Appl. Pharmacol.*, **72**, 159–168

Brenner, B. M. and Rector, F. C. Jr. (1986) (Eds). *The Kidney*, 3rd edn, Vols. 1 and 2. Saunders, Philadelphia

Brokenness, K. M. and Pfeiffer, D. R. (1989). Cyclosporin-A-sensitive and insensitive mechanisms produce permeability transition in mitochondria. *Biochem. Biophys. Res. Commun.*, **163**, 561–566

Browning, M. C. and Tune, B. M. (1983). Reactivity and binding of beta-lactam antibiotics in rabbit renal cortex. *J. Pharmacol. Exptl Ther.*, **226**, 640–644

Buchet, J. P., Roels, H., Bernard, A. and Lauwerys, R. (1980). Assessment of renal function of workers exposed to inorganic lead, cadmium or mercury vapour. *J. Occup. Med.*, **22**, 741–750

Burke, M. D., MacIntyre, F., Cameron, D. and Whiting, P. H. (1989). Cyclosporin A metabolism and drug interactions. In Thompson, A. W. (Ed.), *Cyclosporin: Mode of Action and Clinical Application*. Kluwer Academic, Boston, pp. 267–302

Buss, W. E., Stepanek, J. and Bennett, W. M. (1989). A new proposal for the mechanism of cyclosporin A nephrotoxicity. Inhibition of renal microsomal protein chain elongation following in vivo cyclosporin A. *Biochem. Pharmacol.*, **38**, 4085–4093

Cain, K. (1987). Metallothionein and its involvement in heavy metal-induced nephrotoxicity. In Bach, P. H. and Lock, E. A. (Eds), *Nephrotoxicity in the Experimental and Clinical Situation*, Vol. 1. Martinus Nijhoff, Lancaster, pp. 473–532

Charbonneau, M., Strasser, J., Lock, E. A., Turner, M. J. and Swenberg, J. A. (1989). Involvement of reversible binding to α2u-globulin in 1,4-dichlorobenzene-induced nephrotoxicity. *Toxicol. Appl. Pharmacol.*, **99**, 122–132

Choie, D. D. and Richter, G. W. (1980). Effects of lead on the kidney. In Singhal, R. L. and Thomas, J. A. (Eds), *Lead Toxicity*. Urban and Schwarzenberg, Baltimore, pp. 187–212

Clemens, T. L., Hill, R. N., Bullock, L. P., Johnson, W. D., Sultatos, L. G. and Vesell, E. S. (1979). Chloroform toxicity in the mouse: role of genetic factors and steroids. *Toxicol. Appl. Pharmacol.*, **48**, 117–130

Cojocel, C., Dociu, N., Maita, K., Sleight, S. D. and Hook, J. B. (1983). Effects of aminoglycosides on glomerular permeability, tubular reabsorption and intracellular catabolism of the cationic low molecular-weight protein lysozyme. *Toxicol. Appl. Pharmacol.*, **68**, 96–109

Cojocel, C., Hannemann, J. and Baumann, K. (1985). Cephaloridine-induced lipid peroxidation initiated by reactive oxygen species as a possible mechanism of cephaloridine nephrotoxicity. *Biochim. Biophys. Acta*, **834**, 402–410

Curtis, J. J., Luke, R. G., Dubovsky, E., Diethelm, A. G., Whelchel, J. D. and Jones, P. (1986). Cyclosporin in therapeutic doses increases renal allograft vascular resistance. *Lancet*, **ii**, 477–479

Daley-Yates, P. T. and McBrien, D. C. H. (1985). The renal fractional clearance of platinum antitumour compounds in relation to nephrotoxicity. *Biochem. Pharmacol.*, **34**, 1423–1428

Davey, P. G. and Harpur, E. S. (1987). Antibiotics: The experimental and clinical situation. In Bach, P. H. and Lock, E. A. (Eds), *Nephrotoxicity in the Experimental and Clinical Situation*, Vol. 2. Martinus Nijhoff, Lancaster, pp. 643–658

Davidson, I. W. F., Sumner, D. D. and Parker, J. C. (1982). Chloroform: a review of its metabolism, teratogenic, mutagenic and carcinogenic potential. *Drug Chem. Toxicol.*, **5**, 1–87

Davis, J. M., Emslie, K. R., Sweet, R. S., Walker, L. L., Naughton, R. J., Skinner, S. L. and Tange, J. D. (1983). Early functional and morphological changes in renal tubular necrosis due to *p*-aminophenol. *Kidney Int.*, **24**, 740–747

Dawnay, A. B. St. J. and Cattell, W. R. (1987). The measurement of kidney-derived immunologically reactive material in urine and plasma for studying renal integrity. In Bach, P. H. and Lock, E. A. (Eds), *Nephrotoxicity in the Experimental and Clinical Situation*, Vol. 2. Martinus Nijhoff, Lancaster, pp. 593–612

De Broe, M. E., Paulus, G. J., Verpooten, G. A., Roels, F., Buyssens, N., Wedeen, R., Van Hoof, F. and Tulkens, P. M. (1984). Early effects of gentamicin, tobramycin and amikacin on the human kidney. *Kidney Int.*, **25**, 643–652

Dekant, W., Metzler, M. and Henschler, D. (1986). Identification of *S*-1,2,2-trichlorovinyl-*N*-acetylcysteine as a urinary metabolite of tetrachloroethylene: Bioactivation through glutathione conjugation as a possible explanation of its nephrocarcinogenicity. *J. Biochem. Toxicol.*, **1**, 57–72

Dekant, W., Vamvakas, S. and Anders, M. W. (1989). Bioactivation of nephrotoxic haloalkenes by gluta-thione conjugation: Formation of toxic and muta-genic intermediates by cysteine conjugate β-lyase. *Drug Metab. Rev.*, **20**, 43–83

Dekant, W., Vamvakas, S. and Anders, M. W. (1990). Bioactivation of hexachlorobutadiene by glutathione conjugation. *Fd Chem. Toxicol.*, **28**, 285–293

Dentino, M., Luft, F. C., Yum, M. N., Williams, S. D. and Einhorn, L. H. (1978). Long term effect of *cis*-diamminedichloride platinum (CDDP) on renal function and structure in man. *Cancer*, **41**, 1274–1281

DiBona, G. F., McDonald, F. D., Flamenbaum, W. and Oken, D. E. (1971). Maintenance of renal func-tion in salt loaded rats despite severe renal tubular necrosis. *Nephron*, **8**, 205–220

Dobyan, D. C., Levi, J., Jacobs, C., Kosek, J. and Weiner, M. W. (1980). Mechanism of *cis*-platinum nephrotoxicity. II, Morphologic observations. *J. Pharmacol. Exptl Ther.*, **213**, 551–556

Druet, P., Hirsch, F., Pelletier, L., Druet, E., Baran, D. and Sapin, C. (1987a). Mechanisms of chemically-induced glomerulonephritis. In Fowler, B. A. (Ed.), *Mechanisms of Cell Injury: Implications for Human Health*. Wiley, Chichester, pp. 153–173

Druet, P., Jacquot, C., Baran, D., Kleinknecht, D., Fillastre, J. P. and Mery, J. Ph. (1987b). Immunolog-ically mediated nephritis induced by toxins and drugs. In Bach, P. H. and Lock, E. A. (Eds), *Nephrotoxicity in the Experimental and Clinical Situation*, Vol. 2. Martinus Nijhoff, Lancaster, pp. 727–770

Duggin, G. G. (1980). Mechanism in the development of analgesic nephropathy. *Kidney Int.*, **18**, 553–561

Duggin, G. G. and Mudge, G. H. (1976). Analgesic nephropathy: renal distribution of acetaminophen and its conjugates. *J. Pharmacol. Exptl Ther.*, **199**, 1–9

Dworkin, L. D. and Brenner, B. M. (1985). Biophys-ical basis of glomerular filtration. In Seldin, D. W. and Giebisch, G. (Eds), *The Kidney: Physiology and Pathophysiology*. Raven Press, New York, pp. 397–426

Evan, A. P. and Dail, W. G. (1974). The effects of sodium chromate on the proximal tubules of rat kidney: fine structural damage and lysozymuria. *Lab. Invest.*, **30**, 704–715

Feldman, S., Wang, M. Y. and Kaloyanides, J. (1982). Aminoglycosides induce a phospholipidosis in the renal cortex of the rat: an early manifestation of nephrotoxicity. *J. Pharmacol. Exptl Ther.*, **220**, 514–520

Flamenbaum, W., Kotchen, T. A., Nagle, R. and McNeil, J. S. (1973). Effect of potassium on the renin-angiotensin system and $HgCl_2$-induced acute renal failure. *Am. J. Physiol.*, **224**, 305–311

Foulkes, E. C. (1988). On the mechanism of transfer of heavy metals across cell membranes. *Toxicology*, **52**, 263–272

Fowler, B. A. (1972). The morphological effects of dieldrin and methylmercuric chloride on pars recta segments of rat kidney proximal tubules. *Am. J. Pathol.*, **69**, 163–174

Fowler, B. A. (1989). Biological roles of high-affinity metal-binding proteins in mediating cell injury. *Comments Toxicol.* **3**, 27–46

Fowler, B. A., Kimmel, C. A., Woods, J. S., McCon-nell, E. E. and Grant, L. D. (1980). Chronic low level lead toxicity in the rat. III. An integrated assessment of long term toxicity with special refer-ence to the kidney. *Toxicol. Appl. Pharmacol.*, **56**, 59–77

Fowler, B. A., Mistry, P. and Goering, P. L. (1987). Mechanisms of metal-induced nephrotoxicity. In Bach, P. H. and Lock, E. A. (Eds), *Nephrotoxicity in the Experimental and Clinical Situation*, Vol. 2. Martinus Nijhoff, Lancaster, pp. 727–770

Franchini, I., Mutti, A., Cavatorta, A., Corradi, A., Cosi, A., Olivetti, G. and Borghetti, A. (1978). Nephrotoxicity of chromium: remarks on an experi-mental and epidemiological investigation. *Contrib. Nephrol.*, **10**, 98–110

Friberg, L. (1984). Cadmium and the kidney. *Environ. Hlth Perspect.*, **54**, 1–11

Ganote, C. E., Reimer, K. A. and Jennings, R. B. (1975). Acute mercuric chloride nephrotoxicity: an electron microscopic and metabolic study. *Lab. Invest.*, **31**, 633–647

Gartland, K. P. R., Bonner, F. W. and Nicholson, J. K. (1989). Investigations into the biochemical effects of region-specific nephrotoxins. *Mol. Pharmacol.*, **35**, 242–250

Gilbert, D. N., Wood, C. A., Kohlhepp, S. J., Kohnen, P. W., Houghton, D. C., Finkbeiner, H. C., Lindsley, J. and Bennett, W. M. (1989). Poly-aspartic acid prevents experimental aminoglycoside nephrotoxicity. *J. Infect. Dis.*, **159**, 945–953

Glaumann, B. and Trump, B. F. (1975). Studies on the pathogenesis of ischemic cell injury. *Virchows Arch. B Cell Pathol.*, **19**, 303–323

Goldstein, R. S. and Mayor, G. H. (1983). The nephrotoxicity of cisplatin. *Life Sci.*, **32**, 685–690

Goldstein, R. S., Noordewier, B., Bond, J. T., Hook, J. B. and Mayor, G. H. (1981). *Cis*-dichlorodiammi-neplatinum nephrotoxicity: time course and dose response of renal functional impairment. *Toxicol. Appl. Pharmacol.*, **60**, 163–175

Goldstein, R. S., Pasino, D. A., Hewitt, W. R. and Hook, J. B. (1986). Biochemical mechanism of cephaloridine nephrotoxicity: time and concen-tration dependence of peroxidative injury. *Toxicol. Appl. Pharmacol.*, **83**, 261–270

Gonzalez-Vitale, J. C., Hayes, D. M., Cvitkovic, E. and Sternberg, S. S. (1977). The renal pathology in clinical trials of *cis*-platinum (II) diamminedichlor-ide. *Cancer*, **39**, 1362–1371

Gottschalk, C. W., Moss, N. G. and Colindres, R. E. (1985). Neural control of renal function in health and disease. In Seldin, D. W. and Giebisch, G. (Eds), *The Kidney: Physiology and Pathophysiology*. Raven Press, New York, pp. 581–611

Goyer, R. A. (1982). The nephrotoxic effects of lead. In Bach, P. H., Bonner, F. W., Bridges, J. W. and Lock, E. A. (Eds), *Nephrotoxicity: Assessment and Pathogenesis*. Wiley, Chichester, pp. 338–348

Goyer, R. A. (1989). Mechanism of lead and cadmium nephrotoxicity. *Toxicol. Lett.*, **46**, 153–162

Goyer, R. A. and Krall, A. R. (1969). Ultrastructural transformation in mitochondria isolated from kidneys of normal and lead-intoxicated rats. *J. Cell Biol.*, **41**, 393–400

Goyer, R. A. and Rhyne, B. C. (1973). Pathological effects of lead. *Int. Rev. Exptl Pathol.*, **12**, 1–77

Green, T. and Odum, J. (1985). Structure/activity studies of the nephrotoxic and mutagenic action of cysteine conjugates of chloro- and fluoroalkenes. *Chem.–Biol. Interact.*, **54**, 15–31

Greger, R., Lang, F. and Silbernagl, S. (1981). (Eds). *Renal Transport of Organic Substances*. Springer-Verlag, Berlin

Gregg, N. J., Elseviers, M. M., De Broe, M. E. and Bach, P. H. (1989). Epidemiology and mechanistic basis of analgesic-associated nephropathy. *Toxicol. Lett.*, **46**, 141–151

Grieve, E. M., Hawksworth, G. M., Simpson, J. G. and Whiting, P. H. (1990). Effect of thromboxane synthetase inhibition and angiotensin converting enzyme inhibition on acute cyclosporin A nephrotoxicity. *Biochem. Pharmacol.*, **40**, 2323–2329

Griffiths, E. J. and Halestrap, A. P. (1991). Further evidence that cyclosporin A protects mitochondria from calcium overload by inhibiting a matrix peptidyl-prolyl *cis-trans* isomerase. *Biochem. J.*, **274**, 611–614

Gritzka, T. L. and Trump, B. F. (1968). Renal tubular lesions caused by mercuric chloride: Electron microscopic observations of degeneration of the pars recta. *Am. J. Pathol.*, **52**, 1225–1250

Guder, W. G. and Ross, B. D. (1984). Enzyme distribution along the nephron. *Kidney Int.*, **26**, 101–111

Halder, C. A., Holdsworth, C. E., Cockrell, B. Y. and Piccirillo, V. J. (1985). Hydrocarbon nephropathy in male rats: identification of the nephrotoxic components of unleaded gasoline. *Toxicol. Industr. Hlth*, **1**, 67–87

Hall, B. M., Tiller, D. J., Duggin, G. G., Horvath, J. S., Farnsworth, A., May, J., Johnson, J. R. and Shell, A. G. (1985). Post-transplant acute renal failure in cadaver renal recipients treated with cyclosporine. *Kidney Int.*, **28**, 178–186

Hall, S. H., Bushinsky, D. A., Wish, J. B., Cohen, J. J. and Harrington, J. T. (1983). Hospital acquired renal insufficiency: a prospective study. *Am. J. Med.*, **74**, 243–248

Henderson, C. J., Scott, A. R., Yang, C. S. and Wolf, R. C. (1990). Testosterone-mediated regulation of mouse renal cytochrome P-450 isoenzymes. *Biochem. J.*, **266**, 675–681

Hewitt, H. B. (1956). Renal necrosis in mice after accidental exposure to chloroform. *Br. J. Exptl Pathol.*, **37**, 32–39

Hinson, J. A. (1980). Biochemical toxicology of acetaminophen. *Rev. Biochem. Toxicol*, **2**, 103–129

Hoffman, K. J., Streeter, A. J., Axworthy, D. B. and Baille, T. A. (1985). Identification of the major covalent adduct formed *in vitro* and *in vivo* between acetaminophen and mouse liver proteins. *Mol. Pharmacol.*, **27**, 566–573

Hook, J. B., Rose, M. S. and Lock, E. A. (1982). The nephrotoxicity of hexachloro-1:3-butadiene in the rat: Studies of organic anion and cation transport in renal slices and the effect of monoxygenase inducers. *Toxicol. Appl. Pharmacol.*, **65**, 373–382

Humes, H. D., Sastrasinh, M. and Weinberg, J. M. (1984). Calcium is a competitive inhibitor of gentamicin-renal membrane binding interactions and dietary calcium supplementation protects against gentamicin nephrotoxicity. *J. Clin. Invest.*, **73**, 134–147

Ishmael, J. and Lock, E. A. (1986). Nephrotoxicity of hexachlorobutadiene and its glutathione-derived conjugates. *Toxicol. Pathol.*, **14**, 258–262

Ishmael, J., Pratt, I. S. and Lock, E. A. (1982). Necrosis of the pars recta (S3 segment) of rat kidney produced by hexachloro-1:3-butadiene. *J. Pathol.*, **138**, 99–113

Jalili, M. A. and Abbasi, A. H. (1961). Poisoning by ethyl mercury toluene sulphonanilide. *Br. J. Industr. Med.*, **18**, 303–308

Jao, W., Manaligod, J. R., Gerardo, L. T. and Castillo, M. M. (1983). Myeloid bodies in drug-induced acute tubular necrosis. *J. Pathol.*, **139**, 33–40

Jones, T. W., Wallin, A., Thor, H., Gerdes, R. G., Ormstad, K. and Orrenius, S. (1986). The mechanism of pentachlorobutadienylglutathione nephrotoxicity studied with isolated rat renal epithelial cells. *Arch. Biochem. Biophys.*, **251**, 504–513

Kacew, S. (1987). Detection of nephrotoxicity of foreign chemicals with the use of *in vitro* and *in vivo* techniques. In Bach, P. H. and Lock, E. A. (Eds), *Nephrotoxicity in the Experimental and Clinical Situation*, Vol. 2. Martinus Nijhoff, Lancaster, pp. 533–562

Kagi, J. H. R., Vasak, M., Lerch, K., Gilg, D. E. O., Hunziker, P., Bernhard, W. R. and Good, M. (1984). Structure of mammalian metallothionein. *Environ. Hlth Perspect.*, **54**, 93–103

Kahlmeter, G. and Dahlager, J. I. (1984). Aminoglycoside toxicity—a review of clinical studies published between 1975 and 1982. *J. Antimicrob. Chem.*, **13**, (Suppl. A), 9–22

Kaloyanides, G. J. (1984). Aminoglycoside-induced functional and biochemical defects in the renal cortex. *Fund. Appl. Toxicol.*, **4**, 930–943

Kaloyanides, G. J. and Pastoriza-Munoz, E. (1980).

Aminoglycoside nephrotoxicity. *Kidney Int.*, **18**, 571–582

Kaloyanides, G. J. and Ramsammy, L. S. (1989). Aminoglycoside antibiotics inhibit the phosphatidylinositol cascade in renal proximal tubular cells: possible role in toxicity. In Bach, P. H. and Lock, E. A. (Eds), *Nephrotoxicity in vitro to in vivo, Animals to Man*. Plenum, New York, pp. 193–200

Kawaguchi, A., Goldman, M. H., Shapiro, R., Foegh, M. L., Ramwell, P. W. and Lower, R. R. (1985). Increase in urinary thromboxane B₂ in rats caused by cyclosporin. *Transplantation*, **40**, 214–215

Kempson, S. A., Ellis, B. G. and Price, R. G. (1977). Changes in rat renal cortex, isolated plasma membranes and urinary enzymes following the injection of mercuric chloride. *Chem.–Biol. Interact.*, **18**, 217–234

Kincaid-Smith, P. (1978). Analgesic nephropathy. *Kidney Int.*, **13**, 1–4

Kirschbaum, B. B., Sprinkel, F. M. and Oken, D. E. (1981). Proximal tubule brush border alterations during the course of chromate nephropathy. *Toxicol. Appl. Pharmacol.*, **58**, 19–30

Klein, R., Herman, S. P. and Bullock, B. C. (1973). Methyl mercury intoxication in rat kidneys: functional and pathological changes. *Arch. Pathol.*, **96**, 83–90

Kleinman, J. G., Breitenfield, R. V. and Roth, D. A. (1980). Acute renal failure associated with acetaminophen injection: report of a case and review of the literature. *Clin. Nephrol.*, **14**, 201–205

Kluwe, W. M. (1981). The nephrotoxicity of low molecular weight halogenated alkane solvents, pesticides and chemical intermediates. In Hook, J. B. (Ed.), *Toxicology of the Kidney*. Raven Press, New York, pp. 179–226

Kluwe, W. M. and Hook, J. B. (1978). Polybrominated biphenyl-induced potentiation of chloroform toxicity. *Toxicol. Appl. Pharmacol.*, **45**, 861–869

Kosek, J. C., Mazze, R. I. and Cousins, M. J. (1974). Nephrotoxicity of gentamicin. *Lab. Invest.*, **30**, 48–57

Kriesberg, J. I., Bulger, R. E., Trump, B. F. and Nagle, R. B. (1976). Effects of transient hypotension on the structure and function of rat kidney. *Virchows Arch. B Cell Pathol.*, **22**, 121–133

Kuo, C. H. and Hook, J. B. (1982). Depletion of renal glutathione content and nephrotoxicity of cephaloridine in rabbits, rats and mice. *Toxicol. Appl. Pharmacol.*, **63**, 292–302

Kuo, C. H., Maita, K., Sleight, S. D. and Hook, J. B. (1983). Lipid peroxidation: a possible mechanism of cephaloridine-induced nephrotoxicity. *Toxicol. Appl. Pharmacol.*, **67**, 78–88

Lash, L. H., Elfarra, A. A. and Anders, M. W. (1986). Renal cysteine conjugate β-lyase: bioactivation of nephrotoxic cysteine S-conjugates in mitochondrial outer membrane. *J. Biol. Chem.*, **261**, 5930–5935

Lau, S. S., Monks, T. J. and Gillette, J. R. (1984a).

Identification of 2-bromohydroquinone as a metabolite of bromobenzene and 2-bromophenol: Implication for bromobenzene-induced nephrotoxicity. *J. Pharmacol. Exptl Ther.*, **230**, 360–366

Lau, S. S., Monks, T. J., Green, K. E. and Gillette, J. R. (1984b). The role of *ortho*-bromophenol in the nephrotoxicity of bromobenzene. *Toxicol. Appl. Pharmacol.*, **72**, 539–549

Lauwerys, R. and Bernard, A. (1989). Preclinical detection of nephrotoxicity: description of tests and appraisal of health significance. *Toxicol. Lett.*, **46**, 13–29

Lauwerys, R., Roels, H., Bernard, A. and Buchet, J. P. (1980). Renal responses to cadmium in a population living in a non-ferrous area in Belgium. *Int. Arch. Occup. Environ. Hlth*, **45**, 271–274

Lehman-McKeeman, L. D., Rodriguez, P. A., Takigiku, R., Caudill, D. and Fey, M. L. (1989). d-Limonene-induced male rat-specific nephrotoxicity: Evaluation of the association between d-limonene and α2u-globulin. *Toxicol. Appl. Pharmacol.*, **99**, 250–259

Litterst, C. L. (1981). Alterations in the toxicity of *cis*-dichloro-diammineplatinum-II and in tissue localisation of platinum as a function of NaCl concentration in the vehicle of administration. *Toxicol. Appl. Pharmacol.*, **61**, 99–108

Litterst, C. L. and Weiss, R. B. (1987). Clinical and experimental nephrotoxicity of cancer chemotherapeutic agents. In Bach, P. H. and Lock, E. A. (Eds), *Nephrotoxicity in the Experimental and Clinical Situation*, Vol. 2. Martinus Nijhoff, Lancaster, pp. 771–816

Lock, E. A. (1979). The effect of paraquat and diquat on renal function in the rat. *Toxicol. Appl. Pharmacol.*, **48**, 327–336

Lock, E. A. (1987a). Metabolic activation of halogenated chemicals and its relevance to nephrotoxicity. In Bach, P. H. and Lock, E. A. (Eds), *Nephrotoxicity in the Experimental and Clinical Situation*, Vol. 1. Martinus Nijhoff, Lancaster, pp. 429–461

Lock, E. A. (1987b). The nephrotoxicity of haloalkane and haloalkene glutathione conjugates. In DeMatteis, F. and Lock, E. A. (Eds), *Selectivity and Molecular Mechanisms of Toxicity*. Macmillan, London, pp. 59–83

Lock, E. A. (1988). Studies on the mechanism of nephrotoxicity and nephrocarcinogenicity of halogenated alkenes. *CRC Crit. Rev. Toxicol.*, **19**, 23–42

Lock, E. A., Charbonneau, M., Strasser, J., Swenberg, J. A. and Bus, J. S. (1987). 2,2,4-Trimethylpentane-induced nephrotoxicity. II. The reversible binding of a TMP metabolite to a renal protein fraction containing α2u-globulin. *Toxicol. Appl. Pharmacol.*, **91**, 182–192

Lock, E. A. and Ishmael, J. (1981). Hepatic and renal nonprotein sulfhydryl concentration following toxic doses of hexachloro-1,3-butadiene in the rat. The effect of Aroclor 1254, phenobarbitone or SKF 525A treatment. *Toxicol. Appl. Pharmacol.*, **57**, 79–87

Lock, E. A. and Ishmael, J. (1985). Effect of the organic acid transport inhibitor probenecid on renal cortical uptake and proximal tubular toxicity of hexachloro-1,3-butadiene and its conjugates. *Toxicol. Appl. Pharmacol.*, **81**, 32–42

Lock, E. A., Odum, J. and Ormond, P. (1986). Transport of *N*-acetyl-*S*-pentachloro–1,2-butadienylcysteine by rat renal cortex. *Arch. Toxicol.*, **59**, 12–15

Loehrer, P. J. and Einhorn, L. H. (1984). Cisplatin. *Am. J. Int. Med.*, **100**, 704–713

McDowell, E. M., Nagle, R. B., Zalme, R. C., McNeil, J. S., Flamenbaum, W. and Trump, B. F. (1976). Studies on the pathophysiology of acute renal failure: I. Correlation of ultrastructure and function in the proximal tubule of the rat following administration of mercuric chloride. *Virchows Arch. B Cell Pathol.*, **22**, 173–196

McMurtry, R. J., Snodgrass, W. R. and Mitchell, J. R. (1978). Renal necrosis, glutathione depletion and covalent binding after acetaminophen. *Toxicol. Appl. Pharmacol.*, **46**, 87–100

Magos, L. (1982). Mercury-induced nephrotoxicity. In Bach, P. H., Bonner, F. W., Bridges, J. W. and Lock, E. A. (Eds), *Nephrotoxicity: Assessment and Pathogenesis*. Wiley, Chichester, pp. 325–337

Magos, L. and Butler, W. H. (1972). Cumulative effects of methylmercury dicyandiamide given orally to rats. *Fd Cosmet. Toxicol.*, **10**, 513–517

Maunsbach, A. B., Olsen, T. S. and Christensen, E. (1980) (Eds). *Functional Ultrastructure of the Kidney*. Academic Press, London

Mihatsch, M. J., Thiel, G. and Ryffel, B. (1989). Cyclosporin A: action and side effects. *Toxicol. Lett.*, **46**, 125–139

Mitsumori, K., Hirano, M., Veda, K. and Shirasu, K. (1990). Chronic toxicity and carcinogenicity of methylmercury chloride in B6C3F1 mice. *Fund. Appl. Toxicol.*, **14**, 179–190

Mitsumori, K., Maita, K. and Shirasu, K. (1984). Chronic toxicity of methylmercury chloride in rats: pathological study. *Japan. J. Vet. Sci.*, **46**, 549–557

Mohandas, J., Duggin, G. G., Horvath, J. S. and Tiller, D. J. (1981). Metabolic oxidation of acetaminophen (paracetamol) mediated by cytochrome P-450 mixed function oxidase and prostaglandin endoperoxidase synthetase in rabbit kidney. *Toxicol. Appl. Pharmacol.*, **61**, 252–259

Mohandas, J., Marshall, J. J., Duggin, G. G., Horvath, J. S. and Tiller, D. J. (1984). Differential distribution of glutathione and glutathione related enzymes in rabbit kidney. *Biochem. Pharmacol.*, **33**, 1801–1807

Moldeus, P., Andersson, B., Rahimtula, A. and Berggren, M. (1982). Prostaglandin synthetase catalyzed activation of paracetamol. *Biochem. Pharmacol.*, **31**, 1363–1368

Molland, E. A. (1978). Experimental renal papillary necrosis. *Kidney Int.*, **13**, 5–14

Moller, J. V. and Sheikh, M. I. (1983). Renal organic anion transport system: pharmacological, physiological and biochemical aspects. *Pharmacol. Rev.*, **34**, 315–358

Monks, T. J., Highet, R. J. and Lau, S. S. (1988). 2-Bromo-(diglutathion-*S*-yl) hydroquinone nephrotoxicity. Physiological, biochemical and electrochemical determinants. *Mol. Pharmacol.*, **34**, 492–500

Monks, T. J. and Lau, S. S. (1988). Reactive intermediates and their toxicological significance. *Toxicology*, **52**, 1–53

Monks, T. J. and Lau, S. S. (1990a). Nephrotoxicity of quinol/quinone-linked S-conjugates. *Toxicol. Lett.*, **53**, 59–67

Monks, T. J. and Lau, S. S. (1990b). Glutathione conjugation, γ-glutamyl transpeptidase and the mercapturic acid pathway as modulators of 2-bromohydroquinone oxidation. *Toxicol. Appl. Pharmacol.*, **103**, 557–563

Monks, T. J., Lau, S. S., Highet, R. J. and Gillette, J. R. (1985). Glutathione conjugates of 2-bromohydroquinone are nephrotoxic. *Drug Metab. Dispos.*, **13**, 553–559

Mudge, G. H. (1982). Analgesic nephropathy: renal distribution and drug metabolism. In Porter, G. A. (Ed.), *Nephrotoxic Mechanisms of Drugs and Environmental Toxins*. Plenum, New York, pp. 209–225

Murray, B. M., Paller, M. S. and Ferris, T. F. (1985). Effect of cyclosporin administration on renal haemodynamics in conscious rats. *Kidney Int.*, **28**, 767–774

Myers, B. D. (1986). Cyclosporine nephrotoxicity. *Kidney Int.*, **30**, 964–974

Myers, B. D., Ross, J., Newton, L., Luetscher, J. and Perloth, M. (1984). Cyclosporin associated chronic nephropathy. *New Engl. J. Med.*, **311**, 699–705

Nash, J. A., King, L. J., Lock, E. A. and Green, T. (1984). The metabolism and disposition of hexachloro-1:3-butadiene in the rat and its relevance to nephrotoxicity. *Toxicol. Appl. Pharmacol.*, **73**, 124–137

Newton, J. F., Bailie, M. B. and Hook, J. B. (1983b). Acetaminophen nephrotoxicity in the rat. Renal metabolic activation *in vitro*. *Toxicol. Appl. Pharmacol.*, **70**, 433–447

Newton, J. F., Kuo, C. H., Gemborys, M. W., Mudge, G. H. and Hook, J. B. (1982). Nephrotoxicity of *p*-aminophenol, a metabolite of acetaminophen in the Fischer 344 rat. *Toxicol. Appl. Pharmacol.*, **65**, 336–344

Newton, J. F., Yoshimoto, M., Bernstein, J., Rush, G. F. and Hook, J. B. (1983a). Acetaminophen nephrotoxicity in the rat. I. Strain differences in nephrotoxicity and metabolism. *Toxicol. Appl. Pharmacol.*, **69**, 291–306

Odum, J. and Green, T. (1984). The metabolism and

nephrotoxicity of tetrafluoroethylene in the rat. *Toxicol. Appl. Pharmacol.*, **76**, 306–318

Paul, B. B. and Rubinstein, D. (1963). Metabolism of carbon tetrachloride and chloroform by the rat. *J. Pharmacol. Exptl Ther.*, **141**, 141–148

Perico, N., Zoja, C., Benigni, A., Ghilardi, F., Gualandris, I. and Remuzzi, G. (1986). Effect of short-term cyclosporin administration in rats on renin-angiotensin and thromboxane A$_2$: possible relevance to the reduction on glomerular filtration rate. *J. Pharmacol. Exptl Ther.*, **239**, 229–235

Pfaller, W., Kotanko, P. and Bazzanella, A. (1986). Morphological and biochemical observations in rat nephron epithelia following cyclosporin A. *Clin. Nephrol.*, **25**, Suppl. 1, S105–S110

Plaa, G. L. and Larson, R. E. (1965). Relative nephrotoxic properties of chlorinated methane, ethane and ethylene derivatives in mice. *Toxicol. Appl. Pharmacol.*, **7**, 37–44

Pohl, L. R. (1979). Biochemical toxicology of chloroform. *Rev. Biochem. Toxicol.*, **1**, 79–107

Pohl, L. R., George, J. W. and Satoh, H. (1984). Strain differences in chloroform-induced nephrotoxicity: different rates of metabolism of chloroform to phosgene by the mouse kidney. *Drug Metab. Dispos.*, **12**, 304–308

Price, R. G. (1982). Urinary enzymes, nephrotoxicity and renal disease. *Toxicology*, **23**, 99–134

Ramsammy, L. S., Josepovitz, C., Lane, B. P. and Kaloyanides, G. J. (1989). Polyaspartic acid protects against gentamicin nephrotoxicity in the rat. *J. Pharmacol. Exptl Ther.*, **250**, 149–153

Reid, W. D. (1973). Mechanism of renal necrosis induced by bromobenzene or chlorobenzene. *Exptl Mol. Pathol.*, **19**, 197–214

Rhodin, A. E. and Crowson, C. N. (1962). Mercury nephrotoxicity in the rat. *Am. J. Pathol.*, **41**, 297–313

Ridder, G. M., Von Bargen, E. C., Alden, C. L. and Parker, R. D. (1990). Increased hyaline droplet formation in male rats exposed to decalin is dependent on the presence of α2u-globulin. *Fund. Appl. Toxicol.*, **15**, 732–743

Roch-Ramel, F. and Weiner, I. M. (1980). Renal urate excretion: factors determining the action of drugs. *Kidney Int.*, **18**, 665–676

Roman-Franco, A. A., Turiello, M., Albini, B., Ossi, E., Milgrom, F. and Andres, G. A. (1978). Anti-basement membrane antibodies and antigen-antibody complexes in rabbits injected with mercuric chloride. *Clin. Immunol. Immunopathol.*, **9**, 464–481

Rosenberg, B. (1985). Fundamental studies with cisplatin. *Cancer*, **55**, 2303–2316

Rush, G. F., Smith, J. H., Newton, J. F. and Hook, J. B. (1984). Chemically-induced nephrotoxicity: role of metabolic activation. *CRC Crit. Rev. Toxicol.*, **13**, 99–160

Safirstein, R., Miller, P., Dikman, S., Lyman, N. and Shapiro, C. (1981). Cisplatin nephrotoxicity in rats:

defect in papillary hypertonicity. *Am. J. Physiol.*, **241**, F175-F185

Schnellmann, R. G., Cross, T. J. and Lock, E. A. (1989a). Pentachlorobutadienyl-L-cysteine uncouples oxidative phosphorylation by dissipating the proton gradient. *Toxicol. Appl. Pharmacol.*, **100**, 498–505

Schnellmann, R. G., Ewell, F. P. Q., Sgambati, M. and Mandel, L. J. (1987b). Mitochondrial toxicity of 2-bromohydroquinone in rabbit renal proximal tubules. *Toxicol. Appl. Pharmacol.*, **90**, 420–426

Schnellmann, R. G., Lock, E. A. and Mandel, L. J. (1987a). A mechanism of S-(1,2,3,4,4-pentachloro-1,3-butadienyl)-L-cysteine toxicity to rabbit renal proximal tubules. *Toxicol. Appl. Pharmacol.*, **90**, 513–521

Schnellmann, R. G., Monks, T. J., Mandel, L. J. and Lau, S. S. (1989b). 2-Bromohydroquinone-induced toxicity to rabbit renal proximal tubules: The role of biotransformation, glutathione and covalent binding. *Toxicol. Appl. Pharmacol.*, **99**, 19–27

Scoble, J. E., Senoir, J. C. M., Chou, P., Varghese, Z., Sweny, P. and Moorhead, J. F. (1979). *In vitro* cyclosporin toxicity. *Transplantation*, **47**, 647–650

Seldin, D. W. amd Giebisch, G. (1985) (Eds). *The Kidney: Physiology and Pathophysiology*, Vols 1, 2. Raven Press, New York

Short, B. G., Burnett, V. L., Cox, M. G., Bus, J. S. and Swenberg, J. A. (1987). Site-specific renal cytotoxicity and cell proliferation in male rats exposed to petroleum hydrocarbons. *Lab. Invest.*, **57**, 564–577

Short, B. G., Burnett, V. L. and Swenberg, J. A. (1989). Elevated proliferation of proximal tubule cells and localisation of accumulated α2u-globulin in F-344 rats during chronic exposure to unleaded gasolene or 2,4,4,-trimethylpentane. *Toxicol. Appl. Pharmacol.*, **101**, 414–431

Silverblatt, F. J. and Kuehn, C. (1979). Autoradiography of gentamicin uptake by the rat proximal tubular cells. *Kidney Int.*, **15**, 335–345

Silverblatt, F., Turek, M. and Bulger, R. (1970). Nephrotoxicity due to cephaloridine: a light and electron microscopic study in rabbits. *J. Infect. Dis.*, **122**, 33–44

Simmons, C. F., Bogusky, R. T. and Humes, H. D. (1980). Inhibitory effects of gentamicin on renal mitochondrial oxidative phosphorylation. *J. Pharmacol. Exptl Ther.*, **214**, 709–715

Smeesters, C., Chaland, P., Giroux, L., Moutquin, J. M., Etienne, P., Douglas, F., Corman, J., St-Louis, G. and Daloze, P. (1988). Prevention of acute cyclosporin A nephrotoxicity by a thromboxane synthetase inhibitor. *Trans. Proc.*, **20**, (Suppl. 2), 663–669

Smith, J. H. (1986). Role of renal metabolism in chloroform nephrotoxicity. *Comments Toxicol.*, **1**, 125–144

Smith, J. H. and Hook, J. B. (1984). Mechanism of chloroform nephrotoxicity. III. Renal and hepatic microsomal metabolism of chloroform in mice. *Toxicol. Appl. Pharmacol.*, **73**, 511–524

Smith, J. H., Maita, K., Sleight, S. D. and Hook, J. B. (1983). Mechanism of chloroform toxicity. I. Time course of chloroform toxicity in male and female mice. *Toxicol. Appl. Pharmacol.*, **70**, 467–479

Smith, J. H., Maita, K., Sleight, S. D. and Hook, J. B. (1984). Effect of sex hormone status on chloroform nephrotoxicity and renal mixed function oxidases in mice. *Toxicology.*, **30**, 305–316

Spry, L. A., Zenser, T. V. and Davis, B. B. (1986). Bioactivation of xenobiotics by prostaglandin H synthase in the kidney: Implication for therapy. *Comments Toxicol.*, **1**, 109–123

Stevens, J. L. (1985). Cysteine conjugate β-lyase activities in rat kidney cortex. Subcellular localisation and relationship to the hepatic enzyme. *Biochem. Biophys. Res. Commun.*, **129**, 499–504

Stevens, J. L. and Jones, D. P. (1989). The mercapturic acid pathway: biosynthesis, intermediary metabolism and physiological disposition. In Dolphin, D., Poulson, R. and Avramovic, O. (Eds), *Glutathione: Chemical, Biochemical and Medical Aspects*, Part B. Wiley, New York, pp. 45–85

Stonard, M. D. (1987). Proteins, enzymes and cells in urine as indicators of the site of renal damage. In Bach, P. H. and Lock, E. A., *Nephrotoxicity in the Experimental and Clinical Situation*, Vol. 2. Martinus Nijhoff, Lancaster, pp. 563–592

Stonard, M. D. (1990). Assessment of renal function and damage in animal species. *J. Appl. Toxicol.*, **10**, 267–274

Swenberg, J. A., Short, B. G., Borghoff, S., Strasser, J. and Charbonneau, M. (1989). The comparative pathobiology of α2u-globulin nephropathy. *Toxicol. Appl. Pharmacol.*, **97**, 35–46

Taugner, R., Winkel, K. and Iravani, J. (1966). Zur Lokalisation der Sublimatanreicherung in der Rattenniere. *Virchows Arch. Pathol. Anat.*, **340**, 369–388

Tisher, C. C. (1976). Anatomy of the kidney. In Brenner, B. B. and Rector, F. C. Jr (Eds), *The Kidney*, Saunders, Philadelphia, p. 5.

Tulkens, P. M. (1986). Experimental studies on nephrotoxicity of aminoglycosides at low doses. *Am. J. Med.*, **80**, (Suppl 6B), 105–114

Tune, B. M. (1982). Nephrotoxicity of cephalosporin antibiotics. Mechanisms and modifying factors. In Porter, G. A. (Ed.), *Nephrotoxic Mechanisms of Drugs and Environmental Toxins*. Plenum, New York, pp. 151–164

Tune, B. M. (1986). The nephrotoxicity of cephalosporin antibiotics—structure-activity relationships. *Comments Toxicol.*, **1**, 145–170

Tune, B. M., Fravert, D. and Hsu, C.-Y. (1989). The oxidative and mitochondrial toxic effects of cephalosporin antibiotics in the kidney. A comparative study of cephalosporin and cephaloglycin. *Biochem. Pharmacol.*, **38**, 795–802

Tune, B. M. and Hsu, C.-Y. (1990). Mechanisms of beta-lactam antibiotic nephrotoxicity. *Toxicol. Lett.*, **53**, 81–86

Tune, B. M., Sibley, R. K. and Hsu, C.-Y. (1988). The mitochondrial respiratory toxicity of cephalosporin antibiotics. An inhibitory effect on substrate uptake. *J. Pharmacol. Exptl Ther.*, **245**, 1054–1059

Vallee, B. L. and Ulmer, D. D. (1972). Biochemical effects of mercury, cadmium and lead. *Ann. Rev. Biochem.*, **41**, 92–128

Vander, A. J., Mouw, D. R., Cox, J. and Johnson, B. (1979). Lead transport by renal slices and its inhibition by tin. *Am J. Physiol.*, **236**, F373-F378

Vandewalle, A., Farman, N., Morin, J. P., Fillastre, J. P., Hatt, P.-Y. and Bonvalet, J.-P. (1981). Gentamicin incorporation along the nephron: autoradiographic study on isolated tubules. *Kidney Int.*, **19**, 529–539

Vandoren, G., Mertens, B., Heyns, W., Van Baelen, H., Rombauts, W. and Verhoeven, G. (1983). Different forms of α2u-globulin in male and female rat urine. *Eur. J. Biochem.*, **134**, 175–181

Venkatchalam, M. A., Bernard, D. B., Donohoe, J. F. and Levinsky, N. G. (1978). Ischemic damage and repair in the rat proximal tubule: differences among the S1, S2 and S3 segments. *Kidney Int.*, **14**, 31–49

Walker, P. D. and Shah, S. V. (1987). Gentamicin enhanced production of hydrogen peroxide by renal cortical mitochondria. *Am. J. Physiol.*, **253**, C495-C499

Walker, R. J. and Duggin, G. C. (1988). Drug nephrotoxicity. *Ann. Rev. Pharmacol. Toxicol.*, **28**, 331–345

Webb, J. L. (1966). Mercurials. In Webb, J. L. (Ed.), *Enzyme and Metabolic Inhibitors*, Vol. 2. Academic Press, New York, pp. 729–983

Webb, M. (1977). Metabolic targets of toxicity. In Brown, S. S. (Ed.), *Clinical Chemistry and Chemical Toxicology of Metals*. Elsevier/North Holland Biomedical Press, Amsterdam, pp. 51–64

Weiner, I. M. (1985). Organic acids and bases and uric acid. In Seldin, D. W. and Giebisch, G. (Eds), *The Kidney: Physiology and Pathophysiology*, Vol. 2. Raven Press, New York, pp. 1703–1724

Whiting, P. H. and Thomson, A. W. (1989). Pathological effects of cyclosporin A in experimental models. In Thomson, A. W. (Ed.), *Cyclosporin: Mode of Action and Clinical Application*. Kluwer, Boston, pp. 303–323

Wold, J. S. (1981). Cephalosporin nephrotoxicity. In Hook, J. B. (Ed.), *Toxicology of the Kidney*. Raven Press, New York, pp. 251–266

Wolf, R. C., Berry, P. N., Nash, J., Green, T. and Lock, E. A. (1984). Role of microsomal and cytosolic glutathione S-transferases in the conjugation of hexachlorol:3-butadiene and its possible relevance to toxicity. *J. Pharmacol. Exptl Ther.*, **228**, 202–208

Yuen, C.-T., Corbett, C. R. R., Kind, P. R. N., Thompson, A. E. and Price, R. G. (1987). Isoenzymes of urinary *N*-acetyl β-ᴅ glucosaminidase in patients with renal transplants. *Clin. Chim. Acta*, **164**, 339–350

Zalme, R. C., McDowell, E. M., Nagle, R. B., McNeil, J. S., Flamenbaum, W. and Trump, B. F. (1976). Studies on the pathophysiology of acute renal failure. II. A histochemical study of the proximal tubule of the rat following administration of mercuric chloride. *Virchows Arch. B Cell Pathol.*, **22**, 197–216

FURTHER READING

Bernard, A. and Lauwerys, R. R. (1991). Proteinuria: changes and mechanisms of toxic nephropathies. *Critical Reviews in Toxicology*, **21**, 373–404

Commandeur, J. N. M. and Vermeulen, N. P. E. (1992). Molecular and biochemical mechanisms of chemically induced nephrotoxicity: a review. In Marnett, L. J. (Ed.), *Frontiers in Molecular Toxicology*, American Chemical Society, Washington DC

Hook, J. B. and Goldstein, R. S. (1993). *Toxicology of the Kidney*. 2nd edn. Raven Press, New York

Seldin, D. W. and Giebisch, G. (1985). Renal Pharmacology. In *The Kidney*. Raven Press, New York, pp. 2097–2162

22 Systemic Pulmonary Toxicity

James P. Kehrer

INTRODUCTION

An increasing number of drugs and chemicals are being identified which produce lung damage following systemic administration. Many of these compounds exhibit a remarkable selectivity for lung tissue, while others damage the lung in conjunction with other organs. The organ specificity of some lung toxins can be altered by modifying the route of administration or inhibiting certain enzyme pathways. Several reviews have appeared which discuss details of the toxicity of most of these chemicals (Kehrer and Kacew, 1985; Cooper et al., 1986; Yost et al., 1989; Israel-Biet et al., 1991; Martin, 1991).

Sites of Lung Injury

The lung is a heterogeneous organ containing over 40 different cell types (Sorokin, 1970). Each of these cells is a potential site of toxic damage, although in practice only a few are significant foci for systemic lung toxins. This relative selectivity is a consequence of various factors, including uptake (both active and passive), metabolism, (different cells contain different enzymes and/or isozymes) (Baron et al., 1988), cellular defence systems and relative exposure (for example, endothelial cells see more of a blood-borne toxin). Lung tissue can also be specifically targeted by certain xenobiotics because the concentration of oxygen available (pO_2, 100 mmHg at the alveolar level) is up to 100 times greater than in other tissues and can facilitate redox cycling and/or other oxidative processes initiated by several lung-toxic xenobiotics.

Among the most prominent lung cells attacked by various toxins are the capillary endothelial cells, non-ciliated bronchiolar epithelial cells (Clara cells), ciliated bronchiolar epithelial cells, and both type I and type II alveolar epithelial cells. Damage to any lung cell results in a sequence of events culminating in either repair, death or some abnormal state. The tissue pathology associated with cell damage and repair includes alveolar and interstitial oedema, inflammation, the deposition of excess or abnormal collagen (fibrosis), the breakdown of connective tissue (emphysema) and the loss of mechanisms designed to clear foreign substances from bronchi and alveoli. This sequence of events appears to be controlled by various cytokines (Brandes and Finkelstein, 1990; Kelley, 1990) either released into the interstitial space or via cell–cell interactions. This latter factor is particularly important in terms of epithelial cell–fibroblast interactions which control lung repair processes and the development of fibrosis (Adamson et al., 1990; Witschi, 1991). It also appears likely that cytokines such as tumour necrosis factor and interleukin I participate in protecting lung tissue from oxidative injury (Berg et al., 1990).

GENERAL MECHANISMS OF INJURY AND METHODS OF ASSESSING LUNG DAMAGE

The lung was once considered to do nothing more than exchange gases and other volatile materials between the blood and the environment. Today it is realized that the lung also serves as an important site for metabolism of certain xenobiotics as well as endogenous substances, including phospholipids, serotonin, angiotensin and other vasoactive substances. This metabolic activity, along with its massive surface area, cellular heterogeneity and the fact that it receives virtually the entire output of the heart, has made the lung a particularly common target organ for toxicity.

Although specific mechanisms by which the lung is targeted for injury are not established for many toxins, some general principles have been developed. Systemically administered xenobiotics can damage lung tissue as the result of direct toxicity or following metabolic activation (Boyd, 1982). This activation can occur in the lung itself, or in other tissues followed by transport of the toxic species to the lung. The parent molecule or activated metabolites can produce damage by covalent binding, redox cycling, changing ion gradients, depleting energy or a variety of other mechanisms. These concepts are illustrated in Figure 1.

The heterogeneous nature of lung tissue has resulted in the development of a variety of techniques to assess and quantify injury. Each method has advantages and disadvantages, and the choice is usually based on the type of toxin being used, the expected injury and convenience. For example, the end-result of many toxic insults to lung tissue is fibrosis. The presence or absence of damaged cells and fibrotic tissue (which consists of excess and abnormal collagen) can be assessed histopathologically. More commonly, fibrosis is assessed by measuring total lung hydroxyproline, an amino acid which is found primarily in collagen and can be quantified by a simple colorimetric assay (Witschi *et al.*, 1985).

Other methods which have been used to assess lung damage include measurements of vascular permeability (i.e. using ^{125}I-labelled albumin, which is trapped in lung tissue as permeability increases), oedema (i.e. wet/dry weight ratios), respiratory rates, changes in the composition of bronchoalveolar lavage fluid (i.e. enzyme leakage or infiltrating cells) (Henderson, 1989), the clearance of inhaled particles, morphometric analysis and a number of biochemical parameters, including RNA and DNA synthesis (Witschi, 1975). This last measure has proved to be a useful means of quantifying lung cell proliferation, and provides an indirect index of the extent of the initial injury (Kehrer and Witschi, 1980; Martin and Witschi, 1985). Analysing lung tissue by autoradiography following the administration of radioactive thymidine has also proved to be useful in determining the kinetics of proliferation of different lung cell types following a toxic insult.

An unresolved problem with quantifying lung injury is how best to express the data. Changes seen when biochemical data are expressed per lung may disappear when expressed per mg protein or DNA because of toxin-induced changes in lung size. Problems can also occur since some lesions are quite focal and changes may not be evident when analysing whole lung or examining a limited number of tissue sections.

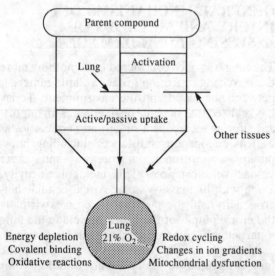

Figure 1 Mechanisms of organ selectivity by systemic lung toxins. A parent compound can directly attack lung tissue or be metabolically activated by the lung or other tissues. The activated metabolite and/or the parent compound may be actively or passively accumulated in lung tissue. Once in the lung, the toxic species may disrupt various functions by covalent binding, redox cycling, oxidative reactions or other unknown mechanisms. These reactions may deplete cellular energy, change ion gradients or disrupt mitochondrial function, thereby producing further cell injury

SYSTEMIC LUNG TOXINS

Paraquat

Background

Paraquat (1,1'-dimethyl-4,4'-bipyridylium dichloride) was first synthesized in 1882 and has been used as a redox indicator (under the name 'methyl viologen') in chemical laboratories since 1933. Its herbicidal properties were discovered in 1959, and since 1962 paraquat has been marketed in over 130 countries as a highly effective contact herbicide (Smith, 1987). The first detailed report of lung toxicity in humans appeared in 1966 (Bullivant). Since that time, numerous accidental and intentional cases of paraquat toxicity have been reported, and intensive research has been conducted to elucidate the mechanisms and test potential treatments for this fatal toxin.

Pathology

Paraquat is a highly water-soluble substance (Figure 2). Aqueous solutions of this chemical are irritating to most biological systems. Oral ingestion usually results in lesions of the mucosal lining of the mouth and throat as well as nausea

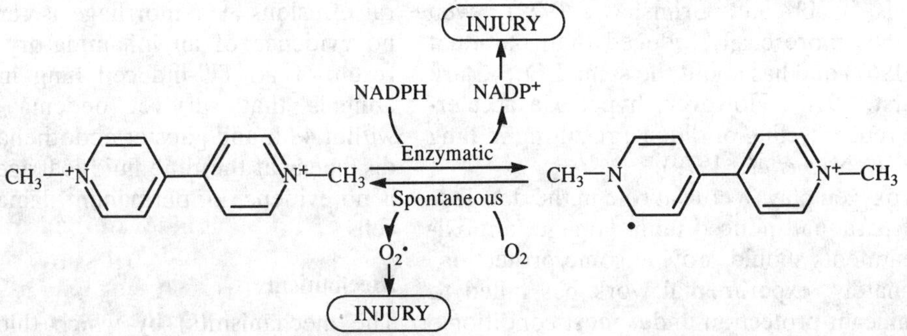

Figure 2 Paraquat redox cycling. Paraquat is actively accumulated by lung tissue, where it is reduced by cellular reductases, which results in the depletion of NADPH. In the presence of oxygen the reduced form of paraquat spontaneously donates an electron to oxygen, which results in the formation of the superoxide anion

and vomiting (Fairshter *et al.*, 1976). Systemic symptoms of toxicity such as diarrhoea and decreased kidney function rapidly ensue, but, unless a massive dose has been ingested, usually disappear in a day or so and the patient looks and feels well. This is deceiving, however, as within a week it becomes apparent that severe lung damage is gradually developing.

Although some species differences are evident, experimental studies in animals treated parenterally or orally with single or multiple doses of paraquat have revealed extensive lung damage characterized by destructive and proliferative phases which are independent of each other (Smith, 1987). During the destructive phase, damage to type I and II alveolar epithelial cells is the first morphological change observed. Damage to the pulmonary capillaries can be seen within 48 h but is much less extensive. There is also some early necrosis of terminal bronchiolar cells.

The destructive stage is associated with alveolar and interstitial oedema and the collapse of lung parenchyma. During the proliferative phase, which is not always preceded by the destructive phase, cells migrate into the alveolar spaces. Many of these mature into fibroblasts and synthesize the excess and abnormal collagen characteristic of intraalveolar fibrosis seen in paraquat poisoning. Although research has concentrated on the lung lesion produced following systemic paraquat treatments, this herbicide is also toxic to the lung when inhaled or instilled intratracheally. The lesion produced is very similar to that following parenteral treatments (Popenoe, 1979; Wyatt *et al.*, 1981).

Mechanisms

The actual mechanism by which paraquat damages the lung is not known despite almost three decades of intensive research. Paraquat will readily accept an electron from NADPH and, under aerobic conditions, is rapidly reoxidized, with the resultant formation of the superoxide or other oxygen radicals (Figure 2). This reaction sequence could lead to cell damage from NADPH depletion (Ilett *et al.*, 1974; Rose *et al.*, 1976; Witschi *et al.*, 1977), free radical generation and lipid peroxidation (Bus *et al.*, 1976), or some combination of these factors. Most data now favour the loss of NADPH as a central factor in cell death. This could result directly from NADPH depletion or be a secondary consequence of impairing the numerous pathways dependent on this vital cofactor (Smith, 1987).

The pulmonary specificity of paraquat is due to its active uptake into the lung and the availability of high concentrations of oxygen relative to other tissues (Rose *et al.*, 1974). Oxygen rapidly reoxidizes paraquat reduced by endogenous enzyme systems. The reoxidation process is accelerated by hyperoxia and slowed by hypoxia, thereby increasing or decreasing the toxicity of paraquat (Fisher *et al.*, 1973; Rhodes *et al.*, 1976). The uptake process occurs via diamine and polyamine transport systems located in the alveolar epithelial and Clara cells of the bronchioles. These systems take up paraquat because of the critical distance between quaternary nitrogens. Diquat (1,1'-ethylene-2,2'-bipyridylium), a closely related herbicide, is not accumulated by lung tissue (Rose and Smith, 1977) and does not produce significant lung damage under normoxic conditions (Cobb and Grimshaw, 1979), even though it is more easily reduced than paraquat (Boon, 1967) and has about the same LD_{50} (Clark and Hurst, 1970). However, hyperoxia accelerates the redox cycling of diquat, resulting in lung damage (Kehrer *et al.*, 1979).

Since oxygen plays a crucial role in the development of paraquat-induced lung damage, antioxidant treatments should provide some protection. Unfortunately, experimental work has failed to find significant protection under most conditions, and treatment continues to rely on adsorbents to prevent paraquat absorption from the gastrointestinal tract, and haemoperfusion or haemodialysis to remove circulating paraquat. The identification of the specific lung system involved in actively accumulating paraquat suggests that its inhibition may provide a new therapeutic strategy (Smith, 1987), but this has not yet been established clinically, and paraquat poisoning remains a serious and often fatal toxicity.

Thioureas

Background

Substances such as phenylthiourea and α-naphthylthiourea (ANTU) produce massive pulmonary oedema and pleural effusion in rats (Dieke *et al.*, 1947). The toxicity of low doses of ANTU is quite specific for the lung (Cunningham and Hurley, 1972) and it has been a popular model for investigations on the pathophysiology of pulmonary oedema. Lethal doses of ANTU range from as low as 7 mg kg^{-1} in some rat strains to over 4000 mg kg^{-1} in primates and chickens (Dieke and Richter, 1946). No human cases of toxicity have been reported. This tremendous species variation, and the fact that rats will consume ANTU in food, led to the development and use of this chemical as a rat poison.

Lung Pathology

The morphological changes associated with thiourea-induced lung toxicity are primarily localized to the endothelium of pulmonary capillaries and venules (Cunningham and Hurley, 1972). Light and electron microscopic studies reveal the presence of gaps in the endothelium and occasional blebs protruding into the capillary lumen. These gaps allow the leakage of a fibrin-rich fluid, resulting in pulmonary oedema and often massive pleu-

ral effusions. Haemorrhage is rare and there is no evidence of an inflammatory response as a result of ANTU-induced lung injury. In those animals that survive, oedema resolves itself within 48 h and gaps at endothelial cell junctions disappear at the time fluid leakage ceases. There is no evidence of permanent damage to any lung cells.

Mechanisms

The mechanism(s) by which thioureas damage lung tissue are not known. The presence of specific binding sites has been suggested, and differences in the number of these binding sites might explain the observed age and species variations in pulmonary toxicity (Gregory, 1970). More likely, metabolic activation may be a necessary step in the pulmonary toxicity of the thioureas. ANTU and thiourea covalently bind to lung proteins, while a non-toxic oxygen analogue, α-naphthylurea, does not (Boyd and Neal, 1976; Hollinger *et al.*, 1976). Binding occurs *in vitro* under both aerobic and anaerobic conditions, is associated with a reduction in glutathione (GSH), and is temperature dependent, which suggests that it is mediated by an activated metabolite (Boyd and Neal, 1976; Hollinger and Giri, 1979; Lee *et al.*, 1980). *In vivo*, both binding and toxicity are increased in animals depleted of GSH, which suggests that GSH may have reacted with and subsequently detoxified a reactive species.

Although most evidence supports the metabolic activation of thioureas to a lung-toxic, oxidative species, this issue has not been completely resolved. Treatments with mixed-function oxidase inducers or inhibitors have no consistent effects on ANTU-induced lung toxicity (Van den Brink *et al.*, 1976). Pulmonary flavin monooxygenase (FMO) can metabolize various thioureas to oxidation products which are more reactive than the parent molecule (Nagata *et al.*, 1990), and it is possible that FMO is the source of the toxic species.

Treatment of rats with small, non-lethal doses of the thioureas produces a profound tolerance to subsequent doses as much as 100 times the usual lethal level. This resistance, known as tachyphylaxis, appears within 24 h, lasts up to 2 weeks, is dose-related, and can be induced with some non-toxic, structurally related, antithyroid drugs (Richter, 1946; Carroll and Noble, 1949). Tachyphylaxis is accompanied by decreases in covalent binding which could be due to changes in specific binding sites or metabolic activation (Boyd and Neal, 1976). However, a more thorough understanding of tachyphylaxis is needed to determine the mechanism of thiourea-induced lung injury.

Butylated Hydroxytoluene

Background

Butylated hydroxytoluene (3,5-di-*t*-butyl-4-hydroxytoluene, BHT) is a synthetic antioxidant widely used as an additive to foods, drugs and cosmetics. At low doses it is relatively non-toxic to all mammalian species. At doses several orders of magnitude greater than those ingested by humans a variety of toxic effects have been identified, including damage to heart, reproductive organs, adrenal glands, kidney and liver. BHT also produces a haemorrhagic disorder in rats and a diffuse lung lesion which occurs only in mice (Witschi *et al.*, 1989). Although receiving the U.S. designation 'Generally Recognized as Safe' (GRAS) in 1958, BHT is highly lipid-soluble and has been detected in human fat stores (Malkinson, 1983). Recent studies have questioned its safety, since it can induce hepatic mixed function oxidase activity and appears capable of both promoting and inhibiting tumour development (Witschi *et al.*, 1989). These findings have prompted the recommendation that the acceptable daily intake (as defined by the FAO/WHO) be decreased from 0.5 mg kg^{-1} day^{-1} to 0.05 mg kg^{-1} day^{-1} (Haigh, 1986).

Lung Pathology

The pulmonary toxicity attributed to BHT was first reported by Marino and Mitchell (1972). Doses over 250 mg kg^{-1} produced a reversible thickening of the alveolar septa, congestion and disruption of the normal lung architecture. Subsequent work with BHT showed that damage occurred following either oral or intraperitoneal dosing (Witschi and Lock, 1978) and, although there were large differences in the LD$_{50}$ values between different strains of mice, lung damage was seen at similar doses (Kehrer and DiGiovanni, 1990).

Detailed histological and cell kinetic analyses have been performed on the lung lesion produced in mice treated with BHT. These studies have shown that type I alveolar epithelial cells are the initial site of damage (Adamson *et al.*, 1977). Vacuolization and necrosis of type I cells is evident within 24 h, resulting in a virtually denuded alveolar basement membrane. This is followed sequentially by type II alveolar cell proliferation and the re-epithelialization of the alveolar surface (Hirai *et al.*, 1977). Capillary endothelial cells also begin to display damage one day after treatment with BHT (Smith, 1984) and they, along with the interstitial cells, begin to divide and infiltrate damaged areas of the lung on day 5 (Adamson *et al.*, 1977). At low BHT doses, repair of the lesion is virtually complete within 2 weeks and there is no residual damage. At higher doses there is deposition of excess collagen characteristic of pulmonary fibrosis.

Pulmonary fibrosis, which results from treatment of mice with single high doses of BHT, is moderate but persists for at least 1 year (Haschek *et al.*, 1982). Several agents, including oxygen (Haschek and Witschi, 1979), radiation (Haschek *et al.*, 1980) and prednisolone (Kehrer *et al.*, 1984), enhance the development of fibrosis in BHT-treated mice. The mechanism responsible for this enhancement is not clear, although it has been proposed that inhibition of the normal re-epithelialization process is a major factor (Haschek and Witschi, 1979).

Mechanism

The local production of an activated metabolite via mixed function oxidase activity appears to be the mechanism by which BHT damages mouse lung tissue (Kehrer and Witschi, 1980). A phenolic ring with a methyl group at the 4-position and an *ortho*-alkyl group are needed to produce lung damage. Mizutani *et al.* (1982) suggested that quinone methides or closely related metabolites play a role in BHT-induced lung damage. However, rats are able to produce as much or more quinone methide than mice but are resistant to the lung-damaging effects. Recently, studies by Bolton and Thompson (1991) showed that the unique species and organ specificity of BHT is caused by the greater capacity of mice than that of rats to metabolize BHT to its *t*-butyl hydroxylated form followed by a two-electron oxidation of this metabolite to the corresponding quinone methide, which is highly lung-toxic (Figure 3).

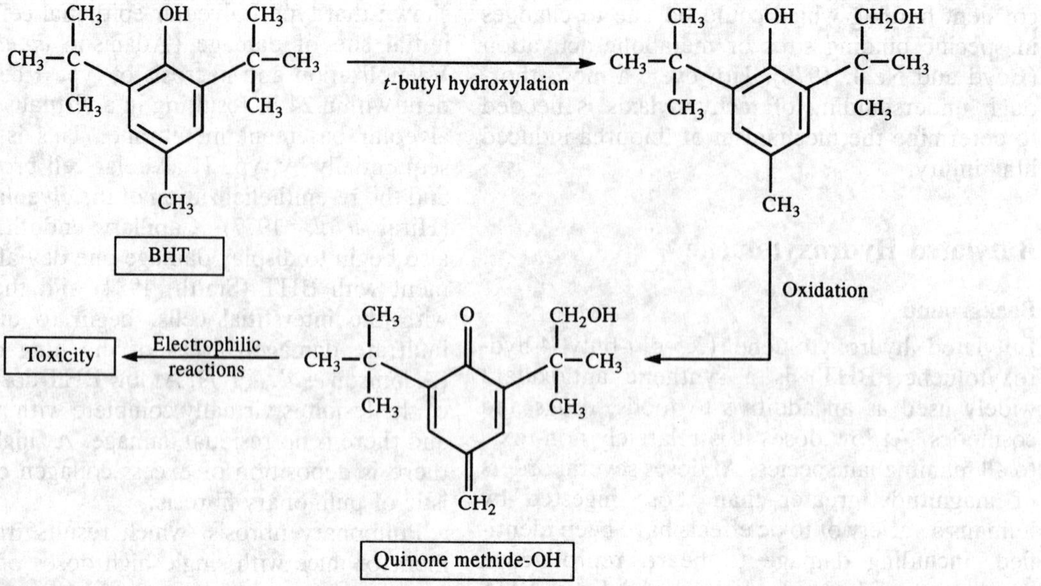

Figure 3 Metabolic activation of butylated hydroxytoluene (BHT). BHT is hydroxylated by lung tissue. The hydroxylated metabolite is oxidized, forming the highly electrophilic quinone methide. This material, which is a major product in mouse lung tissue, is responsible for the observed toxicity

Trialkylphosphorothioates

Background

The trialkylphosphorothioates are a group of chemicals found as contaminants in commercial preparations of many organophosphorus pesticides. At low doses these compounds produce a delayed mortality in mammals, following oral or parental administration, which is independent of cholinesterase inhibition (Imamura and Gandy, 1988). Pathological changes are most prominent in the lung (Aldridge *et al.*, 1979; Verschoyle and Cabral, 1982), and damage to this organ is believed to be the cause of death (Imamura and Gandy, 1988).

O,O,S-trimethyl phosphorothioate   *O,S,S-trimethyl phosphorodithioate*

Figure 4 Structures of two lung-toxic phosphorothioates

Lung Pathology

Two of the most extensively studied trialkylphosphorothioates that produce lung damage are *O,O,S*-trimethyl phosphorothioate (OOS) and *O,S,S*-trimethyl phosphorodithioate (OSS) (Figure 4). All strains of rats tested exhibit evidence of damage to type I alveolar epithelial cells within 48 h of treatment with OOS, often resulting in the exposure of the basement membrane (Dinsdale *et al.*, 1982; Verschoyle and Cabral, 1982). This is followed by hypertrophy and hyperplasia of type II alveolar epithelial cells and massive interstitial thickening. Inflammatory cells infiltrate the alveolar interstitium, and alveolar oedema develops with the presence of numerous alveolar macrophages. If the animal survives this acute phase, the alveolar oedema resolves and lung morphology returns to a nearly normal appearance within 14 days. At the bronchiolar level, significant alterations to Clara cells are evident (Gandy *et al.*, 1984a,b). However, recent data suggest that the changes seen in Clara cells are not a direct toxic effect of the phosphorothioates but rather an indirect response to injury elsewhere in the lung (Imamura and Gandy, 1988). Similar damage, with the additional development of a moderate level of fibrosis, is produced in mice treated with OSS (Kehrer *et al.*, 1986a; Kehrer and Lee, 1987), indicating that the response to phosphorothioates is not species-specific.

Mechanisms

The mechanisms by which trialkylphosphoro-thioates damage lung tissue are not fully established. The phosphorothioates are well absorbed and distributed throughout the body. There is no accumulation by lung relative to other tissues. These compounds are extensively metabolized to reactive species, and the depletion of glutathione (Imamura and Hasegawa, 1984) and covalent binding of labelled material to lung, liver, kidneys and ileum has been found (Imamura and Gandy, 1988). Although the specific source and nature of the toxic species is not known, some studies have suggested that the active toxicant is an *S*-oxide (Nemery and Aldridge, 1988a). Metabolism probably occurs in various organs, and lung specificity is the result of relatively high rates of activation by this organ coupled with low rates of detoxication (Nemery and Aldridge, 1988b). Pretreatment of rats with inhibitors or inducers of drug metabolism protects against OOS-induced lung injury (Imamura *et al.*, 1983). Less consistent results were observed in mice (Kehrer *et al.*, 1986a), and the overall role of mixed-function oxidase (MFO) activity in phosphorothioate metabolism and toxicity is uncertain.

Furans

Background

There are at least 13 furan derivatives that have been found to produce acute lung damage in laboratory animals following inhalation or systemic administration (Boyd, 1980). These chemicals occur naturally in the environment, are used in industry and research, and are found in food and drugs. Most investigations on lung damage following systemic treatment with furans have focused on 4-ipomeanol, which is the 'lung oedema factor' in sweet potatoes infected with the common mould *Fusarium solani*, and nitro-furantoin, a widely used urinary tract antiseptic.

Lung Pathology

Pulmonary bronchiolar necrosis is the primary pathological lesion seen with systemic exposure to various lung-toxic furans. 4-Ipomeanol produces massive alveolar or interstitial oedema, pleural effusion, congestion and haemorrhage in animals within 6–24 h after its systemic administration (Boyd, 1980). Functional changes are caused by swelling and necrosis of the Clara cells (Sabo *et al.*, 1983). Damage is restricted to these cells in the smaller airways at low doses but includes the cells of the larger airways at higher doses.

Although the lung is the primary site of 4-ipomeanol-induced toxicity in most vertebrates, damage occurs in the livers of hamsters and the kidneys of mice (Dutcher and Boyd, 1979; Boyd and Dutcher, 1981). Liver damage is also the major toxic effect in birds, which lack both the ciliated and non-ciliated bronchiolar cells of other vertebrate species (Buckpitt *et al.*, 1982). Many other furan derivatives have been found to produce bronchiolar cell necrosis following their systemic administration. Included are analogues of 4-ipomeanol, furan itself, and sulphur- and nitrogen-containing analogues of furans (Boyd, 1980).

The pulmonary toxicity of nitrofurantoin is a potentially serious side-effect in patients treated with standard doses of this widely used urinary antiseptic. Signs of nitrofurantoin-induced lung damage usually occur within a month of beginning treatment, and include fever, cough, dyspnoea, cyanosis, pulmonary infiltrates and pleural effusion. When nitrofurantoin is discontinued, these symptoms rapidly subside, although radiographic abnormalities may persist for 2–6 weeks. In an occasional patient the disease becomes chronic, culminating in pulmonary fibrosis.

Mechanisms

The toxicity of 4-ipomeanol is due to its bioactivation to an electrophilic species by cytochrome *P*-450 found in Clara cells (Boyd, 1982; Gram, 1989). The metabolite formed is highly reactive, and will covalently bind to lung tissue *in vivo* (Boyd and Burka, 1978) and to microsomal proteins *in vitro* (Boyd *et al.*, 1978). Protection against the toxicity of 4-ipomeanol is provided by pulmonary GSH and other sulphydryl compounds which can react with this metabolite (Boyd *et al.*, 1982).

The furan moiety is clearly necessary for the lung toxicity induced by 4-ipomeanol and related chemicals. Analogues in which the furan is replaced by methyl or phenyl substituents are not toxic to the lung (Boyd, 1976). Clara cells have the greatest metabolic capacity for 4-ipomeanol in mammalian systems, which indicates that the pulmonary toxicity of this chemical is directly related to its site of metabolism. Altering the metabolism of 4-ipomeanol through the use of drug metabolism inducers shifts the target organ for toxicity from lung to liver (Jones *et al.*, 1983).

The mechanism(s) by which nitrofurantoin damages lung tissue are not known. Bronchiolar, hepatic or renal necrosis seen with other furans is not evident with nitrofurantoin, which suggests that it is not bioactivated to an electrophilic metabolite and that its mechanism of toxicity is significantly different. The initial damage appears to be part of a hypersensitivity reaction and the disorder is more prominent in atopic individuals (Israel-Biet *et al.*, 1991). The rarer fibrotic response may be a consequence of direct toxicity, perhaps as the result of redox cycling of nitrofurantoin (Sasame and Boyd, 1979; Martin, 1983). This might lead to the production of superoxide radicals, the depletion of NADPH and lung damage. Oxidative changes in lung tissue from rats treated with nitrofurantoin support this concept (Suntres and Shek, 1992).

Antineoplastic Agents

Background

Lung toxicity has been reported after treatment with many cytotoxic drugs (Table 1). The mechanisms of these toxicities have not been conclusively established for any agent, and the incidence is often poorly documented, since many cases of lung injury are subclinical. The most significant lung toxicity is seen with 1,3-bis-(2-chloroethyl)-1-nitrosourea (BCNU, or carmustine), bleomycin and methotrexate (Powis and Hacker, 1991). These agents, along with cyclophosphamide, are discussed below as examples of the various types of lung pathology and mechanisms that have been identified.

Lung Pathology

Bleomycin is a unique anticancer drug because it does not affect the bone marrow. It does, however, elicit lung damage in up to 10 per cent of treated patients, with mortality from pulmonary toxicity occurring in 1–2 per cent (Hay *et al.*, 1991). Histologically, bleomycin-induced lung damage is characterized by alveolar accumulation of proteinaceous material, alveolar and interstitial oedema, metaplasia of the alveolar epithelium and proliferation of fibroblasts without inflammation (Bedrossian *et al.*, 1973). The initial

Table 1   Lung-toxic anticancer drugs

Agent	Incidence[a]
Nitrosoureas	
carmustine (BCNU)	20–30%
lomustine (CCNU)	Uncertain but
semustine (methyl CCNU)	less than
chlorozotocin	BCNU
Antibiotics	
bleomycin	4–10%
mitomycin c	3–12%
neocarzinostatin	Rare
Alkylating agents	
busulfan	4% (subclinical up to 46%)
chlorambucil	Rare
cyclophosphamide	<1%
ifosfamide	<1%
melphalan	Rare
procarbazine	Rare
Antimetabolites	
cytarabine	Rare
6-mercaptopurine	Rare
methotrexate	8%
azathioprine	Rare
cytosine arabinoside	Rare
fludarabine monophosphate	Rare
Miscellaneous	
teniposide (VM–26)	Rare
vinblastine	3–4% hypersensitivity
vincristine	3–4% hypersensitivity
vindesine	Rare

[a] A rare incidence means that only a limited number of case reports exist.

injury after systemic injections of bleomycin is to pulmonary capillary endothelial cells (Lazo *et al.*, 1990). Electron microscopy reveals subsequent damage to type I alveolar epithelial cells and the appearance of abnormal and increased numbers of type II cells (Adamson, 1976). A similiar, but more rapid and extensive, lesion is produced following intratracheal treatments, which has made this the preferred route for most animal studies. However, other cytotoxic agents also damage the lung following intratracheal administration (Kehrer *et al.*, 1986b), and this route of administration may not completely mimic the damage that occurs after systemic treatment.

The lung pathology seen in patients with BCNU-induced pulmonary damage resembles that for bleomycin (Weiss *et al.*, 1981). In contrast, cyclophosphamide induces a severe interstitial pneumonitis and pulmonary fibrosis (Fraiser *et al.*, 1991). Although occurring in less than 1 per cent of treated patients, this problem is often dose-limiting and life threatening. Cyclophosphamide-induced injury to alveolar cells is characterized by type II cell hyperplasia, interstitial oedema and hyperplasia, and alveolar septal thickening. One week after an acutely lung-toxic dose in mice (100 mg kg^{-1}) the alveoli are re-epithelialized and there is a gradual increase in the deposition of excess collagen, which continues for up to 1 year (Morse *et al.*, 1985).

Histologically, methotrexate-induced lung damage differs from that caused by other cytotoxic agents. An inflammatory reaction is prominent, with the presence of mononuclear cells and eosinophils in the interstitial infiltrate. Discontinuation of therapy with methotrexate usually results in the resolution of lung injury. These findings suggest that this disorder is due to a hypersensitivity reaction. The development of fibrosis is apparently rare, although nearly 70 case reports have appeared (Bedrossian *et al.*, 1979).

Mechanisms

The mechanisms underlying cytotoxic drug-induced pulmonary toxicity are poorly understood. Animal models are inadequate for most of these drugs, since lung injury may take months or even years to become evident. It seems likely that the lung-damaging process is the end-result of a complex series of events which is dependent on several endogenous factors, including activation and deactivation processes, and lung cytokines. Risk factors for developing lung damage include treatment with multiple drugs, the presence of existing lung damage, and cotreatment with hyperoxia and/or radiation. Existing lung damage may be particularly critical for BCNU, which is capable of eliciting only minimal changes in normal lung tissue (Kehrer and Klein-Szanto, 1985).

The risk of lung injury associated with hyperoxia or radiation treatments in patients given various anticancer drugs has mechanistic implications. High oxygen concentrations enhance the toxicity of bleomycin (Berend, 1984), cyclophosphamide (Hakkinen *et al.*, 1982), BCNU (Kehrer and Paraidathathu, 1984) and mitomycin c (Ginsberg and Comis, 1982). This could be the result of additive toxicities, the inhibition of

normal repair processes or a biochemical effect of the drug, such as the inhibition of protective enzyme systems. For example, the inhibition of glutathione reductase by BCNU (Kehrer, 1983) might be a factor in the lung toxicity of this drug. However, clinical doses of BCNU only minimally inhibit glutathione reductase and there appears to be significant excess capacity of this enzyme.

The pulmonary toxicity of anticancer drugs is not due to their accumulation by lung tissue. An enhanced capacity to repair damage may exist in resistant animals, or organ-specific metabolic pathways may be a factor. For example, bleomycin-induced lung damage in different strains and species appears to be inversely related to levels of bleomycin hydrolase activity, which may detoxify bleomycin in resistant animals (Lazo *et al.*, 1990). However, tissues such as muscle, which have even lower levels of bleomycin hydrolase activity, fail to develop damage. This suggests that other factors are involved in the lung-damaging process, and data are available that indicate a role for transforming growth factor β in bleomycin-induced lung fibrosis (Hoyt and Lazo, 1988).

Bleomycin appears to require both a metal ion (usually iron) and oxygen to exert its cytotoxicity. The bleomycin–metal complex generates reactive oxygen species near the nucleus and damages DNA. The oxygen requirement may contribute to targeting the lung for damage, and would explain the enhanced toxicity seen with hyperoxia. This mechanism of injury suggests that various types of antioxidant or iron chelation therapy should be protective against lung damage, but numerous studies have failed to confirm this hypothesis (Hay *et al.*, 1991).

Cyclophosphamide requires bioactivation to exert both its therapeutic and toxic effects. The cytochrome *P*-450 system is clearly capable of such metabolism, but recent data suggest that co-oxidation via the prostaglandin H synthase system (which is found in high concentrations in the lung) is responsible for the lung damage this drug produces (Smith and Kehrer, 1991). Acrolein may be the lung-toxic metabolite, but additional work is needed to prove this hypothesis.

Pyrrolizidine Alkaloids

Background

The pyrrolizidine alkaloids (PAs) are a group of chemicals found in a variety of plant species throughout the world. Plants containing these alkaloids cause significant mammalian morbidity and mortality, including human (Schoental, 1982). Fatal disorders include necrosis or veno-occlusive disease of the liver, and pulmonary lesions in the parenchyma and vasculature as well as pulmonary hypertension (Huxtable, 1980; Mattocks, 1986). Neurological, haematological and gastrointestinal syndromes have also been described (McLean, 1970).

Lung Pathology

Lung lesions become evident several days after systemic treatment with a PA such as monocrotaline, derived from plants of the genus *Crotalaria*. The initial sites of lung damage are the endothelial cells lining the arteries, capillaries and veins. Thrombi appear on the surface of these cells, which then develop an increased permeability resulting in intra-alveolar and interstitial oedema and pleural effusion (Huxtable, 1979). This is followed by focal necrosis of the alveolar walls, damage to interstitial cells, endothelial and alveolar cell proliferation, medial thickening and intimal hyalinosis of arteries, and pulmonary arterial hypertension (Valdiva *et al.*, 1967; McLean, 1970). The normal active uptake of biogenic amines, such as serotonin and noradrenaline (norepinephrine), by pulmonary endothelial cells is inhibited following PA treatment (Hilliker *et al.*, 1984), an effect which may contribute to pulmonary hypertension.

Mechanisms

The PAs require metabolic activation in order to produce either hepatotoxicity or pneumotoxicity (Yost *et al.*, 1989). In contrast to other lung toxins, most of this metabolism occurs in the liver. The oxidation of PAs to pyrrolic compounds is the proximate source of toxic species. This occurs in the hepatic endoplasmic reticulum and requires both oxygen and NADPH. Both the cytochrome *P*-450 mixed-function oxidase and the MFO enzymes are able to metabolize the PAs, but the contribution of *P*-450 is more important (Williams *et al.*, 1989). Once formed, the PA pyrroles have two electrophilic centres and act as bifunctional alkylating agents. This results in significant DNA–DNA and DNA–protein cross-links in liver (Petry *et al.*, 1984), although a role for this action in the toxicity of PAs is not clear.

The lung itself appears incapable of metabolizing PAs to pyrrolic derivatives. Thus, lung damage develops subsequent to the transport of toxic species from the liver where they are formed. This suggests that these 'reactive' metabolites are relatively stable and damage lung primarily because it is next in line in the circulation and has a large capillary bed with which to interact. Monocrotaline, the most extensively studied PA, is mainly hepatotoxic, presumably since this is the site of metabolic activation. However, at lower doses which produce minimal hepatic damage, lung injury and pulmonary hypertension develops (Yost *et al.*, 1989). In contrast, the oxidized form, monocrotaline pyrrole, readily produces an acute lung lesion which leads to death in from hours to weeks when injected intravenously, depending on the dose.

Metals

Background

During recent years concern regarding heavy metal pollution has increased and chronic exposure continues to constitute a major health hazard. The indiscriminate use of heavy metals in industry and agriculture has resulted in the presence of these pollutants in air, soil and water. The consequences to the lung associated with the inhalation of heavy metals are well documented (Goyer, 1991). However, lung damage also occurs as the result of systemic exposure to a few heavy metals, particularly organometallic complexes.

Lung Pathology

Relatively few studies are available which describe lung injury after the systemic administration of heavy metals. Nickel carbonyl, a volatile, colourless organometallic liquid, produces severe pulmonary damage in many species, including man, following systemic administration. The alveolar region is primarily affected, with maximum damage evident 4–6 days following exposure (Hackett and Sunderman, 1968). The earliest changes are swelling of the alveolar endothelium by 6 h. This disappears in 2 days, when damage to type I alveolar epithelial cells and hypertrophy and hyperplasia of type II alveolar cells become evident. These cellular changes are accompanied by evidence of focal fibrosis.

Methylcyclopentadienyl manganese tricarbonyl (MMT), and its demethylated derivative (CMT), have been used as a replacement for tetraethyl lead in petrol and are two additional lung-toxic organometallic compounds. Mice, rats and hamsters develop lung damage characterized by both alveolar and bronchiolar epithelial cell necrosis within 1 day following the systemic administration of MMT (Hakkinen and Haschek, 1982).

Cadmium is highly lung-toxic when inhaled. Chronic exposure produces bronchitis, pulmonary fibrosis and alveolar damage, which may progress to emphysema, while acute exposure can produce a chemical pneumonitis and oedema (Goyer, 1991). Systemically, daily administration of cadmium for 7 days produces some biochemical evidence of lung injury (Kacew et al., 1976). Morphologically, cadmium-injected mice showed emphysematous-like lesions with distended alveoli within 4 h (Chowdhury et al., 1982). Necrotic changes were not evident, however, and lung morphology returned to normal within 24 h. Fetal lung tissue obtained from dams exposed systemically to cadmium exhibited a specific retardation of lung growth and histological changes characteristic of the respiratory distress syndrome (Chernoff, 1973; Daston and Grabowski, 1979).

The systemic administration of beryllium results in a deleterious effect on regenerating liver (Witschi, 1970). Although the inhalation of beryllium produces metabolic and morphological evidence of lung damage (Goyer, 1991), the influence of parenteral beryllium treatment on pulmonary function has not been reported.

Parenterally administered vanadium accumulates in the lung and produces histopathological changes, including widespread intra-alveolar haemorrhage and limited necrosis of regional alveolar septae (Sharma et al., 1980; Wei et al., 1982). Intratracheal instillation of vanadium also produces lung damage characterized by acute interstitial pneumonitis (Henderson et al., 1979). Evidence thus suggests that systemic as well as intratracheal vanadium alters lung function.

Mechanisms

The mechanisms by which metals or organometallic compounds induce lung damage have not been extensively studied. Among the organometallics, MMT and CMT are metabolized by MFO enzymes (Hanzlik et al., 1980), and the most recent data suggest that lung metabolism is responsible for the production of toxic species (Clay and Morris, 1991). Metabolism may also be involved in nickel carbonyl-induced lung damage. This highly water-insoluble compound readily penetrates to the alveoli, and nickel metal has been detected within alveolar cells. Other metals may damage lung by mechanisms similar to those by which they damage cells in other tissues.

Amphiphilic Agents

Background

A variety of compounds with different therapeutic indications have been found to induce a pulmonary lipidosis in animals (Table 2). The common feature of these drugs is that they are both cationic and amphiphilic. Although only amiodarone and chlorphentermine have been proven to induce this disorder in man, the potential exists for many other amphiphilic drugs to induce pulmonary lipidosis.

Lung Pathology

Pulmonary lipidosis is associated with dramatic morphological and biochemical changes, but is

Table 2 Amphophilic agents which produce pulmonary phospholipidosis

Drug	Therapeutic use
Chlorphentermine	Anorectic
Cloforex	Anorectic
Fenfluramine	Anorectic
1-Chloramitriptyline	Antidepressant
Fluoxetine	Antidepressant
Imipramine	Antidepressant
Iprindole	Antidepressant
Amiodarone	Antiarrhythmic
Triparonol	Hypocholesterolaemic
AY–9944	Hypocholesterolaemic
Chlorcyclizine	Antihistamine
Bromhexine	Secretolytic
Chloroquine	Antimalarial
Citalopram	Antidepressant/Serotonin uptake to inhibitor

reversible and seems to produce minimal functional impairment. Morphological examination of lungs obtained from rats treated orally with chlorphentermine reveals the presence of large phospholipid-rich macrophages, or foam cells, resting mainly on the alveolar walls (Kacew and Narbaitz, 1977). Ultrastructural investigation of these foam cells demonstrated the presence of inclusions or myelinoid bodies (Hruban, 1984). Further studies demonstrated that the myelinoid bodies were lysosomal in origin and concentrated material phagocytized within the cell. In particular, the myelinoid bodies were storage vesicles rich in phospholipids of membranes whose digestion was impaired by these drugs.

The pulmonary toxicity with the antiarrhythmic drug amiodarone has an incidence of 4–6 per cent (Israel-Biet *et al.*, 1991). In contrast to the pulmonary injury observed with other amphiphilic agents, the lesion caused by amiodarone often results in clinically significant aberrations, including dyspnoea and dry cough. Occasionally fever and a general malaise occur. Radiographically, a diffuse reticulonodular infiltrate is evident as well as pleural effusion.

The lung toxicity of amiodarone has been replicated in animals and appears to be dose-dependent. The duration of therapy is also a factor because of the exceptionally long half-life of this drug in the bloodstream. In general, symptoms resolve upon discontinuation of the drug, although a permanent pulmonary fibrosis is possible, particularly if treatment is continued. The reversibility of the phospholipidosis seen with other drugs occurs more readily, with a return to normal lipid levels within 2 weeks, although some biochemical changes may persist for longer periods of time.

Mechanisms

Drug-induced pulmonary phospholipidosis is caused by a greatly slowed turnover of lung phospholipids which permits phagocytic cells to accumulate large quantities of lipids. The lung serves as a target organ because it synthesizes and secretes large amounts of phospholipids as part of the pulmonary surfactant. The inhibition of lysosomal phospholipases is believed to be responsible for drug-induced pulmonary phospholipidosis (Reasor, 1987). This could result from the interaction of these drugs with phospholipases, phospholipids, or both. Most evidence, however,

indicates that cationic amphiphilic drugs complex with negatively charged phospholipids as the initial step in this disorder. This impairs the ability of lipases to degrade the phospholipids.

Some additional direct toxicity may explain the lung dysfunction associated with amiodarone. Electron microscopy has revealed cellular damage in addition to phospholipidosis. The amphiphilic nature of amiodarone, together with its ability to accumulate in lung to very high levels, may explain its increased toxic potential relative to other drugs in this category. The mechanism of this injury is unclear, although one study has shown changes consistent with an oxidative mechanism (Kennedy *et al.*, 1988). Other evidence indicates that there is a hypersensitivity component to amiodarone-induced lung injury. Damage can occur after relatively low total doses, and the lung cell changes seen are similar to those characteristic of hypersensitivity pneumonitis. Furthermore, corticosteroid treatment is usually effective in reversing the lung lesion (Israel-Biet *et al.*, 1991).

Miscellaneous Chemicals

Background

Certain hydrocarbons, oleic acid and 3-methylindole have been found to produce acute lung damage following their systemic administration. A number of other chemicals have also been reported to produce lung damage following their systemic administration. Since the mechanisms of lung injury induced by some of these agents differ from those of the better known toxins, a brief description of the pathology of the lesion and the purported mechanism is presented for some selected toxins.

Pathology and Mechanisms

Hydrocarbons

The direct toxicity of simple aromatic and aliphatic hydrocarbons to lung tissue following their systemic administration appears to be low, and has received little attention (Smith and Bend, 1981). There are, however, reports that some hydrocarbons can be bioactivated by pulmonary cytochrome *P*-450s. The known localization of these enzymes within Clara and type II alveolar epithelial cells suggested that damage to these lung cell types might be evident following treatment with various hydrocarbons. Available data support this concept, with damage to Clara cells a uniform finding with these types of compounds.

Any hydrocarbon that is metabolically activated in liver has the potential to undergo similar activation and subsequent cell damage in lung. Studies with carbon tetrachloride have concentrated on the liver because of the dramatic lesion that develops in that organ. However, pulmonary Clara cells also have the capacity to activate carbon tetrachloride (Boyd *et al.*, 1980) and damage to these cells, as well as type I and II alveolar epithelial and pulmonary endothelial cells, has been reported (Gould and Smuckler, 1971; Stewart *et al.*, 1979; Hollinger, 1982).

A highly specific Clara cell lesion is seen following systemic administration of 1-nitronaphthalene, naphthalene, 2-methylnaphthalene, pennyroyal oil and 1,1-dichloroethylene (Mahvi *et al.*, 1977; Griffin *et al.*, 1981; Forkert and Reynolds, 1982; Gordon *et al.*, 1982; Johnson *et al.*, 1984). Most of these chemicals are also hepatotoxic and, until recently, a significant body of evidence suggested that reactive metabolites from the liver were responsible for determining the overall level of injury in the lung. Studies in isolated-perfused lung have now shown, however, that, at least for naphthalene, Clara cell necrosis can be mediated entirely by lung processes (Kanekal *et al.*, 1990).

Oleic acid
Intravenously administered oleic acid has been used as a model of the 'chemical phase' of lung damage which occurs following an embolism due to fat. Evidence of lung damage becomes evident within hours after treatment. The lung lesion is initially characterized by capillary obstruction and both endothelial and type I cell necrosis (Derks and Jacobvitz-Derks, 1977). This is followed by interstitial and intra-alveolar oedema, a marked proliferation of type II cells and the development of a diffuse fibrotic lesion. The precise mechanism of this injury remains unclear, but is likely to be the result of a complex series of events initiated at the lung endothelium and involving various mediators, including prostaglandins and cytokines.

3-Methylindole
3-Methylindole (3MI) is a ruminal fermentation product of L-tryptophan that causes pulmonary oedema and emphysema in a number of species (Yost *et al.*, 1989). Non-ruminant species, such as rat and mouse, which were originally thought to be resistant to this toxicity, are now known also to be sensitive when given a sufficient dose. However, the susceptibility of humans to this toxicant, which is found in cigarette smoke and human faeces, and can be absorbed from the intestine into the systemic circulation, is not known (Yost *et al.*, 1989).

Lungs from animals treated with 3MI show extensive necrosis of type I alveolar cells and bronchiolar epithelium (Huang *et al.*, 1977). This is followed by proliferation of type II cells to repopulate the alveolar epithelium. Other tissues show no evidence of damage. 3MI is rapidly metabolized by the MFO system in both lung and liver systems (Yost *et al.*, 1989) and at least ten metabolites are excreted in the urine (Hammond and Carlson, 1979). An activated metabolite appears to be responsible for the lung damage produced by 3MI. Covalent binding is most extensive in lung tissue (Bray *et al.*, 1984); is dependent on time, temperature, oxygen and NADPH; and is inhibited by carbon monoxide, non-protein sulphydryls and inhibitors of drug metabolism, which also prevent the lung damage (Hanafy and Bogan, 1980; Nocerini *et al.*, 1983). The source of the toxic species is likely to be metabolism within lung (Yost *et al.*, 1989). Although cytochrome *P*-450 has been postulated as the major pathway by which 3MI is bioactivated to an electrophilic metabolite (Hanafy and Bogan, 1980), co-oxidation via the prostaglandin H synthase system also appears capable of producing reactive 3MI metabolites (Formosa and Bray, 1988).

REFERENCES

Adamson, I. Y. R. (1976). Pulmonary toxicity of bleomycin. *Environ. Hlth Perspect.*, **16**, 119–126

Adamson, I. Y. R., Bowden, D. H., Côté, M. G. and Witschi, H. P. (1977). Lung injury induced by butylated hydroxytoluene. Cytodynamic and biochemical studies in mice. *Lab. Invest.*, **36**, 26–32

Adamson, I. Y. R., Hedgecock, C. and Bowden, D. H. (1990). Epithelial cell-fibroblast interactions in lung injury and repair. *Am. J. Pathol.*, **137**, 385–392

Aldridge, W. N., Miles, J. W., Mount, D. L. and Verschoyle, R. D. (1979). The toxicological properties of impurities in malathion. *Arch. Toxicol.*, **42**, 95–106

Baron, J., Burke, J. P., Guengerich, F. P., Jakoby, W. B. and Voigt, J. M. (1988). Sites for xenobiotic activation and detoxication within the respiratory tract: implications for chemically induced toxicity. *Toxicol. Appl. Pharmacol.*, **93**, 493–505

Bedrossian, C. W. M., Luna, M. A., Mackay, B. and Lichtiger, B. (1973). Ultrastructure of pulmonary bleomycin toxicity. *Cancer*, **32**, 44–51

Bedrossian, C. W. M., Miller, W. C. and Luna, M. A. (1979). Methotrexate-induced diffuse interstitial pulmonary fibrosis. *S. Med. J.*, **72**, 313–318

Berend, N. (1984). The effect of bleomycin and oxygen on rat lung. *Pathology*, **16**, 136–139

Berg, J. T., Allison, R. C., Prasad, V. R. and Taylor, A. E. (1990). Endotoxin protection of rats from pulmonary oxygen toxicity: possible cytokine involvement. *J. Appl. Physiol.*, **68**, 549–553

Bolton, J. L. and Thompson, J. A. (1991). Oxidation of butylated hydroxytoluene to toxic metabolites. Factors influencing hydroxylation and quinone methide formation by hepatic and pulmonary microsomes. *Drug Metab. Disp.*, **19**, 467–472

Boon, W. R. (1967). The quaternary salts of bipyridylium—A new agricultural tool. *Endeavour*, **26**, 27–32

Boyd, M. R. (1976). Role of metabolic activation in the pathogenesis of chemically induced pulmonary disease: mechanism of action of the lung-toxic furan, 4-ipomeanol. *Environ. Hlth Perspect.*, **16**, 127–138

Boyd, M. R. (1980). Biochemical mechanisms in pulmonary toxicity of furan derivatives. In Hodgson, E., Bend, J. R. and Philpot, R. M. (Eds), *Reviews in Biochemical Toxicology*, Vol. 2. Elsevier/North-Holland, New York, pp. 71–101

Boyd, M. R. (1982). Metabolic activation of pulmonary toxins. In Witschi, H. P. and Nettesheim, P. (Eds), *Mechanisms in Respiratory Toxicology*, Vol. 2. CRC Press, Boca Raton, Florida, pp. 85–112

Boyd, M. R. and Burka, L. T. (1978). *In vivo* studies on the relationship between target organ alkylation and the pulmonary toxicity of a chemically reactive metabolite of 4-ipomeanol. *J. Pharmacol. Exptl Ther.*, **207**, 687–697

Boyd, M. R., Burka, L. T., Wilson, B. J. and Sasame, H. A. (1978). *In vitro* studies on the metabolic activation of the pulmonary toxin, 4-ipomeanol, by rat lung and liver microsomes. *J. Pharmacol. Exptl Ther.*, **207**, 677–686

Boyd, M. R. and Dutcher, J. S. (1981) Renal toxicity due to reactive metabolites formed *in situ* in the kidney: Investigations with 4-ipomeanol in the mouse. *J. Pharmacol. Exptl Ther.* **216**, 640–646

Boyd, M. R. and Neal, R. A. (1976). Studies on the mechanism of toxicity and of development of tolerance to the pulmonary toxin, alpha-naphthylthiourea (ANTU). *Drug Metab. Disp.*, **4**, 314–322

Boyd, M. R., Statham, C. N. and Longo, N. S. (1980). The pulmonary Clara cells as a target for toxic chemicals requiring metabolic activation; studies with carbon tetrachloride. *J. Pharmacol. Exptl Ther.*, **212**, 109–114

Boyd, M. R., Stiko, A., Statham, C. N. and Jones, R. B. (1982). Protective role of endogenous pulmonary glutathione and other sulfhydryl compounds against lung damage by alkylating agents. Investigations with 4-ipomeanol in the rat. *Biochem. Pharmacol.*, **31**, 1579–1583

Brandes, M. E. and Finkelstein, J. N. (1990). The production of alveolar macrophage-derived growth-regulating proteins in response to lung injury. *Toxicol. Lett.*, **54**, 3–22

Bray, T. M., Carlson, J. R. and Nocerini, M. R. (1984). *In vitro* covalent binding of 3-[^{14}C] methylindole metabolites in goat tissues. *Proc. Soc. Exptl Biol. Med.*, **176**, 48–53

Buckpitt, A. R., Statham, C. N. and Boyd, M. R. (1982). *In vivo* studies on the target tissue metabolism, covalent binding, glutathione depletion, and toxicity of 4-ipomeanol in birds, species deficient in pulmonary enzymes for metabolic activation. *Toxicol. Appl. Pharmacol.*, **65**, 38–52

Bullivant, C. (1966). Accidental poisoning by paraquat: Report of two cases in man. *Br. Med. J.*, **1**, 1272–1273

Bus, J. S., Aust, S. D. and Gibson, J. E. (1976). Paraquat toxicity: Proposed mechanism of action involving lipid peroxidation. *Environ. Hlth Perspect.*, **16**, 139–146

Carroll, K. K. and Noble, R. L. (1949). Resistance to toxic thioureas in rats treated with anti-thyroid compounds. *J. Pharmacol. Exptl Ther.*, **97**, 478–483

Chernoff, N. (1973). Teratogenic effects of cadmium in rats. *Teratology*, **8**, 29–32

Chowdhury, P., Louria, D. B., Chang, L. W. and Rayford, P. L. (1982). Cadmium-induced pulmonary injury in mouse: A relationship with serum antitrypsin activity. *Bull. Environ. Contam. Toxicol.*, **28**, 446–451

Clark, D. G. and Hurst, E. W. (1970). The toxicity of diquat. *Br. J. Industr. Med.*, **27**, 51–55

Clay, J. and Morris, J. B. (1991). Pulmonary activation and toxicity of methylcyclopentadienyl manganese tricarbonyl (MMT) and cyclopentadienyl manganese tricarbonyl (CMT). *Toxicologist*, **11**, 231

Cobb, L. M. and Grimshaw, P. (1979). Acute toxicity of oral diquat (1,1'-ethylene-2,2'-bipyridinium) in cynomolgus monkeys, *Toxicol. Appl. Pharmacol.*, **51**, 277–282

Cooper, J. A. D. Jr, White, D. A. and Matthay, R. A. (1986). Drug-induced pulmonary disease. Part 1. Cytotoxic drugs; Part 2. Noncytotoxic drugs. *Am. Rev. Resp. Dis.*, **133**, 321–340; 488–505

Cunningham, A. L. and Hurley, J. V. (1972). Alpha-naphthyl-thiourea-induced pulmonary oedema in the rat: A topographical and electron-microscope study. *J. Pathol.*, **106**, 25–35

Daston, G. P. and Grabowski, C. T. (1979). Toxic effects of cadmium on the developing rat lung. I.

Altered pulmonary surfactant and the induction of respiratory distress syndrome. *J. Toxicol. Environ. Hlth*, **5**, 973–983

Derks, C. M. and Jacobvitz-Derks, D. (1977). Embolic pneumopathy induced by oleic acid. A systematic morphologic study. *Am. J. Pathol.*, **87**, 143–157

Dieke, S. H., Allen, G. S. and Richter, C. P. (1947). The acute toxicity of thioureas and related compounds to wild and domestic Norway rats. *J. Pharmacol. Exptl Ther.*, **90**, 260–270

Dieke, S. H. and Richter, C. P. (1946). Age and species variation in the acute toxicity of alpha-naphthyl thiourea. *Proc. Soc. Exptl Biol. Med.*, **62**, 22–25

Dinsdale, D., Verschoyle, R. D. and Cabral, J. R. P. (1982). Cellular responses to trialkylphosphoro-thioate-induced injury in rat lung. *Arch. Toxicol.*, **51**, 79–89

Dutcher, J. S. and Boyd, M. R. (1979). Species and strain differences in target organ alkylation and toxicity by 4-ipomeanol. Predictive value of covalent binding in studies of target organ toxicities by reactive metabolites. *Biochem. Pharmacol.*, **28**, 3367–3372

Fairshter, R. D., Rosen, S. M., Smith, W. R., Glauser, F. L., McRae, D. M. and Wilson, A. F. (1976). Paraquat poisoning: New aspects of therapy. *Q. J. Med.*, **45**, 551–565

Fisher, H. K., Clements, J. A. and Wright, R. R. (1973). Enhancement of oxygen toxicity by the herbicide paraquat. *Am. Rev. Resp. Dis.*, **107**, 246–252

Forkert, P.-G. and Reynolds, E. S. (1982). 1,1-Dichloroethylene-induced pulmonary injury. *Exptl Lung Res.*, **3**, 57–68

Formosa, P. J. and Bray, T. M. (1988). Evidence for metabolism of 3-methylindole by prostaglandin H synthase and mixed-function oxidases in goat lung and liver microsomes. *Biochem. Pharmacol.*, **37**, 4359–4366

Fraiser, L., Kanekal, S. and Kehrer, J. P. (1991). Cyclophosphamide toxicity. Characterising and avoiding the problem. *Drugs*, **42**, 781–795

Gandy, J., Ali, F. A. F., Hasegawa, L. and Imamura, T. (1984a). Morphological alterations of rat lung bronchiolar epithelium produced by various trialkyl phosphorothioates. *Toxicology.*, **32**, 37–46

Gandy, J., Fukuto, T. R. and Imamura, T. (1984b). Sequential and dose-dependent alterations in rat bronchiolar epithelium during *O,O,S*-trimethyl phosphorothioate induced delayed toxicity. *J. Pathol.*, **143**, 127–137

Ginsberg, S. J. and Comis, R. L. (1982). The pulmonary toxicity of antineoplastic agents. *Sem. Oncol.*, **9**, 34–51

Gordon, W. P., Forte, A. J., McMurtry, R. J., Gal, J. and Nelson, S. D. (1982). Hepatotoxicity and pulmonary toxicity of pennroyal oil and its constituent terpenes in the mouse. *Toxicol. Appl. Pharmacol.*, **65**, 413–424

Gould, V. E. and Smuckler, E. A. (1971). Alveolar injury in acute carbon tetrachloride intoxication. *Arch. Int. Med.*, **128**, 109–117

Goyer, R. A. (1991). Toxic effects of metals. In Amdur, M. O., Doull, J. and Klaassen, C. D. (Eds), *Casarett and Doull's Toxicology: The Basic Science of Poisons*, Macmillan, New York, pp. 623–680

Gram, T. E. (1989). Pulmonary toxicity of 4-ipomeanol. *Pharmacol. Ther.*, **43**, 291–297

Gregory, A. R. (1970). Inhalation toxicology and lung edema receptor sites. *Am. Industr. Hyg. Assoc. J.*, **31**, 454–459

Griffin, K. A., Johnson, C. B., Breger, R. K. and Franklin, R. B. (1981). Pulmonary toxicity, hepatic, and extrahepatic metabolism of 2-methylnaphthalene in mice. *Toxicol. Appl. Pharmacol.*, **61**, 185–196

Hackett, R. L. and Sunderman, F. W. Jr (1968). Pulmonary alveolar reaction to nickel carbonyl. *Arch. Environ. Hlth*, **16**, 349–362

Haigh, R. (1986). Safety and necessity of antioxidants: EEC approach. *Fd Chem. Toxicol.*, **24**, 1031–1034

Hakkinen, P. J. and Haschek, W. M. (1982). Pulmonary toxicity of methylcyclopentadienyl manganese tricarbonyl: nonciliated bronchiolar epithelial (Clara) cell necrosis and alveolar damage in the mouse, rat, and hamster. *Toxicol. Appl. Pharmacol.*, **65**, 11–22

Hakkinen, P. J., Whiteley, J. W. and Witschi, H. R. (1982). Hyperoxia, but not thoracic X-irradiation, potentiates bleomycin- and cyclophosphamide-induced lung damage in mice. *Am. Rev. Resp. Dis.*, **126**, 281–285

Hammond, A. C. and Carlson, J. R. (1979). The metabolism and disposition of 3-methylindole in goats. *Life Sci.*, **25**, 1301–1306

Hanafy, M. S. M. and Bogan, J. A. (1980). The covalent binding of 3-methylindole metabolites to bovine tissue. *Life Sci.*, **27**, 1225–1231

Hanzlik, R. P., Bhatia, P., Stitt, R. and Traiger, G. J. (1980). Biotransformation and excretion of methyl-cyclopentadienyl manganese tricarbonyl in the rat. *Drug Metab. Disp.*, **8**, 428–433

Haschek, W. M., Klein-Szanto, A. J. P., Last, J. A., Reiser, K. M. and Witschi, H. P. (1982). Long-term morphologic and biochemical features of experimentally induced lung fibrosis in the mouse. *Lab. Invest.*, **46**, 438–449

Haschek, W. M., Meyer, K. R., Ulrich, R. L. and Witschi, H. P. (1980). Potentiation of chemically induced lung fibrosis by thorax irradiation. *Int. J. Radiat. Oncol. Biol. Phys.*, **6**, 449–455

Haschek, W. M. and Witschi, H. P. (1979). Pulmonary fibrosis—a possible mechanism. *Toxicol. Appl. Pharmacol.*, **51**, 475–487

Hay, J., Shahzeidi, S. and Laurent, G. (1991). Mechanisms of bleomycin-induced lung damage. *Arch. Toxicol.*, **65**, 81–94

Henderson, R. F. (1989). Bronchoalveolar lavage: a tool for assessing the health status of the lung. In McClellan, R. O. and Henderson, R. F. (Eds), *Con-*

cepts in Inhalation Toxicology. Hemisphere Publishing Corporation, New York, pp. 415–444

Henderson, R. F., Rebar, A. H. and Denicola, D. B. (1979). Early damage indicators in the lungs. IV. Biochemical and cytologic response of the lung to lavage with metal salts. *Toxicol. Appl. Pharmacol.*, **51**, 129–135

Hilliker, K. S., Imlay, M. and Roth, R. A. (1984). Effects of monocrotaline treatment on norepinephrine removal by isolated, perfused rat lungs. *Biochem. Pharmacol.*, **33**, 2690–2692

Hirai, K. I., Witschi, H. P. and Côté, M. G. (1977). Electron microscopy of butylated hydroxytoluene-induced lung damage in mice. *Exptl Molec. Pathol.*, **27**, 295–308

Hollinger, M. A. (1982). Biochemical evidence for pulmonary endothelial cell injury after carbon tetrachloride administration in mice. *J. Pharmacol. Exptl Ther.*, **222**, 641–644

Hollinger, M. A. and Giri, S. N. (1979). ^{14}C-Thiourea binding in the rat lung. *Res. Commun. Chem. Pathol. Pharmacol.*, **26**, 609–612

Hollinger, M. A., Giri, S. N. and Hwang, F. (1976). Binding of radioactivity from ^{14}C-thiourea to rat lung protein. *Drug Metab. Disp.*, **4**, 119–123

Hoyt, D. G. and Lazo, J. S. (1988). Alterations in pulmonary mRNA encoding procollagens, fibronectin and transforming growth factor-beta precede bleomycin-induced pulmonary fibrosis in mice. *J. Pharmacol. Exptl Ther.*, **246**, 756–771

Hruban, Z. (1984). Pulmonary and generalized lysosomal storage induced by amphiphilic drugs. *Environ. Hlth Perspect.*, **55**, 53–76

Huang, T. W., Carlson, J. R., Bray, T. M. and Bradley, B. J. (1977). 3-Methylindole-induced pulmonary injury in goats. *Am. J. Pathol.*, **87**, 647–666

Huxtable, R. J. (1979). New aspects of the toxicology and pharmacology of pyrrolizidine alkaloids. *Gen. Pharmacol.*, **10**, 159–167

Huxtable, R. J. (1980). Problems with pyrrolizidines. *TIPS.*, **1**, 299–303

Ilett, K. F., Stripp, B., Menard, R. H., Reid, W. D. and Gillette, J. R. (1974). Studies on the mechanism of the lung toxicity of paraquat: Comparison of tissue distribution and some biochemical parameters in rats and rabbits. *Toxicol. Appl. Pharmacol.*, **28**, 216–226

Imamura, T. and Gandy, J. (1988). Pulmonary toxicity of phosphorothioate impurities found in organophosphate insecticides. *Pharmacol. Ther.*, **38**, 419–427

Imamura, T. and Hasegawa, L. (1984). Role of metabolic activation, covalent binding, and glutathione depletion in pulmonary toxicity produced by an impurity of malathion. *Toxicol. Appl. Pharmacol.*, **72**, 476–483

Imamura, T., Hasegawa, L., Gandy, J. and Fukuto, T. R. (1983). Effect of drug metabolism inducer and inhibitor on *O*,*O*,*S*-trimethyl phosphorothioate-induced delayed toxicity in rats. *Chem.-Biol. Interact.*, **45**, 53–64

Israel-Biet, D., Labrune, S. and Huchon, G. J. (1991). Drug-induced lung disease: 1990 review. *Eur. Resp. J.*, **4**, 465–478

Johnson, D. E., Riley, M. G. I. and Cornish, H. H. (1984). Acute target organ toxicity of 1-nitronaphthalene in the rat. *J. Appl. Toxicol.*, **4**, 253–257

Jones, R. B., Statham, C. N. and Boyd, M. R. (1983). Effects of 3-methylcholanthrene on covalent binding and toxicity of 4-ipomeanol in inducible and non-inducible (B6D2) mice. *Toxicology.*, **28**, 183–191

Kacew, S., Merali, Z. and Singhal, R. L. (1976). Comparison of the subacute effects of cadmium exposure upon nucleic acid, cyclic adenosine 3′,5′-monophosphate and polyamine metabolism in lung and kidney cortex. *Toxicol. Appl. Pharmacol.*, **38**, 145–156

Kacew, S. and Narbaitz, R. (1977). A comparative ultrastructural and biochemical study between the effects of chlorphentermine and phentermine on rat lung. *Exptl Molec. Pathol.*, **27**, 106–120

Kanekal, S., Plopper, C., Morin, D. and Buckpitt, A. (1990). Metabolic activation and bronchiolar Clara cell necrosis from naphthalene in the isolated perfused mouse lung. *J. Pharmacol. Exptl Ther.*, **252**, 428–437

Kehrer, J. P. (1983). The effect of BCNU (carmustine) on tissue glutathione reductase activity. *Toxicol. Lett.*, **17**, 63–68

Kehrer, J. P. and DiGiovanni, J. (1990). Comparison of lung injury induced in 4 strains of mice by butylated hydroxytoluene. *Toxicol. Lett.*, **52**, 55–61

Kehrer, J. P., Haschek, W. M. and Witschi, H. P. (1979). The influence of hyperoxia on the acute toxicity of paraquat and diquat. *Drug. Chem. Toxicol.*, **2**, 397–408

Kehrer, J. P. and Kacew, S. (1985). Systemically applied chemicals that damage lung tissue. *Toxicology.*, **35**, 251–293

Kehrer, J. P. and Klein-Szanto, A. J. P. (1985). Enhanced acute lung damage in mice following administration of 1,3-bis(2-chloroethyl)-1-nitrosourea. *Cancer Res.*, **45**, 5707–5713

Kehrer, J. P., Klein-Szanto, A. J. P., Sorensen, E. M. B., Pearlman, R. and Rosner, M. H. (1984). Enhanced acute lung damage following corticosteroid treatment. *Am. Rev. Resp. Dis.*, **130**, 256–261

Kehrer, J. P., Klein-Szanto, A. J. P., Thurston, D. E., Lindenschmidt, R. C. and Witschi, H. R. (1986a). *O*,*S*,*S*-trimethyl phosphorodithioate-induced lung damage in rats and mice. *Toxicol. Appl. Pharmacol.*, **84**, 480–492

Kehrer, J. P., Lee, Y.-C. C. and Smith, R. D. (1986b). Effect of intratracheally administered anticancer drugs on lung hydroxyproline content. *Toxicol. Lett.*, **30**, 63–70

Kehrer, J. P. and Lee, Y.-C. C. (1987). Pulmonary hydroxyproline content and production following treatment of mice with *O*,*S*,*S*-trimethyl phosphorodithioate. *Toxicol. Lett.*, **38**, 321–327

Kehrer, J. P. and Paraidathathu, T. (1984). Enhanced

oxygen toxicity following treatment with 1,3-bis(2-chloroethyl)-1-nitrosourea. *Fund. Appl. Toxicol.*, **4**, 760–767

Kehrer, J. P. and Witschi, H. P. (1980). Effects of drug metabolism inhibitors on butylated hydroxytoluene-induced pulmonary toxicity in mice. *Toxicol. Appl. Pharmacol.*, **53**, 333–342

Kelley, J. (1990). Cytokines of the lung. *Am. Rev. Resp. Dis.*, **141**, 765–788

Kennedy, T. P., Gordon, G. B., Paky, A., McShane, A., Adkinson, N. F. Jr, Peters, S. P., Friday, K., Jackman, W., Sciuto, A. M. and Gurtner, G. H. (1988). Amiodarone causes acute oxidant lung injury in ventilated and perfused rabbit lungs. *J. Cardiovasc. Pharmacol.*, **12**, 23–36

Lazo, J. S., Hoyt, D. G., Sebti, S. M. and Pitt, B. R. (1990). Bleomycin: A pharmacologic tool in the study of the pathogenesis of interstitial pulmonary fibrosis. *Pharmacol. Ther.*, **47**, 347–358

Lee, P. W., Arnau, T. and Neal, R. A. (1980). Metabolism of alpha-naphthylthiourea by rat liver and rat lung microsomes. *Toxicol. Appl. Pharmacol.*, **53**, 164–173

McLean, E. K. (1970). The toxic actions of pyrrolizidine (Senecio) alkaloids. *Pharmacol. Rev.*, **22**, 429–483

Mahvi, D., Bank, H. and Harley, R. (1977). Morphology of naphthalene-induced bronchiolar lesion. *Am. J. Pathol.*, **86**, 559–571

Malkinson, A. M. (1983). Review: Putative mutagens and carcinogens in foods. III. Butylated hydroxytoluene (BHT). *Environ. Mutagen.*, **5**, 353–362

Marino, A. A. and Mitchell, J. T. (1972). Lung damage in mice following intraperitoneal injection of butylated hydroxytoluene. *Proc. Soc. Exptl Biol. Med.*, **140**, 122–125

Martin, F. M. and Witschi, H. P. (1985). Cadmium-induced lung injury: cell kinetics and long-term effects. *Toxicol. Appl. Pharmacol.*, **80**, 215–227

Martin, W. J. (1983). Nitrofurantoin: Evidence for the oxidant injury of lung parenchymal cells. *Am. Rev. Resp. Dis.*, **127**, 482–486

Martin, W. J. (1991). Pharmacologic and other chemical causes of interstitial lung disease. *Chest*, **100**, 241–243

Mattocks, A. R. (1986). *Chemistry and Toxicology of Pyrrolizidine Alkaloids*, Academic Press, Orlando, Florida

Mizutani, T., Ishida, I., Yamamoto, K. and Tajima, K. (1982). Pulmonary toxicity of butylated hydroxytoluene and related alkylphenols: structural requirements for toxic potency in mice. *Toxicol. Appl. Pharmacol.*, **62**, 273–281

Morse, C. C., Sigler, C., Lock, S., Hakkinen, P. J., Haschek, W. M. and Witschi, H. P. (1985). Pulmonary toxicity of cyclophosphamide: a 1-year study. *Exptl Molec. Pathol.*, **42**, 251–260

Nagata, T., Williams, D. E. and Ziegler, D. M. (1990). Substrate specificities of rabbit lung and porcine liver flavin-containing monooxygenases: differences due to substrate size. *Chem. Res. Toxicol.*, **3**, 372–376

Nemery, B. and Aldridge, W. N. (1988a). Studies on the metabolism of the pneumotoxin *O,S,S*-trimethyl phosphorodithioate—I. Lung and liver microsomes. *Biochem. Pharmacol.*, **37**, 3709–3715

Nemery, B. and Aldridge, W. N. (1988b). Studies on the metabolism of the pneumotoxin *O,S,S*-trimethyl phosphorodithioate—II. Lung and liver slices. *Biochem. Pharmacol.*, **37**, 3717–3722

Nocerini, M. R., Carlson, J. R. and Breeze, R. G. (1983). Effect of glutathione status on covalent binding and pneumotoxicity of 3-methylindole in goats. *Life Sci.*, **32**, 449–458

Petry, T. W., Bowden, G. T., Huxtable, T. J. and Sipes, I. G. (1984). Characterization of hepatic DNA damage induced in rats by the pyrrolizidine alkaloid monocrotaline. *Cancer Res.*, **44**, 1505–1509

Popenoe, D. (1979). Effects of paraquat aerosol on mouse lung. *Arch. Pathol. Lab. Med.*, **103**, 331–334

Powis, G. and Hacker, M. P. (Eds) (1991). *Toxicity of Anticancer Drugs*. Pergamon Press, New York

Reasor, M. J. (1987). Role of the alveolar macrophage in the induction of pulmonary phospholipidosis: pharmacologic and toxicologic considerations. In Hollinger, M. A. (Ed.), *Current Topics in Pulmonary Pharmacology and Toxicology*, Vol. 2. Elsevier, New York, pp. 43–71

Rhodes, M. L., Zavala, D. C. and Brown, D. (1976). Hypoxic protection in paraquat poisoning. *Lab. Invest.*, **35**, 496–500

Richter, C. P. (1946). Biological factors involved in poisoning rats with alpha-naphthylthiourea. *Proc. Soc. Exptl Biol. Med.*, **63**, 364–372

Rose, M. S. and Smith, L. L. (1977). Tissue uptake of paraquat and diquat. *Gen. Pharmacol.*, **8**, 173–176

Rose, M. S., Smith, L. L. and Wyatt, I. (1974). Evidence for energy-dependent accumulation of paraquat into rat lung. *Nature.*, **252**, 314–315

Rose, M. S., Smith, L. L. and Wyatt, I. (1976). The relevance of pentose phosphate pathway stimulation in rat lung to the mechanism of paraquat toxicity. *Biochem. Pharmacol.*, **25**, 1763–1767

Sabo, J. P., Kimmel, E. C. and Diamond, L. (1983). Effects of the Clara cell toxin, 4-ipomeanol, on pulmonary function in rats. *J. Appl. Physiol.*, **54**, 337–344

Sasame, H. A. and Boyd, M. R. (1979). Superoxide and hydrogen peroxide production and NADPH oxidation stimulated by nitrofurantoin in lung microsomes: Possible implications for toxicity. *Life Sci.*, **24**, 1091–1096

Schoental, R. (1982). Health hazards of pyrrolizidine alkaloids. A short review. *Toxicol. Lett.*, **10**, 323–326

Sharma, R. P., Oberg, S. G. and Parker, R. D. R. (1980). Vanadium retention in rat tissues following acute exposures to different dose levels. *J. Toxicol. Environ. Hlth*, **6**, 45–54

Smith, B. R. and Bend, J. R. (1981). Metabolic interactions of hydrocarbons with mammalian lung. *Rev. Biochem. Toxicol.*, **3**, 77–122

Smith, L. J. (1984). Lung damage induced by butylated hydroxytoluene in mice. Biochemical, cellular, and morphologic characterization. *Am. Rev. Resp. Dis.*, **130**, 895–904

Smith, L. L. (1987). The mechanism of paraquat toxicity in the lung. *Rev. Biochem. Toxicol.*, **8**, 37–71

Smith, R. D. and Kehrer, J. P. (1991). Cooxidation of cyclophosphamide as an alternative pathway for its bioactivation. *Cancer Res.*, **51**, 542–548

Sorokin, S. P. (1970). The cells of the lungs. In Nettesheim, P., Hanna, M. G. Jr. and Deatherage, J. W. Jr. (Eds), *Morphology of Experimental Respiratory Carcinogenesis*. AEC Symposium Series, Atomic Energy Commission, Vol. **21**, 3–44

Stewart, B. W., Le Mesurier, S. M. and Lykke, A. W. J. (1979). Correlation of biochemical and morphological changes induced by chemical injury to the lung. *Chem.–Biol. Interact.*, **26**, 321–338

Suntres, Z. E. and Shek, P. N. (1992). Nitrofurantoin-induced pulmonary toxicity. In vivo evidence for oxidative-stress mediated mechanisms. *Biochem. Pharmacol.*, **43**, 1127–1135

Valdivia, E., Lalich, J. J., Hayashi, Y. and Sonnad, J. (1967). Alterations in pulmonary alveoli after a single injection of monocrotaline. *Arch. Pathol.*, **84**, 64–76

Van Den Brink, H. A. S., Kelly, H. and Stone, M. G. (1976). Innate and drug-induced resistance to acute lung damage caused in rats by alpha-naphthylthiourea (ANTU) and related compounds. *Br. J. Exptl Pathol.*, **57**, 621–636

Verschoyle, R. D. and Cabral, J. R. P. (1982). Investigation of the acute toxicity of some trimethyl and triethyl phosphorothioates with particular reference to those causing lung damage. *Arch. Toxicol.*, **51**, 221–231

Wei, C., Al Bayati, M. A., Culbertson, M. R., Rosenblatt, L. S. and Hansen, L. D. (1982). Acute toxicity of ammonium metavanadate in mice. *J. Toxicol. Environ. Hlth*, **10**, 673–687

Weiss, R. B., Poster, D. S. and Penta, J. S. (1981). The nitrosoureas and pulmonary toxicity. *Cancer Treat. Rev.*, **8**, 111–125

Williams, D. E., Reed, R. L., Kedzierski, B., Ziegler, D. M. and Buhler, D. R. (1989). The role of flavin-containing monooxygenase in the N-oxidation of the pyrrolizidine alkaloid senecionine. *Drug Metab. Disp.*, **17**, 380–386

Witschi, H. P. (1970). Effects of beryllium on deoxyribonucleic acid-synthesizing enzymes in regenerating rat liver. *Biochem. J.*, **120**, 623–634

Witschi, H. P. (1975). Exploitable biochemical approaches for the evaluation of toxic lung damage. *Essays Toxicol.*, **6**, 120–191

Witschi, H. (1991). Role of epithelium in lung repair. *Chest.*, **99**, 22S–25S

Witschi, H. P., Kacew, S., Hirai, K.-I. and Côté, M. G. (1977). *In vivo* oxidation of reduced nicotinamide-adenine dinucleotide phosphate by paraquat and diquat in rat lung. *Chem.–Biol. Interact.*, **19**, 143–160

Witschi, H. P. and Lock, S. (1978). Toxicity of butylated hydroxytoluene in mouse following oral administration. *Toxicology*, **9**, 137–146

Witschi, H., Malkinson, A. M. and Thompson, J. A. (1989). Metabolism and pulmonary toxicity of butylated hydroxytoluene (BHT). *Pharmacol. Ther.*, **42**, 89–113

Witschi, H. P., Tryka, A. F. and Lindenschmidt, R. C. (1985). The many faces of an increase in lung collagen. *Fund. Appl. Toxicol.*, **5**, 240–250

Wyatt, I., Doss, A. W., Zavala, D. C. and Smith, L. L. (1981). Intrabronchial instillation of paraquat in rats: Lung morphology and retention study. *Br. J. Industr. Med.*, **38**, 42–48

Yost, G. S., Buckpitt, A. R., Roth, R. A. and McLemore, T. L. (1989). Mechanisms of lung injury by systemically administered chemicals. *Toxicol. Appl. Pharmacol.*, **101**, 179–195

FURTHER READING

Gardner, D. E., Crapo, J. D. and Massaro, E. J. (1988). *Toxicology of the Lung*. Raven Press, New York

Jones, R. B., Matthes, S., Shepall, E. J., Fisher, J. H., Stermmer, S. M., Dufton, S. M., Stephens, J. K. and Bearman, S. I. (1993). Acute lung injury following treatment with high-dose cyclophosphamide, cisplatin, and carmustine. *Journal of the National Cancer Institute*, **85**, 640–647

Shapiro, C. L., Yeap, B. Y., Godleski, J., Jochelson, M. S., Shipp, M. A., Skarin, A. T. and Canellos, G. P. (1991). Drug-related pulmonary toxicity in non-Hodgkin's Lymphoma. *Cancer*, **68**, 699–705

Young, L. and Adamson, I. Y. R. (1993). Epithelial-fibroblast interactions in bleomycin-induced lung injury and repair. *Environmental Health Perspectives*, **101**, 56–61

23 Pulmonary Hypersensitivity Responses

Hilton C. Lewinsohn and Heather D. Burleigh-Flayer

INTRODUCTION

Hypersensitivity reactions are aberrations of normal host defence processes (Daul and de Shazo, 1982). Exposure of the respiratory system to harmful organic and inorganic dusts, vapours, gases, and fumes through inhalation can produce hypersensitivity reactions of two main clinical types, namely (1) hypersensitivity pneumonitis and (2) allergic rhinitis and asthma. Allergic rhinitis and asthma are associated with exposure to chemicals whereas hypersensitivity pneumonitis is an inflammatory reaction caused by certain protein antigens, e.g. farmer's lung is caused by exposure to *Micropolyspora faeni*.

We restrict our discussion mainly to the effects of exposure to industrial chemicals. In this chapter we deal with the role of industrial and domestic chemicals against the general background of these pulmonary disorders, and review the magnitude of the problem and its effect on morbidity and mortality. The use of animal models in the study of the pathogenesis of these diseases and laboratory methods for predicting respiratory sensitization are briefly discussed.

Definition of Hypersensitivity Pneumonitis

Hypersensitivity pneumonitis (extrinsic allergic alveolitis) is defined by Salvaggio (1987) as a 'descriptive phrase that characterizes a spectrum of lymphocytic and granulomatous interstitial and alveolar filling pulmonary disorders associated with intense and often prolonged exposure to a wide range of inhaled organic dusts and related occupational antigens'.

The disorder affects the distal portions of the lung (peripheral airways) and is characterized by alveolar and interstitial cell infiltration, with accompanying fever and breathlessness 4–12 h after exposure. The lesions are characterized by mononuclear cell alveolar filling and interstitial infiltrates with a predominance of T lymphocytes and macrophages with evolution into granuloma formation (Salvaggio, 1987). Alveolar macrophages in the infiltrates are 'activated', and suppressor/cytotoxic T lymphocytes predominate (Stankus *et al.*, 1978; Leatherman *et al.*, 1984). High levels of serum-precipitating antibodies to the offending organic dust antigen are found. The levels of IgG, IgA and IgM in both serum and bronchial washings are elevated, but not IgE (Patterson *et al.*, 1976).

Salvaggio (1987) states that any organic dust of appropriate particle size is capable of inducing a hypersensitivity pneumonitis if exposure is sufficiently intense and/or prolonged. He points out that many particulate antigens that produce the disease may themselves be immunological adjuvants. It has been shown experimentally that thermophilic actinomycetes, which are the main source of antigen in many forms of hypersensitivity pneumonitis (farmer's lung, bagassosis, and mushroom worker's lung), have marked adjuvant effects on antibody production and cell-mediated hypersensitivity (Bice *et al.*, 1975).

The various forms of hypersensitivity pneumonitis, also known as extrinsic allergic alveolitis, have been well described in the occupational medical literature and are usually known by names related to the type of exposure or the occupation in which exposure occurs, i.e. farmer's lung, mushroom worker's lung, bird fancier's disease. The diagnosis of hypersensitivity pneumonitis relies on the history and physical examination (Montenaro, 1992). Patients present with cough, fever, malaise, and arthralgias. There may be hypergammaglobulinaemia and a raised erythrocyte sedimentation rate.

Definition of Asthma

Scadding (1985) proposed the following definition of asthma after considering the deliberations of the Ciba Foundation Guest Symposium in 1958 and the suggested definition of the American Thoracic Society:

Asthma is a disease characterized by wide

variations over short periods of time in resistance to flow in the airways of the lungs.

According to Merchant (1990), in the published report of the *Workshop on Environmental and Occupational Asthma*, asthma may affect as many as 20 million Americans. He states that mortality has doubled in the past decade, is twice as great among black Americans and that asthma is responsible for increasing hospitalizations with an estimated annual medical cost of four billion dollars. The United States National Heart, Lung and Blood Institute (NHLBI) estimated in 1989 that asthma affected approximately ten million Americans and people with asthma experience well over 100 million days of restricted activity annually. Asthma is more prevalent among children than adults. Of the ten million Americans with asthma NHLBI estimates that about three million are under 18 years of age. Overall there is no difference in asthma prevalence by sex: 4.0 per cent for both males and females.

It is not possible to quantify the proportion of occupationally or environmentally-induced cases. According to Chan-Yeung (1990) in Japan it is estimated that 15 per cent of cases of asthma in men result from occupational exposure. The same author reports that in the USA, analysis of the 1978 Social Security Disability Survey showed that 7.7 per cent of the respondents identified asthma as a personal medical condition, and 1.2 per cent (15.4 per cent of all those with asthma) attributed it to workplace exposure.

The Workshop on Occupational and Environmental Asthma decided to use a broad and inclusive definition and adopted the one proposed by Newman Taylor in 1980 (quoted in Merchant, 1990):

Variable airway narrowing causally related to exposure in the (working) environment to airborne dusts, gases, vapors or fumes.

Occupational asthma is a disorder where there is generalized obstruction of the airways, usually reversible and caused by inhalation of substances or materials that the individual handles or uses, or which are incidentally present at the workplace or in the environment. Some patients with asthma have a special liability to Type I IgE-mediated hypersensitivity reactions. It used to be customary to refer to allergy in defining asthma, but

these cases are in the minority and not only they but other patients with asthma and some with other respiratory disorders show abnormal bronchoconstrictor responsiveness to many physical and chemical stimuli. This has been called non-specific bronchial or airway reactivity or non-specific bronchial hyper-responsiveness. Postma *et al.* (1989) define airway hyper-responsiveness as an exaggerated bronchoconstrictive reaction on exposure to a small quantity of a non-specific, non-allergenic stimulus to the airways. Quantitative tests may use physical agents, such as cold air and non-isotonic aqueous aerosols, but most test for enhanced responses to pharmacological bronchoconstrictors such as histamine or methacholine. The smallest dose that induces a specified diminution in expiratory airflow is determined.

Agents used as stimuli to measure hyper-responsiveness include:

Histamine	Prostaglandin D_2
Methacholine	Prostaglandin $F_{2\alpha}$
Acetylcholine	Leukotriene C_4, D_4, E_4
Adenosine	β-Adrenergic blockers
Serotonin	Cold air
Bradykinin	Hyperventilation of dry air
Sulphur dioxide	Hypo-/hyperosmolar stimuli

Two tests used to indirectly measure the calibre of the airways are the peak expiratory flow rate (PEFR) and the forced expiratory volume in one second (FEV_1). The values of the 'best test', usually after three efforts have been made, are accepted. Eiser (1987) states that asthma can generally be diagnosed readily from a combination of history, examination, spirometry, diurnal variation in airways obstruction and its relief with bronchodilators. In these circumstances bronchial challenge is not necessary. The actual dose of a bronchoconstrictor (provocative dose) producing a fall of 20 per cent in the baseline FEV_1 ($PD_{20}FEV_1$) can be derived by linear interpolation from the dose–response curve. This widely accepted measurement is useful in the assessment of bronchial hyper-responsiveness. Eiser (1987) concludes that the $PD_{20}FEV_1$ 'appears to be a simple measure and probably clinically useful particularly in the longitudinal studies of the same individuals', and further points out that 'it is the most convenient index for most clinical and epidemiological purposes at present'. The same author concludes that 'it is a simple way of differentiating asthmatic from non-asthmatic in doubtful cases and correlates with the clinical state of an asthmatic. The results obtained from inhalation of methacholine, histamine and cold air are reproducible, even when repeated at 30 minute intervals.'

HISTORICAL BACKGROUND

Occupational lung diseases have been recognized since at least 1556 when Agricola in his treatise on mining described a lung disease that was probably silicosis. Bernardino Ramazzini (1713) was probably the first to describe the relationship between the breathlessness of sifters and millers of grain and their working conditions.

According to Massoud (1964) the term 'byssinosis' was first used by Proust in 1877 for the symptoms of breathlessness described by textile workers. According to O'Holloren (1992), the harmful effects of platinum salts were described among photographic workers in Chicago in 1911 by Karasek. Skin reactivity and asthmas produced by exposure to extracts of castor beans were noted in castor bean mill workers more than 50 years ago (Figley and Elrod, 1928). The work of Pepys (1963) on farmer's lung did much to increase awareness of hypersensitivity diseases of the lungs due to fungi and organic dusts. In recent years occupational asthma has been recognized as an important and common cause of morbidity in a number of industries. The list of substances capable of causing asthma in the workplace is now long and being added to almost monthly in the scientific literature.

CAUSES OF PULMONARY HYPERSENSITIVITY RESPONSES

More than 200 organic and inorganic compounds are known to cause occupational asthma. Substances causing pulmonary hypersensitivity responses can be derived from animal, vegetable, or chemical agents. Some animal handlers are known to suffer from asthma and this may prevent such people from continuing in their chosen professions. Laboratory animal allergy (LAA) can affect all levels of laboratory workers from the person handling animals and cleaning cages

to the research scientist in charge of important projects. It would appear that allergic reactions may develop in about 15–20 per cent of laboratory animal workers, of whom less than half develop asthma (Newman Taylor, 1981). Newman Taylor states that there is a considerable excess of atopics among animal handlers who develop asthma, but not among those who develop other reactions. He comments that those with asthma, unlike those who develop urticaria, are very likely to have positive skin prick tests and specific IgE antibody to animal extracts, particularly urine.

Vegetable causes of asthma are numerous and may affect spice factory workers, bakers, or woodworkers. A variety of allergenic materials have been incriminated.

Chemical causes of occupational asthma may include 'micromolecular' chemicals and are likely to become an increasing problem in the future as their use increases.

PREDISPOSING FACTORS

In atopic workers some industrial processes involving exposure to high molecular weight compounds pose a risk for sensitization and the development of asthma (Chan-Yeung, 1990). These processes include those with potential for exposure to detergent enzymes, platinum salts, flour dust, locusts, animal dander, and gum acacia. Chan-Yeung comments also that atopic status does not seem to be an important factor in exposure to western red cedar and low molecular weight compounds, such as isocyanates. Development of asthma can be influenced by the periodicity of exposure and whether it is intermittent or continuous. Intermittent high-level exposures may be important in isocyanate-induced asthma.

There may be a latent interval of from a few weeks to years before sensitization develops and allergic reactions occur. In industries, such as platinum refining, sensitization occurs within 1–3 years. The role of cigarette smoking in the development of occupational sensitization and asthma is not known (Chan-Yeung, 1990).

MECHANISMS TO EXPLAIN THE PULMONARY HYPERSENSITIVITY RESPONSE

Most industrial agents causing occupational asthma have known or suspected allergic properties, although occupational asthma may also occur through reflex, inflammatory, and pharmacological mechanisms. Proving that a specific agent causes occupational asthma by an immunological mechanism can be problematical. Similarly, the immunological tests of hypersensitivity might help pinpoint a putative allergen but will not prove causation, short of bronchoprovocation testing with the suspected and control agents. Bronchial hyper-reactivity is present in the majority of subjects with occupational asthma, but approximately one-third of those with asthma may show no evidence of excessive reactivity of the airways. This would suggest that direct irritation is not the only mechanism involved in this form of asthma. It has been suggested that bronchial reactivity may be genetically determined and, as such, predisposes to the development of occupational asthma. However, most of the evidence indicates that the hyper-reactivity is the result of the asthma rather than the cause of it.

High molecular weight compounds, such as those present in laboratory animal dander and urine, plant dusts, and enzymes, can induce allergic bronchoconstriction by producing specific IgE and sometimes specific IgG antibodies. Thus, skin testing is often positive (when performed), as are radioallergosorbent testing, enzyme-linked immunosorbent assay and sometimes precipitin tests. Low molecular weight compounds, such as isocyanates, anhydrides, plicatic acid in red cedar dust, and metal salts, may serve as haptens, combining with protein molecules to act as allergens.

Certain clinical characteristics will distinguish allergic from non-allergic asthma. This is particularly important when differentiating an occupational from a non-occupational cause. The latent period from first exposure to the development of symptoms in an individual with an allergen-induced asthma may be long. Re-exposure to the offending agent at low concentrations may cause a recurrence of symptoms. There is also a strong likelihood of an allergic background in an employee who becomes sensitized to an agent in the workplace. In contrast, agents that cause reflex bronchoconstriction (sulphur dioxide, ozone, etc.) or act as direct pharmacological agents affect more employees without respect to atopic background, appear to be dose-related, and do not require a latent period before the onset of symptoms.

The asthmatic response to an allergen can be manifested immediately, with significant airway constriction within the first hour. A late response may occur 4–6 h after initial exposure. This has been termed a biphasic response. A response with both immediate and late airway constriction or recurrent airway constriction can occur, particularly in the evening hours and lasting over many days (Rubinstein *et al.*, 1987).

It has been postulated that an asthma-like illness can occur in persons after a single exceedingly high exposure to an environmental irritant. This has been termed reactive airways dysfunction syndrome (RADS) because a characteristic finding is hyper-reactivity (hyper-responsiveness) of airways (Brooks and Lockey, 1981; Brooks *et al.*, 1985; Boulet, 1988). Individuals develop an asthma-like illness following a single exposure to unusually high levels of an irritant vapour, fumes or smoke. In a number of instances, the high-level exposure was from an accident occurring in the workplace, a road or rail accident with release of spilled chemicals, or a situation where poor ventilation and a limited air exchange were present in the work area. In all cases, symptoms developed within a few hours, and often minutes, after exposure. It seems that acute high-level, uncontrolled irritant exposure can lead to an asthma-like syndrome in some individuals with long-term sequelae and chronic airways disease. Non-immunological mechanisms seem to be operative in the pathogenesis of reactive airways dysfunction syndrome.

The clinical criteria for the diagnosis of reactive airways dysfunction syndrome are:

- A documented absence of previous respiratory complaints or disease.
- The onset of symptoms after one specific exposure incident or accident.
- Exposure to an irritant gas, smoke, fume, or vapour which was present in an unusually high concentration.
- The onset of symptoms occurred within 24 h after the exposure.
- Symptoms simulated asthma with cough, wheezing and dyspnoea predominating.

- Pulmonary function tests usually showed air-flow obstruction.
- Methacholine challenge testing was positive or a clinical history suggested hyper-reactive airways.
- Other pulmonary diseases have been ruled out.

CLINICAL FEATURES OF OCCUPATIONAL ASTHMA

Symptoms vary considerably in their pattern. Typically, a worker with occupational asthma presents with dyspnoea, chest tightness, cough and wheezing occurring at work or within several hours after leaving work. The respiratory symptoms are often accompanied by rhinitis and/or conjunctivitis. Improvement in these symptoms on weekends, vacations or while away from the usual workplace is an important clue. Following the onset of asthma, continued exposure may result in the development of constant and unremitting symptoms that no longer have a relationship to work.

It should be recognized that many patients initially may present with recurrent attacks of 'bronchitis' with cough, sputum production and rhinitis as the predominant symptoms. These symptoms in an otherwise healthy non-smoker should raise the suspicion that they may be related to the work environment. Patients who do develop symptoms immediately after exposure, whenever they work with the same material, will usually recognize the causal relationship themselves. A large number of substances, particularly small molecular weight organic and inorganic compounds (approximately 1000 daltons) may cause late asthmatic reactions. The respiratory symptoms frequently occur after working hours during the evening and at night, but not during the working hours. It is usual for symptoms to gradually become worse as the week continues, and sometimes recovery takes several days or even weeks after exposure ceases.

It is essential to take a detailed occupational history and to attempt to characterize the type of work done, the workplace conditions (such as exhaust ventilation) and the materials used or handled in the workplace. It should be remembered that exposure may occur to agents that are present in the workplace but which are not necessarily used or handled by the patient and are introduced by fellow workers at nearby work stations. If the patient is not sure of the agents present in the workplace, then the employer should be contacted and asked for Material Safety Data Sheets for all the agents used in the work area. In the USA this information must be provided to the worker and to medical personnel requiring it to treat the employee according to the provisions of the Occupational Safety and Health Administration's Hazard Communication Standard. Furthermore, the employer must disclose all the ingredients in a mixture to the physician and cannot claim trade secrecy. The physician may be asked to sign a confidentiality agreement not to disclose the proprietary information provided.

If the plant has an industrial hygienist, then exposure levels should be obtained for the agents to which the employee is exposed. Inquiries should be made to find out if other workers in the same work area or job also have similar complaints. The presence of symptoms in a disproportionate number of workers may provide a clue. It is important to ask if the patient has been involved in any accidental exposures or spills, or in the cleanup operations following an accident or spill.

There is no substitute for a good history in making the diagnosis of occupational asthma, but objective tests are required. Detailed measurement of lung function on a single occasion away from work is a poor method of diagnosing occupational (or non-occupational) asthma. Longitudinal measurements over a defined time interval are a good method for assessing chronic loss of lung function in a group, but a poor method of making the diagnosis of occupational asthma in individuals. The simplest method of confirming occupational asthma is supervised before- and after-shift measurement of lung function, but it is very insensitive. Measurement can be made more sensitive if it is made on the first day back at work after a vacation, but this is surprisingly difficult to achieve. Bronchial provocation tests using samples of the chemicals or materials found in the workplace may be required in some cases.

Evidence that asthma is work-related may be obtained by a 'stop–resume' work test during which the patient's daily symptoms, use of medications and lung function are monitored over a period of time. Prolonged recordings of the peak expiratory flow rate over a period of 3–4 weeks at work, and every 2 h from waking to sleeping at home, by the patient using a portable peak flow meter, have been found very useful in discerning a causal relationship between lung function and exposure. This programme is fraught with potential problems. False negative results may be obtained because the patient may be on concurrent treatment with disodium cromoglycate or corticosteroids. Individuals with persistent airways obstruction, who have less than 20 per cent change in their lung function during the day or week that testing was being performed, may be missed. The worker's compliance to frequent lung function monitoring may be poor, especially in a busy workplace. False positive results may appear because the measurements are being made in an unsupervised manner. There is always the possibility that the worker will falsify the results, especially if compensation is involved.

In the occasional patient with a compelling history of work-related asthma, a specific inhalation provocation test may be necessary to establish or exclude the diagnosis of occupational asthma. When necessary, this test should be performed by experienced personnel in a hospital where resuscitation facilities are available and where frequent observations can be made. Such facilities are generally only available in academic institutions. The tests are time-consuming and expensive. They are usually performed on a research basis and not supported by third-party paying agencies. The worker is exposed to the suspected agent at levels and under conditions that mimic those in the workplace. Changes in lung function are compared with those elicited with an appropriate placebo. Care must be taken not to exceed the concentrations that are met at work.

The main indications for specific inhalational challenge are: (1) occupational asthma suspected but the suspect agent is not a recognized cause; (2) more than one recognized causative agent in the workplace; and (3) absolute confirmation is necessary because the patient may have to change his or her job.

A method for performing this test has been perfected whereby the patient is exposed to the suspected allergen in a similar manner to that which would occur at work, but in a setting where effects can be controlled and lung function can

be measured. A 15 per cent or greater fall in timed vital capacity is sufficient to demonstrate a cause-and-effect relationship, provided no such fall followed a control test using an inert substance.

Non-specific pharmacological agents may be used to provoke bronchoconstriction. They include methacholine, histamine and carbachol. Methacholine increases parasympathetic tone in bronchial smooth muscle, resulting in bronchoconstriction. The objective of these tests is to determine the minimum exposure (i.e. dose) of the test agent (e.g. methacholine) that can precipitate a 20 per cent fall in FEV_1. This concentration is known as the PD_{20} (provocative dose producing a 20 per cent fall in FEV_1). All current subjects with asthma respond to methacholine inhalation, whereas only 75–80 per cent will respond to the various physiological stimuli (exercise, cold air) to the point of resulting in a PD_{20}. Pharmacological challenges with methacholine or histamine can produce significant airway narrowing in some subjects without asthma, whereas this will not occur with exercise or cold air. The primary clinical indication for inhalation challenge with methacholine, histamine, etc. is to identify the presence of bronchial reactivity, an essential component of the asthmatic state.

Most patients presenting with asthma have classic symptoms and bronchial challenges are not necessary for diagnostic purposes. However, patients may present with cough as their only symptom or with atypical dyspnoea without physical findings and with normal spirometry. In these situations a bronchial challenge may be a useful clinical test. A negative methacholine challenge rules out current bronchial asthma and would guide the clinician to consider other causes of bronchial disease such as tumour, bronchiectasis, or possible chronic bronchitis. Bronchial challenge may be useful in identifying workers who are at risk for occupational asthma because of pre-existing bronchial responsiveness.

IMMUNOLOGICAL TESTING

Skin Tests

Skin testing has become the standard method for demonstrating the presence of skin-sensitizing IgE antibodies. The prick test has been found to be the most satisfactory of the epicutaneous skin tests, with more sensitivity and less variability in comparison with the scratch test. Skin testing for allergens is indicated in patients with asthma whose disease began before the age of 40 years and in selected older individuals. Skin testing detects antigen-specific IgE antibodies, yields information of a semiquantitative nature that is more sensitive than radioallergosorbent testing (RAST), correlates with allergic symptoms and signs, gives supportive evidence for instituting immunotherapy, and is superior to available RAST in the diagnosis of life-threatening ana-phylaxis. The results are immediately available and are more cost effective than RAST.

Radioallergosorbent Testing (RAST)

RAST is capable of detecting minute quantities of allergen-specific IgE antibodies that circulate in the serum of allergic patients. It is widely avail-able in a kit form for laboratory use. This test is preferred when skin testing is not meaningful as in dermatographia or existing widespread skin disease. RAST, however, has been marketed for substances not proven to be allergenic, such as aspirin, radiocontrast dyes, etc. Inappropriate selection and interpretation of RAST results may occur.

PULMONARY FUNCTION TESTS

Periodic pulmonary function test monitoring is effective in determining abnormalities in most types of occupational asthma. Pre- and post-shift, as well as serial tests throughout the week, are helpful in distinguishing reflex, pharmacological, and allergic asthma. Findings can include a gen-eralized airway obstruction (FEV$_1$/FVC (forced vital capacity) per cent <70), significant pre- to post-shift changes (>10 per cent change in FEV$_1$), or observation of a more rapid than normal yearly decline in spirometric values of exposed workers. The results of the pulmonary function tests need to be correlated with the clinical history and physical examination, as well as the immunolog-ical evaluation. When doubt exists about an underlying causative agent, or when a new pre-viously unconfirmed allergen and/or other cause of occupational asthma has been suspected, a spe-cific bronchoprovocation inhalation test may be indicated.

PROGNOSIS

Many patients with occupational asthma do not recover completely after cessation of exposure even though their condition is frequently improved. The persistence of symptoms is accompanied by the presence of non-specific bronchial hyper-reactivity demonstrated by methacholine or histamine inhalation challenge tests. As these people did not have asthma before they were exposed to the causative agent, it is fair to assume that their symptoms are the result of occupational exposure. Exposure to the offending agent altered the reactivity of the air-ways in these individuals by some unknown mech-anism.

The factors that affect the prognosis are dur-ation of exposure before onset of symptoms, dur-ation of symptoms before diagnosis, age, race, smoking habits, atopic status, type of asthmatic reaction induced by inhalation challenge, pul-monary function, and non-specific bronchial reac-tivity at the time of diagnosis.

People with persistent asthma after cessation of exposure are commonly diagnosed late and have more severe disease at the time of diagnosis than those who have recovered. Continued exposure to the offending agent in sensitized patients leads to further deterioration in lung function and increase in non-specific bronchial reactivity.

CLINICAL MANAGEMENT

When the causal relationship between asthma and the occupational agent has been established the worker should be removed from exposure. The employer should re-evaluate the manufacturing process and eliminate the use of the offending agent if possible. If this is not possible then the employer should attempt to find the employee an alternative job or a job in another area of the plant away from the offending agent. The employer must take measures to control exposure by means of engineering controls and industrial hygiene monitoring of the workplace. If the levels of exposure cannot be further reduced and the employee cannot be transferred to another job or area in the plant, adequate personal protective equipment must be provided.

Serial measurement of specific IgE antibodies, if present initially, may be useful for monitoring exposure after preventive measures have been instituted. Affected workers who are allowed to continue in the same environment should be followed regularly by their physicians. Their lung function and non-specific reactivity should be monitored regularly. Besides the use of respiratory protective devices, they may require the use of prophylactic medications, such as disodium cromoglycate, beclomethasone dipropionate, and β-adrenergic agonists. However, there are no data to show that prophylactic medications prevent the development of chronic persistent asthma.

The treatment of an acute episode of occupational asthma does not differ from that of any other form of acute asthma attack.

PREVENTIVE OCCUPATIONAL HEALTH AND SAFETY MEASURES

Efficient environmental controls of processes involving sensitizing materials must be installed. Safety measures to minimize the risk of exposure to high concentrations after accidents and spills must be implemented. This may entail the use of personal protective equipment together with adequate supervision and training. Workers and management may require specific education and training by experts in the subject of pulmonary responses to inhaled chemicals, vapours, fumes, gases and particulates that are capable of stimulating an asthmatic response. Good housekeeping practices are essential to minimize any exposure risk. Product formulations may have to be changed if the ingredients are demonstrated to be associated with the production of pulmonary reactions to them. Substitution of harmful agents by innocuous ones may have to be considered. It may be prudent to identify job applicants or workers with pre-existing asthma and advise them that their workplace is known to contain materials or products that have been associated with the development of occupational asthma. They should be offered alternative employment if it is available because it would be impossible in most instances to differentiate between an asthmatic

attack due to the workplace or an exacerbation of their pre-existing problem. Atopy may be an important predisposing factor in occupational asthma caused by high molecular weight compounds but not in that caused by low molecular weight compounds.

ANIMAL MODELS

Animal models of occupational asthma and hypersensitivity pneumonitis have been developed by investigators in an attempt to further understand these disease states. In 1961, Parish and colleagues produced hypersensitivity pneumonitis in guinea pigs and rabbits sensitized to mouldy hay. Many other investigators have developed animal models of hypersensitivity pneumonitis, most typically in the rabbit (Jones, 1970; Richerson *et al.*, 1971; Kawai *et al.*, 1972; Major *et al.*, 1972). However, many of these models have used antigens not commonly related to the disease, adjuvants, and/or intratracheal administration as the route of exposure.

Some models of hypersensitivity pneumonitis were developed to evaluate Type III immune injury while others were developed to evaluate Type IV injury. Richerson (1972) showed that guinea pigs could be immunized in a manner to favour either a Type III or a Type IV reaction. Wilkie *et al.* (1973), through passive transfer experiments, noted both Type III and Type IV reactions. These investigators also reported an increase in respiratory rate in immunized guinea pigs following a challenge. Leach *et al.* (1987) demonstrated hypersensitivity pneumonitis in rats where no adjuvants or conjugation were used to produce a response. In this model, the number of external haemorrhagic foci in the lungs of sensitized animals was directly related to the exposure concentration as well as to alveolar macrophage accumulation, alveolar haemorrhage, pneumonitis, and macrophage IgG and complement.

Asthma in guinea pigs was first reported by Ratner *et al.* (1927) as a result of inhalation exposure to horse dander. The guinea pig model has been successful in producing anaphylaxis by exposure to other high molecular weight complex biological materials (Patterson and Kelly, 1974) and purified proteins (Yagura *et al.*, 1971; Yamamura *et al.*, 1974).

An animal model developed by Karol *et al.* (1978) was the first in which an asthmatic reaction to small airborne chemicals was demonstrated. In this model, animals were sensitized by inhalation exposure to the material for 3 h a day for 5 days. Following a rest period of approximately 2 weeks, animals were challenged by inhalation exposure. The respiratory parameters of the animals were monitored during the challenge to determine if a response occurred. An immunological mechanism of this response was confirmed by determination of antibodies in the sera of animals. This animal model can also be used to investigate agents producing hypersensitivity pneumonitis. Monitoring of pulmonary function of the animals can be extended for up to 24 h to detect the onset of delayed responses. Remote temperature telemetry has also been incorporated into the model as fever is a feature of hypersensitivity pneumonitis.

Recently, screening techniques have been investigated for the determination of a chemical's ability to act as a respiratory sensitizer. Wass and Belin (1990) proposed that there is a correlation between the ability of a chemical to react with mucosal surface proteins and its potential to produce respiratory tract diseases such as asthma. These investigators developed an *in vitro* model to assess the reactivity of a lysine-containing peptide in biologically relevant conditions using high pressure liquid chromatography. Strong reactions occurred for those substances known to act as haptens (e.g. isocyanates and anhydrides) while no reaction was observed for chemicals that do not have sensitizing properties (e.g. simple acids, bases, and solvents). They propose that this method could be used for the screening of potential respiratory sensitizers.

Sarlo and Clark recently (1992) proposed a tier approach for evaluating the respiratory allergenicity of low molecular weight chemicals that uses both *in vitro* and *in vivo* methods. Four tiers of testing are involved in this multilevel approach:

Tier 1 involves evaluating the structure–activity information to ascertain whether the chemical can react covalently with proteins, and a literature search to find out if the chemical belongs to a family of chemicals that are known to be respiratory sensitizers.

Tier 2 consists of an experiment performed to determine if the chemical can covalently bind to protein to form a conjugate under *in vitro* conditions.

Tier 3 uses guinea pigs that are injected with the chemical and their sera are tested for antibodies to evaluate the immunogenicity of the chemical.

Tier 4 involves a guinea pig inhalation study as described by Karol (1983).

SUMMARY

There are still many gaps in our knowledge of asthma. The prevalence of occupational asthma in various occupational settings is largely unknown. The techniques currently available in epidemiological studies for identifying subjects with occupational asthma are not satisfactory. There is no validated health history questionnaire available for asthma or occupational asthma. Cross-sectional studies are likely to underestimate the true prevalence of occupational asthma as workers who develop it tend to leave the jobs that cause it. Studies should be designed to answer the following questions.

- What is the incidence of occupational asthma in industry?
- Is there a dose relationship in sensitization?
- Can the level of exposure be determined below which sensitization does not occur?
- What are the predisposing host factors?
- Can affected workers return to the same job with reduced levels of exposure without detriment to their health?

The use of bronchial challenge tests in the field to identify subjects with asthma should be properly assessed, but this test may not be more informative than a well-designed questionnaire.

Whether non-specific bronchial hyper-reactivity is a predisposing host factor in occupational asthma can only be answered by a prospective study following pre-employment examination.

The methods used to confirm occupational asthma are unsatisfactory. Specific provocation tests are time-consuming and not without discomfort to the patient. Research should be done to develop immunological means of confirming sensitization to occupational agents.

The American Thoracic Society (1993) published a revised version of its guidelines for the evaluation of impairment and disability in patients with asthma which 'takes into consideration not only impairment related to reduced lung function but other parameters, such as the degree of airway hyperresponsiveness and the type and amount of medication required to control symptoms, which are important reflections of the severity of asthma.' The Society's statement provides detailed advice for the use of spirometry and measurement of airway responsiveness by means of methacholine or histamine inhalation test using standardized methods. Routine exercise testing in the investigation of asthma is not recommended.

The American Thoracic Society's guidelines only briefly touch upon the special considerations for subjects with occupational asthma. It is recommended that employees with a temporary impairment or disability are to be 'considered 100 per cent impaired on a permanent basis for the job that caused the illness and for other jobs with exposure to the same causative agent'. The guidelines recommend that 'assessment for long-term impairment or disability should be carried out every 2 years after the removal from exposure when improvement has been shown to plateau'.

The American Thoracic Society 'does not address the methods of identification of the cause of asthma'. The pathogenic mechanisms in asthma in general, and in occupational asthma in particular, remain unknown.

REFERENCES

American Thoracic Society's Ad Hoc Committee on Impairment/Disability Evaluation in Subjects with Asthma (1993). Guidelines for the evaluation of impairment/disability in patients with asthma. *Am. Rev. Respir. Dis.*, **147**, 1056

Bice, D., McKarron, K., Hoffman, E. O. *et al* (1975). Adjuvant properties of *Micropolyspora faeni*. *Int. Arch. Allergy Appl. Immunol.*, **55**, 267

Boulet, L. P. (1988). Increase in airway responsiveness following acute exposure to respiratory irritants. *Chest*, **94**, 376

Brooks, S. M. and Lockey, J. (1981). Reactive airways dysfunction syndrome (RADS). A newly defined occupational disease. *Am. Rev. Resp. Dis.*, **123** (Suppl.), A133 (abstract)

Brooks, S. M., Weiss, M. A. and Bernstein, I. L. (1985). Reactive airways dysfunction syndrome (RADS). Persistent airways hyperreactivity after high level irritant exposure. *Chest*, **88**, 376

Chan-Yeung, M. (1990). Occupational asthma. Workshop on environmental and occupational asthma (Guest Ed. Merchant, J. A.) *Chest*, **98** (Suppl.), 145S

Daul, C. B. and de Shazo, R. D. (1982). Hypersensitivity reactions; understanding their role in disease. *Postgrad. Med.*, **72**, 136

Eiser, N. M. (1987). Bronchial provocation tests. In Nadel, J. A., Pauwels, R. and Snashall, P. D. (Eds), *Bronchial Hyperresponsiveness; Normal and Abnormal Control, Assessment and Therapy*. Blackwell Scientific Publications, Boston, MA, Chapter 7

Figley, K. D. and Elrod, R. H. (1928). Epidemic asthma due to castor bean dust. *JAMA*, **90**, 79

Jones, B. (1970). Experimental pathology relating to 'farmers' lung', *Tubercle*, **51**, 218

Karol, M. H. (1983). Concentration-dependent immunologic response to toluene diisocyanate (TDI) following inhalation exposure. *Toxicol. Appl. Pharmacol.*, **68**, 229

Karol, M. H., Ioset, H. H., Riley, E. J. and Alarie, Y. (1978). Hapten-specific respiratory hypersensitivity in guinea pigs. *Am. Ind. Hyg. J.*, **39**, 546

Kawai, T., Salvaggio, J. and Harris, J. (1972). Cell-mediated immunity in experimental hypersensitivity pneumonitis. *Clin. Res.*, **20**, 511

Leach, C. L., Hatoum, N. S., Ratajczak, H. V., Zeiss, C. R., Roger, J. C. and Garvin, P. J. (1987). The pathologic and immunologic response to inhaled trimetallic anhydride in rats. *Toxicol. Appl. Pharmacol.*, **87**, 67

Leatherman, J. W., Michael, A. F., Schwartz, B. A. and Hoidal, J. R. (1984). Lung T-cells in hypersensitivity pneumonitis. *Ann. Intern. Med.*, **100**, 390

Major, P. C., Lapp, N. L. and Burrell, R. (1972). Immunopathology and pathophysiology in experimental hypersensitivity pneumonitis. *Fed. Proc.*, **31**, 664

Massoud, A. (1964). The origin of the term byssinosis. *Br. J. Industr. Med.*, **21**, 162

Merchant, J. A. (1990). Opening remarks. Workshop on Environmental and Occupational Asthma (Guest Ed. Merchant, J.A.) *Chest*, **98** (Suppl.) 145S

Montanaro, A. (1992). Isocyanate asthma. In Bardana, E. J., Montanaro, A. and O'Hollaren, M. T. (Eds), *Occupational Asthma*. Hanley & Belfus, Philadelphia, USA, pp. 179–188

Newman Taylor, A. J. (1981). Laboratory animal allergy. In Slovak, A. J. M. (Ed.), *Occupational Asthma: Proceedings of the Society of Occupational Medicine Research Panel Symposium*, 10 December 1981. Society of Occupational Medicine, 11 St Andrew's Place, Regents Park, London NW1 4LE, UK

O'Hallaren, M. T. (1992). Asthma due to metals and

metal salts. In Bardana, E. J., Montanaro, A. and O'Hallaren, M. T. (Eds), *Occupational Asthma.* Hanley & Belfus, Philadelphia, USA, pp. 179–188

Parish, W. E. (1961). The response of normal and sensitized experimental animals to products of mouldy hay. *Acta Allergol.,* **16**, 78

Patterson, R. and Kelly, J. F. (1974). Animal models of the asthmatic state. *Ann. Rev. Med.,* **25**, 53

Patterson, R., Schatz, M., Fink, J. N. *et al.* (1976). Pigeon breeders' disease. I. Serum immunoglobulin concentrations; IgG, IgM, IgA and IgE antibodies against pigeon serum. *Am. J. Med.,* **60**, 144

Pepys, J., Jenkins, P. A., Festenstein, G. N., Gregory, P. H., Lacey, M. E. and Skinner, F. A. (1963). Farmer's lung: thermophilic actinomycetes as a source of 'farmer's lung' hay antigen. *Lancet,* **ii**, 607

Postma, D. S., Koeter, G. H. and Sluiter, H. J. (1989). Pathophysiology of airway hyperresponsiveness. In Weiss, S. T. and Sparrow, D. (Eds), *Airway Responsiveness and Atopy in the Development of Chronic Lung Disease.* Raven Press, New York, Chapter 2

Ramazzini, B. (1713). *De morbis artificum diatriba* (Discourse on the disease of workers)

Ratner, B., Jackson, H. C. and Gruehl, H. L. (1927). Respiratory anaphylaxis. *Am. J. Dis. Child,* **23**, 48

Richerson, H. B. (1972). Acute experimental hypersensitivity pneumonitis in the guinea pig. *J. Lab. Clin. Med.,* **79**, 745

Richerson, H. B., Cheng, F. H. F. and Bauserman, S. C. (1971). Acute experimental hypersensitivity pneumonitis in rabbits. *Am. Rev. Resp. Dis.,* **104**, 568

Rubinstein, I., Levison, H., Slutsky, A. S., Hak, H., Wells, J., Zamel, N. and Rebuck, A. S. (1987). Immediate and delayed bronchoconstriction after exercise in patients with asthma. *N. Engl. J. Med.,* **317**, 482

Salvaggio, J. E. (1987). Robert A. Cooke Memorial Lecture: Hypersensitivity pneumonitis. *J. Allergy Clin. Immunol.,* **79**, 558

Sarlo, K. and Clark, E. D. (1992). A tier approach for evaluating the respiratory allergenicity of low molecular weight chemicals. *Fund. Appl. Toxicol.,* **18**, 107–114

Scadding, J. G. (1985). Definition and clinical categorization. In Weiss, E. B., Segal, M. S. and Stein, M. (Eds), *Bronchial Asthma; Mechanisms and Therapeutics,* 2nd edn. Little, Brown and Company, Boston, pp. 3–13

Stankus, R. P., Cashner, F. and Salvaggio, J. E. (1978). Bronchopulmonary macrophage activation in the pathogenesis of hypersensitivity pneumonitis. *J. Immunol.,* **120**, 685

Wass, U. and Belin, L. (1990). An *in vitro* method for predicting sensitizing properties of inhaled chemicals. *Scand. J. Work Environ. Health,* **16**, 208

Wilkie, B., Pauli, B. and Gygax, M. (1973). Hypersensitivity pneumonitis: experimental production in guinea pigs with antigens of *Micropolyspora faeni. Pathol. Microbiol.,* **39**, 393

Yagura, T., Miyagawa, T. and Yamamura, Y. (1971). Experimental allergic asthma in guinea pigs. In Serafini, U., Frankland, A. W., Masala, C. and Jamar, J. M. (Eds), *New Concepts in Allergy and Clinical Immunology, Proceedings of the VII International Congress of Allergology,* Florence, 1970. Excerpta Medica, Amsterdam, pp. 266–274

Yamamura, Y., Yagura, T. and Miyake, T. (1974). Experimental allergic asthma in guinea pigs. In Yamamura, Y., Frick, O. L., Horiuchi, Y., Kishimoto, S., Miyamoto, T., Naranjo, P. and deWek, A. (Eds), *Allergology, Proceedings of the VIII International Congress of Allergology.* American Elsevier Publishing Co., New York, pp. 509–515

FURTHER READING

Bernstein, I. L., Chan-Yeung, M., Malo, J-L. and Berstein, D. I. (1993). *Asthma in the Workplace.* Marcel Dekker, Inc., New York

Briatiro-Vangusa, C., Braun, C. L. J., Cookman, G., Hofman, T., Kimber, I., Loveless, S. E., Morrow, T., Pauluhn, J. Sorensen, T. and Niesson, H. J. (1994). Respiratory allergy: hazard identification and risk assessment. *Fundamental and Applied Toxicology,* **23**, 145–158

Holgate, S. T,. Austin, K. F., Lichtenstein, L. M. and Kay, A. B. (1993). *Asthma: Physiology, Immunopharmacology, and Treatment.* Academic Press, London

Selgrade, M. K., Zeiss, C. R., Karol, M. H., Sarlo, K., Kimber, I., Tepper, J. S. and Henry, M. C. (1994). Workshop on status of test methods for assessing potential of chemicals to induce respiratory allergic reactions. *Inhalation Toxicology,* **6**, 303–319

Sharma, O. P. (1989). *Hypersensitivity Pneumonitis.* Karger, Basel

24 Ophthalmic Toxicology

Bryan Ballantyne

INTRODUCTION

The eye may be a target or route for toxicity under various circumstances (Figure 1).
(1) Direct contact of a material with the eye may produce

(a) A peripheral sensory irritant effect.
(b) Injury and/or inflammation of the eye and surrounding structures (primary irritation).
(c) Initiate a sensitization reaction (allergic conjunctivitis).
(d) Deep eye injury with materials that penetrate surface structures.

(2) Materials having high toxic or pharmacological potency may be absorbed from the surface periocular vessels and, following nasolachrymal drainage, from the nasal mucosa and alimentary tract and exert systemic toxicity.
(3) Materials absorbed by other routes of exposure, or their metabolites, may reach the eye through the systemic circulation and thus exert toxic effects on the eye and its adnexa (systemic toxicity to the eye).

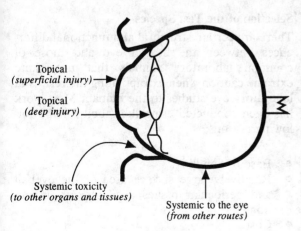

Figure 1 The eye in local and systemic toxicity

PRIMARY IRRITANT EFFECTS ON THE EYE

Chemical injuries to the eye are common, but in the majority of cases are preventable. Injury by direct contact with a chemical may present clinically from occupational and domestic incidents, with the majority usually occurring from substances being handled in an uncontrolled manner in the home. For example, in one study (Kersjes *et al.*, 1987) 84.4 per cent of chemical eye injuries originated in the home; these cases were predominantly accidental exposures in children. Overall, most injuries were from acidic or alkaline solutions. Industrial eye accidents accounted for 14.2 per cent.

The time to onset and severity of chemically-induced eye injury varies with different groups of chemicals and certain specific chemicals. For example, severe eye injury is rapid in onset with alkaline materials (Smally *et al.*, 1992), whereas certain persistent dyestuffs (e.g. gentian violet) may have a latency of several days to the onset of corneal injury (Ballantyne *et al.*, 1973). Although the eye-injuring potential of many liquids or solids is well known, it should be appreciated that many irritant vapours or gases may produce eye injury; examples include tetramethyl butanediamine (Ballantyne *et al.*, 1992), 2-formyl-3,4-dihydro-2*H*-pyran (Myers *et al.*, 1993) and acrolein (Hathaway *et al.*, 1991). Of practical occupational importance is the fact that some vapours, notably of amines, may produce transient visual disturbances at concentrations without injurious sequelae. Thus, glaucopsia (or blue-grey vision) is a temporary disturbance of vision caused by exposure to certain amine vapours. This results from a slight increase in corneal thickness with fogging of vision and haloes appearing around bright objects (Jones and Kipling, 1972). On removal from exposure, vision returns to normal, without subsequent eye injury, in a few hours. While not leaving any permanent harmful effects on the eye, the symptoms of glaucopsia are incapacitating and impair efficient work performance and may predispose to physical accidents. Materials known to produce glaucopsia incude *N*-ethyl piperidine, *N*-methyl morpholine, *N*-ethyl morpholine, tetramethyle-thylenediamine and dimethylamine (Mellerio and Weale, 1966). Triethylamine is also known to cause glaucopsia (Akesson *et al.*, 1986) and the effects have been shown to be quantitatively cor-related with corneal oedema visualized by slit lamp microscopy and an increase in cornea thick-ness measured by pachymetry (Akesson *et al.*, 1985). Similar findings have been described for dimethylamine (Stahlbom *et al.*, 1991).

The eye may be contaminated locally by a chemical or formulation either accidentally or, as in the case of ophthalmic medical preparations, deliberately. There is thus a need to know the potential for materials to produce eye injury by acute or repeated topical contamination of the eye in order that appropriate warnings may be given (e.g. in product safety literature and on labels), that advice may be given about first-aid and medical management, and that recommenda-tions may be given for protective measures when using or handling a particular material or formu-lation. Such considerations applying clearly to industrial and agricultural chemicals, domestic materials and other commercial preparations. For ophthalmic medicinal products this potential to produce injury is required to ensure that the in-use preparation does not cause structural and/or functional injury to the outer or deeper eye structures following acute or repeated deliberate applications to the eye.

The testing of chemicals and formulations for their eye-injuring potential by direct contact with the eye and surrounding structures has, until recently, been simplistic in methodology and con-ducted as acute tests. Basically, after exposure of the eye to the test material (as solid, liquid, vapour, aerosol, etc.), the visible ocular and perioocular tissues are examined for signs of inflammation and/or injury. In addition to macro-scopic evidence of inflammation and injury, cer-tain pharmacological effects may be seen, e.g. midriasis and cycloplegia with anticholinergics. More recently, and considered at the end of this section, methods have been proposed to quantify the response of the test system. Additionally, and because of the nature of the test and its associated discomfort and stress, there have been a prolifer-ation of alternative methods suggested for deter-mining or predicting the eye-injuring potential of chemicals by topical contamination of the eye. A very large number of eye irritation tests have been conducted and published over the past few decades and, in the absence of fully validated alternatives, conventional eye irritation studies continue to be undertaken, but at a decreasing rate. The following section is devoted to a description of the conduct and interpretation of standard eye irritation tests. This is followed by a brief summary of the use of alternatives for assessing the topical eye-injuring potential of materials.

In Vivo Eye Irritation Tests

Most studies are conducted as single dose (acute) procedures. Although clinical reports of eye injury to humans from chemicals have long been reported, it was not until the early 1940s that eye irritation testing as a laboratory animal procedure became formalized (Draize *et al.*, 1944). As noted above, the basis of all variants on acute eye irri-tation tests is exposure to the test chemical fol-lowed by periodic inspection for signs of ocular and periocular injury and/or inflammation to determine their onset, progression and resol-ution. Some of the more important features of these studies are summarized below. Differences exist in the details of specific protocols recom-mended by various regulatory agencies; these have been discussed in detail by Daston and Free-berg (1991).

Selection of the Test Species

There are certain structural and functional differ-ences between the human eye and those of common laboratory animals that necessitate extreme caution when extrapolating the results of laboratory eye studies to the human. Most work has been conducted using the rabbit for the fol-lowing reasons:

- Ease of handling.
- Relatively large surface area of the eyeball and periocular tissues available for inspec-tion.
- Cost.
- There is a large background literature on the ocular effects of chemicals and drugs on the rabbit eye.

- This species is recommended in many regulatory protocols.

Cited disadvantages include the following:

(1) The rabbit has a nictitating membrane; some authorities believe that this structure removes irritant from the surface of the eye, others consider it acts as a trap (Buehler and Newmann, 1964).

(2) The tearing mechanism is less effective in the rabbit than the human (Buehler and Newmann, 1964), a factor of importance in relation to the degree and duration of contact of the foreign material with the eye.

(3) The pH and buffering capacity of the aqueous humor differ in humans and rabbits (Carpenter and Smyth, 1946), which possibly explains why the rabbit eye is more susceptible to chemically-induced iritis.

(4) The rabbit has a slow blink reflex (Mann *et al.*, 1948).

(5) Both the thickness and the histology of the cornea differ between rabbit and human (Carpenter and Smyth, 1946). The rabbit corneal thickness averages 0.37 mm and that of the human 0.5 mm (Marzulli and Simmon, 1971). Histological differences include the corneal epithelium being several layers thinner in the rabbit, and Bowman's membrane is an order of magnitude thinner; both these factors facilitate the penetration of irritants. Also, the area of eye occupied by cornea is 25 per cent in the rabbit but only 7 per cent in humans.

(6) The rabbit eye is more easily anaesthetized by irritants than is the human eye and hence more susceptible to reduction of the protective blinking reflex (Daston and Freeberg, 1991).

Comparative observations, using a variety of materials, have shown that the eye of primates responds differently from that of the rabbit, the rabbit usually having a more marked reaction (Buehler and Newmann, 1964). Other comparative tests on the rabbit, monkey and human have demonstrated that the ocular reactions in the monkey may be more akin to that of the human (Beckley *et al.*, 1969). Thus for critical purposes, such as the testing of ophthalmic preparations, confirmatory studies may be required to be undertaken in non-human primates.

Material to be Tested

For most purposes it is usually recommended that 0.1 ml of liquid or 100 mg of solid be used and placed in the inferior conjunctival sac. In some cases, for example where the test material is suspected of producing eye injury, 0.01 or 0.005 mg or ml of test material may be used. It should be noted that 0.1 ml is close to the maximum volume that can be accommodated in the inferior conjunctival sac and the use of smaller volumes has been suggested to be more appropriate for comparison with the practical aspects of splash contamination of the human eye. Griffith *et al.* (1980) determined the dose-respone relationship for several chemicals of varying irritant potential using different volumes applied to the cornea and compared the results with known human eye irritancy. They found a dose-volume of 0.01 ml produced irritation in the rabbit eye which was most consistent with that observed in humans. Others have confirmed the reliability of the low volume test for determining eye irritating potential (Walker, 1985; Williams, 1985; Freeberg *et al.*, 1986; Allgood, 1989). Also, the low volume eye irritation test in rabbits correlated well with the conventional Draize procedure (Blein *et al.*, 1991).

For exposure to gases, vapour, aerosol or smoke, appropriate exposure chambers with sampling and analytical facilities are required. Because acute ocular irritancy with aerosols may vary with particle size (Punte *et al.*, 1963), it is important that samples be taken for particle size as well as concentration measurements. Also, for practical purposes, it may be necessary to measure ocular irritation as a function of particle size. To reduce the numbers of animals used, eye irritation observations should be routinely incorporated into acute and repeated exposure studies involving airborne materials.

When formulations are tested it is ideal to know if any eye injury produced results from the active ingredient alone, vehicle or formulation. To reduce the number of tests necessary, from a product safety viewpoint only the formulation may need to be tested. Clearly, also for product safety purposes, if a formulation produces eye injury it may be necessary to determine if the in-use dilution of that material is irritant (Ballantyne and Swanston, 1977).

It follows that if a material is required to be

tested in solution, a non-irritant solvent should be chosen, e.g. saline, polyethylene glycol 300, propylene glycol or glyceryl triacetate (Ballantyne *et al.*, 1972).

The Test Procedure

Animals are required to be acclimated for about 1 week before testing to ensure recovery from stress caused by transportation, including corneal dehydration. Animals are housed in cages designed to prevent accidental eye injury, including the use of wire mesh floors in place of sawdust or wood chippings. On the day before testing, animals are examined to ensure the absence of ocular abnormalities.

Studies have been conducted to determine the smallest number of animals that can be used to adequately characterize the eye irritant potential of chemicals. DeSousa *et al.* (1984) examined the ability of two-, three-, and five-animal subsets to predict accurately the outcome of six-animal tests for a large number of petrochemicals, and found that the three-rabbit subsets were 93 per cent accurate in predicting the six-rabbit irritation tests. A similar finding was obtained by Talsma *et al.* (1988) and confirmed by Bruner *et al.* (1992). However, if the findings from a particular three-animal test show a wide variability, then it may be necessary to undertake additional testing.

Materials are usually placed into the inferior conjunctival sac (larger amounts) or onto the surface of the cornea, after which the lids are gently held together for a few seconds. One eye is used for testing in each animal, with the contralateral eye serving as a control. It is now generally considered that application of test material to the surface of the cornea, rather than into the conjunctival sac, is a more practical method for mimicking the actual exposure conditions of accidental eye exposure, except for ophthalmic medicinal preparations which may be instilled into the inferior conjunctival sac (Chan and Hayes, 1985). Special devices for applying measured amounts of test material to the eye have been described (Buehler and Newmann, 1964; Battista and McSweeney, 1965).

Eyes are examined periodically after applying test material. According to the Draize protocol, eyes are inspected at 1, 24, 48 and 96 h, and if necessary at 7 days. The Organization for Economic Cooperation and Development (OECD) guidelines specify 1, 24, 48 and 72 h postexposure, with observations up to 21 days at the investigators discretion. Early observations are essential to detect initial signs of injury and their progression. A minimum of 1 week of observation is required to ensure that any latent injury is detected. Eyes should be examined under standard conditions of illumination.

The use of local anaesthetics has been proposed as a means to alleviate discomfort in eye irritation tests. However, some authorities consider that local anaesthetics may exacerbate ocular irritation. Also, there is some evidence that they may, to variable extents, delay corneal healing and may themselves produce corneal injury and hence potentiate irritation (Datson and Freeberg, 1991). Additionally, local anaesthetics inhibit the blink reflex. Etter *et al.* (1992) have reviewed corneal injury caused by local anaesthetics and have shown experimentally that oxybuprocaine produced a concentration-related increase in corneal permeability. Also, Lapalus *et al.* (1990) found that oxybuprocaine was cytotoxic *in vitro* to corneal epithelial cells.

Standard recommendations for the first-aid management of chemically-induced eye injury include the use of extensive ocular irrigation (Herr *et al.*, 1991). While postexposure irrigation of the eye generally reduces or prevents eye irritation, in some cases increased irritation has been observed after water irrigation (Gaunt and Harper, 1964). Because of this, some regulations have recommended that subgroups of animals be used to determine the efficacy of eye irrigation on the development and severity of eye injury, e.g. the OECD guidelines specify a second group of animals with irrigation 30 s postexposure (OECD, 1987).

The effect of other therapeutic procedures can be incorporated into conventional eye irritation studies; for example the use of anti-inflammatory preparations (Ballantyne *et al.*, 1976). This may involve simple direct visual determination of efficacy or more sophisticated methods such as measurement of aqueous humour prostaglandins (Spampinato *et al.*, 1991).

Scoring of Ocular Lesions

Various schemes have been proposed for grading and scoring the ocular lesions seen in standard eye irritation tests. That introduced by Draize has probably been the one used most frequently (Draize *et al.*, 1944; Draize, 1959), particularly in product development. The Draize system assigns values to effects seen in the cornea, iris and conjunctiva, usually at several specified periods (Table 1). There are three major concerns with this scoring system:

(1) Only certain effects in the three tissues are described. Thus, the cornea is graded separately for opacity and area of involvement; the iris is considered as a whole; there are separate grades for conjunctival hyperaemia, chemosis and discharge. This restriction of the effects recorded may give an incomplete description of the ocular reaction to a chemical.

(2) The range of grades differs with the effect recorded. Corneal effects, both opacity and area of involvement, are graded 0–4; the iris is graded 0–2; effects on the conjunctiva are graded 0–3 for discharge and hyperaemia and 0–4 for chemosis. This non-uniformity in grading can clearly lead to difficulties during interpretation of the numerical scores.

(3) Results are not reported as scores as seen but as arithmetically-derived biased (weighted) numbers derived from the scores as seen (Table 1). For example, corneal scores are a product of grades for opacity and area involved and a bias factor of 5; iris is scored five times the grade observed; the conjunctival score is twice the sum of the grades for hyperaemia, chemosis and discharge. Thus, for a possible total maximum score of 110 points, 73 per cent is derived from the corneal score, 18 per cent from the conjunctiva and 9 per cent from the iris; i.e. there is scoring bias ratio of 8:2:1 with respect to the cornea, conjunctiva and iris.

The Draize approach was modified by the US Food and Drug Administration (FDA) for enforcing the Hazardous Substances Labelling Act. The FDA system (Table 2) does not differentiate between opacity of the cornea and area of involvement, and the scores reported are the actual grades observed and not arithmetically biased total scores. To facilitate the scoring between different laboratories, and to obtain better reproducibility, colour photographs equivalent to scores have been published (Food and Drug Administration, 1965). In the system by Ballantyne and Swanston (1977) grades for lachrymation, blepharitis, chemosis, conjunctival hyperaemia, iritis, keratitis and corneal neovascu-

Table 1 System for scoring ocular lesions

Cornea	
(A) Opacity[a]	
No opacity	0
Scattered or diffuse area, iris details clearly visible	1
Easily discernible translucent areas, iris details slightly obscured	2
Opalescent areas, iris details not visible, pupil size barely discernible	3
Opaque, iris invisible	4
(B) Area of cornea involved	
One-quarter or less, but not zero	1
Greater than one-quarter, but less than half	2
Greater than half, but less than three-quarter	3
Greater than three-quarter, up to whole area	4

Corneal score = (A) × (B) × 5 (maximum total score = 80)

Iris	
(A) Normal	0
Folds above normal, congestion, swelling, circumcorneal injection (any or all), iris still reacting to light	1
No reaction to light, haemorrhage, gross destruction	2

Iris score = (A) × 5 (maximum total score = 10)

Conjunctivae	
(A) Vessels normal	0
Vessels definitely injected above normal	1
Diffuse, deep crimson red, individual vessels not readily discernible	2
Diffuse beefy red	3
(B) No chemosis	0
Any swelling above normal (includes nictitating membrane)	1
Obvious swelling with partial eversion of lids	2
Swelling with lids about half closed	3
Swelling with lids about half closed to completely closed	4
(C) No discharge	0
Any amount of discharge different from normal	1
Discharge with moistening of the lids and hairs adjacent to lids	2
Discharge with considerable moistening around the eyes	3

Conjunctival score = [(A) + (B) + (C)] × 2 (maximum total score = 20)

Total maximum score (cornea + iris + conjunctiva) = 110

[a] Degree of density (most dense area taken for reading).

Source: Draize *et al.* (1944).

Table 2 System for grading ocular lesions according to the US Food and Drug Administration

Cornea	
No ulceration or opacity	0
Scattered or diffuse areas of opacity; details of iris visible	(1)[a]
Discernible translucent areas; iris slightly obscured	2
Nacreous areas; details of iris not visible; pupil barely discernible	3
Complete corneal opacity; iris not discernible	4
Iris	
Normal	0
Markedly deepened folds, congestion, swelling, moderate circumcorneal injection (any or a combination), iris still reacting to light	(1)[a]
No reaction to light; haemorrhage; gross destruction	2
Conjunctivae	
Vessels normal	0
Some vessels definitely injected	1
Diffuse, crimson red, individual vessels not easily discernible	(2)[a]
Diffuse beefy red	3
No swelling	0
Any swelling above normal	1
Obvious swelling with partial eversion of lids	(2)[a]
Swelling with lids about half closed	3
Swelling with lids more than half closed	4

[a] Figures in parenthesis are the lowest grades considered positive.

larization are scored (Table 3). To obtain a more uniform approach, each effect is recorded on a six-point scale (0–5).

Recording, Presentation and Interpretation of Information

The conventional eye irritation study is a subjective evaluation of macroscopic observations and it is therefore not surprising that there has been considerable inconsistency between results obtained from different laboratories using even the same test protocol (Russell and Hoch, 1962; Weil and Scala, 1971). Such differences arise from a variety of factors, including variable training methods in different laboratories, use of groups with different population sizes, differences in age, strain and sometimes sex of animal. Many of the effects seen, such as pannus formation, keratoconus, conjunctival haemorrhages and corneal neovascularization, are not easily scored.

Table 3 Grades for scoring ocular lesions

Effect	Grade	Observation
Lachrymation	0	Normal
	1	Slight excess at lower tarsal margin
	2	Slight wetting of periorbital hair
	3	Obvious wetting of lid margins and periorbital hair
	4	Gross wetting of periorbital hair
	5	Gross wetting of hair with fluid running down face
Blepharitis	0	Eyelids normal
	1	Slight reddening of lid margins
	2	Diffuse redness and slight swelling of lid margin
	3	Diffuse redness of lids with moderate swelling of lids
	4	Diffuse bright redness with marked thickening and deformity of lids
	5	Diffuse bright redness with marked thickening and irregular deformity of lid margins; contracted palpebral fissure
Chemosis	0	No swelling of conjuctivae or nictitating membrane
	1	Minimal swelling with no eversion of lids
	2	Moderate swelling with slight eversion of lids
	3	Moderate swelling with moderate eversion of lids; swollen tissues encroaching over periphery of cornea
	4	Marked swelling and eversion with tissues almost completely obliterating the cornea
	5	Gross swelling and eversion of lids with complete obliteration of cornea
Congestion of conjunctiva and nictitating membrane	0	Vessels normal
	1	A few injected vessels
	2	Diffuse and moderate injection of blood vessels
	3	Diffuse and marked dilatation, but individual vessels still discernible
	4	Diffuse and gross dilatation with individual vessels barely discernible
	5	Diffuse intense redness with no discernible vessels

continued

Table 3 (continued)

Effect	Grade	Observation
Sloughing	0	Absent
	1	Patchy detachment of film
	2	Diffuse detachment of fine membrane
	3	Diffuse detachment of fine film with slight contamination of lacrimal fluid
	4	Obvious stripping of membrane with moderate contamination of lacrimal fluid
	5	Gross detachment of membrane and gross contamination of lacrimal fluid
Iritis	0	Normal iris
	1	Slight injection of blood vessels of iris
	2	Slight thickening of folds with diffuse and moderate injection; still reacting to light
	3	Moderate thickening of folds with diffuse and moderate congestion; slight reduction in response to light
	4	Diffuse and gross erythema with obvious thickening; sluggish reaction to light
	5	No reaction to light, distorted pupil, gross inflammatory change with haemorrhages
Keratitis	0	Normal cornea
	1	Just detectable haziness of cornea
	2	Obvious opacity of cornea (local or general) but iris clearly visible
	3	Local or general opacity of cornea almost obscuring vision of the iris
	4	Local or general opacity of the cornea totally obscuring the iris
	5	Gross opacification of the cornea with deformity and/ or ulceration
Vascularization of cornea	0	Avascular
	1	Localized ingrowth of vessels for 1–2 mm
	2	Generalized in growth of vessels for 1–2 mm

continued

Table 3 (continued)

Effect	Grade	Observation
	3	Generalized ingrowth of vessels for 3–4 mm
	4	Ingrowth of vessels to within 1–2 mm of centre of cornea, but without confluence
	5	Complete vascularization of the cornea with confluence of vessels at the centre of cornea

Source: Ballantyne *et al*. (1977).

Such effects, however, are significant and are usually tabulated separately or as footnotes.

The numerical system involves tabulating scores as a function of the time of inspection; values for individual animals should be presented as well as group mean scores. An example scored according to the Draize method is shown in Table 4. In some instances only cumulative scores are given; because of the variability between animals and resultant interpretational difficulties, this is a practice to be avoided. An alternative method is to record both average scores and ranges (Table 5). For illustrative purposes, and provided the range of responses is not wide, graphical methods may be used to compare different concentrations of the same material or the same dose of different materials; an example is shown in Figure 2. Response–duration histograms (Macrae *et al.*, 1970), showing the relative numbers of animals having different reactions at each inspection

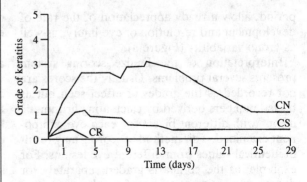

Figure 2 Graphical representation of the average grade of corneal injury versus time from dosing rabbits (10 per group) with 0.1 ml of 5 per cent solutions of 2-chloroacetophenone (CN), *o*-chlorobenzylidene malononitrile (CS) or dibenz[*b,f*]-1,4-oxazepine (CR). Corneal injury graded by the scoring system shown in Table 3

Table 4   Results of an eye irritation study with 5 per cent (w/v) 2-chloroacetophenone dissolved in polyethylene glycol 300; scored and presented by the method of Draize *et al.* (1944)

Rabbit number	Tissue scored[a]	1 h	24 h	48 h	72 h	96 h	7 days
1	Cornea	0	30	45	45	60	60
	Iris	0	5	5	5	5	5
	Conjunctiva	14	14	14	10	10	6
	Total	14	49	64	60	75	71
2	Cornea	0	15	15	30	15	15
	Iris	0	5	5	5	5	5
	Conjunctiva	12	12	12	10	8	4
	Total	12	32	32	45	28	24
3	Cornea	0	30	45	45	45	30
	Iris	0	5	5	5	5	5
	Conjunctiva	16	14	12	10	6	2
	Total	16	49	62	60	55	37
4	Cornea	0	30	45	45	45	45
	Iris	0	5	5	5	5	5
	Conjunctiva	14	14	18	14	12	2
	Total	14	49	68	64	62	52
5	Cornea	0	30	30	45	45	45
	Iris	0	5	5	5	5	5
	Conjunctiva	16	14	16	10	8	6
	Total	16	49	51	60	58	56
6	Cornea	0	30	30	45	55	45
	Iris	0	5	5	5	5	5
	Conjunctiva	16	12	10	10	8	2
	Total	16	47	45	60	68	52
Mean scores	Cornea	0	27.5	35.0	42.5	44.2	40.0
	Iris	0	5.0	5.0	5.0	5.0	5.0
	Conjunctiva	14.7	13.3	13.7	10.7	8.7	3.7
Mean total scores		14.7	45.8	53.7	58.2	57.9	48.7

[a] Maximum tissue scores: cornea 80, iris 10, conjunctiva 20.
Maximum possible total score, 110.

Source: Scored and presented by the method of Draize (1944).

period, allow a ready appreciation of the rate of development and resolution of eye injury, as well as group variability (Figure 3).

Interpretation of the Draize scoring system presents several problems. Usually the scores are not recorded as the grades of effect seen but as biased numbers derived by calculating arithmetic means with different biases for each eye component examined. This method of scoring may result in identical values from different eye lesions. For example, as the cornea is graded separately for degree of opacity and area of involvement, and because this is presented as a biased product, small focal lesions scattered over the surface of the cornea may obtain a score identical to that produced from small localized dense lesions in

one quadrant. This emphasizes the need to record each effect individually.

There have been attempts to reduce the Draize and other scoring systems to a single numerical value for the rating of irritancy. These schemes involve further arithmetic manipulation of scores, taking the situation even further away from the biological response. Several authors give a scale of rating. Kay and Calandra (1962) described seven ratings from minor to severe. Such rating schemes usually have fixed standards and do not give any indication of the nature, severity or duration of eye lesions. While such ratings may have some value in product development, they are not sufficiently precise for regulatory purposes or publication of data, and do not provide the clini-

Table 5 Eye irritation test conducted with 5 mg solid chloroacetophenone using six rabbits

Effect[a]	Time of inspection								
	10 min	1 h	6 h	1	2	3	days 4	7	14
Lacrimation									
Mean	1.8	2.8	2.7	2.4	1.7	2.3	1.8	1.2	0.6
Range	1–3	2–4	2–3	1–3	1–2	1–3	1–3	1–2	0–2
Blepharitis									
Mean	1.1	2.0	2.1	2.7	3.0	3.0	2.9	2.5	1.0
Range	1–2	2	1–4	2–4	2–4	2–4	2–4	2–3	0–2
Chemosis									
Mean	1.9	3.0	3.3	2.7	2.3	2.2	1.6	1.0	0
Range	1–3	2–5	3–4	2–4	2–3	1–3	1–2	0–2	
Hyperaemia									
Mean	2.1	2.5	2.3	3.2	3.2	3.1	3.0	2.4	0.9
Range	2–3	2–3	2–3	3–4	3–4	3–4	2–4	1–4	0–2
Sloughing									
Mean	0	0	0	1.7	2.0	1.5	1.0	0.9	0.3
Range				1–4	1–3	1–2	0–3	0–2	0–3
Iritis									
Mean	0	0	0.3	1.4	1.6	1.7	1.5	1.2	0
Range			0–2	1–2	1–2	1–3	1–3	0–3	
Keratitis									
Mean	0	0	0.9	2.1	2.4	2.8	3.1	3.9	4.0
Range			0–2	2–3	2–4	2–4	2–4	2–5	1–5
Corneal vessels									
Mean	0	0	0	0	0	0	0	0.5	2.3
Range								0–1	0–4

[a] Effects scored by the method shown in Table 3.

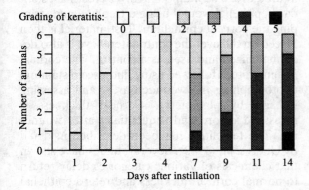

Grading of keratitis: ☐ 0 ☐ 1 ▦ 2 ▦ 3 ■ 4 ■ 5

Figure 3 Response–duration histogram for the development of corneal injury in the rabbit eye following instillation of 2 per cent crystal violet in water. Scoring system according to that shown in Table 3

cal description of eye injury to be expected from contamination of the eye with a particular chemical.

Schemes where the precisely defined grades of effects are presented as a function of time allow a ready appreciation of the onset, duration, resolution, severity and nature of adverse effects on the eye. The FDA system requires that results shall be presented in this way and defines, for regulatory purposes, what constitutes a positive response. A tissue is regarded as having given a positive reaction if there is, at any reading, opacity or ulceration of the cornea, iritis, obvious chemosis with partial eversion of the lids, or a diffuse deep crimson red coloration of the conjunctiva with individual vessels not discernible. A material is considered irritant if four or more animals in a test group of six rabbits show a positive reaction in any tissue. A material which has produced lesions of the cornea and/or iris that have not cleared by the seventh day, is considered a severe eye irritant.

Ancillary Methods

Certain ancillary procedures have been proposed or adopted to obtain a more precise evaluation of the presence and nature of eye injury during the conduct of *in vivo* eye irritation tests.

Use of Fluorescein Staining

Normal corneal epithelium presents a lipophilic barrier to fluorescein but when breached allows fluorescein to penetrate into the underlying stroma. Detection of the presence of fluorescein staining is a valuable guide to early corneal injury. One or two drops of 2 per cent fluorescein are applied directly to the cornea and washed off a few seconds later with isotonic saline. The injured area retains more dye than the intact epithelium and appears a brighter yellow in colour. This is facilitated by examination under ultraviolet light or by using a blue filter in a slit-lamp microscope. Yellowish-green areas stained by fluorescein indicate regions where the dye has penetrated epithelial lesions and diffused into normal tissues. Rose Bengal has been recommended as a stain for areas of degenerate epithelial cells and Alcian Blue for the demonstration of mucus.

Corneal Permeability Studies

Because corneal epithelial damage may increase the rate of penetration of fluorescein through the cornea, the presence of fluorescein in the aqueous humor may give an indication of whether corneal permeability has been increased An increased accumulation in the anterior chamber may be detected by a 'fluorescein flare' in the aqueous humor when a blue filter is used in the slit-beam path of the biomicroscope. Measurement of fluorescein has been used as a basis for quantifying corneal permeability (Maurice, 1967, 1968). Sulphorhodamine B is preferred to fluorescein because of its lower lipid solubility at physiological pH and its decreased permeability in the undamaged cornea, and because the red wavelength emitted by rhodamine allows better quantifiable discrimination (Maurice and Singh, 1986). Changes in fluorescein concentrations in aqueous humor can be quantified using a fluorophotometer attached to a slit-lamp biomicroscope. This gives an objective test for eye injury (Easty and Mathalone, 1969). Etter and Wildhaber (1985) used fluorimetry to quantify corneal permeability to fluorescein in mice following treatment with a series of surfactants. They found good agreement between fluorescein penetration and *in vivo* irritancy.

Slit-Lamp Biomicroscopy

Slit-lamp examination of the eyes is a valuable aid for detecting early and minimal corneal changes and allows a more precise evaluation of the structural condition of the cornea, iris, lens and aqueous humor, e.g. the presence of a flare in the aqueous humor due to excess protein (McDonald *et al.*, 1972). A system of scoring changes seen during biomicroscopy of the eye has been described (Baldwin *et al.*, 1973).

Measurement of Corneal Thickness

The *in vivo* measurement of corneal thickness is an objective approach to determining injury to the cornea, particularly in the early stages of injury. This measurement may be an alternative to standard eye irritation tests rather than supplementary to these studies (this is considered later under the section devoted to alternatives to standard eye irritation tests, pp. 513–519).

Corneal Epithelial Healing Rate

Following injury of the corneal epithelium, re-epithelialization occurs and corneal thickness increases; toxic substances may, however, retard the normal rate of healing. It has been proposed that the measurement of corneal thickness and healing rate can be used as a method for the evaluation of potential eye irritants, particularly with ophthalmic preparations applied to the injured eye. The method involves creating a standard epithelial wound using a trephine and stripping the corneal epithelium. Test material is then placed on the eye; the contralateral eye is also de-epithelialized and used as a control. The corneal healing rate is followed using fluorescein staining, photographing the wounded area, and assessing its size by planimetry. Corneal thickness is measured before and sequentially after wounding. The technique has been described in detail by Ubels *et al.* (1982). Several studies have shown that chemicals of various categories delay return to normal corneal thickness and retard epithelial healing rate (Ubels *et al.*, 1982; Green *et al.*, 1989; Fujihara *et al.*, 1993).

Histopathology

At the end of the observation period the animals are killed, the treated eyes are removed, processed for histology and a detailed examination is undertaken. In some instances the pathogenesis of the ocular lesions are studied after sequential killing during the inspection period.

Alternatives to Conventional Eye Irritation Tests

Criticism of eye irritation tests has come from scientists, informed persons and self-interest groups. The primary basis for the criticism is the discomfort and deliberate injury to the eye produced in standard tests and apparent trivial misuse by testing products such as cosmetic formulations. These pressures, both informed and uninformed and compounded by media hype, and the concern expressed by many practising toxicologists, have led to a proliferation of investigations in an attempt to modify the conventional approach and reduce discomfort, or to replace eye irritation tests with alternative methods. As a consequence there has been a proliferation of publications in which authors report what they consider to be suitable alternatives having the ability to predict *in vivo* eye injury. Some of these approaches have merit in being biologically and mechanistically based but others display a lack of understanding of basic biological principles and the mechanism of induction of eye injury. At the time of writing there is a general opinion that no one method, particularly *in vitro*, can reliably predict the eye irritating potential of a differing series of chemical classes. Several methods, taken together, may predict eye irritating potential but ultimately for high risk situations the results require confirmation (particularly if negative) by *in vivo* procedures. Total reliance on many of the alternative procedures, as currently practised and validated, is unlikely to be helpful in, for example, litigation involving human eye injury from a material judged to be non-irritating by such procedures. Also, and paradoxically inhibitory to alternative procedures, many regulatory authorities support the need for alternative tests for ocular irritancy but do not currently accept the results from these procedures for the purposes of human health hazard evaluation and relevant regulatory actions. Reinhardt (1990) has stressed the need for regulatory bodies to lower their threshold for acceptance of *in vitro* tests.

Alternatives to conventional *in vivo* eye irritations tests can conveniently, although not mechanistically, be subdivided into *in vivo* alternatives, *in vitro* alternatives and the use of non-biological models (Table 6). Some illustrative examples are given below.

Table 6 Classes of approaches for alternatives to conventional eye irritation techniques

In vivo threshold irritant methods
Isolated ocular preparations
Isolated non-ocular preparations
In vitro cytotoxicity assays
Non-biological models
Analogy

In Vivo Alternatives

These methodologies, while using whole animals, aim at significantly reducing discomfort by employing lower doses of test material and increasing the sensitivity of detection of injury by the use of non-invasive objective techniques. Most methods have the advantage of monitoring a functional physiological system with quantifiable evaluations.

Measurement of Corneal Thickness

Measurement of the thickness of the cornea *in vivo* is a particularly sensitive method for the detection of early corneal injury. Corneal oedema can result, for example, from epithelial and/or endothelial damage, an increase in intraocular pressure, and the inhibition of Na^+/K^+-ATPase; such factors may be found in various types of chemically-induced corneal injury (Chan and Hayes, 1985). The procedure offers several advantages, including the following:

(1) Quantitative information is obtained which may be subjected to statistical analysis for comparative evaluation of different materials.

(2) The method is non-invasive and causes the minimum of discomfort to animals.

(3) Increases in corneal thickness occur at concentrations below those causing macroscopic evidence of eye irritancy.

(4) Examination of the concentration-response curve allows predictions of irritant potency.

Corneal thickness may be measured *in vivo* by a simple optical device attached to a slit-lamp biomicroscope or by means of ultrasonic probe devices, both of which show good reproducibility (Chan and Hayes, 1985; Martins *et al.*, 1992). Optical pachymeters have the advantage that no contact with the surface of the cornea is necessary.

Several studies have shown a good predictive correlation for eye irritancy. Thus, Burton (1972) found that measured changes in corneal thickness agreed well with subjectively assessed eye irritation and that persistent corneal injury was associated with a greater degree of corneal thickening. Conquet *et al.* (1977) reached similar conclusions. Jacobs and Martens (1989) also found a good correlation between mean proportionate corneal swelling and corneal opacity and hyperaemia scores.

Increases in corneal thickness are concentration-related (Ballantyne *et al.*, 1975; 1976), and can be measured at concentrations below those producing macroscopic evidence of irritant effects on the cornea or conjunctiva (Figure 4). The method can also be used to detect increases in corneal thickness from exposure to vapour (Ballantyne *et al.*, 1976). With minor irritants, increases in corneal thickness are small and the concentration–effect curve plateaus around those concentrations just producing macroscopic evidence of eye injury; moderate eye irritants produce a concentration-related increase in corneal thickness below and above the irritant threshold; severe eye irritants produce concentration-related linear increases in corneal thickness up to the macroscopically visible irritation concentration and then show an abrupt increase with a marked change in the slope of the concentration–effect curve (Ballantyne *et al.*, 1975; Figure 5). Thus, the shape and slope of the concentration-effect curve can be used to predict the potential severity of eye irritation of a test material. As increases in corneal thickness can be measured at concentrations significantly lower than those that cause a macroscopic irritant effect, the procedure may be carried out with little discomfort to the animal. Also, Martins *et al.* (1992) showed a high sensitivity with good correlation and reproducibility between corneal thickness and clinical observations for irritancy, and they consider that the method may be used with low application volumes without loss of sensitivity.

Intraocular Pressure Measurements

Increases in intraocular pressure (IOP) can result from a variety of causes, including obstruction of the aqueous outflow tract, increase in aqueous humour production from the ciliary body, and increase in aqueous humour solute (Chan and Hayes, 1985). However, it is also common experience that when the eye is exposed to an irritant material there is also an increase IOP followed by recovery; the magnitude of the increase in IOP and its duration usually depend on the severity of the irritant response (Ballantyne *et al.*, 1972; Walton and Heywood, 1978).

IOP can be measured by cannulation of the anterior chamber but this approach has several disadvantages including the development of leaks, general anaesthesia is required, it is not suitable for long-term measurements, and it is

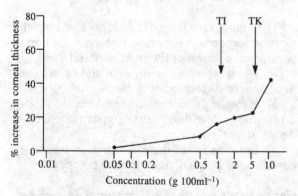

Figure 4 Peak increase in corneal thickness as a function of concentration of dibenz[*b*,*f*]-1,4-oxazepine applied to the rabbit cornea (in polyethylene glycol 300). It can be seen that increases in thickness occur at concentrations below that which is threshold for irritation to the conjunctiva (TI) and even lower than that producing macroscopic evidence of corneal injury (TK, threshold for keratitis)

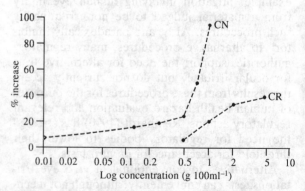

Figure 5 Increases in corneal thickness as a function of concentration of 2-chloroacetophenone (CN) and dibenz[*b*,*f*]-1,4-oxazepine (CR) applied to the eye. For CN, the more irritant material, increases in corneal thickness can be measured at lower concentrations than for the less irritant CR. Also, at any given concentration, the proportionate increase in corneal thickness is greater for CN than for CR

invasive (Ballantyne *et al.*, 1977). Tonometric methods which involve either measuring the amount of corneal deformation produced by a standard force applied to the eye (identation tonometry) or measuring the force required to produce a standard degree of corneal flattening (applanation tonometry) are more appropriate; the latter technique has many advantages over indentation methods (Ballantyne *et al.*, 1977). The rabbit is a suitable animal model because of the large volume of background information now available for this species on the influence of topical irritants on IOP.

Increase in IOP with a given material will depend on the total dose applied to the eye, i.e. the response will vary with both concentration and the volume applied (Figure 6). Thus, for comparative evaluation of different materials, the conditions should be similar with respect to dosing. Also, if materials are to be tested in solution, then solvents without an effect on IOP should be used, e.g. saline, polyethylene glycol 300, glyceryl triacetate, tri(2-ethylhexyl)phosphate, corn oil and 1,1,1-trichloroethane (Ballantyne *et al.*, 1972, 1977).

Increases in IOP can usually be measured within a few minutes of exposing the eye to an irritant. The time taken for the IOP to return to control values depends on the concentration of the test material, its irritant potential, and the ability to penetrate the cornea to produce deeper structural and/or functional injury. Times vary from around an hour to several days. It follows

that measurements should be made early and followed by sequential measurements. In general, the increase in IOP at a specific postexposure time is greater the more irritant the material (Figure 7). Also, as with corneal thickness measurements, mild or moderately irritant materials produce a linear increase in IOP with incremental increases in concentration whereas with severely irritant materials at low concentrations there is a shallow dose–response curve which then shows an abrupt change to a steep curve at higher concentrations (Figure 8). Comparison of the magnitude of changes and the slopes on the dose–response curves can also be

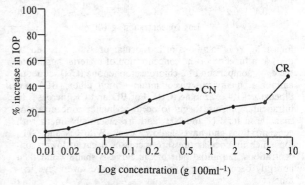

Figure 7 Proportionate increase in peak intraocular pressure in the rabbit eye resulting from the instillation of 0.1 ml solutions of differing concentrations of 2-chloroacetophenone (CN), and dibenz[*b*,*f*]-1,4-oxazepine (CR). The magnitude of the increases in pressure can be readily compared. For the more irritant CN, increases in IOP are measured at lower concentrations

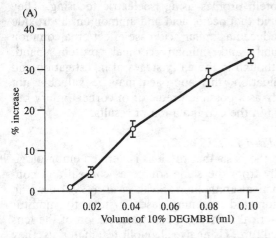

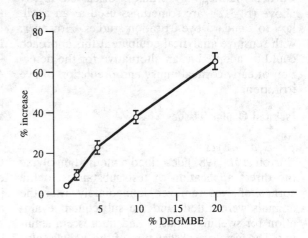

Figure 6 Increases in intraocular pressure (at 10 min) produced by diethylene glycol monobutyl ether (DEGMBE). (A) Increase as a function of volume of test material (40 per cent DPGME). (B) Increase related to instillation of 0.1 ml of different concentrations of DPGME. In both instances the increases are dose dependent

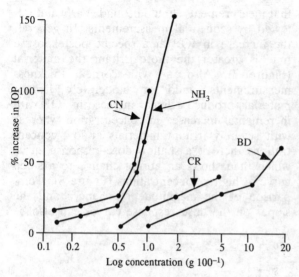

Figure 8 Peak increases in intraocular pressure (around 10 min) as a function of the concentration of material applied to the eye. Comparison of 2-chloroacetophenone (CN), aqueous ammonia, diethylene glycol mono-*n*-butyl ether (BD) and dibenz[*b,f*]-1,4-oxazepine (CR). For BD and CR increases in intraocular pressure begin to occur at higher concentrations than those for CN and NH₃ and are essentially linear with concentrations and have shallow slopes. With CN and NH₃, for which intraocular pressure increases occur at lower concentrations, the initial part of the curve is shallow and then abruptly becomes steep; these materials are severe eye irritants.

used to predict the likely severity of irritation which will be produced by a given material.

Corneal Permeability Studies

Corneal permeability studies, discussed briefly above (p. 512), are sometimes used as an ancillary to standard eye irritation studies. However, with sensitive analytical equipment this approach could be adopted as an alternative for the detection of early corneal injury and prediction of eye irritation.

Isolated Ocular Tissues

Enucleated Eyes

Burton *et al.* (1981) described a method involving the direct application of test substances to the cornea of eyes removed immediately after the animals were killed, and the subsequent evaluation for swelling, opacity and fluorescein staining. The histological structure of the eye was also examined. The eye is mounted on a clamp in a temperature controlled superfusion chamber with

isotonic saline being dripped onto the corneal surface. After a 30–45 min equilibration period, the test material is applied and then washed off. Eyes are subsequently inspected macroscopically, then with a slit-lamp biomicroscope, the corneal thickness is measured, and fluorescein staining observed. Price and Andrews (1985) measured corneal thickness in enucleated rabbit eyes and found the method to be a reliable predictor of eye irritation. In a comparative study using the isolated ocular preparation and involving several laboratories, Whittle *et al.* (1992) found that in overall rating the predictive value of the test and the conformity of results between different laboratories were good. A 10 s exposure allowed most irritant substances to be identified and a 60 s exposure increased the corneal response and could therefore be useful for testing products of potential low irritancy.

Isolated Cornea

Gautheron *et al.* (1992) used the isolated cornea from bovine eyes, held in place by a specially designed holder having compartments in front of and behind the mounted cornea and an incubation chamber. Corneal injury was assessed by opacity, measured by light transmission, and fluorescein permeability from the anterior to posterior chamber of the corneal holder. The results were found to give a good assessment of ocular irritating potential. Using a different approach, Eurell *et al.* (1991) have presented preliminary work with cryomicrotome sections of rabbit and human corneas to assess the effects on corneal protein profiles using isoelectric focusing. They found that acetic acid and ammonium hydroxide produced a similar acid/base effect on a common rabbit and human corneal protein band. Although in the early stages of investigation and validation, this approach may be valuable not only as a possible predictor of corneal injury but also in the extrapolation of results.

Isolated Lens

On the basis that the lens is derived embryologically from the same source as corneal and conjunctival epithelium, Sivak *et al.* (1992) used an automated scanning laser system to monitor spherical aberration and transmission of the lens in culture. Using five alcoholic test materials, they consider that this method of measuring lens damage compared favourably with standard

Draize scores. Clearly this work is at an early stage of development.

Isolated Non-Ocular Preparations

Chorioallantoic Membrane

The chorioallantoic membrane (CAM) of the hen's egg is highly vascular and has been used to determine irritant responses as a predictor for eye irritation. It is a borderline *in vivo/in vitro* system not conflicting with ethical and legal standards (Leupke, 1985). Basically, the test involves the use of fresh fertile eggs from which the shell is gently removed from around the air cell on day 10 of incubation. The vascular CAM is exposed by removing the inner membranes and test substance is dripped onto the membrane. The blood vessels and albumin are subsequently scored for irritant effects (hyperaemia, haemorrhage, coagulation) at 0.5, 2 and 5 min post-treatment. Details of methodology and scoring having been presented by Leupke (1985) who found a good correlation with the Draize irritation scores. Blein *et al.* (1991) found the method to be too sensitive with undiluted materials but with tenfold dilutions there was a reasonable correlation with *in vivo* eye irritation results; under these conditions this gave good discrimination between mild, moderate and severe irritants. Bagley *et al.* (1989) found that the CAM assay for surfactants correctly classified these materials and they showed that the method had high sensitivity, specificity and predictive value.

Martins *et al.* (1992) used a combined approach of the excised bovine eye and CAM assay to assess the eye irritating potential of chemicals; corneal injury was assessed by opacity, fluorescein stain and epithelial detachment. The combined assay was developed to simulate both corneal injury (bovine eye) and mucosal response (CAM). They found a limited correlation using this dual approach with fewer than 40 per cent of the substances tested being in agreement with *in vitro* results. In contrast, Van Erp and Weterings (1990) found a good correlation between the combined assay and *in vivo* results.

Other Tissues

A good correlation was found between haemolysis of bovine erythrocytes, blocking of spontaneous ileal contractions, and *in vivo* eye irritation by various surfactants (Muir *et al.*, 1983).

Cytotoxicity Assays

Cytotoxicity assays measure loss of some cellular or intercellular structure and/or functions, including cell death. They are generally simple to perform, reproducible, and have a clearly defined endpoint. In view of this, many investigators have used cytotoxicity assays as the basis for the development of *in vitro* 'predictive' alternative approaches to eye irritation studies. However, predictability based on comparison with *in vivo* standard eye irritation tests may be variable for a variety of reasons, including the fact that the assay systems are continually exposed whereas *in vivo* there are biological protective mechanisms in operation. Some assays may not be universally capable of detecting all chemical classes of irritants because of the endpoint used.

A variety of cell lines have been used including corneal epithelial cells, lung fibroblasts, Chinese hamster ovary cells, canine renal cells, HeLa cells and microorganisms. In each case where non-ocular cells lines have been used, authors have attempted to justify the reason for choosing that line. For example, the use of canine renal cells was justified by Shaw *et al.* (1991) on the basis that the integrity of the corneal epithelial cells depends on tight and desmosomal junctions, which are also seen in established canine renal epithelial cells and form an impermeable barrier. They may thus be used to detect chemicals that cause an increase in transepithelial permeability. These workers used fluorescein leakage to determine injury to tight junctions and neutral red release to detect renal cell membrane injury. A very large number of endpoints for cytotoxicity assays have been described, some examples of which are given in Table 7.

A kaleidoscope of assays have been described, and a few are given below as illustrative examples.

Crystal Violet Staining

Itagaki *et al.* (1991) employed a simple technique using cultured HeLa S3 cells or SIRC cells (an established line of rabbit corneal cells) in the presence of serial dilutions of the test material. After the incubation period, crystal violet was used to stain residual viable cells. The IC_{50} was calculated, i.e. the concentration of test material inhibiting growth of cells by 50 per cent. Using various surfactants they found good correlations

Table 7 Examples of endpoint measurements used in cytotoxicity assays for assessing alternative methods of testing for eye irritation

Method	Basis/Endpoint	Reference
Microphysiometry	Metabolic rate measurement	Bruner *et al.* (1991)
Uridine uptake inhibition	Membrane damage	Shopsis and Sathe (1984)
Neutral Red uptake	General cytotoxicity	Borenfreund and Puerner (1987)
Neutral Red release	Cell membrane injury	Rohde (1992)
Leucine incorporation	General cytotoxicity	Sina *et al.* (1992)
Total protein	General cytotoxicity	Riddell *et al.* (1986)
Fluorescein leakage	Cell membrane injury	Rohde (1992)
Colony forming efficiency	Lethal cytotoxicity	North-Root *et al.* (1982)
MTT dye reduction	Mitochondrial damage	Sina *et al.* (1992)
Crystal violet staining	Lethal cytotoxicity	Itagaki *et al.* (1991)
Alkaline phosphatase release	Membrane injury	Scaife (1985)
Intracellular ATP	General metabolic toxicity	Kemp *et al.* (1985)

between the IC_{50} and the maximum *in vivo* eye irritation scores for the materials tested.

Silicone Microphysiometer
This is a light-addressable potential sensor device which can be used to indirectly measure the rate of production of acidic metabolite from cells placed in a biosensor flow chamber. The endpoint calculated is the MRD_{50}, i.e. the concentration of test material required to reduce the metabolic rate by 50 per cent (Bruner *et al.*, 1991). Mouse fibroblasts have been used as the test cell. Bagley *et al.* (1992) found that the MRD_{50} for a variety of materials correlated well with the maximum average score for *in vivo* eye irritation.

Microtox Test
This test utilizes changes in luminescence from *Photobacterium phosphoreum*, which is generated through a process linked to respiration by NADH and flavin mononucleotide (Bulich, 1979). Light output is measured photometrically before and after the addition of the test substance and an EC_{50} value calculated, i.e. 50 per cent reduction in light emission. Bagley *et al.* (1992) found that, in general, test substances with the highest *in vivo* irritation gave the lowest EC_{50} values.

Neutral Red Uptake Assay
In this procedure cells, usually mouse fibroblasts or Chinese hamster ovary cells, are exposed to the test material and then to neutral red. Retention of neutral red indicates cell viability. Bagley *et al.* (1992) found that, in general, the concentration of test material required to reduce neutral red uptake decreased as the *in vivo* irritant potential of the test material increased. Attention needs to be paid to the technical aspects of incubation as emphasized by Blein *et al.* (1991) who found that correlation with materials with an extreme pH were underestimated because of the buffering effect of the culture medium and that volatile materials were also underestimated probably because of loss of material.

Several inter-test comparisons have been undertaken. Sina *et al.* (1992) compared leucine incorporation, MTT dye reduction and neutral red uptake in corneal epithelial cells and Chinese hamster lung fibroblasts. None of the endpoint target cell combinations accurately predicted *in vivo* eye irritation in this series but the MTT dye reduction method gave the best overall correlation.

Cytotoxicity assays assess the effect of test material on a particular aspect of cell or intercellular function, or of lethal cytotoxicity. They, therefore, give a measure of potential to cause cell and tissue injury and as such may be used as a screen for predicting tissue injury, including eye injury. The appropriate choice of the test cell and endpoint indicator for certain chemical classes may give reasonable prediction of the potential for eye irritation. The choice of the screening cytotoxicity assay, or assays, should in part be determined by past experience, the likely mechanism for an irritant response, and the chemistry of the material tested.

Non-Biological Methods

One example is the use of synthetic protein membranes based on the fact that protein denaturation may be a factor in corneal injury with several materials. The reactive component is a synthetic protein-globulin matrix. In one series the predictability of ocular irritation was 89 per cent and in another 93 per cent (Soto and Gordon, 1990).

Prediction by Analogy

Computer-Based Modelling

As might be anticipated, there have been proposals that computer-based, structure–activity relationships could be used as a basis for predicting the eye irritating potential of a chemical. Sugai *et al.* (1990) used a quantitative structure–activity relation (QSAR) to analyse the correlations between chemical structure and eye irritation in rabbits. They claimed an accuracy of 86.3 per cent in classifying chemicals with respect to eye irritancy, and state that QSAR is of value in predicting eye irritation. Although the approach could be a useful adjunct with chemicals in a class of known irritancy, it would be a brave (or foolish) person who would risk potential litigation from a product safety evaluation based solely on QSAR.

Prediction Based on Skin Irritation

It has been proposed that materials shown to be primary skin irritants should also be regarded as being eye irritants, and therefore do not require to be tested for ocular irritancy. Such an approach is overcautious in that some skin irritants have been shown not to be eye irritants but the converse is of more concern as materials might be mistakenly classified as non-irritant to the eye. Several studies have shown that there may not be a good correlation between skin and eye irritating potential and that some eye irritants are not skin irritants (Rhodes, 1987). Kennedy and Banerjee (1992) studied 72 fibre finish materials and found a 10.5 per cent error in predicting that a severe skin irritant was a severe eye irritant, and noted a poor predictive association between the skin and eye irritancy for the compounds they studied. Williams (1984) reviewed 60 materials which were severe irritants or corrosive to the skin: 39 were severe eye irritants, six were moderate eye irritants and 18 were mild or non-irritant. He concluded that to suggest that materials are eye irritants on the basis of their skin irritating effects could be misleading.

There is no simple relation between skin and ocular irritancy and in several cases it may be misleading to predict one from the other (Daston and Freeberg, 1991).

General Comments

At the present time, no single alternative test, or combinations of them, can completely predict the eye irritating potential of all substances. Expectations for a uniform test should be discouraged (Reinhardt, 1990). However, an appropriate tiered scheme may be of value in significantly reducing *in vivo* eye irritation testing. Approaches to such schemes have been proposed (Reinhardt, 1990; Jackson and Rutty, 1985). Such schemes should consider a sequential approach to include the following:

(1) Consideration of the physical and chemical characteristics of the test material, along with comparison of materials in the same chemical class whose *in vivo* eye irritating potential are known.

(2) Use of appropriate cytotoxicity studies based on known predictivity for specific chemical classes.

(3) Confirmation of the potential for corneal injury using *in vitro* enucleated eye and/or corneal preparations.

(4) In critical cases, such as high volume chemicals or ophthalmic preparations, ultimate confirmation may be necessary using *in vivo* studies with objective measurements.

SENSORY IRRITATION OF THE EYE

Stimulation of corneal and conjunctival chemoceptors will cause local pain or discomfort and the associated reflexes of increased lacrimation and blepharospasm. These effects are biologically protective in that they give a warning of exposure to a potentially noxious material and some degree of protection from further exposure. Pain, excess lacrimation and blepharospasm also impair vision and are distracting, predisposing to physical accidents and impeding efficient working conditions. Considerations of the peripheral sensory effects on the eye are of importance, for example, in assessing workplace safety and may need to be taken into account in assigning workplace exposure guidelines. Also, from a product safety viewpoint, it is important to know if there is an adequate margin (of safety) between the exposure conditions producing sensory irritation of eye and those leading to eye injury.

It is important to note that some materials may give little, or no, sensory warning on contact with the eye, e.g. bis(2-chloroethyl)sulphate, dimethylsulphoxide and methyl bromide. Clearly with such chemicals there is a need to emphasize the requirement for protective and precautionary measures.

Objective aspects of the sensory irritant response, e.g. blepharospasm, may be studied in experimental animals. However, subjective aspects (e.g. discomfort and pain) require carefully controlled studies in human volunteers. Peripheral sensory irritation of the eye, and other tissues, is considered in detail in Chapter 20.

THE EYE AS A TARGET FOR SYSTEMIC TOXICITY

There are many materials, including drugs and industrial chemicals, that can produce structural and/or functional injury to the eye following systemic distribution after absorption from different sites of exposure. Some representative examples are summarized in Table 8. Observations for injury to the eye are clearly required in toxicological studies of materials that are used medicinally, as food additives, and as industrial chemicals with potential for exposure in the home or workplace. The necessity to undertake, at least, routine examination of the eye in general toxicology studies has been stressed by Barnett and Noel (1969).

As shown in Table 8, a great diversity of toxicopathological effects can be produced at various sites in the eye. With some substances there may be highly site-specific effect, in others a series of sites within and related to the eye may be affected

Table 8 Examples of systemic toxicity to the eye

Chemical	Effect
Methanol	Retinopathy Retrobulbar optic neuropathy
Chloroquine	Retinopathy Corneal opacities
Methylhydrazine	Corneal endothelial injury
Chlorpropamide	Corneal opacities Lens opacities
Dimethylsulphoxide	Corneal opacity
Methylphenyltetrahydropyridine	Retinopathy
Oxygen	Retrolental fibroplasia
Methotrexate	Blepharoconjunctivitis Optic neuropathy
Corticosteroids	Cataract Glaucoma Visual field defects
Chlorpromazine	Keratopathy Cataract

by the same chemical. With multiple site systemic ocular toxicity, the combination of lesions varies with different chemicals and chemical classes. The potential to induce systemic toxicity to the eye depends on a variety of factors.

(1) Total absorbed dose and its determinants, notably frequency, duration and magnitude of environmental exposure dose.

(2) Route of exposure, depending on whether the parent molecule or a metabolite is responsible for the ocular injury.

(3) The biotransforming capacity of the eye. Watkins *et al.* (1991) have reviewed the xenobiotic transforming capacity of ocular tissues and experimentally extended the biochemical database. The role of ocular metabolism in the mechanism of ocular toxicity from xenobiotics is, in general, poorly understood but clearly is a factor to be considered in all cases of ocular toxicity.

With any specific chemical, the potential for producing ocular injury, the site of action and the severity may have markedly different conditions for its genesis.

Systemic toxic effects on the eye may be seen during general toxicology studies, providing the protocol allows for examination of the eye. Investigations into specific aspects may require satellite or additional studies for which more sophisticated monitoring procedures are necessary. Depending on the lesion(s) produced these may include the use of slit-lamp biomicroscopy, light microscopy with special stains and histochemical preparations, transmission or scanning electron microscopy, angiography, tonometry, electroretinography, visual evoked potentials and electrooculography. Electroretinography is a valuable supplement to histopathology in studies of retinal toxicity (Maertins *et al.*, 1993). Also, isolated tissue preparations have been employed, e.g. the retina and lens (Chiou, 1992). Specific lesions may be subject to a spectrum of investigational techniques. Investigation of lenticular toxicity has included the use of various forms of microscopy, biochemical investigations, metabolic studies and the following of morphological and biochemical changes by magnetic resonance imaging and spectroscopy (Schleich *et al.*, 1985), trytophan fluorescence spectroscopy (Lerman and Moran, 1988) and scanning lens monitoring (Mitton *et al.*, 1990). Lens biochemical changes that have been investigated include aldose reductase, sorbitol dehydrogenase, phosphofructokinase, glutathione reductase, glutathione, NADH, NADPH, calcium, cholesterol, phospholipids and protein (Chiou, 1992).

In some cases, experimental studies may not detect certain aspects of systemic toxicity. For example, workers overexposed to styrene may develop dyschromatopsia (Gobba *et al.*, 1991). Styrene vapour concentrations of the order of 25 ppm can lead to impairment of colour vision (Fallas *et al.*, 1992).

Some illustrative examples of materials producing systemic toxicity to the eye are briefly summarized below.

Anti-Neoplastic Agents

Various cancer chemotherapeutic agents have been reported to affect ocular function. Tamoxifen produces retinopathy with refractile opacities in the macular and perimacular areas and a high proportion of patients on carmustine develop retinal effects including infarction, periarteritis and macular oedema (Gerner, 1989; Chiou, 1992). In addition to retinopathy, tamoxifen has also been reported to produce keratopathy (Vinding &

Nielsen, 1983). Like other retinotoxic drugs such as chloroquine and imipramine, tamoxifen is amphiphilic. It has been postulated that amphiphilic materials bind with polar lipids causing abnormal metabolism of such lipids with resultant accumulation in intracellular lysosomes (Lullman *et al.*, 1975), i.e. drug-induced phospholipidosis. Retinal pathology shows lesions in the neuroretina (nerve fibre layer and inner plexiform layer), with the paramacular region being particularly susceptible, possibly because it is highly vascularized and its proximity to the macular area (Kaiser-Kupfer *et al.*, 1981). Ocular complications of systemic cancer chemotherapy are not uncommon, affecting various components of the eyeball, optic nerve and extraocular muscles; the subject has been extensively reviewed by Imperia *et al.* (1989).

Aliphatic Alcohols

Ingestion of ethanol can reduce intraocular pressure and affect extraocular muscle activity. Acute alcoholic intoxication results in various disturbances of vision, including nystagmus, diplopia, temporary convergent strabismus and possibly transient change in colour vision. Chronic alcoholism causes a toxic amblyopia, which may be related to vitamin B complex deficiency (Grant, 1986). Of concern is that ocular malformations may be produced in the offspring of mothers who abuse alcohol during gestation. Up to 90 per cent of children suffering from the foetal alcohol syndrome have eye abnormalities, with two malformations being typical: hypoplasia of the optic nerve head and increased tortuosity of retinal vessels (Stromland, 1989). Serious disturbances of vision may result. Ocular complications of the foetal alcohol syndrome have been reviewed by Grant (1986).

Butyl 2-Chloroethyl Sulphide

In the rat, systemically absorbed butyl 2-chloroethyl sulphide causes swelling of the inner retinal layers, mitochondrial swelling, and disarray of the outer segments of the photoreceptors. Radiolabelled material is found in the retina, choroid, sclera, lens and cornea. Structural effects were preceded by an increase in thiobarbituric acid-reactive products, an indicator of lipid peroxidation (Klain *et al.*, 1991).

Aconitine

Aconitine is the principal constituent of aconite, a herbal remedy used in the Far East. In a methodologically integrated study, Kim *et al.* (1991) showed that the material produced myelo-optic neuropathy in rabbits. Principal findings were a delay in onset and peak latency of the visual evoked potential with reduction in amplitude, and histopathological evidence of myelin injury to the visual pathway, spinal cord and peripheral nerves.

Drugs of Abuse

Drug abusers have a significant incidence of ocular complications (Gastaud *et al.*, 1989). Marijuana causes conjunctival hyperemia and a decrease in intraocular pressure (Green, 1982). Other ocular side-effects include diplopia and blepharospasm. The ocular toxicology of marijuana has been reviewed by Green and McDonald (1987).

Developmental Defects

One special aspect of ocular systemic toxicity is that of developmental defects occurring during gestation as a result of maternal exposure; foetal exposure may have been to the parent molecule or a metabolite. One example, the foetal alcohol syndrome has been mentioned. A further dramatic example is the ocular teratogensis produced experimentally in the rat by exposure to nickel carbonyl. Sunderman *et al.* (1975) found that on exposure to the vapour for 15 min on days 7 or 8 of gestation ocular abnormalities were produced, including anophthalmia or microphthalmia, with a low incidence of extraocular anomalies. As nickel carbonyl can cross the alveolar membrane and blood–brain barrier, they believe that it may cross the foetomaternal barriers.

THE EYE AS A PORTAL FOR SYSTEMIC TOXICITY

Most materials are unlikely to produce systemic toxicity by topical application to the eye (Brown and Muir, 1971), principally because of the small volume that can be accommodated on the surface of the eye and in the conjunctival sac, even following deliberate instillation. Furthermore, lachrymation and blepharospasm may reduce the degree of contamination. For materials of high toxicity or pharmacological potency, sufficient material may be absorbed to produce systemic toxicity. Some sources of exposure with a potential for systemic toxicity may be novel. For example, Nir *et al.* (1992) investigated kohl, an eye cosmetic encountered in Israel, which is frequently applied to infants. They found that the lead content of various samples of kohl varied from 17.3 per cent to 79.5 per cent; blood lead levels were high in infants exposed to kohl (11.2 μg dl^{-1} versus controls of 4.3 μg dl^{-1}; $p < 0.001$).

The absorption of some therapeutic substances by topical application to the eye may be effective enough to be used as a therapeutic route of exposure. For example, Pillion *et al.* (1992) found that glucagon eye drops, containing 0.25 per cent saponin, produced a rapid dose-related increase in blood D-glucose in the rat. Chiou *et al.* (1990) also showed that glucagon may be readily absorbed following ocular instillation, and this could be facilitated by permeation enhancers. Similar work with insulin showed that while plain insulin eye drops had little effect on blood glucose, when combined with permeation enhancers the blood glucose level was markedly reduced in both normal and hyperglycaemic diabetic rabbits (Chiou *et al.*, 1990). Development work has also been conducted with oxytocin and vasopressin (Chiou *et al.*, 1991). Although poorly absorbed as such by the ocular route, the addition of polyoxyethylene-20-stearyl ether markedly enhanced their absorption.

Sites of Absorption

Materials contaminating the eye come into contact with conjunctival blood vessels, pass through the nasolachrymal drainage system into the nasal cavity, and then through to the naso- and oropharynx to be swallowed. The relative contribution of eye, nasal mucosa and alimentary tract to the absorbed dose may vary with the chemical species.

Absorption can occur through the conjunctival blood vessels, and this may be facilitated by materials that also produce a conjunctival hyperaemia. Absorption from this site is also influenced by rate of lachrymation, blepharospasm and patency of the nasolachrymal drainage system.

In many cases the nasal mucosa, with its large surface area and high vascularity, may be a major site of absorption of materials applied to the eye. It is well appreciated that many pharmacologically active materials are absorbed following introduction into the nasal cavity (Chien, 1985). For drugs having a high biological activity via the nasal route and for those with a significant first-pass metabolism by the peroral route, the nasal mucosa may offer a useful route for dosing. Hydrophobicity may be an important determinant for nasal mucosal absorption; for example, the hydrophobic drugs alprenolol and propranolol are well absorbed from the nasal mucosa (Duchateau *et al.*, 1986; Hussain *et al.*, 1980) whereas hydrophilic metaprolol is not well absorbed (Duchateau *et al.*, 1986). The rate of drainage of a material from the conjunctival sac into the nasal cavity depends on a number of factors including the rates of lachrymation and blinking, both of which may be increased with irritant materials. Also, the volume of material instilled will determine the amount transferred. Lachrymation and instilled fluid dynamics in the rabbit eye in relation to drainage from the eye have been investigated by Chrai *et al.* (1973). The drainage capacity of the eye exceeds the normal rate of lachrymation; therefore, drops placed in the conjunctival sac will be rapidly transferred to the nasal cavity (Shell, 1982). Reducing the rate of drainage may decrease systemic absorption. For example, Zimmerman *et al.*, 1984) studied the effects of eyelid closure and manual nasolachrymal occlusion on the absorption of topically applied timolol and on permeation into the eye of topically applied fluorescein. They found, with both eyelid and nasolachrymal occlusion, that the plasma concentration of timolol was significantly reduced and fluorescein in the anterior chamber was increased compared with ordinary eyedrop procedures. For timolol, Chang and Lee (1987) found that the nasal mucosa was about 2.5 times more effective than the conjunctival mucosa in contributing to the total systemic absorption.

Several studies have indicated that topically applied materials reach the alimentary tract and may be absorbed. Thus, Wilensky *et al.* (1967) found that after ecothiopate (echothiophate) and diisopropyl phosphorofluoridate (isofluorphate) had been instilled into the eye, the greatest inhibition of cholinesterase outside the eye was in the intestine. Also, in humans, anticholinesterases applied to the eye produced symptoms of intestinal distress (Humphreys and Holmes, 1963). Anderson (1980) studied the systemic absorption of adrenaline and dipiveprin applied topically to the eye, and found that a high concentration of material was present in the intestinal wall and in the faeces. She suggested that the alimentary tract is not only a major elimination route but is probably also a major absorption pathway.

Illustrative Examples

The potential for industrial and domestic chemicals to produce systemic toxicity following topical contamination of the eye is well known but the major human experience comes from the use of ophthalmic preparations deliberately applied to the eye. Several examples are given below to illustrate the diversity of toxicity that may be produced by this route.

Cyanides

Low molecular weight cyanides can readily diffuse across biological membranes and toxicity may be produced if they are instilled into the conjunctival sac. They are so active by this route that it may be possible to calculate LD_{50} values by experimental instillation into the conjunctival sac. Table 9 compares the acute lethal toxicity of hydrogen and sodium cyanide by contamination of the eye with the lethal toxicity produced by other routes of exposure. It can be seen that by the ocular route, at least in the experimental mammal, these cyanides are lethally potent, with HCN being as toxic as when given by intravenous injection, and more toxic than by the peroral and percutaneous routes.

Timolol

L-Timolol is a non-selective beta-adrenoceptor antagonist used in the treatment of glaucoma, and usually available in preparations of 0.25–0.5 per cent. The use of timolol as eye drops has been associated with a number of serious adverse effects to several body systems (Table 10). It has been shown that the oxidation of timolol exhibits genetic polymorphism, with poor metabolizers having higher plasma timolol concentrations and intensified β-blockage (Huupponen *et al.*, 1991).

Systemic absorption following ocular instillation has been demonstrated in several studies. Kaila *et al.* (1985) instilled 20 μl 0.5 per cent

Table 9 Acute lethal toxicity of hydrogen cyanide (HCN) and sodium cyanide (NaCN) by different routes of administration in the female rabbit

Route	HCN		NaCN	
	LD_{50} (mg kg^{-1})	Time to death (min)	LD_{50} (mg kg^{-1})	Time to death (min)
Transocular	1.04 (0.96–1.13)	4–6	5.06 (4.4–6.10)	4–10
Intravenous	0.59 (0.55–0.65)	2.5–5.5	1.23 (1.11–1.34)	2–12
Intraperitoneal	1.95 (1.60–2.60)	6.9	2.79 (2.48–3.09)	5–26
Peroral	2.56 (2.14–3.05)	30–50	5.11 (4.62–5.66)	13–26
Percutaneous	6.89 (6.43–7.57)	25–260	14.62 (13.75–15.35)	105–345

Values in parentheses are 95% confidence limits.

Source: Ballantyne (1983, 1987).

Table 10 Systemic adverse effects associated with the topical application of timolol to the eye

System	Effect
Cardiovascular	Arrythmias
	Bradycardia
	Cardiac failure
	Hypotension
	Raynaud's plenomenon
Pulmonary	Asthma (exacerbation)
	Bronchospasm
	Dyspnoea
CNS	Confusion
	Depression
	Dizziness
	Hallucinations
	Aggravation of myasthenia gravis
Gastrointestinal	Diarrhoea
	Nausea
	Vomiting
Genital	Impotence
	Decreased libido
Skin	Alopecia
	Uticaria
	Maculopapular rash
Metabolic	Hyperkalaemia
	Altered diabetic hyperglycaemic response

timolol into the conjunctival sac of six volunteers; at 8 min all but one had measurable plasma timolol concentrations (>25 pg ml^{-1}). They also found that nasolachrymal occlusion reduced but did not eliminate systemic absorption of the drug (Kaila *et al.*, 1980). Chang and Lee (1987) found that 75 per cent of a 25 μl dose appeared in the blood stream of the rabbit, and that the nasal mucosa was 2.5 times more effective than the conjunctiva in contributing to systemic absorption of timolol.

Recommendations have been made to reduce the incidence of adverse effects from ocularly applied timolol; these include reduced medication, eyelid closure and nasolachrymal occlusion (Fraunfelder and Meyer, 1987).

Sulphonamides

Several cases of Stevens–Johnson syndrome have been described following the use of ophthalmic preparations containing sulphacetamide (Rubin, 1977; Anderson and Covinsky, 1986). In some, but not all cases, there may have been previous exposure to oral sulphonamides.

Chloramphenicol

Several cases of aplastic anaemia have been reported from the topical use of chloramphenicol ophthalmic preparations (Rosenthal and Blackman, 1965; Carpenter, 1975; Abrahams *et al.*, 1980; Fraunfelder *et al.*, 1982), a few of which were fatal (Abrahams *et al.*, 1980; Fraunfelder *et al.*, 1982). The response has been seen with ointments and drops. Fraunfelder *et al.* (1982) suggest that physicians must carefully weigh the risk–benefit ratio for lethal events that occur for 1 in 30 000 to 50 000 cases, and use chloramphenicol only in cases with organisms resistant to other antibiotics.

Cyclopentalate

Cyclopentalate, a potent anticholinergic drug, is used in ophthalmology to produce rapid mydriasis and cycloplegia. Signs of CNS effects, usually developing within minutes or less than an hour, have included ataxia, dysarthria, disorientation, hallucinations, amnesia and drowsiness; the effects are particularly notable in children although they have been described in adults (Awan, 1976; Shihab, 1980). Gastrointestinal effects (vomiting, distension and ileus) were noted in premature twin neonates given cyclopentalate eyedrops for eye examination after receiving oxygen. Blood samples taken 24 h after instillation of eyedrops gave plasma values of 2 and 22 μg ml^{-1} (Bauer *et al.*, 1973). In a study of 40 patients and a double-blind trial involving 35 subjects, Birkhorst *et al.* (1963) showed a statistically significant incidence of reactions in 5 of 40 patients and 8 of 35 trial subjects.

Proparacaine

Proparacaine is a topical local anaesthetic used to alleviate discomfort during eye examinations. Cydulka and Betzelos (1990) reported a case of tonic-clonic convulsions in a 28-year-old woman following the instillation of two drops of 0.5 per cent proparacaine hydrochloride.

General Comments

The above examples clearly illustrate the potential for materials with high biological activity to be absorbed systemically following application to the eye. They draw particular attention to the need to examine for systemic toxicity following ocular contamination so that appropriate precautionary statements can be made and appropriate protective measures recommended.

REFERENCES

Abrahams, S. M., Degnan, T. J. and Vineiguerra, V. (1980). Marrow aplasia following topical application of chloramphenicol eye ointment. *Arch. Int. Med.*, **140**, 576–577

Akesson, B., Floren, I. and Skerfring, S. (1985). Visual disturbances after human response to triethylamine. *Br. J. Industr. Med.*, **42**, 848–850

Akesson, B., Bengtsson, M. and Floren, I. (1986). Visual disturbance after industrial triethylamine exposure. *Int. Arch. Occup. Environ. Health*, **57**, 297–302

Allgood, G. S. (1989). Use of animal eye test data and human exposures for determining the ocular irritant potential of shampoos. *J. Toxicol. Cut. Ocular Toxicol.*, **8**, 321–326

Anderson, J. A. (1980). Systemic absorption of topical ocularly applied epinephrine and dipiveprin. *Arch. Ophth.*, **98**, 350–353

Anderson, L. and Covinsky, J. O. (1986). Stevens-Johnson syndrome. *Hosp. Ther.*, 66–72

Awan, K. J. (1976). Systemic toxicity of cyclopentolate hydrochloride in adult following topical ocular instillation. *Ann. Ophthal.*, **8**, 803–806

Bagley, D. M., Kong, B. M. and deSalva, S. J. (1989). Assessing the eye irritation potential of surfactant-based materials using the chorioallantoic membrane vascular assay (CAMVA). In Goldberg A. M. (Ed.), *In Vitro Toxicology: New Directions*. Liebert, New York, pp. 265–272

Bagley, D. M., Brunner, L. H., deSalva, O., Cottin, M., O'Brien, K. A. F., Uttley, M. and Walker, A. P. (1992). An evaluation of five potential alternatives *in vitro* to the rabbit eye irritation tests *in vivo*. *Toxicol. In Vitro*, **6**, 275–284

Baldwin, H. A., McDonald, T. O. and Beasley, C. H. (1973). Slit-lamp examination of experimental animal eyes. Grading scales and photographic evaluation of induced pathological conditions. *J. Soc. Cosmet. Chem.*, **24**, 181–195

Ballantyne, B. (1983). Acute systemic toxicity of cyanides by topical application to the eye. *J. Toxicol. Cut. Ocular Toxicol.*, **2**, 119–129

Ballantyne, B. (1987). Toxicology of cyanides. In Ballantyne, B. and Marrs, T. C. (Eds), *Clinical Experimental Toxicology of Cyanide*. Wright, Bristol, pp. 41–127

Ballantyne, B. and Swanston, D. W. (1977). The scope and limitations of acute eye irritation tests. In Ballantyne, B. (Ed.), *Current Approaches in Toxicology*. Wright, Bristol, pp. 139–157

Ballantyne, B., Gazzard, M. F. and Swanston, D. W. (1972). Effects of solvents and irritants on intraocular pressure in the rabbit. *J. Physiol. (Lond.)*, **266**, 12P–14P

Ballantyne, B., Gazzard, M. F. and Swanston, G. W. (1973). Eye damage caused by crystal violet. *Br. J. Pharmacol.*, **49**, 181–182

Ballantyne, B., Gazzard, M. F., Swanston, D. W. and Williams, P. (1975). The comparative ophthalmic toxicology of 1-chloroacetophenone (CN) and dibenz(b.f)-1-4-oxazepine (CR). *Arch. Toxicol.*, **34**, 183–201

Ballantyne, B., Gazzard, M. F. and Swanston, D. W. (1976). The ophthalmic toxicology of dichloromethane. *Toxicology*, **6**, 173–187

Ballantyne, B., Gazzard, M. F. and Swanston, D. W. (1977). Applanation tonometry in ophthalmic toxicology. In Ballantyne, B. (Ed.), *Current Approaches in Toxicology*. Wright, Bristol, pp. 158–192

Ballantyne, B., Sun, J. D., Nachreiner, D. J., Myers, R. C., Neptun, D. A. and Garman, R. H. (1992). Acute and 9-day repeated vapor exposure toxicity of tetramethylbutanediamine (TMBDA) in rats. *Toxicologist*, **12**, 45

Barnett, K. C. and Noel, P. R. E. (1969). The eye in general toxicity studies. In Pigott, P. V. (Ed.), *Evaluation of Drug Effects on the Eye*. Association of Medical Advisors in the Pharmaceutical Industry, London, pp. 15–28

Battista, S. P. and McSweeney, E. S. (1965). Approaches to a quantitative method for testing eye irritation. *J. Soc. Cosmet. Chem.*, **16**, 119–131

Bauer, C. R., Trottier, M. C. T. and Stein, L. (1973). Systemic cyclopentalol (cyclogyl) toxicity in the newborn infant. *Pediat. Pharm. Ther.*, **82**, 501–505

Beckley, J. H., Russell, T. J. and Rubin, L. F. (1969). Use of the rhesus monkey for predicting human responses to eye irritants. *Toxicol. Appl. Pharmacol.*, **15**, 1–9

Birkhorst, R. D., Weinstein, G. W., Baretz, R. M. and Clahane, A. C. (1963). Psychotic reaction induced by cyclopentalate (Cyclogyl). *Am. J. Optom.*, **56**, 1243–1245

Blein, O., Adolphe, M., Lakhdai, B. J., Cambar, J., Gubanski, G., Castelli, D., Contic, C., Hubert, F., Latrille, F., Masson, P., Clouzeau, J., Le Bigot, J. F., De Silva, O. and Dossou, K. G. (1991). Correlation and validation of alternative methods to the Draize eye irritation test (OPAL project). *Toxicol. In Vitro*, **5**, 555–557

Borenfreund, E. and Puerner, J. A. (1987). Short-term quantitative *in vitro* cytotoxic assay involving an S–9 activating system. *Cancer Lett.*, **34**, 243–248

Brown, V. K. M. and Muir, C. M. C. (1971). Some factors affecting the acute toxicity of pesticides to mammals when absorbed through the skin and eye. *Int. Pest Control*, **4**, 16–21

Bruner, L. H., Kain, D., Roberts, D. A. and Parker, R. D. (1991). Evaluation of seven *in vitro* alternatives for ocular safety testing. *Fund. Appl. Toxicol.*, **17**, 136–149

Bruner, L. H., Parker, R. D. and Bruce, R. D. (1992). Reducing the number of rabbits in the low-volume eye test. *Fund. Appl. Toxicol.*, **19**, 330–335

Buehler, L. V. and Newmann, E. A. (1964). A comparison of eye irritation in monkeys and rabbits. *Toxicol. Appl. Toxicol.*, **6**, 701–710

Bulich, A. A. (1979). Use of luminescent test for determining toxicity in aquatic environments. In Markings, L. L. and Kimerle, R. A. (Eds), *Aquatic Toxicology*. American Society for Testing and Materials, Philadelphia, pp. 98–106

Burton, A. B. G. (1972). A method for the objective evaluation of eye irritation. *Food Cosmet. Toxicol.*, **19**, 471–480

Burton, A. B. G., York, M. and Lawrence, R. S. (1981). The *in vitro* assessment of severe eye irritants. *Food Cosmet. Toxicol.*, **19**, 471–480

Carpenter, G. (1975). Chloramphenicol eye drops and marrow aplasia. *Lancet*, **ii**, 326–327

Carpenter, C. P. and Smyth, H. F., Jr. (1946). Chemical burns of the rabbit cornea. *Am. J. Ophthal.*, **29**, 1363–1372

Chan, P.-K. and Hayes, A. W. (1985). Assessment of chemically induced ocular irritation: a survey of methods. In Hayes, A. W. (Ed.), *Toxicology of the Eye, Ear, and Other Special Senses*. Target Organ Toxicology Series, Raven Press, New York, pp. 103–143

Chang, S.-C. and Lee, V. H. L. (1987). Nasal and conjunctival contributions to the systemic absorption of topical timolol in the pigmented rabbit. *J. Ocular Pharmacol.*, **3**, 159–169

Chien, V. W. (1985). *Transnasal System Medication: Fundamentals, Development Concepts and Biomedical Assessment*. Elsevier, Amsterdam

Chiou, G. C. Y. (1992). Toxic responses in the eye and visual system. *Toxicol. Methods*, **2**, 139–167

Chiou, G. C., Shen, Z.-F. and Zheng, Y-Q (1990). Adjustment of blood sugar levels with insulin and glucagon eye drops in normal and diabetic rabbits. *J. Ocular Pharmacol.*, **6**, 237–241

Chiou, G. C., Shen, Z.-F. and Zheng, Y-Q. (1991). Systemic absorption of oxytocin and vasopressin through eye of rabbit. *J. Ocular Pharmcol.*, **7**, 351–359

Chrai, S. S., Patton, R. F., Mehta, A. and Robinson, J. R. (1973). Lacrimation and instilled fluid dynamics in rabbit eye. *J. Pharm. Sci.*, **62**, 1112–1211

Conquet, P., Durand, G., Laillier, J. and Plazonnet, B. (1977). Evaluation of ocular irritation in the rabbit: objective versus subjective assessment. *Toxicol. Appl. Pharmac.*, **39**, 129–134

Cydulka, R. K. and Betzelos, S. (1980). Seizures following the use of proparacaine hydrochloride eye drops. *J. Emerg. Med.*, **8**, 131–133

Daston, G. P. and Freeberg, F. E. (1991). Ocular irritation testing. In Hobson, D. W. (Ed.), *Dermal and Ocular Toxicology: Fundamentals and Methods*. CRC Press, Boca Raton, pp. 509–539

DeSousa, D. J., Rouse, A. A. and Smolon, W. J. (1984). Statistical consequences of reducing the number of rabbits utilized in eye irritation testing data on 67 petrochemicals. *Toxicol. Appl. Pharmac.*, **76**, 234–242

Draize, J. H. (1959). *Appraisal of the Safety of Chemicals in Food, Drugs and Cosmetics*. Association of Food and Drug Officials in the United States, Baltimore, pp. 49–52

Draize, J. H., Woodward, G. and Calvery, H. O. (1944). Method for the study of irritancy and toxicity of substances application topically to the skin and mucus membranes. *J. Pharmacol. Exp. Ther.*, **82**, 377–389

Duchateau, G. S. M. J. E., Znidema, J., Albers, W. M. and Merkus, F. W. H. M. (1986). Nasal absorption of alprenol and metaprolol. *Int. J. Pharmaceutics*, **34**, 131–136

Easty, D. A. and Mathalone, M. B. R. (1969). Toxicity of 1,8,9-triacetoxyanthracene to the cornea in rabbits. *Br. J. Ophthalmol.*, **53**, 819–823

Etter, J.-C. and Wildhaber, A. (1985). Biopharmaceutical test of ocular irritation in the mouse. *Food Chem. Toxicol.*, **23**, 321–323

Etter, J.-C., Gloor, S. and Mayer, J. M. (1992). The aggressiveness of local anaesthetics towards the eye with the development of an ocular irritation test. *Pharm. Acta Helv.*, **67**, 242–249

Eurell, T. E., Sinn, J. M., Gerding, P. A. and Alder, C. L. (1991). *In vitro* evaluation of ocular irritation using corneal protein profiles. *Toxicol. Appl. Pharmacol.*, **108**, 374–378

Fallas, C., Fallas, J., Maslard, P. and Dally, S. (1992). Subclinical ipairment of colour vision among workers exposed to styrene. *Br. J. Indust. Med.*, **49**, 679–682

Food and Drug Administration (1965). *Illustrated Guide for Grading Eye Irritation by Hazardous Substances*. Government Printing Office, Washington, DC

Fraunfelder, F. T., Bagby, G. C., Jr. and Kelly, D. J. (1982). Fatal aplastic anemia following topical administration of ophthalmic chloramphenicol. *Am. J. Ophthal.*, **93**, 356–360

Fraunfelder, F. T. and Meyer, S. M. (1987). Systemic reactions to ophthalmic drug preparations. *Med. Toxicol.*, **2**, 287–293

Freeberg, F. E., Nixon, G. A., Reer, P. J., Weaver, J. E., Bruce, R. D., Griffith, J. F. and Sanders, L. W. (1986). Human and rabbit eye response to chemical insult. *Fund. Appl. Tox.*, **7**, 626–634

Fujihara, T., Nakaro, T. and Hikado, M. (1993). Effects of ofloxain eye drops and eye ointment on corneal re-epithelialization. *J. Toxicol. Cutan. Ocular Toxicol.*, **12**, 67–73

Gastaud, P., Baudouin, C., de Galleani, B. and Fredj-Reggrobellet, D. (1989). Ocular manifestations of drug absorption. *J. Toxicol. Cutan. Ocular Toxicol.*, **8**, 291–309

Gaunt, I. F. and Harper, K. M. (1964). The potential irritancy to the rabbit eye mucosa of certain commercially available shampoos. *J. Soc. Cosmetic Chem.*, **15**, 209–230

Gautheron, P., Dukic, M., Alix, D. and Sina, J. F. (1992). Bovine corneal opacity and permeability test: an *in vitro* assay of ocular irritation. *Fund. Appl. Toxicol.*, **18**, 442–449

Gerner, E. W. (1989). Ocular toxicity of tamoxofen. *Am. J. Ophthalmol.*, **21**, 420–423

Gobba, F., Galassi, C., Imbriani, M., Ghittori, S., Omdela, S. and Cavalleri, A. (1991). Acquired dyschromatopsia among styrene-exposed workers. *J. Occup. Med.*, **33**, 761–765

Grant, W. M. (1986). *Toxicology of the Eye*, 3rd edn. Charles C. Thomas, Springfield, Illinois

Green, K. (1982). Marijuana and the eye—a review. *J. Toxicol., Cutan. Ocular Toxicol.*, **1**, 3–32

Green, K. and McDonald, T. F. (1987). Ocular toxicology of marijuana: an update. *J. Toxicol., Cutan. Ocular Toxicol.*, **6**, 309–334

Green, K., Johnson, R. E., Chapman, J. M., Nelson, E. and Cheeks, L. (1989). Surfactant effects on the rate of rabbit corneal epithelial healing. *J. Toxicol., Cutan. Ocular Toxicol.*, **8**, 253–269

Griffith, J. F., Nixon, G. A., Bruce, R. D., Reer, P. J. and Bannan, E. A. (1980). Dose-response studies with chemical irritants in the albino rabbit eye as a basis for selecting optimum testing conditions for predicting hazards to the human eye. *Toxicol. Appl. Pharmacol.*, **55**, 501–513

Hathaway, G. J., Proctor, N. H., Hughes, J. P. and Fischman, M. C. (1991). *Chemical Hazards of the Workplace*. Van Nostrand Reinhold, New York, p. 65

Herr, R. D., White, G. L., Jr., Bernhisel, K., Manilis, N. and Swanson, E. (1991). Clinical comparison of ocular irrigation fluids following chemical injury. *Am. J. Emerg. Med.*, **9**, 228–231

Humphreys, J. A. and Holmes, J. H. (1963). Systemic effects produced by ecothiophate iodide in treatment of glaucoma. *Arch. Ophthalmol.*, **69**, 737–743

Hussain, A., Kiri, S. and Bawarshi, S. (1980). Nasal absorption of propranolol from different dosage forms by rats and dogs. *J. Pharm. Sci.*, **69**, 1411–1413

Huupponen, R., Kaila, T., Lahder, K., Salminen, L. and Jisalo, E. (1991). Systemic absorption of ocular timolol in poor and extreme metabolizers of debrisoquine. *J. Ocular Pharm.*, **7**, 183–187

Imperia, P. S., Lazarus, H. M. and Lass, J. H. (1989). Ocular complications of systemic cancer chemotherapy. *Surv. Ophthal.*, **34**, 209–230

Itagaki, H., Hagino, S., Kato, S., Kobayashi, T. and Umeda, M. (1991). An *in vitro* alternative to the Draize eye irritation test: evaluation of the crystal violet staining method. *Toxicol. In Vitro*, **5**, 139–143

Jackson, J. and Rutty, D. A. (1985). Ocular tolerance assessment-integrated tier policy. *Food Chem. Toxicol.*, **23**, 309–310

Jacobs, G. A. and Martens, M. A. (1989). An objective method for the eye irritation *in vivo*. *Food Chem. Toxicol.*, **27**, 255–258

Jones, W. T. and Kipling, M. D. (1972). Glaucopsia-blue gray vision. *Br. J. Industr. Med.*, **29**, 460–461

Kaila, T., Huupponen, M. and Salminen, L. (1980). Effect of eyelid closure and nasolacrimal duct occlusion on the systemic absorption of ocular timolol in human subjects. *J. Ocular Pharmacol.*, **2**, 365–369

Kaila, T., Salminen, L. and Huupponen, M. (1985). Systemic absorption of ocularly applied timolol. *J. Ocular Pharmcol.*, **1**, 79–83

Kaiser-Kupfer, M. I., Kupfer, C. and Rodrigues, M. M. (1981). Tamoxifen retinopathy—a clinicopathological report. *Ophthalmologica*, **88**, 89–93

Kay, J. H. and Calandra, S. C. (1962). Interpretation of eye irritation tests. *J. Soc. Cosmet. Chem.*, **13**, 281–289

Kemp, R. B., Meredith, R. W. J. and Gamble, S. H. (1985). Toxicity of commercial products on cells in culture: a possible screen for the Draize eye irritation test. *Food Chem. Toxicol.*, **23**, 267–270

Kennedy, G. L. and Banerjee, A. K. (1992). Relationship between eye and skin irritation in rabbits using a series of textile fibre finishes. *J. Appl. Toxicol.*, **12**, 281–284

Kersjes, M. P., Reifler, D. M., Maurer, J. R., Trestrail, J. H. and McCoy, J. (1987). A review of chemical eye burns referred to the Blodgett Regional Poison Center. *Vet. Hum. Toxicol.*, **29**, 453–455

Kim, S.-H., Kim, S.-D., Kim, S.-Y. and Kurak, J. S. (1991). Myelo-optic neuropathy caused by aconitine in rabbit model. *Jap. J. Ophthal.*, **35**, 417–427

Klain, G. J., Omage, S. T., Schuschereba, S. T. and McKinney, C. M. (1991). Ocular toxicity of systemic and topical exposure to butyl–2-chloroethyl sulfide. *J. Toxicol. Cutan. Ocular Toxicol.*, **10**, 289–302

Lapalus, P., Ettarche, M., Fredj-Reggrobellet, D., Jambru, D. and Elena, P. P. (1990). Cytotoxicity studies in ophthalmology. *Lens Eye Toxicol. Res.*, **7**, 231–242

Lerman, S. and Moran, M. (1988). Acrylamide and iodide fluorescein studies on whole human lenses and their protein extracts. *Current Eye Res.*, **7**, 403–410

Leupke, N. P. (1985). Hen's egg chorioallantoic membrane test for irritating potential. *Food Chem. Toxicol.*, **23**, 287–291

Lullman, H., Lullman-Rauch, R. and Wasserman, O. (1975). Drug-induced phospholipidoses. *Crit. Rev. Toxicol.*, **4**, 185–218

Macrae, W. S., Willinsky, M. D. and Basu, P. K. (1970). Corneal injury caused by aerosol irritant projectors. *Canad. J. Ophthal.*, **5**, 3–11

Maertins, T., Kroetlinger, F., Sander, E., Pauluhn, J. and Machemar, L. (1993). Electroretinography assessment of early retinopathy in rats. *Arch. Toxicol.*, **67**, 120–125

Mann, I., Pirie, A. and Pullinger, R. D. (1948). An experimental and chemical study of the reaction of the anterior segment of the rabbit eye to chemical injury, with specific reference to chemical warfare agents. *Br. J. Ophthalmol.*, **13** (Suppl.)

Martins, T., Pauluhn, J. and Machemer, L. (1992). Analysis of alternative methods for determining ocular irritancy. *Food Chem. Toxicol.*, **30**, 1061–1068

Marzulli, F. N. and Simmon, M. E. (1971). Eye irritation from topically applied drugs and cosmetics: preclinical studies. *Am. J. Optom.*, **48**, 61–79

Maurice, D. M. (1967). The use of fluorescein in ophthalmological research. *Invest. Ophthalmol*, **6**, 464–477

Maurice, D. M. (1968). The penetration of drugs across the cornea. In Pigott, P. V. (Ed.), *Evaluation of Drug Effects on the Eye*. Association of Medical Advisors in the Pharmaceutical Industry, Baltimore, pp. 49–51

Maurice, D. and Singh, T. (1986). A permeability test for acute corneal toxicity. *Toxicol. Lett.*, **31**, 125–130

McDonald, T. O., Baldwin, H. A. and Beasley, C. H. (1972). Slit-lamp examination of experimental animal eyes. I. Technique of illumination of the normal animal eye. *J. Soc. Cosmet. Chem.*, **24**, 163–180

Mellerio, J. and Weale, R. A. (1966). Hazy vision in amine plant operatives. *Br. J. Indust. Med.*, **23**, 153–154

Mitton, K. P., Dzizloszyhski, T., Weerheim, J., Trevithick, J. R. and Sivak, J. G. (1990). Modelling cortical cataractogenesis. X. Evaluation of lens optical function by computer-based image analysis using an *in vitro* rat lens elevated glucose model. In Lerman, S. and Tripathi, R. C. (Eds), *Ocular Toxicology*. Marcel Dekker, New York, pp. 211–228

Muir, C. K., Flower, C. and Van Abbe, N. J. (1983). A novel approach to the search for *in vitro* alternatives to *in vivo* eye irritation testing. *Toxicol. Lett.*, **18**, 1–5

Myers, R. C., Christopher, S. M., Nachreiner, D. J., Losco, P. L. and Ballantyne, B. (1993). Acute toxicity and primary irritancy of acrolein dimer. *Toxicologist*, **13**, 152

Nir, A., Tamir, A., Zelnik, N. and Ianui, T. C. (1992). Is eye cosmetic a source of lead poisoning. *Isr. J. Med. Sci.*, **28**, 417–421

North-Root, H., Yackvich, F., Demetrulias, J., Gacula, M., Jr. and Heinze, J. E. (1982). Evaluation of an *in vitro* cell toxicity test using rabbit corneal cells to predict the eye irritation potential of a surfactant. *Toxicol. Lett.*, **14**, 207–212

OECD (1987). (Organization for Economic Cooperation and Development). *Acute Eye Irritation and Corrosion*. OECD Publication and Information Center, Washington, DC

Pillion, C. L., McCracken, D. L., Yang, M. and Atchison, J. A. (1992). Glucagon administration to the rat vie eye drops. *J. Ocular Pharmacol.*, **8**, 349–358

Price, J. B. and Andrews, I. J. (1985). The *in vitro* assessment of eye irritation using isolated eye. *Food Chem. Toxicol.*, **23**, 313–315

Punte, C. L., Owens, E. J. and Gutentag, P. J. (1963). Exposure to ortho-chlorobenzylidene malononitrile. *Arch. Environ. Health.*, **6**, 366–374

Reinhardt, C. A. (1990). *In vitro* predictive tests for eye irritation. *Toxicol. In Vitro*, **4**, 242–245

Rohde, B. H. (1992). *In vitro* methods in ophthalmic toxicology. In Chiou, G. C. Y. (Ed.), *Ophthalmic Toxicology*, Raven Press Ltd, New York, pp. 109–165

Rhodes, C. (1987). Interpreting acute and irritant responses. *Chem. Industr. (Lond.)*, **19**, 685–688

Riddell, R. J., Clothier, R. H. and Balls, M. (1986). An evaluation of three *in vitro* cytotoxicity assays. *Food Chem. Toxicol.*, **24**, 469–477

Rosenthal, R. C. and Blackman, A. (1965). Bone marrow hypoplasia following the use of chloramphenicaol eye drops. *J. Am. Med. Assoc.*, **191**, 136

Rubin, Z. (1977). Ophthalmic sulfonamide induced Stevens–Johnson syndrome. *Arch. Derm.*, **113**, 235–236

Russell, K. and Hoch, S. (1962). Product development

by rabbit eye irritation. *Proc. Sci. Sec. Toilet Goods Assoc.*, **37**, 27–32

Scaife, M. C. (1985). An *in vivo* cytotoxicity test to predict the ocular irritancy potential of detergent products. *Food Chem. Toxicol.*, **23**, 253–258

Schliech, T., Matson, G. B. and Willis, J. A. (1985). Surface coil phosphorus-31 NMR studies of the intact eye. *Expt. Eye Res.*, **40**, 343–355

Shaw, A. J., Balls, M., Clothier, R. H. and Bateman, N. D. (1991). Predicting ocular irritancy and recovery from injury using Madin–Darby canine kidney cells. *Toxicol. In Vitro*, **5**, 569–571

Shell, J. W. (1982). Pharmacokinetics of topically applied ophthalmic drugs. *Surv. Ophthal.*, **26**, 207–218

Shihab, Z. M. (1980). Psychotic reactions in an adult after topical cyclopentalate. *Ophthalmologia*, **181**, 228–230

Shopsis, C. and Sathe, J. (1984). Uridine uptake inhibition as a cytotoxic test: correlation with the Draize test. *Toxicology*, **29**, 195–296

Sina, J. F., Ward, G. J., Laszeh, M. A. and Gautheron, P. D. (1992). Assessment of cytotoxic assays as predicators of ocular irritation of pharmaceuticals. *Fund. Appl. Toxicol.*, **18**, 515–521

Sivak, J. G., Stuart, D. D., Herbert, K., Van Oostram, J. A. and Segal, L. (1992). Optical properties of the cultured bovine ocular lens as an *in vitro* alternative to the Draize eye toxicity test: preliminary validation for alcohols. *Toxicol. Methods*, **2**, 280–294

Smally, A. J., Binzer, A., Dolin, S. and Viano, D. (1992). Alkaline chemical keratitis: eye injury from airbags. *Ann. Emerg. Med.*, **21**, 1400–1402

Soto, R. J. and Gordon, V. C. (1990). An *in vitro* method for estimating ocular irritation. *Toxicol. In Vitro*, **4**, 332–335

Spampinato, S., Marino, A., Bucolo, C., Canossa, M., Bachetti, T. and Mangiafico, S. (1991). Effect of sodium naproxene eye drops on rabbit ocular inflammation induced by sodium arachidonate. *J. Ocular Pharm.*, **7**, 125–133

Stahlbom, B. Lundh, T., Floren, Z. and Akesson, B. (1991). Visual disturbance in man as a result of occupational exposure to trimethylamine. *Br. J. Industr. Med.*, **48**, 26–29

Stromland, K. (1989). Ocular involvement in the fetal alcohol syndrome. *Surv. Ophthal.*, **31**, 277–284

Sugai, S., Murata, K., Kitagaki, T. and Tomik, I. (1990). Studies on eye irritation caused by chemicals in rabbits. I. A quantitative structure-activity relationship approach to primary eye irritation of chemicals in rabbits. *J. Toxicol. Sci.*, **15**, 248–262

Sunderman, F. W. Jr., Allpass, P. R., Mitchell, J. M., Baselt, R. C. and Albert, D. M. (1975). Eye malformations in rats: induction by prenatal exposure to nickel carbonyl. *Science*, **203**, 550–553

Talsma, D. M., Leach, C. L., Hatoum, N. S. (1988). Reducing the number of rabbits in Draize eye irritation tests: a statistical analysis of 155 structures conducted over 6 years. *Fund. Appl. Toxicol.*, **10**, 146–153

Ubels, J. L., Edelhauser, H. R. and Shaw, D. (1982). Measurement of corneal epithelial healing rates and corneal thickness for evaluation of ocular toxicity of chemical substances. *J. Toxicol., Cut. Ocular Toxicol.*, **1**, 133–146

Van Erp, Y. H. M. and Weterings, P. J. J. M. (1990). Eye irritation screening for classification of chemicals. *Toxicol. In Vitro*, **4**, 267–269

Vinding, T. and Nielson, N. V. (1983). Retinopathy caused by treatment with tamoxifen at low dosage. *Arch. Ophthalmol.*, **61**, 45–50

Walker, A. P. (1985). A more realistic animal technique for predicting human eye response. *Food Cosmet. Toxicol.*, **23**, 175–178

Walton, R. M. and Heywood, R. (1978). Applanation tonometry in the assessment of eye irritation. *J. Soc. Cosmet. Chem.*, **29**, 365–368

Watkins, J. R., Wirthwein, P. D. and Sanders, R. A. (1991). Comparative study of phase II biotransformation in rabbit ocular tissue. *Drug Metab. Dispos.*, **19**, 708–713

Weil, C. S. and Scala, R. A. (1971). Study of intra and interlaboratory variability on the results of rabbit eye and skin irritation tests. *Toxicol. Appl. Pharmacol.*, **19**, 276–360

Whittle, E., Basketter, D. and York, M. (1992). Findings of an interlaboratory trial of the enucleated eye method as an alternative eye irritation test. *Toxicol. Methods*, **2**, 30–41

Wilensky, J. G., Dettbarn, W.-D. and Rosenberg, P. (1967). Effect of ocular instillation of ecothiophate iodide and isofluorophate on cholinesterase activity of various rabbit tissues. *Am. J. Ophthalmol.*, **64**, 398–404

Williams, S. J. (1984). Prediction of ocular irritation potential from dermal irritation test results. *Food Chem. Toxicol.*, **22**, 157–161

Williams, S. J. (1985). Changing concept of ocular irritation evaluation: pitfalls and progress. *Food Chem. Toxicol.*, **23**, 189–194

Zimmerman, J., Kooner, K. S., Kandarakis, A. S. and Ziegler, L. P. (1984). Improving the therapeutic index of topically applied ocular drugs. *Arch. Ophthalmol.*, **102**, 551–553

FURTHER READING

Chiou, G. C. Y. (1992). *Ophthalmic Toxicology*. Raven Press, New York

Grant, W. M. and Schuman, J. S. (1993). *Toxicology of the Eye*. 4th edn. Charles C. Thomas, Springfield, Illinois

Symposium (1994). Ocular effects of organophosphate exposure. *Journal of Applied Toxicology*, **14**, 103–154

25 Fundamentals of Cardiotoxicology

Steven I. Baskin and Edward U. Maduh

INTRODUCTION

Heart damage can be produced by the administration of many therapeutic drugs and by exposure to a variety of chemicals. Potentially cardiotoxic drugs include antineoplastic agents, antibiotics, antidepressant agents, antimalarials and emetine, analgesics, anti-arrhythmics, anaesthetics, barbiturates, sympathomimetic amines, antihypertensives and cardiac glycosides. Cardiotoxic chemicals, to which individuals may be exposed, include alcohol, marijuana, nicotine, endotoxins, insecticides, fungicides, heavy metals, chlorinated solvents, fluorocarbons and the natural toxins produced by certain animals and plants. The list of cardiotoxins discussed is not inclusive. This chapter is organized by discipline and then by examples from major cardiac poisons exemplified by digitalis glycosides, halohydrocarbons and the organophosphates. The brief bibliography should provide a basis for most topics covered.

EMBRYOLOGY

Cardiac embryology provides a foundation for macroscopic and microscopic structures and an understanding of congenital malformations. It also forms a basis for elucidating susceptibility of the cardiovasculature to toxic insults that can occur from gestation to any point through life. Cardiocytes, the extracellular matrix, and coronary vasculature illustrate structure—function relationships which can be affected by poisons.

Early Cardiac Formations

Chemicals that come in contact with the embryo during the third and fourth weeks of its existence are likely to disturb major events of cardiac formation. The precardiac mesoderm is tracked from the lateral plate mesoderm into the precardiac plate which lies anterior to the forming brain. The tissue of the plate will condense and begin to form the bilateral heart tubes as the expansion of the cranial neural folds reverses the orientation of the developing heart.

The myocardial tissue condenses into paired heart tubes which lie along the lateral portions of the anterior intestinal portal. As these paired heart tubes form, the other cell type found in the primitive heart, endocardial cells, appear as cells between the endothelium of the gut and form the myocardium. At about 17 days gestation in the human, the paired heart tubes begin to fuse at the midline of the embryo. It has been demonstrated that embryos in which fusion has been physically prevented will develop bilateral hearts. The normal outcome of the fusion process is a single, tubular heart which consists of an outer myocardial cell layer, an inner endothelial cell layer, and an intervening layer of extracellular matrix.

After formation of the tubular heart, the first ineffective contractions of the myocardium occur. Successively, more caudal cells produce an effective contractile wave which passes down the myocardium from the atrium to the outflow tract. An obvious external change in the tubular heart is a looping process which brings the embryonic atria into a rostral and dorsal position in relationship to the ventricle. This process begins shortly after the completion of the fusion process and is seen first as a displacement of the ventricular region to the right of the embryonic midline. The looping results from the addition and stabilization of materials in the extracellular matrix. In the presence of hyaluronidase, the cardiac extracellular matrix is degraded so that the heart tube consist of the two cell layers without the intervening extracellular matrix. Although these embryos are smaller than untreated controls, heart looping is completely normal. Thus, cardiac looping appears to be an intrinsic mechanism within the myocardium.

Together with the formation of the looped heart tube, cells within the endothelium undergo developmental changes resulting in the formation of progenitors of the heart valves and septa.

These changes are greatly dependent on inter-actions between cells and the extracellular environment and may be critical in normal devel-opment. Defects of myocardial formation induced by xenobiotic exposure may be lethal to the embryo at an early stage and the embryo would be unlikely to survive the first weeks of gestation. Valve development is first signalled by an increased synthesis of extracellular matrix in the atrioventricular (AV) canal and heart outflow tracts.

Extracellular Matrix

Increased synthesis of extracellular matrix at the canal results in the formation of projections called the endocardial cushions. The endothelium of the outflow tract forms a fluted appearance as the increased mass of extracellular matrix mushrooms at all sides. Components of the extracellular matrix include hyaluronic acid, chondroitin sul-phate proteoglycans, and the glycoproteins col-lagen (type I) and fibronectin. Other basement membrane-associated components such as lami-nin, type IV collagen, and heparan sulphate pro-teoglycan can also be found in the developing matrix. Endothelial cells overlying the endocard-ial cushions in the AV canal start (28 day in the human) to hypertrophy and extend filopodial projections into the underlying extracellular matrix. Thus, a portion of the AV canal endo-thelium undergoes an epithelial—mesenchymal cell transformation to become the precursors of the fibroblasts of the valves and membranous septa of the heart.

A series of studies have shown that the epi-thelial—mesenchymal cell transformation which takes place in the AV canal is the result of a specific multifactorial myocardial stimulus. Trans-forming Growth Factor beta (TGFb) is a mole-cule that can effect growth inhibition of stimu-lation and phenotypic change. It has been found that TGFb, in combination with a ventricular explant, can invoke invasion of a collagen gel by endothelial cells from the AV canal. Further-more, a blocking antibody against TGFb is cap-able of preventing mesenchymal cell formation by AV canal explants. Immunocytochemical descriptions of the distribution of TFGb in the mouse heart show that the only TGFb reactivity was found in forming AV valves. It appears that the regional specificity of AV canal myocardium

induction is provided by the specific synthesis of a member of the TGFb family of molecules. The nature of a cofactor which is common to the AV canal and ventricular extracellular matrix is not known.

Subsequent to the extracellular matrix signals, activated endothelial cells enlarge, orient their Golgi in a specific pattern and extend filopodia into the extracellular matrix. Heparan sulphate proteoglycan appears on the surface of activated endothelial cells and then mesenchymal cells actively produce type I collagen. Once cardiac mesenchyme has been produced in the AV canal, it translocates across the endocardial cushions by attaching to and migrating onto the components of the extracellular matrix. Cell migration on extracellular matrix components is a result of repeated cycles of attachment to and detachment from components of the extracellular matrix. As fibronectin is a significant component of the car-diac extracellular matrix, it is likely that one potential mechanism of migration is via receptors for fibronectin. Additional components of the extracellular matrix include collagens I and IV and laminin. The defined attachment mechanisms to these molecules have been demonstrated. Carbohydrates also play a significant role in cell migration. The basis for selection of specific extracellular matrix receptors during cell migration appears to be that receptor—cytoskele-tal linkage is not produced until a receptor binds its specific extracellular ligand. Chemicals which either antagonize or mimic specific mechanisms of cell-extracellular matrix binding may have pro-found effects on mesenchymal cell migration.

Developing Cardiac Valve

During contraction, the tubular heart functions as a primitive effective valve. The cushions adhere and fuse in the midline of the AV canal. This divides the flow into two portions and pro-duces a midline structure called the septum inter-medium. The two orifices which remain will become the mitral and tricuspid openings.

The outflow tract is also called the *bulbus cordis*. This region is further subdivided into conal and truncal areas based on relationships to the conus and pulmonary trunk of the adult heart. Along with the formation of mesenchyme in the AV endocardial cushions, the outflow tract of the tubular heart also undergoes a series of similar changes. Shortly after the initial appearance of mesenchyme in the AV canal, mesenchyme is also found in the extracellular matrix of the outflow tract. Cardiac neural crest cells provide the cells which form within the extracellular matrix of the outflow tract into two dominant projections in the outflow tract lumen, the conotruncal ridges. Division of the outflow tract is accomplished by fusion of the ridges in a pattern which advances from the aortic sac towards the common ventricle against the blood flow. The neural crest cells appear to play a role for the development of the septum. The ridges assume a spiral course during their fusion. This spiral provides an appropriate anatomical relationship between the right and left ventricles and the aorta and pulmonary trunk so that postnatal blood flow is separated into two parallel pumping systems. The myocardial wall undergoes a similar spiral rotation during septation. The advancing outflow tract septation subsequently continues into the developing ventricles to the extent that the septum is aligned with a portion of the septum intermedium and the muscular ventricular septum. It is likely that errors in alignment or timing of the fusion of the septum with the ventricles might produce commonly found ventricular septal defects.

Cell-to-cell Communication

Cardiocytes (myocardial cells or fibres or myocytes) are structurally linked by cell to cell contacts (junctions) and form a complex network in which the angle of orientation differs in various myocardial layers. Two general categories of cardiocytes exist. Contractile cells constitute the bulk of the myocardium, while specialized cells comprise the sinoatrial node, atrioventricular node and bundle of His, and the Purkinje conduction pathway. Binucleation occurs during postnatal development. Contractile filaments which comprise about 55 per cent of the cell's volume, while mitochondria comprise about 30 per cent. During pressure-overload hypertrophy the growth of contractile filaments surpasses that of the mitochondria resulting in a decreased mitochondrial/myofibril volume ratio. In contrast, thyroxine-induced cardiac enlargement is characterized by excessive mitochondrial growth.

Cardiocytes are bounded by a plasmalemma similar to that of other cells. Two specialized regions of the plasmalemma are seen in cardiocytes: the transverse tubules and the intercalated discs. Myocytes obtained from adult rats with cardiac hypertrophy showed a reaquisition of the neonatal pattern of extracellular matrix receptors. These data are correlated with the patterns of extracellular matrix molecule formation which occur in the heart during development and disease. The primary function of collagenous extracellular matrix in the heart appears to be the construction of a distensible network between the myocytes. Myocyte-capillary interactions in the endomysium maintain patency of the capillaries during systole. The distribution of extracellular matrix receptors on cardiac myocytes changes during development and may be sensitive to drug and chemical toxicity. The ability of myocytes to attach to specific types of extracellular matrix molecules may reflect responses found in the extracellular matrix of the heart during physiological or pathological changes.

At birth, the heart must respond to a change in circulation and undergoes an increase in both blood pressure and volume. Various components of the extracellular matrix including fibronectin and collagens are present but not well organized at this stage. In response to models of hypertrophy produced by both rapid pressure overload and in gradual volume overload, the rate of type III collagen synthesis undergoes a rapid increase. This is followed by a gradual increase in the amount of type I collagen. The mass of collagen may increase at either a greater or similar rate to the increase in myocardial mass depending on the hypertrophic model, which implies that the differential response has a physiological basis. The initial response to either pressure or volume increase is to synthesize and secrete the more elastic form of collagen to permit greater compliance. Subsequent addition of a stiffer type I collagen would reduce the compliance as is seen in the hypertrophied myocardium.

BIOCHEMICAL BASIS

Cardiovascular energy metabolism and oxidative phosphorylation, ion balance, excitation—contraction, catecholamine release and metabolism, and gap junctions are important sites of toxicological action. The reduction of pyruvate to lactate is catalysed by lactate dehydrogenase (LDH) and results in regeneration of NAD. In the myocardium, as opposed to skeletal muscle, the LDH isoenzyme has a low affinity for pyruvate and therefore little pyruvate is reduced to lactate except in the ischaemic heart in which pyruvate levels can become quite high. Under normal conditions, when the heart is well oxygenated, it is primarily ADP that regulates ATP production. The heart is extremely sensitive to ADP and any increase results in an immediate increase in ATP production. As a result, the rate of oxidative phosphorylation closely matches the rate of energy utilization.

Metabolic Poisons

The sequence of electron carriers in the electron transport system NAD, FMN, ubiquinone, cytochromes b, c_1, c, a, and a_3 in the heart are affected by a series of metabolic poisons. Electron transport inhibitors block specific carriers. Rotenone, a plant toxin, blocks transport at complex I. Amytal and piericiden (the antibiotic) compete with ubiquinone and block transport at complexes I and II. Antimycin A blocks transport at complex II whereas hydrogen cyanide, hydrogen peroxide and carbon monoxide block the transfer of electrons from cytochrome to oxygen at complex IV.

Highly reactive species of partially reduced oxygen may be formed. Molecules with unpaired electrons are very unstable, highly reactive and referred to as free radicals. One of the most toxic species involved in oxygen free radical damage is the superoxide radical O_2^-. The unpaired valence electrons makes these radicals highly reactive and able to donate an electron or accept a hydrogen atom from methylene groups of polyunsaturated fats in phospholipid membranes. This can lead to the production of organic peroxides and the formation of more free radicals, initiating a chain reaction resulting in lipid peroxidation of membranes and destruction of the cell. The susceptibility to lipid peroxidation is dependent on the overall balance between oxidative stress and the antioxidant capacity of the cell. The introduction of reactive intermediates arising from metabolism of xenobiotics disrupts this balance resulting in oxidative stress leading to severe cellular damage.

Chemicals that partially inhibit Na^+/K^+ ATPase such as ouabain and digoxin may cause the potential voltage difference across the membrane to become slightly less negative. An abrupt drop in the potential difference to a threshold level results in propagation of an action potential which initiates cardiac arrhythmias. The slow channels maintain the plateau of the action potential, and the closing of the slow channels initiates repolarization of the membrane.

Cell Ca^{2+}

Two major ways that agents can interfere with excitation—contraction coupling are through actions on energy liberation or storage and on the mechanisms that regulate intracellular calcium. In addition to regulation of calcium transients for excitation—contraction, the myocardial cell must maintain a calcium gradient at the sarcolemma. Calcium-binding proteins such as calmodulin and parvalbumin may also serve as a calcium buffering system along with mitochondria to maintain low intracellular Ca^{2+} during calcium overload. The mitochondria appear to act as long-term buffers that are able to accumulate relatively large amounts of calcium in a slow process. Ca^{2+}/Na^+ exchange at the sarcolemma also plays an important role in excitation—contraction. When excitation frequency is increased the Na^+/K^+ pump lags behind the rate of entry of sodium through fast and slow channels. The increased intracellular Na^+ increases Ca^{2+}/Na^+ exchange and intracellular Ca^{2+} increases accounting for the increased contractility. Inhibition of Na^+/K^+ ATPase by compounds such as cardiac glycosides promotes this mechanism by increasing intracellular Na^+.

Catecholaminergic Systems

Catecholamines elicit multiple changes in myocardial contractility and heart rhythm. The effects on contraction are mediated through activation of β-adrenergic receptors by the endogenous catecholamines noradrenaline (norepinephrine) and adrenaline (epinephrine), and pharmaceutical agonists such as isoprenaline (isoproterenol). The positive inotropic effects are readily blocked by β-antagonists like propranolol. Binding of catecholamine to beta-receptors dramatically increases the intracellular levels of cAMP. Agonist-bound β-receptor interacts with a GDP-bound G_s protein to cause an exchange reaction to form GTP-bound G_s protein. Noradrenaline (norepinephrine) also stimulates α-adrenergic receptors which lead to the hydrolysis of phosphatidylinositol. The resulting inositol triphosphate increases calcium release from the sarcoplasmic reticulum and enhances contraction. Diacylglycerol is also a product of phosphatidyl-inositol hydrolysis and stimulates protein kinase C. Protein kinase C can lead to changes in the phosphorylation of ionic channels responsible for the pacemaker currents of the sinoatrial node and increases heart rate. These are some of the biochemical changes which may be responsible of cardiac arrhythmias observed with catecholamines.

Cholinergics

Stimulation of cholinergic receptors by acetylcholine results in a depression of contractility. This is especially true in the catecholamine-stimulated myocardium. In contrast to adrenergic stimulation, nitric oxide and cGMP appear to be second and or third intracellular messengers responsible for negative inotropic effects of cholinergic stimulation. However, evidence is lacking that would support a direct effect of cGMP mediating decreased cardiac contractility.

The ability of the heart to beat as a syncytium is dependent on intercellular communication through gap junctions that permit the passage of ions and small molecules between cells and provides a low resistance pathway for conduction of an action potential throughout the myocardium. Opening and closing of the junctional channel is reversibly influenced by intracellular Ca^{2+} and hydrogen ions but the sensitivity to H^+ is considerably greater than to Ca^{2+}. It appears that physiological changes in pH affect electrical coupling but only unphysiologically high concentrations of Ca^{2+} such as those associated with cell death block junctional conductance. A low sensitivity to Ca^{2+} would be essential in the cardiac myocyte in order to avoid junctional closing during the high Ca^{2+} transients occurring during muscle cell contraction. Stimulation of β-receptors or administration of the intracellular messenger 8-bromo-cAMP increases conductance through gap junctions. As conduction velocity in the myocardium is inversely related to the resistance in the conduction pathway, the increase in gap junctional conductance should result in increased velocity of an electrical impulse through the myocardium. This will enhance synchronization of myocardial cells during positive chronotropic activation by catecholamines. The increase in conductance may be the result of phosphorylation of the gap junction protein as they contain probable sites for phosphorylation by a cAMP-dependent kinase.

The Anthracyclines

Anthracyclines are antineoplastic agents whose usefulness is limited by their cardiotoxicity. Treatment with anthracyclines produces both acute and chronic cardiac effects, and the toxicity is complicated by the fact that there is considerable individual variation in response. Acutely, anthracyclines at higher concentrations show a strong negative inotropic effect that is dose dependent. The negative inotropic action probably stems from the disruption of electron transport and oxidative phosphorylation and subsequent free radical formation and lipid peroxidation. The primary pathological effect, shown in children with leukaemia, is a cardiomyopathy that results in congestive heart failure.

Adriamycin (doxorubicin hydrochloride) and the analogue daunorubicin are believed not only to intercalate with DNA but also to cause DNA strand breaks and slow the rate of DNA synthesis. The binding of adriamycin to cardiac DNA leads to a decrease in mRNA and polyribosome levels and a subsequent drop in protein synthesis. The effects on DNA may not be critical to cardiac muscle cells because they do not normally undergo division. However, DNA synthesis is important in mitochondria for the maintenance of membrane proteins. Although DNA binding and subsequent inhibition of protein synthesis could be devastating and may account for chronic adriamycin cardiomyopathy, it does not appear to be the mechanism responsible for the acute effects of adriamycin.

Many aspects of the cardiotoxicity of adriamycin and other anthracyclines can be attributed to the production of the free radical form of the anthracycline. The centre of the adriamycin molecule contains a quinone structure. The quinone nucleus of anthracyclines has been shown to be reduced to the semiquinone radical species at mitochondrial complex I, probably by the NADH dehydrogenase flavin, which leads to the formation of superoxide (O_2^-). Extra-mitochondrially, superoxide is also formed by the NADPH reduction of the anthraquinone to semiquinone. It was found that sarcosomes treated with adriamycin generate high levels of hydroxyl radicals. Apparently, adriamycin is reduced by an NADPH-dependent quinone reductase. The reduced quinone or semiquinone reduces oxygen via superoxide to hydrogen peroxide. Catalase is effective in blocking the formation of free radicals but superoxide dismutase is not, suggesting that the adriamycin semiquinone reacts with hydrogen peroxide to produce hydroxyl radicals.

The free radical species in adriamycin toxicity and subsequent lipid peroxidation came from recognition of protection from cardiac effects provided by the free radical scavenger α-tocopherol, which reduce the toxicity of adriamycin. The semiquinone form of adriamycin can lead to lipid peroxidation by facilitating the transfer of electrons from compounds such as NADH and NADPH to oxygen produce superoxides which in turn form toxic hydroxyl radicals, peroxy radicals and hydrogen peroxide. These highly reactive radicals donate electrons to the methylene groups of phospholipids and form organic peroxides which in turn form more organic radicals causing additional lipid peroxidation. The heart may be especially susceptible because the radical formation is greater in the heart.

Increased tissue calcium was associated with adriamycin cardiotoxicity. Ca^{2+} movement from the fast exchanging compartment is reduced. It has been proposed that such effects could result from adriamycin binding to membranes and the disruption of calcium transport. The calcium antagonists, prenylamine and verapamil, can protect against acute adriamycin toxicity presumably by preventing a rise in intercellular Ca^{2+}. However, verapamil has also been found to increase the accumulation of adriamycin in cardiac muscle cells which may explain the increased cardiac toxicity associated with it. Despite this, verapamil has been used in clinical trials in an attempt to reduce adriamycin toxicity. The effectiveness of Ca^{2+} antagonists is likely to result from tempering the Ca^{2+} overload by inhibiting the uptake of extracellular Ca^{2+}. Chronic adriamycin treatment causes intracellular Ca^{2+} deficiency. Rapid exchange of Ca^{2+} from the sarcoplasmic reticulum is critical to the normal function of contractile proteins and calcium movement from this fast exchanging compartment is reduced by adriamy-

cin. This is a probable cause of contractile depression. At the same time adriamycin induces cellular accumulation of Ca^{2+}.

Adriamycin and its primary metabolite doxorubicinol inhibit not only Na^+/K^+ ATPase, but also Ca^{2+} ATPase of the sarcolemma and Mg-dependent ATPase. The altered cationic pump action correlated with an increased resting tension of the contracting cardiac muscle. Activity of membrane-bound enzymes can be directly affected or the modified activity could be a compensatory response of transport ATPases to ion leakage resulting from membrane damage. Acutely, adriamycin has been shown to increase actomyosin ATPase activity, with subsequent treatments resulting in a decline in actomyosin ATPase activity.

Allylamine

Allylamine is a primary alkylamine that serves as an intermediate in the synthesis of a variety of pharmaceuticals and other commercial products. The relatively specific and potent cardiovascular effects of allylamine is known. Research on the vascular effects of allylamine was spurred by the observation that hydralazine protected the heart from allylamine, presumably through its action on arterial tone. Benzylamine oxidase (BzAO) protected against allylamine. The proposed mechanism was that allylamine was metabolized by BzAO to acrolein, and that acrolein was the reactive agent producing cardiovascular damage. Acrolein is a highly reactive aldehyde and is the critical metabolite in hepatotoxicity resulting from metabolism of allyl alcohol by alcohol dehydrogenase. The role of acrolein in allylamine toxicity was also seen in isolated muscle cells. Cultured aortic muscle cells are more susceptible to the toxic effects of allylamine than fibroblasts or endothelial cells from vascular tissue. BzAO inhibitors protect cultured aortic myocytes from allylamine toxicity. The increased sensitivity of vascular muscle cells appears to result from their high BzAO activity which leads to rapid acrolein production in the presence of allylamine. The myocardium is directly affected by allylamine. Despite being lower in BzAO activity and having only a fraction of the capability of vascular tissue for metabolizing allylamine to acrolein the myocardium appears to be highly sensitive to allylamine toxicity. Myocardial lesions have been found to precede vascular lesions following allylamine treatment. Damage can be produced in the *in vivo* heart within 24 h of a single exposure. The possibility exists that the direct myocardial effects of allylamine may be more damaging to the heart than the vacular effects. As with the vasculature of the heart, isolated myocardial cells are much more sensitive to allylamine than heart fibroblasts and the sensitivity appears to be an enhanced metabolism of allylamine to acrolein by BzAO. Allylamine or a metabolite bind to mitochondria from rat aorta and heart, and the cytotoxicity of allylamine may be the result of mitochondrial injury through inhibition of electron transport at succinoxidase state III or complex II.

Halogenated Hydrocarbons

Hearts of cats anaesthetized with chloroform were found to be sensitized to adrenaline (epinephrine)-induced arrhythmias which could result in sudden death. Since that time the depressant and sensitizing effects of various chlorinated, fluorinated and brominated hydrocarbons on the myocardium have been thoroughly described. In addition to directly affecting the heart, halogenated hydrocarbons have an effect on these other systems which in turn can feedback on the heart and modulate or even produce myocardial effects. The underlying mechanisms at the subcellular and molecular level of the myocardium responsible for attenuated contractility and sensitization to catecholamines have not been well elucidated. Despite the role of extracardiac factors, the primary locus of the depressant and sensitizing action of halogenated hydrocarbons is the heart itself because carbon tetrachloride and 1,1,1-trichloroethane depress contractility in isolated cardiac myocytes and sensitize them to the toxicity of isoprenaline (isoproterenol). The observed reduction in oxygen consumption is probably a secondary manifestation of halogenated hydrocarbon exposure. The lower the vapour pressure the lower the dose required to affect the heart.

The action of halocarbons on the heart could result from impaired gap junctional intercellular communication among cardiac myocyte. Halothane and ethrane reversibly inhibit molecular and electrical coupling between cultured cardiac myocyte. Impaired coupling by halothane and

ethrane reduce conducting channels rather than decrease unitary conduction which would slow conduction velocity within the syncytium and reduce synchronization of force. Inhibition of gap junctional intercellular communication in the myocardium could be a common mechanism by which the large class of halogenated hydrocarbons induce their depressant and arrhythmic effects on the *in vivo* heart. This is supported by the recent observation that ten halogenated hydrocarbons, including carbon tetrachloride, 1,1,1-trichloroethane and tetrachloroethane, reversibly inhibit intercellular communication. Interestingly, the concentrations calculated to effectively block intercellular communication in 50 per cent (EC_{50}) of the myocardial cells correlated with the octanol/water partition coefficients of the ten compounds. The disordering effect produced by halothane between the C–9 and C–18 positions of the phospholipid membrane disrupts the gap junctions and blocks intercellular communication. The action of halogenated hydrocarbons on gap junctions may account for the correlation observed between vapour pressure and the ability to sensitize the heart to arrhythmias.

DIGITALIS

Cardiac glycosides, illustrated by digitalis, are one of the most widely prescribed group of cardiac drugs, yet they can induce considerable toxicity owing to their low toxic-to-therapeutic ratio. The toxicity of digitalis may occur by the same mechanism that produces therapeutic effects. The positive inotropic effect of digitalis has been proposed to correlate with inhibition of Na^+/K^+ ATPase. The inhibition of Na^+/K^+ ATPase is from the binding of the glycoside to a subunit of the transport protein on the outside of the cell membrane. The increased Ca^{2+} enhances cardiac contractility but excessive inhibition of Na^+/K^+ ATPase leads to Ca^{2+} overload probably through the inability of the Ca^{2+}/Na^+ exchange mechanism to maintain the intracellular Ca^{2+} equilibrium. The combination of Ca^{2+} overload and a decrease in the Na^+ and K^+ gradients and subsequent depolarization of the membrane could increase cardiac automaticity, which can lead to arrhythmias. The toxic as well as lethal actions of digitalis have been known since its early use. Many of the central nervous system (CNS) effects that are associated with chronic exposure may not be observed with acute digitalis poisoning and nausea, vomiting and central respiratory depression may be predominant. Cardiac symptoms include bradycardia, tachycardia, conduction disturbances, sinus arrest, paroxysmal atrial tachycardia (PAT), atrial flutter and fibrillation, ventricular ectopic pacemaker activity, premature ventricular contraction (PVC), ventricular tachycardia and fibrillation, asystole and cardiac arrest. Digitalis toxicity is associated with almost every known disturbance of cardiac rhythm. Certain dysrhythmic events are more prominent. In addition to these digitalis-induced arrhythmias, ST segment depression of the electrocardiograph (ECG) is generally observed. Sinus bradycardia is often observed during digitalis therapy and this effect may be enhanced in patients with myocardial insufficiency who respond to therapeutic doses with improved ventricular function. First, second and even third degree AV block are observed. Second (Mobitz I and II) and third degree block are generally indicative of intoxication. Advanced second degree block (Mobitz II) can result in conduction ratios of 2 : 1, 3 : 1 or 4 : 1. These AV conduction disturbances are often accompanied by AV junctional escape beats or junctional pacemakers that are slower than the atrial rate.

Cardiac glycosides have been associated with a variety of ventricular rhythms including premature beats (often bigeminal, trigeminal and multifocal ventricular premature beats), ventricular tachycardia and ventricular fibrillation. Ventricular ectopic activity is one of the most frequent and earliest electrophysiological signs of intoxication. Premature ventricular contractions (PVCs) are probably the most common cardiac glycoside-induced arrhythmia. Digitalis-induced ventricular tachycardia is associated with a relatively high mortality. Cardiotonic steroids are known to elicit several toxic effects in isolated cardiac preparations. These toxic actions include: (1) dysrhythmic activity, (2) contracture (an increase in resting or diastolic tension), and (3) a decline in contractility which follows the positive inotropic effect.

It is generally accepted that digitalis-induced inhibition of sarcolemmal Na^+/K^+ ATPase, the membrane Na^+ pump, is causally related to the direct cardiotoxic actions. Cardiotonic steroids have other actions which contribute to their inotropic and/or toxic effects. For example, studies have indicated that these cardenolides may affect, either directly or indirectly, slow inward Ca^{2+} current.

Some digitalis-induced arrhythmias are mediated by increased automaticity, indicating that the observed extrasystolic events do not require previous membrane depolarization. It is possible that cardiotonic steroid toxicity also elicits abnormal automaticity. Additionally, data indicate that toxic concentrations of digitalis elicit conditions which predispose to reentry or circus movement, i.e. slow impulse propagation, unidirectional block, and a short refractory period. Digitalis intoxication can elicit numerous alterations in the pacemaker function of the SA node. Studies in isolated tissue indicate that direct cardiac effects may be contributory. Toxic concentrations of ouabain decrease maximum diastolic potential, action potential amplitude, and upstroke velocity in rabbit AV node. In isolated cardiac muscle, toxic concentrations of digitalis produce a decline in developed tension and an increase in resting tension (contracture).

Ethyl Alcohol

Acute ethanol exposure decreases heart contractility. In the intact animal, this depression is in part the effect of ethanol on the sympathetic nervous system, but ethanol also has a direct effect on the myocardium. The depressant effect is due primarily from abnormalities in ion movement, specifically Ca^{2+}, although K^+ and Na^+ transport ATPases are also inhibited by ethanol. Alcohol also interferes with Ca^{2+} binding to troponin. Ca^{2+} regulation of troponin interaction with myosin is impaired. This in turn inhibits the interaction of myosin with actin and muscle contraction is inhibited. Myocardial ATP is also reduced by ethanol exposure but this is probably related to the altered Ca^{2+} transport. Ethanol exposure has been reported to increase membrane fluidity and alter the lipid and protein composition of cardiac mitochondrial membranes. Physical changes in mitochondrial membranes produced by ethanol correlate with reduced contents of cytochromes, reduced iron-sulphur clusters in the electron transport chain and decreased oxidation of substrates by mitochondria. Alteration in membrane composition could also be the basis of inhibition of ion transport. Structure and fluidity changes in cardiac membranes would alter the activity of transport proteins imbedded in the membrane and thereby alter the flux of Ca^{2+}, Na^+ and K^+ across the membranes. The cellular effects of ethanol exposure are not limited to the myocardium and occur to varying degrees in other organs of the body.

Cocaine

Abuse of cocaine results in myocardial infarction, ventricular tachycardia and fibrillation, myocarditis and sudden death. Large doses of cocaine increase Ca^{2+} uptake by isolated heart cells and the increased uptake is associated with cell toxicity. Lower doses of cocaine depress cardiac contractility in isolated heart cells and the depression is associated with decreased intracellular Ca^{2+} transients during stimulated contraction. The effect is reversible and the Ca^{2+} pool of the sarcoplasmic reticulum is not affected. Cocaine blocks reuptake of catecholamines at the synapses. Increased catecholamines at myocardial β-adrenergic receptors increases cAMP and activates cAMP-dependent protein kinase which results in phosphorylation of the calcium channel of the sarcoplasmic reticulum. Noradrenaline (norepinephrine) also stimulates α-adrenergic receptors leading to inositol triphosphate-induced Ca^{2+} release from sarcoplasmic reticulum. The stimulation of beta-receptors by noradrenaline would also lead to tachycardia. The role of increased Ca^{2+} in cocaine toxicity is supported by the finding that Ca^{2+} channel antagonists prevent ventricular arrhythmias induced by cocaine. Inhibition of fast Na^+ channels in the sarcolemma has also been implicated in the action of cocaine. When an action potential impulse is propagated the opening of fast Na^+ channels is inhibited, conduction is impaired and arrhythmias may result.

Biological Toxins

A number of toxins from animals alter cardiac inotrophy or chronotropy by their effects on ion movement and subsequent changes in membrane potentials. The most notable of these are the puffer fish toxin, tetrodotoxin, and the shellfish toxin, saxitoxin. Although chemically different, these two toxins have similar effects on fast Na^+ channels. It has been postulated that a guanidinium group on tetrodotoxin binds to a negative charge near the opening of the fast Na^+ channel. This binding does not actually block the channel but induces a conformational change that reduces the fast influx of Na^+ during contraction. A cytosolic binding site for tetrodotoxin has been suggested and at this site, it inhibits the movement of Na^+ through fast channels in a fashion similar to the effect of local anaesthetics. The cytosolic binding site in the frog for tetrodotoxin may simply be a precursor of the membrane-binding protein. Smooth muscle and cardiac muscle are relatively insensitive to tetrodotoxin and saxitoxin compared with nerve fibres. This sensitivity is attributable to binding affinities of membrane proteins associated with fast Na^+ channels for tetrodotoxin and saxitoxin. Na^+ channels isolated from skeletal or cardiac muscle have about a 20–60-fold lower affinity for these toxins than Na^+ channels in the brain.

Batrachotoxin is secreted from the skin of a Columbian frog (*Pyllobates aurotaenia*) and like tetrodotoxin and saxitoxin is primarily a nervous tissue toxin but it can induce ventricular arrhythmias and fibrillation. The mechanism for this effect is an increase in resting Na^+ permeability. The increase in Na^+ permeability reduces the resting potential of the membrane resulting in depolarization. The increase in Na^+ permeability also causes an increase in Ca^{2+} from sodium—calcium exchange, and positive inotrophy ensues. The Na^+ channel antagonist, tetrodotoxin, blocks the Na^+ channels opened by batrachotoxin.

Sea anemone toxin has a positive inotropic effect on the mammalian heart associated with an increase in intracellular concentrations of Na^+, Ca^{2+} and a decrease in intracellular K^+. The positive inotropic effect is accompanied by a prolonged action potential and a decreased velocity of depolariztion. Apparently sea anemone toxin affects the repolarization of the heart and induces enhanced contractility by delaying the inactivation of fast Na^+ channels.

ELECTROPHYSIOLOGY

Electrical properties of cardiac muscle determine most of the mechanical properties of the heart. The heart is an effective blood pump because the entire venticle is rapidly activated within

10–20 ms, by the rapidly conducting specialized pathways, e.g. the Purkinje fibre system, and by propagation through the myocardium. The heart acts as a syncytium and it does not contract tetanically. The mechanical active state is almost maximally developed because of the long duration plateau component of the ventricular cardiac action potential.

Mechanisms of Toxicity

Some cardiotoxic chemicals and biotoxins discussed above act on the heart by affecting the electrical properties of the cell membrane or on other steps of the excitation—contraction coupling sequence. Some drugs antagonize the slow channels and thereby depress inotrophy or even completely uncouple contraction from excitation. Toxins, such as the Japanese puffer fish poison tetrodotoxin (TTX), selectively block the fast Na^+ channels in the heart causing cardiac arrest. Substances such as tetraethylammonium (TEA^+) ion depress the kinetics of activation of the K^+ channels, thereby prolonging the cardiac AP and having important repercussions on the physiology of the heart. Veratridine prolongs the action potential by a different mechanism, namely by depressing the kinetics of spontaneous inactivation of the voltage-activated fast Na^+ channels, i.e. the closing of the inactivation gate is slowed. Other compounds can directly or indirectly, via a metabolic action, affect the release or uptake of Ca^{2+} from the sarcoplasmic reticulum. The transmembrane resting potential in atrial and ventricular myocardial cells is about -80 mV. The resting potential in Purkinje fibres is somewhat greater (approximately -90 mV) and in the nodal cells is lower (approximately -60 mV).

The intracellular ion concentrations are maintained in a different way from those in the extracellular fluid: active ion transport mechanisms expend metabolic energy to transport specific ions against their concentration or electrochemical gradients. These ion pumps are located within the cell membrane. The Na^+/K^+ ATPase is specifically inhibited by the cardiac glycosides, acting on the outer surface. The enzyme/pump is also inhibited by sulphydryl reagents, such as N-ethymaleimide, mercurial diuretics and ethacrynic acid, thus suggesting that SH groups are important for activity. Other inhibitors of the Na^+/K^+ ATPase include oligomycin, chloropromazine free radical, phlorizin, local anaesthetics and ethanol (acutely).

Excitability and action potential generation are almost unaffected at shorter times. However, over a period of many minutes, depending on the ratio of volume to surface area of the cell, the resting membrane potential (E_m) slowly declines because of the gradual dissipation of the ionic gradients. The progressive depolarization depresses the rate of rise of the action potential, and hence propagation velocity, and eventually excitability is lost.

Because of the Ca^{2+}/Na^+ exchange reaction, whenever the cell gains Na^+, e.g. from the action of ouabain, the cell will also gain Ca^{2+} because the exchange reaction becomes depressed as the Na^+ electrochemical gradient is reduced. This effect is thought to be the mechanism of the positive inotropic action of cardiac glycosides. There is a continual leak of Na^+ inward and K^+ outward even in a resting cell and the system would slowly run down if active pumping were blocked, e.g. by cardiac glycosides. In the presence of ouabain (short-term exposure only) to inhibit the pump, the resting potential or net diffusion potential (Ediff) is determined by the ion concentration gradients for K^+ and Na^+ and by the relative permeability for K^+ and Na^+. The depolarizing afterpotential is more prevalent and prominent in the presence of cardiac glycosides. Digitalis may tend to produce ectopic pacemaker activity by this mechanism. In vascular smooth muscle of the dog coronary arteries, however, the cardiac glycosides were found to increase the inward Ca^{2+} current. The depolarizing afterpotential is depressed by Ca^{2+} antagonist drugs like verapamil.

The depolarizing afterpotential is produced by a mixed conductance (non-selective) Na^+/K^+ channel that is activated by Ca^{2+} ion abnormally released from SR extra loaded with Ca^{2+}. Inhibition of the inward L_{Ca} by Ca^{2+} antagonists would cause less Ca^{2+} loading in the sarcoplasmic reticulum, and hence less Ca^{2+} release to activate this ion channel.

Any drug or toxic chemical that affects the resting potential, e.g. depolarizes, will have important repercussions on the cardiac action potential. Depolarization reduces the rate of rise of the action potential, and thereby also slows its velocity of propagation. This, of course, will slow the spread of excitation throughout the heart and will interfere with the heart's ability to act as an efficient blood pump. This effect is progressive as a function of the degree of depolarization. If the myocardial cells and Purkinje fibers were depolarized to approximately -50 mV by any means, the rate of rise goes to zero and all excitability (and contraction) is lost, leading to cardiac arrest. Hyperpolarization usually produces only a small increase in rate of rise. A larger hyperpolarization may actually slow down the velocity of propagation because the critical depolarization required to bring the membrane to its threshold potential is increased. In fact, large hyperpolarizations can lead to propagation block.

If the fast Na^+ channels are either blocked by TTX or voltage inactivated or elevated, the addition of some positive inotropic agents, such as catecholamines or histamine, restores excitability and induces slowly-rising action potentials by increasing the number of slow channels available for voltage activation. The resting potential also affects the duration of the cardiac action potential. With polarizing current, depolarization lengthens the action potential, whereas hyperpolarization shortens it. In contrast, when K^+ is used to depolarize the cells, depolarization shortens the action potential.

The slow channels are also selectively sensitive to acidosis. The slow channels are blocked by verapamil-type of agents but not by the TTX-type agents. The slow channels do not allow Li^+ to pass through whereas the fast channels do. The slow channels are kinetically slow, turning on, turning off and recovering much more slowly than the fast Na^+ channels. The voltage range over which the slow channels inactivate is different from that of the fast Na^+ channels, and the threshold potential is also different for both.

Because of some of these special properties of the slow channels, namely their metabolic dependence and sensitivity to acidosis, the myocardial cells can exert control over their Ca^{2+} influx. Thus, under adverse conditions such as transient regional ischaemia, the number of functional slow channels decreases, and so Ca^{2+} influx and force of contraction diminish. There are agents such as the cardiac glycosides that increase the force of contraction of the heart without increasing the Ca^{2+} current. The mechanism of action of the digitalis compounds on force of contraction is generally proposed as partial inhibition of the Na^+/K^+ ATPase and Na^+/K^+ pump leading to an elevated Na_i^+ and therefore a higher Ca_i^{2+} by the Ca/Na exchange reaction. The higher Ca_i also may load the sarcoplasmic reticulum with more Ca^{2+} for subsequent release.

Inhibitors of metabolism and hypoxia can produce a great number of non-specific toxic effects on the heart. For example, lowering of the ATP level will depress the rate of Na^+/K^+ pumping, and the cells may depolarize. This is not always the case. For example, very little depolarization is produced after 1 h of severe hypoxia. On the other hand, with more prolonged and severe metabolic interference, the myocardial cells depolarize. In the case of ischaemia, in addition to the resultant hypoxia, other factors are involved, including K^+ accumulation in the interstitial space, which itself produces depolarization. Metabolic inhibition and lowering of the ATP level (in hypoxia, the ATP level declines to about 25 per cent of the control value within 20 min. Metabolic inhibition may lower the cyclic AMP level because ATP is the substrate for adenylate cyclase. This, in turn, could affect the activity of cAMP-protein kinase and the number of available slow channels in the myocardial membrane. This reduces or abolishes the inward slow current, and so depresses or blocks the slow AP.

With hypoxia and ischaemia, a profound acidosis is rapidly produced. Metabolic poisons, such as cyanide that block oxidative metabolism and thereby promote anaerobic glycolysis and lactic acid production, may do the same. Acidosis is known to depress contractility with only little effect on the normal cardiac AP and one mechanism for this effect is the selective blockade of the slow channels at acid pH. Blockade of the slow channels inhibits the Ca^{2+} influx which passes through these channels, and depresses the contractions, causing excitation—contraction uncoupling. Acidosis also depresses metabolism.

Acidosis protects against the deleterious effects of hypoxia, with respect to the degree of recovery of contractility that occurs after a period of hypoxia. The mechanism of this protective effect of acidosis was suggested to be the blockade of the slow channels by acidosis, thus inhibiting Ca^{2+} influx and sparing ATP usage.

The effects of some metabolic poisons, such as valinomycin or dinitrophenol (an uncoupler of oxidative phosphorylation), may be reversed or partially prevented by elevation of glucose several fold above the normal level.

High doses of catecholamines are known to produce cardiomyopathies and arrhythmias. One proposed mechanism for this catecholamine-induced myocardial necrosis is a direct effect on the heart resulting from an increased Ca^{2+} influx through the slow channels.

With respect to a possible mechanism for the deleterious effects of catecholamines on the heart, activation of the beta-adrenergic receptor leads to stimulation of the adenylate cyclase and elevation of the cyclic AMP level. The latter activates cyclic AMP-dependent protein kinase and an increased state of phosphorylation of the slow channels could result. This would make a greater fraction of the slow channels become available for voltage activation. The Ca^{2+} influx per beat would increase, and possibly could lead to Ca^{2+} overload of the myocardial cells. Ca^{2+} overload occurs because the Ca^{2+} influx is greater than the efflux.

The methylxanthines, such as caffeine, theophylline, aninophylline and methylisobutyl xanthine (MIX), in high concentration (e.g. 10 mM) have been reported to destroy the membranes of the sarcoplasmic reticulum.

Okadaic acid is a protein phosphatase inhibitor isolated from marine sponges (*Halichondria*). This toxin produces positive inotropy and has been shown to increase the duration of the cardiac action potential. Okadaic acid may act to prevent the dephosphorylation of the Ca^{2+} channel protein to increase calcium channel opening.

Agents that depress Ca^{2+} influx through excitable membranes have been termed Ca^{2+} antagonists. The Ca^{2+} antagonists also block the Ca^{2+} slow channels of vascular smooth muscle cells, and so act as vasodilators and anti-anginal agents. Their action on the myocardial cells cause negative inotropic effects. Some of these drugs, particularly those that have use dependency, possess some antiarrhythmic properties. Verapamil and D600 are use dependent, i.e. the effect is more pronounced and more rapid in onset with higher frequencies of stimulation. Nifedipine is about ten times more potent than verapamil in blocking slow channels in cardiac muscle. Diltiazem, the third major class of organic Ca^{2+} antagonist drugs, structurally resembles diazepam.

Papaverine, a vasodilating drug that has some structural similarities to verapamil, also blocks myocardial slow channels. However, papaverine has at least one other effect, namely it acts as a phosphodiesterase inhibitor and thereby elevates cyclic AMP. The slow channel blocking effect predominates in determining the overall response of cardiac muscle to this drug. The vasodilating effect can result from both properties of papaverine, namely phosphodiesterase inhibition and Ca^{2+} slow channel blockade. Because the Ca^{2+} antagonists depress or block Ca^{2+} influx into the myocardial cells, they produce excitation–contraction uncoupling.

Various heavy metal cations, such as Mn^{2+}, Co^{2+} and La^{3+}, also act as Ca^{2+} antagonists and blockers of Ca^{2+} influx. These cations are believed to compete with Ca^{2+} ions for binding sites on the outer surface of the membrane, including sites on the slow channels. Heavy metals can demyelinate nerve fibres (Pb^{2+}). Mitochondria of several tissues are affected by heavy metals, such as Pb^{2+} and Hg^{2+}, including inhibiting Ca^{2+} accumulation and inhibiting oxidative phosphorylation. Many enzymes are sensitive to heavy metals and to anions such as F^- ion. Manganese (Mn^{2+}) and cobalt (Co^{2+}) ions, in concentrations of about 1 mM, are known to block the slow channels.

Considerable Co^{2+} cardiomyopathy was caused by beer products which contained added Co^{2+} used as a foam stabilizer. Cobalt causes several symptoms including contracture, myocytolysis, and disintegration of the myofibrils. Ischaemic lesions (sequelae of thrombosis) have also occurred.

Lanthanum (La^{3+}) ions, at concentrations of approximately 1 mM, also selectively (relatively) block Ca^{2+} slow channels, like Mn^{2+} and Co^{2+}. La^{3+} displaces Ca^{2+} from binding sites on the outer surface of the cell membrane. The Ba^{2+} depolarization occurs rapidly in cells, like heart cells, in which HgCl content is relatively low.

Cadmium (Cd^{2+}), an environmental pollutant, produces significant cardiotoxic effects. Cd^{2+} depresses contractility of the heart and this effect is often thought to be a Ca^{2+}-antagonistic action. It appears that Cd^{2+} acts on SH groups.

In perfused neonatal rat papillary muscle, Cd^{2+} (0.5 mM) was more potent than Zn^{2+}, Mn^{2+} or even La^{3+} in depressing contractile force. In isolated perfused rat hearts, Cd^{2+} ($3 \times 10^{-5}M$) caused a progressive increase in the P–R interval of the ECG, and then partial or complete A-V block (Wenckebach Type I block). Heart rate was decreased. Rats given Cd^{2+} in their drinking water also developed prolonged PR intervals and other signs of marked changes in cardiac conduction before other overt signs of Cd^{2+} poisoning appeared. Histological examination revealed hypertrophy and vacuolization in the cells of the His–Purkinje system.

Vanadate exerts its inotropic effects by some mechanism other than by inhibition of the Na^+/K^+ pump, namely by altering the duration of the action potential. Also, in contrast to the cardiac glycosides, vanadate in high doses did not produce arrhythmias. Vanadate also was reported to stimulate adenylate cyclase. Agents that affect the K^+ channels in all excitable membranes, including heart cells, include tetraethylammonium ion (TEA$^+$, 5–15 mM), aminopyridines, Ba^{2+} ion (0.05–2.0 mM), Cs^+ ion (1–10 mM), Rb^+ ion (1–10 mM) and local anaesthetics (10^{-5} to 10^{-3}M). Most of these agents depress both the resting potassium conductance (gK) and the excitable K^+ channels (depress the voltage-dependent activation of gK). The kinetics of turn-on of the K^+ channels is also slowed.

TEA$^+$ blocks the voltage-dependent K^+ channels from the inner surface of the membrane by lodging inside the activation gate of the channel. The suppression of K^+ activation by TEA$^+$ is use-dependent because the TEA$^+$ molecule can only enter the K^+ channel to bind when the gate is open.

The aminopyridines are effective in squid giant axon when applied to either internal or external membrane surfaces. The aminopyridine molecules bind to closed K^+ channels but are released from open channels in a voltage-dependent manner.

The digitalis compounds exert potent effects on the heart, including their well known positive inotropic action. The cardiac glycosides increase the maximal force generated and the rate at which the force is developed. There is a fine line between the therapeutic effects (e.g. for congestive heart failure) of the cardiac glycosides and their toxic effects. It is widely believed that the therapeutic and toxic effects act by the same mechanism. The major specific action of the cardiac glycosides is the inhibition of the Na^+/K^+ ATPase and Na^+/K^+ pump in the cell membrane. Although there is some degree of variability from tissue to tissue with respect to the dose – response curves, in general 50 per cent inhibition of the

enzyme occurs at 10^{-7} to 10^{-6} M ouabain, and nearly 100 per cent inhibition occurs at 10^{-4} M.

The therapeutic effect of digitalis on cardiac contractility is presumably the partial inhibition of the Na^+/K^+ pump; the therapeutic action of digitalis is to make more Ca^{2+} available to the myofilaments.

The toxic effect of the cardiac glycosides is presumably a greater degree of inhibition of the Na^+/K^+ pump that causes the ionic gradients to run down too far and cause a Ca^{2+} overload. The Ca^{2+} overload produces a number of deleterious functional and morphological changes and the decrease of the Na^+ and K^+ gradients leads to a partial depolarization and all of its repercussions. In addition, overloading the sarcoplasmic reticulum with Ca^{2+} causes uncontrolled Ca^{2+} release and resulting delayed afterdepolarizations (DADs) and triggered arrhythmias.

Release of catecholamines from nerve terminals, another effect of the cardiac glycosides, could contribute to their overall cardiotoxicity. The catecholamines may act primarily to increase Ca^{2+} influx and cause Ca^{2+} overload. The therapeutic positive inotropic effect of digitalis is not dependent on catecholamine release.

The cardiac glycosides do not increase the inward slow current in myocardial cells but instead, at high doses, they act to depress the slow current. In vascular smooth muscle of dog coronary arteries, the inward slow current (Ca^{2+} influx) is greatly increased by the cardiac glycosides. This action may explain the known coronary vasoconstrictor effect of the cardiac glycosides, which also could contribute to their cardiotoxicity.

The cardiac glycosides also could have an internal site of action that may contribute to their therapeutic or toxic actions on the heart. The sarcoplasmic reticulum has ouabain-sensitive ATPase activity. Glycoside inhibition of the sarcoplasmic reticulum ATPase could result in lowering of Na^+ and Ca^{2+} in the sarcoplasmic reticulum and may interfere with normal excitation–contraction coupling.

The cardiac glycosides can also induce cardiac arrhythmias which lead to death. One mechanism proposed for the genesis of the arrhythmias from glycosides is the increase in incidence and magnitude of the depolarizing afterpotentials that follow the hyperpolarizing afterpotential followed by a spike. The depolarizing afterpotential, if it reaches the threshold potential, triggers a spike. This mechanism is a possible basis for generation of ectopic foci. Cardiac glycosides increase the automaticity of ectopic pacemakers (Purkinje fibres) owing to the increase in slope of the pacemaker potential. Ectopic impulse generation can be exposed in early digitalis intoxication by vagal stimulation that allows time for the ectopic impulse to escape. Although the early digitalis toxicity results from an enhanced ectopic pacemaker mechanism, as the toxicity increases and further depolarization occurs, conduction velocity is depressed. Part of the effect of digitalis on automaticity is mediated by the autonomic nervous system, and β-adrenergic blocking agents provide some protection against the digitalis-induced arrhythmias. Digitalis also has the effect of slowing the heart rate (in patients with congestive heart failure who have reflex tachycardia) and very dramatically slows the ventricular rate in the case of atrial fibrillation. The slowing of the heart rate is mediated in part by the vagus nerve and in part by a direct action on the heart. In the neural portion, digitalis reduces the heart rate secondary to an improvement in cardiac output. Pacemaker suppression by acetylcholine is enhanced by digitalis and pacemaker stimulation by noradrenaline (norepinephrine) is reduced. In the direct effect, digitalis prolongs the refractory period of the AV node to decrease the portion of 'concealed' impulses that may pass through the node during atrial fibrillation or flutter.

Local anaesthetics block excitable membranes without appreciably affecting the resting potential. The tertiary amine local anaesthetics, e.g. lignocaine (lidocaine) and procaine, presumably penetrate through the membrane in the unionized form and block from inside in the ionized form; thus, they are about equally effective when applied to either side of the membrane. The quarternary amine local anaesthetics, which penetrate less readily because of their net charge, block much more effectively when applied inside. Local anaesthetics depress both the resting and voltage-activated membrane conductances, including the fast inward Na^+ current, inward slow current, and K^+ outward current. These drugs act as non-specific membrane stabilizers.

Several local anaesthetics, e.g. lignocaine (lidocaine) and procainamide, have also been used as cardiac antiarrhythmic agents. Procainamide depresses the excitability of the atrium and ventricle to electrical stimulation. Conduction is slowed and pacemaker potentials (phase 4 depolarization) are suppressed. The drug usually prolongs the functional refractory period more than the action potential. The ECG changes, reflecting these effects of the drug, include widening of the QRS complex and prolongation of the P–R and Q–T intervals. Ventricular extrasystoles are suppressed. These properties of local anaesthetic agents contribute to their antifibrillatory and antiarrhythmic qualities. Contractility of the heart is also depressed. The effects of procainamide are much like those of quinidine.

Phenytoin, another antiarrhythmic agent, abolishes ventricular tachycardias due to ectopic foci and can antagonize digitalis arrhythmias. In low concentrations, phenytoin depresses pacemaker activity in Purkinje fibres and has a similar effect on the sinoatrial nodal cells when used in higher concentrations. Phenytoin produces less depression of contractility than comparable antiarrhythmic concentrations of procainamide or quinidine. With respect to cardiotoxicity, phenytoin has caused fatal cardiac arrest by oversuppression of automaticity. Lignocaine (lidocaine) has similarly depressed automaticity.

Quinidine is the *d*-isomer of quinine found in the cinchona tree; both alkaloids have antimalarial activity. They are depressant to contractions of skeletal muscle and cardiac muscle, having significant effects on the heart. Quinidine is used in the treatment of atrial fibrillation and other cardiac arrhythmias. It depresses excitability of the heart, prolongs the functional refractory period and decreases conduction velocity. Quinidine decreases the slope of the pacemaker potential of the SA node, i.e. it depresses automaticity of the heart. Ectopic pacemaker activity is also suppressed by quinidine, perhaps from both its depression of automaticity and to its elevation of the threshold potential, and it is this action that is probably most responsible for its antiarrhythmic effect. Quinidine acts to abolish premature action potentials initiated by a re-entrant or ectopic pacemaker. This gives the drug its antiarrhythmic properties. Quinidine also exerts an anticholinergic action, preventing the cardiac slowing produced by vagal stimulation. The cardiac actions of quinidine are essentially identical to those produced by procainamide. Quinidine may cause cardiac asystole or ventricular tachycardia and fibrillation.

Amiodarone, an antiarrhythmic, antianginal agent, increases coronary flow, reduces oxygen consumption of the heart and antagonizes the actions of catecholamines.

Pentobarbitone (pentobarbital) is a commonly used general anaesthetic agent in experimental animals. It causes a marked depression of myocardial contractility (30 mg kg^{-1} intravenously). Pentobarbitone depresses (reversibly) both the Na$^+$ and K$^+$ conductance activation that occur during excitation in squid axon. The anionic form of the drug appears to be the active form when inserted into the lipid bilayer of membranes.

The general anaesthetic halothane has a negative inotropic effect. Halothane inhibits Ca^{2+} uptake by the sarcoplasmic reticulum in mechanically skinned mycardial fibres of rabbit papillary muscle, and in microsomal fractions is consistent with the myocardial depression. Halothane has also been reported to inhibit the actomyosin ATPase and to alter the conformation of proteins. The effects of halothane on the membrane electrical properties seem to vary from one species to another and from one tissue of the heart to another.

Methyoxyflurane has a negative chronotropic action similar to that of halothane with the exception that there is an initial brief positive chronotropic effect. Purkinje fibres phase 4 depolarization is depressed by halothane but enhanced by methyoxyflurane and cyclopropane. The effects of these agents were reversible.

Enflurane and methoxyflurane substantially reduces postdrive hyperpolarization in isolated canine Purkinje fibres. This effect is reversible. These effects of the anaesthetics resemble those of cardiac glycosides and it is possible that enflurane and methoxyflurane inhibit electrogenic Na$^+$/K$^+$ ATPase and a pump potential. Halothane affects the functioning of the Ca^{2+} slow channels. The effect of halothane is to shorten the cardiac action potential and to depress automaticity. Halothane inhibits the Ca^{2+} slow channels or enhances the kinetics of K$^+$ activation.

Chlorinated solvents are sources of exposure in industry and in the laboratory, e.g. carbon tetrachloride and chloroform. The most toxic chlorinated solvent is trichloroethylene. The primary action of the chlorinated solvents is depression of myocardial contractility which reduces cardiac output, coronary flow and blood pressure. Inhalation of chlorinated solvents can lead to circulatory shock and cardiac arrest. The chlorinated solvents sensitize the heart to arrhythmias. Various fluorocarbons are used as propellants in aerosols such as those for administering bronchodilator drugs. These fluorocarbons are capable of producing cardiac arrhythmias and of depressing contractility.

Polychlorinated biphenyls (PCBs) are widely used in industry and are major environmental contaminants. Significant amounts of PCBs are found in fish and humans, the highest concentrations being in adipose tissue. The addition of PCBs to mitochondria isolated from bovine heart causes inhibition of several mitochondrial enzymes and oxidative phosphorylation.

Overdoses of tricylic antidepressants (TCA), such as amitriptyline, nortriptyline and doxepin, are frequently seen. These drugs have cardiotoxic effects which may be mediated through an anticholinergic action. Imipramine enhances myocardial contractility and heart rate at low doses but at higher doses it depresses contractility, lowered heart rate, markedly lowers the blood pressure, decreases the coronary blood flow and diminished cardiac output. The cardiac electrophysiological symptoms in patients include sinus tachycardia, cardiac arrhythmias, bundle-branch block, and A-V block. Cardiac arrest and hypotension can also occur.

Phenothiazines, such as chlorpromazine, have a direct effect on the heart depressing myocardial contractility and cardiac output. Hypotension commonly occurs. Several of its effects are similar to imipramine and quinidine. Chlorpromazine decreases peripheral vascular resistance and impairs cardiovascular reflex mechanisms. Focal interstitial myocardial necrosis occurs with mucopolysaccharide deposition, particularly near the conduction system. Cardiac catecholamine depletion may occur because the catechol phenothiazines may cause cardiac arrhythmias. The ECG changes include S-T segment alterations, prolongation of P-R and Q-T intervals, decrease in T-wave amplitude, appearance of prominent U-waves, and conduction disturbances.

The anthracycline antineoplastic adriamycin (doxorubicin hydrochloride) produces cardiomyopathy in most regions of the heart. The cardiomyopathy becomes severe and often fatal when cumulative dose levels are reached of greater than

500 mg m^{-2} of body surface area. Adriamycin causes serious cardiac dysrhythmias and a certain incidence of sudden death. ECG changes have been observed in 9–26 per cent of the patients. The acute cardiotoxic effects include arrhythmias. The chronic cardiotoxic effects include congestive heart failure.

Adriamycin was reported, from microelectrode studies, to enhance automaticity of latent pacemaker cells in the His–Purkinje system. It could cause re-entrant arrhythmias as well as arrhythmias based on accelerated automaticity.

Another anticancer agent, cyclophosphamide, also causes heart damage including myocardial necrosis and ECG changes. Dogs given cyclophosphamide (500 mg kg^{-1}) show ECG evidence of myocardial damage, including falling QRS voltage, prolonged Q–T interval and T-wave changes, and death from acute pulmonary oedema. Cyclophosphamide is metabolized by the liver to produce highly toxic active (alkylating) metabolites. Capillary damage and thrombosis was also observed in the heart of a patient treated with cyclophosphamide and who died of acute heart failure.

Many antibiotics produce myocardial depressant effects. Aminoglycoside antibiotics, gentamycin and neomycin, depress $^{45}Ca^{2+}$ uptake and contractility in vascular smooth muscle and depress contractility of cardiac muscle. In isolated perfused guinea pig hearts, gentamycin, in concentrations greater than 0.4 mM produces dose-dependent decreases in left ventricular developed pressure and rate of developed pressure with time (dP/dt) within 5 min. Contractions were abolished at 6.4 mM. Other antibiotics are known to increase ionic permeability in various cell membranes and artificial lipid bilayer membranes. Valinomycin, gramicidin D and amphotericin B increase ion permeability.

Insecticides exert toxic effects on membranes. DDT is known to produce hyperactivity and convulsions. In peripheral nerves, DDT prolongs the depolarizing afterpotential. These effects are from inhibition of both Na$^+$ inactivation (veratridine-like) and K$^+$ activation (TEA$^+$-like) during excitation. Allethrin (a pyrethroid) also increases the depolarizing afterpotentials and induces repetitive afterdischarges. Pyrethroids stimulate Na$^+$ entry through the Na$^+$ channels but act on a different site from BTX and GTX. Aldrin *trans*-diol, a metabolite of the insecticide dieldrin (a cyclodiene) and possibly its active form, depresses and blocks the nerve action potential by suppressing the inward fast Na$^+$ currents.

Cardiac toxicity is common in patients treated with emetine for amoebiasis. The mitochrondria of the myocardial cells become damaged and there is necrosis of some heart cells. Changes include sinus tachycardia, arrhythmias, Q-T interval prolongation, precordial T-wave inversion and conduction disturbances. Ventricular fibrillation may occur.

The cardiotoxic site of action of the salicylates may be on the inner surface of the membrane. In cardiac Purkinje fibres, salicylate (10 mM) depresses the iK$_2$$^+$ (outward potassium) pacemaker current and automaticity.

Ethanol is a myocardial depressant when administered acutely. Cardiomyopathy with dilated heart failure may occur. Intoxicating amounts of ethanol cause leakage of the myocardial cell components. Cardiac arrhythmias and thromboembolism may also occur in alcoholics, independent of malnutrition.

Nicotine stimulates then paralyzes autonomic ganglia and neuromuscular junctions and has potent local anaesthetic-type action on nerve membranes. Nicotine exerts a greater effect on the K$^+$ conductance mechanism at the lower concentrations, nicotine prolongs the action potential and possibly gives rise to repetitive afterdischarges.

L-delta-9-tetrahydrocannabinol ($\triangle$-9-THC), the pharmacologically active substance in marijuana, has different effects on the heart in humans compared with other mammals. In human patients, the intravenous administration of $\triangle$-9-THC, in a dose approximating that delivered by one marijuana cigarette, increased heart rate and cardiac pump performance (increases in heart rate were prevented by propranolol), caused premature ventricular contractions as a result of enhanced ventricular automaticity and ventricular ectopy, and facilitated SA conduction and AV nodal conduction, as indicated by decrease in the A–H interval and in A–V nodal refractoriness.

Gram-negative bacterial endotoxin released from the ischaemic splanchnic bed during circulatory shock may have a direct effect on the heart causing depression of contractility. Depressed inotropic and chronotropic responses of the heart result from the release of noradrenaline (norepinephrine), tyramine or histamine which may occur during shock. Ca-ATPase activity and Ca^{2+} uptake following endotoxin shock could result in heart failure. A myocardial depressant factor isolated from the plasma of haemorrhagic-shocked cats was reported to decrease contractility and prolong the action potential plateau.

E. coli endotoxin can cause severe circulatory shock within 18 h and depress cardiac force development.

Tetrodotoxin (TTX) and saxitoxin, the toxins isolated from the Japanese puffer fish and from the California newt (*Taricha torosa*), respectively, block the fast Na^+ channels in most excitable membranes. In nerve, TTX has an ED_{50} of approximately 10^{-8} M. In skeletal muscle and cardiac muscle, the ED_{50} is approximately 10^{-7} M. In Purkinje fibres, 10^{-5} to 10^{-4} M are needed for complete blockade.

Veretridine, grayanotoxins, batrachotoxin, sea anemone toxin and scorpion toxin depolarize by opening and/or slowing the inactivation of Na^+ channels. The veratrum alkaloids are steroidal plant bases belonging to the genus *Veratrum*. Aconitine is a steroidal alkaloid found in the plant, *Aconitum napellus*. The veratrine alkaloids, in particular veratridine, also have an effect similar to that of grayanotoxin, increase Na^+ permeability resulting in depolarization. Veratridine, as well as batrachotoxin, grayanotoxin and aconitine, alter the voltage dependence of the activation curve for fast Na^+ channels.

Grayanotoxins (GTX) are the toxic tetracyclic diterpenoids from *Rhododendran ericacea*, which act to increase Na^+ permeability, perhaps by opening the voltage-dependent Na^+ channels.

Batrachotoxin (BTX) is a steroidal alkaloid (pyrrole carboxylic ester) found in the skin secretions of the Columbian frog (*Pyllobates aurotaenia*). The LD_{50} for rabbits is approximately 1 mg. Ventricular arrhythmias and fibrillation cause death because of an increase in resting Na^+ permeability. BTX was shown to decrease the resting potential of dog Purkinje fibres and cat ventricular myocardial cells.

A series of neurotoxins has been isolated from the sea anemone (*Anemonia sulcata*). One of these sea anemone toxins (ATX-II) has been purified and sequenced. ATX-II is a small polypeptide containing 47 amino acides (MW about 50 000) and crosslinked by three disulphide bridges. It has potent effects because it releases neurotransmitters from the nerve terminals owing to its depolarization. The positive inotropic effect of ATX-II results from holding open the Na^+ channels. Another anemone toxin obtained from the tentacles of the Bermuda anemone (*Condylactis gigantea*) is a polypeptide of MW 13 000. Condylactis toxin (CTX) greatly prolongs the repolarizing phase of the action potential of lobster and crayfish giant axons.

Two polypeptide toxins have been isolated from corals (*Goniopora*). The first toxin acts similarly to the sea anemone toxin (ATX), namely by slow inactivation of the fast Na^+ channels. The second toxin stimulates Ca^{2+} influx as it competes for binding on the dihydropyridine binding site.

Several toxins have been isolated from bee venom. One of these is the polypeptide apamin. This toxin blocks the Ca^{2+}-activated K^+ conductance channel. It has also been reported that apamin blocks the Ca^{2+} slow channels in cardiac muscle. A second bee venom toxin is melittin which is a polypeptide. This toxin inhibits adenylate cyclase and two types of protein kinases.

Several toxins have been isolated from the venom of the scorpion, *Androctonus australis*, hector. These toxins are single chain proteins composed of 63 or 64 amino acids and eight half-cystine residues. One of these toxins, scorpion toxin 1, has been shown to slow the closing of the Na^+ channel and the opening of the K^+ channel in giant axons of crayfish and lobster. In squid giant axon, the toxin blocks both Na^+ and K^+ conductances, and induces fibrillation at high concentrations. Another scorpion (*Leirus quinquestriatus*) venom was found to decrease Na^+ conductance (by 60 per cent), to slow Na^+ inactivation and to reduce K^+ activation in myelinated nerve fibres of *Xenopus*.

Two polypeptide toxins scorpions, Tityus-q toxin (*Tityus serrulatus*) and Centruoides toxin (*Centruroides suffisus*) have been examined. Tityus-q toxin shifts the voltage dependence of activation and inactivation of the fast Na^+ channel in the negative direction. Centruroides toxin selectively blocks the sarcolemmal fast Na^+ channels compared with the T-tubular Na^+ channels in skeletal muscle.

Ervatarnine, an alkaloid of the Australian tree, *Ervatarnina orientalis*, produces a frequency-dependent block of fast Na^+ channels and slow Na^+ channels. Evatarnine is a competitive inhibitor of BTX, indicating that a common receptor site blocks the cardiac action potential and slows the rate of reactivation of the Na^+ channel.

Volvatoxin A, a cardiotoxic protein from a mushroom (*Volvariella volvacea*), produces systolic cardiac arrest. It makes the sarcoplasmic reticulum membrane leaky to Ca^{2+} ion so that it cannot adequately sequester the myoplasmic Ca^{2+}. A cariotoxin isolated from the venom of the Indian cobra (*Naja nigricollis*) is a polypeptides and causes systolic arrest. It depresses Ca^{2+} accumulation by the sarcoplasmic reticulum through inhibition of the Ca^{2+}-ATPase and release of previously sequestered Ca^{2+}. The toxin also depresses Ca^{2+} accumulation by isolated mitochrondria. Ultrastructural damage observed with this cobra cardiotoxin included disruption of the cell membrane, vacuolated mitochrondria and disrupted myofibrils and contracture bands.

Palytoxin, isolated from zoanthids (genus *Palythoa*), is a potent marine toxin. It depolarizes cells; the depolarization is Na^+-dependent. Palytoxin produces contracture, associated with Ca^{2+} uptake, of isolated cardiac muscle in below nanmolar concentrations. It may selectively inhibit a catecholamine-stimulated Na^+/K^+ ATPase and thus resembles some of the biochemical toxic actions of cardiac glycosides.

Ciguatoxin, an oxygenated polyether synthesized by a dinoflagellate, increases Na^+ permeability and depolarization by activation of the fast Na^+ channels. Goniopora toxin (GPTX), isolated from a coral (*Goniopora* spp.), shows positive inotropic effects by stimulating Na^+ influx and slowing inactivation of the fast Na^+ channels.

Maitotoxin (MTX), a large molecular weight non-protein toxin isolated from a dinoflagellate (*Gambierdiscus toxicus*), is thought to be an activator of the voltage-dependent Ca^{2+} channels. MTX increases Ca^{2+} influx, produces a positive inotropic and chronotropic effect, and contracts smooth muscle. MTX is also reported to stimulate IP3 production in rat aortic smooth muscle cells. MTX exerts an arrhythmogenic effect and causes irreversible rounding of the cells. Cholera toxin is secreted by the bacteria *Vibrio cholera*. It is composed of two types of subunits (A and B). The B subunits have been shown to bind to ganglioside GM1 in the cell membrane, followed by insertion of the A subunits into the cell. The A subunit of cholera toxin ADP-ribosylates the GTP-binding protein and results in a maintained activation of the adenylate cyclase, with the consequent accumulation of cyclic AMP.

Pertussis toxin is a bacterial exotoxin produced by *B. pertussis* which contains an A and a B chain. The B chain binds to glycoprotein surface receptors and facilitates the insertion of the A chain into the cell. Pertussis toxin ADP-ribosylates the $\triangle$-subunit of G-proteins leading to the inhibition of adenylate cyclase. Pertussis toxin blocks open K^+ ion channels in the heart.

Bretylium, an antifibrillatory and antiarrhythmic drug, is reported to produce K^+ channel blockade in heart cells. Bethanidine was found, like bretylium, to inhibit potassium channel blockade but increased the slow Ca^{2+} current and thus showed a positive inotropic effect.

Spiders produce numerous toxins some of which are non-competitive antagonists of glutamate receptors, particularly the L-quisqualate-sensitive glutamate receptors, in both invertebrates and vertebrates. The venom from North American spider (*Argiope trifasciata* and *A. lobata*) also shows similar effects on glutamate receptors. It has been suggested that orgiotoxin produces open-channel block of the glutamate receptor channel.

Several oraneid spider venoms also block transmission at the frog motor endplate (nicotinic AChR), and they inhibit glutamate binding. Other toxins (AG1 and AG2) from *Agelenopsis* produce block of neuronal and cardiac Ca^{2+} channels. Changes in the electrical properties of the cell membrane produced by the cardiotoxic agents have important repercussions on the mechanical activity of the heart and its usefulness as a blood pump. The electrical activity exerts tight control over the mechanical activity. Block of the slow channels by some agents selectively depresses the force of contraction directly by reducing the Ca^{2+} influx but electrical activity remains nearly normal (excitation–contraction uncoupling). Depression of velocity of propagation greatly weakens the heart because the entire heart must be activated quickly for the heart to be effective as a pump. Depressed conduction velocity can give rise to re-entrant arrhythmias that may lead to ventricular fibrillation. Non-uniform changes in duration of the action potential by cardiotoxic agents also predisposes to the development of dysrhythmias and fibrillation. The changes in the electrical properties of the cell membrane produced by many cardiotoxic substances can lead indirectly to changes in the ultrastructure of the cells.

TOXIC CARDIOPATHOLOGY

Toxic injury to the heart and its cells may be acute or chronic, depending on the time that the tissue is exposed to the injurious agent. Acute injury, in many instances, is lethal injury whereas chronic injury allows for a chronic adaptive response; the final outcome may or may not be lethal.

Another subdivision of injury is focused on the cardiac structure that is particularly responsive to the injury. Such cardiac structures are the myocardium, endocardium, intramural and extramural vessels, epicardium and pericardium, lymphatics and the neural elements or the conduction system. Within these tissue components, the myocytes, the endothelial cells, smooth muscle cells, fibroblasts, nerve fibres and the Purkinje and conduction fibres play a selective role as each of these elements can show specific sensitivity to one or other toxic agent. The majority of these agents affect the myocytes or the capillary system. Toxic injuries occur to certain cell structures, subcellular organelles: mitochondria, plasma membrane or contractile proteins.

Acute injury to the heart may be followed by necrosis. It is then called 'acute lethal injury'. Two basic forms of cardiac muscle cell necrosis are distinguishable: contraction band necrosis and coagulation necrosis.

Contraction band necrosis, often seen in focal injury or at the periphery of larger areas of necrotic tissue, is characterized by agglutination of a series of Z-lines and their attached myofibrils which then form a tangle of enmeshed filaments. In coagulation necrosis, mitochondria show swelling and flocculent densities in the matrix space. The nucleus passes through stages of extreme condensation of nuclear chromatin (pyknosis) and dissolution of the nucleus (karyorrhexis and karyolysis). Drugs with the ability to form ion channels disturb the ability of the plasma membrane to maintain the internal environment of cells and volume control. In cells within the normal range, a limited capacity for compensation can be detected; however, in toxic dosage and in combination with other mechanisms, those agents that increase Na^+ influx or inhibit Na^+/K^+-ATPase may initate cell damage. Among the agents are some that create Na^+-specific channels (carboxylic acid ionophores). Examples of agents that inhibit Na^+/K^+-ATPase are cardiac glycosides (*Digitalis purpurea*) and aglycones (oleandrin, neriine and bufodienolides). Morphologically, ouabain, aconitine, veratrum, polypeptides (scorpion venom, anthopleurin-A), grayanotoxin, batrachotoxin and ciguatoxin alter the volume control leading to increased cell swelling, mitochondrial swelling, formation of blebs on the cell surface (particularly of endothelial cells) and subsequently alteration of the bioenergetic mechanism. Chronic administration of mercuric chloride increases both systolic and end-diastolic pressure in the heart, while exerting structural and functional damage to renal tubular cell.

Adrenergic bronchial dilators have caused sudden cardiac arrest at a high dose. Toxic cardiomyopathies have been reported with isoprenaline (isoproterenol), adrenaline (epinephrine), noradrenaline (norepinephrine), salbutamol, terbutaline, ephedrine, metaproterenol, and others.

Some compounds affecting energy metabolism produce mitochrondrial changes. Depending on the severity of the toxic alteration they reveal a sequence of alterations such as contraction of the inner matrix, swelling, disruption of cristae and alteration of inner membranes and formation of flocculent densities in the matrix space. Those toxic agents which directly affect energy metabolism are related to rapid cell death associated with loss of ionic homeostasis and loss of ATP. Rotenone and iodoacetate are examples. Compounds such as cyanide, thyroid hormone, dinitrophenol, paraquat and emetine interfere with energy metabolism. Acriflavine binds to mitochondrial DNA. Others, such dihydrotachysterol and sodium phosphate, induce intracellular calcification. Calcification precipitates are frequently seen in mitochondria. Anthracyclines produce nuclear and nucleolar lesions or massive dilatation of the sarcoplasmic reticulum. Cyanide exists in a number of forms and inhibits cytochrome oxidase. Acute lethal injury produces all the stages of coagulation necrosis described above.

Carbon monoxide poisoning is caused by deprivation of oxygen and oxidative phosphorylation. The toxicity of carbon monoxide is directly related to the affinity of carbon monoxide for haemoglobin and the low dissociation rate. Dinitrophenol is an uncoupler of oxidative phosphorylation. Morphologically, swelling of mitochrondria seems to be the main expression of sublethal doses of dinitrophenol whereas toxic doses result in acute coagulation necrosis. Thyroxine has both acute and chronic effects on the heart. Morphologically, swelling of mitochrondria and contraction band necrosis have been reported. Other agents that affect mitochondria are acriflavine, mercury, dihydrotachysterol, cobalt, lead and sodium phosphate. Sodium iodoacetate (IAA) and fluoride (glycolysis inhibitors) also affect ATP production.

Ultrastructural changes as a consequence of acute free radical injury have been noted. Acute changes following Adriamycin, carbon tetrachloride and 1,3,7,8-tetrachloro-dibenzo-*p*-dioxin (TCDD) administration include changes to mitochondria and perioxosomes. Intravascular thrombosis and necrotizing vasculitis have been linked to drug abuse, such as cocaine. Fenoldopam mesylate, a dopaminergic vasodilator, produces vacuoles in arterial smooth muscle cells at low doses. Many autophagic vacuoles are also found in smooth muscle cells as well as myofibrillar inclusions. At high doses, medial necrosis and haemorrhages occur in the small arteries and arterioles. Iron toxicity of the heart can be both acute and chronic. In acute toxicity, the prominent toxic effect is on the vascular and capillary endothelium which may lead to hypovolaemic shock. Toxic doses of iron also cause mitochondrial swelling and fatty changes in both endothelial cells and myocardium. Thiazides cause necrotizing vasculititis.

Several drugs have their action on the conduction system, e.g. the antidepressant drugs imipramine and metapramine. Imipramine and metapramine produce increases in conduction time and a conduction block at higher doses. Morphological changes in the conduction system following acute and chronic ethanol intoxication are evidence of cell injury, with degeneration of sinus node cells and increased interstitial fibrosis.

Pyridostigmine affects the cardiac parasympathetic nervous system: an alteration of the cytochrome-c oxidase in mitochrondria is proposed as a mechanism of action. 6-Hydroxydopamine (OHDA), a catecholamine depleting agent, causes chemical denervation; acute and chronic inflammation is seen with acute toxic and subchronic exposures, respectively. Both compounds

which affect the innervation of the heart are accompanied by morphological changes in the myocardium, such as increase in collagen. Ultrastructurally, myocyte vacuolization is noted with a widened gap junction. The cytoplasm shows myofibrillar degeneration.

The chief morphological alteration seen in the endocardium is endocardial fibrosis. Fibrosis of the endocardium has been seen after administration of drugs such as methylsergide, ergotamine and serotonin. Serotonin-related fibrosis occurs as a consequence of neoplasms that secrete excessive amounts of serotonin.

Two different morphological drug reactions occur in the pericardium: haemorrhage and pericarditis. Haemorrhage has been reported with minoxidil, theobromine and with anticoagulants. Treatment with hydralazine and procainamide has been complicated by pericarditis.

Subacute toxic injury produces a variable morphological picture. Drugs that have been associated with hypersensitivity myocarditis are: α-methyldopa, hydrochlorothiazide, sulphadiazine sulphisoxazole, sulphonylureas, chloramphenicol, *p*-aminosalicylic acid (PAS), amitriptyline, carbamazepine, indomethacin, penicillin, phenindione, phenylbutazone, oxyphenbutazone, tetracycline, phenytoin, acetazolamide, ampicillin, chlorthalidone, streptomycin and spironolactone.

In acute toxic myocarditis, interstitial oedema is prevalent along with necrosis of myocardial cells. Ultrastructurally, extensive myocytolysis is present. Toxic myocarditis may be accompanied by inflammatory cells. Chronic exposure to organophosphates leads to membrane alteration caused by modifications to the phospholipid/phosphorus and phospholipids, and chronic myocardial damage. Structurally, the changes described under chronic myocardial damage are seen.

Monensin, an ionophorous antibiotic derived from *Streptomyces cinnamonensis*, has both acute and chronic effects. In more subchronic conditions, lipoidosis of myocytes develops. The morphological changes in the heart consist of mitochondrial swelling and lysis of mitochondrial cristae and swelling of the T-tubular system. Swollen mitochondria develop large spherical dense bodies thought to be related to calcium. Contraction bands develop in myofilaments and disruptions of the myofilaments are seen.

The term 'chronic' injury implies that the tissue and its cells survive the toxic consequences and have time to adjust to the injury; the tissue changes seen are a result of such adjustments. A common tissue reaction of chronic injury is the development of fibrosis. In the heart, fibrosis progresses as interstitial fibrosis. Interstitial fibrosis encases single myocytes with bundles of collagen fibres that spread in the space between capillary basement membrane and myocyte basement membrane. Rapid turnover of fresh collagen is laid down as an early response to injury, mainly as type III collagen. Cardiac myocyte hypertrophy, cardiac myocyte atrophy, myofibrillar lysis and myocyte inclusions and storage, characterize the chronic adaptation to toxic injury.

Myofibrillar alteration accompanies a whole host of acute, subacute and chronic forms of myocardial injury. There are different forms of myofibrillar altration. Some acute forms show focal regions of lysis while more chronic forms of myofibrillar loss may represent depressed maintenance of myofilaments under conditions of chronic metabolic or toxic stress. Myofibrillar loss is an important diagnostic sign of cardiomyopathy and is not related to any specific cause. Myofibrillar lysis, either acute or chronic, is prominent in anthracycline toxicity.

In genetic diseases, selected structures in the heart are affected: e.g. the conduction system in chronic oxalosis, alkaptonuria and homocysteinuria; the myocardium in congestive cardiomyopathy of Fabry's disease; hypertrophic cardiomyopathy in type II (Pompe's) glycogen storage disease; restrictive cardiomyopathy in Gaucher's disease.

Ethanol has both acute and toxic effects on heart muscle, particularly the cells of the sinus node. Both chronic and acute exposure produce destructive changes in dark and clear sinus node conducting myocytes. Acute exposure of the myocardium to high levels of ethanol produces disruption of mitochondrial cristae, dilation of the sarcoplasmic reticulum and separation of the intercalated disc. The major toxic breakdown product of ethanol is acetaldehyde which produces morphological changes such as contraction bands, mitochondrial swelling and cristal disarray, as well as myofibrillar disorganization (Z-band).

Antipsychotic and antidepressant drugs can induce a toxic cardiomyopathy which ultrastructurally is characterized by lateral cell separation, changes in the lateral orientation of Z-bands, Z-band attachment to the plasma membrane, and disruption of myofilaments. Drugs such as trifluoperazine (TFP), amitriptyline, calmidazolium and thioridazine are inhibitors of calmodulin. The effect of these drugs can be enhanced by lowering extracellular Ca^{2+}. The mechanism of cell injury in antipsychotic and antidepressant drugs has been suggested to result from an increase in proteolysis as intracellular calcium normally inhibits proteolysis.

Amiodarone is an arrhythmogenic drug which also produces myelinoid inclusion bodies in the heart, as well as other tissues. The increasing accumulation of myelinoid bodies is accompanied by mitochondrial swelling and swelling of the rough endoplasmic reticulum leading to cell death. Amiodarone decreases lipid mobility.

Furazolidone is reported to produce a chronic cardiomyopathy in poultry affecting primarily the myocytes. The most important anomaly reported is myofibrillar lysis. The affected cells appear pale and empty, lacking myofibrils. The distribution varies from focal to diffuse.

Metals

Chronic iron loading under high oxygen tension had a stimulating effect on lipofuscinogenesis in cultured myocytes. In chronic iron overload, a cardiomyopathy develops. Iron overload produces degenerative changes in myocytes ranging from mitochondrial abnormalities to excessive numbers of autophagocytic vacuoles, and accumulation of cytoplasmic ferritin.

Chronic arsenic intoxication has been associated with intimal thickening of small and medium-sized arteries of the heart and extremities and also has been linked with the development of toxic pericarditis.

Cadmium inhibits enzymes that contain sulphhydryl groups and its binds to ligands that include carboxyl-, cysteinyl-, histidyl-, hydroxyl- and phosphatyl-groups. Cadmium interferes with the uptake of other metals such as copper and zinc. External cadmium inhibits the early outward current in myocardial mouse cells in a totally reversible manner. Chronic cadmium toxicity is related to hypertension.

Cobalt-related cardiomyopathy occurred as a sudden outbreak in beer drinkers. Histologically, myocyte vacuolization, accumulation of fat droplets and glycogen, and myofibrillar loss are seen.

In acute copper chloride poisoning, there is acute damage to the capillary endothelium leading to cellular oedema of the capillary wall and acute loss of fluid from the vacular space. Chronic exposure to mercury chloride reveals significant cardiovascular effects with ultrastructural changes mainly related to an increased leakiness of the plasma membrane.

Long-term treatment with corticosteroids may be accompanied by an arteritis of medium to small-sized arteries. High doses of corticosteroids are associated with focal myocardial necrosis.

MATERIALS IN FOODSTUFFS

Few cardiotoxins that cause direct damage the heart are found naturally in food; most are of a secondary nature. Other toxins can produce damage as a result of hypersensitivity. The result of chronic effects on the heart, atherosclerosis, angina pectoris and potentially mycardial infarction, are linked to elevated cholesterol in the diet and to cholesterol formed metabolically in the liver.

Dietary levels of cadmium and sodium have been linked with an increased incidence of hypertension and resulting coronary heart disease. Grains and cereals, meat, fish and poultry, fruits and vegetables are dietary sources of cadmium, but shellfish have the highest levels. Cadmium administration has also been linked with atherosclerosis and changes in blood lipids in pigeons and rats.

Sodium involvement in the induction and maintenance of hypertension has been documented, and stimulation of sodium excretion has been the primary medical treatment for hypertension in humans and animals. Sodium is believed to act through changes in intravascular volume, hormone regulation or membrane potential. Caffeine and the other methyl xanthines, theophylline (in tea) and theobromine (in cocoa), stimulate the CNS and cardiac muscle increasing cardiac output. Systolic pressure is more affected than diastolic pressure. The effects on heart rate and blood pressure are acute but appear to be related to the release of calcium from the sarcoplasmic reticulum.

Ethanol has also been linked with hypertension. It decreases contraction force and produces arrhythmias, ventricular fibrillation and cardiomegaly.

Cobalt

In the mid-1960s cobalt sulphate (1 ppm) was added to beer to enhance the stability of the foam. Cardiomyopathy was noted among heavy beer drinkers in Quebec, Nebraska and Belgium. Forty per cent of those diagnosed died of congestive heart failure. Cobalt cardiomyopathy has been shown to result from combination with lipoic acid and blocking oxidative decarboxylation of Krebs cycle intermediates, pyruvate and alpha-ketoglutarate.

Ethanol

Excessive chronic alcohol consumption leads to slowly developing cardiomyopathy as evidenced by progressive congestive heart failure. Morphologically, cardiomegaly, myocardial cellular degeneration, hypertrophy and lysis, as well as possible interstitial fibrosis are seen. Lipid droplets accumulate in the myofibrils from altered triglyceride/fatty acid metabolism.

Other Substances

Brominated vegetable oils, so treated to increase the lipid density, cause similar microscopic changes. Heart weight is increased from extensive fatty infiltration involving the entire myocardium. Degeneration is accompanied by interstitial oedema with fibre disarray, cell lysis and focal necrosis. Protein deficiency (Kwashiorkor) also leads to a similar cardiomyopathy and decreased contractility. An endemic cardiomyopathy in China has been linked to a diet deficient in selenium and has been called Keshan disease. Death due to cardiomyopathy results from pulmonary congestion due to decreased myocardial capacity.

During the development of atherosclerosis, the tunica intima of an artery or vein becomes thickened through lipid deposition which becomes covered by connective tissue fibres that form a plaque. The narrowing of the vessel and the concomitant decrease in blood flow leads to the symptoms of angina pectoris. As the plaque increases in size and thrombosis occurs, a blockage of flow can occur. In a coronary artery, this leads to myocardial infarction, the death of heart muscle from ischaemia. Deficiencies in dietary magnesium, copper, vanadium, selenium and chromium have been linked to increased hypercholesterolaemia.

The higher the serum cholesterol in a population, the higher the risk of atherosclerotic heart disease. The relative amounts of low density lipoprotein to high density lipoprotein are also indicative of increased risk. A number of dietary risk factors are involved in the development of hypercholesterolaemia, including the intake of saturated and unsaturated fats, cholesterol, total calories, alcohol and fibre. It is the high serum cholesterol and not dietary intake *per se* which is the main cause for concern. Once intake is about 200–300 mg per day, additional consumption has little additional effect on serum levels.

Cillus cereus contamination has been linked to myocardial fatty degeneration and resulting heart failure. Ciguatera, the most common foodborne toxin-related illness in the USA, leads to bradycardia among a host of other non-cardiac symptoms and occurs following ingestion of fish contaminated with a number of dinoflagellate-derived toxins. Ergotamine, a contaminant of mouldy grain, causes a profound vasoconstriction and can trigger thrombosis. Histamine in spoiled seafood leads to constriction of the coronary arteries. Scombroid poisoning from inadequately preserved tuna or bonita has a histamine component. Tyramine, in red wine and some cheeses, has been linked with cardiac arrhythmia and sudden death in persons taking monamine oxidase inhibitors. Vomitoxin and deoxynivalenol, from *Fusarium graminearum*-infected wheat, has caused calcified pericarditis and monosodium glutamate has been linked to arhythmia.

ORGANOPHOSPHATES

The pharmacology of the cholinesterase inhibitors as it relates to the heart has been largely attributed to the actions of excess acetylcholine. The toxic effects of excess acetylcholine result in cardiac slowing, arrhythmias, and eventally cardiac death (e.g. asystole). Compounds that increase acetylcholine levels by antagonizing cholinesterase at the cardiac site will also produce arrhythmias followed by cardiac death. Cholinesterase inhibitors affect peripheral nerves that impinge on the heart, CNS centres that regulate heart rhythm, and lung function that may produce pulmonary complications. Excess acetylcholine at these sites may be the primary reason that cardiac toxicity occurs.

A correlation has been found between signs of toxicity from an organophosphate (soman) and changes in several biochemical parameters. An anticholinesterase (dimethoate) was found to induce severe ECG disturbances (Q–T lengthening, S–T depression, and T-wave inversion) and cardiac failure. The ECG effects on the myocardium were independent of its anticholinesterase action. A correlation could exist between the organophosphorus-induced arrhythmias and the concentration of fatty acids. However, compounds that stimulate muscarinic receptors increase cGMP levels in intact myocardium. Organophosphate-induced arrhythmias may result from mechanisms different from muscaranic stimulation.

Electrophysiological studies have shown that the cardiac arrhythmias caused by VX (pinacolyl methylphosphonofluoridate) may be due to Na^+/K^+ ATPase inhibition. Hypernatraemia and hyperkalaemia have been observed following insecticide misuse in humans with gradual recovery over as long as 5 days. Sinus bradyarhythmia occurred followed by complete atrioventricular blockade. Ventricular extrasystoles were also observed. These arrhythmias may not differ from the torsade arrhythmias described in humans.

During convulsive periods, additional U-waves are observed which may be due to hypoxia or anoxia. Analysis of the literature suggests that cholinesterase inhibitors can exert a ventricular rhythm change that may not be dependent on anoxia. Anoxia can further exaggerate ventricular rhythm disturbances and may complicate interpretation of an ECG pattern.

A direct pathological lesion on the atrium has been described in the heart following acute poisoning with sarin, parathion, trichlorfon or malathion. Fatty infiltration, dilation of blood vessels and haemorrhage of cardiac tissue occurred following malathion intoxication in humans. This lesion may be the result of peripheral increases in vascular resistance.

It may be important to note that all acetylcholinesterase inhibitors do not demonstrate the same cardiac effects. The vagal effects of the organophosphates are potentiated by the addition of exogenous acetylcholine. The bradycardia may lead to cardiac arrest. Ventricular escape may occur after 30–60 s (20–30 beats/min) or death may ensue. Cholinesterase inhibitors may exert their cardiovascular (i.e. blood pressure) effects, in part, through cardioinhibitory vasomotor and respiratory centres. Tachycardia, as well as bradycardia, has been described in humans following organophosphate poisoning.

In the atria, both acetylcholinesterase and butyrylcholinesterase function to modulate the chronotropic effect of acetylcholine. It is suggested that organophosphates decrease atrial rates by inhibiting both acetylcholinesterase and butyrylcholinesterase activity. Butyrylcholinesterase may be more important for the decreased rate induced by acetylcholine, and acetylcholinesterase may be more important for the amplitude of atrial contractions caused by acetylcholine.

In addition to the atrial effects of cholinergic agents, cholinergic stimulation of the ventricles has been observed. It was reported that DFP produces ventricular premature complexes, 'torsade de pointes' in humans.

It is interesting to note that both adrenergic and antiadrenergic substances have been claimed to provide benefit in organophosphate poisoning. This apparent contradiction may reflect an effort to balance temporal changes in transmitter concentrations. Observed decreases in blood pressure appear to be a much more serious toxic effect of these compounds.

Reports in the literature suggest that organophosphorus compounds can manifest their toxicity by affecting cardiac systems. These toxic effects may differ depending on which organophosphate is administered, the dose, route of administration, and other factors such as the pharmacological preparation and species observed. Sinus bradycardia may occur initially, but the more serious event is ventricular in origin. It may take approximately 2 days to 2 weeks for this ventricular cardiac effect to appear. A method of treatment for these arhythmias is not well established. Historically, atropine has been employed as a treatment for organophosphate poisoning. However, atropine administered under hypoxic conditions following organophosphate exposure may induce serious ventricular arrhythmias. The clinical data indicate that these responses are observed in only a portion of the cases. The reasons for this occurrence in only a portion of the cases are not known. Mechanisms proposed for this cardiac toxicology include calcium overload to the heart or inhibition of the sodium pump.

The opinions or assertions contained herein are the private views of the authors and are not to be construed as official or as reflecting the views of the US Army or the US Department of Defense.

FURTHER READING

Acosta, Jr., D. (Ed.) (1992). *Cardiovascular Toxicology*. Raven Press, New York

Balazs, T. (Ed.) (1981). *Cardiac Toxicology*, vols I and II. CRC Press, Boca Raton

Baskin, S. I. (Ed.) (1991). *Principles of Cardiac Toxicology*. CRC Press, Boca Raton

Benowitz, N. L. (1992). Cardiotoxicity in the workplace. *Occupational Medicine*, **7**, 464–478

Shephard, J. T. And Vanhoutte, P. M. (1979). *The Human Cardiovascular System: Facts and Concepts*. Raven Press, New York

Sperelakis, N. (1984). *Physiology and Pathophysiology of the Heart*. Martinus Nijhoff Publishing, Boston

26 Hepatotoxicity

Richard H. Hinton and Paul Grasso

INTRODUCTION

The liver has many metabolic roles and is, accordingly, affected by a very large number of xenobiotics. However, the liver also has an immense capacity for self-repair so that the majority of lesions observed in the liver reverse rapidly on cessation of treatment. Nevertheless the liver's defences can be overwhelmed. Liver failure from paracetamol (acetaminophen) overdose is familiar to most clinical toxicologists whereas repeated liver damage may lead to cirrhosis. Also, while liver cancer is rare in Western Europe and North America it is common in other parts of the world. Non-dose-dependent side-effects on the liver affecting up to 5 per cent of patients are common with many classes of drug and may be sufficiently severe to require cessation of treatment. Hence understanding hepatotoxicity is vital to clinical as well as academic toxicologists.

In any discussion of hepatotoxicity it is necessary to remember Paracelsus' dictum that it is the dose that makes the poison. One of the major roles of the liver is to protect the body against naturally occurring toxins present, for example, in plants or produced by the body's own intestinal flora. Exposure to small amounts of such materials results in changes in the liver which permit efficient removal of the toxin. These changes are called adaptive because they do not compromise the ability of the liver to perform its other vital functions. As the dose of the compound is increased there may come a point when other functions are compromised and this is defined as the toxic phase of the response. However, before considering this and other aspects of the action of chemicals on the liver it is necessary to discuss briefly the structure and metabolic roles of the liver.

ANATOMY AND PHYSIOLOGY OF THE LIVER

The liver is a large organ making up about 3.5 per cent of the body weight of an adult rat or 2 per cent of the body weight of an adult human. The overall shape of the liver differs markedly between species. In rats and mice the liver is divided into several distinct lobes; the human liver, on the other hand, is divided into two poorly differentiated lobes. The liver lies immediately under the diaphragm, is covered in a thin capsule and is supported mechanically by attachments to the diaphragm and by the blood vessels. The liver has a complex blood supply. Approximately 80 per cent of the blood is derived from the portal vein. This drains the duodenum, small intestine and a portion of the colon. The remaining 20 per cent of the blood supply comes from the hepatic artery. Blood leaves the liver by the very short hepatic veins which join the ascending vena cava. The liver acts as an exocrine gland, secreting bile. This bile is conducted down the extrahepatic bile duct into the intestine. In the majority of species, but not in the rat, a portion of the bile secreted from the liver is stored and concentrated in the gall bladder, a blind-ended sac attached to the bile duct. As will be seen later in the Chapter, the organization of the bulk of the liver substance, the parenchyma, means that no lymph is formed in most of the liver. Lymph is, however, formed in the connective tissues of the portal tracts and is drained by a duct which connects with the lymphatics that drain the intestine and from there it passes to the thoracic duct. The portal vein, hepatic artery, extrahepatic bile duct and the major lymphatics all enter the liver substance at a single point, the porta hepatis. The hepatic veins, however, leave at different points, the number and location of which vary with the species. These various connections are summarized in Figure 1.

Organization of Vessels and Nerves within the Liver

As mentioned in the last section the portal vein, the hepatic artery, the extrahepatic bile duct and the major liver lymphatics enter the liver together at the porta hepatis. Once within the liver the

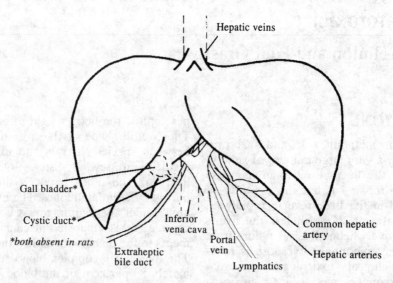

Figure 1   Diagram showing the blood supply to the liver and the drainage of bile and lymph

vessels branch to form the portal tree (Figure 2). At all branch points there is bifurcation of all types of vessel. This has two consequences. First, all branches of the portal tree from the largest to the smallest contain all four types of vessel (Figure 3). Second, there are few anastomoses between vessels. Hence any blockage of a branch of the hepatic artery, which provides oxygenated blood to the liver, will result in destruction of an area of the liver (hepatic infarct), blockage of a

branch of the portal vein will result in a similar lesion known as a pseudo-infarct or Zahn's infarct which is distinguished by atrophic cells, while blockage of a branch of the bile duct will result in local cholestasis. Hepatic infarcts and pseudo-infarcts are normally associated with thrombosis at distant sites and are rare in experimental animals although, as discussed in a later section, local cholestasis may play a role in bile duct proliferation, but this is purely speculative.

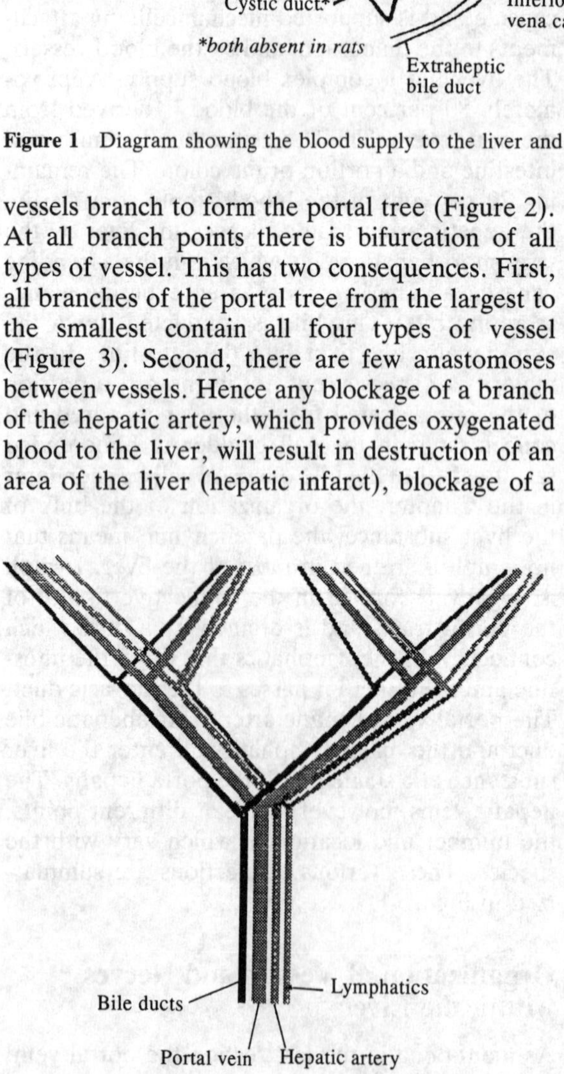

The organization of vessels within the portal tract is more complex than is apparent at first sight. As will be seen from Figure 3 each portal tract contains a single branch of the portal vein and of the hepatic artery but may contain several bile ducts of varying diameter and several lymphatics. Each bile duct is surrounded by a group of blood vessels termed the peribiliary plexus which are supplied from the hepatic artery and which will eventually drain into the portal vein. This is shown in Figure 4. The result is a 'contraflow' system which is assumed to be concerned with the resorption of nutrients lost into the bile, although this is also speculative (Jones *et al.*, 1980). In some species, such as humans and rat, the bile ducts themselves branch often forming blind ended pouches (Yamamoto *et al.*, 1985) which may be involved in bile storage and modification, but there is no certainty on this point.

As the portal tree divides the vessels gradually become smaller. From the smallest veins (terminal hepatic venules) small vessels bud off and

Figure 2   Diagram showing branching of the portal tree within the liver substance. Note that even the smallest branches contain branches of all four types of vessel

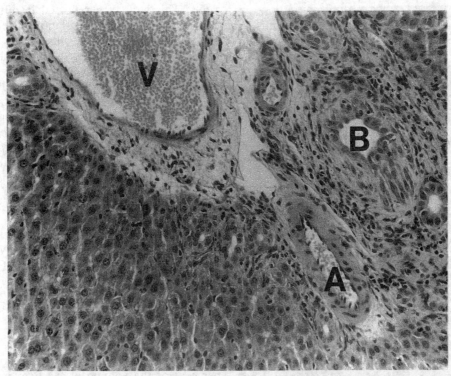

Figure 3 Light micrograph of a middle-sized branch of the portal tree showing branches of the portal vein (V) and the hepatic artery (A) and several bile ducts (B) of various size. The lymphatics are not shown as these small, thin, walled vessels cannot be identified with any certainty under the light microscope

pass to the edge of the portal tract discharging their blood into the capillaries which, in the liver, are termed sinusoids (Figure 5). Similar branches probably arise from the terminal hepatic arterioles but a part of the flow from the hepatic artery is believed to pass through the peribiliary plexus before reaching the parenchyma. As will be discussed later bile is first formed by discharge into channels between hepatocytes termed bile canaliculi. These empty directly into bile ducts as shown in Figure 5. Lymphatic vessels are only found within the portal tracts and around the larger branches of the hepatic veins so that no connections with the parenchyma are necessary.

The liver is only lightly innervated. Most fibres are unmyelinated and from the autonomic nervous system. It is generally assumed that these fibres, which run in the portal tracts up to their smallest branches, are involved in the regulation of blood flow and possibly of bile flow. However, small fibres have been found in the parenchyma contacting hepatocytes (Friedman, 1982) and, because hepatocytes are electrically coupled through the gap junctions, it is reasonable to assume that all hepatocytes may be influenced by signals from the sympathetic nervous system though the effect of this is at the moment obscure.

Organization of the Hepatic Parenchyma

The bulk of the liver is composed of a single type of cell, the hepatocyte. These are assembled into sheets (sometimes termed muralia) each a single cell thick which bifurcate and fuse to give a most complex network. Through this network run the liver capillaries, termed sinusoids. Between cells within the wall run small branching channels called bile canaliculi (Figure 6). The relationship between these vessels is shown schematically in Figure 7.

The liver sinusoids are lined by endothelial cells. Unlike the endothelia of normal capillaries these cells do not form a continuous barrier but are penetrated by fenestrations (Figures 8 and 9) which allow a free exchange of proteins between the blood within the sinusoids and the 'Space of

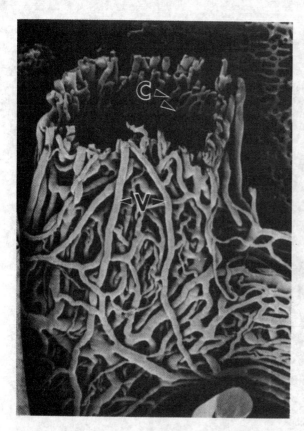

Figure 4 Scanning electron micrograph of a corrosion cast of the peribiliary plexus of inner blood capillaries and outer venules in the rabbit. This network of vessels is most prominant in the larger ducts but extends into the smallest of the portal canals. From Ohtani (1979)

Disse' which lies between the endothelial cell and the hepatocyte. A few small bundles of collagen fibres are occasionally seen in the space of Disse which assist in providing mechanical stability to the liver. Within the sinusoids are Kupffer cells, fixed macrophages which form attachments both to the walls of the endothelial cell and, by means of processes pushed through the fenestrations, to the hepatocytes. The principal role of the Kupffer cells is to remove particulate material which may have been absorbed from the intestine and their position and structure, particularly the numerous processes which may extend right across sinusoids, are adapted to this role.

As blood enters the parenchyma from the portal tract and is drained through branches of the hepatic vein, hepatocytes lying close to portal tracts receive blood with a much higher oxygen content than hepatocytes lying close to the central veins. This is in turn reflected in differences in function and a marked variation in sensitivity to certain toxins. It is thus unfortunate that there is no generally agreed system for labelling the different zones. The two most common nomenclatures are shown in Figure 10. Neither is ideal for toxicologists. A concept of cylinders (circles in thin section) encircling the portal tract to define a periportal area and branches of the hepatic vein to define a centrilobular area corresponds most closely with the distributions of lesions within the liver (Figure 11) and with differences in oxygen tension.

STRUCTURE AND FUNCTION OF THE DIFFERENT TYPES OF CELL IN THE LIVER

Hepatocytes

Structure of Hepatocytes

Hepatocytes (Figure 12) form approximately 90 per cent of the volume of the liver parenchyma but are only 60 per cent of the total cell number. They are large cells approximately cuboidal in shape. The nucleus is normally placed centrally; markedly eccentric nuclei are only seen in severely damaged cells. Approximately 20 per cent of the cytoplasm consists of mitochondria which are actually not spheres or blunt cylinders, as they appear in thin section, but long and often branching tubular structures. Scattered amongst the mitochondria are peroxisomes which normally form only 2 per cent of the volume of the cytoplasm. Normal rat liver peroxisomes can be identified by the crystalloid core, which consists of uric acid oxidase but this is absent from primates, including humans.

Hepatocytes contain a highly developed endoplasmic reticulum which, as usual, is continuous with the outer nuclear membrane. In rodent liver rough surfaced endoplasmic reticulum elements may either be wrapped around mitochondria, an arrangement especially associated with periportal cells, or arranged in small stacks, an arrangement characteristic of cells in the centrilobular region. At high magnifications it is seen that the ribosomes are arranged with great regularity along most rough endoplasmic reticulum (RER) elements. Partial loss of ribosomes (RER

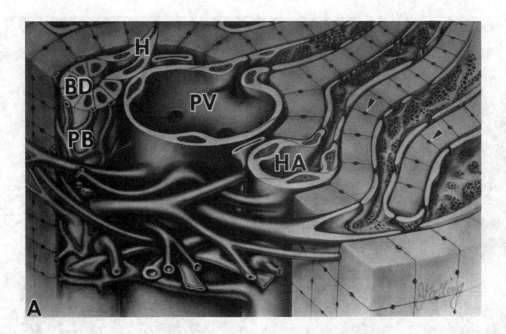

Figure 5   Diagram showing the principal features of a portal canal and connections to the parenchyma. Portal veins (PV) and hepatic arteries (HA) empty either directly into or via small branch vessels. Bile duct (BD) lining cells contact hepatocytes directly, the junction zone being termed the canal of Hering (H). From Jones *et al*. (1980)

degranulation), leading to a 'moth-eaten' appearance is an early sign of hepatotoxicity.

While the RER consists predominantly of sheets of membrane, which on ultrathin sectioning gives the characteristic paired membranes, the smooth surfaced endoplasmic reticulum is predominantly arranged as tubules which, on sectioning, give small circles of ellipses of membrane which are often difficult to identify. In well fed animals smooth surfaced endoplasmic reticulum is largely associated with deposits of the storage polysaccharide glycogen. On treatment with many chemicals the smooth endoplasmic reticulum proliferates with, in extreme cases, masses accumulating in the centre of the cell marginalizing other organelles.

The Golgi apparatus in hepatocytes is small and, in undamaged cells, invariably located close to the bile canaliculus. The stack of membranous sacs (dictyosomes) of the Golgi apparatus is, however, merely the centre of a much more complex series of membranes (Figure 13). The central sacs are connected to a complex of membranous tubules which interleave with elements of the smooth endoplasmic reticulum. Closely associated with the Golgi apparatus in function are the

membranes of the endosome compartment where proteins taken up by endocytosis are sorted. The final stages of sorting following exocytosis also appear to be associated with 'extreme trans-Golgi' elements which do not form part of the main membrane stack. The Golgi apparatus also forms the centre for a system of microtubules which act as 'railroads' for transferring vesicles to or from the sinusoidal surface of the cell. The lysosomes are believed to bind to this network because in normal hepatocytes they are always located close to the Golgi apparatus.

The plasma membrane of the hepatocytes is divided into two domains. As mentioned earlier bile is discharged into small channels between hepatocytes, the bile canaliculi (Figure 12). At the edge of the bile canaliculi the membranes of the hepatocytes are sealed together by tight junctions which almost entirely prevent the passage of both soluble and membrane-bound proteins in to or out of the bile canaliculus by diffusion between the cells. Close to the bile canaliculi are the intermediate junctions which provide an anchoring point for actin microfilaments, some of which are organized to form a contractile belt around the bile canaliculus (the

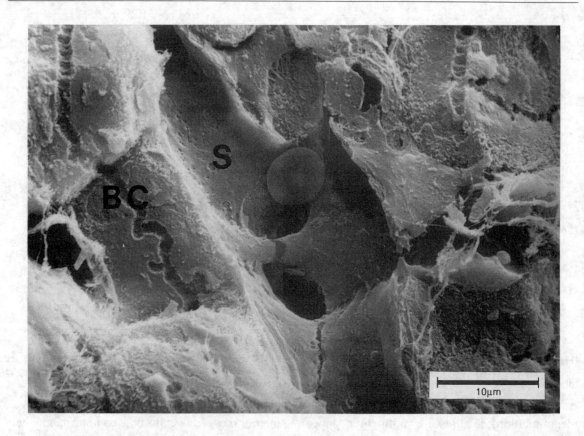

Figure 6   Scanning electron micrograph showing the bile canaliculi (BC) and the sinusoids (S). Tight junction complexes, not visible at this magnification, separate the two types of vessel from each other (courtesy Dr S. Singh and Miss D. Chescoe)

terminal web). Away from the bile canaliculus the cells are joined by 'spot welds' formed by desmosomes. These act as anchorage points for the intermediate filaments of cytokeratin which cross the cell giving it mechanical strength and which also anchor the nucleus in place.

Functions of Hepatocytes

Hepatocytes have many functions. The liver serves both as an exocrine and an endocrine gland. The exocrine secretion of the liver is bile. The formation of bile is a complex topic (Klaasen and Watkins, 1984; Erlinger, 1988). The critical factor in bile formation is the secretion of bile acids and bile salts, detergents important for the emulsification of fat in the intestine. Of the other major components of bile, water appears to enter passively across the tight junctions whereas phospholipids and cholesterol are extracted from the bile canalicular membrane by the detergent action of the bile salts. In some species, such as rat and dog, IgA antibodies are secreted into bile by a process involving uptake of the IgA at the sinusoidal surface of the cell, sorting in the endosome compartment and release into bile by exocytosis. Bile also has an excretory function. Conjugates, both of endogenous materials such as bilirubin and of xenobiotics, are secreted into bile in a process that will be described later in this section. There is also, as mentioned earlier, a slow discharge of lysosomes into bile.

In its second role, as an endocrine gland, the liver secretes almost all the major proteins of plasma with the exception of the immunoglobulins. In addition the liver plays a central role in lipid metabolism, taking up chylomicrons arriving in the blood from the intestine and re-packaging their lipid with a new group of proteins to form very low density lipoprotein (VLDL) particles which are then exported from the liver. The trans-

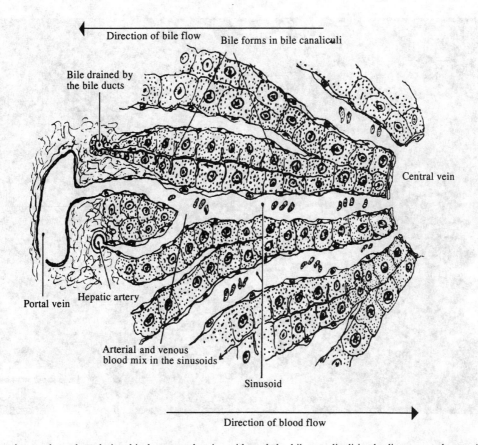

Figure 7 Drawing to show the relationship between the sinusoids and the bile canaliculi in the liver parenchyma. Adapted from Ham (1974)

port of proteins through the exocytic pathway is especially sensitive to changes in intracellular ATP. This is reflected in the accumulation of fat in the damaged liver and in the fall in plasma proteins and disturbances in blood clotting that follow long-standing liver damage.

In addition to forming the bulk of the plasma proteins, the liver is also responsible for their recycling. Most proteins in plasma are glycoproteins possessing a terminal sialic acid on their sugar side chains. Removal of this sialic acid exposes a galactose residue which binds avidly to a receptor on the hepatocyte plasma membrane. Following binding, the proteins are taken up by endocytosis and transferred to lysosomes for digestion. Non-glycosylated plasma proteins, such as albumin, are taken up by using other, less well characterized receptors. The liver is also responsible for recycling old red blood cells. This task is carried out principally by Kupffer cells. Aged red blood cells are recognized because the

removal of sialic acid residues from their cell surface glycoproteins reveal galactose residues which are recognized by a receptor. Following binding the cells are taken up by phagocytosis and their proteins digested. The haem residues are passed to hepatocytes for re-use or degradation.

In addition to these roles the liver acts as the centre of intermediary metabolism in the body. The role of the liver in the metabolism of exogenous lipid has already been discussed. In addition the liver provides a central store of sugar, in the form of glycogen, and is also a major site for the conversion of sugars to lipids and for conversion of amino acids to sugars and lipids. This may have marked consequences. For example, in rats the metabolic demands of lactation result in a 30 per cent increase in liver weight, exacerbating the toxicity of liver-enlarging agents such as BHT (Hinton *et al.*, 1990). In addition the liver is the main, or in the case of humans almost the sole, site of *de novo* cholesterol synthesis. The result

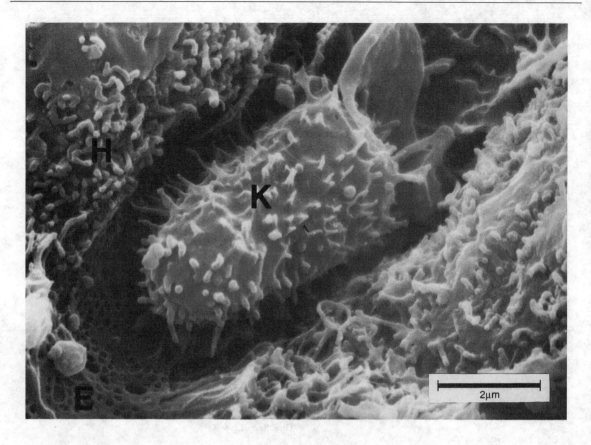

2μm

Figure 8   Scanning electron micrograph showing the relationships between hepatocytes (H), sinusoid endothelial cells (E) and Kupffer cells (K), showing a sieve plate (courtesy Dr S. Singh and Miss D. Chescoe)

is that liver damage causes marked disturbances in endocrine function, for example liver cirrhosis results in feminization in men and masculinization in women (Johnson and Alberti, 1985).

The final function of the liver is in the modification and excretion of a variety of hydrophobic compounds. These reactions involve both endogenous body constituents, such as haem or steroids, as well as nutrients absorbed with the diet or produced by the body's own microflora. In general the physiological role of the reactions is to prepare the compounds for excretion. The enzymes involved are conventionally divided into two groups. Phase 1 reactions involve chemical modification of the reactant normally by oxidation whereas phase 2 reactions are biosynthetic, generally involving conjugation with a hydrophilic moiety such as glucuronic acid or glutathione. Under most circumstances the role of these enzymes is protective and results in the

removal of potentially harmful materials from the body. However, under some circumstances, the metabolites are markedly more toxic than the parent compound (see Chapter 3).

By far the most important group of enzymes involved in phase 1 reactions are the cytochromes *P*-450. These are a large group of enzymes which catalyse a wide variety of reactions (Table 1). The cytochromes *P*-450 are classified into families and subfamilies according to their amino acid sequences, for example cytochrome *P*-450IVA1 is the first member of subfamily A of family 4. There is, however, only limited correlation between the classification of the cytochromes *P*-450 and their substrate specificities (Table 2) and while there are structural analogies between the *P*-450s of different mammalian species it is unclear how far these correlate with the function of the enzymes. The number of isoforms of cytochrome *P*-450 is very large. Some are present

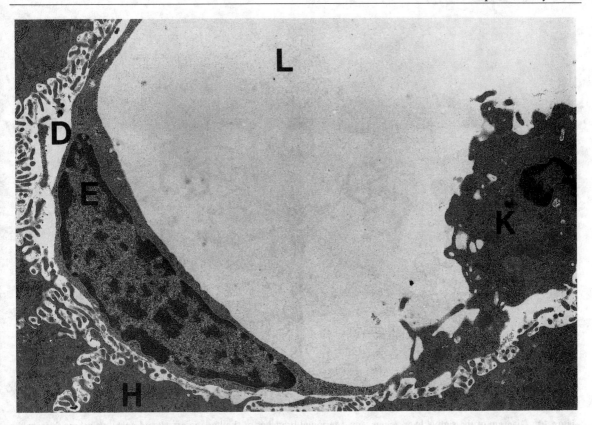

Figure 9 Transmission electron micrograph showing the relationship between hepatocytes (H), sinusoid endothelial cells (E), Kupffer cells (K), the space of Disse (D) and the sinusoid lumen (L) (courtesy Dr S. Singh and Miss D. Chescoe)

constitutively while others are only synthesized in response to inducing agents. Thus the response of animal populations to a xenobiotic may be altered by prior exposure to other chemicals and the situation is further complicated by the fact that outbred populations, such as humans, may show considerable genetic polymorphism.

In spite of the variation in the reactions catalysed by the various isoforms of cytochrome P-450 all function in a similar way (Figure 14); the iron atom of the haem cycles between the ferrous and ferric states. The substrate initially binds to the enzyme in the ferric state. The enzyme–substrate complex then receives an electron from NADPH in a reaction catalysed by a second enzyme, NADPH-cytochrome P-450 reductase reducing the iron to the ferrous state. Molecular oxygen is then bound to the complex. A second electron is transferred to the complex either from NADPH or cytochrome b_5. This results in activation of the oxygen molecule which is split, one atom becoming bound to the substrate, the other binding

hydrogen ions to form water. At the same time the iron atom is reoxidized to the ferric state. The precise sequence of reactions here is uncertain, as is frequently the case for reactions involving free radicals, but this is of little significance for toxicologists. Finally, the oxidised substrate is released from the enzyme, completing the cycle.

Although the cytochromes P-450 normally act as oxygenases they are also capable of acting as reductases, for example on azo compounds, aromatic amines and haloalkanes. Reductase activity is only observed at low oxygen tensions, as found in the centrilobular zone of the liver. Reduction occurs because, in the absence of oxygen, the two electrons received from NADPH can be transferred to certain substrates. Because the electrons are transferred singly to the substrate, reduction inevitably results in the formation of free radical intermediates which may be released from the enzyme, for example by bond cleavage. Hence, although the reductive reactions may be protec-

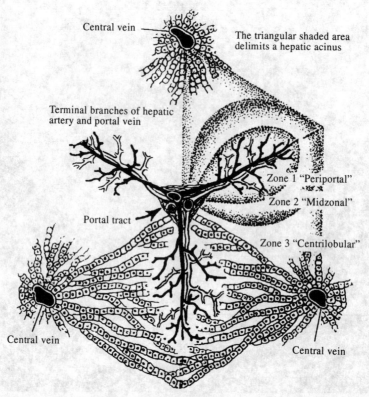

Central vein

The triangular shaded area
delimits a hepatic acinus

Terminal branches of hepatic
artery and portal vein

Zone 1 "Periportal"

Zone 2 "Midzonal"

Portal tract

Zone 3 "Centrilobular"

Central vein

Central vein

Figure 10 Diagram of the simple liver acinus, small terminal branches of the hepatic artery and portal vein branch from the portal tract. These deliver blood into sinusoids which drain into the central vein. Zone 1 receives well oxygenated blood and nutrient-rich blood from the portal tracts. As the blood passes through the parenchyma both nutrient and oxygen concentrations fall, being lowest around the central veins. Adapted from Ham (1974)

tive, they sometimes result in the generation of highly reactive, and hence toxic, products.

Although the cytochromes *P*-450 have evolved to remove potentially toxic material from the body they may, as mentioned in the previous paragraph, actually form toxic intermediates. In general this can be explained by specific features of the chemical structure of the substrate and examples of such reactions will be found in a later section. However, toxicity may also be associated with premature release of oxygen from the cytochrome. This has been demonstrated even with chemicals, such as benzphetamine, which are capable of being hydroxylated. In such cases the oxygen may be released from the enzyme either in the form of the superoxide radical or as a peroxide, resulting in tissue damage. Even with genuine substrates there is a very slight release of superoxide and peroxide from certain isoforms particularly cytochrome *P*-450IIE1. Such isoforms are called 'poorly coupled'.

Although there are several other phase 1 drug metabolizing enzymes in the liver there is little evidence that they play a significant role in the pathogenesis of liver damage. Again, although the liver is the principal location of the phase 2 drug metabolizing enzymes listed in Table 3, these reactions generally remain 'as intended' purely protective; the metabolism of aromatic amines (see later) is a notable exception. It should, however, be noted that there are marked variations in levels of phase 2 enzymes between species of animals and even among individuals (Table 4) and that this may result in major differences in toxicity. For example the chromone FPL 52757 is markedly hepatotoxic in the dog and mildly hepatotoxic to some individual humans but has no effect on other species because it is not detoxified by *N*-acetylation; it causes bile duct necrosis (Eason *et al.*, 1982).

The mechanisms by which compounds are excreted into bile are still not perfectly under-

(A)

(B)

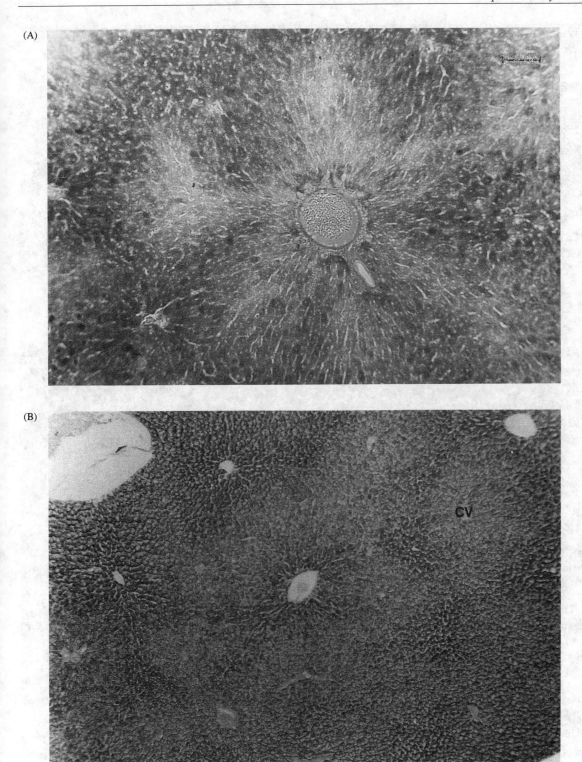

Figure 11 Micrographs showing loss of glycogen from (A) the periportal area and (B) the centrilobular zone. Animals were treated respectively with chlorpromazine (Mullock *et al.*, 1983) and fenofibrate (Price, 1985). Glycogen loss is indicated by pale staining

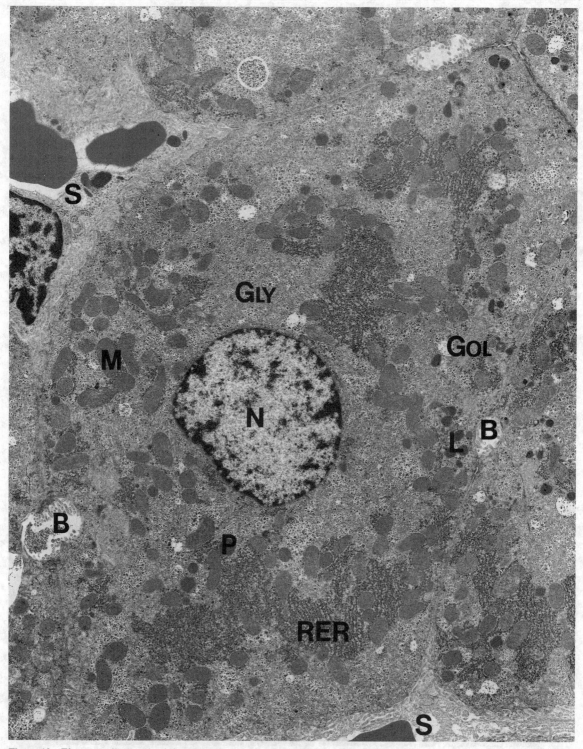

Figure 12   Electron micrograph of the normal structure of a hepatocyte showing the large centrally placed nuclei (N), rough (RER) and smooth (S) endoplasmic reticulum, mitochondria (M), peroxisomes (P). Note that the lysosomes (L) and Golgi apparatus (Gol) are located close to the bile canaliculus (B). Gly indicates areas of glycogen traversed to smooth endoplasmic reticulum. (Courtesy Dr S. C. Price)

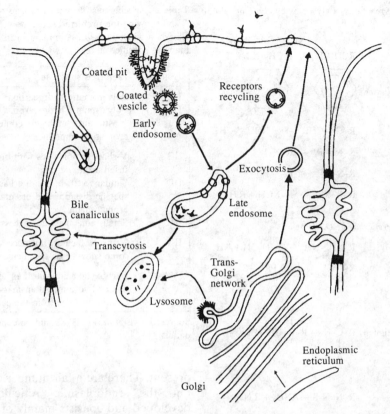

Figure 13 Scheme showing the relationship between the central stack of the Golgi apparatus and associated elements

stood. However, transporters have been identified both for unmodified compounds and conjugates (Vore, 1993). Of particular interest are the so-called P-glycoproteins which catalyse the ATP-dependent transfer into bile of a range of lipophilic, weakly basic polycyclic compounds including a number of agents used in cancer chemotherapy. An increase in these transporters is responsible for the phenomenon of multidrug resistance. In addition an ATP-dependent transporter has now been identified which transports a range of organic anions such as glutathione and glucuronide conjugates and a separate ATP transporter for bile acids, and it would appear likely that other transporters remain to be discovered.

Sinusoid Endothelial Cells

The smallest blood vessels in the liver, the sinusoids, are lined by endothelial cells specialized in structure to assist in the liver's major roles of removal of waste materials from the blood and of blood formation. In the majority of tissues the capillaries form a continuous barrier preventing blood components from coming directly into contact with the cells of the tissue. However, in the liver the endothelial cells which line the smallest blood vessels are pierced by fenestrations about 100 nm in diameter, sometimes called sieve plates (Figure 8) which allow all components of the plasma, but not blood cells, to make direct contact with the hepatocytes. It is for this reason that the smallest blood vessels in the liver are termed sinusoids, not capillaries. Apart from the possession of sieve plates, the sinusoidal endothelial cells present few features of interest to toxicologists. As with other endothelial cells, there would appear to be active uptake of material by pinocytosis, but the nature of the materials absorbed is not known. The cells contain only small numbers of mitochondria and the endoplasmic reticulum is not well developed. The Golgi apparatus and the lysosomal system account for a considerably greater proportion of the cell volume than in hepatocytes.

Table 1   Examples of reactions catalysed by cytochromes *P*-450

(A) *Oxidative Mode*

Aliphatic hydoxylation	$RCH_2CH_3 \rightarrow R\ CH_2{\cdot}CH_2OH$

Aromatic hydoxylation

Epoxidation $R{-}CH{-}CHR' \rightarrow \quad RCH{-\!\!-}CHR$

N-Oxidation $R{-}NH{-}R' \rightarrow R{-}N{-}R'$

S-Oxidation $R{-}S{-}R' \quad \rightarrow R{-}S{-}R'$

Dealkylation $R{-}X{-}R' \quad \rightarrow R{-}XOH + R'H$

Where X may be O,NH or S

Deamination $R{-}CH_2{-}NH_2 \rightarrow R{-}CH_2OH + NH_3$

Desulphuration $RR'PR'' \quad \rightarrow RR'PR'' + S$

Oxidative dehalogenation $R{-}\underset{H}{\overset{X}{C}}{-}H \rightarrow R{-}\overset{X}{C}{-}OH \rightarrow R{-}\overset{O}{C}{-}H$

(B) *Reductive Mode*

Azo reduction $R{-}N{=}N{-}R' \rightarrow RNH_2 + R'NH_2$

Aromatic nitro reduction

Reductive dehalogenation $R{-}\underset{X}{\overset{X}{C}}{-}X \rightarrow R{-}\underset{X}{\overset{X}{C}}{-}H + HX$

Where X is any halogen

(Adapted from Sipes and Gandolfi (1991))

Kupffer Cells

Kupffer cells are fixed macrophages which are found within the sinusoids (Figures 8 and 9). They are attached both to the endothelial cells and, via processes extending through the fenestrations in the endothelial cells, to hepatocytes. Like all macrophages, Kupffer cells are actively phagocytic, removing particulate material such as bacteria or bacterial fragments (endotoxins) which may have entered the blood from the intestine. Kupffer cells are also largely responsible for the recycling of 'old' red blood cells and cooperate with hepatocytes in the metabolism of haem. The structure of Kupffer cells is similar to that of other macrophages. Phagolysosomes are prominent and numerous filamentous elements are

Table 2   Specificities of major isoforms of cytochrome *P*-450 showing the preferred substrate conformations. Clearly a wider range of compounds can be metabolized than are specified here.

Isoform	Preferred substrate
IA1	Polyaromatic hydrocarbons
IA2	Polyaromatic hydrocarbons with amine substituents, multi-ringed heterocyclic aromatic compounds
IIB	V-shaped molecules with one or more non-fused aromatic rings
IID	Similar to 2B but with a basic nitrogen at a specific distance and orientation from an aromatic ring
IIE	Small molecules, not necessarily planar
IIIA	Large molecules, not necessarily planar, some show cross-specificity with 1A1 and 2B
IVA	Carboxylic acids and their esters, usually with one or two unfused aromatic rings at a certain distance from the carboxylate group

Source: Lewis *et al.* (1993) should be consulted for further details.

present. There are a fair number of mitochondria but the endoplasmic reticulum is poorly developed and consists mainly of rough surfaced elements.

Fat-storing (Ito) Cells

Fat-storing cells are found between hepatocytes, there being one fat-storing cell per 20 hepatocytes. It has been suggested that they are specialized fibroblasts. The role of these cells is obscure (Brouwer *et al.*, 1988). The 'fat' droplets which are their most prominent feature contain about 40 per cent vitamin A dissolved in triglyceride. A well-developed RER and Golgi apparatus suggest a secretory function. The nature of the material secreted is uncertain but there is increasing evidence that fat-storing cells secrete components for the sparse matrix of connective tissue found in the space of Disse and that transdifferentiation of these cells may play an important role in hepatic fibrosis (see later).

Other Cell Types of the Liver

Most biochemical tests are carried out on liver homogenates and, when interpreting these, one must bear in mind that blood vessels make up

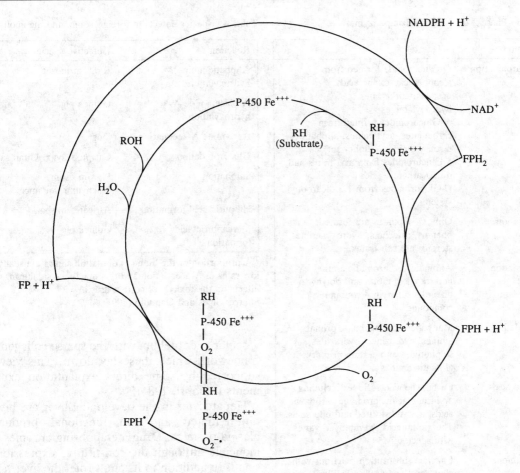

Figure 14 Diagrams showing changes in the oxidation states of iron and oxygen during metabolism of a xenobiotic by cytochrome *P*-450. The inner ring shows varying states of cytochrome *P*-450, the outer ring the states of the flavoprotein (FP) NADPH – cytochrome *P*-450 reductase

about 5 per cent of the hepatic parenchyma so that blood plasma and cells may contribute significantly when measurements are made on the homogenates. Furthermore, even the normal liver generally shows some small inflammatory foci and these may increase greatly in treated animals, again emphasizing the necessity for biochemical studies on poorly characterized hepatotoxins to be accompanied by histological examination of the tissue. Blood cells and inflammatory cells cannot, however, be thought of as normal components of the liver. There is, however, a final cell type, the pit cell, whose status is less clear. Pit cells are rarely observed although there are about 500 000 per gram of rat liver (Wisse *et al.*, 1989). These cells are located on, or embedded in, the endothelial lining and possess numbers of small granules. Isolated pit cells have natural killer (NK) activity (i.e. they recognize and kill tumour cells *in vitro*) and they morphologically resemble a population of NK cells, the large granular lymphocytes, in the blood although the two populations do not seem to be identical.

DEVELOPMENT OF THE LIVER

The Embryonic Liver

The liver develops as a diverticulum of the foregut. Clusters of cells grow from this into a mesenchymal stroma in which has developed a plexus of small blood vessels. The intimate relationship between blood vessels and hepatocytes is thus established from the very origins of the organ. Throughout foetal life the liver consists of sheets

Table 3 Phase 2 drug metabolizing enzymes

Reaction	Substrates
Glucuronidation	*O*-Glucuronide formed from alcohols, carboxylic acids, unsaturated ketones, hydroxylamines *N*-Glucuronides formed from carbamates, arylamines, aliphatic tertiary amines, sulphonamides *S*-Glucuronides from aryl thiols and dithiocarbamic acids *C*-Glucuronides from 1,3 dicarbonyl systems
Sulphation	Only *O*-sulphates are formed; phenols, catechols, hydroxylamines, steroids are substrates
Methylation	Aliphatic and aromatic amines, *N*-heterocycles, mono and polyhydric phenols, sulphydryl-containing compounds
Acetylation	Many including aromatic primary amines, hydrazines, hydrazides, sulphonides and certain primary aliphatic amines
Amino acids	Carboxylic acid residues including arylacetic acids, aromatic carboxylic acids, aryl-substituted and bile acids. The amino acid(s) employed varies with species
Glutathione	Enzymic substitution reactions with alkyl, aryl and aralkyl halides Enzymic addition reactions with alkenes, aryl and alkyl epoxides Non-enzymic addition reactions with many free radicals and reactive intermediates

Source: Sipes and Gandolfi (1991).

Table 4 Species defects in foreign compound metabolism

Reaction	Defective species
Aliphatic amine *N*-hydroxylation	Rat, marmoset
Arylacetamide *N*-hydroxylation	Guinea pig
Arylamine *N*-acetylation	Dog[a]
Glucuronidation	Cat, lion, lynx, Gunn rat
Sulphation	Pig, opossum, brachymorphic mice
Hippuric acid formation	African fruit bat
Mercapturic acid formation	Guinea pig

[a] A proportion of the human population shows unusually low rates of *N*-acetylation and this may have significant effects on the toxicity of certain drugs.
Source: Sipes and Gandolfi (1991).

of hepatocytes two cells thick, unlike the single cell muralia found in adult life. The development of the blood supply to the foetal liver is extremely complex (MacSween and Scothorne, 1987). The development of the ductular system is equally complex but is of more relevance to toxicologists. Bile canaliculi between hepatocytes are seen very early in development. The bile ducts themselves develop much later. It has been suggested (MacSween and Scothorne, 1987) that bile duct lining cells differentiate from immature hepatocytes through contact with the connective tissue of the developing portal tracts whereas mature hepatocytes differentiate from cells in contact with the

vascular endothelium with the sparse collagenous framework which these lay down. This view is supported by some direct explantation experiments (Shiojiri, 1984).

Hepatocytes in the developing liver are highly differentiated and are functional producing plasma proteins. Drug metabolizing enzymes are inducible although the constitutive expression is small. In addition to its adult role, the liver takes on a second temporary role as the main organ for haematopoiesis. Cells deriving from the yolk sac settle in the liver and rapidly dominate the histological picture (Figure 15). All cell lineages are represented although erythropoietic activity is dominant (Moore and Johnson, 1976). In humans the role of the liver as the major haematopoietic organ passes to the bone marrow in the fifth month of gestation but in rats and mice this change occurs in the first three weeks after birth.

Changes in the Liver with Age

There are only minor structural or ultrastructural changes in the liver after birth. The proportion of connective tissue increases to accommodate the increasing weight of the organ. In rats, blood flow through the liver diminishes over the first 12 months of life (Van Bezooijen, 1984). Also in rats there is a marked increase in bile duct hyperplasia with age, possibly as a consequence of spontaneous infections. In both humans and

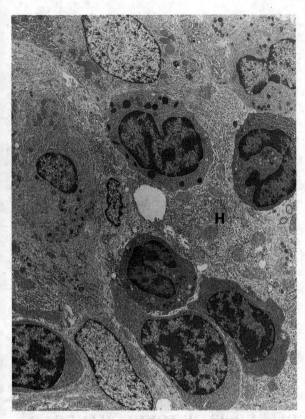

Figure 15 Electron micrograph of the liver of a foetal rat showing very large numbers of immature blood cells between the hepatocytes (H). (Courtesy S. C. Price)

experimental animals the 'age pigment' lipofuscin, which is thought to represent lysosomes filled with an indigestible material consisting largely of peroxidized lipid, accumulates in hepatocytes in later life. There is also a marked increase in nuclear ploidy and in the number of binucleate cells which occurs in mice and, to a lesser extent, in some strains of rats (Johnston *et al.*, 1968, Grice and Burek, 1984). In mice, ageing animals show significant numbers of hexadecaploid nuclei. Of much more significance to toxicologists are significant metabolic alterations, especially in the enzymes which metabolize xenobiotics.

As noted in the previous section, the liver of a newborn rat is underdeveloped and, in particular, has much less drug metabolizing capacity than normal liver. Different drug metabolizing enzymes develop at different rates. Cytochromes *P*-450IA develop before birth, reach maximal activity before weaning (3 weeks) and decline thereafter (Lum *et al.*, 1985). Total cytochrome

P-450 and the amount of mRNA for phenobarbitonel (phenobarbital) inducible isoenzymes IIB1, IIB2, IIC3 and IIIA1 reach adult levels approximately 3 weeks after birth and then stabilize (Omiecinski *et al.*, 1990). However, the activity of benzphetamine *N*-demethylase, which is markedly inducible by phenobarbitone does not stabilize until the animals are over 7 weeks of age (Lum *et al.*, 1985). It is unclear whether this is due to other, unidentified, late-developing isoforms of cytochrome *P*-450 catalysing this reaction or to age-dependent variations in the half-life of the *P*-450 proteins.

In addition to changes in the constitutive expression of genes for drug metabolizing enzymes there are also changes in their inducibility. Many but not all isoforms of cytochrome *P*-450 are inducible in the foetal rat (Marie and Cresteil, 1989). Following birth there are also marked changes in inducibility. The phenobarbitone (phenobarbital)-induced form (*P*-450IIB2) is highly inducible 2 weeks after birth (Giachelli and Omiecinski, 1987) but the degree of inducibility declines later as constitutive expression increases. The main methylcholanthreneinducible isoforms (*P*-450IA) show high constitutive expression early in life but later this constitutive expression declines and the inducibility increases (Ioannides and Parke, 1990).

Changes in hepatic enzyme levels also occur in the ageing animal. Both constitutive expression of drug metabolizing enzymes and their inducibility declines with age (Schmucker and Wang, 1981). Superoxide dismutase and catalase activity also decrease (Mote *et al.*, 1990), and there is a reduced response to peroxisome proliferators (Hinton *et al.*, 1986). The hyperplasia which is so marked in young rats treated with phenobarbitone (phenobarbital) or peroxisome proliferators is much reduced in the ageing animal (Schmucker and Wang, 1981; Hinton *et al.*, 1986). There is thus, in ageing animals, a generalized loss in the capacity of the liver both to metabolize xenobiotics and to protect itself against damaging products of metabolism such as superoxide free radicals.

ADAPTIVE CHANGES IN THE LIVER

Because of its many roles the liver is continuously changing even in histological appearance. Glycogen is stored following meals and used at night.

Fat accumulates transiently, drug metabolizing enzymes alter depending on the composition of the diet. In the small animals normally used in toxicology studies even the size of the liver shows significant variation. For example, a 'normal' rat, mouse or chicken liver is significantly larger than that of their germ-free counterparts (Gordon, 1959). Accordingly it is necessary, before considering the action of hepatotoxins, to identify the changes in the liver that occur naturally in the course of an animal's life.

One would not expect major changes in bile secretion in the normal life of an animal. Changes in the synthesis of plasma proteins will occur following haemorrhage and, more importantly for toxicologists, as a result of inflammation in any part of the body. In the former case there is a compensatory increase in synthesis of normal blood proteins. In the latter case a reaction termed the 'acute phase response' occurs and the liver synthesizes and secretes into the plasma a distinct range of proteins, the acute phase respondents, some of which are barely detectable in normal plasma (Kushner, 1982), in addition to the normal plasma proteins. The intermediary metabolism in the liver is affected by pancreatic, adrenal, pituitary, thyroidal and sex hormones, among others (van Thiel, 1982). The interactions are extremely complex and result *inter alia* in the establishment of marked diurnal rhythms (Belanger, 1988; Feuers and Scheving, 1988). This emphasizes the need for strict standardization of conditions in toxicological studies. Generally, however, although hormones at natural levels will not cause morphological change in the liver apart from affecting glycogen content, marked changes are found in the liver during lactation. In rats the weight of the organ increases by over 30 per cent and this is associated with a marked increase in lipogenesis (Williamson, 1980).

The most marked changes in the liver occur in response to xenobiotics. Even for humans the metabolic load imposed by nutrients derived from food normally far exceeds that caused by synthetic chemicals. Ingestion of xenobiotics may, potentially, result in two processes in the liver: first induction of a number of specific groups of enzymes and second a burst of mitosis. The enzymes affected are principally the 'drug metabolizing' enzymes discussed in the previous section. Enzymes for phase 1 and phase 2 meta-

bolism are induced in parallel. In rats and mice and, to a lesser extent, hamsters there may also be induction of the peroxisomal fatty acid oxidases. This will be discussed in more detail later in this chapter. At the relatively low concentrations which occur naturally, increases in liver enzymes are paralleled by proliferation of smooth endoplasmic reticulum and/or peroxisomes depending on the localization of the enzymes. The control of enzyme induction is not clearly understood but in the case of the Ah receptor (Nebert and Gonzalez, 1987) and of the receptor for 'peroxisome proliferators' (Green, 1993) it appears that inducers bind directly to a DNA-binding receptor. A simple mechanism like this would result in an equally simple dose–response relationship with no distinct threshold; this is generally the situation observed in practice. The control of cell division is even less well understood but it is clear that it parallels, not follows, enzyme induction. Changes in the size of the liver occur naturally in the course of an animal's life but persistent enlargement is associated with an increased risk of cancer (see later).

DIAGNOSIS OF TOXIC CHANGES IN THE LIVER

Diagnosis of liver damage depends principally on the gross pathology and on histological examination of the tissue. The significance of liver enlargement is discussed later in this chapter. There is no single guide to the histopathology of the livers of experimental animals and it is usually necessary to consult both textbooks of general pathology such as that by McGee *et al.* (1992), descriptive texts such as that by Greaves (1990) and atlases such as that by Gopinath *et al.* (1987). Special stains may be useful in the diagnosis of some types of liver damage. Loss of glycogen and certain types of fat accumulation are useful early indicators of liver damage and may be confirmed by staining by the periodic acid Schiff technique and with oil red O, respectively. Pigmented inclusions may be characterized by stains for iron (Perls' Prussian Blue) and lipofuscin (Schmorl's stain). The initial stages of fibrosis may require confirmation with a reticulin stain. Mallory bodies are eosinophilic inclusions characteristic of human alcoholic liver disease and a number of other conditions which predispose to cirrhosis;

they are now known to consist of bundles of intermediate filaments. There is, however, no connection between these and the development of cirrhosis in experimental animals. Mallory bodies are found, for example, in the livers of mice treated with, for example, griseofulvin, colchicine or dieldrin (Meierhenry *et al.*, 1981) and should probably be regarded simply as a marker of hepatocellular damage.

Electron microscopy frequently provides the earliest indications of toxic changes in hepatocytes, degranulation and vacuolation of the RER being a particularly useful indicator. The electron microscope is also invaluable in detecting proliferation of smooth endoplasmic reticulum, peroxisomes and mitochondria although minor changes in these organelles should not, in themselves, be taken as indicators of hepatotoxicity. Mitochondrial damage is also readily detected under the electron microscope, but careful comparison with control sections is needed as these organelles are exquisitely sensitive to postmortem change. A comprehensive guide to ultrastructural pathology has been produced by Ghadially (1982).

Biochemical tests are much less valuable for the diagnosis of liver damage although biochemical studies on the liver itself may be invaluable in determining the mechanism of change. In particular, increases in drug metabolizing enzymes do not, in themselves, indicate damage to the liver. A fall in hepatic glucose-6-phosphatase activity, which parallels a reduction in glycogen, or in reduced glutathione, indicate stress on the liver. ATP levels can be used to quantify acute toxic stress but are not useful in subacute or chronic studies.

Whereas measurement of enzymes and other proteins in blood is important in the diagnosis of human liver disease, such measurements have limited value in work with small laboratory animals. In general the same enzymes are measured in studies on experimental animals as are measured for the diagnosis of liver disease in rats and mice. However, it should be noted that alanine transaminase is a better indicator of liver damage than aspartate transaminase. Gamma glutamyl transpeptidase is a poor marker for cholestasis in rat whereas secretory IgA and free secretory component provide excellent markers in rats but do not change in humans.

ACTIONS OF TOXINS ON THE LIVER

In 1964 a classic review of experimental toxic injury to the liver attempted a comprehensive list of hepatotoxins (Rouiller, 1964). This covered nine published pages. Advances in our knowledge of the deleterious effects of natural and synthetic chemicals make compilation of a similar list impossible within the bounds of a text book such as this. Accordingly it is necessary to group hepatotoxins. Ideally this should be by their mechanism of action, but this is often not known. Conventionally, classification is by the part of the liver lobule affected, but this can vary markedly between species, for example the pyrrilozidine alkaloid retrorsine produces centrilobular necrosis in rats, mice and guinea pigs, periportal necrosis in hamsters, and focal necrosis in chickens and monkeys (White *et al.*, 1973). The site of toxicity may also be influenced by alterations in the activity of drug metabolizing enzymes. For example the sesquiterpenoid ngaione produces midzonal necrosis in untreated rats, periportal necrosis in rats pretreated with phenobarbitone (phenobarbital) but centrilobular necrosis if the animals have been pretreated with inhibitors of cytochrome *P*-450 (Kelly, 1985). Accordingly, in this article we have employed a hybrid system, grouping by chemical class where it appears possible to relate this directly to the mechanism of action, but where this is not possible, grouping by site of action.

Acute Toxic Damage to Hepatocytes

Toxins not Requiring Activation by Specific Enzymes

Agents Affecting Lipid and Lipoprotein Metabolism

The role of the liver in detoxifying potentially dangerous chemicals requires that hepatocytes have an exceptional capacity to take up xenobiotics. When one remembers the numerous metabolic roles of the liver it is not surprising that it is affected by inhibitors of the basic pathways of metabolism, particularly those affecting lipid metabolism. As has been mentioned earlier, the liver plays a central role in fat metabolism both repackaging dietary lipid from the intestine for use by peripheral tissues and engaging in the *de novo* synthesis of fatty acids from sugars and amino acids. It would seem that these processes are especially sensitive to metabolic changes because accumulation of large droplets of fat in the liver (steatosis) is amongst the most common signs of acute hepatotoxicity.

It should be noted that fat accumulation in the liver does not always indicate liver damage. Following partial hepatectomy there is a massive importation of fat into the liver but there is no evidence of hepatocyte misfunction (Bucher and Malt, 1971). In rats fed high fat diets (Ashworth *et al.*, 1961) or made hyperphagic by hormonal manipulation (Meyer and Hartoft, 1960), and in rats treated with the 'peroxisome proliferators' discussed later, fat accumulates in numerous small droplets, quite distinct from the large droplets of 'toxic' fat discussed earlier in this section.

While the 'metabolic fat' discussed in the previous paragraph accumulates in small droplets and is principally found in the periportal zone, the action of hepatotoxins results in accumulation of lipid in large droplets and principally in the centrilobular zone. It is clear that there is more than one mechanism for accumulation of fat in the liver but it seems likely that interference in the formation of VLDL particles plays a major role (Zimmerman, 1978). The protein synthesis inhibitor cycloheximide induces the development of a fatty liver that is correlated with loss of apoprotein B, which forms the core of the VLDL particle (Mori, 1983). In animals treated with ethionine, which decreases hepatic ATP levels apparently by sequestering adenine (Okazaki *et al.*, 1968), the lipoprotein particles are found in the endoplasmic reticulum but not in the Golgi apparatus (Mori, 1983). Transfer from the endoplasmic reticulum to the Golgi apparatus is known to be exceptionally sensitive to low ATP levels (Farquehar and Palade, 1981). Colchicine interferes even further along the export pathway, causing depolymerization of the microtubule network that guides secretory vesicles from the Golgi apparatus to the plasma membrane (Mori, 1983). It would appear that many other toxins also cause steatosis by interfering with lipoprotein metabolism. Puromycin, like cycloheximide, is an inhibitor of protein synthesis. A similar mechanism was proposed for tetracycline toxicity but later work suggests an interference in the assembly of lipoprotein particles (Deboyser *et al.*, 1989). Choline deficiency, treatment with orotic acid and administration of phosphorus also inhibit the release of VLDL particles by mechanisms that are not fully understood.

Inhibition of lipoprotein export is, of course, only one mechanism responsible for accumulation of fat in the liver. Fat accumulation is also caused by necrogenic toxins, such as carbon tetrachloride (see later). Fat accumulation also occurs in animals treated with valproic acid (Olson *et al.*, 1987) and, at high doses, with perfluorodecanoic acid and related compounds (Borges *et al.*, 1993). In these cases fat accumulation appears to result from inhibition of fatty acid oxidation. Fat accumulation also occurs in the human liver following alcohol abuse but the mechanism remains obscure (Andrews and Snyder, 1991).

Effects on Lysosomes

Compounds may affect lysosomes in two ways. First, indigestible material may reach lysosomes and accumulate there causing enlargement and interference in cellular function. Second, compounds may cross the lysosomal membrane and be trapped as a result of the difference in pH between lysosomes and the cytoplasm. The former route is rarely a major problem for toxicologists. Up to 5 per cent of liver lysosomes are discharged into the bile each day (Godfrey *et al.*, 1981) so, in general, materials do not accumulate in lysosomes. However, it would appear that there are circumstances in which fusion of lysosomes with the bile canalicular membrane is prevented and enormously enlarged lysosomes may accumulate in patients with haemochromatosis, Wilson's disease and the various lysosomal disorders (Watts, 1986). It would also appear that spontaneous changes may occur, because in ageing animals, including humans, lipofuscin granules, lysosomal residual bodies containing material with the staining properties of polymerized, peroxidized lipid, accumulate and this process may be accelerated in experimental animals by treatment with 'peroxisome proliferators' (Hinton *et al.*, 1986) and with an imidazole antifungal drug (Nishikawa *et al.*, 1984). Enlargement and labilization of hepatocyte lysosomes has also been observed in rats treated with the food dye neutral red (Abraham *et al.*, 1967), although the mechanism of action has not been determined. Accumulation of material in the lysosomes of Kupffer cells may result in reticuloendothelial blockade and even in cell death (see later).

The acidity of the interior of lysosomes is below pH 5 whereas the cytosol is essentially neutral, having a pH of 7.2. As a result weak bases may be trapped in lysosomes. Taking, as an example, a simple amine with a pK of 8.2: at pH 7.2, 10 per cent of the molecules of this material will be in the non-ionized form and therefore capable of dissolving in phospholipid membranes. Such a material may diffuse across the lysosomal membrane but, at the pH of the interior of the lysosome, less than 0.1 per cent of the compound will be in the non-ionized form, effectively trapping it within the lysosome. Such weak bases accumulate in lysosomes and, as they concentrate, water enters the lysosomes to maintain an osmotic balance resulting in a marked distention of these organelles. The type compound here is monensin which has been much used in cell biology experiments, but similar effects will be produced by any compound with a pK of between 7 and 9.5. Damage by this mechanism requires a high concentration of the compound and, because of the other biological activities of amines, this type of lysosomotrophy is rarely a practical problem although some such effect may contribute to the antimalarial effects of quinine derivatives (Abraham *et al.*, 1967).

Other Metabolic Inhibitors
Although the principal symptom of the action of many direct hepatotoxins affects fat metabolism there are numerous exceptions. Galactosamine, for example, is capable of mimicking galactose to the extent that it is converted into UDP-galactosamine, but the galactosamine cannot be donated to glycoproteins. Thus uridine is effectively sequestered and the resulting depletion of UTP and UDP-sugars has major metabolic consequences. Depending on the dose the result is either irreversible acute hepatitis or chronic hepatitis and cirrhosis (Medline *et al.*, 1970). Other compounds affect quite different systems. The fungal toxin phalloidin prevents the depolymerization of fungal microfilaments. This results, by mechanisms that remain uncertain, in cholestasis and centrilobular hepatocellular necrosis (Read, 1985). The fungal toxin phomopsin is directly cytotoxic but also interferes with cell division, preventing normal liver repair (Kelly, 1985). Another group of compounds, exemplified by griseofulvin, 3,5-diethoxycarbonyl-1,4-dihydrocollidine, inhibit ferrochelatase resulting in an increase in porphyrin deposits (De Matteis *et al.*, 1987). Similar deposits are seen in the livers of animals treated with hexachlorobenzene and the antiarthritic agent 3-[2(2,4,6-trimethylphenyl)-thiothyl]-4-methylsydnone (Greaves, 1990), and in humans with a hereditary deficiency of ferrochelatase (Bloomer, 1988). Alteration in the metabolism of porphyrins is also implicated in the toxicity of arsenic (see next section).

Metals, Near Metals and their Compounds
Several metals are toxic to the liver. In some cases this is a reflection of their general toxicity. High doses of a number of transition metals result in liver damage, possibly from redox cycling. Copper is especially notable. Liver damage from excess copper has been reported in experimental animals, domestic animals and in humans (Stokinger, 1981). Sheep are particularly susceptible (Kelly, 1985). Wilson's disease (Sternlieb and Scheinberg, 1985), a hereditary condition probably involving a defect in the transfer of copper from hepatic lysosomes to bile, produces all the symptoms of copper intoxication. Bedlington terriers also show a hereditary disease with symptoms of copper intoxication which probably involves a defect in copper excretion (Su, 1982).

Other transition elements are capable of causing liver damage. Salts of iron, cobalt and mercury cause liver damage in experimental animals under extreme conditions and, as with copper, hereditary human diseases notably haemochromatosis, cause symptoms of iron intoxication at normal dietary levels (Powell, 1985). In general, however, the liver is less susceptible to transition metal toxicity than other tissues such as the kidneys. This is not because sulphur-binding metals such as copper, zinc, gold, bismuth and mercury do not reach the liver but because the metals induce binding proteins, called metallothioneins, which sequester the metals resulting in their inactivation, and in the case of the liver, exit from the tissue (Ham, 1986).

Several of the less common metals and semimetals are hepatotoxins. Beryllium may induce granulomatous lesions in the liver although its main toxic action is directed against the lung (Stokinger, 1981). Arsenic and its compounds induce hepatocellular damage, indicated by fatty change, particularly in the centrilobular zone. Electron microscopy showed vesicularization of the endoplasmic reticulum and intracellular damage indicated by an increase in autophagosomes (Ishinishi *et al.*, 1980) and mitochondrial swelling (Fowler *et al.*, 1977). Biochemical studies suggest that interference in the assembly of haemoproteins and redox cycling consequent on the release of free haem may contribute to the toxicity (Albores-Medina *et al.*, 1989). Fatty liver is also induced by antimony administration (Stokinger, 1981).

Lanthanides cause hepatic changes (Arvela, 1979) although this is of limited practical importance as these elements are not absorbed by the gut. The lighter members of the series localise to the liver and, in large amounts, induce a fatty liver while the heavier elements show less preference for the liver and cause focal necrosis without fatty change. Electron microscopy shows changes in the nuclei and the endoplasmic reticulum after treatment with the lighter lanthanides but there is much less indication of systematic morphological changes after administration of the heavier elements in the series. The similarity in ionic radius of calcium and the lanthanides, first pointed out by Lettvin *et al.* (1964), suggests a possible mechanism of toxicity. There are, indeed, effects of lanthanides on other tissues which can be directly related to calcium antagonism but, as discussed by Arvela (1979), there are many other interactions which may explain the hepatotoxicity. It is of interest, for example, that hepatic damage caused by praseodymium is antagonized by silybin, an agent which also antagonizes the RNA-polymerase inhibiting toxins phalloidin and alpha-amanitin (Tuchweber *et al.*, 1976). In addition to these effects some lanthanides affect Kupffer cell function (see later).

The metalloid selenium is both an essential nutrient and a potential toxicant. Excess doses of selenium cause liver atrophy, necrosis and haemorrhages both in experimental (Rouiller, 1964) and farm animals (Hogberg and Alexander, 1986). In general, selenites are more toxic than selenates or selenium salts.

Toxins Requiring Metabolic Activation

The effects of the direct-acting hepatotoxins described in the previous section may be modulated by age or by previous exposure of the animal to other agents and there is no easy way to predict interactions. The toxicity of materials which act by the production of active metabolites will always be affected because, as discussed earlier, the concentrations of the drug metabolizing enzymes change with age and may show remarkable changes with previous exposure. In principle it is possible to predict these interactions given knowledge of the isoforms of cytochrome *P*-450 induced by various agents and which isoforms are responsible for the production of active metabolites but as many agents induce more than one isoform of cytochrome *P*-450 and are metabolized in more than one way prediction has been difficult in practice. Recent developments in computer modelling (Lewis *et al.*, 1992), which allow attention to be concentrated on the isoforms producing active metabolites, may improve the situation.

Low Molecular Weight Haloalkanes, Haloalkenes and Haloacetic Acids

Although chloroform and carbon tetrachloride are often considered as the typical hepatotoxin, their mechanism of action is still not fully understood. In both cases it would seem that the initial reaction is a splitting of a carbon-chlorine bond to yield a free radical intermediate. It is likely that more than one isoform of cytochrome *P*-450 is capable of catalysing this reaction and both oxidative and reductive cleavage (Figure 16) has been demonstrated (Andrews and Snyder, 1991; Testai *et al.*, 1992). At low doses the products formed by oxidative cleavage are completely removed by glutathione but even in the presence of glutathione there is some binding of products of the reductive pathway to cell components *in vitro* (Testai *et al.*, 1992) This may explain the protein-binding intermediates found in animals treated with chloroform at doses which do not cause overt hepatotoxicity. At high doses, the rate of production of free radicals rises, depleting glutathione and permitting a range of secondary reactions whose nature may vary with the oxygen tension (Andrews and Snyder, 1991) but clearly involve lipid peroxidation. As most isoforms of cytochrome *P*-450 are concentrated in the centrilobular zone of the liver the damage is greatest in this area. Accordingly, as the dose of the toxin is increased there is increased disruption of both smooth and rough surfaced endoplasmic reticulum, damage to mitochondria and the Golgi apparatus and fat accumulation followed by swelling, hydropic degeneration and frank centrilobular necrosis.

There is no simple method for predicting the

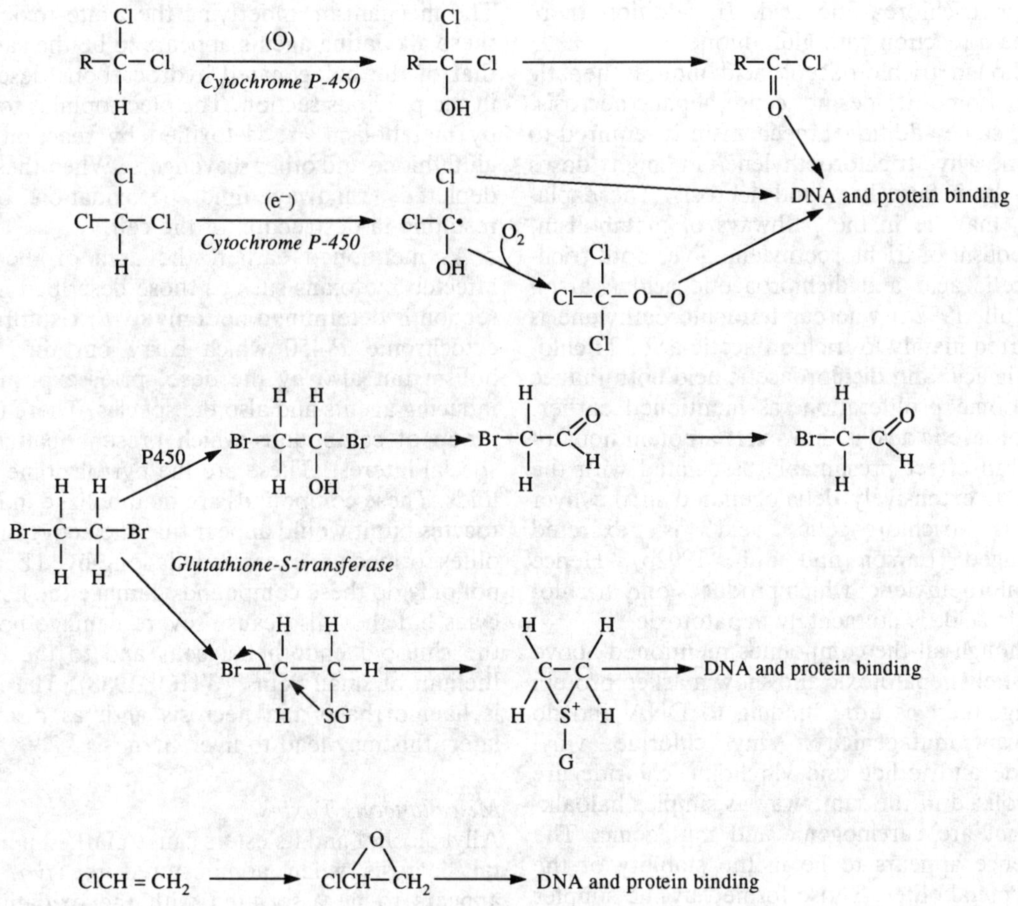

Figure 16 Scheme for the oxidation of haloalkanes and haloalkenes

toxicity for predicting the relative toxicity of haloalkanes from their structure. As can be seen from Figure 16, there are several alternative pathways of metabolism and, with all except the simplest compounds, all pathways will contribute in some degree to the metabolism. A few generalizations may be made. Carbon–fluorine bonds are extremely stable so that fluoroalkanes show little hepatotoxicity. Methyl and ethyl chloride, bromide and iodide are extremely reactive compounds but do not result in damage to the liver, probably because of spontaneous reactions with nucleoophiles in the gut contents or in the blood. Metabolism of haloalkanes by a cytochrome *P*-450 either by the oxidative or the reductive pathway results in extremely reactive intermediates which react strongly with proteins of the endoplasmic reticulum but which are too short lived to enter the nucleus in significant numbers.

Accordingly all haloalkanes cause liver damage of the type described at the end of the last paragraph. However, the episulphonium ions produced by reaction of a haloalkane with glutathione are considerably more stable and are capable of alkylation of DNA; accordingly chemicals such as 1,2-dichloroethane act as initiating agents as well as causing hepatocellular necrosis.

While metabolism of the saturated haloalkanes appears to involve cleavage of a carbon–halogen bond it is likely that the initial reaction for haloethylenes is oxidation of the double bond resulting in formation of an epoxide (Figure 16). These epoxides may degrade in different ways. Major reactions in all cases are rearrangement to form an aldehyde and the formation of a cysteine conjugate. In the case of the more highly substituted haloethylenes the first reaction may involve migration of a halogen between the carbons, forming trichloroacetic acid. In addition there may be a reaction with glutathione.

Although trichloroacetic acid induces hepatic pero-oxisomes it does not cause hepatic necrosis. Hence some additional mechanism is required to explain why trichloroethylene in high doses causes both fatty liver and necrosis. The explanation may lie in the pathways of metabolism. Metabolism of trichloroethylene gives both trichloroacetic acid and dichloroacetic acid (Larson and Bull, 1992a) whereas tetrachloroethylene is converted mainly to trichloroacetic acid. Trichloroacetic acid and dichloroacetic acid both induce peroxisome proliferation, as mentioned earlier. Dichloroacetic acid is, however, a potent hepatotoxin, an effect presumably associated with the fact it is extensively dehalogenated in the liver whereas trichloroacetic acid is excreted unchanged (Larson and Bull, 1992b). Hence tetrachloroethylene, which produces only trichloroacetic acid, is not acutely hepatotoxic.

Although all the compounds mentioned above are acutely hepatotoxic and show marked protein binding, there is little binding to DNA and no significant mutagenicity. Vinyl chloride, vinyl bromide and iodide and vinylidine chloride are metabolized in the same way as simpler haloalkenes but are carcinogenic and mutagenic. The difference appears to lie in the stability of the active metabolites. Those formed by the simpler haloalkenes are highly unstable and have not been detected directly, whereas with the vinyl halides it would seem that the half-life of the epoxide is sufficient to allow it to interact with other cell components, including DNA.

Alkylating Agents other than Haloalkanes or Haloalkenes

The agents discussed in the previous paragraph cause alkylation of proteins in the cytosol but do not have any significant effect on DNA. This is not the case with the majority of the compounds which are metabolized by the cytochromes *P*-450 to produce active metabolites. Accordingly compounds such as polycyclic aromatic amines, the aflatoxins or the simple nitrosamines are potent genotoxins and initiating agents. However, although these compounds are generally thought of simply as hepatocarcinogens, and are discussed here under that heading it is important to remember that, at high doses, all the compounds discussed on pp. 644–646 are potent hepatotoxins.

The mechanism underlying the acute toxicity of these alkylating agents appears to be the same as that of the halogenated hydrocarbons described in the previous section. The electrophiles formed by metabolism are detoxified by reaction with glutathione and other scavengers. When these are depleted, runaway lipid peroxidation occurs resulting in destruction of the cell.

As mentioned earlier, the area of the liver affected by toxins such as those described in this section is determined not only by the isoforms of cytochrome *P*-450 which carry out the metabolism but also by the dose, prior exposure to inducing agents and also the species. There is one group of compounds which present features of special interest. These are the pyrrolizidine alkaloids. These compounds are metabolized in hepatocytes but it would appear that the active metabolites formed are exceptionally long-lived because not only do these compounds damage the hepatocytes but they also cause severe damage both to the sinusoid endothelial cells and to the endothelium of small veins (WHO, 1988). The result is haemorrhage and necrosis and, as discussed later, this may lead to liver cirrhosis.

Miscellaneous Toxins

Allyl alcohol and its esters cause marked periportal necrosis when administered *in vivo*. This appears to be associated with the oxidation of allyl alcohol to acrolein by aldehyde dehydrogenase. The actual mechanism by which acrolein damages hepatocytes is not known but damage is markedly increased in the presence of oxygen and is also facilitated by Kupffer cells (Przybocki *et al.*, 1992).

Chronic Damage to the Liver

Fibrosis and Cirrhosis

Repair of the liver parenchyma normally occurs by regeneration. However repeated injury, for example by alcohol abuse in humans or repeated carbon tetrachloride administration in experimental animals, may eventually cause fibrotic changes in the parenchyma.

Repair by fibrosis may also be observed following administration of single doses of certain compounds, notably the pyrrolizidone alkaloids (WHO, 1988). In addition, repair by fibrosis may be observed in the small spontaneous granulomatous lesions observed in laboratory rats and in similar lesions induced by highly immunogenic materials such as bacterial cell walls or pig intestinal alkaline phosphatase (PAP) (Dijkhuis *et al.*, 1989).

There is strong immunohistochemical evidence that the fibroblast-like cells in small PAP-induced granulomas are derived from fat storing cells (Dijkhuis *et al.*, 1989). As stated earlier, fat storing cells synthesize collagen and proliferate when stimulated by factors derived from Kupffer cells (Zerbe and Gresher, 1988) and it is extremely likely that these cells will be stimulated in viral infections or by foreign carbohydrates or proteins. The reason why pyrrolizidone alkaloids induce fibrosis is unknown but, as discussed earlier, the acute effect of these compounds is a haemorrhagic necrosis associated with damage to branches of the hepatic vein. Damage associated with blood clots is normally repaired by fibrosis in extrahepatic tissues and it is possible that this is also the case in the liver.

It is also not clear why repeated insults to the liver by carbon tetrachloride, ethyl alcohol and other compounds results in repair by fibrosis. It could be that fibrosis requires that the repeat insult should occur before the earlier damage is fully repaired. In the early stages of injury to hepatocytes fibrosis is observed together with an increase in reticulin fibres in the space of Disse. Fat-storing cells from the fibrotic liver show a markedly greater capacity both for collagen synthesis and for cell proliferation than the equivalent cells from normal liver (Dijkhuis *et al.*, 1989). There would thus appear to be two factors which may contribute to the development of further fibrotic change on continued insult. First, it is likely that the sparse reticulin network in the space of Disse plays the role of a basement membrane in guiding liver regeneration and changes to these reticulin fibres associated with collapse of the parenchyma may prevent repair by regeneration. Second, as proliferation of all cells depends on secretion of growth factors from neighbouring cells, changes in the secretion of these factors or in the sensitivity of the target cells may change the balance between regeneration of hepatocytes and proliferation and transformation of fat-storing cells. It is important to stress the word balance; repair by regeneration continues in parallel with development of fibrosis and plays a critical role in the development of the cirrhosis.

The processes which lead from fibrosis to cirrhosis are much better understood. With continued bouts of cell death and fibrous repair the fibrous septa extend and form links between adjacent central veins and between portal tracts and central veins. Capillaries develop in these tracts and enlarge to form veins allowing blood to flow directly from the portal tract to the central vein, thereby bypassing the parenchyma, and death of the parenchymal cells. This results in further cell death followed by further fibrous repair. The condition is self-sustaining and the liver is reorganized into nodules of cells separated by connective tissue septa. The circulation in the nodules is highly disturbed so that foci of cell loss alternate with areas of regeneration. Overall, however, there is a progressive loss of liver substance leading finally to hepatic failure and death.

Hepatocarcinogenesis

Hepatocellular adenomas and carcinomas are frequently observed in experimental studies. These tumours may be induced both by genotoxic and non-genotoxic agents. Furthermore, any treatment which causes chronic hepatocellular damage or which results in a persistant increase in the size of the liver is likely to promote the action of a genotoxic carcinogen and, in fact, many of these regimens will actually increase the incidence of liver cancer on their own. In the past there has been much emphasis on determining whether particular chemicals are genotoxic and elaborate protocols using a combination of several promotors, such as that described by Moslen *et al.*, (1985), have been devised to increase the sensitivity of assays for liver carcinogenesis. Recently more emphasis has been placed on the role of so-called promotors (Ames *et al.*, 1987; Cohen and Ellwein, 1991). To pursue this question would raise issues far outside the scope of the current chapter.

The stages in development of liver cancer appear to be the same in spontaneous tumours and in tumours induced by genotoxic and non-genotoxic carcinogens. The first detectable changes are the development of foci of altered cells (Pitot, 1990). These are small groups of cells, sometimes visible using conventional staining techniques but generally only detectable by histochemical techniques. The early foci are extremely heterogeneous in their enzyme composition.

These early foci do not appear committed to tumour development and, under some experimental conditions (see later) may reverse completely. It is, nevertheless, thought that some foci of altered cells do progress to the second stage of liver carcinogenesis, the development of distinct hyperplastic foci that compress the surrounding tissue. Small hyperplastic foci can, again, reverse completely but larger foci develop into adenomas and, in some cases, to carcinomas. The morphology of liver carcinomas is very varied but tumours induced by non-genotoxic agents generally remain well differentiated, even in metastases, while those induced by the more potent genotoxins may be very anaplastic.

The incidence of cancer in the liver, as in many other tissues, is influenced by many factors (see above). Conventionally discussion is divided between considerations of initiators, that is compounds where a single treatment is sufficient to start the processes which lead to cancer, and promotors, compounds not carcinogenic on their own but which increase the incidence of cancer following treatment with an initiator. This is simplistic when applied to the liver because the classic hepatic 'promotors' are almost all carcinogens in their own right when administered to mice over a lifetime. We consider the compounds under two major headings: compounds which appear to act as direct mutagens and 'non-genotoxic' carcinogens, which in turn are split into compounds which cause chronic liver damage and compounds which cause persistent liver enlargement. It should be noted, however, that both classes of non-genotoxic hepatocarcinogen strongly promote the action of genotoxic agents and theoretical considerations suggest that the enlarged or damaged liver which results from the action of non-genotoxic hepatocarcinogens may be especially susceptible to the action of genotoxic agents.

Mutagenic Hepatocarcinogens

Aminoaryl, Nitroaryl and Azoaryl Compounds

Examples of aromatic amines which increase the incidence of cancer in humans and experimental animals are given in Table 5. The majority of the compounds contain two aromatic rings; aromatic amines with a single ring either do not increase cancer incidence or are very weak carcinogens. It is also noted that there is a marked interspecies variation in the target organ with liver cancer generally being found only in mice. The mechanism of action (King *et al*, 1988) appears to involve *N*-oxidation by cytochromes *P*-450IA1 and IA2 to form the corresponding hydroxylamine. Once formed these can yield the reactive nitrenium ion at an acidic pH or oxidation (Figure 17). Alternatively, there may be further metabolism to form the *N*-hydroxy sulphate or *N*-hydroxyl acetyl derivatives. Spontaneous decomposition of these again results in the formation of nitrenium ions and of DNA and protein adducts. Acetylation or sulphation appears an absolute requirement in the case of *N*-acetylated or *N*-arylated amines. It is likely that the greater potency of the polycyclic aromatic amines and their derivatives as carcinogens results from their ability to facilitate the formation of nitrenium ion by delocalization of its excess electrons. It should be noted that the cytochromes *P*-450 which oxidize aromatic amines have marked structural specificity (Williams and Weisburger, 1991). For example 1-acetylaminofluorene and 3-acetylaminofluorene are not carcinogenic, unlike 2-acetylaminofluorene. The three corresponding hydroxylamines are equally carcinogenic. The difference arises because the liver is unable to metabolize the 1 and 3 isomers. As there are marked interindividual variations in the human population in the ability to *N*-hydroxylate arylamines it would seem likely that there will be equally marked differences in sensitivity to these compounds.

Nitro-analogues of carcinogenic aromatic amines also lead to tumour formation (Williams and Weisburger, 1991). These compounds may be reduced by rather weakly active mammalian enzymes and by gut bacteria to hydroxylamines which can then be further metabolized as described in the previous paragraph. As the nitro reductases are much less specific than the cytochromes *P*-450 which oxidize aromatic amines it appears possible that these compounds may be more widely toxic. In practice this does not seem to be the case. While 1-hydroxyamino naphthalene is carcinogenic, 1-nitronaphthalene is not, presumably because the rate of reduction of the nitro group to the carcinogenic hydroxylamine is much lower than the rate of reduction of the hydroxylamine to an amino group. 1-Naphthylamine is not oxidised by *P*-450IA and so there can be no reformation of the hydroxylamine whose steady state concentration is therefore extremely

Table 5 Organs affected by carcinogenic aromatic amines in different species

	Mouse	Rat	Dog	Human
Benzidine	Liver Zymbal gland	Mammae	Bladder	Bladder
4-Aminobiphenyl	Liver Bladder Endothelia	Mammae Intestine	Bladder	Bladder
2-Naphthylamine	Liver	?Bladder	Bladder	Bladder
3,3'-Dichlorobenzidine	Liver	Mammae Zymbal gland Leukaemia	Bladder Liver	—
4,4'Thiodianiline	Liver Thyroid	Liver Thyroid Ear canal Uterus	—	—
o-Anisidine	Bladder	Bladder	—	—
4-Cl-o-Phenylenediamine	Liver	Bladder	—	—
p-Cresidine	Bladder Liver Nasal cavity	Bladder Liver Olfactory neuroblastoma	—	—

Source: IARC (1982, 1987).

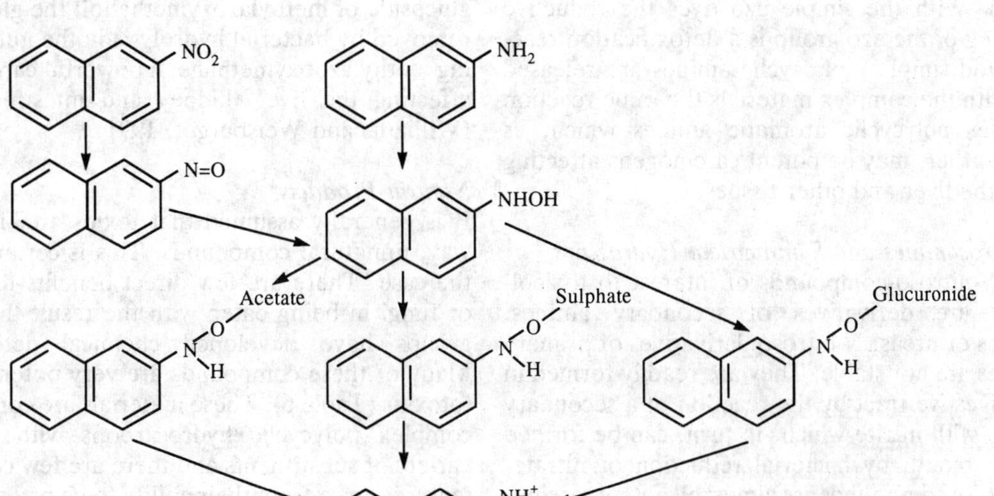

Figure 17 Scheme for the metabolism of aromatic amines

low. However, the effects of equivalent nitroaryl and aminoaryl compounds may sometimes be very different: 2,4-diaminotoluene is a potent carcinogen whereas 2,6-diaminotoluene is consistently negative (Cunningham *et al.*, 1991). 2,6-Dinitrotoluene is, however, a much more potent carcinogen than 2,4-dinitrotoluene (King *et al.*,

1988). As discussed earlier, part of the explanation may lie in the fact that 2,4-diaminotoluene is a potent hepatotoxin and hence increases cancer incidence by a non-genotoxic mechanism. All in all, the varying toxicities of aromatic amines and nitro compounds show the difficulty of predicting toxicity from chemical structures even when the metabolic pathways linking the compounds are well understood.

Aromatic azo compounds can be divided into two distinct groups (Williams and Weisburger, 1991). In the first group are simple compounds consisting of two aromatic groups joined together by an azo bond. These compounds include hepatocarcinogens such as dimethylaminoazobenzene (butter yellow). Carcinogens in this group have an amino group attached to one of the aromatic rings and are metabolized in exactly the same way as the amines described above. The azo group bridging the two rings allows efficient delocalization of the electrons in the nitrenium ion. The carcinogenicity of these compounds is influenced by two factors. First, the azo bond may be reduced, yielding non-carcinogenic or very weakly carcinogenic monocyclic aromatic amines. Second, compounds containing polar constituents such as sulphonic acid residues are usually not carcinogenic.

Complex azo dyes consist of polycyclic structures generally linked by more than one azo group. With the simple azo dyes the reductive splitting of the azo group is a detoxification reaction and simple monocyclic amines are released but with the complex materials the same reaction releases polycyclic aromatic amines which, as seen earlier, may be potent carcinogens affecting both the liver and other tissues.

N-*Nitrosamines and Symmetrical Hydrazines*

The *N*-nitroso-compounds of interest to toxicologists are derivatives of secondary amines, amides or ureas; *N*-nitroso derivatives of primary amines are not stable. They are readily formed in the digestive tract by the reaction of a secondary amine with nitrite which, in turn, can be formed in the mouth by bacterial reduction of nitrate. *N*-nitroso compounds are almost all potent carcinogens. The target organ, however, differs between species and between compounds. Nitroso derivatives of alkylureas, alkylamides and esters are exceedingly potent carcinogens but normally the liver is not the major target organ. These unstable compounds decompose spontaneously yielding alkylating agents on contact with aqueous solutions, especially of a neutral or alkaline pH. *N*-Nitroso derivatives of linear secondary amines such as dimethyl nitrosamine or of cyclic amines such as morpholine require metabolism and are thus much more likely to affect the liver. Such *N*-

nitrosamines are activated by hydroxylation on a carbon adjacent to the nitrogen (Figure 18). This results in cleavage of the carbon–nitrogen bond yielding first a diazonium and then a carbonium ion both of which are potent alkylating agents. Although such metabolism is theoretically possible for all *N*-nitrosamines in the livers of all species there is, as already mentioned, a marked variation in sensitivity. Discussion of the reasons for these differences may be found in specialist monographs (Bartsch *et al.*, 1987; O'Neill *et al.*, 1991).

Metabolism of dialkylhydrazines can yield products identical to those produced by *N*-nitrosamines (Figure 18). As substituted hydrazines are more uncommon both in nature and in industry than secondary amines much less is known about their toxicity. However, there are indications that there is likely to be the same variation in target organ as with the *N*-nitrosamines (Williams and Weisburger, 1991). Probably the most important compound in this class is cycasin, a compound found in cycad flour. Cycasin is the glucoside of methylazoxymethanol: the glucose is removed by bacterial hydrolysis in the gut releasing methylazooxymethane, a powerful carcinogen affecting the liver, kidney and intestinal tract (Williams and Weisburger, 1991).

Natural Products

It is generally assumed that toxins are, in some way, unnatural compounds. This is certainly not the case. There are few direct benefits to plants or fungi in being eaten with the result that both groups have developed chemical deterrents. Many of these compounds are very potent hepatotoxins (Table 6). These materials are commonly complex polycyclic hydrocarbons with a wide variety of substituents and there are few common features apart from their ability to be metabolized to electrophiles. The mechanisms by which they cause liver damage and liver cancer are the same as the synthetic chemicals discussed earlier. The more potent hepatotoxins are considered in some detail by Kelly (1985) and structure–activity relationships in general are discussed by Ashby and Tennant (1988).

Non-mutagenic Hepatocarcinogens

A considerable number of the chemicals which increase the incidence of tumours in the liver give no evidence for mutagenicity in either prokary-

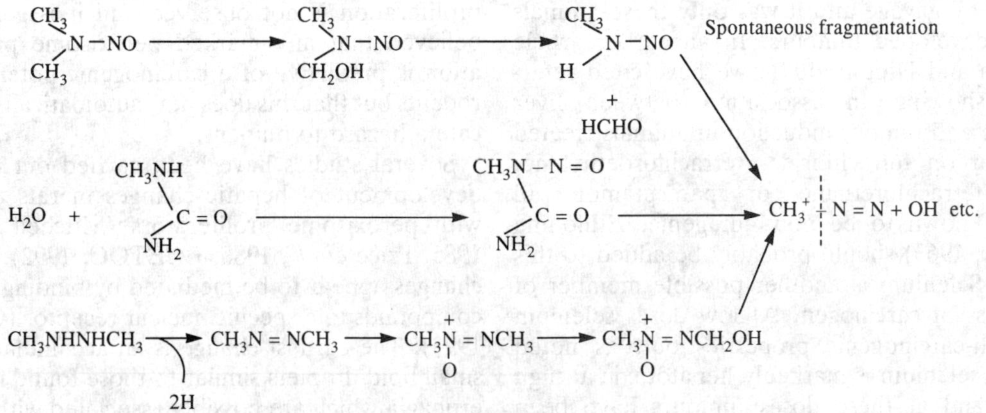

$$CH_3\text{-}N(CH_3)\text{-}NO \longrightarrow CH_3\text{-}N(CH_2OH)\text{-}NO \longrightarrow CH_3\text{-}N(H)\text{-}NO \quad \text{Spontaneous fragmentation}$$

$$+$$
$$HCHO$$

$$H_2O + \underset{NH_2}{\overset{CH_3NH}{C}}=O \longrightarrow \underset{NH_2}{\overset{CH_3N-N=O}{C}}=O \longrightarrow CH_3^+ \!\mid\! N = N + OH \text{ etc.}$$

$$CH_3NHNHCH_3 \xrightarrow{\;-2H\;} CH_3N = NCH_3 \longrightarrow \underset{O}{\overset{+}{CH_3N}} = NCH_3 \longrightarrow \underset{O}{\overset{+}{CH_3N}} = NCH_2OH$$

Figure 18 Scheme for the metabolism of *N*-nitrosamines and dialkylhydrazines

Table 6 Natural products that show marked hepatotoxicity. These plant and fungal products have been responsible for widespread loss of cattle and, especially, sheep. The list is intended to demonstrate the range of sources and effects on the liver and is in no way exhaustive. In particular it should be noted that where soil contains abnormal amounts of trace components such as selenium there may be marked concentrations in growing plants and resultant toxicity

Chemical	Chemical class	Source species	Action
Methylazoxymethanol	Aglycone of glycoside	Cycadales (plants)	Alkylating agents
Ngaione	Furanosesquiterpenoid	Myoporaceae (plants)	Zonal necrosis
Trematoxin	Glycoside	Ulmaceae (plants)	Periportal necrosis
Aflatoxins	Bisfuranocoumarins	*Aspergillus* (fungi)	Alkylating agents
Phomopsin	Not characterized	Moulds on *Lupinus* spp.	Mitotic arrest
Sporidesmin	Not characterized	Moulds on dead ryegrass	Cholestasis
'Many compounds'	Pyrrolizidine alkaloids	Many plants	Alkylating agents Cirrhosis Endothelial damage[a]
Lantadenes (identical to Icterogenin)	Triterpenes	*Lantana camera* *Lippia rehmanni*	Cell enlargement Cholestasis

[a] Petasitenine also induces endothelial cell tumours.

Source: Kelly (1985).

otic (Ashby and Tennant, 1988; Ashby *et al.*, 1989) or eukaryotic (Williams *et al.*, 1989) tests. The mechanism by which they increase cancer incidence is not known. On initial examination they fall into at least four distinct groups but, as discussed at the end of this section, it is possible that with three of the groups the underlying superficial dissimilarities belie an underlying connection: persistent enlargement of the liver (Grasso and Hinton, 1991). The first group, however, is mechanistically distinct.

Agents Causing Chronic Damage to the Liver
There is a close association between chronic tissue damage and the induction of cancer (Butterworth *et al.*, 1991, Grasso *et al.*, 1991). Eschenbrenner and Miller in 1945 showed that chloroform increased liver cancer at doses which were hepatotoxic but not at lower doses. More recently the link between cell proliferation and carcinogenesis has been emphasised by Klaunig *et al.* (1986) who demonstrated that rats treated with chloroform by gavage or in the drinking water showed the same very small amount of DNA binding, but liver damage only developed in rats

treated by gavage and it was only these animals which developed tumours. In an earlier article (Grasso and Hinton, 1991) we have cited references showing an association between liver damage and tumour induction in animals treated with carbon tetrachloride, tetrachloroethylene, 1,1,2,2-tetrachlorethane or paracetamol, all agents known to be non-mutagenic. Ethionine (Farber, 1963) should probably be added to this group. Selenium is another possible member of this class of carcinogen. At low doses selenium has anti-carcinogenic properties but, as noted earlier, selenium is markedly hepatotoxic at high doses, and at these doses tumours have been observed (IARC, 1975; Fishbein, 1978).

Compounds Causing Peroxisome Proliferation
Proliferation of peroxisomes in the liver of rats and mice treated with a number of lipid-lowering drugs was noted in the 1960s but it was only in the late 1970s, when a connection with increased cancer incidence was noted (Cohen and Grasso, 1981; Reddy and Lalwani, 1984) that much interest was taken in these compounds. Since then compounds in this group have been extensively studied. The results have been extensively surveyed by the European Chemical Industry Ecology and Toxicology Centre (ECETOC, 1992).

Although there are marked variations in potency between different peroxisome proliferators the development of hepatic changes are remarkably uniform. It should first be noted that marked peroxisome proliferation is only found in old world rodents (Family Muridae). There are marked differences even within this family with rats and mice responding much more vigorously than hamsters. It is unlikely that other species are totally non-responsive. The most potent peroxisome proliferators are reported to have some effect on rhesus monkeys (Lalwani et al., 1985) and there may even be a marginal change in human patients (R. H. Hinton and S. C. Price, unpublished data). It is, however, reasonable to conclude that peroxisome proliferation is probably metabolically important to rats and mice but is vestigial outside this family of animals. Neither animal studies nor exceedingly comprehensive epidemiological surveys (Committee of Principal Investigators, 1978) in human populations have given any evidence that these materials increase cancer incidence in species where peroxisome proliferation is not observed and it is generally believed that any marked peroxisome proliferation is predictive of a carcinogenic potential in rodents but that this does not, automatically, indicate a hazard to humans.

Several studies have been carried out on the development of hepatic changes in rats treated with peroxisome proliferators (Mitchell et al., 1985; Price et al., 1986; ECETOC, 1992). These changes appear to be mediated by binding of the compounds to a specific nuclear receptor (Green, 1993). The earliest change is an accumulation of small lipid droplets similar to those found in hyperphagia which are possibly associated with alterations in fatty acid metabolism (Mitchell et al., 1986). Within a few hours induction of the oncogenes c-*myc* and c-*fos* is noticed (Bentley et al., 1987) and messenger RNAs for a specific cytochrome P-450 (P-450IVA1, previously known as cytochrome P-452) and for the peroxisomal proteins accumulate (Milton et al., 1990). Consequent on these changes are a burst of cell division, which occurs 2–3 days after first administration of diets, and the accumulation of specialized peroxisomes lacking a uricase rich core, smooth endoplasmic reticulum and a specific, cytosolic, epoxide hydrolase (Meijer and de Pierre, 1987).

In an earlier section the distinction was made between adaptive and toxic changes. It is likely that the changes mentioned above are essentially adaptive, permitting for example oxidation of peroxidized fatty acids. Treatment for 1 month or more results in changes clearly indicative of toxicity, namely the accumulation of enlarged lysosomes filled with material with the staining properties of lipofuscin and, at least in some cases, an increase in cell turnover (Price et al., 1986; Cattley et al., 1987). Dose–response experiments suggest that with each compound there is a distinct threshold for these latter effects suggesting they represent the result of some form of metabolic overload. More prolonged treatment results in the development of foci of altered cells. These foci differ from those formed spontaneously or in response to microsomal inducers such as phenobarbitone (phenobarbital) in that they lack γ-glutamyl transpeptidase and fetal-type glutathione *S*-transferase activity (Rao et al., 1982; Sato, 1989). These foci and at least some of the hyperplastic nodules which develop on more prolonged treatment reverse on withdrawal of the compound (Mompon et al., 1987) but if treatment is continued well differentiated hepatocellular carcinomas appear which occasionally show metastases, particularly to the lungs.

Compounds Inducing Microsomal Oxidases

While compounds causing proliferation of peroxisomes may be treated as a single group, this is not the case for compounds which induce microsomal enzymes. Furthermore, there has been considerable controversy about the mechanism of carcinogenesis by certain compounds, such as the food dye safrole, which are potent inducers of microsomal oxidases but are also weakly mutagenic in certain *in vitro* tests. In the following discussion we will attempt to group the compounds but the classification is very tentative.

First, it should be noted that phenobarbitone (phenobarbital) (IARC, 1987) and other compounds such as butylated hydroxytoluene (Inai *et al.*, 1988) which induce cytochrome *P*-450IIB isoforms almost invariably increase the incidence of liver cancer in mice when administered at high doses. These compounds all cause massive liver enlargement, are potent promotors of the action of genotoxic carcinogens, and give negative results in both *in vivo* and *in vitro* mutagenicity tests. In general these compounds do not increase cancer incidence in species other than mice, although Rossi *et al.* (1977) did report an increase in rats following 3 years administration of phenobarbitone (phenobarbital). It is generally believed that with this group of compounds an increase in liver tumours in mice alone does not indicate any risk to humans. This attitude has recently been supported by studies showing high spontaneous rates of oncogenes in the livers of strains of mice susceptible to liver cancer (Anderson *et al.*, 1992).

At first sight the polyhalogenated aromatic and alicyclic hydrocarbons would appear to form a second group but, in fact, these compounds fall into two or more distinct subclasses. The first group is formed by TCDD (2,3,7,8-tetrachlorodibenzo-*p*-dioxin) and the planar polychlorinated and polybrominated biphenyls (PCBs and PBBs) and related compounds. These induce a group of enzymes controlled by the Ah locus, which include cytochrome *P*-450IA1 and IA2 (Nebert and Gonzalez, 1987). These compounds increase the fat in the liver and cause alterations in the RER, changes which are not observed with the non-planar PCBs which are phenobarbitone

(phenobarbital) type inducers (Kohli *et al.*, 1979). TCDD, PCBs and PBBs all increase the incidence of liver cancer (IARC, 1987). It is of interest that another group of inducers which act on the Ah locus, the polycyclic aromatic hydrocarbons, neither affect liver size nor cause any increase in liver tumours, although they are potent carcinogens.

The second group of halogenated hydrocarbons which increase the incidence of liver tumours are heavily substituted alicyclic compounds. The following have been assessed as hepatocarcinogens (IARC, 1979a, 1987):

- Aldrin/dieldrin
- Lindane
- 2,4,5-T
- 2,4,6-T
- Chlordane
- Chlordecone
- Mirex/Photomirex/Kepone
- Toxaphene

These compounds induce a poorly characterized spectrum of cytochrome *P*-450s. They also produce massive liver enlargement and it is of interest that whereas alpha, beta, gamma and delta hexachlorocyclohexane are all effective inducers of cytochromes *P*-450, only the alpha isomer (lindane) is a hepatocarcinogen, and that it is by far the most potent in causing liver enlargement (Grasso and Hinton, 1991). There is generally little liver damage apart from some accumulation of fat, although in mice treated with dieldrin Mallory bodies accumulate in the cytoplasm (Meierhenny *et al.*, 1981).

With two hepatocarcinogens, the food dyes Ponceau MX (Grasso and Gray, 1977) and safrole (Crampton *et al.*, 1977), the increase in microsomal enzymes reverses on prolonged administration of the compound. Electron microscopic examination, however, shows continued proliferation of the endoplasmic reticulum and enlargement of lysosomes. Such 'hyperplastic, hypoactive' endoplasmic reticulum has also been observed in rats treated with dieldrin but not in mice treated with the same material (Tennekes *et al.*, 1979) and it is likely that the carcinogenicity of Ponceau MX and safrole is attributable to other factors.

There is no evidence for a direct mechanistic relationship between induction of microsomal oxidases and development of cancer. A common feature to all the compounds discussed in this section is continued liver enlargement with little liver damage. This is also observed with other groups of non-genotoxic hepatocarcinogens and will be discussed later. It should also be noted that most of the compounds discussed in this section are only weak carcinogens when administered on their own but all are potent promotors of the action of genotoxic carcinogens.

Compounds Causing Mitochondrial Proliferation
Methapyriline and certain close analogues (Reznik-Schuller and Lijinsky, 1981) cause marked proliferation of mitochondria and liver enlargement in short-term studies and cancer in the longer term. The effects seem to be specific to rats (see Copple *et al.*, 1992). It is of interest that other close analogues of methapyriline cause peroxisome proliferation (Reznik-Schuller and Lijinsky, 1982). Although methapyriline is negative in most *in vivo* and *in vitro* mutagenicity tests there is binding to cell proteins and suppression of mitochondrial protein and DNA synthesis (Lijinsky and Muschik, 1982; Copple *et al.*, 1992). However the relationship of these observations to carcinogenesis remains obscure.

Hormones
Certain types of combined oral contraceptive appear to increase very slightly, but significantly, the risk of cancer incidence in human patients (IARC, 1987). The tumours produced are typical of those induced by non-mutagenic hepatocarcinogens in experimental animals being normally benign, well differentiated and, in some cases, they appear to regress on cessation of treatment (Klatskin, 1977). In animal trials, increases in liver tumours have been observed with ethinyl-oestradiol, the progestins ethynodiol diacetate, norethisterone and norethynodrel as well as various oestrogen–progestin combinations (IARC, 1979b) but there is no evidence for mutagenicity. Several oestrogens are capable of promoting the action of mutagenic carcinogens (IARC, 1979c) and to increase mitotic activity in the liver (Williams, 1982). Other short- and medium-term effects on the liver include induction of a specific group of cytochromes *P*-450 (Nebert and Gonzalez, 1987) and a persistent hepatomegaly.

Other Compounds or Treatments
The incidence of liver cancer, like that of other tumours, in rodents is affected by diet. Increased incidences have been found in rats induced to eat hypercaloric diets whereas the incidence of tumours falls when food consumption of the animals is restricted (Cheney *et al.*, 1983; Pollard and Luckert, 1989). The incidence of liver tumours is also increased in rats receiving a choline deficient diet (Mikol *et al.*, 1983). The increase is not caused by the associated liver damage as an increase in hepatic tumours is also found in rats following transient choline deficiency in early life (Ghosal *et al.*, 1987). Choline deficiency results in hypomethylation of DNA (Wainfen *et al.*, 1989). DNA methylation is important for maintaining the accuracy of post-synthetic repair and cell differentiation and it is thought that DNA hypomethylation, in itself, increases the risk of cancer.

Liver Enlargement and Carcinogenesis
Recent surveys of non-genotoxic carcinogens (Grasso *et al.*, 1991, Hildebrand *et al.*, 1991) indicate that these agents fall into two distinct groups: those agents whose action results in persistent tissue damage and therefore continued cell division and those that cause persistent tissue enlargement but no evidence of cell damage. With these agents there is a mitotic burst immediately after initiation of treatment but with continued treatment the target tissue remains enlarged but the rate of cell division returns to normal. The actions of this group of agents on the liver closely resembles the effects of trophic hormones such as TSH on their target tissues. It has already been made clear that certain hepatocarcinogens fall clearly in to the first group. There is equally strong evidence that other hepatocarcinogens fall in to the second group.

Following initiation of treatment with agents which induce microsomal or peroxisomal enzymes or with certain steroid hormones there is a burst of mitosis in the liver (Schulte-Hermann, 1974; Michalopoulos, 1991). This burst is self-limiting and by 1 week after commencement of treatment the rate of mitosis falls to normal levels. Molecular biological studies, however, suggest that the liver is not in a normal state. Using peroxisome proliferators, it has been demonstrated that there is continued expression of certain proto-oncogenes at an elevated level (Bentley *et al.*, 1987). Both peroxisomal and microsomal inducers indicate that there is a reduction in the number of receptors for a major liver growth factor (TGF-α) on the surface of hepatocytes (Michalopoulos, 1991). Using phenobarbitone (phenobarbital), it has been demonstrated that there is an elevated secretion of the inhibitory growth factor TGF-β (Jirtle *et al.*,

1991). There are also alterations in the nucleus. In the adolescent rat most cells are either binucleate diploids or mononucleate tetrapolods. On treatment with compounds such as phenobarbitone (phenobarbital) or clofibrate the majority of cells become mononucleate tetraploids. If the compounds are removed from the diet the changes are reversible but the changes reappear on subsequent administration of the compounds (Ahmed *et al.*, 1990).

Thus study of the enlarged liver suggests that there is a continued drive for division which is inhibited by downregulation of receptors and secretion of inhibitory growth factors. It is likely that the initial events in neoplasia relate to defects in these inhibitory mechanism because the foci of altered cells and even the hyperplastic nodules which form in response to the agents under consideration reverse on cessation of treatment (Mompon *et al.*, 1987). However, it is becoming clear that microsomal inducers and peroxisome proliferators stimulate the growth of different groups of cells because the foci of altered cells induced by the two groups of compounds differ markedly in their morphology and enzymology (Pitot, 1990) and oncogene expression (Anderson *et al.*, 1992) and also because the same differences are observed when the agents are used as promotors following treatment with genotoxic carcinogens (Pitot, 1990).

Toxic Damage to Sinusoid Endothelial Cells

Sinusoid endothelial cells may be damaged by direct-acting liver toxins or as a result of the release of toxic metabolites from neighbouring hepatocytes. The destruction of sinusoid endothelial cells will cause haemorrhage or, if there is also damage to hepatocytes, haemorrhagic necrosis. There are few toxins which appear to act directly on the endothelium. Sinusoidal endothelial cells do, however, appear to be affected by allyl formate earlier than any other cell types (Haenni, 1964) and light microscopic studies suggest a similar lesion may be produced by urethane (Doljanski and Rosin, 1944) and alloxan (du Bois, 1954). Pyrrolozidine alkaloids cause destruction of the endothelial cells of sinusoids and branches of the hepatic vein, apparently due to a metabolite produced in the hepatocytes (WHO, 1988). In this case the damage to endo-

thelial cells is clear because of the effects on the venous endothelium but it is likely that similar but milder 'by-stander' damage will occur with other toxins. Certain genotoxic carcinogens such as thioacetamide and butter yellow cause enlargement and hyperactivity of endothelial cells (Simon and Rouiller, 1964).

The numbers of tumours arising from endothelial cells (angiosarcomas) can be increased by certain compounds. The most notable of these is vinyl chloride which in animals produces a range of tumours including angiosarcomas, especially in the liver. In humans exposure to vinyl chloride is associated with an increase in a range of tumours in addition to hepatic angiosarcomas (IARC, 1987). Vinyl chloride is a potent mutagen and it is not known why exposure should be associated with this particular tumour. Vinyl chloride is metabolized in hepatocytes by *P*-450 isoenzymes which, as discussed earlier, gives rise to products with protein and DNA binding capacity that are detoxified by glutathione. There is no obvious reason why the sinusoid endothelial cells should be the targets.

Angiosarcoma in humans has also been associated with exposure to arsenic (Lander *et al.*, 1975). Most early effects of arsenic are, however, on hepatocytes and these have been discussed earlier. Angiosarcomas have also been found in patients treated with colloidal thorium dioxide (thorotrast) which was, at one stage, employed as an X-ray contrast media (Swarm, 1967) and is probably associated with accumulation of the radioactive material in the neighbouring Kupffer cells (discussed in the next section).

Toxic Damage to Kupffer Cells

Particulate material taken up by Kupffer cells that is not digestible by lysosomal enzymes may be retained in the liver for very long periods. If the material is radioactive this may have serious consequences. Colloidal thorium dioxide (thorotrast) was used as an X-ray contrast medium up to 1945. Thorium is radioactive, emitting alpha particles. Patients exposed to thorotrast retained thorium in the liver for many years and have developed a range of tumours both in the liver and at other sites of accumulation. Liver tumours have included tumours arising from hepatocytes (hepatomas), from bile duct lining cells (cholangiomas) and from endothelial cells (angiosarcomas)

(Swarm, 1967). Uptake of 'indigestible' material may also result in loss of Kupffer cell function and reticuloendothelial blockade, for example gadolinium chloride (Bouma and Smit, 1989), dextran sulphate (Laskin, 1989) and carrageenen (Abraham *et al.*, 1972) are taken up by Kupffer cells and inhibit their function.

Kupffer cells may also modulate the effects of xenobiotics on hepatocytes. This may occur through processing of the toxin, for example it would appear that the uptake of colloidal beryllium into Kupffer cells and the subsequent release of the free ion plays a significant role in the toxicity of this metal (Skilleter, 1987). Alternatively, the interaction may be complex, for example inactivation of Kupffer cells attenuates the toxicity of paracetamol (acetaminophen) (Laskin, 1989) and of allyl alcohol (Przybocki *et al.*, 1992) whereas activation of Kupffer cells enhances the toxicity of carbon tetrachloride (Sipes *et al.*, 1989). In the brain much of the damage following ischaemic injury results from the secondary effects mediated through glial cells and it is interesting to speculate that inappropriate release of mediators from Kupffer cells may, likewise, exacerbate hepatic damage.

Toxic Damage to Bile Duct Lining Cells

A small number of compounds are specifically toxic to the bile duct lining cells (Tables 7 and 8). This does not appear to be due to a special susceptibility of these cells to the action of the toxin but rather to the concentration of compounds as they pass down the biliary tree. Toxic changes are, therefore, normally confined to middle and large sized ducts. In two cases, the mycotoxin sporidesmin (Mortimer, 1963; Kelly, 1985) and the antiasthmatic FPL 52757 (Eason *et al.*, 1982) toxicity is due to the parent compound.

Table 8   Compounds that cause damage to hepatocytes and bile duct proliferation

Compound	Reference
Ethionine	Farber (1963)
Tannic acid	Korpassy (1961)
Thioacetamide	Ambrose *et al.* (1949)
Flectol H	Panner and Packer (1961)
Allyl alcohol and allyl formate	Haenni (1964)
Butter yellow[a]	Buyssens (1962)
Pyrrolizidine alkaloids	WHO (1988)
Stilbamidine	Seager and Castelnuovo (1947)
Aflatoxin A1	Busby and Wogan (1984)
Coumarin[a]	Evans *et al.* (1989)

[a] These compounds increase the incidence of cholangiocarcinoma in rats.

Table 7   Compounds that cause bile duct necrosis and bile duct proliferation without hepatocellular damage

Compound	Species	Reference
Alpha-naphthylisothiocyanate	Rats, mice	Goldfarb *et al.* (1962)
Sporidesmin	Sheep[a]	Kelly (1985)
FPL 52757	Dogs[b]	Eason *et al.* (1982)
Dibutyl tin	Rats, mice[c]	Barnes and Magee (1958)
Arsenic III or V compounds[d]	Rats, dogs	Byron *et al.* (1967) Ishinishi (1980)
Tilidine fumarate	Rats	McGuire *et al.* (1986)
Oxamniquine	Rats[e]	Gregory (1983)
Methylene dianiline	Rats	Kanz *et al.* (1992)

[a] Direct injection of the alkaloid into rabbit gall bladder also produces a lesion (Worker, 1960).
[b] Bile duct damage in rats may be produced by retrograde infusion (Eason *et al.*, 1982).
[c] Development of the lesion probably depends on interaction with pancreatic enzymes (Aldridge, W. M., personal communication).
[d] Arsenic III and V compounds also induce damage to hepatocytes in the centrilobular area.
[e] Not dogs, mice or hamsters and probably (Chvedoff *et al.*, 1984) not humans.

However, with other compounds such as alpha naphthylisothiocyanate (ANIT) the actual toxin is a metabolite produced by the hepatocytes (Horky *et al.*, 1971; Connolly *et al.*, 1988b). The pattern of change is consistent with a toxin, possibly a glutathione conjugate (Carpenter-Deyo *et al.*, 1991) escaping from the bile ducts and, indeed, electron microscopy shows opening of the tight junctions between bile duct lining cells (Connolly *et al.*, 1988a). In addition to damage to the bile duct lining cells there is also marked portal oedema and haemorrhage presumably from damage to the small blood vessels of the peribiliary plexus. In mice there is destruction of the gall bladder epithelium (Connolly *et al.*, 1988b). Acute lesions heal rapidly; in rats total biliary necrosis produced by ANIT resolves within 7 days with restoration of the normal architecture (Plaa and Priestley, 1976). Chronic treatment with such agents will lead to lethal liver failure if the dose is sufficient to prevent repair of the vessels but if repair is possible bile duct proliferation occurs.

Di- and trialkyl tin salts also cause bile duct damage but by a completely different mechanism. The lesion is only found in species in which there are anastomoses between the bile duct and the pancreatic ducts (WHO, 1990) and consists of an ascending cholangitis that affects initially the extrahepatic portion of the bile duct (Barnes and Magee, 1958). The mechanism of damage is not understood.

Bile Duct Proliferation

Idiopathic or Infectious

It should be noted that spontaneous bile duct proliferation occurs in hamsters and in many strains of rat in the second year of life (Greaves, 1990) and that bile duct changes, up to and including cholangiocarcinoma, are sometimes observed in ageing dogs and cats (Kelly, 1985). The lesions cannot be distinguished from those consequential on bile duct damage described in the next section. Marked bile duct proliferation may follow infection with certain liver flukes, such as *Fasciola hepatica* that infests the bile ducts. It is believed that the changes following such infestations result from damage to the duct by the parasite (Kelly, 1985) and hence have a similar pathogenesis to the lesions described in the next section.

Consequences of Bile Duct Damage

Repeated exposure to toxins affecting the bile ducts results in marked proliferation. With chronic treatment the initial damage caused by the toxin resolves by fibrosis. After a short time heavily vascularised immature connective tissue is seen between the ducts. The bile ducts are embedded in dense connective tissue. Histochemical staining shows that the blood vessels of the peribiliary plexus no longer abut directly onto the basement membrane of the duct but are separated from it by a ring of connective tissue (Kelly *et al.*, 1991). It would seem that development of this type of bile duct proliferation involves two processes. First, the process exemplifies the 'rule' that acute injuries tend to heal by regeneration but that chronic injuries heal by fibrosis. However, the proliferation of ducts and the separation of the vulnerable blood vessels from the ducts suggest that this is an adaptive change that increases the ability of the liver to excrete cytotoxic materials into the bile.

Proliferation Associated with Periportal Damage

Hyperplasia of the bile ducts and ductules occurs with a number of hepatotoxins including ethionine, tannic acid, thioacetamide, allyl formate, butter yellow, lasiocarpine and stilbamidine. With these compounds, unlike the materials discussed in the previous section, damage to bile ducts appears proportional to the degree of hepatocellular damage (Rouiller, 1964). In other cases, exemplified by the antioxidant butylated hydroxytoluene, a very mild bile duct proliferation is observed at doses below those required to cause frank periportal necrosis (Powell *et al.*, 1986). In some cases bile duct proliferation with these agents resembles that described in the previous section, namely well-defined bile ducts often surrounded by fairly dense connective tissue grouped within distinct portal tracts. In other cases a different pattern is observed. In the minimal lesion small bile ducts with little associated connective tissue appear to grow into the parenchyma. With other agents (Fausto *et al.*, 1987), exemplified by the hepatocarcinogens ethionine, 2-acetylaminofluorene and 3'-methyl-4-dimethylaminoazobenzene, the proliferating cells no longer form distinct ducts but are found as strings of so-called oval cells. These have now been isolated and found to be a mixed population, a portion of which are committed bile duct lining cells while others have the potential to differentiate into either hepatocytes or bile duct lining cells (Fausto, 1990). It is thought possible that these cells, which possibly arise from a small population of stem cells present in the normal liver, are associated with the process of carcinogenesis (Fausto, 1990).

Cholestasis

The word cholestasis means simply the absence of bile flow and covers several distinct pathological conditions. First, there is mechanical obstruction of the extrahepatic duct from either gall stones (cholelithiasis) or external pressure, for example carcinoma of the head of the pancreas. Second, there is obstruction of intrahepatic bile ducts, normally as a result of inflammation. Finally, changes in hepatocytes may interfere with the initial secretion of bile into the bile canaliculi, either by inhibiting the secretion of bile acids and bile salts (the fluid component of bile enters by passive diffusion) or by altering the permeability of the tight junctions which prevent materials passed into the bile canaliculus from returning to the plasma. In experimental animals treatment with agents causing biliary obstruction result in proliferation of bile ducts and focal necrosis in the liver parenchyma. Treatment with cholestatic agents which affect hepatocytes, on the other hand, does not generally cause damage to hepatocytes or bile duct lining cells although bile plugs may be observed in bile canaliculi and ducts.

The most common form of gall stone is composed of cholesterol and calcium salts, often arranged in alternating layers (Karran *et al.*, 1985). 'Pigment stones' also occur, especially in Asiatic countries, and consist largely of salts of bilirubin. The two types of stone are thought to form by different mechanisms. Biliary cholesterol is dissolved in the interior of mixed micelles formed by phospholipids and bile acids and salts. Normal human bile is technically supersaturated in cholesterol but this does not normally crystallize. It is thought that crystallization may be provoked by the formation of nucleation centres, short-term fluctuations in cholesterol secretion and changes in the stability of bile micelles with changes in bile salt composition (Heaton, 1985). Formation of pigment stones is associated with infection of the biliary tree: the β-glucuronidase

secreted abundantly by bacteria such as *Escherichia coli* breaks down bilirubin glucuronides and causes precipitation of free acid (Karran *et al.*, 1985). There is probably a threshold to this process as normal bile contains an inhibitor of β-glucuronidase (Godfrey *et al.*, 1981). Cholelithiasis is not normally observed in preclinical studies but an increase in gall stones has been reported in patients treated with clofibrate (Committee of Principal Investigators, 1978).

The normal cause of intrahepatic biliary obstruction in experimental animals is damage to bile duct lining cells. Compounds causing such damage have been considered earlier. There are, however, a few materials which appear to cause intrahepatic obstruction by a distinctive mechanism. In geeldikkop, a photosensitizing disease of sheep in South Africa that results from an interaction between sporidesmin and a component of *Tribulus terrestis*, the bile duct becomes blocked with crystalline material of unknown composition (Kelly, 1985). Similar crystals have been observed in sheep intoxicated by other phytotoxins. It has been suggested that the spontaneous bile duct proliferation observed in some strains of ageing mice may also be associated with obstruction by a crystalloid material (Lewis, 1984). Treatment of rats with benzofuran also causes symptoms of intrahepatic cholestasis but, in this case, there is no evidence of damage to the bile duct (Connelly, 1988). At autopsy gross dilation of the extrahepatic bile duct was noted and it would appear possible that spasm of the sphincter of Oddi may play a role in inducing cholestasis with this material.

Whereas intrahepatic obstructive jaundice is a relatively minor problem in experimental animals, it is a major problem in clinical practice (Read, 1985). The response to phenothiazines is typical of this lesion. The response is confined to a small minority of patients who may show marked hypersensitivity. Patients affected are jaundiced and liver biopsies show portal tract inflammation, sometimes with a high eosinophil content, and some damage to hepatocytes. An immunological mechanism has long been suspected but cannot be proven. It is of interest that bile duct lining cells are a major target in autoimmune disease and that, following liver transplantation, the bile ducts are especially liable to rejection (Welsh and Male, 1989). Investigation of these conditions has been hampered by the fact that, even after immunological manipulation, it has proved impossible to reproduce the condition in experimental animals.

As mentioned earlier, the formation of bile is a complex process and it is, therefore, not surprising that there are many classes of compound that induce intrahepatic cholestasis by interference with bile secretion (Oelberg and Lester, 1986; Kukongviriyapan and Stacey, 1991; Plaa, 1991). The classic agents, in this case, are anabolic and contraceptive steroids. The mechanism of action of these compounds remains obscure. There is a lag phase of approximately 12 hours before the establishment of cholestasis. There are some indications for both interference in the uptake of bile acids into hepatocytes and for alterations in membranes which might affect tight junction structure. It remains unclear how far the mechanism of cholestasis by steroids correlates with the mechanism of cholestasis by D-ring glucuronide conjugates of oestrogens or testosterone. Unlike the parent steroids, the effect of these compounds is immediate and clearly dose-dependent. In this case there is evidence for a direct competition with bile acids at the bile canalicular plasma membrane.

In addition to steroids and their glucuronides many other classes of compound induce cholestasis at the canalicular level. The monohydroxy bile acid lithocholate is cholestatic, probably after conjugation with taurine. Studies show that taurolithocholate inhibits taurocholate uptake into hepatocytes but cytological examination of the livers of treated animals shows dilation of the Golgi apparatus and loss of microvilli from bile canaliculi which would appear to be independent events. The reason why the immunosuppressive drug cyclosporin A can induce cholestasis is equally obscure. Cholestasis following the intake of manganese is observed in both humans and experimental animals. It has been demonstrated that the mechanism requires interaction of manganese and bilirubin at the bile canalicular membrane but why, given that bilirubin excretion is responsible for only a tiny proportion of bile flow, this should result in cholestasis remains obscure.

The compounds mentioned in the last few paragraphs are only a small proportion of those capable of causing cholestasis through their action on hepatocytes. As the compounds described are 'the best understood' it will be clear how limited is our present knowledge of the mechanisms of

cholestasis at the canalicular level, despite the availability of animal models. It is to be hoped that the development of *in vitro* techniques such as the use of hepatocyte doublets and microanalytical techniques may assist solution of these problems in the future.

The reduction of bile flow is a serious toxicological problem but an increase in bile flow (choleresis) is without any serious consequences. Passage of water into bile appears to occur by passive diffusion across the tight junctions between hepatocytes. Normally this is governed by the rate of secretion of bile acids and bile salts. The administration of large doses of compounds whose metabolites are excreted into bile will result in an increase in bile flow and, often, dilation of bile canaliculi. On their own, these are changes without long-term implications.

Acknowledgements

The authors are grateful to Professor L. J. King, Dr S. Cottrell, Dr C. Ioannides, Dr D. Lewis and Dr J. Fowler for advice on specialized points and to Dr S. C. Price, Dr S. Singh and Miss D. Chescoe for provision of electron micrographs.

REFERENCES

Abraham, R., Golberg, L. and Grasso, P. (1967). Hepatic response to lysosomal effects of hypoxia, neutral red and chloroquine. *Nature (Lond.)*, **5097**, 194–196

Abraham, R., Golberg, L. and Coulster, F. (1972). Uptake and storage of degraded carageenan in lysosomes of the reticulo endothelial cells of the rhesus monkey *Macaca mulatta*. *Exp. Mol. Pathol.*, **17**, 77–93

Ahmed, R. S., Price, S. C., Grasso, P. and Hinton, R. H. (1990). Hepatic nuclear and cytoplasmic effects following intermittent feeding of rats with di(2-ethylhexyl)phthalate. *Food Chem. Toxicol.*, **28**, 427–434

Albores-Medina, A. Vebrian, M. E., Bach, P. H., Connelly, J. C., Hinton, R. H. and Bridges, J. W. (1989). Sodium arsenite induced alterations in bilirubin excreteion and heme metabolism. *J. Biochem. Toxicol.*, **4**, 73–78

Ambrose, A. M., Deeds, F. and Rather, L. J. (1949). Toxicity of thioacetamide in rats. *J. Ind. Hyg. Toxicol.*, **31**, 158–161

Ames, B. N., Magraw, R. and Gold, L. S. (1987). Ranking possible carcinogenic hazards. *Science*, **236**, 271–280

Anderson, M., Stanley, L., Devereux, T., Reynolds,

S. and Maronpot, R. (1992). Oncogenes in mouse liver tumours. In Klein-Szanto, A. J. P., Anderson, M. W., Barrett, J. C. and Slaga, T. J. (Eds), *Comparative Molecular Carcinogenesis*. Wiley-Liss, New York, pp. 187–201

Andrews, L. S. and Snyder, R. (1991). Toxic effects of solvents and vapors. In Amdur, M., Doull, J. and Klaassen, C. D. (Eds), *Casarett and Doull's Toxicology*. Pergamon Press, New York, pp. 681–722

Arvela, P. (1979). Toxicity of the rare earths. *Prog. Pharmacol.*, **2**, 69–114

Ashby, J. and Tennant, R. W. (1988). Chemical structure, *Salmonella* mutagenicity and extent of carcinogenicity as indicators of genotoxic carcinogenesis among 22 chemicals tested in rodents by the U.S. NCI//NTP. *Mutation Res.*, **204**, 17–115

Ashby, J., Tennant, R. W., Zeiger, E. and Stasiewicz, S. (1989). Classification according to chemical structure, mutagenicity to Salmonella and level of carcinogenicity of a further 42 chemicals tested for carcinogenicity by the U.S. National Toxicology program. *Mutation Res.*, **223**, 73–103

Ashworth, C. I., Saunders, E. and Arnold, N. (1961). Hepatic lipids, fine structural changes in the liver cells after high fat, high cholesterol and choline deficient diets in rats. *Am. Med. Assoc. Arch. Pathol.*, **72**, 625–636

Barnes, J. M. and Magee, P. N. (1958). The biliary and hepatic lesion produced experimentally by dibutyltin salts. *J. Path. Bacteriol.*, **75**, 267–279

Bartsch, I. K., O'Neill, I. K. and Schulte-Hermann, R. (1987) (Eds). The relevance of N-nitroso compounds to human cancer: exposure and mechanisms. International Agency for Research in Cancer, Lyon

Belanger, P. M. (1988). Chronobiological variation in the hepatic elimination of drugs and toxic chemical agents. *Ann. Rev. Chronobiology*, **4**, 1–46

Bentley, P., Bieri, F., Mitchell, F. E., Wlachter, F. and Staubli, W. (1987). Investigation on the mechanism of liver tumour induction by peroxisome proliferators *Arch. Toxicol.*, **10** (Suppl.), 157–161

Bloomer, J. R. (1988). The liver in protoporphyria. *Hepatology*, **8**, 402–407

Borges, T., Glauert, H. P. and Robertson, L. W. (1993). Perfluorodecanoic acid noncompetitively inhibits the peroxisomal enzymes enoyl-CoA hydratase and 3-hydroxyacyl-CoA dehydrogenase. *Toxicol. Appl. Pharmacol.*, **118**, 8–15

Bouma, J. M. W. and Smit, M. J. (1989). Gadolinium chloride selectively blocks endocytosis by Kupffer cells. In Wisse, E., Knook, D. L. and Decker, K. (Eds), *Cells of the Hepatic Sinusoid*, vol. 2. Kupffer Cell Foundation, Amsterdam, pp. 132–133

Brouwer, A., Wisse, E. and Knook, D. L. (1988). Sinusoidal endothelial and perisinusoidal fat storing cells. In Arias, I. M., Jakoby, W. B., Popper, H., Schachter, D. and Shafritz, D. A. (Eds), *The Liver, Biology and Pathobiology*, 2nd edn. Raven Press, New York, pp. 665–682

Bucher, N. L. R. and Malt, R. A. (1971). *Regeneration of Liver and Kidney*, Little Brown & Co., Boston

Busby, W. F. and Wogan, G. K. (1984). Aflatoxin. In Searl, C. E. (Ed.), *Chemical Carcinogens*, 2nd edn. American Chemical Society, Washington, p. 974

Butterworth, B. E., Slaga, T. J., Farland, W. and McClain, M. (Eds) (1991). Chemically induced cell proliferation: implications for risk assessment. Wiley-Liss, New York

Buyssens, N. (1962). La proliferation des canaux bilaires et la formation de structures tubulaires au cours des affections hepatiques en pathologie humaine et expèrimentale. *Rev. Belge Pathol. Med. Exptl.*, **29**, 1–115

Byron, W. R., Bierbower, G. W., Brower, J. B. and Hansen, W. H. (1967). Pathologic changes in rats and dogs from two year feeding of sodium arsenite or sodium arsenate. *Toxicol. Appl. Pharmacol.*, **10**, 132–147

Carpenter-Deyo, L., Marchand, D. H., Jean, P. A., Roth, R. A. and Reed, D. J. (1991). Involvement of glutathione in 1-naphthylisothiocynanate (ANIT) metabolism and toxicity to isolated hepatocytes. *Biochem. Pharmacol.*, **42**, 2171–2180

Cattley, R. C., Conway, J. G. and Popp, J. A. (1987). Association of persistent peroxisome proliferation and oxidative injury with hepatocarcinogenicity in female F344 rats fed di(2-ethylhexyl)phthalate for 2 years. *Cancer Lett.*, **38**, 15–22

Cheney, K. E., Liu, R. K., Smith, G. S., Meredith, P. J., Mickey, M. R. and Walford, R. L. (1983). The effect of dietary restriction of varying duration on survival, tumor patterns, immune function and body temperature in B10C3F1 mice. *J. Gerontol.*, **38**, 420–430

Chvedoff, M., Faccini, J. M., Gregory, M. H., Hull, R. M., Monro, A. M., Perraud, J., Quinton, R. M. and Reinert, H. H. (1984). The toxicology of the schistosomicidal agent oxamniquine. *Drug Dev. Res.*, **4**, 229–235

Cohen, A. J. and Grasso, P. (1981). Review of the hepatic response to hypolipidaemic drugs in rodents and assessment of its toxicological significance to man. *Food Cosmet. Toxicol.*, **19**, 585–605

Cohen, S. M. and Ellwein, L. B. (1991). Genetic errors, cell proliferation and carcinogenesis. *Cancer Res.*, **51**, 6493–6505

Committee of Principal Investigators (1978). Cooperative trial in the primary prevention of ischaemic heart disease using clofibrate. *Br. Heart J.*, **40**, 1069–1118

Connelly, J. C. (1988). *The toxicity of some oxygen heterocycles*, PhD Thesis, University of Surrey

Connolly, A. K., Price, S. C., Connelly, J. C. and Hinton, R. H. (1988a). Early changes in bile duct lining cells and hepatocytes in rats treated with a-naphthylisothiocyanate. *Toxicol. Appl. Pharmacol.*, **93**, 208–219

Connolly, A. K., Price, S. C., Stevenson, D., Connelly, J. C. and Hinton, R. H. (1988b). Factors influencing the toxicity of alpha-naphthylisothiocyanate towards bile duct lining cells. In Guillouzo, A. (Ed.), *Liver Cells and Drugs*. Colloque INSERM/ John Libby Eurotext, pp. 191–196

Copple, D. M., Rush, G. F. and Richardson, F. C. (1992). Effects of methapyrilene measured in mitochondria isolated from naive and metapyrilene-treated rat and mouse hepatocytes. *Toxicol. App. Pharmacol.*, **116**, 10–16

Crampton, R. F., Gray, T. J. B., Grasso, P. and Parke, D. V. P. (1977). Long-term studies on chemically induced liver enlargement in the rat. II. Transient induction of microsomal enzymes leading to liver damage and nodular hyperplasia produced by safrole and Ponceau MX. *Toxicology*, **7**, 307–326

Cunningham, M. L., Foley, J., Marnpot, R. R. and Matthews, H. B. (1991). Correlation of hepatocellular proliferation with hepatocarcinogenecity induced by the mutagenic noncarcinogen:carcinogen pair— 2,6 and 2,4 diaminotoluene. *Toxicol. Appl. Pharmcol.*, **107**, 562–567

Deboyser, D., Goethals, F., Krack, G. and Robertfroid, M. (1989). Investigation into the mechanism of tetracycline-induced steatosis: study in isolated hepatocytes. *Toxicol. Appl. Pharmacol.*, **97**, 473–479

De Matteis, F., Gibbs, A. H. and Holley, A. E. (1987). Occurrence and biological properties of N-methyl protoporphyrin. *Ann. N.Y. Acad. Sci.*, **514**, 30–40

Dijkhuis, F. W. J., Jonker, A. M., Koudstaal, J. and Hardonck, M. J. (1989). In Wisse, E., Knook, D. I. and Decker, K. (Eds), *Cells of the Hepatic Sinusoid*, vol. 2. Kupffer Cell Foundation, Rijswijk, pp. 76–79

Doljanski, L. and Rosin, A. (1944). Studies on the early changes in the livers of rats treated with various toxic agents with especial reference to the vascular lesions. 1. The histology of the rat's liver in urethane poisoning. *Am. J. Pathol.*, **20**, 945–959

du Bois, A. M. (1954). Actions de l'intoxication alloxanique sur la foie de cobaye. *Z. Zellforsch. Mikroskop. Anat.*, **40**, 485–604

Eason, C. T., Clark, B., Smith, D. A. and Parke, D. V. (1982). The mechanism of hepatotoxicity of a chromone carboxylic acid (PPL 52757) in the dog. *Xenobiotica*, **12**, 155–164

ECETOC (1992). *Peroxisome Proliferators*, ECETOC, Brussels

Erlinger, S. (1988). Bile flow. In Arias, I. M., Jakoby, W. B., Popper, H., Schachter, D. and Shafritz, D. A. (Eds), *The Liver, Biology and Pathobiology*, 2nd edn. Raven Press, New York, pp. 553–572

Eschenbrenner, A. B. and Miller, E. (1945). Induction of hepatomas in mice by repeated oral administration of chloroform with observations on sex differences. *J. Natl. Cancer Inst.*, **5**, 251–260

Evans, J. G., Appleby, E. C., Lake, B. G. and Conning, D. M. (1989). Studies on the induction of cholangiofibrosis by coumarin in the rat. *Toxicology*, **55**, 207–224

Farber, E. (1963). Ethionine carcinogenesis. *Adv. Cancer Res.*, **7**, 383–474

Farquehar, M. G. and Palade, G. E. (1981). The Golgi apparatus (1954–1981)—from artefact to centre stage. *J. Cell Biol.*, **91**, 77s–103s

Fausto, N. (1990). Oval cells and liver carcinogenesis: an analysis of cell lineages using oncogene transfection techniques. In *Mouse Liver Carcinogenesis: Mechanisms and Species Comparisons*. Alan R. Liss, New York, pp. 325–334

Fausto, N., Thompson, N. L. and Braun, L. (1987). Purification and culture of oval cells from rat liver. In Pretlow, T. G. II and Pretlow, T. P. (Eds), *Cell Separation: Methods and Selected Applications*. Academic Press, New York, pp. 45–77

Feuers, R. J. and Scheving, L. E. (1988). Chronobiology of hepatic enzymes. *Ann. Rev. Chronobiol.*, **4**, 209–256

Fishbein, L. (1978). Selenium. In Fishbein, L., Furst, A. and Mehlman, M. A. (Eds), *Advances in Modern Environmental Toxicology*, vol. *11, Genotoxic and Carcinogenic Metals: Environmental and Occupational Occurrence and Exposure*. Princeton Scientific Publishing, Princeton, NJ, pp. 31–59

Fowler, B. A., Woods, J. S. and Schiller, C. M. (1977). Ultrastructural and biochemical effects of prolonged oral arsenic exposure on liver mitochondria in rats. *Environ. Health Perspect.*, **19**, 197–204

Friedman, M. I. (1982). Hepatic nerve function. In Arias, I., Popper, A. H., Schachter, D. and Shafritz, D. A. (Eds), *The Liver, Biology and Pathobiology*. Raven Press, New York, pp. 663–673

Ghadially, F. N. (1982). *Ultrastructural Pathology of the Cell and Matrix*, 2nd edn. Butterworth, London

Ghosal, A. K., Rushmore, T. H. and Farber, E. (1987). Initiation of carcinogenesis by a dietary deficiency of choline in the absence of added carcinogens. *Cancer Lett.*, **37**, 289–296

Giachelli, C. M. and Omiecinski, C. J. (1987). Developmental regulation of cytochrome P450 genes in the rat. *Mol. Pharmacol.*, **31**, 477–484

Godfrey, P. P., Warner, M. J. and Coleman, R. (1981). Enzymes and proteins in bile: variations in output in rat cannula bile during and after depletion of the bile salt pool. *Biochem. J.*, **196**, 1116

Goldfarb, S., Singer, E. J. and Popper, H. (1962). Experimental cholangitis due to alpha-naphthyl isothiocyanate (ANIT). *Amer. J. Pathol.*, **40**, 685–698

Gopinath, C., Prentice, D. E. and Lewis, D. J. (1987). *Atlas of Experimental Toxicological Pathology*. MTP Press, Lancaster

Gordon, H. A. (1959). Morphological and physiological characterisation of germfree life. *Ann. N.Y. Acad. Sci.*, **78**, 208–220

Grasso, P. and Gray, T. J. B. (1977). Long-term studies on chemically-induced liver enlargement in the rat. III. Structure and behaviour of the hepatic nodular lesions induced by Ponceau MX. *Toxicology*, **7**, 327–342

Grasso, P. and Hinton, R. H. (1991). Evidence for and possible mechanisms of non-genotoxic carcinogenesis in rodent liver. *Mutation Res.*, **248**, 271–290

Grasso, P., Sharratt, M. and Cohen, A. J. (1991). Role of persistent, non-genotoxic tissue damage in rodent cancer and relevance to humans. *Ann. Rev. Pharmacol. Toxicol.*, **31**, 253–287

Greaves, P. (1990). *Histopathology of Preclinical Toxicity Studies*. Elsevier, Amsterdam

Green, S. (1993). The molecular mechanisms of peroxisome proliferator action. In Gibson, G. G. and Lake, B. (Eds), *Peroxisomes: Biology and Importance in Toxicology and Medicine*. Taylor and Francis (in the press)

Gregory, M., Monro, A., Quinton, M. and Woolhouse, N. (1983). The acute toxicity of axamniquine in rats, sex-dependent hepatotoxicity. *Arch. Toxicol.*, **54**, 247–255

Grice, H. C. and Burek, J. D. (1984). Age-associated (geriatric) pathology. In *Current Issues in Toxicology*. Springer Verlag, Berlin, pp. 57–107

Haenni, B. (1964). Les effets de l'intoxication aigüe au formate d'allyl. *Pathol. Microbiol.*, **27**, 974

Ham, A. W. (1974). *Histology* 7th edn, J. B. Lippincott, Philadelphia and Toronto

Ham, D. H. (1986). Metallothioneins. *Ann. Rev. Biochem.*, **55**, 913–951

Heaton, K. W. (1985). Bile salts. In Wright, R., Millward-Sadler, G. H., Alberti, K. G. M. M. and Karran, S. (Eds), *Liver and Biliary Disease: Pathophysiology, Diagnosis, Management*, 2nd edn. Bailliere Tindall, London, pp. 277–299

Hildebrand, B., Ashby, J., Grasso, P., Sharatt, M., Bontinck, W. J. and Smith, E. (Eds) (1991). Early indicators of non-genotoxic carcinogenesis. *Mutation Res.*, **248**, 211–376

Hinton, R. H., Mitchell, F. E., Mann, A., Chescoe, D., Price, S. C., Nunn, A., Grasso, P. and Bridges, J. W. (1986). Effects of phthalic acid esters on the liver and thyroid. *Environ. Health Perspect.*, **70**, 195–210

Hinton, R. H., Price, S. C., MacFarlane, M., Cottrell, S., Bremmer, J. H., Bomhardt, E. M. and Grasso, P. (1990). Effects of butylated hydroxytoluene administered prior to and during pregnancy and lactation in adult and neonatal rats. *Toxicologist*, **10**, 297

Hogberg, J. and Alexander, J. (1986). Selenium. In Handbook on the toxicology of the metals (Friberg, L., Nordberg, G. F. and Vouk, V. B. eds), 2nd edn., Vol. 2, Elsevier, Amsterdam, pp. 482–520

Horky, J., Grasso, P. and Goldberg, L. (1971). Influence of phenobarbital on histological and biochemical changes in experimental intrahepatic cholestasis. Exp. Path. Bd. 5, 200–211

IARC (1975). Selenium and selenium compounds. In *IARC monographs on the evaluation of carcinogenic risk of chemicals to man*, vol. 9. IARC, Lyon, pp. 245–260

IARC (1979a). Some halogenated hydrocarbons. *IARC monographs on the evaluation of carcinogenic risk of chemicals to man*, vol. 20. IARC, Lyon

IARC (1979b). Sex hormones. *IARC monographs on the evaluation of carcinogenic risk of chemicals to man*, vol. 21, IARC, Lyon

IARC (1982). Some aromatic amines, anthraquinones and nitroso compounds and inorganic fluorides used in drinking water and dental preparations. *IARC monographs on the evaluation of carcinogenic risk of chemicals to man*, vol. 27. IARC, Lyon

IARC (1987). In *IARC monographs on the evaluation of carcinogenic risk of chemicals to man*, Suppl. 7. IARC, Lyon, pp. 272–310

Inai, K., Kobuke, T., Nambu, S., Takemoto, T., Kou, E., Nishina, H., Fulihara, M., Yomehara, S., Suehiro, S., Tsuya, T., Horiuchi, K. and Tokuoka, S. (1988). Hepatocellular tumorigenicity of butylated hydroxytoluene administered orally to B6C3F1 mice. *Japn. J. Cancer Res.*, **79**, 59–58

Ioannides, C. and Parke, D. V. (1990). The cytochrome P450 I gene family of microsomal hemoproteins and their role in the metabolic activation of chemicals. *Drug Metab. Rev.*, **22**, 1–86

Ishinishi, N., Tomita, M. and Hisanaga, A. (1980). Study in chronic toxicity of arsenic trioxide with special reference to the liver damage. *Fukuoka Iyaku Zasshi*, **71**, 27–40

Jirtle, R. I., Meyer, S. A. and Brockenbrough, J. S. (1991). Liver tumour promoter phenobarbital: a biphasic modulator of hepatocyte proliferation. In Butterworth, B. E., Slaga, T. J., Farland, W. and McClain, M. (Eds), *Chemically Induced Cell Proliferation: Implications for Risk Assessment*. Wiley-Liss, New York, pp. 209–216

Johnston, D. G. and Alberti, K. G. M. M. (1985). The liver and endocrine function. In Wright, R., Millward-Sadler, G. H., Alberti, K. G. M. M. and Karran, S. (Eds), *Liver and Biliary Disease: Pathophysiology, Diagnosis, Management*, 2nd edn. Baillière Tindall, London, pp. 161–188

Johnston, I. R., Mathias, A. P., Pennington, I. and Ridge, D. (1968). The fractionation of nuclei from mammalian liver by zonal centrifugation. *Biochem. J.*, **109**, 127–135

Jones, A. L., Schmcuker, D. L., Renston, R. H. and Murakami, T. (1980). The architecture of bile secretion: a morphological perspective of physiology. *Dig. Dis. Sci.*, **25**, 609–629

Kanz, M. F., Kaphalia, L., Kaphalia, B., Romagnoli, E. and Nsari, G. A. S. (1992). Methylene dianiline: acute toxicity and effects on biliary function. *Toxicol. Appl. Pharmacol.*, **117**, 88–97

Karran, S. and McLaren, M. (1985). Physical aspects of hepatic regeneration. In Wright, R., Millward-Sadler, G. H., Alberti, K. G. M. M. and Karran, S. (Eds), *Liver and Biliary Disease: Pathophysiology, Diagnosis, Management*, 2nd edn. Baillière Tindall, London, pp. 233–250

Karran, S., Lane, R. H. S., Townend, I. and de la Hunt, M. (1985). Calculous disease and cholecystitis. In, Wright, R., Millward-Sadler, G. H., Alberti, K. G. M. M. and Karran, S. (Eds), *Liver and Biliary Diseas: Pathophysiology, Diagnosis, Management*, 2nd edn. Baillière Tindall, London, pp. 1433–1462

Kelly, W. R. (1985). The liver and biliary system. In Jubb, K. V. F., Kennedy, P. C. and Palmer, N. (Eds), Pathology of domestic animals, 3rd edn. Academic Press, Orlando, pp. 239–312

Kelly, J., Price, S. C. and Hinton, R. H. (1991). Development of bile duct proliferation in rats treated with alphanaphthylisothiocyanate. *Hum. Exp. Toxicol.*, **10**, 498–499

King, C. M., Romano, L. J. and Schuetzle, D. (Eds) (1988). *Carcinogenic and Mutagenic Responses to Aromatic Amines and Nitroarenes*. Elsevier, New York

Klaasen, C. D. and Watkins, J. B. (1984). Mechanisms of bile formation, hepatic uptake and biliary excretion. *Pharmacol. Rev.*, **36**, 1–67

Klatskin, G. (1977). Hepatic granulomata, problems in interpretation. *Mt. Sinai J. Med.*, **44**, 798–812

Klaunig, J. E., Ruch, R. J. and Pereira, M. A. (1986). Carcinogenicity of chlorinated methane and ethane compounds administered in drinking water to mice. *Environ. Health Perspect.*, **69**, 89–96

Kohli, K. K., Gupta, B. N., Albro, P. W., Mukhtar, H. and McKinney, J. D. (1979). Biochemical effects of pure isomers of hexachlorobiphenyl: fatty livers and cell structure. *Chem. Biol. Interac.*, **25**, 139–156

Korpassy, B. (1961). Tannins as hepatic carcinogens. *Progr. Exptl. Tumor Res.*, **2**, 245–290

Kukongviriyapan, V. and Stacey, N. H. (1991). Chemical induced interference with hepatocellular transport, role in cholestasis. *Chem. Biol. Interac.*, **77**, 245–261

Kushner, I. (1982). The phenomenon of the acute phase response. *Ann. N.Y. Acad. Sci.*, **389**, 39–48

Lalwani, N. D., Reddy, M. K., Ghosh, S., Barnard, S. D., Molello, J. A. and Reddy, J. K. (1985). Induction of fatty acid ω-oxidation and peroxisome proliferations by DC–040, a new hypolipidaemic agent. *Biochem. Pharmacol.*, **34**, 3473–3482

Lander, J. J., Stanley, R. J., Sumner, H. W., Boswell, D. C. and Aach, R. D. (1975). Angiosarcoma of the liver associated with Fowler's solution. *Gastroenterology*, **68**, 1582–1586

Larson, J. L. and Bull, R. J. (1992a). Species differences in the metabolism of trichloroethylene to the carcinogenic metabolites trichloroacetate and dichloracetate. *Toxicol. Appl. Pharmacol.*, **115**, 278–283

Larson, J. L. and Bull, R. J. (1992b). Metabolism and lipoperoxidative activity of trichloroacetate and dichloroacetate in rats and mice. *Toxicol. Appl. Pharmacol.*, **115**, 268–277

Laskin, D. L. (1989). Potential role of activated macrophages in chemical and drug-induced injury. In Wisse, E., Knook, D. L. and Decker, K. (Eds),

Cells of the Hepatic Sinusoid, vol. 1. Kupffer Cell Foundation, Amsterdam, pp. 284–287

Lettvin, J. Y., Pickard, W. F., McGulloch, W. F. and Pitts, W. S. (1964). A theory of passive ion flux through axon membranes. *Nature*, **202**, 1338–1339

Lewis, D. F. V., Ioannides, C. and Parke, D. V. (1992). Validation of a novel molecular orbital approach (COMPACT) for the prospective safety evaluation of chemicals, by comparison with rodent carcinogenicity and *Salmonella* mutagenicity data as evaluated by the U.S. NCI/NTP. *Mutation Res.*

Lewis, D. F. V., Ioannides, C. and Parke, D. V. (1993). Quantitative structure activity relationships. (submitted for publication)

Lewis, D. J. (1984). Spontaneous lesions of the mouse biliary tract. *J. Comp. Pathol.* **94**, 263–271

Lijinsky, W. and Muschik, G. M. (1982). Distribution of the liver carcinogen mathapyrilene in Fischer rats and its interaction with macromolecules. *J. Cancer Res. Clin. Oncol.*, **103**, 69–73

Lum, P. Y., Walker, S. and Ioannides C. (1985). Foetal and neonatal development of cytochrome P450 and cytochrome P448 catalysed mixed function oxidase systems in the rat: induction by 3-methylcholanthrene. *Toxicology*, **35**, 307–317

McGee, J. O'D., Isaacson, P. G. and Wright, N. A. (1992). *Oxford Textbook of Pathology*. Oxford University Press, Oxford

McGuire, E. J., DiFonzo, C. J., Martin, R. A. and de la Iglesia, F. A. (1986). Evaluation of the chronic toxicity and carcinogenesis in rodents of the synthetic analgesic, tilidine fumarate. *Toxicology*, **39**, 149–163

MacSween, R. N. M. and Scothorne, R. J. (1987). Developmental anatomy and normal function. In MacSween, R. N. M., Anthony, P. P. and Scheuer, P. J. (Eds), *Pathology of the Liver*, 2nd edn. Churchill Livingstone, Edinburgh, pp. 1–45

Marie, S. and Cresteil, T. (1989). Phenobarbital-inducible gene expression in developing rat liver: relationship to hepatocyte function. *Biochem. Biophys. Acta*, **1009**, 221–228

Medline, A., Schaffner, F. and Popper, H. (1970). Ultrastructural features of galactosamine-induced hepatitis. *Exp. Mol. Pharmacol.*, **12**, 201–211

Meierhenry, E. F., Ruebner, B. H., Gershwin, M. E., Hsieh, L. S. and French, S. W. (1981). Mallory body formation in hepatic nodules of mice ingesting dieldrin. *Lab. Invest.*, **44**, 392–396

Meijer, J. and de Pierre, J. D. (1987). Hepatic levels of cytosolic, microsomal and 'mitochondrial' epoxide hydrolase and other drug meatbolising enzymes after treatment with xenobiotics and endogenous compounds. *Chem. Biol. Interac.*, **62**, 249–269

Meyer, J. S. and Hartoft, W. S. (1960). Hepatic lipid produced by hyperphagia in albino rats. Relationship to dietary choline and casein. *Am. J. Path.*, **36**, 365–381

Michalopoulos, G. (1991). Control of hepatocyte proliferation in regeneration and augmentative hepatomegaly and neoplasia. In Butterworth, B. E., Slaga, Mich T. J., Farland, W. and McClain, M. (Eds), *Chemically Induced Cell Proliferation: Implications for Risk Assessment*. Wiley-Liss, New York, pp. 227–236

Mikol, Y. B., Hoover, K. L., Creasia, D. and Poirier, L. A. (1983). Hepatocarcinogenesis in rats fed methyl-deficient, amino acid defined diets. *Carcinogenesis*, **4**, 1619–1629

Milton, M. N., Elcombe, C. R. and Gibson, G. G. (1990). On the mechanism of induction of cytochrome P450IVA1 and peroxisome proliferation in rat liver by clofibrate. *Biochem. Pharmacol.*, **40**, 2727–2732

Mitchell, F. E., Bridges, J. W. and Hinton, R. H. (1986). Effects of mono(2-ethylhexyl)phthalate and its straight chain analogues mono-n-hexyl phthalate and mono-n-octyl phthalate on lipid metabolism in isolated hepatocytes. *Biochem. Pharmacol.*, **35**, 2941–2947

Mitchell, F. E., Price, S. C., Hinton, R. H., Grasso, P. and Bridges, J. W. (1985). Time and dose response study of the effects of rats of the plasticiser di(2-ethylhexyl)phthalate. *Toxicol. Appl. Pharmacol.*, **81**, 371–392

Mompon, P., Greaves, P., Irisarri, E., Monro, A. M. and Bridges, J. W. (1987). A cytochemical study of the livers of rats treated with diethylnitrosamine/phenobarbital, with benzidine/phenobarbital, with phenobarbital or with clofibrate. *Toxicology*, **46**, 217–236

Moore, M. A. S. and Johnson, G. R. (1976). Hemopoietic stem cells during embryonic development and growth. In Cairnie, A. B., Lala, P. K. and Osmond, D. G. (Eds), *Stem Cells of Renewing Cell Populations*. Academic Press, New York

Mori, M. (1983). Ultrasstructural changes of hepatocyte organelles induced by chemicals and their relationship to fat accumulation in the liver. *Acta Pathol. Jpn.*, **33**, 911–922

Mortimer, P. H. (1963). The experimental intoxication of sheep with sporidesmin, a metabolic product of *Pithomyces chartarum*. IV. Histological and histochemical examinations or orally-dosed sheep. *Res. Vet. Sci.*, **4**, 166–185

Moslen, M. T., Ahluwalia, M. B. and Farber, E. (1985). 1,2-Dibromoethane initiation of hepatic nodules in Sprague-Dawley rats selected with Solt-Farber system. *Arch. Toxicol.*, **58**, 118–119

Mote, P. L., Grizzle, J. M., Walford, R. L. and Spindler, S. R. (1990). Age related down regulation of hepatic cyctochrome P1–450, P2–450, catalase and CuZn-superoxide dismutase RNA. *Mech. Age. Devel.*, **53**, 101–110

Mullock, B. M., Hall, D. E., Shaw, L. J. and Hinton, R. H. (1983). Immune responses to chlorpromazine in rats – detection and relation to hepatotoxicity. *Biochem. Pharmacol.*, **32**, 2733–2738

Nebert, D. W. and Gonzalez, F. E. (1987). P450 genes, structure, evaluation and regulation. *Ann. Rev. Biochem.*, **56**, 945–993

Nishikawa, S., Hara, T., Miyazaki, E. and Ohkuro, T. (1984). Studies on the safety of KW–1414: acute toxicity in mice and rats and oral subacute and chronic toxicity studies in rats. *Clin. Report*, **18**, 281–305

Oelberg, D. G. and Lester, R. (1986). Cellular mechanisms of cholestasis. *Ann. Rev. Med.*, **37**, 297–317

Ohtani, O. (1979). The peribiliary portal system in the rabbit liver. *Arch. Histol. Jpn.*, **42**, 153–167

Okazaki, K., Shull, K. H. and Farber, E. (1968). Effects of ethionine on adenosine triphosphate levels and ionic composition of liver cell nuclei. *J. Biol. Chem.*, **243**, 4661–4666

Olson, M. J., Handler, J. F. and Thurman, R. G. (1987). Mechanism of zone-specific hepatic steatosis caused by valproate: inhibition of ketogenesis in periportal regions of liver lobule. *Mol. Pharmacol.*, **30**, 520–525

Omiecinski, C. J., Hassett, C. and Costa, P. (1990). Developmental expression and *in situ* localization of the phenobarbital inducible hepatic mRNAs for cytochromes CYP2B1, CYP2B2, CYP2C6 and CYP3A1. *Mol. Pharmacol.*, **38**, 462–470

O'Neill, I. K., Chen, J. and Bartsch, H. (1991). *Relevance to human cancer of N-nitroso compounds, tobacco smoke and mycotoxins*. International Agency of Research on Cancer, Lyon

Panner, B. J. and Packer, J. T. (1961). Hepatic alterations in rats fed 1,2 dihydro-2,2,4-trimethylquinoline, Flectol H. *Proc. Soc. Exptl. Biol. Med.*, **106**, 16–19

Pitot, H. C. (1990). Altered hepatic foci: their role in murine hepatocarcinogenesis. *Ann. Rev. Pharmacol. Toxicol.*, **30**, 465–500

Plaa, G. L. (1991). Toxic responses of the liver. In Amdur, M., Doull, J. and Klaassen, C. D. (Eds), *Casarett and Doull's Toxicology*. Pergamon Press, New York, pp. 334–353

Plaa, G. L. and Priestley, B. G. (1976). Intrahepatic cholestasis induced by drugs and chemicals. *Pharmacol. Rev.*, **28**, 207–273

Pollard, M. and Luckert, P. H. (1989). Spontaneous diseases in aging Lobund-Wistar rats. In Snyder, D. L. (Ed.), *Dietary Restriction and Aging*. Alan R. Liss, New York, pp. 51–60

Powell, C., Connelly, J. C., Jones, S. M., Grasso, P. and Bridges, J. W. (1986). Hepatic responses to the administration of high doses of BHT to the rat: their relevance to hepatocarcinogenicity. *Fd. Chem. Toxicol.*, **24**, 1331–1143

Powell, L. W. (1985). Haemochromatosis and related iron storage diseases. In Wright, R., Millward-Sadler, G. H., Alberti, K. G. M. M. and Karran, (EDs), *Liver and Biliary Diseas, Pathophysiology, Diagnosis, Management*. Baillière Tindall, London, pp. 963–982

Price, S. C. (1985). Mechanisms of toxicity of the hypolipidaemic compounds. PhD Thesis, University of Surrey

Price, S. C., Hall, D. E. and Hinton, R. H. (1985). Peroxisome proliferation does not follow lipid accumulation in the livers of chlorpromazine-treated rats. *Toxicol. Lett.*, **25**, 11–18

Price, S. C., Hinton, R. H., Mitchell, F. E., Hall, D. E., Grasso, P., Blane, G. F. and Bridges, J. W. (1986). Time and dose study on the response of rats to the hypolipidaemic drug fenofibrate. *Toxicology*, **41**, 169–191

Przybocki, J. M., Reuhl, K. R., Thurman, R. G. and Kauffman, F. C. (1992). Involvement of nonparenchymal cells in oxygen-dependent hepatic injury by allyl alcohol. *Toxicol. Appl. Pharmacol.*, **115**, 57–63

Rao, M. S., Lalwani, N. D., Scarpelli, D. G. and Reddy, J. K. (1982). The absence of gamma-glutamyl transpeptidase activity in putative preneoplastic lesions in hepatocellular carcinoma induced in rats by the hypolipidaemic peroxsisome proliferator Wy–14,643. *Carcinogenesis*, **3**, 1231–1233

Read, A. E. (1985). The liver and drugs. In Wright, R., Millward-Sadler, G. H., Alberti, K. G. M. M. and Karran, S. (Eds), *Liver and Biliary Disease: Pathophysiology, Diagnosis, Management.* Baillière Tindall, London, pp. 1003–1032

Reddy, J. K. and Lalwani, N. D. (1984). Carcinogenesis by hepatic peroxisome proliferators—evaluation of the risk of hypolipidaemic drugs and industrial plasticisers to humans. *CRC Crit. Rev. Toxicol.*, **12**, 1–58

Reznic-Schuller, H. M. and Lijinsky, W. (1981). Morphology of early changes in liver carcinogenesis induced by methapyriline. *Arch. Toxicol.*, **49**, 79–83

Reznic-Schuller, H. M. and Lijinsky, W. (1982). Ultrastructural changes in the liver of animals treated with methapyrilene and some analogues. *Ecotoxicol. Environ. Safety*, **6**, 328–335

Rossi, L., Ravera, M., Repetti, I. and Santi, L. (1977). Long-term administration of DDT or phenobarbital sodium in Wistar rats. *Int. J. Cancer*, **19**, 179–185

Rouiller, Ch. (1964). Experimental toxic injury to the liver. In Rouiller, Ch. (Ed.), *The Liver, Morphology, Biochemistry, Physiology*, vol. 2. Academic Press, New York, pp. 335–476

Sato, K. (1989). Glutathione transferases as markers of preneoplasia and neoplasia. *Adv. Cancer Res.*, **52**, 205–255

Schmucker, D. L. and Wang, R. K. (1981). Effects of aging and phenobarbital on the rat liver drug-metabolising system. *Mech. Age. Devel.* **15**, 189–202

Schulte-Hermann, R. (1974). Induction of liver growth by xenobiotic compounds and other stimuli. *CRC Crit. Rev. Toxicol*, **3** 97–158

Seager, L.D. and Castelnuovo, G. (1947). Toxicity of 'Stilbamidine'. A study of the effects of chronic intoxication. *Am. Med. Assoc. Arch. Pathol*, **44**, 287–296

Shiojiri, N. (1984). The origin of intrahepatic bile duct lining cells in the mouse. *J. Embryol. Exp. Morphol.*, **79**, 25–39

Simon, G. and Rouiller, Ch. (1963). Les effets de l'intoxication aigüe à la thioacetamide sur la foie de rat. Etude au microscope electronique. Cited by Rouiller (1964)

Sipes, J. G., El Sisi, A. E., Simm, W. W. (1989) In Wisse, E., Knook, D. L. and Decker, K. (Eds), *Cells of the Hepatic Sinusoid*, vol. 2. Kupffer Cell Foundation, Amsterdam, pp. 91–93

Sipes, I. G. and Gandolfi, A. J. (1991). Biotransformation of toxicants. In Amdur, M. O., Doull, J. and Klaasen, C. D. (Eds), *Cassarett and Doull's Toxicology*, 4th edn. Pergamon Press, New York, pp. 88–126

Skilleter, D. N. (1987). Beryllium. In Fishbein, L., Furst, A. and Mehlman, M. A. (Eds). *Advances in Modern Environmental Toxicology*, vol. 11, *Genetoxic and Carcinogenic Metals: Environmental and Occupational Occurrence and Exposure*. Princeton, NJ, Princeton Scientific Publishing, pp. 61–86

Sternlieb, I. and Scheinberg, I. H. (1985). Wilson's disease. In Wright, R., Millward-Sadler, G. H., Alberti, K.G.M.M. and Karran (Eds), *Liver and Biliary Disease, Pathophysiology, Diagnosis, Management*. Baillière Tindall, London, pp. 949–961

Stokinger, H. E. (1981). The Metals. In Clayton, G. D. and Clayton, F. F. (Eds), *Patty's Industrial Hygiene and Toxicology*, 3rd edn, vol. 2A. Wiley Interscience, New York, pp. 1493–2060

Su, L.-C. (1982). A defect of biliary excretion of copper in copper laden Bedlington terriers. *Am. J. Physiol*, **243**, G231–G236

Swarm, R. L. (Conference chairman) (1967). Distribution, retention and late effects of thorium dioxide. *Ann. NY Acad. Sci.* **145**, 523–558

Tennekes, H. A., Wright, A. S. and Dix, K. M. (1979). The effect of dieldrin, diet and other environmental components on enzyme function and tumour incidence in the liver of CF-1 mice. *Arch. Toxicol.* Suppl. **2**. 197–212

Testai, E., Gemma, S. and Vittozzi, L. (1992). Bioactivation of chloroform in hepatic microsomes from rodent strains susceptible or resistant to CHC13 carcinogenicity. *Toxicol. Appl. Pharmacol*, **114**, 197–203

Tuchweber, B., Trost, W., Salas, M. and Sieck, R. (1976). Prevention of praesodymium-induced hepatoxicity by silbin. *Toxicol. Appl. Pharmacol*, **38**, 559–570

Van Bezooijen, C. F. A. (1984). Influence of age-related changes in rodent liver morphology and physiology on drug metabolism. A review. *Mech. Aging*, 1–22

Van Thiel, D. H. (1982) Endocrine Function in Arias, I., Popper, H., Schachter, D. and Shafritz, D. A. (Eds), *The Liver, Biology and Pathobiology*. Raven Press, New York, pp. 717–744

Vore, M. (1993). Canalicular transport: discovery of

ATP-dependent mechanisms. *Toxicol. Appl. Pharmacol*, **118**, 2–7

Wainfen, E., Dizik, M., Stender, M. and Christman, J. K. (1989). Rapid appearance of hypomethylated DNA in livers of rats fed cancer-promoting, methyl-deficient diets. *Cancer Res.* **49**, 4094–4097

Watts, R. W. E. (1986). *Lysosomal Storage Diseases, Biochemical and Clinical Aspects*. Taylor and Francis, London

Welsh, K. and Male, D. (1989). Transplantation and rejection. In Roitt, I., Brostofff, J. and Male, D. (Eds), *Immunology* 2nd edn. Gower Medical Publishing, London, pp. 24. 1–24.10

White, I. N. H., Mattocks, A. R. and Butler, W. H. (1973). The conversion of the pyrrolizidine alkaloid retrorsine to pyrrolic derivatives *in vivo* and *in vitro* and its acute toxicity to various animal species. *Chem. Biol. Interact.* **6**, 207–218

Williams, G. M. (1982). Sex hormones and liver cancer. *Lab. Invest*, **46**, 352–353

Williams, G. M., Mori, H. and McQueen, C. A. (1989). Structure activity relationships in the rat hepatocyte DNA-repair test for 300 chemicals. *Mutation Res.*, **221**, 263–286

Williams, G. M. and Weisburger, J. H. (1991) Chemical carcinogenesis. In Amdur, M., Doull, J. and Klaassen, C. D. (Eds), *Casarett and Doull's Toxicology*. Pergamon Press, New York, pp. 127–200

Williamson, D. H. (1980) Integration of metabolism in the tissues of the lactating rat. *FEBS Lett.*, **117**, K93–K105

Wisse, E., Geerts, A., Bouwens, L., van Bossuyt, H., Vanderkerken, K. and van Goethem, F. (1989). Cells of the hypatic sinusoid Anno 1988: an attempt to review the IVth International Kupffer cell symposium. In Wisse, E., Knook, D. I. and Decker, K. (Eds), *Cells of the Hepatic Sinusoid*, vol. 2. Kupffer Cell Foundation, Rijswijk, pp. 1–9

WHO (1988). *Environmental Health Criteria 80, Pyrrolizidine alkaloids*. World Health Organization, Geneva

WHO (1990). *Environmental Health Criteria, Tributyltin compounds*. World Health Organization, Geneva

Worker, N. P. (1960). Effect of injection of a hepatotoxin directly into the gall bladder of rabbits. *Nature*, **185**, 785–786

Yamamoto, K., Fisher, M. M. and Phillips, M. J. (1985). Hilar biliary plexus in human liver: a comparative study of the intrahepatic bile ducts in man and animals. *Lab. Invest.*, **52**, 103–106

Zerbe, O. and Gresner, A. M. (1988). Proliferation of fat-storing cells is stimulated by secretions of Kupffer cells from normal and injured liver. *Exp. Mol. Path.*, **49**, 87–101

Zimmerman, H. J. (1978). Hepatotoxicity, the adverse effects of drugs and other chemicals on the liver. Appleton Century Crofts, New York

FURTHER READING

Foa, V., Emmett, E. A., Maroni, M. and Colombi, A. (1987). Parts II and III. Biochemical indices of liver toxicity. In *Occupational and Environmental Chemical Hazards*. Ellis Horwood, Ltd., Chichester

Meeks, R. G., Harrison, S. D. and Bull, R. J. (1991). *Hepatotoxicology*. CRC Press, Boca Raton, Florida

Plaa, G. L. (1991). Toxic responses of the liver. *Casarett and Doull's Toxicology*. 4th edn. Pergamon Press, New York, pp. 334–354

27 Toxicology of the Pancreas

Joan M. Braganza

INTRODUCTION

The exocrine pancreas is a target for toxicity from oxygen free radicals as well as reactive intermediates from xenobiotics. The evidence suggests that this vulnerability may underlie all forms of acquired pancreatic disease and that differences in clinicopathological expression reflect variation in degree/duration of oxidative stress and the chemical species involved. This 'radical' departure from standard teaching (Howat and Sarles, 1979; Gyr et al., 1984; Go et al., 1986; Johnson, 1987; Case, 1990) requires an appreciation of evolutionary and anatomical links between pancreas and liver as well as an understanding of free radical biology and pathology (Braganza, 1991).

NORMAL PANCREAS

Evolution

Phylogeny

The human arrangement of the hepatopancreaticoduodenal complex is a relatively recent phylogenetic development compared with the primitive nature of drug metabolizing enzymes (Bridges, 1980) (Figure 1).

Embryology

The pancreas develops through two evaginations of the foregut during the fifth week of gestation: ventral, initially bilobed, from the lateral aspect of the hepatic bud; and dorsal. Duct systems appear in each outgrowth by the sixth week and open into the gut tube. By the next week the duodenum rotates to become a retroperitoneal organ. The two anlagen of the pancreas then fuse, so that the dorsal bud forms the bulk of the gland while the ventral bud forms the inferior aspect of the 'head' and the uncinate process. The duct of the larger dorsal bud (duct of Santorini) opens directly into the gut through a tiny orifice on the minor duodenal papilla; while, a fraction distally, the major papilla is the entry point for the bile

duct and duct of the ventral pancreas (duct of Wirsung). In 10–80 per cent of humans these two ducts may fuse into a common channel, the ampulla of Vater: smooth muscle surrounding the lower end of each duct and of the ampulla forms the sphincter of Oddi. During the seventh week of gestation the duct systems of the pancreas fuse and the section of dorsal duct between the site of fusion and the minor duodenal papilla usually withers away. In some 5 per cent of individuals fusion fails to occur and gland drainage relies largely on Santorini's duct. This condition, 'pancreas divisum', is recognizable by endoscopic retrograde cholangiopancreatography (ERCP).

Pancreatic acini—the secretory units—bud off the distalmost cells of the elongating duct system. A lobular arrangement is seen in the fourth month and acinar cells are functional a month later, as shown by abundant rough endoplasmic reticulum (RER) and zymogen (enzyme precursor) granules. Enzyme secretion begins in the 26th week of gestation to coincide with the emergence of the trypsinogen activator, enterokinase, in the duodenum. Endocrine cells of the pancreas also seem to originate from the duct system. They soon detach and adopt an islet arrangement.

Structure

Applied Anatomy

The human pancreas is a solid glandular organ, some 20 cm long and just under 100 g in weight. It lies deep in the upper abdomen, usually in a transverse plane at the level of the first lumbar vertebra. The 'head' of the gland abuts the medial aspect of the duodenum while its 'tail' abuts the splenic hilum. It is surrounded by a thin condensation of retroperitoneal connective tissue. The anterior surface of the 'head' is covered by the transverse colon and coils of small intestine. The stomach lies in front of the 'neck' and 'body' of the gland, separated by the lesser sac.

The pancreas is closely related to a number of

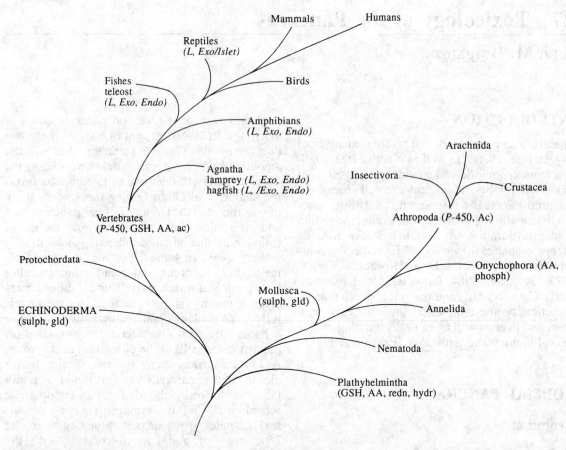

Figure 1 Phylogenetic tree to show that xenobiotic metabolizing enzymes were present in animals well before the different components of the hepato/exocrine/endocrine pancreas separated. Conjugating reactions: with GSH (glutathione), AA (amino acids), sulph (sulphate), glu (glucose) and gld (glucuronic acid). Primitive degradation reactions: redn (reduction) and hydr (hydrolysis). Drug-metabolizing enzymes: *P*-450 (cytochrome *P*-450 dependent), Ac (acetylation). L = liver, Exo = exocrine pancreas, Endo = endocrine pancreas, Islet = Islet arrangement. Source: reproduced with permission from Braganza, 1991

important blood vessels: behind it lie the aorta, inferior vena cava, superior mesenteric artery and portal vein; along its upper border are the hepatic and splenic arteries. Large vessels from the arteries contribute to the gland's high vascularity. Venous drainage is into the portal vein. Lymphatics on the surface of the pancreas lead into a complex system of lymph nodes. The pancreas has extrinsic and intrinsic innervation; the former consists of afferent and efferent parasympathetic fibers from the vagus nerves, as well as a network of sympathetic fibres.

Microanatomy

The traditional view was that acini (Latin 'acinus' = berry) were tagged to the duct system like grapes on a stem, but recent reconstruction studies show that, in fact, ductal and acinar elements divide dichotomously to form branched structures with anastomotic loops (Go *et al.*, 1986). A variable proportion of the gland's blood supply passes directly to pancreatic islets and hormone-enriched blood may then enter acinar lobules before draining into veins. An insular–acinar 'portal' circulation would favour zonality of pancreatic exocrine function, in the same way as the simple hepatic acinus describes a microcirculatory functional unit in the liver. This concept would rationalize the higher levels of pancreatic enzymes in 'peri-insular acini', which display changes associated with hyperactivity. Neighbouring acini are separated by distinct basal laminae composed of collagen type IV, while collagen type I and fibronectin are present in connective tissues surrounding lobules, ducts and blood vessels.

Structure–Function Relationships

The acinar cell is histologically polarized in that the lower portion with RER membranes is basophilic and the apical portion with zymogen granules is eosinophilic. The RER manufactures intra-membranous, digestive and lysosomal enzymes. Sieving in the Golgi complex is incomplete, so that lysosomal enzymes are present in normal pancreatic juice (Go *et al.*, 1986). The luminal plasma membrane projects microvilli consisting of bundles of microfilaments. These contain actin, myosin, tropomyosin, α-actinin and villin. Microvilli are anchored to a terminal web, an extension of the inner leaflet of the plasma membrane. Freeze-fracture studies show that the bulk of zymogen granules are located near the apical plasma membrane in readiness for exocytosis, but also that vesicles impinge against the basolateral membrane of the acinar cell, apparently for discharge directly into the interstitial space. Lumina of acini contain aggregates of protein fibrils.

Ductal cells are equipped to secrete a bicarbonate-rich fluid: they have abundant mitochondria and immunostainable carbonic anhydrase activity. The 'fuzzy coat' lining ductal epithelium is caused by mucus secreted by interspersed cells. Endocrine cells are also scattered in ductal epithelium and secrete VIP (vasoactive intestinal polypeptide) and substance P.

Acinar Cell

Enzyme Synthesis and Growth Regulation

High rates of amino acid influx in the rat pancreas are mediated by at least four transporters in the basolateral membrane, while amino acid efflux is mediated by at least two further transporters and activated by trans-exchange with extracellular amino acids (Mann *et al.*, 1989). Within the RER amino acids are combined in specific sequences to yield different enzymes; those specifications are stored in chromosomes using messenger RNA as the informing molecule. Gene transcription and translation steps have been identified (Go *et al.*, 1986). Diet and endocrine status are among many factors that interact to alter enzyme synthesis profiles. Recent work in rats shows that at least some of those changes are brought about by signal transduction mechanisms akin to those involved when the regulated secretory pathway is

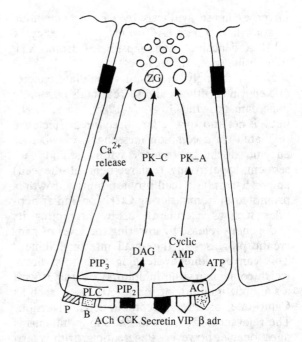

Figure 2 Plasma membrane receptors and intracellular chemical messengers involved in signal transduction by the regulated secretory pathway in the acinar cell. Abbreviations as defined in text

activated by occupancy of specific plasma membrane receptors (Musa, 1989).

These membrane receptors fall into two main classes (Figure 2), of which one mainly accommodates secretin and VIP and the other accommodates mainly CCK (cholecystokinin-pancreozymin) and ACh (acetylcholine) (Go *et al.*, 1986; Johnson, 1987; Case, 1990). The CCK receptor has high affinity (K_d for CCK-8 65 pM) and low affinity (K_d 15 nM) subtypes. Synthetic CCK receptor antagonists include glutaramic acid derivatives (e.g. CR-1392, CR-1409, CR-1505 from Rotta Research Laboratories, Milan, Italy), benzodiazepine derivatives (e.g. L-364, 718 from Merck, Sharp & Dohme Research Laboratories, West Point, Pennsylvania, USA) and a series of CCK analogues. The acinar cell membrane also has receptors for somatostatin, insulin, epidermal growth factor and pirenzepine (low affinity, M_2B subtype). Occupation of the CCK-type receptor increases the synthesis of several proteolytic enzymes, acting preferentially via increased cytoplasmic Ca^{2+}. Hyperthyroidism extends the effect to include heightened synthesis of amylase and lipase. Occupation of the secretin-type receptor increases lipase synthesis by causing activation of adenylate cyclase (AC) which generates cyclic AMP (adenosine monophosphate) from ATP (adenosine triphosphate).

Not surprisingly, factors that stimulate pancreatic enzyme synthesis and secretion also promote pancreatic growth (Go *et al.*, 1986; Musa, 1989), but it is not known whether these three effects are regulated via a common messenger, or whether enzyme discharge triggers synthesis and subsequent hypertrophy (enlargement of the cell) and/or hyperplasia (cell proliferation). Growth is promoted by administering CCK (or similar peptides such as caerulein), or by promoting its endogenous release by lowering the level of pancreatic proteases in the small intestinal lumen. This can be done by feeding with soya flour, which contains trypsin inhibitors; treatment with a synthetic inhibitor of serine proteases, such as Camostate; or by pancreatoduodenal diversion. The relevance of the feedback loop in humans is questionable, however. Pancreatic growth is also evoked by hormones (glucocorticoids, insulin, epidermal growth factor), the bile salt-binding resin cholestyramine, occlusion of the main pancreatic duct, pancreatic trauma, and dietary deprivation of essential amino acids followed by free access. Whatever the stimulant to growth may be, the polyamine biosynthetic pathway is ultimately involved.

Regulated Secretory Pathway

Proteins synthesized in the RER are transported vectorially to the cisternal space through signal-transport sequences. Thereafter transport is believed to follow the zymogen granule packaging and exocytosis model of Jamieson and Palade (1977), in which lysosomal and food digestion enzymes are largely separated from each other in different membrane-bound compartments. As in other secretory cells (Berridge, 1984), signal transduction is accomplished through a system of intracellular messengers (Figure 2). Occupation of the CCK-type receptor leads via a G-protein (guanine nucleotide binding protein) to activation of phospholipase C (PLC) producing inositol 1,4, 5-triphosphate (PIP$_3$) and diacylglycerols (DAG) from precursor inositol 4,5-bisphosphate (PIP$_2$), preferentially. Those chemical messengers mobilize Ca^{2+}, probably from the RER (Case, 1990), or activate protein kinase C (PKC), respectively (Figure 2). The rise in cytosolic Ca^{2+} activates

calmodulin (CAM) and thereby protein kinase (PK), and phosphatase (PP). Recent studies suggest that occupancy of the low-affinity CCK receptor evokes inhibition of secretion. Signal transduction after occupation of secretin/VIP receptors is accomplished via an increase in cyclic AMP which, in turn, activates protein kinase A (PKA). Both pathways alter levels of stimulatory (G$_s$) and inhibitory (G$_i$) proteins and thus modulate protein phosphorylation. Very recent studies suggest that biological free radicals provide a further network of intracellular signal transducers in a variety of secretory cells and that the pancreatic acinar cell will prove to be no exception. Examples of such reactive species include the nitric oxide radical derived from arginine (Moncada *et al.*, 1991; Shreck and Baeuerle, 1992) and 4-hydroxynonenal which is a product of free radical oxidation of lipids (Rossi *et al.*, 1990).

The methylation of membrane phospholipids, by transfer of methyl groups from methionine via sulphadenosyl methionine (SAMe) also seems to be very important for signal transduction in a variety of cells (Hirata and Axelrod, 1980). Thus, it has been shown that the binding of catecholamine to its receptor activates methyl transferases, resulting in methylation of phosphatidylethanolamine to generate phosphatidylcholine. In the process membrane fluidity increases, allowing lateral mobility of the β-adrenergic receptor, so that it can interact with a G-protein coupling factor and AC to generate cyclic AMP, as in Figure 2. *In vitro* studies also showed that when SAMe was present in the incubation medium, treatment with PLC was accompanied by methylating enzyme-facilitated flip-flop realignment of membrane phospholipids with increased membrane fluidity. The potential application of these findings to signal transduction in the acinar cell is denied by meagre information (Johnson, 1987).

It is not known exactly how zymogen granules are shunted to the apical plasma membrane and exocytosed but it seems that microtubule/myosin phosphorylation is involved in the first process; that membrane proteins in zymogen granule membrane, apical membranes or both are necessary for the fusion event; that G-proteins, other Ca^{2+} dependent proteins and probably also the 'wild' variant of the newly identified cystic fibrosis transmembrane regulator (CFTR) interact to facilitate enzyme discharge; and that an increase in membrane fluidity is probably a prerequisite for that final event (Johnson, 1987; Case, 1990; Marino and Gorelick, 1992; Morgan and Burgoyne, 1992; Padfield *et al.*, 1992; Trezise *et al.*, 1993).

The pancreas has inherent safety devices against autodigestion. The most potent enzymes (proteolytic, phospholipase A_2) are synthesized as zymogens; enzymes that travel down the regulated pathway are constrained within membrane enclosed granules; the trypsinogen activator enterokinase is located in another organ, the duodenum; a low molecular weight trypsin inhibitor is co-secreted and can trap as much as 20 per cent of potential trypsin activity; and, should any trypsin become prematurely activated within the gland, it quickly activates an inhibitor-resistant protease mesotrypsin, which in turn inactivates trypsinogen and other zymogens to curtail the activation cascade (Go *et al.*, 1986).

Non-regulated Secretory Pathway

There is evidence for a constitutive, non-regulated facility for protein discharge from acinar cells (Arvan and Castle, 1987) through pathways which seem to be preferentially located in the basolateral membrane, and lead directly into the interstitium and bloodstream (Figure 3). As a backup mechanism, plasma contains safeguards against premature activation of pancreatic proteases that enter via the 'endocrine' route. These include α_1 protease inhibitor, whose primary function is to protect against leucocyte-derived elastase: it completely inactivates proteases and also binds to proelastase, acting as a transporter. Some activity is regained when the enzymes are off-loaded to α_2 macroglobulin, a disadvantage offset by the rapid removal of complexes in the reticuloendothelial system. Lipocortins are potential endogenous inhibitors of phospholipase A_2, but none was identified in a preliminary study of rat pancreas (T. Nevalainen, personal communication).

Ductal Cells

Bicarbonate Secretion

Secretin and VIP are the main stimuli of ductal HCO_3^- secretion although other agonists, notably CCK, can potentiate their action. Signal transduction involves cyclic AMP which increases the open-state probability of a Cl^- channel on the lumenal plasma membrane. Recent evidence suggests that CFTR plays a pivotal role in this regard (Reader, 1992). The active secretion of bicarbonate into the duct system results from the coordinated action of a $Cl^--HCO_3^-$ exchange protein spanning the lumenal membrane; intracellular carbonic anhydrase, which generates H_2CO_3 from CO_2 that has diffused into the cell; and three proteins in the basal plasma membrane (sodium potassium exchanger, hydrogen sodium antiporter, potassium channel) (Johnson, 1987; Case, 1990; Raeder, 1992). Na^+ seems to enter the duct via intercellular spaces.

Mucus Secretion

Different cells secrete highly sulphated mucin, weakly sulphated neutral mucin, sialomucin, or sulphomucin (Go *et al.*, 1986). Following mucin synthesis, glysosylation occurs in the Golgi apparatus. Thereafter glycoproteins are packaged in synthetic granules and propelled along microtubules for exocytosis. Cholinergic agonists and prostaglandins are secretagogues while bile salts may owe their effectiveness to a local response mediated by receptors on the cell surface.

Pancreatic Juice

Phases of Secretion

Interdigestive secretion varies with phases of upper gastrointestinal motility. The digestive pattern is evoked by food, hormonal and neural stimuli. The coordination between secretion and motility may help to protect the intestinal lining from its secretions; and to ensure that duodenal pressure does not exceed that in the pancreatic duct.

Composition

The human pancreas secretes between 0.7 and 2.5 l of pancreatic juice each day (Lentler, 1981). The juice, pH 7.5–8.8, is isotonic with serum. Its bicarbonate concentration rises with flow rate to a maximum of 130–150 mmol l^{-1} at a rate of 300 ml h^{-1}: the sum of HCO_3^- and Cl^- is constant at around 154 mmol l^{-1}. Na^+ is the principal cation (139–143 mmol l^{-1}); the concentration of Ca^{2+} varies between 2.2 and 4.6 mmol l^{-1}. Digestive enzymes account for most of the high protein content, 4.8–5.3 g l^{-1}, while traces of albumin, globulin and mucoprotein account for the remain-

Normal

Pancreatitis

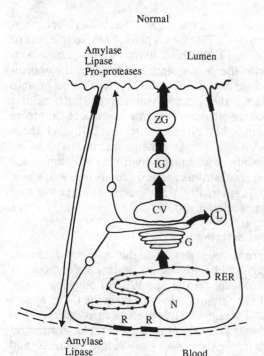
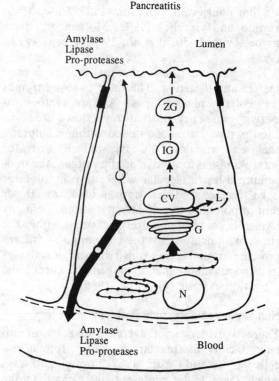

Figure 3 Non-regulated vesicular pathway into the interstitium via the basolateral membrane: a minor secretion route in the normal acinar cell (Arvan and Castle, 1987) but seemingly used preferentially in pancreatitis. R = plasma membrane receptor; N = nucleus; RER = rough endoplasmic reticulum; G = Golgi stacks; L = lysosome; CV = condensing vacuole; IG = intermediate granule; ZG = zymogen granule. Source: reproduced with permission from Braganza, 1992

der. There are more than 20 different enzymes including inactive precursors of serine proteases (three forms of trypsinogen, two of chymotrypsinogen, two of proelastase, and kallikreinogen) and exopeptidases (four forms of procarboxypeptidase, and phospholipase A_2); and lipase, colipase, cholesterol ester hydrolase, amylase, RNAse and DNAse (Howat and Sarles, 1979; Go *et al.*, 1986). The concentration of lipids is very low, 5.2 mg l^{-1}. Other constituents include lysosomal enzymes, lactoferrin and a 'pancreatic stone protein' (Go *et al.*, 1986) which helps to solubilize Ca^{2+}.

ABNORMAL PANCREAS: OBSERVATIONS AND TRADITIONAL INTERPRETATIONS

Diseases and Definitions

Acute pancreatitis, chronic pancreatitis and pancreatic cancer are the main acquired diseases of

the exocrine pancreas (Howat and Sarles, 1979; Go *et al.*, 1986; Weatherall *et al.*, 1988). The gland is affected in kwashiorkor (Go *et al.*, 1986; Braganza, 1991) and by the ageing process (Braganza, 1992) but these conditions tend to be painless. It is already damaged at birth in the congenital disease cystic fibrosis (Go *et al.*, 1986; Braganza, 1991); and is involved in the congenital metal storage diseases, haemochromatosis and Wilson's disease.

Pancreatitis commonly manifests as a severe attack of upper abdominal pain accompanied by a sharp rise in blood levels of pancreatic enzymes. The suffix 'itis' implies inflammation and, indeed, hordes of inflammatory cells are a histological feature of the worst forms of clinical or experimental pancreatitis; however, animal studies show that this is not the primary event (Go *et al.*, 1986; Braganza, 1988a, 1991; Uden *et al.*, 1990a). Whatever the inciting agent or the route of attack may be, the fundamental problem is a metabolic blockade to exocytosis. Blood and urinary levels of enzymes, including zymogens, not activated proteases (Goekas *et al.*, 1981; Shorrock, 1988), rise sharply, presumably having entered via the non-regulated secretory pathway (Figure 3). Thereafter lysosomal and zymogen compartments coalesce (Go *et al.*, 1986; Case, 1990), presumably to remove redundant cellular material, and acinar cells dedifferentiate into tubular complexes (Sarles *et al.*, 1984). Studies of human acute pancreatitis suggest a similar evolution (Durie *et al.*, 1985; Gudgeon *et al.*, 1990). Inflammation is clearly a secondary event; so 'pancreastasis' is a better descriptor than 'pancreatitis' of the earliest metabolic aberrations (Braganza, 1990a, 1991).

Another definition (Weatherall *et al.*, 1988), 'sudden wholesale necrosis of pancreatic acinar cells', is unacceptable because clinical recovery is rapid with normalization of blood enzyme levels by 72 h in the majority of patients. Histology of the pancreas from such cases, or from animal models of self-limiting pancreatitis, shows moderate interstitial oedema, a sprinkling of inflammatory cells and foci of fat necrosis. In a proportion of cases, and in certain animal models, the condition deteriorates to haemorrhagic pancreatic necrosis (HPN) and death from multisystem organ failure is the usual outcome. The overall death rate in humans is 20 per cent.

Pancreatitis may strike a gland that was previously normal and will return to normal when, and if, it recovers from the active lesions of oedema and/or haemorrhage and/or necrosis. The term 'acute pancreatitis' describes this situation and the same term is applied if recovery is complete following future attacks (Figure 4). Alternatively, the attack or recurrence may occur against a background of chronic destruction, in which case the pathology is proof after the superimposed lesions of active damage, and associated abdominal pain, which punctuate the clinical course of the disease, have healed. The term 'chronic pancreatitis' describes this. In the early stages of this disease diagnosis is facilitated by the dual approach of pancreatic function testing to detect reduction in exocrine secretory capacity, and ERCP to identify distortion of the pancreatic duct system (Braganza, 1988c). The established disease has the characteristic triad of steatorrhoea, intraductal calculi and diabetes. It is noteworthy that pancreatic cancer and cystic fibrosis may present with, or be complicated by,

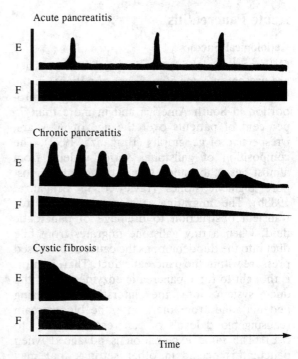

Figure 4 Exocrine pancreatic disease. Profiles of blood enzymes and pancreatic secretory capacity in acute pancreatitis, chronic pancreatitis and cystic fibrosis. E = enzyme levels; F = pancreatic function. Source: reproduced from Uden *et al.* (1990a) with permission

acute or chronic pancreatitis (Howat and Sarles, 1979; Go *et al.*, 1986; Braganza, 1991).

Hospital admissions and other statistics suggest a true increase in frequency of pancreatic diseases in developed countries in the past 50 years (Howat and Sarles, 1979; Go *et al.*, 1986). In the case of acute pancreatitis this is reflected in mortality statistics. Chronic pancreatitis is damaging and, although it does not usually result in death directly, reduces lifespan from associated problems such as diabetes and maldigestion. The cardinal problem in pancreatic cancer is the long presymptomatic period of tumour growth. Death follows within 6 months of the first symptom in most patients; hence mortality statistics give incidence as well as prevalence rates. Since 1940 the age-adjusted death rate from pancreatic cancer has doubled in England and Wales, trebled in the USA and quadrupled in Japan.

Acute Pancreatitis

Aetiological Factors

Gallstones are the overriding risk factor. They are present in some 50 per cent of patients in the USA and Europe, but in a much higher proportion in South America and in more than 75 per cent of patients over the age of 80 years, irrespective of geography (Braganza, 1992). The composition of gallstones varies widely, from almost pure cholesterol stones through to almost pure pigment stones (reviewed in Braganza, 1988b). The 'migrating gallstone theory' regards transient obstruction to drainage of pancreatic fluid, when a tiny gallstone migrates from bile duct into the duodenum, as the cause of increased pressure within the pancreatic duct. That, in turn, is thought to force pancreatic enzymes out of the duct system into the interstitium (causing oedema) and from there into the bloodstream (causing blood levels of pancreatic enzymes to rise). The same explanation is advanced when pancreatitis occurs in other settings that may increase ductal pressure (Table 1, Braganza, 1988a, 1991). This explanation is supported by the ease with which oedematous pancreatitis is produced experimentally when the pancreatic duct is clamped transiently (Saluja *et al.*, 1989), and even more easily when secretin is simultaneously infused (Sanfey *et al.*, 1986).

Certain agents seem to initiate the human disease by compromising the pancreatic microcirculation, while others may do so by interfering with the metabolism of the acinar cell. Experimental models are available to simulate these situations (Table 1).

The following conditions may damage the pancreas by more than one route, sequentially or concurrently: an alcoholic debauch (which increases duodenal and sphincter pressure while also affecting the metabolism of pancreatic acinar cells); cardiopulmonary bypass surgery (which could compromise the pancreatic microcirculation but also involves prolonged exposure to volatile anaesthetics which might be the true precipitant); renal transplantation (when the same considerations apply with the additional possibility of drug-mediated toxicity); and pancreatic hyperstimulation, as may follow exposure to an insecticide, diazinon (Go *et al.*, 1986), or a scorpion bite (Go *et al.*, 1986) (which not only increases ductal pressure but alters acinar cell

metabolism). The last condition can be reproduced experimentally by those noxae of which the insecticide has anticholinesterase properties; and the venom evokes the release of neurotransmitters from cholinergic terminals within the gland (Go *et al.*, 1986). A similar state can be provoked by infusing supramaximal doses of CCK or caerulein which cause damage through interactions with the low-affinity CCK receptor (Braganza, 1991).

Progression and Pathophysiology

Investigators have been preoccupied by HPN and, in particular, its relationship to gallstones. It is generally assumed that the gland is cannabalized by its own prematurely activated enzymes, especially elastase which would rationalize hemorrhage, and phospholipase A_2 which would explain cellular necrosis. Active enzymes have indeed been found in the gland, ascitic fluid and bloodstream of patients or animals with HPN. A popular theory (Figure 5) fails to explain, however, why the experimental transpancreatic passage of bile, via an intestinal loop for many months, resulted in complete activation of pancreatic enzymes but not HPN (Robinson and Dunphy, 1963). Another theory revolves around bacterial toxins in infected bile or duodenal fluid, but evidence of infection is lacking at the time of presentation in most patients. Both concepts cannot explain the development of HPN when the inciting agent enters by the microcirculation or from within the acinar cell. Proposals to overcome these problems include thrombosis of pancreatic capillaries due to massive edema of the gland, activation of trypsinogen by lysosomal cathepsin B (Steer and Meldolesi, 1987), and altered fluidity of intracellular membranes, jeopardizing calcium compartmentation (reviewed in Braganza, 1986). Tubular complexes representing dedifferentiated acini are reversible in edematous pancreatitis (Bockman, 1981) but persist until acini are effaced in HPN, as exemplified in a pancreas allograft model (Knoop *et al.*, 1989).

Treatment and Outcome

The following agents have not proved useful in controlled clinical trials: the high molecular weight antiprotease aprotinin (Trasylol), glucagon, and plasma. Infusions of dextran, plasma or albumin nevertheless remain the mainstay of treatment in acute pancreatitis and their value

Table 1 Acute pancreatitis: agents/routes[a]

	Human	Experimental
Ductal	Migrating gallstone	Duct clamp ± secretin
	Pancreas divisum	[a]Duodenal obstruction ± infection
	Ampullary cancer	[a]Retrograde bile ± enzyme
	Duodenal diverticulum	[a]Prograde bile ± aspirin/ethanol
	Afferent loop obstruction	
Arterial	Hypothermia	Ischaemia-reperfusion
	Translumbar aortography	Oleic acid infusion into artery
	Vasculitis	[a]Glass beads into splenic artery
	Serum triglycerides > 20 mmol/l	
Acinar	Trauma	[a]CDE diet
	Virus (mumps, HIV, Hepatitis B)	Drugs
	Hypercalcaemia, porphyria	Chemicals
	Chronic renal failure	
	Inflammatory bowel disease	
	Surfeit after fast	
	Anorexia nervosa	
	? Pregnancy	
	Total parenteral nutrition	
	Essential fatty acid deficiency	
	Reye's syndrome	
	Haemolytic uraemic syndrome	
	Drugs and chemicals	
Mixed	Alcoholic debauch	[a]Pancreas allograft
	Cardiopulmonary bypass	Supramaximal CCK, etc.
	Post-renal transplant	Insecticide
	Insecticide	Scorpion bite
	Scorpion bite	

[a] Typically HPN; see text.

Source: reproduced with permission from Braganza, 1991

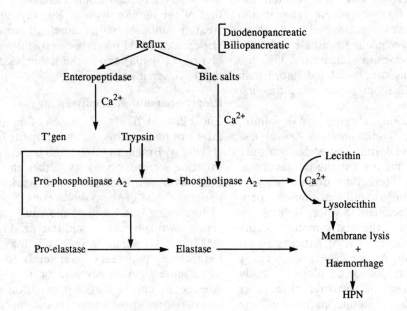

Figure 5 Traditional explanation for gallstone-related pancreatitis. HPN = haemorrhagic pancreatic necrosis

may not lie simply in the expansion of the intravascular compartment. Low molecular weight inhibitors of serine proteinases (e.g. Gabexate, Camostate) are proving useful in animal models when given prophylactically (Ohshio *et al.*, 1989). Other experimental measures include the use of CCK-receptor antagonists to prevent further acinar stimulation by endogenous hormones (Modlin *et al.*, 1989); or repeated exchange transfusion (Blower, 1989) to remove active enzyme/protein complexes.

Chronic Pancreatitis

Aetiological Factors

In developed countries the disease is regarded as synonymous with alcoholism. Yet, alcohol on its own is a weak risk factor: some 17 years of drinking more than 150 g alcohol daily usually precedes the first symptom, so that the peak age at presentation is in the third or fourth decade (Howat and Sarles, 1979). The paradox that a few patients report after drinking less than 50 g alcohol daily for less than 2 years is said to indicate that there is no threshold for alcohol toxicity to the pancreas and/or that certain individuals are genetically predisposed and/or that pancreatic injury reflects the sum of toxicities from alcohol, cigarette smoke and diets that either contain too much or too little fat and protein (Howat and Sarles, 1979). In Brazil, it is claimed that 100 per cent of patients have alcoholic disease, whereas only 45 per cent of cases in Manchester, UK, fall into this category, as strictly defined (more than 50 g per day for 12 months preceding the first symptom).

Hyperparathyroidism, chronic renal failure, renal transplantation, inflammatory bowel disease and exposure to certain drugs/chemicals are other accepted risk factors but the interaction is not straightforward. Hereditary disease (autosomal dominant pattern with incomplete penetrance) has been documented where several siblings may be involved; the first symptom occurs in childhood and 20 per cent of patients go on to develop pancreatic cancer. There is no ready explanation when the disease develops in family members but without an ancestral history, or when it follows the alcoholic pattern in one member and is idiopathic in another. In recent years a link has been shown between old age and calcifying chronic pancreatitis (Braganza, 1992).

The same disease but with much higher prevalence, familial clustering, presentation in the first decade, and accelerated course to pancreatic calculi and diabetes is found in several countries of tropical zones. These peculiarities suggest the disease-promoting effect of indigenous genetic and environmental factors (Braganza, 1988d). There is some evidence for the former insofar as the diabetes component is concerned. The good geographic match between the distribution of the disease and the growth/consumption of cassava (tapioca, manioc), which contains cyanogenic glycosides, led to the hydrogen cyanide toxicity theory (McMillan and Geevarghese, 1979), that there is inadequate detoxification of this poison by impoverished malnourished people because of low dietary protein, and hence sulphur amino acid intake. The main problems with this attractive theory are that certain populations who subsist on cassava do not develop chronic pancreatitis; that among natives of the tropical belt who do, there are many who have not consumed cyanogenic foods in excess; and that whereas some patients develop the full-blown disease, others have insulin-requiring diabetes but without calcific chronic pancreatitis.

There is no reproducible animal model for chronic pancreatitis but a histological picture of fibrosis and tubular complexes, very similiar to that of the human disease, is easily produced by treating animals with dimethylbenzanthracene (Bockman, 1981) or carbon tetrachloride (Veghelyi *et al.*, 1950a) and in the latter instance intraductal concrements occur.

Progression and Pathophysiology

The classical mode of presentation is with an attack of pancreatitis, followed by further attacks (Figure 4, Braganza, 1991) and steady erosion of exocrine secretory capacity, although the rate of progress is unpredictable and varies between patients. Most of them develop background pain of increasing intensity but the cause of the pain is unknown and may be multifactorial (Braganza, 1990b, 1991). Viable acinar cells may be a prerequisite as pancreatic pain tends to disappear when more than 90 per cent of acini are killed. Anecdotal reports suggest that chronic pancreatitis may predispose to pancreatic cancer (Howat and Sarles, 1979; Balakrishnan, 1987).

As the earliest abnormality at light microscopic level is the ductal protein plug and, because ducts become more distorted over time and ductal calculi and strictures develop (Figure 6), ductal elements are traditionally regarded as the focus and ductal obstruction as the cause of the disease, with the proviso that a congenital deficiency of pancreatic stone protein confers vulnerability (Go *et al.*, 1986). The ductal theory is undermined by the recent discovery of free anastamoses between lumina of pancreatic ducts and acini.

Electron microscopic and secretory studies show that acinar cells bear the brunt of the early injury. They are larger than normal, with large nuclei and nucleoli, expanded RER and highly developed Golgi, which explains heightened protein synthesis and increased secretion of protein and calcium (reviewed by Braganza, 1986). Acinar cells also show signs of damage such as

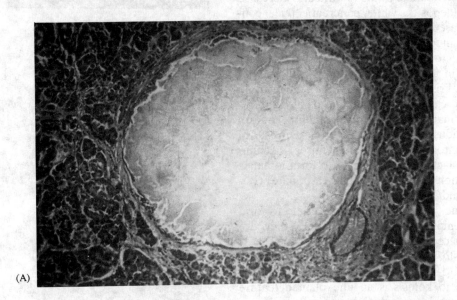

(A)

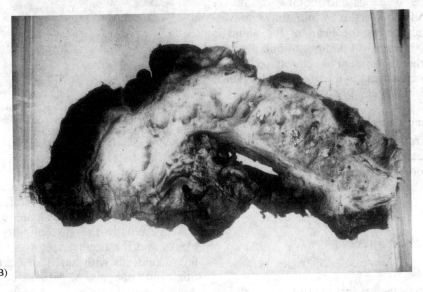

(B)

Figure 6   (A) Ductal protein plug in the early stage of chronic pancreatitis and (B) the typical end-stage of a fibrosed gland with distorted ducts containing calculi

microvesicles containing fat or zymogen material, dilated RER, and excessive amounts of lipofuscin (Sandilands *et al.*, 1990). In keeping with these changes, secretory profiles show increased amounts of lysosomal enzymes (Go *et al.*, 1986) and especially of lactoferrin (Balakrishnan *et al.*, 1988) relative to digestive enzymes, with subnormal amounts of trypsin inhibitor and pancreatic stone protein. Duct cells are also involved but to a much lesser extent: in the early stages they show increased numbers of mitochondria and increased lipofuscin deposits, while pancreatic juice contains increased amounts of duct-derived products especially mucoproteins (Harada *et al.*, 1981). Levels of lactoferrin and mucoprotein are particularly high in the tropical variant (Nagalotimath, 1980; Balakrishnan *et al.*, 1988) which would explain the early development of pancreatic calculi (Heckmann, 1971). Recent studies confirm that the nidus of a pancreatic stone consists of shed cells around which protein fibrils, calcium, mucin and lactoferrin aggregate to form a matrix for deposition of calcite (calcium carbonate) (Pitchumoni and Viswanathan, 1987).

Over time, acinar cells dedifferentiate to form tubular complexes (Figure 7) before they are finally replaced by fibrous tissue. Islets may show nesidioblastosis even when patients are frankly diabetic (Go *et al.*, 1986; Balakrishnan, 1987). Resistance to ketosis is an unexplained feature when diabetes develops and requires insulin. A possible role for bile reflux in initiating/aggravating duct strictures in the head of the gland is suggested by histological findings of bile pigment throughout the duct system or sequestered within pancreatic parenchyma in a few cases (Braganza, 1986; Sandilands *et al.*, 1990).

Treatment and Outcome

Pain control requires addictive analgesics or near-total pancreatectomy, because duct drainage procedures do not afford long-term relief. Steatorrhea and diabetes are managed along standard lines.

Cancer of the Pancreas

Aetiological Factors

Established risk factors include old age, high fat/protein diets and tobacco smoke. A series of reports suggests that volatile chemicals may also

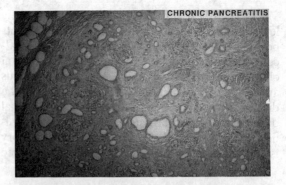

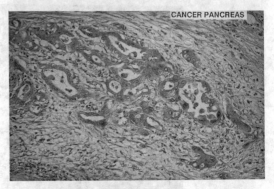

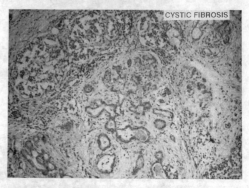

Figure 7 Tubular complexes: a typical histological feature of chronic pancreatitis, pancreatic cancer and cystic fibrosis. They appear transiently after oedematous acute pancreatitis and persist until gland destruction in HPN

be involved. Alcoholism remains under suspicion as a risk factor but excessive coffee consumption is probably not a factor. A genetic predisposition is suggested by the susceptibility of American blacks and the occurrence of the disease in siblings, kindreds with hereditary chronic pancreatitis and patients with ataxia telangiectasia. Animal models fall into two main classes, as discussed below.

Progression and Pathophysiology

Pancreatic ductal cells are generally regarded as being the source of most human pancreatic cancers (Howat and Sarles, 1979; Go *et al.*, 1986) but there is some evidence that acini, which dedifferentiate into tubular complexes (Figure 7), may be the progenitor in a number of cases (Moossa, 1980; Bockman, 1981; Parsa *et al.*, 1985). Most tumours lie in the 'head' of the gland, a predilection that is not entirely explained by the relatively greater amount of ductal epithelium. It has been suggested that reflux of a biliary carcinogen or procarcinogen, directly or via the duodenum, into the pancreatic duct may explain this propensity (Howat and Sarles, 1979; Go *et al.*, 1986). The tumour quickly obstructs the pancreatic and/or bile duct. Pain, diabetes, weight loss and recurrent thrombosis are other common associations, and the last of these may be linked to a highly expressed plasminogen activator on cancer cells (Steven and Al-Ahmad, 1984; Steven *et al.*, 1986).

A multistep evolution of human pancreatic cancer is accepted. Genotoxic agents, whether chemical, virus or other, damage nucleophilic oxygen as well as nitrogen atoms of DNA bases. The most reactive groups are the *N*-7 of guanine and *N*-3 and *N*-7 of adenine. Damage is quickly repaired by specific enzymes but multiple 'hits', epigenetic agents (tumour promoters) and genetically determined defects in DNA repair are just some of many factors that favour mutation. Cultured human pancreatic explants provide a tool to study these aspects (Scarpelli *et al.*, 1987). Biochemical studies show the DNA-damaging effects of certain nitrosamines as well as formaldehyde, while immunohistochemical studies indicate persistence of O^6-methyl guanine in target cell nuclei after treatment with alkylating nitrosamines. Acquisition of the cancer phenotype involves activation of oncogenes: in the case of the pancreas the c-*K-ras* oncogene seems to be preferentially activated by mutation at codon 12 (Almoguera *et al.*, 1988; Parsa *et al.*, 1988). Oncogenes, in turn, cause increased expression of receptors for growth factors on plasma membranes of cells, leading to activation of the growth-promoting ornithine pathway. Other characteristic features include loss of certain cell surface proteins (Scarpelli *et al.*, 1987) and increased expression of others, notably a plasminogen activator-like protease (Steven and Al-Ahmad, 1984; F. Steven, personal communication), along with increased expression of an intracellular multidrug-resistance (MDR) gene product P-glycoprotein (Goldstein *et al.*, 1989), and an early increase in the ratio of lysosomal to digestive hydrolases in pancreatic juice (Go *et al.*, 1986).

Treatment and Outcome

Ampullary tumours reveal themselves early by an attack of pancreatitis or painless jaundice, and are hence essentially curable by surgery. Otherwise the 5-year survival of pancreatic cancer is less than 2 per cent.

Pancreas in Miscellaneous Systemic Diseases

Cystic Fibrosis

The gene on chromosome 7 has now been identified. In 68 per cent of patients a single mutation, F508, associated with pancreatic involvement, results in deletion of a TTT triplet which predicts loss of a phenylalanine residue in the specified protein (Riordan *et al.*, 1989). A stylized reconstruction indicated that the protein spans the membrane, that the defective mutation occurred within the intracytoplasmic portion at the ATP-binding site, and, furthermore, that its amino acid sequence was homologous to several bacterial transport proteins as well as to the MDR glycoprotein of cancer cells. These predictions have been confirmed and, although it is not known for certain how the protein normally functions nor whether it is restricted to the plasma membrane or also involves membranes of intracellular organelles, its central role as a chloride ion channel is verified while a role, interchangeable and interacting with MDR (Trezise *et al.*, 1993), as a transporter of various macromolecules is strongly suggested (Marino and Gorelick, 1992). These developments do not yet make it easier to understand why cysts and fibrosis involve the pancreas, and also eventually the lungs which are normal at birth, why neonates have such high levels of trypsinogen and other pancreatic enzymes in blood (Figure 4) at a time when normal amounts of enzyme are recovered from the duodenum (Waters *et al.*, 1990), and why patients with the disease may show classical features of acute or chronic pancreatitis, including dedifferentiation of acini into tubular complexes (Figure 7) and occasionally pancreatic calculi, or why young adults with the disease may develop pancreatic cancer (reviewed by Uden *et al.*, 1990a). A similar pattern of cysts and fibrosis in pancreas and lung can be produced by exposing animals to carbon tetrachloride while rearing them on a diet deficient in methionine (Veghelyi *et al.*, 1950a, b).

Metal Storage Diseases

In the iron storage disease haemochromatosis pancreatic damage is associated with lysosomal overactivity, painless atrophy of acini fibrosis and diabetes. The histological features of Wilson's disease are similar and pancreatic exocrine secretory capacity is impaired (Dreiling and Grateron, 1983).

Kwashiorkor

This disease of underprivileged communities, especially in the tropical belt, causes characteristic lesions in many organs but the pancreas is a particular target with loss and vacuolization of acinar cytoplasm with fibrosis and sometimes tubular/cystic complexes (Veghelyi and Kemeny, 1962; Golden and Ramdath 1987; Golden, 1991).

PANCREAS: TARGET FOR OXYGEN RADICAL TOXICITY

Oxygen Free Radicals: the Paradox

Free Radical Biology

Free radicals (denoted as $^\bullet$ to indicate the unpaired electron) are products of normal cellular metabolism and molecular oxygen is their chief source (Autor, 1982; Dormandy, 1983; Slater, 1984; Halliwell and Gutteridge, 1985). Up to 10 per cent of O_2 in cells is normally metabolized down the univalent pathway yielding successively the superoxide anion free radical, $O_2^{-\bullet}$; hydrogen peroxide, $H_2O_2^\bullet$; the hydroxyl free radical, $OH^\bullet$; and finally H_2O. Free transition metals favour the interaction between $O_2^{-\bullet}$ and H_2O_2 to yield $OH^\bullet$ (Fenton reaction). Oxygen free radicals are involved in a wide range of vital cellular functions: respiration, lysosomal scavenging, metabolism of diverse endogenous and exogenous (xenobiotic) lipids via the microsomal cytoch-

rome *P*-450 system, production of prostaglandins and leukotrienes from arachidonic acid (C20:4), and signal transduction though regulation of these and other second messengers, e.g. by activating guanylate cyclase or PK-C. Oxygen radicals, and also certain lipid oxidation fragments, provide chemotactic signals as well as being part of the lethal chemical substances of phagocytic cells (Weissman, 1983; Venge and Lindbom, 1985; Arfors and Dol Maestro, 1986; Weiss, 1989). Free radicals are also involved in the immune response in that activated macrophages release interleukin I and tumour necrosis factor, which seem to require reactive oxygen species as obligate intracellular signal transducers (Schreck and Baeuerle, 1991); and, furthermore, certain free radical oxidation products (FROPs), for example aldehydes, alter the structure and thereby the immunogenicity of membrane domains/gamma globulin. Perhaps most importantly, oxygen radicals ensure that cells have a finite lifespan (Dormandy, 1988).

Any threat from excessive free radical activity is curbed by inherent defences, of which structural organization is the most important. Other strategies include controlled production rates, especially of $OH^\bullet$, feedback regulation loops (e.g. inhibition of cytochromes *P*-450 by lipid peroxides, and inhibition of the latter by PK-C), an interlinked system of preventive and chain-breaking antioxidants along with systems for their regeneration (Dormandy, 1983; Slater, 1984; Halliwell and Gutteridge, 1985, 1986; Scott, 1988; Braganza, 1991), and prompt disposal of FROPs. Thus caeruloplasmin (ferroxidase I), apolactoferrin and transferrin trap transition metals. Superoxide dismutase (SOD) catalyses the production of H_2O_2 from $O_2^{-\bullet}$ while catalase and the selenoenzyme glutathione (GSH) peroxidase remove H_2O_2. The latter also removes lipid/drug peroxides. There is evidence that selenium-independent GSH peroxidases and GSH transferases provide a backup facility in states of selenium deficiency (Diplock 1984), while cells of exocrine glands secrete an additional peroxidase (Guyan *et al.*, 1986). GSH reconstruction is facilitated by vitamin E, acting with a strong reductant such as vitamin C. The levels of several enzymes increase when oxidant load increases. The second line of antioxidant defence is afforded by interactions between many micronutrients (Figure 8, Braganza, 1991).

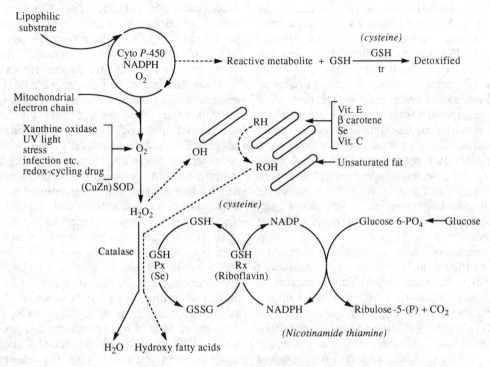

Figure 8   Schematic representation of free radical producing and quenching mechanisms in cells. Source: reproduced with permission from Braganza, 1991

In contrast to an abundance of defences against oxygen radicals, GSH is the only significant opposition to non-biological radicals that are produced on bioactivation of drugs and chemicals via the microsomal cytochrome *P*-450 system (Orrenius and Moldeus, 1984; Orrenius, 1985). Furthermore, whereas GSH is continually recycled in these reactions, it is lost to the cell through conjugation with reactive metabolites. Cysteine is the rate-limiting component for GSH synthesis. It draws on methionine, an essential amino acid, which acts through its metabolite SAMe to methylate numerous substrates, including membrane phospholipids, while feeding into energy-generating and growth-regulating pathways (Maeda *et al.*, 1986; Drugs, 1989).

Ascorbate has been shown to be the most effective antioxidant in plasma, completely protecting lipoproteins from peroxidative damage induced by aqueous peroxyl radicals and the oxidants released from activated neutrophils (Frei *et al.*, 1990). Metal sequestration, primarily by caeruloplasmin, also facilitates antioxidant defence within extracellular fluid (Dormandy, 1983; Halliwell and Gutteridge, 1986). Vitamin E is the

main lipid-soluble antioxidant in plasma with β-carotene assisting in hypoxic states. The melanin content of skin affords protection against UV light-induced oxidants. Secretory epithelia are protected by mucus which traps OH˙ (Cross *et al.*, 1984). Bile is a disposal route for FROPs (Braganza *et al.*, 1983) and metabolites of xenobiotics complexed to bile salts (Rozman and Hanninen, 1986); the latter may undergo an enterohepatic circulation (Rozman and Hanninen, 1986). Considering these points and that bile salts are potent inducers of cellular free radical activity (Craven *et al.*, 1986), it is perhaps not surprising to find that bilirubin is a powerful antioxidant (Stocker *et al.*, 1987).

Free Radical Pathology

An excess of pro-oxidant over antioxidant forces in cells, 'oxidative stress' (Sies, 1985), may arise in three main ways (Braganza, 1989; 1991): (1) because of an absolute increase in cellular oxidant load, whether through overactivity of an intrinsic source and/or an extrinsic source (Halliwell and Gutteridge, 1985; Pryor, 1986; Boucher *et al.*, 1988), (2) because of an absolute dietary deficiency of antioxidants, or (3) because of an imbalance in favour of radicals, although their production rates and antioxidant levels are still 'normal'. OH• is the major threat because of its extreme reactivity: the target is dictated by the presence of metal protein catalysts (site-specificity) to drive the Fenton reaction (Halliwell and Gutteridge, 1986). Oxygen radicals are just one of many potential tissue-damaging agents; others include proteases, cytotoxic protein and lipid fragments, cytolytic properties of the complement cascade and macrophage/neutrophil-derived toxins (Venge and Lindbom, 1985). In human disease it may be impossible to identify a temporal sequence or to dissect out these different components.

The sequelae of oxidative stress are unpredictable and differ from organ to organ and even within cells of the same organ. This is because of several factors (Cohen, 1986): (1) the complement of radical-generating and quenching systems, (2) differences in biomembrane phospholipid composition, (3) the available excretory routes for FROPs, (4) the population of resident macrophages and immune systems which could amplify and perpetuate free radical damage, and (5) tissue-specific biochemistry, i.e. damage is linked with perturbation of particular biochemical process or pathway. With regard to the last factor, it is interesting to note that certain cellular processes which have a 'house-cleaning' or protective role may have considerable reserve, i.e. they are not rate-limiting until the level is greatly depressed. This seems to be the case with GSH and GSH-reductase/peroxidase systems. By contrast, a pathway may be rate-limiting because of some unusual metabolic demand of a tissue: glucose metabolism by the brain is an example. When redox cycling drugs (e.g. adriamycin, paraquat) or chemicals that undergo bioactivation are the cause of oxidative stress, the route of entry is another important consideration. Whereas ingested agents would first encounter the liver, inhaled agents that bypass the pulmonary circulation would not be so discriminatory (Braganza, 1991).

Oxidative stress compromises cellular integrity in several ways: by (1) depleting energy-generating systems, (2) reducing the bioavailability of SAMe and GSH, (3) disrupting ionic, especially calcium, homoeostasis, (4) oxidizing biomembranes, and (5) interacting with critical cellular macromolecules (Slater, 1984; Orrenius, 1985; Sies, 1985; Braganza, 1989, 1991). The first four effects contribute to cellular necrosis and the last has implications for carcinogenesis. The links between free radicals and cancer are extremely complex (McBrien and Slater, 1983; Halliwell and Gutteridge, 1985; Dormandy, 1988). Organic radicals have genotoxic potential while oxygen species and lipid oxidation fragments may be epigenetic. Free radical attack on PUFA follows one of two main pathways (Figure 9) depending on membrane lipid composition and perhaps also on cell complement of different antioxidants. Thus microsomal, mitochondrial and plasma membranes contain an abundance of linoleic acid, (C18:2), an attack on which causes isomerization to a protein-stabilized non-peroxide conjugated diene isomer (9 cis, 11 trans LA) (Dormandy, 1988; Smith *et al.*, 1992). Free radical attack on more highly unsaturated fatty acids, e.g. C20:4, as in membranes of phagocytosing cells, initiates the vicious cycle of lipid peroxidation, generating a constellation of friable products. Cancer cells tend to show high levels of the linoleic acid isomer, which would favour immortalization as the isomer reduces cell membrane fluidity (Dormandy, 1988). Paradoxically, they contain low levels of lipid peroxidation products and high levels of vitamin E: both may be linked to high levels of cellular PK-C evoked by oncogene-stimulated expression of membrane receptors for growth factors.

Radical-induced stimulation of collagen synthesis would promote fibrosis while production of clastogenic factors would favour the immune response: the combination would allow disease chronicity unless counter-regulating factors were equally activated. Many of those are derived from activated neutrophils and macrophages drawn into the area by lipid oxidation fragments that enter the extracellular space. It is known that a small proportion of the chemical arsenal of activated phagocytes normally escapes outside the confines of the phagocytic vacuole (Weiss, 1989). That arsenal includes: collagenase, elastase and phospholipase A_2, oxygen metabolites, myeloperoxidase which catalyses the interaction between H_2O_2 and halides to yield the potent oxidant hypochlorous acid (HOCl), platelet and complement activating factors, cachectin, and thromboxanes and leukotrienes. The wholesale discharge of these chemicals into the extracellular

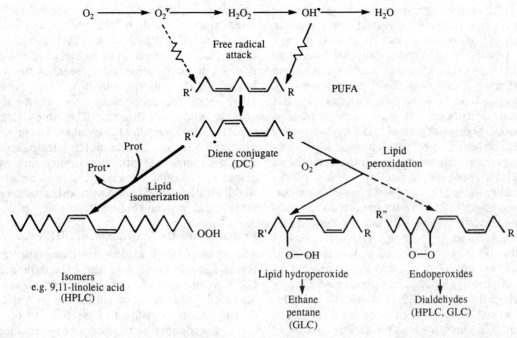

$$O_2 \longrightarrow O_2^{\overline{\cdot}} \longrightarrow H_2O_2 \longrightarrow OH^{\bullet} \longrightarrow H_2O$$

Figure 9 Schematic pathways following free radical attack on polyunsaturated fatty acids (PUFA) and methods to detect some end-products. HPLC = high performance liquid chromatography; GLC = gas liquid chromatography. Source: reproduced with permission from Braganza, 1991

space, termed 'frustrated phagocytosis', tends to occur when the primary chemotactic stimulus is overwhelming and particularly when detergents/crystals/cell casts are the chemoattractants. Multisystem organ failure follows when key methionine residues in α_1 protease inhibitor are inactivated by OH$^{\bullet}$ and HOCl.

Free radical involvement in human disease is inferred when increased levels of FROPs are found in accessible biological material, using a panel to overcome the non-specificity of individual markers (Smith and Anderson, 1987; Smith *et al.*, 1992); and the argument is strengthened if the condition is ameliorated by treatment with antioxidants and/or substances, such as GSH or ATP, that are known to be depleted on a free radical attack (Miquel *et al.*, 1989). Lipid-based markers are the most popular (Figure 9). FROPs of circulating lipoproteins and those that result from an attack on vulnerable amino acids, as in GSH, matrix components, gamma-globulin and CAM, have been characterized but these tend to be research tools. The redox state in tissues, as reflected in blood cell fractions, is a useful pointer to oxidative stress. Impaired redox potential is characterized by low ratios of GSH/GSSG; ATP/

ADP; NADPH/NADP; and ascorbic acid to its oxidized metabolites. Morphological clues to oxidative stress include ultrastructural findings of membrane blebbing, cytoplasmic microvesiculation, disorganized/dilated ER, and excessive amounts of the malondialdehyde-condensation product lipofuscin (Braganza, 1991).

Oxidative Stress in Experimental Acute Pancreatitis

Oedematous Pancreatitis

Pretreatment with the antioxidant enzymes SOD and catalase confers protection in animal models of oedematous pancreatitis, including hyperstimulation, ischaemia/reperfusion injury, transient duct clamping, and oleic acid perfusion models (Sanfey *et al.*, 1986; Braganza, 1988a, 1990a, 1991). It follows that oxygen free radicals initiate 'pancreastasis' (Figure 3). Allopurinol, which stimulates pancreatic secretion in dogs (Horiuchi *et al.*, 1989), also ameliorates (Sanfey *et al.*, 1986; Wisner and Renner, 1988); hence it is assumed that xanthine oxidase, which is inhibited by the drug, is the source of excessive free radical activity. The enzyme exists as the dehydrogenase but in adverse states is converted to the oxidase through the action of a calcium-dependent protease. However, allopurinol can curb oxidative stress in many other ways, not least by scavenging OH$^•$ (Parks, 1988). Activated leucocytes do not seem to be involved in the pancreastasis stage but doubtless contribute, not least through platelet activation (Dabrowsky *et al.*, 1989; Dabrowsky and Gabryelewicz, 1992), to changes in pancreatic and lung microvasculature in the established case (Guice *et al.*, 1989a; McEntee *et al.*, 1989).

In theory there are many ways in which oxidative stress might interfere with exocytosis: by activating guanylate cyclase and altering the balance between G_i and G_s proteins (Arfors and Del Maestro, 1986), by interfering with microtubular transport systems (Irons, 1986) and actin (Clarkson *et al.*, 1986), by reducing membrane fluidity through production of 9,11 LA$'$ (Dormandy, 1988), as well as attacking vulnerable enzymes in the methionine trans-sulphuration pathway (Davies *et al.*, 1986b), thereby reducing membrane phospholipid methylation (Figure 10). It may be that different mechanisms operate in different animal models (O'Konski and Pandol, 1990). However, observations in the choline-deficient, DL-ethionine-supplemented dietary model (CDE) (Rao *et al.*, 1976) suggest that impaired membrane phospholipid methylation may be a critical factor. Oxygen free radicals, especially OH$^•$, have been implicated in the earliest exocytosis paralysis/oedematous phase (Nonaka *et al.*, 1989), but not thereafter. Cell casts are visible beneath the plasma membrane of acinar cells by 48 h, by which time myriads of leucocytes have invaded the pancreatic interstitium and, from that point onwards, the gland contains substantial amounts of active elastase although at the outset there is very little by way of active trypsin. Death from HPN follows by the fifth day. Studies of hepatocytes treated with DL-ethionine show that this analogue follows the metabolic pathway of the natural amino acid methionine (Figure 10) but does not readily donate its ethyl group in the way that SAMe donates its methyl group: the adenine moeity is thus trapped, depleting cells of ATP and jeopardizing protein and PIP$_3$ synthesis (Trimble, 1982). Molecular biology studies of the pancreas in the CDE model indicate that the defect in signal transduction involves 'interference with some coupling event that normally allows receptor interaction to result in phospholipase C stimulation' (Steer and Meldolesi, 1987). A reduction in membrane phospholipid methylation could be relevant if methylation were essential for membrane fluidity and that, in turn, were to be a prerequisite for proper alignment between the enzyme and its substrate. This interpretation would also explain why the combined deprivation of methionine and choline potentiates pancreatic damage compared with that from either agent alone: the choline–betaine pathway contributes to the limited capacity to resynthesize methionine from homocysteine (Figure 10).

Free Radicals Do Not Rationalize HPN

The zymogens of human pancreatic proteases (Guyan *et al.*, 1988), and also phospholipase A$_2$ (T. Nevalainen *et al.*, unpublished data), are not activated, nor is pancreatic trypsin inhibitor destroyed, on exposure to high doses of the primary or secondary metabolites of oxygen. Hence, it is very unlikely that oxygen free radicals directly activate pancreatic zymogens to initiate HPN. Instead, many observations suggest that activated phagocytes may be the primary source of those activated enzymes in HPN (Braganza, 1988a), and also the main cause of multisystem organ failure through frustrated phagocytosis (Braganza *et al.*, 1986a; Braganza, 1988a; Rinderknecht, 1988; Braganza, 1991). In this scheme (Figure 11), the discharge of excessive amounts of FROPs into the pancreatic interstitium, as part of the reversal in secretory polarity (Figure 3), is envisaged as the chemoattractant (Venge and Lindbom, 1985). Interstitial oedema is expected as part of the inflammatory response, and would be magnified when platelets are activated (Dabrowski *et al.*, 1989). The self-limiting nature of panacreatitis in several animal models may then be attributed to restoration of exocytosis through mobilization of natural antioxidant reserves. When the block to exocytosis is complete, however, the load of FROPs diverted into the interstitium should be much higher, with a correspondingly higher chemotactic drive. It is not difficult to see that this situation, when accompanied by the presence of crystals, cell casts, or apoptosis—as in bile reflux (Go *et al.*, 1986; Blower, 1989), CDE (Rao *et al.*, 1976), and pancreas allograft (Knoop *et al.*, 1989) models of HPN respectively—sets the scene for frustrated phagocytosis.

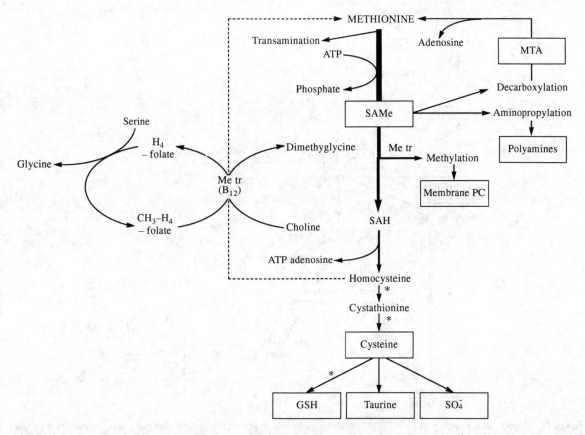

Figure 10 Pathways of methionine metabolism. SAMe = sulphadenosylmethionine; MTA = methylthioadenosine; SAH = sulphadenosylhomocysteine; GSH = glutathione; SO_4^- = inorganic sulphate; CH_3-H_4-folate = methyltetrahydrofolate; Me tr = methyl transferases. Source: reproduced with permission from Braganza, 1991

Secondary, but rapid (Geokas *et al.*, 1981; Durie *et al.*, 1985; Shorrock, 1988; Gudgeon *et al.*, 1990) activation of trypsinogen and pancreatic phospholipase A_2 by platelet-activated plasmin and thrombin respectively (Rinderknecht, 1988), would overwhelm enzyme inhibitors and hasten death.

Therapeutic Strategy

Figure 11 also indicates the points at which different therapeutic manoeuvres should help. Any strategy directed at point 1, e.g. use of CCK receptor antagonists in hyperstimulation models (Modlin *et al.*, 1989), should be most effective but countered by a limited application. The use of allopurinol in the ischaemia/reperfusion injury model is an example of therapy directed at point 2, i.e. to inhibit a putative intracellular source of free radicals. The short half-lives of antioxidant enzymes precludes success of therapies directed at point 3, and attempts to stabilize the enzymes,

e.g. by complexing with polyethylene glycol (Guice *et al.*, 1989b), may make the molecule too large to enter cells. Studies of the CDE model strongly suggest that strategies directed at overcoming the exit block of pancreatitis, by increasing membrane fluidity, may be useful. Treatment with SAMe would seem to be a good way to do this (Hirata and Axelrod, 1980; Maeda *et al.*, 1986; Focus, 1989; Scott *et al.*, 1992) (Figure 10). Varied reports concerning SAMe uptake into cells suggest, however, that its metabolite methlythioadenosine (MTA) (Figure 10), may be preferable, especially as the presence of many receptors for adenosine on acinar cell membranes (Yamagishi, 1986) should ensure that this metabolite is actively taken up into the gland. A very recent report documents protection in the CDE model by a synthetic vitamin C analogue, given at intervals by interperitoneal injection, at the time of starting the diet or 3 h later (Nonaka *et al.*, 1991).

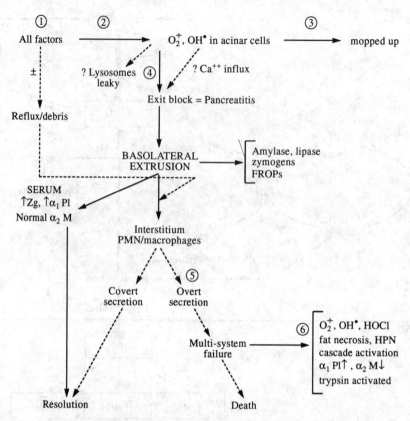

Figure 11 Hypothesis for pathogenesis of HPN indicating, by numbers, points at which therapeutic strategies may be directed. See text for explanation. Note that although α_1 protease inhibitor levels increase in the blood, there is no proof that the inhibitor is active. Source: reproduced with permission from Braganza, 1988

Vitamin C in small doses may act as a pro-oxidant but in larger doses combats oxidative stress by helping to refurbish GSH from GSSG, indirectly by facilitating the recycling of vitamin E and possibly also directly; by reacting with certain organic species, e.g. acetylacrolein which is a vinylogue of methylglyoxal (McBrien and Slater, 1983); and, perhaps most important in the context of HPN, by reacting with HOCl and so protecting α_1 protease inhibitor from destruction (Winterbourn, 1985; Halliwell *et al.*, 1987). Albumin, thiol groups, methionine and urate also protect this inhibitor to greater or lesser extents. The further recruitment/activation of phagocytes can perhaps be prevented by strategies directed at point 5. The drug 5-aminosalicyclic acid (5-ASA) has this capacity and it also protects against OH$^\bullet$ and HOCl (Miyachi *et al.*, 1987); these advantages will have to be weighed against possible drug toxicity (see later). Fructose 1,6-diphosphate, a high energy intermediate of glycolysis, also

inhibits generation of oxygen free radicals by stimulated canine and human neutrophils and could prove useful in pancreatitis (Sun *et al.*, 1990). *N*-Acetylcysteine (NAC) is a precursor of GSH (Figure 10) which combats leucocyte-derived oxidants. When frustrated phagocytosis has already caused activation of different cascades—including platelet, complement, kinin and trypsinogen—existing therapeutic options are heroic, e.g. repeated exchange transfusions (Blower, 1989), rather than practical or efficacious. However, it is interesting to note the beneficial effect of hypertonic saline-dextran infusions in bile-induced HPN in dogs (Horton *et al.*, 1989): those substances protect in a non-specific manner against certain oxygen free radicals (Halliwell and Gutteridge, 1986). It remains to be seen whether inhibitors of platelet-activating factor and/or a global serine protease inhibitor such as Camostate (which should inhibit trypsin, chymotrypsin, elastase, thrombin, plasmin, kallikrein, C_1-esterase, etc.) are useful at this stage: experimental studies show that this type of inhibitor can be toxic at high doses. Anti-cytokines are also being considered (Braganza, 1991).

Oxidative Stress in Human Pancreatitis

Pancreastasis and Phagocyte-Activation Sequence

Analysis of blood (Durie *et al.*, 1985; Gross *et al.*, 1990; Chaloner *et al.*, 1991; Scott *et al.*, 1993) and urine (Gudgeon *et al.*, 1990) samples from patients in the early stages of acute pancreatitis offer indirect support for this sequence (Braganza, 1988a, 1990a,b, 1991). Proof comes from *in vitro* studies of pancreatic fragments taken surgically from patients recovering from a first attack. There was a profound reduction in discharge of labelled proteins into the incubation medium on stimulation with carbamylcholine but a greater than normal release in unstimulated conditions (Adler and Kern, 1984), findings compatible with blockade of the regulated secretory pathway (Figure 2) and compensatory overactivity of the alternate vesicular route (Figure 3).

Recent studies of admission blood samples provide clear evidence of oxidative stress early in the course of human acute pancreatitis: high serum levels of lipid oxidation markers and very low levels of several antioxidants, especially ascorbic acid and selenium (Chaloner *et al.*, 1991; Scott *et al.*, 1993). Oxidative stress within the vascular compartment is likely to reflect an extension of that problem which seems to trigger secretory dysregulation within pancreatic acinar cells (Figure 3), as well as the extracellular discharge of oxidants from activated phagocytes.

The brisk leucocyte response, as high as that in septic states, the sharp rise in C-reactive protein levels from hepatic synthesis stimulated by macrophage-derived factors, and high interleukin-6 levels, are just some of many observations (Gyr *et al.*, 1984; Pancreatic Society, 1990) indicating phagocyte involvement at a very early stage in the human disease. These findings cannot incriminate leucocytes as the initiator of HPN or major contributor to multisystem organ failure. Recent papers on the appearance and origin of plasma neutrophil elastase–α_1 protease inhibitor complexes (Gross *et al.*, 1990) and active phospholipase A_2 support these connections, however

(Buchler *et al.*, 1989). Further support comes from the non-pancreatitis shock lung syndrome (Travis, 1983), and from the dramatic effects of treatment with NAC in patients with pancreatitis-associated shock lung and renal failure (Braganza *et al.*, 1986a; Braganza, 1991).

All these observations suggest that the intravenous administration of a non-specific promoter of exocytosis, together with antioxidants that can protect plasma α_1 protease inhibitor from leucocyte-derived oxidants might offer first-line treatment in human pancreatitis (Figure 11) (Braganza, 1990a,b, 1991). The ability of methionine to abort the course of HPN in the CDE animal model (Rao *et al.*, 1976) and of SAMe to protect in the allograft HPN model (Scott *et al.*, 1992), suggests that SAMe could be effective. This compound has the additional advantages of increasing cell levels of ATP to maintain redox potential, and of GSH to combat leucocyte-derived antioxidants. Other agents are available to help the last action (e.g. NAC, synthetic vitamin C analogue, 5-ASA) and could also find clinical application (Braganza, 1991; Scott *et al.*, 1993). Selenium has multifarious roles as an intracellular and plasma antioxidant (Sies, 1985) and has already proved to be effective in ameliorating the course of human acute pancreatitis (Kuklinski, 1992). It is likely that global antioxidant supplementation will be superior to any agent in isolation (Sharer *et al.*, 1993).

Recurrent (Non-Gallstone) Pancreatitis

Against this background (see earlier) the time course of enyzme profiles versus exocrine secretory capacity in patients with recurrent (non-gallstone) pancreatitis (Figure 4) could be interpreted as indicating different patterns of pancreatic oxidative stress: episodic in recurrent acute pancreatitis, persistent but subject to exacerbations in chronic pancreatitis (Uden *et al.*, 1990a). The reversibility of tubular complexes in the former and their persistence in the latter (Figure 7) supports this notion.

These deductions are strengthened by high levels of FROPs (Figure 9) in duodenal juice and/ or serum, collected in the asymptomatic interval between painful attacks, from patients with recurrent (non-gallstone) pancreatitis (Guyan *et al.*, 1990). Whereas the subgroup with chronic pancreatitis had similar levels to those with acute pancreatitis of the diene conjugation product 9,

11 LA', they had substantially higher levels of a lipid peroxidation marker. These data suggested a greater shortfall in lipid anti-peroxidants in the face of increased antioxidant demand, principally from induced cytochromes *P*-450, in the chronic pancreatitis subgroup. The reasons for incriminating cytochromes *P*-450 are discussed later. Home dietary inventories from patients with idiopathic disease, who had not changed their diets or lifestyles between attacks, revealed significantly lower intakes of selenium and vitamin C than for age- and sex-matched controls (Rose *et al.*, 1986). Female patients also ingested lower amounts of many other antioxidants (Figure 8). Selenium was the best discriminator overall, and consideration of this factor alongside theophylline clearance, a marker of cytochrome *P*-450I induction, gave a discriminant line (Figure 12) to separate data from controls (with higher intakes of selenium for any given level of theophylline clearance) and chronic pancreatitis patients (Rose *et al.*, 1986). Data from patients with acute pancreatitis were in the borderline zone (Braganza *et al.*, 1986c). A similar demarcation emerged when blood 9,11 LA', and selenium concentrations replaced theophylline clearance and selenium intake, respectively, in a discriminant analysis (Uden *et al.*, 1990a), which suggested that this trace element may help to curb the isomerization pathway of free radical attack on lipids (Figure 9).

When these studies were extended to include a group of enzyme-induced controls, i.e. patients with epilepsy on treatment with anticonvulsant drugs, the lower intakes of methionine and vitamin C emerged as the key factors identifying patients with chronic pancreatitis (Uden *et al.*, 1988). These findings suggest the importance of reactive intermediates from drugs and chemicals in generating oxidative stress in chronic pancreatitis compared with oxygen free radicals in several experimental models of acute pancreatitis and the human conditions that they stimulate (Table 1). GSH is the main defence against organic species and the rate-limiting component for its synthesis, cysteine, draws on the essential amino acid methionine which is also required for numerous other cellular functions (Figures 8 and 10). The multifarious roles of vitamin C in combating oxidative stress have also been discussed (see earlier). Several other observations helped to formulate a scheme (Figure 13) on which antioxidant supplemental therapy might be based. (1) In a temperate zone (Manchester, UK) as well as a tropical zone (Madras, India), blood levels of selenium (Braganza *et al.*, 1988a; Guyan *et al.*, 1989; Uden *et al.*, 1990a; Yadar *et al.*, 1991; Uden *et al.*, 1992) and vitamin C (the bioactive form measured by HPLC) (Uden *et al.*, 1992a; Kay *et al.*, 1990) were significantly lower than in local controls, with extremely low ascorbic acid levels in those with calcific disease. These changes were found whether or not the patient had pancreatic exocrine malfunction. (2) Those patients (Uden *et al.*, 1992), and others (Kalvaria *et al.*, 1986), also had subnormal levels of vitamin E and β-carotene with very low levels on exocrine pancreatic failure. (3) Leucocytes from Swedish patients (Martensson and Bolin, 1986) admitted with an alcohol-induced exacerbation of chronic pancreatitis, showed low GSH/GSSG ratios but high methionine levels, indicating oxidative stress and a metabolic blockade in the trans-sulphuration pathway (Figure 10), respectively. (4) Isolated experimental selenium deficiency caused dilation of the RER in pancreatic acinar cells, followed by cell dedifferentiation and replacement fibrosis, as also caused by isolated zinc deficiency (Go *et al.*, 1986). Copper deficiency also tended to attack acinar cells selectively. When a relatively non-toxic copper-chelating agent was used to accomplish this in rats and normal diets were resumed some 8 weeks later, there was wide-

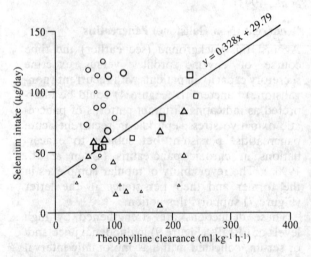

Figure 12 Discriminant analysis of theophylline clearance and selenium intake data. The smallest symbols indicate unsaturated fatty acid intakes of less than 20 g day^{-1}; intermediate sized symbols, 21–40 g day^{-1}; and large symbols more than 40 g day^{-1}. (○) Controls; (□) acute pancreatitis; (△) chronic pancreatitis

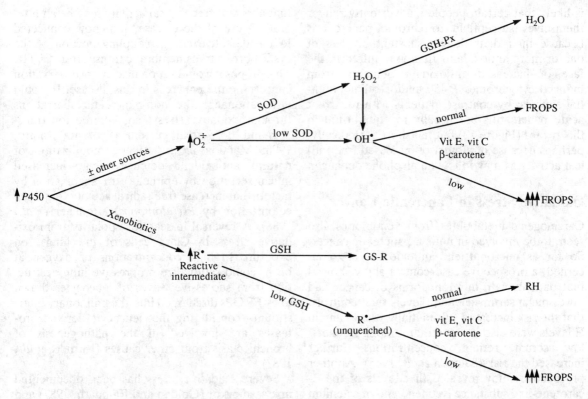

Figure 13 Proposed explanation for increased levels of free radical oxidation products in duodenal juice from patients with recurrent (non-gallstone) pancreatitis. See text for explanation. Source: reproduced from Guyan *et al.* 1990 by kind permission of Pergamon Press Ltd, Headington Hill Hall, Oxford OX3 0BW, UK

spread transdifferentiation into cells that were morphologically and functionally indistinguishable from hepatocytes (Rao *et al.*, 1988). The effects of experimental methionine deficiency were shown to vary with degree and duration, and confounding factors. Mild protracted deficiency resulted in pancreatic fibrosis (Veghelyi *et al.*, 1950b; Veghelyi and Kemeny, 1962); more severe deficiency accelerated toxicity from carbon tetrachloride (Veghelyi *et al.*, 1950a) causing vacuolation of pancreatic acinar cells and cystic dilatation of acini, while profound deficiency, along with dietary choline depletion, resulted in HPN (Rao *et al.*, 1976).

Considering all these points, the wide differences in antioxidant intake profiles between patients (Braganza *et al.*, 1986c; Rose *et al.*, 1986; Uden *et al.*, 1988) and that antioxidant defence can only be as strong as the weakest link in a complex chain (Figure 8) (Scott, 1988; Braganza, 1991), it seemed that a supplement of preventive and chain-breaking items was more likely to suc-

ceed than any single component. Accordingly different doses of selenium ACE (Wassen International, Leatherhead, UK) with or without methionine (Evans Ltd, Horsham, UK) were given in a long-term exploratory study (Braganza, 1991). Doses and combinations which controlled symptoms varied widely between patients (Sandilands *et al.*, 1990; Braganza *et al.*, 1987, 1988b, 1991). The combination that most frequently afforded long-term relief proved its value in preventing further painful attacks and controlling background pain through a 20-week double-blind, placebo-controlled trial (Uden *et al.*, 1990b). That combination, which provided daily doses of 600 μg organic selenium, 9000 IU β-carotene, 0.54 g vitamin C, 270 IU vitamin E and 2 g methionine, normalized blood antioxidant profiles (Uden *et al.*, 1992). Ongoing studies indicate that these doses may be required for 6 months, followed by a 50 per cent dose reduction and further reductions thereafter gauged by blood level of relevant items and also of FROPs. It is likely that certain people inadvertently render themselves susceptible to chronic pancreatitis because their diets deliver substantially less of one or more antioxidants than is required in the face of increased antioxidant demand, from induced cytochromes *P*-450 and/or other potential sources; by contrast, patients with recurrent acute pancreatitis are usually in equilibrium in this regard (Figure 12) but fall short periodically, perhaps because of a burst of increased free radical activity as may follow an alcoholic debauch.

Oxidative Stress in Pancreatic Cancer

Carcinogenic metabolites from xenobiotics also seem to be involved in human pancreatic cancer. So far as micronutrient antioxidants are concerned, a prospective case–control study showed that patients with different forms of cancer had lower mean serum selenium levels than controls, that the risk increased substantially when vitamin E levels were also low and that, among smokers, low serum retinol concentrations further increased the risk (Salonen *et al.*, 1985). Another prospective study revealed that levels of the β-carotene-like substance lycopene and of selenium were significantly lower in patients who went on to develop pancreatic cancer than in controls (Burney *et al.*, 1989). An increased incidence of pancreatic cancer has recently been noted in patients with pernicious anaemia but unfortunately levels of GSH-peroxidase and methionine were not measured: those antioxidant defence systems would be expected to be jeopardized (Figures 8 and 10). If antioxidant lack, relative or absolute, does play a part in the pathogenesis of this tumour, then the emphasis would have to be on prophylaxis rather than therapy. The highly complex interactions between the various micronutrient antioxidants on the one hand and between those items and carcinogenesis on the other (McBrien and Slater, 1983; Griffin, 1979) make it unlikely that any simple recipe will succeed.

Oxidative Stress in Other Pancreatic Diseases

Increased levels of FROPs have been registered in body fluids and target organs of patients with cystic fibrosis (reviewed by Uden *et al.*, 1992a). The lack of correlation between those levels and conventional indices of disease severity suggests that aberrant free radical activity may be an integral feature of the disease, somehow connected to the defective energy-coupling portion of the cystic fibrosis transmembrane transporter, CFTR. This proposal would rationalize every observation concerning the pancreas in this disease. It would also rationalize the non-pancreatic aberrations through oxidative stress (e.g. altered ion transport and short-circuit current) (Scott and Rabito, 1988; Matalon *et al.*, 1989), mobilization of natural antioxidant defences (e.g. increased mucin secretion by epithelia), or aggravation by factors that increase free radical activity (e.g. lung colonization by *Pseudomonas*) (Boucher *et al.*, 1988). A reversal in secretory polarity from oxidative stress in Clara cells of the lungs, on exposure to high concentrations of oxygen at birth, could rationalize progressive lung destruction from successive waves of leucocytes drawn in by FROPs discharged into the pulmonary interstitium—considering that leucocyte-derived proteases are involved in the pathogenesis of bronchiectasis from other causes (Burnett *et al.*, 1987).

Severe oxidative stress has been documented in kwashiorkor (Golden and Ramdath, 1987) and seems to represent the combined effects of increased free radical load from infective agents, dietary/atmospheric contaminants, strong ultraviolet rays, etc. in conjunction with poor dietary antioxidant intake. Iron-catalysed free radical production plays an important part in the tissue injury of haemochromatosis (Gutteridge *et al.*, 1985) and it is likely that copper-catalysed reactions are similarly involved in Wilson's disease.

PANCREAS: TARGET FOR TOXICITY FROM DRUGS AND CHEMICALS

Drug-Metabolizing Enzymes

Background

This has been covered in Chapters 3 and 6. Briefly, the conversion of a lipophilic drug that easily traverses membranes into a polar hydrophilic compound that is readily eliminated from cells is usually a two-stage process. In phase I an electrophilic group is inserted or revealed through the action of a microsomal electron-transport system of monoxygenases. In phase II the substituent group is conjugated with an amino acid, GSH or glucuronic acid. The various enzymes involved are collectively termed drug-metabolizing enzymes but, in fact, they metabolize a wide range of xenobiotics and also endogenous lipids (sterols, prostaglandins, bile acids, bilirubin, cholesterol, etc.). The terminal component of the phase I system, cytochrome *P*-450, exists in multiple molecular forms that were formerly classified according to substrate/species but nowadays by gene families (Roman numerals I, II, III, IV, XIA, XIB, XVII, XIX, XXI) with subfamilies indicated by capital letters (A–E) and individual genes by Arabic numerals 1 to 13 (Nebert *et al.*, 1987; Guengerich, 1989). It is recognized that the intrinsic level and inducibility of certain isoenzymes is genetically determined (Idle and Smith, 1979).

Studies of hepatocytes show that a xenobiotic traverses the plasma membrane along pathways shared by bilirubin and other organic anions, such as sulphobromophthalein, BSP, and, likewise, is transported by GSH-S-transferase B (ligandin) to the SER for phase I reactions. The ingredients are oxygen, NADPH, the flavoprotein NADPH cytochrome *P*-450 oxido-reductase, the hemoprotein cytochrome *P*-450, membrane phospholipids (Wade, 1986) and the trace element selenium (Correia and Burk, 1976). Phospholipids are vital because they hold substrate–enzyme complexes in optimal configuration, while stabilizing the active site region of the cytochrome. As regards selenium, there is increasing evidence of its importance in ensuring substrate–enzyme complexing through mechanisms independent of GSH peroxidase (Correia and Burk, 1976). On insertion of activated oxygen into the lipophilic substrate, a hydroxylated polar metabolite is generally produced which dissociates and moves into the aqueous environment of the cell where, if required, it becomes more polar through conjugation with GSH, glucuronic acid, sulphate, bile acids, etc. Polarity, size and charge are just some of the characteristics that determine the route of excretion, whether into bile or urine (Smith, 1973).

Hepatic Enzyme Induction

On exposure to xenobiotics, hepatocytes adapt by increasing the activities of appropriate cytochromes *P*-450. Two broad patterns of response are recognized: phenobarbitone-type (phenobarbital-type) and 3-methyl-cholanthrene (3-MC) type (Bowman and Rand, 1980; Schenkman and Kupfer, 1982; Hodson and Levi, 1987). The earliest event is an increase in mRNA, followed by increased haem synthesis through heightened activity of mitochondrial enzymes. The phenobarbitone-type response is characterized by expansion of SER membranes so that cell size increases and by the time the response reaches its peak, which may take a week or more, the weight of the liver may increase substantially; involvement of many isoenzymes of the broad *P*-450 II subfamily; and absence of potentiation by subsequent exposure to inducers of the 3-MC type. Characteristics of the 3-MC-type response include a narrow spectrum of enzyme activity; lack of change in SER area, microsomal protein, hepatocyte or liver weight; a short time to maximal effect; potentiation by phenobarbitone-type inducers; and a change in the enzyme's absorption peak for light from 450 nm to 448 nm. The metabolism of xenobiotics via cytochromes *P*-450 generally also ensures that they are 'detoxified'. On chronic exposure to xenobiotics, cells adapt by increasing levels of ancillary systems (reviewed in Braganza, 1988b, 1991). Thus an increase in GSH-S-transferase B results in more efficient extraction of substrate from plasma, as reflected in a fall in serum bilirubin levels and rapid early-phase disappearance of injected BSP. Evidence for accelerated phase II reactions can be obtained in several ways, e.g. by noting an increase in urinary D-glucaric acid, organic sulphate or mercapturic acid excretion. Furthermore, SER expansion that accompanies the phenobarbitone-type response results in increased production of very low density lipoprotein, albumin and γ-glutamyl-transpeptidase so that serum values may exceed the upper limits of the references ranges. For the same reason, the concentration of phospholipid in bile may increase.

Inheritance, species, sex and age are among many host factors that govern the level of enzyme induction. Of dietary factors, PUFA, especially C18:2 (as in corn, peanut and linseed oil), is a potent inducer of cytochromes *P*-450I (formerly called *P*-448) (Wade, 1986; Parker *et al.*, 1986). Other dietary inducers include volatile constituents from roasted freshly ground coffee, brassica vegetables, and barbecued foods. Other environmental sources include addictions (e.g. alcoholism, cigarettes), vehicle emissions, occupation (e.g. halogenated hydrocarbons), hobbies, prescribed drugs, and domestic chemicals.

Extra-hepatic Enzyme Induction

The contribution by extra-hepatic enzymes to the overall disposition of xenobiotics *in vivo* is small, even in the presence of enzyme induction. Nevertheless, drug metabolism in extra-hepatic sites may be toxicologically very significant (reviewed in Braganza, 1991). In the past few years there has been an escalation of interest in pancreatic cytochromes *P*-450. It is now known that these exist in adults of many species, that their distribution within acini, or ducts, or both varies between species (Baron *et al.*, 1983), and that pancreatic monooxygenases in animals and humans are inducible (Weibkin *et al.*, 1984; Foster *et al.*, 1993). Furthermore, on treating animals with certain substrates, e.g. nitrosamines, during the peak phase of DNA synthesis, the cells that evolve resemble hepatocytes both structurally and functionally (Rao *et al.*, 1983).

Enzyme Induction is a Double-edged Tool

It is paradoxical that a defence reaction, enzyme induction, may have deleterious consequences. This threat arises because the cellular load of oxygen radicals inevitably increases, and, more importantly, because certain chemicals undergo bioactivation to highly toxic species, so that prior enzyme induction amplifies the risk. If antioxidants are simultaneously denied, through dietary manipulation, the risk increases further. Selenium deprivation causes newly synthesized haem to be wasted down the bilirubin pathway instead of being incorporated into cytochrome *P*-450 (Correia and Burk, 1976). It is noteworthy that not all cytochrome *P*-450 inducers are primarily metabolized by that system. Thus, alcohol is largely metabolized via cytosolic dehydrogenases, and cytochromes *P*-450IIE assists only when intake increases substantially over long periods. However, even small doses of alcohol are potent inducers of that subfamily, so that they increase the yield of, and hence potential damage from, reactive intermediates of chemicals to which the animal may be simultaneously exposed, and which are processed by the same system (Sato *et al.*, 1980; Strubelt, 1980; Koop *et al.*, 1985). Those chemicals include nitrosamines, paraceta-

mol (acetaminophen) estrogens, ketones, aliphatic and halogenated hydrocarbons.

Pancreatic Disease: Casualty of Detoxification

Evidence for Liver and Pancreas Induction

Table 2 summarizes many observations from patients with pancreatic disease at Manchester, UK. They are collectively best interpreted as indicating liver as well as pancreatic enzyme induction, and include aspects that have been discussed in previous reviews (Uden, *et al.*, 1990a; Braganza, 1986, 1988a,b,d, 1991). *In vivo* studies of cytochromes *P*-450 showed no differences between patients and controls with regard to debrisoquine hydroxylation status (*P*-450II subfamily); a modest increase in antipyrine clearance (*P*-450II subfamily); but unequivocal increase in theophylline clearance (*P*-450I subfamily) (Acheson, 1987; Acheson *et al.*, 1989). These conclusions applied to most if not all patients with chronic pancreatitis, to some 50 per cent with gallstone-related acute pancreatitis, and to the majority with recurrent (non-gallstone) acute pancreatitis, and to the few with pancreatic cancer who reported relatively early. Recent studies showed increased theophylline clearance in tropical patients—at Madras (Chaloner *et al.*, 1990) and also Trivandrum, South India (J. M. Braganza and V. Balakrishnan, unpublished data)—than in local controls. However, the clearance values in those patients were much lower than in the Manchester patients, which underlined the need to consider antioxidant status, rather than enzyme induction alone.

Ultrastructural studies showed an increase in SER volume density in hepatocytes (Soames *et al.*, 1988) and RER/SER volume density in acinar cells (Tasso *et al.*, 1973) from European patients with 'early' chronic pancreatitis. Immunocytochemistry of surgically obtained tissue fragments, using a panel of mono-specific antibodies against different cytochromes *P*-450, provided proof of enzyme induction (Foster *et al.*, 1993). Control liver and/or pancreas material from cadaver organ donors and biopsy fragments from patients with chronic pancreatitis or pancreatic cancer were graded by an arbitrary scoring system in which 0 indicated no induction and 4 indicated heavy induction of all cells. The results are summarized

Table 2 Pancreas: target for chemical toxicity

	Liver	Pancreas
Compatible with enzyme induction	↑ Size hepatocyte ↑ SER ↑ VLDL to serum ↑ Phospholipid to bile ↑ Drug metabolism 　　BSPk₁ 　　Antipyrine clearance 　　Theophylline clearance 　　Urine DGA ↑ Cytos P450	↑ Size acinar cell ↑ RER ↑ Protein to PJ ↑ Calcium to PJ ? Pancreatic 　Contribution ↑ Cytos *P*-450
Suggest oxidative stress	↑ Microvesicular fat ↑ Lipofuscin ↑ FROPs in serum ↑ FROPs in bile	↑ Microvesiculation ↑ Lipofuscin 'Pancreastasis' 'Tubular complexes' ↑ Lysosomal enzymes in PJ
and Mobilization of natural antioxidants	↑ Ferroxidase I in serum	↑ Lactoferrin in PJ ↑ Mucin in PJ

Source: reproduced with permission from Braganza, 1991

in Figure 14. The following additional points emerged. (1) There was evidence of enzyme zonality in the normal liver: the isoenzymes *P*-450IIIA1 (pregnenelone-inducible form) and NADPH oxido-reductase showed centrilobular preference; *P*-450IA2 (polycyclic aromatic hydrocarbon-inducible form) showed a periportal preference; *P*-450IIE (alcohol-inducible form) was evenly distributed; and the phase II marker, an isoenzyme of GSH-transferase (GST 5–5), showed wide variability in distribution and expression. Bile duct cells showed lower levels than hepatoytes of certain enzymes but more uniform distribution of GST 5–5. (2) Liver enzyme induction in patients with chronic pancreatitis and pancreatic cancer was associated with loss of zonality. The order of enzyme increase was broadly similar in each disease: *P*-450IIIA1 > *P*-450IA2 > *P*-450IIE = oxido-reductase, and a maximal score of 4 was attained for at least one enzyme in each patient with each disease. GST 5–5 scores did not increase substantially. (3) There was no zonality in the normal pancreas where ductal cells generally showed lower levels of the enzymes than acinar cells. (4) Pancreatic acinar but not ductal cells displayed clear enzyme induction in chronic pancreatitis, although the order of change differed slightly from that in

hepatocytes: *P*-450IIIA1 = oxido-reductase > *P*-450IA2 > *P*-450IIE. A similar sequence emerged in pancreatic cancer except that in this case enzyme induction was found whether the tumor cells still had an acinar or ductal phenotype or whether the distinction could not be made. A maximal score of 4 was attained for one or other enzyme in every patient from each diagnostic subgroup. Changes in GST 5–5 levels were, however, generally less impressive. (5) Certain, as yet unidentified, cells of pancreatic islets from normal adults contained very high levels of *P*-450IA2. As this was not a feature in babies or children, it presumably reflected an inductive response to xenobiotics encountered in day-to-day living. There was clear induction of one or more enzymes in islets of chronic pancreatitis as well as pancreatic cancer groups.

A few other studies have been published on immunocytochemical localization of drug-metabolizing enzymes in the normal human pancreas (McManus *et al.*, 1987; Sasano and Sasano, 1988) but not in the diseased gland.

Evidence for Oxidative Stress in Liver and Pancreas

Table 2 also summarizes observations that are best interpreted as indicating oxidative stress in

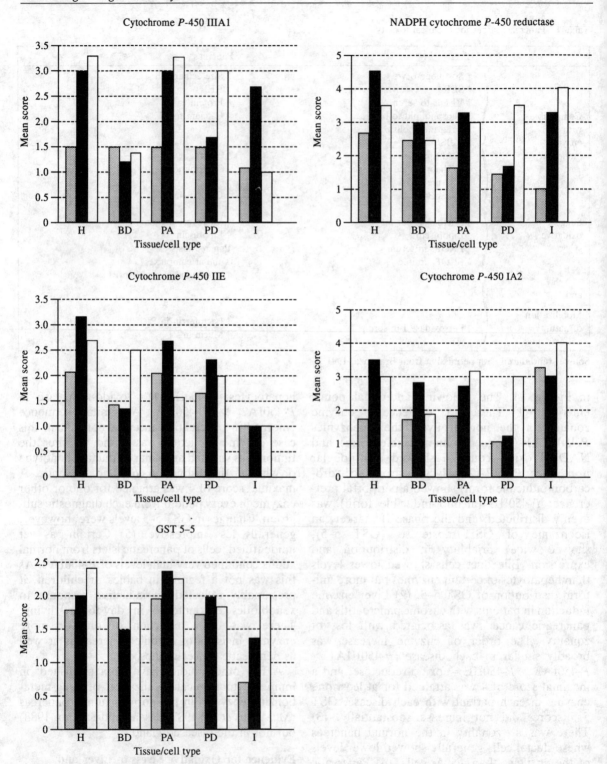

Figure 14   Summary of immunohistochemical findings using a panel of monospecific antibodies against different drug-metaboli-zing enzymes in subjects with and without exocrine pancreatic disease. Source: reproduced with permission from Foster *et al.*, 1993. ( ) Control; (■) chronic pancreatitis; (□) cancer pancreas. H = hepatocyte; BD = bile duct; PA = pancreatic acinar cell; PD = pancreatic duct cell; I = islet cell

liver and pancreas from patients with pancreatic disease. The importance of antioxidant lack in precipitating hepatic oxidative stress is further underlined by the rapid early-phase disappearance of injected BSP as well as the high levels of bilirubin in secretin-stimulated bile, with dramatic surges in the first 24 h of admission with acute-on-chronic pancreatitis, as these changes are reminiscent of those that accompany enzyme induction in selenium-deficient animals (Correia and Burk, 1976; Diplock, 1984). With regard to pancreatic involvement it is noteworthy that lactoferrin levels were several times higher in tropical patients with non-alcoholic chronic pancreatitis than in their European counterparts with alcoholic disease (Balakrishnan *et al.*, 1988).

Integrated Scheme

It is difficult to dismiss the various changes listed in Table 2 as non-specific responses to tissue damage because of the uniform direction of change despite the following differences: putative etiological factors, exocrine secretory capacity, endocrine status, duration of symptomatic illness, and antecedent treatment. These arguments also make it impossible to rationalize the changes as being secondary to pancreatic disease or its treatment. Instead the evidence suggests that the aberrations may be linked to disease pathogenesis. Furthermore, it seems that the gland can be damaged from reactive intermediates generated *de novo* through induced pancreatic cytochromes *P*-450, and also from stable metabolites that are generated via induced hepatic cytochromes *P*-450, if they entered the gland in refluxed bile or in the bloodstream (Figure 15) (Braganza, 1988a; Sandilands *et al.*, 1990). Studies of nasal epithelia from patients with cystic fibrosis showed similar levels of drug-metabolizing enzymes as in controls (J. Foster *et al.*, unpublished data). Preliminary data from kwashiorkor-affected tissues indicated low enzyme levels (Golden, 1991), which is not surprising considering that low dietary protein intakes impair enzyme synthesis, and that severe oxidative stress destroys cytochromes *P*-450 (Schenkman and Kupfer, 1982).

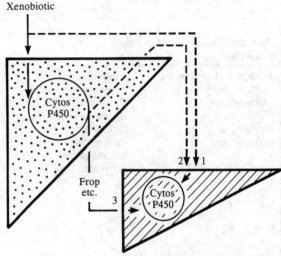

Hepatopancreatic interrelationships

i.e. casualties of heightened, but unmitigated oxidative–detoxification reactions

Figure 15 Possible routes of pancreatic injury from toxic metabolites of drugs/chemicals. See text for discussion. Source: reproduced with permission from Braganza, 1991

Chemicals in Non-neoplastic Pancreatic Disease: Human

Acute Pancreatitis

Table 3 is taken from a recent textbook (Braganza, 1991) and represents a synthesis of reviews (Nakashima and Howard, 1977; Mallory and Kern, 1980; Lendrum, 1981; Thomas, 1982; Guérin *et al.*, 1982; Dobrilla *et al.*, 1984; Laugier and Sarles, 1984), along with more recent information from case reports uncovered by computer-assisted searches. The interpretation of a proposed link is sometimes confounded by an association between concurrent disease and the pancreatic lesion—e.g. a three-way connection between azathioprine, Crohn's disease and pancreatitis; and the more recently documented three-way relationship between HIV infection, pancreatic lesions, and treatment with pentamidine or ddi (Schwartz and Brandt, 1989). In other cases the interpretation is not possible because of insufficient clinical and biochemical detail. Table 4 (from Braganza, 1991) attempts to understand drug-induced acute pancreatitis in the absence of a confounding influence—from pharmacological properties (Smith, 1973; Bowman and Rand, 1980; Schenkman and Kupfer, 1982; Halliwell

Table 3 Drugs and human pancreatitis[a]

Definite	Probable	Possible	?
No other factor	−	±	−/?
Temporal sequence	+	+	±/?
Rechallenge	+	−	−/?
Frusemide (Furosemide)	Azathioprine	Acetaminophen	Amphetamines
Methyldopa	5-Aminosalicylic acid	L-Asparaginase	β-Blockers
Metronidazole	Chlorothiazide	(paracetamol)	Cimetidine
Oestrogens	Dideoxyinosine	Calcium excess	Cholestyramine
Tetracycline	Diphenoxylate	Chlorthalidone	Clofibrate
Valproic acid	Pentamidine	Cytosine-ara	Clonidine
	Nitrofurantoin	Corticosteroids	Cyproheptidine
	Sulphonamides	Erythromycin	Dextropropoxyphene
		Ethacrynic acid	Diazoxide
		Indomethacin	Enalapril
		Isoniazid	Histamine
		6-Mercaptopurine	Isotretinoin
		Metronidazole	Meprobromate
		Procainamide	Phenformin
		Rifampicin	Warfarin
		Salicylates	
		Sulindac	
		Theophylline	
		Vinblastine	

[a] Note: − no information; + clear information; ± conflicting evidence; ? questionable interpretation from insufficient information; −/?, +/? some articles with information, others giving insufficient or questionable information.
Source: reproduced with permission from Braganza, 1991

Table 4 Possible mechanisms of drug toxicity in human acute pancreatitis

Possible mechanism	Drugs
Impeded protein synthesis/transport/secretion	Alcohol, L-asparginase, azathioprine, caerulein/CCK, calcium infusion, cobalt chloride, colchicine, corticosteroids, cytosine-ara, ddi, DL-ethionine, 6-mercaptopurine, pentamidine, phenylalanine, puromycin, sulphonamides, tetracycline, theophylline, vinblastine
P-450 induction	Alcohol, corticosteroids, isoniazid, meprobromate, rifampicin, valproic acid
Toxic metabolite Via P-450	Alcohol, azathioprine, indomethacin, isoniazid, methyldopa, metronidazole, nitrofurantoin, oestrogens, paracetamol, sulindac, valproic acid
Via other route	Chlorothiazide, chlorthalidone, ethacrynic acid, procainamide, sulphonamides
Increased triglycerides	Alcohol, β-blocker, corticosteroids, istoretinoin, oestrogens
Impeded drainage	Alcohol, dextropropoxyphene, diphenoxylate
Haptene formation	Alcohol, 5-aminosalicylic acid, isoniazid, procainamide, sulphonamides
No clues	Amphetamines, cholestyramine, cimetidine, clonidine, cyproheptidine, diazoxide, enalapril, histamine, phenformin, salicylates, warfarin

Source: reproduced with permission from Braganza, 1991

and Gutteridge, 1985; Hodson and Levi, 1987); by analogy with drug toxicity in the liver (Plaa and Hewitt, 1982; Trimble, 1982; Cohen, 1986); and by considering likely mechanisms in the genesis of other forms of acute pancreatitis (Table 1). Of course, an agent can injure the pancreas in more than one way, as exemplified by ethyl alcohol (Table 4).

With regard to injury from bioactivated drug metabolites, a case report of α-methyldopa-associated severe acute pancreatitis affecting ectopic as well as entopic pancreas denied alternate explanations (Bembow, 1988). The principle of pharmacogenetics (Idle and Smith, 1979) could explain why the most persuasive case reports linking frusemide (furosemide) and pancreatitis involved American blacks (Buchanan and Cane, 1977): other negroid races have been reported to possess higher intrinsic levels of certain cytochromes *P*-450. Prior induction of cytochromes *P*-450 by an extrinsic agent is equally important. This connection is recognized in the case of paracetamol (acetaminophen) or carbon tetrachloride-associated acute liver toxicity. Reports on drug- or chemical-related acute pancreatitis sometimes mention alcohol but seldom, if ever, whether the patient was a smoker or whether the diet contained substantial amounts of C18:2 fatty acids. Antioxidant status, perhaps the most important consideration of all, is significant by lack of mention in any report. Finally, two case reports that have a bearing on pathogenesis and treatment are worth discussing. One of them concerned a man who died within 12 h of consuming a large amount of theophylline and who showed all the neurological manifestations ascribed to blockade of adenosine receptors (Burgan *et al.*, 1982). The authors concluded that he did not have pancreatitis at autopsy because there was no histological evidence of inflammation. His blood amylase level was ten times the upper limit of normal 5 h after tablet ingestion and had doubled within the next 3 h, increments that typically accompany the pancreastasis phase of experimental pancreatitis (Figure 3). Blockade of adenosine receptors on plasma membranes of pancreatic acinar cells (Yamagishi, 1986) would be expected to compromise cell stores of SAMe and ATP (Figure 10). The second report (Deprez *et al.*, 1989), if confirmed, undermines the potential usefulness of 5-ASA in curbing the phagocyte activation component of acute pancreatitis.

The following inhaled chemicals have been mentioned in the context of acute pancreatitis: dimethylformamide (Chary, 1974), pentachlorophenol (as part of a wood preservative which also contained zinc naphthanate) (Cooper and MacCauley, 1982), trichloroethylene, volatile petrochemical products and diesel/petrol exhaust fumes (Braganza *et al.*, 1986b). It is recognized that many aliphatic/halogenated hydrocarbons undergo bioactivation and hence that prior enzyme induction magnifies tissue damage (Sato *et al.*, 1980; Strubelt, 1980; Plaa and Hewitt, 1982; Koop *et al.*, 1985). As little as 30 g alcohol may thus precipitate an attack of pancreatitis some 10 h later on exposure to those chemicals in home or work environment. A genuine link between inhaled hydrocarbons and acute pancreatitis would rationalize the observation that postoperative pancreatitis, after halogenated hydrocarbon anaesthetics, occurred even when the operation was nowhere near the gland (Howat and Sarles, 1979; Go *et al.*, 1986).

Chronic Pancreatitis

Alcoholism, cyanogenic glycosides, drugs such as azathioprine, oestrogens and sodium valproate, and high fat/protein diets are among the accepted environmental risk factors. A comprehensive review of alcohol-related hepatotoxicity (Leiber, 1988) applies equally to potential ways in which alcohol might injure the pancreas. In the case of the liver the emphasis has shifted away from mitochondrial damage to cytochrome *P*-450IIE-mediated production of reactive intermediates from drugs/chemicals to which the animal is simultaneously exposed. Induction of these isoenzymes could rationalize the resistance to ketosis when patients become diabetic, because ketones would be more rapidly processed. It is also important to note that the main metabolite of alcohol, acetaldehyde, tends to form adducts with constituents of the cytoskeleton and plasma membrane: the former would jeopardize secretion and could thus provoke a reversal in secretory polarity (in acinar cell as well as insulin-secreting cell), while the latter could generate chemotactins. Acetaldehyde itself may be further converted to acrolein which is extremely cytotoxic. Computer-assisted discriminant analysis of factors contributing to accelerated theophylline clearance in patients at Manchester, UK (Acheson *et al.*, 1989) picked out cigarette useage as the major influence, with a contribution from dietary protein and other factors. Each of the drugs incriminated in chronic pancreatitis is metabolized to reactive intermediates. Recent studies of European patients suggest an aetiological connection between regular inhalation of volatile chemicals, usually in the occupational environment, and chronic pancreatitis in non-alcoholics (Braganza *et al.*, 1986b; Dossing *et al.*, 1985), as well as in ex-alcoholics (Braganza *et al.*, 1986b). Those chemicals included paints, solvents and thinners; diesel/petrol fumes; and degreasing agents and dyes. This suspicion has now been confirmed in a large case–control study at Manchester, UK (McNamee *et al.*, 1993). A similar range of chemicals emerged in several patients with non-gallstone recurrent acute pancreatitis or pancreatic cancer (Figure 16).

The difficulties with the cassava hypothesis for tropical chronic pancreatitis have been discussed. Pancreatic toxicity was seen as an inadequate detoxification of hydrogen cyanide released from the cyanogenic glycosides linamirin, [2-(β-D-glucopyranosyl-oxy)isobutyronitrile] and lotaustralin (methyl linamirin) in cassava. An alternative suggestion (Braganza, 1988d) that the non-cyanide portion may be responsible was based on experimental damage to other organs (Ballantyne, 1987). It is supported by recent reports that in rats another plant nitrile, 1-cyano-2-hydroxy-3-butene(nitrile), depleted pancreatic GSH, and that subtle differences in nitrile structure spared the pancreas but caused liver and kidney damage (Wallig *et al.*, 1988). A study of xenobiotic exposure at Madras, India, where few people subsist on cyanogenic foods, revealed that many patients with chronic pancreatitis were in regular close contact with smoke (from firewood, vehicle emissions or cigarettes) and also petrochemical products, especially kerosene fumes from lamps or cookers (Braganza *et al.*, 1990). These links, if validated by case–control studies, could rationalize cardiomyopathy in those patients, considering that similar effects accompany kerosene toxicity in experimental animals (Rai and Singh, 1980), and also the decline in disease incidence in Kerala, India, in the past few years in line with electrification. Although there are no reports of kerosene metabolism by the pancreas, studies of the liver strongly suggest damage by toxic metabolites (Starek and Kaminski, 1982), one of which is acrolein which is also produced from acetaldehyde and allyl alcohol. The regular use of C18:2 fatty acids in cooking oil (linseed, peanut) would facilitate prior enzyme induction as would polycyclic aromatic hydrocarbons in smoke. Enzyme induction and antioxidant lack would be expected to accelerate damage from nitriles or kerosene.

Experimental Non-neoplastic Pancreatic Injury

Individual references are given in Table 5, which is taken from a recent review (Braganza, 1991). Some agents (asterisked) generate toxic metabolites, whether oxygen radicals, organic intermediates or both. Similar studies of hepatic injury show that a combination of items potentiates damage, e.g. coadministration of ethyl alcohol and high corn oil diets to rats increases the production of lipid radicals within microsomes (McCay and Reinke, 1987). The pancreas seems to be much more sensitive than the liver to damage from toxic metabolites, judging by studies with carbon tetrachloride where 0.07 g (100 g body weight)$^{-1}$ was sufficient to induce pancreatic lesions but twice as much was needed to cause hepatic injury. Pancreatic lesions were similar to those of human chronic pancreatitis (Veghelyi *et al.*, 1950a), except that features compatible with enzyme induction (Table 2) were lacking—which is not surprising considering that toxic metabolites from carbon tetrachloride tend to destroy cytochromes *P*-450 (Schenkman and Kupfer, 1982). Differences in the distribution of pancreatic cirrhosis nodules in different glands were ascribed to possible differences in blood supply (Veghelyi *et al.*, 1950a; Veghelyi and Kemeny, 1962), which in turn could reflect variations in islet-acinar 'portal' circulation especially now that certain cells in pancreatic islets have been shown to contain easily inducible cytochromes *P*-450 (Figure 14).

When pancreatic injury is caused by interference with protein synthesis in the RER, it is hardly likely that antioxidants will find use in prophylaxis or treatment. However, where a reactive intermediate is involved, GSH precursors and/or vitamin C could be useful.

Chemicals in Cancer of the Pancreas

Human Cancer

Risk factors revealed by demographic studies would be rationalized through involvement of pancreatic cytochromes *P*-450 (Figure 14). While immunocytochemical studies cannot pinpoint the location of induced cytochromes *P*-450, whether in the SER, plasma membrane or nuclear membrane, involvement of the last group poses a major threat because of its proximity to DNA.

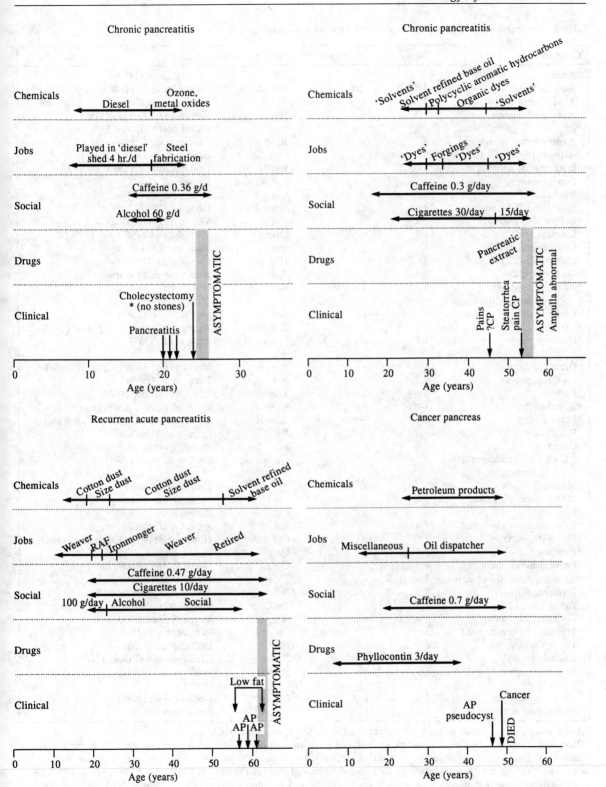

Figure 16 Examples of xenobiotic exposure histories in patients at Manchester, UK

Table 5 Chemicals and non-neoplastic experimental pancreatic injury

Chemical[a]	Injury[b]	Preparation[c]	Species	Reference
*Abrin	3,5	i,v	Rat	Barbieri *et al.* (1979)
*Acetaldehyde	3	i,iv	Rat, dog	Majumdar *et al.* (1986)
*Allyl alcohol	3	i	Rat	Nizze *et al.* (1979)
Aminoacids: lysine	1,3	i	Rat	Kitajima and Kishino (1985)
phenylalanine				Bieger and Kern (1975)
Amino methyl-α-carboline	4	i	Rat	Takaya *et al.* (1985)
*Azathioprine	5	ii	Dog	Broe and Cameron (1983)
β Adrenergic agonists	5	i	Rabbit	De Dios *et al.* (1989)
*Bendamustin	4	i	Rat, mouse	Horn *et al.* (1985)
Bile salts	1	ii	Cat	Hong *et al.* (1988)
Caerulein, CCK, etc	1	i,iv	Several	Go *et al.* (1986)
*Carbon tetrachloride	2,3,4	i	Rat	Veghelyi *et al.* (1950a)
*Chlorothiazide	1,3	i	Mouse	Cornish *et al.* (1961)
Colbaltous chloride	5	i	Rat	Kern and Kern (1969)
*Corn oil (20%)	4	i	Hamster	Parker *et al.* (1986)
*Corticosteroid	1,3,4	i	Rabbit	Benscome and Lazarus (1956)
*1-Cyano-2-hydroxy-3-	3,6	i	Rat	Wallig *et al.* (1988)
butene (nitrile)				
Cyclosporin	5	i	Rat	Mueller *et al.* (1988)
*Cythion	3	i	Teleost	Wallig *et al.* (1988); Ray *et al.* (1984)
*Diazinon	1,3	i	Guinea pig, dog	Frick *et al.* (1987)
Dibutylin dichloride	1	i	Rat	Merkord and Henninghausen (1989)
*2,4-dinitrophenol	1,3	i,iv	Rat	Letko *et al.* (1989)
*Endrin	4	i	Teleost	Datta and Ghose (1975)
*DL-Ethionine	1–6	i,iv	Several	Go *et al.* (1986); Rutledge *et al.* (1987)
*Ethyl alcohol	2–6	i–iv	Several	Go *et al.* (1986); Wilson *et al.* (1986)
Fenofibrate	3	i	Rat	Price *et al.* (1986)
Galactose	3	i	Rat	Putzke and Bienengraber (1967)
1,2,4,5,7,8-Hexachloro(9H)-	3	i	Guinea pig	De Caprio *et al.* (1987)
xanthene				
Modofinil	5	i	Rat	Chariot *et al.* (1987)
Monosodium glutamate	5	i	Rat	Lee and Sheen (1988)
Oleic acid	1	ii	Cat	Sanfey *et al.* (1986)
Palmitoylpentachlorophenol	3,6	i	Rat	Ansari *et al.* (1987)
Pancreatic enzymes	1	ii	Cat	Hong *et al.* (1988); Letko *et al.* (1989)
*Paraquat	3,4	i	Carp	Benedeczky *et al.* (1986)
*Petrochemicals: crude	4	i	Chick	Nwokolo and Ohale (1986)
diesel oil	3	i	Trout	Poirer *et al.* (1986)
Tetracycline	5	i,iii	Pigeon	Tucker and Webster (1972)
Puromycin	1,3	i	Rat	Longnecker (1991)
Toxin: paradysentery	3,4	i	Rat	Veghelyi *et al.* (1950a)
Tricothecene (mycotoxin)	3	i	Pig	Pang *et al.* (1986)
Triethyl citrate	6	i	Rat	Ohtaki *et al.* (1985)
Uraemia toxins	3,5	i	Rat	Krempien and Grosser (1987)
Venom: scorpion	1	i	Several	Williams *et al.* (1982); Murthy *et al.* (1989)
sand viper	1,3	i	Rat	Hodhod *et al.* (1989)
Vinblastine/vincristine	3,4,5	i	Mouse	Nevalainen (1975)

[a] Asterisked items are known to generate oxygen radicals and/or reactive intermediates.
[b] Pattern of injury: 1 = 'acute pancreatitis', i.e. reduced secretion into duct + increased serum enzymes; 2 = 'chronic pancreatitis', i.e. cirrhosis equivalent; 3 = 'toxic', i.e. detected by ultrastructural (microvesiculation ± lipofuscin ± membrane blebbing ± dilated disorganised ER) and/or functional changes (leakage of LDH, etc.); 4 = 'degenerative', i.e. loss of staining polarity ± tubular complexes ± cysts ± atrophy; 5 = reduced protein and/or phospholipid synthesis and/

Notes to table 5 (continued)

or reduced protein secretion; 6 = 'miscellaneous', including immune, vascular, apoptotic (macrophage-initiated), P-450-mediated, etc.
[c] Preparation: i = whole animal; ii = isolated perfused gland; iii = gland slices; iv = dispersed acini; v = subcellular fraction.

Source: Reproduced with permission from Braganza, 1991

Cigarette smoke is the clearest association. It is recognized that each puff of smoke delivers 10^{15} free radicals in the gas phase (e.g. oxides of nitrogen) and 10^{14} free radicals in the tar phase (e.g. from benzo[a]pyrene). Smoke contains two main classes of potentially genotoxic chemicals—polycyclic aromatic hydrocarbons (Freudenthal and Jones, 1976) and nitrosamines (Lijinsky, 1987), and several potential epigenetic agents (Williams, 1984), including catechols and phenolic compounds. Simple alkylating agents tend to cause point mutations in DNA whereas complex adducts, as derived from benzo[a]pyrene and certain nitrosamines, can cause frameshifts.

Chemicals inhaled in the work environment are other potential sources of genotoxins. Suspected agents include coal-tar (Registrar General, 1958; Redmond et al., 1976) and coal-pitch (Turner and Grace, 1938; Dorken, 1964); benzene (Wocka-Marek et al., 1987), benzidine and β-naphthylamine (Mancuso and El-Attar, 1967); methylene chloride (Friedlander et al., 1978); petroleum products (Lin and Kessler, 1981; Norell et al., 1986); paints, varnishes, thinners, solvents and degreasing agents (Lin and Kessler, 1981; Norrel et al., 1986). Many of these substances are produced during the fractionation of petroleum. This process yields natural gas (C_{1-2}), used for fuel and in the chemical industry; liquefied or bottled gas (C_{3-4}), used as fuel gas, for the synthesis of rubber compounds and in the petrochemical industry; petroleum ether (C_{4-5}), for solvents and to anaesthetize small animals; gasolenes (C_{6-10}) in cleaning fluids, solvents, and for refining stock; kerosenes (C_{5-16}), used as jet, tractor and gas turbo-fuels and in lamps and stoves in underdeveloped countries; gas-oil (C_{9-16}), used as diesel or furnace oil; lubricating stocks ($C_{>17}$), for white oils, lubricating oils and greases; waxes ($C_{>20}$), for ceiling wax; and bottoms ($C_{>20}$), used as heavy fuel oil, road oil and asphalt. Suspicion that chronic pancreatitis in tropical zones may increase the risk for pancreatic cancer (Balakrishnan, 1987) would be rationalized if smoke and kerosene fumes were to be involved: the mutagenicity of airborne particles from a kerosene heater has been demonstrated (Yamanaka and Maruoka, 1984). Similarly, it is not difficult to see why chronic pancreatitis in temperate zones may be a forerunner of pancreatic cancer since aliphatic/aromatic halogenated hydrocarbons, as in solvents, degreasing agents, paint thinners, etc., seem to be involved in each condition (Figure 16) (McNamee et al., 1993). These hydrocarbons, whose potential genotoxicity is recognized (Schwartz and Brandt, 1989) are ubiquitous (Aviado et al., 1976; Nicholson and Moore, 1979) in the polluted atmosphere of industrialized and traffic-congested cities.

Other suspected risk factors for pancreatic cancer could be rationalized through promotion of cytochromes P-450 activity. Thus, the increased susceptibility of American blacks may be due to a higher intrinsic level of certain cytochromes P-450 (Idle and Smith, 1979). The interaction between genetic and environmental factors influencing cytochromes P-450 may explain the occurrence of pancreatic cancer in siblings and kindreds with hereditary chronic pancreatitis. It would also rationalize the report of pancreatic cancer in a chemical worker and his son who were exposed to vinyl chloride and other substances (Reiner et al., 1977). The association between high fat diets and pancreatic cancer may reflect the steady increase in consumption of PUFA, especially C18:2, in corn-oil by Western societies in the past 50 years (Hollander and Tarnawski, 1986). Although coffee has been exonerated in large-scale studies it is impossible to be sure that it does not play a part in individual cases, through numerous volatile chemicals in roasted coffee (Gianturco et al., 1966), e.g. when the disease developed simultaneously in husband and wife who consumed vast amounts of margarine and coffee essence (Ferguson and Watts, 1980). Continued suspicion that alcohol may be a risk factor is understandable now that its inducing effect on cytochrome P-450IIE is appreciated. It is hardly surprising that these potential interactions could not be dissected out in the study relating expression of different pancreatic cytochromes *P*-450 (Figure 14) and exposure to xenobiotics (Foster *et al.*, 1993). Failure or inability to document prior exposure to enzyme inducers or antioxidant status could also explain discrepant results concerning chemicals and human pancreatic cancer in some studies (Li *et al.*, 1969; Hoar and Pell, 1981; Mack and Paganini-Hill, 1981; Gold *et al.*, 1985).

Experimental Cancer

The inhalation route of xenobiotic entry, which may be very relevant to the pathogenesis of human pancreatitis and also pancreatic cancer, has not been used in experimental studies although the methodology is well documented (Witschi and Brain, 1985). Cancer experiments have largely focused on a ductal phenotype tumour as produced by the nitrosamine, *N*-nitrosobis (2-hydroxy-propyl) amine (BOP), in hamsters (Go *et al.*, 1986; Pour and Lawson, 1984); and an acinar phenotype tumour from *O*-diazoacetyl-L-serine, azaserine, in rats (Go *et al.*, 1986, Longnecker *et al.*, 1984) (Table 6). Transgenic mouse models have recently been described involving either an elastase enhancer/promoter–SV40 T-antigen construct (Ornitz *et al.*, 1987), or an elastase enhancer/promoter–*myc* oncogene construct (Sandgren *et al.*, 1990). The former has an acinar phenotype while the latter may have a ductal or mixed phenotype. The *in vitro* model of carcinogenesis (Parsa *et al.*, 1985) using foetal rat or foetal/adult human pancreas explants would, however, appear to be the most versatile for the study of pancreatic drug-metabolizing enzymes and their inducibility, especially now that antibodies to specific *P*-450s are available.

The spectrum of cancer precursor lesions in BOP and azaserine models includes the atypical acinar cell focus consisting of cells with increased size of nucleus, prominent nucleolus, increased mitotic index, cytoplasmic basophilia and reduced zymogen content; atypical acinar cell nodule, similar in all respects except that it is larger; acinar cell adenoma with size more than 3 mm and a tendency to capsule formation; cystic ductal complex with one or more luminal spaces lined by flattened epithelium containing some cells that possess zymogen granules; tubular ductal complex with small lumina; and finally, carcinoma-in-

situ. The last three lesions and papillary hyperplasia are characteristic of BOP-induced lesions in hamsters, whereas the first three are typical of cancer in rats following exposure to any carcinogen (Go *et al.*, 1986).

Several oxidized derivatives of dipropylnitrosamine (Figure 17) can produce pancreatic cancer in hamsters but BOP is the most pancreas-specific and carcinogenic potency lies in the order MOP > BOP > HPOP > BHP (Table 7). HPOP exists as a tautomeric mixture of the open chain and cyclic forms (Figure 17); so it is not surprising that the cyclic form, NDMM, which is a derivative of morpholine, also has carcinogenic potential. It resembles the endocrine cell toxin streptozotocin, which may help to rationalize the variable effects on exocrine cancer yield when this drug is given along with BOP. Structure–activity relationships have been defined for these nitrosamines (Moossa, 1980; Pour and Lawson, 1984). Thus, the presence of a keto or hydroxy group in the β-position on an aliphatic chain proved to be a prerequisite for pancreatic carcinogenicity; the addition of a second β-keto group increased activity and specificity for the pancreas; the replacement of a 2-oxo chain with a methyl group diminished pancreas specificity as did prolongation of the aliphatic chain; and carboxylation at the 3-position was associated with complete loss of pancreatotropism. HPOP and MOP seem to be more proximate carcinogens, but the ultimate carcinogen is unclear. The bulk of BOP metabolism occurs in the liver by a microsomal cytochrome *P*-450-dependent system, and to a much lesser extent by a cytosolic system which utilizes NADH or NADPH (Boux *et al.*, 1983). There is agreement that substantially less BOP is metabolized in the pancreas, and that exocrine cell cytosol may be the predominant site, with little (Kokkinakis and Scarpelli, 1989) or no (Boux *et al.*, 1983) contribution from microsomes.

These data suggest that carcinogenic metabolites produced in the liver may enter the gland by way of the bloodstream, and in certain circumstances through bile reflux (Ruckert *et al.*, 1981). This concept, which has also been proposed for human pancreatic disease (Braganza, 1983, 1986, 1988a) is supported by the greater damage to pancreatic DNA after *in vivo* than *in vitro* treatment of animals with BOP and MOP (Curphey *et al.*, 1987), and the observation that interruption of the hepatic blood supply reduced the DNA-

Table 6 Main animal models for pancreatic cancer

Model	Hamster	Rat
Carcinogen	BOP	Azaserine
Tumour phenotype	Ductal	Acinar
Tumour histogenesis	?	Acinar
Proximate carcinogen(s)	HPOP, MOP, other	Diazoacetate
Activator	P-450-dependent/other	Pyridoxal-dependent
Location	Microsomal/cytosolic	?
GSH/GSSG change	$\times 19/\times 14$	?
DNA damage	O^6 methylguanine	N^7-carboxy-methyl-guanine
Potential liver contribution	+++	±
Promoters effects	Similar (see text)	Similar (see text)
Effect of BOP		
Pancreas cancer yield	> 80%	Nil
Metabolising capacity		
Liver microsomes NADH/NADPH	+++++/+	±/++
Cytosol NADH/NADPH	+/+	±/±
Pancreas microsomes NADH/NADPH	±/+	ND/ND
Cytosol NADH/NADPH	±/+	ND/+
DNA damage		
Whole organ	++++	+
Duct/acinar cell	+++/+	+/+
DNA repair efficiency		
Whole organ	?	?
Duct/acinar cell	+/+++	++++/+++++
Mutagenicity		
Via liver S9	?	?
Via acinar cell	+	+
Via pancreas	+	++
Protein synthesis reduction	Nil	Nil
Effect of azaserine		
Pancreas cancer yield	Nil	> 80%
Metabolizing capacity	+++	+++
DNA damage		
Whole organ	+++	+++
Duct/acinar cell	−/++	−/+++
DNA repair efficiency	?	?
Mutagenicity (via acinar)	+	+
Protein synthesis reduction	+	++

damaging effect of MOP *in vivo* (Schaeffer *et al.*, 1984). In any case, oxidative stress is shown by the 14-fold increase in GSH and 19-fold increase in GSSG in the pancreas after BOP treatment (Toyooka *et al.*, 1989). BOP was found to damage DNA in cells isolated from the whole pancreas, hence largely acinar, in doses as low as 0.5 µg ml^{-1} (Levin *et al.*, 1984) and HPOP was marginally less potent. Damage to duct cells was substantially higher than to acinar cells when these were examined separately (Lawson and Nagel, 1988) and DNA repair efficiency was also much lower in ductal cells. Several specific methylated and hydroxypropylated DNA bases were identified after BOP and HPOP treatment. However, levels of O^6-methyl guanine best reflected their relative carcinogenic potency (Kokkinakis and Scarpelli, 1989); while O^6 and N^7-alkyl guanine adducts persisted much longer in ductal than acinar cells (Bax *et al.*, 1990). Mutagenicity does not seem to have been tested via liver fractions. Studies of pancreatic S-9 fractions from control and polychlorinated-biphenyl-induced hamsters showed mutagenicity in strain TA100 by BOP

Table 7   Pancreatic cancer and chemicals (1)

	Abbreviation	Species
Nitrosamines		
N-Nitrosobis (2-hydroxy-propyl) amine	BHP	Hamster, rat
N-Nitrosobis (2-oxopropyl)-amine	BOP	Hamster
N-Nitroso (2-hydroxy-propyl)-(2-oxopropyl) amine	HPOP	Hamster, rat
N-Nitrosodimethylamine	DMN	Rat
N-Nitroso-2, 6-dimethyl-morpholine	NDMM	Hamster
N-Nitrosomethyl (2-oxopropyl) amine	MOP	Hamster
N-Methyl-N-nitrosourea	MNU	Guinea pig, human
N-Methyl-N-nitrosourethane	MNUT	Guinea pig
N-Nitroso (2-oxopropyl) propylamine	NOPPA	Guinea pig
N^d-(N-Methyl-N-nitrosocarbamoyl)-L-ornithine	MNCO	Hamster, rat
N-Nitroso dimethylamine	DMN	Rat, human
4-(Methylnitrosaminol)-1-(3-pyridy)-1-butanone 'Tobacco specific'	NNK	Rat
Other		
2-Acetylaminofluorene	AAF	Rat, dog
Azaserine	—	Rat
4-Hydroxyquinoline-1-oxide	4-HAQ	Rat

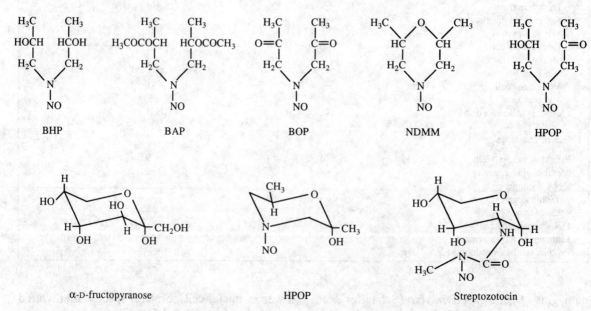

Figure 17   Chemical structure of some oxidized derivatives of dipropylnitrosamine and, for comparison, chemical structure of islet cell toxins such as streptozotocin. For abbreviations see Table 7

and HPOP but not by NDMM or BHP (Mori *et al.*, 1986). NDMM was mutagenic in a study with strain TA1535 as detector (Scarpelli *et al.*, 1980); and use of Chinese hamster V79 cells as target showed that BOP was a more potent mutagen that HPOP (Mangino *et al.*, 1985). However, carcinogenic or mutagenic potential was not reflected in protein synthesis which was unchanged by BOP treatment (Zucker *et al.*, 1986). Finally, it is noteworthy that treatment of pregnant animals with BOP caused a different spectrum of tumours in maternal and foetal tissues (Pour, 1986).

Azaserine (Figure 18) produces precursor

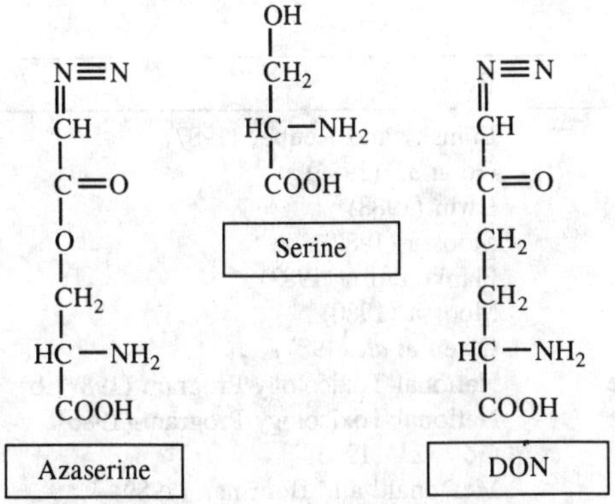

Figure 18 Chemical structure of the amino acid serine, the genotoxin azaserine, and a related compound (DON)

lesions of the acinar phenotype in rats. As in the case of BOP, this carcinogen requires metabolic activation but seemingly via a pyridoxal-dependent reaction yielding diazoacetate: the structurally similar 6-diazo-5-oxo-L-norleucine (DON) was much less effective (Lilja *et al.*, 1981). The reaction results in N^7-carboxymethylguanine in addition to the more usual O^6 guanine adduct (Go *et al.*, 1986). The degree of pancreatic DNA damage is the same in *in vitro* and *in vivo* studies which indicates that another organ, such as the liver, is not required for metabolic activation and does not contribute substantially to carcinogenicity (Curphey *et al.*, 1987). Persistence of DNA damage, indicating delay in repair, has been shown by studies of rat acinar cells in primary culture (Steinmetz and Mirsalis, 1984). The frequency of mutation in V79 cells increased in direct culture with azaserine but without further increase on co-culture with rat acinar cells.

High PUFA, especially C18:2, diets as well as factors that promote pancreatic growth (Dowling *et al.*, 1987) increased tumour yield in BOP and azaserine models. The confusing literature on the effect of various hormones has been reviewed (Skett, 1987). From the information in Table 6, it is clear that species specificity of BOP and azaserine is best explained in terms of differences in pancreatic DNA damage/repair efficiency. With regard to ductal versus acinar phenotype, the facts are consistent with a hypothesis that the acinar cell may be the cell of origin for tumour induction in both species (Moore *et al.*, 1983), but that species-dependent factors influence subsequent development so that the tumour acquires

features of duct cells in hamsters but retains acinar cell features in rats.

Tables 7 and 8 summarize information regarding pancreatic chemical carcinogens: individual references are given only for those substances that were not mentioned in previous reviews (Moossa, 1980; Longnecker *et al.*, 1984; Go *et al.*, 1986). The rapidly expanding literature on the influence of antioxidant treatment in experimental cancer will have to await a future review.

The real question is whether these animal models are relevant to human pancreatic cancer. Very recent reports describe pancreatic cancers in rats, including a ductal phenotype lesion, from a tobacco-specific nitrosamine (Rivenson *et al.*, 1988; Pour and Rivenson, 1989). A dearth of reports on polycyclic aromatic hydrocarbon-induced experimental cancer is not surprising, considering that the inhalation route has not been tested, nor the effect of concurrent exposure to halogenated species, and especially to alcohol. The most abundant DNA adducts in human as well as experimental pancreatic cancer involve O^6 methyl-guanine. Other clear parallels relate to the positive association between high fat diets and pancreatic cancer yield, and evidence of a liver contribution to xenobiotic metabolism of potential carcinogens. Finally, the question of histogenesis has been raised for ductal phenotype lesions in man (Bockman, 1981; Iwanig and Jamieson, 1982), as well as in the BOP hamster model.

Summary: Target for Toxicity

Of the drugs and chemicals incriminated/suspected in the aetiology of pancreatic cancer, chronic pancreatitis and acute pancreatitis, several are known to undergo bioactivation. The paradox that the pancreas bears the brunt of injury, although the liver is clearly involved to the same extent (Table 2), may result from a much greater endowment of GSH and ancillary detoxification symptoms therein. Observations in patients with alcoholic chronic pancreatitis show that overt signs of liver damage may be delayed for a decade after the first symptom of pancreatic damage (Howat and Sarles, 1979). Involvement of liver cytochromes *P*-450 in the pancreatic cancer setting may explain why hepatic metastases are often present at the time of clinical presentation in the human disease. The spectrum of pancreatic injury inducible by the same toxin, e.g.

Table 8 Pancreatic cancer and chemicals (2)

Chemicals	Species	Reference
Acrolein	Rat	Lijinsky and Reuber (1987)
Aflatoxin	Monkey	Go et al. (1986)
2-Amino-5-nitrophenol	Rat	Irwin (1988)
Azinphos-methyl	Rat	Moossa (1980)
Azo dyes: yellow 3	Rat	Plankenhorn (1983)
Benzo[a]pyrene	Several	Moossa (1980)
1-3-Butadiene	Rat	Owen et al. (1987)
Chlorendic acid	Rat, mouse	National Toxicology Program (1987a,b)
Chlorinated paraffins	Rat, mouse	National Toxicology Program (1986)
Clofibrate	Rat	Go et al. (1986)
2,6-Dichloro-p-pheny-lenediamine	Rat	McDonald and Boorman (1989)
Dimethylaminobenzenes	Rat	Moossa (1980); Watari (1985)
7,12-Dimethylbenz[a]-anthracene	Rat, mouse	Go et al. (1986); Moossa (1980)
Dimethylhydrazine	Rabbit	Moossa (1980)
4-Fluoro-4-aminobiphenyl	Rat	Moossa (1980)
N-2-Fluor-enylacetamide	Rat	Moossa (1980)
2,7-Fluor-enylenebisacetamide	Rat, mastomys	Moossa (1980); Hoch-Ligeti et al. (1985)
2-Mercaptobenzthiazole	Rat, mouse	Dieter (1988)
Methylazoxymethanol acetate	Guppy	Fournie et al. (1987)
3-Methylcholanthrene	Mouse	Moossa (1980)
Nafenopin [2-methyl-2-(p-1,2,3,4-tetrahydro-1-naphthyl)-phenoxy propionic acid]	Rat	Go et al. (1986)
Nitrofen [2-4-dichloro-1 (4-nitrophenoxy) benzene]	Rat	Go et al. (1986)
Toluene	Rat, mouse	National Toxicology Program (1987c)

DL-ethionine or ethyl alcohol, underlines the need to consider dose, species, confounding factors and a multiplicity of potential tissue-damaging agents, including products of activated phagocytes and the immune response. Finally, the mystery of ketone resistance in diabetics with chronic pancreatitis, especially in tropical zones, may be resolved if induced cytochromes *P*-450IIE are implicated, as this isoenzyme family seems to process ketones.

HORIZONS

The bulk of information presented in this chapter suggests that the regulated secretory pathway in pancreatic acinar cells is exquisitely sensitive to oxidative stress, and that this vulnerability plays a major part in each of the acquired pancreatic diseases (Braganza, 1991). There are clues as to the pathogenesis of oxidative stress in these diseases as well as in certain congenital diseases (Table 9) (Braganza, 1991). The predominance of cytochromes *P*-450 as a source of excessive free radical activity should not come as a surprise when one considers that this is a very primitive acquisition in phylogenetic terms (Figure 1). Hence, evidence of chemical damage to pancreatic acinar cells in lower vertebrates, e.g. the toxicity of weedkillers in teleosts, or diesel oil in trout (Table 5), should not be disregarded as irrelevant to human pancreatic disease. The similarity in patterns of pancreatic damage from toxic metabolites or antioxidant deficiency, e.g. vacuolation of cytoplasm and dilated ER on exposure to many toxins as well as from isolated trace metal deficiency, or production of pancreatic hepatocytes by a particular regimen of BOP treatment or copper deficiency, can be reconciled with the realization that each manoeuvre would precipitate oxidative stress. These similarities underline the importance of considering antioxidant status, enzyme induction as well as concurrent exposure to a drug/chemical that undergoes bioactivation in pancreatic toxicology. These three factors can probably be considered as components of disease aetiology (Rothman, 1986), insofar as pancreatic disease is concerned (Table 9). The inhalation route may be especially important with regard to the second and third component, while the first component has implications for treatment and, more importantly, for prophylaxis.

Table 9 Summary: a 'radical' approach to pancreatic disease

DISEASE	FREE RADICALS			ANTIOXIDANTS		OXIDATIVE STRESS		
	Load	Source	Type	Supply	Type ↓	Pattern	Speed	Degree
ACUTE PANCREATITIS								
– edematous duct/artery	↑	XO	$O_2(1)$	N or ↓	Vit C + GSH items	episodic	rapid	mild
xenobiotics	↑	P-450	$O_2(1)$ + organic					
idiopathic	↑	mixed						
mixed	↑	mixed						
– HPN	↑↑	PMN/MO	$O_2(2)$	↓↓		often fatal		severe
CHRONIC PANCREATITIS								
– alcoholism	↑↑	P450IIE ADH		N or ↓	Vit C ± methionine ± selenium	constant + bursts	gradual	moderate
– idiopathic	↑↑	P450s		N or ↓				
cigarette smoke		P450IA2						
volatile chemicals		P450IIE	$O_2(1)$ + organic					
C18:2 oil/fat		P450I						
– tropical	↑↑			↓↓	Vit C ± β-carotene ± SAA ± selenium	constant	rapid	severe
wood smoke		P450I						
cassava		P450 ?						
kerosene		P450 ?						
C18:2 oil		P450I						
CANCER PANCREAS	↑↑	P450IIIA1 P450IA2 P450IIE	$O_2(1)$ + genotoxins	N or ↓	?	constant	gradual	moderate
CYSTIC FIBROSIS								
– childhood	↑	CFTR	$O_2(1)$	N	Vit C ± selenium	constant	gradual	mild
– adult	↑↑	PMN/MO pseudo-monas	$O_2(2)$ $O_2(1)$	varied		bursts	rapid	severe
KWASHIORKOR	↑↑	mixed	$O_2(1,2)$ organic	N or ↓	all	constant	rapid	severe
METAL STORAGE	↑	Fenton	$O_2(1)$	?	?	constant	gradual	moderate

Abbreviations: PMN = polymorphonuclear cells; MO = macrophages, XO = xanthine oxidase; $O_2(1)$ = primary metabolites of oxygen; $O_2(2)$ = secondary metabolites; HPN = haemorrhagic pancreatic necrosis; CFTR = cystic fibrosis transmembrane regulator gene.
Source: reproduced with permission from Braganza, 1991

Acknowledgements

It is a pleasure to acknowledge the expertise and good humour of Miss Carroline Thorpe during the preparation of this chapter. I appreciate further secretarial help from Miss L. Batty. I thank Mrs S. Roe of the Medical Illustrations Department at the hospital for preparing the figures.

REFERENCES

Acheson, D. W. K. (1988). The pharmacokinetics of theophylline and antipyrene and the pharmacogenetics of debrisoquine metabolism in patients with exocrine pancreatic disease. MD Thesis, University of London, UK

Acheson, D. W. K., Hunt, L. P., Rose, P., Houston, J. B. and Braganza, J. M. (1989). Factors affecting the accelerated clearance of theophylline and antiyprine in patients with exocrine pancreatic disease. *Clin. Sci.*, **76**, 377–387

Adler, G. and Kern, H. F. (1984). Fine structural and biochemical studies in human acute pancreatitis. In Gyr, K. E., Singer, M. V. and Sarles, H. (Eds). *Pancreatitis – Concepts and Classification.* Exerpta Medica, Oxford, pp. 37–42

Almoguera, C., Shibata, D., Forrester, K., Martin, J., Arnheim, N. and Perucho, M. (1988). Most human carcinomas of the exocrine pancreas contain mutant *c-K-ras* genes. *Cell* **53**, 549–554

Anon (1989). Focus on S-adenosye-L-methromone. In *Drugs*, **38**, 389–416

Ansari, G. S., Kaphalia, B. S., Boor, P. J. (1987). Selective pancreatic toxicity of palmitoylpentachlorophenol. *Toxicology*, **46**, 57–63

Arfors, K. E., and Del Maestro, R. (Eds) (1986). Free radicals in the microcirculation. *Acta Physiol. Scand.*, **126** (suppl. 548)

Arvan, P. and Castle, J. D. (1987). Phasic release of newly synthesised secretory proteins in the unstimulated rat exocrine pancreas. *J. Cell Biol.*, **104**, 243–252

Autor, A. P. (Ed.) (1982). *Pathology of Oxygen.* Academic Press, London

Aviado, D. M., Zakhari, S., Simaan, J. A. and Ulsamev, A. G. (1976). *Methyl Chloroform and Trichloroethylene in the Environment.* CRC Press, Ohio

Balakrishnan, V. (Ed.) (1987). *Chronic Pancreatitis in India.* St. Joseph's Press, Trivandrum

Balakrishnan, V., Sauniere, J. F., Hariharan, M. and Sarles, H. (1988). Diet, pancreatic function and chronic pancreatitis in South India and France. *Pancreas*, **3**, 30–35

Ballantyne, B. (1987). Toxicology of cyanides. In Ballantyne, B. and Marrs, T. C. (Eds) *Clinical and*

Experimental Toxicology of Cyanides. Wright, Bristol, pp. 41–126

Barbieri, A., Gasperi-Campani, A., Derenzini, M., Betts, C. M. and Stirpe, F. (1979). Selective lesions of acinar pancreatic cells in rats poisoned by abrin. *Virchows Arch. Cell. Pathol.*, **30**, 15–24

Baron, J., Kawabata, T. T., Redick, J. A. *et al.* (1983). Localization of carcinogen metabolising enzymes in human and animal tissue. In Rydstrom, J., Montelios, J. and Bengtsson, M. (Eds), *Extrahepatic Drug Metabolism and Chemical Carcinogenesis.* Elsevier, Oxford, pp. 73–82

Bax, J., Pour, P. M., Nagel, D. L., Lawson, T. A., Woutersen, R. A. and Scherer, E. (1990). Longterm persistence of DNA alkylation in hamster tissues after N-nitrosobis(2-oxopropyl)amine. *J. Cancer Res. Clin. Oncol.*, **116**, 149–155

Bembow, E. W. (1988). Simultaneous acute inflammation in entopic and ectopic pancreas. *J. Clin. Pathol.* **41**, 430–434

Bencosme, S. A. and Lazarus, S. S. (1956). Pancreas of cortisone-treated rabbits. *Arch Pathol*, **62**, 285–295

Benedeczky, I., Nemcsok, J. and Halasy, K. (1986). Electron microscopic analysis of the cytopathological effect of pesticides in the liver, kidney and gill tissues of carp. *Acta Biol. (Szeged)*, **32**, 69–91

Berridge, M. J. (1984). Inositol trisphosphate and diacylglycerol as second messengers. *Biochem. J.* **220**, 345–360

Bieger, W. and Kern, H. F. (1975). Studies on intracellular transport in the rat exocrine pancreas. I. Inhibition by aromatic amino acids *in-vitro. Virchows Arch. Pathol. Anat.* **367**, 289–305

Blower, A. L. (1989). Treatment of acute necrotising haemorrhagic pancreatitis by whole blood exchange transfusion. *MD Thesis*, University of Manchester, UK

Bockman, D. E. (1981). Cells of origin of pancreatic cancer. *Cancer*, **47**, 1528–1534

Borch, K., Kullman, E., Hallhagen, S., Ledin, T and Ihse, J. (1988). Increased incidence of pancreatic neoplasia in pernicious anaemia. *World J. Surg.*, **12**, 866–870

Boucher, R. C., van Scott, M. R., Willumsen, N., Jackson Stutts, M. (1988). Mechanisms and cell biology of airway epithelial injury. *Am. Rev. Respir. Dis.*, **138**, S41–S44

Boux, L. J., Leung, K.-H., Sweet, M. and Archer, M. C. (1983). Enzymatic reduction of β-ketonitrosamines. *Carcinogenesis*, **4**, 1495–1498

Bowman, W. C. and Rand, M. J. (1980). *Textbook of Pharmacology*, 2nd edn. Blackwell, London

Braganza, J. M. (1983). Hypothesis. Pancreatic Disease: casualty of hepatic detoxification? *Lancet*, **ii**, 1000–1003

Braganza, J. M. (1986). The pancreas. In Pounder, R. (Ed.), *Recent Advances in Gastroenterology*, Vol. 6. Churchill Livingstone, London, pp. 251–280

Braganza, J. M. (1988a). Free radicals and pancreatitis.

In Rice-Evans, C. and Dormandy, T. L. (Eds), *Free Radicals: Chemistry, Pathology and Medicine*. Richelieu Press, London, pp. 357–381

Braganza, J. M. (1988b). The role of the liver in exocrine pancreatic disease. *Int. J. Pancreatol*, **3**, S19-S42

Braganza, J. M. (1988c). Pancreatic function tests. In Weatherall, D. J., Ledingham, J. G. G. and Warrell, D. (Eds), *The New Oxford Textbook of Medicine*, 2nd Edn. University Press, Oxford, pp. 12.12–12.15

Braganza, J. M. (1988d). Oxidant stress: common denominator in the pathogenesis of temperate zone and tropical chronic pancreatitis? Proceedings of World Health Organisation Symposium on malnutrition-related diabetes, The Wellcome Tropical Institute, London July 1988. In Alberti, K. G. G. M., Keen, H. and Parry, E. O. (Eds), *Malnutrition-related Diabetes*. University Press, Oxford

Braganza, J. M. (1989). Towards antioxidant therapy for gastrointentinal disease. Royal Society of Medicine Current Medical Literature. *Gastroenterology*, **8**, 99–106

Braganza, J. M. (1990a). Experimental acute pancreatitis. *Current Opinion in Gastroenterology*, **6**, 763–768

Braganza, J. M. (Ed.). (1990b). Pancreas. *Current Opinion in Gastroenterology*, **6**

Braganza, J. M. (Ed.) (1991). *The Pathogenesis of Pancreatitis*. Manchester University Press, Manchester

Braganza, J. M. (1992). The pancreas. In Brocklehurst, J. C., Tallis, R. and Fillit, J. (Eds). *Textbook of Geriatric Medicine and Gerontology*. 4th Edn, Churchill Livingstone, London, pp. 527–535

Braganza, J. M., Wickens, D. G., Cawood, P., Dormandy, T. L. (1983). Lipid peroxidation (free radical oxidation) products in bile from patients with pancreatic disease. *Lancet*, **ii**, 375–379

Braganza, J. M., Holmes, A. M., Moreton, A. R., Stalley, L., Ku, R. and Kishen, R. (1986a). Acetylcysteine to treat complications of pancreatitis. *Lancet*, **i**, 914–915

Braganza, J. M., Jolley, J. E. and Lee W. R. (1986b). Occupational volatile chemicals and pancreatitis: a link? *Int. J. Pancreatol.*, **1**, 9–19

Braganza, J. M., Fraine, E., Rose, P., Martin, H. (1986c). Dietary antioxidants, unsaturated fat, cytochrome P450, and pancreatitis. *Proc. Int. Assoc. Pancreatol.*, São Paulo, 1986

Braganza, J. M., Jeffrey, I. J. M., Foster, J. and McCloy, R. F. (1987). Recalcitrant pancreatitis: eventual control by antioxidants. *Pancreas*, **2**, 489–494

Braganza, J. M., Hewitt, C. and Day, J. P. (1988a). Serum selenium concentration in chronic pancreatitis: lowest values during painful exacerbations. *Trace Elements Med.*, **5**, 79–84

Braganza, J. M., Thomas, A. and Robinson, A.

(1988b). Antioxidants to treat chronic pancreatitis in childhood? *Int. J. Pancreatol.* **3**, 209–216

Braganza, J. M., John, S., Padmayalam, I., Mohan, V., Viswanathan, M., Chari, S. and Madanagopalan, M. (1990). Xenobiotics and tropical chronic pancreatitis. *Int. J. Pancreatol.*, **7**, 231–245

Bridges, J. W. (1980). The role of the drug-metabolizing enzymes. In *Environmental Chemicals, Enzyme Function and Human Disease. Ciba Foundation Symposium* 76 (new series), Excerpta Medica, Amsterdam, pp. 5–17

Broe, P. J. and Cameron, J. (1983). Azathioprine and acute pancreatitis: studies in an isolated perfused canine pancreas. *J. Surg. Res.*, **34**, 159–163

Buchanan, N., Cane R. D. (1977). Frusemide-induced pancreatitis. *Lancet*, **ii**, 1417

Buchler, M., Malfertheiner, P., Schadlich, H., Nevalainen, T. J., Friess, H., Beger, H. G. (1989). Role of phospholipase A_2, in human acute pancreatitis. *Gastroenterology*, **97**, 1521–1526

Burgan, T. H. D., Gupta, I. and Bate, C. H. (1982). Fatal overdose of theophylline simulating acute pancreatitis. *Br. Med. J.*, **284**, 939–940

Burney, P. G. J., Comstock, G. W. and Morris, J. S. (1989). Serologic precursors of cancer: serum micronutrients and the subsequent risk of pancreatic cancer. *Am. J. Clin. Nutr.*, **49**, 895–900

Burnett, D., Chambra, A., Hill, S. L. and Stockley, R. A. (1987). Neutrophils from subjects with chronic obstructive lung disease show enhanced chemotoxis and extracellular proteolysis. *Lancet*, **ii**, 1043–1046

Case, R. M. (Ed.) (1990). The exocrine pancreas. *Proceedings of the 10th BSG Smith Kline, French International Workshop*, Dublin, 1989. Swan Press, London

Chaloner, C., Sandle, L. N., Mohan, V., Snehalatha, C., Viswanathan, M. and Braganza, J. M. (1990). Evidence for induction of cytochrome P450I in patients with tropical chronic pancreatitis. *Int. J. Clin. Pharmacol. Ther. Toxicol.*, **28**, 235–240

Chaloner, C., Shiel, N., Schofield, D., Bottiglieri, T. and Braganza, J. M. (1991). Evidence for early oxidative stress in human acute pancreatitis and clues to its correction. *Digestion*, **49** (Supplement with Proceedings of the European Pancreatic Club, Lund 1991), 14

Chariot, J., Appia, F., Vaille, C. and Roze, C. (1987). Effect of modafinil on pancreatic exocrine secretion in rats. A comparison with adrafinil and related drugs. *Fundam. Clin. Pharmacol.*, **1**, 243–252

Clarkson, T. W., Sager, P. R. and Syversen, T. L. M. (Eds) (1986). *The Cytoskeleton: a Target for Toxic Agents*. Plenum Press, London

Chary, S. (1974). Dimethylformamide: a cause of acute pancreatitis? *Lancet*, **ii**, 356

Cohen, J. M. (Ed.) (1986). *Target Organ Toxicity*. CRC Press, Florida

Cooper, R. G. and MacCaulay, M. B. (1982). Pentachlorophenol pancreatitis. *Lancet*, **i**, 517

Cornish, A. L., McLellan, J. T. and Johnston, D. N. (1961). Effects of chlorothiazide on the pancreas. *N. Engl. J. Med.*, **256**, 673–675

Correia, M. A. and Burk, R. F. (1976). Hepatic heme metabolism in selenium-deficient rats: effect of phenobarbitone. *Arch. Biochem. Biophys.*, **177**, 624–644

Craven, P. A., Pfanstiel, J. and DeRuberts, F. R. (1986). Role of reactive oxygen in bile salt stimulation of colonic epithelial proliferation. *J. Clin. Invest.*, **77**, 850–859

Cross, C., Halliwell, B. and Allen, A. (1984). Antioxidant protection: a function of tracheobronchial and gastrointestial mucus. *Lancet*, **i**, 1328–1330

Curphey, T. J., Coon, C. I., Schaeffer, B. K. and Longnecker, D. S. (1987). *In vivo* and *in vitro* genotoxicity of selected compounds towards rodent pancreas. *Carcinogenesis*, **8**, 1033–1037

Dabrowski, A., Gabryelewicz, A. and Chyczewski, L. (1989). Effect of platelet-activating factor antagonist on oxygen radicals in caerulein-induced acute pancreatitis in rats. *Digestion*, **43**, 136

Dabrowski, A. and Gabryelewicz, A. (1992). Oxidative stress: an early phenomenon characteristic of acute experimental pancreatitis. *Int. J. Pancreatol.*, **12**, 193–195

Datta, S. K. and Ghose, K. C. (1975). Toxic effect of endrin on the hepatopancreas of a teleost, *Cyprinus carpio*. *Indian Biol.*, **17** 37–41

Davies, D. S., Tee, L. B. G., Hampden, C. and Boobis, A. R. (1986). Acetaminophen toxicity in isolated hepatocytes. In Kocsis, J. J., Jollow, D. J., Witmer, C. M., Nelson, J. O. and Snyder, R. (Eds), *Biological Reactive Intermediates III*. Plenum Press, London, pp. 993–1003

DeCaprio, A. P., Briggs, R., Gierthy, J. F., Kim, J. C. S., and Kleopfer, R. D. (1987). Acute toxicity in the guinea pig and *in vitro* 'dioxin-like' activity of the environmental contaminant 1, 2, 4, 5, 7, 8-hexachloro(9H)xantheine. *J. Toxicol. Environ. Health*, **20**, 241–248

De Dios, I., Calvo, J., San Roman, J. I., Plaza, M. A., and Lopez, M. A. (1989). Beta$_1$ and beta$_2$ adrenergic agonists in exocrine pancreatic secretion in the rabbit. *Arch. Int. Physiol. Biochim*, **97**, 37–43

Diem, K. and Lentner, C. (Eds) (1970). *Geigy Scientific Tables*, 8th Edn. Ciba Geigy, Basle, pp. 651–653

Dieter, M. P. (1988). Toxicology and carcinogenesis of 2-mercaptobenzothiazole (CAS No 149-30-4) in F344/N rats and B6C3F$_1$, mice. (Gavage studies). *Natl Toxicol. Program Tech. Rep. Ser.*, **332**, 172

Deprez, P., Descamps, C. H. and Flasse, R. (1989) Pancreatitis induced by 5-aminosalicylic acid. *Lancet*, **ii**, 445–446

Diplock, A. T. (1984). The glutathione-S-transferases in selenium deficiency. In Rotilio, G. and Bannister, J. V. (Eds), *Life Chemistry Reports, suppl 2*. Harwood Academic Publications, London, pp. 381–385

Dobrilla, G., Chilovi, F. and Amplatz, S. (1984).

Drug-induced acute pancreatitis. In Banks, P. A. and Bianchi Porro, G. (Eds), *Acute Pancreatitis*. Masson Italia, Milano, pp. 23–41

Dorken, H. (1964). Einige daten bei 280 patienten mit pankreaskrebs. *Gastroenterologia*, **102**, 47–50

Dormandy, T. L. (1983). An approach to free radicals. *Lancet*, **ii**, 1126–1128

Dormandy, T. L. (1988). In praise of peroxidation. *Lancet*, **ii**, 1126–1128

Dossing, M., Jacobson, O. and Rasmussen, S. N. (1985). Chronic pancreatitis possibly caused by occupational exposure to organic solvents. *Hum. Toxicol.* **4**, 237–240

Dowling, R. H., Folsch, U and Riecken, E-O. (Eds) (1987). Enteropancreatic adaptation: new approaches. *Gut*, **28** (suppl. 1)

Dreiling, D. A. and Grateron, H. (1983). Studies in pancreatic secretion. VII. Pancreatic function in patients with Wilson's disease. *Mt. Sinai J. Med*, **50**, 335–337

Drugs (1989). Focus on S-adenosyl-L-methionine, *Drugs*, **38**, 389–416

Durie, P. R., Gaskin, K. G., Ogilvy, J. E., Smith, C. R., Forstner, C. G. and Largman, C. (1985). Serial alterations in the form of immunoreactive pancreatic cationic trypsin in plasma from patients with acute pancreatitis. *J. Paediatr. Gastroenterol. Nutr.*, **4**, 199–207

Ferguson, L. J. and Watts. J. McK. (1980). Simultaneous cancer of the pancreas occurring in husband and wife. *Gut*, **21**, 537–540

Foster, J. R., Idle, J. R., Hardwick, J. P., Bars, R., Scott, P. and Braganza, J. M. (1993). Induction of drug metabolising enzymes in human pancreatic cancer and chronic pancreatitis. *J. Pathol.*, **169**, 457–463

Fournie, J. W., Hawkins, W. E., Overstreet, R. M. and Walker, W. W. (1987). Exocrine pancreatic neoplasms induced by methylazoxymethanol acetate in the guppy *Poecilia reticulata*. *J. Natl. Cancer Inst.*, **78**, 715–725

Frei, B., Stocker, R., England, L. and Ames, B. N. (1990). Ascorbate: the most effective antioxidant in human blood plasma. In Emerit, I., Packer, L. and Auclair, C. (Eds). *Antioxidants in Therapy and Preventive Medicine*. Plenum Press, New York, pp. 155–163

Freudenthal, R. I. and Jones, P. W. (Eds) (1976). *Polynuclear Aromatic Hydrocarbons: Chemistry, Metabolism and Carcinogenesis*. Raven Press, New York

Frick., T. W., Dalo, S., O'Leary, J. F. *et al.* (1987). Effects of the insecticide, diazinon, on pancreas of dogs, cat and guinea pig. *J. Environ. Pathol. Toxicol. Oncol.*, **7**, 1–12

Friedlander, B. R., Hearne, T. and Hall, S. (1978). Epidemiologic investigation of employees chronically exposed to methylene chloride. *J. Occup. Med.*, **20**, 657–666

Geokas, M. C., Largman, C. and Durie, P. R., (1981). Immunoreactive forms of cationic trypsin in plasma and ascitic fluid of dogs in experimental pancreatitis. *Am. J. Pathol.*, **105**, 31–39

Gianturco, M. A., Giammarino, A. S., and Friedel, P. (1966). Volatile constituents of coffee. *Nature*, **210**, 1358

Go, V. L. W., Gardner, J. D., Brooks, F. P., Lebenthal, E., DiMagno, E. P. and Scheele, G. A. (Eds) (1986). *The Exocrine Pancreas*. Raven Press, New York

Gold, E. B., Gordis, L., Diener, M. D., Seltser, R., Boitnott, J. K., Bynum, T. E. and Hutcheon, D. F. (1985). Diet and other risk factors for cancer of the pancreas. *Cancer*, **55**, 460–467

Golden, M. H. N. (1991). The exocrine pancreas in severe malnutrition. In Braganza, J. M. (Ed.). *The Pathogenesis of Pancreatitis*, Manchester University Press, Manchester, pp. 139–155

Golden, M. H. N., and Ramdath, D. (1987). Free radicals in the pathogenesis of kwashiorkor. *Proc. Nutr. Soc.*, **46**, 53–68

Goldstein, J., Galski, H., Fojo, A. *et al.* (1989). Expression of a multidrug resistance gene in human cancers. *J. Natl Cancer Inst.*, **81**, 116–124

Griffin, A. C. (1979). Role of selenium in the chemoprevention of cancer. *Adv. Cancer Res.*, **29**, 419–442

Gross, V., Scholmerich, J. and Leser, H. G. (1990). Granulocyte elastase in assessment of severity of acute pancreatitis. *Dig. Dis. Sci.*, **35**, 97–105

Gudgeon, A. M., Heath, D. I., Hurley, P. *et al.* (1990). Trypsinogen activation peptides assay in the early prediction of severity of acute pancreatitis. *Lancet* i, 4–8

Guengerich, F. P. (1989). Characterization of human microsomal cytochrome P-450 enzymes. *Annu. Rev. Pharmacol. Toxicol.*, **29**, 241–264

Guérin, J. M., Timbourtine, O. and Segresta, J. M. (1982). Pancreatites iatrogènes medicamenteuses. *Thérapie*, **37**, 207–217

Guice, K. S., Oldham, K. T., Caty, M. G., Johnson, K. J. and Ward, P. A. (1989a). Neutrophil-dependent oxygen-radical mediated lung injury associated with acute pancreatitis. *Ann. Surg.*, **210**, 740–747

Guice, K. S., Oldham, K. T. and Johnson, K. J. (1989b). Failure of antioxidant therapy (polyethylene glycol-conjugated catalase) in acute pancreatitis. *Am. J. Surg.*, **157**, 145–149

Gutteridge, J. M. C., Rowley, D. A., Griffiths, E. and Halliwell, B. (1985). Low molecular weight iron complexes and oxygen radical reactions in idiopathic haemochromatosis. *Clin. Sci.*, **68**, 463–469

Guyan, P. M., Butler, J., Braganza, J. M. and Stevens, F. S. (1986). Evidence for a reoxidizing enzyme in human pancreatic juice. *Biochem. Soc. Trans.*, **14**, 890–891

Guyan, P. M., Braganza, J. M. and Butler, J. (1988). The effect of oxygen metabolites on the zymogens of human pancreatic proteases. In Rice-Evans, C. and Dormandy, T. (Eds), *Free Radicals: Chemistry, Pathology and Medicine*. Richelieu Press, London, pp. 471–474

Guyan, P. M., Yadav, S. and Miller, P. (1989). Micronutrient antioxidants in chronic pancreatitis: comparison of blood levels in temperate and tropical zones. *Digestion*, **43**, 147

Guyan, P. M., Uden, S. and Braganza, J. M. (1990). Heightened free radical activity in pancreatitis. *Free Radical Biol. Med.*, **8**, 347–354

Gyr, K. E., Singer, M. E. and Sarles, H. (Eds) (1984). *Pancreatitis—Concepts and Classification*. Excerpta Medica, Oxford

Halliwell, B. and Gutteridge, J. M. C. (1985). *Free Radicals in Biology and Medicine*. Clarendon Press, Oxford

Halliwell, B. and Gutteridge, J. M. C. (1986). Oxygen free radicals and iron in relation to biology and medicine: some problems and concepts. *Arch. Biochem. Biophys.*, **246**, 501–514

Halliwell, B., Wasil, M., and Grootvelt, M. (1987). Biologically significant scavenging of the myeloperoxidase-derived oxidant hypochlorous acid by ascorbic acid. *FEBS Letts*, **213**, 15–18

Harada, H., Ueda, O., Kochi, F., Kobayashi, T. and Komazawa, P. (1981). Comparative effects on viscosity and concentration of protein and hexosamine in pure pancreatic juice. *Gastroenterol. Jpn*, **16**, 623–631

Heckmann, A. M. (1971). Association of lactoferrin with other proteins as demonstrated by changing electrophoretic mobility. *Biochim. Biophys. Acta.*, **251**, 380–387

Hirata, F. and Axelrod, J. (1980). Phospholipid methylation and biological signal transmission. *Science*, **209**, 1082–1090

Hoar, S. K. and Pell, S. A. (1981). A retrospective cohort study of mortality and cancer incidence among chemists. *J. Occup. Med.*, **23**, 485–490

Hoch-Ligeti, C., Wagner, B. P., Deringer, M. K. and Stewart, H. L. (1985). Tumour induction in *Praomys (Mastomys) natalensis* by N,N'-2,7-fluorenylenebisacetamide. *J. Natl Cancer Inst.*, **74**, 909–915

Hodhod, S., Swelam, N., Tash., F. and El-Asmar, M. F. (1989). Effect of *Cerastes cerastes* (Egyptian sand viper) venom on rat pancreas. *Egypt J. Biochem*, **7** 19–38

Hodson, E., and Levi, P. E. (1987). *A Textbook of Modern Toxicology*. Elsevier, Oxford

Hollander, D. and Tarnawski, A. (1986). Dietary essential fatty acids and the decline in peptic ulcer disease—a hypothesis. *Gut*, **27**, 239–242

Hong, S. S., Case, R. M. and Kim, K. H. (1988). Analysis in the isolated perfused cat pancreas of factors implicated in the pathogenesis of pancreatitis. *Pancreas*, **3**, 450–458

Horiuchi, A., Iwatsuki, K., Yonekura, H., Chiba, S., and Oguchi, H. (1989). Allopurinol stimulates pancreatic exocrine secretion in the dog. *Pancreas*, **4**, 179–184

Horn, U., Haertl, A., Guettner, J. and Hoffmann, H. (1985). Toxicity of the alkylating agent bendamustin. *Arch. Toxicol.* **8** (suppl.), 504–506

Horton, J. W., Dunn, C. W., Burnweit, C. A. and Walker, P. B. (1989). Hypertonic saline-dextran resuscitation of acute canine bile-induced pancreatitis. *Am. J. Surg.*, **158**, 48–56

Howat, H. T. and Sarles, H. (Eds). (1979). *The Exocrine Pancreas*. W. B. Saunders, London

Idle, J. R. and Smith, R. C. (1979). Polymorphism of oxidation at carbon centres of drugs and their clinical significance. *Drug Metab. Rev.*, **9**, 301–319

Irons, R. D. (1986). The role of reactive intermediates in sulphydryl-dependent immunotoxicity: interference with microtubule assembly and microtubule-dependent cell function. In Kocsis, J. J., Jollow, D. J., Witmer, C. M., Nelson, J. O. and Snyder, R. (Eds), *Biological Reactive Intermediates III*. Plenum Press, London, pp. 645–656

Irwin, R. D. (1988). Toxicology and carcinogenesis studies of 2-amino-5-nitrophenol (CAS No 121–88–0) in F344/N rats and B6C3F1 mice (gavage studies). *Gov. Rep. Announce Index (US)*, **88**, 836–766

Iwanig, V. and Jamieson, D. (1982). Comparison of secretory protein profiles in developing rat pancreatic rudiments and rat acinar tumour cells. *J. Cell Biol.*, **95**, 742–746

Jamieson, J. D., and Palade, G. E. (1977). Production of secretory proteins in animal cells. In Brinkley, B. R. and Porter, K. R. (Eds), *International Cell Biology*. Rockefeller University Press, New York pp. 308–317

Johnson, L. R., (Ed.) (1987). *Physiology of the Gastrointestinal Tract*, 2nd edn. Raven Press, New York, pp. 1089–1208

Kalvaria, I., Labadrios, D., Shephard, G. S., Vesser, L. and Marks, I. N. (1986). Biochemical vitamin E deficiency in chronic pancreatitis. *Int. J. Pancreatol.*, **1**, 119–128

Kay, P. M., Schofield, D., Bilton, D., Snehalatha, C., Mohan, V. and Braganza, J. M. (1991). Vitamin C deficiency: key risk factor for calcifying chronic pancreatitis in temperate and tropical zones? *Gut*, **32**, A1201

Kern, H. F., and Kern, D. (1969). Elektronenmikroskopische Untersuchungen über die Wirkung von Kobaltchlorid auf das exokrine Pankreasgewebe des Meerschweinchens. *Virchows Arch. Cell Pathol.*, **4** 54–70

Kitajima, S., and Kishino, Y. (1985). Pancreatic damage produced by injecting excess lysine in rats. *Virchows Arch. Cell Pathol.*, **49**, 295–305

Knoop, M., McMahon, R. F. T., Braganza, J. M., and Hutchinson, I. V. (1989). Acute pancreatitis after experimental pancreatic transplantation. *Am. J. Surg.*, **158**, 452–458

Kokkinakis, D. M. and Scarpelli, D. G. (1989). DNA alkylation in the hamster induced by two pancreatic carcinogens. *Cancer Res.*, **49**, 3184–3189

Koop, D. R., Crump, B. L., Nordbloom, G. D. and Coon, M. J. (1985). Immunochemical evidence for induction of the alcohol-oxidizing cytochrome P-450 of rabbit liver microsomes by diverse agents: ethanol, imidazole, trichloroethylene, acetone, pyrazole and isoniazid. *Proc. Natl Acad. Sci. USA*, **82**, 4065–4069

Krempien, B. and Grosser, G. (1987). Ultrastructure and protein synthesis of the exocrine rat pancreas in acute and chronic uremia. *Verh. Dtsch. Ges. Pathol.*, **71**, 102–107

Kuklinski, P. (1992). Akute Pankreatitis—eine 'Free Radical Disease'. Letalitätssenkung durch natriumselenit (Na_2SeO_3)-therapie. *Z. Gesamte Inn. Med.* **47**, S.165–167

Laugier, R. J. and Sarles, H. (1984). Toxic pancreatitis. *Drugs Pharm. Sci.*, **21**, 487–503

Lawson, T. and Nagel, D. (1988). The production and repair of DNA damage by N-nitrosobis (2-oxopropyl)amine and azaserine in hamster and rat pancreas acinar and duct cells. *Carcinogenesis*, **9**, 1007–1010

Lee, K. T. and Sheen, P. C. (1988). The effect of monosodium L-glutamate on the rat pancreatic acinar cells. *Nutr. Rep. Int.*, **38**, 789–798

Lendrum, R. (1981). Drugs and the pancreas. *Adverse Drug Reactions Bull.*, **90**, 328–331

Letko, G., Falkenberg, B. and Wilhelm, W. (1989). Effects of trypsin, chymotrypsin and uncoupling on survival of isolated acinar cells from rat pancreas. *Int. J. Pancreatol.*, **4**, 431–441

Levin, J. Phillips, B. and Iqbal, Z. M. (1984). DNA damage in isolated hamster and rat pancreas cells by pancreatic carcinogens. *Chem. Biol. Interact.*, **48**, 59–67

Li, F. P., Fraumeni, J. F., Mantel, N. and Miller, R. W. (1969). Cancer mortality amongst chemists. *J. Natl Cancer Inst.*, **43**, 1159–1164

Lieber, C. S. (1988). Biochemical and molecular basis of alcohol-induced injury to liver and other tissues. *N. Engl. J. Med.*, **319**, 1639–1650

Lijinsky, W. (1987). Structure-activity relations in carcinogenesis by N-nitroso compounds. *Cancer Metasis. Rev.*, **6**, 301–356

Lijinski, W. and Reuber, M. D. (1987). Chronic carcinogenesis studies of acrolein and related compounds. *Toxicol. Ind. Health*, **3**, 337–345

Lilja, H. S., Longnecker, D. S., Curphey, T. J., Daniel, D. S. and Adams, W. O. (1981). Studies of DNA damage in rat pancreas and liver by DON, ethyl diazoacetate and azaserine. *Cancer Lett.*, **12**, 139–146

Lin, R. S. and Kessler, II (1981). A multifactorial model for pancreatic cancer in man. *JAMA*, **245**, 147–152

Longnecker, D. S. (1991). Pathology of pancreatitis. In Braganza, J. M. (Ed.), *The Pathogenesis of Pan-*

creatitis. Manchester University Press, Manchester, pp. 3–18

Longnecker, D. S., Wiebkin, P., Schaeffer, B. K. and Roebuck, B. D. (1984). Experimental carcinogenesis in the pancreas. *Int. Rev. Exp. Pathol.*, **26**, 177–229

McBrien, D. C. H. and Slater, T. F. (1983). *Protective Agents in Cancer*. Academic Press, London

McCay, P. B. and Reinke, L. A. (1987). Detection of reactive free radicals in liver of ethanol-fed rats: potentiating effect of high fat diets. In Paoletti, R., Kritchevsky, D. and Holmes, W. L. (Eds), *Drugs Affecting Lipid Metabolism*. Springer-Verlag, Berlin, pp. 81–192

McDonald, M. M. and Boorman, G. A. (1989). Pancreatic hepatocytes associated with chronic 2,6-dichloro-p-phenylenediamine administration in Fischer 344 rats. *Toxicol. Pathol.*, **17**, 1–6

McEntee, G., Leahy, A., Cottell, D., Dervan, P., McGeeney, K. and Fitzpatrick, J. M. (1989). Three-dimensional morphological study of the pancreatic microvasculature in caerulein-induced pancreatitis. *Br. J. Surg.*, **76**, 853–855

Mack, T. M. and Paganini-Hill, (1981). Epidemiology of pancreas cancer in Los Angeles. *Cancer*, **47**, 1474–1483

McManus, M. E., De la Hall, P., Stupans, I., Burgess, W., Brennan, J. and Birkett, D. J. (1987). Immunohistochemical localization and distribution of NADPH–cytochrome P450 reductase in human tissues. *Proceedings of 7th International symposium on microsomes and drug oxidation, 1987*, Miners, J. O. (Ed.), Taylor and Francis, London, pp. 20–27

McMillan, D. E., and Geevarghese, P. H. (1979). Dietary cyanide and tropical malnutrition diabetes. *Diabetes Care*, **2**, 202–208

McNamee, R., Braganza, J. M. and Cherry, N. (1993). A case referent study of chronic pancreatitis and occupational exposure to hydrocarbons. *Gut*, **34** (abstract in press)

Maeda, N. Kon, K., Sekiya, M. *et al.* (1986). Increase of ATP level in human erythrocytes induced by S-adenosyl-L-methionine. *Biochem. Pharmacol.*, **35**, 625–629

Majumdar, A. P. N., Vesenka, D., Dubick, M. A., Yu, G. S. M., DeMorrow, J. M. and Geokas, M. C. (1986). Morphological and biochemical changes of the pancreas in rats treated with acetaldehyde. *Am. J. Physiol.*, **250**, G598-G606

Mallory, A., and Kern, F. (1980). Drug-induced pancreatitis. A critical review. *Gastroenterology*, **78**, 813–820

Mancuso, T. F. and El-Attar, A. A. (1967), Cohort study of workers exposed to betanaphthylamine and benzidine. *J. Occup. Med.*, **9**, 277–282

Mangino, M., Scarpelli, D. and Hollenberg, P. F. (1985). Activation of N-nitrosobis(2-oxopropyl) amine and N-nitroso(2-hydroxypropyl)-(2-oxopropyl)amine to mutagens for V79 cells by isolated hamster and rat pancreatic acinar cells. *Cancer Res.*, **45**, 5219–5224

Mann, G. E., Norman, P. S. R. and Smith, I. C. H. (1989). Amino acid efflux in the isolated perfused rat pancreas: trans-stimulation by extracellular amino acids. *J. Physiol.*, **416**, 485–502

Marino, C. R. and Gorelick, F. S. (1992). Scientific advances ibn cystic fibrosis. *Gastroenterology*, **103**, 681–693

Martensson, J. and Bolin, T. (1986). Sulphur amino acid metabolism in chronic relapsing pancreatitis. *Am. J. Gastroenterol*, **81**, 1179–1184

Matalon, S., Beckman, J. S., Duffey, M. E. and Freeman, B. A. (1989). Oxidant inhibition of epithelial active sodium transport. *Free Radical Biol. Med.* **6**, 557–564

Mason, W. T. and Satelle, D. B. (1988). The secretory event. *J. Exp. Biol.*, 139

Mekord, J. and Hennighausen, G. (1989). Acute pancreatitis and bile duct lesions in rat induced by dibutyltin dichloride. *Exp. Pathol.*, **36**, 59–62

Miquel, J., Quintanilha, A. T. and Weber, H. (1989). *Handbook of Free Radicals and Antioxidants in Biomedicine*. CRC Press, Florida

Miyachi, Y., Yoshioka, A., Simamura, S. and Nima, Y. (1987). Effect of sulphasalazine and its metabolites on the generation of reactive oxygen species. *Gut*, **28**, 190–195

Modlin, I. M., Bilchik, A. J., Zucker, K. A., Adrian, T. E., Sussman, J. and Graham, S. M. (1989). Cholecystokinin augmentation of 'surgical' pancreatitis. Benefits of receptor blockade. *Arch. Surg.*, **124**, 574–578

Moncada, S., Palmer, R. M. J. and Higgs, A. (1991). Nitric oxide: physiology, pathophysiology, and pharmacology. *Biol. Rev.*, **43**, 109–142

Moore, M. A., Takahashi, M., Ito, N. and Bannasch, P. (1983). Early lesions during pancreatic carcinogenesis induced in the Syrian hamster by DHPN or DOPN. II. Ultrastructural findings. *Carcinogenesis*, **4**, 439–448

Moossa, A. R. (Ed.) (1980). *Tumours of the Pancreas*. Williams & Wilkins, London

Morgan, A. and Burgoyne, R. D. (1992). Exo 1 and Exo 2 proteins stimulate calcium-dependent exocytosis in permeabilised adrenal chromaffin cells. *Nature*, **355**, 833–836

Mori, Y., Yamazaki, H., Toyoshi, K., Maruyama, H. and Konishi, Y. (1986). Activation of carcinogenic N-nitrosopropylamines to mutagens by lung and pancreas S9 fractions from various species and humans. *Mutation Res.*, **160**, 159–169

Mueller, M. K., Bergmann, K., Degenhardt, H., Kloeppel, G., Loehr, M., Coone, H. J. and Goebell, H. (1988). Differential sensitivity of rat exocrine and endocrine pancreas to cyclosporine. *Transplantation*, **45**, 698–700

Murthy, K. R. K., Medh, J. D., Dave, B. N., Vakil, Y. E. and Billimoria, F. R. (1989). Acute pancreatitis and reduction of hydrogen ion concentration in gastric secretions in experimental acute myocarditis produced by Indian red scorpion, *Buthus tamaulus*, venom. *Indian J. Exp. Biol.*, **27**, 242–244

Musa, O. A. (1989). Regulation of pancreatic enzymes synthesis. *PhD Thesis*, University of Manchester, UK

Nagalotimath, S. J. (1980). Pathology of calcific pancreatitis with diabetes. In Podolsky, S. and Viswanathan, M. (Eds). *Secondary Diabetes: the Spectrum of the Diabetes Syndromes*. Raven Press, New York, pp. 117–145

Nakashima, Y. and Howard, J. M. (1977). Drug-induced acute pancreatitis. *Surg. Gynecol. Obstet.*, **145**, 105–109

National Toxicology Program (1986). Toxicology and carcinogenesis studies on chlorinated paraffins (C_{12}, 60 per cent chlorine) (CAS No 63449–39–8) in F344/N rats and B6C3F mice. (Gavage studies). *Natl Toxicol. Program Tech. Rep. Ser.*, **308**, 206

National Toxicology Program (1987a). Toxicology and carcinogenesis studies of chlorendic acid (CAS No 115–28–6) in F344/N rats and B6C3F mice (feed studies). *Natl Toxicol. Program Tech. Rep. Ser.*, **304**, 225

National Toxicology Program (1987b). Toxicology and carcinogenesis studies on chlorendic acid (CAS No 115–28–6) in F344/N rats and B6C3F1 mice (feed studies). *Gov. Rep. Announce Index (US)*, **87**, (746), 576

National Toxicology Program (1987c). Toxicology and carcinogenesis of commercial grade 2, 4 (80 per cent)—and 2, 6 (20 per cent)—Toluene diisocyanate (CAS No 26471–62–5) in F344/N rats and B6C3F1 mice. (Gavage studies). *Gov. Rep. Announce Index (US)*, **87**, (708), 208

Nebert, D. W., Adesnik, M., Coon, M. J. *et al.* (1987). The P-450 gene superfamily. Recommended nomenclature. *DNA*, **6**, 1–11

Nevalainen, T. J. (1975). Cytotoxicity of vinblastine and vincristine to pancreatic acinar cells. *Virchows Arch. Cell Pathol.*, **18**, 119–127

Nicholson, W. J. and Moore, J. A. (1979). Health effects of halogenated aromatic hydrocarbons. *Ann. NY Acad. Sci.*, **320**

Nizze, H., Lapis, K. and Kovács, L. (1979). Allyl alcohol-induced changes in rat exocrine pancreatitis. *Digestion*, **19**, 359–369

Nonaka, A., Manabe, T. and Asano, N. (1989). Direct ESR measurement of free radicals in mouse pancreatic lesions. *Int. J. Pancreatol.*, **5**, 203–211

Nonaka, A., Manabe, T. and Tobe, T. (1991). Effect of a new synthetic ascorbic acid derivative, as a free radical scavenger, on the development of acute pancreatitis in mice. *Gut*, **32**, 528–532

Norell, S., Ahlbom, A., Olin, R., Erwald, R., Jacobson, G., Lindberg-Navier, I. and Wiechel, K. L. (1986). Occupational factors and pancreatic cancer. *Br. J. Ind. Med.*, **43**, 775–778

Nwokolo, E. and Ohale, L. O. C. (1986). Growth and anatomical characteristics of pullet chicks fed diets contaminated with petroleum. *Bull. Environ. Contam. Toxicol.*, **37**, 441–447

Ohshio, G., Saluja, A. K., Leli, U., Sengupta, A. and Steer, M. L. (1989). Esterase inhibitors prevent lysosomal enzyme redistribution in two non-invasive models of experimental pancreatitis. *Gastroenterology*, **96**, 853–859

Ohtaki, T., Yamada, S., Azegami, J. and Imai, K. (1985). Acute toxicity tests of triethyl citrate in rats. *Iyakuhin Kenkyu*, **16**, 214–219

O'Konski, M. S. and Pandol, S. J. (1990). Effects of caerulein on the apical cytoskeleton of the pancreatic acinar cell. *J. Clin. Invest.*, **86**, 1649–1657

Ornitz, D. N., Hammer, R. E., Messing, A., Palmiter, R. D. and Brinster, R. L. (1987). Pancreatic neoplasia induced by SV40 T-antigen expression in acinar cells of transgenic mice. *Science*, **238**, 188–193

Orrenius, S. (1985). Biochemical mechanisms of toxicity. *Trends Pharmacol. Sci.* (FEST supplement), 15–20

Orrenius, S. and Moldeus, P. (1984). The multiple roles of glutathione in drug metabolism. *Trends Pharmacol. Sci.*, **5**, 432–435

Owen, P. E., Glaister, J. R., Gaunt, I. F. and Pullinger, D. H. (1987). Inhalation toxicity studies with 1,3-butadiene: 3. Two year toxicity/carcinogenicity study in rats. *Am. Ind. Hyg. Assoc. J.*, **48**, 407–413

Padfield, P. J., Balch, W. E. and Jamieson, J. D. (1992). A synthetic peptide of the rab3a effector domain stimulates release from permeabilised pancreatic acini. *Proc. Natl Acad. Sci. USA*, **89**, 1656–1660

Pancreatic Society of Great Britain and Ireland. (1990). Selected abstracts. *Gut*, **31**, A486–488

Pang, V. F., Adams, J. H., Bearsley, V. R., Buck, W. B. and Haschek, W. M. (1986). Myocardial and pancreatic lesions induced by T-2 toxin, a trichothecene mycotoxin, in swine. *Vet. Pathol.*, **23**, 310–319

Parker, G., Branigan, S., Houston, J. B. and Braganza, J. M. (1986). Potent induction of cytochromes P448 by corn oil in Syrian golden hamsters. *Gut*, **27**, A603

Parks, D. A. (1988). Ischaemia-reperfusion injury: a radical view. *Hepatology*, **8**, 680–682

Parsa, I., Longnecker, D. S., Scarpelli, D. G., Pour, P., Reddy, J. K. and Lefkowitz, M. (1985). Ductal metaplasia of human exocrine pancreas and its association with carcinoma. *Cancer Res.*, **45**, 1285–1290

Parsa, I., Pour, P. M. and Cleary, C. M. (1988). Amplification of c-Ki-ras-2 oncogene sequences in human carcinoma of pancreas. *Int. J. Pancreatol.*, **3**, 45–52

Pitchumoni, C. S. and Viswanathan, K. V. (1987). DC plasma emission spectroscopic analysis of pancreatic calculi. *Int. J. Pancreatol.*, **2**, 149–158

Plaa, G. and Hewitt, W. R. (1982). *Toxicology of the Liver*. Raven Press, New York

Plankenhorn, L. J. (1983). Carcinogenicity of azo dyes: acid black 52 and yellow 3 in hamsters and rats. Vol 3. *Gov. Rep. Announce Index (US)*, **84**, 45

Poirer, A., Laurenchin, F., Baudin, F., Bodennec, G. and Quentel, C. (1986). Experimental poisoning of the rainbow trout, *Salmo giardneri* Richardson, by engine diesel oil: mortalities, hematological changes, histology. *Aquaculture*, **55**, 115–137

Pour, P. M. (1986). Induction of exocrine pancreatic, bile duct, and thyroid gland tumors in offspring of Syrian hamster treated with N-nitrosobis(2-oxopropyl)amine during pregnancy. *Cancer Res.*, **46**, 3663–3666

Pour, P. M. and Lawson, T. (1984). Pancreatic carcinogenic nitrosamines in Syrian hamsters. *IARC Sci. Publ. 57* (N-nitroso Compounds: Occurrence, Biological Effects and Relevance to Human Cancer), pp. 683–688

Pour, P. M. and Rivenson, A. (1989). Induction of a mixed ductal–squamous–islet cell carcinoma in a rat treated with a tobacco-specific carcinogen. *Am. J. Pathol.*, **134**, 627–631

Price, S. C., Hinton, R. H., Mitchell, F. E., Hall, D. E., Grasso, P., Glane, G. F. and Bridges, J. W. (1986). Time and dose study on the response of rats to the hypolipidaemic drug fenofibrate. *Toxicology*, **4**, 169–191

Pryor, W. A. (1986). Oxy radicals and related species. *Ann. Rev. Physiol.*, **48**, 657–667

Putzke, H. P. and Bienengraber, A. (1967). Die galaktose-induzierte Pankreas Dystrophie bzw Pankreatitis. *Beitr. Pathol. Anat.*, **135**, 333–349

Raeder, M. G. (1992). The origin of and subcellular mechanisms causing pancreatic bicarbonate secretion. *Gastroenterology*, **103**, 1674–1684

Rai, U. C. and Singh, D. S. K. (1980). Cardiopulmonary changes in mongrel dogs after exposure to kerosene smoke. *Indian J. Exp. Biol.*, **18**, 1263–1266

Rao, K. N., Tuma, J. and Lombardi, B. (1976). Acute haemorrhagic pancreatic necrosis in mice. *Gastroenterology*, **70**, 720–726

Rao, M. S., Subbarao, M. S., Luetteke, N. and Scarpelli, D. G. (1983). Further characterization of carcinogen-induced hepatocyte-like cells in hamster pancreas. *Am. J. Pathol.*, **110**, 89–94

Rao, M. S., Dwividi, R. S., Subbarao, B. *et al.* (1988). Almost total conversion of pancreas to liver in the adult rat: a reliable model to study transdifferentiation. *Biochem. Biophys. Res. Commun.*, **156**, 131–136

Ray, A. K. and Bhattacharya, S. (1984). Histopathological changes in the hepatopancreas of the fresh water airbreathing teleost *Anabas testudineus* (Bloch) exposed to acute and chronic levels of Cythion. *J. Curr. Biosci.*, **1**, 170–174

Redmond, C. K., Strobino, B. R. and Cypress, R. H. (1976). Cancer experience among coke by-product workers. *Ann. NY Acad. Sci.*, **271**, 102–106

Registrar General's Decennial Supplement (1958). England and Wales 1951, Part II, Occupational Mortality. Her Majesty's Stationery Office, London

Reiner, R. R., Fraumeni, J. F., Ozols, R. F. and Bender, R. (1977). Pancreatic cancer in father and son. *Lancet*, **i**, 911

Rinderknecht, H. (1988). Fatal pancreatitis, a consequence of excessive leucocyte stimulation? *Int. J. Pancreatol.*, **3**, 105–112

Riordan, J. R., Rommens, J. M., Kerem, B. *et al.* (1989). Identification of the cystic fibrosis gene: cloning and characterization of complementary DNA. *Science*, **245**, 1066–1073

Rivenson, A., Hoffmann, D., Prokopcsyk, B., Amin, S. and Hecht, S. S. (1988). Induction of lung and exocrine pancreatic tumours in F344 rats by tobacco-specific and areca-derived nitrosamines. *Cancer Res.*, **48**, 6912–6917

Robinson, T. M. and Dunphy, J. E. (1963). Continuous perfusion of bile and protease activators through the pancreas. *JAMA*, **183**, 530–533

Rose, P., Fraine, E., Hunt, L. P., Acheson, D. W. K. and Braganza, J. M. (1986). Dietary antioxidants and chronic pancreatitis. *Hum. Nutr. Appl. Nutr.*, **40C**, 151–164

Rossi, M. A., Fidale, F., Esterbauer, H. and Dianzani, M. U. (1990). Effect of 4-hydroxyalkenals on hepatic phosphatidylinositol-4,5-biphosphate-phospholipase C. *Biochem. Pharmacol.*, **39**, 1715–1719

Rothman, K. J. (1986). *Modern Epidermiology*. Little Brown, Boston

Rozman, K. and Hanninen, O. (Eds) (1986). *Gastrointestinal Toxicology*. Elsevier, Amsterdam

Ruckert, K., Pracht, B. and Kloppel, G. (1981). Differences in experimental pancreatic carcinogenesis induced by oral or subcutaneous administration of 2,2'-dihydroxydi-n-propyl nitrosamine in duct-ligated hamsters. *Cancer Res.*, **41**, 4715–4719

Rutledge, P. L., Saluja, A. K., Powers, R. E. and Steer, M. L. (1987). Role of oxygen-derived free radicals in diet-induced haemorrhagic pancreatitis in mice. *Gastroenterology*, **93**, 41–47

Salonen, J., Salonen, R., Lappetelainen, R., Maenpaa, P., Alfthan, G. and Puska, P. (1985). Risk of cancer in relation to serum concentrations of selenium and vitamins A and E: matched case-control analysis of prospective data. *Br. Med. J.*, **290**, 417–420

Saluja, A., Saluja, M., Villa, A., Leli, U., Rutledge, P., Meldolesi, J. and Steer, M. (1989). Pancreatic duct obstruction in rabbits causes digestive zymogen and lysosomal enzyme co-localization. *J. Clin. Invest.*, **84**, 1260–1266

Sandgren, E. P., Quaife, C. J., Paulovich, A. G., Palmiter, P. D. and Brinster, R. L. (1990). Pancreatic neoplasia in transgenic mice. *Proc. Am. Assoc. Cancer Res.*, **31**, 479–480

Sandilands, D., Jeffrey, I. J. M., Haboubi, N. Y.,

MacLennan, I. A. M. and Braganza, J. M. (1990). Abnormal drug metabolism in chronic pancreatitis. *Gastroenterology*, **98**, 766–772

Sanfey, H., Sarr, M. G., Bulkley, G. B. and Cameron, J. L. (1986). Oxygen-derived free radicals and acute pancreatitis: a review. *Acta Physiol. Scand.*, **126** (suppl. 548) 109–118

Sasano, H. and Sasano, N. (1988). Extra adrenal immunohistochemical distribution of steroid 21-hydroxylase in human. *Tohoku J. Exp. Med.*, **154**, 21–28

Sato, A., Nakajima, R. and Koyama, Y. (1980). Effects of chronic ethanol consumption on hepatic metabolism of aromatic and chlorinated hydrocarbons in rats. *Br. J. Ind. Med.*, **37**, 382–386

Scarpelli, D. G., Rao, M. S., Subbarao, V., Beversluis, M., Gurka, D. P. and Hollenberg, P. F. (1980). Activation of nitrosamines to mutagens by postmitochondrial fraction of hamster pancreas. *Cancer Res.*, **40**, 67–74

Scarpelli, D. G., Reddy, J. K. and Longnecker, D. S. (Eds) (1987). *Experimental Pancreatic Carcinogenesis*. CRC Press, Florida

Schaeffer, B. K., Weibkin, P., Longnecker, D. S., Coon, C. I. and Curphey, T. J. (1984). DNA damage produced by N-nitroso-methyl(2-oxopropyl)amine (MOP) in hamster and rat pancreas: a role for the liver. *Carcinogenesis*, **5**, 565–570

Schenkman, J. B. and Kupfer, D. (Eds) (1982). Hepatic cytochrome P450 mono-oxygenase system. *International Encyclopedia of Pharmacology and Therapeutics*, section 108. Pergamon Press, Oxford

Schreck, R. and Baeuerle, P. A. (1991). A role for oxygen radicals as second messengers. *Trends in Cell Biology*, **1**, 39–42

Schwartz, M. S. and Brandt, L. J. (1989). The spectrum of pancreatic disorders in patients with the acquired immune deficiency syndrome. *Am. J. Gastroenterol.*, **84**, 459–462

Scott, G. (1988). Antioxidants: can man improve on nature? In Rice-Evans, C. and Dormandy, T. L. (Eds), *Free Radicals: Chemistry, Pathology and Medicine*. Richelieu Press, London, pp. 103–130

Scott, J. A. and Rabito, C. A. (1988). Oxygen radicals and plasma membrane potential. *Free Radical Biol. Med.*, **5**, 237–246

Scott, P. D., Bruce, C., Schofield, D., Shiel, N., Braganza, J. M. and McCloy, R. F. (1993). Vitamin C status in patients with acute pancreatitis. *Br. J. Surg.*, **80**, 750–754

Scott, P. D., Knoop, M., McMahon, R. F. T., Braganza, J. M. and Hutchinson, I. V. (1992). S-Adenosyl-1-methionine protects against haemorrhagic pancreatitis in partially immunosuppressed pancreatico-duodenal transplant recipients. *Drug Investigation*, **4** (Supplement 4), 69–77

Shorrock, K. (1988). An investigation into the induction and pathogenesis of hyperstimulation pancreatitis. *MD Thesis*, University of Sheffield, UK

Sies, H. (Ed.) (1985). *Oxidative Stress*. Academic Press, London

Skett, P. (1987). Hormonal regulation and sex differences of xenobiotic metabolism. *Prog. Drug Metab.*, **10**, 85–140

Slater, T. F. (1984). Free radical mechanisms in tissue injury. *Biochem. J.*, **222**, 1–15

Smith, C. V. and Anderson, R. E. (1987). Methods for determination of lipid peroxidation in biological samples. *Free Rad. Biol. Med.*, **3**, 341–344

Smith, G. N., Taj, M. and Braganza, J. M. (1991). Identification of a conjugated diene component of duodenal bile as 9Z, 11E-octadecadienoic acid. *Free Radical Biol. Med.*, **10**, 13–21

Smith, R. L. (1973). *The Excretory Function of Bile*. Chapman and Hall, London

Soames, A. R., Foster, J. F., Haboubi, N. Y. and Braganza, J. M. (1988). Liver ultrastructure in non-alcoholic pancreatic disease. *Clin. Sci.*, **74** (suppl. 18), 20P

Starek, A. and Kaminski, M. (1982). Toxicity of certain petroleum derivatives used as dielectrics in electromachining. V. Morphological, cytoenzymic and biochemical changes in the liver of rats chronically exposed to kerosene hydrocarbons. *Med. Pr.*, **33**, 38–53

Steer, M. L. and Meldolesi, J. (1987). The cell biology of experimental pancreatitis. *N. Engl. J. Med.*, **316**, 144–150

Steinmetz, K. L. and Mirsalis, J. C. (1984). Induction of unscheduled DNA synthesis in primary cultures of rat pancreatic cells following *in vivo* and *in vitro* treatment with genotoxic agents. *Environ. Mutagen*, **6**, 321–330

Steven, F. S. and Al-Ahmad, R. K. (1984). Guanidinobenzoatase as a marker for tumour cells. In Peters, M. (Ed.), *Protides of the Biological Fluids*. Pergamon Press, Oxford, pp. 351–354

Steven, F. S., Griffin, M. M., Wong, J. L. H. and Itzhaki, S. (1986). Evidence for inhibitors of the cell surface protease guanidinobenzoatase. *J. Enzyme Inhib.*, **1**, 127–137

Stocker, R., Glazer, A. N. and Ames, B. N. (1987). Antioxidant activity of albumin-bound bilirubin. *Proc. Natl. Acad. Sci. USA*, **84**, 5918–5922

Strubelt, O. (1980). Interactions between ethanol and other hepatotoxic agents. *Biochem. Pharmacol.*, **29**, 1445–1449

Sun, J., Farias, L. A. and Markov, A. K. (1990). Fructose 1–6 diphosphate prevents intestinal ischaemic reperfusion injury and death in rats. *Gastroenterology*, **98**, 117–126

Takaya, S., Nakatsuru, Y., Ohgaki, H., Sato, S. and Sugimura, T. (1985). Atrophy of salivary glands and pancreas of rats fed on diet with amino-methyl-α-carboline. *Proc. Jpn Acad.*, **61**, 277–280

Tasso, F., Stemmelin, N., Sarles, H. *et al.* (1973). Comparative morphometric study of the human pancreas in its normal state and in primary chronic calcifying pancreatitis. *Biomedicine*, **18**, 134–144

Thomas, F. B. (1982). Drug-induced pancreatitis: fact versus fiction. *Drug Therapy Hospital*, **7**, 60–72

Timbrell, J. A. (1982). *Principles of Biochemical Toxicity*. Taylor & Francis, London

Toyooka, T., Furukawa, F. and Suzuki, T. (1989). Determination of thiols and disulfides in normal rat tissues and hamster pancreas treated with N-nitrosobis(2-oxypropyl)amine using 4-(aminosulfonyl)-7-fluoro-2,1,3-benzoxadiazole-4-sulfonate. *Biomed. Chromatogr.*, **3**, 166–172

Travis, J. (1983). Oxidants and antioxidants in the lung. *Am. Rev. Resp. Dis.*, **135**, 773

Trezise, A. E. O., Romano, P. R., Gill, D. R., Hyde, S. C., Sepulveda, F. V., Buchwald, M. and Higgins, C. F. (1993). The multidrug resistance and cystic fibrosis genes have complementary patterns of epithelial expression. *EMBO J.* (in press)

Tucker, P. C. and Webster, P. D. (1972). Effects of tetracycline on pancreatic protein synthesis and secretion. *Clin. Res.*, **20**, 76

Turner, H. M. and Grace, H. G. (1938). An investigation into cancer mortality among males in certain Sheffield trades. *J. Hyg.*, **38**, 90–94

Uden, S., Acheson, D. W. K., Reeves, J., Worthington, H., Hunt, L. P., Brown, S. and Braganza, J. M. (1988). Antioxidants, enzyme induction and chronic pancreatitis; a reappraisal following studies in patients on anticonvulsants. *Eur. J. Clin. Nutr.*, **42**, 562–569

Uden, S., Bilton, D., Guyan, P. M., Kay, P. M. and Braganza, J. M. (1990a). Rationale for antioxidant therapy in pancreatitis and cystic fibrosis. In Emerit, I., Packer, L. and Auclair, C. (Eds), *Antioxidants in Therapy and Preventive Medicine*. Plenum Press, London, pp. 555–572

Uden, S., Bilton, D., Nathan, L., Hunt, L. P., Main, C. and Braganza, J. M. (1990b). Antioxidant therapy for recurrent pancreatitis: placebo-controlled trial. *Aliment. Pharmacol. Ther.*, **4**, 357–371

Uden, S., Schofield, D., Miller, P. F., Day, J. P., Bottiglieri, T. and Braganza, J. M. (1992). Antioxidant therapy for recurrent pancreatitis: biochemical profiles in a placebo-controlled trial. *Aliment. Pharmacol. Therap.*, **6**, 229–240

Veghelyi, P. V., Kemeny, T. T., Bozsonyi, J. and Sos, J. (1950a). Toxic lesions of the pancreas. *Am. J. Dis. Child*, **80**, 390–403

Veghelyi, P. V., Kemeny, T. T., Bozsonyi, J. and Sos, J. (1950b). Dietary lesions of the pancreas. *Am. J. Dis. Child*, **79**, 658–665

Veghelyi, P.V., Kemeny, T. T. and Sos, J. (1950c). Bronchial changes in experimentally induced cystic degeneration of the pancreas. *Am. J. Dis. Child*, **79**, 846–854

Veghelyi, P. V. and Kemeny, T. T. (1962). Protein metabolism and pancreatic function. In de Reuck, A. V. S. and Cameron, M. P. (Eds), *Ciba Foundation Symposium on the Exocrine Pancreas*. J. & A. Churchill, London, pp. 329–349

Venge, P. and Lindbom, A. (Eds) (1985). *Inflammation: Basic Mechanisms, Tissue Injury, and Clinical Models*. Almqvist & Wiksell, Stockholm

Wade, A. E. (1986). Effects of dietary fat on drug metabolism. *J. Environ. Pathol. Toxicol. Oncol.*, **6**, 161–189

Wallig, M. A., Gould, D. H. and Fettman, M. J. (1988). Comparative toxicities of the naturally occurring nitrile 1-cyano-3,4-epithiobutane and the synthetic nitrile *n*-valeronitrile in rats: differences in target organs, metabolism and toxic mechanisms. *Food Chem. Toxicol.*, **26**, 149–157

Watari, C. (1985). Ultramicromorphology of experimental pancreatic damage by carcinogens in response to glycyrrhizin of licorice extract. *Wakan Iyaku Gakkaishi*, **2**, 164–165

Waters, D. L., Dorney, S. F. A., Gaskin, K. J., Gruca, M. A., O'Halloran, M. and Wilcken, B. (1990). Pancreatic function in infants identified as having cystic fibrosis in a neonatal screening programme. *N. Engl. J. Med.*, **332**, 303–308

Weatherall, D. G., Ledingham, J. G. G. and Worrall, D. (Eds) (1988). *The New Oxford Textbook of Medicine*, 2nd edn. University Press, Oxford

Weibkin, P., Schaeffer, B. K., Longnecker, D. S. and Curphey, T. J. (1984). Oxidative and conjugative metabolism of xenobiotics by isolated rat and hamster acinar cells. *Drug Metab. Dispos.*, **12**, 427–431

Weiss, S. J. (1989). Tissue destruction by neutrophils. *N. Engl. J. Med.*, **320**, 365–375

Weissman, G. (Ed.) (1983). *Advances in Inflammation Research*, vol. 5. Raven Press, New York, pp.

Williams, G. (1984). Modulation of chemical carcinogenesis. *Fundam. Appl. Toxicol.*, **4**, 325–344

Williams, J. A., Gallagher, S. and Sankaran, H. (1982). Scorpion toxin-induced amylase secretion in guinea pig pancreas: evidence for a new neurotransmitter. *Proc. Soc. Exp. Biol. Med.*, **170**, 384–389

Wilson, J. S., Korsten, M. A., Leo, M. A. and Lieber, C. S. (1986). New technique for the isolation of functional rat pancreatic mitochrondria and its application to models of pancreatic injury. *J. Lab. Clin. Med.*, **107**, 51–58

Winterbourn, C. C. (1985). Comparative reactivities of various biological compounds with myeloperoxidase-hydrogen peroxide-chloride, and similarity of the oxidant to hypochlorite. *Biochem. Biophys. Acta*, **840**, 204–210

Wisner, J. R. and Renner, I. G. (1988). Allopurinol attenuates caerulein-induced acute pancreatitis in rats. *Gut*, **29**, 926–929

Witschi, H. P. and Brain, D. (Eds) (1985). *Toxicology of Inhaled Materials*. Springer-Verlag, New York

Wocka-Marek, T., Kalemba, K., Zajac-Nedza, M., Zygan, U. and Braszcznyska, Z. (1987). Evaluation of health status of workers employed in benzene processing and ethylbenzene manufacture. Clinical Symptoms and lesions of the internal organs. *Pol. Tyg. Lek.*, **42**, 1519–1523

Yamagishi, F. (1986). Existence of adenosine A₂/Ra-receptors in exocrine glands of the dog pancreas. *Shinshu Igaku Zasshi*, **34**, 213–223

Yamanaka, S. and Maruoka, S. (1984). Mutagenicity of the extract recovered from airborne particles outside and inside a home with an unvented kerosene heater. *Atm. Environ.*, **18**, 1485–1487

Zucker, P. F., Chan, A. M. and Archer, M. C. (1988). Cellular toxicity of pancreatic carcinogens. *J. Natl Cancer Inst.*, **76**, 1123–1127

FURTHER READING

Banerjee, A. K., Patel, K. J. and Grainger, S. L. (1989). Drug-induced acute pancreatitis: a critical review. *Medical Toxicology and Adverse Drug Experiences*, **4**, 186–198

Jenson, R. T. (1992). Pancreatic pathology. *Yale Journal of Biology and Medicine*, **45**, 465–469

McNamee, R., Braganza, J. M., Hogg, J., Leck, I., Rose, P. and Cherry, N. M. (1994). Occupational exposure to hydrocarbons and chronic pancreatitis. *Occupational and Environmental Medicine*, **51**, 631–637

Pietri, F. and Clavel, F. (1991). Occupational exposure and cancer of the pancreas. *British Journal of Industrial Medicine*, **48**, 583–587

Scarpelli, D. G. (1989). Toxicology of the pancreas. *Toxicology and Applied Pharmacology*, **101**, 543–554

28 Toxicology of Skeletal Muscle

Karl E. Misulis, Mary Ellen Clinton and Wolf-D. Dettbarn

INTRODUCTION

Muscle toxicology has been the subject of extensive research over the past 40 years. This has not only added to our ability to care for affected patients but has also contributed to our understanding of basic muscle physiology. This chapter will review clinical and experimental toxicology of skeletal muscle.

The mechanisms of toxicity of drugs and chemicals are very diverse but there are some common underlying themes. The mechanisms of attack can be divided into four basic areas: (1) disruption of normal membrane function, (2) altered energy generation with changes in mitochondrial function,(3) altered protein turnover, and (4) disruption in movement or metabolism of cellular materials.

Damage to the muscle fibre membrane may impair muscle activation by depolarization. The depolarization causes inactivation of voltage-dependent sodium channels, thereby raising the threshold for activation. Therefore, neuromuscular transmission may fail. The normal neuromuscular junction has 1-to-1 transfer of action potentials from the nerve to the muscle across a broad range of frequencies. When the threshold is changed, this transfer breaks down. Damage to the sarcolemma causes an influx of extracellular Ca^{2+}. Damage to the mitochrondria causes inhibition of ATP generation causing reduced activity of calcium pumps that either extrude or sequester Ca^{2+}. This again results in an increase in Ca^{2+} intracellular concentration. Sarcoplasmic Ca^{2+} regulates many processes; some of these are modulation of enzyme activity, muscle contraction, and protein and phospholipid turnover. A change in sarcoplasmic Ca^{2+} homeostasis can lead to loss of control of these processes.

Thus, an increase in sarcoplasmic Ca^{2+} can cause phospholipase A_2 activation, triggering the eicosanoid cascade with lipoxygenase activity causing sarcolemmal damage, while activation of proteases leads to myofilament damage. Studies of these mechanisms have only just begun and may lead to new approaches in the treatment of myotoxicity.

Alterations in protein turnover are particularly common in patients with elevated levels of some hormones, for example, corticosteroid administration or hyperthyroidism.

In this chapter, we will discuss some of the more important toxins which produce clinically important myopathies in humans.

ETHANOL MYOPATHY

Clinical Syndromes

Ethanol has been known to cause injury to muscle since Jackson's initial description in 1822. There are two syndromes related to exposure to ethanol itself. One is acute and the other chronic (Hed *et al.*, 1962; Pittman and Decker, 1971).

The acute form of alcoholic myopathy is associated with binge drinking superimposed on a history of intermittent or chronic excess ethanol drinking. Symptoms begin abruptly and may be severe including very painful, generalized muscle pain and swelling with rhabdomyolysis. In a more mild form of the acute syndrome there may be focal or diffuse myalgias, tenderness, swelling, or painful muscle cramps. Acute alcoholic myopathy tends to recur either because of individual susceptibility or because of personal drinking patterns. Elevation in creatine kinase (CK) is virtually always present and myoglobinuria is common. Resolution occurs over 2 weeks following cessation of ethanol (Hed *et al.*, 1955, 1962; Fahlgren *et al.*, 1957; Perkoff *et al.*, 1966). The disorder is usually self-limiting, with avoidance of ethanol being the mainstay of treatment and prevention. If it occurs, rhabdomyolysis and the associated potassium, phosphate and calcium disturbances require treatment.

The chronic myopathy will be discussed later.

Myopathies associated with alcoholism are caused by other factors. These include vitamin deficiencies, especially thiamine; disturbances of electrolytes, including potassium, phosphorus and magnesium; endocrinopathies, diabetic and hypothyroid; and mechanical compression. These will not be covered in detail.

Pathology of Ethanol Myopathy

The acute form of alcoholic myopathy includes histological features of necrosis, phagocytosis and regenerating fibres with relative sparing of the sarcolemmal membrane (Hed *et al.*, 1955; Ekbom, 1964; Perkoff, 1966; Martin *et al.*, 1982). Infrequently there may be tubular aggregates (Chui *et al.*, 1975). Type I fibres are preferentially affected (Haller, 1985; Martinez *et al.*, 1973). Ultrastructurally, intracellular fluid increases and myofibrils become separated by clear, fluid-filled spaces. The sarcomeric Z-discs and A- and I-bands become irregular, and I-bands become discontinuous. Mitochondrial cristae appear disrupted even in well preserved fibres (Klinkerfuss *et al.*, 1967; Kahn and Meyer, 1970; Martinez *et al.*, 1973). Permanent residual changes including nests of regenerating fibres can be seen at 2 months following the acute syndrome (Haller, 1985).

In the chronic form of ethanol-induced myopathy, light microscopic changes may be normal or minimal. Electron microscopy shows enlarged intermyofibrillar spaces and increased glycogen and lipid deposition. Myofilaments may be discontinuous, and the sarcoplasmic reticulum may be hyperplastic or vacuolated. Mitochondrial structure is preserved, but the perimeters and diameters are reduced (Del Villar Negra *et al.*, 1984). Morphometric examination of fibre types reveals a selective atrophy of type IIB fibres. In more severely affected muscle, fibre types I and IIA may also be atrophic but type IIBs remain disproportionately smaller (Kiessling *et al.*, 1973, 1975; Hanid *et al.*, 1981; Slavin *et al.*, 1983; Martin *et al.*, 1985). These changes are associated with ethanol intakes of more than 100 g per day for more than 3 years. The degree of atrophy progresses in those who continue to drink while in those who remain free of ethanol there is a progressive resolution of the atrophy over a period of up to 18 months (Martin *et al.*, 1985).

Pathophysiology of Ethanol Myopathy

Factors which may account for the myopathy of alcoholism include those which affect membranes and membrane transport, intermediary metabolism, and organelle function. There may be additional toxic effects of the metabolites of ethanol. It is likely that ethanol produces its toxicity through more than one mechanism. The following is a summary of those which have been studied.

Membrane concentrations of cholesterol, total phospholipid, and phospholipid esters are normal (Sunnasy *et al.*, 1983), but membrane fluidity, including that of the sarcoplasmic reticulum, is altered with ethanol (Ferguson *et al.*, 1984; Ohnishi, 1985). Short-term exposure increases fluidity by disordering acyl chains of phospholipids in the hydrophobic membrane core. Prolonged exposure is associated with an increase in the membrane content of cholesterol and a corresponding decrease of fluidity to less than that of membranes never exposed to ethanol (Goldstein and Chin, 1981). Alterations in resting membrane Na^+ permeability, enzyme–substrate binding, membrane phospholipids, insulin-stimulated amino acid transport, and temperature optima of enzymes may play a role in membrane characteristics of ethanol administration (Ferguson *et al.*, 1984).

Disruption of ion transport and membrane function probably contributes to alcoholic myopathy. Acutely, ethanol suppresses membrane Na^+–K^+ ATPase activity. This allows for increased membrane Na^+ permeability. ATPase activity increases with chronic ethanol administration. Likewise, there is a corresponding drop in oxygen consumption with acutely administered ethanol that increases when it is given chronically. Furthermore, the cell resting potential is lowered by ethanol administration in naive animals but becomes elevated with sustained ethanol intake (Rubin, 1979; Ferguson *et al.*, 1984; Blachley *et al.*, 1985).

Sarcoplasmic reticulum Ca^{2+} permeability is altered by ethanol *in vitro*. Ethanol increases the channel size but not the affinity of the Ca^{2+} gate so that passive Ca^{2+} permeability increases (Ohnishi, 1985). Excess permeability of the sarcoplasmic reticulum even in the resting state may result in negative inotropism of muscle and hence weakness. This effect is not as marked in animals receiving ethanol chronically as it is in those who are naive to ethanol. These two phenomena represent adaptive responses to chronic ethanol administration, and they suggest that derangements of ion transport may be important in the development of the acute myopathy.

Nutritional status is important in the pathogenesis of the acute myopathy of ethanol. The usual clinical history in acute myopathy is one of days to weeks spent drinking ethanol in large amounts while personal care including feeding is neglected (Hed *et al.*, 1955, 1962; Fahlgren *et al.*, 1957; Perkoff *et al.*, 1966). In a study of food deprivation, rats were given a tube-fed normal diet, vitamin and mineral supplementation while simultaneously taking ethanol by inhaling vapour for 3 weeks. Blood ethanol levels were maintained at 100–300 mg dl^{-1}. Half the group had food abruptly withdrawn while ethanol was continued for all. Serum CKs rose between 1 and 3 days. Myoglobinuria developed in 14 of 45 of the starved rats. Muscle histology showed necrosis in the starved group while in the group receiving ethanol but fed, muscle histology was normal. Creatine kinase rose linearly in all animals but was significantly higher in the starved group (Haller and Knochel, 1980).

For chronic myopathy, however, nutrition does not seem to play a significant role. Studies similar to those in the acute myopathy have not been performed because of the duration of ethanol exposure needed to produce the chronic myopathy. In patients admitted for social complications of ethanol abuse or for voluntary rehabilitation there has been poor correlation between nutritional status and myopathy (Martin *et al.*, 1985; Urbano-Marquez *et al.*, 1989).

Interruption of intermediary metabolism probably has a role in the pathogenesis of the ethanol myopathy. Glucose uptake and utilization, gastrointestinal absorption, and gluconeogenesis are reduced in the presence of ethanol and are especially marked when starvation is added as a factor (Reitz, 1979; Cook *et al.*, 1988). Muscle metabolism is specifically altered especially with acute alcoholic intake and in the acute alcoholic myopathy. There is decreased glucose uptake, lowered lactate production, and a reduction in the activity of virtually all glycolytic enzymes (Perkoff, 1971; Hed *et al.*, 1977; Chui *et al.*, 1978; Martin *et al.*, 1984a; Trounce *et al.*, 1987). The observation of increased glycogen—glycogen

accumulation seen ultrastructurally (Hanid *et al.*, 1981)—correlates with the failure of glycolysis.

The acute form of alcoholic myopathy may be precipitated in part by a massive failure of energy production because of the unavailability of glucose. The dual mechanisms of impaired gluconeogenesis combined with a failure of membrane transport and glycolytic enzyme dysfunction could play a major role in producing the myonecrosis characteristic of the acute myopathy. Chronic ethanol intake blocks muscle glycogenolysis, which may account for the preferential type IIB muscle fibre atrophy characteristic of chronic alcoholics. Type IIB fibres are fast twitch fibres which depend almost exclusively on glucose utilization as a substrate for energy production.

Lipid metabolism is altered with ethanol exposure. The mechanisms and their importance in the pathogenesis of the myopathy are uncertain. Triglyceride is the major accumulating lipid in muscle exposed chronically to ethanol as with most myopathies and correlates with the total amount of ethanol consumed over years (Sunnasy *et al.*, 1983). β-Oxidation by mitochondria is reduced with chronic ethanol exposure. The interruption of oleate metabolism may cause mitochondrial toxicity by uncoupling oxidative phosphorylation (Lange and Sobel, 1983). Carnitine levels are normal in muscle chronically exposed to ethanol but lipid transport, itself, has not been studied in alcoholism (Trounce *et al.*, 1987).

Protein metabolism is poorly studied in ethanol-exposed muscle. There is, however, a diminished protein synthesis (Rubin, 1979), a lower protein to DNA ratio (Martin *et al.*, 1984b), and a reduced insulin induced amino acid transport (Rubin and Rottenberg, 1982). Actomyosin contractility is reduced with ethanol exposure (Puszkin and Rubin, 1975; Rubin *et al.*, 1976), and there are alterations in regulation of the relaxing system related to troponin (Puszkin and Rubin, 1976).

Ethanol has a limited effect on mitochondria. Defects in structure have been mentioned above. Metabolic derangements include uncoupling of oxidative phosphorylation (Lange and Sobel, 1983). In studies on muscle of alcoholics by Martin *et al.* (1982), labelling studies on mitochondria were normal and there was normal activity of marker enzymes for mitochondria including glutamate dehydrogenase, succinate dehydrogenase and maleate. In later work, the mitochondrial markers isocitrate dehydrogenase, MAO, and cytochrome oxidase were found not to be different in alcoholics with proximal wasting than in controls (Trounce *et al.*, 1987). Myofibrillary Ca-ATPase, however, is reduced in alcoholics with the greatest amount of atrophy (Martin *et al.*, 1984a).

Ethanol is promptly metabolized first to acetaldehyde, then to acetate and finally to acetyl CoA. The effects of acetaldehyde, the major metabolite of ethanol, are similar both qualitatively and quantitatively to those of the parent substance. Concentrations of acetaldehyde are low compared with ethanol, but the metabolism of acetaldehyde can be blocked experimentally thereby producing higher concentrations. In such settings, protein synthesis, mitochondrial respiration, and muscle contractility are reduced in similar proportions to that seen with ethanol alone (Weishaar *et al.*, 1978).

Electrolyte disturbances may be seen in association with alcoholism and may contribute to its muscle toxicity. Hypokalaemic myopathy may occur in alcoholism and is discussed in detail below. Usually, however, hypokalaemia in the alcoholic represents a redistribution of K^+ into the intracellular compartment rather than a total body reduction in K^+ (Haller and Knochel, 1984).

Magnesium deficiency is common in alcoholics with mean total body deficits of 1.15 mEq kg^{-1} (Flink, 1986). This may be associated with muscle weakness but no known pathological changes in muscle. Hypomagnesaemia may cause impairment of magnesium-dependent enzymes involved in intermediary metabolism, and potentially may affect magnesium-dependent contractile proteins.

Hypophosphataemia occurs in chronic alcoholics and may produce a myopathy. The myopathy associated with it occurs in the setting of re-feeding when the alcoholic is brought into hospital for treatment of the dependency state or complications of alcoholism. The mechanism of the latter phenomena is best explained as the rapid utilization of available but deficient amounts of phosphorus as a result of a carbohydrate load (Haller *et al.*, 1984).

Acute Alcoholic Rhabdomyolysis

Acute rhabdomyolysis typically occurs in alcoholics with a life-long history of abuse,

although it can occur after a single binge. In some patients, the myopathy presents during the phase of withdrawal, but this is much less common. The clinical presentation is one of pain and swelling in the muscles which develops over the course of minutes to a few hours. Brief muscle cramps are frequently superimposed on the diffuse steady pain. The cramps usually last less than a minute, but may result in local exacerbation of the steady pain for several hours.

The most serious sequela of the rhabdomyolysis is renal failure. The muscle necrosis results in release of large amounts of enzymes into the blood, such as creatine kinase, lactate dehydrogenase (LDH), and others. Myoglobin is greatly increased in the blood and is excreted in the urine, giving the urine of these patients a dark orange or brown colour. The nephropathy is thought to be the result of the large load of myoglobin (Koffler *et al.*, 1976). If untreated, the renal failure may be fatal. Therefore, plasmapheresis is used to reduce the serum myoglobin and thereby protect the kidneys. Haemodialysis is not effective in preventing the nephropathy. Vigorous hydration is also very helpful, and may be especially of benefit with maintenance of adequate urine output. Hyperphosphataemia and hyperkalaemia are commonly associated with rhabdomyolysis and are likely because of the renal failure. There is evidence that treatment with potassium before an inciting event may actually reduce the rhabdomyolysis, but after the event, administration of either potassium or phosphate can result in a clinical worsening.

The muscle swelling with acute alcoholic myopathy is the result of damage to the muscle membrane, so that there is influx of very large amounts of fluids. The muscle mass of the body is so large that many litres may be deposited here. The clinical result is massive swelling of the extremities and face. The oedema is confined to the muscles, so that oxygen and carbon dioxide diffusion are not affected. The major complication of this extremity oedema is the development of compartment syndromes. When the oedema is sufficient to tamponade blood supply to a myofascial compartment, there is the risk of further ischaemia and necrosis. This can only be prevented by fasciotomy.

The mechanisms of damage due to ethanol are not completely understood. Hypotheses have included ischaemia, interference with glycolytic enzyme activity, direct effect of ethanol on muscle membrane, and primary sarcolemmal membrane damage. This latter hypothesis is supported by the findings of Knutsson and Katz (1967) and Mayer (1973). Experimental data in humans and animals regarding the relative roles of alcohol and the usually associated malnutrition have been conflicting (Dimberg *et al.*, 1967; Song and Rubin, 1972; Rubin *et al.*, 1976; Haller and Drachman, 1980; Haller and Knochel, 1980). Summarizing many studies, it appears that with normal caloric and vitamin administration, mild myopathy can develop with heavy ethanol intake, but that for dramatic changes to occur, the ethanol must be administered in the setting of poor nutrition. Pre-existing hypophosphataemia has also been implicated in experimental animals.

Treatment of Acute Rhabdomyolysis

Rhabdomyolysis results from muscle injury. Minimum muscle injury causes membrane leaks of all muscle enzymes including CK, LDH, aldolase, myoglobin and others. Myoglobinaemia causes renal failure by precipitation of pigment in the renal tubules. Urinary myoglobin is seen as darkly stained urine, but the level of urinary myoglobin does not correlate with serum myoglobin levels. Serum CK is more commonly measured than is myoglobin. CKs above 45 000 mU ml^{-1} are associated with myoglobinaemia and the greater likelihood of renal failure. Factors that predispose to myoglobin precipitation and hence renal failure are acidosis, dehydration and hypotension. Treatment of rhabdomyolysis hinges on dilution of the myoglobin with saline, diuresis with osmotic agents or loop diuretics, alkalinization of the urine with bicarbonate and treatment of electrolyte disturbances.

Treatment of rhabdomyolysis by dilution of the urine may take massive amounts of saline. During the acute phase of myoglobinuria, 2–3 days, muscle continues to release myoglobin. In addition, muscle membrane mechanisms function poorly so that muscle takes on large amounts of saline at the expense of the intravascular space. Owing to this third space phenomenon, the involved muscles may become hugely and unpreventably oedematous. Hence, very large amounts of fluids are necessary to dilute the pigment, an average of 13 l day^{-1} over 3 days. Intravascular pressure monitors are often a necessary guide to monitoring volume status. Alkalinization of the

urine to pH 7.5 is helpful in preventing renal tubular precipitation of myoglobin. Acetazolamide controls the alkalaemia.

Metabolic derangements that require specific attention include hypocalcaemia accompanied by hyperphosphataemia in the first 3 days. These are best managed conservatively. Hypocalcaemia is followed by transient hypercalcaemia. Dilution alone is usually sufficient treatment. Hyperkalaemia seen early in rhabdomyolysis may be severe and is attributed both to release of intracellular potassium and to oliguria.

Haemodialysis does not prevent renal failure but is necessary if anuria develops. Plasmapheresis has the potential for removing substantial amounts of myoglobin and hence reducing the risk of renal failure. Fasciotomies of involved restricted muscle spaces may become necessary to prevent compression neuropathies, most commonly in the anterior compartment of the lower leg.

Acute Hypokalaemic Myopathy in Alcoholics

While potassium has been implicated in the development of the acute alcoholic myopathy described above, there is also an acute myopathy in alcoholics which is integrally linked to the level of potassium (Martin *et al.*, 1971). This has different clinical features from those described above. The cardinal clinical findings are the acute development of weakness, but without pain, cramps and muscle swelling. Acute hypokalaemia myopathy in alcoholics is completely reversed by the administration of potassium, unlike the disorder described above. Pathological changes also differentiate this myopathy from that above. The acute weakness is associated with vacuoles in the muscle fibres with both types I and II fibres being approximately equally affected. Also, there are not the changes in phosphorylase, ATPase, and oxidative enzymes observed with alcoholic rhabdomyolysis. The mechanisms of muscle damage with hypokalaemic myopathy are not completely known, but may involve ischaemia. On the basis of their studies in dogs, Knochel and Schlein (1972) hypothesized that hypokalaemia resulted in vasoconstriction, thereby infarcting the skeletal muscle. This study showed that the effect of hypokalaemia was enhanced by exercise, during which the expected vasodilation did not occur, thereby exacerbating the ischaemia.

Chronic Alcoholic Myopathy

In addition to the acute myopathies associated with alcoholism, there have been reports of a chronic myopathy in alcoholics (Ekbom *et al.*, 1964; Klinkerfuss *et al.*, 1967; Perkoff *et al.*, 1967). The described syndrome is the gradual onset of weakness with early involvement of the lower extremities. The upper extremities become weaker later. This might be expected on the basis of chronic changes in asymptomatic patients with heavy ethanol intake. However, many of the electromyographic and histological changes reported in the muscles of alcoholic patients could be explained by a peripheral neuropathy. In fact, some of the reports described a myopathy superimposed on a pre-existing peripheral neuropathy. When a neuropathy is present, the typical findings of myopathy are difficult to distinguish from effects of the neuropathy, unless the myopathic features are quite severe. In addition, some of the features which the authors attributed to myopathy are commonly seen in patients with pure neuropathies. It is reasonable to conclude that at least some of the patients reported as chronic alcoholic myopathy actually have neuropathy (Faris and Reyes, 1971; Rossouw *et al.*, 1976).

DRUG-INDUCED MYOPATHIES

Opiates

Generalized and focal myopathies have been ascribed to heroin injection (Richter *et al.*, 1971). In the generalized form, the patients presented with diffuse severe weakness with muscle tenderness and oedema several hours after injection with impure heroin. Pathological findings were muscle fibre necrosis with oedema and focal haemorrhage. Non-specific findings included myoglobinuria and increased serum levels of muscle enzymes. Some of these patients developed renal failure, presumably from the myoglobinuria. Since these initial reports, other cases have been reported.

The same group reported focal myopathy after heroin injection (Pearson and Richter, 1979). The rhabdomyolysis was localized to the region of the injection.

More recently, other opiates have been reported to produce myopathies. Pentazocine (Talwin) was shown to produce focal muscle necrosis following intramuscular injection (Choucair and Ziter, 1984; Hertzman *et al.*, 1986). In one family, the frequent injection of pentazocine into the proximal muscles of several members of the same family mimicked limb-girdle muscular dystrophy (Choucair and Ziter, 1984).

The mechanism of necrosis is not known and, in fact, may not be due to the heroin *per se*. The necrosis may be a direct effect of other substances in the injection, or perhaps an allergic reaction to one of the substances.

Drugs Affecting Microtubules

The predominant drugs active on microtubules which produce neuromuscular toxicity are colchicine, vincristine and vinblastine. The two latter vinca alkaloids produce their toxicity mainly in the peripheral nerves. The peripheral neuropathy may be dose-limiting. Colchicine has prominent CNS effects with acute intoxication, although a myopathy may also be seen.

While all of these drugs interact with microtubules, their specificity of action is different. Certain regions are preferentially affected by some of these agents but not others (Goldschmidt and Steward, 1989).

Colchicine

Colchicine is used predominantly for the treatment of gout and as an adjunct for treatment of other collagen vascular disorders. With acute intoxication, most of the symptoms are due to involvement of the CNS, and patients may develop failure of multiple organs. However, chronic therapy produces a myopathy in some patients which is very similar to that produced by other microtubule-toxins (Davies *et al.*, 1988; Wallace and Singer, 1988). The myopathy is clinically more significant than that due to vincristine, which has predominant effects on the peripheral nerves (Riggs *et al.*, 1986).

The myopathy has been reported after single or multiple acute intoxications but is more commonly seen with chronic administration (Kuncl and Duncan, 1988).

Typical presenting signs are the subacute onset

of progressive proximal weakness. The weakness can be very variable, with some patients only mildly affected and others being unable to ambulate. The occurrence of these symptoms in patients treated with colchicine suggests the diagnosis, but the differential diagnosis includes polymyositis and axonal neuropathy unrelated to the colchicine. In the patients of Kuncl and Duncan (1988), all those with myopathy had some degree of renal insufficiency.

Diagnosis rests on clinical suspicion, with a history of colchicine administration. Electromyography (EMG) shows myopathic changes most prominent in proximal muscles. Signs of axonal neuropathy are also seen in most patients. CK is uniformly elevated and may be mildly elevated in patients on colchicine without clinical signs of myopathy. However, the neuropathy is likely to be less clinically significant than the myopathy. Biopsy is characteristic, with vacuoles which are found on electron microscopy to be autophagic vacuoles. The vacuoles are both central and subsarcolemmal.

The pathogenesis of colchicine myopathy is thought to result from disruption of microtubules (Paulson and McClure, 1975; Kuncl and Wiggins, 1988). Colchicine binds tubulin, the basic subunit of microtubules, and thereby prevents polymerization into microtubules. This may interfere with movement of lysosomes thereby resulting in accumulation. Colchicine is an amphiphilic molecule; however, its effect in this regard is relatively weak. The relative contribution of membrane alterations to the toxicity of colchicine is not known, but is probably relatively minor.

Discontinuation of colchicine treatment is associated with rapid improvement in clinical and pathological findings, although the CK may remain elevated for more than a year (Riggs *et al.*, 1986). No specific treatment is available or required.

As mentioned previously, patients with renal failure have an increased incidence of colchicine myopathy, owing to reduced plasma clearance. This is most common in patients with gout. Similarly, liver failure is expected to increase the incidence of myopathy. This would be especially true in patients treated with colchicine for disorders which commonly involve the liver, e.g. amyloidosis and primary biliary cirrhosis (Kaplan *et al.*, 1986; Zemer *et al.*, 1986; Cohen *et al.*, 1987).

Recently, methods to reduce the toxicity of colchicine in patients who receive the drugs have been sought. Scherrmann *et al.*, (1989) showed that rabbits immunized against colchicine had increased tolerance to the lethal effects of an acute overdose. At 3 mg kg^{-1} the mortality of the immunized animals was 17 per cent of the non-immunized animals. However, the protective effect was dose-limited. At 6 mg kg^{-1}, all of the animals died regardless of whether they received the immunizations or not.

Vincristine

Vincristine is a chemotherapeutic agent used widely for treatment of a variety of tumours. The main neurologic side-effect of vincristine is an axonal peripheral neuropathy. In many patients this is dose-limiting. The main symptoms of the neuropathy are sensory loss and dysaesthesias with weakness developing distally. However, in addition to this neuropathy, vincristine has been implicated in producing a myopathy. This is much milder than the neuropathy and not frequently clinically recognized. This condition is characterized by progressive weakness. Muscle biopsy has shown the characteristic changes of denervation, with fibre type grouping and increased variation in fibre size. In addition, occasional foci of necrosis have been observed (Bradley *et al.*, 1970).

The most common method of administration of vincristine is by intravenous infusion at intervals no closer than 1 week. However, recently many chemotherapeutic agents are being given by continuous infusion over several days. The pattern of toxicity with this regimen is currently under study. One report mentioned that two of nine patients treated with 5-day infusions of vincristine (total dose 4 mg m^{-2}) developed severe muscle pain near the end of the infusion (Pinkerton *et al.*, 1988).

In animals, administration of high doses of vincristine resulted in profound weakness which was due to muscle effects; the peripheral nerves were spared during the relatively short duration of this study (Slotwiner *et al.*, 1966).

Vincristine produces neuropathy by interference with microtubule formation; however, the mechanism of myopathy is not completely understood.

Vincristine should be used with caution in patients with pre-existing peripheral neuropathy. This has especially been demonstrated for patients with hereditary peripheral neuropathy. The incidence of dose-limiting neuropathy is greatly increased in these patients (McGuire *et al.*, 1989).

Just as for colchicine, mechanisms to prevent the neuropathy and myopathy from vincristine are being investigated. Favaro *et al.* (1988) showed that administration of 50 mg kg^{-1} of gangliosides reduced the deterioration in the compound action potential of rabbits administered vincristine. The dose of vincristine was 0.2–0.25 mg kg^{-1} week^{-1}, high by human standards. Vincristine myopathy was not mentioned in this study.

Amiodarone

Amiodarone is a new antiarrhythmic which has been used extensively only in the past few years. Recently, it has been found to produce a prominent neuromyopathy (Meier *et al.*, 1979; Jacobs and Costa-Jussa, 1985).

The pathological changes are membrane and lipid inclusions in both peripheral nerves and muscles of affected patients. The inclusions may persist for 2 years following discontinuation of the drug (Alderson *et al.*, 1987). This results, in part, from the very long half-life of amiodarone, but also may be dependent on limitations of repair mechanisms in the muscle.

Clinically, the neuropathy is more significant than the myopathy. The myopathy is relatively mild in most instances. There is no specific treatment, other than discontinuation of the drug.

Barbiturates

Administration of barbiturates may produce a rhabdomyolysis indistinguishable from that associated with heroin injection. In addition, subcutaneous administration may cause focal necrosis of the adjacent muscle (Pollard, 1973). However, these conditions are usually not serious enough to warrant specific treatment. By recognizing these disorders, clinicians can frequently avoid needless additional laboratory evaluation.

Clofibrate

Clofibrate is an agent used to lower serum levels of lipids in patients at risk for atherosclerotic vascular disease. Some patients administered clofib-

rate have developed increased CK without clinically evident myoglobinuria (Langer and Levy, 1968). These changes resolved after the clofibrate was discontinued. This complication is more common in patients with incipient renal failure, as they develop higher concentrations of the drug in the blood (Pierides *et al.*, 1975).

The mechanism of action of clofibrate is not know but is probably a direct effect on the muscle membrane.

Chloroquine

Chloroquine has been used for years for the treatment of malaria and, more recently, for some connective tissue disorders, e.g. scleroderma, systemic lupus erythematosus (SLE) and rheumatoid arthritis.

Whisnant *et al.* (1963) described patients with the gradual development of progressive proximal weakness which was more marked in the lower extremities. Histological examination revealed vacuolar degeneration. Symptoms gradually improved after discontinuation of chloroquine therapy. Since this initial report, several authors have confirmed these findings. Type I fibres are preferentially involved. Segmental necrosis is the result of overdevelopment of autophagic vacuoles with markedly increased lysosomal protease activity (Kumamoto *et al.*, 1989).

Laboratory findings relating to the myopathy include mildly elevated CK and myopathic changes on EMG (MacDonald and Engel, 1970; Estes *et al.*, 1987).

This diagnosis of chloroquine myopathy is often clouded by the simultaneous presence of chloroquine neuropathy. The neuropathy has both axonal and demyelinating features, but the predominant pathology is demyelination. Human biopsies have revealed segmental demyelination with regions of remyelination. There were cytoplasmic inclusions in the Schwann cells and some other supporting cells, but these were not seen within the axons (Tegner *et al.*, 1988).

The cause of death in many patients with acute chloroquine poisoning is the development of a severe cardiomyopathy. Therefore, many patients with chloroquine poisoning have electrocardiographic abnormalities in association with abnormalities in blood pressure and heart rate.

Treatment of chloroquine poisoning is mainly supportive, including mechanical ventilation and pharmacological treatment of systemic hypotension. Recently, diazepam has been demonstrated to be helpful in both patients and animals (Riou *et al.*, 1988a,b).

Recently, chloroquine has been implicated in patients with defects in neuromuscular transmission. Robberecht *et al.* (1989) described a patient being treated with chloroquine for reticular erythematosus mucinosis. The patient developed a myasthenic syndrome which was associated with failure of neuromuscular transmission on repetitive stimulation and single fibre EMG. After discontinuation of the chloroquine, the patient continued to have a decremental response to repetitive stimulation and jitter was at the upper limit of normal, indicating that the patient had a pre-existing neuromuscular transmission abnormality. The authors concluded that chloroquine exacerbated the conduction failure.

Sghirlanzoni *et al.* (1988) reported a young woman who developed a myasthenic syndrome 6 weeks after beginning chloroquine therapy for SLE. Pathological examination showed the vacuolar myopathy described above and, in addition, membranous bodies in the distal motor nerves. Symptoms resolved within 6 months following discontinuation of the chloroquine.

Emetine

Emetine is the main constituent of ipecacuanha, a drug commonly used to induce vomiting in patients after ingestion of many toxic substances. Short-term administration is safe; however, long-term administration has been associated with diffuse weakness and muscle pain. Patients subjecting themselves to long-term emetine administration have taken it usually for weight control, but this drug is also occasionally used for amoebiasis (Bennett *et al.*, 1982).

Pathological changes include diffuse atrophy without inflammation. The atrophy was most prominent in type II fibres. Some fibres had a moth-eaten appearance on oxidative stains.

The skeletal myopathy is frequently associated with a cardiomyopathy (Kuntzer *et al.*, 1989; Lachman *et al.*, 1989). Electrocardiographic abnormalities have included T-wave inversion with prolongation of the Q–T interval.

Emetine has been found to reduce the quantal content of the endplate potential at low doses (Alkadhi, 1987). At higher doses, there was a postsynaptic effect in addition to this presynaptic effect. The postsynaptic effect was a reduction in permeability of the ionic channel regulated by the acetylcholine receptor.

Drug-Induced Hypokalaemic Myopathy

Many drugs cause wasting of potassium by the kidneys, with resultant predisposition to the development of muscle necrosis. This is similar to the hypokalaemic myopathy associated with alcoholism. These drugs include amphotericin B, licorice, and azathioprine.

Amphotericin produced hypokalaemia by wasting due to renal damage (Drutz *et al.*, 1970). Licorice produces a syndrome resembling primary aldosteronism characterized by hypokalaemia which responds to administered potassium plus discontinuation of exposure. The same effect is produced by carbenoxolone, a derivative of licorice administered for gastric ulcer.

Amphiphilic Drug Myopathy

Amphiphilic drugs are those which have both hydrophobic and hydrophilic regions. The amphiphilic nature of many drugs is thought to be a common thread connecting their potential for producing myopathies (Drenckhahn and Lullman-Rauch, 1979; Hruman, 1984; Kuncl and Wiggins, 1988).

The two regions of the drugs produce muscle damage in distinct ways. The hydrophobic region inserts into the muscle membrane. This increases the permeability and results in deterioration of surface membrane stability. Resultant increases in endocytosis and phagocytosis produce a necrotizing myopathy.

The hydrophilic regions of the internalized drugs disturb the pH in the lysosomes, thereby inhibiting lysosomal enzyme activity (Hostetler and Richman, 1982). This results in a vacuolar myopathy, which has some features in common with myopathies in patients resulting from congenital lysosomal enzyme deficiency. Pathologically, this has the appearance of patchy muscle fibre necrosis, with non-necrotic fibres having subsarcolemmal vacuoles. The drugs which are most likely to produce these effects are those with greater water solubility.

The two types of muscle damage, necrotizing and vacuolar myopathy, may be produced by the same drugs, although specific agents, dose and duration of exposure may result in a predominance of one type of damage over the other.

Many drugs are amphiphilic but some are more likely to produce myopathy than others. These include chloroquine, hydroxychloroquine, doxorubicin and amiodarone. Kuncl and Wiggins (1988) summarized these drugs. A portion of a table from their review is redrawn in Table 1.

Focal Myopathies

We have already mentioned some important causes of focal myopathies, such as local injections of opiates. Many other substances can produce focal muscle damage, mainly by intramuscular injection. One of the most common causes are local anaesthetics. Local anaesthetics are frequently administered to block pain. The injections are given into the tissue in the region of the damaged nerve. Care is taken not to inject directly into the nerve as this would exacerbate damage. As a result, the predominant location of injection is the muscle. In most patients this produces local pain which is relatively mild and self-limiting. After injection into superficial muscle, there may be local pitting, the result of focal necrosis and subsequent scarring (Parris and Dettbarn, 1989).

The necrosis which occurs in skeletal muscle following intramuscular injection is similar to that used by researchers for the study of muscle regeneration (Benoit and Belt, 1970; Sadeh *et al.*, 1985). Bupivacaine, a local anaesthetic, has been used extensively to produce muscle necrosis. As will be detailed below, this necrosis is followed

by regeneration from satellite cells. The necrosis is felt to be calcium-dependent (Steer *et al.*, 1986). Lignocaine (lidocaine) produces focal necrosis which is similar to that produced by bupivacaine. The frequent combination of lidocaine plus adrenaline (epinephrine) severely potentiated the muscle damage. The effect of adrenaline is to produce vasoconstriction, thereby slowing clearance of the lignocaine from the region (Yagiela *et al.*, 1982). No specific treatment is needed for focal damage from local anaesthetic injection. In most instances the muscles will heal without significant neurological sequelae.

ENDOCRINE MYOPATHIES

Normal muscle metabolism is influenced by neural input, the amount of work performed, and circulating hormones. While all of the circulating factors have not been identified, the influence of several hormones has been well described. Muscle dysfunction occurs by either excess or deficiency of these hormones. The most common of these disorders will be discussed.

Corticosteroids

Corticosteroid Excess

Syndromes of corticosteroid excess may be from either exogenous administration or endogenous overproduction (Ruff and Weissmann, 1988).

The most common systemic effects of corticosteroid excess are fluid retention, hypertension, capillary fragility, and occasionally an euphoric

Table 1 Amphiphilic drug myopathy. Source: adapted from Kuncl and Wiggins (1988), used by permission

Drug	Clinical use	Muscle	Nerve	Heart
Chlorpromazine	Psychosis	+	−	−
Imipramine	Depression	+	−	−
Procainamide	Arrhythmia	+	−	−
Quinacrine	Malaria	+	−	−
Amiodarone	Arrhythmia	+	+	−
Chloroquine	Malaria, SLE	+	+	+
Colchicine	Gout	+	+	+
Doxorubicin	Tumours	+	+	+
Hydroxychloroquine	Malaria, SLE	+	+	+

Actions of selected amphiphilic drugs. These are the drugs currently available in the USA. Other drugs are available elsewhere.

Muscle, nerve, and heart headings indicate whether these regions are affected by the drug. Damage occurs in other organs, but is not reviewed here.

mood. There is redistribution of fat, with accumulation in the face, abdomen, and top of the back. The development of corticosteroid myopathy is heralded by the development of wasting and progressive weakness of the proximal muscles. The legs are usually affected more than the arms, such that the predominant complaints are the inability to rise from a chair or to walk up stairs. While some patients may develop myalgias, the muscle involvement is usually painless.

Laboratory studies are usually unrevealing, with normal CK and aldolase. Biopsy reveals atrophy of mainly type II (fast) fibres with preservation of type I (slow) fibres. Fibre necrosis and inflammation are not present. Nerve conduction velocities are normal, but the amplitude of the compound muscle action potential may be reduced especially in proximal muscles (Kimura, 1983). EMG is usually normal because evaluation of motor units is performed at low levels of tension production when few units are discharging. At this level of recruitment, the units are predominantly type I (slow).

Corticosteroids are prescribed for a variety of medical conditions for control of either inflammation or oedema. These include rheumatoid arthritis, brain tumours, inflammatory myopathies, myasthenia gravis, dermatitis, and many others. Most patients tolerate the medications well, with no muscular effects. However, some develop corticosteroid myopathy which is especially worse with high dose or long duration of administration.

The diagnosis of corticosteroid myopathy is especially difficult in patients who are being treated for neuromuscular disorders. When a patient with polymyositis or myasthenia gravis becomes weaker while being treated with prednisone, the weakness can be from either an effect of the steroid or the disease being refractory to the medication. The differentiation between these possibilities is facilitated by muscle biopsy and EMG, but often a definitive diagnosis is only possible by observing the effect of reducing the dose of steroid. If the patient becomes stronger, the aetiology was most likely steroid myopathy, while if the weakness becomes more profound, then stronger immunosuppressants or other therapy are indicated for the underlying disease.

The mainstay of treatment of steroid myopathy is reducing the dose. This is not possible in all patients; however, keeping the dose at a minimum lessens the risk of myopathy. Alternatives include using a non-fluorinated steroid or changing to an alternate-day regimen (Ruff and Weissmann, 1988). Phenytoin may be helpful, but this is not widely used (Gruener and Stern, 1972). Exercise is also helpful in preventing steroid myopathy or reversing the effects when already developed (Horber *et al.*, 1985). Anabolic steroids and protein loading have not been helpful (Ruff and Weissmann, 1988).

The pathophysiology of steroid myopathy is not completely known but is probably related to decreased muscle protein synthesis (Goldberg *et al.*, 1980). At high doses, protein degradation is also increased. This is exacerbated by reduced intake of protein, a concern because many patients treated with steroids have reduced protein and calorie intake. Protein synthesis is probably impaired because of altered translation of DNA in the nucleus (Baxter, 1976). The reason for the predominance of effect on type II fibres is not known, especially as type I fibres have higher numbers of glucocorticoid receptors (Shoji and Pennington, 1977).

Corticosteroid Deficiency

Approximately 25–50 per cent of patients with corticosteroid deficiency (Addison's disease) have complaints of muscle pain and weakness. The diagnosis is confirmed by measuring corticosteroid levels. EMG, CK and biopsy are usually normal (Ruff and Weissman, 1988).

The weakness is due to impaired carbohydrate metabolism and abnormalities in serum electrolytes, particularly hyperkalaemia.

Treatment of myopathy caused by corticosteroid deficiency is replacement of hormone and reduction of serum potassium levels.

Some patients with corticosteroid deficiency develop hyperkalaemic periodic paralysis. This is different from familial hyperkalaemic periodic paralysis in that the levels of potassium required to produce weakness are much greater in patients with Addison's disease than the familial syndrome. This is because the degree of hyperkalaemia in familial periodic paralysis is much less than that required to produce weakness in normal patients, indicating that the defect is in more than potassium metabolism.

Thyroid Disorders

Thyroid disorders are frequently mentioned as causing myopathies; however, the most common symptoms are systemic. Thyrotoxic myopathy is present in patients who are hyperthyroid for long periods of time. In addition to thyrotoxic myopathy, hyperthyroidism is occasionally associated with other muscle conditions, including a form of periodic paralysis and myasthenia gravis.

Hyperthyroidism

Patients with hyperthyroidism frequently develop proximal muscle weakness with wasting. The shoulder girdle muscles are usually affected more than the pelvic girdle. Myalgias may be present, but are infrequently a prominent feature. Deep tendon reflexes are normal or hyperactive. Patients may be aware of fasciculations and myokymia, but these are also not common or prominent features.

Diagnosis is usually dependent on clinical suspicion, with clues from the other signs of hyperthyroidism. These are goitre, tremor, eye signs, and warm, moist skin. The eye signs are exophthalmos and deficits in eye movements; this being due to infiltrative ophthalmopathy. This disorder involves increased retro-orbital tissue and is thought to be autoimmune. Cardiac findings are tachycardia, widened pulse pressure, and occasional atrial fibrillation. The symptoms also include nervousness, increased sweating, fatigue, weight loss, insomnia, and occasionally diarrhoea.

EMG is frequently interpreted as normal, but careful examination usually reveals low amplitude, short duration motor unit potentials with early recruitment (Kimura, 1983). In patients with these abnormalities, the EMG may reveal fasciculations and myokymia. Serum CK and LDH are typically normal or low.

Muscle biopsy is normal or shows only non-specific changes, such as fatty infiltration and decreased muscle fibre size. Nerve terminals may be damaged, contributing to the exacerbation of myasthenia gravis by hyperthyroidism (Ruff and Weissmann, 1988).

The diagnosis of thyrotoxic myopathy must include consideration of other muscle disorders including those also associated with hyperthyroidism. These include myasthenia gravis and a form of periodic paralysis. Periodic paralysis can usually be differentiated on clinical grounds. Myasthenia gravis is differentiated by testing neuromuscular junction transmission.

Thyrotoxic periodic paralysis is thought to be due to the depolarization of the muscle fibre membrane resulting in reduced membrane excitability. The reason for the periodic exacerbations is not known but in thyrotoxic individuals relatively small shifts in electrolytes, such as potassium, may result in ineffective muscle activation. In many respects, thyrotoxic periodic paralysis resembles hypokalaemic periodic paralysis. Histological examination of muscle reveals a vacuolar myopathy in both, although it is not as severe as in familial hypokalaemic periodic paralysis. However, thyrotoxic periodic paralysis is not merely an exacerbation of familial periodic paralysis, because patients with the latter disorder do not have exacerbations of their disease by exogenous thyroid hormone administration (Ruff and Weissmann, 1988). Treatment of thyrotoxic periodic paralysis is merely the treatment of the hyperthyroidism. In the vast majority of patients, their muscle disorder recovers after they have become euthyroid.

The excess thyroxine causes increased protein degradation in the muscle, thereby producing atrophy (Fliam *et al.*, 1978). Also, the muscle is relatively insulin-resistant, contributing to the glycogen depletion. Other changes in the muscle include alteration in contractile characteristics of the muscles. The fibre-type proportions shift so that there is an increase in the proportion of fast oxidative–glycolytic fibres at the expense of both slow oxidative and fast glycolytic. The predominance of this effect on slow muscle produces a reduction in twitch contraction time (Fitts *et al.*, 1984). This change in fibre type is due to alterations in myosin ATPase activity, and a shift in the isoforms of myosin.

Membrane excitability is reduced, with muscle fibre membrane depolarization and an increased threshold for activation. These effects exacerbate neuromuscular transmission, especially in patients with myasthenia gravis, a disorder of transmission (Gruener *et al.*, 1975).

The only effective treatment of thyroid myopathy is correction of the hyperthyroid state. The muscle symptoms resolve after the patient becomes euthyroid.

Hypothyroidism

Hypothyroidism is not specifically a toxic myopathy but is included here for comparison with thyrotoxic myopathy. Hypothyroidism is frequently associated with proximal muscle weakness and spasms. In contrast to hyperthyroidism, reflexes are usually prolonged in duration, owing to a delayed relaxation phase.

EMG may show increased insertional activity with occasional repetitive discharges. Low-amplitude polyphasic motor unit potentials have been seen and CK may be increased.

With hypothyroidism, skeletal muscle has an increased proportion of slow fibres at the expense of fast fibres. This is essentially the reverse of the fibre-type change in hyperthyroidism. Ultrastructural studies show glycogen accumulation. Some patients develop muscles which appear hypertrophic. The aetiology of this is not clear. It may be the result of a combination of increased size of muscle fibres and increased connective tissue.

The differential diagnosis of weakness associated with hypothyroidism includes peripheral neuropathy. This is usually not a prominent clinical feature of hypothyroidism.

The pathophysiology of hypothyroid myopathy is probably related to effects on carbohydrate metabolism and β-adrenergic receptor number. Impaired glycogenolysis results in glycogen accumulation. The insulin-resistant state associated with hypothyroidism also probably contributes to the muscle fatigue. The reduction in the number of β-adrenergic receptors further impairs glycogenolysis through reducing stimulation by adrenaline.

The only effective treatment of hypothyroid myopathy is administration of replacement hormone.

Parathyroid Hormone

Parathyroid dysfunction may be associated with myopathies, but the pathophysiology of these disorders is probably a combination of the effects of calcium and vitamin D metabolism. Parathyroid hormone (PTH) is a peptide hormone which binds to membrane receptors and stimulates cyclic AMP production. While muscle is not a primary target of PTH, it has effects on this tissue as well. These are increased intracellular calcium, activation of calcium-dependent proteases, and reduction in sensitivity of calcium binding to troponin (Ruff and Weissmann, 1988).

Hyperparathyroidism and Vitamin D Intoxication

A minority of patients with hyperparathyroidism develop proximal muscle weakness and atrophy. Physical examination reveals brisk tendon reflexes. Laboratory evaluation shows elevated calcium and depressed phosphorus. CK and aldolase are typically normal. The degree of muscle weakness does not correlate well with the serum calcium. Hypercalcaemia is frequently asymptomatic, but with very high levels patients may develop nausea, vomiting, anorexia, constipation, and ultimately confusion. Patients with severe hypercalcaemia frequently develop nephrolithiasis or urolithiasis. Acute renal failure from nephrocalcinosis is less common.

Diagnosis of hyperparathyroidism is frequently suspected when an elevated calcium and depressed phosphorus are found on routine testing. Assay for PTH shows elevated levels in hyperparathyroidism, depressed levels in vitamin D intoxication. Some neoplasms, such as bronchogenic lung cancer, produce a PTH-like substance which produces many of the same symptoms as primary hyperparathyroidism.

Treatment of hyperparathyroidism consists of identifying the underlying cause and correcting it. In cases of primary hyperparathyroidism this is surgical removal of the parathyroid glands. Reduction in PTH levels is not always possible, especially in patients with tumour-production of PTH-like hormone. In this case, treatment with mithramycin 25–50 g kg^{-1} intravenously is often effective. Administration of phosphorus (1–1.5 g day^{-1}) may also suppress serum calcium levels. In patients with vitamin D intoxication, prednisone may also be helpful.

Hypoparathyroidism

Most of the symptoms of hypoparathyroidism are from hypocalcaemia. Patients typically present with tetany, a result of the repetitive discharge of peripheral nerves and muscle fibres. The tetany is due to increased excitability of the nerve membrane when calcium concentration is reduced. This effect is further enhanced by hypomagnesaemia, a frequent accompaniment of hypocalcaemia in hypoparathyroidism.

Diagnosis is suspected by the finding of both

hypocalcaemia and hypomagnesaemia. Measurement of PTH levels confirms the diagnosis.

Pseudohypoparathyroidism

Pseudohypoparathyroidism is characterized by the same clinical features as true hypoparathyroidism, but the levels of PTH are normal or increased. The electrolyte abnormalities of hypocalcaemia, hypophosphataemia, and often hypomagnesaemia are present. The pathophysiological basis of pseudohypoparathyroidism is reduced sensitivity of the cells to PTH.

Pituitary Hormones

Growth Hormone and Somatomedins

Acromegaly is caused by increased growth hormone production. Elevated growth hormone induces increased production of somatomedins by the liver. Somatomedins at least partially mediate the physiological actions of growth hormone. Patients with acromegaly frequently have entrapment neuropathies. The most common of these is the compression of the median nerve, carpal tunnel syndrome. In addition to mononeuropathies, patients with acromegaly also develop muscle weakness. This weakness is in spite of increased muscle mass.

Muscle biopsy shows focal necrosis with vacuolar degeneration. Both fast and slow muscle fibres are hypertrophied.

The pathophysiological basis of myopathy due to growth hormone excess probably results from both reduced actomyosin ATPase activity and decreased membrane excitability (Ruff and Weissmann, 1988).

INTRODUCTION TO EXPERIMENTAL MYOPATHIES

Experimental myopathies have been produced in animals for the study of clinically important toxic myopathies, muscular dystrophies, and muscle development. Many of these studies have concentrated on muscle necrosis and the regeneration of muscle fibres following insult.

The value of the experimental myopathies is twofold: (1) they resemble toxic myopathies seen in humans, and (2) they allow the study of basic toxic mechanisms and help in the development of treatment regimens.

ACETYLCHOLINESTERASE INHIBITORS

A well-known symptom of poisoning by acetylcholinesterase inhibitors (AChE-Is) is muscular weakness. This may persist for months following exposure. This weakness has been attributed to neurotoxic effects leading to demyelination of nerve axons. More recent evidence suggests that changes in neuromuscular transmission as a result of exposure to AChE-I can lead to functional and morphological changes at the neuromuscular junction and the muscle itself (Ecobichon, 1982). These changes are thought to be caused by repeated and prolonged endplate depolarizations leading to supercontractions and destruction of subjunctional myofibrils.

Transmission at the neuromuscular junction originates through an action potential at the nerve terminal triggering release of acetylcholine (ACh) into the synaptic cleft. The ACh interacts with ACh receptors (AChR) at the postsynaptic membrane initiating a depolarization which is the endplate potential (EPP). Once the EPP reaches a critical amplitude of 40–50 mV, a propagated muscle action potential triggers the contraction of the muscle fibre. The interaction of ACh with the AChR is terminated by ACh hydrolysis through acetylcholinesterase (AChE).

By preventing ACh hydrolysis with AChE-Is, neuromuscular transmission is modified by prolonging the interaction of ACh with the AChR, leading to repetitive discharges of the nerve terminals and generalized fasciculations.

So-called facilitatory drugs, such as the AChE-Is of the carbamate and organophosphate type have a number of characteristic actions at the neuromuscular junction. Following injection, a single impulse can cause repetitive activity, also called postdrug repetition (PDR). Asynchronous firing of nerve terminals can also be seen in the absence of nerve stimulation, giving rise to fasciculations. Transmission of these responses leads to twitch potentiation, so-called postdrug potentiation (PDP). The effects depend on the frequency of stimulation. At low frequencies, the twitch tension is potentiated because of repetitive firing of the muscle fibres. At high rates of stimulation, the muscle is unable to maintain a tetanic contraction (Karczmar, 1967; Riker and Okamoto, 1969; Hobbiger, 1976; Hartman *et al.*, 1986).

Critical inhibition of AChE causes death, primarily through respiratory failure, generally arising from central impairment of respiration, bronchoconstriction, and failure of neuromuscular transmission in the diaphragm and intercostal muscles. The relative importance of central versus peripheral events varies with the species of animal and the distribution (lipid solubility) and stability of the AChE-I.

Acetylcholinesterase Inhibition and Muscle Necrosis

Histochemical Changes

Light microscopic changes
Injection of an AChE-I at a dose that causes fasciculations produces morphological changes in skeletal muscles of rats. These begin as focal areas in the subjunctional region of the muscle fibre (Preusser, 1967; Fischer, 1968; Ariens *et al.*, 1969; Laskowski *et al.* 1977) progressing to a generalized breakdown with a loss of staining quality and phagocytosis. Only a small segment of fibre lengths is affected. Progressively greater lengths of muscle fibres are affected with time (Fenichel *et al.*, 1972; Wecker *et al.*, 1978; Patterson *et al.*, 1987).

Following the first light microscopic changes such as localized eosinophilia, swelling of the sarcoplasm, and loss of striations in several muscle fibres, a complete but localized necrosis is observed (Gupta *et al.*, 1987b). These changes are demonstrated in Figure 1.

All lesions are limited to the direct subjunctional region of the muscle (Ariens *et al.*, 1969; Patterson *et al.*, 1987). Depending on the time of sacrifice after the initial injection, the longer the delay, the greater the local damage and the spatial extent of the lesions. The diaphragm muscle among all the muscles tested has the highest number of lesions per 1000 muscle fibres, followed by the soleus. The fast-twitch extensor digitorum longus (EDL) appears to be the least affected of the muscles tested. The repair of these lesions is rapid as few lesions are seen within a week following the injection (Ariens *et al.*, 1969; Gupta *et al.*, 1985a, 1986, 1987a,b). Coinciding with the onset of histological changes there is a significant increase in the blood level of creatine kinase indicating destruction of muscle membrane (Dettbarn *et al.*, 1987).

Ultrastructural Changes
Within 30 min after the injection of an AChE-I the first changes are seen in motor nerve terminals. The most frequent morphological changes are swollen mitochondria, myelin figures, membrane enclosures and larger number of coated vesicles. In the subsynaptic area and the surrounding muscle fibre, vesicular structures are seen in the primary and secondary subsynaptic cleft. The cleft vesicles have a similar appearance to synaptic vesicles but vary in diameter. Changes in the subsynaptic folds vary in degree of severity within the same muscle. Normal subsynaptic clefts with few cleft vesicles are seen side by side with subsynaptic clefts with many cleft vesicles and a widening of the cleft itself, as shown in Figure 2 (Salpeter *et al.*, 1979; Kawabuchi, 1982; Laskowski *et al.*, 1977; Meshul *et al.*, 1985).

Supercontraction of subjunctional sarcomeres is always present as well as disruption of cytoarchitectural organization. Mitochondria show swelling leading to lysis of the central cristae followed by total destruction. Myelin figures beneath the endplate are frequently observed while the region more distal to the endplate is less affected. The nucleoli of the muscle cell nucleus are enlarged and move to the periphery of the nucleus. There is an increase in the number of sacroplasmic ribosomes with subsequent dilation of the sarcoplasmic reticulum and loss of striation of the myofibrils, followed by total destruction of the myofilaments and fragmentation of Z-bands.

Reversible AChE Inhibitors and Myopathies

Long-term treatment of rats with prostigmine sulphate for 42–150 days caused degeneration of postsynaptic folds, mainly in red muscle fibre and less so in white muscle (Engel *et al.*, 1973). The postsynaptic membrane profile concentration was decreased by 29 per cent in red muscle fibres and by 10 per cent in white muscle fibres. The mean miniature EPP amplitude was decreased by 29 per cent. Frequency, quantum content and muscle resting membrane potential were not affected by neostigmine (Engel *et al.*, 1973; Hudson *et al.*, 1985, 1986).

In acute experiments, prostigmine, as well as physostigmine, in concentrations between 0.2 and 0.6 mg kg^{-1} cause muscle fibre necrosis, not unlike that seen with less reversible inhibition of

(A)

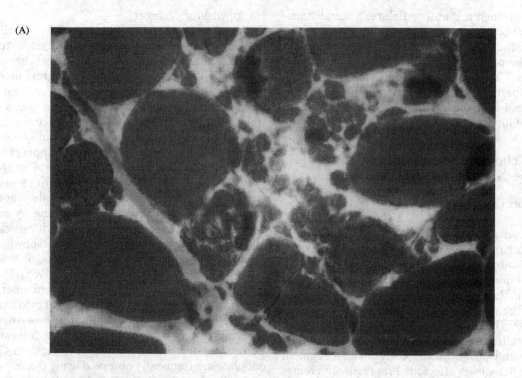

(B)

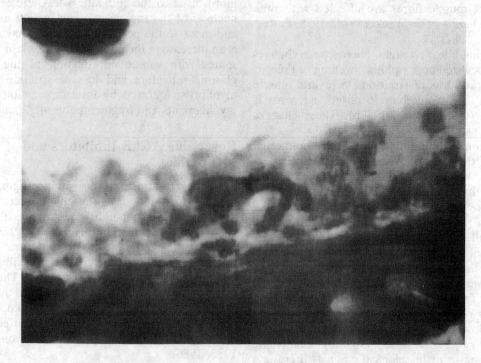

Figure 1 Light micrograph of a cross-section of a rat skeletal muscle following subcutaneous injection with diisopropyl phosphorofluoridate, an organophosphate acetylcholinesterase inhibitor. (A) Four muscle fibres undergoing phagocytosis with some surrounding fibres appearing normal. (B) Muscle fibre undergoing phagocytosis under the region of the endplate, as indentified by the AChE stain. The fibre below the damaged one appears normal. Source: Patterson *et al.* (1987), used with permission.

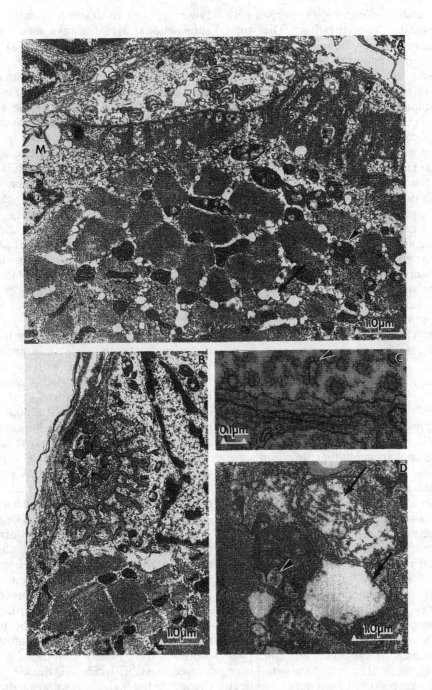

Figure 2 Electron micrograph of endplate region from a rat after injection with paraoxon, an organophosphate inhibitor of acetylcholinesterase. (A) Motor endplate displaying disrupted subsynaptic organization including dilated sarcoplasmic reticulum and T tubules (arrow), abnormal mitochondria (arrowhead), and whorls of membrane (M) beneath the subsynaptic folds. The nerve terminals often contained dilated mitochondria. (B) Mildly affected endplate displaying minor dilatation of sarcoplasmic reticulum and a few abnormal mitochondria. (C) At 30 min, coated vesicles (arrowhead) were frequently encountered near the nerve terminal membrane. (D) Three types of abnormal mitochondria were encountered: the least affected (arrowhead) contained clear patches between cristae; a second type of mitochondrion was dilated and contained severely disrupted cristae (arrow); a third type (double arrow) contained one region that was severely dilated and free of cristae. All three may be stages in the same pathological process. Source: Laskowski *et al*. (1977), used by permission

AChE. The number of necrotic fibres rises with increasing inhibitor concentration. The total number of necrotic fibres, however, is less than that caused by irreversible AChE-I because pronounced muscle fasciculations are seen only for about 30 min after reversible inhibition of AChE. The same symptoms can be observed for over 6 h after irreversible inhibition of the enzyme. Repeated application of the reversible inhibitor, i.e. three times during a given 1.5-h period, leads to prolonged fasciculations and an increased number of lesions (Kawabuchi *et al.*, 1976; Wecker *et al.*, 1978).

Rats when given sublethal doses of pyridostigmine through a gastric tube develop focal necrosis and marked changes in the motor endplate region of skeletal muscle (Gebbers *et al.*, 1986). Myopathic changes were also seen when rats were fed pyridostigmine subchronically. In this case, more changes were seen in the postjunctional area than in the presynaptic terminals. With prolonged feeding (15 days) of a similar dose of pyridostigmine, no increase in the pathology was seen, suggestive of adaptation to the inhibitor (Bowman *et al.*, 1989).

Selective Susceptibility of Muscles

Following exposure to AChE-I, the slow-twitch soleus muscle is more affected than the fast-twitch muscle. This seems to imply that slow fibres are more vulnerable to AChE-I than fast fibres. In the diaphragm muscles, however, fast-twitch, intermediate and slow-twitch fibres are equally affected and it appears that the damage is not selective for any given muscle fibre type. Rather than a selectivity of fibre type, the severity of signs is related to muscle activity pattern (Rash and Elmund, 1988). Both soleus and diaphragm are consistently active either as antigravity or respiratory muscles. In addition to this firing pattern, PDR is imposed on them by the AChE-I. The EDL muscle is only activated during ambulation. Following AChE-I treatment, movement is reduced during the acute toxicity period. There are other data supporting this synergistic effect of AChE-I and muscle activity. In the absence of AChE-I, prolonged high frequency stimulation produces severe alterations in pre- and postsynaptic mitochondria. The severity of these changes is related to frequency and duration of stimulation (Rash and Elmund, 1988). The histopathology is similar to that seen after AChE-I-induced PDR;

however, supercontraction of sarcomeres in the subjunctional areas, always seen with AChE-I, are absent (Rash and Elmund, 1988). The importance of activity pattern is demonstrated by the fact that during stimulation of muscle the threshold concentration for AChE-I to induce neuromuscular lesions is reduced (Rash and Elmund, 1988). Other mechanisms that may contribute to the lesser sensitivity of the EDL to the AChE-I may be found in pharmacokinetic variables that influence delivery of specific inhibitors, differences between muscles in location and accessibility of AChE to the agent, and selective distributions of enzymes hydrolyzing or binding organophosphates in serum and muscle. Selectivity of AChE for central or peripheral neural actions may be another reason for differences in muscle response (Dettbarn, 1984a,b; Meshul *et al.*, 1985; Misulis *et al.*, 1987b).

Mechanisms of Necrosis

As muscle necrosis is always seen in the vicinity of the endplate, the necrosis is probably caused by increased contractile activity in individual muscle fibres (Leonard and Salpeter, 1982; Meshul *et al.*, 1985; Patterson *et al.*, 1987). The extreme vesiculation and disruption of the sarcoplasmic reticulum (SR) under the endplate as well as the swollen mitochondria may reflect overloading of the muscle Ca^{2+}-binding capacity which could result in high sarcoplasmic Ca^{2+} levels leading to the necrosis (Salpeter *et al.*, 1979). The control of intracellular Ca^{2+} concentration is of great importance to muscle fibres because a transient rise in Ca^{2+} leads to contraction. An increased net influx of Ca^{2+} forces the mitochondria and SR to maintain Ca^{2+} homeostasis by sequestering the excessive amounts of this ion. This is an energy-consuming process utilizing ATP and creatine phosphate. Shortage of energy will ultimately cause the free sarcoplasmic Ca^{2+} to rise, triggering events leading to muscle damage.

Studies have clearly established a relationship between AChE-I-induced muscle lesions and changes in the high-energy phosphate compounds (Gupta and Dettbarn, 1987). Levels of ATP and creatine phosphate are significantly reduced in EDL, soleus, and hemi-diaphragm muscles coinciding with the appearance of muscle necrosis.

The onset of damage to the muscle fibres is probably determined by a number of factors, such as the variability of energy supplies in the form of glycogen, creatine phosphate, and ATP. The time course of the necrosis, as reported earlier, correlates with the reduced levels of ATP and creatine phosphate, the reduction of which may have been the result of an increased demand for energy and a low rate of ADP phosphorylation caused by an increased level of sarcoplasmic Ca^{2+}. During AChE-I or carbamylcholine-induced twitch potentiation and prolonged fasciculations, an increased influx of Ca^{2+} was observed in the region of the endplate (Salpeter *et al.*, 1979).

Adaptation to Repeated Exposure to AChE-I

Only a slight increase in the number of lesions is seen when repeated injections of AChE-I are given. A reduction of lesions as well as total protection against the AChE-I is achieved with prolonged treatment.

Rats adapt to repeated exposure to low doses of AChE-I and survive a cumulative concentration of several-fold the acute 50 per cent lethal dose. During treatment with diisopropyl phosphorofluoridate (DFP), a recovery of AChE activity from less than 15 per cent to 75 per cent of control is seen. Simultaneously, a significant decrease in binding sites of the nicotinic AChR, with no change in affinity constant, is observed (Gupta *et al.*, 1986).

The induction of tolerance to the toxicity of AChE-I may be caused by several mechanisms including: (1) downregulation of acetylcholine receptors at the neuromuscular junction, (2) modification in ACh release from the nerve terminal, and (3) rapid *de novo* synthesis of AChE in skeletal muscles.

Prevention of Myopathy

Protection against the necrotic action has been achieved by rapid reactivation of the phosphorylated AChE with pyridine-2-aldoxime methyl chloride (2-PAM). Blocking of PDR may be another mechanism for prevention or treatment of organophosphate intoxication. Thus by lowering the amount of ACh accumulation at the neuromuscular junction, signs of toxicity such as antidromic nerve activity and muscle fasciculations can be prevented or reduced.

Immediate reactivation of the phosphorylated AChE with 2-PAM following exposure to AChE-I of the organophosphate type prevents neuromuscular lesions (Laskowski *et al.*, 1977; Wecker *et al.*, 1978). Neuromuscular blocking agents that in low concentrations block presynaptic receptors involved in release of ACh, can prevent neuromuscular toxicity. These compounds, such as *D*-tubocurarine or atropine, do not interfere with normal neuromuscular transmission but block PDR and thus prevent hyperstimulation of the muscle (Patterson *et al.*, 1988).

Human Toxicity

Acetylcholinesterase inhibitors are routinely administered to patients with myasthenia gravis, a disorder of neuromuscular transmission. In this disease, the patient makes antibodies to the ACh receptor. Binding of these antibodies to the receptors increases their turnover, thereby decreasing the number of available receptors. Therefore, quanta of ACh released from the presynaptic terminal are less effective in producing activation of the postjunctional membrane. To increase the stimulation produced by release of acetylcholine, AChE-Is such as pyridostigmine are administered. The decreased breakdown of ACh results in improved neuromusucular transmission, and clinical improvement.

Lesions similar to those found in rat skeletal muscle have been reported in muscles from humans either exposed to AChE-I as pesticides or following suicide attempts (DeReuck and Willems, 1975; Ahlgren *et al.*, 1979; Wecker *et al.*, 1986). Chronic exposure may also result in a necrotizing myopathy. One patient reported by Ahlgren *et al.* (1979) developed a myopathy with prolonged exposure to diazinon. This patient developed cholinergic symptoms but had normal nerve conduction velocities, suggesting that the muscle changes were not secondary to peripheral nerve involvement. More recently, a reversible paralysis of proximal limb, neck, and respiratory muscles has been described following a massive dose of AChE-I during suicide attempts. All patients were maintained with a life support system. Paralysis of neck and proximal lower limb muscles, as well as of the respiratory muscles, appeared after an acute cholinergic crisis but before the expected onset of delayed neuropathy (Senanayake and Karalliedde, 1987). It is likely that the neuromuscular dysfunction described in these patients was related to the neuromuscular necrosis.

Conclusions

The muscle damage induced by AChE-Is depends on a functional innervation and free available ACh receptors (Wecker and Dettbarn, 1976; Leonard and Salpeter, 1979). The damage depends on the duration of a critical inhibition of AChE (less than 30 per cent of control) and muscle fasciculations. The muscle damage appears to be caused by increased accumulation of free sarcoplasmic Ca^{2+} either from intracellular stores such as sarcoplasmic reticulum or mitochondria and increased uptake of extracellular Ca^{2+} during prolonged muscle activity. The fact that in *in vivo* studies pretreatment with *D*-tubocurarine or atropine (Patterson *et al.*, 1987) or using a Ca^{2+} channel blocker such as diltiazem (Meshul, 1989) either prevented or reduced the neuromuscular damage rules out release of intracellular Ca^{2+}. Other support comes from *in vitro* studies showing that muscle damage is prevented in the absence of extracellular Ca^{2+} (Leonard and Salpeter, 1979). Both observations rule out direct effects of the AChE-I on muscle as a cause for the myopathy. It is suggested that the AChE-I-induced repetitive muscle activity reduces ATP and creatine phosphate leading to failure of Ca^{2+} sequestration into the mitochondria and sarcoplasmic reticulum. The ultimate increase in free sarcoplasmic Ca^{2+} may activate phospholipase A_2 and proteases which compromise sarcolemma and myofibrillar structures.

LOCAL ANAESTHETICS

Clinical Syndromes

Local anaesthetics may produce muscle damage after intramuscular injection. The regional injection of these agents is usually for peripheral nerve blockade or analgesia in joints. Much of the drug infiltrates into surrounding muscle. Bupivacaine, a local anaesthetic, has been observed to produce muscle necrosis in patients as well as in laboratory tests. In humans, injection of bupivacaine in and adjacent to skeletal muscle has produced focal necrosis, evident on physical examination as dimpling (Parris and Dettbarn, 1989). This improves over approximately 2 months, as the muscle regenerates. Injection of bupivacaine behind the eye for regional anaesthesia produced transient diplopia in some patients. This is thought to result from transient muscle dysfunction. This is most probably related to focal necrosis from the bupivacaine (Porter *et al.*, 1988).

Laboratory studies of muscle necrosis due to bupivacaine have not concentrated so much on possible human exposure, but rather have used bupivacaine-induced degeneration and regeneration as clues to mechanisms of muscle damage in other conditions, such as Duchenne muscular dystrophy (Cullen and Fulthorpe, 1975; Duncan, 1978).

While most of the reports of local anaesthetic-induced muscle necrosis have described the effects of bupivacaine, lignocaine (lidocaine) and other agents of this class have the same potential.

Pathological Findings

Histological examination of human muscles has not been reported, to our knowledge; however, animal studies have been revealing. Injection of skeletal muscle with bupivacaine produces an intense inflammatory necrosis (Figure 3). The ultrastructural appearance of the muscle may be completely destroyed. This is followed by regeneration of the muscle within approximately 7–14 days.

The appearance of the necrosis is similar to that produced by a variety of other agents, such as snake venoms (Gutierrez *et al.*, 1986) and chemicals, such as calcium ionophores. Systemic toxicity of bupivacaine may be increased when administered in combination with other local anaesthetics (Lalka *et al.*, 1978).

Pathophysiology

The muscle regenerates from satellite cells which apparently remain intact during the necrosis (Carlson, 1973; Mong, 1988). The regenerated muscle differs from the original muscle in that there is a greater amount of connective tissue and increased variation in fibre size. The efficacy of muscle regeneration is better in the slow soleus than in the fast EDL, and is better in younger than older animals (Sadeh, 1988).

The necrosis caused by local anaesthetics results from activation of calcium-dependent proteases (Steer *et al.*, 1986; Steer and Mastaglia, 1986). The activation of proteases is thought to be via increased synthesis of prostaglandin E_2,

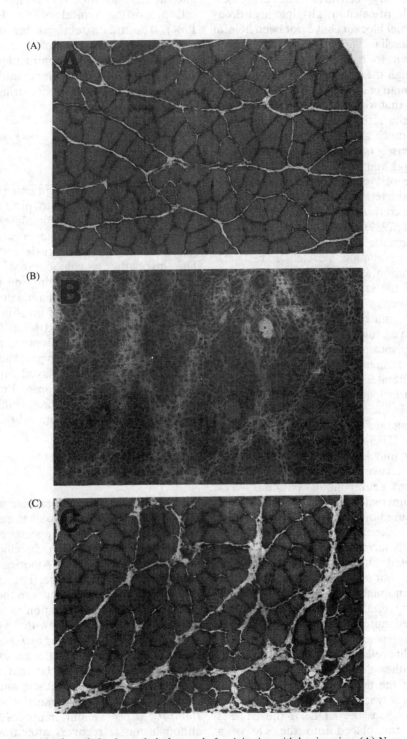

Figure 3 Light micrograph of rat skeletal muscle before and after injection with bupivacaine. (A) Normal cross-section. (B) Three days after injection. Necrosis of virtually all fibres is prominent. (C) Cross-section of muscle 2 weeks after injection. The fibres have regenerated, with resultant pathological changes of increased variation in fibre size, increased central nucleoli, and increased connective tissue. Haematoxylin and eosin stain

which subsequently activates the proteases. Despite the role of calcium, physiological doses of calcium channel blockers have not been helpful (Steer and Mastaglia, 1986). High dose verapamil has been shown to reduce calcium-dependent necrosis, although these levels are not attainable in humans (Zeman *et al.*, 1985).

It was shown that with initial reinnervation, the histochemical characteristics are different, such that there is a much greater proportion of fibres which stain intensely on actomyosin ATPase reaction (Hall-Craggs and Seyan, 1975). These have the appearance of type II fibres. However, the contraction characteristics do not conform to a frank fibre type conversion (Misulis *et al.*, 1987a; Clinton *et al.*, 1989). In many respects, the regenerating muscle has characteristics in common with developing muscle. In fact, the muscle regeneration after necrosis is thought to follow many of the same processes which occur during development.

Regenerating muscle had some fibre-type grouping; however, this was not marked, suggesting that the bupivacaine-induced muscle necrosis left the neural elements relatively intact. Eventually, the regenerated muscle had differentiated into the three principal histochemical fibre types: I, IIA and IIB. In the absence of innervation, the muscle did regenerate but without differentiation into fibre types (Hall-Craggs and Seyan, 1975). The regenerated muscles were smaller, suggesting that adequate recovery of contractile protein amounts requires neural input. Within 1 week after necrosis, innervated fibres regained ATPase activity as measured by actomyosin ATPase reaction. However, denervated muscles failed to develop this early increase.

The regenerated muscle not only has replaced the muscle fibres but also the number of satellite cells returns to normal. That is, during proliferation and reorganization of satellite cells to replace destroyed muscle fibres, there is sufficient proliferation to replace the satellite cells. The number of satellite cells is controlled by the innervating nerve rather than being an endogenous characteristic of the muscle. The normal soleus has approximately twice the proportion of nuclei being satellite cells as the EDL. If the EDL is made necrotic and placed into the site of a removed soleus, then after regeneration, the proportion of satellite cells is the same as in the native soleus. Similarly, the necrotic soleus put into the EDL location regenerates with a satellite cell proportion typical of the EDL (Schultz, 1984). These data reinforce the hypothesis that regenerating skeletal muscle is not differentiated and its biochemical and contractile characteristics will be controlled by the innervating nerve. This condition is similar to that occurring during development.

SEROTONIN

Serotonin (5-hydroxytryptamine) has been administered to animals to produce an experimental myopathy which simulates many of the changes seen in Duchenne muscular dystrophy (Mendell *et al.*, 1976; Christie and Modi, 1984). The myopathy is characterized by numerous mononuclear cells infiltrating the interfibre connective tissue. The inflammatory cells are observed in the vicinity of myofibres undergoing degeneration. Christie and Modi (1984) showed that the mononuclear cells were predominantly macrophages. Other cell types, such as polymorphonuclear leukocytes, played little or no role in the inflammatory response. Presumably, the purpose of the macrophage infiltration is to degrade and remove muscle debris.

VENOMS

A variety of snake venoms can cause skeletal muscle necrosis similar to that seen with local anaesthetics. This has importance for clinical practice as well as research. Specifically, the crotalinae snakes of Central America may produce mainly focal muscle damage. The muscle necrosis is similar to that described for the local anaesthetics; however, regeneration is often slow and incomplete, especially with venoms from *Bothrops asper* and *Bothrops jararacussu* (Gutierrez *et al.*, 1986). Part of the reason for the impaired regeneration may be that these venoms have distinct effects on muscle and vasculature. Block of some of the haemorrhagic effect of the *Bothrops asper* venom improves regeneration, although muscle recovery after this treatment is still not to the extent seen in muscles injected with bupivacaine. The reason for this discrepancy is most probably that the mechanism of necrosis is different from that of bupivacaine, so that the ability of the satellite cells to recover is less.

Other toxins also produce muscle necrosis but have better regeneration than is seen with the two *Bothrops* venoms. These are notexin, taipoxin, and isolated *B. asper* myotoxin (Harris *et al.*, 1975; Harris and Maltin, 1982; Gutierrez *et al.*, 1984). These toxins do not produce the haemorrhage seen with those described above.

REFERENCES

Adler, A. J., Fillipone, E. J. and Berlyne, G. M. (1985). Effect of chronic alcohol intake on muscle composition and metabolic balance of calcium and phosphate in rats. *Am. J. Physiol.*, **249**, E584-E588

Ahlgren, J. D., Manz, H. J. and Harvey, J. C. (1979). Myopathy of chronic organophosphate poisoning. A clinical entity? *South Med. J.*, **72**, 555–559

Alderson, K., Griffin, J. W., Cornblath, D. R., Levine, J. H., Juncl, R. W. and Griffith, L. S. C. (1987). Neuromuscular complications of amiodarone therapy. *Neurology*, **37** (Suppl.), 355

Alkadhi, K. A. (1987). Effects of emetine and dehydroemetine at the frog neuromuscular junction. *Eur. J. Pharmacol.*, **138**, 257–264

Anderson, R., Cohen, M., Haller, F., Elms, J., Carter, N. W. and Knockel, J. P. (1980). Skeletal muscle phosphorus and magnesium deficiency in alcohol myopathy. *Miner. Electrolyte Metab.*, **4**, 106–112

Ariens, A. T., Meeter, E., Wolthuis, O. L., van Benthem, R. M. J. (1969). Reversible necrosis at the endplate region in striated muscles of the rat poisoned with cholinesterase inhibitors. *Experientia*, **25**, 57–59

Baxter, T. (1976). Glucocorticoid hormone action. *Pharmacol. Ther.*, **2**, 605

Bennett, H. S., Spiro, A. J., Pollack, M. A. and Zucker, P. (1982). Ipecac-induced myopathy simulating dermatomyositis. *Neurology*, **32**, 91

Benoit, P. W. and Belt, W. D. (1970). Destruction and regeneration of skeletal muscle after treatment with a local anaesthetic. *J. Anat.*, **107**, 547–556

Blachley, J. D., Johnson, J. H. and Knochel, J. P. (1985). Review: the harmful effects of ethanol on ion transport and cellular respiration. *Am. J. Med. Sci.*, **89**, 22–26

Bowman, P. J., Schuschereba, S. T., Johnson, T. W., Woo, F. J., McKinney, L., Wheeler, C. R., Frost, D. and Korte, J. W. (1989). Myopathic changes in diaphragm of rats fed pyridostigmine bromide subchronically. *Fund. Appl. Toxicol.*, **13**, 110–117

Bradley, W. G., Lassman, L. P., Pearce, G. W. and Walton, J. N. (1970). The neuromyopathy of vincristine in man. Clinical, electrophysiological and pathological studies. *J. Neurol. Sci.*, **10**, 107

Carlson, B. M.(1973). The regeneration of skeletal muscle—a review. *Am. J. Anat.*, **137**, 119–150

Choucair, A. K. and Ziter, F. A. (1984). Pentazocine abuse masquerading as familial myopathy. *Neurology*, **34**, 524–527

Christie, K. N. and Modi, B. V. (1984). Some histochemical observations on invasive cells in a myopathy induced in rats with 5-hydroxytryptamine. *Neuropathol. Appl. Neurobiol.*, **10**, 447–460

Chui, L. A., Neustein, L. H. and Munsat, T. L. (1975). Tubular aggregates in subclinical alcoholic myopathy. *Neurology*, **25**, 405–412

Chui, L. A., Munsat, T. L., and Craig, J. R. (1978). Effect of ethanol on lactic acid production by exercised normal muscle. *Muscle Nerve*, **1**, 56–61

Clinton, M. E., Misulis, K. E. and Dettbarn, W-D. (1989). Acceleration of reinnervation and conversion of slow to fast twitch with denervated regenerating muscle. *Soc. Neurosci. Abstr.*, **15**, 1359

Cohen, A. S., Rubinow, A., Anderson, J. J., Skinner, M., Mason J. H., Libbey, C. and Kayne, H. (1987). Survival of patients with primary (AL) amyloidosis: colchicine-treated cases from 1976 to 1983 compared with cases seen in previous years (1961 to 1973). *Am. J. Med.*, **82**, 1182–1190

Cook, E. B., Preece, J. A., Tonbin, S. D. M., Sugden, M. C., Cox, D. J. and Palmer, T. N. (1988). Acute inhibition by ethanol of intestinal absorption of glucose and hepatic glycogen synthesis on glucose refeeding after starvation in the rat. *Biochem. J.*, **254**, 59–65

Cullen, M. J. and Fulthorpe, J. J. (1975). Stages in fibre breakdown in Duchenne muscular dystrophy. *J. Neurol. Sci.*, **24**, 179

Davies, H. O., Hyland, R. H., Morgan, C. D. and Laroye, G. J. (1988). Massive overdose of colchicine. *Can. Med. Assoc. J.*, **138**, 335–336

Del Villar Negra, A., Marino Angulo, J. and Rivera-Pomar, J. M. (1984). Skeletal muscle changes in chronic alcoholic patients. A conventional, histochemical ultrastructural and morphometric study. *Acta Neurol. Scand.*, **70**, 185–196

DeReuck, J. and Willems, J. (1975). Acute parathion poisoning: myopathic changes in the diaphragm. *J. Neurol.*, **208**, 309–314

Dettbarn, W-D. (1984a). Pesticide induced muscle necrosis: mechanisms and prevention. *Fund. Appl. Toxicol.*, **4**, S18-S26

Dettbarn, W-D. (1984b). Consequences of acetylcholinesterase inhibition in fast and slow muscles of rat. In *Cholinesterases, 2nd International Symposium on Cholinesterases*, Bled, Yugoslavia. Walter de Gruyter, Berlin, New York, pp. 401–414.

Dettbarn, W-D., Vreca, I. and Sket, D. (1987). Correlation of organophosphate induced myopathy with blood creatine kinase level and residual cholinesterase activity in muscle. *18th FEBS Meeting*, Ljubljana, Yugoslavia

Dimberg, R., Hed, R., Kallner, G. and Nygren, A.

(1967). Liver–muscle enzyme activities in the serum of alcoholics on a diet poor in carbohydrates. *Acta Med. Scand.*, **181**, 227

Drenckhahn, D. and Lüllmann-Rauch, R. (1979). Experimental myopathy induced by amphiphilic cationic compounds including several psychotropic drugs. *Neuroscience*, **4**, 549–562

Drutz, D. J., Fan, J. H. and Tai, T. Y. (1970). Hypokalemic rhabdomyolysis and myoglobinuria following amphotericin B therapy. *JAMA* **211**, 824

Duncan, C. J.(1978). Role of intracellular calcium in promoting muscle damage: a strategy for controlling the dystrophic condition. *Experientia*, **34**, 1531

Ecobichon, D. J. (1982). Organophosphorus ester insecticides. In Ecobichon, D. J. and Joy, R. M. (eds), *Pesticides and Neurological Diseases*. CRC Press, Bocaraton-Florida, pp. 115–223

Ekbom, K., Hed, R., Kirstein, L. and Astrom, K. E. (1964). Muscular affectations in chronic alcoholism. *Arch. Neurol.*, **10**, 449

Engel, A. G., Lambert, E. H. and Santa, T. (1973). Study of long-term anticholinesterase therapy. Effects on neuromuscular transmission and motor endplate fine-structure. *Neurology*, **23**, 1273–1281

Estes, M. L., Ewing-Wilson, D., Chou, S. M., Mitsumoto, H., Hanson, M., Shirey, E. and Ratliff, N. B. (1987). Chloroquine neuromyotoxicity: clinical and pathologic perspective. *Am. J. Med.*, **82**, 447–455

Fahlgren, H., Hed, R. and Lundmark, C. (1957). Myonecrosis and myoglobinuria in alcohol and barbiturate intoxication. *Acta Med. Scand.*, **158**, 405–412

Faris, A. A. and Reyes, M.G. (1971). Reappraisal of alcoholic myopathy. Clinical and biopsy study on chronic alcoholics without muscle weakness or wasting. *J. Neurol. Neurosurg. Psychiatry*, **34**, 86

Favaro, G., DiGregorio, F., Panozzo, C. and Fiori, M. G. (1988). Ganglioside treatment of vincristine-induced neuropathy. An electrophysiologic study. *Toxicology*, **49**, 325–329

Fenichel, G. M., Kibler, W. B., Olson, W. H. and Dettbarn, W-D. (1972). Chronic inhibition of cholinesterase as a cause of myopathy. *Neurology*, **22**, 1026–1033

Ferguson, E. R., Blachley, J. D., Carter, N. W. and Knochel, J. P. (1984). Derangements of muscle composition, ion transport and oxygen consumption in chronically alcoholic dogs. *Am. J. Physiol.*, **246**, F700-F709

Fischer, G. (1968). Inhibierung und Restitution der Acetylcholinesterase an der motorischen Endplatte in Zwerchfell der Ratte nach Intoxikation mit Soman. *Histochemie*, **16**, 144–149

Fitts, R. H., Brimmer, C. J., Troup, J. P. and Unsworth, B. R. (1984). Contractile and fatigue properties of thyrotoxic rat muscle. *Muscle Nerve*, **7**, 470–477

Fliam, K. E., Li, J. B. and Jefferson, L. S. (1978).

Effects of thyroxine on protein turnover in rat skeletal muscle. *Am. J. Physiol.*, **235**, E231

Flink, E. B. (1986). Magnesium deficiency in alcoholism. *Alcoholism Clin. Exp. Res.*, **10**, 590–594

Gebbers, J. O., Lötscher, M., Kobel, W., Portmann, R. and Laissue, J. A. (1986). Acute toxicity of pyridostigmine in rats: Histological findings. *Arch. Toxicol.*, **58**, 271–275

Goldberg, A. L., Tischler, M, DeMartino, G. and Griffith, G. (1980). Hormonal regulation of protein degradation and synthesis in skeletal muscle. *Fed. Proc.*, **39**, 31

Goldschmidt, R. B. and Steward, O. (1989). Comparison of the neurotoxic effects of colchicine, the vinca alkyloids, and other microtubule poisons. *Brain Res.*, **486**, 133–140

Goldstein, D. B. and Chin, J. H. (1981). Interaction of ethanol with biological membranes. *Fed. Proc.*, **40**, 2073–2076

Gruener, R. G. and Stern, L. Z. (1972). Diphenylhydantoin reverses membrane effects in steroid myopathy. *Nature*, **235**, 54

Gruener, R. G., Stern, L. Z., Payne, C. and Hannapel, C. (1975). Hyperthyroid myopathy. Intracellular electrophysiological measurements in biopsied human intercostal muscle. *J. Neurol. Sci.*, **24**, 339–349

Gupta, R. C. and Dettbarn, W-D. (1987). Alterations of high-energy phosphate compounds in the skeletal muscles of rats intoxicated with DFP and soman. *Fund. Appl. Toxicol.*, **8**, 400–407

Gupta, R. C., Patterson, G. T. and Dettbarn, W-D. (1985). Mechanisms involved in the development of tolerance to DFP toxicity. *Fund. Appl. Toxicol.*, **5**, S17-S28

Gupta, R. C., Patterson, G. T. and Dettbarn, W-D. (1986). Mechanisms of toxicity and tolerance to diisopropylfluorophosphate at the neuromuscular junction of rat. *Toxicol. Appl. Pharmacol.*, **84**, 541–550

Gupta, R. C., Patterson, G. T and Dettbarn, W-D. (1987a). Biochemical and histochemical alterations following acute soman intoxication in the rat. *Toxicol. Appl. Pharmacol.*, **87**, 393–402

Gupta, R. C., Patterson, G. T. and Dettbarn W-D. (1987b). Acute tabun toxicity: biochemical and histochemical changes in brain and skeletal muscle of rat. *Toxicology*, **46**, 329–341

Gutierrez, J. M., Ownby, C. L. and Odell, G. V. (1984). Skeletal muscle regeneration after myonecrosis induced by crude venom and a myotoxin from the snake *Bothrops asper*. *Toxicon*, **22**, 719

Gutierrez, J. M., Chavez, F., Mata, E. and Cerdas, L. (1986). Skeletal muscle regeneration after myonecrosis induced by *Bothrops asper* (Terciopelo) venom. *Toxicon*, **24**, 223–231

Hall-Craggs, E. C. B and Seyan, H. S. (1975). Histochemical changes in innervated and denervated skeletal muscle fibres following treatment with bupivacaine (Marcain). *Exp. Neurol.*, **46**, 345–354

Haller, R. G. (1985). Experimental acute alcoholic myopathy—a histochemical study. *Muscle Nerve*, **8** 195–203

Haller, R. G. and Drachman, D. D. (1980). Alcoholic rhabdomyolysis: an experimental model in the rat. *Science*, **208**, 412–415

Haller, R. G. and Knochel, J. P. (1980). Experimental alcoholic rhabdomyolysis—a histological study. *J. Neuropathol. Exp. Neurol.*, **39**, 358

Haller, R. G., and Knochel, J. P. (1984). Skeletal muscle disease in alcoholism. *Med. Clin. North Am.*, **68**, 91–103

Haller, R. G., Carter, N. W., Ferguson, E. and Knochel, J. P. (1984). Serum and muscle potassium in experimental alcoholic myopathy. *Neurology*, **34**, 529–532

Hanid, A., Slavin, G., Mair, W., Sowter, C., Ward, P. and Levi, J. (1981). Fibre type changes in striated muscle of alcoholics. *J. Clin. Pathol.*, **34**, 991–995

Harris, J. B and Maltin, C. A. (1982). Myotoxic activity of the crude venom and the principal neurotoxin, taipoxin, of the Australian taipan *Oxyuranus scutellatus*. *Br. J. Pharmacol.*, **76**, 61

Harris, J. B., Johnson, M. A. and Karlsson, E. (1975). Pathological responses of rat skeletal muscle to a single subcutaneous injection of a toxin isolated from the venom of the Australian tiger snake, *Notechis scutatus*. *Clin. Exp. Pharmacol. Physiol.*, **2**, 383

Hartman, G. S., Fiamengo, S. A. and Riker, F. D. (1986). Succinylcholine: mechanisms of fasciculation and their prevention by *d*-tubocurarine or diphenylhydantoin. *Anesthesiology*, **65**, 405–413

Hed, C., Larsson, H. and Wahlgon, F. (1955). Acute myoglobinuria. *Acta Med. Scand.*, **152** 459–463

Hed, R., Lundmark, C., Fahlgren, H. and Orell, S. (1962). Acute muscular syndrome in chronic alcoholism. *Acta Med. Scand.*, **171**, 585

Hed, R., Lindbland, L. E., Nygren, A. and Sunblad, L. (1977). Forearm glucose uptake during glucose tolerance tests in chronic alcoholics. *Scand. J. Clin. Lab. Invest.*, **37**, 229–233

Hertzman, A, Toone, E. and Resnik, C. S. (1986). Pentazocine induced myocutaneous sclerosis. *J. Rheumatol.*, **13**, 210–214

Hobbiger, F. (1976) Pharmacology of anticholinesterase drugs. In Zaimis, E. (Ed.), *Handbook of Experimental Pharmacology*. Springer, Berlin, Heidelberg, New York, **42**, 487–582

Horber, F. F., Scheidegger, J. R., Grunig, B. E. and Frey, F. J. (1985): Experience that prednisone-induced myopathy is reversed by physical training. *J. Clin. Endocrinol. Metab*, **61**, 83–88

Hostetler, K. Y. and Richman, D. D. (1982). Studies on the mechanism of phospholipid storage induced by amantadine and chloroquine in madrin darby canine kidney cells. *Biochem. Pharmacol.*, **31**, 3795–3799

Hruman, Z. (1984). Pulmonary and generalized lysosomal storage induced by amphiphilic drugs. *Environ. Health Perspect.*, **55**, 53–57

Hudson, C. S., Foster, R. E. and Kahng, M. W. (1985). Neuromuscular toxicity of pyridostigmine bromide in the diaphragm, extensor digitorum longus, and soleus muscles of the rat. *Fund. Appl. Toxicol.*, **5**, S260–S269

Hudson, C. S., Foster, R. E. and Kahng, M. W. (1986). Ultrastructural effects of pyridostigmine on neuromuscular junctions in rat diaphragm. *Neurotoxicology*, **7**, 167–186

Jackson, J. (1822). On a peculiar disease resulting from the use of ardent spirits. *N. Engl. J. Med.*, **XI**, 351–353

Jacobs, J. M. and Costa-Jussa, F. R. (1985). The pathology of amiodarone neurotoxicity. II. Peripheral neuropathy in man. *Brain*, **108**, 753–769

Kahn, L. B. and Meyer, J. S. (1970). Acute myopathy in chronic alcoholism: a study of 22 autopsy cases, with ultrastructural observations. *Am. J. Clin. Pathol.*, **53** 516

Kaplan, M. M., Alling, D. W., Zimmerman, H. J. *et al.* (1986). A prospective trial of colchicine for primary biliary cirrhosis. *N. Engl. J. Med.*, **315**, 1448–1454

Karczmar, A. G. (1967). Neuromuscular pharmacology. *Ann. Rev. Pharmacol.*, **7**, 241–276

Kawabuchi, M. (1982). Neostigmine myopathy is a calcium ion-mediated myopathy initially affecting the motor end-plate. *J. Neuropath. Exp. Neurol.*, **41**, 289–314

Kawabuchi, M., Osame, M., Igata, A. and Kanaseki, T. (1976). Myopathic changes at the endplate region induced by neostigmine methylsulfate. *Experientia*, **32**, 623–625

Kiessling, K. H., Pilstrom, L., Karlsson, J. and Piel, K. (1973). Mitochondrial volume in skeletal muscle from young and old, untrained and trained healthy men and from alcoholics. *Clin. Sci.*, **43**, 547–554

Kiessling, K. H., Pilstrom, L., Bylund, A. C., Piehl, K. and Saltin, B. (1975). Effects of chronic ethanol abuse on structure and enzyme activities of skeletal muscle in man. *Scand. J. Clin. Lab. Invest.*, **35**, 601–607

Kimura, J. (1983). Myopathies. In *Electrodiagnosis in Diseases of Nerve and Muscle: Principle and Practice*. F. A. Davis, Philadelphia, pp. 527–548

Klinkerfuss, G., Bleisch, V., Dioso, M. M. and Perkoff, G. T. (1967). A spectrum of myopathy associated with alcoholism. II. Light and electron microscopic observations. *Ann. Intern. Med.*, **67**, 493

Knochel, J. P. (1980). Hypophosphatemia in the alcoholic. *Arch. Intern. Med.*, **140**, 613–615

Knochel, J. P. and Schlein, E. M. (1972). On the mechanism of rhabdomyolysis in potassium depletion. *J. Clin. Invest.*, **51**, 1750

Knutsson, E. and Katz, S. (1967). The effect of ethanol on the membrane permeability to sodium and potassium ions in frog muscle fibers. *Acta Pharmacol.*, **25**, 54

Koffler, A., Friedler, R. M. and Massry, S. G. (1976). Acute renal failure due to non-traumatic rhabdomyolysis. *Ann. Intern. Med.*, **85**, 23

Kumamoto, T., Araki, S. Watanabe, S., Ikebe, N. and Fukuhara, N. (1989). Experimental chloroquine myopathy: morphological and biochemical studies. *Eur. Neurol.*, **29**, 172–178

Kuncl, R. W. and Duncan, G. (1988). Chronic human colchicine myopathy and neuropathy. *Arch. Neurol.*, **45**, 245–246 (letter)

Kuncl, R. W. and Wiggins, W. W. (1988). Toxic myopathies. *Neurol. Clin.*, **6**, 593–619

Kuntzer, T. Bogousslavsky, J., Deruaz, J. P., Janzer, R. and Regli, F..(1989). Reversible emetine-induced myopathy with ECG abnormalities: a toxic myopathy. *J. Neurol.*, **236**, 246–248

Lachman, M. F., Romeo, R. and McComb, R. B. (1989). Emetine identified in urine by HPLC, with fluorescence and ultraviolet/diode array detection, in a patient with cardiomyopathy. *Clin. Chem.*, **35**, 499–502

Lalka, D., Vicuna, N., Burrow, S. R. *et al.* (1978). Bupivacaine and other amide local anesthetics inhibit the hydrolysis of chloroprocaine by human serum. *Anesth. Analg.*, **57**, 534–539

Lange, L. G. and Sobel, B. E. (1983). Mitochondrial dysfunction induced by fatty acid ethyl esters, myocardial metabolites of ethanol. *J. Clin. Invest.*, **72**, 724–731

Langer, T. and Levy, R. I. (1968). Acute muscular syndrome associated with administration of clofibrate. *N. Engl. J. Med.*, **279**, 856

Laskowski, M. D., Olson, W. H. and Dettbarn, W-D. (1977). Initial ultrastructural abnormalities at the motor endplate produced by a cholinesterase inhibitor. *Exp. Neurol.*, **57**, 13–33

Leonard, J. P. and Salpeter, M. M. (1979). Agonist-induced myopathy at the neuromuscular junction is mediated by calcium. *J. Cell Biol.*, **82**, 811–819

Leonard, J. P. and Salpeter, M. M. (1982). Calcium mediated myopathy at neuromuscular junctions of normal and dystrophic muscle. *Exp. Neurol.*, **76**, 121–138

MacDonald, R. D. and Engel, A. G. (1970). Experimental chloroquine myopathy. *J. Neuropathol. Exp. Neurol.*, **29**, 479–499

McGuire, S. A., Gospe, S. M. Jr and Dahl, G. (1989). Acute vincristine neurotoxicity in the presence of hereditary motor and sensory neuropathy type I. *Med. Pediatr. Oncol.*, **17**, 520–523

Martin, F., Ward, K., Slavin, G., Levi, J. and Peters, T. J. (1985). Alcoholic skeletal myopathy: a clinical and pathological study. *Q. J. Med.*, **55** 233–521

Martin, F. C., Slavin, G., Levi, A. J. and Peters, T. J. (1984a). Glycogen content and activities of key glycolytic enzymes in muscle biopsies from control

subjects and patients with chronic alcoholic skeletal myopathy. *Clin. Sci.*, **66**, 69–78

Martin, F. C., Slavin, G., Levi, A. J. and Peters, T. J. (1984b). Investigation of the organelle pathology of skeletal muscle in chronic alcoholism. *J. Clin. Pathol.*, **37**, 448–454

Martin, F. C., Slavin, G. and Levi, A. J. (1982). Alcoholic muscle disease. *Br. Med. Bull.*, **38**, 53–56

Martin, J. B., Craig, J. W., Eckel, R. E. and Munger, J. (1971). Hypokalemia myopathy in chronic alcoholism. *Neurology*, **21**, 1160–1168

Martinez, A. J., Hooshmand, H. and Faris, A. A. (1973). Acute alcoholic myopathy. Enzyme histochemistry and electron microscopic findings. *J. Neurol. Sci.*, **20**, 245–252

Mayer, R. F. (1973). Recent studies in man and animal of peripheral nerve and muscle dysfunction associated with chronic alcoholism. *Ann. NY Acad. Sci.*, **215**, 370

Meier, C., Kauer, B., Muller, U. and Ludin, H. P. (1979). Neuromyopathy during chronic amiodarone treatment: a case report. *J. Neurol.*, **220**, 231–239

Mendell, J. R., Silverman, L. M., Verrill, H. L., Parker, J. M. and Olson, W. H. (1976). Imipramine-serotonin induced myopathy. *Neurology*, **26**, 968–974

Meshul, C. K. (1989). Calcium channel blocker reverses anticholinesterase induced myopathy. *Brain Res.*, **497**, 142–148

Meshul, C. K., Boyne, A. F., Deshpande, S. S. and Albuquerque, E. X. (1985). Comparison of the ultrastructural myopathy induced by anticholinesterase agents at the endplates of rat soleus and extensor muscles. *Exp. Neurol.*, **89**, 96–114

Misulis, K. E., Clinton, M. E. and Dettbarn, W-D. (1987a). Local and systemic effects of muscle regeneration on motor axon reinnervation. *Soc. Neurosci. Abst.*, **13**, 1619

Misulis, K. E., Clinton, M. E., Dettbarn, W-D. and Gupta, R. C. (1987b). Differences in central and peripheral neural actions between soman and diisopropylfluorophosphate organophosphorus inhibitors of acetylcholinesterase. *Toxicol. Appl. Pharmacol.*, **89**, 391–398

Mong, F. S. F. (1988). Satellite cells in the regenerated and regrafted skeletal muscles of rats. *Experientia*, **44**, 601–603

Ohnishi, S. T. (1985). Chronic alcohol ingestion alters the calcium permeability of sarcoplasmic reticulum of rat skeletal muscle. *Memb. Biochem.*, **6**, 33–47

Parris, W. C. and Dettbarn, W.-D. (1989). Muscle atrophy following nerve block therapy. *Anesthesiology*, **69**, 289

Patterson, G. T., Gupta, R. C., Dettbarn, W-D. (1987). Diversity of molecular form patterns of acetylcholinesterase in skeletal muscle of rat. *Asia Pac. J. Pharmacol.*, **2**, 265–273

Patterson, G. T., Gupta, R. C., Misulis, K. E. and Dettbarn, W.-D. (1988). Prevention of diisopropylphosphorofluoridate (DFP)-induced skeletal muscle fibre lesions in rat. *Toxicology*, **48**, 237–244

Paulson, J. C. and McClure, W. O. (1975). Microtubules and axoplasmic transport. Inhibition of transport by podophyllotoxin: an interaction with microtubule protein. *J. Cell Biol.*, **67**, 461–467

Pearson, J. and Richter, R. W. (1979). Addiction to opiates: neurologic aspects. In Vinken, P. J. and Bruyn, G. W. (Eds). *Handbook of Clinical Neurology*, Vol. 37. North Holland, Amsterdam, pp. 365–400

Perkoff, G. T. (1971). Alcoholic myopathy. *Ann. Rev. Med.*, **22**, 125–132

Perkoff, G. T., Hardy, P. and Velez-Garcia, E. (1966). Reversible acute muscular syndrome in chronic alcoholism. *N. Engl. J. Med.*, **274**, 1277–1285

Perkoff, G. T., Dioso, M. M., Bleisch, V. and Klingerfuss, G. (1967). A spectrum of myopathy associated with alcoholism. I. Clinical and laboratory features. *Ann. Intern. Med.*, **67**, 481–492

Pieredis, A. M., Alvarez-Ude, F. and Kerr, D. N. S. (1975). Clofibrate-induced muscle damage in patients with chronic renal failure. *Lancet*, **2**, 1279

Pinkerton, C. R., McDermott, B., Philip, T. *et al.* (1988). Continuous vincristine infusion as part of a high dose chemoradiotherapy regimen: drug kinetics and toxicity. *Cancer Chemother. Pharmacol.*, **22**, 271–274

Pittman, J. G. and Decker, J. W. (1971). Acute and chronic myopathy associated with alcoholism. *Neurology*, **21**, 293

Pollard, R. (1973). Surgical implications of some types of drug dependence. *Br. Med. J.*, **1**, 784

Porter, J. D., Edney, D. P., McMahon, E. J. and Burns, L. A. (1988). Extraocular myotoxicity of the retrobulbar anesthetic bupivacaine hydrochloride. *Invest. Ophthalmol. Vis. Sci.*, **29**, 163–174

Preusser, H. J. (1967). Die Ultrastruktur der motorischen Endplatte im Zwerchfell der Ratte und Veränderungen nach Inhibierung der Acetylcholinesterase. *Z. Zellforsch. Mikrosk. Anat.*, **80**, 436–457

Puszkin, S. and Rubin, E. (1975). Adenosine diphosphate effect on contractility of human muscle actomyosin: inhibition by ethanol and acetaldehyde. *Science*, **188**, 1319–1320

Puszkin, S. and Rubin, E. (1976). Effects of ADP, ethanol, and acetaldehyde on the relaxing complex of human muscle and its adsorption by polystyrene particles. *Arch. Biochem. Biophys.*, **177**, 574–584

Rash, J. E. and Elmund, J. K. (1988). Pathophysiology of anticholinesterase agents. *Final Report to US Department of Defense, DAMD17-84-C-4010*

Reitz, R. C. (1979). Effects of ethanol on the intermediary metabolism of liver and brain. In Majchrowicz, E. and Noble, E. P. (Eds), *Biochemistry and Pharmacology of Ethanol*. Vol. 1. Plenum Press, New York, pp. 353–360

Richter, R. W., Challenor, Y. B., Pearson, J., Kagen, L. J., Hamilton, L. L. and Ramsey, W. H. (1971).

Acute myoglobinuria associated with heroin addiction. *JAMA*, **216**, 1172

Riggs, J. E., Schochet, S. S. Jr, Gutmann, L., Crosby, T. W. and DiBartolomeo, A. G. (1986). Chronic human colchicine neuropathy and myopathy. *Arch. Neurol.*, **43**, 521–523

Riker, W. F. Jr and Okamoto, M. (1969). Pharmacology of motor nerve terminals. *Ann. Rev. Pharmacol.*, **9**, 173–208

Riou, B., Rimailho, A., Galliot, M., Bourdon, R. and Huet, Y. (1988a). Protective cardiovascular effects of diazepam in experimental acute chloroquine poisoning. *Intensive Care Med.*, **14**, 610–616

Riou, B., Barriot, P., Rimailho, A. and Baud, F. J. (1988b). Treatment of severe chloroquine poisoning, *N. Engl. J. Med*, **318**, 1–6

Robberecht, W., Bednarik, J., Bourgeois, P., van Hees, J. and Carton, H. (1989). Myasthenic syndrome caused by direct effect of chloroquine on neuromuscular junction. *Arch. Neurol.*, **46**, 464–468

Rossouw, J. E., Keeton, R. G. and Hewlett, R. H. (1976). Chronic proximal muscular weakness in alcoholics. *S. Afr. Med. J.*, **50**, 2095

Rubin, E. (1979a). Alcoholic myopathy in heart and skeletal. *N. Engl. J. Med.*, **301**, 28–33

Rubin, E. (1979). Metabolic and pathological changes in muscle during acute and chronic administration of ethanol. In Majchrowicz, E. and Noble, E. P. (Eds). *Biochemistry and Pharmacology of Ethanol*. Vol. 1. Plenum Press, New York, pp. 623–639

Rubin, E. and Rottenberg, H. (1982). Ethanol induced injury and adaptation in biological membranes. *Fed. Proc.*, **41**, 2465–2471

Rubin, E., Katz, A. M., Lieber, C. S., Stein, E. P. and Puszkin, S. (1976). Muscle damage produced by chronic alcohol consumption. *Am. J. Pathol.*, **83**, 499–515

Ruff, R. L. and Weissman, J. (1988). Endocrine myopathies. *Neurol. Clin.*, **6**, 575–592

Sadeh, M. (1988). Effects of aging on skeletal muscle regeneration. *J. Neurol. Sci.*, **87**, 67–74

Sadeh, M., Czyzewski, K. and Stern, L. Z. (1985). Chronic myopathy induced by repeated bupivacaine injections. *J. Neurol. Sci.*, **67**, 229–238

Salpeter, M. M., Kasprzak, H., Feng, H. and Fertuck, H. (1979). Endplates after esterase inactivation *in vivo*: correlation between esterase concentration, functional response and fine-structure. *J. Neurocytol.*, **8**, 95–115

Scherrmann, J. M., Utrizberea, M., Pierson, P. and Terrien, N. (1989). The effect of colchicine-specific active immunization on colchicine toxicity and disposition in the rabbit. *Toxicology*, **56**, 213–222

Schultz, E. (1984). A quantitative study of satellite cells in regenerated soleus and extensor digitorum longus muscles. *Anat. Rec.*, **208**, 501–506

Senanayake, N. and Karalliedde, L. (1987). Neurotoxic effects of organophosphorus insecticides. An intermediate syndrome. *N. Engl. J. Med.*, **361**, 761–763

Sghirlanzoni, A., Mantegazza, R., Mora, M., Pareyson, D. and Cornelio, F. (1988). Chloroquine myopathy and myasthenia-like syndrome. *Muscle Nerve*, **11**, 114–119

Shoji, S. and Pennington, R. J. T. (1977). Binding of dexamethasone and cortisol to cytosol receptors in rat extensor digitorum longus and soleus muscles. *Exp. Neurol.*, **57**, 342

Slavin, G., Martin, F., Ward, P., Levi, J. and Peters, T. J. (1983). Chronic alcohol excess is associated with selective but reversible injury to 2B muscle fibres. *J. Clin. Pathol.*, **36**, 772–777

Slotwiner, P., Song, S. K. and Anderson, P. J. (1966). Spheromembranous degeneration of muscle induced by vincristine. *Arch. Neurol.*, **15**, 172

Song, S. K. and Rubin, E. (1972). Ethanol produces muscle damage in human volunteers. *Science*, **175**, 327

Steer, J. H. and Mastaglia, F. L. (1986). Protein degradation in bupivacaine-treated muscles: the role of extracellular calcium. *J. Neurol. Sci.*, **75**, 343–351

Steer, J. H., Mastaglia, F. L., Papadimitriou, J. M. and van Bruggen, I. (1986). Bupivacaine-induced muscle injury. Role of extracellular calcium. *J. Neurol. Sci.*, **73**, 205–217

Sunnasy, D., Cairns, S. R., Slavin, G. and Peters, T. J. (1983). Chronic alcoholic skeletal muscle myopathy: a clinical, histological and biochemical assessment of muscle lipid. *J. Clin. Pathol.*, **36**, 778–784

Tegner, R., Tome, F. M., Godeau, P., Lhermitte, F. and Fardeau, M. (1988). Morphologic study of peripheral nerve changes induced by chloroquine treatment. *Acta Neuropathol.*, **75**, 253–260

Trounce, I., Byrne, E., Dennett, X., Santamaria, J., Doery, J. and Peppard, R. (1987). Chronic alcoholic proximal wasting: physiological, morphological, and biochemical studies in skeletal muscle. *Aust. NZ J. Med.*, **17**, 413–419

Urbano-Marquez, A., Estruch, R., Navarro-Lopez, F., Grau, J. M., Mont, L. and Rubin, E. (1989). The effects of alcoholism on skeletal and cardiac muscle. *N. Engl. J. Med.*, **320**, 409–415

Wallace, S. L. and Singer, J. Z. (1988). Review: systematic toxicity associated with the intravenous administration of colchicine—guidelines for use. *J. Rheumatol.*, **15**, 495–499

Wecker, L. and Dettbarn, W-D. (1976). Paraoxon induced myopathy: muscle specificity and acetylcholine involvement. *Exp. Neurol.*, **51**, 281–291

Wecker, L., Kiauta, T. and Dettbarn, W-D. (1978). Relationship between acetylcholinesterase inhibition and the development of a myopathy. *J. Pharmacol. Exp. Ther.*, **206**, 97–104

Wecker, L., Mrak, R. E. and Dettbarn, W-D. (1986). Evidence of necrosis in human intercostal muscle following inhalation of an organophosphate insecticide. *Fund. Appl. Toxicol.*, **6**, 172–174

Weishaar, R., Bertuglia, S., Ashikawa, K., Sarma, J. S. M. and Bing, S. J. (1978). Comparative effects of chronic ethanol and acetaldehyde exposure on myocardial function in rats. *J. Clin. Pharm.*, **18**, 377–386

Whisnant, J. P., Espinosa, R. E., Kierland, R. R. and Lambert, E. H. (1963). Chloroquine neuromyopathy. *Mayo Clin. Proc.*, **38**, 501

Yagiela, J. A., Benoit, P. W. and Fort, N. F. (1982). Mechanism of epinephrine enhancement of lidocaine-induced skeletal muscle necrosis. *J. Dent. Res.*, **61**, 686–690

Zeman, R. J., Kameyama, T., Matsumoto, K., Bernstein, P. and Etlinger, J. D. (1985). Regulation of protein degradation in muscle by calcium – evidence for enhanced nonlysosomal proteolysis associated with elevated cytosolic calcium. *J. Biol. Chem.*, **260**, 13619–13624

Zemer, D., Pras, M., Sohar, E., Modan, M., Cabili, S. and Gafni, J. (1986). Colchicine in the prevention and treatment of the amyloidosis of familial Mediterranean fever. *N. Engl. J. Med.*, **314**, 1001–1005

FURTHER READING

Ballantyne, B. (1988). Xenobiotic-induced rhabdomyolysis. In Ballantyne, B. (Ed.), *Perspectives in Basic and Applied Toxicology*, Wright, London, pp. 70–153

Kunel, R. W. and George, E. B. (1993). Toxic neuropathies and myopathies. *Current Opinions in Neurology*, **6**, 695–704

Mastaglia, F. L. and Walton, Lord (1992). *Skeletal Muscle Pathology*. Churchill Livingstone, Edinburgh

29 The Toxicology of Bone and Cartilage

A. B. G. Lansdown

INTRODUCTION

Bone and cartilage are highly specialized tissues providing an essential framework and functional rigidity to the vertebrate body. They are structurally complex, comprising discrete cell types embedded in prominent matrices. Cartilage predominates in the early embryonic skeleton but this is progressively replaced by bone with advancing age. Skeletal tissues undergo a programmed sequence of cell division, differentiation, macromolecular synthesis, resorption and remodelling under the control of intrinsic factors, nutrient availability and conditions in the microenvironment. This implies that development at any one time is a manifestation of the interaction between the genotype of the individual and extraneous factors, which may include conditions of toxic importance.

Although cartilage and bone subserve major supportive roles in the body, they are metabolically active tissues and become increasingly subject to resorption and remodelling as the occasion demands. This physiological role involves maintenance of circulating levels of zinc, calcium and manganese in response to hormonal and nutritional changes. Although dentine, as found in teeth, is similar to bone, it is more stable and less susceptible to metabolic and nutritional alterations.

The complex developmental patterns in cartilage and bone, their role in maintaining mineral homoeostasis and their sensitivity to hormonal and age-related changes suggest that both tissues will be particularly vulnerable to toxic changes resulting from foreign substances assimilated into the body. Numerous congenital abnormalities involving cartilage and bone are described in the medical and veterinary literature, and pathological conditions, including chondrodystrophy, osteoporosis, osteoarthroses and Paget's disease, are well documented, but in many cases their causation is unclear.

Although toxicology as we know it today represents an accumulation of knowledge compiled over nearly 50 years, surprisingly little refers to the specific action of environmental or xenobiotic materials on cartilage, bone or teeth. That which is available is widely scattered. This chapter aims to collate as far as possible information as to how representative substances influence bone structure or function, with reference to their action on biochemical pathways or hormonally mediated changes.

EMBRYOLOGY, STRUCTURE AND FUNCTION

Embryology

Cartilage and bone are mesodermal structures with a common origin in the early embryo (Hall, 1970). Control of the process whereby a cell enters a chondrogenic or osteogenic pathway is imperfectly understood, although factors in the microenvironment, including oxygen level, cell-to-cell influences and, maybe, chemical modulators, are possibly contributory (Hall, 1968; Owen, 1970). While the major macromolecules of the intercellular matrices are probably similar, the relative amounts present in the two tissues differ appreciably, which implies the existence of precise control mechanisms (Jackson, 1970). It is conceivable that a form of 'negative feedback' mechanism operates (Scarano and Augusti-Tocco, 1967).

Bone exists in two main forms in the vertebrate skeleton: endochondrial bone, which comprises all parts of the post-cranial skeleton, and intramembranal bone, which is found in certain elements of the skull. Endochrondrial bone is preformed in cartilage which becomes ossified as the individual ages. Membrane bones, in contrast, develop directly from condensations of osteoblasts in the cranial mesenchyme. Subsequently they anastomose to form the vault of the adult skull.

In characteristic endochondrial bones, development proceeds from a condensation of prechondroblasts in the mid-shaft blastema (diaphysis of long bones). An extracellular matrix composed largely of mucopolysaccharide (chondroitin sulphate) is secreted, giving the tissue a metachromatic property. Subsequent development sees an elongation of the cartilage rudiment proximally and distally, and the formation of a perichondral sheath in the mid-shaft region. The perichondrium becomes the site of osteoblastic activity and mineralization which extends to replace the greater part of the cartilagenous model. Cartilage persists at the terminal aspects of the elements to form the epiphyses. In due course, ossification appears in these regions also. Capillary channels from the surrounding connective tissue 'invade' the epiphyseal cartilages, allowing the migration of osteoblasts and osteocytes. Through later embryogenesis and adolescent stages, a band of proliferating cartilage remains, separating diaphyseal and epiphyseal ossifications, this region being the metaphyseal growth plate which is responsible for extension of the element to its genetically predetermined adult proportions. Many examples are available to show that toxic conditions impairing body growth inhibit cell proliferation in this region.

Experiments conducted with cultured bone and limb explants have demonstrated that full development of joints and joint cavities is dependent upon appropriate movement and muscle action. In the absence of these influences, adjacent bones tend to fuse and articular surfaces form imperfectly (Hamburger and Waugh, 1940). In experimental models where spinal damage is induced surgically, or where neuromuscular paralysis is produced by toxins, joint deformities develop (Drachmann and Sokoloff, 1966).

Collagen

Collagen is an essential component of connective tissues, including cartilage and bone. It consists of polypeptide chains twisted in a coiled-coil formation (Herring, 1968; Speakman, 1971). These fibres are extracellular and are held in a triple helix formation by means of covalent bonds and various cross-linkages involving calcium, copper, protein and mucopolysaccharides (Matthews, 1965; Katsura and Davidson, 1966).

In bone and cartilage, collagen forms a structural matrix binding calcium, phosphate and other mineral ions (Weinstock *et al.*, 1967).

Occasionally, mineral ions which have no known functional role are taken up, competing with essential ions such as calcium for binding sites (Herring, 1968). Hydroxyproline is a major component of collagen and is used as a marker for collagen synthesis under normal and pathological conditions (Firschein, 1967, 1969; Oberg *et al.*, 1969). Also, as a close relationship exists in bone development between collagen synthesis and mineralization, radiolabelled proline uptake is available as a monitor for toxic changes leading to impaired mineralization. It can be used to study the repair of bone injury, as in fractures and metabolic diseases (Shtacher and Firschein, 1967).

Dentine

Dentine, such as occurs in tooth enamel, consists of a dense organic matrix composed of collagen, mucopolysaccharide, lipid and protein. Human dentine consists of 72 per cent inorganic matter (Clarke *et al.*, 1965). Dentine is robust and is more resistant to toxic change than are other skeletal tissues. Even so, it is known to bind foreign metal ions such as strontium (Curzon and Spector, 1980).

Physiological Aspects of Cartilage and Bone

Bone is considerably denser and more vascular than cartilage, and exhibits a rich mineral deposit consisting mainly of calcium and phosphorus. The calcium exists partly as a labile form which can be released in response to physiological or hormonal change, and partly as a structural component of the bone (Talmage, 1969). The disposition or mobilization of labile calcium is probaby modulated by a delicately balanced feedback mechanism involving parathyroid hormone, thyrocalcitonin and vitamin D, which influence the synthetic or catabolic activity of osteocytes and osteoclasts (Reynolds *et al.*, 1974). Newly formed bone is more susceptible to resorption than established bone and responds more readily to depression in calcitonin or increases in parathyroid hormone release. Depression in calcitonin leads to increased parathyroid hormone secretion triggering a release of labile calcium. Presumably hypercalcaemia, through nutritional causes, toxic changes or age-related effects, evokes calcitonin release from the thyroid, leading to enhanced ossification patterns. The control mechanisms are poorly understood.

In late adolescence or adulthood, minimal cartilage remains in the skeleton other than in the rib cage and in the articular regions. Articular cartilages are a robust form of hyaline cartilage and contain abundant collagen. They are bathed in synovial fluid which reduces friction. Under normal circumstances articular cartilages are moulded to the bone extremities and show a low tendency to mineralize, except in osteoarthritic conditions, which may or may not be mediated by toxic factors in the environment or by drugs (Mansfield, 1983). Normal articular cartilages exhibit a low mitotic rate at maturity, such that with advancing age and cell loss there is a progressive thinning of the articular surface and discomfort. Reduced synovial fluid production through nutritional or toxic alteration is a further potential cause of pathological changes leading to arthroses, as seen commonly in old age (Bullough and Goodfellow, 1968; Freeman *et al.*, 1975) Osteoarthrosis is a complex condition and, according to some, one that almost certainly involves an immunological component (Glynn, 1978).

TOXIC DAMAGE IN CARTILAGE AND BONE

A toxic substance may act to induce structural or functional damage at any age from early embryogenesis through to advanced geriatric stages. The effect will be a manifestation of the nature of the insult, its specificity of action, and the developmental and functional state of the tissue at the time. A wide range of nutritional constituents, environmental chemicals and therapeutic agents are capable of adversely influencing cartilage or bone at some stage, leading to transitory or irreversible changes. Of these, a significant proportion impair the availability or metabolism of essential nutrients such as calcium, phosphate or zinc. Others influence enzyme systems or biosynthetic pathways. A third category illustrated induces hormonal changes.

Early Developmental Changes

Toxic compounds inducing skeletal abnormalities in early embryogenesis may act at any of the following stages: induction; chondrogenesis; osteogenesis; growth. Abnormality at one stage may evoke disturbances at subsequent stages. Whereas induction of mesenchymal cells to undergo chondrogenesis or osteogenesis is essentially a feature of the early embryo, osteogenesis and growth associated with modelling and remodelling occur through most of an individual's lifetime.

In the induction process it is held that oxygen tension is important (Hall, 1968). Hypoxia is a known cause of circulatory disturbances leading to oedema with alterations in anion–cation balance, and changes in sugar, lactic acid and free amino acid concentration (Grabowski, 1966). In hypoxia calcium is taken up prematurely by chondroblasts, which leads to abnormalities in perichondral differentiation and mineralization. Oxygen levels in the embryo may be influenced by a number of teratogens, including trypan blue, dinitrophenol, lactic acid and calcium chloride. These cause metabolic imbalances and skeletal deformity (Grabowski, 1964; Kaplan and Johnson, 1968). Vascular changes, rarefaction of cell populations, blisters and oedema resulting from hypervitaminosis A, bis azo-dyes and deficiencies in linoleic or pantothenic acids are other recorded causes of local oxygen deficiency leading to deformities in early bone formation (Marin-Padilla, 1966; Turbow, 1966; Morriss and Steele, 1974; Sandor and Amels, 1975).

More specific defects were observed in embryos exposed to nitrogen mustard (Sweeney and Watterson, 1969; Salzgeber, 1979). This alkylating agent exhibits a predilection for mesenchymal tissue causing reduced mitotic activity and chromosomal abnormality. Mitotic inhibition and necrosis leading to abnormal cartilage formation underlie rib and limb-bud deformities.

Vitamin A exerts a specific influence on mesenchymal differentiation and has been variously implicated in defects of cellular metabolism, migration and mitotic activity (Marin-Padilla, 1966; Kochhar, 1968; Morriss and Steele, 1974). In various embryonic systems hypervitaminosis A has induced chondrodystrophy in the cephalic and axial mesoderm leading to failure in the closure of the vertebral column, with resulting exencephaly, craniorachischisis and spina bifida. Cellular shrinkage, oedema and prominent intercellular spaces were recorded. As an alternative mechanism, vitamin A is implicated in mucopolysaccharide synthesis. At different stages hyper- and hypovitaminosis lead to deformities associated with abnormal cartilage (Wolbach, 1947; Fell and Mellanby, 1952).

It is suggested that vitamin A may be involved in the sulphation of polysaccharides, or in the metabolic turnover of mucopolysaccharides (Wolf and Varandani, 1960; Pasternak and Thomas, 1968). Experimental studies have indicated that the influence of vitamin A on bone development relates closely to its concentration, the genotype of the target tissue and its developmental stage (Kochhar, 1967; Nolen, 1969; Robens, 1970; Biddle and Fraser, 1976).

Among the important skeletal deformities associated with hypervitaminosis A is that of cleft palate (Kochhar and Johnson, 1965; Kochhar, 1968). The mechanism for cleft palate as seen in numerous teratological studies is controversial, but may involve a failure in mucopolysaccharide synthesis or in the horizontalization of the palatine shelves (Asling *et al.*, 1960; Loevy, 1962; Ross and Walker, 1967). Cleft palate has regularly been reported in rodent embryos emposed to X-irradiation, cortisone, prednisolone, dexamethasone and triamcinolone. While it is tempting to speculate that the mechanism for cleft palate formation by the various teratogens is similar, this may not be so (Kochhar *et al.*, 1968; Andrew and Zimmerman, 1971).

Salicylates have long been known as a cause of chondrodystrophy and skeletal abnormality in teratological studies. They are known to inhibit a number of enzyme systems, notably those involved in the sulphation of polysaccharides in cartilage development (Whitehouse and Bostrom, 1961; Larsson and Bostrom, 1965; Grisolia *et al.*, 1968; McArthur and Smith, 1969). Although skeletal deformities are known to occur in human babies through prenatal aspirin, the concentrations have been at suicidal levels (Jackson, 1948; *British Medical Journal*, 1963). Skeletal deformities resulting from salicylate exposure relate closely to the concentration, stage in pregnancy of exposure and species genotype (Warkany and Takacs, 1959; Larsson *et al.*, 1963; Eriksson, 1971). Impaired chondrogenesis in the vertebrae and long bones is a cause of defective ossification and growth (Lansdown, 1970). In the older embryo/foetus salicylates inhibit ossification and metastatic mineralization in soft tissues, possibly by inhibiting oxidative phosphorylation (Whitehouse, 1963; Somogyi *et al.*, 1969). This means that individuals exposed to high levels of salicylate become subject to hypocalcinosis (Cotty and Harris, 1968). In another study Berry and Nickols (1979) demonstrated that tooth development was impaired in mice exposed to salicylate prenatally, which suggests a toxic effect on odontoblast activity.

Toxic Alterations in Late Embryogenesis and Post-natal Growth

Many toxic agents affecting cartilage or bone in these later developmental stages do so by their action on the availability of essential nutrients, or by inhibiting biosynthetic pathways. For convenience, these toxic substances may be grouped as follows: (1) agents that precipitate a general nutritional insufficiency; (2) toxicity leading to the deficiency or excess of specific nutrients; (3) situations resulting in an imbalance of nutrients; (4) the presence of substances of dubious nutritional value which impair essential metabolic pathways.

Table 1 illustrates the major nutrients deemed necessary for normal development in skeletal tissues. In several cases the importance of a substance will vary according to the development stage. Others, such as vitamin A, are essential for normal growth but are detrimental if present in insufficient amounts or in excess.

Proteins and Amino Acids

Protein deficiency is an acknowledged cause of growth retardation in humans and in animal models. Many examples exist to show that protein and/or calorie insufficiency leads to reduced ossification and collagen synthesis (Frandson *et al.*, 1954; Reddy *et al.*, 1972; Krishnamachari and Iyengar, 1975). In these situations the changes are usually irreversible and catch-up growth fails to occur even in the presence of growth hormone and protein-sufficient diets later (Toews and Lee, 1975). Frank abnormalities may not occur, but human babies subject to prenatal malnutrition fail to grow normally after refeeding (Dickerson and Hughes, 1972).

Table 1 Major nutrients necessary for normal development in skeletal tissue

Nutrient	Major function in bone	Deficiency	Excess
Vitamin C	Maintains intercellular matrix of cartilage, bone and teeth; essential in collagen synthesis	Degenerative changes, rickets	?
Vitamin A	Mucopolysaccharide synthesis	Cartilage defects	Excess growth
Vitamin D	Promotes growth and mineralization of bone; controls calcium uptake in the intestinal mucosa	Rickets, osteomalacia	?
Calcium	Bone and tooth formation	Stunted growth, osteoporosis, rickets	?
Phosphorus	Bone and tooth formation	Calcium loss, weakness in bone	Skeletal erosion
Sulphur	Mucopolysaccharide synthesis	Chondrodystrophy	Stunted growth
Magnesium	Enzyme activation	Growth failure	?
Iron	Enzyme activation	Reduced energy	?
Fluoride	Maintenance of bone structure	Bone and tooth decay	?
Zinc	Enzyme constituent	Reduced growth	?
Copper	Enzyme constituent	Skeletal changes	?
Manganese	Enzyme constituent	Skeletal changes	?

Many amino acids are important in skeletal growth but those containing sulphur are particularly relevant. It is evident that in certain cases a deficiency of only one amino acid may be as damaging as a more general form of protein deficiency (Zamenhof *et al.*, 1974; Hurley, 1977). The importance of individual amino acids in development is demonstrated by use of specific antagonists. Thus, ethionine is a well-known antagonist for methionine; affected foetuses develop a marked impairment in bone growth (Lee *et al.*, 1955).

Vitamins

Among the vitamins necessary for normal development in cartilage or bone, vitamins A and D are recognized, as are niacin, riboflavin and folic acid. The importance of the last three of these is well illustrated in teratological experiments using specific inhibitors such as 6-aminonicotinamide, galactoflavine and α-methyl pteroylglutamic acid, respectively. Embryos exposed to these substances at sensitive stages develop cleft palate, abnormal bone fusions, micrognathia, defective mineralizations and growth retardation (Chamberlain and Nelson, 1963; Hurley, 1977).

In addition to its action in the early embryo, hypervitaminosis A has been shown to act on later stages of development, causing a variety of skeletal defects, particularly involving the skull region (Cohlan, 1953; Masi *et al.*, 1966; Giroud, 1968). These may be attributable to impaired mitotic activity (Morriss, 1972). Vitamin A and related compounds (retinoids) are also known to cause degenerative changes in cartilage and bone, possibly due to their ability to promote a premature release of lysosomal hydrolases (Goodman *et al.*, 1974).

Recently there has been considerable interest in the action of retinoids in the remodelling of growing bone. Experiments in rodents have shown that they can activate the catabolism of bone, with the result that soft tissues become pathologically mineralized. Interestingly, there is a difference in response to the various analogues. Rat tissues exhibit a greater response than do mouse tissues to the active compounds. In bones taken from more mature young exposed to toxic retinoids, the main toxic changes include increased radiolucency, a marked narrowing of diaphyses and increased tendency to fracture (Turton *et al.*, 1985). Histologically these changes were characterized by a greatly increased periosteal osteoclast activity but with a greater tendency to mineralization in endosteal aspects. Resulting bones were denser and narrower than normal, with metaphyseal plate regions being prematurely ossified (Teelmann, 1989). Limited observations reported in non-rodent species show that the vitamin A analogues cause changes in the bone shaft regions and in other tissues, leading to such manifestations as exostoses, hyperostoses and spondylitis (Clarke, 1970; Cho *et al.*, 1975; Mahrle and Berger, 1982).

Vitamin D or ergocalciferol is best known for its capacity to prevent rickets in early childhood.

Deficiency is recognized by retarded growth, particularly in the long bones, skull and sternal cartilages (Sevastikoglou *et al.*, 1970). Hypovitaminosis is accompanied by hypophosphataemia and hypocalcaemia; long bones inadequately mineralize and diaphyses form imperfectly. In human babies, hypoplasia in tooth enamel is a further complication (Rosen *et al.*, 1974). Although vitamin D has an acknowledged role in mineralization and calcium metabolism, its action is imperfectly understood. It has an indirect action on the parathyroid gland and may be involved in alkaline phosphatase and citrate metabolism (Sevastikoglou *et al.*, 1970). Although an essential nutrient, vitamin D can be toxic in bone, favouring the removal of 'lime salts' (Carlsson, 1952). The interaction between vitamin D and parathyroid hormone is not understood but a synergistic action has been suggested (Goldhaber, 1963). It seems that, at optimal levels, vitamin D can regulate calcium and phosphate uptake, whereas a deficiency activates a demineralization process (Ornoy *et al.*, 1968, 1969). It is also reported that hypervitaminosis enhances magnesium uptake (Ornoy *et al.*, 1968).

Minerals

At least 21 mineral elements are essential in optimal mammalian development, and, of these, at least half are essential in structural development and function of bone or cartilage. Mineral requirements differ according to the age of an individual, its health and its hormonal status. As bone growth progresses, so requirements for calcium and phosphate increase. The availability of both minerals may be markedly influenced by dietary factors. Phytates, oxalates, fats and substances which create an alkaline medium in the intestine can impair calcium uptake, and in severe cases lead to a hypocalcaemia. Ions such as strontium, lead, aluminium, beryllium and iron may block calcium channels with the same effect. All these situations are capable of producing a rachitogenic effect in young bone, although the mechanism may be more complex than a competition for ion-binding sites in the intestinal mucosa. For example, in a 'strontium rickets' situation it is suggested that there may be a deactivation of vitamin D_3 or an inhibition of the mineralization process (Corradino *et al.*, 1971). Strontium ingestion was shown to cause a pronounced reduction

in levels of calcium-binding protein in intestine and absorption of radiolabelled calcium.

Lead is metabolized by bone in a similar way to calcium: it is readily taken up by osteocytes, and is concentrated in bone, forming a reservoir from which to induce toxic effects on tissues such as the brain and kidneys (Roser, 1983). Evidence presented by Pounds and Rosen (1986) suggests that lead is bound in bone in several forms, since only part is available to EDTA chelation. Whereas lead is known to inhibit calcium uptake, Moore (1979) noted that other minerals such as zinc, copper and magnesium blocked lead uptake.

Among cations, fluorides, phosphates and phosphonates are known to impair calcium uptake in growing bone (Clarke and Bélanger, 1967). The importance of a correct calcium:phosphate ratio in growing bone is well recognized. High phosphate leads to extraskeletal calcium binding with osteoporosis developing, as calcium is mobilized to maintain homoeostasis (Spencer *et al.*, 1975). Polyphosphonates and diphosphates inhibit the formation of calcium hydroxyapatite through their adsorption to bone matrix (Francis, 1969). In contrast, fluoride tends to alter the structural and physical properties of bone by changing the pattern of calcium binding. Apatite crystals are smaller and less numerous than usual, and although the actual lengths of bones were not significantly altered, fluoride has been shown to increase their flexibility (Shambaugh and Petrovic, 1968). Some evidence was presented here that fluoride actually increased the tensile strength of some bones, although the mechanism is not known.

Calcium availability for mineralization is influenced by other substances that selectively bind to it. Dyes such as alizarin, calcein blue, DCAF and tetracycline are readily absorbed in bone and may be used as markers of growth in experimental studies (Rahn and Perrin, 1970). These are of small toxicological significance. However, tetracycline may inhibit ossification in growing bone if present at sufficiently high levels (Rolle, 1967). Other evidence suggests that tetracycline enhances the intracellular uptake of calcium by osteoblasts and osteocytes, leading to a premature mineralization. In cultured bone explants tetracycline was shown in inhibit collagen synthesis by blocking the uptake of proline and its incorporation into protocollagen, an effect which is possibly related to an interaction between tetracycline and the ferrous ion required in the oxidation process (Halmé *et al.*, 1969).

Zinc, copper, magnesium and manganese are important at trace levels in bone and cartilage development. In most cases skeletal deformities are recorded where these minerals are deficient in the diet, rather than present at excessive levels. For zinc and magnesium, at least, intestinal uptake seems to be controlled by a negative feedback mechanism. Zinc is important in mineralizing and growing bone, as it forms an essential component of alkaline phosphatase; thus, circulating deficiency due to the presence of cycloheximide or actinomycin D tends to diminish bone growth (Yamaguchi and Yamaguchi, 1986; Yamaguchi and Takahashi, 1983). As in the case of calcium, intestinal uptake of zinc is inhibited by the presence of ion-binding agents such as phytate, histidine, EDTA and some other amino acids, as well as competing metal ions, including lead, cobalt, nickel, chromium, mercury and cadmium (Yamaguchi and Yamaguchi, 1986). Alcohol is a further recorded antagonist to zinc uptake and metabolism (Eckhardt *et al.*, 1981).

Manganese seems to be an enigma in bone development. It is important in fetal chondrogenesis and in otolith mineralization in the inner ear but its action is not understood (Tsai and Everson, 1967; Gamble *et al.*, 1971). Manganese deficiency is a cause of perosis and thickened diaphyses, possibly as a consequence of its interaction with alkaline phosphatase (Wolbach and Hegsted, 1953; Leach *et al.*, 1969). It is unclear whether manganese and zinc interact.

Copper is potentially important as an enzyme constituent in collagen cross-linking and in the mineralization process. Copper deficiency at the former stage results in an increased level of soluble collagen, with a reduced tendency to bind mineral ions. Lathyrogenic compounds obtained from certain plants seem to interact with copper cross-linking in collagenesis, which results in abnormal bone formation in avian and mammalian embryos (Herring, 1968).

Although strontium may be important in early mineralization of bone, at high concentrations it competes with calcium for binding sites. Limited information is available to demonstrate that strontium displaces calcium in mineralizing tissues to produce pathological changes (Lansdown *et al.*, 1972; Curzon and Spector, 1980), although the toxicological problems associated with strontium in its radioactive form, ^{90}Sr, have been well publicized. In this last situation it is more likely that the toxic changes in bone and other tissues are attributable to the high-energy beta-emission rather than to the strontium ion. Similar conclusions are no doubt true for other radioactive bone-seeking elements such as plutonium, radium and phosphorus. Of interest, too, are studies of the binding of calcium, yttrium and thorium ions by bone sialoprotein. This may have implications in both calcification and the unusual distribution of certain radioactive cations in bone (Williams and Peacocke, 1965).

DISCUSSION

In routine toxicity studies cartilage and bone tend to be less frequently damaged than the liver, kidney or endocrine organs. However, teratological abnormalities involving bone are a common observation, particularly where test compounds adversely influence mitosis, synthetic pathways or differentiation patterns.

Toxic agents influencing these skeletal tissues either may act through a direct influence on the cell or its local environment, or may influence more general aspects involving nutritional pathways, hormonal profiles or general metabolic activities, involving bone or cartilage as part of a more complex change, affecting several other organ systems. Obviously, the skeletal tissues, like those of other systems, are highly vulnerable to toxic or environmental change during their developmental phases. Resulting damage is likely to persist throughout an individual's life, occasionally leading to disability.

Many of the toxic situations relevant to cartilage, bone or tooth involve essential nutrients such as calcium and phosphate. The effects range from inhibition in intestinal uptake and blockage by ionic competition in intra- or extracellular binding sites, to inhibition or inactivation of enzyme pathways. Failure in mucopolysaccharide synthesis and bone growth or abnormalities are commonly seen in tissues exposed to toxic agents in developmental phases, whereas osteoporosis, alterations in remodelling and other structural or physiological change frequently result from toxic change during adulthood.

Evidence is presented in this chapter to show that bone is tolerant to a number of changes resulting from toxic insult. Substances such as strontium, tetracycline, some xenobiotic metal elements, selenium and fluorescent dyes which show an affinity for calcium become readily bound in mineralizing tissues, but, except in extreme circumstances (concentration of toxin and period of exposure, etc.), the tissues rarely show evidence of histological change. Subtle changes seen by histochemistry or electron microscopy are rarely reflected as physiological or structural abnormality. However, this storage phenomenon may have toxic implication for other tissues, as, for example, where a reservoir of toxic material such as lead builds up. Gradual release of bound lead can result in brain damage.

Despite more than 50 years' research, much still remains to be learned concerning inherent control mechanisms in bone growth and physiological change. It has been a popular tissue for anatomists and pathologists to study, presumably because of its comparative durability and resistance to biodegradation. It is fascinating that after more than 2000 years scientists are speculating as to the significance of toxic changes in bone in the remains of people from ancient dynasties in Egypt, China and elsewhere. The ancient bones of the inhabitants of Qumran still bear the traces of dye from their plant food, bound to calcium deposits (Stecholl *et al.*, 1971).

REFERENCES

Andrew, F. D. and Zimmerman, E. F. (1971). Glucocorticoid induction of cleft palate in mice: no correlation with inhibition of mucopolysaccharide synthesis. *Teratology*, **4**, 31–38

Asling, C. W., Nelson, M. M., Dougherty, H. L., Wright, H. V. and Evans, H. M. (1960). The development of cleft palate resulting from maternal pteroylglutamic (folic) acid deficiency during the latter half of gestation in rats. *Surg. Gynec. Obstet.*, **111**, 19–28

Berry, C. L. and Nickols, C. D. (1979). The effects of aspirin on the development of the mouse third molar. A potential screening system for weak teratogens. *Arch. Toxicol.*, **42**, 185–190

Biddle, F. G. and Fraser, F. C. (1976). Genetics of cortisone-induced cleft palate in the mouse—embryonic and maternal effects. *Genetics*, **84**, 743–754

British Medical Journal (1963). Salicylates and congenital malformations. *Br. Med. J.*, **1**, 352

Bullough, P. and Goodfellow, J. (1968). The significance of the fine structure of articular cartilage. *J. Bone Jnt Surg.*, **50**, 852–857

Carlsson, A. (1952). On mechanism of skeletal turnover of lime salts. *Acta Physiol. Scand.*, **26**, 200–211

Chamberlain, J. G. and Nelson, M. M. (1963). Congenital abnormalities in the rat resulting from single injections of 6-aminonicotinamide during pregnancy. *J. Exptl Zool.*, **153**, 285

Cho, D. Y., Frey, R. A., Guffy, M. M. and Leipold, H. W. (1975). Hypervitaminosis A in the dog. *Am. J. Vet. Res.*, **36**, 1597–1603

Clarke, I. and Belanger, L. (1967). The effects of alterations in dietary magnesium on calcium, phosphate and skeletal metabolism. *Calc. Tiss. Res.*, **1**, 204–218

Clarke, L. (1970). The effect of excess vitamin A on long bone growth in kittens. *J. Comp. Pathol.*, **80**, 625–638

Clarke, R. D., Smith, J. G. and Davidson, E. A. (1965). Hexosamine and acid glycosaminoglycans in human teeth. *Biochim. Biophys. Acta*, **101**, 267–272

Cohlan, S. Q. (1953). Excessive intake of vitamin A as a cause of congenital anomalies in the rat. *Science*, **117**, 535–536

Corradino, R. A., Ebel, J. G., Craig, P. H., Taylor, A. N. and Wasserman, R. H. (1971). Calcium absorption and vitamin D_3-dependent calcium-binding protein. Inhibition by dietary strontium. *Calc. Tiss. Res.*, **7**, 81–92

Cotty, V. F. and Harris, A. F. (1968). The effect of acetylsalicylic acid on mineralization. *Arch. Int. Pharmacodyn.*, **174**, 28–31

Curzon, M. E. J. and Spector, P. C. (1980). Strontium uptake by rat enamel from various strontium salts. *J. Dent. Res.*, **59**, 1988

Dickerson, J. W. T. and Hughes, P. C. R. (1972). Growth of the rat skeleton after severe nutritional intrauterine and post-natal retardation. *Resuscitation*, **1**, 163–170

Drachmann, D. B. and Sokoloff, L. (1966). The role of movement in embryonic joint development. *Devel. Biol.*, **14**, 401–420

Eckhardt, M. J., Harford, T. C., Kaelber, C. T., Parker, E. S., Rosenthal, L. S., Ryback, R. S., Salmoiraghi, G. C., Vanderveen, E. and Warren, K. R. (1981). Health hazards associated with alcohol consumption. *J. Am. Med. Assoc.*, **246**, 648–666

Eriksson, M. (1971). Salicylate-induced foetal damage late in pregnancy. *Acta Pediat. Scand. Suppl.*, **211**, 1–24

Fell, H. B. and Mellanby, E. (1952). Metaplasia produced in cultures of chick ectoderm by high vitamin A. *J. Physiol.*, **119**, 470–488

Firschein, H. E. (1967). Collagen turnover in calcified tissues. *Arch. Biochem. Biophys.*, **119**, 119–123

Firschein, H. E. (1969). Collagen and mineral dynamics in bone. *Clin. Orthop. Rel. Res.*, **66**, 212–225

Francis, M. D. (1969). The inhibition of calcium hydroxyapatite crystal growth by polyphosphonates and polyphosphates. *Calc. Tiss. Res.*, **3**, 151–162

Frandson, A. M., Nelson, M. M., Sulon, E., Becks, H. and Evans, H. M. (1954). The effects of various levels of dietary protein on skeletal growth and endochondrial ossification in young rats. *Anat. Rec.*, **119**, 247–265

Freeman, P. A., Lee, P. and Bryson, T. W. (1975). Total hip joint replacement in osteoarthritis and poly arthritis. A statistical study of the results. *Clin. Orthop.*, **95**, 224–230

Gamble, C. T., Hansard, S. L. and Moss, B. R. (1971). Manganese utilization and placental transfer in the gravid gilt. *J. Anim. Sci.*, **32**, 84–87

Giroud, A. (1968). Nutrition of the embryo. *Fed. Proc.*, **27**, 163–184

Glynn, L. E. (1978). The immunological pathogenesis of rheumatoid arthritis. *Med. J. Aust.*, **1/2**, 77–78

Goldhaber, P. (1963). Some chemical factors influencing bone resorption in tissue culture. In Sognnaes, R. F. (Ed.), *Mechanism of Hard Tissue Destruction*. American Association for the Advancement of Science, Washington, D.C., p. 609

Goodman, D. S., Smith, J. E., Hembry, R. M. and Dingle, J. T. (1974). Comparison of the effects of vitamin A and its analogues upon rabbit ear cartilage in organ culture and upon growth of the vitamin A-deficient rat. *J. Lipid Res.*, **15**, 405–414

Grabowski, C. T. (1964). The etiology of hypoxia-induced malformations in the chick embryo. *J. Exptl Zool.*, **157**, 307–326

Grabowski, C. T. (1966). Physiological changes in the bloodstream of chick embryos emposed to teratogenic doses of hypoxia. *Devel. Biol.*, **13**, 199–213

Grisolia, S., Santos, I. and Mendelson, J. (1968). Inactivation of enzymes by aspirin and salicylates. *Nature*, **219**, 1252

Hall, B. K. (1968). *In vitro* studies on the mechanical evocation of adventitious cartilage in the chick. *J. Exptl Zool.*, **168**, 283–306

Hall, B. K. (1970). The origin of cartilage and bone from common stem cells. *Calc. Tiss. Res.*, **4** (Suppl.), 147

Halmé, J. Kivirikko, K. I., Kaittla, I. and Saxèn, L. (1969). Effect of tetracycline on collagen biosynthesis in cultured embryonic bones. *Biochem. Pharmacol.*, **18**, 827–836

Hamburger, V. and Waugh, M. (1940). The primary development of the skeleton in nerveless and poorly innervated limb transplants of chick embryos. *Physiol. Zool.*, **13**, 367–380

Herring, G. M. (1968). The chemical structure of tendon, cartilage, dentine and bone matrix. *Clin. Orthop.*, **60**, 261–299

Hurley, L. S. (1977). Nutritional deficiencies and excesses. In Wilson, J. G. and Fraser, F. C. (Eds), *Handbook of Teratology*, Vol. 1. Plenum Press, New York, pp. 261–308

Jackson, A. V. (1948). Toxic effects of salicylate on the foetus and mother. *J. Pathol. Bacteriol.*, **60**, 587–593

Jackson, S. F. (1970). Environmental control of macromolecular synthesis in cartilage and bone: morpho-

genetic response to hyaluronidase. *Proc. Roy. Soc. Lond. B*, **175**, 405–453

Kaplan, S. and Johnson, E. M. (1968). Oxygen consumption in normal and trypan blue treated embryos. *Teratology*, **1**, 369–374

Katsura, N. and Davidson, E. A. (1966). Studies on porcine costal cartilage protein-polysaccharide complex. I. Enzymic degradation *Biochim. Biophys. Acta*, **121**, 120–127

Kochhar, D. M. (1967). Teratogenic activity of retinoic acid. *Acta Pathol. Microbiol. Scand.*, **70**, 398–404

Kochhar, D. M. (1968). Studies of vitamin A-induced teratogenesis: effects on embryonic mesenchyme and epithelium and on incorporation of ^{3}H-thymidine. *Teratology*, **1**, 299–310

Kochhar, D. M. and Johnson, E. M. (1965). Morphological and autoradiographic studies of cleft palate induced in rat embryos by maternal hypervitaminosis A. *J. Embryol. Exptl Morphol.*, **14**, 223–238

Kochhar, D. M., Larsson, K. S. and Bostrom, H. (1968). Embryonic uptake of S^{35} sulphate: change in level following treatment with some teratogenic agents. *Biol. Neonate*, **12**, 41–53

Krishnamachari, K. A. V. R. and Iyengar, L. (1975). The effect of maternal malnutrition on the bone density of the neonate. *Am J. Clin. Nutrit.*, **28**, 482–486

Lansdown, A. B. G. (1970). Histological changes in the skeletal elements of developing rabbit foetuses following treatment with sodium salicylate. *Fd Cosmet. Toxicol.*, **8**, 647–653

Lansdown, A. B. G., Grasso, P. and Longland, R. C. (1972). Reduced foetal calcium without skeletal malformations in rats following high maternal doses of a strontium salt. *Experientia*, **28**, 558–559

Larsson, K. S. and Bostrom, H. (1965). Teratogenic action of salicylates related to the inhibition of mucopolysaccharide synthesis. *Acta Paediat. Scand.*, **54**, 43–48

Larsson, K. S., Ericsson, B. and Bostrom, H. (1963). Salicylate-induced skeletal and vessel malformations in mouse embryos. *Acta Morphol. Neerl.-Scand.*, **6**, 35–44

Leach, R. M., Muenster, A. M. and Wien, E. M. (1969). Studies on the role of manganese in bone formation. *Arch. Biochem. Biophys.*, **133**, 22–28

Lee, C. M., Wiseman, B. A., Kaplan, S. A. and Warkany, J. (1955). Effects of ethionine injections on pregnant rats and their offspring. *Arch. Pathol.*, **59**, 232–237

Loevy, H. (1962). Developmental changes in the palate of normal and cortisone-treated Strong-A mice. *Anat. Rec.*, **142**, 375–390

McArthur, J. N. and Smith, M. J. H. (1969). The determination of the binding of salicylate to serum proteins. *J. Pharm. Pharmacol.*, **21**, 589–594

Mahtle, G. and Berger, H. (1982). DMBA-induced tumours and their prevention by aromatic retinoid (Ro. 10–9359). *Arch. Dermatol. Res.*, **272**, 37–47

Mansfield, J. R. (1983). Food allergies: clinical aspects

and natural allergens. In Conning, D. M. and Lansdown, A. B. G. (Eds), *Toxic Hazards in Food*, Croom-Helm, London, pp. 275–291

Marin-Padilla, M. (1966). Mesodermal alterations induced by hypervitaminosis A. *J. Embryol. Exptl Morphol.*, **15**, 261–269

Masi, P. L., Frumento, F. and Parrini, C. (1966). Malforme congenite maxillo-dentali nella, prole di topi trattati con ipervitaminosi A. *Riv. Ital. Stomat.*, **21**, 1129–1136

Matthews, M. B. (1965). The interaction of collagen and acid mucopolysaccharides. A model for connective tissue. *Biochem. J.*, **96**, 710–716

Moore, M. R. (1979). Diet and lead toxicity. *Proc. Nutrit. Soc.*, **38**, 243–250

Morriss, G. M. (1972). Morphogenesis of the malformations induced in rat embryos by maternal hypervitaminosis A. *J. Anat.*, **113**, 241

Morriss, G. M. and Steele, C. E. (1974). The effect of excess vitamin A on the development of rat embryos in culture. *J. Embryol. Exptl Morphol.*, **32**, 505–514

Nolen, G. A. (1969). Variations in responses to hypervitaminosis A in three strains of the albino rat. *Fd Cosmet. Toxicol.*, **7**, 209–214

Oberg, T., Fajers, C.-M., Friberg, U. and Lohmander, S. (1969). Collagen formation and growth in the mandibular joint of the guinea pig as revealed by autoradiography with ³H-proline. *Acta Odont. Scand.*, **27**, 452–442

Ornoy, A., Menczel, J. and Nebel, L. (1968). Alterations in the mineral composition and metabolism of rat foetuses and their placentas induced by maternal hypervitaminosis D₂. *Israel J. Med. Sci.*, **4**, 827–832

Ornoy, A., Nebel, L. and Menczel, Y. (1969). Impaired osteogenesis of foetal long bones: Induced by maternal hypervitaminosis, D₂. *Arch. Pathol.*, **87**, 563–571

Owen, M. (1970). The origin of bone cells. *Int. Rev. Cytol.*, **28**, 213–238

Pasternak, C. A. and Thomas, D. B. (1968). Metabolism of sulfated mucopolysaccharides in vitamin A deficiency. *Am. J. Clin. Nutrit.*, **22**, 985–990

Pounds, J. G. and Rosen, J. F. (1986). Cellular metabolism of lead: a kinetic analysis in cultured osteoblastic bone cells. *Toxicol. Appl. Pharmacol.*, **83**, 531–545

Rahn, B. A. and Perrin, S. M. (1970). Calcein blue as a fluorescent label in bone. *Experientia.*, **26**, 519

Reddy, G. S., Sastrip, J. G. and Rao, B. S. (1972). Radiographic photodensitometric assessment of bone density changes in rats and rabbits subjected to nutritional stresses. *Indian J. Med. Res.*, **60**, 1807–1815

Reynolds, J. J., Holick, M. F. and Deluca, H. F. (1974). The effects of vitamin D analogues on bone resorption. *Calc. Tiss. Res.*, **15**, 333–339

Robens, J. (1970). Teratogenic effects of hypervitaminosis A in the hamster and the guinea-pig. *Toxicol. Appl. Pharmacol.*, **16**, 88–99

Rolle, G. (1967). Histochemical study of ribonucleoproteins and mucopolysaccharides in developing bone of normal and tetracycline-treated chick embryos. *Anat. Rec.*, **158**, 417–432

Rosen, J. F. (1983). The metabolism of lead in isolated bone cell populations: interactions between lead and calcium. *Toxicol. Appl. Pharmacol.*, **71**, 101–112

Rosen, J. F., Roginski, M., Nathenson, G. and Finberg, L. (1974). 25-Hydroxyvitamin D, plasma levels in mothers and their premature infants with neonatal hypocalcaemia. *Am. J. Dis. Child.*, **127**, 220

Ross, L. M. and Walker, B. E. (1967). Movement of palatine shelves in untreated and teratogen-treated mouse embryos. *Am. J. Anat.*, **121**, 509–522

Salzgeber, B. (1979). Mechanisms of limb teratogenesis: malformations in chick embryo induced by nitrogen mustard. In Persaud, T. V. N. (Ed.), *Advances in the Study of Birth Defects*, Vol. 1. MTP, Lancaster, pp. 141–162

Sandor, S. and Amels, D. (1975). The early malformative syndrome. *Morphol. Embryol. (Bucharest)*, **21**, 21

Scarano, E. and Augusti-Tocco, G. (1967). Biochemical pathways in embryos. In Florkin, M. and Stotz, E. H. (Eds), *Comprehensive Biochemistry*, Vol. 28. Elsevier, Amsterdam, pp. 55–112

Sevastikoglou, J. A., Ray, R. D., Hjertquist, S.-O. and Bergquist, E. (1970). Vitamin D and skeletal metabolism. *Acta Orthop. Scand., Suppl.*, **136**, 1–85

Shambaugh. G. E. and Petrovic, A. (1968). Effects of sodium fluoride on bone. *J. Am. Med. Assoc.*, **204**, 964–973

Shtacher, G. and Firschein, H. E. (1967). Collagen and mineral kinetics in bone after fracture. *Am. J. Physiol.*, **213**, 863–866

Somogyi, A., Berczi, I. and Selye, H. (1969). Inhibition by salicylates of various calcifying connective tissue reactions. *Arch. Int. Pharmacodyn.*, **177**, 211–223

Speakman, P. T. (1971). Proposed mechanism for the biological assembly of collagen triple helix. *Nature*, **229**, 241–243

Spencer, H., Kramer, L. and Norris, C. (1975). Calcium absorption and balances during high phosphate intake in man. *Fed. Proc.*, **34**, 888

Stecholl, S. H., Goffer, Z., Haas, N. and Nathan, H. (1971). Red stained bones from Qumran. *Nature*, **231**, 469–470

Sweeney, R. M. and Watterson, R. L. (1969). Changing body wall and rib defects after local application of nitrogen mustard to different mediolateral portions of rib-forming levels of two-day chick embryos. *Teratology*, **2**, 199–220

Talmage, R. V. (1969). Calcium homeostasis—calcium transport–parathyroid action. The effects of parathyroid hormone on the movement of calcium between bone and fluid. *Clin. Orthop.*, **67**, 211–223

Teelmann, K. (1989). Retinoids: toxicology and teratogenicity to date. In Mackie, K. (Ed.), *Pharmacology and Therapeutics* special issue on *Retinoids*. Pergamon Press, Oxford, pp. 29–44.

Toews, J. G. and Lee, M. (1975). Retarded skeletal maturation in the progeny of rats malnourished during pregnancy and lactation. *Nutrit. Rep. Int.*, **11**, 223–230

Tsai, H. C. and Everson, G. J. (1967). Effect of manganese deficiency on acid mucopolysaccharides in cartilage of guinea pigs. *J. Nutrit.*, **91**, 447–452

Turbow, M. M. (1966). Trypan blue-induced teratogenesis of rat embryos cultivated *in vitro*. *J. Embryol. Exptl Morphol.*, **15**, 387–395

Turton, J. A., Hicks, R. M., Gwynne, J., Hunt, R. and Hawkey, C. M. (1985). Retinoid toxicity. In *Retinoids, Differentiation and Disease*, Ciba Foundation Symposium 113. Pitman, London, pp. 220–251

Warkany, J. and Takacs, E. (1959). Experimental production of congenital malformations in rat by salicylate poisoning. *Am. J. Pathol.*, **35**, 315–331

Weinstock, A., King, P. C. and Wuthier, R. E. (1967). The ion-binding characteristics of reconstituted collagen. *Biochem. J.*, **102**, 983–988

Whitehouse, M. W. (1963). Some effects of salicylates upon connective tissue metabolism. In Dixon, A. St. J., Martin, B. K., Smith, M. J. M. and Wood, P. H. N. (Eds), *Salicylates*. Little Brown, Boston, pp. 55–64

Whitehouse, M. W. and Bostrom, H. (1961). Studies on the action of some anti-inflammatory agents in inhibiting the biosynthesis of mucopolysaccharide synthesis. *Biochem. Pharmacol.*, **7**, 136–150

Williams, P. A. and Peacocke, A. R. (1965). The binding of calcium and yttrium ions to a glycoprotein from bovine cortical bone. *Biochem. J.*, **105**, 1177–1185

Wolbach, S. B. (1947). Vitamin A deficiency and excess in relation to skeletal growth. *J. Bone Jnt Surg.*, **29**, 171–192

Wolbach, S. B. and Hegsted, D. M. (1953). Perosis: epiphyseal cartilage in choline and manganese deficiencies in the chick. *Arch. Pathol.*, **56**, 453

Wolf, G. and Varandani, P. T. (1960). Studies on the function of vitamin A in mucopolysaccharide synthesis. *Biochim. Biophys. Acta*, **43**, 501–512

Yamaguchi, M. and Takahashi, K. (1983). Calcitonin inhibits the increase in bone acid phosphatase activity by high dose of zinc in rats. *Toxicol. Lett.*, **19**, 155–158

Yamaguchi, M. and Yamaguchi, R. (1986). Action of zinc on bone metabolism in rats. Increases in alkaline phosphatase activity and DNA content. *Biochem. Pharmacol.*, **35**, 773–777

Zamenhof, S., Hall, S. M., Grauel, L., Van Marthens, E. and Donahue, M. J. (1974). Deprivation of amino-acids and prenatal brain development in rats. *J. Nutrit.*, **104**, 1002–1007

FURTHER READING

Jones, G. and Sambrook, P. N. (1994). Drug induced disorders of bone metabolism. *Drug Safety*, **10**, 480–489

Yiamouyiannis, J. A. (1993). Fluoridation and Cancer. *Fluoride*, **26**, 83–96

30 Cutaneous Toxicology

Steven J. Hermansky

INTRODUCTION

This chapter describes the general principles of the toxicological responses of the skin to cutaneously encountered xenobiotics. This discussion will be augmented by an abbreviated description of the methods used in the predictive testing currently used to identify potential cutaneous irritants and sensitizers. However, because of the large amount of information available, there will be no attempt to make these discussions complete. Several comprehensive references are available (Hobson, 1991; Marzulli and Maibach, 1991c).

When addressing the effect of chemical substances on the skin, there are several fundamental factors to be considered. These include such variables as humidity, temperature, air currents (wind), exposure to radiation (including light), nutrition of the organism, friction, pressure, trauma (lacerations) and, perhaps, electromagnetic current. These variables influence the overall appearance and function of the skin, as well as the response of the skin to toxic insult. Physical agents (friction, pressure, electrical currents, and trauma), thermal factors (excessive heat and cold), and living organisms (bacteria and parasitic insects) produce pathological responses in the skin. Most of the literature deals with the toxic responses of the skin to chemicals as a series of discrete, mechanistically-based entities. In reality, there can be several concurrent, pathological processes which influence the immediate response of the skin to chemicals. This confounds the diagnosis and treatment of skin ailments. For example, chemical irritants have been shown to increase the allergic contact dermatitis response and, thus, may have profound effects on the diagnosis of skin ailments (McLelland et al., 1991). Furthermore, physical trauma to the skin such as pressure or friction can alter the response of the skin to chemical irritants while the converse is also true (Susten, 1985). Genetic factors can also influence an individual's susceptibility to irritation following chemical exposure (Ishii et al., 1990).

This chapter will deal primarily with the effects of chemicals, natural or synthetic, on the skin and will not, in general, address the interaction of the resulting toxicological responses with other pathological processes.

Toxic changes in the skin are of significant importance to the organism because the skin is one of the largest organs of the body and possesses functions vital to survival. In humans, the skin comprises approximately 10 per cent of the normal body weight. The skin is constantly exposed to environmental conditions and, consequently, possesses several important functions related to the interaction of an organism with its surroundings. These include protection from adverse conditions, regulation of body temperature and a role in the retention or loss of body water (Rongone, 1987). Several biochemical functions have also been attributed to the skin including metabolism, melanin production, and protein and lipid synthesis and metabolism (Rongone, 1987; Lerner and McGuire, 1961; Johnson and Fusaro, 1972). The skin is also known to act as a storage depot for glucose (primarily when blood glucose concentrations are elevated).

The skin displays several toxicological responses to chemical and/or physical insult. Responses that are produced by entirely different insults and resulting from fundamentally different changes in the skin often appear outwardly to be very similar. Therefore, the classification of skin ailments has historically been by morphology (appearance) rather than by mechanism. The functional changes produced by an insult to the skin and the impact of these changes on the behaviour and survival of the organism are not well understood.

A significant number of environmentally-related diseases and injuries involve the skin. Skin problems constitute approximately 34 per cent of all occupational diseases but may be as high as 70 per cent in some occupations (Mathias, 1985; Hogan and Lane, 1986; Suskind, 1990). These statistics are based on reported incidences of skin diseases and injuries and generally omit lacerations, burns and reactions of short duration. Thus, actual numbers have been estimated to be anywhere from 10- to 50-fold higher than medically reported (Mathias, 1985).

In addition to occupational hazards, a recent survey indicated that greater than 10 per cent of the general population claimed to have experienced adverse reactions to cosmetics and toiletries in the preceding 5 years (DeGroot, 1987). Generally, the incidence of non-occupational adverse reactions of the skin to xenobiotics is unknown. However, owing to the potential for exposure to a wide variety of chemicals, it can be speculated that non-occupational exposure to xenobiotics results in a significant amount of adverse reactions. The cosmetics industry recognizes these reactions and is constantly attempting to minimize the risk of sensitization but less often of irritation (DeGroot *et al.*, 1988).

STRUCTURE OF THE SKIN

The skin is a heterogeneous organ that consists of two different layers derived from separate germ cell lines (Figure 1). The thin, outermost layer, or epidermis, is comprised primarily of loose connective tissue. The innermost layer, or dermis, is of variable thickness that contains both connective and adipose tissue. Normal skin also contains appendages, blood vessels and neuronal components.

Epidermis

This outer layer of the skin is a stratified cellular tissue derived from the ectoderm and has no direct blood supply. Therefore, the epidermis must be completely penetrated and the dermis injured for bleeding to occur. The epidermis receives all of its nutrients from the dermis. The primary cells of the epidermis (keratinocytes) are constantly evolving and forming a cornified, protective barrier or stratum corneum (the horny scales). The stratum corneum is several layers thick and composed of flattened keratinocytes that are no longer viable or metabolically active. The intercellular spaces in the stratum corneum are filled by a matrix of materials including ceramides (a class of lipids that do not contain glycerol). This combination of cells and intercellular components plays a key role in the protective nature of the epidermis.

Beneath the stratum corneum are several layers

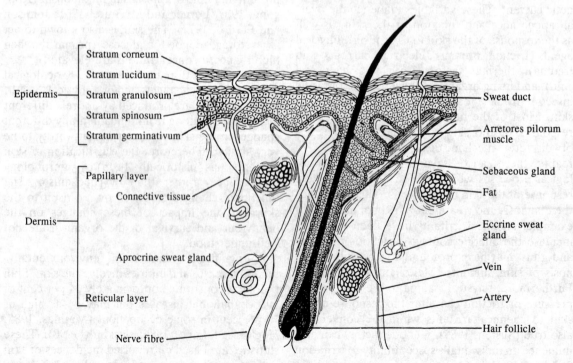

Figure 1   Schematic representation of the structure of human skin

of viable, extremely metabolically active keratinocytes which form the remainder of the epidermis. Lying adjacent to the dermis is the innermost or basal cell layer (the stratum germinativum) which consists of a single layer of columnar epithelial cells. Presumably, keratinization begins in this layer by synthesis of fibrous prekeratins. When the cells of the basal cell layer divide, they travel outward to become part of the prickle cell layer (the stratum spinosum) which is several cell layers thick. By the time the cells reach the outermost areas of this layer, aggregated filaments extend the length of the cell. As the cells move closer to the surface of the skin, they form protein aggregates and keratohyalin granules and increase in size to form the stratum granulosum which is two to four cell layers thick. In this layer, the number of cytoplasmic granules increase and the nuclei of the cells either break apart or are dissolved and the cells die.

Between the outermost layer (the stratum corneum) and the stratum granulosum lies the stratum lucidum which varies in size and appearance. The stratum lucidum is most prominent in thick skin such as that found in the ball of the foot. Eleidin, presumably a product resulting from the transformation of keratohyalin, is found in this layer and is transformed into keratin as the stratum corneum is formed. The stratum corneum, which is continually being worn away, is constantly replaced in this manner. In the stratum corneum, the keratinocytes are filled with a filamentous network of keratins. The keratins are buried in an array of mucus and lipids encapsulated by a chemical-resistant cell membrane. It has been estimated that it takes 26–28 days for a cell from the basal cell layer to progress through the layers of the skin to the outermost region of the stratum corneum (Rongone, 1987).

Approximately 10 per cent of the cells of the epidermis are Langerhans cells which are dendritic cells primarily responsible for antigen recognition (Emmett, 1991; Kalish, 1991)

Dermis

Beneath the thin, protective epidermis is the much thicker dermis. This inner layer of the skin is derived from the mesoderm and is composed of connective tissue, fibroblasts, collagen and elastic fibres. The dermis serves as a supporting unit for the epidermis and constitutes 90–95 per cent of the mass of human skin. The dermis is composed of two layers. The papillary layer (so named because of its prominent papillae) is the outer, thinner layer that contains a finer network of collagen fibres than the inner, or reticular layer.

Capillaries are prominent around the papillae of the outer layer of the dermis. The exchange of nutrients and waste products between the blood and epidermis occurs by diffusion through the large surface area of this section of the dermis. Although not completely understood, it appears that the dermis may also serve as a reservoir of nutrients for the epidermis.

The predominant cell in the dermis is the fibroblast which synthesizes fibrous proteins and several granular substances including hyaluronic acid and mucopolysaccharides. The dermis also contains several other cell types including macrophages, histiocytes, mast cells and fat cells. Blood vessels, nerve fibres and nerve endings that are associated with the skin are also located in the dermis.

Appendages Associated With the Skin

Two types of skin, differentiated by their structure and cutaneous appendages, are recognized. Glabrous skin, found only in the palms and soles, has a thick, highly protective stratum corneum as well as sweat glands and encapsulated nerve endings. Hairy skin, found throughout the rest of the body, has a relatively thin stratum corneum and contains hair follicles, sweat glands and sebaceous glands but does not contain encapsulated nerve endings. Sweat glands secrete an aqueous solution (sweat) that aids the body in cooling by evaporation. There are two types of sweat glands. The eccrine sweat glands are located over the entire surface of the body and have ducts that lead directly to the epidermal surface. Secretion by the eccrine sweat glands is under autonomic control and sweating is induced by emotional or thermal stimuli or in response to certain tastes. Apocrine sweat glands are located only in the areas of the axilla, genitalia and nipples and have a duct that leads to a hair canal. The secretory product of the apocrine sweat glands is initially odourless but it acquires odour following degradation by bacteria found on the surface of the skin. There is no known function of the apocrine sweat glands except for possible communication within or between species (as a sex attractant or as a territorial marker).

Sebaceous glands are generally associated with hair follicles and, as with hair follicles, are found over the entire surface of the body except for the glabrous skin of the palms of the hands and soles of the feet. Sebaceous glands are under hormonal control and excrete sebum, a mixture consisting primarily of lipid breakdown products, into the hair canal. The process of sebum secretion, termed holocrine secretion, does not account for all lipids found on the surface of the skin. Some lipids are contributed by the desquamation of keratinocytes from the stratum corneum. Therefore, the quantity of lipids on the surface of the skin is dependent on the local concentration and activity of the sebaceous glands as well as the amount of desquamation in the area. In areas where the sebaceous glands are numerous and actively secreting sebum, nearly 90 per cent of the lipids on the surface of the skin can be derived from sebum. The primary function of sebum is as an antibacterial agent, but the lipid components may also act as a waterproofing compound (primarily in hairy mammals) and may prevent the loss of water from the epidermis in humans (Monteiro-Riviere, 1991).

Hair follicles have three primary layers including the inner root sheath, outer root sheath and the connective tissue sheath. Hair follicles undergo regular phases of growth (anagen) and atrophy (catagen) separated by periods of inactivity (telogen). The phases of hair growth are generally recognized to be under complex hormonal control. The cells of the deepest part of the hair follicle (sometimes termed the germinal matrix) are one of the most metabolically active areas of the body (Emmett, 1991). Therefore, the response of the skin to a cutaneously encountered xenobiotic may be affected by the amount and growth of hair present at the site of contact. For this reason, hair growth should be synchronized within animals in a cutaneous toxicity study. This is best accomplished by clipping all animals the day before treatment (and at regular intervals during a repeated study) which induces a new hair growth cycle in all animals. This is especially important in studies of tumour initiation and promotion where metabolism can be critical to the outcome of the study (Monteiro-Riviere, 1991).

The nails and hair are important to the forensic toxicologist in the identification of poisonings,

particularly involving arsenic (Blanke and Poklis, 1991). In addition, piloerection, where the hair tends to stand vertical to the plane of the skin, is an important effect of some neuroactive agents. This condition is produced following stimulation of the adrenergic receptors and resulting contraction of the arretores pilorum muscle (Weiner, 1980). Other than these specific examples, these appendages are not generally of major concern to the toxicologist and will not be addressed further in this chapter.

FUNCTION OF THE SKIN

As stated earlier, the skin is the primary location where an organism interfaces with the physical, chemical and biological environments (Suskind, 1977). It is vulnerable to toxic effects from agents encountered in the environment, especially those that may be absorbed into and through the skin. Thus, the primary function of the skin is not absorption but rather the protection of the body (Zesch, 1987; Suskind, 1990).

The keratinized stratum corneum, which exists as a layer of loosely packed, dead epidermal cells, acts as a diffusion barrier against the absorption of chemicals into the skin (Dugard, 1987). Chemicals encountered by the intact skin may slowly pass into and then through this diffusion barrier and be gradually released into the body, eventually producing toxicity. The intact stratum corneum also provides a significant defence against the loss of water from the body. Additionally, the dermis contains an abundance of water that is systemically available during times of water deprivation. The dermal blood supply is substantially larger than that required for the metabolic activity of the skin. Therefore, radiation of heat from the body, controlled by the rates of blood flow to the skin, as well as the evaporation of sweat, aid in the thermal regulation of the body. Elastic and collagen fibres provide the skin with a physical barrier against trauma (Suskind, 1990) and a barrier to invasion by microorganisms (related, in part, to the secretory products of the sebaceous glands).

Melanin, produced by melanocytes, is found in varying concentrations in the skin. Following production by the melanocyte, the melanin is transferred to keratinocytes in a specialized organelle (the melanosome). These organelles are normally broken down in light-skinned people but not in dark-skinned people. It is unknown if pigmentation plays a significant role in modifying chemical damage to the skin. However, melanin certainly plays a major role in the protection against ultraviolet radiation (Emmett, 1991) and is also known to act as an oxygen scavenger. It may also decrease the concentration of mutagenic and carcinogenic reactive oxygen species found in the skin (Nordland *et al.*, 1989).

The skin, particularly the epidermis, is capable of metabolizing significant amounts of chemicals. This can have a protective effect in metabolizing potentially harmful xenobiotics to less toxic metabolites or a detrimental effect by activating less toxic compounds to more toxic metabolites (for example, proximate carcinogens can be metabolized to highly reactive ultimate carcinogens). The metabolic activity of the skin may also produce harmful results by changing an innocuous chemical into a hapten and inducing allergic contact dermatitis. Thus, the metabolizing capability of the skin is important to the pharmacology and toxicology of externally contacted xenobiotics and cannot be discounted in the evaluation of the potential health effects of environmental compounds.

The maintenance of an intact and fully functional skin is essential to survival. Alteration of the skin by any of several mechanisms, induced by physical, biological or chemical means, can have serious implications for the health and well-being of the organism.

DERMATOLOGICAL EFFECTS OF TOXIC AGENTS

Cutaneous exposure of humans or animals to a xenobiotic substance may result in a toxicological reaction or dermatosis (defined as any pathological process of the skin). Toxic agents can include medicinal compounds, food constituents, environmental agents (natural or synthetic contaminants), and a host of other sources. Exposure can be accidental, suicidal, or homicidal (Espinoza and Fenske, 1988). Effects of cutaneous exposure may be apparent immediately or may develop after days, weeks or years and the severity may vary from mild 'subjective irritation' where no gross or histological changes are observed (for example, the burning and stinging experienced

following the topical application of astringents) to life-threatening effects (Bruner, 1991). By a wide margin, the most common reactions to agents that contact the skin are inflammatory reactions to irritants, allergens and photosensitizers (Suskind, 1990).

In general, a chemical substance must be absorbed into at least the outermost layers of the skin to produce a reaction and, as discussed above, the skin (especially the stratum corneum) has evolved several protective mechanisms to retard the movement of chemicals. The rate and extent of absorption and subsequent skin reaction depend on several externally determined or extrinsic factors and two primary intrinsic factors that are determined by characteristics of the skin (Dugard, 1983). The extrinsic factors are often related to the chemistry of the substance in contact with the skin and include chemical concentration, molecular size, ionization and polarity (which affect lipid solubility), pK_a and pH of the chemical (Wester and Maibach, 1985; Berner *et al.*, 1988).

Environmental variables are also considered extrinsic factors and can play an important role in the irritation potential of a chemical. For example, low environmental humidity or increased humidity and warmth secondary to occlusion may enhance the irritation potential of a chemical (Rothenborg *et al.*, 1977). Other extrinsic properties may be related to the vehicle in which the chemical is dissolved or suspended when it contacts the skin. These factors can include the partition coefficient of the chemical between the stratum corneum and the vehicle; antioxidants and preservatives within the vehicle; the corrosive properties of the vehicle; and several other properties of the vehicle that affect the chemical or the skin (Zesch, 1987; Suskind, 1990). The intrinsic factors are related to the properties of the skin and are primarily concerned with a diffusion constant for the chemical and the thickness (number of cell layers) of the stratum corneum. Intrinsic factors can be related to genetic background, age, sex, race, concomitant disease states, neurological factors, dietary state of the individual and medication (Mathias, 1987) as well as the location in the body where the chemical contact occurs.

It is generally recognized that the skin reactivity of children may be higher than in adults (Marcussen, 1963). Conversely, the skin of the elderly is often dry and irritated (itchy) and may be slower to react to an irritant (or the irritation may be less perceptible) than in younger adults. The mechanisms of these age differences are poorly understood but decreased water content and altered lipid composition may be important in the decreased reactivity of elderly skin (Elias, 1981). Furthermore, epidermal proliferation tends to be decreased in the elderly resulting in changes to the stratum corneum and overall epidermal thickness.

Clinically, black skin appears to be less irritable than white skin (Weigand and Gaylor, 1974). However, comparisons between black and white skin irritation based on visual evaluation of skin changes may not be valid because of the difficulty in identifying erythema in black skin. Black skin may contain a thicker (more cell layers) stratum corneum and altered electrical skin resistance compared with white skin (Lammintausta and Maibach, 1988) but differences in irritability may be more perceived than real.

While it has been suggested that women are more susceptible to skin irritation than men (especially to soaps and detergents), this is most likely related to the greater exposure to irritants (both in frequency and quantity) and not to any real difference in skin irritability. However, clinical experience has suggested that women may have an increased susceptibility to skin irritation during the premenstrual period (Lammintausta and Maibach, 1988).

Most skin irritation appears to be due to solids (primarily powders) and liquids that contact the skin. Skin irritation from contact with airborne particles or vapours is possible but rarely described. This may be due to the fact that irritation from airborne substances may be missed clinically (Lammintausta and Maibach, 1988). Most skin irritation resulting from contact with a liquid or powder is attributed to chemical reactions but the physical characteristics (including sharp and/or rough edges) of the particles within a powder or suspension may play an important role in the irritability of the substance. The repeated damage to the outer layers of the skin by such particles can also significantly increase a concurrent chemically-induced irritation, which can confound the diagnoses and treatment of skin ailments.

While the diagnosis of dermatological reactions and/or toxicity is difficult because of the similar appearance of many types of skin changes, it is most useful for this discussion to classify these effects by their mechanism of action. Cutaneous reactions can be immunologically mediated, non-immunologically mediated, or mediated by unknown mechanisms.

Irritant Dermatitis

Irritant dermatitis resulting from the contact of the skin with chemicals is the most common form of xenobiotic-induced skin irritation. Nevertheless, the exact nature of this injury is not well defined (Agner and Serup, 1987). In general, the concentration of the chemical, circumstances of contact (for example, occlusive conditions and length of time of exposure) and presence of other, physically acting agents may be more important than how deeply the offending agent diffuses into the skin (Zesch, 1987). Therefore, virtually any chemical substance, under the appropriate conditions, can produce cutaneous irritation. In both humans and laboratory animals, erythema (redness) and oedema (swelling) are the most common signs of contact irritation (especially in animals). Vesiculation, scaling, and thickening of the epidermis can also be observed (Table 1 lists a number of irritant-induced clinical responses that may be observed on the skin of laboratory animals).

Chemical Burns

Following contact of the skin with an irritant, a continuum of effects occurs, but two general patterns of reactions can be identified. The first involves the contact of the skin with a corrosive agent of sufficient strength (often an acidic or alkaline solution) to cause an active and rapid response (often rapid cell death). In this 'primary irritation', pain, heat and erythema are often

Table 1   Selected irritant-induced responses that may be observed in animals

Exfoliation: dandruff-like surface scales
Excoriations: superficial scratches or cracks on the skin
Fissures: deep cracks in the surface of the skin
Ulcer: open sore
Erythema: reddened skin
Oedema: raised, swollen skin
Eschar: scab formation
Ecchymosis: haemorrhage into the skin or bruising
Necrosis: areas of dead skin

observed clinically. Microscopic changes can include varying degrees of tissue destruction, vascular permeability changes (often resulting in oedematous changes) and inflammatory cell infiltration. The extreme of this type of injury is often described as a 'chemical burn' and the exact appearance of the lesion (both on gross and microscopic observation) varies with the offending agent. Eliminating the chemical from contact with the skin is imperative to limiting the amount of tissue damage. This is usually best accomplished by repeatedly washing the affected area with copious amounts of soap and water. However, some xenobiotics may react vigorously with water (for example, calcium oxide) which could result in further tissue damage.

A knowledge of the chemistry of the compounds that may contact the skin is useful to the prevention of serious injury. Specific therapeutic interventions, based on the chemistry of the compounds, are required for many cutaneous irritants. Therefore, it is important for industrial health and safety personnel and medical practitioners as well as individuals handling these substances to be aware of the potential dangers and recommended treatment in the case of accidental exposure. Every employer in the USA is required by the US Labor Code, Section 6390, to maintain a Material Safety Data Sheet (MSDS) for each substance located and used at the work site (Adams, 1990). These documents provide information on the precautions for the use of a substance and recommendations for treatment in case of accidental exposure. Unfortunately, the MSDS is not a comprehensive reference and substances in mixtures at a concentration of less than 1 per cent are not required to be listed at all. Nevertheless, the MSDS indicates initial emergency procedures and usually lists a telephone number to gain additional information.

Cumulative Dermatitis

At the other end of the cutaneous irritation scale is repeated contact of the skin with mildly to moderately irritating substances (often termed marginal irritants). This type of chemical contact often results in slow, insidious changes in the skin that may result in thickening with or without wrinkling and/or changes in pigmentation. Many of the changes observed are the indirect effects of cutaneous inflammation and may not result from direct cellular damage caused by the chemi-

cal. Frequent and extensive exposure to a marginal irritant may produce a form of desensitization known as 'hardening' (Rothenborg *et al.*, 1977; Lammintausta and Maibach, 1988). This reaction appears to be chemical-specific and the biological mechanisms are unclear but thickening of the skin following repeated chemical exposure may be an important factor.

Microscopic changes that occur following repeated contact of the skin to marginal irritants include thickening of the entire epidermis (hyperplasia) and hyperkeratosis (thickening of the stratum corneum). This type of pathological change may be referred to as cumulative insult dermatitis and the cause may be difficult to elucidate because of the many factors usually involved and often low acute irritancy of the offending agent(s).

A list of some common microscopic changes that may be observed following exposure to irritants is presented in Table 2.

Characterization of Skin Irritation

The concept of irritation or inflammation has a very long history mainly because of its close relationship to the perennial human problem of infection. Egyptian scrolls, dated perhaps as early

Table 2 Selected microscopic changes that may be observed following exposure to irritants

Hyperkeratosis: thickening or overgrowth of the stratum corneum
Parakeratosis: retention of the nuclei in a thickened stratum corneum
Acanthosis: increased thickness of the epidermal layer of the skin
Epidermitis: inflammation, as evidenced by the presence of inflammatory cells, in the epidermis
Dermal oedema: presence of excess intercellular fluid in the skin
Dermatitis: inflammation, as evidenced by the presence of inflammatory cells, in the dermis
Folliculitis: inflammation of the hair follicles
Ulceration: loss of outer layer(s) of the skin, exposing the dermis or subcutaneous tissue
Congestion: swelling of the small blood vessels supplying the skin resulting in decreased blood flow to the affected area
Hydropic degeneration: presence of excess intracellular fluid within the cells of the epidermis
Dermal haemorrhage: presence of blood (fluids and cells) in the extravascular space of the dermis
Dermal fibrosis: abnormal formation of fibrous connective tissue

as 2650 BC, have several references to a word indicating inflammation that is associated with wounds (Ryan and Manjo, 1977). It was not until medical advances in the late nineteenth and early twentieth centuries that the separation of the inflammatory response from infections occurred.

The current description of the response of the skin to an irritant has evolved in the past 100 years and continues to change as advances in technology allow further insight into the process. One of the most important concepts, initially grasped in the late 1800s, is that the inflammatory response is a process and not a state.

In 1889, Julius Cohnheim described inflammation as a series of changes to the affected area including redness, swelling, pain, warmth and altered function. Each of these descriptors was accompanied by a discussion of microscopic changes and causative factors that have been modulated by modern medicine but not significantly altered. While these descriptions were intended to describe general inflammation, they describe skin inflammation in response to irritation equally well.

Attempts in the past century to further characterize skin irritation have led to greater awareness of the causes of irritation and specific cutaneous changes following contact with an irritant. It is now clear that the initial changes in the skin can be related to a chemical mediator (for example, histamine, serotonin or the kinins) released into the vasculature in response to chemical contact or direct vascular damage caused by various mechanisms (e.g. a thermal or chemical burn).

Several authors have attempted to characterize the sequence of events following the contact of a chemical irritant with the skin. Steel and Wilhelm (1966, 1970) described skin irritation produced by organic solvents in terms of three phases of the response. These authors considered the first phase of irritant inflammation to be an increased permeability and blood flow to the region between 0 and 2 h. The increased blood flow and permeability appeared to occur simultaneously. Inflammatory cells generally infiltrated the area within 5 min. The initial erythematous response faded rapidly and vascular permeability slowly returned to normal by 90 min. The second phase of irritation occurred between 2 and 10 h after exposure and was defined as a return to normal vascular permeability accompanied by leukocytosis and the return of erythema (increased blood flow to the area). The third phase of the irritant response occurred sometime between 10 and 36 h and consisted of increased vascular permeability.

Recent studies do not support the concept that chemical irritation can be separated into distinct phases (Patrick *et al.*, 1985; Agner and Serup, 1987). The irritation of a chemical and the resulting effects on the skin appear to be related to the specific irritant applied. Furthermore, skin irritation appears to be produced by multiple mechanisms resulting in variable patterns of response.

As indicated earlier, the ability of a compound to provoke irritation is related to chemical stability, purity, and unique chemical properties (Mathias, 1987). Several factors including sunlight, temperature and oxidation (extrinsic factors) may alter a chemical, rendering it more or less irritating. Furthermore, alterations of intrinsic factors within an individual or population may contribute to the apparent irritability of a chemical (Agner and Serup, 1989a). Variations in these factors are especially important with marginal irritants and can partially account for the wide range of reported reactions to certain compounds.

Allergic Contact Dermatitis

Definition and Description

Allergic contact dermatitis, or dermatitis venenata, is the result of an elaborate interaction between the complicated pathophysiological mechanisms of Type IV cell-mediated immunity and environmental sensitizers (allergens). Characteristic structural changes in the skin are induced following the contact of the skin with an allergen (Schmidt, 1989). While skin changes due to irritant dermatitis are generally produced by a direct interaction of the chemical with the constituents of the skin, allergic dermatitis results when the chemical elicits an immune reaction that, in turn, results in changes in the skin. The diffusion of the compound into the skin is often the determining parameter in whether a compound will produce allergic dermatitis (Zesch, 1987).

Chemicals that are potential allergens are continually being developed and introduced into the human environment. Therefore, allergic contact dermatitis can be expected to continue to be a dermatological problem, especially in the workplace. Allergens may be simple chemicals (haptens) that must interact with a chemical within the organism before becoming allergenic or they may be complicated chemicals or biological substances that elicit the allergenic responses without chemical modification. Allergic contact dermatitis remains one of the most common occupational diseases that may become debilitating if the causative agent is not identified and exposure controlled (Nethercott and Holness, 1989; Slavin and Ducomb, 1989). The condition is notable because of the extremely low concentration of chemical required to induce a reaction.

The period between initial contact with the causative agent and the development of skin sensitivity (the induction period) may be as little as 2 or 3 days for strong sensitizers like poison ivy or as long as several years for a weak sensitizer like chromate. Following a short sensitization period, if sufficient allergen remains from the initial contact, a spontaneous reaction may occur at the site of exposure. This is demonstrated by the presence of an allergic reaction following the first exposure to poison ivy. Once the sensitivity to an allergen has been established, it generally persists for many years. Following the initial development of sensitivity, the time between re-exposure to the causative agent and the occurrence of clinically observable effects is generally between 12 and 48 h but may be as short as 4 h or as long as 72 h. Thus arises the term 'delayed hypersensitivity' (Slavin and Ducomb, 1989). For reasons that are not entirely clear but possibly related to particular intrinsic factors, an individual may be repeatedly exposed to an allergen and not develop sensitivity to the substance for many years while other individuals develop sensitivity following a single or very short exposure period to the same substance. The time between initial exposure and development of sensitivity is termed the 'refractory period' (Emmett, 1991).

Acute contact dermatitis is characterized by papules and sharply demarcated erythema. Blisters are also produced following the release of cytotoxic compounds by white blood cells attracted to the affected site. Therefore, the vesicle fluid is not antigenic and contact of this fluid with unexposed areas of the skin will not result in additional dermatitis (Slavin and Ducomb, 1989). Oedema may also occur in areas of loose tissue.

Acute (short-term) and chronic (long-term) allergic contact dermatitis are gradations of the same condition. As allergic contact dermatitis increases in duration (usually from repeated exposure to the causative agent), the prevalence of blisters in the affected area decreases. The blisters are gradually replaced by the formation of a crust (scaling) and/or lichenification (thickening of the epidermis). Erythema may or may not persist during chronic allergic dermatitis. The key element in the formation of subchronic or chronic allergic dermatitis is recurrent exposure to the causative agent. If the agent can be identified and exposure eliminated, the disease state will resolve. Unfortunately, because of the wide range of potential exposure to antigenic compounds including metals and metal-containing compounds, cosmetics, deodorants, clothing dyes, food additives, adhesives, oils, plants or animals and their products (lanolin) and fragrances to name just a few, this is often an extremely difficult if not monumental task. The success of corticosteroids in treating allergic contact dermatitis has generally eliminated this condition from the list of serious disorders. However, owing to the difficulty of identifying and eliminating allergens as well as the prevalence of potential allergens, this skin reaction is a potentially serious disease that will continue to be a major cause of cutaneous eruptions (Menne and Nieboer, 1989). Furthermore, exposure via the skin to potentially allergenic chemicals has also been suggested as a major route of sensitization for respiratory allergy (Kimber and Cumberbatch, 1992).

Chemistry of Haptens

Haptens are low-molecular-weight environmental chemicals that form covalent bonds with cutaneous carrier proteins or other cellular macromolecules. When this carrier molecule is a normal endogenous entity, as is usually the case, the resulting chemical complexes are no longer identified by the system as 'self'. Therefore, this now foreign molecule is perceived as an intruder (the allergen) and elicits an allergic reaction. Examples of commonly occurring haptens include metals (nickel, cobalt and chromium), quinones, aldehydes, and acrylates (Benezra, 1987; DeGroot, 1987).

The majority of haptens that are skin sensitizers have electrophilic properties. Thus, they are able to accept electron pairs from nucleophiles such as amino (NH_2) and thiol (SH) groups that are found in cutaneous proteins (Benezra, 1987). Some potential haptens must be transformed by metabolism or reaction with light before they are able to bind to cutaneous proteins and become allergenic. These compounds constitute a special class of allergic sensitizers and are often termed 'prohaptens'. A unique subgroup of prohaptens that must react with light to become allergenic belong to the class of photoreactive chemicals termed 'photosensitizers' or 'photoallergens' (see below). When photoallergens react with light, they often form free radicals which rapidly react with cutaneous proteins, forming the allergen.

Other Allergens

Other allergens may contain long, hydrophobic side chains that appear to form hydrophobic bonds within cell membranes. Examples of compounds that are this type of allergen include lanolin and the extremely allergenic pyrocatechols found in the *Rhus* genus of plants which includes poison ivy.

Light-induced Cutaneous Toxicity

The most biologically active spectrum of light is found from 290 nm to 700 nm. This spectrum can be further defined as ultraviolet or UV (290–400 nm) and visible (400–700 nm). The UV spectrum is generally further divided into UV-A (315–400 nm), UV-B (280–315 nm) and UV-C (220–280 nm). UV-C wavelengths do not naturally occur on the surface of the earth as this spectrum is absorbed in the stratosphere, predominantly by ozone. Generally, the longer the wavelength, the deeper the light penetrates into the skin (Stern, 1986; Kornhauser *et al.*, 1991). The wavelengths of light found in the UV-B spectrum are generally considered the primary source of toxic changes in the skin. However, the UV-A spectrum is increasingly believed to play an important role in the effect of light on the skin. The specific wavelengths responsible for a particular biological response are termed the 'action spectrum' for that effect (Kaidbey, 1991). The action spectrum for several light-induced cutaneous reactions have been clearly identified.

There are several effects which result from the exposure of the skin to light whether the light is natural or manmade (thus, the UV light found in tanning booths is no safer than UV light created by the sun). In some cases, xenobiotics play a role

in these effects while in others, the interaction of light with the normal components of the skin is responsible. In either case, adverse reactions of the skin to light (UV or visible) is termed photosensitization (Emmett, 1991).

Photosensitization not Related to Xenobiotics

The exposure of the unprotected skin to UV light (from sunlight or artificial sources) can result in several toxic responses of the skin. These include short-term, generally reversible effects such as sunburn (erythema) and tanning (enhanced pigment darkening) as well as long-term, generally irreversible effects such as premature skin ageing (actinic elastosis) and the development of skin cancer.

Exposure of the skin to UV-B radiation can selectively alter the immunological function of the skin (photoimmunotoxicity). This can alter the immune response to contact allergens and microorganisms (such as Herpes simplex types I and II). Furthermore, the altered immunological function induced by UV-B light exposure can facilitate the development and growth of skin cancer. Altered immune response related to UV-B light exposure, associated with concurrent chemical exposure, may result in a complex relationship of light and chemicals on the alteration of immune system function (Krutmann and Elmets, 1988).

Photosensitization Related to Xenobiotic Exposure

Xenobiotics localized within the skin can interact with light (generally UV but, perhaps, visible as well) and produce adverse reactions in the skin in many ways. These include phototoxicity, photoallergy, depigmentation, induction of endogenous photosensitizers, and induction of photosensitivity disease states (Emmett, 1979). Of these, the most frequently observed are phototoxicity and photoallergy (Emmett, 1991).

Phototoxicity
Phototoxicity is defined as a non-immunological, light-induced dermatitis to a photoactive chemical (Marzulli and Maibach, 1991a). The skin response in phototoxicity is likened to an exaggerated sunburn. After local absorption or distribution to the skin following systemic absorption from distant sites, the chemical reacts with light and the resulting light-altered compound pro-

duces skin irritation. It is possible that many phototoxic reactions are caused by the production of free radicals which cause lipid peroxidation and localized inflammation (Hayes, 1989). As with any chemical irritant, erythema, oedema and desquamation may occur with or without hyperpigmentation. The affected area of the skin is generally limited to areas exposed to light (i.e. areas not covered by clothing). The severity of phototoxic reactions is usually dose-related. Furthermore, phototoxic reactions can be elicited in most individuals who are exposed to an adequate amount of the compound and the appropriate action spectrum. A list of potential phototoxic agents is presented in Table 3.

Photoallergy
Photoallergy is similar to allergic contact dermatitis with the exception that the xenobiotic must react with light prior to becoming allergenic. The role of light in the production of a photoallergen is most likely to be one of two types of reactions. The absorption of light by the chemical may, in itself, produce a potent allergen. Conversely, the absorption of light by the chemical may produce a reactive intermediate (hapten) that combines with cellular constituents resulting in an altered cellular component that is an allergen (Emmett, 1991). Clinically, photoallergy generally presents as dermatitis on light-exposed areas which often spreads to areas not exposed to light (i.e. photoallergy may occur in areas covered by clothing). The severity of a photoallergic reaction may not appear to be dose-related (the skin reactions may be very severe with relatively low exposure) and the reaction does not necessarily develop in all individuals exposed to the offending' agent and appropriate action spectrum. A list of potential photoallergenic agents is presented in Table 4.

Table 3 Selected phototoxic agents

Tetracyclines (antibiotics)
Sulphonamides (antibiotics)
Chlorpromazine (antipsychotic agent)
Anthracene (constituent of many dyes)
Porphyrins (animal and plant respiratory pigments)
Psoralens (photochemotherapy agents for psoriasis)
Cadmium sulphide (colourant in tattoos)
Certain dyes
Coal tar
Perfumes

Table 4 Selected potentially photoallergenic agents

Sulphonamides (antibiotics)
Phenothiazines (antipsychotic agents)
Coumarins (anticoagulants)
Anilides (components in medicines and dyes)
Aftershave lotions
Sunscreen agents (*p*-aminobenzoic acid derivatives)

Cutaneous Carcinogenesis

Skin cancer is the most common form of cancer in humans. The principal cause of skin cancer in humans is UV radiation (Suskind, 1990). There are three primary types of skin cancer: carcinomas of the epidermal-basal and squamous cells, sarcomas of the mesodermal elements, and melanomas. Squamous cell carcinomas are most often associated with chronic exposure to UV light (Hogan and Lane, 1986). The production of skin cancer by chemicals has been known for more than 200 years (Potter, 1963) and it is apparent that several chemicals modulate the carcinogenic effects of UV light (Emmett, 1973). Additionally, a past history of trauma or frostbite to the light-exposed area may also play a role in the development of skin cancer (Hogan and Lane 1986; Rustin *et al.*, 1984). Prevention and early detection are the foundations of skin cancer treatment. Chemical carcinogenesis is covered in other areas of this book and will not be addressed in detail here.

Acne-like Eruptions

Acne is a well known effect of several cutaneous toxins (Espinoza and Fenske, 1988). Testosterone, chlorinated compounds and topical steroids are known to produce eruptions in humans similar to acne vulgaris. Although the potential of cosmetics to cause acne may be somewhat exaggerated (Jackson, 1991), a skin lesion termed 'acne cosmetica' has been described for acne-like eruptions caused by cosmetics. Like acne vulgaris, these reactions are initiated by the proliferation of the epithelium of the sebaceous gland and formation of a keratin cyst resulting in the development of a pustule filled with fatty compounds and other products of sebaceous origin.

Chloracne

The skin reaction termed 'chloracne' may be one of the most sensitive measures of exposure to specific toxins known (Tindall, 1985; Poland and Glover, 1977). Chloracne, with accompanying, specific epidermal changes, is the most characteristic and frequently observed lesion resulting from primate, including human, exposure to the halogenated aromatic hydrocarbon class of toxins (Crow, 1970; Taylor, 1974). Owing to the specific cause of the lesion, chloracne is rarely observed in clinical practice (Zugerman, 1990). In humans, this 'hallmark' of chlorinated hydrocarbon exposure is characterized by prominent, dense, large blackheads (comedones), abscesses and skin-coloured cystic lesions (Taylor, 1979). Almost every follicle in the affected area may be involved. The skin of the face, frequently areas near the eyes and behind the ears, is usually involved first. Severe chloracne may involve the trunk, arms, legs, face, neck and back and is frequently refractory to treatment and scarring may be severe. Chloracne may appear as early as 1–3 weeks after the first exposure or may not manifest itself for several months. Mild cases clear up spontaneously within a few months while severe cases persist for as long as 30 years (Scientific Review Committee of the American Academy of Clinical Toxicology, 1985). The lesion is so specific that if there is no medical history of chloracne, the likelihood of significant exposure or adverse health effects from halogenated aromatic hydrocarbons, specifically 2,3,7,8-tetrachlorodibenzo-*p*-dioxin (TCDD), is considered remote (Council on Scientific Affairs, 1982).

EVALUATING CHEMICALS FOR POTENTIAL ADVERSE EFFECTS ON THE SKIN

It is essential that the toxicologist, healthcare professional and industrial hygienist understand the importance of the 'prior-to-use safety assessment' as the cornerstone of control of cutaneous hazards. This necessitates the evaluation of initial acute toxicity screening in animals followed by a tier of tests for safety dictated by the potential for and conditions of human exposure to the chemical. The tier assessment includes single and repeated exposure of laboratory animals and human subjects. Therefore, a discussion of the techniques of such safety assessment follows. While animals should always be exposed to

chemicals before humans (Klecak, 1991), human testing will be discussed first.

Human Testing

The diagnostic or predictive tool used most often for irritant or allergic contact dermatitis is patch testing (Slavin and Ducomb, 1989; Marzulli and Maibach, 1991b). The test is always performed on normal skin that is free of injury or disease. In predictive testing with untested chemicals, it is best to start with diluted solutions of the chemical and utilize an unoccluded test site. The first application should be limited to 30 min or 1 h to minimize the risk to the subjects (Patrick and Maibach, 1991). As with most *in vivo* cutaneous techniques, comparison of the results between tests is extremely difficult because of the subjective nature of evaluating cutaneous irritation, effect of environmental and genetic differences between individuals and groups, effect of the specific vehicle, application technique and exposure period. Human studies with untested chemicals should always be conducted and monitored by medical personnel with ample experience in the appropriate discipline and informed consent must be obtained under all circumstances.

Patch testing procedures have the potential to produce adverse effects. For example, patch tests causing serious irritation may rarely result in scarring or permanently altered pigmentation of the site. Rarely, the patch testing procedure alone may be the cause of sensitization to a chemical. Therefore, the necessity of diagnostic or predictive patch testing must be carefully evaluated before the studies are initiated.

Sensitization Patch Testing

For patch testing to be a reasonably reliable tool in the identification of contact allergens, meticulous attention to detail must be maintained. The method involves the application of a small amount of one or several suspected allergens in relevant concentrations and in appropriate vehicles. The occurrence of the disease is then documented, in miniature, at the site of application. A standardized procedure for patch testing was developed in Scandinavia and has been widely used in diagnosing contact allergies (Hjorth, 1991). Generally, a single application is sufficient for diagnosis of an allergic contact dermatitis. However, in predictive tests as part of pre-exposure testing, several occlusive patches are applied for 2 days as an induction to sensitization followed by a 2-week rest period and then challenge with a patch at a different skin site (Marzulli and Maibach, 1973). There are several alterations to these basic procedures for predictive tests in humans (Marzulli and Maibach, 1991b).

The most common site for diagnostic patch testing is the back but the lateral or inner side of the upper arm, the thighs, or the legs may also be used (Hjorth, 1991). A small aluminium cup fixed to a strip of tape (the Finn chamber) is currently the patch used most frequently throughout the world (Adams, 1990). A patch composed of a cellulose allergen-bearing disc attached to a polyethylene-coated aluminium paper backing is also often used (Slavin and Ducomb, 1989). Using these patches, 50–55 diagnostic tests can be performed on the back of the patient at the same time. For proper diagnostic evaluation, the chemical-treated patches must remain on the skin for at least 24 h but often are left on the skin for 48–96 h owing to the latency of many skin reactions.

Following the exposure period, the patch is removed and 20–30 min allowed to elapse prior to the evaluation of the sites to allow non-specific, mechanical irritation to subside. A positive reaction can include erythema, oedema, and, perhaps, vesicles at the application site. Local reactions that are irritant in nature will subside after several hours while a true allergic reaction will persist for several days (Slavin and Ducomb, 1989). The test sites should also be evaluated 7–10 days after patch removal as some reactions do not occur for 96 h or a week after exposure.

Both false-positive and false-negative reactions occur as several factors can influence the result. These include both intrinsic and extrinsic factors. For example, chemical concentration, current treatment with anti-inflammatory medications, UV light exposure, reaction to the adhesive tape used in the patch, and hyperexcited skin states can alter the results of a diagnostic or predictive patch test (Oxholm and Maibach, 1990).

Photopatch testing involves similar techniques to patch testing except that the treated site is exposed to a source of UV light following the application of the test substance.

Irritant Patch Testing

The potential of a chemical to produce cutaneous irritation is difficult to evaluate because all chemicals are irritating under some conditions. Indeed, merely increasing the water content of the skin by occlusion with impermeable tape often results in mild to moderate irritation (Olson, 1991). The changes in the skin resulting from the application of a mild irritant may be difficult to detect on gross examination but they may result in significant alteration in function.

Original study designs for irritant patch testing in humans recommended the use of application periods of up to 48 h (Kooyman and Snyder, 1942; Draize *et al.*, 1944; Justice *et al.*, 1961; Rostenberg, 1961). More recent study designs have recommended shorter exposure times and a 4-h application period has been adopted by the National Academy of Sciences (1977). Patches, bandages or chambers are utilized to apply the test substance to the skin. Increasing the degree of occlusion will generally increase the severity of irritation and the use of highly occlusive tape to hold the patch in place can significantly affect the results of a study. Accordingly, the area of chemical exposure should be clearly marked to differentiate irritation or skin damage produced by the tape from that produced by the test chemical.

While it may be sufficient to evaluate some compounds of limited human exposure utilizing a single exposure study design, compounds proposed for consumer use are often tested utilizing cumulative (repeated exposure) irritation assays. Some chemicals that are non-irritating following a single contact with the skin may be highly irritating following repeated contact with the skin. A consumer product that has been reported to be irritating can be separated into individual ingredients and the irritating component identified by the use of cumulative patch testing. The study design for these assays, including length of exposure period and number of treatments, varies between investigators (Patrick and Maibach, 1991). The specific study design (duration of contact, concentration of chemical, location of exposure, etc.) used in cumulative patch testing is often customized to the expected exposure pattern or suspected irritability and toxicity of the chemical.

Several modifications of patch testing have

been developed for specific applications. The scarification test, in which the epidermis is abraded using the bevel of a needle, was developed to evaluate the irritability of compounds that may be applied to damaged skin (Patrick and Maibach, 1991). The soap chamber test was developed to compare the potential for soaps to produce drying and flaking which are effects not normally produced using conventional patch testing methodology (Frosch and Klingman, 1979). Flex washing tests or elbow crease washing tests do not involve the use of a patch and have been used by some investigators primarily for evaluating the irritation produced by soaps and detergents. These tests have been used as a replacement for the arm immersion test originally proposed by Kooyman and Snyder (1942). Many other variations of irritant testing have been utilized for miscellaneous purposes and, undoubtedly, more will be developed in the future.

Patch tests often over- or underestimate the irritant potential of a chemical. This is as a result of the wide variability in the susceptibility of individuals to develop irritation (intrinsic factors) as well as the multitude of possible exposure conditions, especially with a consumer product (extrinsic factors). Thus, the selection of subjects for testing and conditions of exposure must be controlled and carefully evaluated when assessing the results of irritant patch testing.

Evaluation of Patch Test Results

Patch tests are generally evaluated visually by assigning grades of irritation to the occluded area. The clinician focuses on the centre of the patch for purposes of reproducible and accurate grading. The grades, based primarily on erythema, generally consist of a zero for no response and a 1–4 or 5 for increasingly inflamed sites. This scale does not include vesicular, bullous or eschar formation. Therefore, more detailed grading systems with up to 16 possible grades have been proposed (Patrick and Maibach, 1991).

Several other mechanisms of evaluating the results of patch testing have been developed. These are briefly discussed below.

Animal Testing

When animals are used as models for human exposure to chemicals, the differences and similarities between species are important factors to consider. While the relationship of animal dose–response data to human toxicity is not always clear, an understanding of the potential for toxicity is essential to the development of human exposure guidelines. An important objective is to establish a relationship between animal data and epidemiological findings. This task is extremely difficult because of the poor availability of reliable data on the toxicity and irritability of most chemicals in humans. When both animal data and epidemiological findings exist for a chemical, the correlation of the information can aid in the assessment of laboratory data as it relates to humans.

Sensitization Testing in Animals

The most widely accepted animal model for predictive sensitization studies is the guinea pig (Middleton, 1978). There are several variations of the tests designed to evaluate the allergenic potential of chemicals. A summary of the study designs that utilize guinea pigs is presented in Table 5. This chapter will deal only with the general descriptions and principles of the tests.

To assess the potential sensitization properties of a chemical, guinea pigs are treated with an initial dose or several doses of the chemical (the induction phase) by intradermal and/or cutaneous application. Following a sensitization or incubation phase of approximately 2 weeks, the animals are treated with a second dose or series of doses of the same test chemical (the challenge phase). The chemical concentration and application site are often different between the induction and challenge phases. Sensitization is evaluated by examining the skin reaction following the challenge phase compared with any skin reaction immediately following the induction phase. The difference in the reaction between the two applications accounts for non-specific skin irritation caused by the chemical. The relevance of the results of the tests to human exposure must be evaluated based on the severity and repeatability of the biological properties of the reaction. Often the number of animals that respond is a more important indicator of the sensitizing potential of a chemical than the severity of individual reactions. Practical experience is the best guide in this endeavour as laboratory experiments may be conducted under extreme or unrealistic conditions. A fundamental understanding of the test

Table 5 Summary of guinea pig sensitization tests

Name of the study design	Induction phase	Challenge phase	Sensitivity
Draize	ID	ID	Low
Freund's complete adjuvant	ID[a]	T-U	Medium
Optimization	ID	ID and T-O	High
Open epicutaneous	T-U	T-U	High
Split adjuvant	T-O[b]	T-O	High
Buehler	T-O	T-O	High
Maximization	ID[a] and T-O	T-O	High

[a] Mixed with Freund's complete adjuvant (FCA).
[b] FCA injected into the sensitization site.
ID = intradermal injection; T-O = occluded topical application; T-U = unoccluded topical application.

procedures along with the potential for false-positive and false-negative findings is also required.

Intradermal Techniques

Draize *et al.* (1944) were the first to describe standardized irritation and sensitization tests. The Draize sensitization test is the simplest, most inexpensive predictive test to perform (Botham *et al.*, 1991). However, the test has several drawbacks including a high incidence of false negatives with weak sensitizers (Marzulli and Maguire, 1982). Furthermore, the test recommends a consistent induction concentration of 0.1 per cent injected intradermally without regard to use pattern or exposure potential of the chemical (Klecak, 1991). The Draize test is no longer routinely used in testing laboratories and is being replaced by other techniques.

The optimization test is highly sensitive but more difficult and time consuming to perform than other tests. Because of this, the optimization test is not used as often as other, equally sensitive tests.

In the Freund's complete adjuvant test, the test substance is mixed with Freund's Complete Adjuvant (FCA; a mixture of heat-killed *Mycobacterium tuberculosis*, paraffin oil and mannide monooleate) prior to intradermal injection for induction. The use of FCA increases the immunological response and aids in the detection of weak sensitizers (Henningsen, 1991). The test utilizes three injections of this mixture at different sites during the induction phase. In the challenge phase, the test substance is generally applied epidermally (non-occluded) in a range of non-irritating concentrations. This test is considered as sensitive as the optimization test and is of low cost to perform (Stampf *et al.*, 1982). The primary drawback to this test is the use of intradermal induction doses. The intradermal induction bypasses the effect of the stratum corneum to limit the absorption of potential sensitizers. Furthermore, the use of FCA may cause the sensitizing potential of the test chemical to be overestimated.

Epicutaneous Techniques

The open epicutaneous test utilizes an induction phase of repeated applications of an undiluted test substance (which may be a formulation of a final product for consumer exposure) over several weeks. The challenge phase is separated into initial and rechallenge phases. Klecak *et al.* (1977) found this test to be a sensitive, highly predictive test. However, this is the only test that requires an induction phase dose–response and, therefore, requires the use of more animals than other tests.

The Buehler test was designed to reproduce a human patch test in animals and, therefore, allows variation of conditions to optimize the detection of moderate to strong sensitizers prior to testing in humans. This test utilizes induction and challenge phases of occluded epidermal doses of the test substance which may be allergenic chemicals or final product formulations. The results of this test can be very difficult to read and interpret, especially when low concentrations of test chemicals are used. This is primarily because of the high incidence of inflammatory reactions in both control and treated animals. This test may result in false-negative results but these problems may be related to poor study conduct and may not be attributable to the design of the test (Robinson *et al.*, 1989, 1990). Performed correctly, the Buehler test is relatively expensive but is able to detect weak sensitizers (Botham *et al.*, 1991).

Methods that Require Intradermal and Epicutaneous Treatment

The split adjuvant technique requires that the skin be meticulously shaved and cleaned followed by placing dry ice onto the treatment site prior to induction. This technique employs an induction phase over 9 days where FCA is injected into the treatment site twice on the fourth day. The test substance for both the induction and challenge phases is applied epicutaneously and the site is occluded. The combination of occlusion and FCA treatment allows this test to detect weak sensitizers. This technique is not currently being used by many laboratories.

The guinea pig maximization test is the most widely used test in Europe and is generally considered to be very sensitive (Botham *et al.*, 1991). The induction phase of this test employs the simultaneous injection of FCA alone, test material in saline, and test material in FCA into three different locations in close proximity to each other. This is followed 7 days later by epicutaneous application of the test substance on a filter paper. The filter paper is occluded and held into place with tape and an adhesive bandage. The filter paper and bandaging are then left in place for 48 hours. The challenge phase, conducted with the test substance applied epicutaneously for 24 hours, is performed 2 weeks after the epidermal induction phase. The maximization test is considered to have good predictive value in humans but does not lend itself well to use with final product formulations (Klecak, 1991). The maximization test may result in false-positive results. Indeed, the original classification scheme for the test did not allow for a test substance to be classified as a non-sensitizer; the lowest rating (0) corresponded to a weak sensitizer (Botham *et al.*, 1991).

Other Predictive Tests for Sensitizers

While the guinea pig tests remain the industry standard for evaluation of the sensitization potential of a compound, new techniques are continually evaluated. Of these, the most promising appears to be the mouse ear swelling test (MEST).

The mouse has been studied extensively as a model for delayed-type hypersensitivity (Nakano and Nakano, 1978; Tanaka, 1980; Johnson *et al.*, 1984). In 1968, the technique of measuring the swelling of the mouse ear as an indicator of delayed-contact hypersensitivity was developed (Asherson and Ptak, 1968). This is a quantitative test as the swelling of the ear is measured using a micrometer.

The MEST has received considerable attention and is considered by many authors to be an acceptable alternative animal model to the guinea pig tests in predicting the sensitization potential of chemicals in humans (Gerberick and Ryan, 1989; Henningsen, 1991). However, the test is not yet accepted by government agencies as an alternative to the guinea pig tests. The MEST is generally performed by injecting an abdominal site with FCA once and topically applying the test chemical to the same site (the induction phase) for several consecutive days beginning the day of FCA injection. A week after the final abdominal induction dose, a challenge dose of the test chemical is applied to the left ear of the mice with the right ear serving as a control. At 24 and 48 h after the challenge dose, the mice are lightly anaesthetized and the thickness of both ears measured with a micrometer. The test is evaluated by comparing the thickness of the left ear with that of the right ear. Mice are considered positive if the challenged ear is more than 20 per cent thicker than the control ear (Gad *et al.*, 1986; Henningsen, 1991).

The MEST is less expensive and may be more sensitive than the guinea pig models. This has been questioned because of the unpredictable reactivity of the mouse to certain sensitizers (Cornacoff *et al.*, 1988). The results of the MEST can also be difficult to interpret correctly as the tools that measure the thickness of the ears can have significant variation especially when handled by different technicians. Furthermore, when measuring oedematous swelling, the pressure exerted on the surface of the ear can have a much greater impact on the measurement obtained than when measuring swelling produced by cellular infiltrates. This problem can be largely avoided if high-precision, electronic calipers are utilized (Henningsen *et al.*, 1984).

Irritation Testing in Animals

It is generally recognized that human skin and the skin of other animals are different and do not always react to chemicals in the same manner. Overall, the skin of laboratory animals is more easily irritated than the skin of humans although this is not always the case (Phillips *et al.*, 1972; Olson, 1991). Animal testing will reliably detect moderate to strong irritants but the degree of irritation often correlates poorly with the degree of skin response in humans. Therefore, comprehensive experimental protocols are required to establish the degree of risk to humans. Comprehensive animal testing can also aid in the identification of adequate labelling of chemical containers and suggest appropriate protective clothing for use in the workplace.

A low acute oral or inhaled toxicity may indicate that extensive cutaneous testing is not required as the skin is generally a more effective barrier to absorption than the intestinal tract or lungs. This generalization is not always true and the degree of human exposure and chemistry of the compound must be carefully considered when making testing decisions. For obvious reasons, the evaluation of a compound for irritability in animals does not need to be performed with strongly alkaline or acidic substances. Severe skin irritation can be presumed with these compounds and specific precautionary measures recommended without the results of animal testing. Only limited irritation testing may need to be performed when the substance will not come into direct and close contact with the skin (Gelbke, 1987).

Selection of Animal Species

Selection of the proper species and strain of animals for use in a toxicology study of any design is very important to the usefulness (predictive value) of the results (Rao and Huff, 1990). The albino rabbit remains the species of choice in acute and repeated application irritation testing. Several authors (Davies *et al.*, 1972; Motoyoshi *et al.*, 1979; McCreesh and Steinberg, 1987) have addressed the use of other species including guinea pigs, hairless mice, albino rats and miniature swine in cutaneous irritation testing. Considerable interspecies variability has been identified. The skin of rabbits is generally identified as the most sensitive of the species tested while human skin is one of the least sensitive. The reactivity of the skin of the albino rat is considered to be similar to the reactivity of human skin. Thus, the albino rat is becoming increasingly utilized in repeated cutaneous toxicity studies.

Single Application Irritation Testing (Draize Test)

The test described by Draize *et al.* in 1944, or slight modifications of this test, is the most widely used test for predicting the potential skin irritation of chemicals and chemical mixtures. The authors divided the various elements of irritation into distinct categories for grading (Table 6). In this test, the hair is clipped from the back of a rabbit and four distinct areas for the application of test substances are identified. Two of the four areas are abraded by making four epidermal incisions in the appropriate areas. All four areas are covered by gauze that is held in place with adhesive tape and the test substance is applied to the appropriate areas under the gauze. The entire trunk of the rabbit is wrapped in impervious cloth or plastic to hold the patches in place and decrease the evaporation of volatile test substances. The rabbits generally remain wrapped for 24 h after treatment and are evaluated for irritation at the time of unwrapping and 24 and

Table 6 Evaluation of skin reactions as described by Draize *et al.* (1944)

Skin reaction	Score
Erythema and eschar formation	
Very slight erythema (barely perceptible)	1
Well-defined erythema	2
Moderate to severe erythema	3
Severe erythema (beet redness) to slight eschar formation	4
Total possible erythema score	4
Oedema formation	
Very slight oedema (barely perceptible)	1
Slight oedema (edges of area well defined by definite raising)	2
Moderate oedema (area raised approximately 1 mm)	3
Severe oedema (raised 1 mm and extending beyond the area of exposure)	4
Total possible oedema score	4
Total possible score for primary irritation	8

48 h after being unwrapped. Generally, four test substances are evaluated in a series of six rabbits.

The Draize test for dermal irritation has been criticized for various reasons. The original purpose of the test was to identify substances that would not be irritating to human skin and was primarily designed to eliminate false negatives. While the occurrence of false positives is undesirable in the development of new consumer products, they are infinitely preferable to the occurrence of false negatives which could lead to disastrous results when an undetected irritant is added to consumer products. Several aspects of the standardized Draize test, including the abrasion of the skin and time of exposure, are disputed. This has resulted in several modifications to the method. As with the evaluation of patch testing in humans, the subjective nature of the evaluation of the treatment areas results in significant variations between laboratories as well as between technicians (Weil and Scala, 1971). This impedes the comparison of results between laboratories and makes the job of the risk assessor more difficult.

Repetitive Application Irritation Testing
The use of repeated cutaneous applications over at least 7–14 days appears to be better able to predict the irritability of a test substance than a single application. This is especially true if the material is designated for use in a consumer product that will remain in contact with the skin for extended periods or if there will be repeated applications of the material. Additionally, the repeated application test to assess irritability can be combined with an assessment for systemic toxicity by the cutaneous route. In this case, three or more groups of five to ten animals per sex (generally albino rats or rabbits) are used with each group receiving a different dose of the test substance daily for 2, 3, 4 or 13 weeks (weekend doses may be omitted). An additional group of animals is handled similarly but treated with the vehicle or, when no vehicle is used, with water to serve as a control group. The fur is removed from the back of the animals with a veterinary clipper and the test chemical is applied directly to the back. The animal is then wrapped with an occlusive dressing and returned to its home cage for a period of 6 h. The wrapping is removed and the back gently wiped with a damp or dry cloth. The animals are observed daily for signs of

cutaneous irritation (Table 1) and graded for the presence of erythema and oedema (Table 6). At termination of the study, both treated and untreated skin are collected and evaluated microscopically for signs of irritation. A list of common microscopic changes observed following the application of irritating test substances is presented in Table 2.

An evaluation of repetitive application studies using mild to severe irritants indicates that several haematology and clinical chemistry parameters may be affected by chemically-induced skin irritation (Weaver *et al.*, 1990, 1991, 1992; Hermansky *et al.*, 1993). These changes, summarized in Table 7, do not appear to be related to systemic toxicity of the chemical but correlate well with the degree of cutaneous irritation. The relationship of these parameters to cutaneous irritation is not clear but may be related to the vascular and fluid balance alterations that may occur following cutaneous irritation. Regardless of the cause of these changes, their consistent occurrence emphasizes the relationship of the skin to the overall health of the organism. It is also essential that the risk assessor be aware of these irritation-induced changes when evaluating the findings of repeated cutaneous application studies.

Table 7 Clinical pathology measurements that may be affected by cutaneous irritation

Decreased values
  Haemoglobin concentration
  Haematocrit
  Erythrocyte count
  Serum calcium concentration
  Serum inorganic phosphorus concentration
  Serum creatinine concentration

Increased values
  Total leukocyte count
  Neutrophil count
  Platelet count (rabbit only)
  Serum globulin concentration (rabbit only)
  Serum glucose concentration (rat only)

Parameters that are variably affected
  Mean corpuscular volume (MCV)
  Mean corpuscular haemoglobin (MCH)
  Total serum protein concentration
  Serum albumin concentration

METHODS OF EVALUATING *IN VIVO* IRRITATION RESULTS

As discussed above, the interpretation of both human and animal cutaneous testing relies heavily on visual scoring of areas of the skin treated with the test substance. The subjectiveness of visually graded results in human patch testing and acute and repeated exposure studies in animals (Table 6) makes it very difficult to compare tests graded by different individuals and laboratories. This confounding experimental variable has led to complications for the toxicologist and risk assessor in evaluating the potential human hazard of cutaneous exposure to chemicals.

Therefore, methods other than visual scoring or grading of skin inflammation have been developed to aid in the interpretation of patch testing in dark-skinned humans as well as in an attempt to decrease the subjective nature of visually grading skin irritation in all tests. Blood flow to the skin must generally increase threefold or greater to be detected visually and reactions produced by mild or moderate irritants or weak sensitizers may not be detected by visual evaluation alone. Finally, the importance of differentiating an allergic reaction from an irritant reaction, especially in human diagnostic patch testing, cannot be overstated and methods of greater sensitivity than visual grading may increase the ability to differentiate these reactions.

Several methods developed for the evaluation of patch testing results have been examined in considerable detail. Contact thermography is the imaging of the temperature of an area of the skin where an irritant has been applied (Ring, 1986). The methodology is based on the premise that the greater the degree of irritation, the higher the relative temperature of the affected skin (that is, irritation and inflammation are fundamentally related). However, contact thermography has shown that different irritants produce lesions of different temperatures in humans. For example, croton oil produces a warm lesion while sodium lauryl sulphate results in the formation of a cold lesion (Agner and Serup, 1988). Because changes in the temperature of the affected skin are now known to be irritant-specific, thermography is not considered a useful method for quantifying the degree of irritation. Recent use of infrared thermography has shown promise in the differen-

tiation of allergic and irritant responses but more research is needed (Baillie *et al.*, 1990).

Another method of evaluating skin inflammation caused by irritant or allergic dermatitis is laser Doppler flowmetry or velocimetry (Staberg *et al.*, 1984). The instrument is equipped with a hand-held probe that emits a laser light onto the skin and measures blood flow through the area. This technique is generally considered more sensitive than visual scoring in detecting erythema in humans (Wahlberg and Wahlberg, 1984). However, the technique often produces poor correlation with visual scoring. This is based partially on the dependence of visual scoring on parameters other than blood flow (i.e. blistering) as well as the fact that mild irritants often produce erythematous reactions with a disproportionately low increase in blood flow (Gawkrodger *et al.*, 1991).

Transepidermal water vapour loss, measured with an evaporimeter (Lammintausta *et al.*, 1987), has also been used to evaluate patch tests. The technique, which evaluates the function of the stratum corneum as a barrier to water loss, is generally more sensitive to irritant dermatitis (indicating epidermal damage) than to allergic dermatitis. The technique has, therefore, been evaluated in humans as a method of differentiating irritant and allergic dermatitis. However, the variable severity of an allergic reaction does not allow this test to differentiate between allergic and irritant responses in all cases (Agner and Serup, 1989b).

Another technique that has been used in the evaluation of skin irritation is the erythema index which quantifies the inflammatory response by comparing the reflection of red and green light from the skin (Diffey *et al.*, 1984). Skin thickness measurements have also been used to evaluate oedematous reactions (Olson, 1991). Based on the observation that repeated exposure to irritants often results in an increased roughness and brittleness of the skin, measurements of physical changes to the cells of the stratum corneum following exposure to irritants have been evaluated (Olson, 1991). The loose, outer layer of cells of the stratum corneum are obtained from humans by non-invasive techniques (washing the site) and the cells are evaluated for shape, size and morphology under a light microscope. Because of the greater availability of intact skin samples, this technique appears to have more promise in animal testing.

To the risk assessor, a quantitative, objective measure of cutaneous inflammation remains a highly desirable goal. Alternative methods of evaluating inflammation in animals include many of the same methods used for evaluating the results of irritation patch testing in humans. However, owing to several factors, including the thick and variable patterns of fur growth in most species (especially rabbits), these measurements have generally been unsatisfactory in animals.

Because of availability of intact animal skin samples at study termination (following euthanasia), other methods of evaluating irritation, not currently practical for humans, have been developed for use in animal irritation studies. Evaluations of morphometry (the measurement of structural forms) on cells obtained from the full thickness of skin can be utilized in animals. Measurements of the average total cell volume, nuclear size and shape, as well as calculated parameters (e.g. the nuclear/cytoplasmic ratio) can be obtained with this method. Additionally, special fluorescent stains can be utilized to observe and grade the roughness of the surface of the skin.

Several biochemical markers have been evaluated as potential indicators of the degree of irritation. These include enzyme activity, tissue or serum concentration of prostaglandins and/or leukotrienes, and acute phase reactant proteins (Olson, 1991). Ideally, as with any clinical test, the biological sample should be easy to obtain, objectively measured and the results should be consistent and repeatable. Results of studies with the above markers have generally been unsuccessful at identifying inflammation. As techniques and instrumentation improve, an acceptable biochemical marker for evaluating cutaneous inflammation may be identified, resulting in enhanced evaluation and interpretation of the *in vivo* assessment of cutaneous irritation, preferably, in both animals and humans.

IN VITRO ASSAYS

The *in vivo* procedures employing animals used by the toxicologist and risk assessor to measure the potential of a material to produce cutaneous irritation have been increasingly challenged. The validity of these evaluations as they relate to humans, as well as the use of animals in these procedures, have been questioned. As a result, attempts to measure the irritant potential of test substances using *in vitro* techniques have significantly increased. Several recent technological developments have made the *in vitro* growth of skin as well as measurement of relevant structural and/or functional alterations in the cultured skin possible. While a complete description of the methods and applications of these techniques is beyond the scope of this chapter, a description of the general principles is warranted. It appears that cutaneous irritation is an area where alternative methods to whole animal predictive testing may soon play a substantial role in risk assessment (van den Heuvel and Fiedler, 1990).

The purpose of developing *in vitro* techniques to predict the potential irritability of a test substance can be: (1) to evaluate specific aspects of the irritation or sensitization process, (2) to provide supplemental information to *in vivo* evaluations for the risk assessor, or (3) to replace an *in vivo* procedure (Hobson and Blank, 1991). Furthermore, *in vitro* tests may be more cost effective and, if designed and used properly, provide more objective and meaningful results than whole animal studies.

In reducing the number of animals used for toxicological experiments and predictive testing, *in vitro* methods have particular value (Gad, 1990; Purchase, 1990). The primary ethical considerations for the toxicologist, industry and governmental agencies is the protection of human health. Therefore, the change from *in vivo* to *in vitro* techniques requires a comprehensive process of evaluation of the performance characteristics of the *in vitro* methodology. This process of proving the effectiveness of a new procedure is termed 'validation'. The validation of any new toxicological technique, whether or not it be an *in vitro* process, requires an exhaustive comparison of the new technique with results obtained in previous or concurrent studies using established techniques of evaluation as well as comparison with existing relevant epidemiological data in humans. The selection of the test substances for the validation work must be done carefully and should represent a wide range of both chemical and toxicological classes. Based on the legal and ethical implications, this validation and the subsequent move from *in vivo* to *in vitro* techniques must be a careful, deliberate process (van den Heuvel and Fiedler, 1990). The final acceptance or rejection of an *in vitro* test depends on the ability to utilize the results and the confidence in the decisions based on the information provided by the procedure (Soto and Gordon, 1991).

A validation scheme for alternative methods has been devised and includes three stages (Scala, 1986). The first stage develops a mechanistic relationship between the alternative assay and the endpoint of interest in the target organ and can involve the evaluation of up to a hundred chemicals. The accuracy and dependability of the assay procedures are determined in the second stage. Therefore, problems with the methodology are detected, evaluated and, if possible, corrected during this stage. The third and final stage is performed after the new assay has gained considerable regulatory and scientific acceptance. This phase involves many laboratories and the testing of up to more than 1000 chemicals.

Ideally, the validation of an *in vitro* technique should be performed, at least partially, using human data. There are generally little or no human toxicological data available on enough compounds to evaluate and validate an *in vitro* technique satisfactorily. However, there is a substantial amount of data available on the cutaneous irritability of a multitude of chemicals and chemical mixtures. Researchers attempting to develop new *in vitro* techniques can access this information and compare the results of their models with the known findings of these chemicals in humans (Bason *et al.*, 1992). Indeed, individual reputations and the future of entire companies have been staked in an attempt to develop a reliable and economical *in vitro* alternative to predictive irritation testing in animals.

Types of *In Vitro* Alternative Methods

Several different types of *in vitro* models have been developed to predict the cutaneous irritancy and sensitization potential of compounds (Parish, 1986; Hobson and Blank, 1991). Structure–activity and biochemical models currently appear to have limited value but increased mechanistic knowledge and technological advances may increase the usefulness of these models in the future. Computerized structure–activity models may have some applications but have not received a great deal of industrial or regulatory accept-

ance. These models generally depend on the correlation of a toxic endpoint (in this case, cutaneous irritation or sensitization) with specific chemical functional groups and/or a measured parameter of the molecule (e.g. rotational freedom of the functional group within the molecule). Based on an accumulated database of known chemicals, untested chemicals are evaluated for the potential to produce the toxic endpoint by comparison with the known chemicals of similar structural features. Obviously, these models rely heavily on the molecular interactions involved in production of the toxic endpoint. As the knowledge of molecular mechanisms of irritation and sensitization increases, the use of these databases for structure–activity modelling will also increase in accuracy and dependability. This methodology will undoubtedly have greater use in the future and the scientific interest in structure–activity models continues to be intense.

The biochemical events that are involved in the production of an irritant response are exceedingly complex and not well understood. It is clear that irritants from different chemical classes produce cutaneous changes leading to inflammation by vastly different mechanisms. Thus, development of an accurate structure–activity model for irritation of a wide range of chemicals is a monumental task. Similarly, production of a biochemical model to accurately predict the potential irritancy of chemicals and chemical mixtures is a considerably difficult undertaking. Current biochemical models emphasize the interaction between the irritant and an endogenous molecule of the skin. The interaction would, presumably, be required to initiate the irritant response. However, the identification of even one of probably many biochemical events responsible for initiating irritation is difficult. Current biochemical models utilize mixtures of carefully selected organic chemicals organized into separate sections to simulate layers of the skin (Gordon *et al.*, 1989). The test substance is added to the system and several parameters including chemical reactivity are evaluated.

Mechanistically-based computer or biochemical models used to predict the irritancy potential of a specific class of chemicals may provide valuable information in the selection of new chemicals for future work within that class. These models also add useful information on the mechanisms of irritation and inflammation and are currently being used to a limited extent in pharmacology and toxicology.

Cell culture methodology has recently been adapted to *in vitro* irritation assays involving both cutaneous and ocular irritancy. Potential irritancy is evaluated by measuring the cytotoxicity of the chemical in a cell culture. Owing to the many cell varieties found in normal skin, the major complication encountered with this methodology has been the selection of the appropriate cell type(s) for use in the system. Furthermore, the effect of the stratum corneum in protecting viable cells of the epidermis from irritants is not taken into account by a cell culture model (Hobson and Blank, 1991). Several cell types have been evaluated as models for cutaneous irritation with significant differences being identified (Gajjar and Benford, 1990). The most frequently used cell type is the keratinocyte and an established line of human epidermal keratinocytes is now available commercially (Clonetics Corporation, San Diego, CA).

Many of the problems with cell culture systems are overcome by utilizing skin tissue models. Epidermal slices obtained from either human or animal sources have been evaluated as models for irritancy (Oliver and Pemberton, 1985). These systems show some promise as successful alternatives to *in vivo* testing especially with the possibility of combining the test system with *in vitro* evaluations of skin penetration (Hobson and Blank, 1991).

Undoubtedly, the most recent addition to the *in vitro* irritation assays, the skin equivalent models, have generated the most interest. Skin equivalent models are differentiated human keratinocyte cultures grown on an artificial membrane system (Hobson and Blank, 1991). Several of these skin equivalent systems are currently commercially available. The mechanisms that have been developed to create these systems are as elaborate as they are variable. Skin equivalent models are produced using patented methods that involve complex processes to induce cellular development and differentiation. The final product is a very close approximation of human skin tissue that may include a stratum corneum on the surface and, at the base, proteins similar to a basement membrane. Even special pigmented equivalents are available. These models are becoming increasingly sophisticated and representative of human skin tissue but they continue to lack dermal appendages such as sweat glands and hair follicles. While the physical approximation to human skin is clear, the relevance of information obtained using the skin equivalent models to humans is unclear but very promising. There is currently a vast amount of work being performed in several laboratories throughout the world with these models. The results of these studies will undoubtedly help define the abilities and limitations of the skin equivalent models.

A relatively new technique, the silicon microphysiometer (Parce *et al.*, 1989), is currently being evaluated for use as a tool for *in vitro* evaluation of cellular response following exposure to a chemical. The instrument indirectly measures cell metabolism by non-invasively determining the rate of acid metabolite production (Bruner *et al.*, 1991). The methodology takes advantage of the hypothesis that changes in the biological, chemical, or physical environment of a cell should be reflected by fluctuations of molecular concentrations within the cell. Therefore, molecular fluctuations identified in cells following exposure to a chemical should correlate with the potential of the chemical to produce irritation. Utilizing human epidermal keratinocytes, preliminary studies with this model have provided excellent correlation with *in vivo* ocular irritancy data and work into ocular irritation as well as cutaneous irritation is proceeding (Bruner *et al.*, 1991).

ACKNOWLEDGEMENT

Thanks to Susan M. Christopher, BS, for her skilful artwork in Figure 1.

REFERENCES

Adams, R. M. (1990). Patch testing for occupational allergens and the evaluation of patients with occupational contact dermatitis. *Allergy Proc.*, **11**, 117–120

Agner, T. and Serup, J. (1987). Skin reactions to irritants assessed by polysulfide rubber replica. *Contact Derm.*, **17**, 205–211

Agner, T. and Serup, J. (1988). Contact thermography for assessment of skin damage due to experimental irritants. *Acta Derm. Venereol. (Stockh.)*, **68**, 192–195

Agner, T. and Serup, J. (1989a). Seasonal variation of skin resistance to irritants. *Br. J. Dermatol.*, **121**, 323–328

Agner, T. and Serup, J. (1989b). Skin reactions to irritants assessed by non-invasive bioengineering methods. *Contact Dermatitis*, **20**, 352–359

Asherson, G. L. and Ptak, W. (1968). Contact and delayed hypersensitivity in the mouse. I. Active sensitization and passive transfer. *Immunology*, **15**, 405–416

Baillie, A. J., Biagioni, P. A., Forsyth, A., Garioch, J. J. and McPherson, D. (1990). Thermographic assessment of patch-test responses. *Br. J. Dermatol.*, **122**, 351–360

Bason, M. M., Harvell, J., Realica, B., Gordon, V. and Maibach, H. I. (1992). Comparison of in vitro and human in vivo dermal irritancy data for four primary irritants. *Toxic. in Vitro*, **6**, 383–387

Benezra, C. (1987). Molecular aspects of allergic contact dermatitis. *Acta Derm. Venereol. (Stock.)*, **134** (Suppl.), 62–63

Berner, B., Wilson, D. R., Guy, R. H., Mazzenga, G. C., Clarke, F. H. and Maibach, H. I. (1988). The relationship of pK_a and acute skin irritation in man. *Pharmaceut. Res.*, **5**, 660–663

Blanke, R. V. and Poklis, A. (1991). Analytical/forensic toxicology. In Amdur, M. O., Doull, J. and Klaassen, C. D. (Eds), *Toxicology, The Basic Science of Poisons*, 4th edn, Pergamon Press, New York, NY, pp. 905–923

Botham, P. A., Basketter, D. A., Maurer, T., Mueller, D., Potokar, M. and Bontinck, W. J. (1991). Skin sensitization—a critical review of predictive test methods in animals and man. *Food Chem. Toxicol.*, **29**, 275–286

Bruner, L. H., Miller, K. R., Owicki, J. C., Parce, J. W. and Muir, V. C. (1991). Testing ocular irritancy *in vitro* with the silicone microphysiometer. *Toxic. in Vitro*, **5**, 277–284

Bruner, R. H. (1991). Pathological processes of skin damage related to toxicant exposure. In Hobson, D. W. (Ed.), *Dermal and Ocular Toxicology Fundamentals and Methods*. CRC Press, Boca Raton, FL, pp. 73–109

Cornacoff, J. B., House, R. V. and Dean, J. H. (1988). Comparison of a radioisotopic incorporation method and the mouse ear swelling test (MEST) for contact sensitivity to weak sensitizers. *Fund. Appl. Toxicol.*, **10**, 40–44

Council on Scientific Affairs (1982). Health effects of agent orange and dioxin contaminants. *JAMA*, **248**, 1895–1897

Crow, K. D. (1970). Chloracne. *Trans. St. Johns Hosp. Dermatol. Soc.*, **56**, 77–99

Davies, R. E., Harper, K. H. and Kynoch, S. R. (1972). Interspecies variation in dermal reactivity. *J. Soc. Cosmet. Chem.*, **23**, 371–381

DeGroot, A. C. (1987). Contact allergy to cosmetics: causative ingredients. *Contact Derm.*, **17**, 26–34

DeGroot, A. C., Nater, J. P., der Lende, B. and Rijken, B. (1987). A large-scale enquiry into adverse effects of cosmetics. *Ned. T. Geneeskd*, **131**, 863–865

DeGroot, A. C., Beverdam, E. G. A., Ayong, C. T., Coenraads, P. J. and Nater, J. P. (1988). The role of contact allergy in the spectrum of adverse effects caused by cosmetics and toiletries. *Contact Derm.*, **19**, 195–201

Diffey, B. L., Oliver, R. J. and Farr, P. M. (1984). A portable instrument for quantifying erythema induced by ultraviolet radiation. *Br. J. Dermatol.*, **111**, 663–672

Draize, J. H., Woodard, G. and Calvery, H. O. (1944). Methods for the study of irritation and toxicity of substances applied to the skin and mucous membranes. *J. Pharmacol. Exp. Therap.*, **82**, 377–390

Dugard, P. H. (1983). Skin permeability theory. In Marzulli, F. N. and Maibach, H. I. (Eds). *Dermatotoxicology*. Hemisphere Publishing Corporation, Washington, DC, pp. 91–116

Dugard, P. H. (1987). Skin permeability theory in relation to measurements of percutaneous absorption in toxicology. In Marzulli, F. N. and Maibach, H. I. (Eds), *Dermatotoxicology*, 3rd edn. Hemisphere Publishing Corporation, Washington, DC, pp. 95–120

Elias, P. M. (1981). Lipids and the epidermal permeability barrier. *Arch. Dermatol. Res.*, **270**, 95–117

Emmett, E. A. (1973). Drug photoallergy. *Crit. Rev. Toxicol.*, **2**, 211–255

Emmett, E. A. (1979). Phototoxicity from endogenous agents. *Photochem. Photobiol.*, **40**, 429–436

Emmett, E. A. (1991). Toxic responses of the skin. In Amdur, M. O., Doull, J. and Klaassen, C. D. (Eds), Casarett and Doull's *Toxicology, The Basic Science of Poisons*, 4th edn, Pergamon Press, New York, NY, pp. 463–483

Espinoza, C. G. and Fenske, N. A. (1988). Dermatological manifestations of toxic agents. *Ann. Clinical Lab. Sci.*, **18**, 148–154

Frosch, P. J. and Klingman, A. M. (1979). The soap chamber test. A new method for assessing the irritancy of soaps. *J. Am. Acad. Dermatol.*, **1**, 35–41

Gad, S. C. (1990). Recent developments in replacing, reducing, and refining animal use in toxicologic research and testing. *Fund. Appl. Toxicol.*, **15**, 8–16

Gad, S. C., Dunn, B. J., Dobbs, D. W., Reilly, C. and Walsh, R. D. (1986). Development and validation of an alternative dermal sensitization test: the mouse ear swelling test (MEST). *Toxicol. Appl. Pharmacol.*, **84**, 93–114

Gajjar, L. and Benford, D. J. (1990). Comparison of cultured keratinocytes and fibroblasts as models for irritancy testing *in vitro*. *Toxic. in Vitro*, **4**, 280–283

Gawkrodger, D. J., McDonagh, A. J. G. and Wright, A. L. (1991). Quantification of allergic and irritant patch test reactions using Laser-Doppler flowmetry and erythema index. *Contact Derm.*, **24**, 172–177

Gelbke, H. P. (1987). Concept for the sequential testing of industrial chemicals. *J. Toxicol. Sci.*, **12**, 253–258

Gerberick, G. F. and Ryan, C. A. (1989). A predictive

mouse ear-swelling model for investigating topical phototoxicity. *Food Chem. Toxicol.*, **27**, 813–819

Gordon, V. C., Kelly, C. P. and Bergman, H. C. (1989). An *in vitro* method for determining dermal irritation. *Toxicologist*, **9**, 6

Hayes, J. A. (1989). Systemic responses to toxic agents. In Marquis, J. K. (Ed.), *A Guide to General Toxicology*, 2nd edn. Karger, New York, pp 24–61

Henningsen, G. M. (1991). Dermal hypersensitivity: immunologic principles and current methods of assessment. In Hobson, D. W. (Ed.), *Dermal and Ocular Toxicology Fundamentals and Methods*, CRC Press, Boca Raton, FL, pp. 153–192

Henningsen, G. M., Koller, L. D., Exon, J. H., Talcott, P. A. and Osborne, C. A. (1984). A sensitive delayed-type hypersensitivity model in the rat. *J. Immunol. Methods*, **70**, 153–165

Hermansky, S. J., Weaver, E. V., Neptun, D. A. and Ballantyne, B. (1993) Clinical pathology changes related to cutaneous irritation in the Fischer 344 rat and New Zealand White rabbit

Hjorth, N. (1991). Diagnostic patch testing. In Marzulli, F. N. and Maibach, H. I. (Eds), *Dermatotoxicology*, 4th edn. Hemisphere Publishing Corporation, Washington, DC, pp. 441–451

Hobson, D. W. (Ed.) (1991). *Dermal and Ocular Toxicology Fundamentals and Methods*, CRC Press, Boca Raton, FL

Hobson, D. W. and Blank, J. A. (1991). *In vitro* alternative methods for the assessment of dermal irritation and inflammation. In Hobson, D. W. (Ed.), *Dermal and Ocular Toxicology Fundamentals and Methods*. CRC Press, Boca Raton, FL, pp. 323–368

Hogan, D. J. and Lane, P. (1986). Dermatologic disorders in agriculture. *State Art Rev. Occup. Med.*, **1**, 285–300

Ishii, N., Ishi, H., Ono, H., Horiuchi, Y., Nakajima, H. and Aoki, I. (1990). Genetic control of nickel sulfate delayed-type hypersensitivity. *J. Invest. Dermatol.*, **94**, 673–676

Jackson, E. M. (1991). Cosmetics: substantiating safety. In Marzulli, F. N. and Maibach, H. I. (Eds), *Dermatotoxicology*, 4th edn. Hemisphere Publishing Corporation, Washington, DC, pp. 835–845

Johnson, J. A. and Fusaro, R. M. (1972). Role of skin in carbohydrate metabolism. *Adv. Metab. Disord.*, **6**, 1–55

Johnson, K. W., Holsapple, M. P., White, K. L. Jr and Munson, A. E. (1984). Assessment of delayed contact hypersensitivity in mice. *Toxicologist*, **4**, 109

Justice, J. D., Travers, J. J. and Vinson, L. J. (1961). The correlation between animal tests and human tests in assessing product mildness. *Proceedings of the Scientific Section of the Toilet Goods Association*, **35**, 12–17

Kaidbey, K. (1991). The evaluation of photoallergic contact sensitizers in humans. In Marzulli, F. N. and Maibach, H. I. (Eds), *Dermatotoxicology*, 4th edn.

Hemisphere Publishing Corporation, Washington, DC, pp. 595–605

Kalish, R. S. (1991). Recent developments in the pathogenesis of allergic contact dermatitis. *Arch. Dermatol.*, **127**, 1558–1563

Kimber, I. and Cumberbatch, M. (1992). Dendritic cells and cutaneous immune responses to chemical allergens. *Toxicol. Appl. Pharmacol.*, **117**, 137–146

Klecak, G. (1991). Identification of contact allergens: predictive tests in animals. In Marzulli, F. N. and Maibach, H. I. (Eds), *Dermatotoxicology*, 4th edn. Hemisphere Publishing Corporation, Washington, DC, pp. 363–413

Klecak, G., Geleick, H. and Frey, J. R. (1977). Screening of fragrance materials for allergenicity in the guinea pig. I. Comparison of four testing methods. *J. Soc. Cosmet. Chem.*, **28**, 53–64

Kooyman, D. J. and Snyder, F. H. (1942). Tests for the mildness of soaps. *Arch. Dermatol. Syphilol.*, **46**, 846–855

Kornhauser, A., Wamer, W. and Gilers, A. Jr (1991). Light-induced dermal toxicity: effects on the cellular and molecular level. In Marzulli, F. N. and Maibach, H. I. (Eds). *Dermatotoxicology*, 4th edn. Hemisphere Publishing Corporation, Washington, DC, pp. 527–569

Krutmann, J. and Elmets, C. A. (1988). Recent studies on mechanisms in photoimmunology. *Photochem. Photobiol.*, **48**, 787–798

Lammintausta, K. and Maibach, H. I. (1988). Exogenous and endogenous factors in skin irritation. *Int. J. Dermatol.*, **27**, 213–222

Lammintausta, K., Maibach, H. I. and Wilson, D. (1987). Human cutaneous irritation: induced hyporeactivity. *Contact Derm.*, **17**, 193–198

Lerner, A. B. and McGuire, J. S. (1961). Effect of alpha and beta melanocyte stimulating hormones on skin colour in man. *Nature*, **189**, 176–179

McCreesh, A. H. and Steinberg, M. (1987). Skin irritation testing in animals. In Marzulli, F. N. and Maibach, H. I. (Eds), *Dermatotoxicology*, 3rd edn. Hemisphere Publishing Corporation, Washington, DC, pp. 153–172

McLelland, J., Shuster, S., Matthews, J. N. S. (1991). 'Irritants' increase the response to an allergen in allergic contact dermatitis. *Arch. Dermatol.*, **127**, 1016–1019

Marcussen, P. V. (1963). Primary irritant patch test reactions in children. *Arch. Dermatol.*, **87**, 378–382

Marzulli, F. N. and Maibach, H. I. (1973). Antimicrobials: experimental contact sensitization in man. *J. Soc. Cosmet. Chem.*, **24**, 399–421

Marzulli, F. N. and Maguire, H. C. Jr (1982). Usefulness and limitations of various guinea pig test methods in detecting human skin sensitizers—validation of guinea pig tests for skin hypersensitivity. *Food Cosmet. Toxicol.*, **20**, 67–74

Marzulli, F. N. and Maibach, H. I. (1991a). Phototoxicity of topical and systemic agents. In Marzulli,

F. N. and Maibach, H. I. (Eds), *Dermatotoxicology*, 4th edn. Hemisphere Publishing Corporation, Washington, DC, pp. 581–594

Marzulli, F. N. and Maibach, H. I. (1991b). Contact allergy: predictive testing in humans. In Marzulli, F. N. and Maibach, H. I. (Eds) *Dermatotoxicology*, 4th edn. Hemisphere Publishing Corporation, Washington DC, pp. 415–439

Marzulli, F. N. and Maibach, H. I. (Eds) (1991c). *Dermatotoxicology*, 4th edn. Hemisphere Publishing Corporation, Washington, DC

Mathias, C. G. T. (1985). The cost of occupational skin disease. *Arch. Dermatol.*, **121**, 332–341

Mathias, C. G. T. (1987). Clinical and experimental aspects of cutaneous irritation. In Marzulli, F. N. and Maibach, H. I. (Eds), *Dermatotoxicology*, 3rd edn. Hemisphere Publishing Corporation, Washington, DC, pp 173–190

Menne, T. and Nieboer, E. (1989). Metal contact dermatitis: a common and potentially debilitating disease. *Endeavour*, **13**, 117–122

Middleton, J. D. (1978). Predictive animal tests for delayed dermal hypersensitivity in man. *Soap Perfum. Cosmet.*, **51**, 201–205

Monteiro-Riviere, N. A. (1991). Comparative anatomy, physiology, and biochemistry of mammalian skin. In Hobson, D. W. (Ed.), *Dermal and Ocular Toxicology Fundamentals and Methods*. CRC Press, Boca Raton, FL, pp. 3–72

Motoyoshi, K., Toyoshima, Y., Sato, M. and Yoshimura, M. (1979). Comparative studies on the irritancy of oils and synthetic perfumes to the skin of rabbit, guinea pig, rat, miniature swine and man. *Cosmet. Toiletries*, **94**, 41–42

Nakano, K. and Nakano, Y. (1978). Suppressor cells in antigenic competition in contact allergy in mice. *Immunology*, **34**, 981–987

National Academy of Sciences, Committee for the Revision of NAS Publication 1138 (1977). *Principles and Procedures for Evaluating the Toxicity of Household Substances*. National Academy of Sciences, Washington, DC, pp. 23–59

Nethercott, J. R. and Holness, D. L. (1989). Occupational allergic contact dermatitis. *Clin. Rev. Allergy*, **7**, 399–415

Nordland, J. J., Abdel-Malek, Z. A., Boussy, R. E. and Rheinis, L. A. (1989). Pigment Cell Biology: An Historical Review. *J. Invest. Dermatol.* **92** (4 Supp.), 53–60

Oliver, G. J. A. and Pemberton, M. A. (1985). An *in vitro* epidermal slice technique for identifying chemicals with potential for severe cutaneous effects. *Food Chem. Toxicol.*, **23**, 229–232

Olson, C. T. (1991). Evaluation of the dermal irritancy of chemicals. In Hobson, D. W. (Ed.), *Dermal and Ocular Toxicology Fundamentals and Methods*. CRC Press, Boca Raton, FL, pp. 125–151

Oxholm, A. and Maibach, H. I. (1990). Causes, diagnosis, and management of contact dermatitis. *Comp. Therapy*, **16**, 18–24

Parce, J. W., Owicki, J. C., Kercso, K. M., Sigal, G. B., Wada, H. G., Muir, V. C., Bousse, L. J., Ross, K. L., Sikic, B. I. and McConnell, H. M. (1989). Detection of cell-affecting agents with a silicon biosensor. *Science*, **246**, 243–247

Parish, W. E. (1986). Evaluation of *in vitro* predictive tests for irritation and sensitization. *Food Chem. Toxicol.*, **24**, 481–494

Patrick, E. and Maibach, H. I. (1991). Predictive skin irritation tests in animals and humans. In Marzulli, F. N. and Maibach, H. I. (Eds), *Dermatotoxicology*, 4th edn. Hemisphere Publishing Corporation, Washington, DC, pp. 201–222

Patrick, E., Maibach, H. I. and Burkhalter, A. (1985). Mechanisms of chemically induced skin irritation. *Toxicol. Appl. Pharmacol.*, **81**, 476–490

Phillips, L. II, Steinberg, M., Maibach, H. I. and Akers, W. A. (1972). A comparison of rabbit and human skin response to certain irritants. *Toxicol. Appl. Pharmacol.*, **21**, 369–382

Poland, A. and Glover, E. (1977). Chlorinated biphenyl induction of amyl hydrocarbons hydroxylase activity: a study of the structure activity relationships. *Mol. Pharmacol. Toxicol.*, **22**, 517–554

Potter, M. (1963). Percivall Pott's contribution to cancer research. *Natl Cancer Inst. Monogr.*, **10**, 1–13

Purchase, I. F. H. (1990). Strategic considerations in industry's use of *in vitro* toxicology. *Toxic. in Vitro*, **4**, 667–674

Rao, G. N. and Huff, J. (1990). Refinement of long-term toxicity and carcinogenesis studies. *Fund. Appl. Toxicol.*, **15**, 33–43

Ring, E. J. J. (1986). Skin temperature measurements. *Bioeng. Skin*, **2**, 15–30

Robinson, M. K., Stotts, J., Danneman, P. J., Nusair, T. L. and Bay, P. H. S. (1989). A risk assessment process for allergic contact sensitization. *Food Chem. Toxicol.*, **27**, 479–487

Robinson, M. K., Nusair, T. L., Fletcher, E. R. and Ritz, H. L. (1990). A review of the Buehler guinea pig skin sensitization test and its use in a risk assessment process for human skin sensitization. *Toxicology*, **61**, 91–107

Rongone, E. L. (1987). Skin structure, function, and biochemistry. In Marzulli, F. N. and Maibach, H. I. (Eds), *Dermatotoxicology*, 3rd edn. Hemisphere Publishing Corporation, Washington, DC, pp. 1–70

Rostenberg, A. (1961). Methods for the appraisal of the safety of cosmetics. *Drug Cosmet. Ind.*, **88**, 592

Rothenborg, H. W., Menne, T. and Sjolin, K. E. (1977). Temperature dependent primary irritant dermatitis from lemon perfume. *Contact Derm.*, **1**, 37–48

Rustin, M. H. A., Chanbers, T. J. and Munro, D. D. (1984). Post-traumatic basal cell carcinomas. *Clin. Exp. Dermatol.*, **9**, 379–383

Ryan, G. B. and Manjo, G. (1977). *Inflammation*. The Upjohn Company, Kalamazoo, MI

Scala, R. A. (1986). Theoretical approaches to validation. In Goldberg, A. M. (Ed) *Progress in In Vitro Toxicology*. Mary Ann Liebert Inc., New York

Schmidt, G. (1989). Buchbesprechungen. *Dermatol. Mon. Schr.*, **175**, 214–219

Scientific Review Committee of the American Academy of Clinical Toxicology (1985). Commentary on 2,3,7,8-tetrachlorodibenzo-*p*-dioxin (TCDD). *Clin. Toxicol.*, **23**, 191–204

Slavin, R. G. and Ducomb, D. F. (1989). Allergic contact dermatitis. *Hosp. Practice*, **24**, 39–51

Soto, R. J. and Gordon, V. C. (1991). Evaluation of an *in vitro* dermal irritation assay. *Toxicologist*, **10**, 79

Staberg, B., Kemp, P. and Serup, J. (1984). Patch test responses evaluated by cutaneous blood flow measurements. *Arch. Dermatol.*, **120**, 741–743

Stampf, J. L., Benezra, C. and Asakawa, Y. (1982). Stereospecificity of allergic contact dermatitis (ACD) to enantiomers. Part III. Experimentally induced ACD to natural sesquiterpene dialdehyde polygodial in guinea pigs. *Arch. Dermatol. Res.*, **274**, 277–281

Steel, R. H. and Wilhelm, D. L. (1966). The inflammatory reaction in chemical injury, I. Increased vascular permeability and erythema induced by various chemicals. *Br. J. Exp. Pathol.*, **45**, 612–623

Steel, R. H. and Wilhelm, D. L. (1970). The inflammatory reaction in chemical injury, III. Leucocytosis and other histological changes induced by superficial injury. *Br. J. Exp. Pathol.*, **51**, 265–279

Stern, W. K. (1986). Photosensitivity: II. Testing. *Clinics Dermatol.*, **4**, 88–97

Suskind, R. R. (1977). The Environment and the skin. *Environ. Health Perspect.*, **20**, 27–44

Suskind, R. R. (1990). Environment and the skin. *Med. Clin. N. Am.* **74**, 307–324

Susten, A. S. (1985). The chronic effects of mechanical trauma to the skin: a review of the literature. *Am. J. Indust. Med.*, **8**, 281–288

Tanaka, K. (1980). Contact sensitivity in mice induced by toluene diisocyanate (TDI). *J. Dermatol.*, **7**, 277–280

Taylor, J. A. (1974). Chloracne—a continuing problem. *Cutis*, **13**, 585–591

Taylor, J. A. (1979). Environmental chloracne: update and overview. *Ann. NY Acad. Sci.*, **320**, 295–307

Tindall, J. P. (1985). Chloracne and chloracnegens. *J. Am. Acad. Dermatol.*, **13**, 539–558

Van den Heuvel, M. J. and Fielder, R. J. (1990). Acceptance of *in vitro* testing by regulatory authorities. *Toxic. In Vitro*, **4**, 675–679

Wahlberg, J. E. and Wahlberg, E. (1984). Patch test irritancy quantified by laser Doppler flowmetry. *Contact Derm.*, **11**, 257–258

Weaver, E. V., Gill, M. W., Van Miller, J. P. and Ballantyne, B. (1990). Correlation of clinical pathology and irritancy from percutaneous toxicity studies in the albino rabbit. *Toxicology*, **10**, 57

Weaver, E. V., Gill, M. W., Neptun, D. A., Hermansky, S. J., Wagner, C. L. and Ballantyne, B. (1991). Comparison of clinical pathology and irritancy from percutaneous toxicity studies in the Fischer 344 rat. *Toxicology*, **11**, 291

Weaver, E. V., Hermansky, S. J., Neptun, D. A., Losco, P. E. and Ballantyne, B. (1992). Comparison of the New Zealand White Rabbit and the Fisher 344 rat as animal models for repeated cutaneous toxicity studies. *Toxicology*, **12**, 108

Weigand, D. A. and Gaylor, J. R. (1974). Irritant reaction in Negro and Caucasian skin. *South Med. J.*, **67**, 548–551

Weil, C. S. and Scala, R. A. (1971). Study of intra- and interlaboratory variability in the results of rabbit eye and skin irritation tests. *Toxicol. Appl. Pharmacol.*, **19**, 276–360

Weiner, N. (1980). Norepinephrine, epinephrine and the sympathomimetic amines. In Gilman A. G., Goodman, L. S. and Gilman, A. (Eds), *The Pharmacological Basis of Therapeutics*, 6th edn. Macmillan Publishing Co., Inc., New York, NY, pp. 138–175

Wester, R. and Maibach, H. I. (1985). Structural activity correlations. In Maibach, H. I. and Bronaugh, R. L. (Eds), *Percutaneous Absorption*. Marcel Dekker, New York, pp. 107–123

Zesch, A. (1987). The adverse reactions of vehicles and externally applied drugs. *Acta Derm. Venereol. (Stockh.)*, **134** (Suppl.) 22–29

Zugerman, C. (1990). Chloracne. Clinical manifestations and etiology. *Dermatologic Clinics*, **8**, 209–213

FURTHER READING

Adams, R. M. (1990). *Occupational Skin Disease*. 2nd edn. W. B. Saunders Co., Philadelphia

Fenske, R. A. (1993). Dermal exposure assessment techniques. *Annals of Occupational Hygiene*, **37**, 687–706

Hobson, D. W. (1991). *Dermal and Ocular Toxicology*. CRC Press, Boca Raton, Florida

Marzuilli, F. N. and Maibach, H. (1991). *Dermatotoxicology*, 4th edn. Hemisphere Publishing Corporation, New York

31 Ototoxicity

Andrew Forge and Ernest S. Harpur

INTRODUCTION

In writing this chapter we have elected not to present a comprehensive and systematic account of the toxic effects of chemicals on the inner ear, such as can be found elsewhere (Harpur, 1986). Rather, we have attempted to present sufficient information to permit the reader, otherwise unfamiliar with this somewhat neglected aspect of toxicology, to understand ototoxic processes. In fact the ear comprises a number of morphologically distinct tissues but is often referred to as if it were just two organs—those subserving, first, the sense of hearing, and second, the sense of balance.

The term 'ototoxicity' is sometimes used to refer to the process by which chemicals, the vast majority of which are drugs, cause damage to either of these senses. We restrict its use to damage caused to the peripheral end-organs of hearing and balance in the inner ear. Although when drug-induced loss of hearing or dysequilibrium was first observed it was believed to result from injury to central pathways, it is now well established that in all known cases of ototoxic injury the lesion is in the peripheral end-organs.

We believe that an understanding of the basic structure and function of the organs of hearing and balance and of the methods which have been used, or are currently available, for their study is the *sine qua non* for full comprehension of ototoxicity. Thus, we begin with an account of the anatomy and physiology of the inner ear and then summarize techniques by which each of these may be studied. We attempt to explain why the inner ear is a selective target, focusing on the kinetics of ototoxic drugs in inner ear fluids and tissues and current understanding of the physiological and biochemical mechanisms underlying ototoxic processes.

ANATOMY AND PHYSIOLOGY OF THE INNER EAR

The inner ear, depicted in a simple diagram in Figure 1, comprises the hearing organ, the cochlea and the organs of balance, the vestibular system. It is formed of a system of membranous canals (the membranous labyrinth) enclosed in bony channels in the base of the skull. The complete enclosure of the inner ear structures within the bone means that they are not exposed directly to potentially damaging environmental agents. The bony channels forming the inner ear are filled with perilymph, which is similar in composition to cerebrospinal fluid, i.e. sodium is the predominant cation. The fluid within the membranous canals is endolymph (Figure 1). This is an unusual extracellular fluid, as it has a high potassium concentration ($\sim$140 mM). Ototoxic agents reach the inner ear predominantly through the blood supply, but access is also possible from the middle ear cavity via the membrane covering the round window at the base of the cochlea.

Neurosensory Epithelia

Vestibular System

The vestibular system consists of the three semicircular canals, organized in three mutually orthogonal planes, and two sac-like structures—the utricle and the saccule. The neuroepithelia of the vestibular system containing the sensory cells are contained in the maculae of the utricle and the saccule, and the cristae, which are located within swellings, the ampullae, at one end of each semicircular canal. The vestibular neuroepithelia are organized in two-dimensional arrays of sensory and supporting cells. There are two types of sensory 'hair' cells distinguished by their shape and innervation pattern. The functional differences between these cell types is not yet clear, but they are distributed differentially. The cells which predominate in the central regions of the neuroepithelia are designated Type 1, while the majority of cells at the periphery are Type 2s.

717

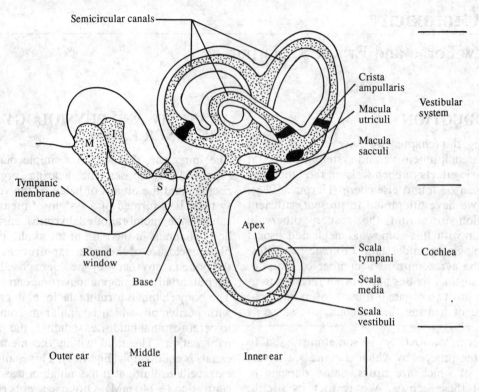

Figure 1 Schematic drawing of the middle and inner ear. Efficient transmission of airborne sound to the fluid-filled inner ear is effected by the ossicles of the middle ear, the malleus (M), incus (I) and stapes (S). The representation of the inner ear structures is highly simplified. The five sensory structures of the vestibular system—the three cristae ampullaris and the two maculae of the utricle and saccule—are shown. In the cochlea the neurosensory epithelium, or organ of Corti, rests on the basilar membrane which divides the scala tympani from the scala media

Cochlea

The cochlea is coiled in a spiral, the number of turns from base to apex varying with species. The centre of the spiral, the modiolus, contains the nerve and blood supply of the cochlea. In the cochlea the membranous canal divides the bony channel into three compartments (Figures 1 and 2): the scala vestibuli and the scala tympani, which contain perilymph, and the scala media, which contains endolymph. The scalae vestibuli and tympani connect at the apex of the cochlea. In cross-section the membranous canal is almost triangular in shape (Figure 2). Separating the scala media from the scala vestibuli is Reissner's membrane (the vestibular membrane). The partition between scala tympani and scala media is formed by the acellular basilar membrane, upon which rests the cochlear neuroepithelium, the organ of Corti. Within the organ of Corti are the sensory hair cells and various supporting cells. The hair cells are arranged in parallel rows along

the length of the spiral and again there are two types (Figure 3): a single row of inner hair cells (IHCs) and 3–5 rows (depending on the species) of outer hair cells (OHCs). In the guinea-pig, the animal most studied, on average there are approximately 2000 IHCs and 7000 OHCs along the length of the organ of Corti (Coleman, 1975; Thorne and Gavin, 1984). In man there are about 3000 IHCs and 9000 OHCs (Wright *et al.*, 1987). Overlying the organ of Corti and the hair cells is another acellular, fibrous structure, the tectorial membrane.

During sound stimulation, the stapes footplate displaces fluid along the scala vestibuli and scala tympani, resulting in displacement of the basilar membrane towards and away from the scala media. The movement of the basilar membrane leads to excitation of the sensory cells. There are a number of systematic dimensional variations of the basilar membrane and organ of Corti along the length of the spiral which affect the mechan-

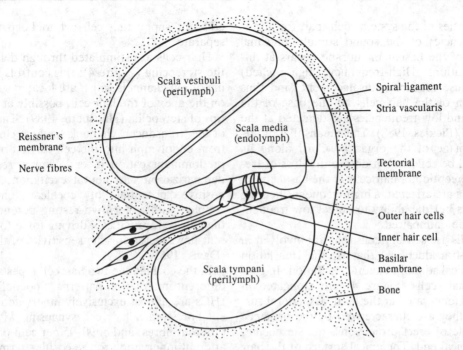

Figure 2 Simplified drawing of a transverse section through a single turn of the cochlea, illustrating the division by membranous partitions into three compartments filled either with perilymph or the potassium-rich endolymph which is formed by the ion-transporting epithelium of the stria vascularis. The neurosensory epithelium (organ of Corti) comprises the hair cells and the synaptic terminals of the auditory nerve together with various supporting cells (not shown)

Labels on figure:
Scala vestibuli (perilymph)
Spiral ligament
Stria vascularis
Scala media (endolymph)
Reissner's membrane
Nerve fibres
Tectorial membrane
Outer hair cells
Inner hair cell
Basilar membrane
Scala tympani (perilymph)
Bone

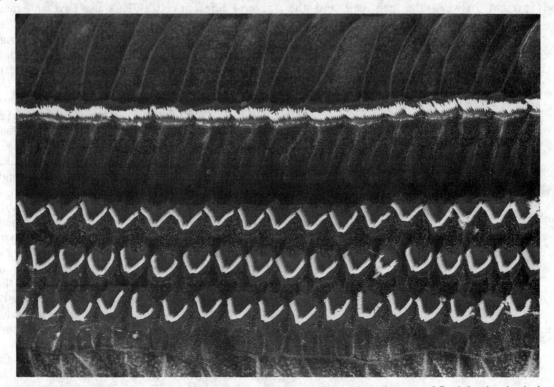

Figure 3 Scanning electron micrograph of the surface of a basal turn of the guinea-pig organ of Corti showing the single row of inner hair cells and three rows of outer hair cells with their distinctive pattern of W-shaped stereocilia. ×1200

ical properties of the system such that, for different frequencies of the sound stimuli, maximal vibration of the basilar membrane occurs at different locations. High-frequency (high-pitched) sounds cause maximum displacement, and thus stimulation of the hair cells, at the base of the cochlea, and low frequencies are detected at the apical end (Pickles, 1988). This means that differential damage of the organ of Corti along its length will be reflected in differential loss of frequency perception; if hair cells at the basal end of the cochlea are affected, a high-frequency hearing loss results but the ability to detect low frequencies may be unimpaired.

Hair cells are sensory cells that are involved in 'mechano-transduction'—that is, the translation of mechanical stimuli to neural excitation. In general the hair cells (Figure 4) are elongated in shape and innervated at the their basolateral surface, but they are characterized by the presence of a bundle of erect projections, the stereocilia, at their apical end. The apical surface of the hair cell is bathed in endolymph, into which the stereocilia project, while the body of the cell is surrounded with perilymph (Figure 5). Tight junctions present between the hair cell and the

adjacent supporting cell act to keep the fluids separate.

Hair cells are stimulated through deflection of the stereocilia (Figure 4); this controls the opening of ion channels which are located somewhere on the apex of the hair cell, possibly at the distal tips of stereocilia (Hudspeth, 1989). The opening of the 'transducer' channels leads to current flow from endolymph into the cell carried by K^+, the predominant cation in endolymph, resulting in depolarization and neural excitation. The high positive potential of cochlear endolymph, coupled with a negative resting potential inside the hair cell, provides a driving force for the current flow, increasing the sensitivity of the system (Davis, 1965)

In the cochlea the two hair cell types show very different innervation patterns (Spoendlin, 1973). IHCs are almost exclusively innervated by afferent fibres, each hair cell synapsing with several different fibres, and c. 90–95 per cent of the total afferent innervation to the cochlea terminates on IHCs. In contrast, only 5 per cent of the cochlear afferent innervation terminates on OHCs and each afferent fibre in the OHC region innervates several different cells. OHCs also have an extensive direct efferent innervation. Among IHCs, efferent nerves synapse with the afferent endings beneath the sensory cell. This innervation pattern, as well as other functional data, suggests that the IHC is the primary receptor cell for acoustic information. OHCs, on the other hand, may have a modulatory or effector role. Recording of the neural activity of individual cochlear afferent nerves in response to sound shows that each nerve is extremely sensitive to one particular frequency, its 'characteristic frequency'. This high degree of sensitivity or 'tuning' of the nerve to a particular frequency is physiologically vulnerable and it has been found that ototoxic agents which cause the loss of OHCs but leave the IHCs apparently intact also cause a loss of sharp neural tuning. It has also been shown that there is an active process associated with the tuning of the nerves which is manifested by the emission of acoustic signals from the ear in response to stimulating input sounds (otoacoustic emissions) (Kemp, 1978).

It has been shown that it is possible to isolate OHCs from the cochlea and maintain them in short-term culture (Brownell *et al.*, 1984). Such isolated OHCs have so-called 'motile' properties;

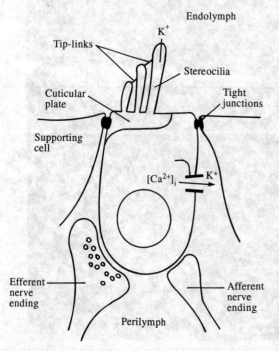

Figure 4 Generalized drawing of sensory hair cell showing the direction of K^+ flow associated with transduction

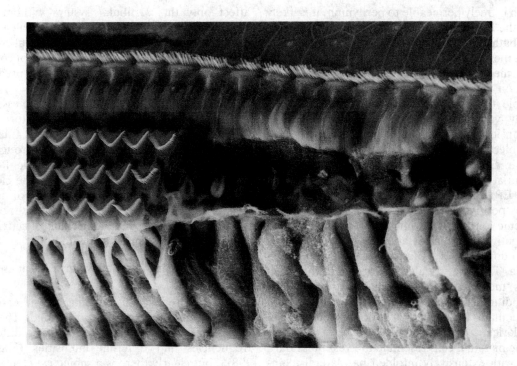

Figure 5 Basal turn of guinea-pig organ of Corti, showing the inner hair cells and, central left, the normal pattern of outer hair cells. To their right is a discrete lesion, of unknown aetiology, in which there is complete destruction of outer hair cells. The organ of Corti has fractured during processing, revealing the internal cellular architecture of the organ of Corti. On the left can be seen the cylindrical cell bodies of the third row of outer hair cells behind the supporting cells. The surfaces of the sensory and supporting cells unite to form a diffusional barrier between perilymph, which surrounds the bodies of the cells, and endolymph, which bathes their apical surfaces. In the region of hair cell loss it is seen that the supporting cells have expanded and maintained the integrity of this barrier. SEM ×1300

reversible changes in length can be elicited by a number of different conditions (Zenner *et al.*, 1985; Ashmore, 1987). It is therefore thought that OHCs *in vivo* actively modulate the movement of the basilar membrane in response to sound, leading to amplification of the signal reaching the IHC and increasing sensitivity.

Non-sensory Epithelia

In addition to the neuroepithelia there are ion-transporting epithelia in both the cochlea and the vestibular system: the stria vascularis and the dark cell regions, respectively. These are involved in the local production of endolymph and, since the apical surfaces of the sensory hair cells in both the cochlea and the vestibular system are bathed in endolymph, any agent which injures the endolymph-forming tissues will affect the trans-

duction process and reduce hair cell responsiveness to stimuli.

The dark cell regions are located around the utricular macula and at the base of the saddle-shaped cristae (but not in the saccule). They consist of a single layer of cells directly overlying connective tissue. The basolateral surfaces of the dark cells form extensive infoldings that enclose numerous mitochondria and contain high levels of Na^+/K^+-ATPase. The general morphology of dark cells is consistent with cells engaged in active ion transport and the dark cells are presumed to be directly involved in the production and maintenance of vestibular endolymph. Tight junctions between the cells separate endolymph at the apical surface of the cell from the intercellular spaces of the epithelium. As there appears to be no permeability barrier between the dark cell epithelium and the underlying connective tissue, which is freely permeable to perilymph, it is likely that the basolateral surfaces of the dark cells are also bathed in perilymph.

In the cochlea, along the lateral wall of the scala media, is located the stria vascularis. This rests on the spiral ligament, which is freely permeable to perilymph. The stria vascularis is a highly vascularized ion-transporting epithelium responsible for the maintenance of both the ionic and electrical characteristics of cochlear endolymph. Endolymph has a high positive electrical potential of 80–100 mV, the endocochlear potential (EP). This comprises two components, a highly positive potential generated by active electrogenic ion transport into the scala media, and a negative potential of about -40 mV resulting from diffusion of potassium out of the scala media. The stria vascularis is formed of three cell types: the marginal, intermediate and basal cells. In addition, and unusually for an epithelium, it also contains a complex network of intraepithelial capillaries.

The marginal cells resemble the vestibular dark cells with extensively infolded basolateral membranes on which Na^+/K^+-ATPase and adenyl cyclase are localized. Presumably they are ultimately responsible for the maintenance of endolymph. The intermediate cells are enclosed entirely within the corpus of the stria, reaching neither the apical surface nor the basal limit of the tissue. The majority of intermediate cells appear to be melanocytes in which all stages of melanogenesis can be identified. One function of these cells may be to protect the stria in periods of adverse conditions. The basal cells, which form a tight junctional network, separate the stria from the underlying spiral ligament, which is freely permeable to perilymph.

METHODS OF STUDY

Physiology and Function

Techniques for assessing the activity of the inner ear have largely been developed for the cochlea. Physiological investigation of the vestibular system is difficult to perform, especially with experimental animals, and there are no widely used sensitive tests of vestibular function. In the context of ototoxicity this is probably not a significant drawback. There are no agents known to affect only the vestibular system without also being potentially damaging to the cochlea, and chemical agents which are cochleotoxic also have effects in the vestibular system. (Noise, of course, which some define as an ototoxic agent, predominantly affects the cochlea.)

The functioning of the cochlea can be assessed at a number of different levels. Auditory cues detected by the cochlea evoke responses at higher brain centres which can be monitored through the specific reflexes which are elicited (the Preyer reflex) or by behavioural audiograms; the electrical activity associated with the passage of neural signals in the brainstem can be monitored; or the electrophysiological and biomechanical activity of the cochlea itself can be evaluated.

The Preyer Reflex and Behavioural Response Audiometry

The Preyer reflex is a twitching of the external pinna of the ear in response to sound. The test can be refined by presenting tones of different frequencies and different intensities (Harpur, 1981), but clearly there is a subjective element in determining whether there is a response and the twitching is elicited only at quite high sound pressure levels, so that quite significant losses in hearing acuity can accrue before any effect on the reflex is noticeable. This test, therefore, is not generally recommended other than to derive some crude evaluation.

More sophisticated and sensitive estimation of the ability of an animal to 'hear' can be obtained through behavioural response audiometry to derive behavioural audiograms (Stebbins *et al.*, 1981). For these, an animal is trained to perform some task when sounds are presented. The threshold of the response—that is, the lowest sound pressure level at which a response is elicited—can be determined for a number of different frequencies over the frequency range to which the animal is sensitive. Any change in the threshold concomitant with the administration of some ototoxic agent can then be evaluated. Such procedures have the advantage that repeated testing of the same animal is possible, allowing pre-administration and post-administration thresholds to be compared and the progression of alteration to be followed.

Brainstem Auditory Evoked Responses (BAER)

The stimulation of the auditory nerve following reception of a sound in the cochlea leads to successive stimulations of a number of centres along the auditory neural pathway in the brainstem to the auditory cortex. The electrical activity associated with such stimulations can be recorded with electrodes placed on the skull as a succession of waves of different amplitudes and latencies. The recording of these evoked responses is a non-invasive procedure that can potentially be used repeatedly in an individual subject (Finitzo-Hieber, 1981), thereby allowing examination of the progression of a hearing impairment following an ototoxic insult. Consequently, BAER recording is finding increasing use, although it should be pointed out that the level of sound necessary to produce a response may be somewhat higher than the actual auditory threshold, so that initial stages of a progressive hearing loss, or a relatively small impairment of hearing, may not be detectable. It has been shown that permanent increases in BAER thresholds at particular frequencies correlate with loss of hair cells at appropriate locations in the cochlea, and that it is possible to monitor transient, i.e. recoverable, changes in hearing acuity using this procedure (Schmidt *et al.*, 1990).

Physiological and Biomechanical Activities of the Cochlea

A number of different parameters of cochlear functioning can be monitored: the resting endocochlear potential, or various sound-evoked responses that derive from the activity of particular parts of the transduction pathway. Assessment of changes to each of these can be used to make some kind of differentiation of the possible locations of lesions caused by injurious agents.

(1) *Endocochlear potential (EP)* As noted above, the EP provides a driving force for current flow through the hair cells, and a decline in the level of EP decreases the sensitivity of the organ of Corti to sound stimuli and therefore results in deterioration of auditory threshold. EP can be monitored via a potassium-filled glass electrode inserted into the scala media either through the round window membrane and the basal coil of the organ of Corti, or through the lateral wall. Alterations of the EP generally reflect an effect on the stria vascularis, which is responsible for the generation and maintenance of EP.

(2) *Cochlear microphonic potential (CM)* The modulation of current flow through the hair cells during transduction is associated with an alternating extracellular electrical potential that mimics exactly the original sound stimulus, i.e. the frequency and polarity of CM follows precisely that of the stimulus (hence 'microphonic'). CM predominantly derives from the activity of the outer hair cells. By varying the frequency of the acoustic stimulus the CM originating from different regions of the cochlea can be assessed. The sound level at each frequency required to produce a constant CM output, or the amplitude of CM in relation to sound intensity at each frequency, can be measured.

(3) *Compound action potential (CAP)* Neural excitation following sound stimulation results in the generation of action potentials in the auditory nerve. The gross activity of all the neural units responding to the particular sound stimulus can be recorded remotely from electrodes placed close to the round window as the compound action potential. The CAP is a measure of the actual ultimate output from the cochlea, and consequently it has been argued that it is the most meaningful measure for rapid assessment of the functional effects of potentially ototraumatic agents (Liberman, 1990).

The recording of EP, CM and CAP are invasive techniques. In general, these procedures are used acutely and the animal has to be sacrificed after the recording has been made. This means that in examination of ototoxic agents, pre- and post-administration levels of these potentials, or the progression of any alteration, cannot be made unless this occurs over a time-period sufficiently short for the animal to be maintained under anaesthesia, which may be the case with some agents, such as diuretics, which produce acute effects on EP. It also means that determination of abnormality must be made by comparison with untreated control subjects. However, these disadvantages can be overcome by permanently implanting a round window electrode for recording CM and CAP. With such a procedure long-term, continuous electrophysiological assessment of the effects of ototoxic agents in individual conscious animals has been successfully undertaken (Aran and Darrouzet, 1975).

(4) *Otoacoustic emissions (OAEs)* As well as electrical responses, sound stimuli also elicit active mechanical responses. These are thought to derive from stimulus-induced activity of the OHCs that influences the movement of the basilar membrane. The active mechanical response leads to the emission of sounds from the ear, a 'cochlear echo' or otoacoustic emission (Kemp, 1978) that is detected in the external ear canal some microseconds after the stimulating input signal. OAEs provide a non-invasive, yet very sensitive, objective means to assess cochlear function which merely involves the insertion of a small probe consisting of a microphone and loudspeaker assembly into the external ear canal. This procedure can be used repeatedly and reproducibly in individual subjects and is finding increasing clinical application especially for testing cochlear function in new-born babies. There are a number of different types of OAE signal depending upon the stimulus parameters used and for studies of animals the most useful is the acoustic distortion product (ADP). By using a variety of stimulating frequencies, ADPs of different frequencies, i.e. emissions from different regions of the cochlea, can be obtained, enabling assessment of the active mechanical responses along the length of the cochlea. Recording of ADP has recently been shown to be a sensitive, reproducible method for assessment of ototoxic effects in the cochleae of animals (Brown *et al.*, 1989).

Structural Examinations

Examination of the inner ear structures by light or electron microscopy is widely used in assessing the effects of ototoxic agents. For the vestibular system, in the absence of reliable functional tests, such procedures may be the only ready means to evaluate ototoxic injury, and in the cochlea they allow assessment of the location and extent of lesions and correlation of this with information on functional deficits.

The most straightforward means for assessing the neuroepithelia of the inner ear is to examine the features at the surface in whole mounts of the tissue. Following fixation, either by direct perfusion using the round and oval windows to gain access to the labyrinth, or after intravital perfusion of the whole animal, the bone enclosing the inner ear is picked away and the neuroepithelia dissected out. The organ of Corti is removed in segments, usually sequentially from apex to base, which can be examined by light microscopy using either phase-contrast or differential interference contrast microscopy or, after appropriate additional processing (Davies and Forge, 1987), by scanning electron microscopy (SEM), as shown in Figures 3 and 5. Hair cells are easily recognized by their distinctive hair bundles and it becomes possible to draw up a 'cyto-cochleogram', essentially a map depicting the position of each hair cell along the entire length of the organ of Corti. The location and number of damaged or missing hair cells can then be accurately determined and related to physiological data from the same cochlea if this is available (Figure 6). In general, light microscopy is best used to quantify and map the extent of missing hair cells once the damage caused by an ototoxic agent has stabilized, although by focusing beneath the surface to examine the larger cell organelles, some assessment of possible damage to hair cells which are still present in the organ of Corti can be made. It is also possible to examine details of the stereociliary bundles using light microscopy (Liberman, 1990), but with SEM it is also possible to assess more subtle alterations at the surface of the organ of Corti. Thus, some of the earliest events in the progression of damage to the hair cells can be identified or relatively minor alterations, especially to the stereociliary bundle, which would not be visible by light microscopy but may have quite significant functional implications, can be assessed. Recently, high-resolution SEM has shown the presence of fine fibrils between stereocilia, 'tip-links', which may be intimately involved in the transduction process (Pickles *et al.*, 1984), and which may be damaged without there being any other significant alterations to the stereociliary bundle (Osborne and Comis, 1990). However, SEM only allows study of the cell surface and in some situations effects on the cell body may precede any detectable abnormalities at the apical surface (Harpur and Bridges, 1979; Forge, 1985).

These 'surface specimen techniques' can also be applied to the vestibular neuroepithelium, but phase-contrast and differential interference contrast microscopy are more difficult to apply here, because of the relative thickness of the tissue and because these tissues, particularly the cristae, are not flat. Furthermore, the sensory cells are not organized in a recognizable pattern as they are in

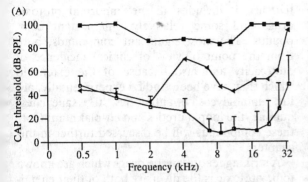

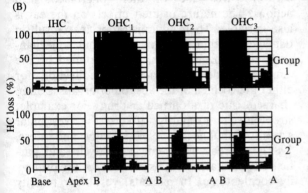

Figure 6 (A) Auditory compound action potential (CAP) thresholds in guinea-pigs, plotted as a function of the frequency of the pure tone stimuli. The control data are the mean and standard error in a population of 17 untreated animals. Also shown are individual responses in two animals, recorded 24 h following treatment with gentamicin 12 mg kg^{-1} day^{-1} for 10 days. Note that in animal 1 there is marked threshold elevation at all frequencies, whereas in animal 2 thresholds at the lowest frequencies are close to normal. (B) Hair cell loss (as a percentage of total number of hair cells) in the 2 animals with significant threshold shifts (Figure 6A). These cell counts were obtained, using light microscopy, by examining as surface preparations the entire organ of Corti dissected out in segments. Note the selective loss of outer hair cells. In animal 2, the hearing loss (Figure 6A) corresponds to loss of outer hair cells in the upper basal turn. It is clear that although the outer hair cells are present in the lower basal turn, their function is severely impaired, as indicated by the threshold elevations at very high frequencies (Figure 6A). In animal 1 the profound threshold elevation at all frequencies corresponds to extensive loss of outer hair cells in all turns except at the apex. However, even in this animal there is very little loss of inner hair cells.

the organ of Corti, and it is almost impossible to distinguish between the two types of vestibular hair cell from their surface characteristics. Thus, maps of the vestibular neuroepithelia equivalent to a cochleogram cannot be drawn up. Only a rather more general assessment of hair cell loss is possible. For more accurate determination of

the extent and location of hair cell loss it is necessary to cut serial sections for light microscopy (Aran *et al.*, 1982), where the two hair cell types can be identified from their morphology.

Sectioning is also an alternative method for examining cochlear tissues. For light microscopy, the intact cochlea is usually decalcified prior to embedding and sections of the whole cochlea in a plane parallel to the central axis of the spiral (the modiolus) are obtained. For electron microscopy it is more usual to dissect out the tissues from the cochlea prior to embedding. Sectioning has the advantage that it allows examination of tissues other than the neuroepithelium— in particular, the stria vascularis—which may be sites of action for ototoxic agents or which are affected as damage following the initial ototoxic insult progresses. Furthermore, when sections of the entire cochlea are taken, the tissues are retained in their original relationship. This allows assessment of more gross changes in tissue arrangement—for example, swelling or collapse of Reissner's membrane occurring as a consequence of interference with the mechanisms that maintain the volume of cochlear fluids. It is also possible to obtain 'cytocochleograms' from cochlear sections by examining serial sections, reconstructing the length of the cochlear spiral and determining the absolute distance from the apex or base of any particular hair cell. This technique is far more laborious than surface examination of whole mounts but is favoured in some laboratories (Liberman, 1990) because damage to hair cells can be evaluated from effects other than those occurring at the surface, and it is possible to examine the non-sensory tissues at the precise locations where hair cells are affected and thereby obtain a more integrated view of the effects of damaging agents.

The different means for assessing inner ear structure, light microscopy of whole mounts, SEM, light microscope sections and thin sections for electron microscopy, provide different kinds of information. In order to obtain as much information as possible from the limited amount of material the inner ear provides, techniques have been developed for combining some of these procedures for examination of the same piece of tissue in different ways. Thus, it is possible to embed tissue for sectioning after examination by SEM (Hunter-Duvar, 1978), or embed the whole cochlea in plastic and cut the resulting block in such a way that the surface of the organ of Corti can be viewed prior to taking transverse sections of the same regions for light or electron microscopy (Spoendlin and Brun, 1974; Liberman, 1990).

Methods to Examine the Direct Effects of Ototoxic Agents

Many studies of the effects of ototoxic agents involve examination of structure and/or function after systemic application of the agent, a situation which mimics clinical conditions. However, such a regimen has many obvious disadvantages, not least that it is difficult to separate the initial interaction of the agent from the ensuing sequelae.

Perfusion of the fluid spaces of the inner ear with ototoxic substances provides one means of assessing direct effects (Nuttall, 1981; Bobbin and Ceasar, 1987). In an anaesthetized animal, the cochlea is exposed and two small holes are made in the bony wall over the perilymphatic scalae. A solution of salts of similar composition to perilymph and containing the substance under study is gently pumped into the cochlea through one hole and flows out from the other. The effects can be determined by simultaneous monitoring of CM, CAP and/or OAE, and the reaction can be terminated at some specified point to examine the attendant structural correlates by perfusion of fixative.

Examination of the direct effects of ototoxic agents at a cellular level is also possible. Recently procedures have been developed for isolating hair cells from the cochlea (Brownell *et al.*, 1984; Zajic and Schacht, 1987) or vestibular system and maintaining them in short-term culture, and for culturing explants of the developing organ of Corti (Richardson and Russell, 1991). These systems allow direct access to the hair cells and examination of the immediate effects of ototoxic agents by physiological, biochemical and cell biological methods. Increasingly such approaches are being adopted in efforts to understand the molecular basis of the interaction of ototoxic agents with the sensory cells of the inner ear.

OTOTOXIC DRUGS

Many drugs are known to be toxic to the inner ear (Table 1). Although Table 1 is not an exhaustive list, it includes all the important ototoxic drugs and some relatively unimportant compounds. The most significant compounds, both from the point of view of clinical incidence of ototoxicity and also because of the extent to which they have been studied experimentally, are the aminoglycoside antibiotics, the salicylates, quinine, the loop diuretics and *cis*-platinum. Only these compounds will be discussed further in this chapter.

A striking feature of the drugs which are known to be ototoxic is the diversity both of their chemical structures and of their pharmacological actions. The nature of their effects on the ear is also variable. Their administration may result in damage to either auditory or vestibular mechanisms, or both. However, as exemplified by the aminoglycoside antibiotics, a predilection for either the cochlea or the vestibular organs is often characteristic of a particular drug. For example, streptomycin primarily affects the vestibular system (Schuknecht, 1957; Walby and Kerr, 1982), whereas neomycin, kanamycin and particularly amikacin (Cazals *et al.*, 1983) are primarily cochleotoxic. In patients, vestibular toxicity can give rise to symptoms such as dizziness or vertigo and can be objectively detected as a decrease in the nystagmic response (eye movements) induced by caloric or rotational stimulation of the vestibular end-organs. Although the lesion may be permanent, most subjects can adequately compensate with time for the loss of vestibular function.

Auditory effects range from potentially transient symptoms such as diplacusis, tinnitus or a mild reduction in auditory acuity to total and permanent deafness. Salicylates and other nonsteroidal anti-inflammatory agents commonly cause tinnitus which is reversible when the drug is stopped and is only rarely associated with permanent hearing loss (Chapman, 1982). Therapeutic doses of quinine characteristically cause tinnitus, but excessive doses of quinine or chloroquine may result in permanent deafness (Toone *et al.*, 1965; McKenzie *et al.*, 1968). Large intravenous doses of the loop diuretics such as ethacrynic acid or frusemide (furosemide) may cause a transient hearing impairment, although the deafness may be permanent (Rybak, 1988), particularly if the patient is uraemic or is also administered an aminoglycoside antibiotic (Mathog and Klein, 1969). The anti-tumour drug *cis*-platinum

Table 1 Compounds known to be causes of or implicated in ototoxicity[a]

Classification	Compounds
Systemic administration	
Antibiotics	
Aminoglycosides	Amikacin, dibekacin, dihydrostreptomycin, framycetin, gentamicin, kanamycin, neomycin, netilmicin, paromomycin, ribostamycin, sisomicin, streptomycin, tobramycin
Others	Ampicillin, capreomycin, chloramphenicol, colistin (polymyxin E), erythromycin, minocycline, polymyxin B, rifampicin, vancomycin, viomycin
Anti-inflammatory agents	Fenoprofen, ibuprofen, indomethacin, naproxen, phenylbutazone, **salicylates**
Antimalarials	Chloroquine, **quinine**
Antitumour agents	
Cytotoxics	Actinomycin, bleomycin, ***cis*-platinum**, nitrogen mustards (e.g. mustine)
Hypoxic cell radiosensitizers	Misonidazole
Beta-blockers	Practolol, propranolol
Contraceptives	Medroxyprogesterone
Loop diuretics	Bumetanide, ethacrynic acid, frusemide (furosemide), piretanide
Tricyclic antidepressants	Imipramine
Topical application in the middle ear *(absorption through the round window membrane)*	
Quaternary ammonium compounds	Benzalkonium chloride, benzethonium chloride, chlorhexidine
Iodine disinfectants	Iodine–potassium iodide (Lugol's) solution in 70 per cent alcohol, iodophor (Iodopax) solution in 70 per cent alcohol, povidone–iodine solution and scrub
Others	Bonain's solution (cocaine, phenol and thymol), formaldehyde–gelatin (absorbable gelatin sponge), lignocaine

[a] The compounds discussed in this chapter are shown in bold type.

frequently causes tinnitus and permanent hearing loss which appears to be dose-related (Vermorken *et al.*, 1983).

Hearing loss induced by aminoglycosides may develop suddenly during therapy or, more commonly, the onset can be gradual and progress even after dosage has been discontinued. On occasions the hearing loss may not even appear until some time after the drug administration has stopped. With the progressive permanent lesions which are a feature of aminoglycoside and *cis*-platinum ototoxicity, audiometric assessment reveals a hearing loss which is initially confined to high frequencies (Fausti *et al.*, 1984), but which eventually may involve frequencies in the speech range and result in a permanent disability. The degree of vestibular or auditory impairment with aminoglycosides may depend upon the drug itself, the unit or total dose, the route and period of administration and the patient's age or pathological state; for example, the risk is substantially increased by impaired renal function (Jackson and Arcieri, 1971). The situation is further complicated in that the aminoglycosides, to varying degrees, and *cis*-platinum are nephrotoxic. For an extensive review of risk factors associated with ototoxicity, see Harpur (1986).

Location and Nature of Ototoxic Lesions

Cochlea

Histopathological studies of the lesions in the inner ear of animals have contributed much to our understanding of drug-induced ototoxicity. Permanent hearing loss caused by ototoxic drugs such as the aminoglycoside antibiotics and *cis*-platinum always seems to be associated with loss of hair cells in the organ of Corti. Although effects are somewhat variable between drugs and between species of animals (Harpur, 1987), it has usually been found that the cochlear lesion originates in the first row of outer hair cells of the basal turn of the organ of Corti (Wersall, 1981). The damage then progresses to affect the other rows of outer hair cells, and to involve cells near the apex of the cochlea. The inner hair cells are usually damaged only in regions where there is extensive loss of outer hair cells (McDowell, 1982). In agreement with clinical findings, this progression of hair cell damage is paralleled by a hearing loss which is initially confined to high frequencies (Stebbins *et al.*, 1981), but eventually may involve all frequencies. The hair cells in the organ of Corti are, in general, much more sensitive to damage than the supporting cells (Wersall, 1981). In this context, it is interesting to note that the selective vulnerability of the hair cells compared with the supporting cells is preserved when cultures of the organ of Corti are directly exposed to ototoxic agents *in vitro* (Richardson and Russell, 1991). Degeneration of the neural innervation of the organ of Corti is a secondary event, following the death of the hair cells (Hawkins and Johnsson, 1981; Wersall, 1981).

The stria vascularis is now known to be the primary site in the cochlea for the ototoxic action of the loop diuretics. Intravenous administration of ethacrynic acid or frusemide to guinea-pigs and rats causes transient morphological changes in the stria vascularis, the time-course of which parallels the loss and recovery of electrical activity in the cochlea (Brummett *et al.*, 1977; Bosher, 1980a, b; Pike and Bosher, 1980). It is not known whether the hair cell loss in the organ of Corti produced by high doses or repetitive administration of ethacrynic acid (Mathog *et al.*, 1970; Johnsson and Hawkins, 1972; Crifo, 1973) results from a direct action on hair cells or is secondary to prolonged changes in the stria vascularis.

It has also been postulated that the degeneration of hair cells in the organ of Corti caused by aminoglycosides may occur secondary to drug effects on other tissues in the cochlea, notably the spiral ligament, the stria vascularis, Reissner's membrane or the region of the outer sulcus (Haw-

kins *et al.*, 1972; Johnsson and Hawkins, 1972; Hawkins, 1973). However, the exact time sequences of the damage to these tissues and hair cell degeneration is not known (Hawkins, 1973), so that a cause-and-effect relationship is speculative. Certainly, direct damage to hair cells by ototoxic drugs cannot be excluded.

It is apparent from animal studies that co-administration of a loop diuretic with an aminoglycoside antibiotic produces greatly augmented cochlear damage compared with that caused by the loop diuretic alone. Administration of a large intravenous dose of ethacrynic acid or frusemide shortly before a single, non-ototoxic dose of kanamycin rapidly produces depression of cochlear function which is permanent and associated with extensive hair cell destruction (West *et al.*, 1973; Brummett *et al.*, 1975). The interaction also occurs with other loop diuretics, such as bumetanide and piretanide, but not with diuretics which have a different mechanism of action, such as hydrochlorazide or mannitol (Brummett *et al.*, 1974). All aminoglycoside antibiotics have been found to interact with the loop diuretics (Brummett, 1981a), as have the non-aminoglycoside, ototoxic antibiotics viomycin and polymixin B (Davis *et al.*, 1982) and the anti-tumour drug *cis*-platinum (Brummett, 1981b).

Vestibular System

In the vestibular system damage is seen initially in the hair cells of the cristae ampullaris and then progresses to affect cells on the sides of the cristae (Wersall, 1981). The most vulnerable cells are the Type 1 sensory cells, although in more severe lesions the Type 2 cells are also destroyed. Degeneration of the cells in the macula utriculi and macula sacculi occurs at a later stage. As in the cochlea, the supporting cells and nerve fibres survive the hair cells but eventually they too may be destroyed (Wersall, 1981).

THE BASES OF SELECTIVITY FOR THE INNER EAR

Selective Distribution — Pharmacokinetics

The reason why a number of therapeutic agents are selectively toxic to the inner ear has been the focus of much attention. However, despite extensive study, particularly of the aminoglycosides, it remains essentially unexplained. One of the earliest hypotheses for the selective ototoxic effect of the aminoglycoside antibiotics was their preferential accumulation in inner ear fluids. They are polycationic hydrophilic molecules and are eliminated from the body in an unchanged state, almost exclusively through the kidneys. Their nephrotoxic potential is attributable, at least in part, to the very high concentrations they achieve in the renal cortex (Kaloyanides and Pastoriza-Munoz, 1980). Studies have been conducted in animals to examine a possible relationship between ototoxicity and the concentration of aminoglycosides in the fluids and tissues of the cochlea.

The relevance of the presence of a drug in perilymph or endolymph for a toxic effect on the hair cells can be deduced from inspection of Figures 2 and 5. The intercellular spaces surrounding the hair cells of the organ of Corti (Figure 5) are filled with a fluid identical with and continuous with perilymph. A drug present in the perilymph of the scala tympani would readily penetrate the basilar membrane (Masuda *et al.*, 1971) and gain access to the lateral membranes of the hair cells and the synaptic regions at their base. The principal boundaries between endolymph and perilymph, formed by selectively permeable membranes and tight junctions between adjacent cells, appear to be Reissner's membrane, the lateral wall of the scala media (notably the stria vascularis) and the network formed by the apical surfaces of the hair cells and adjacent supporting cells in the organ of Corti. Penetration of a drug into endolymph across these boundaries would be a prerequisite for access to the hair-bearing (apical) ends of the hair cells. However, if the aminoglycosides exert their effect directly on the hair cells, it is not known whether this takes place at the apical membranes or the basolateral membranes of the cells.

Perilymph Kinetics

The only consistent findings of the various studies in animals are that the peak concentration after extravascular injection occurs much later in perilymph (about 4 h) than in serum (about 15–30 min) and that the disappearance of the drug initially occurs more slowly from perilymph. For example, the disappearance half-life ($t_{1/2}$) of kanamycin from guinea-pig perilymph was 15 h, compared with 80 min in serum (Stupp *et al.*, 1973).

A number of other early findings have not been borne out by subsequent studies. It was originally claimed (Voldrich, 1965; Stupp *et al.*, 1973) that, after single doses, aminoglycosides achieved very high concentrations in perilymph, in contrast to other organs; that the perilymph kinetics were non-linear (i.e. there was a disproportionate increase in perilymph concentration with increasing dose); that the penetration into, and the long $t_{1/2}$ in, perilymph was peculiar to ototoxic drugs; that there was a correlation between ototoxic potential and $t_{1/2}$ in perilymph; and that after multiple doses the long $t_{1/2}$ in perilymph is the determinant of accumulation in perilymph. More recent evidence from carefully controlled studies suggests that none of these claims are tenable. Most workers have found that even with very high doses of aminoglycosides the peak concentration in perilymph is about an order of magnitude below the peak concentration in serum (Toyoda and Tachibana, 1978; Harpur *et al.*, 1981), which is turn is less than the peak concentration in the kidney (Toyoda and Tachibana, 1978). Furthermore, perilymph kinetics are linear, at least for gentamicin (Federspil, 1981) and ribostamycin (Harpur *et al.*, 1981).

Penetration into perilymph and a long $t_{1/2}$ there is apparently not a unique feature of aminoglycosides (Federspil, 1981). Brummett and Fox (1982) reported no differences in the single-dose kinetics of a number of aminoglycosides to explain differences in their ototoxic potential, but after multiple dosing differences were seen in the extent of accumulation in perilymph. It is important to distinguish between the accumulation in perilymph resulting from impaired renal elimination rather than local effects on the ear. Thus, in any study of aminoglycoside kinetics after multiple dosing, it is necessary to measure renal function or to measure serum accumulation as well as perilymph accumulation.

The situation is complicated in that most aminoglycosides are nephrotoxic and their nephrotoxic potential does not necessarily parallel their ototoxic potential. After multiple dosing of guinea-pigs for 4 weeks all aminoglycosides studied, except netilmicin, accumulated in serum and all accumulated in perilymph, although netilmicin accumulated to a much smaller extent than others. Brummett *et al.* (1978) found netilmicin to be less ototoxic than gentamicin and concluded that the major factor limiting the ototoxic action of netilmicin was its lack of accumulation in the cochlea. They attributed accumulation of gentamicin to a greater degree of nephrotoxicity with this drug. However, Brummett and Fox (1982) showed for a number of aminoglycosides that there was no direct correspondence between accumulation in plasma and in perilymph. Furthermore, the extent of accumulation in perilymph did not relate to the ototoxic potencies of the drugs. For example, Fox *et al*. (1980) showed that gentamicin C_1 was less ototoxic than gentamicin, although their perilymph concentrations after long-term treatment were the same. They therefore attributed the lesser ototoxicity of gentamicin C_1 compared with gentamicin to a difference in intrinsic toxic potency (Fox *et al*., 1980).

Most workers have relied on comparison of the peak level after a single dose and after multiple dosing to determine the extent of accumulation (Brummett and Fox, 1982), despite the fact that the time of peak level may change after multiple dosing (Toyoda and Tachibana, 1978; Harpur and Gonda, 1982). Harpur and Gonda (1982) studied the full kinetic profile of ribostamycin in perilymph and serum after a single dose and after the last of 14 multiple doses under conditions of unchanged renal function. There was no accumulation of the drug in perilymph despite a long $t_{1/2}$ (15 h) after a single dose. This was attributable to a marked increase in the rate of transfer from perilymph to serum after multiple dosing. It was the first time any evidence was presented for such a change. Hawkins (1973) has discussed evidence that aminoglycosides damage the capillaries and pericapillary tissue in the lateral wall of cochlea. However, knowledge of perilymph flow in the cochlea and potential sites for elimination of exogenous molecules from cochlea fluids is insufficient to permit any further theory to be formed about how aminoglycosides could increase or reduce their own elimination from perilymph.

Endolymph Kinetics

Some early reports (Stupp *et al*., 1973; Federspil, 1981) suggested that the concentration of aminoglycosides in guinea-pig endolymph, after a single dose, is similar to that found in perilymph. However, collection of endolymph which is uncontaminated by either perilymph or blood is very difficult and these early studies were almost certainly technically flawed. Watanabe *et al*. (1971), on the other hand, found no kanamycin in endolymph after a single dose or even after multiple dosing for 1 week, when levels in perilymph had accumulated 4–5-fold. After 2 weeks of multiple dosing a small amount of drug was detectable in endolymph, at which time electrophysiological changes were also present. It cannot, therefore, be concluded that the presence of kanamycin in endolymph accounted for the electrophysiological changes, since one or more effects of the drug might have caused these changes and simultaneously increased the permeability of the scala media to kanamycin—that is, they may have been coincident but independent occurrences. Tran Ba Huy *et al*. (1981, 1983b) studied the kinetics of gentamicin in endolymph and perilymph during and after constant infusions of the drug. Although the drug was detectable in perilymph 45 min after the start of an infusion and continued to rise for up to 48 h, no drug was detectable in endolymph until after 10 h and this showed very little further accumulation. After a 48 h infusion the drug persisted in endolymph for up to 15 days without significantly declining. It was thought that the slow elimination of the drug might be accounted for by slow release of the drug from binding sites in cochlear tissues such as the stria vascularis and the organ of Corti.

Kinetics in Cochlear Tissues

It has been suggested (Desrochers and Schacht, 1982) that the crucial sites for determining ototoxicity are the cochlear tissues, not the perilymph. However, studies of the distribution of radiolabelled dihydrostreptomycin within the cochlea (Balogh *et al*., 1970; Nilsson Tammela and Tjalve, 1986) do not suggest that selective toxicity can be explained by selective tissue localization of the drug. Furthermore, chronic administration of neomycin to guinea-pigs produced a very high concentration of the drug in renal tissue compared with levels in the organ of Corti and stria vascularis, which were approximately equal and no greater than levels in the heart, liver, lung or spleen—tissues which do not show toxicity (Desrochers and Schacht, 1982).

The possibility that ototoxicity correlates better with the levels of the drug in inner ear tissues than inner ear fluids has prompted several recent investigations. Tran Ba Huy *et al*. (1986) found that, in contrast to other tissues which do not show toxicity, uptake of gentamicin in inner ear tissues and the renal cortex were both rapid and saturable. However, the ratio between gentamicin concentrations in the inner ear tissues and those in plasma was always less than unity. Redistribution of the drug into secondary cellular compartments was evidenced by the complex multiphase elimination kinetics. The half-lives of elimination from cochlear tissues were extremely long, varying from 10 h to 30 days, depending on the duration of drug administration. It was felt that redistribution of the drug into susceptible cells or cellular compartments was an important factor in the development of the delayed toxicity.

Some aminoglycoside antibiotics are more cochleotoxic than vestibulotoxic, and vice versa. The possibility that this could result from selective distribution into the affected tissue has been tested. Tran Ba Huy and Deffrennes (1988) thought that the predilection of gentamicin to affect the vestibular apparatus was explained by a greater affinity for vestibular than cochlear tissues. However, they obtained their data *in vitro* using homogenates of organ of Corti and vestibular maculae. *In vivo* pharmacokinetic studies (Dulon *et al.*, 1986) of a number of drugs with varying vestibulotoxic and cochleotoxic potentials indicate that their toxicity is not related to different tissue concentrations. Dulon *et al.* (1986) found similar cochlear and vestibular drug levels for amikacin, gentamicin and netilmicin—drugs which exhibit quite different cochleotoxic and vestibulotoxic potentials. However, it should be remembered that the tissues that were examined are heterogeneous and the possibility of selective uptake in specific cell populations cannot be discounted. Tran Ba Huy and Deffrennes (1988) have also studied the binding of gentamicin to tissue homogenates prepared from organ of Corti taken from either the base or the apex of the cochlea. They found no difference in uptake into the two tissues and concluded that this was not a basis for the selective vulnerability of tissues at the base of the cochlea.

Kinetics of Aminoglycoside–Loop Diuretic Interactions

Orsulakova and Schacht (1981) studied the distribution of radiolabelled ethacrynic acid in the mouse cochlea. Ethacrynic acid was present mainly in the stria vascularis but prior administration of neomycin increased the ethacrynic acid content of both endolymph and cochlear tissues. The increase in the concentration of ethacrynic acid in tissues caused by neomycin was thought to result from an effect of neomycin on membrane integrity and cellular permeability. It was also thought to explain the ototoxic potentiation which occurs when the two drugs are administered together.

An alternative hypothesis is that ethacrynic acid markedly increases the penetration of gentamicin into endolymph (Tran Ba Huy *et al.*, 1983a). Since aminoglycosides seem to penetrate very slowly into endolymph when administered on their own, the increased penetration into endolymph in the presence of ethacrynic acid could explain the very rapid development of hair cell damage after administration of aminoglycoside–loop diuretic combinations.

Summary

The concentrations of aminoglycosides achieved in the fluids and tissues of the inner ear are not high compared, for example, with the kidney. Although long half-lives have been demonstrated in cochlear fluids and tissues, accumulation following multiple dosing is variable and, in the absence of renal impairment, is modest (Toyoda and Tachibana, 1978; Harpur *et al.*, 1981). Penetration of aminoglycosides into endolymph is delayed and might be an important determinant of toxicity to the hair cells. Brummett and Fox (1982) pointed out that the concentration of aminoglycosides in perilymph associated with complete hair cell destruction following chronic drug administration, was 5/1000 the cytotoxic drug concentration *in vitro*. They concluded that the cytotoxic effect of aminoglycosides on the hair cells is highly selective and not simply a result of preferential accumulation of the drug in perilymph. In the absence of a clear relationship between ototoxicity and the concentration of drug in perilymph or cochlear tissues, a knowledge of pharmacokinetics in the cochlea does not at present satisfactorily explain this selective organ toxicity.

Physiological and Biochemical Mechanisms

Aminoglycosides

Aminoglycosides are positively charged molecules which would not normally be expected to cross the cell membrane. Their toxic side-effects are also quite specific. Besides the inner ear, only the kidney and the neuromuscular junction are affected, and in the inner ear itself it is the sensory cells—particularly, the outer hair cells—which are vulnerable. Consequently, any hypothesis which attempts to explain the ototoxic nature of these drugs must take these factors into account.

It has been suggested that aminoglycosides interfere with glucose uptake and/or metabolism in the organ of Corti. It has been reported that there is less glycogen in the outer hair cells of the basal turn of the cochlea, the region most susceptible to aminoglycoside damage, than in the more apical hair cells, and that there is a depletion of glycogen granules, as assessed from electron microscopy of thin sections, after aminoglycoside treatment. However, this idea does not explain the specific nature of the ototoxic action *vis à vis* other tissues. There is no evidence that carbohydrate metabolism is any different in the organ of Corti from elsewhere in the body. Furthermore, it provides no indication of how the drug might enter the cell to inhibit intracellular biochemistry.

From early morphological studies of aminoglycoside ototoxicity it was concluded that one of the initial effects of the drug was to cause fusion of stereocilia (Wersall, 1981). Consequently, it was suggested that the stereocilia may be a primary site of drug action, the cationic aminoglycoside disrupting the negatively charged cell coat over the stereociliary surface, enabling the membranes of adjacent stereocilia to come closely together, so leading to their fusion. More recently, a loss of the stereociliary glycocalyx of cochlear hair cells soon after systemic administration of aminoglycoside has been reported (De Groot and Veldman, 1988). However, this effect was similar on both outer and inner hair cells, whereas it is outer hair cells that are preferentially lost from the organ of Corti following aminoglycoside treatment. Furthermore, during aminoglycoside-induced hair cell degeneration, extensive alterations to the cell body may precede obvious

morphological effects at the apical surface (Harpur and Bridges, 1979; Forge, 1985).

Nevertheless, acute effects of aminoglycosides at the apical surface of hair cells have been demonstrated directly in the lateral line systems of fish and reptiles (which contain hair cells phylogenetically related to those in the mammalian inner ears), and in cultured explants of the mammalian organ of Corti. Here two separate effects of the direct application of aminoglycosides have been identified: an increase in stereociliary stiffness which is dependent upon the presence of calcium and may involve some interaction at the membrane surface, and a blocking of the transduction channels (which may be located at the tips of the stereocilia—Hudspeth, 1989), which is inhibited by calcium. However, both these effects are reversible, their occurrence does not coincide with any obvious hair cell degeneration and they do not appear to affect one hair cell type preferentially. Hair cell degeneration in the cultured explants occurs at much higher concentrations of the drug (*c.* 1 mM) than those at which reversible effects on the stereocilia occur (*c.* 50 μM), and is preceded by the formation of large membranous blisters at the cell apex. The formation of these blisters, which rapidly follows the application of the drug at this higher concentration, suggests some effect on lipid metabolism. Thus, while aminoglycosides potentially may act at the stereocilia and/or transduction channels, it is thought that these actions are probably independent of those which produce hair cell degeneration.

The most complete hypothesis to date to account for the ototoxicity of the aminoglycosides envisages a specific, irreversible interaction of the drug with a particular cell membrane phospholipid, phosphatidylinositol 4′,5′-bisphosphate (PhIP$_2$) (Schacht, 1986). This phospholipid is a 'second messenger' molecule that activates a cascade of intracellular biochemical pathways involved in the control of intracellular calcium levels. Although it is present in the membranes of most cells, neural tissues, including the ear, and the kidney, show a much more active metabolism of phosphoinositides than do other tissues such as the liver or lung, and it has been demonstrated *in vivo* that neomycin inhibits the turnover of phosphoinositides in both the kidney and the inner ear. From *in vitro* studies of lipid bilayers and monolayers it has also been shown that the interaction of the aminoglycosides with PhIP$_2$ is qualitatively different from their interaction with other anionic phospholipids and that they bind irreversibly. In addition, the extent to which different aminoglycosides alter the surface pressure of monomolecular films of $PhIP_2$, a measure of how well each one binds, correlates with the 'intrinsic' ototoxicity of each as determined by the concentration of drug perfused into the perilymph that is necessary to depress CM potential: e.g. neomycin has the greatest effect on surface pressure and is the most effective in suppressing CM, while amikacin is less 'ototoxic' and causes much less disturbance of the phospholipid monolayer.

Although $PhIP_2$ seems a likely candidate as a specific binding site for aminoglycosides in the inner ear, this alone cannot completely explain aminoglycoside ototoxicity. The phospholipid is located on the inner leaflet of the plasma membrane, so the drug has to cross the membrane to reach it. Other experiments using perfusion of the cochlea have indicated that there may be an initial, reversible, calcium-inhibited step, and that an energy-dependent process precedes irreversible binding. A three-stage process to describe the interaction of aminoglycosides with the hair cell has therefore been proposed (Schacht, 1986). First, there is an initial reversible binding of the drug, possibly to anionic phospholipids exposed at the extracellular surface of the membrane. Second, an energy-dependent step by which the drug crosses the membrane. Third, a specific irreversible binding to $PhIP_2$. Once the drug is bound, those reactions dependent upon phosphoinositide turnover would be inhibited. In addition, the interaction with membrane phospholipids may also affect membrane permeability, enabling the subsequent direct entry of the drug into the cell. Once inside, the drug could have effects on various cell processes, including, for example, carbohydrate metabolism.

These effects of aminoglycosides have been determined from *in vitro* studies with phospholipids and with intact cochleae. More recently competitive binding between calcium and neomycin, energy-dependent uptake of the drug and binding to $PhIP_2$ have all been demonstrated in isolated outer hair cells, which indicates that these aspects of the process apply to the presumed cochlear target cell for the aminoglycosides. They have also been demonstrated in the vestibular neuroepithelia *in vitro*. It has also been shown that $PhIP_2$ is involved in the active motile responses of outer hair cells, and it has been suggested that it is the second messenger system through which the direct efferent nerve supply to the outer hair cells acts. There may therefore be a much higher level of $PhIP_2$ metabolism in outer than in inner hair cells, which would account for differential susceptibilities, but there is no direct evidence for this.

However, turnover of $PhIP_2$ has not been demonstrated as an early event after systemic application of the drug. It has also been found that when isolated hair cells are incubated with gentamicin, cell viability is unimpaired (Dulon *et al.*, 1989). This may imply that additional, as yet unidentified factors, are involved in the ototoxic response. It has been reported very recently that isolated hair cells can be killed with gentamicin that has been exposed to a drug-metabolizing extract from liver cells (Huang and Schacht, 1990), which suggests that a product of aminoglycoside metabolism rather than the drug itself might in fact be the active agent, but it is generally considered that aminoglycosides are excreted from the body without being metabolized and the putative metabolite has not been characterized, nor has its *in vivo* ototoxic potential been assessed. As yet, therefore, the *in vivo* ototoxicity of the aminoglycosides is not fully understood.

cis-Platinum

cis-Platinum (*cis*-dichlorodiammine platinum II or *cis*-DDP), like the aminoglycosides, is a highly charged molecule. It, too, is nephrotoxic as well as ototoxic. It induces a progressive loss of hair cells, the extent of which correlates with the dose of drug administered (Hoeve *et al.*, 1988), that occurs following repeated injections of relatively low drug doses (1 mg kg^{-1} daily) administered by intramuscular, intraperitoneal or subcutaneous routes, and after a single intravenous high dose (10–12.5 mg kg^{-1}) (Laurell and Engstrom, 1989b; Laurell and Bagger-Sjoback, 1991a,b). The pattern of hair cell damage in the cochlea also resembles that of the aminoglycosides, with outer hair cells in the basal turn preferentially affected.

As yet, however, there is no consistent idea of the basis of *cis*-DDP's ototoxicity. It has been reported (McAlpine and Johnstone, 1990) that a rapid deterioration in the auditory nerve response threshold is produced when *cis*-DDP is present in the scala media at concentrations of about 5 μM, but no effect is apparent with perilymphatic perfusion at drug concentrations of less than 3 mM. This suggests that one possible site of the drug action is at the apical end of the hair cells, and from other characteristics of the response to a single systemic administration it has been concluded that the drug blocks transduction channels. However, as with similar experiments with aminoglycosides, it is difficult from these results to explain differential effects on inner and outer hair cells. Nor is it known whether and how they might be related to hair cell degeneration. In recent studies (Saito *et al.*, 1991) incubation of isolated hair cells with concentrations of *cis*-DPP as high as 1 mM for up to 6 h did not impair cell viability. Thus, at present neither the site of drug action nor the mechanisms that cause cell death are known.

Salicylates

Salicylates produce a loss of hearing sensitivity and tinnitus (the perception of sound in the absence of acoustic signals, or 'ringing in the ears'). These effects are almost entirely reversible, disappearing with termination of the drug administration.

Early experimental studies indicated that one action of salicylates was upon the cochlear blood supply. Constriction of the vessels in the spiral ligament, stria vascularis and the vessels lying beneath the basilar membrane was observed after systemic administration (Hawkins, 1976). This may occur as a consequence of the effects of salicylate upon prostaglandin synthesis. It has therefore been argued that the acute suppression of the CAP, also reported to occur after salicylate treatment, may be related to a salicylate-induced ischaemia. However, there has been no consistent explanation put forward as to precisely how such an effect might produce a relatively specific effect on CAP. Moreover, an interference with the blood supply to the stria might be expected to lead to a diminution of the EP, which declines rapidly during anoxia, but EP does not appear to be affected by salicylates (Puel *et al*, 1989; Stypulkowski, 1990). Although effects on the vasculature should not be discounted, and may be a confounding factor, there is at present more compelling evidence that salicylates act directly upon the outer hair cells. Indeed, the studies from which this conclusion derives provide an excellent illustration of how the different techniques for

examination of the cochlea can be used to delineate the site of drug action.

Salicylates are known to enter perilymph rapidly after administration. Potentially, therefore, they might act on the bodies of inner or outer hair cells, the synapses, or the nerves, all of which are directly exposed to perilymph, but histological examination of the cochlea after systemic drug treatment has shown abnormalities to occur specifically in outer hair cells (Douek *et al.*, 1983). In addition, otoacoustic emissions, which derive from the active responses of outer hair cells, are reversibly suppressed in humans after aspirin ingestion (Long *et al.*, 1986; Martin *et al.*, 1988), and acoustic distortion products have been shown to be depressed in experimental studies in animals (Stypulkowski, 1990). CM is also affected, although it has been variously reported to be depressed (Puel *et al.*, 1990) or to rise (Stypulkowski, 1990). Furthermore, following systemic administration (Stypulkowski, 1990) and with perilymphatic perfusion (Puel *et al.*, 1989, 1990) CAP responses to low-intensity stimulation are suppressed but those to high-intensity signals are unaffected. This, too, suggests an effect on the OHC, as the CAP response to signals of low intensity is thought to be elicited after amplification of the signal reaching the IHC through the active processes associated with the outer hair cell (Kim, 1986). It has also been demonstrated *in vitro* that the fast motile responses of isolated OHCs that are normally elicited by electrical stimulation are reversibly inhibited by salicylate.

This last observation suggests that, *in vitro* at least, salicylates affect the OHCs directly. This is probably also the case *in vivo*. As noted above, EP is not affected after systemic administration or with perilymphatic perfusion of salicylate (Puel *et al.*, 1990; Stypulkowski, 1990), which indicates that the observed depression of OHC function is not an indirect effect of a reduction in the driving current to the hair cells. Furthermore, although it is well known that salicylates inhibit prostaglandin synthesis, the perilympathic perfusion of agents which are more potent than salicylates in this regard do not affect cochlear function (Puel *et al.*, 1990).

It is therefore considered that salicylates may interact directly at the basolateral membrane of the OHCs, leading to inhibition of the active mechanical response. Salicylates are known to affect membrane permeability—in particular, causing an increase in K^+ and decrease in Cl^- conductance—and it has been argued (Stypulkowski, 1990) that this occurs in the cochlea. Numerous K^+ channels have been localized to the basolateral membrane of the OHC (Ashmore and Meech, 1986). There is, however, no direct evidence that salicylates have any action upon these.

While an action of salicylates on the active processes of the outer hair cells would produce the observed loss in hearing sensitivity, it is not clear whether the tinnitus that also occurs is a separate or a related phenomenon. Some clinical evidence suggests that tinnitus is the more prevalent effect and does not always coincide with hearing loss. It has been shown that following systemic salicylate administration there is an increase in the spontaneous firing rate of auditory neurones (Evans and Borerwe, 1982), i.e. neural stimulation in the absence of an acoustic signal. As salicylate enters perilymph, it has access to and could act directly upon the afferent nerve synapses, but in other systems salicylates usually decrease and eventually block neural excitation (Neto, 1980). Furthermore, it is neurons which respond normally to high frequencies that are affected (Evans and Borerwe, 1982), whereas low-frequency fibres do not show an increased spontaneous firing rate (Stypulkowski, 1990), and the perceived tinnitus in humans is reported to be of high frequency; it is difficult to see why only high-frequency fibres should be affected by perilymphatic salicylate acting upon synapses. As an alternative there have been suggestions that the effects of salicylate upon the active processes of the hair cells is directly related to the production of tinnitus, or may affect the mechanical relationship of the OHCs and IHCs in such a manner so as to stimulate activity in the inner hair cells at the basal end of the cochlea (Stypulkowski, 1990). However, at present such explanations are entirely speculative and the mechanisms underlying the development of tinnitus after salicylate administration are still not understood.

Quinine

The effects of quinine resemble those of salicylate. It produces a reversible hearing loss and tinnitus that disappears upon withdrawal of the drug, and the degree of threshold shift correlates closely with, and can be used as a predictor of, the concentration of the drug in blood plasma (Alvan *et al.*, 1991). It has been reported that quinine also causes constriction of cochlear capillaries (Hawkins, 1976), which was thought to be the basis of its ototoxicity and to indicate a similar mechanism of action to salicylate. More recently, it has been considered that quinine may act directly upon OHCs to affect cochlear mechanics, but its mechanism of action may be different from that of salicylate.

Electron microscopy of thin sections of the organ of Corti fixed at the time of maximal effect following systemic application of the drug has shown swelling of the lateral cisternae, an organized endoplasmic reticulum immediately inside the lateral plasma membrane, in outer hair cells (Karlsson *et al.*, 1991a). Perilymphatic perfusion of quinine (Puel *et al.*, 1990) has been shown to produce a depression of CM and CAP, but the effect is different from that of salicylate, because quinine affects CAP across all stimulus intensities as opposed to just the low-intensity responses which salicylate suppresses. As EP is unaffected, these results indicate a direct effect on outer hair cells. Studies using isolated hair cells (Karlsson and Flock, 1990) have shown quinine to initiate slow changes in shape (whereas salicylate inhibits fast motile responses), and direct examination of the organ of Corti in intact cochlea preparations has shown quinine to affect the micromechanics of the organ of Corti (Karlsson *et al.*, 1991b).

Thus, the hearing loss due to quinine may result from a direct effect on the outer hair cells affecting their slow contractile properties and thereby the vibrational characteristics of the basilar membrane. It is known that quinine induces and enhances muscular contraction by affecting the availability of intracellular calcium released from the sarcoplasmic reticulum and it has been argued that quinine may act similarly on outer hair cells affecting intracellular calcium levels, possibly mediated by some event at the lateral cisternae that follows an initial action of the drug at the lateral plasma membrane.

Agents Affecting the Non-sensory Epithelia

Loop Diuretics

All the so-called 'loop' diuretics, including ethacrynic acid, frusemide (furosemide), bumetanide and piretanide, whose primary diuretic action is in the ascending limb of Henle's loop, cause temporary hearing loss and decline in CAP through an action upon the stria vascularis that inhibits maintenance of EP. The effects occur very rapidly following systemic administration of large doses. When frusemide is administered by intravascular injection, EP begins to decline within seconds and reaches a nadir after about 2–3 min (Lee and Harpur, 1985); with ethacrynic acid the effect is somewhat slower, and when this agent is administered by intraperitoneal injection, the maximum decline may not occur until 15–30 min post injection (Forge, 1981). The effects are almost entirely reversible, EP being almost fully recovered within 4–6 h. The maximum reduction in EP, which can fall to −40 mV, the potassium diffusion potential (Lee and Harpur, 1985), and the time required for recovery of EP are directly proportional to the dose of drug administered (Rybak *et al.*, 1991). The decline in EP coincides with the development of an extensive oedema in the stria vascularis that can cause the tissue to swell to almost twice its normal thickness. This, too, is reversible, the stria regaining a normal morphology approximately in parallel with the recovery of EP.

The development of oedema indicates that diuretics interfere with the normal ion transport processes in the stria, and the rapid onset of their effects suggests that they gain direct access to their site of action through entry from the strial vasculature. This mode of entry would give direct access to the basolateral membranes of the marginal cells. Alterations to marginal cells are among the earliest detectable responses observed in structural studies, and it has been demonstrated that loop diuretics inhibit Na^+/K^+-ATPase and adenyl cyclase in the stria; these enzymes are present predominantly in the basolateral membranes of the marginal cells. However, it has been shown that the concentration of diuretic that will completely abolish the positive component of EP is 1–2 orders of magnitude lower than that required for the inhibition of strial Na^+/K^+-ATPase or adenyl cyclase. Thus, in the cochlea the primary action of the diuretics is not upon these enzymes. In the kidney a $Na^+/K^+/Cl^-$ cotransporter has been characterized as a site of diuretic action. In the vestibular dark cell layer, whose physiology can be examined more directly than the stria because it is composed only of 'marginal'-type cells, diuretics have been shown to act at the basolateral membranes to affect Cl^- transport by interaction with a $Na^+/K^+/Cl^-$ cotransporter (Marcus and Marcus, 1989).

Aminoglycoside Antibiotics

In addition to their effects on the organ of Corti (see above), the aminoglycoside antibiotics also affect the stria vascularis. Originally, Hawkins (1973) reported atrophy of the stria several weeks after a course of chronic aminoglycoside administration and suggested that the primary action of these drugs was in fact upon the stria, with effects in the organ of Corti and the loss of hair cells occurring subsequently. Although it is now generally accepted that the hair cells are a primary site of aminoglycoside action, there is evidence that the stria also is affected in the initial stages of the response of the cochlea to these drugs; immediately following the end of a course of aminoglycoside treatment alterations to the stria can be seen at the same time as the earliest effects in the organ of Corti are apparent (Forge and Fradis, 1985). However, as both the organ of Corti and the stria show drug-induced abormalities at these earliest stages, it is not possible to determine the relative chronology of these events, or whether effects in the stria and the organ of Corti are related or occur independently. The lateral wall of the cochlea has been shown to contain a high level of $PhIP_2$, higher in fact than that of the organ of Corti, and thus it is possible that the stria may be directly susceptible to the drugs if, as discussed above, this phospholipid serves as the target for aminoglycoside action. However, there is no direct evidence for an interaction between aminoglycoside and strial tissues.

Following the end of aminoglycoside treatment, over the period during which loss of outer hair cells from the organ of Corti progresses, the stria becomes thinner. This decrease in thickness is due to an atrophy almost exclusively of marginal cells (Forge *et al.*, 1987). Some cells are lost by a process which shows morphological attributes of apoptosis, a process of controlled cell death, but the majority of marginal cells remain but with much reduced volume. Such alteration might be expected to affect EP and the ionic profile of endolymph, but EP appears to be maintained at close to normal levels for up to 4 weeks after the end of aminoglycoside treatment (Harpur, unpublished results). Thus, the functional consequences of the effects of aminoglycoside ototoxicity on the stria are not clear. Obviously, the reorganization in the organ of Corti resulting from the loss of hair cells and their replacement by supporting cells that occurs fol-

lowing aminoglycoside treatment will have profound effects on cochlear physiology. This might
be expected to influence the activity of the stria,
but as yet there is no indication of whether and
how there might be an interrelationship between
effects in the stria and in the organ of Corti.

cis-*Platinum*

Cis-DPP causes a decline in EP, indicating an
action in the stria, and has been reported to cause
strial atrophy, but the effects appear to vary,
depending upon the dose of drug administered
(Laurell and Engstrom, 1989a). Following a
single intravenous high dose (10–12.5 mg kg^{-1})
EP begins to decline within 1 day and becomes
permanently lost in parallel with the loss of hair
cells that also ensues. However, with lower doses
of the drug given repeatedly (e.g. daily injections
of *c.* 2 mg kg^{-1} for 10–14 days) by subcutaneous
or intramuscular routes, although hair cell loss
occurs, EP does not show any immediate alteration. Ultimately strial atrophy develops several
days or weeks after the end of the chronic treatment. The target for the drug action in the stria
is not known, but the differing responses to the
different dosing regimens suggests that effects in
the stria and in the organ of Corti are independent of each other and that the stria may be less
susceptible to damage from *cis*-DPP than are the
outer hair cells.

Role of Metabolism

There is no compelling evidence that any ototoxic
drug must first be metabolically activated. However, there has long been controversy about the
possible role of metabolism in the ototoxicity of
ethacrynic acid. It has been argued that ethacrynic acid requires biotransformation to its cysteine
conjugate to exert its ototoxic effect. This hypothesis largely rested on the evidence (Brown,
1975) that (1) the cysteine conjugate of ethacrynic
acid was more potently ototoxic than ethacrynic
acid and (2) there was an irreducible latency to
the onset of ototoxicity with ethacrynic acid but
not with its cysteine adduct. Furthermore, Koechel (1981) demonstrated a correlation between
the rate at which thiol conjugates liberate ethacrynic acid *in vitro* and their ototoxic potential in
guinea-pigs as well as their diuretic potency in
dogs. Analogues of ethacrynic acid which lack

sulphydryl reactivity also lack ototoxicity and are
only weakly saluretic.

The cysteine conjugate of ethacrynic acid is a
product of the primary conjugation of ethacrynic
acid with glutathione (Klaassen and Fitzgerald,
1974), so that the biotransformation of ethacrynic
acid to its cysteine conjugate may be modulated
by altering tissue levels of reduced glutathione
(GSH). It was, therefore, unexpected that the
acute ototoxic effect of ethacrynic acid in guinea-
pigs was not affected either by administration of
N-acetyl-L-cysteine or after profound depletion
of GSH, caused by administration of buthionine
sulphoxamine (Lazenby *et al.*, 1988). Hoffman *et
al.* (1988), on the other hand, found that
depletion of GSH by administration of buthionine
sulphoxamine rendered the cochlea very sensitive
to the ototoxic effect of ethacrynic acid and kanamycin in combination. Although this latter study
provided no information about the protective role
of GSH in the ototoxicity of ethacrynic acid or
kanamycin alone, Hoffman *et al.* speculated that
GSH could protect the cochlea from compounds
whose mechanism of ototoxicity involved generation of free radical species.

It has been shown that the sulphydryl-containing radioprotectant WR 2721 provided some protection against kanamycin-induced ototoxicity in
the guinea-pig (Pierson and Moller, 1981). This
effect of WR 2721 was attributed to its scavenging
free radical species in the cochlea. However,
there is no evidence for metabolism of aminoglycosides in any species and it seems highly improbable that the generation of free radicals could be
involved in the ototoxicity of aminoglycosides.
Furthermore, it has been shown that *N*-acetyl
cysteine augmented rather than protected against
the ototoxicity of kanamycin in the guinea-pig
(Bock *et al.*, 1983). An alternative explanation is
that kanamycin could inactivate an endogenous
free radical trap which has been shown to exist
in the cochlea (Pierson and Gray, 1982), although
even this is speculation.

Recently it was shown that the viability of isolated cochlear hair cells *in vitro* was compromised
by gentamicin only when a hepatic metabolizing
fraction was present (Huang and Schacht, 1990).
It was concluded that gentamicin was cytotoxic
only after conversion to an active metabolite. If
metabolism is required for aminoglycosides to
exert their ototoxic effect, then it may be that
the intact cochlea is capable of metabolism of

aminoglycosides, since it has been shown that hair cells in intact cochlear culture are vulnerable to aminoglycoside-induced injury without addition of a hepatic fraction (Richardson and Russell, 1991).

Thus, the role of metabolism in the ototoxicity of ethacrynic acid remains unresolved. It also remains to be seen what part, if any, metabolism plays in the ototoxicity of aminoglycosides *in vivo*.

REFERENCES

Alvan, G., Karlsson, K. K., Hellgren, U. and Villen, T. (1991). Hearing impairment related to plasma quinine concentration in healthy volunteers. *Br. J. Clin. Pharmacol.*, **31**, 409–412

Aran, J.-M. and Darrouzet, J. (1975). Observation of click-evoked compound VIII nerve responses before, during and over seven months after kanamycin treatment in the guinea pig. *Acta Otolaryngol.*, **79**, 24–32

Aran, J.-M., Erre, J.-P., Guilhaume, A. and Aurousseau, C. (1982). The comparative ototoxicities of gentamicin, tobramycin and dibekacin in the guinea pig. A functional and morphological cochlear and vestibular study. *Acta Otolaryngol. Suppl.*, **300**, 1–30

Ashmore, J. (1987). A fast motile response in guinea pig outer hair cells: the cellular basis of the cochlear amplifier. *J. Physiol.*, **388**, 323–347

Ashmore, J. F. and Meech, R. W. (1986). Ionic basis of the resting potential in outer hair cells isolated from guinea pig cochlea. *Nature*, **322**, 368–371

Balogh, K., Hiraide, F. and Ishii, D. (1970). Distribution of radioactive dihydrostreptomycin in the cochlea: an autoradiographic study. *Ann. Otol.*, **79**, 641–652

Bobbin, R. P. and Ceasar, G. (1987). Kynurenic acid and gamma-D-glutamyl-aminomethylsulfonic acid suppress the compound action potential of the auditory nerve. *Hearing Res.*, **25**, 77–81

Bock, G. R., Yates, G. K., Miller, J. J. and Moorjani, P. (1983). Effects of *N*-acetylcysteine on kanamycin ototoxicity in the guinea pig. *Hearing Res.*, **9**, 255–262

Bosher, S. K. (1980a). The nature of the ototoxic actions of ethacrynic acid upon the mammalian endolymph system. I. Functional aspects. *Acta Otolaryngol.*, **89**, 407–418

Bosher, S. K. (1980b). The nature of the ototoxic actions of ethacrynic acid upon the mammalian endolymph system. II. Structural-functional correlates in the *stria vascularis*. *Acta Otolaryngol.*, **90**, 40–54

Brown, A. M., McDowell, B. and Forge, A. (1989). Acoustic distortion products can be used to monitor the effects of chronic gentamicin treatment. *Hearing Res.*, **42**, 143–156

Brown, R. D. (1975). Comparison of the cochlear toxicity of sodium ethacrynate, furosemide and the cysteine adduct of sodium ethacrynate in cats. *Toxicol. Appl. Pharmacol.*, **31**, 270–282

Brownell, W. E., Bader, C. R., Bertrand, D. and de Ribeaupierre, Y. (1984). Evoked mechanical responses of isolated cochlear outer hair cells. *Science*, **227**, 194–196

Brummett, R. E. (1981a). Effects of antibiotic-diuretic interactions in the guinea pig model of ototoxicity. *Rev. Infect. Dis.*, **3**, Suppl., 216–223

Brummett, R. E. (1981b). Ototoxicity resulting from the combined administration of potent diuretics and other agents. *Scand. Audiol., Suppl.*, **14**, 215–224

Brummett, R. E. and Fox, K. E. (1982). Studies of aminoglycoside ototoxicity in animal models. In Whelton, A. and Neu, H. C. (Eds), *The Aminoglycosides. Microbiology, Clinical Use and Toxicology*. Marcel Dekker, New York, pp. 419–451

Brummett, R. E., Fox, K. E., Brown, R. T. and Himes, D. L. (1978). Comparative ototoxic liability of netilmicin and gentamicin. *Arch. Otolaryngol.*, **104**, 579–584

Brummett, R. E., Smith, C. A., Ueno, Y., Cameron, S. and Richter, R. (1977). The delayed effects of ethacrynic acid on the stria vascularis of the guinea pig. *Acta Otolaryngol.*, **83**, 98–112

Brummett, R. E., Traynor, J., Brown, R. and Himes, D. (1975). Cochlear damage resulting from kanamycin and furosemide. *Acta Otolaryngol.*, **80**, 86–92

Brummett, R. E., West, B. A., Traynor, J. and Manor, N. (1974). Ototoxic interaction between aminoglycoside antibiotics and diuretics. *Toxicol. Appl. Pharmacol.*, **29**, 97

Cazals, Y., Arna, J.-M., Erre, J.-P., Guilhaume, A. and Aurousseau, C. (1983). Vestibular acoustic reception in the guinea pig: a saccular function? *Acta Otolaryngol.*, **95**, 211–217

Chapman, P. (1982). Naproxen and sudden hearing loss. *J. Laryngol. Otol.*, **96**, 163–166

Coleman, J. W. (1975). Hair cell ratios in the spiral organ of the guinea pig. *Br. J. Audiol.*, **9**, 19–23

Crifo, S. (1973). Ototoxicity of sodium ethacrynate in the guinea pig. *Arch. Otorhinolaryngol.*, **206**, 27–38

Davies, S. and Forge, A. (1987). Preparation of the mammalian organ of Corti for scanning electron microscopy. *J. Microscopy*, **147**, 89–101

Davis, H. (1965). A model for transducer action in the cochlea. *Cold Spring Harbor Symp. Quant. Biol.*, **30**, 181–190

Davis, R. R., Brummett, R. E., Bendrick, T. W. and Himes, D. L. (1982). The ototoxic interaction of viomycin, capreomycin and polymyxin B with ethacrynic acid. *Acta Otolaryngol.*, **93**, 211–217

Desrochers, C. S. and Schacht, J. (1982). Neomycin concentrations in inner ear tissues and other organs of the guinea-pig after chronic drug administration. *Acta Otolaryngol.*, **93**, 233–236

Douek, E. E., Dodson, H. C. and Bannister, L. C. (1983). The effects of sodium salicylate on the cochlea of guinea pigs. *J. Laryngol. Otol.*, **93**, 793–799

Dulon, D., Aran, J.-M., Zajic, G. and Schacht, J. (1986). Comparative uptake of gentamicin, netilmicin and amikacin in the guinea pig cochlea and vestibule. *Antimicrob. Agents Chemother.*, **30**, 96–100

Dulon, D., Zajic, G., Aran, J.-M. and Schacht, J. (1989). Aminoglycoside antibiotics impair calcium entry but not viability and motility in isolated cochlear outer hair cells. *J. Neurosci.*, **24**, 338–346

Evans, E. F. and Borerwe, T. A. (1982). Ototoxic effects of salicylates on the responses of single cochlear nerve fibres and on cochlear potentials. *Br. J. Audiol.*, **16**, 101–108

Fausti, S. A., Rappaport, B. Z., Schechter, M. A., Frey, R. H., Ward, T. T. and Brummett, R. E. (1984). Detection of aminoglycoside ototoxicity by high frequency auditory evaluation: selected case studies. *Am. J. Otolaryngol.*, **5**, 177–182

Federspil, P. (1981). Pharmacokinetics of aminoglycoside antibiotics in the perilymph. In Lerner, S. A., Matz, G. J. and Hawkins, J. E. Jr (Eds), *Aminoglycoside Ototoxicity*. Little Brown, Boston, pp. 99–108

Finitzo-Hieber, T. (1981). Auditory brainstem response in assessment of infants treated with aminoglycoside antibiotics. In Lerner, S. A., Matz, G. J. and Hawkins, J. E. Jr (Eds), *Aminoglycoside Ototoxicity*. Little Brown, Boston, pp. 269–280

Forge, A. (1981). Ultrastructure in the stria vascularis of the guinea pig following intraperitoneal injection of ethacrynic acid. *Acta Otolaryngol*, **92**, 439–457

Forge, A. (1985). Outer hair cell loss and supporting cell expansion following chronic gentamicin treatment. *Hearing Res.*, **19**, 171–182

Forge, A. and Fradis, M. (1985). Structural abnormalities in the stria vascularis following chronic gentamicin treatment. *Hearing Res.*, **20**, 233–244

Forge, A., Wright, A. and Davies, S. J. (1987). Analysis of structural changes in the stria vascularis following chronic gentamicin treatment. *Hearing Res.*, **31**, 253–266

Fox, K. E., Brummett, R. E., Brown, R. and Himes, D. (1980). A comparative study of the ototoxicity of gentamicin and gentamicin C_1. *Arch. Otolaryngol.*, **106**, 44–49

deGroot, J. C. M. J. and Veldman, J. E. (1988). Early effects of gentamicin on inner ear glycocalyx cytochemistry. *Hearing Res.*, **35**, 39–46

Harpur, E. S. (1981). Ototoxicological testing. In Gorrod, J. W. (Ed.), *Testing for Toxicity*. Taylor and Francis, London, pp. 219–240

Harpur, E. S. (1986). Disorders of the ear. In D'Arcy, P. F. and Griffin, J. P. (Eds), *Iatrogenic Diseases*, 3rd edn. Oxford University Press, Oxford, pp. 713–749

Harpur, E. S. (1987). Ototoxicity. Morphological and functional correlates between experimental and clinical studies. In Ballantyne, B. (Ed.), *Perspectives in Basic and Applied Toxicology*. John Wright, Bristol, pp. 42–69

Harpur, E. S. and Bridges, J. B. (1979). An evaluation of the use of scanning and transmission electron-microscopy of the gentamicin-damaged guinea-pig organ of Corti. *J. Laryngol. Otol.*, **93**, 7–23

Harpur, E. S. and Gonda, I. (1982). Analysis of the pharmacokinetics of ribostamycin in serum and perilymph of guinea pigs after single and multiple doses. *Br. J. Audiol.*, **16**, 95–99

Harpur, E. S., Jabeen, F., Kingston, R., Gonda, I., Brammer, K. W. and Gregory, M. H. (1981). Single and multiple dose pharmacokinetics of ribostamycin in serum and perilymph of guinea pigs in relation to its low toxicity. In Brown, S. S. and Davies, D. S. (Eds), *Organ-directed Toxicity, Chemical Indices and Mechanisms*. Pergamon Press, Oxford, pp. 31–36

Hawkins, J. E. Jr. (1973). Ototoxic mechanisms. *Audiology*, **12**, 383–393

Hawkins, J. E. Jr. (1976). Drug ototoxicity. In Keidel, W. D. and Neff, W. D. (Eds), *Handbook of Sensory Physiology*, Vol. 5, Part 3. Springer-Verlag, Berlin, pp. 707–748

Hawkins, J. E. Jr and Johnsson, L.-G. (1981). Histopathology of cochlear and vestibular ototoxicity in laboratory animals. In Lerner, S. A., Matz, G. J. and Hawkins, J. E. Jr (Eds), *Aminoglycoside Ototoxicity*, Little Brown, Boston, pp. 175–195

Hawkins, J. E. Jr, Johnsson, L.-G. and Preston, R. E. (1972). Cochlear microvasculature in normal and damaged ears. *Laryngoscope*, **82**, 1091–1104

Hoeve, L. J., Mertens zur Borg, I. R., Rodenburg, M., Brocaar, M. P. and Groen, B. G. (1988). Correlations between *cis*-platinum dosage and toxicity in a guinea pig model. *Arch. Otorhinolaryngol.*, **245**, 98–102

Hoffman, D. W., Jones-King, K. L., Whitworth, C. A. and Rybak, L. P. (1988). Potentiation of ototoxicity by glutathione depletion. *Ann. Otol. Rhinol. Laryngol.*, **97**, 36–41

Huang, M. Y. and Schacht, J. (1990). Formation of a cytotoxic metabolite from gentamicin by liver. *Biochem. Pharmacol.*, **40**, R11–R14

Hudspeth, A. J. (1989). How the ear's works work. *Nature*, **341**, 397–404

Hunter-Duvar, I. M. (1978). A technique for preparation of cochlear specimens for assessment with the scanning electron microscope. *Acta Otolaryngol., Suppl.*, **351**, 1–23

Jackson, G. G. and Arcieri, G. (1971). Ototoxicity of gentamicin in man: a survey and controlled analysis of clinical experience in the United States. *J. Infect. Dis., Suppl.*, **124**, 130–137

Johnsson, L.-G. and Hawkins, J. E. Jr (1972). Strial atrophy in clinical and experimental deafness. *Laryngoscope*, **82**, 1105–1125

Kaloyanides, G. J. and Pastoriza-Munoz, E. (1980). Aminoglycoside nephrotoxicity. *Kidney Int.*, **8**, 571–582

Karlsson, K. K. and Flock, A. (1990). Quinine causes isolated outer hair cells to change length. *Neurosci. Lett.*, **116**, 101–105

Karlsson, K. K., Flock, B. and Flock, A. (1991a). Ultrastructural changes in the outer hair cells of the guinea pig cochlea after exposure to quinine. *Acta Otolaryngol.*, **111**, 500–505

Karlsson, K. K., Ulfendahl, M., Khanna, S. M. and Flock, A. (1991b). The effects of quinine on the cochlear mechanics in the isolated temporal bone preparation. *Hearing Res.*, **53**, 95–100

Kemp, D. T. (1978). Stimulated acoustic emission from within the human auditory system. *J. Acoust. Soc. Am.*, **64**, 1386–1391

Kim, D. O. (1986). Active and non-linear cochlear biomechanics and the role of outer-hair-cell sub-system in the mammalian auditory system. *Hearing Res.*, **22**, 105–114

Klaassen, C. D. and Fitzgerald, T. J. (1974). Meta-bolism and biliary excretion of ethacrynic acid. *J. Pharmacol. Exptl Ther.*, **191**, 548–556

Koechel, D. A. (1981). Ethacrynic acid and related diuretics: relationship of structure to beneficial and detrimental actions. *Ann. Rev. Pharmacol. Toxicol.*, **21**, 265–293

Laurell, G. and Bagger-Sjoback, D. (1991a). Degeneration of the organ of Corti following intravenous administration of cisplatin. *Acta Otolaryngol.*, **111**, 891–898

Laurell, G. and Bagger-Sjoback, D. (1991b). Dose-dependent inner ear changes after i.v. administration of cisplatin. *J. Otolaryngol.*, **20**, 158–167

Laurell, G. and Engstrom, B. (1989a). The combined effect of cisplatin and furosemide on hearing function in guinea pigs. *Hearing Res.*, **38**, 19–26

Laurell, G. and Engstrom, B. (1989b). The ototoxic effect of cisplatin on guinea pigs in relation to dosage. *Hearing Res.*, **38**, 27–34

Lazenby, C. M., Lee, S. J., Harpur, E. S. and Gescher, A. (1988). Glutathione depletion in the guinea pig and its effect on the acute cochlear toxicity of ethacrynic acid. *Biochem. Pharmacol.*, **37**, 3743–3747

Lee, S. J. and Harpur, E. S. (1985). Abolition of the negative endocochlear potential as a consequence of the gentamicin-furosemide interaction. *Hearing Res.*, **20**, 37–43

Liberman, M. C. (1990). Quantitative assessment of inner ear pathology following ototoxic drugs or acoustic trauma. *Toxicol. Pathol.*, **18**, 138–148

Long, G. R., Tubis, A. and Jones, K. (1986). Changes in spontaneous and evoked otoacoustic emissions and corresponding psychoacoustic threshold micro-structures induced by aspirin consumption. In Allen, J. G., Hall, J. L., Hubbard, A., Neely, S. T. and Tubis, A. (Eds), *Peripheral Auditory Mechanisms*. Springer-Verlag, New York, pp. 213–220

McAlpine, D. and Johnstone, B. M. (1990). The oto-toxic mechanism of cisplatin. *Hearing Res.*, **47**, 191–204

McDowell, B. (1982). Patterns of cochlear degeneration following gentamicin administration in both old and young guinea pigs. *Br. J. Audiol.*, **16**, 123–129

McKenzie, I. F. C., Mathew, T. H. and Bailie, M. J. (1968). Peritoneal dialysis in the treatment of quinine overdose. *Med. J. Aust.*, **1**, 58–59

Marcus, D. C. and Marcus, N. Y. (1989). Transepi-thelial electrical responses to Cl$^-$ of nonsensory region of gerbil utricle. *Biochim. Biophys. Acta*, **987**, 56–62

Martin, G. K., Lonsbury-Martin, B. L., Probst, R. and Coats, A. C. (1988). Spontaneous otoacoustic emissions in a nonhuman primate. 1. Basic features and relations to other emissions. *Hearing Res.*, **33**, 49–68

Masuda, Y., Sando, I. and Hemenway, W. G. (1971). Perilymphatic communication routes in the cochlea. *Arch. Otolaryngol.*, **94**, 240–245

Mathog, R. H. and Klein, W. J. Jr (1969). Ototoxicity of ethacrynic acid and aminoglycoside antibiotics in uraemia. *New Engl. J. Med.*, **280**, 1223–1224

Mathog, R. H., Thomas, V. G. and Hudson, W. R. (1970). Ototoxicity of new and potent diuretics. *Arch. Otolaryngol.*, **92**, 7–13

Neto, F. R. (1980). Further studies on the actions of salicylates on nerve membranes. *Eur. J. Pharmacol.*, **68**, 155–162

Nilsson Tammela, M. and Tjalve, H. (1986). Whole body autoradiography of [^{3}H]-dihydrostreptomycin in guinea pigs and rats: the labelling of the inner ear in relation to other tissues. *Acta Otolaryngol.*, **101**, 247–256

Nuttall, A. L. (1981). Perfusion of aminogylcosides in perilymph. In Lerner, S. A., Matz, G. J. and Hawkins, J. E. Jr (Eds), *Aminoglycoside Ototoxicity*. Little Brown, Boston, pp. 51–61

Orsulakova, A. and Schacht, J. (1981). A biochemical mechanism of the ototoxic interaction between neo-mycin and ethacrynic acid. *Acta Otolaryngol.*, **93**, 43–48

Osborne, M. P. and Comis, S. D. (1990). High resolution scanning electron microscopy of stereocilia in the cochlea of normal, postmortem, and drug-treated guinea pigs. *J. Elect. Microsc. Tech.*, **15**, 254–260

Pickles, J. O. (1988). *An Introduction to the Physiology of Hearing*. Academic Press, London

Pickles, J. O., Comis, S. D. and Osborne, M. P. (1984). Cross-links between stereocilia in the guinea pig organ of Corti, and their possible relation to sensory transduction. *Hearing Res.*, **15**, 103–112

Pierson, M. G. and Gray, B. H. (1982). Superoxide dismutase activity in the cochlea. *Hearing Res.*, **6**, 141–151

Pierson, M. G. and Moller, A. R. (1981). Prophylaxis of kanamycin-induced ototoxicity by a radioprotect-ant. *Hearing Res.*, **4**, 79–87

Pike, D. A. and Bosher, S. K. (1980). The time course of the strial changes produced by intravenous furosemide. *Hearing Res.*, **3**, 79–89

Puel, J.-L., Bledsoe, S. C. Jr, Bobbin, R. P., Ceasar, G. and Fallon, M. (1989). Comparative actions of salicylate on the amphibian lateral line and guinea pig cochlea. *Comp. Biochem. Physiol.*, **93C**, 73–80

Puel, J.-L., Bobbin, R. P. and Fallon, M. (1990). Salicylate, mefenamate, meclofenamate, and quinine on cochlear potentials. *Otolaryngol. Head Neck Surg.*, **102**, 66–73

Richardson, G. P. and Russell, I. J. (1991). Cochlear cultures as a model system for studying aminoglycoside induced ototoxicity. *Hearing Res.*, **53**, 293–311

Rybak, L. P. (1988). Ototoxicity of ethacrynic acid (a persistent clinical problem). *J. Laryngol. Otol.*, **102**, 518–520

Rybak, L. P., Whitworth, C. and Scott, V. (1991). Comparative acute ototoxicity of loop diuretic compounds. *Eur. Arch. Otorhinolaryngol.*, **248**, 353–357

Saito, T., Moataz, R. and Dulon, D. (1991). Cisplatin blocks depolarization-induced calcium entry in isolated cochlear outer hair cells. *Hearing Res.*, **56**, 143–147

Schacht, J. (1986). Molecular mechanisms of drug-induced hearing loss. *Hearing Res.*, **22**, 297–304

Schmidt, S.-H., Anniko, M. and Hellstrom, S. (1990). Electrophysiological effects of the clinically used local anesthetics lidocaine, lidocaine-prilocaine and phenol on the rat's inner ear. *Eur. Arch. Otorhinolaryngol.*, **248**, 87–94

Schuknecht, H. F. (1957). Ablation therapy in the management of Meniere's disease. *Acta Otolaryngol. Suppl.*, **132**, 1–42

Spoendlin, H. (1973). The innervation of the cochlear receptor. In Moller, A. R. (Ed.), *Basic Mechanisms of Hearing*. Academic Press, New York, pp. 185–230

Spoendlin H. and Brun, J.-P. (1974). The block-surface technique for evaluation of cochlear pathology. *Arch. Otorhinolaryngol.*, **208**, 137–145

Stebbins, W. C., McGinn, C. S., Feitosa, M. A. G., Moody, D. B., Prosen, C. A. and Serafin, J. V. (1981). Animal models in the study of ototoxic hearing loss. In Lerner, S. A., Matz, G. J. and Hawkins, J. E. Jr (Eds), *Aminoglycoside Ototoxicity*. Little Brown, Boston, pp. 5–25

Stupp, H., Kupper, K., Lagler, F., Sous, H. and Quante, M. (1973). Inner ear concentrations and ototoxicity of different antibiotics in local and systemic application. *Audiology*, **12**, 350–363

Stypulkowski, P. H. (1990). Mechanisms of salicylate ototoxicity. *Hearing Res.*, **46**, 113–145

Thorne, P. R. and Gavin, J. B. (1984). The accuracy of hair cell counts in determining distance and position along the organ of Corti. *J. Acoust. Soc. Am.*, **76**, 440–442

Toone, E. C. Jr, Hayden, G. D. and Ellman, H. M. (1965). Ototoxicity of chloroquine. *Arthritis Rheum.*, **8**, 475–476

Toyoda, Y. and Tachibana, M. (1978). Tissue levels of kanamycin in correlation with oto- and nephrotoxicity. *Acta Otolaryngol.*, **86**, 9–14

Tran Ba Huy, P., Bernard, P. and Schacht, J. (1986). Kinetics of gentamicin uptake and release in the rat: comparison of inner ear tissues and fluids with other organs. *J. Clin. Invest.*, **77**, 1492–1500

Tran Ba Huy, P. and Deffrennes, D. (1988). Aminoglycoside ototoxicity: influence of dosage regimen on drug uptake and correlation between membrane binding and some clinical features. *Acta Otolaryngol.*, **105**, 511–515

Tran Ba Huy, P., Manuel, C., Meulemans, A., Sterkers, O. and Amiel, C. (1981). Pharmacokinetics of gentamicin in perilymph and endolymph of the rat as determined by radioimmunoassay. *J. Infect. Dis.*, **143**, 476–486

Tran Ba Huy, P., Manuel, C., Meulemans, A., Sterkers, O., Wassef, M. and Amiel, C. (1983a). Ethacrynic acid facilitates gentamicin entry into endolymph of the rat. *Hearing Res.*, **11**, 191–202

Tran Ba Huy, P., Meulemans, A., Wassef, M., Manuel, C., Sterkers, O. and Amiel, C. (1983b). Gentamicin persistence in rat endolymph and perilymph after a two-day constant infusion. *Antimicrob. Agents Chemother.*, **23**, 344–346

Vermorken, J. B., Kapteijn, T. S., Hart, A. A. M. and Pinedo, H. M. (1983). Ototoxicity of *cis*-diamminedichloroplatinum (II): influence of dose, schedule and mode of administration. *Eur. J. Cancer Clin. Oncol.*, **19**, 53–58

Voldrich, L. (1965). The kinetics of streptomycin, kanamycin and neomycin in the inner ear. *Acta Otolaryngol.*, **60**, 243–248

Walby, A. P. and Kerr, A. G. (1982). Streptomycin sulphate and deafness: a review of the literature. *Clin. Otolaryngol.*, **7**, 63–68

Watanabe, Y., Nakajina, R., Oda, R., Uno, M. and Naito, T. (1971). Experimental study on the transfer of kanamycin to the inner ear fluids. *Med. J. Osaka Univ.*, **21**, 257–263

Wersall, J. (1981). Structural damage to the organ of Corti and the vestibular epithelia caused by aminoglycoside antibiotics in the guinea pig. In Lerner, S. A., Matz, G. J. and Hawkins, J. E. Jr (Eds), *Aminoglycoside Ototoxicity*. Little Brown, Boston, pp. 197–214

West, B. A., Brummett, R. E. and Himes, D. L. (1973). Interaction of kanamycin and ethacrynic acid. Severe cochlear damage in guinea pigs. *Arch. Otolaryngol.*, **98**, 32–37

Wright, A., Davis, A., Bredberg, G., Ulehlova, L. and Spencer, H. (1987). Hair cell distribution in the normal human cochlea. *Acta Otolaryngol. Suppl.*, **444**, 4–48

Zajic, G. and Schacht, J. (1987). Comparison of isolated outer hair cells from five mammalian species. *Hearing Res.*, **26**, 249–256

Zenner, H. P., Zimmermann, U. and Schmitt, U. (1985). Reversible contraction of isolated cochlear hair cells. *Hearing Res.*, **18**, 127–133

FURTHER READING

de Oliveira, J. A. A. (1989). *Audiovestibular Toxicity of Drugs, Volumes 1 and 2.* CRC Press, Boca Raton, Florida

Harpur, E. S. (1988). Ototoxicity: morphological and clinical correlations between experimental and clini-cal studies. In Ballantyne, B. (Ed.), *Perspectives in Basic and Applied Toxicology*, Wright, London, pp. 42–69

Huang, M. Y. and Schacht, J. (1989). Drug-induced ototoxicity: pathogenesis and prevention. *Medical Toxicology and Adverse Drug Experiences*, **4**, 452–467

32 Toxicology of the Adrenal, Thyroid and Endocrine Pancreas

John A. Thomas

INTRODUCTION

There are many target organs in the endocrine system that are sensitive to chemical and drug insult (Thomas and Keenan, 1986). Both the male and the female reproductive systems are vulnerable to chemically induced changes. Likewise, the foetus and the neonate can be affected by chemicals and drugs (Thomas, 1989). Gonadal toxicities and teratogenesis are important aspects of endocrine aberrations brought about by either chemicals or drugs (Thomas and Ballantyne, 1990). Reproductive toxicology (see Chapter 39) and developmental toxicology (see Chapter 40) certainly can involve the endocrine system. However, there are other non-gonadal target organs in the endocrine system that can be affected by drugs and chemicals.

The thyroid gland, the adrenal gland and the pancreas can each be affected by various drugs and chemicals (Thomas et al., 1985). In the case of the thyroid and adrenal glands, drugs and synthetic steroids can interfere with their internal secretions either by affecting the glands directly or by interfering with trophic hormone secretion at the level of the adenohypophysis (Table 1). Because numerous drugs and related factors can affect the secretion and/or release of adenohypophyseal hormones, it is important to be aware of such factors or conditions when attempting clinically to assess pituitary function. With the advent of radioimmunoassays (RIA), it is now possible to assess the blood levels of most trophic hormones. Drug-induced alterations of pituitary function tests can lead to misinterpretations and therapeutic misadventures. Indeed, the results of pituitary function can be altered by many endogenous and exogenous agents (Thomas et al., 1989).

It is estimated that nearly 90 per cent of all endocrine toxicities appear in the adrenal gland, the testes and the thyroid gland (Table 2) (Colby, 1988). Some endocrine organs appear to be more sensitive to toxic agents, and this often leads to multiple disruptions in the hormonal balance of the organism. It is not uncommon for chemically induced changes in gonadal function to affect the activity of the thyroid gland. Chemically induced changes in sex steroids can affect pancreatic secretion of insulin. Chemically induced stress leading to an increased secretion of glucocorticoids can also affect insulin secretion, but more importantly can affect adrenocorticotropin (ACTH) levels and hence alter the pituitary–adrenal axis.

The thalidomide tragedy of the 1960s led to the formulation of toxicological testing guidelines for the field of teratology. Thereafter, selected protocols for reproductive and developmental toxicology tests were instituted. Generally, test requirements have not been imposed for other endocrine organs.

Chemically induced changes in the endocrine system can be purposeful. For example, synthetic steroids can effectively suppress pituitary gonadotropins, thereby affording millions of women with a chemical method of birth control. The chemical suppression of excessive endogenous hormone secretion also can be therapeutically achieved in the adrenal and thyroid glands.

PITUITARY

Pituitary–Target Organ Relationships

A knowledge of hormonal feedback systems is of value in attempting to predict the effect(s) of potentially toxic agents on a particular endocrine target organ (Thomas and Keenan, 1986). Although the measurement of specific hormone levels might not be possible for all general toxicological screenings of substances, some bioassays and microscopic techniques may yield useful information. For example, a slowing in animal growth rates, in most instances caused by dimin-

Table 1 Effects of various agents on pituitary secretions

Drug	GH		FSH/LH		TSH		ACTH	
	Basal increase/ decrease	Stimulated beyond basal	Basal increase/ decrease	Stimulated beyond basal	Basal increase/ decrease	Stimulated beyond basal	Basal increase/ decrease	Stimulated beyond basal
Progestins	↓	↓	↓				↓	↓
Oestrogens	↑	↑	↓			↑		↓
Glucocorticoids	↓		↓	↓	↓	↑		↓
Phenothiazines	↓	↓						
L-Dopa		↑						
Phenytoin							↓	↓
Propranolol		↑						
Morphine		↓						
Ethanol		↓						↓

Source: modified from Thomas and Keenan (1986).

Table 2 Incidence of chemically induced endocrine lesions

Order of frequency	Organ	
1	Adrenal gland	⎫
2	Testis	⎬ 90% of total
3	Thyroid gland	⎭
4	Ovary	
5	Pancreas	
6	Pituitary gland	
7	Parathyroid gland	

Source: Colby (1988).

ished nutritional intake, can result from the suppression of pituitary growth hormone (GH) secretion. Similarly, a decrease in adrenal weights following the administration of certain chemicals can be caused by an interference with pituitary ACTH.

Generally, chemically induced changes that affect pituitary–target organ relationships seldom manifest themselves after a single administration of a toxic agent. Rather, compounds that have the potential to exert deleterious effects on the endocrine system ordinarily require longer durations of exposure and repeated administrations. While chemically induced stress can provoke a rapid response in catecholamine secretion and an outpouring of glucocorticoids, other hormonal changes would ordinarily not be so immediate. Agents causing the induction of hepatic microsomal enzyme systems that affect hormone meta-

bolism usually require upwards of a week before hormone changes in the endocrine systems.

It is important to understand some of the more basic or classical hormonal relationships between the adenohypophysis and the respective endocrine target organs (Figure 1). Chemicals, including certain classes of therapeutically effective drugs, can interfere with the release of trophic hormones or can interfere with their synthesis (Thomas and Keenan, 1986). Still other toxic

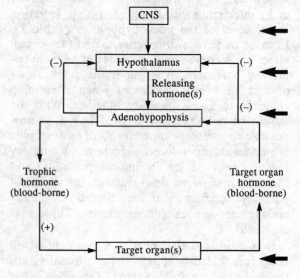

Figure 1 Relationship between adenohypophyseal–hypothalamic axis and hormone target organs

agents can exert inhibitory actions on the biosynthesis of target organ hormone secretions. Thus, there are several sites of actions of different chemicals on the adenohypophyseal–target organ feedback systems.

Depending on the particular chemical, the sites of action may differ in their sensitivity to toxic agents. Target organs such as the gonads are sensitive to toxic substances because rapidly dividing cells are often vulnerable to chemical destruction. Environmental stresses can affect the secretory activity of certain of the hypothalamic-releasing hormones and hence alter pituitary–target organ relationships. Sometimes toxic agents can bind to circulating blood proteins and alter the ratio of free and bound forms of target organ hormones. Such changes in binding can also modify the pituitary–target hormone relationship.

Adenohypophysis

Trophic hormones and their hypothalamic-releasing hormones are shown in Table 3. As the trophic hormones are either protein or glycoprotein in chemical composition, they cannot be measured by standard spectrophotometric procedures. These hormones must either be bioassayed or measured by using RIA (Thomas *et al.*, 1989). Bioassays were useful for certain of the adenohypophyseal hormones but such tests have been replaced by newer and more sensitive RIA. Bioassays, however, might be employed where there is only a secondary interest in determining whether a particular toxicological agent is affecting trophic hormone levels. Sometimes a target organ that is known to be directly influenced by a particular trophic hormone can be examined, and provide general insight into the nature of the chemically induced alterations in the endocrine system. Despite the more complex and involved RIA methodologies, they are of immense value for measuring different hormones (Table 4). RIA represents an analytical approach of great sensitivity, and such techniques have been applied to well over 200 biological substances, many of which cannot be assayed by other techniques. Unlike bioassays that often require large amounts of tissue (or blood), the greater sensitivity of the RIA can be achieved with very small samples of biological fluids.

Some hormones can be measured by competitive assays either by utilizing an immune system or a non-immune system. In the immune system assay the antibody acts as the binding protein (e.g. insulin, ACTH), whereas in the non-immune assay system the binding reagent is often

Table 4 Hormones that can be measured by competitive assays using either immune or non-immune systems

Protein hormones	Steroid hormones
TSH	Aldosterone
ACTH	Cortisol
STH (GH) (growth hormone)	Dihydrotestosterone
FSH	Oestradiol
LH (and HCG)	Oestrone
Oxytocin	Progesterone
Insulin	Testosterone
Prolactin	

Source: modified from Thomas *et al.* (1989).

Table 3 Trophic hormones of the anterior pituitary gland and their respective hypothalamic releasing hormones

Adenohypophyseal trophic hormone	Hypothalamic releasing hormone
ACTH (adrenocortical tropic hormone)	Corticotropic-releasing hormone (CRH)
TSH (thyroid-stimulating hormone)	Thyrothropic-releasing hormone (TRH)
FSH (follicle-stimulating hormone)	Follicle-stimulating releasing hormone (FRH)
LH (luteinizing hormone)	Luteinizing-hormone releasing hormone (LRH)
STH (GH) (growth hormone)	Somatotropin-releasing hormone (SRH) (GRH)
STH (GH) (growth hormone)	Somatotropin-inhibitory hormone (STH) (GIH)
Prolactin	Prolactin-inhibitory hormone (PIH)
Prolactin	Prolactin-releasing hormone (PRH)
MSG (melanocyte-stimulating hormone)	Melanocyte-stimulating releasing hormone (MRH)
MSH (melanocyte-stimulating hormone)	Melanocyte-inhibiting hormone (MIH)

a naturally-occurring protein with a high affinity for the hormone being measured (e.g. cortisol, thyroxine). Monoclonal antibodies are also used in the measurement of various hormones.

The concept of radioassays, whether the binding protein is an antibody or a naturally occurring protein with a high affinity for the hormone to be measured, is the same. Basically, the binding sites are saturated with a radioactive form of the hormone and, subsequently, incubated with the non-radioactive form of the hormone that is to be measured. Competition occurs between the radioactive and the non-radioactive form of the hormone. The ratio of antibody-bound to free (unbound) radioactive hormone is reduced as the concentration of non-radioactive hormone is increased. By using solutions containing known amounts of hormone, a standard curve can be constructed, thus providing a sensitive competitive binding assay for a particular hormone. Other immunoassays can likewise be used.

Measurement of Anterior Pituitary Hormones

Adrenocorticotropin (ACTH)

Modulation of adrenocortical growth and secretory activity is by ACTH. ACTH exerts a number of physiological actions, including maintenance of the adrenal gland and stimulation of adrenal cortical steroid secretion. ACTH can cause depletion of adrenal gland ascorbic acid.

There are several pathological states that can alter ACTH secretion. Furthermore, stress induced from any one of a variety of environmental or chemical stimuli can cause a rapid elevation in ACTH blood levels. There is a diurnal rhythm for the secretion of corticosteroids.

Several methods are available for measuring ACTH but most assays resort to assessing adrenal gland parameters (Thomas *et al.*, 1989). Certainly, the gravimetric assay of adrenal glands represents one of the simplest methods for indirectly evaluating ACTH activity. In hypophysectomized animals (e.g. rats), ACTH injections can maintain the weight of the adrenal glands. ACTH stimulates increases in plasma cortisol and corticosterone and elevates urinary 17-hydroxy-corticosteroids and 17-ketosteroids, which can be used as an index of adrenal cortex function. ACTH causes involution of the thymus gland,

deposition of hepatic glycogen, and leads to a decrease in circulating eosinophils in hypophysectomized rodents. These latter ACTH-induced changes in these biological parameters have also been used to assess ACTH activity.

Radioligand-receptor assays and other immunoassays have been developed for ACTH. These RIAs are very sensitive but can represent a considerable investment of time and expense for routine toxicological assessment of the pituitary–adrenal axis.

Thyroid-Stimulating Hormone (TSH)

Thyroid-stimulating hormone (TSH) is a glycoprotein capable of stimulating the growth and proliferation of cells of the thyroid gland. TSH can produce a number of biochemical and histological changes in the thyroid gland. TSH assays have employed the uptake of ^{32}P in the thyroid glands of baby chicks. Like ACTH, and for routine toxicological assessment of TSH, many tests involve the measurement of target organ secretory responses. The evaluation of TSH often employs the measurement of thyroxine (T_4) and triiodothyronine (T_3).

Several chemicals, environmental factors and pathological states can affect thyroid hormone secretion (Thomas and Bell, 1982; Thomas *et al.*, 1989). Certain foodstuffs and plants contain chemicals (i.e. goitrogens) that can act as antithyroidal agents. Most of these conditions seem to directly affect the thyroid gland rather than interfering with TSH secretion.

TSH can be measured by RIA. Such tests are very sensitive and highly specific but the species from which the antisera are obtained can affect the levels being detected. Cross-reactivity of antisera can occur. There are other physiological and non-physiological factors that can affect the measurement of TSH and thyroid hormones (Table 5).

Somatotrophin (GH)

Somatotrophin (STH) or growth hormone (GH) appears to exert a variety of complex metabolic actions leading to protein anabolism and a stimulation of RNA synthesis. A deficiency in GH leads to a reduction in the incorporation of amino acids into protein. Growth hormone causes a marked stimulation of cartilaginous growth at the epiphyses of long bones. Human recombinant DNA growth hormone has been approved for

Table 5 Factors influencing TSH, T_3 and T_4 levels in rat plasma

Sex of animal
Age of animal
Time of day
Stage of Oestrous cycle
Strain of animal
Environmental temperature
Blood collection technique
Animal handling
Locomotor activity of the animal

therapeutic use by the US Food and Drug Administration (FDA).

Many factors can affect the secretion of GH (Thomas and Thomas, 1988). Hypoglycaemia can cause a sudden and dramatic increase in serum GH. Starvation can affect GH levels, and cold stress or surgical trauma can lead to an increase in serum GH. Drugs and chemicals that affect catecholamine neurotransmission and the autonomic nerve system can influence GH secretion. GH bioassays have utilized body weight gain tests in hypophysectomized female rats. GH has been assayed by measuring the width of the tibial epiphysial growth plate. A sensitive RIA for rat growth hormone and for human growth hormone is available. GH can be measured by one of several immunological methods.

Whether GH is assessed using bioassays or by the more accurate and sensitive RIA, or other immunoassays, the experimental design of either acute or chronic toxicity tests must closely monitor the nutritional status of the animals. Many toxic agents can retard dietary intake and, hence, reduce body weights. Experimental designs employing paired-feeding protocols may help the toxicologist in interpreting GH activity.

THYROID GLAND

An understanding of the physiology of the thyroid is important for understanding its endocrine toxicity (Thomas and Bell, 1982; Thomas and Keenan, 1986). The primary products of the thyroid are the hormones T_4 and T_3. The initial step in the synthesis of these thyroid hormones is the uptake of dietary iodide into the follicular cells of the thyroid in response to thyrotropin (TSH). Following cellular uptake, the iodide is oxidized, possibly through a free radical mechanism, and then combined with the tyrosine components of a protein to form either monoiodotyrosyl or diiodotyrosyl residues. Two molecules of the latter can combine to form T_4 whereas one molecule of each can combine to form T_3. Normally, T_4 predominates over T_3 in the thyroid, although the ratio can be altered under certain pathological conditions.

T_4 and T_3 can be incorporated into thyroglobulin, which is stored in the follicular colloid material of the thyroid gland. In response to TSH, T_4 and T_3 release results from their proteolytic cleavage from thyroglobulin. Normally, thyroglobulin does not enter the circulation. Monoiodotyrosine and diiodotyrosine can also be released at this stage; however, before reaching the circulation they are enzymatically degraded. The liberated iodine in the form of iodide is eventually reincorporated into protein by the thyroid gland.

T_3 and T_4 are transported in the plasma in association with proteins. Although there are species differences in the protein-binding patterns of the thyroid hormones, the primary binding protein in humans is called thyroxine-binding globulin (TBG). It is an acidic glycoprotein with a molecular weight of 40 000 daltons. It binds T_4 with a relatively high binding affinity and T_3 with a lower affinity. A second transport protein called thyroxine-binding pre-albumin, although present in higher amounts than thyroxine-binding globulin, has a lower binding affinity for the thyroid hormones and is considered of secondary importance. In humans, and most other mammals, the thyroid hormones can secondarily bind to albumin.

As a consequence of thyroid plasma protein binding, less than 0.1 per cent of the total plasma thyroid hormones exist in a free or unbound form. Care must be exercised when monitoring thyroid function in a species like the rat which does not possess a TBG (i.e. high affinity binding protein). Therefore, the rat has lower plasma levels of protein-bound thyroid hormone. Also, because it is the free form of the hormone which is available for degradation, it is not unreasonable to expect that the plasma half-life for T_4 would be longer in a species with a TBG than in a species without one. The T_4 plasma half-life in the human, which has a TBG, is 5–9 days; in the rat, which does not have a TBG, the T_4 plasma half-life is only 12–24 h.

There are several biochemical steps in the biosynthesis of T_3 and T_4 where toxic chemicals can interfere with thyroid function. A number of these chemicals/drugs are shown in Table 6. They can be categorized by their mechanism of toxic action(s). Stress is a common factor in conditions leading to reduced T_3 syndromes both in animals and humans. The stress may be either thermal or non-thermal. Cold is well known for its actions in stimulating thyroid gland activity. Decreased serum T_3 in starved rats is primarily the result of diminished thyroid secretion of T_4. Experience with laboratory rats has also revealed that a variety of physical and environmental factors (Table 5) also can alter circulating (i.e. plasma) levels of TBG, T_4 and/or T_3.

Many drugs possess side-effects that can interfere with thyroid gland function (Table 7). Salicylates, anticoagulants, phenytoin and other classes of drugs can reduce thyroid function. Propylthiouracil (PTU), a therapeutic drug used in the treatment of hyperthyroidism, decreases T_3 and T_4. PTU is but one drug in a large chemical class of thyroid inhibitors. Phenoxyisobutyrate derivatives, such as clofibrate, induce morphological changes in the thyroid gland.

Diproteverin, a calcium channel blocking agent with anti-anginal properties, causes hypertrophy of thyroid follicular epithelium. Its actions appear to result from enhanced binding and clearance of

Table 7 Effects of selected pharmacological agents on thyroid activity

Drug/hormone	T_3 uptake	^{131}I uptake	Thyroid-binding globulin levels
Aminosalicylic acid	—	↓	—
Anabolic steroids	↑	—	↓
Anticoagulants (dicoumarol and heparin)	↑	—	—
Antiflammatory agents (phenylbutazone)	↑	↓	—
Indocyanine green (cardio-green)	—	↓	—
Corticosteroids	—	↓	↓
Phenytoin (DPH)	↑	—	—
Oral contraceptives	↓	—	↑
Lithium carbonate	—	↑	—
Phenothiazines	—	↓	↓
Salicylates	↓	—	—
Suphonamides	—	↓	—

Source: modified from Thomas and Keenan (1986).

unconjugated T_4 with a subsequent increase in serum TSH. Amiodarone, an antiarrhythmic drug, often causes thyroid disorders (Rani, 1990). It is an iodine-rich agent which can cause either

Table 6 Chemicals producing abnormal thyroid function

Blockade of iodide trapping	Blockade of iodide oxidation	Mechanism not established
Chlorate	Amphenone	Acetazolamide
Hypochlorite	Carbimazole	Chlorpromazine
Iodate	Cobalt	Chlortrimeton
Nitrate	Methimzole	Thiopentone (thiopental)
Perchlorate	*p*-Aminosalicylate	Tolbutamide
Thiocyanate	Phenylbutazone	
	Phenylinadanedione	
	Propylthiouracil	
	Resorcinol	

Source: modified from Thomas and Keenan (1986).

hypo- or hyperthyroidism after prolonged therapy. Amiodarone has specific inhibitory effects on agonist-stimulated functions in thyroid cells, probably by interfering with TSH–receptor interactions.

A large number of chemical agents influence the binding, distribution and metabolism of thyroid hormones but seldom do they lead to permanent alterations in thyroid function, primarily because of endocrine regulatory mechanisms. Long-term thyroid hormone derangements caused by xenobiotics may lead to follicular cell carcinogenesis (Hill *et al.*, 1989). It is difficult to use the rodent model for studying the effects in humans because rodents lack TBG. TBG serves as an important buffer system in the control of thyroid hormones. Toxicology studies have to consider that chemicals or drugs frequently act at different levels of thyroid hormone synthesis, utilization and excretion. This action is particularly evident when there is a structural relationship between T_3 or T_4 and the chemical or drug (e.g. phenytoin–DPH).

There are both natural and synthetic agents that can affect the thyroid glands (Donaldson, 1980; Thomas and Keenan, 1986). There are several plant toxins that are considered natural goitrogens. Vegetables of the cabbage family such as broccoli, brussel sprouts, cauliflower, horseradish, mustard seed and turnips contain a chemical class of compounds known as glucosinolates. Glucosinolates can be biotransformed into thiocyanates and isothiocyanates which are potent natural goitrogens. Likewise, onions, garlic and chives contain 5-substituted cysteine sulphoxides which are also natural goitrogens. Raw soybeans, especially if there is inadequate iodine uptake, may produce simple goitres. Heating or cooking the soybean destroys the natural goitrogens. Cassava, a starchy plant, contains considerable amounts of hydrogen cyanide that can cause an increased incidence of goitres.

A number of synthetic herbicides can produce alterations in thyroid gland activity (Stevens and Sumner, 1991). There are also a number of chemical classes of herbicides, including chlorinated phenylureas, substituted uracils, pyridazinones and diphenyl ethers. Nitrofen, a halogenated nitrophenol that is a selective pre- and postemergence herbicide, reduces follicular size and colloidal density. Triazines are an important class of herbicides that also suppress thyroid

activity. In animals, long-term feeding studies with amitrole produce thyroid adenomas and adenocarcinomas. Amitrole inhibits thyroid peroxidase, leading to an increased TSH and goitrogenicity (Rani, 1990). Aminothiazole exerts a direct action on the thyroid by inhibiting T_4 synthesis and also accelerates its deiodination. 2,4-D can decrease serum protein-bound iodine. Fungicides (e.g. nabam, zineb and zuram) are capable of inhibiting iodine uptake by the thyroid. Chlorine dioxide, sometimes used as an alternative disinfectant in municipal water supplies, reportedly decreases T_4 levels in primates.

It is obvious that many chemicals and drugs can alter thyroid function. The mechanism of toxicological action varies, ranging from inhibiting the anion pump in the thyroid to reducing T_3 and T_4 synthesis.

ADRENAL GLANDS

The adrenal gland has distinct anatomical zones that exert different hormonal and neural actions. The adrenal medulla secretes adrenaline (epinephrine) and noradrenaline (norepinephrine) in response to sympathetic nerve stimulation, and their release produces systemic effects resembling generalized sympathetic stimulation. The adrenal cortex produces two principal groups of steroid hormones, the mineralocorticoids and the glucocorticoids, although small amounts of androgenic hormones may also be secreted.

The primary mineralocorticoid in humans is aldosterone although deoxycorticosterone also exhibits mineralocorticoid activity. Cortisol, the major glucocorticoid produced in humans, also exhibits a low level of mineralocorticoid activity. The physiological action of aldosterone is to modulate electrolyte levels. It promotes the renal reabsorption of sodium in the ascending portion of the loop of Henle, the distal tubule, and in the collecting tubule. The reabsorption of sodium is also accompanied by the reabsorption of chloride anion. In addition to stimulating the reabsorption of sodium, aldosterone also enhances the urinary excretion of potassium and hydrogen ions. The increased elimination of hydrogen ions can lead to alkalosis and an increased extracellular content of bicarbonate ions, which when combined with an increased extracellular sodium and chloride content, tend to promote the tubular reabsorption of water.

The adrenal cortex is necessary for survival. Without mineralocorticoids, the extracellular fluid potassium concentration rises, and the sodium and chloride content falls. Total lack of aldosterone secretion causes the urinary elimination of 20 per cent of the total body sodium in 1 day. The sodium elimination can cause a dangerous reduction in the extracellular and blood volume which, if not restored, will lead to diminished cardiac output and death.

The glucocorticoids secreted in humans are cortisol or hydrocortisone, although both corticosterone and cortisone possess some glucocorticoid activity. Glucocorticoids regulate carbohydrate, protein and fat metabolism. With carbohydrate metabolism, the glucocorticoids stimulate gluconeogenesis and decrease glucose utilization. Both these effects can lead to increased blood glucose levels. Glucocorticoids produce a marked reduction in cellular protein content, although hepatic protein increases, as does the production of plasma protein by the liver. It is believed that glucocorticoids interfere with the transport of amino acids into extrahepatic cells, and combined with continuing protein catabolism in these cells results in an increase in plasma amino acids. Increased plasma amino acid levels and their subsequent transport into the liver probably promotes gluconeogenesis. The glucocorticoids also promote the mobilization of fatty acids from adipose tissue which elevates plasma fatty acid levels. This effect, plus an increased oxidation of fatty acids in the cells, is probably involved in the switch from glucose utilization to fatty acid utilization as a source of energy during periods of stress.

Corticosteroids are bound to plasma proteins. Corticosteroid-binding globulin (CBG) has a high affinity, but a low binding capacity. Conversely, plasma albumin has a low affinity and a relatively high binding capacity. Physiologically, most of the hormone will be bound to CBG; pharmacological doses quickly overload the total binding site on CBG. Several agents can adversely affect adrenocortical function (Thomas and Keenan, 1986; Colby, 1988). If a compound does not produce detectable morphological damage to the adrenal following repeated administration, it is usually accepted that no adrenotoxicity has occurred. This is not to assume that toxicity will

pass undetected, particularly considering the influence that adrenocortical hormones have on plasma electrolytes, and carbohydrate, protein and fat metabolisms.

The guinea-pig is a particularly useful model to study the actions of chemicals or drugs on the adrenal gland. The guinea-pig has, perhaps, the largest adrenal gland/body weight ratio of any animal model. Besides its large size, it is readily dissected into functional zones. Like humans, the guinea-pig has adrenal glands that are very adept at metabolizing xenobiotics (Colby, 1988).

Among the endocrine target organs, the adrenal cortex seems to be particularly susceptible to chemical insult. A host of agents have been reported to produce morphological or functional lesions in the gland (Table 8). These lesions may be highly localized and in specific anatomical areas of the adrenal cortex. Chemical-induced functional deficits can produce specific physiological deficits. Carbon tetrachloride produces adrenocortical necrosis, but its locus of toxicity is only the innermost region of the gland, i.e. the zona reticularis. On the other hand, spironolactone, a mineralocorticoid antagonist, produces functional lesions in the zona fasciculata of the adrenal cortex. DDT metabolites (e.g. 3-methylsulphonyl-DDE) (Jonsson et al., 1991) exert their adrenotoxicity by specifically binding to a non-extractable residue in the zona fasciculata. Thus, particular agents have a propensity to affect certain subpopulations of cells within the adrenal cortex. While the adrenal medulla can be adversely affected by various chemicals, by far the majority of chemical lesions are associated with the adrenal cortex.

Chemicals or drugs that affect the brain or adenohypophysis leading to changes in ACTH secretion will, of course, alter the secretory rate of adrenal steroids. Likewise, agents affecting the renin–angiotensin system can affect mineralocorticoid secretion. Chemicals can either directly or indirectly affect adrenal cortical function. The response of the adrenal gland to ACTH may be compromised by chemically induced changes on membrane receptors, cyclic nucleotide levels, protein synthesis and other biochemical processes involved in stimulating steroidogenesis. Thus changes in biochemical processes in adrenal cortical secretions caused by chemicals can be mediated by several different mechanisms. The adrenal cortex is vulnerable to many different

Table 8 Compounds producing lesions in the adrenal cortex

Acrylonilrile	7,12-Dimethylbenzanthracene	Polyglutamic acids
ACTH	Ethanol	Pyrazole
Aflatoxin	Etomidate	Spironolactone
Aminoglutethimide	Fluphenazine	Sulphated mucopolysaccharides
Aniline	Hexadimethrine bromide	Suramin
Carbon tetrachloride	Iprindole	Tamoxifen
Chenodeoxycholic acid	Ketoconazole	Tetrachlorvinphos
Chloroform	Mefloquine	Testosterone
Chlorphentermine	Methanol	Thioacetamide
Clotrimazole	Nitrogen oxides	Thioguanine
Cyproterone	Oestrogens	Toxaphene
$o'p'$-DDD	Parathion	Triparanol
Danazol	PBBs, PCBs	Urethane
Phenytoin (DPH)	Polyanthosulphonate + aminocaprionic acid	Zimelidine

Source: Colby (1988).

chemicals and through different processes. The vascularity of the adrenal cortex is excellent so that the delivery of toxic agents is seldom a limiting factor. It is rich in lipids and, hence, fat-soluble toxins are readily assimilated and sequestered in the adrenal gland. The capacity of the adrenal cortex to metabolize foreign substances is, in part, a result of its high concentration of cytochrome *P*-450. Hence, xenobiotics can undergo detoxification. Alternatively, the metabolism of a xenobiotic may also lead to more toxic intermediates. Bioactivation, or producing more active metabolites, may actually be associated with intermediates with greater inherent toxicities. Toxic metabolites tend to be highly reactive with their concentration usually reaching high local levels producing chemical lesions.

The mechanism of toxic action of spironolactone on the adrenal cortex has been studied extensively (Colby, 1988). Spironolactone is a modified steroid that is a mineralocorticoid antagonist. It competes for aldosterone receptors in the kidney and thus is used as a diuretic. Spironolactone has both renal and extrarenal sites of action. Its extrarenal sites of action include the liver, the adrenal cortex and the testes. In the testes, spironolactone is more potent in inhibiting steroidogenesis when compared with several other drugs (Table 9). Aminoglutethimide, a

potent adrenolytic agent, can also inhibit gonadal steroidogenesis. Thus, chemicals or drugs that inhibit adrenal gland steroidogenesis can often inhibit testicular steroidogenesis (Thomas and Keenan, 1986; Brun *et al.*, 1991).

PANCREAS

The pancreas has a role in digestion, and secretes two important hormones, insulin and glucagon. These hormones are synthesized in the islets of Langerhans by *beta* cells (insulin) and *alpha* cells (glucagon). A primary concern, when testing for toxicity of an experimental drug, is the potential for the compound to interfere with the normal functioning of the pancreatic *beta* cells. Often, pancreatic toxicity is heralded by hyperglycaemia and although increased blood glucose might be found during routine clinical chemistry, additional tests are required to pinpoint specific toxicity.

The relationship between insulin and carbohydrate, fat and protein metabolism, can be appreciated by studying diabetes mellitus. In diabetes mellitus, hyperglycaemia results from an impaired utilization of glucose. The failure of glucose to penetrate adipose tissue will mobilize fat, producing a rise in the free fatty acid and triglyc-

Table 9 Inhibitors of steroid secretion

Compound	Relative inhibiting potency *in vitro* (Leydig cells)		
	Testosterone	Progesterone	Cytotoxicity
Ketoconazole	+	+	−
Cycloheximide	+	+	−
Chlorpromazine	++	++	+
Aminoglutethimide	++	+++	−
Spironolactone	++++	−	−

Source: modified from Brun *et al.* (1991).

eride content of plasma and the triglyceride content of the liver. A fatty liver in the diabetic may occur from the absence of lipoprotein synthesis owing to accelerated gluconeogenesis. When glucose oxidation is impaired, fatty acids form the major source of energy; however, this generates an excess of intermediary metabolites, collectively described as ketone bodies (acetone, acetoacetic acid, and β-hydroxybutyric acid), which can lead to the development of metabolic acidosis.

Hyperglycaemia also can lead to the appearance of glucose in the urine (glycosuria) when the blood glucose levels exceed the renal threshold of approximately 180 mg dl^{-1} of blood. At lower blood glucose levels, all the filtered ketose is normally reabsorbed by the renal tubules. Increased blood levels of glucose leading to glycosuria can be caused by emotional stress and the concomitant release of glucose from liver glycogen in response to adrenaline. Glycosuria also can be the consequence of impaired renal tubular function caused by compounds such as the glycoside, or phlorizin. Renal glycosuria, irrespective of the underlying cause, can produce an osmotic diuretic effect which can lead to dehydration and polydipsia. Glycogenolysis and gluconeogenesis are increased in diabetes, generating glucose which further enhances hyperglycaemia.

Characteristics of insulin-dependent (IDDM) and non-insulin-dependent diabetes mellitus (NIDDM) are shown in Table 10. Diabetes mellitus is not a single disease entity. Rather, it represents a heterogeneous group of glucose intolerance pathologies evidenced by expression of fasting hyperglycaemia. It may or may not be

Table 10 Some characteristics of insulin-dependent (IDDM) (type I) and non-insulin-dependent (NIDDM) (type II) diabetes mellitus

Characteristic	IDDM (Type I)	NIDDM (Type II)
Age of onset	Under 30 years	Over 40 years
Type of onset	Abrupt	Gradual
Nutritional status at onset	Undernourished	Obese
Clinical symptoms	Polydipsia, polyphagia and polyuria	Often none
Ketosis	Frequent	Infrequent
Endogenous insulin	Negligible	Present; but relatively ineffective because of obesity
Lipid abnormalities	Hypercholesterolaemia Lipids elevated in ketoacidosis	Cholesterol and triglycerides often elevated
Insulin therapy	Required	Required in only 20–30% of patients
Hypoglycaemic drugs	Should not be used	Efficacious
Diet	Mandatory	Frequently diet alone

Table 11 Diabetogenic agents

Agent	Use	Susceptible species
Alloxan	Experimental diabetes	Several
Streptozotocin	Experimental diabetes; anticancer agent	Several
Cyproheptadine	Antihistamine and anti-5-HT drug	Rodents
Pentamidine	Antitrypanosomal agent	Human
Hexamethylmelamine	Anticancer drug	Rat
Vacor	Rodenticide	Human

Source: modified from Fischer (1985).

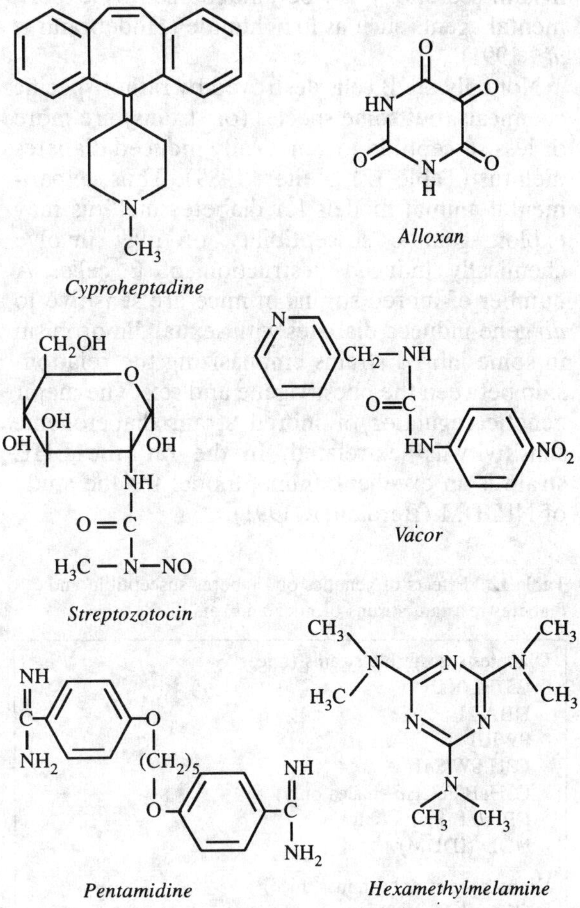

caused by an absolute or relative deficiency of insulin. Thus, NIDDM and IDDM appear to be separate diseases with different aetiologies. IDDM often involves a development of autoimmunity against β-cells. NIDDM involves genes that are associated with obesity and/or insulin resistance and not with genes that affect the immune system.

Several chemicals or drugs can actually be toxic to pancreatic β cells (Figure 2) (Fischer, 1985; Thomas and Keenan, 1986). From a structural view, there are virtually no chemical similarities among these various agents. This suggests different mechanisms of toxic action(s). Alloxan has been used for many years to purposely destroy pancreatic β cells in an effort to produce experimental diabetes. It has an avidity for β cells and concentrates in this target organ. Alloxan destroys β cell function leading to hyperglycaemia and glycosuria in experimental animals. Alloxan is rapidly biometabolized to dialuric acid, a product that undergoes autoxidation to yield amounts of peroxide, superoxide anion and free radicals. On the other hand, the toxic action(s) of streptozotocin may reside in the fact that it contains an *N*-methylnitrosourea moiety. Streptozotocin is also an alkylating agent. Both alloxan and streptozotocin produce damage to pancreatic DNA.

Diabetogenic agents are effective in producing hyperglycaemia in several species including humans (Table 11) (Fischer, 1985; Chatterjee *et al.*, 1991). The pharmacological and toxicological spectrum may differ but their common adverse action resides in their ability to cause varying degrees of destruction of pancreatic β cells. Although alloxan was probably the first agent used to cause β cell necrosis, it has largely been

Figure 2 Chemical structures of diabetes-producing compounds

replaced by the methylnitrosourea analogue, streptozotocin, to produce experimental insulin-dependent diabetes. Cyproheptadine, pentamidine and hexamethylmelamine are also capable of suppressing the function and altering the morphology of insulin-secreting cells. Other drugs, such as phenytoin (DPH) and diazoxide (proglycem) can exert an inhibitory effect on insulin secretion. They may also act by preventing the peripheral utilization of glucose. Conversely, oral hypoglycaemic drugs (e.g. sulphonylureas) can stimulate β cell secretion and are used therapeutically in NIDDM (type II). Cyclosporin, a potent immunosuppressant agent, reduces the requirement for insulin in IDDM (type I), but its mechanism of action on the β cell remains largely unknown. Finally, cholecystokinin, an endogenous hormone that can physiologically enhance insulin secretion, can be antagonized by experimental agents such as loxiglumide (Hildebrand *et al.*, 1991).

Not only are β cells destroyed by rather specific chemicals, but some species (or strains) are more or less susceptible to genetically induced diabetes mellitus (Table 12) (Leiter, 1989). Thus, experimental animal models for diabetes mellitus may exploit genetic susceptibility or may involve chemically induced destruction of β cells. A number of inbred strains of mice are sensitive to *db* gene-induced diabetes with sexual dimorphism in some inbred strains emphasizing the relationship between the obesity gene and sex. The major genetic regulator of inbred strain diabetogenic sensitivity is sex-related. In the rat, the BHE strain is an excellent animal model for the study of NIDDM (Berdanier, 1991).

Table 12 Effects of genetics on diabetes-susceptible and diabetes-resistant strains of mice and rats

Diabetes-susceptible strains (mice)[a]
C57BL/KsJ
DBA/2J
SWR/J
C3H.SW/SnJ
C3HeB/FeCHp (males only)
CBA/Lt (males only)
NOD (IDDM)
Diabetes-resistant strains (mice)[a]
C57BL/6J
129/J
Ma/MYJ
Diabetes-susceptible strains (rats)
BB (IDDM)
BHE
BHE/cdb

[a] Source: modified from Leiter (1989) and Berdanier (1991).

Considerable progress has also been made in culturing pancreatic islet cells, hence affording an important *in vitro* model to study insulin secretion (Takaki, 1989). Insulinoma cell lines have contributed greatly to studies of morphology and function of islet cells, which are relevant to the aetiology of diabetes mellitus. Progress in tissue culture for the transplantation of islet cells across major histocompatibility barriers may lead to replacement therapy for diabetic patients. Artificial pancreas implants in experimental animals may eventually advance to where the concept can be used in diabetic patients requiring islet cell replacement. Recently, a hybrid pancreas consisting of a plastic housing containing a coiled membrane surrounded by living pancreas cells has been shown to be effective in secreting insulin and modulating blood glucose levels.

It is also possible to destroy the α cells of the pancreas somewhat selectively (Thomas and Keenan, 1986). There are species differences with regard to α cell destruction. The injection of cobalt chloride has been shown to produce degranulation and vacuolization of the α cells in rabbits, dogs and guinea pigs. Synthalin A can also selectively cause necrosis of pancreatic α cells.

While attention focuses on those agents that produce destruction of β cells leading to diabetogenic states, there are still many other agents that cause pancreatitis (Banerjee *et al.*, 1989; Steer, 1989). Thus, both endocrine and exocrine function of the pancreas are vulnerable to chemical insult. Drugs and chemicals cause acute pancreatitis, but seldom cause chronic pancreatitis. Acute pancreatitis is often accompanied by increased blood levels of pancreatic enzymes, notably amylase. The exact mechanism in cellular inflammation is not understood, but several factors may be involved (Table 13). Pancreatic duct hypertension may lead to autodigestion and necrosis-induced inflammation of the pancreas. In animals, choline deficiency coupled with the infusion of caevalin (a pancreozymin–cholecystokinin analogue) leads to acute pancreatitis.

A large number of drugs have been associated with acute pancreatitis (Table 14). The cause-and-effect is more definite with some classes of drugs such as the diuretics. Diuretic-induced changes in electrolytes appear to be correlated with acute pancreatitis, particularly in association with hyperamylasaemia. Tetracyclines may exert

Table 13 Possible mechanisms of drug-induced pancreatitis

Mechanism	Drugs implicated
Pancreatic duct constriction	Indomethacin Salicylates (via prostaglandin inhibition) Opiates
Immune suppression	Steroids Azathioprine
Cytotoxic effect	Azathioprine Colaspase (L-asparaginase)
Arteriolar thromboses	Oestrogens
Osmotic effects	Contrast media
Pressure effects	Contrast media
Metabolic effects (ionic changes)	Thiazides
Direct cellular toxicity	Sulphonamides Frusemide (furosemide) Chlorothiazide
Possible hepatic mechanism (via free radicals)	Paracetamol (acetaminophen) Tetracyclines

Source: Banerjee *et al*. (1989).

Table 14 Drugs and other chemicals which have been implicated as causing acute pancreatitis

Definite	Possible
Azathioprine	Bumetanide Anticholinesterases
Cisplatin	Carbamazepine
Colaspase (L-asparaginase)	Chlorthalidone Clonidine
Frusemide (furosemide)	Colchicine
Tetracycline	Corticosteroids Cotrimoxazole
Thiazides	Cyclosporin
Sulphonamides	Cytarabine (cytosine arabinoside) Diazoxide Enalapril
Probable	Ergotamine
Cimetidine	ERCP contrast media
Indomethacin	Ethacrynic acid
Mefenamic acid	Isoniazid
Oestrogens	Isotretinoin (13-*cis*-retinoic acid)

continued

Table 14 (continued)

Definite	Possible
Opiates	Mercaptopurine
Paracetamol (acetaminophen)	Methyldopa Metronidazole
Phenformin	Nitrofurantoin
Valproic acid	Oxphenbutazone
Fonofos	Piroxicam
Diazinon	Procainamide Rifampicin Salicylates Sulindac

Source: modified from Banerjee *et al*. (1989).

a direct pancreotoxicity; azathioprine suppresses the immune system yet has a direct cytotoxic action. Other drugs may also possess a direct cytotoxic action, e.g. valproic acid and possibly L-asparaginase. Allergic reactions are associated with sulphonamides and their pancreotoxicity. It is evident that many drugs can cause acute pancreatitis but the underlying mechanisms are poorly understood (see Chapter 27).

Acknowledgements

The author wishes to express his sincere appreciation to Mrs Betty L. Patton and Ms Manuela K. Nolan for their editorial assistance and comments in the preparation of this chapter.

REFERENCES

Banerjee, A. K., Patel, K. J. and Grainger, S. L. (1989). Drug-induced acute pancreatitis: a critical review. *Med. Toxicol. Adverse Drug Exp.*, **4**, 186–198

Berdanier, C. D. (1991). The BHE rat: an animal model for the study of non-insulin-dependent diabetes mellitus. *FASEB J.*, **5**, 2139–2144

Brun, H. P., Leonard, J. F., Moronvalle, V., Caillaud, J. M., Melcion, C. and Cordier, A. (1991). *Toxicol. Applied Pharmacol.*, **108**, 307–320

Chatterjee, A. K., Varayotha, V., Fischer, L. J. (1991). Interactions of diabetogenic compounds: cyproheptidine and alloxan. *Fund. Appl. Toxicol.*, **16**, 188–197

Colby, H. D. (1988). Adrenal gland toxicity: chemically induced dysfunction. *J. Am. Coll. Toxicol.*, **7**, 45–69

Donaldson, W. E. (1980). Natural toxins. In Hodgson,

E. and Guthrie, F. E. (Eds), *Introduction to Biochemical Toxicology*. Elsevier, New York, pp. 376–388

Fischer, L. J. (1985). Drugs and chemicals that produce diabetes. *TIPS*, (Feb) 72–75

Hildebrand, P., Ensinck, J. W., Ketterer, S., Delco, F., Mossi, S., Bangerter, U. and Beglinger, C. (1991). Effect of cholecystokinin antagonist on meal-stimulated insulin and pancreatic polypeptide release in humans. *J. Clin. Endocrinol. Metab.*, **72**, 1123–1129

Hill, R. N., Erdreich, L. S., Paynter, O. E., Roberts, P. A., Rosenthal, S. L. and Wilkinson, C. F. (1989). Thyroid follicular cell carcinogenesis. *Fund. Appl. Toxicol.*, **12**, 629–697

Jonsson, C. O., Rodriguez, H. R., Lund, B. O., Bergman, A. and Brandt, I. (1991). Adrenocortical toxicity of 3-methylsulfonyl-DDE in mice. *Fund. Appl. Toxicol.*, **16**, 365–374

Leiter, E. H. (1989). The genetics of diabetes susceptibility in mice. *FASEB J.*, **3**, 2231–2241

Rani, C. S. S. (1990). Amiodarone effects on thyrotropin receptors and responses stimulated by thyrotropin and carbachol in cultured dog thyroid cells. *Endocrinol.*, **127**, 2930–2937

Steer, M. L. (1989). Classification and pathogenesis of pancreatitis. *Surg. Clin. N. Am.*, **69**, 467–480

Stevens, J. T. and Summer, D. D. (1991). Herbicides. In Hayes, W. J., Jr and Laws, E. R., Jr (Eds), *Handbook of Pesticide Toxicology*. Academic Press, New York, pp. 1317–1408

Takaki, R. (1989). Culture of pancreatic islet cells and islet hormone producing cell lines morphological and functional integrity in culture. *In Vitro Cell. Devel. Biol.*, **25**, 763–781

Thomas, J. A. (1989). Pharmacology and toxicologic responses in the neonate. *J. Am. Coll. Toxicol.*, **8**, 957–962

Thomas, J. A. and Ballantyne, B. (1990). Occupational reproductive risks: sources, surveillance and testing. *J. Occup. Med.*, **32**, 547–554

Thomas, J. A. and Bell, J. U. (1982). Endocrine toxicology. In Hayes, A. W. (Ed.), *Principles and Methods of Toxicology*. Raven Press, New York, pp. 487–507

Thomas, J. A. and Keenan, E. G. (1986). *Principles of Endocrine Pharmacology*. Plenum Press, New York, pp. 1–294

Thomas, J. A., Korach, K. and MacLaughlin, E. (Eds) (1985), *Endocrine Toxicology, Target Organ Toxicity Series*. Raven Press, New York, pp. 1–340

Thomas, J. A. and Thomas, M. J. (1988). Human growth hormone. In Thomas, J. A. (Ed.), *Drugs, Athletes and Physical Performance*. Plenum Press, New York, pp. 199–215

Thomas, J. A., Thomas, M. J. and Thomas, D. J. (1989). Hormone assays and endocrine function. In Hayes, A. W. (Ed.), *Principles and Methods of Toxicology*, 2nd edn. Raven Press, New York, pp. 677–698

FURTHER READING

Atterwill, C. K. and Flack, J. D. (1992). *Endocrine Toxicology*. Cambridge University Press

Barsano, C. P. and Thomas, J. A. (1992). Endocrine disorders of occupational and environmental origin. *Occupational Medicine*, **7**, 479–502

Thomas, J. A. (1994). Actions of drugs/chemicals on nonreproductive endocrine organs. *Toxic Substances Journal*, **13**, 187–200

Vanderpump, M. P. J. and Tunbridge, W. M. G. (1993). The effects of drugs on endocrine function. *Clinical Endocrinology*, **39**, 389–397

Klara Miller and Clive Meredith

INTRODUCTION

General Concepts in Immunology

The development of the immune system may be considered as a series of adaptive cellular responses leading to some survival advantage of the evolving species. The earliest manifestation of this is phagocytosis, which is found in unicellular organisms and has a defensive as well as a nutritive function. In higher invertebrates a vascular system developed that allowed phagocytosis to proceed by both fixed and circulatory cells, and this defence mechanism was further amplified by a disseminated lymphoid system in primitive vertebrates and by the specialized lymphoid structures that occur in higher forms (lymph nodes, spleen and collections of lymphoid cells within the respiratory and alimentary tracts).

With further evolution there also occurred the development of an elaborate series of substances (e.g. kallikrein system and complement system) that could augment and enhance the efficiency of both the specific and non-specific defence mechanisms, and a complex genetic system controlling the cell surface determinants involved in cellular interactions. These genetically controlled 'antigenic' determinants distinguish one individual of a given species from another, and form the major histocompatibility complex (MHC) antigens.

The cell type responsible for the remarkable specificity of immune responses is the lymphocyte. Lymphocytes, however, do not function in isolation and there are many other contributing cells that are needed for the 'capture' and 'presentation' of antigen to lymphocytes during the initiation of the response (accessory cells), and others, such as mast cells and macrophages, concerned with the execution of the various effector stages of the response. Immune responses not only protect the host against invasive microorganisms such as bacteria and viruses, but also involve homoeostatic and surveillance control. Protection against foreign invaders is provided when the immune system is able to recognize, isolate and neutralize, eliminate or metabolize antigenic material by cellular or humoral effector mechanisms, whereas homoeostatic control is maintained by the removal of effete or damaged cellular elements such as circulating erythrocytes or leucocytes. Surveillance implies the recognition and destruction of abnormal cell types that occur within the body which are affected by certain viruses and chemicals. It has been postulated that failure of the immune system to recognize these mutant cells plays a causal role in the development of neoplastic disease.

The main cell lines involved in immune defence mechanisms are mononuclear phagocytes, antigen-presenting cells (accessory cells) and populations of lymphoid cells (Figure 1). All cell populations arise from stem cells in the bone marrow, as do other cell lines, such as polymorphonuclear leucocytes, which participate in immunological reactions through the release of chemical mediators.

Lymphocytes

Most of the lymphocytes present in blood and lymph and peripheral lymphoid tissue are small round cells with metabolic activity kept at a minimum but with the capacity to change to an active state once the surface receptors have received the appropriate signal. Activated lymphocytes tend to migrate out of the circulation to sites of inflammation or remain sequestered at sites of antigen localization, although some activated lymphocytes are frequently found in the circulation during a vigorous immune response. Lymphocyte motility is greatly increased by activation; and in cultures of mononuclear cells containing a foreign antigen or a mitogenic lectin, blastogenic activation is associated with clustering around macrophages. Comparable cell-attached phenomena occur in tissues *in vivo*, and this is particularly evident in the early stages of a response in the clustering of lymphocytes around dendritic cells or macrophages in lymphoid tissue

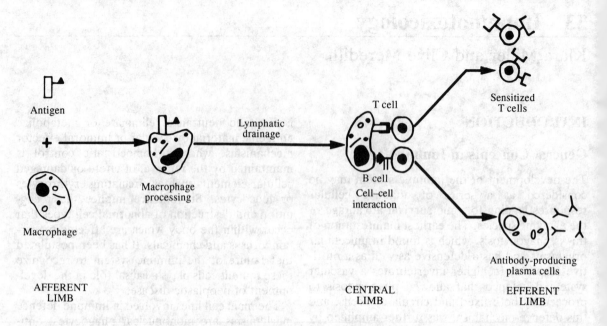

Antigen

Macrophage

Macrophage processing

Lymphatic drainage

T cell

B cell

Cell–cell interaction

Sensitized T cells

Antibody-producing plasma cells

AFFERENT LIMB

CENTRAL LIMB

EFFERENT LIMB

Figure 1   Schematic and very simplified representation of the principal events during the development of an immune response

following the capture of antigen (Austyn, 1987). It is also a feature of the late effector stages, e.g. during graft rejection.

Lymphocytes are functionally heterogeneous and consist of two main populations, T and B, concerned with cell-mediated or humoral immunity, respectively. T cells are generated in the thymus from precursors that have migrated from the bone marrow to the thymus (Boyd and Hugo, 1991). Considerable mitotic activity occurs in the thymus, particularly in the cortex, and the epithelial cells, fibroblasts, dendritic cells and macrophages of the thymus provide a microenvironment essential for differentiation to occur. Hormones secreted by thymic epithelial cells have been shown to have specific effects on the differentiation and functional activity of T cells. Cortical thymocytes have long been known to lack immunobiological activity and this is due to lack of surface structures found on mature cells such as the TCR (T cell receptor) complex. It is probable that part of the considerable death rate of cortical thymocytes is due to some cells failing to rearrange TCR genes effectively. The relatively small numbers of thymocytes in the medullary region are phenotypically and functionally similar to peripheral T cells. It does not follow, however, that these cells are on the way out to the periphery and some medullary thymocytes are known

to remain resident in the thymus for long periods (Nikolic-Zugic, 1991).

About 80 per cent of the lymphocytes in human blood and 60 per cent of lymphocytes in peripheral lymphoid tissue are of T lineage, and most express either the T4 (CD4) or T8 (CD8) surface membrane antigen (cluster differentiation antigens). Cells bearing CD4 (helper cells) are concerned with activation of B cells and macrophages and recognize antigen in association with the MHC Class II molecules, whereas cells bearing CD8 recognize antigen in association with MHC Class I molecules. Cells within the CD4 population will provide 'help' for specific antibody production, whereas others have a different role. Recent studies in the mouse have demonstrated the existence of two functionally distinct T4 cells, TH1 and TH2, with one subset involved in delayed type hypersensitivity reactions (Bottomly, 1988).

Helper TH1 cells are thought to have evolved primarily against extracellular pathogens, whereas T4 cells associated with inflammatory and hypersensitivity reactions are concerned with defence against intracellular pathogens such as mycobacteria. A different T cell population, the T8 population, is thought to have evolved principally to combat virus-infected cells by a direct cell–cell cytotoxic mechanism. CD8[+] T cells also have the capacity to act as 'suppressor' cells. Overactivity of suppressor T cells may result in an inability to respond to an antigenic challenge, while underactivity may allow the development of autoimmune manifestations.

The primary compartment in mammals in which B cells are generated from stem cells is the bone marrow. At least 75 per cent of pre-B cells are deleted; the remainder are released into the periphery in response to unknown signals. It is during this stage that recognition diversity is generated in an antigen-independent fashion (Gallagher and Osmond, 1991). This occurs through rearrangement of heavy chain and then kappa and lambda light chain U-region genes. B lymphocytes bear surface immunoglobulin, and there is a massive production of new B cells daily. Clearly most of the cells will die; otherwise there would be a progressive increase in peripheral B cell numbers. In fact, their survival depends on activation by encounter with antigen. This is most likely to occur at sites such as the spleen or lymph nodes, where antigen-capturing cells such as dendritic cells have removed antigen from blood or lymph and retained it on their surface.

Most antigens are proteins or are haptens complexed with protein. B cells responding to these so-called thymus-dependent antigens do so in co-operation with T cells and this co-operation requires direct cell–cell interaction of antigen-presenting cell, B cell and T helper cell as well as numerous soluble factors. The mitotically activated B cells typically generate subclones, and the various progeny of a single activated B cell may make antibody of IgM, IgG, IgA, IgD and IgE classes. A different population of B cells responds to so-called thymus-independent antigens without the involvement of T cells with a predominantly IgM response. Both antibody-secreting cells (plasma cells) and memory B cells will arise from activated virgin or established B cells (MacLennon and Gray, 1986). IgM and most subclasses of IgG activate complement when they bind to antigen, and if the antigen–antibody complex is on the surface of a foreign cell such as a Gram-negative bacillus, this activation causes cell lysis and cell death. Plasma cells found in mucosa-associated lymphoid tissue of the digestive, respiratory and urinary tracts secrete dimeric IgA which is converted to secretory IgA when secretory component (produced by epithelia) transports the IgA through the mucosal barrier into the lumen or into external secretions such as tears or milk through the internal lymphatic route.

The biological potency of IgE antibodies arises from their unique ability to combine with specific receptors on the surface of mast cells and basophils. This interaction leaves the antigen-binding end of the IgE molecule available for combination with antigen. Bridging by antigen of adjacent IgE antibodies triggers the release of pharmacological mediators, such as histamine, which alter the permeability of adjacent small blood vessels, thereby permitting antibodies of diverse classes and phagocytic cells to accumulate at the local site. These sites include the skin and mucosal surfaces in contact with the external environment. IgE-mediated inflammation is of protective value in parasite infestation, particularly in helminth infections. The major significance of the IgE class is not in protective immunity, however, but as the mediator of immediate hypersensitivity or anaphylaxis (Table 1).

Natural Killer Cells

Some lymphocytes from non-immunized subjects are able to lyse suitable target cells and have been named NK (natural killer) cells (Kimber, 1985). These cells are large granular lymphocytes, non-immunoglobulin-bearing, non-adherent and apparently not of thymic origin. NK cells mediate cytolytic reactions not involving MHC Class I or

Table 1 Pharmacological mediators derived from mast cells or basophils

Mediator	Effects
Histamine	Vasodilation—increased capillary permeability
Enzymes	Proteolytic (tryptase) C3 convertase (glucosaminidase)
Heparin	Anticoagulant
Chemotaxins	Chemotaxis of eosinophils/neutrophils (ECF-A) (NCF)
Thromboxanes	Platelet aggregation
Prostaglandins	Vasodilation; bronchial muscle contraction
Leucotrienes (LTB$_4$)	Vasoactive bronchoconstriction
SRS (LTC$_4$, LTD$_4$)	Chemotactic/chemokinetic

Class II antigen on the target cells. However, the *in vitro* direct cell–cell lysis tests used to identify them do not necessarily reflect their true function, which may include defence against virus infection. NK cells secrete a variety of lymphokines, including interferon, when appropriately stimulated.

Macrophages

Macrophages are defined as phagocytic mononuclear cells and are grouped together on the basis of having a common origin and similar cytochemistry. They are, however, a very heterogeneous group of cells and include the connective tissue histocytes, Kupffer cells and osteoclasts (Loutit *et al.*, 1982). Additionally, the entire glial cell population of the central nervous system is now thought to be made up of cells related to macrophages. The major source of macrophages is the haematopoietic tissue of the marrow (van Furth, 1980) and monocytes are generated from stem cells at a rate of approximately 7×10^6 cells kg^{-1} h^{-1}. They remain circulating in the blood with a half-life of 8–12 h before migrating and undergoing further differentiation to macrophages at different tissue sites. In some sites, such as the peritoneal or pleural cavities, and in the alveolar regions of the lung, they may remain in suspension and are a common source of macrophages for *in vitro* experiments.

Macrophages phagocytose particulates such as plastic or carbon particles and mineral dusts as well as bacteria and protozoa. They also recognize a great range of antigens, not only those of external origin. Their surveillance role includes the removal of effete red cells through glycolipid and phospholipid systems. The hydrolytic enzymes of all mononuclear phagocytes are synthesized in the ribosomes of the endoplasmic reticulum and incorporated into primary lysosomes. After ingestion, fusion of a lysosome with the formed phagocytic vacuole results in killing and digestion of the particulate matter and exoplasmosis of degradation products of the cell surface (Allison, 1967). An oxidative destructive mechanism ('respiratory burst') also operates in addition to attack by lysosomal enzymes.

Macrophages also have other important effector functions such as trophic and antigen-presenting functions. Products secreted include enzymes such as collagenase, arginase and lysozyme, the adhesion molecule fibronectin, growth regulating factors such as interleukin-1 and several important plasma proteins such as α_2-macroglobulin and complement components. As mentioned above, macrophages from different sites display considerable heterogeneity, which includes differences in secretion patterns and antigen-presenting functions, as evidenced by the ability to form clusters with activated T helper cells in the presence of antigen (Inaba and Steinman, 1987). Intracellular antigens are mainly presented in the context of MHC Class I molecules, whereas exogenous antigens associate with MHC Class II molecule, and this is related to differing processing within the cell itself.

Macrophages which are maximally functional in any assay (antimicrobial, tumoricidal and antigen-presenting assays) are referred to as 'activated' macrophages. Activated cells spread more extensively on glass or plastic culture dishes and have a higher density of surface membrane receptors such as the IgG Fc receptor. Agents such as lipopolysaccharide (LPS) have been shown to induce increased production and secretion of interleukin-1 and other cytokines, whereas the lymphocyte product interferon-α induces increased expression of MHC Class II, important in antigen expression. Macrophages which have been 'activated' by the products of an antigen-specific lymphocyte activation are non-specifically more effective in ingesting and killing a wide range of bacteria.

Dendritic Cells

Dendritic cells are non-phagocytic cells found in lymphoid tissues and the interstitial tissue of non-lymphoid organs such as the epithelium. They possess long mobile cytoplasmic processes, have few lysosomes and stain weakly for non-specific esterase. Dendritic or 'interdigitating' cells are found in T areas of spleen, lymph nodes, Peyer's patches and the medullary region of the thymus. Langerhans cells, which also belong to the dendritic family (Austyn, 1987), are found in the epidermis of skin; 'veiled' cells, i.e. cells with bulbous pseudopods, are found in the peripheral lymph and drift into nodes via the afferent lymphatics. Dendritic cells lack most conventional surface markers associated with the macrophage lineage, but expression of MHC Class II is very strong and they play an important role in helper

T cell activation, retaining substantial amounts of antigen on the cell surface and forming clusters with resting T cells. Dendritic cells from all species have proven to be potent stimulators of the autologous mixed leucocyte reaction (MLR) and *in vitro* mitogen- and antigen-induced lymphocyte proliferation (King and Katz, 1990). Follicular dendritic cells (FDC) are found only in B cell follicles in peripheral lymphoid tissues. FDC bind antigen–antibody–complement complexes very strongly and retain them on their surface for long periods, thereby presenting antigens to the B lymphocytes sequestered with the centre.

Cytokines

It is now accepted that the immune system is regulated by a variety of mediators (cytokines) produced by both cells of the immune system and cells of the microenvironment of the immune system (Hamblin, 1988). These cytokines underpin and maintain normal immune function and control the development of the immune response to antigen. Cytokines are secreted polypeptides, and a simple cytokine can affect a number of different cell types.

In recent times the availability of recombinant cytokines and of anticytokine monoclonal antibodies has revolutionized the scope of cytokine research. Dissection of the genomic structure and location of the protein structure of cytokines has been possible, and the term 'interleukin' is now used for cytokine factors produced by cells of the immune system for which the nucleotide sequence is known. However, there are a number of 'interleukins' which are within the general definition but which have retained their original title—e.g. tumour necrosis factor, TNF; the colony stimulating factors (CFSs); and interferon-γ (IFN-γ) (Table 2).

There are a number of general biological effects of cytokines which are important for understanding and interpreting their roles. A single cytokine can affect a number of different cell types (it is said to be pleiotropic). Several cytokines act back on the cells that secreted them (autocrine effect). For example, IL-1 and IL-2 are produced by macrophages and T cells, respectively, and can bind to their receptors on the cells that secreted them, to produce more cytokine secretion. Many cytokines act on neighbouring cells to induce the production of other cytokines (paracrine effects)—an action presumably of great importance in the amplification of the immune response.

A further important biological feature of cytokines is their ability to act synergistically with each other and with other stimulants. This frequently means that minute levels of cytokines, which on their own are ineffective, in combination may produce pronounced biological effects. For example, IL-2 and IL-4 synergize to cause proliferation to T cell clones.

Individual cytokines have biological activities relevant to roles either in normal immune responses or in stress/inflammation responses, or in both of these. IL-1 and IL-2 are important in interactions between antigen-presenting cells and T cells which initiate primary and secondary immune responses to antigen. IL-3 and the CSFs are important in the development of myeloid haemopoietic cells from pluripotent stem cells in response to stress, and it is assumed, although not established, that they play a role in normal haemopoiesis. These same cytokines also play a role in the activation of mature cells during normal immune or inflammatory stimulation. IL-7 is a growth factor for early lymphoid cells of B and T lineage. IL-4, IL-5 and IL-6 are essential for the development of humoral immune responses by B cells. Two cytokines, IL-1 and IL-6, as well as TNF and IL-8, have biological actions important in inflammation, and IL-4 and IL-5 have potent effects on eosinophils and mast cells/basophils, compatible with a role in allergic disease and inflammation.

It is probable that in many normal situations cytokines are released by, and act on, cells in close contact. In such a way, detrimental 'bystander' effects of cytokines would be limited. In contrast, acute or chronic inflammation may be accompanied by their release into the circulation and systemic action. The balance determining whether secreted soluble factors produce a satisfactory limited immune response or tissue-damaging reaction also depends on homoeostatic mechanisms. Continued cellular stimulation may result in continued production of mediators, which then induce a chain of responses which, unchecked, might be damaging. A short half-life of soluble factors is evidence that under normal conditions most are rapidly deactivated by a variety of different processes, thereby ensuring their unavailability for bioactivity. It follows that

Table 2 Cytokines and the target cells of their biological activities

Cytokine	Target
Interleukin-1, IL-1	Diverse including haematopoietic and non-haematopoietic cells
Interleukin-2, IL-2	T cells; B cells; NK cells; macrophages
Interleukin-3, IL-3	Multipotential stem cells; mast cells; granulocytes; monocytes/macrophages; eosinophils; megakaryocytes
Interleukin-4, IL-4	B cells; T cells; mast cells; haematopoietic/progenitor cells; monocytes/macrophages; thymocytes
Interleukin-5, IL-5	Eosinophils; B cells
Interleukin-6, IL-6	B cells; fibroblasts; hepatocytes; thymocytes; T cells; haematopoietic progenitor cells
Interleukin-7, IL-7	Pre-B cells; thymocytes
Interleukin-8, IL-8	Neutrophils
Granulocyte macrophage colony stimulating factor, GM-CSF	Multipotential stem cells; monocyte/macrophages; neutrophils; eosinophils
Macrophage colony stimulating factor, M-CSF	Multipotential stem cells; monocytes/macrophages
Granulocyte colony stimulating factor, G-CSF	Multipotential stem cells; neutrophils
Tumour necrosis factor, TNF Lymphotoxin, LT, TNF-β	Diverse, including: tumour cells; transformed cell lines; fibroblasts; neutrophils; adipocytes; endothelial cells; chondrocytes; hepatocytes; monocytes/macrophages

drugs or toxic agents which act on the mediators themselves, or cells that produce them, may cause damaging immune reactions such as hypersensitivity or chronic immunodeficiency.

IMMUNOTOXICOLOGY

General Concepts

The science of toxicology has developed along 'target' organ-specific lines and the immune system would therefore be regarded as an organ, and chemically induced damage to the immune system subject to these dose–effect and dose–response relationships which are fundamental principles in toxicology. For example, reduction in circulating CD8 T cells, increased production of interleukin-2 or decreased antigen-specific IgA secretion at mucosal membranes would all be considered effects rather than responses as far as toxicologists are concerned.

In toxicology damage to a target organ is related to the concentration of the toxic agent or metabolite in that organ. Certain immune-mediated effects, however, may not conform to this concept. For example, compounds of inorganic mercury and gold damage the kidneys as a secondary consequence of their interaction with the immune system. Thus, despite the fact that the observed toxic response is on the kidneys, the effect is due to the action of the agent on immunocompetent cells.

Conventionally, in dose–response relationships, the proportion of a population, human or animal, exhibiting a specified toxic effect would increase with the degree of exposure to the chemical. However, from the point of view of the immune system dose–response relationships must be considered at a number of levels (Nicklin and Miller, 1990). In a strictly biological sense, individual lymphocytes may function on a quantal basis—that is they may have responded or not responded—but only when a large number of cells react to a drug or chemical may there be a measurable response. Unlike conventional target organ studies, however, minor effects at the level of regulatory cells may have dramatic consequences for the organism as a whole. On the other hand, overtly toxic effects in one effector system may be compensated for by enhanced reactivity in parallel pathways, which makes it difficult to resolve immunotoxic target cell or organ-specific effects with any degree of certainty. Damage might also arise through direct toxic effects (as may well occur during a standard subacute or subchronic toxicity test protocol), leading to effects on primary lymphoid organs and/or generalized immune dysfunction.

Most importantly, consideration must be given not only to the effects of the toxic agent upon and within the immune system as a whole, but also to the effects and constraints imposed by antigen. Antigenic challenge is inseparable from immune reactivity; it occurs continuously and drives the immune mechanism. Without antigen, there is no immune response, and the concept of immunotoxicity becomes meaningless. Thus, not only does antigen add another dimension to the dose–effect or dose–response relationship, but also the requirement of antigen actually separates conventional toxicity from immunotoxicity. Whereas it is perfectly possible to examine the effect of an agent upon lymphoid organ weight, for example, some form of antigen challenge must be considered when evaluating the effect of the chemical or drug on immune reactivity. However, recent advances in molecular biology together with recent knowledge of cytokine regulation of the immune response may provide a means for early detection of altered immune reactivity without the need for *in vivo* antigen challenge.

Background

There is now compelling experimental evidence that the mammalian immune system can be damaged and immune reactivity subsequently altered following exposure to a wide and diverse range of drugs and environmental chemicals (Descotes, 1986) (Table 3). There is also strong evidence that treatment with therapeutic agents, as well as exposure to drugs of abuse, alter immune functions in humans (Dean *et al.*, 1985). There is very limited information concerning chemically induced suppression of immune function and other immunological parameters in humans. Where alterations do exist, the biological consequences in terms of increased susceptibility to infection and to certain forms of cancer are unclear. There is, however, as stated above, a substantial database demonstrating enhanced tumour development in patients undergoing immunosuppressive drug therapy as well as evidence of decreased resistance to infections in subjects with genetic or disease-related immune deficiencies. It is important to keep in mind that epidemiology is a fairly blunt tool and that epidemiological evidence is almost impossible to obtain after environmental exposure, given the diversity of human behaviour and genetic constitution, and the very high background evidence. Some limited human data will be discussed later in this chapter, but the authors believe that clinical data available from patients justify concerns about the potential of chemicals to impair immune function. While it is not legitimate to directly compare the effects of the AIDS virus with the effect of immunotoxic drugs or chemicals, it is worth emphasizing that the ultimate lethality of AIDS is not directly attributable to the viral infection but is a secondary effect resulting from chronically impaired immune function. As immunotoxicologists, it is this impairment of immune function which we seek to characterize in relation to exposure to putative immunomodulatory drugs and chemicals.

Hypersensitivity Reactions

In contrast to immunosuppression, a substantial database exists in both human and laboratory animals for a variety of chemicals and drugs that induce hypersensitivity reactions. The manifestations of this type of immunotoxicity may be allergic reactions, mediated through IgE-based mechanisms, antibody- or immune complex-mediated damage, cell-mediated reactions, including contact sensitization and/or autoimmune responses. The respiratory tract and the skin are the two primary routes of sensitization when environmental and occupational exposure is considered, although allergic reactions to food additives are increasingly reported as a consumer concern.

Autoimmune manifestations, where the immune response is directed against one or more of the body's own constituents, may be chemical- or drug-induced and several experimental animal models for studying autoimmune reactions exist. Metal-induced autoimmunity (e.g. mercury- and gold-induced autoimmunity in rat and mice) clearly demonstrates that a genetic predisposition for the induction of autoreactive cells exists; the popliteal lymph node assay which monitors the ability of chemicals to induce immune activations

Table 3   Examples of chemicals with reported selectivity towards immune cells

Benzene	Organophosphates
Diethylstilboestrol	parathion-methyl
Halogenated aromatic hydrocarbons	parathion
polychlorinated biphenyls	malathion
polybrominated biphenyls	Organotins
dibenzo-*p*-dioxins	di-*n*-octyltin chloride
Hexachlorobenzene	tri-*n*-butyltin oxide
Isocyanates	Trimellitic anhydride
methyl isocyanate	
toluene diisocyanate	
Metals	
chromium	
lead	
nickel	

by measuring increased popliteal lymph node weight after hindfoot pad injections in rats and mice appears a promising indicator of the potential of chemicals and drugs to induce autoimmune manifestations and has been used successfully in several laboratories.

Several recent reviews have appeared specifically on autoimmunity which will not be considered further in the context of this chapter (Kammuller *et al.*, 1989; Merk *et al.*, 1992). It should be pointed out, however, that in chemically induced autoimmunity the adverse response is not restricted to the chemical compound inducing it, but involves responses to self-antigens as well. If the inducing agent is a non-specific stimulator, the adverse immune response may not be directed at all towards the inducing agent, but be confined to anti-self responses.

The extensive human and animal data on occupational and environmental allergens amply demonstrate that allergens comprise a very diverse group of substances. They include biologically derived material, such as plant and animal products, drugs and chemicals, both organic and inorganic in nature. Allergens are frequently classified as those which are complete antigens (of high molecular weight) and those which are haptens (of low molecular weight) and therefore incapable of alone inducing an immune response. Although allergens comprise such an enormous range of materials, the clinical reaction to all allergens has been successfully classified as Types I–IV (Coombs and Gell, 1975). Each requires initial exposure to the chemical for induction/sensitization, and a subsequent exposure to elicit clinical symptoms. Once sensitized to a material,

an individual is at risk of hypersensitivity reactions whenever exposed to the same, or cross-reacting, allergens. Type I reactions are due to the release of pharmacologically active molecules from mast cells or basophils as a result of the allergen cross-linking with its specific IgE (or other cytotropic antibody) present on the surface of the cells. It is of rapid onset, and clinical signs and symptoms include urticaria, bronchoconstriction and anaphylactic shock. Immediate responses, particularly when the respiratory system is involved, can be life-threatening. The late type of mainly humoral mediated reactions (types II and III) occur 4–12 h after the administration of antigen. The responses are caused by IgG or IgM antibodies reacting with the chemical bound to a cell surface (Type II) or by forming immune complexes (Type III), thus inducing complement activation resulting in cytotoxicity or inflammation. Examples of allergens associated with Type II reactions are penicillin and trimellitic anhydride; Type III reactions are generally observed with large-molecular-weight occupational allergens, such as those associated with fungi, plants and other biological materials.

The Type IV reaction is typified by contact dermatitis and is the only type of allergic response which is mediated by cells rather than antibodies. The inflammatory responses result from release of lymphokines from activated T lymphocytes and are characterized by late onset (24–72 h). Contact sensitivity is probably the most frequently encountered toxicological consequence of the interaction of chemicals, and certainly the most thoroughly investigated. With respect to predictive testing of chemicals with the potential to sensitize humans, the guinea-pig has traditionally been used as the animal model.

There are a number of accepted guinea-pig tests for assessing skin-sensitizing potential (Anderson and Maibach, 1985). They vary primarily in the way the guinea-pig is exposed to the compound, the schedule of application during the induction phase and the use of adjuvants. Some assays use epicutaneous application under occlusion (the Buehler test), some require intradermal injection (the Draize test) and others use a combination of both topical application and intradermal injection (e.g. the guinea-pig maximization test). A number include the use of Freund's complete adjuvant to non-specifically enhance the immune response and thereby increase the sensitivity of the assay. After challenge the inflammatory response is assessed by the degree of erythema and oedema manifested as well as the number of animals sensitized. This evaluation is subjective and may be confusing when irritant or coloured chemicals are used. At present seven of these test methods are approved for use by the OECD guidelines (1981) for detecting skin sensitization. The requirement for allergenicity tests extends from chemicals with industrial use to consumer products which may indicate a hazard if allergenic ingredients are present in sufficient concentration.

In recent years alternative methods using the mouse, the classical animal for studying the mechanism of delayed-type hypersensitivity reaction, have been developed. Several predictive tests based on measuring changes in ear thickness have been developed and partially validated (Maisey and Miller, 1986; Gad et al., 1986). Another approach, the murine local lymph node assay (LLNA), based on induction events only (similarly to the PLNA), measures the proliferative activity in the draining lymph nodes following topical application on the ear and intravenous injection of [³H]-thymidine (Kimber et al., 1990). This may be a rapid and cost-effective assay for screening new chemicals and holds much promise for the future. The main benefit of the more quantitative murine test methods, however, would be improved ranking of allergens and better discrimination between allergenic and irritant materials.

The guinea-pig has also been used experimentally as a model to evaluate sensitization potential via the respiratory tract. There is a great need for further research into animal model systems which provide information on both immunological events and functional changes in hypersensitivity reactions following exposure to chemicals via the respiratory tract and the gastrointestinal tract.

Immunosuppression in Human Populations

A few chemicals have been associated with immune alterations in humans (as well as experimental animals) following exposure. There have been two major outbreaks of poisoning due to consumption of rice bran oil contaminated with polychlorinated biphenyls (PCBs); one in Japan in 1968, the other in Taiwan in 1969. The most prominent symptoms in PCB-exposed patients were ocular and dermal abnormalities. Where depression of delayed-type hypersensitivity responses has been demonstrated, plasma PCB concentrations and severity of symptoms have all been found to correlate (Chang et al., 1982). Patients also showed signs of immune suppression such as persistent skin infection, bronchitis-like respiratory symptoms and a moderate decrease in immunoglobulin concentrations, especially the IgM and IgA fractions. It is not clear whether the observed immune suppression is due directly to the toxic effects of these chemicals or is an indirect result of toxicity to other tissues. Abnormalities in hepatic, neural and endocrinological functions as a result of PCB poisoning could affect tissues of the lymphoid system (PCB exposure in laboratory animals has commonly been associated with atrophy of both primary and secondary lymphoid organs). In vitro experiments, however, have demonstrated that the PCBs could affect leucocytes directly.

Substantial human exposure to polybrominated biphenyls (PBBs) occurred when livestock feed in Michigan was contaminated, thereby contaminating the food chain. A number of immune parameters were altered, and are still apparent 15 years following the original incident. It is unclear what influence, if any, these immunological alterations, which include changes in lymphocyte subpopulations, have had on susceptibility to infection in the exposed populations.

There have been several disasters in which TCDD was released into the environment, but evidence of TCDD-related immune alterations in humans is very limited. Nevertheless, there are

numerous data demonstrating its potent immunotoxicity in all the laboratory animal species tests.
However, since TCDD-mediated immunotoxicity
has been shown experimentally to be genetically
linked, it may also be that the genetic variability
that would exist within exposed subject groups
makes it very difficult to determine the differing
susceptibility of the human immune system to
TCDD (Murray and Thomas, 1992).

Exposure of experimental animals to a wide
range of pesticides, including organophosphates,
carbamates and organotin compounds, has
resulted in a variety of immune alterations, some
of which could be correlated with impaired
immune function (Murray and Thomas, 1992).
Of these, a carbamate insecticide, aldicarb, is at
present the subject of extensive laboratory and
clinical investigations. Epidemiologists have
assessed the immune status of otherwise healthy
women who have chronically ingested low levels
of aldicarb-contaminated groundwater, and demonstrated altered numbers of T cells, including
a decreased CD4/CD8 ratio in those individuals
compared with controls. No altered susceptibility
to infection has been observed in this very small
group of individuals, so that it remains difficult
to relate these changes to health risks. However,
in a study of 85 workers exposed to organophosphate pesticides marked impairment of neutrophil chemotaxis and an increased incidence of
respiratory tract infection correlated well with
length of exposure (Hermanowicz and Kossman,
1984). This is one of the few studies showing a
direct association between exposure and a change
in immune status.

Exposure to asbestiform fibres may be considered as one of the few examples of occupational exposure where changes in the immune
status of exposed populations have been well
documented (Miller, 1985). Augmented humoral
immunity and impaired cell-mediated immunity
after asbestos exposure have been reported in
most studies. Studies where T cells were enumer-
ated by use of specific monoclonal antibodies
have found that the number and percentage of T
cells decreased in asbestos-exposed subjects compared with controls, even after correction for age
and smoking histories. Two other studies have
described decreased cytotoxic lymphocyte functions, which raises the possibility of immune alterations beyond the putative effect on lymphocytes.
Furthermore, the finding that impaired T lympho-

cyte function is evident in some asbestos-exposed
subjects with no evidence of fibrosis at the time
of sampling suggests that immune changes might
be involved in the pathogenesis of disease (Miller
and Brown, 1985). Animal studies have also demonstrated that asbestos inhalation activates macrophages in an adjuvant fashion, induces the
secretion of several potentially fibrogenic cytokines such as IL-1 and TNF, and may confer antigenic properties on the macrophage leading to
immune dysregulation (Miller, 1979).

In contrast to human data, there is compelling
evidence in laboratory animals that many chemicals adversely alter the immune systems. As will
be discussed in the following section, many of the
data are flawed and techniques for evaluation of
test results need still to be developed. The problem is further complicated by the interplay
between the immune system and the neuroendocrine systems; the immune system—and the
young thymus, in particular—is known to be
exquisitely sensitive to stress-induced hormonal
changes. Nevertheless, data generated on potential immunotoxicity during evaluation of a new
drug or chemical should improve human risk
assessment.

Approaches to Immunotoxicity Testing

A number of different approaches for evaluating
the immune system of experimental laboratory
animals as a target for toxicity have been published (Vos, 1977; Miller, 1985; Luster *et al.*,
1988). Many of these are intended to be used in
conjunction with a subchronic exposure regimen
and consist of 'tiered' approaches. One tier (Tier
I) would focus on evaluating relevant pathological
and haematological parameters; the second tier,
on evaluating the competence of immune cells.
In 1988 Luster and colleagues published the
results of the US National Toxicology Program
(NTP) interlaboratory programme, whose purpose was to show that selected immunological
assays were validated in the mouse. These assays
are divided into two tiers.

The first tier is meant to provide a screening
mechanism for identification of immunotoxic
compounds; the first tier includes the weight and
histology of spleen and thymus, spleen cellularity,
haematology and functional assays, including the
antibody response to sheep and red blood cells
(a T-dependent antigen).

The second tier assays include enumeration of cell types, including T and B cells, resident peritoneal cells and various stem cells of the bone marrow, further functional assays of cell populations obtained from animals after exposure to the agent, and host resistance assays. These assays are fully described in a recent chapter by White (1992) and will be only briefly described here. Four functional assays were selected in the NTP approach for evaluating cell-mediated immunity: spleen lymphocyte responses to the T lymphocyte mitogen concanavalin A, the mixed leucocyte culture response (MLR), the cytotoxic T lymphocyte assay (CTL) and the delayed hypersensitivity response (DHR) to keyhole limpet haemocyanin.

The response of spleen cells to concanavalin A provides an evaluation of the ability of T lymphocytes to undergo blastogenesis and proliferation; the MLR measures ability to respond to alloantigenic determinants; whereas CTL measures the ability of the spleen cells to recognize allogenic cells, and to proliferate and differentiate into mature cells which are capable of identifying and lysing the foreign cell. In contrast to these assays, where spleen cells remain in culture for as long as 5 days after being removed from the animals, the DHR assay represents a more holistic approach, in which responses are induced *in vivo* during exposure to the test compound. This approach is similar to the assay utilized for evaluation of humoral immunity (Tier I) which measures the spleen IgM and IgG antibody response to the T-dependent antigen, sheep erythrocytes, using a modified haemolytic plaque assay (Jerne and Nordin, 1963). This assay is thought to represent one of the most useful indicators of immunocompetence, unlike the measurement of basal serum immunoglobulin levels, which were found to be of minimum value in indicating immunotoxicity in the mouse (although it is thought to be useful in the rat). Assays which have been selected by the NTP for measuring innate or non-specific immunity (that is, those immunological functions which do not require prior exposure to a specific antigen) include natural killer (NK) activity and evaluation of macrophage function. In evaluating NK activity, an *in vitro* cytotoxicity assay is conducted which utilizes the YAC–1 cell line as the target cell; macrophage assays include measuring phagocytic capacity, and the ability to respond to activation by the cytokine gamma

interferon as evidenced by enhanced capacity to kill tumour cells. The NTP also includes assays of infectious or tumour models to assess changes in host resistance.

Two examples of host resistance models are inoculation of *Listeria monocytogenes* for assessing competence of macrophages and T lymphocytes and the tumour metastasis model using B16F10 melanoma cells. Both mortality and bacterial colony counts, particularly of the spleen and liver, are used to assess host resistance to the bacterium; enumeration of lung tumour nodules and the measurement of DNA synthesis in the lung of tumour-bearing mice are utilized for assessing host resistance in the tumour challenge model. Although it can be argued that the host resistance assays provide a holistic approach to immune function in the animal and thus allow assessment of biologically relevant information, they can be seen as having many parallels with the LD_{50} test; any arguments valid against that assay can be invoked against the host-resistance assay. The use of infectious agents and tumour cells that are relatively safe to handle in an animal house environment, and/or the need for strict isolation procedures, must also be important considerations.

The NTP testing panel, described above, uses an inbred mouse hybrid strain, B6C3F1, rather than the rat, the animal conventionally used by toxicologists (except for eliciting potential hypersensitivity reactions). Toxicologists would obviously prefer to use the rat, and to perform tests for identifying potential immunotoxicants within the context of routine toxicology studies. Such an immunotoxicity screen has been established at the National Institute of Public Health and Environmental Hygiene in the Netherlands, using a tiered approach as part of a subacute or subchronic toxicity study (Vos, 1980). The approach is to make immunopathology the cornerstone for identifying potentially immunotoxic events; only if changes are seen in this tier would more specific immunological investigations be undertaken. It should be noted, however, that this approach recognizes that conventional histology (e.g. haematoxylin and eosin stained paraffin sections), while allowing the pathologist to judge changes in tissue architecture and the morphology of cells within the lymphoid organs, may not give sufficient information about the immune system. Indeed, cells with different functions are known to manifest similar morphology. Consequently, more sophisticated histochemical methods such as enzyme histochemistry, immunocytochemistry and electron microscopy are applied, and assays based on molecular biology such as *in situ* hybridization are also being developed (for review of histopathological techniques, see Schuurman *et al.*, 1992).

An example is the use of immunoperoxidase and monoclonal antibody techniques to visualize the distribution of defined lymphocyte subsets and macrophages within frozen tissue sections. The successful application of this tiered approach is best demonstrated in the very fine studies conducted on tributyltin oxide (TBTO). Short-term (subacute) studies showed that high doses of TBTO had an effect on lymphoid tissue weight and morphology, as well as on numbers of circulating T cell and serum immunoglobulin levels. These findings were repeated and extended to include host resistance assays, including resistance to the parasite *Trichinella spiralis*. Immune parameters, including host resistance, were significantly affected at dose levels at which there was no evidence of general toxicity. The Institute then conducted a 2 year study administering TBTO at 0, 0.5, 5 and 50 mg per kg diet. Decreases in serum IgE levels and decreased resistance to *T. spiralis* were observed at 5 and 50 mg again in the absence of general toxicity, demonstrating conclusively that the characteristic toxic effect of TBTO is on the immune system (Vos *et al.*, 1990).

Such studies are by their very nature costly, time-consuming and, unless carefully designed, potentially wasteful of animals. Since it is not practical to evaluate all immunologically relevant parameters during toxicity studies, the challenge facing the immunotoxicologist is to identify which tests would be most appropriate to assess and predict the immunotoxic potential of chemicals in the rat. Some recent progress has been made at a recent international workshop (International Workshop on Immunotoxicology and Immunotoxicity of Metals, 1989: Dayan *et al.*, 1990), where methods for assessing potential immunotoxicity during conventional toxicity studies were put forward. The meeting concluded that the inclusion of some immune-related parameters (haematology, blood chemistry, organ weights and histopathology) could be included without difficulty in standard protocols for screening

chemicals and that selected functional assays be recommended for compounds for which some immunotoxic properties were implied (Tables 4 and 5). Chemicals suspected of having effects on immune function on the basis of prior studies, structure–activity relationships or other information could also be evaluated further by selected functional assays, even if negative results were obtained in the morphological and haematological assays. These recommendations reflect the present lack of method standardization and validation (although there has been some recent progress in the interlaboratory studies carried out under the auspices of IPCS), as well as criteria for evaluation of test results. This is due in part to the diverse nature of the immune system itself and the present emphasis on functional reserves or redundancy, concepts not always given similar emphasis in other complex target organ systems

Table 4   Immune system-related parameters that can be evaluated in repeat dose toxicity studies in rats for chemicals and drugs for which no *a priori* immunotoxic potential has been identified

Haematology	Relative and absolute differential white blood cell counts (lymphocytes, monocytes, granulocytes, abnormal cells)[a]
	Bone marrow cellularity (nucleated count and smear)[b]
Blood chemistry	Albumin/globulin ratio[a]
	Serum immunoglobulin classes[b]
Organ weights	Thymus[c]
	Spleen[c]
	Lymph nodes (local and distant to application site, e.g. for oral route, mesenteric and popliteal lymph nodes)[b]
Histopathology	Thymus[a]
	Spleen[a]
	Lymph nodes (local and distant to application site)[a]
	Bone marrow
	Peyer's patches[c] (oral) or bronchus-associated lymphoid tissue (inhalation)[c]

[a] Relevant parameters already included in most toxicity test guidelines.
[b] Relevant parameters but method not yet standardized and validated.
[c] Relevant parameters not yet included in some toxicity test guidelines.

Table 5 Functional methods available or requiring development in rodents to assess immunotoxicity (selected assays would be strongly recommended for compounds for which some immunotoxic properties were implied)

Category parameter assessed	Rat
Cell-mediated immunity	
mixed leucocyte response	1
mitogen proliferation	2
delayed hypersensitivity response	2
T lymphocyte cytotoxicity	1
Antibody-mediated immunity	
antibody plaque forming cell response	2
serum antibody titre to specific antigen (ELISA)	2
Natural resistance	
natural killer cell cytotoxicity	2
macrophage: phagocytosis and intracellular killing	3
polymorphonuclear leucocyte function	1
Host resistance assessment models	
influenza virus	1
Listeria monocytogenes	2,4
tumour models	1
Plasmodium trichinella	2,4

1. Further development required.
2. Method(s) currently available, but not standardized or validated in interlaboratory comparison.
3. Method standardized and validated.
4. Preferred method(s).

such as, for example, the nervous system; in part, to the lack of concordance between laboratories.

Clearly, if immunotoxicology is to play a significant role in the safety evaluation of drugs and chemicals, it is important that it can offer tests which are sensitive, specific and reproducible. The current status of testing in animals indicates that further methods and techniques for evaluation of test results must be developed. In the opinion of the authors newer molecular biology methods, including the use of gene probes, may provide a means for the early identification of suspected immunotoxic effects of chemicals. Accordingly, we conclude with a brief description of the development and application of this new technology as applied to immunotoxicity assessment.

Molecular Immunotoxicology

Molecular immunotoxicology has been extremely fortunate in that a considerable proportion of the efforts in molecular biology over the last decade have been directed towards a better understanding of the immune system and the role of cyto-kines in the induction and direction of immune responses. This has resulted in a large number of immunoregulatory cytokines and growth factors being cloned at both cDNA and genomic level, most often of mouse or human origin, thus enabling molecular analysis of gene expression to be performed at the level of DNA, RNA or protein (Berger and Kimmel, 1987). Analysis of DNA and the intricate control systems within DNA relates to what the cell is programmed to perform; analysis of polypeptides or proteins allows the identification of events which can have occurred as a result of DNA programming or as a result of change in environment, perhaps in response to external stimuli. Such analysis has been used, for example, to demonstrate that cyclosporin A inhibits the full expression of IL-2 receptor molecules on the T lymphocyte membrane. However, the most direct form of analysis is the expression of mRNA species within the cell. Since most mRNA species are relatively short-lived, existing only for the purpose of conveying information from nucleus to cytoplasm, the analysis of mRNA can pinpoint precisely what a cell is doing at any point in time and the way in which it is responding to external stimuli.

Analysis of modulated mRNA expression can be applied to at least three situations which are relevant to immunotoxicological testing. First, the analysis can be conducted on *in vivo* exposed animals: tissues such as spleen, thymus, lymph glands can be removed and gross analysis for specific mRNAs can be conducted. Second, analysis can be performed on *ex vivo* material: tissue or cells taken from exposed animals can be stimulated or manipulated *in vitro* to determine the effects of pre-exposure *in vivo* on the ability of cells to generate characteristic patterns of mRNA expression. Finally, analysis can be performed exclusively *in vitro*, where defined cell populations (e.g. alveolar or peritoneal macrophages) can be preincubated with test compound before stimulation and expression analysis.

In terms of overall strategy, this molecular immunotoxicological analysis is relatively straightforward. From cells or tissue exposed to test compound, RNA is extracted, purified and immobilized on a membrane support. Bound mRNA species are detected with probes derived from complementary cDNAs or oligonucleotides; these probes are radiolabelled or coupled to enzyme–substrate detection systems. After stringent washing to reduce background and eliminate non-specific binding, the membrane is subjected to autoradiography or other detection systems, whence the presence of specific mRNAs can be confirmed and semiquantitative analysis performed by densitometry (Figure 2) (Cheley and Anderson, 1984).

Application of Molecular Immunotoxicology in *in vitro* Systems

Cytokines, as stated earlier, underpin and maintain normal immune function and control the development of the immune response. All cytokines are important, but some are more important than others. For example, IL-1 and IL-2 appear to be involved in a variety of intercellular communication and can be considered as central to the development of the immune response, whereas others appear to have more specialized roles—e.g. IL-5 in the development of eosinophilia in parasitic infection. In developing *in vitro* screening systems we have sought to analyse expression of those cytokines upon which the immune response is pivoted, although in certain cases analysis of certain more peripheral cytokines may be indicated (for details see Meredith, 1992).

At present, because the majority of cDNA probes are of human or mouse origin, rat immune cell populations can only be analysed with probes that will cross-hybridize—e.g. where there is sufficient homology in amino acid sequence between the species. There are situations where cDNA probes will cross-hybridize: for example, we have successfully used murine IL-1 probes on rat mRNA (there is 83 per cent homology in predicted amino acid sequence) whereas for others (e.g. IL-3) there appears to be a lack of homology between species.

One line of criticism which has been levelled at this type of *in vitro* analysis is that not all immunotoxic compounds exert their effects by direct modulation of expression of a few key cytokines. However, this is to miss the point: the value of these *in vitro* systems does not simply lie in analysing the molecular mechanisms of cytokine modulation by immunopharmacological agents. Since cytokine expression is essential for the development of immune responses both *in vivo* and *in vitro*, it is possible to establish patterns of expression for *in vitro* models of immune activation—e.g. macrophage stimulation by lipopolysaccharide (LPS), mitogen/alloantigen stimulation of lymphocyte cultures. The effect of test chemicals on these characteristic patterns of cytokine expression can then be monitored following *in vivo* or *in vitro* exposure. Under these conditions, analysis of cytokine and related mRNAs becomes a semiquantitative marker of immunotoxicity. We have applied this type of analysis to the compounds azathioprine and tributyltin oxide

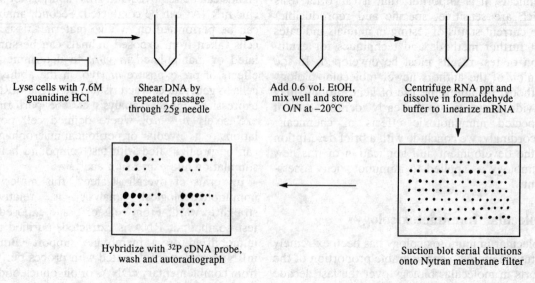

Lyse cells with 7.6M
guanidine HCl

Shear DNA by
repeated passage
through 25g needle

Add 0.6 vol. EtOH,
mix well and store
O/N at –20°C

Centrifuge RNA ppt and
dissolve in formaldehyde
buffer to linearize mRNA

Hybridize with ^{32}P cDNA probe,
wash and autoradiograph

Suction blot serial dilutions
onto Nytran membrane filter

Figure 2 Schematic representation of the technique used to analyse specific mRNA expression in macrophage or lymphocyte populations

(TBTO) and we can demonstrate inhibition of the expression of mRNAs for IL-2 and IL-2 receptor in mixed lymphocyte cultures en route to the development of cytotoxic T cells. The use of a highly specific probe for cytotoxic T cells, based on the DNA sequence for a serine esterase unique to this cell population (Lobe *et al.*, 1986), allows confirmation of the ultimate development of failure of development of functional cytotoxic lymphocytes. The inclusion of determination of expression of a high-turnover housekeeping gene such as actin or a metabolic gene, e.g. G3PDH, allows discrimination between those compounds which exert a selective immunotoxicity and compounds which act via a non-specific cytotoxic mechanism.

On the basis of our experience in the field of molecular immunotoxicity, we would propose the following simple experiments for the investigation of the immunomodulatory potential of a drug or chemical.

(1) Ability to induce expression of monokine mRNAs (e.g. IL-1α/β, IL-6, TNFα) in cultured macrophages.

(2) Ability to modulate expression of these monokine mRNAs in LPS-stimulated cultured macrophages.

(3) Ability to induce expression of lymphokine mRNAs (e.g. IL-2, IL-4, IL-2rec, IL-6, IL-10, 1FN-γ) in cultured splenocytes.

(4) Ability to modulate expression of those lymphokine mRNAs in cultured splenocytes stimulated with alloantigen or mitogen. Analysis of mRNAs specific to cytotoxic T cells (proteases or lipases).

(5) Analysis of total cytokine mRNA levels in selected cells or tissues e.g. spleen, thymus, lymph nodes, alveolar/peritoneal macrophages following *in vivo* exposure.

(6) Analysis of *ex vivo* cells as in (2) and (4).

This structure is liable to modification, as the amount of data available expands and indicates priorities to be evaluated; there may also be specialized assays which merit inclusion in a preliminary screen. At present, however, it represents a framework within which pertinent information can be obtained and which can point the way to other more specific experiments. Furthermore, it is likely that economical and political pressure will dictate that a significant proportion of screening tests for immunotoxicity be performed *in vitro* with a consequent reduction in the number and severity of laboratory animal experiments.

Clearly, if immunotoxicology is to play a significant role in the safety evaluation of drugs and chemicals, it is important that it can offer tests which are sensitive, specific and reproducible. In this laboratory our ongoing research programme is attempting to establish such tests by the application of molecular biological techniques to the analysis of immune cell populations. It is beyond dispute that molecular analysis of the modulation of gene expression is a very powerful technique. However, it is the manner in which this technology is harnessed and applied to problems in immunotoxicology which will not only determine its value as a potential immunotoxicological screening system but also give insight into the biochemical mechanisms which underlie immunotoxic effects.

ACKNOWLEDGEMENTS

Research in Molecular Immunotoxicology in the authors' laboratory is supported by the Commission of European Communities to whom our thanks are due.

REFERENCES

Allison, A. C. (1967). Lysosomes and disease. *Sci. Am.*, **217**, 62–72

Anderson, K. E. and Maibach, H. I. (Eds) (1985). *Current Problems in Dermatology*, Vol. 14, *Contact Allergy Predictive Tests in Guinea Pigs*. Karger, Basel

Austyn, J. M. (1987). Lymphoid dendritic cells. *Immunology*, **62**, 161–170

Berger, S. L. and Kimmel, A. R. (Eds) (1987). *Guide to Molecular Cloning Techniques* (issued as Vol. 152 of *Methods in Enzymology*). Academic Press, London

Bottomly, K. (1988). A functional dichotomy in CD4+ T lymphocytes. *Immunol. Today*, **9**, 268–274

Boyd, R. L. and Hugo, P. (1991). Towards an integrated view of thymopoiesis. *Immunology Today*, **12**, 71–79

Chang, K. J., Hsieh, K. H., Tang, T. Y., Tung, T. A. and Lee, T. P. (1982). Immunological evaluation of patients with PCB poisoning. Evaluation of delayed-type skin hypersensitivity and its relation to clinical studies. *J. Toxicol. Environ. Hlth*, **9**, 217–223

Cheley, S. and Anderson, R. (1984). A reproducible microanalytical method for the detection of specific RNA sequences by dot-blot hybridisation. *Anal. Biochem.*, **137**, 15–19

Coombs, R. R. A. and Gell, P. G. H. (1975). Classification of allergic reactions responsible for clinical hypersensitivity disease. In Gell, P. G. H., Coombs, R. R. A. and Lachmann, P. J. (Eds), *Clinical Aspects of Immunology*. Blackwell Scientific, Oxford, pp. 761–781

Dayan, A. D., Hertel, R. F., Hesseltine, E., Kazantzis, G., Smith, E. and Van der Venne, M. T. (Eds) (1990). *Immunotoxicity of Metals and Immunotoxicology*. IPCS Joint Symposia No. 15. Plenum Press, New York

Dean, J. H., Luster, M. I., Munson, A. E. and Amos, H. (1985) (Eds). *Immunotoxicology and Immunopharmacology*. Raven Press, New York

Descotes, J. (1986). *Immunotoxicology of Drugs and Chemicals*. Elsevier, Amsterdam

Gad, S. C., Dunn, B. J., Dobbs, D. W., Reilly, C. and Walsh, R. D. (1986). Development and validation of an alternative dermal sensitisation test: the mouse ear swelling test (MEST). *Toxicol. Appl. Pharmacol.*, **84**, 93–114

Gallagher, R. B. and Osmond, D. G. (1991). To B or not to B: that is the question. *Immunology Today*, **12**, 1–3

Hamblin, A. S. (1988). *Lymphokines*. IRL Press, Oxford

Hermanowicz, A. and Kossman, S. (1984). Neutrophil function and infectious disease in workers occupationally exposed to phospho-organic pesticides: role of mononuclear derived chemotactic factor for neutrophils. *Clin. Immunol. Immunopathol.*, **23**, 13–22

Inaba, K. and Steinman, R. H. (1987). Resting and sensitised T lymphocytes exhibit distinct stimulatory (antigen presenting cell) requirements for growth and lymphokine release. *J. Exptl Med.*, **165**, 1403–1417

Jerne, N. K. and Nordin, A. A. (1963). Plaque formation in agar by single antibody producing cells. *Science*, **140**, 405–408

Kammuller, M. E., Bloksma, N. and Seinen, W. (1989) (Eds). *Autoimmunity and Toxicology: Disregulation Induced by Drugs and Chemicals*. Elsevier, Amsterdam

Kimber, I. (1985). Natural killer cells. *Med. Lab. Sci.*, **42**, 60–77

Kimber, I., Hilton, J. and Botham, P. A. (1990). Identification of contact allergens using the murine local lymph node assay: comparisons with the Buehler occluded patch test in guinea pigs. *J. Appl. Toxicol.*, **10**, 173–180

King, P. D. and Katz, D. R. (1990). Mechanisms of dendritic cell function. *Immunology Today*, **11**, 206–211

Lobe, C. G., Finlay, B. B., Paranchych, W., Paetkau, V. H. and Bleackley, R. C. (1986). Novel serine proteases encoded by two cytotoxic T-lymphocyte-specific genes. *Science*, **232**, 858–861

Loutit, J. F., Nisbet, N. W., Marshall, M. J. and Vaughan, J. M. (1982). Versatile stem cells in bone marrow. *Lancet*, **II**, 1090–1093

Luster, M. I., Munson, A. E., Thomas, P. T., Holsapple, M. P., Fenters, J., White, K. L. Jr, Laver, L. D. and Dean, J. H. (1988). Development of testing battery of assess chemical-induced immunotoxicity. *Fund. Appl. Toxicol.*, **10**, 2–19

MacLennon, I. C. M. and Gray, D. (1986). Antigen-driven selection of virgin and memory B cells. *Immunol. Rev.*, **91**, 61–68

Maisey, J. and Miller, K. (1986). Assessment of the ability of mice fed on vitamin A supplemented diet to respond to a variety of potential contact sensitisers. *Contact Dermatitis*, **15**, 17–23

Meredith, C. (1992). Molecular immunotoxicology. In Miller, K., Turk, J. L. and Nicklin, S. (Eds), *Principles and Practice of Immunotoxicology*. Blackwell Scientific, Oxford, pp. 344–357

Merk, H. F., Gleichmann, E. and Gleichmann, H. (1992). Adverse immunological effects of drugs and other chemicals; methods to detect them. In Miller, K., Turk, J. L. and Nicklin, S. (Eds), *Principles and Practice of Immunotoxicology*. Blackwell Scientific, Oxford, pp. 86–103

Miller, K. (1979). Alterations in the surface-related phenomena of alveolar macrophages following inhalation of crocidolite asbestos and quartz dusts. *Environ. Res.*, **20**, 162–182

Miller, K. (1985). Review: Immunotoxicology. *Clin. Exptl Immunol.*, **61**, 219–223

Miller, K. and Brown, R. C. (1985). The immune system and asbestos-associated disease. In Dean, J. H., Luster, M. I., Munson, A. E. and Amos, H. (Eds), *Immunotoxicology and Immunopharmacology*. Raven Press, New York, pp. 429–440

Murray, M. J. and Thomas, P. T. (1992). Toxic consequences of chemical interactions with the immune system. In Miller, K., Turk, J. L. and Nicklin, S. (Eds), *Principles and Practice of Immunotoxicology*. Blackwell Scientific, Oxford, pp. 65–85

Nicklin, S. and Miller, K. (1990). Dose-effects and dose responses in immunotoxicology: Problems and conceptional considerations. In Dayan, A. D., Hertel, R. F., Hesseltine, E., Kazantzis, G., Smith, E. and Van der Venne, M. T. (Eds), *Immunotoxicity of Metals and Immunotoxicology*. IPCS Joint Symposia No. 15. Plenum Press, New York, pp. 43–56

Nikolic-Zugic, J. (1991). Phenotype and functional stages in the intrathymic development of $\alpha\beta$T cells. *Immunology Today*, **12**, 65–70

Schuurman, H. J., de Weger, R. A., van Loveren, H., Krajnc-Franken, M. A. M. and Vos, J. G. (1992). Histological approaches of immunotoxicology. In Miller, K., Turk, J. L. and Nicklin, S. (Eds), *Principles and Practice of Immunotoxicology*. Blackwell Scientific, Oxford, pp. 279–303 van Furth, R. (1980). Origins and kinetics of mononuclear phagocytes. In van Furth, R. (Ed.), *Mononuclear Phagocytes, Functional Aspects*. Martinus Nijhoff, Boston, pp. 1–10

Vos, J. G. (1977). Immunosuppression as related to toxicology. *CRC Crit. Rev. Toxicol.*, **5**, 67–101

Vos, J. G. (1980). Immunotoxicity assessment: screening and function studies. *Arch. Toxicol. Suppl.*, **4**, 95–108

Vos, J. G., de Klerk, A., Krajnc, E. I., van Loueren, H. and Rozing, J. (1990). Immunotoxicity of bis(tri-n-butyltin) oxide in the rat: Effects on thymus-dependent immunity and on non-specific resistance following long-term exposure in young versus aged rats. *Toxicol. Appl. Pharmacol.*, **105**, 144–155

White, K. L. Jr (1992). Specific immune function assays. In Miller, K., Turk, J. L. and Nicklin, S. (Eds), *Principles and Practice of Immunotoxicology*. Blackwell Scientific, Oxford, pp. 304–323

FURTHER READING

Dean, J. H., Luster, M. I., Muson, A. E. and Ames, H. (1985). *Immunotoxicology and Immunopharmacology*. Raven Press, New York

Luster, M. I. and Rosenthal, G. J. (1993). Chemical agents and the immune response. *Environmental Health Perspectives*, **100**, 219–226

Newcombe, D. S., Rose, N. R. and Bloom, J. C. (Eds) (1992). *Clinical Immunotoxicology*. Raven Press, New York

34 Haematotoxicology

John Amess

INTRODUCTION

This chapter will consider the effect of drugs and toxins on the bone marrow and cellular compartment of the blood. Lymphopoiesis has not been considered, and extensive lists of drugs and toxins affecting the haemopoietic system have not been included.

BONE MARROW FAILURE

The term 'bone marrow failure' refers to a reduction in circulating blood cells which has arisen primarily as a result of a failure of bone marrow precursor cells to produce mature cells, rather than the production of abnormal cells which have a shortened survival or the production of normal cells which are subjected to an abnormal environment. In bone marrow failure the cells remaining in the marrow appear morphologically normal, or near normal. The stroma of the marrow also appears morphologically normal.

There are two major groups of bone marrow failure—the aplastic anaemias, where the failure lies in the pluripotent stem cell, and the single-cell cytopenias, where the failure possibly lies in one or other of the committed cell lines. There is overlap between these groups, for single-cell failure may progress to total marrow failure and, following partial recovery, aplastic anaemia may continue with a prolonged period of single-cell deficiency. Aplastic anaemia will be considered in the first instance; selective neutropenia and thrombocytopenia will be discussed later in the chapter.

APLASTIC ANAEMIA

Aplastic anaemia is defined as a syndrome of unexpected pancytopenia (anaemia, leucopenia and thrombocytopenia) with marrow hypoplasia, in which normal haemopoietic marrow is replaced by fat cells. Abnormal cells are not found in either the peripheral blood or the bone marrow. However, there may be mild dyserythropoiesis in the bone marrow and consequent macrocytosis in the peripheral blood. While a similar picture regularly occurs in patients receiving cytotoxic chemotherapy or radiotherapy for malignant disease, such patients, normally, quickly recover and are not considered to have aplastic anaemia. Although, in general, the development and recovery of aplasia following exposure to cytotoxic drugs are predictable, there are exceptions. Repeated or prolonged exposure to small doses of alkylating agents, particularly busulphan, may lead to a prolonged and unpredictable aplasia.

Aplastic anaemia is the most devastating form of haemopoietic failure in man, and its pathogenesis, diagnosis, treatment and prognosis have been reviewed by Gordon-Smith (1989). In order to address the prognosis and therapeutic approach, aplastic anaemia may be categorized as mild or severe. Severe aplastic anaemia has been defined by the International Aplastic Anemia Study Group as (1) a marrow of less than 25 per cent normal cellularity or a marrow of less than 50 per cent normal cellularity with less than 30 per cent haemopoietic cells; (2) at least two of the following three peripheral blood values: granulocytes less than $0.5 \times 10^9\ l^{-1}$, platelets less than $20 \times 10^9\ l^{-1}$, or anaemia with reticulocytes less than 1 per cent (corrected for haematocrit) (Camitta et al., 1979). Mild aplastic anaemia may be defined as marrow hypoplasia with pancytopenia not severe enough to meet the preceding criteria. The incidence of aplastic anaemia in developed temperate countries is probably of the order of 3–6 per million of population per annum. In the Far East, China and Japan the incidence appears to be rather higher than in the West, perhaps because of the higher prevalence of hepatitis, the more widespread use of chloramphenicol and the extensive use of insecticides.

Possible Pathogenetic Mechanisms

The pathogenesis of most cases of aplastic anaemia has been enigmatic. In some patients direct damage to stem cells, whether dose-dependent or idiosyncratic, by poisons, toxins or drugs appears likely. However, there is increasing evidence that immune mechanisms play an important role in the pathogenesis of aplastic anaemia (Marmont, 1987). As many as 43 per cent of cases of acquired aplastic anaemia have been considered to be idiopathic and 26 per cent associated with chloramphenicol. These percentages may vary from study to study, depending on how extensive and detailed a history is obtained and on how strong an association is required to suggest a possible aetiological role. Unfortunately, even a strong association between exposure to an agent and the development of aplastic anaemia does not necessarily elucidate its pathogenesis.

Drug-induced Aplastic Anaemia

A wide variety of drugs have been implicated in the development of aplastic anaemia (Nissen-Druey, 1989; Adamson and Erslev, 1990), but in the majority of instances the number of cases for individual drugs is small and epidemiological evidence weak (International Agranulocytosis and Aplastic Anemia Study, 1986).

Chloramphenicol

Perhaps most attention has been given to chloramphenicol—a nitrobenzene compound with a dichloracetamide side-chain. This antibiotic was introduced into general use in 1949 and it was predicted, on the basis of the similarity of its structure to that of amidopyrine (a drug notorious for producing blood dyscrasias) that it would cause haematological toxicity. In fact, amidopyrine most commonly produced an immune agranulocytosis, although aplastic anaemia has been reported. The first case of blood dyscrasia following chloramphenicol was described in 1950 and was fatal aplastic anaemia (Rich *et al.*, 1950). The actual risk of developing fatal aplastic anaemia after being treated with chloramphenicol is low, about 1 in 20 000–30 000 (Modan *et al.*, 1975). This is 10–20 times the risk of developing fatal idiopathic aplastic anaemia in unexposed individuals.

The toxic effect of chloramphenicol on marrow function appears at two levels. The first is a dose-dependent, reversible marrow suppression which is seen in many, if not all, exposed patients. This has been ascribed to mitrochondrial damage (Yunis *et al.*, 1980) and will be considered further in the section dealing with sideroblastic anaemia. The second is the development of sustained aplastic anaemia which appears weeks or months after exposure to the drug and does not appear to be related to the dose, duration or route of administration. The mechanism of chloramphenicol-induced aplastic anaemia is unknown. A minority of patients develop severe aplastic anaemia at doses which are tolerated by a majority of individuals without evidence of bone marrow suppression. The individual increased susceptibility suggests abnormal pharmacokinetics of the drug or a conditioned action on hypersensitive haemopoietic cells. Single reports give supportive evidence for a predisposition to aplastic anaemia. There have been a few case reports of identical twins developing aplastic anaemia after chloramphenicol exposure. It has also been shown that aplastic anaemia from any cause is linked to certain histocompatibility antigens (Chapius *et al.*, 1986; Odum *et al.*, 1987). On the basis of *in vitro* studies of DNA synthesis in marrow from patients who have recovered from chloramphenicol-induced aplasia and from their relatives, Yunis (1976) also postulated a genetic predisposition to the development of this syndrome. However, Howell and co-workers (1975) were unable to demonstrate that granulocyte–macrophage colony-forming units (CFU-GM) grown from patients who had recovered from chloramphenicol-induced aplasia were more sensitive to exposure to chloramphenicol, *in vitro*, than CFU-GM from normal patients. Thus, while a genetic predisposition to chloramphenicol-induced aplastic anaemia might exist, the nature of the proposed defect is unknown.

Several other factors have been considered in the pathogenesis of chloramphenicol-induced aplastic anaemia. This may be related to previous bone marrow damage, because mice pretreated with busulphan and, therefore having 'residual marrow damage' have been claimed to be more sensitive to dose-related marrow suppression by chloramphenicol than are controls (Morley *et al.*, 1976). This toxicity, however, is probably different from that resulting in true aplastic anaemia. It has also been suggested that drugs may act on haemopoiesis indirectly by damaging regulatory cell populations or immunological mechanisms. The toxicity of chloramphenicol *in vitro* can be reversed by the action of lithium on colony-stimulating factor (CSF)-producing cells, and chloramphenicol has been shown to inhibit the growth of cultured marrow stromal cells. Lymphocytes from patients who have recovered from chloramphenicol-induced aplastic anaemia can be stimulated *in vitro* by the drug, which indicates that immune mechanisms may play a role. The immunological aspects of aplastic anaemia have recently been reviewed by Marmont (1987).

Phenylbutazone and Non-steroidal Anti-inflammatory Agents

Phenylbutazone and its analogue, oxyphenbutazone, have been widely implicated in the production of aplastic anaemia (Inman, 1977). These pyrazolones share some structural similarities to chloramphenicol and to amidopyrine. The incidence of aplastic anaemia following exposure to phenylbutazone is probably similar to that seen with chloramphenicol (*Lancet* Editorial, 1986). As in the case of chloramphenicol, fatal cases have been observed after doses which are well tolerated by many other individuals and have also been reported after the second of two short courses. Phenylbutazone is now only available for the treatment of ankylosing spondylitis.

Other non-steroidal anti-inflammatory drugs have also been reported as causing aplastic anaemia. Benoxaprofen (Opren), a propionic acid derivative, was associated with a number of cases before its withdrawal from the market on the basis of toxicity. The indole derivatives, indomethacin and sulindac, have both been associated with aplastic anaemia but the risk factor for these drugs seems to be less than for phenylbutazone or chloramphenicol (International Agranulocytosis and Aplastic Anemia Study, 1986).

Gold Salts

Gold salts deserve a special mention. Aplastic anaemia is a rare, but often fatal, complication of gold salt therapy. In a study of adverse drug reactions it was estimated that 1.6 deaths occur per 10 000 prescriptions written for gold compounds (Girdwood, 1974). Neither the total dose of gold nor other known side-effects of gold therapy appear to be predictive for the development of aplasia. Persistence with gold injections

in the face of a falling neutrophil count may lead to aplasia or aplasia may appear without warning. However, gold salts are one of the few drugs for which careful monitoring of blood counts may prevent the development of aplasia.

In the past the pathogenesis of gold-related aplastic anaemia has been ascribed to gold being a direct marrow toxin. Gold may be removed from the body by chelation with dimercaprol (British anti-Lewisite, BAL), penicillamine or acetylcysteine. There is no evidence that removal of gold in this way accelerates recovery and it is possible to detect gold in the marrow of patients who have recovered from gold-induced aplasia. Bone marrow transplantation of a small number of patients with suitable donors has resulted in successful engraftment and long-term survival. Recently haematological recovery from gold-induced aplasia has been reported after immunosuppressive treatment with anti-human thymocyte globulin (ATG) or very-high-dose corticosteroids. Recent studies have suggested an immune-mediated mechanism of action by gold salts. Gold salts accumulate in macrophages in the synovia of patients with arthritis, and *in vitro* they have been shown to interfere with various macrophage–T cell interactions. The ATG eliminates suppressor T cells that are preventing normal stem cell growth and differentiation. While a direct link between suppression of marrow function by gold salts and recovery after ATG therapy has not been made, gold cannot simply be considered a direct 'marrow toxin'.

Other Drugs Linked to Aplastic Anaemia

Among other drugs listed as having a strong link with the development of aplastic anaemia are antithyroid drugs (methimazole, carbimazole, propylthiouracil), anticonvulsants (diphenylhydantoin, trimethadione), sulphonamides, antimalarials (mepacrine, amodiaquine, pyrimethamine) and antidiabetic agents (chlorpropamide, tolbutamide) (de Gruchy, 1975; Adamson and Erslev, 1990).

A still unsolved problem is the role of phenothiazines in producing aplastic anaemia. On the basis of Pisciotta's work, these drugs are listed as aetiological agents of aplastic anaemia in many reviews. He found that bone marrow from previously afflicted individuals showed a lower colony growth than normal and a subnormal uptake of [^{3}H]-thymidine *in vitro* (Pisciotta,

1973). Phenothiazine-associated aplastic anaemia, even though occurring in a minority of exposed individuals, is dose-dependent. Moderate degrees of bone marrow hypoplasia recover if the exposure is stopped early. Paradoxically, patients developing leucopenia to the first course of phenothiazine eventually tolerate the drug when it is readministered.

Chemical-induced Aplastic Anaemia

Many of the compounds causing aplastic anaemia contain benzene or other organic compounds. Benzene is present in many commercial solvents, coal derivatives and petroleum products. Insecticides are often applied in a petroleum-based medium, and therefore the precise component which is involved in aplastic anaemia due to insecticides or solvents is often unclear.

Benzene

Benzene is widely used in industry; it constitutes 1 per cent of unleaded petrol sold in the USA and 5 per cent of that sold in Europe. It is also a prominent component of tobacco smoke. Current federal regulations in the USA limit a safe exposure to one part per million during an 8 h day, 5 days a week, a level still considered by some to be unsafe. Benzene can cause marrow suppression and occasionally leukaemia in laboratory animals. Studies in rats have suggested that the haematologically toxic compounds in benzene poisoning are various breakdown products, particularly *para*-benzoquinone (Kalf, 1987). These products apparently suppress DNA synthesis in differentiated precursor cells and inhibit proliferation of progenitor cells and microenvironmental cells. The most common haematological abnormality developing in man after exposure to benzene is pancytopenia due to a hypoplastic marrow or a hyperplastic marrow with myelodysplasia (Goldstein, 1983). The subsequent development of leukaemia in patients with myelodysplasia has occurred frequently enough for benzene to be considered as being leukaemogenic.

The incidence of haematological problems increases with intensity and duration of exposure. Episodic exposure may result in transient blood changes with no apparent residual effects. Although removal of a haematologically affected subject from a benzene-containing environment may result in the disappearance of peripheral blood abnormalities, the effect on the long-term risk of aplasia or leukaemia is not known. Patients who develop refractory anaemia or leukaemia may have clonal chromosome abnormalities in their bone marrow, commonly deletions of chromosomes 5 and/or 7 (Heim and Mitelman, 1986). Even in the absence of such specific karyotype abnormalities, there appears to be an increased incidence of aneuploidy and chromosome aberrations in haematologically normal workers exposed to benzene concentrations of 5–25 ppm when compared with normal controls. This suggests that genetic damage to haemopoietic cells may occur in the absence of any overt haematological signs, and if an analogy can be drawn with other chemically induced leukaemias and preleukaemic states, particularly those following cytotoxic therapy, a latent period of up to 10 or more years may elapse before the clinical emergence of an aberrant haemopoietic clone (see Secondary Leukaemic Syndromes, pp. 798–799).

Other Chemicals

Insecticides have been associated with aplastic anaemia. Gamma-benzene hexachloride (lindane) has especially been implicated. Because insecticides are often distributed in an aerosol, it is difficult to estimate the level of exposure. They may be incorporated into soaps and powders that are used for many purposes around the house, so that the user is not fully aware of their presence.

Exposure to toluene, in industry, or among glue sniffers or glue users, is also considered to be hazardous.

Hair Dyes

Aplastic anaemia has been described after the use of hair dyes (Hopkins and Manoharan, 1985), but in view of their widespread use there is little firm evidence that they are an aetiological factor (Jouhar, 1976).

Radiation-induced Aplastic Anaemia

Radiation-induced aplastic anaemia is discussed in Chapter 55.

PURE RED CELL APLASIA (PRCA)

Pure red cell aplasia is characterized by anaemia, reticulocytopenia and erythroid hypoplasia in the bone marrow without abnormalities in the myeloid and megakaryocytic series (Sieff, 1983; Erslev, 1990). Acute pure red cell aplasia is most frequently preceded by a viral infection, particularly by members of the parvovirus family. However, PRCA has been reported in association with a wide variety of drugs and chemicals (Erslev, 1990). It is usually of acute onset and is reversible with discontinuation of the drug or chemical.

The pathogenesis of PRCA occurring with most of the drugs is unknown. However, in one case of PRCA associated with phenytoin it was demonstrated that the drug exerted its effect by specifically inhibiting DNA synthesis, probably at the step of deoxyribotide formation (Yunis *et al.*, 1967). In a more recent study an IgG inhibitor was demonstrated in the serum of a patient receiving phenytoin, and the inhibitor suppressed autologous and allogeneic erythroid burst-forming unit growth in the presence of the drug (Dessypris *et al.*, 1985). Studies to demonstrate antibodies in sera of patients developing PRCA while on drugs have failed in most cases.

MEGALOBLASTIC ANAEMIA

The megaloblastic anaemias are a group of disorders characterized by the distinctive appearance of the developing red cells in the bone marrow. These are megaloblasts which differ from the normoblast, the normal red cell precursor, in several respects. They are larger and, in a stained preparation, the nuclear pattern tends to have a finely stippled appearance rather than the coarser clefts in the normoblast nucleus. In addition, they tend to retain cytoplasmic basophilia as the cell matures. There are also morphological abnormalities of granulopoiesis and, on occasions, megakaryocytes. The characteristic granulocyte changes are the presence of giant metamyelocytes and hypersegmented neutrophils (Figure 1). The megaloblastic anaemias have recently been reviewed by Chanarin (1990).

Megaloblastic anaemia is most commonly the result of either vitamin B_{12} or folate deficiency but may arise as a result of abnormal metabolism of these or interference with DNA synthesis by drugs and chemicals. In megaloblastic anaemia there is ineffective production of blood cells. If the causative process is chronic, then the predominant change is the presence of macrocytosis, which is usually recognized by the presence of a raised mean corpuscular volume (MCV). Eventually the process leads to the development of anaemia, leucopenia and thrombocytopenia. In the rapid development of severe megaloblastic anaemia, as seen in very ill patients, cytopenias rather than macrocytosis are the presenting haematological features (Chanarin, 1990).

It is likely that the morphological changes seen in the megaloblast relate to the abnormally slender and elongated chromosomes present in megaloblastic anaemia and to the large number of chromosome breaks that are present. This would suggest that the morphological changes are related to the way formed DNA is assembled within the cell. It has recently been proposed that hypomethylation inhibits the establishment of DNA supercoils and affects the orientation of DNA helix formation (Zacharias *et al.*, 1988). However, the generally held view is that megaloblastic anaemia is due to an unbalanced nucleic acid synthesis. This concept and how normal mammalian DNA is replicated and the nature of the DNA defect in megaloblastic anaemia have been reviewed by Hoffbrand and Wickramasinghe (1982).

Biochemical Basis of Megaloblastic Anaemia

Megaloblastic anaemia develops in situations of defective DNA synthesis related to a reduced supply of one or other of the four immediate precursors of DNA: the deoxyribonucleoside triphosphates, adenine (dATP) and guanine (dGTP) (purines), and thymine (dTTP) and cytosine (dCTP) (pyrimidines). Folate deficiency principally impairs synthesis of dTTP, since folate is needed in the form of 5,10-methylene tetrahydrofolate polyglutamate as coenzyme in thymidylate synthesis, a rate-limiting reaction in DNA synthesis. The integrity of this reaction may be tested by the deoxyuridine (dU) suppression test (Wickramasinghe and Matthews, 1988). During this reaction, the folate coenzyme is oxidized to the dihydrofolate state and the enzyme dihydrofolate reductase (DHFR) is required to return the folate to tetrahydrofolate (THF) (Figure 2). DHFR is inhibited by methotrexate, by pyrimethamine and, in bacteria but only weakly in human tissues, by trimethoprim (see below). Vitamin B_{12}, as methylcobalamin, is required for the con-

(A)

(B)

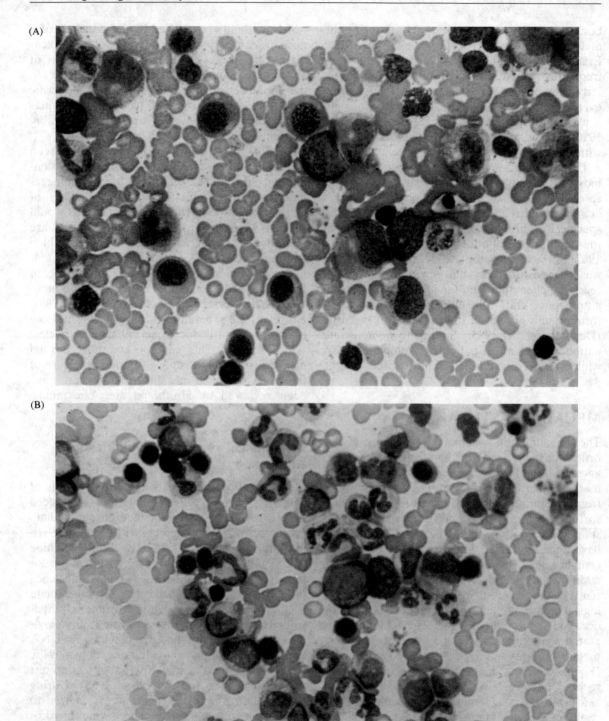

Figure 1 (A) A bone marrow aspirate demonstrating megaloblastic erythropoiesis and giant metamyelocytes from a female patient who had been ventilated with 50 per cent nitrous oxide:50 per cent oxygen for 4 days. (B) A bone marrow aspirate demonstrating normoblastic erythropoiesis with residual giant metamyelocytes and hypersegmented neutrophils from the same patient as Figure 1A, 7 days after discontinuing ventilation with nitrous oxide:oxygen mixture

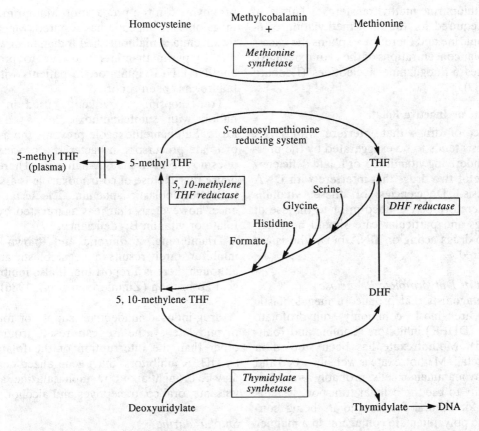

Figure 2 Outline of the intracellular interconversion of reduced folates after the uptake of 5-methyl THF from plasma. The steps involved in the biosynthesis of thymidylate. Abbreviations: THF, tetrahydrofolate; DHF, dihydrofolate

version of methyl THF, which enters bone marrow and other cells from plasma, to THF. Methylcobalamin is required for the transmethylation of homocysteine to methionine, methyl THF being the usual methyl donor. *S*-Adenosylmethionine (SAM) is required as a cofactor and methionine synthetase as enzyme in this reaction. Reduced folates, other than methyl THF, are the correct substrates for polyglutamate addition needed to keep folate inside the cells and to form the various polyglutamate derivatives, including the 5,10-methylene coenzyme required for thymidylate synthesis. The exact substrate for folate polyglutamate function may be THF or formyl THF.

Drug-induced Megaloblastic Change

Treatment with any drug which either directly or indirectly affects cellular DNA biosynthesis can result in megaloblastic bone marrow change and

the characteristic blood count and film changes. Many of these drugs are cytotoxic drugs used in the treatment of malignant disease. These drugs and their sites of action have been reviewed by Scott and Weir (1980). They include drugs that interfere with DNA biosynthesis by blocking DNA assembly, ribonucleotide reduction, pyrimidine precursor biosynthesis, purine precursor biosynthesis, thymidylate biosynthesis and mechanisms unknown.

Drugs that less commonly precipitate the development of megaloblastic change frequently interfere with vitamin B_{12} or folate metabolism. Before these are discussed, it should be noted that there have been recent developments in explaining the occasional and unexpected toxicity of azathioprine, the frequently used purine antagonist. Azathioprine has recently been shown to cause acute myelosuppression, with associated megaloblastic change. These patients have now been shown to have inherited extremely low levels of thiopurine methyltransferase. This is an enzyme required for the thiol methylation of 6-mercaptopurine and therefore explains the excess intracellular concentrations of the cytotoxic active metabolites 6-thioguanine nucleotides (Lennard *et al.*, 1989).

Inadequate or Inactive Folate

The effect of drugs that interfere with DNA biosynthesis tends to be exaggerated by the presence of underlying vitamin B_{12} or folate deficiency or the use of two drugs that interfere with DNA biosynthesis. Deficiencies of these vitamins should therefore be excluded prior to the use of such drugs and particular care should be taken when two drugs acting on DNA biosynthesis are administered.

Inhibition of Dihydrofolate Reductase

Folate antagonists that produce a megaloblastic anaemia are most commonly dihydrofolate reductase (DHFR) inhibitors (Lambie and Johnson, 1985). Methotrexate has been studied in greatest detail. Methotrexate is well absorbed and retained by mammalian cells, probably as a result of its ability to use the cellular transport systems intended for natural folates and its being converted into polyglutamate conjugates in a manner similar to folates. In addition, it has a very high affinity for mammalian DHFR. Methotrexate, when given in high doses, results in the rapid appearance of megaloblastic changes. However, its prolonged use, at low levels, has also been found to lead to severe megaloblastic anaemia. The effects of methotrexate, as well as of other DHFR inhibitors, are reversed by supplying fully reduced folate such as formyl THF (folinic acid).

Other DHFR inhibitors, which include pyrimethamine, triamterene and trimethoprim, have a much lower affinity for human DHFR while retaining a strong affinity for bacterial or plasmodial DHFR. Nevertheless, when there is associated folate deficiency or poor renal function, or when drugs are used in combination, these components can cause megaloblastic anaemia which has proved fatal.

Pyrimethamine, when used alone, has been shown to cause megaloblastic change but only at high doses and prolonged use. When used in combination with co-trimoxazole, it may also cause the development of megaloblastic change and in combination with dapsone, for malarial prophylaxis in the preparation Maloprim, severe megaloblastic anaemia has resulted. Megaloblastic anaemia in malnourished Indian farm workers, due to pyrimethamine, and due to proguanil, another DHFR inhibitor, in patients with renal failure, has been reported.

Trimethoprim is frequently used in combination with sulphamethoxazole as co-trimoxazole. Sulphamethoxazole prevents the assembly of folate precursors in bacteria, a process which does not occur in mammalian cells. There is evidence that the use of co-trimoxazole is associated with megaloblastic anaemia. The usual experience, however, is that it is aggravated by either folate or vitamin B_{12} deficiency.

Triamterene, a diuretic and known DHFR inhibitor, rarely results in megaloblastic anaemia. although there is a report that it also inhibits folic acid absorption (Zimmerman *et al.*, 1986).

A drug-induced inadequate supply of folate for thymidylate synthetase can result from causes other than the interruption of the folate cycle by DHFR inhibitors. Such generalized deficiency may be brought about by sulphasalazine, anticonvulsants, oral contraceptives and alcohol.

Sulphasalazine

Sulphasalazine is a drug widely used in the treatment of ulcerative colitis and rheumatoid arthritis. Most patients receiving more than 2.5 g daily have evidence of a haemolytic process due to oxidant damage to red cells. In addition, megaloblastic anaemia has been associated with sulphasalazine and it has been reported that two-thirds of patients taking the drug have megaloblastic marrow changes. The mechanism of action is unclear. However, aspects of folate metabolism have been shown to be altered by this drug. Malabsorption of folate has been demonstrated by a number of methods (Swinson *et al.*, 1981). In addition to an effect on folate absorption, there are reports that sulphasalazine inhibits several enzymes in the rat concerned with folate metabolism and human intestinal brush border folate conjugase.

Anticonvulsant Drugs

The anticonvulsant drug most commonly associated with the development of megaloblastic anaemia is phenytoin, but other drugs such a primidone, phenobarbitone and other barbiturates have been implicated. The reason for the development of megaloblastic change may be due to folate deficiency or in some subjects as a direct result of the toxic effect of the drug (Chanarin, 1990).

The explanation for the development of folate deficiency in patients taking anticonvulsant drugs is probably the summation of a number of facets that each tend towards a negative folate balance. The dietary folate intake among those on anticonvulsants has been reported to be only two-thirds of that consumed by a control group. Another mechanism that may influence folate status by anticonvulsants is enzyme induction. Phenytoin has also been reported to promote urinary excretion of newly absorbed folate given as folic acid. If this occurred with endogenous plasma methyl THF, it would be another explanation for the presence of a low serum folate.

Oral Contraceptives

The incidence of megaloblastic anaemia in women taking oral contraceptives for long periods of time is low (Lindenbaum *et al.*, 1975). These authors have demonstrated a reversible interference with nucleic acid synthesis in the cervical epithelium of contraceptive users, similar to that seen in patients with megaloblastic anaemia. They proposed that this effect could be due to drug interference with folate cofactor interactions. Equally, it is possible that these agents cause an increased turnover of folate cofactors, as has been shown for phenytoin. However, if oral contraceptives have an effect on folate metabolism, then it is small (Chanarin, 1990).

Haematological Complications of Alcohol

There are two main mechanisms to account for the effect of alcohol on haemopoiesis: first, the direct toxic effect of ethanol, or its metabolic products, on developing haemopoietic cells and perhaps their progeny in the peripheral blood, and, second, the additional effect of folate deficiency, which is largely nutritional in origin. The haematological complications of alcoholism have been reviewed by Chanarin (1990), and the metabolism and metabolic effects of alcohol by Lieber (1980).

Folate Deficiency and Alcohol

Folate deficiency is frequently associated with the chronic ingestion of alcohol. There is, however, a marked contrast between alcoholics from deprived backgrounds, particularly the so-called 'skid row' alcoholics in the USA, who show a high incidence of megaloblastic bone marrow change and anaemia which is largely due to folate deficiency, and those from a higher income group, where such changes are less common.

The main causes for folate deficiency are an inadequate diet and alcohol in the form of spirits. Beer drinkers have a lower incidence of folate deficiency, owing to the significant folate content of beer. Other mechanisms for the development of folate deficiency have been postulated but either they remain unproven or their significance is uncertain (Scott and Weir, 1980; Chanarin, 1990).

The Direct Toxic Effects of Alcohol

The commonest change in the peripheral blood is macrocytosis. Although folate deficiency may be a contributory factor, it appears likely that the macrocytosis results from a direct toxic effect of alcohol on the bone marrow. Anaemia is variable, being present in only 11 of 84 patients in the UK (Wu *et al.*, 1975) and about 50 per cent of malnourished alcoholics in the USA taking more than 100 g of ethanol daily, 19 per cent of whom died. Leucopenia was present in 6 per cent and thrombocytopenia in 55 per cent (Savage and Lindenbaum, 1986).

Growth of erythroid colonies from marrow progenitor cells is suppressed by concentrations of alcohol present *in vivo*. Acetaldehyde is a more potent suppressor than ethanol. Pluripotential stem cells are not affected and granulocyte progenitors are more resistant than erythroid progenitors. Ethanol-associated thrombocytopenia is brought about by suppressing thrombopoiesis at the level of the maturing megakaryocyte. Granulopoiesis appears to be affected by suppression at the level of CFU-GM and by inhibition of GM-CSF.

The morphological evidence that alcohol and its metabolites have a direct effect on the bone marrow cells includes the development of cytoplasmic and nucleolar vacuoles, ringed sideroblasts as well as megaloblastic changes (Figure 3). When sideroblastic change is present, the peripheral erythrocytes are typically of dimorphic appearance, normochromic and hypochromic cells. Megaloblastic marrow changes occur after

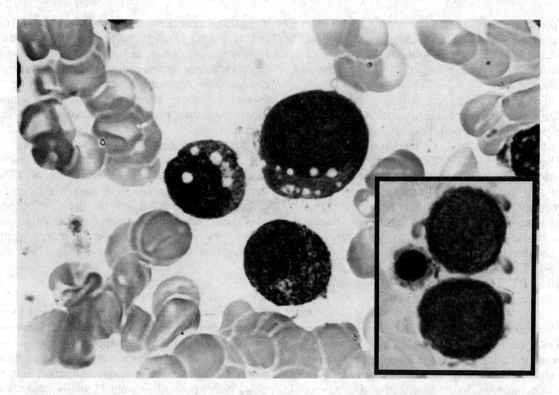

Figure 3 A bone marrow aspirate from an alcoholic female patient, showing cytoplasmic vacuolation in both erythroid and granulocyte precursors. The insert is a Perl's stain for iron on the above marrow aspirate, which shows two basophilic erythroblasts and a late erythroblast. The latter has a ring of cytoplasmic iron-containing granules—i.e. ring sideroblast.

4–10 days of high alcohol intake and revert to normal after ceasing alcohol, without other therapy. If the subject continues to imbibe alcohol, the megaloblastic change persists, even if dietary folate is sufficient to reverse megaloblastosis secondary to pure folate deficiency. Pancytopenia and megaloblastic bone marrow change have also been described in patients receiving amino acid–ethanol mixtures given as parenteral nutrition.

The deoxyuridine suppression test on bone marrows from alcoholic patients is normal despite megaloblastosis, an indication that the megaloblastosis does not arise through impairment of vitamin B_{12}–folate pathways.

The evidence that these changes are due to the direct toxic effect of alcohol rests on the relatively rapid disappearance of these phenomena on alcohol withdrawal alone. Alcohol withdrawal leads to a reticulocytosis, reaching a peak after 7 days and, where there is uncomplicated anaemia, to a rise in haemoglobin. In the absence of splenomegaly, the platelets increase and the white cell count rises. The bone marrow changes disappear within a few days.

Haemolytic anaemia may occur in alcoholic liver disease but is not considered to be due to a direct effect of alcohol on circulating erythrocytes. Three types of haemolytic anaemia in patients with liver disease were discussed by Cooper (1980). The first is the chronic mild haemolysis associated with chronic cirrhosis and congestive splenomegaly. The second haemolytic syndrome is that occurring in association with hypertriglyceridaemia in patients with alcohol-induced acute fatty liver. It is thought that the haemolytic process is primarily due to acute portal hypertension with acute congestive splenomegaly. The third type of haemolytic syndrome discussed is spur cell anaemia, which is seen in severe liver disease, especially alcoholic cirrhosis. The red cells are characteristically spiculated and are haemolysed in the spleen. Membrane cholesterol is markedly increased without elevation of membrane phospholipid, which results in a raised cholesterol/phospholipid ratio.

The emphasis has been on the effect of alcohol on erythropoiesis and erythrocytes. However, alcohol also affects both leucocyte and platelet numbers and function. Liu (1980) reviewed studies dealing with the mechanisms for the increased incidence and severity of infection observed in alcoholics. Among the multiple factors included are abnormalities in the number and function of granulocytes, macrophages and lymphocytes. Alcohol may also induce thrombocytopenia and abnormal platelet function.

Inadequate or Inactive Vitamin B₁₂

The interruption of the folate cycle by drugs such as methotrexate causes a decrease in the supply of folate for thymidylate synthetase. It is less obvious that blocking the vitamin B_{12}-dependent conversion of methyltetrahydrofolate brings about a similar result. However, vitamin B_{12} deficiency, as seen with pernicious anaemia, may cause severe megaloblastic anaemia. Thus, inactivation of cellular vitamin B_{12} or interference with its supply would be expected to lead to megaloblastic change. The following drugs interfere with vitamin B_{12} in one or other of these ways: nitrous oxide, metformin, cholestyramine, *para*-aminosalicylate, neomycin and colchicine.

Inactivation of Cellular Vitamin B₁₂: Nitrous Oxide

In 1956 Lassen and his co-workers described bone marrow depression in patients with tetanus ventilated with a mixture of 50 per cent nitrous oxide and 50 per cent oxygen for periods of 4–17 days. Megaloblastic change was referred to in some of the pathology reports. The megaloblastic change was later shown to be due to inactivation of vitamin B_{12} by nitrous oxide (Amess *et al.*, 1978). It had been shown previously that nitrous oxide oxidizes cob(I)alamin to cob(III)alamin and cob-(II)alamin. Since methylcobalamin must be in the fully reduced cob(I)alamin form for biological activity, the reaction between nitrous oxide and vitamin B_{12} impairs the methionine synthetase reaction and, in some circumstances, causes the haematological and neurological features of vitamin B_{12} deficiency.

Megaloblastic haemopoiesis can be demonstrated by bone marrow aspiration in some patients after as little as 2 h nitrous oxide exposure. This morphological change has been supported by an abnormal deoxyuridine suppression test (Nunn *et al.*, 1986). Megaloblastic change has been described on exposure for less than 1 h in patients receiving intensive care. This, however, is not manifest in routine blood counts, nor are the effects seen clinically. Prolonged nitrous oxide inhalation for several days leads to severe megaloblastic anaemia with pancytopenia and, in some, death. Occasionally intermittent nitrous oxide exposure has been used to allow procedures that cause undue discomfort—for example, daily physiotherapy in a patient with painful contractures. Thus, nitrous oxide/oxygen mixture given three times a day for 15–30 min has caused megaloblastic anaemia after 24 days and again after 14 days (Nunn *et al.*, 1982).

Intermittent exposure to nitrous oxide may be abused in those with access to the gas, such as dentists and operating theatre personnel, in whom neurological signs and symptoms, as seen with vitamin B_{12} deficiency, have been described. In some cases the neuropathy has been accompanied by typical blood changes of a megaloblastic anaemia (Blanco and Peters, 1983). Two out of twenty asymptomatic dentists regularly involved in administering nitrous oxide for dental analgesia had slightly abnormal deoxyuridine suppression tests. These two subjects had normal blood counts but their blood films showed hypersegmented neutrophils and their bone marrow smears showed mildly megaloblastic erythropoiesis and the presence of giant metamyelocytes (Sweeney *et al.*, 1985).

A different situation is encountered when nitrous oxide is given to patients with undiagnosed subclinical vitamin B_{12} deficiency. Two such patients presented with subacute combined degeneration of the spinal cord 8 weeks after receiving a nitrous oxide anaesthetic for 90 min (Schilling, 1986). Similarly, two patients have been reported who, after cardiac surgery, developed severe megaloblastic bone marrow change associated with unsuspected mild vitamin B_{12} deficiency. One patient received nitrous oxide/oxygen for the duration of the operation and the other was ventilated with nitrous oxide/oxygen for 24 h (Amess *et al.*, 1981).

Malabsorption of vitamin B₁₂

Impaired vitamin B_{12} absorption may occur in diabetic patients treated with oral hypoglycaemic agents of the biguanide group; this is sometimes accompanied by megaloblastic anaemia. Vitamin

B_{12} malabsorption may also occur with the administration of cholestyramine, colchicine, neomycin, *para*-aminosalicylic acid and potassium supplements.

Miscellaneous

There are case reports suggesting that acyclovir, lithium, nitrofurantoin, tetracycline, arsenic and even an aspirin-containing preparation have been associated with megaloblastic anaemia (Scott and Weir, 1980).

SIDEROBLASTIC ANAEMIA AND MITOCHONDRIAL DAMAGE

Sideroblastic anaemias are characterized by the presence of a variable number of hypochromic cells in the peripheral blood and an excess of iron in the bone marrow, many of the developing erythroblasts containing iron granules (sideroblasts) arranged in a ring around the nucleus. The presence of ring sideroblasts is the diagnostic feature of the anaemia, in which iron accumulates at the site of haem synthesis, the mitochondria. These changes lead to ineffective erythropoiesis. Many drugs and chemicals are capable of causing bone marrow dysfunction through their effect on mitochondrial metabolism. This action may be reflected in interruption of mitochondria-related functions such as haem synthesis, with consequent sideroblastic changes, or ultimately in compromised cellular synthetic machinery and cessation of cellular proliferation. In general, drug-induced bone marrow suppression as a consequence of mitochondrial injury is dose-dependent and reversible on the removal of the offending agent (Yunis and Salem, 1980). In order to understand the pathogenetic mechanisms of drug- or chemical-induced sideroblastic anaemia, haem biosynthesis will be outlined.

Biosynthesis of Haem

The biosynthesis of haem involves a series of mitochondrial and cytoplasmic enzymatic reactions (Figure 4). The first step in haem synthesis consists of condensation of succinate with glycine to form delta-aminoketoadipic acid, which then decarboxylates to yield delta-aminolaevulinic acid (ALA). This reaction is catalysed by the enzyme ALA synthetase, which requires pyridoxal-5-

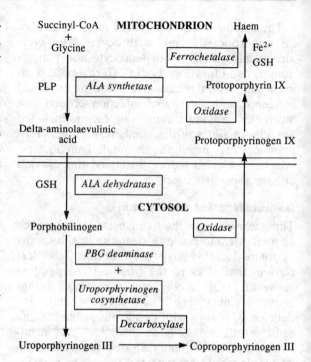

Figure 4 Pathway of haem synthesis. Abbreviations: PLP, pyridoxal phosphate; ALA, delta-aminolaevulinic acid; GSH, glutathione; PBG, porphobilinogen

phosphate (PLP) as a coenzyme. The next step is the condensation of two molecules of ALA to form porphobilinogen through the action of ALA dehydrase, an SH-requiring enzyme. Several steps ensue extramitochondrially, yielding coproporphyrinogen III, which in the mitochondria undergoes a two-step oxidation to protoporphyrin IX. The final step in haem synthesis, occurring within the mitochondria, is the incorporation of iron into protoporphyrin IX to form haem. It is catalysed by the enzyme ferrochelatase, which is an SH-requiring enzyme and is intimately associated with the inner mitochrondrial membrane (Sassa, 1990). The rate of iron uptake by mitochondria in erythroblasts appears to be inversely related to the intracellular concentration of haem. In anaemias with disordered haem synthesis, such as sideroblastic anaemia, iron accumulates in the mitochondria.

Drugs Which Interfere with Haem Synthesis

Sideroblastic bone marrow change has been described in association with a number of drugs or chemicals. These include: the antituberculosis drugs, alcohol, lead, chloramphenicol, lincomycin and penicillamine.

Antituberculosis Drugs

Sideroblastic anaemia has been reported with the use of isoniazid, pyrizinamide and cycloserine. In one patient with sideroblastic anaemia secondary to isoniazid therapy, ALA synthetase activity in bone marrow cells was decreased but could be corrected to near-normal levels by the addition of PLP *in vitro*. Moreover, a dose-dependent inhibition of ALA synthetase in the bone marrow was demonstrated in the same study (Konopka and Hoffbrand, 1979). It is apparent that isoniazid causes sideroblastic anaemia by interfering with the availability of PLP for the synthesis of ALA. A small number of patients taking isoniazid develop sideroblastic anaemia. However, the majority of patients on isoniazid for several months demonstrate a large increase in sideroblastic iron. It has been suggested that there is a genetic or nutritional predisposition to developing sideroblastic change (Yunis and Salem, 1980). In particular, there is a progressive decrease in blood PLP concentration with age and lower levels are seen in blacks. In the majority of patients developing isoniazid-induced sideroblastic anaemia, recovery occurs promptly and fully upon withdrawal of the drug or with pyridoxine administration.

Cycloserine- and pyrazinamide-induced sideroblastic anaemia may also be due to interference with pyridoxine metabolism (Yunis and Salem, 1980).

Alcohol

Alcohol is probably the most common cause of sideroblastic bone marrow abnormalities. The patients are usually severe alcoholics who frequently are also folate deficient. Full-blown sideroblastic anaemia has been reported only in chronically malnourished alcoholics.

The exact pathogenetic mechanisms underlying sideroblastic changes from alcohol have not been fully elucidated. Acute ethanol ingestion inhibits haem synthesis at several enzymatic steps, including ALA dehydrase, uroporphyrinogen decarboxylase, coproporphyrinogen oxidase and ferrochelatase. There is also general agreement that alcohol interferes with haem synthesis through its effect on pyridoxine metabolism (Yunis and Salem, 1980).

Chloramphenicol

Chloramphenicol principally suppresses erythropoiesis in a consistent and dose-dependent manner (Scott *et al.*, 1965). The effect is distinct from and unrelated to the rare complication of aplastic anaemia. Alterations of iron kinetics are detectable early and along with a reticulocytopenia, the serum iron rises and plasma iron clearance is prolonged. These can be accompanied by the development of ring sideroblasts.

The biochemical mechanisms for the development of the erythroid changes remain uncertain. The major adverse effect of chloramphenicol on the function of the differentiated marrow cells is inhibition of mitochondrial protein synthesis, specifically of certain cytochromes and cytochrome oxidase. Associated reduction of haem synthesis appears to occur secondarily, as both ALA synthetase and ferrochelatase, enzymes not known to be synthesized in mitochondria, are inhibited by the drug. The sideroblastic abnormality appears to be part of a defect of erythroid differentiation and proliferation consequent to the generalized mitochondrial disturbance rather than the result of a primary effect on haem synthesis initiated by chloramphenicol.

Bone marrow culture studies have shown that the drug selectively suppresses erythroid differentiation and proliferation. Greater than usual therapeutic doses of chloramphenicol are required for inhibition of *in vitro* granulocyte colony growth, and the inhibition can be blocked by supplemented colony stimulating factor. However, *in vitro* erythroid colony formation (CFU-E) is inhibited by therapeutic concentrations of chloramphenicol and erythropoietin has no protective effect. The drug completely inhibits erythroid burst-forming unit (BFU-E) production when added to murine or human marrow cultures, and proliferation of marrow and spleen CFU-E as well as of BFU-E is also impaired after chloramphenicol administration to mice.

Lead Poisoning

Lead is a toxic metal without any function in the human body. It has a strong affinity for the sulphydryl (–SH) groups, the amino group of lysine, the carboxyl group of glutamine and aspartic acids, and the hydroxyl group of tyrosine. Lead binds to proteins, modifies their tertiary structure and, hence, inactivates enzymatic properties. It appears likely that every enzyme could be inactivated by lead; those enzymes that are rich in SH groups appear to be sensitive to the smallest concentrations. The mitochondria are among the cellular structures that are particularly sensitive to lead. Lead poisoning and its effects have been reviewed by Piomelli (1987).

About 10 per cent of ingested lead is absorbed and about 40 per cent of inhaled lead of small particle size is retained in the body. Much of this lead will pass to the bones, but some will remain in the soft tissues, such as the bone marrow, the blood, the liver, kidney, heart and brain. There is a high concentration of lead in the bone marrow and it is particularly bound to red cells and red cell precursors.

Anaemia is present in the majority of patients with chronic lead poisoning. In adults this is usually a mild microcytic anaemia with an increased reticulocyte count. In children this form of anaemia tends to be more severe, with the red cells being more clearly microcytic, probably owing to associated iron deficiency. Basophilic stippling, although not a reliable index of lead poisoning, is a characteristic finding in the red cells. Red cells with iron-containing aggregates, siderocytes, are also found in the peripheral blood (Figure 5).

Lead toxicity is one of the causes of sideroblastic change in man but its incidence has not been documented. Electron microscopy has shown that there are many grossly swollen mitochondria in the red cell precursors, with ferritin particles and ferruginous micelles accumulating in the mitochondria and also scattered in the cytoplasm. However, ferrokinetic studies show that the degree of ineffective erythropoiesis induced by the inhibited haemoglobin synthesis is not severe and is overshadowed by an increased effective erythropoiesis, presumably in response to the haemolytic component due to the various other disturbances in the mature red cell. Erythroid hypoplasia may occur in prolonged lead exposure and is reflected in a prolonged plasma iron clearance and decreased iron incorporation into new erythrocytes.

The pathogenesis of these morphological changes is complex and not completely understood. The presence of basophilic stippling has been shown by electron microscopy to result from deposition of ribosomal DNA and mitochondrial fragments. Paglia and co-workers (1975) provided a biochemical explanation for the microscopic finding with the demonstration that in lead intoxication there is inhibition of the enzyme pyrimidine-5-nucleotidase, which under normal conditions plays a prominent role in the cleavage of residual nucleotide chains that persist in the cell after nuclear extrusion. The activity of this enzyme is decreased in lead poisoning, even in the absence of detectable basophilic stippling. The defect in pyrimidine-5-nucleotidase probably contributes to the shortening of erythrocyte survival. Individuals genetically defective in this enzyme exhibit marked chronic haemolysis.

Reduced red cell survival may also be due to the effect of lead on the erythrocyte membrane. Membrane alterations from lead are morphologically reflected in crenation of the erythrocyte and, at least in part, are due to changes in the conformation of proteins. These changes in the spatial arrangement of proteins are thought to inhibit ATPase and, hence, are responsible for a marked and selective loss of potassium ions from the cell.

There are so many mechanisms for interference by lead on haem and haemoglobin synthesis, as well as on erythrocyte function and survival, that it is surprising that anaemia is a rather late sign of lead intoxication. The effect of lead on haem synthesis has been extensively studied, *in vitro* and *in vivo*. ALA dehydratase has been shown to be the enzyme most susceptible to inhibition by lead. The activity of both coproporphyrinogen oxidase and ferrochelatase is also inhibited but that of ALA synthetase is increased. This results in decreased haem synthesis, accumulation of ALA and increased ALA excretion in the urine.

Sideroblastic change might be expected with the significant block of haem synthesis seen with lead poisoning. However, lead also competes for intracellular iron-binding sites, so that it may limit intracellular accumulation of iron. Reduced ferrous iron supply to the site of haem synthesis, and in children frequent concomitant iron deficiency, most probably account for the usual absence of the sideroblastic abnormality in lead intoxication.

Aluminium-Induced Microcytic Anaemia

Aluminium overload, which may occur in association with the use of untreated haemodialysis water or of aluminium-containing phosphorus binders in uraemia, may cause a microcytic anaemia by an unknown mechanism (Mladenovic, 1988). Two main mechanisms have been proposed for the development of anaemia. One

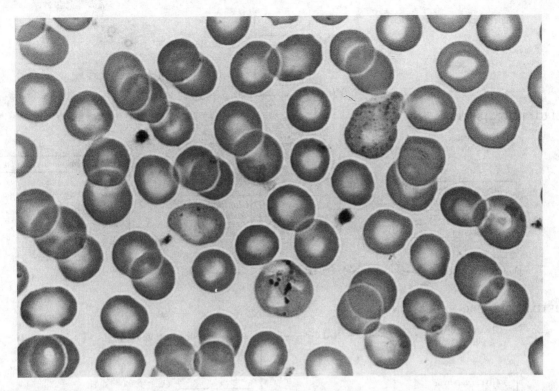

Figure 5 Blood film from a male patient with lead poisoning due to the consumption of aphrodisiacs. There is one erythrocyte containing coarse siderotic granules and another irregularly shaped erythrocyte demonstrating punctate basophilia

possibility is the direct inhibition of haem synthesizing enzymes (McGonigle and Parsons, 1985); alternatively, aluminium may cause anaemia by disruption of iron distribution and metabolism (Mladenovic, 1988). A recent study (Rosenlöf *et al.*, 1990) supports the suggestion that aluminium induces a microcytic anaemia by binding to transferrin and thus interferes with the incorporation of iron into haem (Mladenovic, 1988).

HAEMOLYTIC ANAEMIA

The essential feature of a haemolytic anaemia is a reduction in the life-span of the patient's erythrocytes. The classification and pathophysiology of the haemolytic anaemias have been reviewed (Dacie, 1985).

Haemolytic anaemia may be produced by drugs or chemicals in three main circumstances.

(1) Oxidative haemolysis in patients with normal erythrocytes.
(2) Oxidative haemolysis in patients with erythrocytes that are less able to withstand oxidative stress. This is particularly seen in glucose-6-phosphate dehydrogenase deficiency. These chemical- or drug-induced haemolytic anaemias are the result of the interaction between an extrinsic cause and inborn error of metabolism.

(3) Immune. The patient either produces antibodies against a drug or drug metabolites or the drug induces the production of an autoantibody against a red cell antigen.

Chemical- and Drug-induced Oxidative Haemolysis

Normal erythrocytes are not generally prone to oxidative denaturation by chemicals or drugs, as they are endowed with an impressive array of protective antioxidant and/or redox defence mechanisms (Gordon-Smith 1980; Stern, 1989). These serve to reverse oxidant damage or to prevent it by detoxifying 'oxygen radicals', which include superoxide ($:O_2^-$), peroxide (H_2O_2) and the highly reactive hydroxyl radical ($\cdot OH$). The best-known mechanisms are presented in

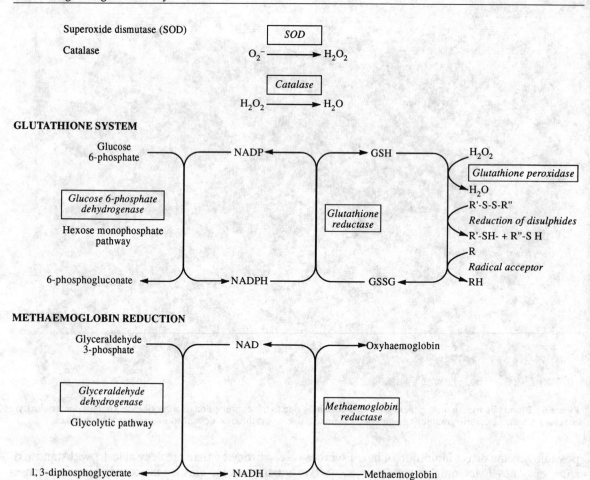

Superoxide dismutase (SOD)

Catalase

$$O_2{}^- \xrightarrow{\ SOD\ } H_2O_2$$

$$H_2O_2 \xrightarrow{\ Catalase\ } H_2O$$

GLUTATHIONE SYSTEM

Glucose 6-phosphate dehydrogenase

Hexose monophosphate pathway

Glutathione reductase

Glutathione peroxidase

Reduction of disulphides

Radical acceptor

METHAEMOGLOBIN REDUCTION

Glyceraldehyde dehydrogenase

Glycolytic pathway

Methaemoglobin reductase

Figure 6　Principal reactions in the erythrocyte for the reduction of oxidized compounds. Abbreviations: $O_2{}^-$, superoxide; NADPH, reduced nicotinamide adenine dinucleotide phosphate; GSH, reduced glutathione: GSSG, oxidized gluthathione

Figure 6. They include superoxide dismutase, catalase, the glutathione system, reduced nicotinamide adenine dinucleotide phosphate (NADPH), methaemoglobin reductase, reduced nicotinamide adenine dinucleotide (NADH), membrane-associated vitamin E and vitamin C. In chemical- or drug-induced oxidative damage of the erythrocyte, all or only some of the mechanisms available for maintaining the reducing environment are mobilized. This partly depends on the site of the oxidative denaturation or the biochemical behaviour of the drug.

Impaired antioxidant defence may occur when there is a congenital deficiency of reducing enzymes, when there is inhibition of these enzymes by other agents or when there is a relative deficiency of these enzymes related to the patient's age (Gordon-Smith, 1980). For example, deficiency of the hexose monophosphate pathway enzyme glucose-6-phosphate dehydrogenase (G6PD) results in the inefficient recycling of glutathione (GSH) and, therefore, suboptimal protection against peroxide and slow reduction of abnormal disulphides. These patients are therefore unusually susceptible to added stress imposed by exogenous oxidant drugs and, even in the absence of exogenous oxidants, the reduced erythrocyte survival seen with some G6PD-deficient variants is associated with the abnormal presence of intermolecular disulphide bonds.

In addition to enzyme deficiencies leading to an increased propensity to drug-induced haemolysis, this also occurs with the unstable haemoglobins Zürich (Hitzig *et al.*, 1960), Hasharon, Haemoglobin H and β-thalassaemia.

Oxidation of the Erythrocyte Membrane

Oxidative damage to the erythrocyte causes alterations in the cell membrane and in haemoglobin, affecting both the haem group and the globin chains. Membrane rigidity and lysis may result, together with methaemoglobin and Heinz body formation. Which of these is most important in damaging erythrocyte function depends on the type and origin of the oxidant stress and on the nature of the failure in reducing antioxidant protective mechanisms.

The phospholipids in the lipid bilayer of the erythrocyte contain unsaturated fatty acids which are subject to peroxidation with subsequent malonyldialdehyde formation. The red cell membrane may be damaged in other ways than oxidation of lipids. On the inner surface of the membrane, reduced glutathione maintains the sulphydryl groups ($-SH$) in the reduced state. Oxidation of these groups leads to the formation of mixed disulphides with increased potassium loss and autohaemolysis *in vitro*, and binding of denatured haemoglobin (Heinz bodies) to the membrane by $-S-S$ bonds causes rigidity of the membrane and intravascular haemolysis.

Oxidation of Haemoglobin

Oxidation of haemoglobin leads to the formation of methaemoglobin and to the denaturation and precipitation of globin as Heinz bodies. The iron in haemoglobin must be in the ferrous state to permit the reversible combination with oxygen. If the iron is oxidized to the ferric form, haemoglobin is converted to methaemoglobin, which cannot serve as an oxygen carrier. Methaemoglobin formation by itself may not be a prerequisite for red cell destruction, as evidenced by the absence of haemolysis in patients with methaemoglobinaemia induced by nitrites or in methaemoglobin reductase deficiency. However, methaemoglobin may be further oxidized to products that cause cellular damage.

The characteristic effect of excessive oxidation of haemoglobin is denaturation of the molecule, with precipitation, condensation and attachment of the denatured protein to the inside of the membrane. The insoluble precipitates are Heinz bodies. The spleen is able to remove the Heinz bodies from erythrocytes without destroying the cells that contain them. In practice, therefore, Heinz bodies are rarely seen in the peripheral blood, except after splenectomy, when the spleen is atrophic or, in chemical- or drug-induced cases when exceptionally large amounts of these agents have been taken. Heinz bodies are not usually discernible in standard Romanowsky stained blood films but are easily visible by the light microscope in unstained 'wet' preparations of blood, and they can be readily stained supravitally by basic dyes (Figure 7). Cells that have had Heinz bodies removed by the spleen often have a characteristic 'bite' appearance (Figure 8). The exact mechanism of Heinz formation has not been unravelled (Gordon-Smith, 1980; Dacie, 1985), but it is apparent that Heinz body formation is not necessarily associated with clinically significant methaemoglobinaemia, although the presence of this with Heinz body formation is suggestive of drug-induced oxidative damage.

Drugs Involved in Oxidative Haemolysis

Currently used drugs that may produce significant haemolysis or methaemoglobinaemia have been previously reviewed (Gordon-Smith, 1980; Dacie, 1985). Although some of the agents have chemical properties in common, great diversity exists in their chemical composition or structure, making it extremely difficult to predict which agent may cause oxidative denaturation in the normal erythrocyte. While there does not appear to be any common pharmacological link to explain their haemolytic property, many of them possess an arylamine nucleus, or, like chloramphenicol, may be converted to aromatic amines by reductive metabolism *in vivo*, so they could be looked at as derivatives of aniline. It is also recognized now that the oxidative damage from aniline is related primarily to its metabolite, phenylhydroxylamine (Harrison and Jollow, 1986).

Oxidative Haemolysis in Normal Subjects

This occurs more commonly in infants than in older children or adults. There are many reasons for this, which include both constitutional and environmental factors. Neonates have a relative deficiency of reducing power compared with older children. This has been attributed to a decreased NADH:methaemoglobin reductase activity, a possible vitamin E deficiency and a relative inability of the liver to metabolize drugs that have been detoxified by glucuronide conjugation.

In addition, infants are exposed to more oxidizing substances than are most adults. Their small

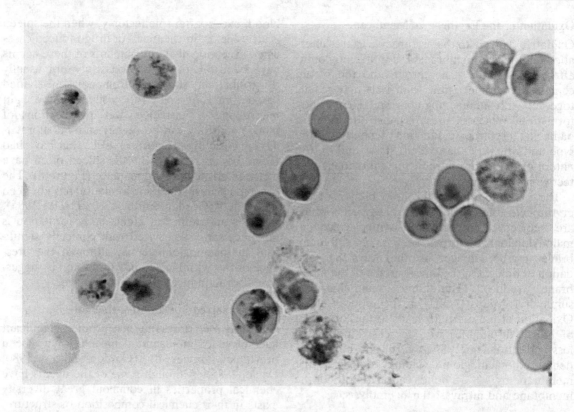

Figure 7 Blood from a male patient with an unstable haemoglobin (Hb Bristol) stained with a supravital stain to demonstrate the presence of Heinz bodies. These are irregular precipitates attached to the erythrocyte membrane

size means that toxic levels of oxidant substances are reached following relatively low dose absorption and infants' high surface area to volume ratio means that substances absorbed through the skin may reach toxic proportions. In infancy absorption of nitrites from the gastrointestinal tract may cause cyanosis due to methaemoglobinaemia. Nitrites are mainly derived from nitrate in drinking-water, particularly well-water, which has been contaminated with excessive amounts of fertilizer, but excessive consumption of spinach which has been left for some time before cooking has been implicated. Nitrates are converted to nitrites by bacteria in the gastrointestinal tract. Carrots may also contain high nitrite and nitrate levels. Ingestion of carrot juice has been recorded as a cause of infantile methaemoglobinaemia. It has been suggested that nitrites produce methaemoglobin by four nitrite ions and four protons reacting with each oxyhaemoglobin tetramer to form methaemoglobin nitrate, oxygen and water.

Methaemoglobinaemia has been described in infants due to absorption through the skin of aniline dyes used as marker inks. An important cause of methaemoglobinaemia and haemolytic anaemia in infants is water-soluble vitamin K analogues.

In adults with normal erythrocytes the use of oxidative drugs in pharmacological dosages may produce methaemoglobinaemia, mild cyanosis, chronic haemolysis with the production of Heinz bodies and 'bite cells' on the blood film. The drugs most commonly producing this haematological picture are dapsone and salazosulphapyridine (Gordon-Smith, 1980).

Powerful oxidants may produce acute intravascular haemolysis, methaemoglobinaemia, intravascular coagulation and renal failure. This severe and often fatal syndrome is usually due to accidental contamination or to a deliberate self-poisoning attempt. Sodium chlorate, a weed killer, and arsine, a by-product of smelting processes, may produce this syndrome. Naphthalene poisoning may also lead to acute haemolytic anaemia.

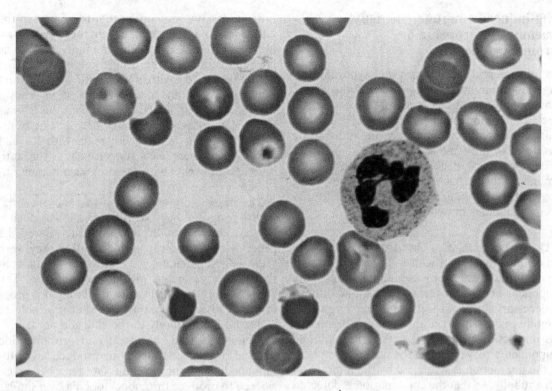

Figure 8 Blood film from a female patient taking sulphasalazine for chronic inflammatory bowel disease. A 'bite' cell and several 'blister' cells are demonstrated

Chloramines, used to sterilize water, are also potent oxidants which have been incriminated in producing Heinz body-positive haemolytic anaemia in patients undergoing dialysis.

Oxidative Haemolysis in G6PD Deficiency

Deficiencies of enzymes in the hexose monophosphate (pentose phosphate) pathway and in the glutathione cycles are the best-recognized causes of individual susceptibility to haemolysis by oxidant drugs, particularly the deficiency of G6PD. Glucose-6-phosphate dehydrogenase deficiency is numerically the most important cause of susceptibility to oxidant stress. In G6PD deficiency inadequate generation of NADPH results in accumulation of oxidized glutathione (GSSG) and probably hydrogen peroxide (Beutler, 1990).

Many different variants of G6PD deficiency have been described, most of them producing no clinical disorder. If it were not for the introduction of oxidant drugs, many so-called deficient patients, particularly from African and Far Eastern communities, would never have come to clinical notice. The clinical features produced by oxi-

dant drugs in patients with G6PD deficiency depend mainly on the G6PD variant.

In patients with Mediterranean or Cantonese variants, because of the extreme instability of the enzyme, the erythrocyte enzyme activity is very low. Accordingly, acute severe intravascular haemolytic anaemia is induced by fava (broad) beans and oxidant drugs. In the African type, A, the enzyme is more stable, so that haemolysis may be self-limiting as the old cells lyse and young cells, with their higher enzyme activity, increase. In the individual variants such as Chicago and Oklahoma, the picture of chronic extravascular haemolysis is exacerbated by the use of oxidant drugs. Haemolysis in G6PD deficiency is dose-dependent but the dose required is usually below pharmacological levels. Nevertheless, severe haemolysis due to exposure to drugs is rare in both the drug-sensitive patients and those with favism, provided that certain drugs are avoided (Dacie, 1985). Oxidant stress is also generated by infection, and red cells in a patient with G6PD deficiency may haemolyse at a much lower dose of oxidant drug than when not infected.

Drug-induced Immune Haemolytic Anaemia, Neutropenia or Thrombocytopenia

The fundamental mechanisms and syndromes of drug-induced immune cytopenia are the same, with certain exceptions, regardless of the cell affected. Immune haemolytic anaemia, neutropenia and thrombocytopenia are therefore to be considered in the same section.

The theoretical background of drug-induced immune cytopenia has recently been reviewed by Rosse (1990). Drugs are able to induce the formation of antibodies in two ways.

(1) *Drug as antigen* The drug itself may be part of the antigenic structure. The evidence suggests that the drug, acting as a hapten, and some component of the cell form a 'neoantigen'; both are necessary for the expression of the antigen, as antibody will not interact unless both are present. This interaction of the drug with the membrane component is very loose. In the case of the platelet, the interaction is stabilized by the interaction with antibody, so that the combination is detected on the cell membrane. In the case of the red cell, the interaction of the drug and the cellular component is not stabilized by reaction with antibody and is usually readily disrupted by washing the cell for *in vitro* testing.

In the past, many of the immune drug-induced cytopenias, which are now considered to be due to hapten-like reactions, were thought to be the result of immune complex interaction. In this situation the cellular compartment acts as an 'innocent bystander' antibody, usually IgM, against a drug–protein complex becoming attached to the cell membrane. However, it is clear that immune complexes are able to mediate destruction of blood cells (Rosse, 1990) and that some drug-induced reactions may be due to this cause. A small proportion of patients taking procainamide have a syndrome resembling systemic lupus erythematosus; in the course of this syndrome anaemia, neutropenia or thrombocytopenia may be seen. In most patients immune complexes are demonstrable in the serum and it has been proposed that these are the cause of cellular destruction.

(2) *Drug as non-antigen* In almost all instances of proven drug-induced immune cytopenia, the drug or one of its metabolites is demonstrated in one way or another to be part of the antigen. An instance in which this was shown not to be the case was the immune haemolytic anaemia caused by the drug α-methyldopa. The antibody reacted with normal red cells without the addition of the drug or any of its known metabolites; it appeared to react with the Rhesus (Rh) protein, as it sometimes had specificity for the Rh antigens and did not react with Rh null cells. All of these facts suggested that the antibody did not react with the drug as a hapten but did not explain the reaction.

The most likely explanation was the one originally proposed by Worlledge and associates (1966). They proposed that the drug altered the proteins of the red cell surface so that they were seen as foreign antigens. Antibody is made to them that cross-reacts with normal antigens. The Rh protein is the one usually exhibiting this property, because it is so antigenic that it is able to stimulate the antibody to the changed antigen.

Mefenamic acid, levodopa and procainamide have also been considered to produce an autoimmune haemolytic anaemia. Gold has been considered to produce thrombocytopenia by a similar mechanism.

Drugs Involved in Immune Cytopenia

A great variety of drugs have been involved in syndromes of drug-dependent immune cellular destruction. Some are more commonly encountered (e.g. quinidine thrombocytopenia, penicillin-induced haemolytic anaemia). Others have been shown to have occurred much less frequently, often only once. The various drugs that have caused drug-dependent haemolytic anaemia, neutropenia and thrombocytopenia have been reviewed (Habibi, 1987; Mueller-Eckhardt, 1987; Rosse, 1990).

The clinical syndrome for immune cytopenia due to a drug, when the drug is part of the antigen, is strikingly similar for the three cell lines affected. In a patient who has not previously taken the offending drug, the onset of immune cytopenia occurs at least 2–3 weeks after commencing the drug. On the other hand, patients may be sensitized after taking the drug for months.

If the patient has been sensitized to the drug by previous ingestion, whether or not immune cytopenia had occurred, cytopenia develops more quickly. If antibody is still present in the serum, the onset of cytopenia may be immediate.

The dose of the drug is usually not important either in bringing about sensitization or initiating cell destruction. Even a small dose of the drug can cause cellular destruction; the quinine in tonic water can cause thrombocytopenia in a patient sensitized to the drug. The reaction to penicillin is an exception to this rule, as large doses of the drug (more than 10 million units daily) must be given before immune haemolytic anaemia is seen. This may relate to the fact that such doses are needed in order to coat the erythrocytes with the drug.

In general, the destruction of the blood cells will continue if the drug continues to be administered. After the drug is stopped, in most instances, the counts begin to improve within a day or two and, will be normal within 10–14 days.

The clinical syndrome when the drug is not part of the antigen is different, as is illustrated by the immune haemolysis initiated by α-methyldopa. The onset of the reaction is dependent on the dose of the drug; patients taking larger doses are more likely to develop haemolysis. The onset is slower and occurs weeks to months after starting the drug. When the drug is discontinued, antibody production and cellular destruction continue for as long as 4–6 months. Readministration of the drug does not necessarily result in a relapse in antibody production. Many patients who take α-methyldopa acquire a positive direct antiglobulin (Coombs) test but few develop haemolytic anaemia. The difference between patients with methyldopa-induced autoantibodies who develop haemolytic anaemia and those who do not is thought to be related to the amount of IgG autoantibody on the red cells and to variations in macrophage recognition of these antibodies.

Immune Haemolytic Anaemia

Drugs are believed to be the cause in 12–24 per cent of all reported cases of immune haemolytic anaemia (Petz and Garratty, 1980). The most commonly reported type has been the autoimmune haemolytic anaemia produced by α-methyldopa described above. The drug-induced immune haemolytic anaemia in which the drug acts as a hapten is rare; with the exception of penicillin and cephalosporin, the drugs reported have caused only a single or at most a few cases (de Gruchy, 1975).

The immune haemolytic anaemia induced by the majority of drugs acting as haptens is primarily due to lysis by complement. Large amounts of antibody may be induced, so that the lysis may be severe and sudden. Since it is mediated primarily by complement, much of the lysis is intravascular and results in haemoglobinaemia and haemoglobinuria. The haemoglobinuria may be so severe as to cause renal failure. The antibody may be IgG or IgM. The subclasses of IgG have not been determined but must include those that fix complement.

The red cells are frequently normal in size and shape, although there may be a spherocytosis. The reticulocyte count is usually elevated, although it may be normal at the onset of the haemolysis, since the marrow may not have had sufficient time to respond. The immune destructive process may rarely affect other cells at the same time.

In most instances the Coombs test is positive only with antisera containing antibodies to complement components (anti-C3d, anti-C4d); IgG or IgM is not detected on the circulating red cells, as the antigen and antibody are removed during washing preparation for the test.

The syndrome seen with penicillin-induced antibody is somewhat different, probably because the drug is firmly attached to the cell. This allows IgG-mediated immune destruction; complement is not usually fixed. In most cases the degree of haemolysis is mild and develops over a period of 1–2 weeks during therapy with the drug. If complement is fixed, relatively severe haemolytic anaemia may result. The Coombs test is usually positive with anti-IgG but occasionally small amounts of C3d or C4d may be detected on the membrane. The serum usually contains a high titre of antibodies to penicillin, mainly to the benzylpenicilloyl group. At least 3 per cent of patients receiving large doses of penicillin will have a positive Coombs test with anti-IgG, but only a few of these will develop haemolytic anaemia.

Few other drugs are like penicillin in affixing to the membrane in such a way that washing does not displace them. Cephalosporins are related to penicillin chemically and they may on occasion cause haemolysis on this basis. Sometimes this is due to antibody specificity for this drug, but more often the antibodies have been previously stimulated by penicillin and cross-react with the related cephalosporins. Cephalosporins can also modify the red cell membrane such that plasma proteins bind non-specifically to red cells, producing a positive Coombs test but without evidence of haemolysis.

Drug-induced haemolytic anaemia may sometimes be caused by more than one mechanism acting simultaneously (Salama and Mueller-Eckhardt, 1987).

DRUG-INDUCED NEUTROPENIA

In general, two patterns may be recognized: (1) a mild to moderate neutropenia with a neutrophil count between 0.5 and 2.0 × 10⁹ 1⁻¹; and (2) severe neutropenia with a neutrophil count less than 0.5 × 10⁹ 1⁻¹. The latter is often referred to as agranulocytosis. A mild non-progressive neutropenia is not uncommonly seen with certain drugs, such as the phenothiazines and antithyroid drugs, after the commencement of treatment. The neutropenia does not progress despite the continued administration of the drug and the count does not fall to low levels. It usually rises rapidly following cessation of the drug and often rises while the drug is still being administered (de Gruchy, 1975). The term 'agranulocytosis' literally means the absence of granulocytes from the peripheral blood. It was introduced in 1922 by Schultz to describe a clinical syndrome characterized by the sudden onset of sore throat, fever and extreme prostration, often associated with necrosis of the mucous membranes, sepsis and death within a few days. The clinical picture was associated with a complete or almost complete absence of neutrophils in the peripheral blood, which was later shown to be due to the antipyretic amidopyrine, which is no longer in use.

Drug-induced agranulocytosis is thought to result from one of two basic mechanisms. The first is immunological and the second mechanism involves direct suppression of haemopoietic stem cell proliferation by the drug. Drugs associated with agranulocytosis have been reviewed (de Gruchy, 1975; Dale, 1990).

Immune Neutropenia

Immune-mediated drug-induced agranulocytosis may be due to immune destruction of neutrophils or immune suppression of granulocyte precursors or may be associated with autoantibody formation. The drugs causing immune neutropenia have been previously reviewed (Rosse, 1990).

Amidopyrine was the first recognized drug to act as a hapten-like drug leading to immune destruction of neutrophils. Since then drug-dependent neutrophil antibodies have been reported with a number of drugs, such as sulphapyridine, propylthiouracil, levamisole and the β-lactam group of antibiotics, which includes the penicillins and cephalosporins. The antibody is usually IgG but occasionally IgM. The bone marrow often shows 'maturation arrest'—that is, few cells beyond the myelocyte stage of development. This is presumably due to the later cells being destroyed either in the bone marrow or peripherally. If the offending drug is stopped, these rapidly reappear in the marrow and in the peripheral blood.

Immune suppression of granulopoiesis in the bone marrow has been reported in a few instances. Much of the evidence to support this concept has been derived from *in vitro* culture experiments. Barrett *et al.* (1976) described a case of amidopyrine-induced agranulocytosis with inhibition of colony formation in the presence of the patient's serum and drug. Kelton *et al.* (1979) similarly demonstrated drug-dependent serum suppression of CFU-GM and CFU-E in a patient developing pancytopenia while taking quinidine but it did not directly affect mature cells. This contrasts with the detection of a quinidine-dependent IgG antibody cytotoxic to mature cells (Eisner *et al.*, 1977). Recently a patient was reported who developed propylthiouracil (PTU)-induced agranulocytosis with evidence of a PTU-dependent antibody reactive not only with mature granulocytes and monocytes, but also with myeloid and erythroid progenitors (Fibre *et al.*, 1986).

Neutropenia Due to Direct Marrow Suppression

The second mechanism, that of direct marrow suppression, has been reviewed by Vincent (1986). It is best exemplified by the agranulocytosis induced by phenothiazines. Agranulocytosis usually occurs in mentally ill patients taking substantial doses of phenothiazines for prolonged periods (Pisciotta, 1973). Agranulocytosis normally occurs suddenly as in the immune variety but is not associated with symptoms of neutrophil lysis. Marrow examination most often shows a reduction in haemopoietic precursors, although blood abnormalities are identical with those seen in the immunological type—i.e. lymphopenia and severe neutropenia. After the patient has recovered, readministration of the drug will not result in immediate neutropenia, but agranulocytosis will recur after a few days if enough drug is given. Laboratory studies suggest that individuals susceptible to chlorpromazine have a latent proliferative defect, possibly genetic, in their marrow cells. A genetic factor is supported by the finding that this drug causes toxicity selectively in whites rather than blacks (Pisciotta, 1973).

The role of specific drug pharmacology in the aetiology of drug-induced agranulocytosis is well illustrated by studies with histamine H-2 antagonists. Metiamide, the first H-2 antagonist used in humans, was found to cause agranulocytosis with an unacceptably high frequency and was withdrawn from clinical practice. Cimetidine, an H-2 blocker in current use, is chemically identical apart from the substitution of a cyanoguanide side-chain for the thiourea side-chain of metiamide. This subtle change has resulted in very few properly documented cases of agranulocytosis with the extensive use of cimetidine. Indeed, patients have been reported where cimetidine has been used successfully in patients with prior metiamide-induced agranulocytosis. This finding may be a reflection of cellular drug uptake; unlike metiamide, radiolabelled cimetidine is not incorporated into bone marrow precursors in rats. It has been shown from studies with murine marrow cultures that pluripotential stem cells may be recruited from the resting state into cell cycle via a histamine H-2 receptor. This transition and also histamine-induced DNA synthesis are blocked by both metiamide and cimetidine *in vitro*. These fundamental changes in cell cycle parameters may account for the failure of proliferation and differentiation of the progenitor cells. The relative safety of cimetidine is probably due to lack of marrow uptake, but it may be anticipated that if plasma levels were elevated then the risk of agranulocytosis would be greater. A case of neutropenia following high-dose cimetidine therapy has been reported in a patient showing no toxicity with conventional doses of cimetidine. Two patients with renal failure have been reported who developed bone marrow hypoplasia due to

accumulation of the H-2 antagonist ranitidine (Amos *et al.*, 1987).

Some drugs would appear to induce agranulocytosis by both immune and direct toxic effects. For example, amodiaquine, an antimalarial drug, has been shown to inhibit CFU-GM from the marrow of a patient with agranulocytosis and, in a separate report, to produce agranulocytosis by a drug-dependent antibody which affects mature cells. Similarly, the mechanism for β-lactam-induced neutropenia could be either immune (see above) or dose-dependent inhibition of the growth of CFU-GM.

DRUG-INDUCED THROMBOCYTOPENIA

As with drug-induced neutropenia, there are two main pathogenetic mechanisms responsible for drug-induced thrombocytopenia. The first is increased destruction of platelets in the peripheral blood. This is nearly always due to an immunological mechanism and is the most commom reason for selective drug-induced thrombocytopenia. Usually the number of megakaryocytes in the marrow is either normal or increased. However, it is possible that antibodies active against platelets can also, at times, be active against megakaryocytes and therefore inhibit platelet production. The second mechanism is decreased production of platelets by the marrow by a direct toxic effect on megakaryocytes. In addition, there is a third uncommon mechanism, due to a direct dose-related non-immune action of a drug on the platelets, which was classically seen with the antibiotic ristocetin. This drug has been shown *in vitro* to cause platelet aggregation and it is probable that the effect *in vivo* is of similar pathogenesis. Ristocetin is no longer used as therapy but in an *in vitro* test for the investigation of von Willebrand's disease.

The drugs causing selective thrombocytopenia have been previously listed (de Gruchy, 1975; Aster and George, 1990). In addition, solvents, including benzene, cresol, naphthalene, spot remover and model aeroplane glue, or insecticides, including chlorophenothane, DDT, chlordane and gamma-benzene hexachloride (lindane), have been associated with marrow-related thrombocytopenia.

Drug-induced Immune Thrombocytopenia

The drugs producing immune thrombocytopenia have been listed (Aster and George, 1990; Rosse, 1990). The immune thrombocytopenia induced by the hapten-like drugs is often rapid in onset and severe, leading to bleeding as a presenting symptom. The platelet count often falls to less than $10 \times 10^9 \, 1^{-1}$ and the marrow usually shows an increase in megakaryocytes. The antibody is usually IgG but IgM antibodies have also been reported. The components of complement may also be found on the platelet membrane, which suggests that complement may play a role in the destruction of platelets.

The stereoisomers quinine and quinidine are perhaps the most common cause of immune thrombocytopenia due to a drug. The specificity of the antibodies can be divided into two major groups. Some antibodies react with only one or other of the stereoisomers, termed non-cross-reactive. On the other hand, some antibodies react with either of the stereoisomers, termed cross-reactive.

The amount of drug needed to elicit the reaction may be very small. Quinine water used in gin and tonic may cause severe thrombocytopenia. The bone marrow is usually normal except for increased numbers of megakaryocytes. Rarely quinidine may cause an immune-mediated aplastic anaemia.

Thrombocytopenia occurring during heparin therapy is being observed with increasing frequency (King and Kelton, 1984). Heparin-dependent platelet antibodies are present in the serum of most patients during the acute episode and it is generally believed that the thrombocytopenia results from immune injury to platelets. Spontaneous bleeding rarely develops in patients with heparin-associated thrombocytopenia, despite the administration of heparin, although platelet counts may fall to less than $20 \times 10^9 \, 1^{-1}$. However, thrombocytopenia following heparin administration is accompanied by the seemingly paradoxical development of thrombosis, with a frequency approaching 20–40 per cent in some studies. Thrombosis can be arterial or venous, often occurring at multiple sites, and may continue to develop unless heparin is discontinued. Thrombocytopenia or thrombosis may recur if heparin is readministered. Several hypotheses have been proposed to explain how heparin causes thromboses in these patients. It has been suggested that serum from some patients with heparin-associated thrombocytopenia may contain antibodies that react with heparin bound to endothelial cells or with heparin sulphate synthesized by endothelial cells. Immune injury to both platelets and endothelial cells may play a part in the development of thrombosis in some patients after heparin therapy.

Gold, which is used in the treatment of rheumatoid arthritis, may cause immune thrombocytopenia. The syndrome bears a close resemblance to the autoimmune haemolytic anaemia seen with α-methyldopa. The onset of the thrombocytopenia is dose-dependent; usually more than 500–1000 mg is given before thrombocytopenia is seen. Furthermore, the onset of the syndrome is often delayed for weeks or months after the start of therapy. Antibody binding to the platelet may be detected in the serum without the addition of the drug. This suggests that the antigen may be an altered integral protein of the membrane and the antibody is produced in response to the altered antigen, as may be the case with alpha-methyldopa (Rosse, 1990). An alternative conclusion is that gold-induced thrombocytopenia, in rheumatoid arthritis patients, may be caused by the induction or the enhancement by gold of platelet-autoantibody formation.

Thrombocytopenia Due to Direct Marrow Suppression

Selective megakaryocyte aplasia or hypoplasia leading to thrombocytopenia is uncommon. The thiazide diuretics, oestrogens and alcohol appear to have a relatively specific effect on platelet production.

SECONDARY LEUKAEMIC SYNDROMES

Exposure to ionizing radiation and to a growing list of drugs and chemicals is associated with an increased risk of developing leukaemia and myelodysplasia. In virtually no instance can a single leukaemogenic event be identified. It has been postulated that multiple factors must occur in precise sequence in order for leukaemia to evolve (Nowell, 1988).

Chemicals/Drugs and Leukaemia

This subject has recently been reviewed by Rosner and Grünwald (1990).

Chemical-induced Leukaemia

Benzene and its cogener toluene have been well documented as agents inducing haemopoietic damage and subsequent leukaemia (Jacobs, 1989). Exposure to benzene has been heavy and prolonged in industries that have a history of inadequate safety precautions. The occupations chiefly affected have been the leather and shoe industries, which use glues containing benzene, and dry cleaning, printing and paint spraying, in which benzene solvents are employed. Nearly all cases of leukaemia have been preceded by a period of hypoplasia or myelodysplasia.

Although acute leukaemia, mostly myeloblastic, predominates in chronic benzene toxicity, there are several reports of chronic myeloid leukaemia, chronic lymphocytic leukaemia and, more recently, hairy cell leukaemia.

Recent reports describe acute leukaemia following exposure to a weed killer, an insecticide, a soil fumigant, solvents including benzene, ethylene oxide, in patients with psoriasis treated with psoralen and ultraviolet light and in hospital multiple drug and chemical exposure. Although cigarette smoking is the major single known cause of cancer mortality, this has not been consistently associated with leukaemia. However, a recent report describes a significant increase in risk of acute myeloblastic leukaemia in association with cigarette smoking (Severson, 1987).

Drug-induced Leukaemia

The extensive use of cytotoxic drugs in combination chemotherapy programmes or as single agents has improved the survival of many patients with malignant disease. However, these patients now live long enough to develop secondary myelodysplasia or acute myeloid leukaemia. Drugs most frequently implicated are alkylating agents such as melphalan, chlorambucil and cyclophosphamide, and other cytotoxic drugs such as procarbazine and the nitrosourea compounds. Therapy-related leukaemic syndromes occur most frequently in long-term survivors of Hodgkin's disease who have previously been treated with both alkylating agent-containing chemotherapy and extensive radiation; the estimated actuarial risk in such patients varies from 6 per cent to 9 per cent, depending on the series. The average time between the diagnosis of the initial tumour and the appearance of the secondary leukaemia varies from 48 months to 68 months. The majority of patients present with the peripheral blood and bone marrow findings consistent with a myelodysplastic syndrome before developing frank acute leukaemia.

Chloramphenicol has been the most frequently incriminated non-cytotoxic drug to be linked with leukaemia (Ellims *et al.*, 1979; Schmitt-Graff, 1981). In a few of these patients the leukaemia was preceded by a period of marrow depression and it is here that the strongest evidence for the causal relationship between the drug and the disease is found, analogous to the case of benzene- or radiation-induced leukaemia.

Phenylbutazone has also been incriminated as causing leukaemia, but in only two patients was well-documented phenylbutazone-associated bone marrow aplasia followed by acute leukaemia.

POLYCYTHAEMIA

Polycythaemia usually refers to an increased number of erythrocytes in the blood. In polycythaemia rubra vera, one of the chronic clonal myeloproliferative disorders, there is often an additional increase in granulocytes and platelets. This has been shown to occur in excess in two heavily irradiated groups of males—patients given Thorotrast and radium chemists. Polycythaemia rubra vera has also been described in participants in a nuclear weapon test (Caldwell *et al.*, 1984).

Tissue hypoxia is the most important cause of the development of secondary polycythaemia. Cobalt and carbon monoxide may lead to the polycythaemia through this mechanism. Polycythaemia was regularly observed, together with other signs, in epidemics of beer drinker's cardiomyopathy in the 1960s. The onset of these epidemics coincided with the introduction of minute amounts of cobalt into some brands of beer to stabilize the 'head'. This effect of cobalt is considered to be secondary to an action on the central nervous system which results in respiratory alkalosis. In turn, this increases the affinity of haemoglobin for oxygen, which is interpreted by

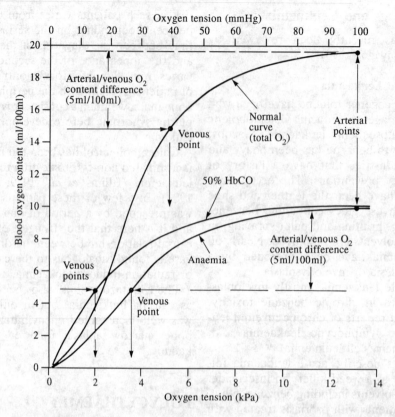

Figure 9 Influences of anaemia and carbon monoxide poisoning on the relationship between oxygen tension and content. The normal curve is constructed for a haemoglobin concentration of 14.4 g dl^{-1}. Assuming an arterial/venous oxygen content difference of 5 ml per 100 ml, the venous PO$_2$ is about 5.3 kPa (40 mmHg). The curve of anaemic blood is constructed for a haemoglobin concentration of 7.2 g dl^{-1}. If the arterial/venous oxygen content difference remains unchanged, the venous PO$_2$ will fall to 3.6 kPa (27 mmHg), a level which is low but not dangerously so. The curve of 50 per cent carboxyhaemoglobin is based on a total haemoglobin (including carboxyhaemoglobin) of 14.4 g dl^{-1}. Assuming an arterial/venous oxygen content difference of 5 ml per 100 ml, the venous PO$_2$ is only 1.9 kPa (14 mmHg), a level which is dangerously low, as it must be associated with a greatly reduced tissue PO$_2$. Arterial PO$_2$ is assumed to be 13.3 kPa (100 mmHg) in all cases. Reproduced by permission from Nunn (1987)

tissue sensors as hypoxia. These then act to increase erythropoietin (Miller *et al.*, 1974).

Carbon monoxide is well known to displace oxygen from combination with haemoglobin, the affinity being approximately 300 times greater than the affinity for oxygen. The presence of carboxyhaemoglobin also causes a leftward shift of the dissociation curve of the remaining oxyhaemoglobin and therefore increased affinity for oxygen by haemoglobin (Figure 9). The disappearance of coal gas from domestic use in many countries has reduced the popularity of carbon monoxide for attempted suicide. However, carbon monoxide poisoning, both accidental and suicidal, accounts for more than 1000 deaths in England and Wales each year. The toxic effect of carbon monoxide is related not only to tissue

hypoxia, but also, more importantly, to the direct tissue toxicity of carbon monoxide (Piantadosi, 1987).

Carbon monoxide is to be found in blood of normal subjects and patients, in trace concentrations, as a result of its production in the body but mainly as a result of the internal combustion engine and smoking. Smoking alone, without lung disease, may result in polycythaemia (Moore-Gillon and Pearson, 1986).

Alcohol has also been implicated as a possible aetiological factor in the development of relative polycythaemia, but only rarely has it been confirmed as the principal cause of polycythaemia in individual patients. The distinguishing feature of relative polycythaemia is the coexistence of a high normal red cell mass with a low normal plasma volume. Perhaps one mechanism tending to increase the red cell mass in heavy drinkers is an increase in hepatic synthesis of erythropoietin by a regenerating liver. A possible reason for the reduction in plasma volume is the inhibition by alcohol of the release of antidiuretic hormone from the pituitary.

Polycythaemia can also occur after renal transplantation when azathioprine and prednisolone are used for immunosuppression. More recently it has been suggested that polycythaemia after renal transplantation is more likely to occur with patients receiving cyclosporin and prednisolone as immunosuppression. Possibly the propensity to develop polycythaemia in these patients is reduced by the bone marrow suppressive effect of azathioprine.

REFERENCES

Adamson, J. W. and Erslev, A. J. (1990). Aplastic anemia. In Williams, W. J., Beutler, E., Erslev, A. J. and Lichtmann, T. A. (eds), *Hematology*, 4th edn, McGraw-Hill, New York, 158–174

Amess, J. A. L., Burman, J. F., Murphy, M. F., Paxton, A. M. and Mollin, D. L. (1981). Severe megaloblastic bone marrow change associated with unsuspected mild vitamin B_{12} deficiency. *Clin. Lab. Haematol.*, **3**, 231–237

Amess, J. A. L., Burman, J. F., Rees, G. M., Nancekievill, D. G. and Mollin, D. L. (1978). Megaloblastic haemopoiesis in patients receiving nitrous oxide. *Lancet*, **ii**, 339–342

Amos, R. J., Kirk, B., Amess, J. A. L., Jones, A. L. and Hinds, C. J. (1987). Bone marrow hypoplasia during intensive care: bone marrow culture studies implicating ranitidine in the suppression of haemopoiesis. *Human Toxicol.*, **6**, 503–506

Aster, R. H. and George, J. N. (1990). Thrombocytopenia due to enhanced platelet destruction by immunologic mechanisms. In Williams, W. J., Beutler, E., Erslev, A. J. and Lichtman, M. A. (Eds), *Hematology*, 4th edn. McGraw-Hill, New York, pp. 1370–1398l

Barrett, A. J., Weller, E., Rozengurt, N., Longhurst, P. and Humble, J. G. (1976). Amidopyrine agranulocytosis: drug inhibition of granulocyte colonies in the presence of patient's serum. *Br. Med. J.*, **ii**, 850–851

Beutler, E. (1990). Glucose-6-phosphate dehydrogenase deficiency. In Williams, W. J., Beutler, E., Erslev, A. J. and Lichtman, M. A. (Eds), *Hematology*, 4th edn. McGraw-Hill, New York, pp. 591–606

Blanco, G. and Peters, H. A. (1983). Myeloneuropathy and macrocytosis associated with nitrous oxide abuse. *Arch. Neurol.*, **40**, 416–418

Caldwell, G. G., Kelley, D. B., Heath, C. W. and Zack, M. (1984). Polycythemia vera among participants of a nuclear weapons test. *J. Am. Med. Assoc.*, **252**, 662–664

Camitta, B. M., Thomas, E. D., Nathan, D. G., Gale, R. P., Kopecky, K. J., Rappeport, J. M., Santos, G., Gordon-Smith, E. C. and Storb, R. (1979). A prospective study of androgens and bone marrow transplantation for treatment of severe aplastic anemia. *Blood*, **53**, 504–514

Chanarin, I. (1990). *The Megaloblastic Anaemias*, 3rd edn. Blackwell Scientific, Oxford

Chapius, B., von Fleidner, V. E., Jeannet, M., Merica, H., Vuagnat, P., Gratwohl, A., Nissen, C. and Speck, B. (1986). Increased frequency of DR2 in patients with aplastic anaemia and increased DR sharing in their parents. *Br. J. Haematol.*, **63**, 51–57

Cooper, R. A. (1980). Hemolytic syndromes and red cell membrane abnormalities in liver disease. *Semin. Hematol.*, **17**, 103–112

Dacie, J. V. (1985). *The Haemolytic Anaemias*, Vol. 1. Churchill Livingstone, Edinburgh

Dale, D. C. (1990). Neutropenia. In Williams, W. J., Beutler, E., Erslev, A. J. and Lichtman, M. A. (Eds), *Hematology*, 4th edn. McGraw-Hill, New York, pp. 806–816

de Gruchy, G. C. (1975). *Drug-induced Blood Disorders*. Blackwell Scientific, Oxford

Dessypris, E. N., Redline, S., Harris, H. W. and Krantz, S. B. (1985). Diphenylhydantoin-induced pure red cell aplasia. *Blood*, **65**, 789–794

Eisner, E. V., Carr, R. M. and MacKinney, A. A. (1977). Quinidine-induced agranulocytosis. *J. Am. Med. Assoc.*, **238**, 884–886

Ellims, P. H., van der Weyden, M. B., Brodie, G. N., Firkin, B. G., Whiteside, M. G. and Faragher, B. S. (1979). Erythroleukemia following drug induced hypoplastic anemia. *Cancer*, **44**, 2140–2146

Erslev, A. J. (1990). Pure red cell aplasia. In Williams, W. J., Beutler, E., Erslev, A. J. and Lichtman, M. A. (Eds), *Hematology*, 4th edn. McGraw-Hill, New York, pp. 430–438

Fibre, W. E., Claas, F. H. J., van der Star-Dijkstra, W., Schaafsma, M. R., Meyboom, R. H. B. and Falkenburg, J. H. T. (1986). Agranulocytosis induced by propylthiouracil: evidence of a drug dependent antibody reacting with granulocytes, monocytes and haemopoietic progenitor cells. *Br. J. Haematol.*, **64**, 363–373

Girdwood, R. H. (1974). Death after taking medicaments. *Br. Med. J.*, **i**, 501–504

Goldstein, B. D. (1983). Clinical hematoxicity of benzene, *Adv. Med. Environ. Toxicol.*, **4**, 51–61

Gordon-Smith, E. C. (1980). Drug-induced oxidative haemolysis. *Clin. Haematol.*, **9**, 557–586

Gordon-Smith, E. C. (1989). Aplastic anaemia—aetiology and clinical features. *Baillière's Clin. Haematol.*, **2**, 1–18

Habibi, B. (1987). Drug-induced immune haemolytic

anaemias. *Baillière's Clin. Immununol. Allerg.*, **1**, 343–356

Harrison, J. H. and Jollow, D. J. (1986). Role of aniline metabolites in aniline-induced hemolytic anemia. *J. Pharmacol. Exptl Ther.*, **238**, 1045–1054

Heim, S., Mitelman, H. (1986). Chromosome abnormalities in the myelodysplastic syndromes. *Clin. Haematol.*, **15**, 1003–1021

Hitzig, W. H., Frick, P. G., Betke, K. and Huisman, T. H. J. (1960). Haemoglobin Zürich: eine neue Hämoglobinanomalie mit sulfonamidinduzierter Innenkörperanämie. *Helv. paediat. Acta*, **15**, 499–514

Hoffbrand, A. V. and Wickramasinghe, R. G. (1982). Megaloblastic anaemia. In Hoffbrand, A. V. (Ed.), *Recent Advances in Haematology*, Churchill Livingstone, Edinburgh, pp. 25–44

Hopkins, J. E. and Manoharan, A. (1985). Severe aplastic anaemia following the use of hair dye: Report of two cases and review of literature. *Postgrad. Med. J.*, **61**, 1003–1005

Howell, A., Andrews, T. M. and Watts, R. W. E. (1975). Bone marrow cells resistant to chloramphenicol in chloramphenicol-induced aplastic anaemia. *Lancet*, **i**, 65–69

Inman, W. H. (1977). Study of fatal bone marrow depression with special reference to phenylbutazone and oxyphenbutazone. *Br. Med. J.*, **i**, 1500–1505

International Agranulocytosis and Aplastic Anemia Study (1986). Risks of agranulocytosis and aplastic anemia. A first report of their relation to drug use with special reference to analgesics. *J. Am. Med. Assoc.*, **256**, 1749–1757

Jacobs, A. (1989). Benzene and leukaemia. *Br. J. Haematol.*, **72**, 119–121

Jouhar, A. J. (1976). Aplastic anaemia and hair dye. *Br. Med. J.*, **i**, 1074

Kalf, G. F. (1987). Recent advances in the metabolism and toxicity of benzene. *CRC Crit. Rev. Toxicol.*, **18**, 141–159

Konopka, L. and Hoffbrand, A. V. (1979). Haem synthesis in sideroblastic anaemia. *Br. J. Haematol.*, **42**, 73–87

Kelton, J. G., Huang, A. T., Mold, N., Logue, G. L. and Rosse, W. F. (1979). The use of in vitro techniques to study drug-induced pancytopenia. *New Engl. J. Med.*, **301**, 621–624

King, D. J. and Kelton, J. G. (1984). Heparin-associated thrombocytopenia. *Ann. intern. Med.*, **100**, 535–540

Lambie, D. G. and Johnson, R. H. (1985). Drugs and folate metabolism. *Drugs*, **30**, 145–155

Lancet Editorial (1986). Analgesics, agranulocytosis and aplastic anaemia: A major case control study. *Lancet*, **ii**, 899–900

Lassen, H. C. A., Henriksen, E., Neukirch, F. and Kristensen, H. S. (1956). Treatment of tetanus. Severe bone-marrow depression after prolonged nitrous-oxide anaesthesia. *Lancet*, **i**, 527–530

Lennard, L., van Loon, J. A. and Weinshilboum, R. M. (1989). Pharmacogenetics of acute azathioprine toxicity: Relationship to thiopurine methyltransferase genetic polymorphism. *Clin. Pharmacol. Ther.*, **46**, 149–154

Lieber, C. S. (1980). Metabolism and metabolic effects of alcohol. *Semin. Hematol.*, **17**, 85–99

Lindenbaum, J., Whitehead, N. and Reyner, F. (1975). Oral contraceptive hormones, folate metabolism and the cervical epithelium. *Am. J. Clin. Nutrit.*, **28**, 346–353

Liu, Y. K. (1980). Effects of alcohol on granulocytes and lymphocytes. *Semin. Hematol.*, **17**, 130–136

McGonigle, R. J. S. and Parsons, V. (1985). Aluminium-induced anaemia in haemodialysis patients. *Nephron*, **39**, 1–9

Marmont, A. M. (1987). Immunological aspects of aplastic anaemia. *Baillière's Clin. Immunol. Allerg.*, **1**, 327–342

Miller, M. E., Howard, D., Stohlman, F. and Flanagan, P. (1974). Mechanism of erythropoietin production by cobaltous chloride. *Blood*, **44**, 339–346

Mladenovic, J. (1988). Aluminium inhibits erythropoiesis *in vitro*. *J. Clin. Invest.*, **81**, 1661–1665

Modan, B., Segal, S., Shani, M. and Sheba, C. (1975). Aplastic anemia in Israel: evaluation of the etiologic role of chloramphenicol on a community-wide basis. *Am. J. Med. Sci.*, **270**, 441–445

Moore-Gillon, J. M. and Pearson, T. C. (1986). Smoking, drinking and polycythaemia. *Br. Med. J.*, **292**, 1617–1618

Morley, A., Trainor, K. and Remes, J. (1976). Residual marrow damage: Possible explanation for idiosyncrasy to chloramphenicol. *Br. J. Haematol.*, **32**, 525–531

Mueller-Eckhardt, C. (1987). Drug-induced immune thrombocytopenia. *Baillière's Clin. Immunol. Allerg.*, **1**, 369–389

Nissen-Druey, C. (1989). Pathophysiology of aplastic anaemia. *Baillière's Clin. Haematol.*, **2**, 37–40

Nowell, P. (1988). Molecular events in tumor development. *New Engl. J. Med.*, **319**, 575–577

Nunn, J. F. (1987). *Applied Respiratory Physiology*, 3rd edn. Butterworths, London, p. 269

Nunn, J. F., Chanarin, I., Tanner, G. and Owen, E. R. T. C. (1986). Megaloblastic bone marrow changes after repeated nitrous oxide anaesthesia. Reversal with folinic acid. *Br. J. Anaesth.*, **58**, 1469–1470

Nunn, J. F., Sharer, N. M., Gorchein, A., Jones, J. A. and Wickramasinghe, S. N. (1982). Megaloblastic haemopoiesis after multiple short-term exposure to nitrous oxide. *Lancet*, **i**, 1379–1381

Odum, N., Platz, P., Morling, N., Jacobsen, N., Jakobsen, B. K., Ryder, L. P. and Svejgaard, A. (1987). Increased frequency of HLA-DPw3 in severe aplastic anaemia (AA), *Tissue Antigens*, **29**, 184–185

Paglia, D. E., Valentine, W. N. and Dahlgren, J. G. (1975). Effects of low-level lead exposure to pyrimidine-5-nucleotidase and other erythrocyte enzymes. Possible role of pyrimidine-5-nucleotidase in the pathogenesis of lead-induced anaemia. *J. Clin. Invest.*, **56**, 1164–1169

Petz, L. D. and Garratty, G. (1980). Drug-induced immune hemolytic anemia. In Petz, L. D. and Garratty, G. (Eds), *Acquired Immune Hemolytic Anemias*, Churchill Livingstone, Edinburgh, pp. 267–304

Piantadosi, C. A. (1987). Carbon monoxide, oxygen transport and oxygen metabolism. *J. Hyperbaric Med.*, **2**, 27–44

Piomelli, S. (1987). Lead poisoning. In Nathan, D. G. and Oski, F. A. (Eds), *Hematology of Infancy and Childhood*, 3rd edn. Saunders, Philadelphia, pp. 389–412

Pisciotta, A. V. (1973). Immune and toxic mechanisms in drug-induced agranulocytosis. *Semin. Hematol.*, **10**, 279–310

Rich, M. L., Ritterhoff, R. J. and Hoffman, R. L. (1950). A fatal case of aplastic anemia following chloramphenicol (Chloromycetin) therapy. *Ann. Int. Med.*, **33**, 1459–1467

Rosenlöf, K., Fyhrquist, F. and Tenhunen, R. (1990). Erythropoietin, aluminium, and anaemia in patients on haemodialysis. *Lancet*, **335**, 247–249

Rosner, F. and Grünwald, H. W. (1990). Chemicals and leukemia. In Henderson, E. S. and Lister, T. A. (Eds), *Leukemia*, 5th edn. Saunders, Philadelphia, pp. 271–287

Rosse, W. F. (1990). Reactions of warm-reacting antibodies: Drug-dependent antibodies. In Rosse, W. F. (Ed.), *Clinical Immunohematology: Basic Concepts and Clinical Applications*. Blackwell Scientific, Boston, pp. 533–553

Salama, A. and Mueller-Eckhardt, C. (1987). On the mechanisms of sensitization and attachment of antibodies to RBC in drug-induced immune hemolytic anemia. *Blood*, **69**, 1006–1010

Sassa, S. (1990). Synthesis of heme. In Williams, W. J., Beutler, E., Erslev, A. G. and Lichtman, M. A. (Eds), *Hematology*, 4th edn. McGraw-Hill, New York, pp. 322–328

Savage, D. and Lindenbaum, J. (1986). Anemia in alcoholics. *Medicine*, **65**, 322–338

Schilling, R. F. (1986). Is nitrous oxide a dangerous anaesthetic for vitamin B_{12}-deficient subjects? *J. Am. Med. Assoc.*, **255**, 1605–1606

Schmitt-Graff, A. (1981). Chloramphenicol-induced aplastic anemia terminating with acute nonlymphocytic leukaemia. *Acta. Haemat.*, **66**, 267–268

Schultz, W. (1922). Ueber eigenartige Halserkrankungen. *Dtsch. Med. Wschr.*, **48**, 1495–1497

Scott, J. L., Finegold. S. M., Belkin, G. A. and Lawrence, J. S. (1965). A controlled double-blind study of the hematologic toxicity of chloramphenicol. *New Eng. J. Med.*, **272**, 1137–1142

Scott, J. M. and Weir, D. G. (1980). Drug-induced megaloblastic change. *Clin. Haematol.*, **9**, 587–606

Severson, R. K. (1987). Cigarette smoking and leukemia. *Cancer*, **60**, 141–144

Sieff, C. (1983). Pure red cell aplasia. *Br. J. Haematol.*, **54**, 331–336

Stern, A. (1989). Drug-induced oxidative denaturation in red blood cells. *Semin. Hematol.*, **26**, 301–306

Sweeney, B., Bingham, R. M., Amos, R. J., Petty, A. C. and Cole, P. V. (1985). Bone marrow toxicity in dentists exposed to nitrous oxide. *Br. Med. J.*, **291**, 567–569

Swinson, C. M., Parry, J., Lumb, M. and Levi, A. J. (1981). Role of sulphasazine in the aetiology of folate deficiency in ulcerative colitis. *Gut*, **22**, 456–461

Vincent, P. C. (1986). Drug-induced aplastic anaemia and agranulocytosis. Incidence and mechanisms. *Drugs*, **31**, 52–63

Wickramsinghe, S. N. and Matthews, J. H. (1988). Deoxyuridine suppression: biochemical basis and diagnostic applications. *Blood Rev.*, **2**, 168–177

Worlledge, S. M., Carstairs, K. C. and Dacie, J. V. (1966). Autoimmune haemolytic anaemia associated with alpha-methyldopa therapy. *Lancet*, **ii**, 135–139

Wu, A., Chanarin, I., Slavin, G. and Levi, A. J. (1975). Folate deficiency in the alcoholic—its relationship to clinical and haematological abnormalities, liver disease and folate stores. *Br. J. Haematol.*, **29**, 469–478

Yunis, A. A. (1976). Pathogenetic mechanisms in bone marrow suppression from chloramphenicol and thiamphenicol. In Hibino, S. (Ed.), *Proceedings of the First International Symposium on Aplastic Anemia*. University Park Press, Tokyo, pp. 321–331

Yunis, A. A., Arimuru, G. K., Lutcher, C. L., Blasquez, J. and Halloran, M. (1967). Biochemical lesion in dilantin-induced erythroid aplasia. *Blood*, **30**, 587–600

Yunis, A. A., Miller, A. M., Salem, Z. and Arimura, G. K. (1980). Chloramphenicol toxicity: pathogenetic mechanisms and the role of pNo2 in aplastic anemia. *Clin. Toxicol.*, **17**, 359–373

Yunis, A. A. and Salem, Z. (1980). Drug-induced mitochondrial damage and sideroblastic change. *Clin. Haematol.*, **9**, 607–619

Zacharias, W., O'Connor, T. R. and Larson, J. E. (1988). Methylation of cytoxine in the 5-position alters the structural and energetic properties of the supercoil-induced Z-helix of B-Z junctions. *Biochemistry*, **27**, 2970–2978

Zimmerman, J., Selhub, J. and Rosenberg, H. (1986). Competitive inhibition of folic acid absorption in rat jejunum by triamterene. *J. Lab. Clin. Med.*, **108**, 272–276

FURTHER READING

Babior, B. M. and Stossel, T. P. (1994). *Hematology: A Pathophysiological Approach*. 3rd edn. Churchill Livingstone, Edinburgh

Irons, R. D. (1985). *Toxicology of the Blood and Bone Marrow*. Raven Press, New York

PART FIVE: SPECIAL TOXICOLOGY

35 Mutagenicity

D. J. Tweats

INTRODUCTION

It has been known for several hundred years that exposure to particular chemicals or complex mixtures can lead to cancer in later life (Doll, 1977), and it has been postulated more recently that chemicals can also induce heritable changes in man, leading to diseases in the next generation (review: ICPEMC, 1983). There has been accumulating evidence that such changes can arise following damage to DNA and resulting mutations (see, e.g., Bridges, 1976; Russell and Shelby, 1985). Therefore, it has become necessary to determine whether widely used chemicals or potentially useful new chemicals possess the ability to damage DNA. In industry such information may be used to discard a new chemical if a safer alternative can be found, to control or eliminate human exposure for a mutagenic industrial compound, or, for a drug, to proceed with development if benefits clearly outweigh risks. Data concerning the mutagenicity of a new chemical have become part of the basic toxicological information package. They are needed for decision-making and to reduce risks that might otherwise be unforeseen.

This chapter provides the background to the structure of DNA; DNA repair; the molecular nature of mutations; links between mutation and cancer; heritable diseases; *in vitro* tests; *in vivo* tests; and likely future developments. Other chapters of this volume are inextricably linked to this subject, including those on metabolism (3), cytogenetic tests (36), carcinogenesis (37), teratogenesis (40) and regulations (42).

DNA Structure

With the exception of certain viruses, the blueprint for all other organisms is contained in code by deoxyribonucleic acid (DNA), a giant macromolecule whose structure allows a vast amount of information to be stored accurately. We have all arisen from a single cell, the fertilized ovum containing two sets of DNA (packaged with pro-

tein to form chromatin), one set from our mother, resident in the nucleus of the unfertilized ovum, the second set from our father via the successful sperm. Every cell in the adult has arisen from this one cell and (with the exception of the germ cell and specialized liver cells) contains one copy of these original chromosome sets.

The genetic code is composed of four 'letters'—two pyrimidine nitrogenous bases, thymine and cytosine, and two purine bases, guanine and adenine—which can be regarded functionally as arranged in codons (or triplets). Each codon consists of a combination of three letters (Figure 1); therefore, 4^3 (64) different codons are possible. Sixty-one codons code for specific amino acids (three produce stop signals), and as only 20 different amino acids are used to make proteins, one amino acid can be specified by more than one codon (Table 1).

As shown in Figure 1, the bases on one strand are connected together by a sugar (deoxyribose) phosphate backbone. DNA can exist in a single-stranded or double-stranded form. In the latter state the two strands are held together by hydrogen bonds between the bases. Hydrogen bonds are weak electrostatic forces involving oxygen and nitrogen atoms. As a strict rule, one fundamental to mutagenesis, the adenine bases on one strand always hydrogen bond to the thymine bases on the sister strand. Similarly, guanine bases pair with cytosine bases. Adenine and thymine form two hydrogen bonds, and guanine and cytosine form three.

Double-stranded DNA has a unique property in that it is able to make identical copies of itself when supplied with precursors, relevant enzymes and cofactors. In simplified terms, two strands begin to unwind and separate as the hydrogen bonds are broken. This produces single-stranded regions. Complementary deoxyribonucleotide triphosphates then pair with the exposed bases under the control of a DNA polymerase enzyme.

A structural gene is a linear sequence of codons which codes for a functional polypeptide, i.e. a linear sequence of amino acids. Individual poly-

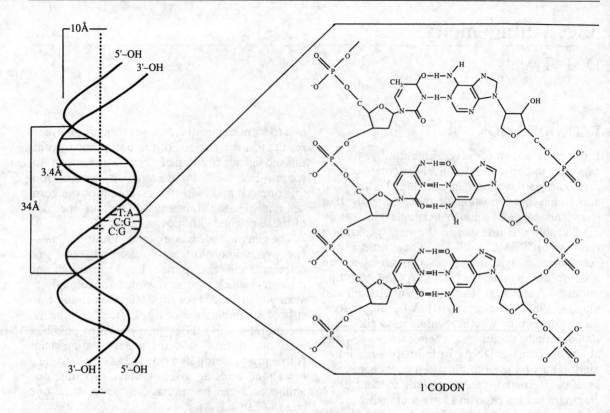

1 CODON

Figure 1   Structure of DNA. From Brusick (1987). Reproduced with permission

peptides may have a structural, enzymatic or regulatory role in the cell. Although the primary structure of DNA is the same in prokaryotes and eukaryotes, there are differences between the genes of these two types of organism, in internal structure, numbers and mechanism of replication. In bacteria there is a single chromosome, normally a closed circle, which is not complexed with protein, and replication does not require specialized cellular structures. In plant and animal cells there are many chromosomes, each present as two copies, as mentioned earlier, and the DNA is complexed with protein. Replication and cell division require the proteinaceous spindle apparatus. The DNA of eukaryotic cells contains repeated sequences of some genes. Also, eukaryotic genes, unlike prokaryotic genes, have non-coding DNA regions called introns between coding regions called exons. This property means that eukaryotic cells have to use an additional processing step at transcription.

Transcription

The relationship between the DNA in the nucleus and proteins in the cytoplasm is not direct. The information in the DNA molecule is transmitted to the protein-synthesizing machinery of the cell via another informational nucleic acid, called messenger RNA (mRNA), which is synthesized by an enzyme called RNA polymerase. Although similar to DNA, m-RNAs are single-stranded, and possess the base uracil instead of thymine and the sugar ribose rather than deoxyribose. These molecules act as short-lived copies of the genes being expressed.

In eukaryotic cells the initial mRNA copy contains homologues of both the intron and exon regions. The intron regions are then removed by enzymes located in the nucleus of the cell. Further enzymes splice the exon regions together to form the active mRNA molecules. In both groups of organisms mature mRNA molecules then pass out of the nucleus into the cytoplasm.

Table 1   Genetic code

UUU ⎫ phenylalanine UUC ⎭	UCU ⎫ UCC ⎬ serine UCA ⎪ UCG ⎭	UAU ⎫ tyrosine UAC ⎭	UGU ⎫ cysteine UGC ⎭
UUA ⎫ leucine UUG ⎭		UAA[a] ⎫ nonsense or UAG[b] ⎭ chain termination	UGA nonsense UGG tryptophan
CUU ⎫ CUC ⎪ leucine CUA ⎪ CUG ⎭	CCU ⎫ CCC ⎬ proline CCA ⎪ CCG ⎭	CAU ⎫ histidine CAC ⎭ CAA ⎫ glutamine CAG ⎭	CGU ⎫ CGC ⎬ arginine CGA ⎪ CGG ⎭
AUU ⎫ AUC ⎬ isoleucine AUA ⎭ AUG methionine	ACU ⎫ ACC ⎬ threonine ACA ⎪ ACG ⎭	AAU ⎫ asparagine AAC ⎭ AAA ⎫ lysine AAG ⎭	AGU ⎫ serine AGC ⎭ AGA ⎫ arginine AGG ⎭
GUU ⎫ GUC ⎪ valine GUA ⎪ GUG ⎭	GCU ⎫ GCC ⎬ alanine GCA ⎪ GCG ⎭	GAU ⎫ aspartic acid GAC ⎭ GAA ⎫ glutamic acid GAG ⎭	GGU ⎫ GGC ⎬ glycine GGA ⎪ GGG ⎭

[a] Also known as the ochre codon.
[b] Also known as the amber codon.

Translation

The next process is similar in both eukaryotes and prokaryotes, and involves the translation of mRNA molecules into polypeptides. This procedure involves many enzymes and two further types of RNA: transfer RNA (tRNA) and ribosomal RNA (rRNA). There is a specific tRNA for each of the amino acids. These molecules are involved in the transportation and coupling of amino acids into the resulting polypeptide. Each tRNA molecule has two binding sites, one for the specific amino acid, the other containing a triplet of bases (the 'anticodon') which is complementary to the appropriate codon on the mRNA.

rRNA is complexed with protein to form a subcellular globular organelle called a ribosome. Ribosomes can be regarded as the 'reading head' which allows the linear array of mRNA codons each to base-pair with an anticodon of an appropriate incoming tRNA/amino acid complex. The polypeptide chain forms as each tRNA/amino acid comes into register with the mRNA codon and with specific sites on the ribosome. A peptide bond is formed between each amino acid as it passes through the reading head of the ribosome (Venitt and Parry, 1984).

A summary of transcription and translation is shown in Figure 2.

Gene Regulation

Structural genes are regulated by a special set of codons, in particular 'promoter' sequences. The promoter sequence is the initial binding site for RNA polymerase before transcription begins. Different promoter sequences have different affinities for RNA polymerase. Some sets of structural genes with linked functions have a

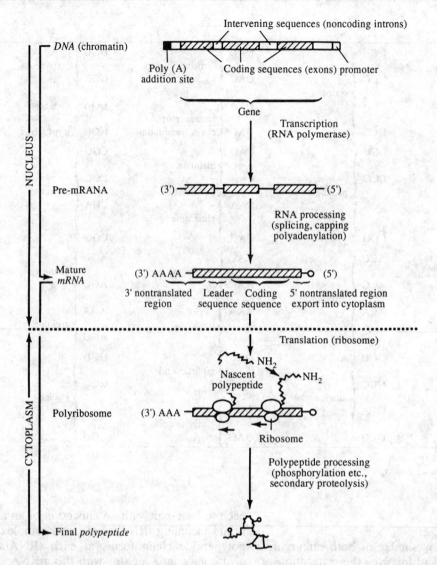

Figure 2 Transcription and translation (eukaryotic cells). From Brusick (1987). Reproduced with permission

single promoter and their co-ordinate expression is controlled by another regulatory gene called an operator. A group of such genes is called an operon. The activity of the operator is further controlled by a protein called a repressor, since it stops the expression of the whole operon by binding to the operator sequence, preventing RNA polymerase from binding to the promoter. Repressors can be removed by relevant chemical signals or in a time-related fashion.

In the ways described above only the genes required at a given moment are expressed. This not only helps to conserve the energy of the cell, but also is critical for correct cellular differen-

tiation, tissue pattern formation and formation of the body plan.

DNA Repair

All living cells appear to possess several different major DNA repair processes (reviews: Walker, 1984; Rossman and Klein, 1988). Such processes are needed to protect cells from the lethal and mutating effects of heat-induced DNA hydrolysis; ultraviolet light; ionizing radiation; DNA reactive chemicals; free radicals, etc. In single-celled eukaryotes such as the yeast *Saccharomyces cerevisiae*, the number of genes known to be involved in DNA repair approaches 100 (Friedberg, 1988). The number in mammalian cells is expected to be at least equal to this and emphasizes the importance of correction of DNA damage.

Some gene products appear to play an isolated role in DNA repair. For example, photoreactivating enzyme uses the energy from photons of visible light wavelengths to split cyclobutyl pyrimidine–pyrimidine dimers induced by ultraviolet (UV) irradiation (Sutherland, 1981). Another example is given by O^6-alkyl guanine-DNA transferase, which can remove the methyl group from O^6-methylguanine in the absence of light (Olsson and Lindahl, 1980).

Excision Repair

Some groups of enzymes (light-independent) are apparently organized to act co-operatively to recognize DNA lesions, remove them and correctly replace the damaged sections of DNA. The most comprehensively studied of these is the excision repair pathway. A diagram illustrating the *E. coli* excision repair pathway is shown in Figure 3 (Husain *et al.*, 1985).

Briefly the pathway can be described as follows:

(1) *Preincision reactions* UvrA protein dimers are formed which bind to the DNA at a location distant from the damaged site. The UvrB protein then binds to the DNA–UvrA complex to produce an energy-requiring topological unwinding of the DNA via DNA gyrase. This area of unwinding is then translocated, again using ATP as an energy source, to the site of the damaged DNA.

(2) *Incision reactions* The UvrC protein binds to the DNA–UvrA,B complex and incises the DNA at two sites—seven bases to the 5' end and three bases to the 3' end of the damage.

(3) *Excision reactions* UvrD protein and DNA polymerase 1 excise the damaged bases and then resynthesize the strand, using the sister strand as a template. The Uvr complex then breaks down, leaving a restored, but nicked, strand.

(4) *Ligation reaction* The nick in the phosphate backbone is repaired by DNA ligase.

A similar excision repair mechanism exists in mammalian cells (see, e.g., Cleaver, 1983). In both cases the process is regarded as error-free and does not lead to the generation of mutations. However, this pathway can become saturated with excessive numbers of damaged DNA sites, forcing the cell to fall back on other repair mechanisms.

Error-prone Repair

Exposure of *E. coli* to agents or conditions that either damage DNA or interfere with DNA replication results in the increased expression of the so-called 'SOS' regulatory network (review: Walker, 1984). Included in this network is a group of at least 17 unlinked DNA damage-inducible (*din*) genes. The *din* gene functions are repressed in undamaged cells by the product of the *lexA* gene (Little and Mount, 1982) and are induced when the LexA protein is cleaved by a process that requires modified RecA protein (RecA*), which then acts as a selective protease (Little, 1984). A diagram showing *din* gene activation is shown in Figure 4. The *din* genes code for a variety of functions, including filamentation, cessation of respiration, etc. Included are the *umuDC* gene products, which are required for so-called 'error-prone' or mutagenic DNA repair (Kato and Shinoura, 1977). The precise biochemical mechanism by which this repair is achieved is still not fully understood. Bacterial polymerase molecules have complex activities, including the ability to 'proof-read' DNA—i.e. to ensure that the base-pairing rules of double-stranded DNA are met. It is hypothesized that Umu proteins may suppress this proof-reading activity, so that base mismatches are tolerated (Villani *et al.*, 1978). Recent evidence suggests that DNA lesions are bypassed, and this bypass step required UmuDC proteins and RecA* protein (Bridges *et al.* 1987). The net result is that random base insertion occurs opposite the lesion which may result in mutation.

Analogues of the *umuDC* genes can be found in locations other than the bacterial chromosome—e.g. plasmid pKM101 (Walker and Dobson, 1979), a derivative of the drug resistance plasmid R46 (Mortelmans and Stocker, 1979), which carried *mucAB* genes (Shanabruch and Walker, 1980) (see pp. 815–816). Mutagenic repair, as controlled by *umuDC*, is not universal even among enterobacteria (Sedgwick and Goodwin, 1985). For instance, *Salmonella typhimurium* LT2 does not appear to express mutagenic repair

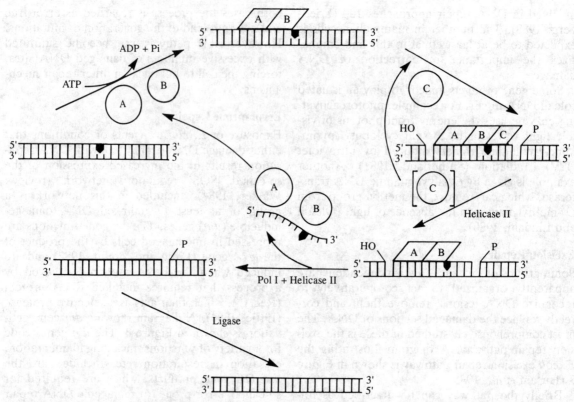

Figure 3   Bacterial excision repair. Redrawn from Husain *et al.* (1985). A, B, C refer to the gene products of the *Uvr*A, B, and C genes, respectively. Pol I = DNA polymerase I

(Walker, 1984). Thus, the usefulness of strains of this species is greatly enhanced by using derivatives containing plasmids with genes coding for error-prone repair (MacPhee, 1973; McCann *et al.*, 1975a,b). For further details see pp. 835–836.

RecA protein is also involved in the major pathway of post-replication repair (Smith and Meun, 1970), which reconstitutes double-stranded DNA containing gaps in one strand, opposite lesions on the other, by recombinational exchange (Rupp *et al.*, 1971). Unlike error-prone repair, post-replication repair is a widespread strategy for surviving DNA damage (Sedgwick and Goodwin, 1985).

With regard to error-prone repair in mammalian cells, understanding is fragmentary. No eukaryotic equivalent of the UmuDC protein is known and the contribution of proof-reading to the fidelity of DNA synthesis in eukaryotes is unclear. Rossman and Klein (1988) concluded that mammalian cells can tolerate DNA lesions by a mechanism that eventually leads to mutation fixation, but the processes by which this occurs

seem inherently different from those used by prokaryotes.

Mismatch Repair

Mispairs that break the normal base-pairing rules can arise spontaneously due to DNA biosynthetic errors, events associated with genetic recombination and the deamination of methylated cytosine (review: Modrich, 1987). With the latter, when cytosine deaminates to uracil, an endonuclease enzyme, *N*-uracil-DNA glycosylase (Lindahl, 1979), excises the uracil residue before it can pair with adenine at the next replication. However, 5-methyl cytosine deaminates to form thymine and will not be excised by a glycosylase. As a result, thymine exists on one strand paired with guanine on the sister strand, i.e. a mismatch. This will result in a spontaneous point mutation if left unrepaired. For this reason methylated cytosines form spontaneous mutation 'hot-spots' (review: Miller, 1985). The cell is able to repair mismatches by being able to distinguish between the

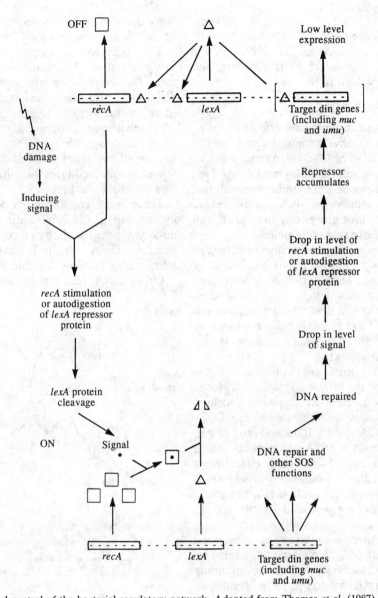

Figure 4 Induction and control of the bacterial regulatory network. Adapted from Thomas *et al.* (1987)

DNA strand that exists before replication and a newly synthesized strand.

The mechanism of strand-directed mismatch correction has been demonstrated in *E. coli* (see, e.g., Wagner and Meselson, 1976). In this organism adenine methylation of d(G–A–T–C) sequences determines the strand on which repair occurs. Thus, parental DNA is fully methylated, while newly synthesized DNA is undermethylated, for a period sufficient for mismatch correction. By this means the organism preserves the presumed correct sequence—i.e. that present on

the original DNA strand—and removes the aberrant base on the newly synthesized strand. Adenine methylation is achieved in *E. coli* by the *dam* methylase, which is dependent on *S*-adenosylmethionine. Mutants (*dam*) lacking this methylase are hypermutable, as would be expected by this model (Marinus and Morris, 1974).

Other 'mutator' genes have been implicated in the mismatch repair pathway, including *mut H*, *mut L* and *mut S* ('mut' for 'mutator'). It appears that the *mut H* product is involved in recognition of the –G–A–T–C– target sequences and possesses endonuclease activity (Modrich, 1987). The *uvrD* gene, which codes for DNA helicase II (catalyses the unwinding of double-stranded DNA), is also involved in this pathway.

The Adaptive Repair Pathway

The mutagenic and carcinogenic effects of alkylating agents such as ethyl methane sulphonate are due to the generation of O^6-alkylguanine residues in DNA, which result in point mutations (see next section). Bacterial and mammalian cells can repair a limited number of such lesions before DNA replication, thus preventing mutagenic and potentially lethal events taking place.

If *E. coli* are exposed to low concentrations of a simple alkylating agent, a repair mechanism is induced that causes increased resistance to subsequent challenge with a high dose. This adaptation response was first described by Samson and Cairns (1977) and has recently been reviewed by Lindahl *et al.* (1988). The repair pathway is particularly well understood.

The signal that provokes induction of the response is one of the minor alkylation products, an alkyl phosphotriester—i.e. a product formed in the sugar phosphate backbone of the DNA molecule (Teo *et al.*, 1986). Induced resistance to cell killing is due to a DNA glycosylase, which releases a spectrum of damaged bases from DNA—in particular, 3-methyladenine—which would otherwise block replication (Karran *et al.*, 1982). This glycosylase is coded by the *alk A*[+] gene.

Induced resistance to mutagenesis is ascribed to the reversion of O^6-alkylguanine to guanine by a transalkylation reaction in which the offending alkyl group is transferred to a cysteine residue of a protein called O^6-alkylguanine-DNA-alkyltransferase. This self-alkylation can only occur once and then the protein become inactivated. This seems costly to the cell, but underlines the importance of removal of these lesions. O^4-Alkyl thymine adducts are repaired in a similar fashion.

The adaptive response is regulated by the *ada* gene (Jeggo, 1979), which also codes for the alkyltransferase. Thus, the Ada protein has two functions—one regulatory, the other as a DNA repair enzyme (Lindahl *et al.*, 1988). Sequencing of the *ada* gene and the alkylated Ada protein has shown that the cysteine that accepts alkyl groups from O^6-alkylguanine is Cys-321, which is

the closest of the 12 cysteines to the C terminus of the 39 kD Ada protein (Demple *et al.*, 1985).

The Ada protein accepts a second alkyl group at Cys-69 in the *N*-terminal part of the Ada protein. This alkyl group is received from the alkylphosphotriester mentioned earlier and is involved in the induction of the adaptive response. The alkyltransferase protein, alkylated at Cys-69, binds to a specific sequence in the promoter regions of the genes induced during the adaptive response and facilitates the initiation of transcription, as shown in Figure 5.

There is no convincing evidence for a similar mechanism of inducible antimutagenic repair in eukaryotic cells, although a constitutive O^6-alkylguanine DNA alkyltransferase is present in human cells (review: Lindahl *et al.*, 1988).

Other DNA repair pathways exist in cells, as

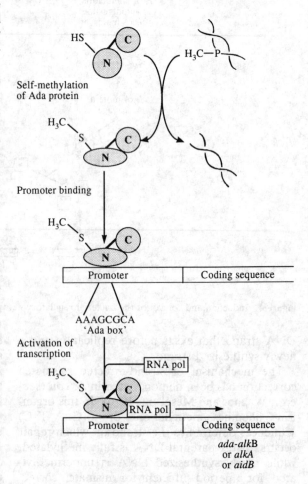

Figure 5 Induction of the *E. coli* adaptive response. Figure kindly provided by B. Sedgwick

described in the references cited in this section. Much still remains to be elucidated in mammalian cells concerning mechanisms and strategies of repair related to mutagenesis.

Plasmids

Plasmids are extrachromosomal genetic elements that are composed of circular double-stranded DNA. In bacteria some can mediate their own transfer from cell to cell by conjugation—i.e. they contain a set of *tra* genes coding for tube-like structures, such as pili, through which a copy of plasmid DNA can pass during transfer.

Plasmids range in size from 1.5 to 200 million daltons. The number of copies per cell differs from plasmid to plasmid. Copy number relates to control of replication and this correlates with size—i.e. small plasmids tend to have large copy numbers per cell. This may relate to a lack of replication control genes (Mortelmans and Dousman, 1986).

Plasmids carrying genes for antibiotic resistance (R factors) can have major clinical significance, as pathogenic strains can acquire resistance rapidly via this means.

Plasmids can be classified into groups (more than 20) according to their incompatibility. Plasmids belonging to the same incompatibility group cannot coexist stably in a single cell. Antibiotic resistance genes can be readily acquired by plasmids if they exist as transposable DNA sequences—i.e. discrete genetic elements which can move to new locations in the genome. These mobile genetic elements are called transposons (Hedges and Jacob, 1974). These possess inverted repeat DNA sequences at their outer ends. They occur in eukaryotes as well as prokaryotes, and much use of these genetic elements is made in genetic engineering techniques (for further information, see Kingsman *et al.*, 1988).

Plasmids and DNA Repair

Many plasmids are known to possess three properties: (1) increased resistance to the bactericidal effects of UV and chemical mutagens; (2) increased spontaneous mutagenesis; and (3) increased susceptibility to UV and chemically induced mutagenesis. Some plasmids possess all three properties; others may possess just one, e.g. increased susceptibility to mutagenesis (review: Mortelmans and Dousman, 1986). Often the pro-

file of activity depends on the DNA repair status of the host cell (Pinney, 1980). Plasmid pKM101 carries DNA repair genes and has been widely used in strains used in bacterial mutagenicity tests.

A genetic map of pKM101 is given in Figure 6. Plasmid pKM101 has lost a 13.8 kilobases fragment of plasmid R46, which carries genes coding for resistance to the antibiotics streptomycin, sulphonamides and tetracycline. This loss increases the safety of handling pKM101 strains relative to those carrying the parent plasmid R46. Both strains retain the gene coding for a β-lactamase resulting in ampicillin resistance. This latter marker is useful for checking for the presence of the plasmid.

R46 induces a tenfold increase in spontaneous mutation of mis-sense base change mutations in wild type strains, but does not affect the background of frameshift mutations. However, in strains that have lost excision repair (e.g. *uvrB⁻* strains) the plasmid also enhances the yield of frameshift mutations (Mortelmans and Stocker, 1976, 1979).

The activities described above are due to the presence of the *muc AB* (mutagenesis, UV and chemical) operon carried by the plasmid. These genes code for two proteins of molecular weight 16 k and 45 kD, respectively (Perry and Walker, 1982). The operon is flanked by inverted repeat DNA sequences, and thus it is likely that these

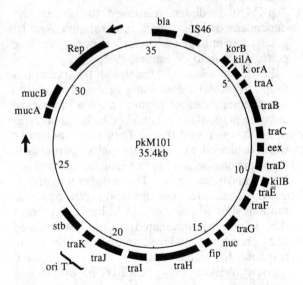

Figure 6 Genetic map of plasmid pKM101. Adapted from Walker (1986)

genes have been introduced into the plasmid DNA from the bacterial chromosome via a transposon (Langer *et al.*, 1981).

pKM101 restores DNA repair and mutagenesis to *E. coli umuC⁻* mutants, and thus *mucAB* are functional analogues of the *umuDC* genes (Walker and Dobson, 1979). It was therefore a surprise when comparisons of the nucleotide sequences of the two operons only showed 52 per cent homology (Perry *et al.*, 1985).

The search for a precise function of the *muc AB* genes has proved frustrating. Studies of the activity of R46 in *Salmonella typhimurium* and *E. coli* have shown that this plasmid protects excision repair defective strains but not those lacking *rec A* (Mortelmans and Stocker, 1976; Tweats *et al.*, 1976). Walker extended these findings, showing that the spontaneous and induced mutator effect was independent of functional excision repair and recombination repair controlled by *rec BC* and *rec L*, but was completely dependent on functional *rec A* and *lex A* genes (Walker, 1977). These findings show that *muc AB* gene products are involved in SOS error-prone repair (see pp. 811–812). Thus, the *muc AB* genes behave as if they are part of the SOS regulon. They contain two binding sites for the Lex A repressor protein (Walker, 1984) and are induced when the RecA protein, activated by DNA damage into its protease form, cleaves the Lex A repressor, allowing induction of the operon (Perry *et al.*, 1982; Little, 1984).

pKM101-mediated resistance to UV is also dependent on the *UvrE⁺* mutator and *Rec L⁺* genes, but mutagenesis is independent of these genes (Todd and Glickman, 1979).

Fowler *et al.* (1979) analysed the mutations found in pKM101-containing strains of *E. coli* to see whether different mechanisms account for the increase in spontaneous and UV-induced mutagenesis. It was found that in both cases mutations were enhanced at A:T base pairs, particularly transversions, which implies that the mechanism is the same in both cases. This is difficult to understand, as spontaneous mutation can occur at random sites whether or not lesions are present (i.e. it may be untargeted), while UV-induced and chemically induced mutations occur in response to specific lesions—i.e. are targeted (review: Walker, 1984). Clearly, no one simple explanation can reconcile these observations.

It is probable that, like the model of action for

UmuDC protein in error-prone repair, bases are inserted opposite non-coding lesions in a two stage process that required Umu DC or Muc AB proteins for the second lesion bypass stage (Bridges *et al.*, 1987). The end result is inhibition of proof-reading by DNA polymerase III, resulting in incorporation of incorrect (mutagenic) bases opposite the lesion. Thus, the products of *muc AB* genes may involve alteration in the function of the polymerase III–enzyme complex. In *E. coli* strains that contain both pKM101 and functional *umu DC⁺* genes both sets of proteins contribute to this function, which results in an increased extent of error-prone repair. In *Salmonella typhimurium* strains the presence of pKM101 installs a fully functioning error-prone repair system (Sedgwick and Goodwin, 1985; Little *et al.*, 1989).

Nature of Point Mutations

The word 'mutation' can be applied to point-mutations which are qualitative changes involving one or a few bases in base sequences within genes, as described below, as well as to larger changes involving whole chromosomes (and thus many thousands of genes), and even to changes in whole chromosome sets (as described in the next chapter).

Point mutations can occur when one base is substituted for another (base substitution). Substitution of another purine for a purine base or of another pyrimidine for pyrimidine is called a transition, while substitutions of purine for pyrimidine or pyrimidine for purine are called transversions (Figure 7A). Both types of base substitution have been identified within mutated genes. These changes lead to a codon change which can cause the 'wrong' amino acid to be inserted into the relevant polypeptide and are known as mis-sense mutations (Figure 7B). Such polypeptides may have dramatically altered properties if the new amino acid is close to the active centre of an enzyme or affects the three-dimensional make-up of an enzyme or a structural protein. These changes, in turn, can lead to change or reduction in function, which can be detected as a change in phenotype of the affected cells.

A base substitution can also result in the formation of a new inappropriate terminator (or non-sense) codon (see Table 1), and are thus known as non-sense mutations. The polypeptide formed

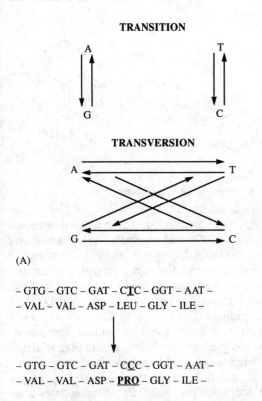

TRANSITION

TRANSVERSION

(A)

– GTG – GTC – GAT – C**T**C – GGT – AAT –
– VAL – VAL – ASP – LEU – GLY – ILE –

↓

– GTG – GTC – GAT – C**C**C – GGT – AAT –
– VAL – VAL – ASP – **PRO** – GLY – ILE –

i.e. a T – C transition results in a change from leucine to proline in the resulting polypeptide.

(B)

– GAC – ACC – G**CC** – **C**GG – CAG – GCC –CTG – AGC –
– ASP – THR – ALA – ARG – GLN – ALA – LEU – SER –

↓

– GAC – ACC – G**CC** – AGG – CCC –TGA –
– ASP – THR – ALA – **GLY** – **ARG** – **PRO** – **STOP**

i.e. deletion of one cytosine base results in a change in reading frame on the DNA which in turn generates a stop codon. The polypeptide produced from this mutated gene will be truncated.

(C)

Figure 7 Nature of DNA point-mutations. (A) Transitions and transversions; (B) mis-sense mutations; (C) frameshift mutations

from such mutated genes will be shorter than normal and is most likely to be inactive. Owing to the redundancy of the genetic code (see Table 1), about a quarter of all possible base substitutions will not result in an amino acid replacement and will be silent mutations.

Bases can be deleted or added to a gene. As each gene is of a precisely defined length, these changes, if they involve a number of bases that is not a multiple of 3, result in a change in the 'reading frame' of the DNA sequence and are thus known as frameshift mutations, as illustrated in Figure 7C. Such mutations tend to have a dramatic effect on the polypeptide of the affected gene, as most amino acids will differ from the point of the insertion or deletion of bases onwards. Very often a new terminator codon is produced, so, again, short inactive polypeptides will result.

Both types of mutation result in an altered polypeptide, which, in turn, can have a marked effect on the phenotype of the affected cell. Much use of phenotypic changes is made in mutagenicity tests.

Base substitutions and frameshift changes occur spontaneously, and can be induced by radiations and chemical mutagens. It is apparent that the molecular mechanisms resulting in these changes are different in each case, but the potential hazards associated with mutagens capable of inducing the different types of mutation are equivalent.

Suppressor Mutations

In some instances a mutation within one gene can be corrected by a second mutational event at a separate site on the chromosome. As a result, the first defect is suppressed and the second mutation is known as a suppressor mutation. Most suppressor mutations have been found to affect genes encoding for transfer RNAs. Usually the mutation causes a change in the sequence of the anticodon of the tRNA. Thus, if a new terminator or nonsense codon is formed as the first mutation, this can be suppressed by a second mutation forming a tRNA species that now has an anticodon complementary to a termination codon. Thus, the new tRNA species will supply an amino acid at the terminator site on the mRNA and allow translation to proceed. Surprisingly most suppressors of this type do not adversely affect cell growth, which implies that the cell can tolerate translation proceeding through termination signals, producing abnormal polypeptides. An alternative explanation is that the particular DNA sequences surrounding normal terminator codons result in a reduced efficiency of suppressor tRNAs (review: Bossi, 1985).

Frameshift suppression is also possible. This

can be achieved by a second mutation in a tRNA gene such that the anticodon of a tRNA molecule consists of 4 bases rather than 3—e.g. an extra C residue in the CCC anticodon sequence of a glycine tRNA gene. This change will allow correction of a +1 frameshift involving the GGG codon for glycine (Bossi, 1985).

Adduct Formation

The discussion of adaptive repair (pp. 814–815) made reference to the fact that some unrepaired alkylated bases are lethal, owing to interference with DNA replication, while others, such as O^6-methylguanine (Figure 8) lead to mutation if unrepaired. These differences indicate that not all DNA adducts (i.e. DNA bases with additional chemical groups, not associated with normal DNA physiology) are equivalent. In fact, some adducts appear not to interfere with normal DNA functions or are rapidly repaired, others are mutagenic and yet others are lethal. Chemicals that form electrophilic species readily form DNA adducts. These pieces of information are hardwon, and the reader is recommended to read reviews of the pioneering work of Brooks and Lawley (review: Lawley, 1989) summarizing work identifying the importance of DNA adduct formation with polycyclic hydrocarbons and the importance of 'minor' products of base alkylation such as O^6-methyl guanine, and, in addition, the work of the Millers in linking attack of nucleophilic sites in DNA by electrophiles to mutagenesis and carcinogenesis (Miller and Miller, 1971).

If a DNA adduct involves the nitrogen or oxygen atoms involved in base-pairing, and the adducted DNA is not repaired, base substitution can result. Adducts can be small, such as the simple addition of methyl or ethyl groups, or they can be very bulky, owing to reaction with multiringed structures, e.g. the metabolites of aflatoxin B_1 (Figure 9). The most vulnerable base is guan-

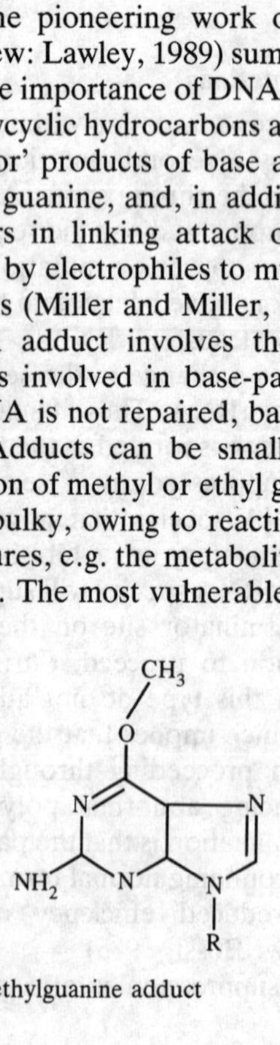

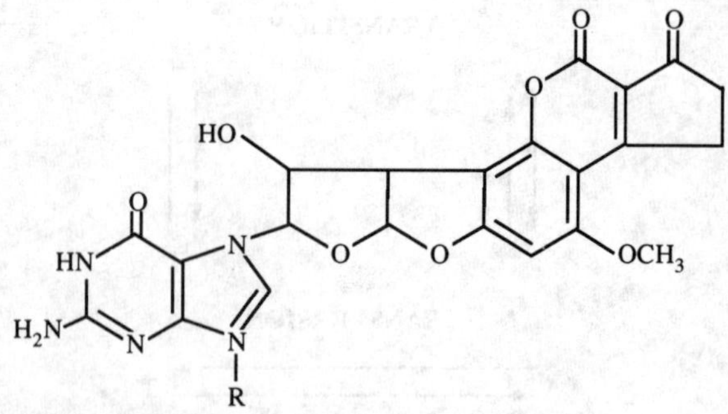

Figure 9 Aflatoxin B1-guanine adduct

ine, which can form adducts at several of its atoms (e.g. N^7, C^8, O^6 and exocyclic N^2) (Venitt and Parry, 1984). Adducts can form links between adjacent bases on the same strand (intrastrand cross-links) and can form interstrand cross-links between each strand of double-stranded DNA.

The induction of frameshift mutation does not necessarily require covalent adduct formation. Some compounds that have a flat, planar structure, such as particular polycyclic hydrocarbons, can intercalate between the DNA strands of the DNA duplex. The intercalated molecules may interfere with DNA repair enzymes or replication and cause additions and deletions of base-pairs. The precise mechanism is still unclear, although several mechanisms have been proposed. Hotspots for frameshift mutation often involve sections of DNA where there is a run of the same base—e.g. the addition of a guanine to a run of 6 guanine residues. Such information led to a 'slipped mispairing' model for frameshift mutation (Streisinger *et al.*, 1966; Roth, 1974). In this scheme single strand breaks allow one strand to slip and loop out one or more base-pairs, the configuration being stabilized by complementary base-pairing at the end of the single-stranded region. Subsequent resynthesis results ultimately in additions or deletions of base-pairs (Miller, 1985).

Particular DNA adducts can result in specific types of point mutation. This has been confirmed by the studies of Jeffrey Miller and others on mutational specificity, using model systems such as the *E. coli lacI* gene. Mutagenic carcinogens such as 4-nitroquinoline-1-oxide (4-NQO) and aflatoxin B_1 (AFB$_1$) are dependent on error-prone repair to generate viable mutants in bacteria (see pp. 811–812). However, each produces a specific pattern of base substitutions. Thus, 4-NQO

Figure 8 O^6 methylguanine adduct

induces mutations only at GC base-pairs and AFB$_1$ induces only GC-to-TA transversions. This provides evidence that most carcinogen-induced mutations are directly targeted (not untargeted as a result of SOS error-prone repair induction) and result from premutational lesions—i.e. adducts (review: Miller, 1985). Miller argues that the specificity of AFB$_1$ results from the following sequence: adduct formation on guanine residues; depurination (which is mutagenic if SOS error-prone repair is induced); bypass of the lesion; followed by preferential adenine incorporation. The net result is GC-to-TA transversion.

Mutations Due to Insertion Sequences

The subject of mutations due to insertion sequences is reviewed in Cullum (1985). Studies of spontaneous mutation in *E. coli* detected a special class of mutations that were strongly polar, reducing the expression of downstream genes (Jordan *et al.*, 1967). These genes mapped as point mutations and reverted like typical point-mutations. However, unlike point-mutations, mutagens did not increase their reversion frequency. Further studies showed that these mutations were due to extra pieces of DNA that can be inserted into various places in the genome. They are not just random pieces of DNA but are 'insertion sequences' 0.7–1.5 kilobases long that can 'jump' into other DNA sequences. They are related to transposons (see p. 815), which are insertion sequences carrying easily detected markers such as antibiotic resistance genes, and Mu phages (bacterial viruses).

The Link between Mutation and Cancer

The change in cells undergoing normal, controlled cell division and differentiation to cells that are transformed, dividing without check, and are undifferentiated or abnormally differentiated, does not appear to occur as a single step—i.e. transformation is multistage. Evidence for this comes from *in vitro* studies, animal models and clinical observations—in particular, the long latent period between exposure to a carcinogen and the appearance of a tumour in the target tissue. There is much evidence for the sequence of events shown in Figure 10—i.e. tumour initiation, promotion, malignant conversion and progression, as summarized by Harris *et al.* (1987). Such a scheme provides a useful working

model but does not necessarily apply to all 'carcinogens' in all circumstances (see Chapters 37 and 38).

Study of Figure 10 shows that there are several points where genetic change appears to play a role. Such change may occur spontaneously, due to rare errors at cell division such as misreplication of DNA or spindle malfunction, or may be induced by exposure to viruses (e.g. acute transforming retroviruses), ionizing and non-ionizing radiations absorbed by DNA (e.g. X-rays; UVC) or particular chemical species capable of covalently interacting with DNA (as discussed earlier) or with vital proteins, such as tubulin, that polymerize to form the cell division spindle apparatus.

Proto-oncogenes as Genetic Targets

Why should DNA damage be inextricably linked to cancer? The answer to this question has become clear during the last 10 years with the study of oncogenes (Bishop, 1987).

In the cancerous state, control of normal growth and differentiation of cells is abnormal. Cancer cells continue to live longer than normal cells, they often abandon normal pattern formation characteristic of organized tissues and they do not maintain the non-dividing status of terminally differentiated cells. It is now appreciated that normal control of these functions lies with a small set of genes termed proto-oncogenes. Abnormal 'activation' of these genes can result in a change in cell behaviour important in the transformation of normal cells to neoplastic cells. In their activated state these genes are known as oncogenes.

Oncogenes were originally discovered in the genome of acute transforming retroviruses (review: Bishop, 1985) and are known in this form as v-oncogenes. Subsequent studies have shown that proto-oncogenes are highly conserved in evolution and can be detected through a range from yeast to human cells. They are expressed during regulated growth, such as embryogenesis, regeneration of damaged tissues and stimulation of cell division by growth factors (Stowers *et al.*, 1987). Activation of cellular proto-oncogenes into c-oncogenes in spontaneous and chemically induced tumours has been extensively studied in recent years.

A variety of mechanisms have been described in which particular proto-oncogenes have become

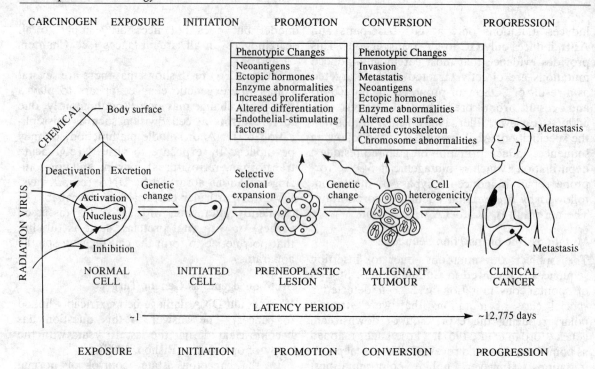

Figure 10　Events leading to neoplasia. From Harris *et al.* (1987). Reproduced with permission and redrawn

activated to form c-oncogenes, as shown in Figure 11. All of these mechanisms involve changes in DNA or in gene position or in gene number. Point mutation falls into the first category; it is of particular relevance to this chapter and is discussed more fully below.

Activation of Proto-oncogenes via Point Mutation

The discovery of the activation of an oncogene by point-mutation has been neatly summarized by Robertson (1983). If the expression of viral oncogenes is compared with that from proto-

c-myc c-abl	Chromosomal translocation →	lg/myc bcr/abl	Murine plasmacytoma Human Burkitt's lymphoma CML
N-myc c-myc c-Ki-ras	Gene amplication →	DM/HSR	Neuroblastoma Small cell lung carcinoma Adrenocortical tumor of mice
c-Ha-ras c-Ki-ras c-N-ras	Point mutation →	12th, 13th, 61st codon mutation	Colon carcinoma Lung carcinoma AML Chemical induced rodent tumors
myc myb erb mos int-1 int-2	Promoter/enhancer insertion →	LTR/c-onc LTR/common Domain	Chronic, non-transforming leukemia virus

Figure 11　Mechanisms of proto-oncogene activation. Adapted from Stowers *et al.* (1987)

oncogenes, the viral genes are grossly 'over-expressed', as these genes have come under the control of powerful viral regulatory elements (LTRs: long terminal repeats). This led to a dosage hypothesis of oncogenesis—i.e. too much of a good thing.

Weinberg and colleagues and Barbacid's group (Reddy *et al.*, 1982; Tabin *et al.*, 1982) analysed the DNA sequence on an oncogene from the EJ human bladder carcinoma cell line, expecting to confirm the dosage hypothesis (i.e. a mutation outside the protein coding sequence of the gene) affecting the regulatory region and enhancing transcription and yield of protein. What they found was a single mutation in the protein coding sequence of the gene, resulting in the substitution of a thymine base for a guanine, with the consequence that valine is incorporated into the protein concerned (called p21) in place of glycine, at the relevant position in the polypeptide. Such a change is likely to change the conformation of the protein, as glycine is the only amino acid without a side chain. Thus, valine is bulkier, and possibly such a change could alter the substrate specificity of the protein. The net result could be increased enzyme activity, as in the case of the gene dosage effect.

The relevant gene in the bladder cancer line is the Harvey-*ras* or H-*ras* oncogene, a member of the *ras* gene family. There are three main members: K-*ras* (K for Kirsten), N-*ras* (N for neuroblastoma) and H-*ras*. The v-oncogene equivalents for H-*ras* and K-*ras* were originally identified in the Harvey and Kirsten murine sarcoma viruses. An equivalent viral analogue of N-*ras* has not yet been identified. In humans these three genes are on three separate chromosomes (11 for H-*ras*, 1 for N-*ras* and 12 for K-*ras*). Each codes for a protein of 21 kD of very similar amino acid sequence (review: Bos, 1988).

It has been found that a substantial number of human tumours (10–15 per cent) contain activated *ras* oncogenes (Barbacid, 1986). It is intriguing that, in all cases so far examined, activation depends on a point-mutation in either codon 12, 13 or 61 of one of the *ras* proto-oncogenes (Table 2), although mutations at other codons have been detected in mutagenized *ras* genes found to be transforming in NIH/3T3 cells *in vitro* (review: Bos, 1988). The p21 protein coded by *ras* genes possesses GTPase activity and is membrane-bound. Mutations at codon 12 will

Table 2 Transforming *ras* genes. From Bos *et al.* (1988)

Gene	Codon	Mutation	Amino acid change
H-*ras*	12	GGC–GTC	gly–val
		GGC–GAC	gly–asp
	61	CAG–AAG	glu–lys
		CAG–CGG	glu–arg
K-*ras*	12	GGT–CGT	gly–arg
		GGT–AGT	gly–ser
		GGT–TGT	gly–cys
		GGT–GAT	gly–asp
		GGT–GTT	gly–val
	13	GGC–GAC	gly–asp
	61	CAA–CAT	glu–his
N-*ras*	12	GGT–AGT	gly–ser
		GGT–GTT	gly–val
		GGT–GAT	gly–asp
	13	GGT–CGT	gly–arg
		GGT–GTT	gly–val
		GGT–GAT	gly–asp

affect the interaction of protein with bound nucleotide or with magnesium and water molecules in the nucleotide binding site. Activating mutations at codons 61 will affect GTP hydrolysis (Burck *et al.*, 1988). The true function of p21 is unknown, but the protein is known to be bound to the inner surface of the plasma membrane. It is suggested that it may have a function in transducing signals from growth factor receptors across the cytoplasm, eventually to the nucleus (see, e.g., Fleischman *et al.*, 1986).

The study of rodent tumours induced by chemical carcinogens has underlined the importance of *ras* genes as vital targets. Point-mutations resulting in activation of *ras* proto-oncogenes in several chemically induced rodent tumours have been described. Barbacid and colleagues have found activated H-*ras* (mutation in codon 12) in the majority of mammary tumours induced by nitroso-methylurea (NMU) (Sukumar *et al.*, 1983). Similarly, activation of H-*ras* (codon 61) is detected in mammary and skin tumours induced by 7,12-dimethylbenz[*a*]anthracene (DMBA) (Quintanilla *et al.*, 1986).

Nitrosomethylurea is an alkylating agent known to induce the formation of O^6-methylguanine in DNA. Such a lesion is consistent with the type of point-mutation (G→A transition) observed at the 12th codon of H-*ras* (Zarbl *et al.*, 1985). The mutation at codon 61 in DMBA-induced tumour cells (mainly A→T transversion) is consistent with the formation of adenine adducts, resulting from DMBA metabolites binding to adenine residues (Quintanilla *et al.*, 1986).

Ras oncogenes are not the only oncogenes that have been demonstrated to be activated by point-mutation—e.g. mutations in the *neu* oncogene have been reported in tumour cells induced by *N*-ethyl-*N*-nitrosourea (Bargmann *et al.*, 1986). However, they do seem to be in the majority. There is a striking correlation between the tissue type affected and the *ras* oncogene activated. Epithelial tumours (skin, breast, liver) tend to have activated H-*ras*, while mesenchymal tumours (lymphomas, fibrosarcomas, renal mesenchyme) have either K-*ras* or N-*ras* activated (Guerrero and Pellicer, 1987).

The number of proto-oncogenes that must be activated in order to convert a normal cell into one that is tumorigenic is unknown at present. Single retroviral oncogenes can induce a rapid onset of neoplasia, while their cellular analogues are involved in a slowly developing multistage disease. The reasons for this difference appear to lie in the regulation of these genes in their different locations. As mentioned earlier, viral genes are driven by powerful regulatory elements, retroviral LTRs, and they can be delivered to a large number of cellular targets, some of which may be undergoing critical stages of growth or differentiation. In contrast, cellular oncogenes are driven by promoters of low-to-moderate strength and can only be involved in the neoplastic process in those cells in which they become activated (Barbacid, 1986). There is evidence that several oncogenes may co-operate to achieve the neoplastic state (Schwartz and Witte, 1988)— usually one connected with the membrane/cytoplasm with one acting as the nucleus.

The evidence that cellular oncogenes have a causative role in neoplasia is compelling. However, several authors inject a note of caution about the oncogene concept. Oncogenes remain to be identified in 75 per cent of human cancers. In the experimental systems where oncogenes have been identified, no evidence that the altered gene had any role in the carcinogenic process has been provided; carcinogenesis appears to result in a combination of genetic and epigenetic alterations affecting the capacity of the cell to overcome its normal proliferative restraints and to escape immunosurveillance. (Barbacid, 1986; Farber, 1987).

Evidence that oncogenes are not the only genes involved in neoplasia has come from the study of heritable cancers and the discovery of 'tumour suppressor' genes.

Tumour Suppressor Genes

Oncogenes act in a dominant manner—i.e. if one copy becomes 'activated', its host cell has taken a step in the neoplastic process. The expression of tumour suppressor genes appears to inhibit neoplastic transformation. However, only one active gene is necessary for suppression; thus, both copies need to be lost or inactivated before the cell becomes neoplastic.

Retinoblastoma is a childhood cancer of the eye (frequency 1 per 20 000 births). Neoplastic cells arise in the fetal retinal layer and about 40 per cent of cases are hereditary. The hereditary disease presents early in life, it often involves both eyes and patients have a high risk of tumours elsewhere, such as in the bone, as they grow older. The sporadic form usually appears later in life and is localized in one eye, and there is not an increased risk of tumours elsewhere. It appears that the normal function of the gene involved (*rb*) is in differentiation of the visual apparatus.

In the hereditary form it can be shown in some cases that peripheral lymphocytes and other cells have lost part of chromosome 13 resulting from a germ line clastogenic (chromosome breakage) event. In sporadic cases only the cells of the tumour have an abnormal pair of chromosomes 13.

These data have been explained by Knudson (review, 1985). Two hits are needed to express the tumour. In the hereditary form the first hit is inherited as the chromosome 13 deletion in all cells. The second occurs randomly in susceptible retinal cells. Because cells in both retinas already carry the first mutation, the risk of tumour formation is equal and high for both eyes. In the sporadic form two chance mutations must occur within the same retinoblast. Because either mutation alone is unlikely, there is a low probability that both events will occur simultaneously in the same cell.

Cavenee and colleagues (1983) have investigated the genetic changes found in retinoblastoma cells. Their findings are summarized in Figure 12. They have found gene loss due to point mutation; gene conversion; chromosome deletion; mitotic recombination; whole chromo-

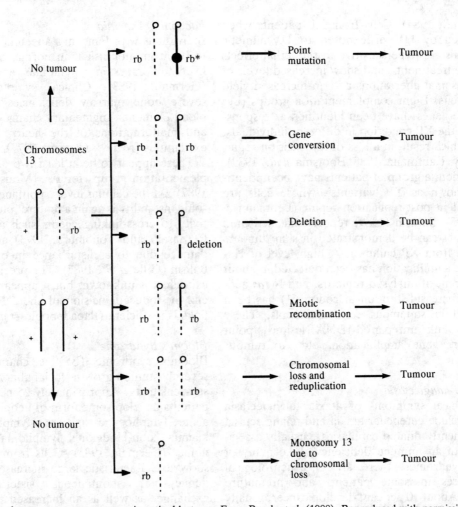

Figure 12 Loss of tumour suppressor genes in retinoblastoma. From Burck *et al.* (1988). Reproduced with permission

some loss and reduplication of the abnormal chromosome; and loss due to aneuploidy.

Wilms' tumour (nephroblastoma), a childhood renal cancer, gives a very similar molecular picture to that seen with retinoblastoma and also results from loss or inactivation of a suppressor gene on chromosome 11 (Koufos *et al.*, 1984; review: Knudson, 1985).

Other tumours that appear to result from deletion or inactivation of suppressor genes include familial adenomatous polyposis (chromosome 5: Bodmer *et al.*, 1987); small-cell lung cancer (chromosome 3: Naylor *et al.*, 1987); colorectal carcinomas (chromosome 5: Solomon *et al.*, 1987); and renal cell carcinoma (chromosome 3: Zbar *et al.*, 1987).

Tumours such as Wilms' and retinoblastoma are heritable conditions resulting in tumours in child-hood. There are other cancer-prone conditions that provide further evidence for the role of DNA changes in cancer induction. These are rare syndromes associated with defects in DNA repair.

Human DNA Repair Deficiency Syndromes

Xeroderma Pigmentosum

Defective DNA repair has been implicated in a variety of genetic disorders (Arlett and Lehmann, 1978). Perhaps the best-studied is xeroderma pigmentosum (XP). Almost all XP patients eventually develop benign and malignant skin tumours (e.g. fibromas, malignant melanomas, basal and squamous cell carcinomas, etc.), particularly if exposed to mild doses of UV (review: Cleaver, 1983). An increased frequency of tumours in unexposed tissues has also been suggested (Kraemer *et al.*, 1984). Cells from XP patients when irradiated by UV or exposed to UV-mimetic chemicals are hypersensitive to the lethal effects of these treatments, and show increased levels of chromosomal aberrations and an increased yield of mutants. Eight complementation groups (i.e. separate genes) have been identified as responsible for the XP condition in different individuals, all of which result in a loss of the excision repair pathway (Kaufmann, 1988; Bootsma *et al.*, 1989). In addition, a group of patients have been identified, known as XP 'variants', whose cells are deficient in post-replication repair (Lehmann *et al.*, 1975). Sarasin (1989) reports that activated oncogenes can be demonstrated in skin tumours isolated from XP children. A high level of Ha-*ras* gene amplification has been detected in about 40 per cent of analysed tumours, and N-*ras* activation (base substitution at codon 61) has been detected in squamous cell carcinomas. These findings link unrepaired DNA lesions, point mutation, gene amplification, etc., to tumour initiation.

Ataxia Telangiectasia

The clinical symptoms of ataxia telangiectasia (AT) include cerebellar ataxia and telangiectasia (permanently dilated capillaries), usually associated with an immune deficiency. Like many of these syndromes, there are also neurological deficiences in some patients and premature ageing. About 10 per cent develop cancer, usually of the lymphoid system (Spector *et al.*, 1982). The cells of AT patients are extremely sensitive to ionizing radiation and to chemicals capable of inducing DNA strand breaks. Indeed, several patients have died as a consequence of exposure to conventional doses of radiotherapy. Cells from AT patients also have spontaneous chromosome instability (review: Heim *et al.*, 1989). The nature of the biochemical deficiency in these cells is not known. However, it appears that DNA synthesis is much more resistant to ionizing radiation than normal, as a result of losing a signal that inhibits DNA synthesis on a damaged DNA template (Painter, 1981). The net result is anomalous processing of DNA lesions. Many AT patients show a stable clonal translocation involving chromosomes 7 and 14 (McKinnon, 1987). However, it is apparent that there are many variants of the disease, indicating genetic and phenotypic heterogeneity (Ziv *et al.*, 1989).

Fanconi's Anaemia

Individuals with Fanconi's anaemia (FA) appear to be at greater risk than normal of developing liver tumors, skin carcinomas and leukaemia (German, 1983). Clinical symptoms include severe bone marrow deficiencies affecting all blood elements, pigmentary changes in the skin, and malformations of the heart, kidneys and extremities (review: Cleaver, 1977).

There appear to be at least two different complementation groups for FA (Moustacchi *et al.*, 1987). At the cellular level, spontaneous chromosome instability is again a feature, plus high sensitivity to cross-linking agents such as mitomycin C (Sasaki and Tonomura, 1973) and oxidative damage due to a disturbance in oxygen metabolism (Gille *et al.*, 1987). The precise biochemical defect is unknown, but it appears that repair enzyme-induced incision of the DNA at crosslinks is inefficient (Papadopoulo *et al.*, 1987).

Bloom's Syndrome

Bloom's syndrome (BS) is characterized by severely stunted growth, facial abnormalities and sun-sensitivity. Approximately 25 per cent of BS patients develop some form of neoplasia, such as acute lymphocytic and non-lymphocytic leukaemia, non-Hodgkin's lymphoma and carcinomas (German, 1983). Cells from BS patients show a characteristic large increase in the frequency of spontaneous sister chromatid exchange, as well as an increased frequency of chromosome breakage (Changanti *et al.*, 1974). It appears that BS results from a mutation in the gene coding for DNA ligase I (review: Lindahl, 1987), which is the main ligase active during DNA replication.

Other Syndromes

Cockayne's syndrome (CS) results in dwarfism, premature senility, retinal pigment degeneration, optic atrophy, deafness, mental retardation and sensitivity to sunlight. Cells from these individuals have normal sensitivity to X-rays but increased sensitivity to UV, which suggests a DNA repair defect (Schmickel *et al.*, 1977). Repair of UV-induced pyrimidine dimers in actively transcribing regions of DNA occurs rapidly. CS cells are specifically deficient in this repair process (Mayne *et al*, 1988).

Patients with Gardner's syndrome develop polyposis, and cancer of the colon and rectum, as well as osteomas and multiple soft-tissue tumours. Fibroblasts from these patients are hypersensitive to UV, X-rays and mitomycin C, which suggests a defect having pleiotropic effects on DNA repair (Little and Nagasawa, 1980). However, further studies have failed to detect any measurable defect in the repair of UV-induced damage (Henson *et al.*, 1983).

Patients with Chediak–Higashi syndrome are sun-sensitive; lymphoblastoid cell lines from these patients are hypersensitive to UV light and the syndrome is frequently accompanied by malignancy (Tanaka and Orri, 1980). However, the cells from these patients exhibit normal levels of unscheduled (excision repair) DNA synthesis after UV irradiation and may thus possess normal excision repair of UV-induced damage.

The overwhelming impression of DNA repair deficiencies in humans is that such deficiencies lead to cancer proneness and serves to underline the centrality of DNA damage to carcinogenesis. However, consideration of Gardner's and Chediak–Higashi syndromes (above) suggests that DNA damage may not be the whole story.

Trichothiodystrophy (TTD) is an autosomal recessive disorder characterized by sulphur-deficient brittle hair. In addition, ichthyosis (scaling of skin), unusual facial appearance and mental and physical retardation are also observed (see, e.g., Price *et al.*, 1980). Severe photosensitivity has been reported for about half of the patients studied. Skin cancer has not been reported for any patient with TTD. Cells from TTD patients show a heterogeneity in the biochemistry of the cellular defects: some have deficiency in excision repair of UV damage and appear to be very similar to XP (complementation group D), while others (without photosensitivity) have no defects in excision repair (review: Lehmann *et al.*, 1988). These authors point out that the findings with TTD challenge the dogma that a defect in excision repair is the underlying cause of cancer in, for example, XP patients. It is possible that the tumours that do arise in XP may result from a combination of an enhanced frequency of somatic mutations *plus* a possible depression of the immune response following solar exposure of XP patients (Bridges, 1981). It is hypothesized that TTD and XP-D represent different defects in the same gene, with diverse clinical symptoms the result (Lehmann *et al.*, 1988).

Genotoxic versus Non-genotoxic Mechanisms of Carcinogenesis

The previous discussions of oncogene activation and human DNA repair deficiencies provide strong evidence for carcinogenesis via genotoxic mechanisms. However, it has been recognized for many years that cancers can arise without biologically significant direct or indirect interaction between a chemical and cellular DNA (see, e.g., Gatehouse *et al.*, 1988). The distinction between non-genotoxic and genotoxic carcinogens has recently been brought into a sharper focus following the identification of a comparatively large number of 'non-genotoxic' carcinogens by the United States National Toxicology Program (Tennant *et al.*, 1987). These include a wide range of chemicals acting via a variety of mechanisms, including augmentation of high 'spontaneous' tumour yields; disruption of normal hormonal homeostasis in hormone-responsive tissues; peroxisome proliferation; proliferation of urothelial cells following damage via induced kidney stones; etc. (Clayson, 1989). This author points out that a major effort is under way to determine whether many of these compounds can elicit similar effects in humans.

Ashby and Tennant (1988) and Ashby *et al.* (1989) stress the significance of their observations that 16 tissues are apparently sensitive to genotoxic carcinogens, while a further 13 tissues are sensitive to both genotoxic and non-genotoxic carcinogens (Table 3). Also, genotoxic carcinogens tend to induce tumours in several tissues of both males and females in both rats and mice. This contrasts with non-genotoxic carcinogens, which may induce tumours at high doses, in one tissue, of one sex, of one species. Although it is most unlikely that all non-genotoxic carcinogens will prove to be irrelevant in terms of human risk, it appears from the analysis above that a proportion of carcinogens identified by the use of near-toxic levels in rodent bioassays are of dubious relevance to the induction of human cancer. For further discussion, see Butterworth and Slaga (1987).

Genetic Damage and Heritable Defects

Concern about the effects of radiations and chemicals on the human gene pool, and the resulting heritable malformations and syndromes,

Table 3 Tissues sensitive to genotoxic and/or non-genotoxic carcinogens

Tissues sensitive primarily to genotoxins	Tissues sensitive to both genotoxins and non-genotoxins
Stomach	Nose
Zymbal gland	Mammary gland
Lung	Pituitary gland
Subcutaneous tissue	Integumentary system
Circulatory system	Kidney
Clitoral gland	Urinary bladder
Skin	Liver
Intestine/colon	Thyroid gland
Uterus	Hematopoietic system
Spleen	Adrenal gland
Tunica vaginalis	Pancreas
Bile duct	Seminal vesicle
Ovary	Urinary tract
Haderian gland	Lymphatic system
Preputial gland	
[Multiple organ sites]	

has steadily risen during this century. The recognition that changes in morphology would result from changes in the hereditary material due to mutations (from the Latin word *mutare*, to change), was adopted by de Vries following observations on the evening primrose, *Oenothera* (de Vries, 1901). Muller went on to demonstrate that X-rays could induce mutations in the germ cells of the fruit fly *Drosophila melanogaster* (Muller, 1927).

Prior to World War II, the only mutagen known was radiation, and thus it was thought that the mutation process required a high activation energy that could only be provided by radiation (Crow, 1989). This attitude changed with the discovery by Auerbach and Robson in the early 1940s that mustard gas was also a potent mutagen for germ cells (Auerbach and Robson, 1946). The discovery of other chemical mutagens soon followed (e.g. urethane, ethylene oxide, epichlorohydrin, etc.) (review: Wassom, 1989). Due to wartime restrictions the work on mustard gas was not published until after the war. The first published report of a chemical mutagen was for allyl-

isothiocyanate from mustard oil (Auerbach and Robson, 1944).

The realization that exposure to particular man-made chemicals and exposure to radiations, particularly following the use of atomic bombs at Hiroshima and Nagasaki (and subsequent nuclear weapon testing above ground), could result in increases in heritable defects in human children led to calls for controls of known hazards and the identification and control of new hazards. Another factor was the impact of drugs, particularly antibiotics, in reducing infant mortality and disease. Thus, the relative contribution made by heritable diseases has increased dramatically in the latter half of the century.

The human gene pool is known to carry many deleterious genes acquired from preceding generations which result in numerous genetic diseases. It is clear that these arise as a result of DNA changes affecting particular chromosomes or genes. They can be grouped as follows:

(1) Chromosome abnormalities, small changes in either number or structure (see Chapter 36).

(2) Autosomal dominant gene mutations, in which a change in only one copy of the pair of genes is sufficient for the condition to be expressed.

(3) Autosomal recessive gene mutations in which both copies of a gene must be mutated for the trait to become manifest.

(4) Sex-linked conditions, which may also be recessive or dominant, where the mutant gene is on an X chromosome and will be expressed at high frequency in males (XY) and at a much lower frequency in females (XX), if the gene acts in a recessive manner.

(5) Polygenic mutations, in which the condition results from the interaction of several genes and may include an environmental component.

Each type of inherited defect is discussed in more detail below, along with the impact each has on the human population.

Autosomal Dominant Mutations

McKusick (1988) describes 1443 human autosomal dominant conditions, with many more listed as probable. Monogenic familial hypercholesterolaemia has a frequency of approximately 2.0 per 1000 live births and is a typical example (Heiberg and Berg, 1976). These patients have abnormally high serum cholesterol levels, which increases the risk of coronary heart disease. Homozygotes usually die from cardiac infarction in the third decade of their lives, while about 50 per cent of heterozygotes die of ischaemic heart disease before the age of 60.

Dominant conditions have a special place in the monitoring of human mutagenesis. The relationship between mutations and birth frequency for such conditions is relatively direct. Any increase in the mutation rate will be reflected in the following generation in an increased birth frequency of children with the condition, born to normal parents (Carter, 1977). Dominant mutations that are not lethal contribute moderately to the total genetic load. Genetic counselling is clear-cut in that affected individuals have a 50 per cent probability of transmitting the trait to their children.

Particular dominant conditions are monitored in populations and are regarded as 'sentinel anomalies' to give an early warning of the impact of induced mutations caused by chemicals or radiations (see, e.g., Czeizel, 1989). Such studies have revealed some surprising findings. To date, no germinal mutagenic effects of chemicals have been documented in humans, including children born to people exposed to very large doses of mutagenic drugs, pesticides, etc., or following self-poisoning (Czeizel, 1986). In addition, large-scale studies of the offspring of survivors exposed to ionizing radiation at Hiroshima and Nagasaki have been essentially negative (Sankaranarayanan, 1988). This contrasts markedly with the identification of human mutagenic carcinogens (see above).

Autosomal Recessive Mutations

McKusick (1988) lists 626 confirmed and a similar number of suspected human conditions that are due to autosomal recessive mutations. A very well studied example is fibrocystic disease of the pancreas (cystic fibrosis). This is a generalized disorder of the mucus-secreting glands of the lungs, pancreas, mouth and gastrointestinal tract, as well as the sweat glands. The latter tend to secrete sweat with a higher concentration of ions than normal. Mucus is more viscous than normal, and as a result dried-up secretions block the glands and their ducts, so that they atrophy and become replaced by scar tissue.

The disease has a high frequency, with an inci-

dence of 1 in 2000 live births in Caucasian populations, and accounts for 1–2 per cent of admissions to children's hospitals. In affected individuals it appears that the channel that transports chloride in and out of epithelial cells is disrupted—in particular, the 'gate' which opens and closes the channel (Frizzell *et al.*, 1987). Because of this defect, chloride is trapped within the cell and excess sodium is absorbed. It is now known that the gene responsible codes for a protein in the membrane of epithelial cells involved in this 'gating' process (Riordan *et al.*, 1989).

Syndromes due to recessive genes are normally rare, because the disease is only expressed when in homozygous form. Thus, normally both parents are heterozygous carriers and do not express the disease. The prevalence of the condition thus depends on the frequency of carriers in any one population.

With regard to the induction of new mutations due to increasing exposure to germ cell mutagens, it may be expected that recessive genes may accumulate in a human population as a result of such exposure. However, this could be masked for many generations until the frequency had risen to such an extent that heterozygotes were relatively common. Then the increased likelihood of the heterozygotes carrying the same recessive gene producing homozygous children would become noticeable via birth statistics. Tracing this back to the causative agent would be almost impossible.

Sex-linked Conditions

As the X chromosome is much larger than the Y chromosome, for many genes on the X chromosome there are no corresponding genes on the Y chromosome. This leads to special patterns of inheritance, particularly with recessive genes. A female with a recessive gene on the X will not show the syndrome, as is the case for normal recessive genes. However, a male with such a gene on his X chromosome will not be able to mask it with the normal copy, as this is not present on his Y chromosome.

McKusick (1988) lists 139 confirmed X-linked conditions, with about 100 others probably due to sex-linked genes. The highest incidence of any of these conditions is Duchenne muscular dystrophy, with a frequency of 0.2 per 1000 live births. This condition results in progressive weakness and wasting of certain muscles, apparently without any defect in the nervous system. The muscle fibres undergo necrosis, to be replaced by fatty and fibrous tissue. Most patients are invalids by 11 and most do not survive beyond 20 years old. The affected boys have high plasma levels of creatine kinase, due to leakage of this enzyme from the dystrophic muscles into the blood. Levels of this enzyme may be raised in women carrying the affected gene.

For many X-linked conditions reproductive fitness is low and often zero. When it is zero, assuming equal mutation rates in the two sexes, the birth frequency of affected males is three times the mutation rate. One-third of patients are affected as a result of new mutations. Only the latter frequency responds quickly to an increase in the mutation rate, and it takes several generations before the full effect of the increase in the proportion of heterozygous women and the increase in frequency of affected male children born to carrier mothers is reached (Carter, 1977).

Polygenic Mutations in Multifactorial Conditions

Hereditary diseases with simple modes of inheritance represent the tip of the iceberg of disease where gene mutations play a part. Cleft lip, anencephaly, spina bifida, diabetes mellitus, etc., all show some genetic determination in their aetiology. In general, individual genes appear to have a small effect and act with varying dominance — i.e. some genes have low penetrance, in that they are only expressed in some individuals.

Insulin-dependent (type I) diabetes mellitus results from the destruction of the insulin-producing β cells of the pancreas due to an autoimmune response. Family studies have indicated that predisposition to the condition is polygenic. The principal genes leading to susceptibility are within the major histocompatibility gene complex (human leukocyte antigen, or HLA, region).

Some progress has been made in identifying amino acid differences resulting from genetic lesions associated with the disease. The HLA-DQβ alleles positively associated with type I diabetes have either alanine, valine or serine at amino acid position 57, while aspartic acid is found in alleles not associated with the disease (Todd *et al.*, 1987).

The polymorphic 5′ region of the insulin gene on chromosome 11p contributes to susceptibility to type I diabetes (reported in Field, 1988).

Non-genetic factors are also associated with the disease — in particular, infection with particular viruses. There is an increased prevalence of type I diabetes in congenital rubella patients and there is an increased frequency of Coxsackie B viral antibodies in newly diagnosed diabetics compared with controls (review: Field *et al.*, 1987). It is possible that viral infection is a stress which catalyses the pathological process which leads to type I diabetes without being a direct component.

The previous discussion illustrates the bewildering complexity surrounding the nature of just one multifactorial disease. Tissue types and the HLA complex seem to play an important role in susceptibility to over 40 diseases (Thomson, 1988) and much more understanding will be reached by using the new DNA technology to study this region in affected individuals.

The total number of diseases and conditions referred to in the preceding sections is considered to represent only a small proportion of the many gene loci in man capable of causing effects detrimental to health (Department of Health, 1989).

Role of Mutations in Other Conditions

Atherosclerosis

Atherosclerosis is a disease characterized by focal intimal thickening of medium- and large-sized arteries (review: Nilsson, 1986). Such lesions can result in cerebral and myocardial infarction. Risk factors for these conditions include hypercholesterolaemia, hypertension, smoking and diabetes. The lesions or plaques develop by gradual accumulation of cells and extracellular material.

The most prevalent cell type within the lesion are smooth muscle cells, and a great many studies have focused on this cell type, its migration into the intima and its response to mitogenic growth factors. Benditt and Benditt (1973) reported evidence of a monoclonal origin of smooth muscle cells in atherosclerotic lesions, suggesting that they originated from proliferation of a single stem cell. These authors suggested that the neoplastic growth characteristics of the stem cell were induced by mutagens or viruses. This theory is only one of many, and the area remains controversial (Nilsson, 1986). The role of locally produced growth factors (see, e.g., Morisaki *et al.*, 1989) and viruses (Pyrzak and Shih, 1987) appear convincing in particular models of the disease.

Ageing

Genetic instability is widely thought to be involved in the process of ageing (review: Kirkwood, 1989). Studies of the accumulation of somatic mutations have shown that there is no simple relationship. There does appear to be an interaction between mutations, defective epigenetic controls affecting gene expression and interaction with other molecular events. There is a correlation between DNA excision-repair capacity and life-span (Hart and Setlow, 1974), accumulation of mutations in human lymphocytes (Morley *et al.*, 1983) and reduced growth potential of cells from patients with human DNA repair-deficiency syndromes, in comparison with repair-proficient controls (Thompson and Holliday, 1983).

Reproductive Effects

If a potent genotoxin is able to cross the placental barrier, it is very likely to interfere with differentiation of the developing embryo and thus possess teratogenic potential. Indeed, many of the better studied teratogens are also mutagenic (Kalter, 1977). However, mutagens form only one class of teratogens and a large proportion of teratogens are not mutagenic. Alternative mechanisms of teratogenesis include cell death, mitotic delay, retarded differentiation, vascular insufficiency, inhibited cell migration, etc. (Beckman and Brent, 1986; Chapter 40).

It is known that much foetal wastage and many spontaneous abortions arise as a result of the presence of dominant lethal mutations in the developing embryo, many of which appear to be due to major chromosomal damage. In addition, impairment of male fertility is also a consequence of exposure to mutagens. A special issue of *Mutation Research* (**229**, No. 2, 1990) is devoted to male-mediated F_1 abnormalities.

GENETIC TOXICOLOGY

Advent of Genetic Toxicology

The previous sections have illustrated the potential impact that unidentified, widely disseminated mutagens could have on cancer frequencies and heritable disease in man. While this concept was growing in the 1950s and 1960s, Barthelmess (1956) and Lederberg (1962) published reviews

and new studies showing that a variety of man-made chemicals could be shown to be mutagenic in various test systems, including those based on micro-organisms.

Several seminal conferences were held in the 1960s with a focus on chemical mutagens—in particular, their effects on germ cells and the risk to future generations (review: Wassom, 1989). Muller, in 1963, expressed similar concerns to the USA Food and Drug Administration (FDA). He made the point that humans were being exposed to a great number of new chemicals, such as food additives, drugs, pesticides, etc., not encountered by previous generations, and thus humans were not specifically adapted to such chemicals by natural selection (Wassom, 1980).

Genetic toxicology became recognized as a formal discipline in May 1969 when the Environmental Mutagen Society was founded in the USA under the chairmanship of Dr Alexander Hollaender, from Oak Ridge National Laboratory, with a group of interested geneticists (as recounted by Wassom, 1989). In the following year the European Environmental Mutagen Society was formed. The primary thrust of these societies was towards estimating risks to germ cells. However, this was broadened in the 1970s when evidence began to accumulate that carcinogenicity and mutagenicity were linked. This new direction was encouraged by the use of *in vitro* metabolic activation systems, capable of producing reactive electrophilic metabolites from procarcinogens (Malling, 1971). From this time onwards newly identified carcinogens were detected first as mutagens or chromosome-damaging agents and subsequently as carcinogens in whole-animal tests. Some examples are shown in Table 4 (Tweats, 1984). An important factor in the history of genetic toxicology was the development of genetically well-defined strains of micro-organisms, carrying mutations in particular genes coding for amino acid biosynthetic enzymes. These, when coupled with an *in vitro* metabolic activation system, derived from rodent liver, provided a quick powerful tool for assessing mutagenicity of novel compounds.

Early analyses of rodent carcinogens and non-carcinogens suggested that almost all carcinogens were also mutagens (Ames *et al.*, 1973a).

From 1973 onwards various national expert committees were formed to advise governments on what approach may be taken to screen new

Table 4 Examples of newly identified carcinogens detected by short-term tests

Compound	Function/Source	Mutagenicity	Carcinogenicity
Furylfuramide (AF-2)	Food preservative	Kada (1973)	Nomura (1975)
Ethylene dibromide	Grain fumigant	Malling (1969)	Olson *et al.* (1973)
2,4-Diaminoanisole	Hair dye component	Ames *et al.* (1975)	NCI (1978a)
Tris-(2,3-dibromopropyl) phosphate	Flame retardant	Prival *et al.* (1977)	NCI (1978b)
Formaldehyde	Fumigant, etc.	Auerbach *et al.* (1977)[a]	Swenberg *et al.* (1980)
Amino acid pyrolysates	Broiled foods	Matsumoto *et al.* (1977)	Sugimura and Sata (1983)
1-Nitropyrene	Diesel exhausts, etc.	Lofroth *et al.* (1980)	Ohgake *et al.* (1982)

[a] Review.

chemicals for potential heritable or carcinogenic risks. Such committees began the task of formulating guidelines.

From 1976 onwards key methods papers were written for what were to become mainline tests in the various national guidelines. The USA EMS monographs published by Plenum Press and edited by Alexander Hollaender (*Chemical Mutagens, Principles and Methods for Their Detection*) were very influential in this regard. These allowed new laboratories to get to grips with the new assays on a sound basis.

In 1976 Italy banned hair dyes found to be mutagenic in the Ames test, a decision that caused a major impact in toxicology, following a paper on the subject by Ames' group (Ames *et al.*, 1975).

Also, from 1976 various countries began to issue national guidelines for mutagenicity testing, including Italy (Comma, 1977), the USA (EPA, 1978) and the UK (DHSS, 1981). In 1984 the European Economic Community issued 'recommendations' for all new drugs at the Product Licence Application stage (EEC, 1984).

Today it is not possible to register a new drug, food additive, etc., or transport a new industrial chemical within the major industrialized nations, without providing basic mutagenicity information.

The field of genetic toxicology is at a crossroads, with exciting new developments on the horizon, with promising new systems, derived from the recent developments in DNA technology, likely to make an impact in the next decade. In addition, the provision of extensive carcinogenicity information plus corresponding mutagenicity tests have clearly shown that not all

carcinogens are mutagens, which opposes the view formed in the 1970s. The importance and status of 'non-genotoxic' carcinogens will become a well-studied topic in the next few years.

The following sections will examine the basis and practicalities of genetic test systems used for screening new chemical entities for genotoxic activity which use mutation as the end-point.

In Vitro Test Systems

The principal tests can be broadly categorized into microbial and mammalian cell assays. In both cases the tests are carried out in the presence and absence of *in vitro* metabolic activation enzymes, usually derived from rodent liver.

In Vitro Metabolic Activation

The target cells for *in vitro* mutagenicity tests often possess a limited (often overlooked) capacity for endogenous metabolism of xenobiotics. However, to simulate the complexity of metabolic events that occur in the whole animal, there is a critical need to supplement this activity.

Choice of Species

A bewildering variety of exogenous systems have been used for one purpose or another in mutagenicity tests. The choice begins with plant or animal preparations. The attraction of plant systems has stemmed from a desire to avoid the use of animals, where possible, in toxicity testing. In addition, plant systems have particular relevance when certain chemicals are being tested, e.g. herbicides.

If animal systems are chosen, preparations derived from fish (see, e.g., Kada, 1981) and birds (Parry *et al.*, 1985, etc.) have been used. However, by far the most widely used and validated are those derived from rodents—in particular, the rat. Hamsters may be preferred as a source of metabolizing enzymes when particular chemical classes are being screened—e.g. aromatic amines, heterocyclic amines, *N*-nitrosamines and azo dyes (Prival and Mitchell, 1982; Haworth *et al.*, 1983).

Choice of Tissue

The next choice is that of source tissue. Preparations derived from liver are the most useful, as this tissue is a rich source of mixed-function oxygenases capable of converting procarcinogens to genetically active electrophiles. However, many extrahepatic tissues (e.g. kidney, lung, etc.) are also known to possess important metabolic capacity which may be relevant to the production of mutagenic metabolites in the whole animal.

Cell-free versus Cell-based Systems

Most use has been made of cell-free systems— in particular, crude homogenates such as 9000 *g* supernatant (S9 fraction) from rat liver. This fraction is composed of free endoplasmic reticulum, microsomes (membrane-bound packets of 'membrane-associated' enzymes), soluble enzymes and some cofactors. Hepatic S9 fractions do not necessarily completely reflect the metabolism of the whole organ, in that they mainly possess phase I metabolism (e.g. oxygenases) and are deficient in phase II systems (e.g. conjugation enzymes). The latter are often capable of efficient detoxification, while the former are regarded as 'activating'. This can be a strength, in that S9 fractions are used in screening tests as a surrogate for all tissues in an animal, some of which may be exposed to reactive metabolites in the absence of efficient detoxification. Many carcinogens are organ-specific in extrahepatic tissues, yet liver S9 fraction will reveal their mutagenicity. The deficiency of S9 fractions for detoxification can also be a weakness, in that detoxification may predominate in the whole animal, such that the potential carcinogenicity revealed *in vitro* is not realized *in vivo*.

Cell-free systems, when supplemented with relevant cofactors, are remarkably proficient, despite their crudity, in generating reactive electrophiles from most procarcinogens. However, they provide at best a broad approximation of *in vivo* metabolism and can fail to produce sufficient quantity of a particular reactive metabolite to be detectable by the indicator cells or they can produce inappropriate metabolites that do not play a role *in vivo* (see Gatehouse and Tweats, 1987, for discussion).

Some of these problems can be overcome by the use of cell-based systems—in particular, primary hepatocytes. Hepatocytes closely simulate the metabolic systems found in the intact liver and do not require additional cofactors for optimal enzyme activity. However, apart from greater technical difficulties in obtaining hepatocytes as opposed to S9 fraction, hepatocytes can effectively detoxify particular carcinogens and prevent their detection as mutagens. Despite these difficulties, hepatocytes have a role to play in mutagenicity screening, in both bacterial and mammalian-based systems (see Tweats and Gatehouse, 1988).

Inducing Agents

The final choice considered here is whether to use 'uninduced' liver preparations or those derived from animals pretreated with an enzyme inducer to promote high levels of metabolic activity. If induced preparations are preferred, which inducer should be used?

It appears that uninduced preparations are of limited use in screening assays, as they are deficient in particular important activities such as cytochrome P-450$_{IA1}$ cytochrome oxygenases. In addition, species and organ differences are most divergent with uninduced enzyme preparations (Brusick, 1987).

The above differences disappear when induced microsomal preparations are used. A number of enzyme inducers have been used, the most popular being Aroclor 1254, which is a mixture of polychlorinated biphenyls (as described by Ames *et al.*, 1975). However, concern about the toxicity, carcinogenicity and persistence of these compounds in the environment has led to the use of alternatives, such as a combination of phenobarbitone (phenobarbital) and β-naphthoflavone (5,6-benzoflavone). This combination results in the induction of a range of mono-oxygenases similar to that induced by Aroclor 1254 (see, e.g., Ong *et al.*, 1980). More selective inducers such as phenobarbitone (cytochrome P-450$_{IIA1}$, P-450$_{IIB1}$) or 3-methylcholanthrene (cytochrome P-450$_{IA1}$) have also been used.

In summary, genetic toxicity tests with both bacterial and mammalian cells are normally carried out with rat liver cell-free systems (S9 fraction) from animals pretreated with enzyme inducers. However, investigations should not slavishly follow this regimen: there may be sound scientifically based reasons for using preparations from different species or different organs, or for using whole cells such as hepatocytes.

Standard Method of S9 Fraction Preparation

The following method describes the production of hepatic S9 mix from rats induced with a combination of phenobarbitone and β-naphthoflavone, and is an adaption of the method described by Gatehouse and Delow (1979).

Male albino rats within the weight range 150–250 g are treated with phenobarbitone sodium 16 mg ml^{-1}, 2.5 ml kg^{-1} in sterile saline, and β-naphthoflavone 20 mg ml^{-1}, 5 ml kg^{-1} in corn oil. A fine suspension of the latter is achieved by sonicating for 1 h. These solutions are dosed by intraperitoneal injection on days 1, 2 and 3.

Phenobarbitone sodium is normally administered between 0.5 and 2 h prior to β-naphthoflavone.

The animals are killed on day 4 by cervical dislocation and the livers removed as quickly as possible and placed on ice-cold KCl buffer (0.01M Na$_2$HPO$_4$ + KCl 1.15%). The liver is cleaned, weighed, minced and homogenized (in an Ultra Turrax homogenizer) in the above buffer to give a 25 per cent (w/v) liver homogenate. The homogenate is stored at 4 °C until it can be centrifuged at 9000 g for 15 min. The supernatant is decanted, mixed and divided into 2 ml volumes in cryotubes. These are then snap-frozen in liquid nitrogen. Storage at −196 °C for up to 3 months results in no appreciable loss of most P-450 isoenzymes (Ashwood-Smith, 1980).

Quality control of S9 batches is usually monitored by ability to activate compounds known to require metabolism to generate mutagenic metabolites. This is a rather crude approach and more accurate data can be obtained by measuring biochemical parameters—e.g. protein, cytochrome P-450 total activity (from crude S9) and related enzyme activities (from purified microsomes) such as 7-ethoxyresorufin-O-deethylase and 7-methoxycoumarin-O-demethylase—to give an indication of S9 batch-to-batch variation and to

set standards for rejecting suboptimal batches (Hubbard *et al.*, 1985). For further details on critical features affecting the use and limitations of S9 fraction, see Gatehouse (1987).

S9 Mix

The S9 fraction prepared as described above is used as a component in 'S9 mix' along with buffers and various enzyme cofactors. The amount of S9 fraction in the S9 mix can be varied, but a 'standard' level of 0.1 ml ml^{-1} of S9 mix (or 10 per cent S9) is often recommended for general screening.

No single concentration of S9 fraction in the S9 mix will detect all classes of genotoxic carcinogen with equal efficiency (Gatehouse *et al.*, 1990). Some mutagens, including many polycyclic aromatic hydrocarbons, are activated to mutagens by higher than normal levels of S9 fraction in the S9 mix (see, e.g., Carver *et al.*, 1985).

The mixed-function oxidases in the S9 fraction require NADPH, normally generated from the action of glucose-6-phosphate dehydrogenase acting on glucose-6-phosphate and reducing NADP, both of which are normally supplied as cofactors. As an alternative, isocitrate can be substituted for glucose-6-phosphate (to be used as a substrate by isocitrate dehydrogenase) (Linblad and Jackim, 1982). Additional cofactors may be added (e.g. flavin mononucleotide), when particular classes of compound such as azo dyes are being tested (Prival *et al.*, 1984), or acetyl coenzyme A when aromatic animes such as benzidine are being tested (Kennelly *et al.*, 1984).

The composition of a 'standard' S9 mix is given in Table 5.

Bacterial Mutation Tests

The study of mutation in bacteria (and bacterial viruses) has had a fundamental role in the science of genetics in the twentieth century. In particular, the unravelling of biochemical anabolic and catabolic pathways, the identification of DNA as the hereditary material, the fine structure of the gene, the nature of gene regulation, etc., have all been aided by bacterial mutants.

As an offshoot of studies of genes concerned with the biosynthesis of amino acids, a range of *E. coli* (see, e.g., Yanofsky, 1971) and *Salmonella typhimurium* strains (see, e.g., Ames, 1971) with relatively well-defined mutations in known genes became available. How these strains became the

Table 5 Composition of standard S9 mix

Constituent	Final Conc. in mix (mM)
Glucose-6-phosphate	5
Nicotinamide adenine dinucleotide phosphate	4
MgCl$_2$.6H$_2$O ⎫	8
⎬ **Salt solution**	
KCl ⎭	33
Phosphate buffer (0.2 M)	100
Distilled water to make up to the required volume	
S9 fraction added at 0.1 ml per ml of S9 mix	

For assays using cultured mammalian cells, phosphate buffer and distilled water are replaced by tissue culture medium, as high concentrations of Na and K salts are toxic to such cells. The concentration of S9 fraction in the S9 mix varies, depending on the relevant assay (see individual sections). Once prepared, S9 mix should be used as soon as possible, and should be stored on ice until required. S9 fraction, once thawed, should not be refrozen for future use.

basis of 'reverse' mutation assays is illuminatingly told by MacPhee (1989). Thus, bacteria already mutant at an easily detectable locus are treated with a range of doses of the test material to determine whether the compound can induce a second mutation that directly reverses or suppresses the original mutations. Thus, for amino acid auxotrophs, the original mutation has resulted in loss of ability to grow in the absence of the required amino acid. The second mutation restores prototrophy—i.e. the affected cell is now able to grow in the absence of the relevant amino acid, if provided with inorganic salts and a carbon source. This simple concept, in fact, underlines the great strength of these assays, for it provides enormous selective power which can identify a small number of the chosen mutants from a population of millions of unmutated cells and cells mutated in other genes. The genetic target—i.e. the mutated DNA bases in the gene in question (or bases in the relevant tRNA genes; see the discussion of suppressor mutations, pp. 817–818)—can thus be very small, just one or a few bases in length.

An alternative approach is to use bacteria to detect 'forward mutations'. Genetic systems which detect forward mutations have an apparent advantage, in that a wide variety of genetic changes may lead to a forward mutation—e.g. point mutation, deletions, insertions, etc. In addition, forward mutations in a number of different genes may lead to the same change in phenotype; thus, the genetic target is much larger than that seen in most reverse mutation assays. However, if a particular mutagen causes rare specific changes, these changes may be lost against the background of more common events (Gatehouse *et al.*, 1990). Spontaneous mutation rates tend to be relatively high in forward mutation systems. Acquisition of resistance to a toxic chemical (e.g. an amino acid analogue or antibiotic) is a frequently used genetic marker in these systems. For instance, the use of resistance to the antibiotic streptomycin preceded the reversion assays in common use today (see, e.g., Newcombe, 1952).

Reversion Tests—Background
There are several excellent references describing the background and use of bacteria for reversion tests (Brusick, 1987; Gatehouse *et al.*, 1990). Three different protocols have been widely used: plate-incorporation assays, treat and plate tests, and fluctuation tests. These methods are described in detail in the following sections. Fundamental to the operation of these tests is the genetic compositions of the tester strains selected for use.

Genetic Make-up of Tester Strains The most widely used strains are those developed by Professor Bruce Ames and colleagues which are mutant derivatives of the organism *Salmonella typhimurium*. Each strain carries one of a number of mutations in the operon coding for histidine biosynthesis. In each case the mutation can be reverted either by base-change or by frameshift mutations. The genotype of the commonly used strains is shown in Table 6.

For the most commonly used strains, the DNA sequence at the site of the original mutation in the relevant histidine gene has been determined (Table 7). With the exception of the TA102 strain (see below), all contain G–C base-pairs at the site of the histidine mutation, and this has some effect on the selectivity of the mutagens detected—i.e. those that act preferentially on these bases.

Description of Mutant Histidine Genes A brief description of these mutations is given below:

hisG46 requires histidine, owing to the loss of the enzyme PR-ATP pyrophosphorylase. The activity of the *hisG* gene is lost, owing to a

Table 6 Genotype of commonly used strains of *Salmonella typhimurium* LT2

Strain	Genotype[a]
TA1535	*hisG*$_{46}$ *rfa* △ *gal chlD bio uvrB*
TA100	*hisG*$_{46}$ *rfa* △ *gal chlD bio uvrB* (pKM101)
TA1537	*hisC*$_{3076}$ *rfa* △ *gal chlD bio uvrB*
TA1538	*hisD*$_{3052}$ *rfa* △ *gal chlD bio uvrB*
TA98	*hisD*$_{3052}$ *rfa* △ *gal chlD bio uvrB* (pKM101)
TA97	*hisD*$_{6610}$ *hisO*$_{1242}$ *rfa* △ *gal chl*^{D} *bio uvrB* (pKM101)
TA102	*his*△(*G*)$_{8476}$ *rfa galE* (pAQ1) (pKM101)

[a] *rfa* = deep rough; *gal E* = UDP galactose 4-epimerase; *chlD* = nitrate reductase (resistance to chlorate); *bio* = biotin; *uvrB* = UV endonuclease component B. △ = deletion of genes following this symbol.
The *his* mutations are discussed in the text.

pAQ1: a plasmid carrying the *hisG*$_{428}$ gene.
pKM101: a plasmid carrying the *mucAB* genes that enhance error-prone repair.

mis-sense base mutation that occurred spontaneously (Ames, 1971) (Table 7). This mutation can be reverted directly or by a variety of suppressor mutations.

hisC3076 requires histidine, owing to loss of imidazole acetolaphosphate transaminase. It

carries a frameshift mutation induced by the mutagen ICR364-OH (Isono and Yourno, 1974), with an additional G–C base-pair in a run of G–C pairs—i.e. a frameshift hot-spot. This mutation is reverted by frameshift mutagens such as 9-aminoacridine, ICR-191 (an acridine with a mustard side-chain) and epoxides of polycyclic hydrocarbons.

hisD3052 requires histidine, owing to the loss of the enzyme L-histidinol dehydrogenase. It carries a frameshift mutation resulting from the deletion of C–G base-pairs in a repetitive C–G hot-spot after treatment with the frameshift mutagen ICR364-OH (Isono and Yourno, 1974) (Table 7). This mutation is reverted well by aromatic nitroso derivatives of aromatic amine carcinogens and by the carcinogenic metabolites of aflatoxin B$_1$ and benzo[*a*]pyrene.

In addition to these mutations, the most recent generation of strains contains further mutations of histidine biosynthetic genes. Strain TA102 contains a genetically engineered multicopy plasmid, pAQ1 (Figure 13), which carries the *hisG428* mutation.

hisG428 is an ochre mis-sense mutation in the gene coding for PR-ATP pyrophosphorylase. Unlike the previously described strains, this

Table 7 Histidine mutations in commonly used *Salmonella* strains

Mutation	Strain	Nature of mutation	Reversion events
his G428	TA102 TA104	w/t CAG–AGC–AAG–CAA–GAG–CTG– mutant CAG–AGC–AAG–TAA (ochre)	All possible transitions and transversions Extragenic suppressors Small deletions (−3, −6)
his G46	TA100 TA1535	w/t GTG–GTC–GA*T–CTC–GGT–ATT– mutant –CCC–	Subset of base-pair substitution events Extragenic suppressors
his D6610	TA97	w/t GTC–ACC–CCT–GAA–GAG–A*TC–GCC mutant GTC–ACA–CCC–CCC–TGA (opal)	Frameshifts
his D3052	TA98 TA1538	w/t GAC–ACC–GCC–CGG–CAG–GCC–CTG–AGC mutant GAC–ACC–GCC–GGC–AGG–CCC–TGA (opal)	Frameshifts
his C3076	TA1537	w/t sequence not known mutant presumed +1 near CCC	Frameshifts

A* = 6-methyldeoxyadenosine.
w/t = wild type.

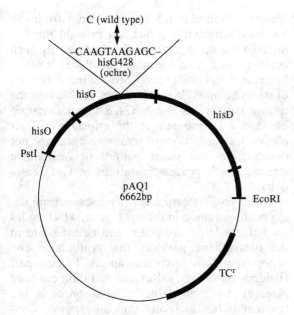

Figure 13 Map of plasmid pAQ1. Redrawn from Levin *et al*. (1982a)

results in a new T–A base-pair within the mutant site (Table 7). This site is flanked by a direct repeat –A–G–A–G–C– sequence which may allow the persistence of a single-stranded region of DNA at this site, which may make it more prone to base change mutagens. As this mutation is carried on a multicopy plasmid (the normal chromosomal *hisG* gene is deleted), a large target (about 30 copies of the gene) is presented for mutation induction. It appears that mutagens that can act by an oxidative mechanism (e.g. bleomycin, X-rays, malondialdehyde, etc.) act preferentially at A–T base-pairs and are thus detected by this strain (Levin *et al.*, 1982a)

An additional frameshift-detecting strain, TA97, has also been introduced recently. This strain carries the *hisD6610* mutation.

hisD6610 results in a run of 6 C–G base-pairs at the site of mutation due to a +1 frameshift and detects substituted triazines, phenothiazines, PR toxin, etc. (Levin *et al.*, 1982b) when present in the correct genetic background.

Additional mutations The success of strains containing the mutations described above stems not only from these mutations, which are highly sensitive to reversion, but also from additional

mutations or deletions affecting other genes. Ames and colleagues realized that many carcinogens (or their metabolites) are large molecules that are not necessarily able to cross the protective cell wall and outer layers of the *Salmonella* cell. Wild-type cells are described as 'smooth' and produce a lipopolysaccharide that acts as a barrier to particular molecules. Ames introduced *rfaE* mutations (deep rough) into the *Salmonella* tester strains, which results in a defective lipopolysaccharide (the lipopolysaccharide is lost down to the ketodeoxyoctanoate-lipid core) and increases permeability to bulky hydrophobic chemicals (Ames *et al.*, 1973b). In addition, these strains with defective cell walls are less pathogenic than their *rfaE+* counterparts.

As mentioned above (pp. 810–815), bacteria possess several major DNA repair pathways. Most of these appear to be error-free and can repair DNA damage without generating mutations. Ames and colleagues constructed a series of strains with a DNA deletion removing the *uvrB* gene coding for a subunit of the first enzyme, the cor-endonuclease I, in the error-free excision repair pathway. This change increases the sensitivity of the tester strains to mutagens by several orders of magnitude. The deletion through *uvrB* also includes the nitrate reductase (*chl*) and biotin (*bio*) genes.

DNA interstrand cross-linking agents (e.g. the quinone mitomycin C, psoralens +UV − light, etc.) require an intact excision repair pathway to generate mutations (see, e.g., Kondo *et al.*, 1970). DNA interstrand cross-links produced by mitomycin C are removed from one strand, along with a small number of adjacent bases, by excision repair. The gap that is left behind is repaired by post-replication repair. The remaining broken cross-link, still attached to the other strand, is probably a secondary premutational lesion which can either be accurately repaired by excision repair, the opposite newly repaired strand being used as a template, or give rise to a mutation through error-prone repair (Cole, 1973). Thus, it is useful to include a strain with an intact excision repair pathway in the test battery. *Salmonella typhimurium* TA102 is such a strain. The relative loss in sensitivity to other types of mutagen due to the *uvrB+* background is offset by the presence of multicopies of the *hisG428* mutation in this strain, as described earlier.

The Use of the Plasmid pKM101. Salmonella typhimurium LT2 strains do not appear to possess classical 'error-prone' repair as found in *E. coli* strains and some other members of the Entero-bacteria (Walker, 1984; Sedgwick and Goodwin, 1985). This is due to a deficiency in *umu D* activity in these *Salmonella* strains (Herrera *et al.*, 1988; Thomas and Sedgewick, 1989). One way to overcome this deficiency and to increase sensitivity to mutagens is to use strains containing a plasmid carrying analogues to the *umu DC* genes.

The first to show enhanced chemical mutagenesis in *Salmonella typhimurium* containing a plasmid was MacPhee (1973), using the *hisG46* strain containing N-group R factor, R205, when testing the mutagen methyl methane sulphonate. This finding led Ames to screen similar plasmids for use in the Ames test. Ames and colleagues selected pKM101, a deletion derivative originally isolated by Mortelmans (1975) of the N-group plasmid R46. The new pKM101-containing strains (TA98 and TA100) were able to detect many carcinogens which were not detected before or were detected with less sensitivity. These included aflatoxin B$_1$, benzo[*a*]pyrene, sterigmatocystin, etc. (McCann *et al.*, 1975a,b). Mortelmans and Dousman (1986) screened a further 33 plasmids and, remarkably, pKM101 still proved to be the most useful plasmid in this regard (for further discussion, see pp. 815–816).

E. coli Tester Strains. Ames and colleagues have made an impressive contribution to mutagenicity testing by the development of the *Salmonella*/microsome test and, in particular, its application in the study of environmental mutagens. In genetic terms, *Salmonella* strains are, in some ways, not the best choice (see, e.g., Venitt and Croften-Sleigh, 1981). The case for *Escherichia coli* strains is eloquently presented in MacPhee (1989). Unlike the *Salmonella* strains, *E. coli* B strains such as the WP2 series developed by Bridges, Green and colleagues (Bridges, 1972; Green and Muriel, 1976) possess the *umuDC*$^+$ genes involved in generating mutations (as described above); they are also part-rough and thus allow many large molecules to enter the cell. MacPhee states that, had these differences been known at the time, the progressive development of the *Salmonella* mutagenicity test would probably not have occurred. Thus, the incorporation of new

mutations and plasmids into the Ames strains to 'increase sensitivity' in fact just brought the *Salmonella* test up to the level that had already been achieved with *E. coli* strains (MacPhee, 1989).

Levin *et al.* (1982a) proposed the incorporation of strain *Salmonella typhimurium* TA102 into the testing battery, as the *hisG428* target mutation has an A–T base-pair at the critical site. This allows the detection of mutagenic agents not detected by the usual battery of *Salmonella* strains, which possess mutations at G–C base-pairs.

The *E. coli* WP2 *trp E* series possess a terminating ochre mutation in the *trp E* gene, which codes for anthranilate synthetase, and enzyme late in the biosynthetic pathway for tryptophan. The ochre mutation involves an A–T base-pair (Bridges *et al.*, 1967). Reverse mutation can take place at the original site of mutation or in the relevant tRNA loci, and thus all types of transition and transversion can be detected. Although error-prone repair is present, strains possessing *uvrA* mutations and mutator plasmids (pKM101 or R46) have advantages, including the detection of some frameshift mutagens.

In addition to being effective general strains for mutagen detection, studies by Wilcox *et al.* (1990) have shown that a combination of *E. coli* WP2 *trp E* (pKM101), which has a functioning excision repair system for the detection of cross-linking agents, and *E. coli* WP2 *trp E uvrA* (pKM101) can be used as alternatives to *Salmonella* TA102 for the detection of oxidative mutagens. The *E. coli* strains have the advantage of lower spontaneous mutation rate and are somewhat less difficult to use and maintain.

Storage and Checking of Tester Strains Detailed instructions for maintenance and confirmation of the phenotypes of the various tester strains are given in Maron and Ames (1983) and Gatehouse *et al.* (1990). Permanent master cultures of tester strains should be stored in liquid nitrogen or in dry ice. Such cultures are prepared from fresh nutrient broth cultures, to which DMSO is added as a cryopreservative. These cultures are checked for the various characteristics before storage as described below. Cultures for use in individual experiments should be set up by inoculation from the master culture or from a plate made directly from the master culture, not by passage from a previously used culture. Passage in this way will inevitably increase the number of pre-existing mutants, leading to unacceptably high spontaneous mutation rates (Gatehouse *et al.*, 1990).

The following characteristics of the tester strains should be confirmed at monthly intervals or if the internal controls of a particular experiment fail to meet the required limits:

- Amino acid requirement.
- Sensitivity to the lethal effects of the high-molecular-weight dye crystal violet for those strains carrying the *rfaE* mutation.
- Increased sensitivity to UV irradiation for those strains carrying the *uvrA* or *uvrB* mutations.
- Resistance to ampicillin for strains carrying pKM101 and resistance to tetracycline for strains carrying pAQ1.
- Sensitivity to diagnostic mutagens. This can be measured very satisfactorily by testing pairs of strains—one giving a strongly positive response, the partner a weak response, as shown in Table 8.

The importance of these checks together with careful experiment-to-experiment controls of spontaneous mutation rates and response to reference mutagens cannot be overstressed; failure to apply them can result in much wasted effort.

Plate Incorporation Assay
Protocol for Dose Ranging and Selection Before carrying out the main tests, it is necessary to carry out a preliminary toxicity dose ranging test. This should be carried out following the same basic protocol as the mutation test, except that instead of scoring the number of mutants on, for example minimal media plates with limiting amounts of a required amino acid, the number of survivors is scored on fully supplemented minimal media. A typical protocol is outlined below:

(1) Prepare a stock solution of the test compound at a concentration of 50 mg ml^{-1} in an appropriate solvent. It may be necessary to prepare a lower concentration of stock solution, depending on the solubility of the test compound.

(2) Make dilutions of the stock solution.

(3) To 2.0 ml aliquots of soft agar overlay medium (0.6 per cent agar and 0.5 per cent sodium chloride in distilled water) containing a trace of histidine and excess biotin and maintained at 45 °C in a dry block, add 100 μl of the tester strain and 100 μl at a solution of the test article. Use only one plate per dilution.

(4) Mix and pour on to dried Vogel and Bonner minimal medium plates as in an Ames test, including an untreated control and a solvent control, if necessary. The final concentrations of test compound will be 5000, 1500, 500, 150 and 50 μg plate^{-1}.

(5) Repeat step (3), using 0.5 ml of 8 per cent S9 mix per 2.0 ml aliquot of soft agar in addition to the test compound and tester strain. The S9 mix is kept on ice during the experiment.

(6) Incubate the plates for 2 days at 37 °C and examine the background lawn of growth with a microscope (×8 eyepiece lens, ×10 objective lens). The lowest concentration giving a depleted background lawn is regarded as a toxic dose.

Table 8 Diagnostic mutagens for checking pairs of strains

Pairs of strains	Mutagen	Response
(a) *S. typhimurium*		
TA1535/TA100	Methyl methane sulphonate	Low/High
TA1538/TA98	4-Nitroquinoline-*N*-oxide	Low/High
TA1537/TA1538	2-Aminofluorene (in the presence of rat liver S9)	Low/High
TA100/TA102	Mitomycin C	Low/High
TA98/TA100	Sodium azide	Low/High
(b) *E. coli* WP2		
uvrA/uvrA (pKM101)	Potassium dichromate	Low/High

High = unequivocal positive response.
Low = weak or negative effect at the same dose in the responsive strain.

This test will also demonstrate excess growth, which may indicate the presence of histidine or tryptophan or their precursors in the test material, which could make testing for mutagenicity impracticable by this method.

When setting the maximum test concentration, it is important to test into the mg plate^{-1} range where possible (Gatehouse *et al.*, 1990), as some mutagens are only detectable when tested at high concentrations. However, for non-toxic, soluble mutagens an upper limit of 5 mg plate^{-1} is recommended (DeSerres and Shelby, 1979). For less soluble compounds at least one dose exhibiting precipitation should be included.

Ames Salmonella/*Plate Incorporation Method*
The following procedure is based on that described by Ames and colleagues (Maron and Ames, 1983), with additional modifications.

(1) Each selected test strain is grown for 10 h at 37 °C in nutrient broth (Oxoid No. 2) or supplemented minimal media (Vogel–Bonner) on an orbital shaker. A timing device can be used to ensure that cultures are ready at the beginning of the working day.

(2) 2.0 ml aliquots of soft agar overlay medium are melted just prior to use and cooled to 50 °C, and relevant supplements added—i.e. L-histidine, final concentration 9.55 μg ml^{-1}, and D-biotin, 12 μg ml^{-1}. (N.B.: If *E. coli* WP2 tester strains are used, the only supplement required is tryptophan 3.6 μg ml^{-1}.) The medium is kept semi-molten by holding the tubes containing the medium in a hot aluminium dry block, held at 45 °C. It is best to avoid water baths as microbial contamination can cause problems.

(3) The following additions are made to each tube of top agar: the test article (or solvent control) in solution (10–200 μl), the test strain (100 μl) and, where necessary, S9 mix (500 μl). The test is carried out in the presence and absence of S9 mix. The exact volume of test article or solvent may depend on toxicity or solubility, as described in the preceding section.

(4) There should be at least three replicate plates per treatment with at least five test doses plus untreated controls. Duplicate plates are sufficient for the positive and sterility control treatments. The use of twice as many negative control plates as used in each treatment group will lead to

more powerful tests from a statistical standpoint (Mahon *et al.*, 1989).

(5) Each tube of top agar is mixed and quickly poured onto dried prelabelled Vogel–Bonner basal agar plates.

(6) The soft agar is allowed to set at room temperature and the plates are inverted and incubated (within 1 h of pouring) at 37 °C in the dark. Incubation is continued for 2–3 days.

(7) Before scoring the plates for revertant colonies, the presence of a light background lawn of growth (due to limited growth of non-revertant colonies before the trace of histidine or tryptophan is exhausted) should be confirmed for each concentration of test article by examination of the plate under low power of a light microscope. At concentrations that are toxic to the test strains, such a lawn will be depleted and colonies may appear that are not true revertants but surviving, non-prototrophic cells. If necessary, the phenotype of any questionable colonies (pseudo-revertants) should be checked by plating on histidine- or tryptophan-free medium.

(8) Revertant colonies can be counted by hand or with an automatic colony counter. Such machines are relatively accurate in the range of colonies normally observed (although calibration against manual counts is a wise precaution). Where accurate quantitative counts of plates with large numbers of colonies are required, only manual counts will give accurate results.

Controls
Positive Controls Where possible, positive controls should be chosen that are structurally related to the test article. This increases the confidence in the results. In the absence of structurally related mutagens, the set of positive controls given in Table 9 can be used. The use of such controls validates each test run and helps to confirm the nature of each strain. Pagano and Zeiger (1985) have shown that it is possible to store stock solutions of most routinely used positive controls (sodium azide, 2-aminoanthracene, benzo[a]pyrene, 4-nitroquinoline oxide) at −20 °C to −80 °C for several months, without loss of activity. This measure can help reduce potential exposure to laboratory personnel.

Untreated/Vehicle Controls Untreated controls omit the test article, but are made up to volume with buffer. The vehicle control is made up to

Table 9 Positive controls for use in plate incorporation assays

Species	Strain	Mutagen	Conc. (µg plate^{-1})[a]
(a) In the absence of S9 mix			
S. typhimurium	TA1535 TA100	Sodium azide	1–5
	TA1538 TA98	Hycanthone methane sulphonate	5–20
	TA1537	ICR 191	1
E. coli	WP2 *uvrA*	Nifuroxime	5–15
(b) In the presence of S9 mix			
E. coli	WP2 *uvrA* (pKM101)		
S. typhimurium	TA1538		
	TA1535	2-Aminoanthracene	1–10
	TA100		
	TA98		
	TA1537	Neutral red	10–20

[a] The concentrations given above will give relatively small increases in revertant count above the spontaneous level. There is little point in using large concentrations of reference mutagens which invariably give huge increases in revertant counts. This would give little information on the day-to-day performance of the assay.

volume with the solvent used to dissolve the test substance. It is preferable to ensure that each of the treated plates contains the same volume of vehicle throughout.

As detailed by Gatehouse (1987), the nature and concentration of solvent may have a marked effect on the test result. Dimethylsulphoxide is often used as the solvent of choice for hydrophobic compounds. However, there may be unforeseen effects, such as an increase in mutagenicity of some compounds—e.g. *p*-phenylenediamine (Burnett *et al.*, 1982)—or a decrease in mutagenicity of others, such as simple aliphatic nitrosamines (Yahagi *et al.*, 1977). It is essential to use fresh batches of the highest purity grade available and to prevent decomposition/oxidation on storage. The products after oxidation, etc., are both toxic and can induce base-pair substitutions in both bacterial and mammalian assays. Finally, DMSO and other organic solvents can inhibit the oxidation of different premutagens by microsomal mono-oxygenases (Wolff, 1977). To reduce the risk of artefactual results, it is essential to use the minimum amount of organic solvent (e.g. <2 per cent w/w) compatible with adequate testing of the test chemical.

It is important to keep a careful check of the number of mutant colonies present on untreated or vehicle control plates. These numbers depend on the following factors:

(1) The repair status of the cell—i.e. excision repair-deficient strains tend to have more 'spontaneous mutants' than repair-proficient cells.

(2) The presence of mutator plasmids. Excision-deficient strains containing pKM101 have a higher spontaneous mutation rate at both base substitution and frameshift loci than excision-proficient strains.

(3) The total number of cell divisions that take place of the cells in the supplemented top agar. This is controlled by the supply of nutrients—in particular, histidine. Rat liver extracts may also supply trace amounts of limiting nutrients, resulting in a a slight increase in the spontaneous yield of mutants in the presence of S9 mix.

(4) The size of the initial inoculum. During growth of the starting culture, mutants will arise. Thus, if a larger starting inoculum is used, more of these 'pre-existing' mutants will be present per plate. In fact, the 'plate mutants' arising as described in point (3) predominate.

(5) The intrinsic mutability of the mutation in question. In practice the control mutation values tend to fall within a relatively precise range for each strain. Each laboratory should determine

the normal range of revertant colonies per plate for each strain. Acceptable ranges are shown in Table 10 (Gatehouse *et al.*, 1990).

Deviations in background reversion counts from the normal range should be investigated. It is possible that cross-contamination, variations in media quality, etc., have occurred that may invalidate particular experiments.

Frequent checks should also be made on the sterility of S9 preparations, media and test articles. These simple precautions can prevent loss of valuable time and resources.

Evaluation of Results   At least two independent assays are carried out for each test article. The criterion for a positive response is a reproducible and statistically significant result at any concentration for any strain. When positive results are obtained, the test is repeated, using the strain(s) and concentration range with which the initial positive results were observed. This range may be quite narrow for toxic agents.

Several statistical approaches have been applied to the results of plate incorporation assays (review: Mahon *et al.*, 1989). These authors make a number of important suggestions to maximize the power of statistical analyses; those that relate to the method of analysis are reproduced below.

(1) Unless it is obvious that the test agent has had no effect, the data should be plotted, to give a visual impression of the form of any dose response and the pattern of variability.

(2) Three methods of analysis—linear regression (see, e.g., Steel and Torrie, 1960); a multiple comparison analysis, Dunnett's method

Table 10   Acceptable negative control counts for the routinely used strains. From Gatehouse *et al.* (1990)

Test strain	Range	References
TA1535	3–37	Kier *et al.* (1986)
TA1537	4–31	Kier *et al.* (1986)
TA98	15–60	Kier *et al.* (1986)
TA100	75–200	Kier *et al.* (1986)
TA97 (TA97a)	90–180	Maron and Ames (1983)
TA102	240–360	Maron and Ames (1983)
WP2 *uvrA* (pKM101)	45–151	Venitt *et al.* (1984)

(Dunnett, 1955); and a non-parametric analysis, Wahrendorf's method (Wahrendorf *et al.*, 1985)—can all be recommended. Each has its strengths and weaknesses, and other methods are not excluded.

(3) Linear regression assumes that variance across doses is constant and that the dose response is linear. If the variance is not approximately constant, then a transformation may be applied or a weighted analysis may be carried out. If the dose response tends to a plateau, then the dose scale may be transformed. If counts decline markedly at high doses, then linear regression is inappropriate.

(4) Dunnett's method, perhaps with a transformation, is recommended when counts decline markedly at one or two high doses. However, when the dose response shows no such decline, other methods may be more powerful.

(5) Wahrendorf's non-parametric method avoids the complications of transformations of weighting and is about as powerful as any other method. However, it is inappropriate when the response declines markedly at high dose.

Preincubation Tests
Some mutagens are poorly detected in the standard plate incorporation assay, particularly those that are metabolized to short-lived reactive electrophiles—e.g. short-chain aliphatic *N*-nitroso compounds (Bartsch *et al.*, 1976) and azo dyes (see, e.g., Prival *et al.*, 1984). It is also possible that some metabolites may bind to components within the agar. Such compounds can be detected by using a preincubation method first described by Yahagi *et al.* (1975) in which the bacteria, test compound and S9 mix are incubated together in a small volume at 37 °C for a short period (30–60 min) before adding the soft agar and pouring as for the standard assay. In this variation of the test, during the preincubation step, the test compound, S9 mix and bacteria are incubated in liquid at higher concentrations than in the standard test, and this may account for the increased sensitivity with relevant mutagens. In the standard method the soluble enzymes in the S9 mix, cofactors and the test agent may diffuse into the bottom agar. This can interfere with the detection of some mutagens—a problem that is overcome in the preincubation method (Forster *et al.*, 1980; Gatehouse and Wedd, 1984).

The test is carried out as follows:

(1) The strains are cultured overnight, and the inocula and S9 mix are prepared as in the standard Ames test.

(2) The soft agar overlays are prepared and maintained at 45 °C prior to use.

(3) To each of 3–5 tubes maintained at 37 °C in a Driblock are added 0.5 ml of S9 mix, 0.1 ml of the tester strain (10–18 h culture) and a suitable volume of the test compound, to yield the desired range of concentrations. The S9 mix is kept on ice prior to use.

(4) The reaction mixtures are incubated for up to 1 h at 37 °C.

(5) 2.0 ml of soft agar is added to each tube. After mixing, the agar and reaction mixture are poured onto previously labelled, dried Vogel–Bonner plates.

(6) Once the agar has set, the plates are incubated for 2–3 days before revertant colonies are scored.

The use of controls is as described for the plate incorporation assay. It is crucial to use the minimum amount of organic solvent in this assay, as the total volume of the incubation mixture is small relative to the solvent component.

This procedure can be modified to provide optimum conditions for particular chemical classes. For instance, preincubation times greater than 60 min plus aeration have been found necessary in the detection of allyl compounds (Neudecker and Henschler, 1985).

Maron and Ames (1983) suggest that the preincubation modification can be used routinely or when inconclusive results are obtained in the standard test. Gatehouse *et al.* (1990) propose that a novel test compound should first be tested in the plate incorporation assay and then, if negative results are obtained, the preincubation assay. This strategy is attractive, as it provides two types of exposure conditions, two levels of S9 fraction (1.8 per cent and 7.1 per cent final concentration) and some degree of repetition of experiments.

Fluctuation Tests

The fluctuation test was originally devised by Luria and Delbruck (1943) to demonstrate that bacterial variants arose by random mutation rather than by adaptation to a selective agent and to measure the rate of spontaneous mutation (Hubbard *et al.*, 1984). The development of the fluctuation test as a sensitive bacterial mutation

assay has owed much to Green and colleagues (see, e.g., Green *et al.*, 1976), who have used Ryan's modification of the test (Ryan, 1955). Further development of the assay in microtitre plates has been reported by Gatehouse (1978) and Gatehouse and Delow (1979).

In the fluctuation test the number of mutants in a series of small independent replicate cultures is determined. Amino-acid-requiring bacteria are treated in a suitable medium either with or without a metabolizing system, with the chemical to be tested and with a trace of the required amino acid. As for the Ames test, this trace allows a few generations of growth, which allows mutation expression following the initial DNA damage. This mixture is then divided into a large number of aliquots—e.g. into 50 test tubes or the 96 wells of a microtitre tray. When the trace of amino acid is consumed, only cells that have reverted at the target gene, thus restoring biosynthesis of the relevant amino acid, can grow. Test tubes or wells containing such a revertant become turbid and the medium in the well or tube becomes acid, as a result of acid release during growth. A pH indicator such as bromocresol purple or bromothymol blue can highlight such changes. The pH of the medium will drop into the range 5.2–6.8 in such cultures, causing a change of the indicator to yellow.

Protocol for the Fluctuation Test The microtitre fluctuation test is carried out as follows for the detection of compounds that do not require metabolic activation:

(1) The strains are grown at 37 °C overnight in Davis–Mingioli minimal media supplemented with the appropriate amino acids (20 μg ml^{-1}) and vitamins (1–10 μg ml^{-1}).

(2) The overnight cultures are subcultured into the same medium and incubated for a further 3 h at 37 °C with agitation (210 rev min^{-1}) to provide log phase cells.

(3) The required concentrations of test article are prepared in replicate in 20 ml of test medium containing a limited amount of the required amino acid (e.g. 1 μg ml^{-1} tryptophan). Each 20 ml is inoculated with 20 μl of one of the 3 h cultures. Untreated solvent and positive controls are included for each strain tested.

(4) Each 20 ml volume is accurately dispensed

in 200 μl aliquots into each well of sterile micro-titre plates (with lids) containing 96 wells.

(5) The plates are sealed in plastic containers. Humidity may be maintained by a 10 per cent solution of the disinfectant Roccal, in each container, which also eliminates fungal contamination.

(6) The containers are incubated for 3 days at 37 °C.

(7) At the end of the incubation period, 20 μl of bromothymol blue is added to each well to detect those in which normal growth has occurred following mutation. In cases where the acidity of the test compound interferes with the use of a pH indicator, positive wells are identified by the size of the bacterial pellet at the base of the well.

(8) The following mutagens may be used as a positive control in this test: E. coli WP2–N-ethyl-N-nitro-N-nitrosoguanidine (ENNG) (0.25 μg ml⁻¹); E. coli WP2 uvrA (pKM101)–ENNG (0.1 μg ml⁻¹).

For the detection of compounds that require metabolic activation the following protocol is used:

(1) The strains are grown and subcultured as described above.

(2) To 3 ml of fluctuation test 'preincubation' medium (glucose 16 mg ml⁻¹, trytophan 0.8 μg ml⁻¹, Davis–Mingioli salts medium) add 1 ml of S9 mix containing 100–300 μl of S9 fraction, 20 μl of a 3 h tester strain culture and test compound in appropriate solvent, and then make up to 5 ml with 0.1 M phosphate buffer (pH 7.4). Untreated, solvent and positive controls are included for each strain tested.

(3) Each 5 ml volume of reaction mixture is dispensed in 50 μl aliquots into each well of a sterile microtitre plate. The plates are incubated in sealed containers overnight at 37 °C

(4) Top up each well on the following day with 150 μl of Davis–Mingioli fluctuation test medium containing 0.8 per cent w/w glucose.

(5) The plates are incubated for a further 3 days at 37 °C in humidified plastic containers.

(6) After a total incubation period of 4 days at 37 °C, pH indicator is added as previously.

The following mutagens are suitable positive controls: E. coli WP2–cyclophosphamide (400 μg ml⁻¹); E. coli WP2 uvrA (pKM101)–2-aminoanthracene (5–20 μg ml⁻¹). Like the plate incorpor-

ation procedure, *Salmonella typhimurium* strains can be used in fluctuation tests.

Evaluation of Results A statistically significant, reproducible increase in the number of positive wells or tubes indicates a mutagenic response. The preferred methods of statistical analysis are reviewed in Robinson *et al.* (1989). The statistical analysis can be made more powerful if there are independent replicates of the control and preferably of some of the treatments. Chi-squared analysis can be used to compare treated groups with control on a 2 × 2 basis—i.e. each dose is compared with the control in turn. A single significant difference should not be regarded as firm evidence of mutagenicity. A consistent result over the same dose range in two or preferably three independent experiments should be sought.

The mutant frequency can be calculated by equating the fraction of replicate cultures containing no mutants to the zero term of the Poisson distribution:

$$m = -\ln{(P_0)}$$

where m = average number of mutants per culture and P_0 = fraction of cultures containing no mutants.

Uses of the Fluctuation Test The fluctuation test is regarded in some instances as more sensitive than the plate incorporation assay, and is particularly useful in detecting mutagens which are only effective at near-lethal doses. It is also suitable for studying samples where the concentrations of mutagens may be low. The technique has been successfully used for studying mutagens in human faeces (Kuhnlein *et al.*, 1981), urine (Falck *et al.*, 1981) food (Levin *et al.*, 1981), water supplies (Forster *et al.*, 1983) and tissue extracts (Parry *et al.*, 1976).

The fluctuation test also offers advantages as outlined for the preincubation test described in the previous section. In the plate incorporation assay the test agent, cofactors and soluble cytosolic soluble fraction of the S9 mix can diffuse out of the agar overlay into the basal agar. This can have several consequences, including the use of initially higher concentrations of test agent in the Ames test, causing problems with highly toxic, weakly mutagenic samples (Hubbard *et al.*, 1984) and difficulties in detecting labile mutagenic metabolites which can quickly become depleted in the plate incorporation assay. Under these circumstances the fluctuation test is the preferred method (Gatehouse and Wedd, 1984).

Antibiotics can provide a difficult challenge in bacterial mutation tests. The fluctuation test can be used to test high concentrations of β-lactam antibiotics which will kill susceptible bacteria only if they are growing and thus synthesizing new cell wall components. In this modification of the test, exposure takes place in buffer or unsupplemented minimal media. Following exposure the cells are removed by filtration and washed. The filters are suspended in fluctuation test medium and the test carried out as normal (Paes and Tweats, 1980).

In the laboratories of Glaxo, Ware, Hertfordshire, UK, the fluctuation test with *E. coli* tester strains has been used for over 10 years, alongside the Ames test, *Salmonella typhimurium* strains being used for the detection of bacterial mutagens. This approach has proved to be very powerful to cover specificity of genetic marker, the need to run tests in liquid and agar, and the need to carry out tests at different concentrations of S9 fraction.

Treat and Plate Tests
Treat and plate assays, in which the agent is incubated with the bacterial tester strain prior to plating, is another test with advantages related to exposure to the test agent in liquid. Thus, the test may be preferred for the detection of labile mutagenic metabolites and for the detection of agents that are only mutagenic at levels close to bactericidal concentrations. In this assay the exposure to the test agent is normally carried out in buffer without nutrients, followed by the selection of mutants on selective agar. Thus, the test can be used when growth stimulation due to the test agent would confound the methods described earlier (Green, 1984; Mahon *et al.*, 1989) and can be used for testing β-lactam antibiotics (Tweats and Paes, 1981).

In this test, care has to be taken concerning background mutation levels. In selecting the inoculum size for exposure to the test agent, it has to be borne in mind that the number of exposed cells should be sufficiently large to detect the small number of mutants induced by the agent at the target locus. However, the inoculum must not be so large that the number of pre-existing mutants is in great excess compared with the

number of induced mutants. In addition, the number of spontaneous mutants present after plating on selective agar should not be so small that there are random major variations in counts between control and treated cultures.

Protocol for the Treat and Plate Test For tests in the absence of metabolic activation the following protocol is used, derived from Green (1984):

(1) Log-phase cultures are prepared as for the fluctuation test, to a titre of approximately 2×10^8 cells ml^{-1}.
(2) The cultures are centrifuged, resuspended in Davis–Mingioli salts media (unsupplemented) (DM) and recentrifuged to wash the cells. The pellet is resuspended in an equal volume of DM.
(3) Three to five concentrations of test agent are added to the washed cultures in labelled universal bottles. Untreated solvent and positive controls are prepared in the same manner.
(4) The universals are incubated at 37 °C for a set period, e.g. 30–60 min.
(5) Treatment may be terminated by centrifugation and washing as in step (2) above, or the cells may be removed by filtration, followed by resuspension in fresh DM medium. Care must be taken to dispose of the unwanted and chemically contaminated filtrate or centrifugation washing. (One method used in the laboratories at Glaxo is to solidify the contaminated liquids with agar. Then the agar is burnt.)
(6) The cell suspension is spread (0.1–0.2 ml) on to minimal media selective agar—e.g. DM medium containing glucose but deficient in tryptophan (0.25 μg ml^{-1}) for the *E. coli* WP2 series. Three to five plates should be used.
(7) In this test, unlike the plate incorporation assay, survival is also measured. The cell suspension is diluted in DM to 10^{-5}–10^{-6}-fold in 0.1–9.9 ml and 0.5–4.5 ml steps. Again 0.1–0.2 ml is spread on to supplemented DM plates containing excess tryptophan (20 μg ml^{-1}). As before, 3–5 plates per group should be prepared.
(8) The plates are incubated at 37 °C for 48–72 h.
(9) The number of colonies per selective plate is calculated, as is the number of colonies on the survival plates.

For tests in the presence of metabolic activation the only modification is to add 1 ml of standard

S9 mix (as described above) to 4 ml of washed bacterial culture suspended in unsupplemented DM medium, then proceed as per the normal method from step (3). Different levels of S9 fraction in the S9 mix can be used if required.

As for the other test protocols described, the test should be repeated for confirmation of results.

Evaluation of Results To determine the mutant frequency for a given treatment, the following calculation should be performed:

$$\frac{\text{No. of mutants per treated plate } - \text{ No. of mutants per control plate}}{\text{No. of viable cells per treated plate}}$$

Green (1984) gives a firm warning against using the following invalid calculation:

$$\text{mutation frequency} = \frac{\text{mutants per treated plate}}{\text{viable cells per treated plate}} - \frac{\text{mutants per control plate}}{\text{viable cells per control plate}}$$

which gives false results. The reasons for this can be understood if spontaneous mutation, under the conditions of the assay, is considered. As explained previously, when there is a trace of the required amino acid in the selective plates, two classes of spontaneous mutant are observed: (a) pre-existing mutants, present in the population at the time of plating; (b) plate mutants which arise during the short period of growth on the plate, which stops when the amino acid is exhausted. In practice, most of the spontaneous mutants that are observed are plate mutants. The number of plate mutants is dependent on the final number of auxotrophic cells which can grow on the selective agar plate and are therefore able to mutate. This number is dependent on the amount of, for example, tryptophan in the selective agar. It is almost independent of the number of cells plated. However, when many cells are plated (within limits of approximately 5×10^4 and 5×10^8), the *same* number of cells will grow on the selective plate containing the limiting tryptophan and will give rise to approximately the same number of plate mutants. Although this danger of miscalculation has been well known for years, occasionally

papers still appear having fallen into this trap—e.g. as pointed out by Paes (1984).

A treat and plate test is regarded as positive if the mutation frequency is statistically significantly increased compared with the control in replicate experiments. The test is discussed in Mahon *et al.* (1989), and the tests for statistical significance are those recommended for mammalian gene mutation assay results, as described by Arlett *et al.* (1989). The latter authors recommend analyses of data by weighted analysis of variance (regression), using either Poisson-derived or empirically-derived weights. Mutation frequency should be tested at each treatment dose for a significant increase over the negative control. A test should be carried out for a significant linear relationship between increasing mutant frequency and increasing dose.

In a treat and plate test, a defined number of cells is treated with a defined level of mutagen for a defined period, and the results are related to survival. Therefore, the test is the method of choice for quantitative measurement of mutagenicity (Green, 1984).

Forward Mutation Tests

Forward mutation is an end-point that may arise from various events, including base substitutions, frameshifts, DNA deletions, etc., as mentioned earlier.

Although bacterial forward mutation systems have not gained the popularity of reverse mutation tests (owing, in part, to lower sensitivity to some mutagens and lack of specificity), they have proved useful on occasion and have their supporters.

Several forward mutation tests have been devised, and a brief mention of two of the more widely used systems is provided below.

The ara *Forward Mutation Test* The L-arabinose resistance test with *Salmonella typhimurium* is based on *ara D* mutants of the L-arabinose operon (Hera and Pueyo, 1986). *ara D* mutants are unable to use L-arabinose as the sole carbon source. The assay scores a change from L-arabinose sensitivity to L-arabinose resistance, which is defined as the ability to grow in a medium containing L-arabinose plus another carbon source such as glycerol.

This phenotypic change reflects forward mutations in at least three different loci in the arabinose operon (Pueyo and Lopez-Barea, 1979).

Strains have been constructed along the same lines as the recommended Ames strains with mutations to remove excision repair and mutations to increase permeability, and including the mutator plasmid pKM101—i.e. *Salmonella typhimurium* BA3 *ara D531, hisG46*, △uvrB *bio* and BA9 *araD531, hisG46* △uvrB, *bio, rfa* (pKM101).

Protocols for the test have included plate incorporation, preincubation, and treat and plate tests (Hera and Pueyo, 1986). In the latter tests the assay does not have the problem of 'plate mutants' as described for reverse mutation tests in the previous section. The recommended procedure has the following outline protocol:

(1) Incubate the test strain of bacteria (10^7–10^8 cells per ml) and the test agent at 37 °C in non-selective DM medium with shaking.

(2) Wash the cells after a 2 h exposure period.

(3) Plate on selective medium (DM salts, 2 mg ml^{-1} glycerol, 2 mg ml^{-1} L-arabinose, 20 μg ml^{-1} L-histidine, 12 μg ml^{-1} biotin) containing an additional supplement of D-glucose, 0.5 mg per plate.

For metabolic activation 30 μl of S9 fraction and appropriate cofactors are included in the initial incubation mixture as the standard level. Different concentrations of S9 fraction can be used as required.

The group who have developed this test recommend that strain BA9 can replace the four strains used in the standard Ames test and that for the mutagens tested to date this strain detects the same range of mutagens as the Ames test strains with equal or better sensitivity. The test does seem suitable for testing complex mixtures such as red wine (Dorado *et al.*, 1988). However, the spontaneous background count using the protocol outlined above is over 500 per plate. If fewer cells are used, false negative results are obtained (Xu *et al.*, 1984).

Versatility of Bacterial Mutation Assays

In the previous subsection the use of bacterial mutation tests to measure the mutagenicity of a complex mixture (red wine) is mentioned. Space does not allow the description of modifications of the standard protocols for special circumstances.

However, the reader is recommended to read the following references if requiring information on the following test situations:

Testing of volatile or gaseous mutagens, which requires the use of closed or sealed containment (e.g. Bridges, 1978; Hirota *et al.*, 1987).

The testing of urine, faeces or body fluids for traces of mutagens, which may require concentration of the relevant fluids using, e.g., XAD–2 columns (review: Combes *et al.*, 1984).

The measurement of the formation of mutagenic nitroso derivatives following nitrosation of compounds likely to be ingested by humans (WHO, 1978; Kirkland *et al.*, 1984).

Detection of mutagens in food (Rowland *et al.*, 1984).

Eukaryotic Mutation Tests

Prokaryotic systems, as described, have proved to be quick, versatile and in many cases surprisingly accurate in identifying potential genetic hazards to man. However, there are intrinsic differences between eukaryotic and prokaryotic cells in the organization of the genome and the processing of the genetic information (see p. 808). Thus, there is a place for test systems based on mammalian cells for fundamental studies to understand the mutation process in higher cells and for the use of such tests for screening for genotoxic effects.

The early work of Muller showed the usefulness of the fruit fly *Drosophila melanogaster* as a higher system for measuring germ line mutations in a whole animal. The *Drosophila* sex-linked recessive lethal test has yielded much useful information (see below, pp. 853–855) and in the 1970s was a popular system for screening chemicals for mutation, but this test failed to perform well in international collaborative trials to study the utility of such tests to detect carcinogens and popularity waned. Another *Drosophila* test devised in the 1980s, the SMART assay (Somatic Mutation and Recombination Test) shows much promise and may revive the popularity of *Drosophila* for screening for genotoxic agents (see pp. 853–855).

There are a number of *in vivo* tests to measure mutation in rodents, such as the mouse specific-locus test (pp. 856–857). These are very useful for fundamental studies of radiation and chemically induced mutation, but they are rather cumbersome, are used in only a small number of expert laboratories, and are used in special circumstances where germ-line damage needs to be measured. This situation is rapidly changing as the new technologies of the last 10–15 years begin to have an impact in the construction of new model systems to measure mutation *in vivo* (see 'Future Developments', pp. 858–860).

In contrast to the situation *in vivo*, there are a number of test systems that use cultured mammalian cells, from both established and primary lines, that now have a large database of tested chemicals in the literature, that are relatively rapid and that are feasible to use for genetic toxicity screening. These are discussed in the next section.

In Vitro Tests for the Detection of Mammalian Mutation

There have been a variety of *in vitro* mutation systems described in the literature, but only a small number have been defined adequately for quantitative studies (Cole *et al.*, 1990). These are based on the detection of forward mutations in a similar manner to the systems described earlier for bacteria (pp. 832–833). A defined large number of cells are treated with the test agent and then, after a set interval, exposed to a selective toxic agent, so that only cells that have mutated can survive. As cultured mammalian cells are diploid (or near-diploid), normally there are two copies of each gene. Recessive mutations can be missed if a normal copy is present on the homologous chromosome. As mutation frequencies for individual genes are normally very low, an impossibly large population of cells would need to be screened to detect cells in which both copies are inactivated by mutation. This problem is overcome by measuring mutation in genes on the X chromosome in male cells where only one copy of the gene will be present, or using heterozygous genes where two copies of a gene may be present but one copy is already inactive through mutation or deletion.

Many genes are essential for the survival of the cell in culture, and thus mutations in such genes would be difficult to detect. However, use has been made of genes that are not essential for cell survival but allow the cell to salvage nucleotides from the surrounding medium. This saves the cell energy, as it does not have to make these compounds from simpler precursors by energy-expensive catabolism. These enzymes are located at the cell membrane. If the cell is supplied with toxic nucleotides, the 'normal' unmutated cells will transport these into the cell and kill the cell. However, if the cells have lost the enzyme as a result of mutation (or chromosomal deletion, rearrangement, etc.), then they will not be able to 'salvage' the exogenous toxic nucleotides and will survive. The surviving mutant cells can be detected by the formation of colonies on tissue culture plates or, in some cases, in the wells of microtitre plates.

One factor to take into account with these tests is that of expression time. Although a gene may be inactivated by mutation, the mRNA existing before the mutational event may decay only slowly, so that active enzyme may be present for some time after exposure to the mutagen. Thus, the cells have to be left for a period before challenging with the toxic nucleotide: this is the expression time, and differs between systems.

The two most popular genes for measuring mutation *in vitro* are those coding for hypoxanthine guanine phosphoribosyl transferase (*Hgprt*) and thymidine kinase (*TK*). The *Hgprt* gene is located on the X chromosome in humans and in the Chinese hamster, from which many useful cell lines have been obtained. This gene has been cloned and sequenced (Konecki *et al.*, 1982; Patel *et al.*, 1986a). In man it is a large gene (44 kilobases) containing 9 exon blocks (Patel *et al.*, 1986a). It appears that for hemizygous loci such as *Hgprt*, large genetic changes such as chromosomal deletions may not be tolerated, as these extend to flanking regions of the target gene, which may contain essential genes. As there is only one copy of such genes in male cells, those containing these changes will be lost. Thus, where the *Hgprt* gene is the genetic target, the changes detected are primarily point mutations (see, e.g., Rossiter *et al.*, 1990).

There is added interest in the *Hgprt* gene, as total deficiency in humans leads to the neurological disorder known as the Lesch–Nyan syndrome, while partial deficiency is associated with forms of gouty arthritis (Kelly and Wyngaarden, 1983). Analysis of Lesch–Nyan patients has shown that point mutations, small deletions and rearrangements have inactivated the *Hgprt* gene in relevant patients (Patel *et al.*, 1986b).

The *TK* gene is autosomal, is of moderate size (11–13 kilobases) and is present on chromosome

11 in the mouse and chromosome 17 in humans. As heterozygotes (TK^+/TK^-) cells are used for screening for mutagenicity, all kinds of genetic events are theoretically detectable, including chromosomal changes.

Apart from direct DNA changes, there is evidence that apparent loss of gene function can occur due to modification of gene expression as a result of DNA methylation. Treatment with 5-azacytidine, which demethylates DNA, can reactivate the expression of some 'mutations' at both *TK* (Harris, 1982) and *Hgprt* (Grant and Worton, 1982) loci.

Chinese Hamster Lines

Chinese hamster cell lines have given much valuable data over the past 15 years but their use for screening is limited by lack of sensitivity, as only a relatively small target cell population can be used, owing to metabolic co-operation (see Cole *et al.*, 1990); however, they are still in use, so a brief description follows.

Chinese hamster CHO and V79 lines have high plating efficiencies and short generation times (less than 24 h). These properties make the lines useful for mutagenicity experiments. Both cell lines have grossly rearranged chromosomal complements, which has an unknown effect on their responsiveness to mutagens (Tweats and Gatehouse, 1988). There is some evidence that Chinese hamster lines are undergoing genetic drift in different culture collections (Kirkland, 1992).

V79 System

The Chinese hamster V79 line was established in 1958 (Ford and Yerganian, 1958). Publication of the use of the line for mutation studies (by measuring resistance to purine analogues due to mutation at the *Hgprt* locus) occurred 10 years later (Chu and Malling, 1968). The V79 line was derived from a male Chinese hamster; hence, V79 cells possess only a single X chromosome.

V79 cells grow as a cell sheet or monolayer on glass or plastic surfaces. If large numbers of cells are treated with a mutagen, when plated out, cells in close contact can link via intracellular bridges. These allow the transfer of cellular components between cells such as messenger RNA. Thus, if a cell carries a mutation in the *Hgprt* gene resulting in the inactivation of the relevant mRNA, it can receive viable mRNA or intact enzyme from adjacent non-mutated cells. Therefore, when the mutated cell is challenged with a toxic purine, it is lost, owing to the presence of active enzyme derived from the imported mRNA. This phenomenon is termed 'metabolic co-operation' and severely limits the sensitivity of lines such as V79 for mutagen detection. This drawback can be overcome to an extent by carrying out the detection of mutant clones in semi-solid agar (see, e.g., Oberly *et al.*, 1987) or by using the 'respreading technique' (see, e.g., Fox, 1981).

The theoretical basis of the V79/*Hgprt* (and CHO/*hgprt*) assay is shown in Figure 14, with 8-azaguanine (8-AG) or preferably 6-thioguanine (6-TG) as the selective agent. The latter purine is more efficient in eliminating sensitive cells than is 8-AZ (see, e.g., Newbold *et al.*, 1975).

The preferred expression time for *Hgprt* mutants is 6–8 days, although care needs to be taken when testing chemicals well into the toxic range, where the 'expression time' needs to be extended to allow recovery.

Preliminary Cytotoxicity Testing An essential first step is to carry out a preliminary study to evaluate the toxicity of the test material to the indicator cells, under the conditions of the main

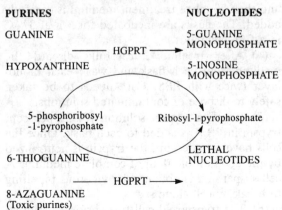

The V79 cell line is derived from a male Chinese hamster and thus possesses XY chromosomes in its karyotype.

The Hgprt gene is located on the X chromosome.

∴ Each cell contains only one functional gene.

∴ One mutational event can render the cell hgprt⁻.

PURINES	NUCLEOTIDES
GUANINE	5-GUANINE MONOPHOSPHATE
HYPOXANTHINE	5-INOSINE MONOPHOSPHATE

HGPRT ⟶

5-phosphoribosyl-1-pyrophosphate   Ribosyl-1-pyrophosphate

6-THIOGUANINE   LETHAL NUCLEOTIDES

HGPRT ⟶

8-AZAGUANINE
(Toxic purines)

HGPRT⁺ cells are killed by 6-thioguanine/8-azaguanine hgprt⁻ cells survive (essential purines are synthesised *de novo*)

Figure 14 The theoretical basis of the V79/Hgprt assay

mutagenicity test. When selecting dose levels, the solubility of the test compound, the resulting pH of the media and the osmolality of the test solutions all need to be considered. The latter two parameters have been known to induce false positive effects in *in vitro* mammalian tests (see, e.g., Brusick, 1986). The experimental procedure is carried out as follows:

(1) Seed T75 plastic tissue culture flasks with a minimum of 2.5×10^6 cells in 20 ml of Eagle's medium containing 20 mM L-glutamine; 0.88 g l^{-1} sodium bicarbonate; 20 mM HEPES; 50 μg ml^{-1} streptomycin sulphate; 50 IU ml^{-1} benzylpenicillin; and 7.5 per cent of fetal bovine serum. The flasks are incubated for 18–24 h at 37 °C in a CO_2 incubator to establish monolayer cultures.

(2) Prepare treatment medium containing various concentrations of test compound—e.g. 19.7 ml of Eagle's medium (without serum) plus 300 μl of stock concentration of compound in a preferred solvent (e.g. water, ethanol, DMSO, etc.). The final concentration of solvent other than water should not exceed 1 per cent v/v. Normally a range of 0–5000 μg ml^{-1} (final concentration) is covered. For a sparingly soluble compound, the highest concentration will be the lowest at which visible precipitation occurs. Similarly, if a compound has a marked effect on osmolality, concentrations should not be used that exceed 500 milliosmoles (mosm) per kg. In addition, a pH range of 6.5–7.5 should not be exceeded.

(3) Each cell monolayer is rinsed with a minimum of 20 ml phosphate buffered saline (PBS) and then 20 ml of treatment medium is carefully added. The flasks are incubated for 3 h at 37 °C in a CO_2 incubator.

(4) After treatment, carefully discard the medium from each flask and wash each monolayer twice with PBS. Care needs to be taken safely to dispose of contaminated solutions.

(5) 10 ml of trypsin solution (0.025 per cent trypsin in PBS) is added to each flask. Once the cells have rounded up, the trypsin is neutralized by the addition of 10 ml of complete medium. A cell suspension is obtained by vigorous pipetting to break up cell clumps.

(6) The trypsinized cell suspension is counted and diluted in complete media before assessing for survival. For each treatment set up five Petri dishes containing 200 cells per dish.

(7) Incubate at 37 °C in a CO_2 incubator for 7–10 days.

(8) The medium is removed and the colonies are fixed and stained, using 5 per cent Giemsa in buffered formalin. Once the colonies are stained, the Giemsa is removed and the colonies are counted.

The method can be repeated including 20 per cent v/v S9 mix.

To calculate percentage survival, the following formula is used:

$$\frac{\text{cell titre in treated culture}}{\text{cell titre in control culture}} \times \frac{\text{mean no. of colonies on treated plates}}{\text{mean no. of colonies on control plates}} \times 100$$

The cloning efficiency (CE) of the control culture is calculated as follows:

$$CE = \frac{\text{mean no. of colonies per plate}}{\text{no. of cells per plate (i.e. 200)}} \times 100$$

In the absence of precipitation or effects on pH or osmolality, the maximum concentration of the main mutagenicity study is a concentration that reduces survival to approximately 20 per cent of the control value.

Procedure for the Chinese Hamster V79/Hgprt Assay The assay usually comprises three test concentrations, each in duplicate, and four vehicle control replicates. Suitable positive controls are ethylmethane sulphonate (−S9) and dimethyl benzanthracene (+S9). V79 cells with a low nominal passage number should be used from frozen stocks to help minimize genetic drift. The procedure described includes a reseeding step for mutation expression.

Steps 1–5 are the same as the cytotoxicity assay. As before, tests can be carried out in the presence and in the absence of S9 mix.

(6) The trypsinized cultures are counted and a sample is assessed for survival as for the cytotoxicity assay. In addition, an appropriate number of cells are reseeded for estimation of mutation frequency at the day 8 expression time. The cells

are transferred to roller bottles (usually 490 cm²) for this stage. The bottles are gassed with pure CO_2, the tops are tightened and the bottles are incubated at 37 °C on a roller machine (approximate speed 0.5–1.0 rev min⁻¹). Usually 10⁶ viable cells are reseeded in 50 ml of Eagle's medium containing serum, but more cells are required at the toxic dose levels.

(7) The bottles are subcultured as necessary throughout the expression period to maintain sub-confluency. This involves retrypsinization and determining the cell titre for each treatment. For each culture a fresh roller bottle is reseeded with a minimum of 10⁶ cells.

(8) On day 8, each culture is again trypsinized, counted and diluted so that a sample cell population can be assessed for cloning efficiency and a second sample can be assessed for the induction of 6TG-resistant cells.

(9) The cell suspension is diluted in complete medium and 2×10^5 cells added per petri dish (10 petri dishes per treatment). 6-Thioguanine is added to the medium at a final concentration of 10 μg ml⁻¹.

(10) The petri dishes are incubated for 7–10 days and the medium is then removed. The colonies are fixed and stained as previously. The colonies (>50 cells per clone) are then counted.

Mutation frequency in each culture is calculated as:

$$\frac{\text{mean no. colonies on thioguanine plates}}{1000 \times \text{mean no. colonies on survival plates}}$$

Data Analysis (see Arlett *et al.*, 1989) A weighted analysis of variance is performed on the mutation frequencies, as the variation in the number of mutations per plate usually increases as the mean increases. Each dose of test compound is compared with the corresponding vehicle control by means of a one-sided Dunnett's test and, in addition, the mutation frequencies are examined to see whether there is a linear relationship with dose.

The criterion employed for a positive response in this assay is a reproducible statistically significant increase in mutation frequency (weighted mean for duplicate treated cultures) over the concurrent vehicle control value (weighted mean for four independent control cultures). Ideally, the response should show evidence of a dose–response relationship. When a small isolated significant increase in mutation frequency is observed in only one of the two duplicate experiments, then a third test should be carried out. If the third test shows no significant effects, the initial increase is likely to be a chance result. In cases where an apparent treated-related increase is thought to be a result of unusually low variability or a low control frequency, comparison with the laboratory historical control frequency may be justified.

Chinese Hamster CHO/Hgprt System Chinese hamster ovary (CHO) cells have 21 or 22 chromosomes with one intact X chromosome and a large acrocentric marker chromosome (Natarajan and Obe, 1982). The use of these cells in mammalian mutation experiments was first reported by Hsie *et al.* (1975), and was refined into a quantitative assay for mutagenicity testing by O'Neill *et al.* (1977a, b). The performance of this system has been reviewed by the US EPA Gene-Tox Program (Li *et al.*, 1988). The experimental procedure for this assay is similar to the V79/Hgprt system already described, and for more detailed descriptions the reader is referred to Li *et al.* (1987).

Mouse Lymphoma L5178Y TK⁺/⁻ Assay
Whereas the Chinese hamster cell systems are regarded as relatively insensitive, the mouse lymphoma L5178Y TK⁺/⁻ test is undoubtedly more sensitive. Unfortunately, there are persistent doubts regarding its specificity—i.e. the ability to distinguish between carcinogens and non-carcinogens (see, e.g., Tennant *et al.*, 1987). However, a great advantage is the ability of these cells to grow in suspension culture in which intracellular bridges do not occur. Thus, the problems of metabolic co-operation are avoided, which allows a large number of cells to be treated for optimum statistical analysis of results.

A candid historical overview of the development of the mouse lymphoma TK⁺/⁻ mutagenicity assay is given by its originator, Clive (1987). Initially methodologies were developed for producing the three TK genotypes (TK⁺/⁺ and TK⁻/⁻ homozygotes and the TK⁺/⁻ heterozygote) and optimizing conditions for isolating the first TK⁺/⁻ heterozygotes (Clive *et al.*, 1972). This first heterozygote was lost; however, it was recognized that subsequent heterozygotes produced distinctly bimodal distributions of mutant-colony sizes, owing to differences in growth rate. These were interpreted in terms of single-gene (large-colony mutants) and viable chromosomal mutations (small-colony mutants). A period of diversification of the mouse lymphoma assay followed and controversy over the significance of small-colony mutants (see, e.g., Amacher *et al.*, 1980).

Following this, a series of cytogenetic studies confirmed the cytogenetic interpretation for small-colony mutants (see, e.g., Hozier *et al.*, 1982). Molecular studies showed that most mutations resulting in small-colony mutants involve large-scale deletions (Evans *et al.*, 1986). A current theory states that, for many compounds, deletion mutants are induced by binding of the compound to complexes between topoisomerase II and DNA (see, e.g., DeMarini *et al.*, 1987; Clive, 1989). Topoisomerases are enzymes that control supercoiling via breakage and reunion of DNA strands; it is the latter step that is disrupted, which leads to chromosome damage and deletions. Further molecular studies (Applegate *et al.*, 1990) have shown that a wide variety of genetic events can result in the formation of $TK^{-/-}$ genotype from the heterozygote, including recombinations and mitotic non-disjunction.

The $TK^{+/-}$ line was originally isolated as a spontaneously arising revertant clone from a UV-induced $TK^{-/-}$ clone. The parental $TK^{+/+}$ cell and the heterozygote were then the only TK-competent mouse lymphoma cells that could be maintained in THMG medium (3 μg ml^{-1} thymidine, 5 μg ml^{-1} hypoxanthine, 0.1 μg ml^{-1} methotrexate and 7.5 μg ml^{-1} glycine) (Clive, 1987). Thus, like most established lines, these cells are remote from wild-type cells. The karyotype of the $TK^{+/-}$ −3.7.2C line has a modal chromosome number of 40 like wild-type, but has a variety of chromosomal rearrangements and centromeric heteromorphisms (Sawyer *et al.*, 1985; Blazak *et al.*, 1986).

The theoretical basis for the mouse lymphoma L5178Y/TK$^{+/-}$ → TK$^{-/-}$ assay is shown in Figure 15.

Two main protocols have been devised for carrying out mutation assays with mouse lymphoma L5178Y cells—i.e. plating the cells in soft agar or a fluctuation test approach. It is the latter that is described in the following section, based

The gene coding for thymidine kinase (TK) is on mouse chromosomes number 11.

The mouse lymphoma L5178Y line is $TK^{+/-}$, i.e. one gene copy is already inactivated by mutation.

∴ Each cell contains only one functional gene.

∴ One mutational event can render the cell tk$^{-/-}$.

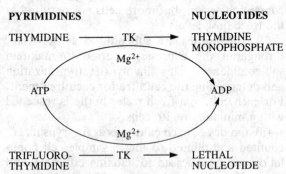

PYRIMIDINES   **NUCLEOTIDES**

$TK^{+/-}$ cells are killed by trifluorothymidine
tk$^{-/-}$ cells survive (thymidine monophosphate can be synthesized *de novo* via thymidylate synthetase etc.)

Figure 15 The theoretical basis of the L5178Y $TK^{+/-}$ mouse lymphoma assay

on Cole *et al.* (1986). The reader is referred to Clive *et al.* (1987) for a full description of the soft-agar method.

Preliminary Cytotoxicity Assay The cells are maintained in RPMI 1640 medium containing 2.0 mM glutamine, 20 mM HEPES, 200 μg ml^{-1} sodium pyruvate, 50 IU ml^{-1} benzylpenicillin, 50 μg ml^{-1} streptomycin sulphate and 10 per cent donor horse serum (heat-inactivated for 30 min at 56 °C). This medium is designated CM10. Conditioned medium is CM10 in which cells have grown exponentially for at least 1 day. Treatment medium contains 3 per cent horse serum and 30 per cent conditioned media (CM3). Medium without serum is known as incomplete medium (ICM). If treatment time exceeds 3 h, treatment is carried out in CM10.

The method is as follows:

(1) The cell titre of an exponentially growing culture of cells in CM10 is determined with a Coulter counter. The cell suspension is centrifuged at 70 *g* for 5 min and the supernatant is reduced such that 3 ml contains approximately 5 × 10^6 cells (3 h treatment) or 2 × 10^6 (treatment >3 h).

(2a) For tests in the absence of S9 mix, treatment groups are prepared by mixing 3 ml of the above cell suspension, 0.1 ml of solution of test compound and 6.9 ml of ICM (3 h treatment) or 6.9 ml of CM10 (treatment >3 h).

(2b) Tests in the presence of S9 mix are carried out in the same way, except the treatment medium contains 10 per cent v/v S9 mix at the expense of ICM—i.e. 3 ml cell suspension, 5.9 ml ICM, 1 ml S9 mix and 0.1 ml test compound solution/vehicle. The composition of the S9 mix is as described earlier (p. 896). It is prepared immediately before required and kept on ice until it is added to the test system. For the vehicle controls, if an organic solvent is used, it should not exceed 1 per cent v/v.

(3) After the treatment period, cells are spun down at 70 g for 5 min and the supernatant is transferred for assessment of pH (pH meter) and osmolality (e.g. using Wescor Vapour Pressure Osmometer). The cell pellet is washed twice in PBS and then resuspended in 10 ml CM10. (All contaminated material and waste should be disposed of safely.)

(4) The cell titre of each culture is counted and a sample diluted in CM10 for assessment of post-treatment survival. For this two 96-well microtitre plates are charged with 200 μl of a diluted cell suspension, using a multi-channel pipette such that each well contains on average 1 cell.

(5) Plates are incubated for 7–8 days at 37 °C and 5 per cent CO_2 in 95 $\pm$ 3 per cent relative humidity.

(6) The plates are removed from the incubator and 20 μl of MTT [3-(4,5-dimethylthiazol-2-yl)-2,5-diphenyltetrazolium bromide] at 5 mg ml^{-1} (in PBS) is added to each well with a multichannel pipette. The plates are left to stand for 1–4 h and are then scored for the presence of colonies with a Titertek mirror-box, which allows direct viewing of the bottom surface of the plates.

(7) Cytotoxicity can also be determined post-treatment as follows: T25 flasks are set up after treatment containing 0.75×10^5 cells per ml in 5 ml CM10. Flasks are incubated with loose lids at 37 °C with 5 per cent CO_2 in 95 $\pm$ 3 per cent relative humidity. Two days later the cell titre of each culture is determined with a Coulter counter.

(8) Following this procedure, various calculations are carried out to aid selection of dose levels for the main mutation assay.

(a) *Cloning efficiency* In microtitre assays calculations are based on the Poisson distribution—i.e.

$$P(o) = \frac{\text{no. of wells without a colony}}{\text{total no. of cells}}$$

$$\text{cloning efficiency (CE)} = \frac{-\ln P_0}{\text{No. of cells per well}} \times 100 \text{ per cent}$$

(b) *Relative survival* Relative survival (S) is calculated as follows:

$$S = \frac{\text{CE of treated group}}{\text{CE of control group}}$$

(c) *Growth* Growth in suspension (SG) is calculated as follows:

$$SG = \frac{\text{cell count after 3 days}}{0.75 \times 10^5}$$

Relative suspension growth (RSG) is calculated as follows:

$$RSG = \frac{\text{SG of treated group}}{\text{SG of control group}} \times 100 \text{ per cent}$$

Selection of Dose Levels The highest test concentration is selected from one of the following options, whichever is the lowest:

- A concentration which reduces survival to about 10–20 per cent of the control value.
- A concentration which reduces RSG to 10–20 per cent of the control value.
- The lowest concentration at which visible precipitation occurs.
- The highest concentration which does not increase the osmolality of the medium to greater than 400 mmol kg^{-1} or 100 mmol above the value for the solvent control.
- The highest concentration that does not alter the pH of the treatment medium beyond the range 6.8–7.5.
- If none of these conditions are met, 5 mg ml^{-1} should be used.

Lower test concentrations are selected as fractions of the highest concentration, usually including one dose which causes 20–70 per cent survival and one dose which causes >70 per cent survival.

Main Mutation Assay The assay normally comprises three test concentrations, a positive control and vehicle control. All treatment groups are set up in duplicate. The expression time is 2 days, unless there are indications that the test agent inhibits cell proliferation, where an additional or possibly alternative expression time should be employed.

Stock cultures are established from frozen ampoules of cells that have been treated with thymidine, hypoxanthine, methotrexate and glycine for 24 h, which purges the culture of pre-existing $TK^{-/-}$ mutants. This cell stock is used for a maximum of 2 months.

Treatment is normally carried out in 50 ml centrifuge tubes on a roller machine. During the expression time the cells are grown in T75 plastic tissue culture flasks. For estimation of cloning efficiency and mutant induction, cells are plated out in 96-well microtitre plates. Flasks and microtitre plates are incubated at 37 °C in a CO_2 incubator as in the cytotoxicity assays.

Cell titres are determined by diluting of the cell suspension in Isoton and counting an appropriate volume (usually 0.5 ml) with a Coulter counter. Two counts are made per suspension.

The experimental procedure is carried out as follows:

(1) On the day of treatment stock solutions for the positive control and the various concentrations of test compound (selected as per the previous section) are prepared.

(2) Treatment is carried out in 30 per cent conditioned media. The serum concentration is 3 per cent (3 h treatment) or 10 per cent (treated >3 h).

(3) Cell suspensions of exponentially growing cells are prepared as in the cytotoxicity assay, except that 6 ml of media required for each treatment culture contains 10^7 cells (3 h treatment) or 3×10^6 cells (>3 h treatment). The number of cells per treatment may be increased if marked cytotoxicity is expected, to allow enough cells to survive (e.g. if 20 per cent survival or less is expected, 2×10^7 cells may be treated).

(4) For tests in the absence of S9 mix, 6 ml of cell suspension, 0.2 ml test compound/vehicle and 13.8 ml ICM (3 h treatment) or 13.8 ml CM10

(treatment >7 h) are mixed in a 50 ml centrifuge tube. For treatments in the presence of S9 mix, 6 ml cell suspension, 11.8 ml ICM, second S9 mix and 0.2 ml of test compound/vehicle are prepared.

(5) After treatment the cells are centrifuged at 70 g for 5 min, and supernatant is discarded and the cell pellet is resuspended in PBS (pH 7). This washing procedure is repeated twice, and finally the cell pellet is resuspended in CM10.

(6) Each culture is counted so that a sample of cells can be assessed for post-treatment survival, and the remaining cell population assessed for estimation of mutation frequency.

(7) For survival estimation, cells are placed into 96-well microtitre trays at a cell density of 1 cell per well as per the cytotoxicity assay.

(8) For mutation estimation, the cells are diluted to a cell density of 2×10^5 cells per ml with CM10 in tissue culture flasks and the culture is incubated at 37 °C in a CO_2 incubator. On day 1 each culture is counted and diluted with fresh medium to a cell density of 2×10^5 cells per ml in a maximum of 100 ml of medium.

(9) On day 2 each culture is counted again and an aliquot of cells taken so that: (a) a sample of the cell population can be assessed for cloning efficiency. Plates are incubated at 37 °C in a CO_2 incubator for 7 days. (b) a sample of the cell population can be assessed for the induction of TFT-resistant cells (mutants). For this 2×10^3 cells are plated per well in 200 μl CM10 containing 4 μg ml^{-1} TFT. TFT and TFT-containing cultures must not be exposed to bright light, as the material is light-sensitive. The plates are incubated for 10–12 days at 37 °C in a CO_2 incubator.

(10) At the end of incubation 20 μl MTT is added to each well. The plates are left to develop for 1–4 h at 37 °C and then scored for colony-bearing wells. Colonies are scored by eye and are classified as small or large.

The calculation for cloning efficiency is made as for the cytotoxicity assay.

Relative total growth (RTG) is a cytotoxicity parameter which considers growth in suspension during the expression time and the cloning efficiency of the end of the expression time as follows:

$$\text{Suspension growth (SG)} = \frac{24 \text{ h cell count}}{2 \times 10^5} \times \frac{48 \text{ h cell count}}{2 \times 10^5}$$

$$RTG = \frac{\text{SG treated culture}}{\text{SG control culture}} \times \frac{\text{CE of treated culture}}{\text{CE of control culture}}$$

Mutation frequency (MF) is calculated as follows:

$$MF = \frac{-\ln P_0 \text{ for mutation plates}}{\text{No. of cells per well} \times CE/100}$$

Data Analysis Data from the fluctuation test described above are analysed by an appropriate statistical method as described in Robinson *et al.* (1989) and p. 842. Data from plate assays are analysed as described in Arlett *et al.* (1989) and p. 844 for treat and plate tests.

Status of Mammalian Mutation Tests
At present the only practical assays for screening new chemical entities for mammalian mutation are the mammalian cell assays described above. The protocols are well-defined, and mutant selection and counting procedures are simple and easily quantified. In general, the genetic endpoints are understood and relevant to deleterious genetic events in humans. For these reasons the assays are still regarded as valuable in safety evaluation (Li *et al.*, 1991). It is, however, recognized that there are still unknown factors and molecular events that influence test results. This can be illustrated by the conclusions of the third UKEMS collaborative trial, which focused on tests with cultured mammalian cells. The following points were made:

- The number of cells to be cultured during expression imposes a severe limitation in the use of surface attached cells.
- The importance of a careful determination of toxicity.
- That S9 levels may need to be varied.
- That the aromatic amine benzidine is mutagenic only at the TK locus in L5178Y TK$^{+/-}$ cells. The most disturbing finding was that benzidine (detectable without metabolism by S9 mix) did not produce detectable DNA adducts (as shown by ^{32}P-post-labelling) in L5178Y cells. Thus, the mechanism for mutagenesis in L5178Y cells by benzidine remains to be elucidated (Arlett and Cole, 1990).

Mutation Tests Using *Drosophila melanogaster*

Drosophila melanogaster, a species of fruit fly, has a special place in mutagenicity screening. The fundamental studies by Muller (1927) on X-rays and by Auerbach and Robson (1944) with mustard gas used *Drosophila* as the indicator organism.

Drosophila has many advantages for use in screening for mutagens. The cells and chromosomes are organized in the same way as mammalian cells. The flies have a short generation time (10 days) and can be easily cultured in large numbers. In genetic terms, the genome is extremely well-characterized and many different marker stocks are available. Systems are available for measuring mutation in both germ and somatic cells (reviews: Wurgler *et al.*, 1986; Mitchell and Combes, 1984).

In recent times *Drosophila* has become well characterized as to its metabolic capability and capacity for DNA repair.

Metabolism
A wide variety of metabolic activation steps can be carried out by *Drosophila* (review: Vogel 1982). The presence of cytochrome *P*-450 in adult flies and larvae has been demonstrated biochemically. Enzymes responsible for phase II reactions are also present—e.g. glutathione *S*-transferase, glucuronyl transferase, etc. Monoamine oxidases appear to be important in activation and deactivation of mutagens in *Drosophila* (Zijlstra and Vogel, 1985).

Larvae also possess enzymes for metabolic activation in first, second and third instar larvae. Studies on enzyme distribution pattern in larvae and adult flies have established that there are significant differences (e.g. Hallstrom *et al.*, 1983), although in practice few differences have been seen in mutation induction with respect to specific classes of chemical (Würgler *et al.*, 1986).

Several tissues appear to be involved in metabolic activity. These include the fat bodies, the Malpighian tubules, various tissues in the digestive tract, and gonadal tissue (Casida, 1969).

It is well known that *Drosophila* has a poor capacity to activate most aromatic hydrocarbons and amines, indicating that the relevant *P*-450 (IA1) forms are, at best, present in low levels. There are interstrain differences in metabolic capacity and the DDT-resistant substrain of the

Oregon R strain appears to have a particularly high activity (Hallstrom, 1986). It is possible that transgenic flies will be developed in the future containing genes coding for mammalian *P*-450 isozymes.

DNA Repair

Photoreactivation, excision repair and postreplication repair have all been detected and studied in *Drosophila* (Boyd *et al.*, 1983).

Several DNA repair-deficient stocks have been isolated and used in mutagenicity screening. These include strains carrying defective excision repair genes, such as *mei-9* or *mus-201* (Vogel *et al.*, 1985) and the *mu*-2 repair defect, which potentiates the induction of terminal deficiencies (Mason *et al.*, 1984). The *mei-9* deficiency considerably enhances sensitivity to spontaneous and mutagen-induced genetic and lethal effects.

Recommended Tests

A variety of tests are available based on particular marker strains (Mitchell and Combes, 1984). As *Drosophila* tests are no longer widely used for screening, brief details only are given here of the classical sex-linked recessive lethal test for germ cell damage and the 'SMART' (Somatic Mutation and Recombination Test) assays. It is possible that the latter tests will revive interest in *Drosophila* for regulatory testing.

Sex-linked Recessive Lethal Test The genetic basis of the test is shown in Figure 16. Adult male wild-type flies are treated with one of a number of doses of the test compound (selected from previous toxicity tests) or the control. This is undertaken either by mixing the chemical with food or by adding it to an aqueous solution of 1.0–5.0 per cent sucrose. For insoluble compounds suspensions may be employed in organic solvents or dispersants diluted in sucrose solutions.

The male flies are mated to 'Muller-5' females whose X chromosomes carry the white apricot (light orange) eye recessive allele (W^a) and the semi-dominant bar-eye character (B). The Bar mutation gives narrow bar-eye phenotype in males (as this is on the X chromosome, it is fully expressed in males, as they are XY). In females it gives bar-eye when both X chromosomes carry the gene and a kidney eye shape in heterozygous females.

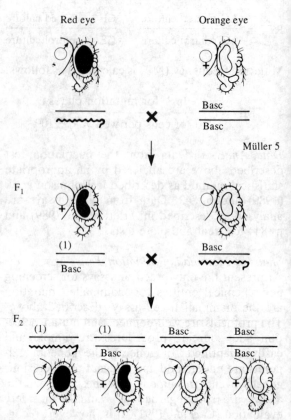

Figure 16 The genetic basis of the *Drosophila melanogaster* sex-linked recessive lethal assay. Redrawn from Würgler *et al.* (1984)

Each male is mated with three different groups of females at 3-day intervals. Sperm development covers a 9-day period and it is known that certain stages are more sensitive than others to particular mutagens. By producing these different broods over this period, different sperm stages are covered. The later broods measure mutations in progressively earlier stages in sperm development at the time of treatment. As shown in Figure 16, the F_1 progeny are mated to obtain the F_2 generation.

Recessive lethal mutations exert their effects only if both copies of the relevant gene are inactivated or if present as a single copy on the X chromosome in males, where the gene cannot be masked by a dominant allele, as there is no corresponding X chromosome. In this latter situation the males carrying the lethal mutation die before maturity. Therefore, if a recessive lethal is induced in X-chromosome-carrying sperm in the parental generation, it will be carried by females in the F_1 generation and will result in loss of wild-type males in the F_2 progeny (distinguishable by their round red eyes). A full description of technical aspects of the assay is given in Würgler *et al.* (1984).

The test predominantly detects gene mutations and small deletions. There are approximately 600–800 genes on every X chromosome which can act as recessive lethals, so low induced mutation frequencies can be detected.

The sex-linked recessive lethal test has been used to screen many hundreds of compounds. In general, the test is reasonably accurate in detecting carcinogens and distinguishing them from non-carcinogens, with the exception of the aromatic hydrocarbons and amines mentioned earlier (Würgler *et al.*, 1986). The popularity of the system has waned in part because of this and because the test is time-consuming and somewhat tedious.

SMART Assays Some of the disadvantages of the sex-linked recessive lethal test are overcome by one-generation tests such as the SMART assays. These include: (a) the wing mosaic system based on the wing hair markers multiple wing hairs (*mwh*) and flare (*flr*) (Graf *et al.*, 1984); (b) the white/white-coral eye mosaic system using two alleles at the white locus (Vogel, 1985). These markers are masked in the parental flies, as they are present in the heterozygous state but become expressed following mutagen treatment as a result of mutation, deletion, recombination, etc., inactivating the sole wild-type gene.

Multiple Wing Hairs/Flare Wing Mosaic System Mitotic recombination between *flr* and the centromere result in two genetically marked daughter cells, one homozygous for *mhw* and the other homozygous for *flr*. During development of the larva and pupa the two cells produce adjacent cell clones. During metamorphosis the cells differentiate into wing blade cells that express the *mwh* and those that express the *flr* phenotype, and the mutant clones become visible as a twin spot. Mitotic recombination between *mwh* and *flr* leads to a *mwh* single spot. In addition, single spots can be produced by gene mutation, deletion, etc. Clones induced early in the development of the larvae result in larger spots than those induced later (Wurgler *et al.*, 1986).

White/White-Coral Eye Mosaic System In this system, advantage is taken of the ability to distinguish the expression of two different alleles at the white eye locus on a sepia-eye color background. Female larvae which are *w/w*^{co} at the white locus are exposed to mutagens. This gene is at the tip of the X chromosome and is a long way from the centromere. As a result there is an ample opportunity for recombination to occur; such an exchange leads to one daughter cell homozygous for *w*^{co} and the other homozygous for *w*. The adjacent clones derived from these two cells form a *w/w*^{co} twin spot in the differentiating eye. Thus, one area of the eye is dark-colored (white-coral) and an adjacent area is white, contrasting with the intermediate color of the heterozygous cells in the rest of the eye. In addition, single mosaic light (or white) spots can also be scored (Vogel, 1985).

Test Performance Studies on more than 350 chemicals have confirmed that these tests detect a broad spectrum of genetic damage; however, mitotic recombination between homologous chromosomes appears to be the event most frequently detected (Vogel, 1991), although compounds showing exclusively recombination or exclusively mutation are rare (Frei, 1991).

In Vivo Mammalian Mutation Tests

Mammalian mutation studies of chemicals in the whole animal have provided fundamental information on mutation parameters in germ cells such as dose response, dose fractionation, sensitivity of various stages in gametogenesis, etc., just as is known for ionizing radiation (Russell, 1989b). This has led to estimations of the possible impact chemical mutagens may have on heritable malformation, inborn errors of metabolism, etc. Today germ cell studies are still required when estimating the heritable damage a mutagen may inflict on exposed human populations.

The existing tests tend to be cumbersome and are not used for routine genetic toxicology screening, and thus only brief descriptions will follow. Reviews of existing data, particularly by Holden (see, e.g., Holden, 1982; Adler and Ashby, 1989), have indicated that most if not all germ cell mutagens also induce DNA damage in somatic cells, as detected by well-established assays such as the rodent micronucleus test (see Chapter 36). The converse is not true—i.e. some mutagens/clastogens can induce somatic cell damage but do not induce germ cell changes, which probably reflects the special protection afforded to the germ cells, such as that provided by the blood-testis barrier. In other words, it appears that germ cell mutagens are a subset of somatic cell mutagens.

In vivo mammalian mutation tests are not restricted to germ cell tests. The mouse spot test described below is, again, a test used first for studying radiation-induced mutation but has also been used for screening chemicals for *in vivo* mutagenic potential. This test has had several proponents but compared with *in vivo* chromosomal assays is not widely used.

Mouse Somatic Spot Test

The mouse spot test was developed 25 years ago by Russell and Major (1957) for assaying radiation damage and was first used for testing chemicals for mutagenicity by Fahrig in 1975. Results of the studies which followed were reviewed under the GENE-TOX program by Russell *et al.* (1981).

A spectrum of genetic alterations ranging from major chromosomal changes to point mutations is detectable. These changes result in the inactivation or loss of gene product at a set of heterozygous loci controlling hair pigmentation (Russell, 1984).

The method involves exposing embryos *in utero* to the test chemical at the time that melanocyte precursor cells migrate from the neural crest to the dermis. After birth the pelts of the pups are examined for clones of mutant cells that result in spots of coloured fur of a different hue from that of the main pelt. As the embryos are heterozygous for several coat colour genes, the coat colour spots result from inactivation of the single remaining wild-type allele exposing the recessive marker gene.

Areas of missing pigment cells can be detected as white patches located near the central midline of the coat. These result from cytotoxicity—i.e. death of the melanocyte precursor cells.

A variety of different heterozygotes have been developed for use in this test (Russell, 1984). The C57BL X T heterozygote is typical and is heterozygous at the b (brown), c^{ch} (café au lait), d ('blue'-grey) and p (lilac-grey) loci. Females are mated when they are 3–6 months old. After confirmation of mating (observation of a vaginal plug), the pregnant dams are treated at 10¼ days (or shortly before if warranted by pharmacokinetic data), when about 200 melanoblasts are targeted. Sensitivity will be lost if dosing takes place too early, as too few melanoblasts are present; if too late, the mutant clones will be too small to be easily visible. As this is a screening test, the intraperitoneal route is usually used.

The pups are observed at birth as per a standard reproductive toxicology test, to gain information about embryotoxicity and teratogenicity. The coats are observed at 12–14 days, when the hairs are short, dense and uniform. Any coat colour spots are noted as to location and size. A second examination is carried out at 25–35 days for late-developing spots. The pelts can be photographed or preserved. Confirmation of the presence of a mutant clone of hairs may be noted by microscopical examination of the hairs.

The GENE-TOX report mentioned earlier established criteria for defining negative results using a multiple-decision procedure developed by Selby and Olson (1981). A result is negative if the spot frequency in an experimental group is not statistically significantly higher than the appropriate control (Fischer's Exact Test) and the induced frequency is less than four times the control frequency. Relatively large group sizes (>155) are required to adequately demonstrate negative results (Russell, 1984). If no effects are seen in all the various parameters (embryotoxicity, teratogenicity included), it may be necessary to check whether the test compound is able to cross the placenta.

The Mouse Specific Locus Test

The mouse somatic spot test is a type of specific locus test. The classical specific locus test was developed independently by Russell at Oak Ridge in the late 1940s (Russell, 1951; 1989b) and Carter in Edinburgh (Carter *et al.*, 1956). The test consists of treatment of parental mice homozygous for a wild-type set of marker loci. The targets for mutation are the germ cells in the gonads of the treated mice. These are mated with a tester stock that is homozygous recessive at the marker loci. The F_1 offspring that result are normally heterozygous at the marker loci and thus express the wild-type phenotype. In the event of a mutation from the wild-type allele at any of these loci, the F_1 offspring express the recessive phenotype.

The test marker strain (T) developed by Russell uses seven recessive loci, viz: *a* (non-agouti), *b* (brown), *c^ch* (chinchilla), *d* (dilute), *p* (pink-eyed dilution), *s* (piebald) and *se* (short-ear). As for the mouse spot test, these genes control coat pigmentation, intensity or pattern, and, for the *se* gene, the size of the external ear.

As the occurrence of mutation is rare even after mutagen treatment, the specific locus test is the ultimate study of mutation, requiring many thousands of offspring to be scored, plus significant resources of time, space and animal husbandry. Because of these constraints it is often difficult to define a negative result, as insufficient animals are scored or all stages of spermatogenesis are not covered. Of the 25 compounds tested in the assay, as reviewed by Ehling *et al.* (1986), 17 were regarded as 'inconclusive' and 8 positive. The scale studies can reach is illustrated by the test of ethylene oxide described by Russell *et al.* (1984), where exposures of 101 000 and 150 000 ppm per hour were used over 16–23 weeks. A total of 71 387 offspring were examined. The spermatogonial stem-cell mutation rate in the treated animals did not differ significantly from the historical control frequency!

With regard to the design of the test, mice are mated when 7–8 weeks old. By this age all germ cell stages are present. The test compound is normally administered by the ip route to maximize the likelihood of germ cell exposure. The preferred dose is just below the toxic level so long as fertility is not compromised. One lower dose should also be included.

In males spermatogonia are most at risk but it is also desirable that later stages also be exposed. Thus, the mice are mated immediately after treatment to 2–4 females. This is continued each week for 7 weeks. Then the first group has completed its rearing of the first set of offspring and is remated. This cycle can be continued for the lifetime of the males. Tests can also be carried out by dosing females, when treatment is carried out for 3 weeks to cover all stages of oogenesis.

The offspring are examined immediately after birth for identification of malformations (dominant visibles) and then at weaning for the specific locus mutations. Presumptive mutant mice are checked by further crosses to confirm their status (Searle, 1984).

Comparison of mutation frequencies is made with the historical database. For definition of a positive result the same principles are recommended as for the mouse spot test (Selby and Olson, 1981). A minimum size of 18 000 offspring per group is recommended by those authors for definition of a negative result.

Of the compounds showing clear-cut positive results, some produce specific locus mutations in the first 7 weeks after treatment, e.g. triethylene-melamine (Cattanach, 1982), whereas others, e.g. procarbazine, induce mutations only in later mating (Ehling, 1984). Most only produce small increases in mutations at the marker loci. However, two 'supermutagens' are now known — ethylnitrosourea (ENU) and chlorambucil. Russell (1989a) states that the mutation frequency obtained from a single ip injection of 6 mg ENU per mouse is 75 000 times greater than that considered to be a maximum permissible level of risk in man from a whole year of exposure to radiation. ENU induces primarily gene mutation in spermatogonia, while chlorambacil apparently induces deletions and other chromosome structural aberrations in postgonial stages (Russell, 1989b).

The specific locus test remains a fundamentally important method for studying heritable mutations. Further modifications of the test harnessing molecular techniques are now being developed (Russell, 1989a).

Dominant Lethal Test

The term 'dominant lethal' is used to describe embryonic death resulting from genetic damage in parental germ cells. The induction of dominant lethals in mice as an indicator of genetic damage was first shown by Kaplan and Lyon (1953). Bateman (1966) suggested the use of the dominant lethal assay for screening for mutagens.

The test is based on observing the viability of uterine implantations. Implantations that die at an early stage can be recognized, as they form a deciduoma or 'mole'. The decidium is a growth of maternal uterine tissue under the stimulus of the implanting egg. Its growth is autonomous, whatever the fate of the egg, until the 11th day of pregnancy, when it stops. Where there is normal growth, fetal tissues overwhelm the decidium.

For early deaths, deciduoma persist unaltered apart from necrosis of the upper part, throughout pregnancy, being shed at birth with the rest of the uterine contents (Bateman, 1984).

The initiating genetic event for early deaths is

predominantly chromosomal damage in the parental germ cells resulting in a dominant lethal mutation (Brewen *et al.*, 1975). The latter authors showed that the types of chromosome aberrations responsible are predominantly double fragments, chromatid interchanges and chromatid deletions (see Anderson, Chapter 36).

The standard mouse dominant lethal assay is performed by treating sexually mature males of proven fertility with single or multiple doses of test compounds (usually ip) and then mating them with three virgin females (8–10 weeks old) for 1 week. The females are changed each week for 8 weeks, as for the specific locus test. This ensures that all stages of the spermatogenic cycle are covered. The females are killed and dissected 17 days later. The corpora lutea, which are equivalent to the number of released ova, are counted and the uterine contents scored for early (moles) and late deaths and for living foetuses. The induction of dominant lethals is calculated by comparing the frequency of pre- and postimplantation loss of zygotes in the experimental groups with the untreated or vehicle control group. The test doses are chosen to be close to the maximum tolerated dose, so long as this does not result in sterility.

Test variations include treating females and mating with untreated males. Another variation which may increase sensitivity, although reducing the overall information that can be obtained from the test, is to treat males for 8 weeks and then mate for 2 weeks after treatment (Green *et al.*, 1975).

The statistical treatment of the data from the test is relatively complex and the reader is referred to Bateman (1984) for details.

The mouse dominant lethal assay enjoyed popularity in the 1960s and 1970s as a screen for germ cell damage. Green *et al.*, (1985) reviewed 450 papers for the GENE-TOX Program (Green *et al.*, 1985). Some compounds positive in the test produce dominant lethals in the first few weeks after treatment, as the damage occurs preferentially in cells of the later (postmeiotic) stages of spermatogenesis, e.g. triethylene melamine, while a small number of compounds induce effects in the later weeks of sampling as the early stages of spermtogenesis are affected—e.g. mercaptopurine, which produces dominant lethals only in the fifth week after treatment (early spermatocytes) (Generoso *et al.*, 1975). It is possible

that dominant lethal induction in spermatogonial cells will be missed, owing to germinal selection (Ehling *et al.*, 1986).

The dominant lethal assay is now much less widely used, as the test is considered to be relatively insensitive (Olesen, 1990).

FUTURE DEVELOPMENTS

Regulatory guidelines for mutagenicity tests, such as the UK Department of Health requirements (1989), are a compromise. There are accepted tests for measuring chromosome damage *in vitro* and *in vivo*; however, the stated tests for point mutation are both *in vitro*. There is no validated test *in vivo* that is in widespread use. Studies of carcinogens have shown that many are tissue-specific in the sites of the induced tumours (see, e.g., Tennant *et al.*, 1987). Thus, there is a need for an *in vivo* mutagenicity test that could, in principle, be applied to any tissue.

With the advent of the new DNA technologies there are several promising approaches that could provide the required animal models.

Use of Tissue-specific Genetic Polymorphisms

The specific locus test described earlier makes use of coat color genes or genes controlling external morphology. It is possible to identify other marker genes in different tissues and then identify loss of function of these genes due to mutation. One such system is a mouse assay that is able to detect mutations in intestinal crypt cells.

The assay is being developed in two forms: one treating young adult mice (Winton *et al.*, 1989) and the second a transplacental assay (like the mouse spot test), where treatment is given on a single occasion (day 9) and the mutant intestinal cell population is measured postnatally (Schmidt *et al.*, 1990). The assay measures changes in the genes coding for glycoprotein/glycolipid in the membranes of the epithelium of the small intestine. These changes can be detected by loss in the ability to bind the lectin *Dolichos biflorus* agglutinin (DBA). Mutations arise at the *Dlb-1^b* locus and mutant cells can be recognized as white unstained patches in otherwise brown peroxidase-stained epithelium of adult small intestine, following histochemical staining.

Most mouse strains possess the *Dlb–I^b* allele (e.g. C57BL/6J), which confers positive binding of the lectin. One of these strains is crossed with mice possessing the *Dlb-I^a* allele (e.g. SWR mice), which does not show DBA binding in intestinal epithelium. The F$_1$ heterozygote (Dlb-I^a/Dlb-I^b) shows DBA binding conferred by the single *Dlb-I^b* allele. Inactivation of this allele by mutation can result in loss of DBA binding ability.

After treatment, the whole of the small intestine is scored for mutant clones. As a result, the test requires only small numbers of animals. It has to date been used to detect only a limited number of mutagens, such as ethylnitrosourea (Schmidt, 1990) and 1,2-dimethylnitrosamine (Winton *et al.*, 1990). However, the latter authors have also tested a dietary mutagen [2-amino-3,8 dimethylimidazo (4,5-*f*) quinoxaline] and this assay could have particular utility in measuring the mutagenicity of food mutagens. The principle used in the test can be applied to other tissues, as suitable genetic polymorphisms are identified.

Restriction Site Mutation Analysis

Restriction site mutation analysis provides a method for detecting DNA base changes in restriction enzyme recognition sites. Restriction enzymes are endonucleases which locate defined short DNA sequences and induce breaks within them. If a point-mutation or deletion occurs, disrupting the recognition sequence for a particular restriction nuclease, the DNA is no longer sensitive to the cutting action of the enzyme at that site.

Parry *et al.* (1990) proposed a method for detecting the changes outlined above, using amplification of DNA sequences from mutagen-exposed cells or tissues using the polymerase chain reaction (PCR) (review: White *et al.*, 1989). This technique allows any known DNA sequence for which DNA primers are available or can be synthesized, to be greatly amplified. In the PCR, DNA is replicated by a heat-resistant DNA polymerase called the *Taq* polymerase and the newly synthesized DNA is heat denatured, after which further polymerization can occur. If nucleotides and cofactors are replenished, further cycles of polymerization and denaturation can take place. The amplified DNA sequence can then be run on a polyacrylamide gel and can be identified as a characteristic band.

As many different DNA restriction nucleases are known, each recognizing a different recognition sequence, it is possible to identify restriction sites within most stretches of nucleotides. Thus, incubation of the DNA with different enzymes will result in cuts in the DNA. If DNA, after successful nuclease attack, is incubated in the PCR, then no amplification will occur, as primer sites will have been lost. Thus with normal wild type DNA no PCR will occur and no amplified product will be observed on the gel. Following mutagen exposure base changes may occur at the restriction sites leading to resistance to nuclease cutting and then the DNA can be amplified by PCR.

Early studies following the principles outlined have been carried out successfully with gene sequences within the *E. coli gpt* gene, either integrated into a human chromosome in mouse/human hybrid cells (Parry *et al.*, 1991), or on a shuttle vector (plasmid) in human cells (Palombo *et al.*, 1991).

The method can in principle be applied to any known DNA sequence within any species, tissue and gene.

Transgenic Models

It has become possible to microinject fertilized mouse eggs with 'foreign' DNA. The incoming DNA becomes integrated into the mouse genome and thus all cells within the developed adult 'transgenic' contain a copy of the new DNA. Two transgenic strains have been developed as models for studying mutation.

The first model, described by Gossen *et al.* (1989), contains a *lac Z* (β-galactosidase) gene from *E. coli* carried by a λ bacteriophage vector. This transcript was microinjected into the pronucleus of (BALB/c × DBA/2) CD2 F$_1$ eggs. The transgenic produced contains 80 copies of the *lac Z* gene per haploid chromosome set.

The second model contains a *lac I* (lac repressor) gene on a λ shuttle vector integrated into the genome of an inbred C57B1/6 mouse (Kohler *et al.*, 1991). In both cases the mouse is treated with the test agent by the ip route or the likely route of human exposure. Multiple daily treatments may be preferred. Genomic DNA is isolated by standard methods from the desired tissue. The λ vector is rescued from the genomic DNA by mixing with *in vitro* λ 'packaging extract', which excises the target λ sector and packages the DNA into a λ phage head. These phages are then used to infect a host *E. coli* strain. For the *lac Z* system a *lac Z⁻ E. coli* C indicator strain is used. For the *lac I* system the *E. coli* SCS–8 indicator strain is used, which has a deleted Lac region and contains a *Lac Z⁻* gene on a *phi 80* insert.

For the λ *lac Z* system the bacteria and the λ phage containing the rescued DNA are incubated in soft agar with a chromagenic reagent (X-gal). After 16 h incubation the lysis plaques produced by the phage are scored. If a phage contains a normal *lac Z* gene, the X-gal is metabolized to a blue-coloured product. If a mutated *lac Z* gene is carried by the phage, the X-gal remains intact and no colour is produced. Thus, scoring consists of counting clear plaques against the background of unmutated blue plaques. The clear plaques are picked off and replated to confirm that they are true mutants.

For the *lac I* system a similar plating routine is carried out. In this case mutants are detected as blue mutant plaques against a background of non-mutant colourless plaques. These can arise as a result of mutations that inactivate the *lac* repressor protein or *lac I* promoter or mutations within the *lac* repressor binding domain, which block repressor binding to the *lac Z* operator. Density of plaques is limited to 50 000 pfu per plate to ensure accuracy in detection of plaques with the mutant phenotype (Kohler *et al.*, 1991).

A summary of the procedure for the *lac Z* system is given in Figure 17.

Early studies with model mutagens in both these systems have shown that increases in mutant frequencies can be detected in both somatic tissue (liver, bone marrow, skin) and germinal cells (testis) (Kohler *et al.*, 1991; Myhr and Kirkland, 1991). Spontaneous background mutant frequencies range from approximately 6×10^{-6} to 28×10^{-6}. Germ cells appear to exhibit lower background rates than do somatic tissue. The mutagens tested induce dose-related increases in mutant frequency in a variety of tissues, although varying rates are observed from tissue to tissue.

Much more validation work on these systems is required to determine responses to a wide range of tissue-specific genotoxic carcinogens and

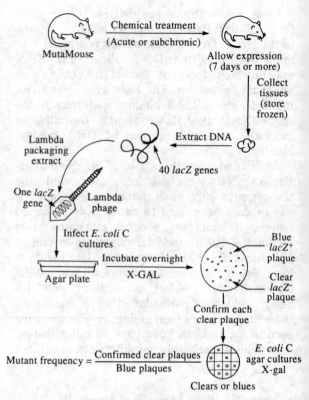

Figure 17 The transgenic MutaMouse LacZ system. Reproduced with permission from D. Kirkland and redrawn

non-carcinogens under a wide variety of conditions. It also remains to be shown that mutational analyses of these transgenes is a true reflection of mutation of resident genes. At present the transgenic models are at best prototypes of more refined systems to come. They do hold the promise of providing a tool to explore mutation rates under a wide variety of conditions and for screening for mutation *in vivo* in important tissues excluded from study by conventional means, e.g. stomach.

REFERENCES

Adler, I.-D. and Ashby, J. (1989). The present lack of evidence for unique rodent germ-cell mutagens. *Mutation Res.*, **212**, 55–66

Amacher, D. E., Paillet, S. C., Turner, G. N., Ray, V. A. and Salsburg, D. S. (1980). Point mutations at the thymidine kinase locus in L5178Y mouse lymphoma cells. 2. Test validation and interpretation. *Mutation Res.*, **72**, 447–474

Ames, B. N. (1971). The detection of chemical

mutagens with enteric bacteria. In Hollaender, A. (Ed.), *Chemical Mutagens, Principles and Methods for Their Detection*, Vol. 1. Plenum Press, New York, pp. 267–282

Ames, B. N., Durston, W. E., Yamasaki, E. and Lee, F. D. (1973a). Carcinogens are mutagens: a simple test system combining liver homogenates for activation and bacteria for detection. *Proc. Natl Acad. Sci. USA*, **70**, 2281–2285

Ames, B. N., Kammen, H. O. and Yamasaki, E. (1975). Hair dyes are mutagenic: Identification of a variety of mutagenic ingredients. *Proc. Natl Acad. Sci. USA*, **72**, 2423–2427

Ames, B. N., Lee, F. D. and Durston, W. E. (1973b). An improved bacterial test system for the detection and classification of mutagens and carcinogens. *Proc. Natl Acad. Sci. USA*, **70**, 782–786

Applegate, M. L., Moore, M. M., Broder, C. B. *et al.* (1990). Molecular dissection of mutations at the heterozygous thymidine canise locus in mouse lymphona cells. *Proc. Natl. Acad. Sci. USA*, **87**, 51–55

Arlett, C. F. and Cole, J. (1990). The third United Kingdom Environmental Mutagen Society collaborative trial: overview, a summary and assessment. *Mutagenesis*, **5** (Suppl), 85–88

Arlett, C. F. and Lehmann, A. R. (1978). Human disorders showing increased sensitivity to the induction of genetic damage. *Ann. Rev. Genet.*, **12**, 95–115

Arlett, C. F., Smith, D. M., Clark, G. M., Green, M. H. L., Cole, J., McGregor, D. B. and Asquith, J. C. (1989). Mammalian cell assays based upon colony formation. In Kirkland, D. J. (Ed.), *UKEMS Subcommittee on Guidelines for Mutagenicity Testing. Report Part III: Statistical Evaluation of Mutagenicity Test Data*. Cambridge University Press, Cambridge, pp. 66–101

Ashby, J. and Tennant, R. W. (1988). Chemical structure, *Salmonella* mutagenicity and extent of carcinogenicity as indices of genotoxic carcinogens among 222 chemicals tested in rodents by the US NCI/NTP. *Mutation Res.*, **204**, 17–115

Ashby, J., Tennant, R. W., Zeiger, E. and Stasiewicz, S. (1989). Classification according to chemical structure, mutagenicity to *Salmonella* and level of carcinogenicity of a further 42 chemicals tested for carcinogenicity by the US National Toxicology Program. *Mutation Res.*, **223**, 73–104

Ashwood-Smith, M. J. (1980). Stability of frozen microsome preparations for use in the Ames *Salmonella* mutagenicity assay. *Mutation Res.*, **69**, 199–200

Auerbach, C., Moutschen-Dahmen, M., and Moutschen, J. (1977). Genetic and cytogenetic effects of formaldehyde and related compounds. *Mutation Res.*, **39**, 317–362

Auerbach, C. and Robson, J. M. (1944). Production of mutations by allyl *iso*thiocyanate. *Nature*, **154**, 81–82

Auerbach, C. and Robson, J. M. (1946) Chemical production of mutations. *Nature*, **157**, 302

Barbacid, M. (1986). Oncogenes and human cancer: cause or consequence? *Carcinogenesis*, **7**, 1037–1042

Bargmann, C. I., Hung, M. C. and Weinberg, R. A. (1986). Multiple independent activations of the *neu* oncogene by a point mutation altering the transmembrane domain of p15. *Cell*, **45**, 649–657

Barthelmess, A. (1956). Mutagenic drugs. *Arzneimittel Forsch*, **6**, 157–168

Bartsch, H., Camus A.-M., and Malaveille, C. (1976). Comparative mutagenicity of *N*-nitrosamines in a semi-solid and in a liquid incubation system in the presence of rat or human tissue fractions. *Mutation Res.*, **37**, 149–162

Bateman, A. J. (1966). Testing chemicals for mutagenicity in a mammal. *Nature*, **210**, 205–206

Bateman, A. J. (1984). The dominant lethal assay in the male mouse. In Kilbey, B. J., Legator, M., Nichols, W. and Ramel, C. (Eds), *Handbook of Mutagenicity Test Procedures*. Elsevier, Amsterdam, pp. 471–483

Beckman, D. A. and Brent, R. L. (1986). Mechanism of known environmental teratogens: drugs and chemicals. *Clin. Perinatol.*, **13**, 649–687

Benditt, E. P. and Benditt, J. M. (1973). Evidence for a monoclonal origin of human atherosclerotic plaques. *Proc. Natl Acad. Sci. USA*, **70**, 1753–1756

Bishop, J. M. (1985). Viral oncogenes. *Cell*, **42**, 23–38

Bishop, J. M. (1987). The molecular genetics of cancer. *Science*, **235**, 305–311

Blazak, W. F., Steward, B. E., Galperin, I., Allen, K. L., Rudd, C. J., Mitchell, A. D. and Caspary, W. J. (1986). Chromosome analysis of trifluorothymidine-resistant L5178Y mouse lymphoma cells colonies. *Environ. Mutagen.*, **8**, 229–240

Bodmer, W. F., Bailey, C. J., Bodmer, J., Bussey, H. J. R., Ellis, A., Gorman, P., Lucibello, F. C., Murday, V. A., Rider, S. H., Scrambler, P., Sheer, D., Soloman, E. and Spurr, N. K. (1987). Localization of the gene for familial adenomatous polyposis on chromosome 5. *Nature*, **328**, 614–616

Bootsma, D., Keijzer, W., Jung, E. G. and Bohrent, E. (1989). Xeroderma pigmentosum complementation group XP-1 withdrawn. *Mutation Res.*, **218**, 149–152

Bos, J. L. (1988). The ras gene family and human carcinogenesis. *Mutation Res.*, **195**, 255–271

Bossi, L. (1985). Informational suppression. In Scaife, J., Leach, D. and Galizzi, A. (Eds), *Genetics of Bacteria*. Academic Press, New York, pp. 49–64

Boyd, J. B., Harris, P. V., Presley, J. M. and Narachi, M. (1983). *Drosophila melanogaster*: a model eukaryote for the study of DNA repair. In Friedberg, E. C. and Bridges, B. A. (Eds), *Cellular Response to DNA Damage*. Alan R. Liss, New York, pp. 107–123

Brewen, J. G., Payne, H. S., Jones, K. P. and Preston, R. J. (1975). Studies on chemically induced dominant lethality. I. The cytogenetic basis of MMS-induced dominant lethality in post-meiotic germ cells. *Mutation Res.*, **33**, 239–250

Bridges, B. A. (1972). Simple bacterial systems for detecting mutagenic agents. *Lab. Pract.* **21**, 413–419

Bridges, B. A. (1976). Short-term screening tests for carcinogens. *Nature*, **261**, 195–200

Bridges, B. A. (1978). On the detection of volatile liquid mutagens with bacteria: experiments with dichlorvos and epichlorhydrin. *Mutation Res.*, **54**, 367–371

Bridges, B. A. (1981). How important are somatic mutations and immune control in skin cancer? Reflections on xeroderma pigmentosum. *Carcinogenesis*, **2**, 471–472

Bridges, B. A., Dennis, R. E. and Munson, R. J. (1967). Differential induction and repair of ultraviolet damage leading to true reversions and external suppressor mutations of an ochre codon in *Escherichia coli* B/r WP2. *Genetics*, **57**, 897–908

Bridges, B. A., Woodgate, R., Ruiz-Rubio, M., Sharif, F., Sedgwick, S. G. and Hubscher, U. (1987). Current understanding of UV-induced base pair substitution mutation in *E. coli* with particular reference to the DNA polymerase III complex. *Mutation Res.*, **181**, 219–226

Brusick, D. (1986). Genotoxic effects in cultured mammalian cells produced by low pH treatment conditions and increased ion concentrations. *Environ. Mutagen.*, **8**, 879–886

Brusick, D. (1987). *Principles of Genetic Toxicology*, 2nd edn. Plenum Press, New York, London

Burck, K. B., Liu, E. T. and Larrick, J. W. (1988). *Oncogenes. An Introduction to the Concept of Cancer Genes*. Springer-Verlag, New York, Berlin, Heidelberg, London, Paris, Tokyo

Burnett, C., Fuchs, C., Corbett, J. and Menkart, J. (1982). The effect of dimethylsulphoxide on the mutagenicity of the hair-dye, *p*-phenylenediamine. *Mutation Res.*, **103**, 1–4.

Butterworth, B. E. and Slaga, T. J. (1987). *Nongenotoxic Mechanisms in Carcinogenesis*. Banbury Report No. 25. Cold Spring Harbor Laboratory, N.Y.

Carter, C. O. (1977). The relative contribution of mutant genes and chromosome abnormalities to genetic ill-health in man. In Scott, D., Bridges, B. A. and Sobels, F. H. (Eds), *Progress in Genetic Toxicology*. Elsevier/North Holland, Amsterdam, pp. 1–14

Carter, T. C., Lyon, M. F. and Philips, R. J. S. (1956). Induction of mutations in mice by chronic gamma irradiation; interim report. *Br. J. Radiol.*, **29**, 106–108

Carver, J. H., Machado, M. L. and MacGregor, J. A. (1985). Petroleum distillates suppress *in vitro* metabolic activation: higher (S9) required in the *Salmonella*/microsome mutagenicity assay. *Environ. Mutagen.*, **7**, 369–380

Casida, J. E. (1969). Insect microsomes and insecticide chemical oxidations. In Gilette, J. R., Conney, A. H.,

Cosmides, G. J. and Estabrook, R. W. (Eds), *Microsomes and Drug Oxidation*, Academic Press, New York, pp. 517–531

Cattanach, B. M. (1982). Induction of specific-locus mutations in female mice by triethylene melamine (TEM). *Mutation Res.*, **104**, 173–176

Cavenee, W. K., Dryja, R. P., Phillips, R. A., Benedict, W. F., Godbout, R., Galie, B. L., Murphree, A. L., Strong, L. C. and White, R. C. (1983). Expression of recessive alleles by chromosomal mechanisms in retinoblastoma. *Nature*, **305**, 779–784

Changanti, R. S. K., Schonberg, S. and German, J. (1974). A many fold increase in sister chromatid exchanges in Bloom's syndrome lymphocytes. *Proc. Natl Acad. Sci. USA*, **71**, 4508–4512

Chu, E. H. Y. and Malling, H. U. (1968). Mammalian cell genetics. II. Chemical induction of specific locus mutations in Chinese hamster cells *in vitro*. *Proc. Natl Acad. Sci. USA*, **61**, 1306–1312

Clayson, D. B. (1989). ICPEMC publication No. 17: Can a mechanistic rationale be provided for nongenotoxic carcinogens identified in rodent bioassays? *Mutation Res.*, **221**, 53–67

Cleaver, J. E (1977). DNA repair processes and their impairment in some human diseases. In Scott, D., Bridges, B. A. and Sobels, F. H. (Eds), *Progress in Genetic Toxicology*. Elsevier/North Holland, Amsterdam, pp. 29–42

Cleaver, J. E. (1983). Xeroderma pigmentosum. In Stanbury, J. B., Wyngaarden, J. B., Fredrickson, D. S., Goldstein, J. C. and Brown, M. S. (Eds), *The Metabolic Basis of Inherited Disease*. McGraw-Hill, New York, pp. 1227–1248

Clive, D. (1987). Historical overview of the mouse lymphoma TK$^{+/-}$ mutagenicity assay. In Moore, M. M., Demarini, D. M., De Serres, F. J. and Tindall, K. R. (Eds), *Mammalian Cell Mutagenesis*. Banbury Report 28. Cold Spring Harbor Laboratory, N.Y., pp. 25–36

Clive, D. (1989). Mammalian cell genotoxicity: A major role for non-DNA targets? *Mutation Res.*, **223**, 327–328

Clive, D., Caspary, W., Kirkby, P. E., Krehl, R., Moore, M., Mayo, J. and Oberly, T. J. (1987). Guide for performing the mouse lymphoma assay for mammalian cell mutagenicity. *Mutation Res.*, **189**, 145–156

Clive, D., Flamm, W. G. and Patterson, J. B. (1972). A mutational assay system using the thymidine kinase locus in mouse lymphoma cells. *Mutation Res.*, **16**, 77–87

Cole, R. S. (1973). Repair of DNA containing interstrand crosslinks in *Escherichia coli*: sequential excision and recombination. *Proc. Natl Acad. Sci. USA*, **70**, 1064–1068

Cole, J., Fox, M., Garner, R. C., McGregor, D. B. and Thacker, J. (1990). Gene mutation assays in cultured mammalian cells. In Kirkland, D. J. (Ed.), *UKEMS Subcommittee on Guidelines for Mutagenic-*

ity Testing. Report Part I revised. Cambridge University Press, Cambridge, pp. 87–114

Cole, J., Muriel, W. J. and Bridges, B. A. (1986). The mutagenicity of sodium fluoride to L5178Y (wild-type and TK+/− 3.7.2c) mouse lymphoma cells. *Mutagenesis*, **1**, 157–167

Combes, R., Anderson, D., Brooks, T., Neale, S. and Venitt, S. (1984). The detection of mutagens in urine, faeces and body fluids. In Dean, B. J. (Ed.), *UKEMS Subcommittee on Guidelines for Mutagenicity Testing. Report Part II: Supplementary Tests.* United Kingdom Environmental Mutagen Society, Swansea, pp. 203–244

Comma, L. (1977). Ministerial Decrees (28 July 1977), (25 August 1977). The testing of pharmaceutical products prior to clinical trials. *Official Gazette* (G.U.) Nos. 216 (9 August 1977) and 238 (1 September 1977). Rome

Crow, J. F. (1989). Concern for environmental mutagens: some personal reminiscences. *Environ. Molec. Mutagen.*, **14**, Suppl. 16, 7–10

Cullum, J. (1985). Insertion sequences. In Scaife, J., Leach, D. and Galizzi, A. (Eds), *Genetics of Bacteria.* Academic Press, New York, pp. 85–96

Czeizel, A. (1986). Self-poisoning as a model for the study of mutagenicity and teratogenicity of chemicals in human beings. In Ramel, C., Lambert, B. and Magnusson, I. (Eds), *Genetic Toxicology of Environmental Chemicals. Part B: Genetic Effects and Applied Mutagenesis.* Alan R. Liss, New York, pp. 237–244

Czeizel, A. (1989). Population surveillance of sentinel anomalies. *Mutation Res.*, **212**, 3–9

DeMarini, D. M., Doerr, C. L., Meyer, M. K., Brock, K. H., Hozier, J. and Moore, M. M. (1987). Mutagenicity of *m*-AMSA and *o*-AMSA in mammalian cells due to clastogenic mechanism: possible role of topoisomerase. *Mutagenesis*, **2**, 349–355

Demple, B., Sedgwick, B., Robins, P., Totty, N., Waterfield, M. D. and Lindahl, T. (1985). Active site and complete sequence of the suicidal methyltransferase that counters alkylation mutagenesis. *Proc. Natl Acad. Sci. USA*, **82**, 2688–2692

Department of Health (1989). *Guidelines for the Testing of Chemicals for Mutagenicity.* Committee on Mutagenicity of Chemicals in Food, Consumer Products and the Environment. Report on Health and Social Security No. 35. HMSO, London

Department of Health and Social Security (1981). *Guidelines for the Testing of Chemicals for Mutagenicity.* Prepared by the Committee on Mutagenicity of Chemicals in Food, Consumer Products and the Environment. Department of Health and Social Security. Report on Health and Social Subjects No. 24. HMSO, London

DeSerres, F. J. and Shelby, M. D. (1979). Recommendations on data production and analysis using the *Salmonella*/microsome mutagenicity assay. *Mutation Res.*, **64**, 159–165

de Vries, H. (1901). *The Mutation Theory*, Verlag von Veit & Co., Leipzig

Doll, R. (1977). Strategy for detection of cancer hazards to man. *Nature*, **265**, 589–596

Dorado, G., Ariza, R. R. and Pueyo, C. (1988). Mutagenicity of red wine in the L-arabinose resistance test with *Salmonella typhimurium*. *Mutagenesis*, **3**, 497–502

Dunnett, C. W. (1955). A multiple comparison procedure for comparing several treatments with a control. *J. Am. Stat. Assoc.*, **50**, 1096–1121

EEC (1984). Methods for the determination of physico-chemical properties, toxicity and ecotoxicity; Annex V to Directive 79/831/EEC. *Official Journal of the European Communities*, No. L251, 131–145

Ehling, U. H. (1984). Methods to estimate the genetic risk. In Obe, G. (Ed.), *Mutations in Man.* Springer, Berlin, pp. 292–318

Ehling, U. H., Chu, E. H. Y., DeCarli, L., Evans, H. J., Hayashi, M., Lambert, B., Neubert, D., Thilly, W. G. and Vainio, H. (1986). Report 8. Assays for germ-cell mutations in mammals, In Montesano, R., Bartsch, H., Vainio, H., Wilbourn, J. and Yamasaki, H. (Eds), *Long-term and Short-term Assays for Carcinogens. A Critical Appraisal.* IARC Scientific Publications, No. 83, Lyon, pp. 245–265

EPA (1978). Proposed Guidelines for Registering Pesticides in the US: Hazard Evaluation: Humans and Domestic Animals. *Federal Register*, **43**, No. 163, 22 August 1978

Evans, H. H., Mencl, J., Horng, M. F., Ricanti, M., Sanchez, C. and Hozier, J. (1986). Locus specificity in the mutability of L5178Y mouse lymphoma cells: the role of multilocus lesions. *Proc. Natl Acad. Sci. USA*, **83**, 4379–4385

Fahrig, R. (1975). A mammalian spot test: induction of genetic alterations in pigment cells of mouse embryos with X-rays and chemical mutagens. *Molec. Gen. Genet.*, **138**, 309–314

Falck, K., Sorsa, M. and Vainio, H. (1981). Use of the bacterial fluctuation test to detect mutagenicity in the urine of nurses handling cytostatic drugs. *Mutation Res.*, **85**, 236–237

Farber, E. (1987). Possible etiologic mechanisms in chemical carcinogenesis. *Environ. Hlth Perspect.*, **75**, 65–70

Field, L. L. (1988). Insulin-dependent diabetes mellitus: A model for the study of multifactorial disorders. *Am. J. Human Genet.*, **43**, 793–798

Field, L. L., McArthur, R. G., Shin, S. Y. and Yoon, J. W. (1987). The relationship between Coxsackie-B-virus-specific IgG responses and genetic factors (HLA-DR, Gm, Km) in insulin-dependent diabetes mellitus. *Diabetes Res.*, **6**, 169–173

Fleischman, L. F., Chahwala, S. B. and Cantley, L. (1986). Ras-transformed cells: altered levels of phosphatidylinositol-4,5-biphosphate and catabolites. *Science*, **231**, 407–410

Ford, D. K. and Yerganian, G. (1958). Observations

on the chromosomes of Chinese hamster cells in tissue culture. *J. Natl Cancer Inst.*, **21**, 393–425

Forster, R., Green, M. H. L., Gwilliam, R. D., Priestley, A. and Bridges, B. A. (1983). Use of the fluctuation test to detect mutagenic activity in unconcentrated samples of drinking water in the United Kingdom. In Jolley, R. L. (Ed) *Water Chlorination, Environmental Impact and Health Effects*, Vol. 14. Ann Arbor Science, Ann Arbor, pp. 1189–1197

Forster, R., Green, M. H. L. and Priestley, A. (1980). Optimal Levels of S9 fraction in Ames and fluctuation tests: apparent importance of diffusion of metabolites from top agar. *Carcinogenesis*, **2**, 1081–1085

Fowler, R. G., McGinty, L. and Mortelmans, K. E. (1979). Spontaneous mutational specificity of drug resistance plasmid pKM101 in *Escherichia coli*. *J. Bacteriol.*, **140**, 929–937

Fox, M. (1981). Some quantitative aspects of the response of mammalian cells *in vitro* to induced mutagenesis. In Marchelonis, J. J. and Hanna, M. G. (Eds), *Cancer Biology Reviews*, Vol. 3. Marcel Decker, New York, Basel, pp. 23–62

Frei, H. (1991). Somatic mutation and recombination tests (SMART) in Drosophila. *Mutation Res.*, **252**, 169–170

Friedberg, E. C. (1988). DNA repair in the yeast *Saccharomyces cerevisiae*. *Microb. Rev.*, **52**, 70–102

Frizzell, R. A., Schonmacher, R. A. and Halm, D. R. (1987). Chloride channel regulation in cystic fibrosis epithelia. *Prog. Clin. Biol. Res.*, **254**, 101–113

Gatehouse, D. (1978). Detection of mutagenic derivatives of cyclophosphamide and a variety of other mutagens in a microtitre[R] fluctuation test, without microsomal activation. *Mutation Res.*, **53**, 289–296

Gatehouse, D. (1987). Guidelines for testing of environmental agents. Critical features of bacterial mutation assays. *Mutagenesis*, **2**, 397–409

Gatehouse, D. G. and Delow, G. F. (1979). The development of a 'Microtitre[R]' fluctuation test for the detection of indirect mutagens and its use in the evaluation of mixed enzyme induction of the liver. *Mutation Res.*, **60**, 239–252

Gatehouse, D. G. and Tweats, D. J. (1987). Letter to the Editor. *Mutagenesis*, **1**, 307–308

Gatehouse, D. and Wedd, D. J. (1984). The differential mutagenicity of isoniazid in fluctuation assays and *Salmonella* plate tests. *Carcinogenesis*, **5**, 391–397

Gatehouse, D. G., Wedd, D. J., Paes, D., Delow, G., Burlinson, B., Pascoe, S., Brice, A., Stemp, G. and Tweats, D. J. (1988). Investigations into the genotoxic potential of loxtidine, a long-acting H_2-receptor antagonist. *Mutagenesis*, **3**, 57–68

Gatehouse, D. G., Wilcox, P., Forster, R., Rowland, I. R., and Callander, R. D. (1990). Bacterial mutation assays. In Kirkland, D. J. (Ed.), *Basic Mutagenicity Tests: UKEMS Recommended Procedures*. Cambridge University Press, Cambridge, pp. 13–61

Generoso, G. M., Preston, R. J. and Brewen, J. G. (1975). 6-mercaptopurine, an inducer of cytogenetic and dominant lethal effects in pre-meiotic and early meiotic germ cells of male mouse. *Mutation Res.*, **28**, 437–447

German, J. (1983). Patterns of neoplasia associated with the chromosome-breakage syndromes. In German, J. (Ed.), *Chromosome Mutation and Neoplasia*. Alan R. Liss, New York, pp. 97–134

Gille, J. J. P., Wortelboer, H. M. and Joenje, H. (1987). Antioxidant status of Fanconi anemia fibroblasts. *Human Genet.*, **77**, 28–31

Gossen, J. A., De Leeuw, W. J. F., Tan, C. H. T., Zwarthoff, E. C., Berends, F., Lohman, P. H. M., Knook, D. L. and Vijg, J. (1989). Efficient rescue of integrated shuttle vectors from transgenic mice. A model for studying mutations *in vivo*. *Proc. Natl Acad. Sci. USA*, **86**, 7971–7975

Graf, U., Wurgler, F. E., Katz, A. J., Frei, H., Juon, H., Hall, C. B. and Kale, P. G. (1984). Somatic mutation and recombination test in *Drosophila melanogaster*. *Environ. Mutagen.*, **6**, 153–188

Grant, S. G., and Worton, R. G. (1982). 5-Azacytidine-induced reactivation of HPRT on the inactive X chromosome in diploid Chinese hamster cells. *Am. J. Human Genet.*, **34**, 171A

Green, M. H. L. (1984). Mutagen testing using Trp[+] reversion in *Escherichia coli*. In Kilbey, B. J., Legator, M., Nichols, W. and Ramel, C. (Eds), *Handbook of Mutagenicity Test Procedures*, 2nd edn. Elsevier, Amsterdam, pp. 161–187

Green, M. H. L. and Muriel, W. J. (1976). Mutagen testing using TRP+ reversion in *E. coli*. *Mutation Res.*, **38**, 3–32

Green, M. H. L., Muriel, W. J. and Bridges, B. A. (1976). Use of a simplified fluctuation test to detect low levels of mutagens. *Mutation Res.*, **38**, 33–42

Green, S., Auletta, A., Fabricant, J., Kapp, R., Manandhar, M., Shen, C.-J., Springer, J. and Whitfield, B. (1985). Current status of bioassays in genetic toxicology – the dominant lethal assay. *Mutation Res.*, **154**, 49–67

Green, S., Moreland, F. M. and Flamm, G. W. (1975). A more refined approach to dominant lethal testing. *Mutation Res.*, **31**, 340

Guerrero, I. and Pellicer, A. (1987). Mutational activation of oncogenes in animal model systems of carcinogenesis. *Mutation Res.*, **185**, 293–308

Hallstrom, I. (1986). Genetic regulation of the cytochrome P-450 system in *Drosophila melanogaster*. In Ramel, C., Lambert, B. and Magnusson, J. (Eds), *Genetic Toxicology of Environmental Chemicals*, Part B. *Genetic Effects and Applied Mutagenesis*. Alan, R. Liss, New York, pp. 419–425

Hallstrom, I., Blanck, A. and Atuma, S. (1983). Comparison of cytochrome P-450 dependent metabolism in different developmental stages of *Drosophila melanogaster*. *Chem.–Bio. Interact.*, **46**, 39–54

Harris, C. C., Weston, A., Willey, J. C., Trivers, G. E. and Mann, D. L. (1987). Biochemical and molecular epidemiology of human cancer: Indicators of carcinogen exposure, DNA damage and genetic predisposition. *Environ. Hlth Perspect.*, **75**, 109–119

Harris, M. (1982). Induction of thymidine kinase in enzyme-deficient Chinese hamster cells. *Cell*, **29**, 483–492

Hart, R. W. and Setlow, R. B. (1974). Correlation between deoxyribonucleic acid excision repair and lifespan in a number of mammalian species. *Proc. Natl Acad. Sci. USA*, **71**, 2169–2173

Haworth, S., Lawlor, T., Mortelmans, K., Speck, W. and Zeiger E. (1983). Salmonella mutagenicity results for 250 chemicals. *Environ. Mutagen., Suppl.*, **1**, 3–142

Hedges, R. W. and Jacob, A. E. (1974). Transposition of ampicillin resistance from RP4 to other replicons. *Molec. Gen. Genet.*, **132**, 31–40

Heiberg, A. and Berg, K. (1976). The inheritance of hyperlipoproteinaemia with xanthomatosis. A study of 132 kindreds. *Clin. Genet.*, **9**, 203–233

Heim, S., Johansson, B. and Mertens, F. (1989). Constitutional chromosome instability and cancer risk. *Mutation Res.*, **221**, 39–51

Henson, P., Fornace, A. J. Jr. and Little, J. B. (1983). Normal repair of ultraviolet-induced DNA damage in a hypersensitive strain of fibroblasts from a patient with Gardner's syndrome. *Mutation Res.*, **112**, 383–395

Hera, C. and Pueyo, C. (1986). Conditions for optimal use of the L-arabinose-resistance mutagenesis test with *Salmonella typhimurium*. *Mutagenesis*, **1**, 267–274

Herrera, G., Urios, A., Aleixandre, V. and Blanco, M. (1988). UV light-induced mutability in *Salmonella* strains containing the *umu DC* or the *muc AB* operon: evidence for a *umu C* function. *Mutation Res.*, **198**, 9–13

Hirota, H., Hayashi, K., Suzuki, Y. and Shimizu, H. (1987). The bubbling method for detecting mutagenic activity in gaseous compounds. *Mutation Res.*, **182**, 359–360

Holden, H. E. (1982). Comparison of somatic and germ cell models for cytogenetic screening. *J. Appl. Toxicol.*, **2**, 196–200

Hozier, J., Sawger, D., Clive, D. and Moore, M. (1982). Cytogenetic distinction between the TK⁺ and TK⁻ chromosomes in L5178Y/TK⁺/⁻ -3.7.2.C mouse lymphoma cell line. *Mutation Res.*, **105**, 451–456

Hsie, A. W., Brimer, P. A., Mitchell, T. J. and Gosslee, D. G. (1975). The dose-response relationship for ethyl methane sulfonate-induced mutation at the hypoxanthine-guanine phosphoribosyl transferase locus in Chinese hamster ovary cells. *Somatic Cell Genet.*, **1**, 247–261

Hubbard, S. A., Brooks, T. M., Gonzalez, L. P. and

Bridges, J. W. (1985). Preparation and characterisation of S9-fractions. In Parry, J. M. and Arlett, C. F. (Eds), *Comparative Genetic Toxicology*. Macmillan, London, pp. 413–438

Hubbard, S. A., Green, M. H. L., Gatehouse, D. and Bridges, J. W. (1984). The fluctuation test in bacteria. In Kilbey, B.J., Legator, M., Nichols, W. and Ramel, C. (Eds), *Handbook of Mutagenicity Test Procedures*, 2nd edn. Elsevier, Amsterdam, pp. 142–161

Husain, I., Van Houten, B., Thomas, D.C., Abdel-Monem, M. and Sancar, A. (1985). Effect of DNA polymerase I and DNA helicase II on the turnover rate of UvrABC excision nuclease. *Proc. Natl Acad. Sci. USA*, **82**, 6774–6778

ICPEMC (1983). Committee 1 Final Report: screening strategy for chemicals that are potential germ-cell mutagens in mammals. *Mutation Res.*, **114**, 117–177

Isono, K. and Yourno, J. (1974). Chemical carcinogens as frameshift mutagens: *Salmonella* DNA sequence sensitive to mutagenesis by polycyclic carcinogens. *Proc. Natl Acad. Sci. USA*, **71**, 1612–1617

Jeggo, P. (1979). Isolation and characterisation of E. coli K-12 mutants unable to induce the adaptive response to simple alkylating agents. *J. Bacteriol.*, **139**, 783–791

Jordan, E., Saedler, H. and Starlinger, P. (1967). Strong polar mutations in the transferase gene of the galactose operon in *E. coli*. *Molec. Gen. Genet.*, **100**, 296–306

Kada, T. (1973). *Escherichia coli* mutagenicity of furyl furamide. *Jap. J. Genet.*, **48**, 301–305

Kada, T. (1981). The DNA-damaging activity of 42 coded compounds in the Rec-assay. In de Serres, F. J. and Ashby, J. (Eds), *Evaluation of Short-term Tests for Carcinogens—report of the International Collaborative Program*. Elsevier/North Holland, Amsterdam, pp. 175–182

Kalter, K. (1977). Correlation between teratogenic and mutagenic effects of chemicals in mammals. In Hollaender, A. (Ed.), *Chemical Mutagens: Principles and Methods for Their Detection*, Vol. 6. Plenum Press, New York, pp. 57–82

Kaplan, W. D. and Lyon, M. F. (1953). Failure of mercaptoethylamine to protect against the mutagenic effects of radiation. II. Experiments with mice. *Science*, **118**, 777–778

Karran, P., Hjelmgren, T. and Lindahl, T. (1982). Induction of a DNA glycosylase for N-methylated purines is part of the adaptive response to alkylating agents. *Nature*, **296**, 770–773

Kato, T. and Shinoura, Y. (1977). Isolation and characterisation of mutants of *Escherichia coli* deficient in induction of mutations by ultraviolet light. *Molec. Gen. Genet.*, **156**, 121–132

Kaufmann, W. K. (1988). Review: *In vitro* complementation of xeroderma pigmentosum. *Mutagenesis*, **3**, 373–380

Kelley, W. N. and Wyngaarden, J. B. (1983). Clinical

syndromes associated with hypoxanthine guanine phosphoribosyltransferase deficiency. In Stanbury, J. B., Wyngaarden, J. B., Frederickson, D. S., Goldstein, J. L. and Brown, M. S. (Eds), *The Metabolic Basis of Inherited Disease*. McGraw-Hill, New York, pp. 1115–1143

Kennelly, J. C., Stanton, C. and Martin, C. N. (1984). The effect of acetyl-CoA supplementation on the mutagenicity of benzidines in the Ames assay. *Mutation Res.*, **137**, 39–45

Kier, L. E., Brusick, D. J., Auletta, A. E., Von Halle, E. S., Brown, M. M., Simmon, V. F., Dunkel, V., McCann, J., Mortelmans, K., Prival, M., Rao, T. K. and Ray, V. (1986). The *Salmonella typhimurium/* mammalian microsomal assay. A report of the US Environmental Protection Agency Gene-Tox Program. *Mutation Res.*, **168**, 69–240

Kingsman, A. J., Chater, K. F. and Kingsman, S. M. (1988). *Transposition*. Forty-third symposium of the Society for General Microbiology. Cambridge University Press, Cambridge

Kirkland, D. (1992). Chromosomal abberation tests *in vitro*: problems with protocol design and interpretation of results. *Mutagenesis*, **7**, 95–106

Kirkland, D., Gatehouse, D., Reed, P., Sullman, S., Vennitt, S., Walters, C. and Watkins, P. (1984). Bacterial mutation assays with nitrosation products. In Dean, B. J. (Ed.), *UKEMS Subcommittee on Guidelines for Mutagenicity Testing. Report Part II: Supplementary Tests*. United Kingdom Environmental Mutagen Society, Swansea, pp. 245–260

Kirkwood, T. B. L. (1989). DNA, mutations and aging. *Mutation Res.*, **219**, 1–7

Knudson, A. G. (1985). Hereditary cancer oncogenes and antioncogenes. *Cancer Res.*, **45**, 1437–1443

Kohler, S. W., Provost, G. S., Fieck, A., Kretz, P. L., Bullock, W. O., Sorge, J. A., Putman, D. L. and Short, J. M. (1991). Spectra of spontaneous and mutagen-induced mutations in the *Lac I* gene in transgenic mice. *Proc. Natl Acad. Sci. USA*, **88**, 7958–7962

Kondo, S., Ichikawa, H., Iwo, K. and Kato, T. (1970). Base change mutagenesis and prophage induction in strains of *Escherichia coli* with different DNA repair capacities. *Genetics*, **66**, 167–217

Konecki, D. S., Brennand, J., Fuscee, J. C., Caskey, C. T. and Chinault, A. C. (1982). Hypoxanthine-guanine phosphoribosyltransferase genes of mouse and Chinese hamster: Construction and sequence analysis of cDNA recombinants. *Nucleic Acids Res.*, **10**, 6763–6775

Koufos, A., Hausen, M. F., Lampkin, B. C., Workman, M. L., Copeland, N. G., Jenkins, N. A. and Cavenee, W. K. (1984). Loss of alleles at loci on human chromosome 11 during genesis of Wilm's tumour. *Nature*, **309**, 170–172

Kraemer, K. H., Myung, M. L. and Scotto, J. (1984). DNA repair protects against cutaneous and internal neoplasia: evidence from xeroderma pigmentosum. *Carcinogenesis*, **5**, 511–514

Kuhnlein, U., Bergstrom, D. and Kuhnlein, H. (1981). Mutagens in feces from vegetarians and non-vegetarians. *Mutation Res.*, **85**, 1–12

Langer, P. J., Sharnabruch, W.G. and Walker, G.C. (1981). Functional organisation of plasmid pKM101. *J. Bacteriol.*, **145**, 1310–1316

Lawley, P. (1989). Mutagens as carcinogens: development of current concepts. *Mutation Res.*, **213**, 3–26

Lederberg, J. (1962). *Bull. Atom. Sci.* (1955); reprinted in Schull, W.S. (Ed.), *Mutations*. University of Michigan Press, Ann Arbor, pp. 237–238

Lehmann, A. R., Arlett, C. F., Broughton, B. C., Harcourt, S. A., Steingrimsdottir, H., Stefanini, M., Taylor, A. M. R., Natarajan, A. T., Green, S. King, M. D., Mackie, R. M., Stephenson, J. B. P. and Tolmie, J. L. (1988). Trichothiodystrophy, a human DNA repair disorder with heterogeneity in the cellular response to ultraviolent light. *Cancer Res.*, **48**, 6090–6096

Lehmann, A. R., Kirk-Bell, S., Arlett, C. F., Paterson, M. C., Lohman, P. H. M., de Weerd-Kastelein, E. A. and Bootsma, D. (1975). Xeroderma pigmentosum cells with normal levels of excision repair have a defect in DNA synthesis after UV-irradiation. *Proc. Natl Acad. Sci. USA*, **72**, 219–223

Levin, D. E., Blunt, E. L. and Levin, R. E. (1981). Modified fluctuation test for the detection of mutagens in food with *Salmonella typhimurium* TA98. *Mutation Res.*, **85**, 309–321

Levin, D. E., Hollstein, M., Christman, M. F., Schwiers, E. A. and Ames, B. N. (1982a). A new *Salmonella* tester strain (TA102) with A–T base pairs at the site of mutation detects oxidative mutagens. *Proc. Natl Acad. Sci. USA*, **79**, 7445–7449

Levin, D. E., Yamasaki, E. and Ames, B. N. (1982b). A new *Salmonella* tester strain, TA97, for the detection of frameshift mutagens. A run of cytosines as a mutational hot-spot. *Mutation Res.*, **94**, 315–330

Li, A. P., Aaron, C. S., Aueltta, A. E., Dearfield, K. L., Riddle, J. C., Slesinski, R. S. and Stankowski, L. F., Jr. (1991). An evaluation of the roles of mammalian cell mutation assays in the testing of chemical genotoxicity. *Regulatory Toxicol. Pharmacol.*, **14**, 24–40

Li, A. P., Carver, J. H., Choy, W. N., Gupta, R. S., Loveday, K. S., O'Neill, J. P., Riddle, J. C., Stankowski, L. F. and Yang, L. C. (1987). A guide for the performance of the Chinese Hamster ovary cell/hypoxanthine guanine phosphoribosyl transferase gene mutation assay. *Mutation Res.*, **189**, 135–141

Li, A. P., Gupta, R. S., Heflich, R. H. and Wassom, J. S. (1988). A review and analysis of the Chinese hamster ovary/hypoxanthine guanine phosphoribosyl transferase assay to determine the mutagenicity of chemical agents. A report of Phase III of the US

Environmental Protection Agency, Gene. Tox. Program. *Mutation Res.*, **196**, 17–36

Linblad, W. J. and Jackim, E. (1982). Mechanism for the differential induction of mutation by S9 activated benzo(*a*)pyrene employing either a glucose-6-phosphate dependent NADPH-regenerating system or an isocitrate dependent system. *Mutation Res.*, **96**, 109–118

Lindahl, T. (1979). DNA glycosylases, endonucleases for apurinic/apyrimidinic sites and base excision repair. *Proc. Nucl. Acid. Res. Mol. Biol.*, **22**, 135–192

Lindahl, T. (1987). Regulation and deficiencies in DNA repair. *Br. J. Cancer*, **56**, 91–95

Lindahl, T., Sedgwick, B., Sekiguchi, M. and Naka-beppu, Y. (1988). Regulation and expression of the adaptive response to alkylating agents. *Ann. Rev. Biochem.*, **57** 133–157

Little, C. A., Tweats, D. J. and Pinney, R. J. (1989). Studies of error-prone DNA repair in *Escherichia coli* K-12 and Ames *Salmonella typhimurium* strains using a model alkylating agent. *Mutagenesis*, **4**, 90–94

Little, J. B. and Nagasawa, H. (1980). Repair of potentially lethal damage in UV-irradiated Gardner's syndrome fibroblasts; Effects on survival and sister chromatid exchanges. *Radiation Res.*, **83**, 474

Little, J. W. (1984). Autodigestion of *lex A* and phage T repressors. *Proc. Natl Acad. Sci. USA*, **81**, 1375–1379

Little, J. W. and Mount, D. W. (1982). The SOS regulatory system of *Escherichia coli*. *Cell*, **29**, 11–22

Lofroth, G., Hefner, E., Alfheim, I. and Moller, M. (1980). Mutagenic activity in photocopies. *Science*, **209**, 1037–1309

Luria, S. E. and Delbruck, M. (1943). Mutations of bacteria from virus sensitivity to virus resistance. *Genetics*, **28**, 491–511

McCann, J., Choi, E., Yamasaki, E. and Ames, B. N. (1975). Detection of carcinogens as mutagens in the *Salmonella*/microsome test assay of 300 chemicals. *Proc. Natl Acad. Sci. USA*, **72**, 5135–5139

McCann, J., Spingarn, N. E., Kobori, J. and Ames, B. N. (1975). Detection of carcinogens as mutagens: Bacterial tester strains with R factor plasmids. *Proc. Natl Acad. Sci. USA*, **72**, 979–983

McKinnon, P. J. (1987). Ataxia-telangiectasia: an inherited disorder of ionising-radiation sensitivity in man. *Human Genet.*, **75**, 197–208

McKusick, V. A. (1988). *Mendelian Inheritance in Man: Catalogs of Autosomal Dominant, Autosomal Recessive and X-linked Phenotypes*, 8th edn. Johns Hopkins University Press, Baltimore

MacPhee, D. G. (1973). *Salmonella typhimurium* hisG46 (R-Utrecht): possible use in screening mutagens and carcinogens. *Appl. Microbiol.*, **26**, 1004–1005

MacPhee, D. G. (1989). Development of bacterial mutagenicity tests: a view from afar. *Environ. Molec. Mutagen.*, **14**, Suppl. 16, 35–38

Mahon, G. A. T., Green, M. H. L., Middleton, B., Mitchell, I. de G., Robinson, W. D. and Tweats, D. J. (1989). Analysis of data from microbial colony assays. In Kirkland, D. J. (Ed.), *Statistical Evaluation of Mutagenicity Test Data*. Cambridge University Press, Cambridge, pp. 26–65

Malling, H. V. (1969). Ethylene dibromide: a potent pesticide with high mutagenic activity. *Genetics*, **61**, S39

Malling, H. V. (1971). Dimethylnitrosamine: Formation of mutagenic compounds by interaction with mouse liver microsomes. *Mutation Res.*, **13**, 425–429

Marinus, M. G. and Morris, R. N. (1974). Biological function for the 6-methyladenine residues in the DNA of *Escherichia coli* K12. *J. Molec. Biol.*, **85**, 309–322

Maron, D. M. and Ames, B. N. (1983). Revised methods for the *Salmonella* mutagenicity test. *Mutation Res.*, **113**, 173–215

Mason, J. M., Strobel, E. and Green, M. M. (1984). *Mu–2* mutator gene in *Drosophila* that potentiates the induction of terminal deficiencies. *Proc. Natl. Acad. Sci. USA*, **81**, 6090–6094

Matsumoto, T., Yoshida, D., Mizusaki, S. and Okamoto, H. (1977). Mutagenic activity of amino acid pyrolysates in *Salmonella typhimurium* TA98. *Mutation Res.*, **48**, 279–286

Mayne, L. V., Mullenders, L. H. F. and Van Zeeland, A. A. (1988). Cockayne's syndrome: a UV sensitive disorder with a defect in the repair of transcribing DNA but normal overall excision repair. In Friedberg, E. C. and Hanawalt, P. C. (Eds), *Mechanisms and Consequences of DNA Damage Processing*. Alan R. Liss, New York, pp. 349–353

Miller, E. C. and Miller, J. A. (1971). The mutagenicity of chemical carcinogens: correlations, problems and interpretations. In Hollaender, A. (Ed.), *Chemical Mutagens, Principles and Methods for Their Detection*, Vol. 1. Plenum Press, New York, pp. 83–120

Miller, J. H. (1985). Pathways of mutagenesis revealed by analysis of mutational specificity. In Scaife, J., Leach, D. and Galizzi, A. (Eds), *Genetics of Bacteria*. Academic Press, New York, pp. 25–40

Mitchell, I. de G. and Combes, R. D. (1984). Mutation tests with the fruit fly *Drosophila melanogaster*. In Venitt, S. and Parry, J. M. (Eds), *Mutagenicity Testing, a Practical Approach*. IRL Press, Oxford, pp. 149–185

Modrich, P. (1987). DNA mismatch correction. *Ann. Rev. Biochem.*, **56**, 435–466

Morisaki, N., Koyama, N., Mori, S., Kanzaki, T., Koshikawa, T., Saito, Y. and Yoshida, S. (1989). Effects of smooth muscle cell derived growth factor (SDGF) in combination with other growth factors on smooth muscle cells. *Atherosclerosis*, **78**, 61–67

Morley, A. A., Trainor, K. J., Seshadri, R. and Ryall, R. G. (1983). Measurement of *in vivo* mutations in human lymphocytes. *Nature*, **302**, 155–156

Mortelmans, K. E. (1975). *Effect of R Plasmids on* Salmonella typhimurium: *UV-killing, UV-mutagenesis and Spontaneous Mutability*. PhD Thesis, Stanford University, California

Mortelmans, K. E. and Dousman, L. (1986). Mutagenesis and plasmids. In de Serres, F. J. (Ed.), *Chemical Mutagens, Principles and Methods for Their Detection*, Vol. 10. Plenum Press, New York, London, pp. 469–508

Mortelmans, K. E. and Stocker, B. A. D. (1976). Ultraviolet light protection, enhancement of ultraviolet light mutagenesis, and mutator effect of plasmid R46 in *Salmonella typhimurium. J. Bacteriol.* **128**, 271–282

Mortelmans, K. E. and Stocker, B.A.D. (1979). Segregation of the mutator property of plasmid R46 from its ultraviolet-protecting property. *Molec. Gen. Genet.*, **167**, 317–328

Moustacchi, E., Papadopoulo, D., Diatoloff-Zito, C. and Buchwald, M. (1987). Two complementation groups of Fanconi's anemia differ in their phenotypic response to DNA-crosslinking treatment. *Human Genet.*, **75**, 45–47

Muller, H. J. (1927). Artificial transmutation of the gene. *Science*, **66**, 84–87

Myhr, B. and Kirkland, D. J. (1991). *In vivo* mutagenesis as detected at the *Lac Z* locus in the mutamouse. Abstract P-7-36, *21st Annual Meeting of the EEMS on Environmental Mutagens—Carcinogens, Prague, 25–31 August 1991*

Natarajan, A. T. and Obe, G. (1982). Mutagenicity testing with cultured mammalian cells: cytogenetic assays. In Heddle, J. A. (Ed.), *Mutagenicity, New Horizons in Genetic Toxicology*. Academic Press, New York, pp. 172–213

National Cancer Institute (NCI) (1978a). *Bioassay of 2,4-Diaminoanisole Sulfate for Possible Carcinogenicity*. NCI Carcinogenesis Technical Report Series No. 84, DHEW, USA publication (NIH) 78–1334. US Government Printing Office, Washington, D. C.

National Cancer Institute (NCI) (1978b). *Bioassay of Tris (2,3-dibromopropyl) phosphate for Possible Carcinogenicity*. NCI Carcinogenesis Technical Report Series No. 76, DHEW USA publication (NIH) 78–1326. US Government Printing Office, Washington, D. C.

Naylor, S. L., Johnson, B. E., and Minna, J. D. and Sakaguchi, A. Y. (1987). Loss of heterozygosity of chromosome 3p markers in small-cell lung cancer. *Nature*, **329**, 451–454

Neudecker, T. and Henschler, D. (1985). Allyl isothiocyanate is mutagenic in *Salmonella typhimurium. Mutation Res.*, **156**, 33–37

Newbold, R. F., Brookes, P., Arlett, C. F., Bridges, B. A., and Dean, B. (1975). The effect of variable serum factors and clonal morphology on the ability to detect hypoxanthine guanine phosphoribosyl transferase (HPRT) deficient variants in cultured Chinese hamster cells. *Mutation Res.*, **30**, 143–148

Newcombe, H. B. (1952). A comparison of spontaneous and induced mutations of *Escherichia coli* to streptomycin resistance and dependence. *J. Cell. Comp. Physiol.*, **39**, Suppl. 1, 13–26

Nilsson, J. (1986). Growth factors and the pathogenesis of atherosclerosis. *Atherosclerosis*, **62**, 185–199

Nomura, T. (1975). Carcinogenicity of the food additive furylfuramide in foetal and young mice. *Nature*, **258**, 610–611

Oberly, T. J., Bewsey, B. J. and Probst, G. S. (1987). A procedure for the CHO/HGPRT mutation assay involving treatment of cells in suspension culture and selection of mutants in soft agar. *Mutation Res.*, **182**, 99–111

Ohgake, H. Matsukura, N., Morino, K. Kawachi, T., Sugimura, T., Morita, K., Tokiwa, H., and Hirota, T. (1982). Carcinogenicity in rats of the mutagenic compounds 1-nitropyrene and 3-nitrofluoranthene. *Cancer Lett.*, **15**, 1–7

Olesen, F. B. (1990). Overview of *in vivo* mammalian testing systems. In Mendelsohn, M. L. and Albertini, R. J. (Eds), *Mutation and the Environment*. Part B: *Metabolism, Testing Methods and Chromosomes*. Wiley-Liss, New York, pp. 171–184

Olson, W. A., Habermann, R. T., Weisburger, E. K., Ward, J. M. and Weisburger, J. H. (1973). Induction of stomach cancer in rats and mice by halogenated aliphatic fumigants. *J. Natl Cancer Inst.*, **51**, 1993–1995

Olsson, M. and Lindahl, T. (1980). Repair of alkylated DNA in *Escherichia coli*: methyl group transfer from O^6-methylguanine to a protein cysteine residue. *J. Biol. Chem.*, **255**, 10569–10571

O'Neill, J. P., Brimer, P. A., Machannoff, R., Hirsch, G. P. and Hsie, A. W. (1977a). A quantitative assay of mutation induction of the hypoxanthine-guanine phosphoribosyltransferase locus in Chinese hamster ovary cells (CHO/HGPRT system): Development and definition of the system. *Mutation Res.*, **45**, 91–101

O'Neill, J. P., Couch, D. B., Machannoff, R., San Sebastian, J. R., Brimer, P. A. and Hsie, A. W. (1977b). A quantitative assay of mutation induction at the hypoxanthine-guanine phosphoribosyltransferase locus in Chinese hamster ovary cells (CHO/HGPRT system): Utilization with a variety of mutagenic agents. *Mutation Res.*, **45**, 103–109

Ong, T., Mukhtar, M., Wolf, C. R. and Zeiger, E. (1980). Differential effects of cytochrome P450-inducers on promutagen activation capabilities and enzymatic activities of S-9 from rat liver. *J. Environ. Pathol. Toxicol.*, **4**, 55–65

Paes, D. J. (1984). Microbial mutagenicity of selected hydrazines (misuse of data). *Mutation Res.*, **136**, 89–90

Paes, D. J. V. and Tweats, D. J. (1980). Bacterial and mutagenicity tests of β-lactam antibiotics. *Mutation Res.*, **74**, 245

Pagano, D. A. and Zeiger, E. (1985). The stability

of mutagenic chemicals stored in solution. *Environ. Mutagen.*, **7**, 293–302

Painter, R. B. (1981). Radioresistant DNA synthesis: an intrinsic feature of ataxia telangiectasia. *Mutation Res.*, **84**, 183–190

Palombo, F., Bignami, M. and Dogliotti, E. (1991). Non-phenotypic selection of *N*-methyl-*N*-nitrosourea induced mutations in human cells. Abstract P-7-7, *21st Annual Meeting of the EEMS on Environmental Mutagens—Carcinogens, Prague, 25–31 August 1991*

Papadopoulo, D., Averbeck, D. and Moustacchi, E. (1987). The fate of 8-methoxy-psoralen-photoinduced DNA interstrand cross-links in Fanconi's anemia cells of defined complementation groups. *Mutation Res.*, **184**, 271–280

Parry, J. M., Arlett, C. F. and Ashby, J. (1985). An overview of the results of the *in vivo* and *in vitro* test systems used to assay the genotoxicity of BZD, DAT, DAB and CDA in the second UKEMS study. In Parry, J. M. and Arlett, C. F. (Eds), *Comparative Genetic Toxicology: The Second UKEMS Collaborative Study*. Macmillan, London, pp. 597–616

Parry, J. M., Shamsher, M. and Skibinski, D. O. F. (1990). Restriction site mutation analysis: a proposed methodology for the detection and study of DNA base changes following mutagen exposure. *Mutagenesis*, **5**, 209–212

Parry, J. M., Tweats, D. J. and Al-Mossawi, M. A. J. (1976). Monitoring the marine environment for mutagens. *Nature*, **264**, 538–540

Patel, P. I., Framson, P. E., Caskey, C. T. and Chinault, A. C. (1986a). Fine structure of the human hypoxanthine phosphoribosyltransferase gene. *Molec. Cell. Biol.*, **6**, 393–403

Patel, P. I., Yang, T. P., Stout, J. T., Konecki, D. S., Chinault, A. C. and Caskey, C. T. (1986b). Mutational diversity at the human HPRT locus. In Ramel, C., Lambert, B. and Magnusson, J. (Eds), *Genetic Toxicology of Environmental Chemicals. Part A: Basic Principles and Mechanisms of Action*. Alan R Liss, New York, pp. 457–463

Perry, K. L., Elledge, S. J., Lichtman, M. R. and Walker, G. C. (1982). Plasmid mediated enhancement of chemical mutagens. In Sugimura, S., Kondo, S. and Takebe, H. (Eds), *Environmental Mutagens and Carcinogens*. University of Tokyo Press, Tokyo, and Alan R. Liss, New York, pp. 113–120

Perry, K. L., Elledge, S. J., Mitchell, B. B., Marsh, L. and Walker, G. C. (1985). *umu DC* and *muc AB* operons whose products are required for UV light- and chemical-induced mutagenesis; Umu D, MucA and Lex A proteins share homology. *Proc. Natl Acad. Sci. USA*, **82**, 4331–4335

Perry, K. L. and Walker G. C. (1982). Identification of plasmid (pKM101)-coded proteins involved in mutagenesis and UV resistance. *Nature*, **300**, 278–281

Pinney, R. J. (1980). Distribution among incompat-ability groups of plasmids that confer UV mutability and UV resistance. *Mutation Res.*, **72**, 155–159

Price, V. H., Odom, R. B., Ward, W. H. and Jones, F. T. (1980). Trichothiodystrophy. Sulfur-deficient brittle hair as a marker for a neuroectodermal symptom complex. *Arch. Dermatol.*, **116**, 1375–1384

Prival, M. J., Bell, S. J., Mitchell, V. D., Peiperl, M. D. and Vaughn, V. L. (1984). Mutagenicity of benzidine and benzidine-congener dyes and selected monoazo dyes in a modified *Salmonella* assay. *Mutation Res.*, **136**, 33–47

Prival, M. J., McCoy, E. C., Gutter, B. and Rosenkranz, H. S. (1977). Tris(2,3-dibromopropyl)phosphate: mutagenicity of a widely used flame retardant. *Science*, **195**, 76–78

Prival, M. J. and Mitchell, V. D. (1982). Analysis of a method for testing azo-dyes for mutagenic activity in *S. typhimurium* in the presence of FMN in hamster liver S9. *Mutation Res.*, **97**, 103–116

Pueyo, C. and Lopez-Barea, J. (1979). The L-arabinose-resistance test with *Salmonella typhimurium* strain SV3 selects forward mutations at several *ara* genes. *Mutation Res.*, **64**, 249–258

Pyrzak, R. and Shih, J. C. H. (1987). Detection of specific DNA segments of Marek's disease herpes virus in Japanese quail susceptible to atherosclerosis. *Atherosclerosis*, **68**, 77–85

Quintanilla, M., Brown, K., Ramsden, M. and Balmain, A. (1986). Carcinogen-specific mutation and amplification of Ha-*ras* during mouse skin carcinogenesis. *Nature*, **322**, 78–80

Reddy, E. P., Reynolds, R. K., Santos, E. and Barbacid, M. (1982). A point mutation is responsible for the acquisition of transforming properties by the T238 human bladder carcinoma oncogene. *Nature*, **300**, 149–152

Riordan, J. R., Rommens, J. M., Kerem, B., Alon, N., Rozmahel, R., Grzeolczak, Z., Zielenski, J., Lok, S., Plavsic, N., Chou, J., Drumm, M. L., Iannuzzi, M. C., Collins, F. S. and Tsui, L. (1989). Identification of the cystic fibrosis gene: cloning and characterization of complementary DNA. *Science*, **245**, 1066–1073

Robertson, M. (1983). Oncogenes and the origins of human cancer. *Br. Med. J.*, **286**, 81–82

Robinson, W. D., Green, M. H. L., Cole, J., Healy, M. J. R., Garner, R. C. and Gatehouse, D. (1989). Statistical evaluation of bacterial/mammalian fluctuation tests. In Kirkland, D. J. (Ed.), *Statistical Evaluation of Mutagenicity Test Data*. Cambridge University Press, Cambridge, pp. 102–140

Rossiter, B. J. F., Muzny, D. M., Hampson, I., Caskey, C. T. and Fox, M. (1990). Induced reversion of a spontaneous point mutation within the Chinese hamster HGPRT gene to the wild-type sequence. *Mutagenesis*, **5**, 605–608

Rossman, T. G. and Klein, C. B. (1988). From DNA damage to mutation in mammalian cells: a review. *Environ. Molec. Mutagen.*, **11**, 119–133

Roth, J. R. (1974). Frameshift mutations. *Ann. Rev. Genet.*, **8**, 319–346

Rowland, I., Rubery, E. and Walker, R. (1984). Bacterial assays for mutagens in food. In Dean, B. J. (Ed.), *UKEMS Subcommittee on Guidelines for Mutagenicity Testing. Report Part II: Supplementary Tests*. United Kingdom Environmental Mutagen Society, Swansea, pp. 203–244

Rupp, W. D., Wilde, C. E., Reno, D. L. and Howard-Flanders, P. (1971). Exchanges between DNA strands in ultraviolet-irradiated *Escherichia coli*. *J. Molec. Biol.*, **61**, 25–44

Russell, L. B. (1984). Procedures and evaluation of results of the mouse spot test. In Kilbey, B. J., Legator, M., Nichols, W. and Ramel, C. (Eds), *Handbook of Mutagenicity Test Procedures*. Elsevier, Amsterdam, pp. 393–403

Russell, L. B. (1989a). Functional and structural analyses of mouse genomic regions screened by the morphological specific locus test. *Mutation. Res.*, **212**, 23–32

Russell, L. B., Cumming, R. B. and Hunsicker, P. R. (1984). Specific-locus mutation rates in the mouse following inhalation of ethylene oxide and the application of the results to estimation of human genetic risk. *Mutation Res.*, **129**, 381–388

Russell, L. B. and Major, M. H. (1957). Radiation induced presumed somatic mutations in the house mouse. *Genetics*, **42**, 161–175

Russell, L. B., Selby, P. B., Von Halle, E., Sheridan, W. and Valcovic, L. (1981). Use of the mouse spot test in chemical mutagenesis: interpretation of past data and recommendations for future work. *Mutation Res.*, **86**, 355–379

Russell, L. B. and Shelby, M. (1985). Tests for heritable genetic damage and for evidence of gonadal exposure in mammals. *Mutation Res.*, **154**, 69–84

Russell, W. L. (1951). X-ray induced mutations in mice. *Cold Spring Harbor Symp. Quant. Biol.*, **16**, 327–336

Russell, W. L. (1989b). Reminiscences of a mouse specific-locus test addict. *Environ. Molec. Mutagen.*, **14** (Suppl. 16), 16–22

Ryan, F. (1955). Spontaneous mutation in non-dividing bacteria. *Genetics*, **40**, 726–738

Samson, L. and Cairns, J. (1977). A new pathway for DNA repair in *E. coli*. *Nature*, **267**, 281–282

Sankaranarayanan, K. (1988). Prevalence of genetic and partially genetic diseases in man and the estimation of genetic risk of exposure to ionizing radiation. *Am. J. Human Genet.*, **42**, 651–662

Sarasin, A. (1989). Molecular mechanisms of mutagenesis in mammalian cells: present and future. *Mutation. Res.*, **220**, 51–53

Sasaki, M. S. and Tonomura, A. (1973). A high susceptibility of Fanconi's anemia to chromosome breakage by DNA cross-linking agents. *Cancer Res.*, **33**, 1829–1836

Sawyer, J., Moore, M. M., Clive, D. and Hozier, J.

(1985). Cytogenetic characterization of the L5178Y TK$^{+/-}$3.7.2C. mouse lymphoma cell line. *Mutation Res.*, **147**, 243–253

Schmickel, R. D., Chu, E. H. and Trosko, J. E. (1977). Cockayne syndrome, a cellular sensitivity to ultraviolet light. *Pediatrics*, **60**, 135–139

Schmidt, G. H., O'Sullivan, J. F. and Paul, D. (1990). Ethylnitrosourea-induced mutations *in vivo* involving the *Dolichos biflorus* agglutinin receptor in mouse intestinal epithelium. *Mutation Res.*, **228**, 149–155

Schwartz, R. C. and Witte, O. N. (1988). The role of multiple oncogenes in hematopoietic neoplasia. *Mutation Res.*, **195**, 245–253

Searle, A. G. (1984). The specific locus test in the mouse. In Kilbey, B. J., Legator, M., Nichols, W. and Ramel, C. (Eds), *Handbook of Mutagenicity Test Procedures*. Elsevier, Amsterdam, pp. 373–391

Sedgwick, S. G. and Goodwin, P. A. (1985). Differences in mutagenic and recombinational DNA repair in enterobacteria. *Proc. Natl Acad. Sci. USA*, **82**, 4172–4176

Selby, P. B. and Olson, W. H. (1981). Methods and criteria for deciding whether specific-locus mutation-rate data in mice indicates a positive, negative or inconclusive result. *Mutation Res.*, **83**, 403–418

Shanabruch, W. G. and Walker, G. C. (1980). Localization of the plasmid (pKM101) gene(s) involved in *recA$^+$lexA$^+$*-dependent mutagenesis. *Molec. Gen. Genet.*, **129**, 289–297

Smith, K. C. and Meun, D. H. C. (1970). Repair of radiation induced damage in *Escherichia coli*. I. Effect of *rec* mutations on post-replication repair of damage due to ultraviolet irradiation. *J. Molec. Biol.*, **51**, 457–472

Solomon, E., Voss, R., Hall, V., Bodmer, W. F., Jass, J. R., Jeffreys, A. J., Lucibello, F. C., Patel, I. and Rider, S. H. (1987). Chromosome 5 allele loss in human colorectal carcinomas. *Nature*, **328**, 616–619

Spector, B. D., Filipovich, A. H., Perry, G. S. and Kersey, J. H. (1982). Epidemiology of cancer in ataxia-telangiectasia. In Bridges, B. A. and Harnden, D. G. (Eds), *Ataxia-telangiestasia—A Cellular and Molecular Link between Cancer, Neuropathology, and Immune Deficiency*. Wiley, New York, pp. 103–138

Steel, R. G. D. and Torrie, J. H. (1960). *Principles and Procedures of Statistics*. McGraw-Hill, New York

Stowers, S. J., Maronpot, R. R., Reynolds, S. H. and Anderson, M. W. (1987). The role of oncogenes in chemical carcinogenesis. *Environ. Hlth Perspect.* **75**, 81–86

Streisinger, G., Okada, Y., Emrich, J., Newton, J., Tsugita, A., Terzaghi, E. and Inouye, M. (1966). Frameshift mutations and the genetic code. *Cold Spring Harbor Symp. Quant. Biol.*, **31**, 77–84

Sugimura, T. and Sata, S. (1983). Mutagens-carcinogens in foods. *Cancer Res.*, Suppl., 2415S–2421S

Sukumar, S., Notario, V., Martin-Zanca, D. and Barbacid, M. (1983). Induction of mammary carcinomas in rats by nitroso-methylurea involves a malignant activation of H-*ras*-1 locus by single point mutations. *Nature*, **306**, 658–661

Sutherland, B. M. (1981). Photoreactivating enzymes. *Enzymes*, **14**, 481–515

Swenberg, J. A., Kerns, W. D., Mitchell, R. I., Gralla, E. J. and Pavkov, K. L. (1980). Induction of squamous cell carcinomas of the rat nasal cavity by inhalation exposure to formaldehyde vapor. *Cancer Res.*, **40**, 3398–3402

Tabin, C. J., Bradley, S. M., Bargmaan, C. I., Weinberg, R. A., Papageorge, A. G., Scolnick, E. M., Dhar, R., Lowy, D. and Chang, E. H. (1982). Mechanism of activation of a human oncogene. *Nature*, **300**, 143–149

Tanaka, H. and Orri, T. (1980). High sensitivity but normal DNA repair activity after UV-irradiation in Epstein-Barr virus-transformed lymphoblastoid cell lines from Chediak–Higashi syndrome. *Mutation Res.*, **72**, 143–150

Tennant, R. W., Margolin, B. H., Shelby, M. D., Zeiger, E., Haseman, J. K., Spalding, J., Caspary, W., Resnick, M., Stasiewicz, S., Anderson, B. and Minor, R. (1987). Prediction of chemical carcinogenicity in rodents from *in vitro* genetic toxicity assays. *Science*, **236**, 933–941

Teo, I., Sedgwick, B., Kilpatrick, M. W., McCarthy, T. C. and Lindahl, T. (1986). The intracellular signal for induction of resistance to akylating agents in *E. coli*. *Cell*, **45**, 315–324

Thomas, H. F., Cole, J. A. and Freeman, B. (1989). Plasmid pKM101 muc⁻- and muc⁺-mediated anthracycline mutagenicity and cytotoxicity in *Salmonella typhimurium*. *Environ. Mutagen.*, **9**, 369–391

Thomas, S. M. and Sedgwick, S. G. (1989). Cloning of *Salmonella typhimurium* DNA encoding mutagenic DNA repair. *J. Bacteriol.*, **171**, 5776–5782

Thompson, K. V. A. and Holliday, R. (1983). Genetic effects on the longevity of cultured human fibroblasts II DNA repair deficient syndromes. *Gerontology*, **29**, 83–88

Thomson, G. (1988). HLA disease association: models for insulin dependent diabetes mellitus and the study of complex human genetic disorders. *Ann. Rev. Genet.*, **22**, 31–50

Todd, J. A., Bell, J. I. and McDevitt, H. O. (1987). HLA-DQβ gene contributes to susceptibility and resistance to insulin dependent diabetes mellitus. *Nature*, **329**, 599–604

Todd, P. A. and Glickman, B. W. (1979). UV protection and mutagenesis in *uvr D*, *uvr E* and *rec L* strains of *Escherichia coli* carrying the pKM101 plasmid. *Mutation Res.*, **62**, 451–457

Tweats, D. J. (1984). The predictive value of batteries of short-term tests for carcinogens. *Fd Add. Contam.*, **1**, 189–197

Tweats, D. J. and Gatehouse, D. G. (1988). Discussion Forum: Further debate of testing strategies. *Mutagenesis*, **3**, 95–102

Tweats, D. J. and Paes, D. J. (1981). A new approach to bacterial mutagenicity tests of β-lactam antibiotics. *J. Pharm. Pharmacol.*, **33**, 76P

Tweats, D. J., Thompson, M. J., Pinney, R. J. and Smith, J. T. (1976). R factor-mediated resistance to ultraviolet light in strains of *Escherichia coli* deficient in known repair functions. *J. Gen. Microbiol.*, **93**, 103–110

Venitt, S. and Crofton-Sleigh, C. (1981). Mutagenicity of 42 coded compounds in a bacterial assay using *Escherichia coli* and *Salmonella typhimurium*. In de Serres, F. J. and Ashby, J. (Eds), *Evaluation of Short-term Tests for Carcinogens. Report of the International Collaborative Program*. Progress in Mutation Research, Vol. 1. Elsevier, New York, pp. 351–360

Venitt, S., Crofton-Sleigh, C. and Forster, R. (1984). Bacterial mutation assays using reverse mutation. In Venitt, S. and Parry, J. M. (Eds), *Mutagenicity Testing, a Practical Approach*, IRL Press, Oxford, Washington D.C., pp. 45–97

Venitt, S. and Parry, J. M. (1984). Background to mutagenicity testing. In Venitt, S. and Parry, J. M. (Eds), *Mutagenicity Testing, a Practical Approach*. IRL Press, Oxford, Washington, D. C., pp. 1–24

Villani, G., Boiteux, S. and Radman, M. (1978). Mechanism of ultraviolet-induced mutagenesis: extent and fidelity of *in vitro* DNA synthesis on irradiated template. *Proc. Natl Acad. Sci. USA*, **75**, 3037–3041

Vogel, E. (1982). Dependence of mutagenesis in *Drosophila* males on metabolism and germ cell stage. In Sugimura, T., Kondo, S. and Takebe, H. (Eds), *Environmental Mutagens and Carcinogens*. University of Tokyo Press, Tokyo, and Alan R. Liss, New York, pp. 183–194

Vogel, E. W. (1985). The *Drosophila* somatic recombination and mutation assay (srm) using the white-coral somatic eye color system. *Prog. Mutation Res.*, **5**, 313–317

Vogel, E. W. (1991). The future of SMART assays: emphasis on the underlying action principles? *Mutation Res.*, **252**, 169

Vogel, E. W., Dusenbery, R. L. and Smith, P. D. (1985). The relationship between reaction kinetics and mutagenic action of monofunctional alkylating agents in higher eukaryotic systems. IV. The effects of the excision defective *mei-9*[L1] and Mus(2)201[D1] mutants on alkylation-induced genetic damage in *Drosophila*. *Mutation Res.*, **149**, 193–207

Wagner, R. and Meselson, M. (1976). Repair tracts in mismatched DNA heteroduplexes. *Proc. Natl Acad. Sci. USA*, **73**, 4135–4139

Wahrendorf, J., Mahon, G. A. T. and Schumacher, M. (1985). A non-parametric approach to the statistical analysis of mutagenicity data. *Mutation Res.*, **147**, 5–13

Walker, G. C. (1977). Plasmid (pKM101)-mediated enhancement of repair and mutagenesis. Dependence on chromosomal genes in *Escherichia coli*. *Molec. Gen. Genet.*, **152**, 93–103

Walker, G. C. (1984). Mutagenesis and inducible responses to deoxyribonucleic acid damage in *Escherichia coli*. *Microbiol. Rev.*, **48**, 60–93

Walker, G. C. (1986). Plasmid biology of pKM101: role of the mucAB genes. In Levy, S. B. and Novick, R. B. (Eds), *Antibiotic Resistance Genes: Ecology, Transfer and Expression*. Banbury Report 24. Cold Spring Harbor Laboratory, N.Y., pp. 313–320

Walker, G. C. and Dobson, P. P. (1979). Mutagenesis and repair deficiencies of *Escherichia coli umu C* mutants are suppressed by the plasmid pKM101. *Molec. Gen. Genet.*, **172**, 17–24

Wassom, J. S. (1980). Mutagenicity research in the United States. *Mutagens Toxicol.*, **9**, 4–15

Wassom, J. S. (1989). Origins of genetic toxicology and the environmental mutagen society. *Environ. Molec. Mutagen.*, **14**, Suppl. 16, 1–6

White, T. J., Arnheim, N. and Erlich, H. A. (1989). The polymerase chain reaction. *Trends Genet.*, **5**, 185–189

Wilcox, P., Naidoo, A., Wedd, D. J. and Gatehouse, D. G. (1990). Comparison of *Salmonella typhimurium* TA102 with *Escherichia coli* WP2 tester strains. *Mutagenesis*, **5**, 285–291

Winton, D. J., Gooderham, N. J., Boobis, A. R., Davies, D. S. and Ponder, B. A. J. (1990). Mutagenesis of mouse intestine *in vivo* using the D1b-1 specific locus test: Studies with 1,2-dimethylhydrazine, dimethylnitrosamine and the dietary mutagen 2-amino-3,8-dimethyl imidazo [4,5-f-] quinoxaline. *Cancer Res.*, **50**, 7992–7996

Winton, D. J., Peacock, J. H. and Ponder, B. A. J. (1989). Effect of gamma radiation of high and low dose rate on a novel *in vivo* mutation assay in mouse intestine. *Mutagenesis*, **4**, 404–406

Wolff, S. (1977). *In vitro* inhibition of mono-oxygenase dependent reactions by organic solvents. *International Conference on Industrial and Environmental Xenobiotics, Prague*

World Health Organization (1978). *The Potential Carcinogenicity of Nitrosatable Drugs*, ed, F. Coulston and J. F. Dunne. WHO Symposium, Geneva, June, 1978. Ablex Publishing Corporation, Norwood, N.J.

Würgler, F. E., Ramel, C., Moustacchi, E. and Carere, A. (1986). Report 12: Assays for genetic activity in *Drosophila melanogaster*. In Montesano, R., Bartsch, H., Vainio, H., Wilborne, J. and Yamasaki, H. (Eds), *Long-term and Short-term Assays for Carcinogens: A Critical Appraisal*. IARC Scientific Publication No. 83, Lyon, pp. 351–393

Würgler, F. E., Sobels, F. H. and Vogel, E. (1984). *Drosophila* as an assay system for detecting genetic changes. In Kilbey, B. J., Legator, M., Nichols, W. and Ramel, C. (Eds), *Handbook of Mutagenicity Test Procedures*, 2nd edn. Elsevier, Amsterdam, pp. 555–601

Xu, L., Whong, W. Z. and Ong, T. M. (1984). Validation of the *Salmonella* (SV50)/L-arabinose-resistant forward mutation assay with 26 compounds. *Mutation Res.*, **130**, 79–86

Yahagi, T., Degawa, M., Seino, Y., Matsushima, T., Nagao, M., Sugimura, T. and Hashimoto, Y. (1975). Mutagenicity of carcinogen azo dyes and their derivatives. *Cancer Lett.*, **1**, 91–96

Yahagi, T., Nagao, M., Seino, Y., Matsushima, T., Sugimura, T. and Okada, M. (1977). Mutagenicities of *N*-nitrosamines in *Salmonella*. *Mutation Res.*, **48**, 121–130

Yanofksy, C. (1971). Mutagenesis studies with *Escherichia coli* mutants with known amino acids (and base-pair) changes. In Hollaender, A. (Ed.), *Chemical Mutagens, Principles and Methods for Their Detection*, Vol. 1. Plenum Press, New York, pp. 283–287

Zarbl, H., Sukumar, S., Arthur, A. V., Martin-Zanca, D. and Barbacid, M. (1985). Direct mutagenesis of Ha-ras-1 oncogenes by *N*-nitroso-*N*-methylurea during initiation of mammary carcinogenesis in rats. *Nature*, **315**, 382–385

Zbar, B., Braunch, H., Talmadge, C. and Linehan, M. (1987). Loss of alleles on the short arm of chromosome 3 in renal cell carcinoma. *Nature*, **327**, 721–724

Zijlstra, J. A. and Vogel, E. W. (1985). The possible involvement of monoamine oxidases in the bioactivation and deactivation of mutagens in *Drosophila melanogaster*. In *Fourth International Conference on Environmental Mutagens, Stockholm, 24–28 June 1988*. Abstract book, p. 106

Ziv, Y., Amiel, A., Jasper, N. G. J., Berkel, A. I. and Shiloh, Y. (1989). Ataxia-telangiectasia: a variant with altered *in vitro* phenotype of fibroblast cells. *Mutation Res.*, **210**, 211–219

FURTHER READING

Ashby, J., Gentile, J. M. Sankaranarayanan, K. and Glickman, B. W. (1994). Report of the international workshop on standardization of genotoxicity procedures. *Mutation Research*, **312**, No. 3, 195–318

Auletta, A. E., Dearfield, K. L. and Cimino, M. C. (1993). Mutagenicity test schemes and guidelines. *Environmental and Molecular Mutagensis*, **21**, 38–45

Brusick, D. J. (1994). *Methods for Genetic Risk Assessment*. Lewis Publishers, Boca Raton, Florida

Li, A. P. and Heflich, R. H. (1991). *Genetic Toxicology*. CRC Press, Boca Raton, Florida

Mitchell, A. D. (1993). Genetic toxicology. In Stacey, N. H. (Ed.), *Occupational Toxicology*. Taylor and Francis, London

36 Cytogenetics

Diana Anderson

INTRODUCTION

There are various types of cytogenetic change which can be detected in chromosomes. These are structural chromosome aberrations (CAs); numerical changes which could result in aneuploidy; and sister chromatid exchanges (SCEs). Chromosome aberration assays are used to detect the induction of chromosome breakage (clastogenesis) in somatic or germinal cells by direct observation of chromosome damage during metaphase analysis, or by indirect observation of micronuclei. Chromosome damage detected in these assays is mostly lethal to the cell during the cell cycle following the induction of the damage. Its presence, however, indicates a potential to induce more subtle chromosome damage which survives cell division to produce heritable cytogenetic changes. Cytogenetic damage is usually accompanied by other genotoxic damage such as gene mutation.

Cytogenetic Damage and Its Consequences

Structural and numerical chromosomal aberrations in somatic cells may be involved in the aetiology of neoplasia and in germ cells can lead to perinatal mortality, dominant lethality or congenital malformations in the offspring (Chandley, 1981), and some tumours (Anderson, 1990).

Chromosome defects arise at the level of the individual chromosome or at the level of the chromosomal set, so affecting chromosomal number.

Individual Chromosome Damage

Damage to individual chromosomes consists of breakage of chromatids, which must result from a discontinuity of both strands of the DNA in a chromatid. How mutagens produce chromosome breakage is not totally understood, but DNA lesions which are not in themselves discontinuities will produce breakage of a chromosome as a consequence of their interference with the normal process of DNA replication. In haploid microorganisms and prokaryotes chromosome breaks are usually lethal, but in diploid eukaryotes this is not so. According to Bender *et al.* (1974), in these organisms chromosome breaks may reconstitute in the same order, probably as a result of an enzyme repair process, resulting in no apparent cytogenetic damage; they may remain unjoined as fragments, which could result in cell death at the next or following mitoses—if, for example, unrejoined fragments are introduced into the zygote via a treated germ cell, the embryo may die at a very early stage from a dominant lethal mutation; or they may rejoin in a different order from the original one, producing chromosomal rearrangements. There are various types of chromosomal rearrangements:

Reciprocal translocations can result from the exchange of chromosomal segments between two chromosomes and, depending on the position of the centromeres in the rearranged chromosomes, different configurations will result.

(1) Asymmetrical exchanges arise when one of the rearranged chromosomes carries both centromeres and is known as dicentric, while the other carries none and is acentric. The cell or zygote carrying this anomaly usually dies, death being caused by segregation difficulties of the dicentric or the loss of the acentric fragment at cell division. Such a translocation contributes to dominant lethality.

(2) Symmetrical exchanges occur when each rearranged chromosome carries just one centromere. This allows the zygote to develop normally, but when such heterozygotes form germ cells at meiosis, about half of their gametes will be genetically unbalanced, since they have deficiencies and duplications of chromosomal material. The unbalanced gametes which survive produce unbalanced zygotes, which results in death shortly before and after birth, or congenital malformations.

Centric fusions (Robertsonian translocations) involve the joining together of two chromosomes, each of which has a centromere at or near one end, to produce a single metacentric or submetacentric chromosome. When Robertsonian translocations are produced in a germ cell and result from breakage and rejoining in the short arms of the two chromosomes, as a consequence of loss of the derived acentric fragments, a genetic deficiency can result. Some Robertsonian translocations are able to survive but others pose a risk. In heterozygotes the two arms of the translocation chromosome may pair with the two separate homologous chromosomes at meiosis but segregate in a disorderly manner. Some of the resultant germ cells lack copies (nullisomy) or carry two copies (disomy) of one or other of the two chromosomes involved, which results in monosomic or trisomic embryos. Monosomics die early but trisomic embryos, which carry three copies of a chromosome, can survive to birth or beyond. If chromosome 21 is involved in the translocation, it can form a translocation trisomy and produce inherited Down syndrome (this differs from non-disjunctional Down syndrome trisomy).

Deletions and deficiencies are produced when two breaks arise close together in the same chromosome. The two ends of the chromosome join when the fragment between the breaks becomes detached. At the next cell division the unattached piece of chromosome is likely to be lost. Large deletions may contribute to dominant lethality. Small deletions are difficult to distinguish from point mutations. Deletions may uncover pre-existing recessive genes. If one gene that is essential for survival is uncovered, it can act as a lethal in a homozygote and as a partial dominant in a heterozygote.

Inversions occur when two breaks occur in the same chromosome. The portion between them is detached and becomes reinserted in the opposite way to its original position, i.e. the gene order is reversed. This need not cause a genetic problem, but imbalanced gametes could result in congenital malformation or fetal death.

Some human neoplasms are associated with specific chromosome changes (Yunis, 1983; Croce, 1987). The mechanisms by which proto-oncogenes become activated to oncogenic forms in tumour cells include, as well as single-point mutations, deletions and translocations of genetic material between chromosomes and gene amplification (Klein and Klein, 1985; Barbacid, 1987; Croce, 1987). The consequence of this genetic change may be the altered production of an otherwise normal gene product. This can occur either by increasing the rate at which messenger RNA is produced from the gene (transcriptional activation) or by post-transcriptional stabilization of the messenger RNA or the final protein product. Both mechanisms have been seen in Burkitt's lymphoma cells (Adams *et al.*, 1983; Minden, 1987) and in mouse plasmacytomas induced by pristane treatment. In these tumours the normal cellular *myc* gene which is involved in the control of cell proliferation is translocated to the immunoglobulin locus. This is highly transcriptionally active during B cell development. This causes an elevated level of the *myc* protein or inability to switch off the gene at the appropriate time, which produces uncontrolled cell proliferation. Thus, chromosome rearrangements may induce neoplasia by activating a potential oncogene that is a proto-oncogene.

Another mechanism operates in the case of human chronic myeloid leukaemia. A proportion of cases of this disease have the 'Philadelphia chromosome', a piece of chromosome 9 carrying a proto-oncogene known as c-*abl* which undergoes reciprocal translocation with a piece of chromosome 22. The c-*abl* gene becomes joined to a gene on chromosome 22, with the resultant production of a fusion protein encoded by both DNA sequences (Shtivelman *et al.*, 1985). The exact mechanism by which this qualitatively altered gene product exerts its effects, causing cell transformation, is not known.

Gilbert (1983) reviews the various types of cytogenetic events which can lead to neoplasia in humans, such as reciprocal translocations, deletions or non-reciprocal rearrangements, with chromatin loss and duplication of whole chromosomes or chromosome segments. Such changes can cause the elimination of tumour suppressor genes, resulting in malignancy (Phillips, 1987).

The tumour state can also be inherited, and retinoblastomas and osteosarcomas develop in children who inherit a defective copy of chromosome 13 from one parent. The defect has been shown to involve a deletion or mutation in a specific gene (Friend *et al.*, 1986). Tumours arise when the normal copy of the same gene on the other chromosomes is lost or mutated in early childhood. This demonstrates that the gene when present in a functional state, has suppressive effects on the development of tumours. Genes on chromosome 11 are also frequently lost in tumours or in children with the Tay–Sachs familial variant of Wilms' tumour (Koufos *et al.*, 1985). It is possible that predisposition is determined by inheritance of a defective allele at the same locus (Department of Health Report, 1989).

Chromosome Set Damage

Accuracy of chromosome replication and segregation of chromosomes to daughter cells requires accurate maintenance of the chromosome complement of a eukaryotic cell. Chromosome segregation in meiosis and mitosis is dependent upon the synthesis and functioning of the proteins of the spindle apparatus and upon the attachment and movement of chromosomes on the spindle. The kinetochores attach the chromosomes to the spindle and the centrioles are responsible for the polar orientation of the division apparatus. Sometimes such segregation events proceed incorrectly and homologous chromosomes separate, with deviations from the normal number (aneuploidy) into daughter cells or as a multiple of the complete karyotype (polyploidy). When both copies of a particular chromosome move into a daughter cell and the other cell receives none, the event is known as non-disjunction.

Aneuploidy in live births and abortions arises from aneuploid gametes during germ cell meiosis. Trisomy or monosomy of large chromosomes leads to early embryonic death. Trisomy of the smaller chromosomes allows survival but is detrimental to the health of an affected person—e.g. Down syndrome (trisomy 21), Patau syndrome (trisomy 13) and Edward syndrome (trisomy 18). Sex chromosome trisomies (Klinefelter's and XXX syndromes) and the sex chromosome monosomy (XO), known as the Turner syndrome, are also compatible with survival.

Aneuploidy in somatic cells is involved in the formation of human tumours. Up to 10 per cent of tumours are monosomic and trisomic for a specific chromosome as the single observable cytogenetic change. Most common among such tumours are trisomy 8, 9, 12 and 21 and monosomy for chromosomes 7, 22 and Y.

Thus, chromosome changes can have severe consequences in cells and whole organisms, and this present chapter will be concerned with cytogenetic assays which measure gross chromosome changes in somatic and germ cells *in vitro* and *in vivo* and in humans.

IN VITRO CYTOGENETIC ASSAYS

The *in vitro* cytogenetic assay is a short-term mutagenicity test for detecting chromosomal damage in cultured mammalian cells.

Cultured cells have a limited ability metabolically to activate some potential clastogens. This can be overcome by adding an exogenous metabolic activation system such as S9 mix to the cells (Ames *et al.*, 1975; Natarajan *et al.*, 1976; Maron and Ames, 1983; Madle and Obe, 1980).

Observations are made in metaphase cells arrested with a spindle inhibitor such as colchicine or colcemid to accumulate cells in a metaphase-like stage of mitosis (c-metaphase) before hypotonic treatment to enlarge cells and fixation with alcohol/acetic acid solution. Cells are then dispersed on to microscope slides and stained and slides are randomized, coded and analysed for chromosome aberrations with high-power light microscopy. Details of the procedure are given in Dean and Danford (1984) and Preston *et al.* (1981, 1987). The UKEMS guidelines (Scott *et al.*, 1990) recommend that all tests be repeated regardless of the outcome of the first test and that, if a negative or equivocal result is obtained in the first test, the repeat should include an additional sampling time. In the earlier version of the guidelines (Scott *et al.*, 1983) a single sampling at approximately 1.5 normal cycle times (−24 h for a 1.5 cell cycle) from the beginning of treatment was recommended, provided that a range of concentrations was used which induced marginal to substantial reductions in mitotic index, usually an indicator of mitotic delay. However, Ishidate (1988a) reported a number of chemicals which gave negative responses with a fixation time of 24 h but which were positive at 48 h. This was when a Chinese hamster fibroblast line (CHO) with a doubling time of 15 h was used. It would appear, therefore, that there are chemicals which can induce extensive mitotic delay at clastogenic doses and may be clastogenic only when cells have passed through more than one cell cycle since treatment (Thust *et al.*, 1980).

A repeat test should include an additional sample at approximately 24 h later but it may only be necessary to score cells from the highest dose at this later fixation time. When the first test gives a clearly positive result, the repeat test need only utilize the same fixation time. The use of other sampling times is in agreement with other guidelines (European Community EEC Directive—European Communities, 1984; American Society for Testing and Materials—Preston *et al.*, 1987; Japanese Guidelines—JMHW, 1984; Joint Directives, 1987; Ishidate, 1988b).

Cell Types

Established cell lines, cell strains or primary cell cultures may be used. The most often used are Chinese hamster cell lines and human peripheral blood lymphocytes. The merits of these two cell lines have been reported (Ishidate and Harnois, 1987; Kirkland and Garner, 1987). The cell system must be validated and consistently sensitive to known clastogens.

Chinese Hamster Cell Lines

Chinese hamster cell lines have a small number of large chromosomes (11 pairs). Chinese hamster ovary cells in which there has been an extensive rearrangement of chromosome material and the chromosome number may not be constant from cell to cell, are frequently used. Polyploidy, endoreduplication and high spontaneous chromosome aberration frequencies can sometimes be found in these established cell lines, but careful cell culture techniques should minimize such effects. Cells should be treated in exponential growth when cells are in all stages of the cell cycle.

Human Peripheral Blood Lymphocytes

Blood should be taken from healthy donors not known to be suffering from viral infections or receiving medication. Staff handling blood should be immunized against hepatitis B and regular donors should be shown to be hepatitis B antigen negative. Donors and staff should be aware of AIDS implications, and blood and cultures should be handled at containment level 2 (Advisory Committee on Dangerous Pathogens, 1984).

Peripheral blood cultures are stimulated to divide by the addition of a T cell mitogen such as phytohaemagglutinin (PHA) to the culture medium. Mitotic activity is at a maximum at about 3 days but begins at about 40 h after PHA stimulation and the chromosome constitution remains diploid during short-term culture (Evans and O'Riordan, 1975). Treatments should commence at about 44 h after culture initiation. This is when cells are actively proliferating and cells are in all stages of the cell cycle. They should be sampled about 20 h later. In a repeat study the second sample time should be about 92 h after culture initiation. Morimoto *et al.* (1983) report that the cycle time for lymphocytes averages about 12–14 h except for the first cycle.

Female donors can give higher yields of chromosome damage (Anderson *et al.*, 1989).

Positive and Negative Controls

When the solvent is not the culture medium or water, the solvent, liver enzyme activation mixture and solvent and untreated controls are used as negative controls.

Since cultured cells are normally treated in their usual growth medium, the solubility of the test material in the medium should be ascertained before testing. Extremes of pH can be clastogenic (Cifone *et al.*, 1987), so the effect of the test material on pH should also be determined, but buffers can be utilized.

Various organic solvents are used, such as dimethyl sulphoxide (DMSO), dimethylformamide, ethanol and acetone. The volume added must not be toxic to cells. Greater than 10 per cent water v/v can be toxic because of nutrient dilution and osmolality changes.

A known clastogen should always be included as a positive control. When metabolic activation is used, a positive control chemical known to require metabolic activation should also be used to ensure that the system is functioning properly. Without metabolic activation, a direct-acting positive control chemical should be used. A structurally related positive control can also be used. Appropriate safety precautions must be taken in handling clastogens (IARC, 1979; MRC, 1981).

Positive control chemicals should be used to produce relatively low frequencies of aberrations so that the sensitivity of the assay for detecting weak clastogens can be established (Preston *et al.*, 1987).

Aberration yields in negative and positive controls should be used to provide a historical database.

Treatment of Cells

When an exogenous activation system is employed, short treatments (about 3 h) are usually necessary because S9 mix is often cytotoxic when used for extended lengths of time. However, cells may be treated with chemicals either continuously up to harvest time or for a short time followed by washing and addition of fresh medium to allow cell cycle progression. Continuous treatment avoids centrifugation steps required with washing of cells and optimizes the endogenous metabolic capacity of the lymphocytes.

When metabolic activation is used, S9 mix should not exceed 1–10 per cent of the culture medium by volume. It has been shown that the S9 mix is clastogenic in CHO cells and mouse lymphoma cells (Cifone *et al.*, 1987; Kirkland *et al.*, 1989) but not in human lymphocytes, where blood components can inactivate active oxygen species which could cause chromosome damage. When S9 mix from animals treated with other enzyme-inducing agents such as phenobarbitone/ beta-naphthoflavone, is used, clastogenesis may be minimized (Kirkland *et al.*, 1989).

Prior to testing, it is necessary to determine the cytotoxicity of the test material, in order to select a suitable dose range for the chromosome assay both with and without metabolic activation. The range most commonly used determines the effect of the agent on the mitotic index (MI), i.e. the percentage of cells in mitoses at the time of cell harvest. The highest dose should inhibit mitotic activity by approximately 50 per cent (EEC Annex V), 75 per cent (UKEMS: Scott *et al.*, 1990) or exhibit some other indication of cytotoxicity. If the reduction in MI is too great, insufficient cells can be found for chromosome analysis. Cytotoxicity can also be assessed by making cell counts in the chromosome aberration test when using cell lines. In the lymphocyte assay total white cell counts can be used in addition to MI. A dose which induces 50–75 per cent toxicity in these assays should be accompanied by a suitable reduction in mitotic index.

If the test material is not toxic, it is recommended by, for example, the EEC (Annex V) that it be tested up to 5 mg ml^{-1}. The UKEMS recommends that chemicals be tested up to their maximum solubility in the treatment medium and not just their maximum solubility in stock solutions.

For highly soluble non-toxic agents, concentrations above 10 mM may produce substantial increases in the osmolality of the culture medium which could be clastogenic by causing ionic imbalance within the cells (Ishidate *et al.*, 1984; Brusick, 1987). At concentrations exceeding 10 mM the osmolality of the treatment media should be measured and if the increase exceeds 50 mmol kg^{-1}, clastogenicity resulting from high osmolality should be suspected and, according to the UKEMS, is unlikely to be of relevance to human risk. The UKEMS also does not recommend the testing of chemicals at concentrations exceeding their solubility limits as suspensions or precipitate.

A minimum of three doses of the test material should be used—the highest chosen as described above, the lowest on the borderline of toxicity and an intermediate one. Up to six doses can be managed satisfactorily, and this ensures the detection of any dose response and that a toxic range is covered. MIs are as required for the preliminary study (at least 1000 cells per culture). It is also useful to score endoreduplication and polyploidy for historical data. Cells from only three doses need to be analysed.

The range of doses used at the repeat fixation time can be those which induce a suitable degree of mitotic inhibition at the earlier fixation time, but if the highest dose reduces the MI to an unacceptably low level at the second sampling time, the next highest dose should be chosen for screening.

A complete assay requires the test material to be investigated at a minimum of three doses together with a positive (untreated) and solvent-only control, all in the presence and absence of a metabolic activation system. The solvent-only control can be omitted if tissue culture medium is used as a solvent. When two fixation times are used in repeat tests, the positive control is necessary at only one time but the negative or solvent control is necessary at both times.

Duplicates of each test group and quadruplicates of solvent or negative controls should be set up. The sensitivity of the assay is improved with larger numbers scored in the negative controls (Richardson *et al.*, 1989).

Scoring Procedures

Prior to scoring, slides should be coded, randomized and then scored 'blind'. Metaphase analysis should only be carried out by an experienced observer. Metaphase cells should be sought under low-power magnification and those with well-spread, i.e. non-overlapping, clearly defined non-fuzzy chromosomes examined under high power with oil immersion. It is acceptable to analyse cells with total chromosome numbers or that have lost one or two chromosomes during processing. In human lymphocytes ($2n=46$) 44 or more centromeres and in CHO cells ($2n=22$; range 21–24) 20 or more centromeres can be scored. Chromosome numbers can be recorded for each cell, to give an indication of aneuploidy. Only cells with increases in numbers (above 46 in human lymphocytes and 24 in CHO cells) should be considered in this category, since decreases can occur through processing.

Recording microscope co-ordinates of cells is necessary and allows verification of abnormal cells. A photographic record is also useful of cells with aberrations. Two hundred cells (100 from each of two replicates) should be scored per treatment group. When ambiguous results are obtained, there may be further 'blind' reading of these samples.

Data Recording

The classification and nomenclature of the International System for Human Cytogenetic Nomenclature (ISCN, 1985) as applied to acquired chromosome aberrations is recommended. Score sheets giving the slide code, microscope scorer's name, date, cell number, number of chromosomes and aberration types should be used. These should include chromatid and chromosome gaps, deletions, exchanges and others. A space for the Vernier reading for comments and a diagram of the aberration should be available.

From the score sheets, the frequencies of various aberrations should be calculated and each aberration should be counted only once. To consider a break as one event and an exchange as two events is not acceptable, since unfounded assumptions are made about mechanisms involved (Revell, 1974).

Presentation of Results

The test material, test cells used, method of treatment, harvesting of cells, cytotoxicity assay, etc., should be clearly stated as well as the statistical methods used. Richardson *et al.* (1989) recommend that comparisons be made between the frequencies in control cells and at each dose level using Fisher's Exact Test.

In cytogenetic assays the absence of a clear positive dose–response relationship at a particular time frequently arises. This is because a single common sampling time may be used for all doses of a test compound. Chromosome aberration yields can vary markedly with post-treatment sampling time of an asynchronous population, and increasing doses of clastogens can induce increasing degrees of mitotic delay (Scott *et al.*, 1990). Additional fixation times should clarify the relationship between dose and aberration yield.

Gaps are by tradition excluded from quantification of chromosome aberration yields. Some gaps have been shown to be real discontinuities in DNA (e.g. Heddle and Bodycote, 1970). Where chromosome aberration yields are on the borderline of statistical significance above control values, the inclusion of gaps could be useful (Anderson and Richardson, 1981). Further details on this approach may be found in the UKEMS guidelines (Scott *et al.*, 1990).

Since chromosome exchanges are relatively rare events, greater biological significance should be attached to their presence than to gaps and breaks.

Chemicals which are clastogenic *in vitro* at low doses are more likely to be clastogenic *in vivo* than those where clastogenicity is detected only at high concentrations (Ishidate *et al.*, 1988). Negative results in well-conducted *in vitro* tests are a good indication of a lack of potential for *in vivo* clastogenesis, since almost all *in vivo* clastogens have given positive results *in vitro* when adequately tested (Thompson, 1986; Ishidate *et al.*, 1988).

IN VIVO CYTOGENETICS ASSAYS

Damage induced in whole animals can be detected in *in vivo* chromosome assays in either somatic or germinal cells by examination of metaphases or the formation of micronuclei. The micronucleus test can also detect whole chromosome loss or aneuploidy in the absence of clastogenic activity and is considered comparable in sensitivity to chromosome analysis (Tsuchimoto and Matter, 1979).

Rats and mice are generally used for *in vivo* studies, with the mouse being employed for bone marrow micronucleus analysis and the rat for metaphase analysis, but both can be used for either. Mice are cheaper and easier to handle than rats, and only a qualitative difference in response has been found between the species (Albanese *et al.*, 1988). Chinese hamsters are also widely used for metaphase analysis because of their low diploid chromosome number of 22. However, there are few other historical toxicological data for this species.

Somatic Cell Assays

Metaphase Analysis

Metaphase analysis can be performed in any tissue with actively dividing cells, but bone marrow is the tissue most often examined. Cells are treated with a test compound and are arrested in metaphase by the administration of colcemid or colchicine at various sampling times after treatment. Preparations are examined for structural chromosome damage. Because the bone marrow has a good blood supply, the cells should be exposed to the test compound or its metabolites in the peripheral blood supply, and the cells are sensitive to S-dependent and S-independent mutagens (UKEMS: Topham *et al.*, 1983).

Peripheral blood cells can be stimulated to divide even though the target cell is relatively insensitive (Newton and Lilly, 1986). It is necessary to stimulate them with a mitogen since the number of lymphocytes which are dividing at any one time is very low. Cells are in G_0 when exposure is taking place, so they may not be sensitive to cell cycle stage specific mutagens and any damage might be repaired before sampling.

Micronuclei

The assessment of micronuclei is considered simpler than the assessment of metaphase analysis. This assay is most often carried out in bone marrow cells, where polychromatic erythrocytes are examined. Damage is induced in the immature erythroblast and results in a micronucleus outside the main nucleus, which is easily detected after staining as a chromatid-containing body. When the erythroblast matures, the micronucleus, whose formation results from chromosome loss during cell division or from chromosome breakage forming centric and acentric fragments, is not extruded with the nucleus. Micronuclei can also be detected in peripheral blood cells (MacGregor *et al.*, 1980). In addition, they can be detected in liver (Tates *et al.*, 1980; Braithwaite and Ashby, 1988) after partial hepatectomy or stimulation with 4-acetylaminofluorene, or they can be detected in any proliferating cells.

Germ Cell Assays

The study of chromosome damage is highly relevant to the assessment of heritable cytogenetic damage. Many compounds which cause somatic cell damage have not produced germ cell damage (Holden, 1982) and, so far, all germ mutagens have also produced somatic damage.

Germ cell data, however, are needed for genetic risk estimation, and testing can be performed in male or female germ cells. The former are most often used, owing to systemic effects in females. Testing in the male is performed in mitotically proliferating premeiotic spermatogonia, but chromosomal errors in such cells can result in cell death or prevent the cell from passing through meiosis. Damage produced in postmeiotic cells, the spermatids or sperm are more likely to be transmitted to the F_1 progeny (Albanese, 1987). In females it is during early fetal development of the ovary that öogonial divisions and prophase stages of meiosis up to arrested diplotene stage occur. Therefore, testing necessitates the use of pregnant mothers at suitable gestation stages. The arrested dictyate öocyte stage is the most commonly tested stage in the adult female. To test other stages during the first or second meiotic divisions demands the use of öocytes undergoing ovulation which occur naturally or are hormone-stimulated. It is thus more difficult technically to test female germ cells.

Heritable Chromosome Assays

Damage may be analysed in the heritable translocation test, which involves the examination in male F_1 animals of diakinesis metaphase 1 spermatocytes for multivalent association (Leonard,

1973, 1975; Cattanach, 1982). Fertilized ova can also be analysed by cytogenetic analysis (Albanese, 1987), or early embryos can be examined by metaphase analysis (Hansmann, 1973). Such techniques are demanding technically, and the heritable translocation assay requires large numbers of animals to attain appropriate sample sizes. Chromosome damage in fertilized ova or early embryos may not be compatible with survival after birth, so it is only the heritable translocation assay which provides absolute evidence of induced heritable effects. In fetal mice which have been exposed transplacentally after exposure of the mother, tissues can be assessed for micronuclei or metaphase analysis. Cole *et al.* (1981) scored micronuclei in polychromatic erythrocytes in the liver or peripheral blood of fetal mice. Such methods have been reviewed by Henderson (1986) and are used to investigate factors which might affect embryos.

Experimental Design—General Features of *In Vivo* Assays

Treatment of Animals

A control group dosed with a vehicle used routinely or an untreated control will be needed in addition to vehicle controls. Water soluble materials can be administered in distilled water or isotonic saline, and the pH may require adjustment if there is a marked deviation from physiological pH. Various substances other than water can be used as controls. Although DMSO is used in *in vitro* studies, it is not wise to use it in animal studies. It is locally irritant and toxic, and increases the penetration through cell membranes, so altering absorption and distribution patterns. Methyl cellulose or carboxymethyl cellulose (0.5 per cent up to 2 per cent w/v) can be used as a water-based vehicle for homogenous suspensions obtained after milling. For those substances that are not miscible with water, corn (maize) oil can be used but this could affect absorption rates. Tween 80 may also aid in the suspension of non-wettable materials. The pH of aqueous solutions may require adjustment if they differ markedly from physiological pH. Routes of administration, such as gavage, intraperitoneal, intradermal or intravenous, can be used with these agents, but for inhalation routes an experienced inhalation toxicologist is required to advise on the most appropriate action.

It is usually necessary to determine the toxicity of the test substance unless this is available from the scientific literature. The test substance is required for regulatory purposes to be tested at the maximum tolerated dose—i.e. a dose which produces some signs of toxicity such as hypoactivity, piloerection, ataxia, ptosis or a change in the body weight. Toxicity of the animals is usually observed over a 14 day observation period. In the case of the micronucleus assay, to determine toxicity to the cells, the ratio between polychromatic and normochromatic erythrocytes (normocytes or NCE) can be measured and, in the case of metaphase analysis, MIs. These values are measured over a period up to 72 h.

The highest dose, when toxicity is not evident, ranges from 2 to 5 g kg^{-1}, according to different regulatory guidelines (see Richold *et al.*, 1990). A single dose level is considered adequate for screening purposes, but for more extensive evaluation, several dose levels are required. Dose values should not normally exceed 10 ml kg^{-1} by the intraperitoneal (ip) and intravenous (iv) route or 20 ml kg^{-1} by the oral route. There is often a tenfold separation between the upper and lowest dose, and there is also an intermediate dose. Sometimes the lowest dose is selected as the most appropriate for man. Less than twofold separation factor for doses should not be considered.

In terms of the route of exposure, there is a need to maximize the chance of absorption or to mimic human exposure. Hayashi *et al.* (1989) in a collaborative study compared the oral and ip routes and found them to be equally sensitive when toxicity is accounted for, and Shelby (1986) argued that the ip route and the route relevant to human exposure could be used sequentially in the evaluation of a compound. However, Ashby (1985) argued against the ip route as being suitable. In general, the oral route is preferable, and dermal or subcutaneous routes are not used unless it is clear that the compound is absorbed or used by these routes.

A concurrent vehicle control group should be included in each experiment at each sampling time in order to compare the treated groups. Untreated controls can by induced when a non-standard vehicle is used. A positive control group should be included to confirm the sensitivity of the assay and check on the scoring. A sufficient dosage of the positive control substance is required to check on any reduced assay sensitivity.

Assays are usually performed only once, but if equivocal results are obtained, another study design or alternative dosage route may be considered for sensitivity optimization.

There are various requirements for animal husbandry and welfare, and in the UK project and personal licences are mandatory for animal experimentation. Various safety precautions are necessary to protect personnel from exposure to suspect mutagens and carcinogens (Ehrenburg and Wachtmeister, 1977; Waters, 1980), and special waste disposal procedures should be observed.

Rodent Micronucleus Test

The rodent micronucleus test can be used as a sensitive screen to assess hazard or for more extensive/qualitative hazard determinations to aid in risk assessment.

Rats and mice can be used and methods are now available to avoid contaminating mast cell granules in rats, which stain in a similar way to micronuclei. Hayashi *et al.* (1983) and McGregor *et al.* (1983) used fluorescent stains and Pascoe and Gatehouse (1986) utilized haematoxylin and eosin. Romagna and Staniforth (1989) used a cellulose column which provides good-quality preparations. Romanowsky-type stains, such as May–Grunwald/Giemsa (Schmid, 1976), are routinely employed for mouse micronuclei or Wright's stain (Albanese and Middleton, 1987).

It is suggested in various international guidelines that 5 males and 5 females be used per group, although only a few quantitative differences in clastogenic responses have been shown to exist between sexes (Henry *et al.*, 1980; Collaborative Study Group for the Micronucleus Test, 1986). The use of two sexes has been debated. The EEC, OECD and EPA recommend the use of both sexes but the UKEMS (Richold *et al.* 1990) and Japanese Guidelines (JMHW, 1984) suggest the use of males only. This obviously reduces animal numbers, and Lovell *et al.* (1989) state that with a group size of 7, there is not a significant loss in test sensitivity if 2000 polychromatic erythrocytes (PCEs) are read.

Since no qualitative differences exist in response to clastogens, even though different strains of rats and mice have different spontaneous frequencies of micronucleated polychromatic erythrocytes (MPEs) (Collaborative Study Group for the Micronucleus Test, 1988), there is no preferred strain. It is appropriate, however, that the spontaneous incidence should not exceed 0.4 per cent (i.e. 4 per 1000 PCEs) (Topham *et al.*, 1983). Young animals of 6–8 weeks for mice and 8–10 weeks for rats should be used to avoid fat deposition in the marrow, since fat in older animals interferes with the clarity of staining.

The experimental unit is the animal and not the cell, but if less than 500 cells are examined clusters of cells might be formed (Albanese and Middleton, 1987; Mirkova and Ashby, 1987). Regulatory guidelines generally require 1000 PCEs scored per animal. Mirkova and Ashby (1987) favour the reading of 2000 PCEs. However, the minimum number of PCEs to score per animal depends upon the spontaneous frequency of micronuclei, the lower the frequency the greater the number of PCEs per animal requiring analysis to detect a specified level of increase in MPEs. Two thousand PCEs should be scored if the control incidence is less than 0.2 per cent. Confirmation of equivocal results could be achieved by extending numbers of PCEs read before a repeat study.

For positive controls, the group size can be smaller (no fewer than 3 animals), using an optimal sampling time with a dose to monitor sensitivity.

To determine toxicity, the PCE:NCE (polychromatophilic erythrocyte: normochromatic erythrocyte) ratio is examined, and alterations in the ratio result from the inhibition of division or maturation of nucleated erythropoietic cells or replenishment of marrow with peripheral blood. A total of 1000 erythrocytes (PCEs and NCEs) should be examined.

For the micronucleus test, either a single-dose study with two harvest times at 24 and 48 h after treatment or a multiple-dose study with two or three doses 24 h apart, followed by a single harvest time 24 h after the last dosing, is currently considered acceptable (UKEMS guidelines: Richold *et al.*, 1990).

A 72 h sampling time was initially required, based on the results with 7,12-dimethylbenzanthracene (Salamone and Heddle, 1983), but responses can be shown at earlier times (Ashby and Mirkova, 1987). Most regulatory authorities, however, require three sampling times, and 24 h is suitable to detect most chemicals which induce micronuclei. MacGregor *et al.* (1987) claim that it is not necessary to sample the marrow of treated animals earlier than 19–24 h after dosing, since the life-span of an immature or RNA positive erythrocyte is between 10–20 h in both rat and mouse (Salamone and Heddle, 1983).

Usually both femurs are removed and cleared of extraneous muscle. From the proximal end the shafts are aspirated with a needle and the marrow flushed out with serum to obtain a homogeneous cell suspension. The cells are concentrated by centrifugation at 800–1000 rpm for 5 min. A small drop of suspension is spread on the smear-free slide and pulled with a cover glass (Schmid, 1976). Another method is to push the marrow onto the slide with a pin inserted in the epiphysial (distal) end. The marrow is mixed with serum to disperse the cells, using the edge of a second slide (Salamone and Heddle, 1983). Alternatively, a fine sable paint brush in physiological saline is inserted into the distal end of the femur and drawn across the slide for up to four strokes with fewer cells at the end of strokes (Albanese and Middleton, 1987).

The scored elements are the micronucleated cells and not the number of micronuclei. The majority of micronuclei are circular but some are oval or ring-shaped. Doubtful shapes should not be scored. Cells which are orange/red after staining should be classed as mature (NCEs); those which are bluish as immature (PCEs). The frequency of micronuclei in NCEs should be 0–1 per 1000. For each animal the number of PCEs, NCEs, micronucleated PCEs and micronucleated NCEs as well as PCE:NCE ratio should be recorded. It is not necessary to record Vernier readings for micronucleated cells. The micronuclei arise from anaphase lag of chromosome fragments, bridged translocations or detached whole chromosomes.

Detailed recommendations on the type of statistical analysis to be carried out on data generated in this assay have been proposed by Lovell *et al.* (1989). The positive and negative control values should fall within the historical control range for the laboratory. If the test material has been administered at the highest dose and there is a negative response, the test material should be classified as negative under the test conditions. No-effect levels could be used in risk evaluation.

Rodent Bone Marrow Metaphase Analysis

Most bone marrow metaphase assays have been carried out in the rat, although mouse and Chinese hamster are also used. It is conducted at doses up to the maximum tolerated (MTD) or for non-toxic substances 2 g kg^{-1} or 5 g kg^{-1}, depending on the regulatory authorities. A dose that causes a 50 per cent reduction in the MI or some other index of cellular toxicity in a preliminary toxicity assay is also used. A single dose may be used for screening purposes but for hazard assessment at least three doses should be used. A dose relevant to man is sometimes included and an intermediate between it and the MTD. Other protocols, including a tenfold and one-third of the MTD have been used (Anderson and Richardson, 1981) but the UKEMS (Richold *et al.*, 1990) recommends that dose levels should be separated by approximately twofold intervals. The OECD guidelines (1983) recommend 5 males and 5 females but the UKEMS (Richold *et al.*, 1990) recommends 7 males per test group only. The OECD recommends that 50 cells per animal be scored (500 per test group) and the UKEMS (Richold *et al.*, 1990) also recommends that this number is scored.

OECD (1984) recommends that cells be sampled at 6, 24 and 48 h after a single dose administration. Cells are also sampled at 6 and 24 h after a multiple administration. The UKEMS debates the use of a 48 h sampling and suggests that it should only be used when there is evidence of mitotic delay. This can be determined during the preliminary toxicity assay.

A mitotic arresting agent such as colchicine or colcemid is dosed to the animals at 2 to 4 h prior to sampling. Methods for satisfactory stained metaphase spreads have been described by Adler (1984). All slides should be coded and randomized. Various readings should be taken of aberrations and recorded for future reference and Good Laboratory Practice audits. The classification criteria of Scott *et al.* (1990) can be used and all aberrations should be described fully in the raw data. For each animal, the number of cells scored, the number of cells with each aberration type, the frequency of aberrations including and excluding gaps should be determined. Recommendations on the statistical analysis of this assay have been made by Lovell *et al.* (1989). The positive and negative control values should fall within the acceptable range for the laboratory for a substance to be considered positive or negative under the conditions of the study.

Germ Cell Cytogenetic Assays

Either mouse or rat can be used but the mouse is generally the preferred species. Normally such assays are not conducted for routine screening purposes.

Spermatogonial metaphases can be prepared by the air-drying technique of Evans *et al.* (1964) for the first and second meiotic metaphase (MI and MII) in the male mouse. This method is not so suitable for rat and hamster. The numbers of spermatogonial metaphases can be boosted if, prior to hypotonic treatment, the testicular tubules are dispersed in trypsin solution (0.25 per cent). At least 1 month between treatment and sample should be allowed to pass in the mouse to allow treated cells to reach meiosis. Brook and Chandley (1986) established that 11 days and 4 h was required for spermatogonial cells to reach preleptotene and 8 days and 10 h to reach zygotene. It takes 4 h for cells to move from MI to MII but test compounds can alter this rate. A search for multivalent formation can be made at MI for the structural rearrangements induced in spermatogonia. Cawood and Breckon (1983) examined the synaptonemal complex at pachytene, using electron microscopy. Errors of segregation should be searched for at the first meiotic division in the male mouse, MII cells showing 19 (hypoploid) and 21 (hyperploid) chromosomes (Brook and Chandley, 1986). Hansmann and El-Nahass (1979), Brook (1982) and Brook and Chandley (1985) describe assays in the female mouse and procedures used for inducing ovulation by hormones and treatment of specific stages of meiosis.

SISTER CHROMATID EXCHANGE ASSAYS

SCEs are reciprocal exchanges between sister chromatids. They result in a change in morphology of the chromosome but breakage and reunion are involved, although the exact mechanism is unclear. They are thought to occur at homologous loci.

In 1958 Taylor demonstrated SCEs, using autoradiographic techniques to detect the disposition of labelled DNA following incorporation of [³H]-thymidine. 5-Bromo-2'-deoxyuridine (BrdU) has now replaced [³H]-thymidine and various staining methods have been used to show the differential incorporation of BrdU between sister chromatids: fluorescent—Hoechst 33258 (Latt, 1973); combined fluorescent and Giemsa (Perry and Wolff, 1974); and Giemsa (Korenberg and Freedlender, 1974). The fluorescent plus Giemsa procedure is recommended in view of the fact that stained slides can be stored and microscope analysis is simpler.

So that SCEs can be seen at metaphase, cells must pass through S phase (Kato, 1973, 1974; Wolff *et al.*, 1974). SCEs appear to occur at the replication point, since SCE induction is maximal at the beginning of DNA synthesis but drops to zero at the end of S phase (Latt and Loveday, 1978).

For SCE analysis *in vitro*, any cell type that is replicating or can be stimulated to divide is suitable. The incorporation of BrdU into cells *in vivo* allows the examination of a variety of tissues (Latt *et al.*, 1980). Edwards *et al.* (1993) suggest that it is necessary to standardize protocols measuring SCE since different responses can be obtained depending on the extent of simultaneous exposure of test compound and BrdU.

Relevance of SCE in Terms of Genotoxicity

SCEs do not appear to be related to other cytogenetic events, since potent clastogens such as bleomycin and ionizing radiation induce low levels of SCE (Perry and Evans, 1975). The mechanisms involved in chromosome aberrations and SCE formation are dissimilar (e.g. Galloway and Wolff, 1979). There is no evidence that SCEs are in themselves lethal events, since there is little relationship to cytotoxicity (e.g. Bowden *et al.*, 1979). It was suggested by Wolff (1977) that they relate more to mutational events due to a compatibility with cell survival. However, there are examples of agents that induce significant SCE increases in the absence of mutation (Bradley *et al.*, 1979) as well as the converse (Connell, 1979; Connell and Medcalf, 1982).

The SCE assay is particularly sensitive for alkylating agents and base analogues, agents causing single-strand breaks in DNA and compounds acting through DNA binding (Latt *et al.*,

1981). The most potent SCE inducers are S-phase-dependent. Painter (1980) reports that agents such as X-irradiation, which inhibits replicon initiation, are poor SCE inducers, whereas mitomycin C, which inhibits replication fork progression, is a potent SCE inducer.

Experimental Design

Established cell lines, primary cell cultures or rodents may be used. Detailed information on *in vitro* and *in vivo* assays may be obtained in reviews of SCE methods by Latt *et al.* (1977, 1981), Perry and Thompson (1984) and Perry *et al.* (1984). The *in vitro* methods will be briefly explored here.

Either monolayer or suspension cultures can be employed, or human lymphocytes. Human fibroblasts are less suitable because of their long cell cycle duration.

The concentration of organic solvents for the test compound should not exceed 0.8 per cent v/v, as higher concentrations could lead to slight elevations in the SCE level (Perry *et al.*, 1984).

For monolayer cultures, the cultures are set up the day before BrdU treatment so that the cells will be in exponential growth before the addition of BrdU or the test compound. After BrdU addition the cells are allowed to undergo the equivalent of two cell cycles before cell harvest. A spindle inhibitor such as colchicine or colcemid is introduced for the final 1–2 h of culture to arrest cells in metaphase, after which the cells are harvested and chromosome preparations are made by routine cytogenetic techniques.

In the absence of metabolic activation, BrdU and the test agent can be added simultaneously and left for the duration of BrdU labelling. Shorter treatments should be used in the presence of metabolic activation or to avoid synergistic effects with BrdU, when cells can be pulse treated for, e.g., 1 h before BrdU addition (see Edwards *et al.* (1993).

Peripheral blood cultures are established in medium containing BrdU and PHA. Colcemid is added 1–2 h before harvest and the cells are harvested between 60 and 70 h post PHA stimulation. Cell harvest and slide preparations are conducted according to routine cytogenetic methods.

Heparinized blood samples may be stored at 4 °C for up to 48 h without affecting the SCE response (Lambert *et al.*, 1982). If the test agent is known to react with serum or red blood cells, the mononuclear lymphocytes may be isolated by use of a Ficoll/Hypaque gradient (Boyum, 1968).

If metabolic activation is not required, treatment is best conducted over the whole of the final 24 h of culture, or if metabolic activation is required, a pulse exposure may be employed to treat cultures at the first S phase at around 24–30 h, or at 48 h for an asynchronous population.

Exposure of cells to fluorescent light during the culture period leads to photolysis of BrdU-containing DNA and a concomitant increase in SCE frequency (Wolff and Perry, 1974). Consequently, SCE cultures should be kept in the dark and manipulated under subdued light conditions such as yellow safe light. Furthermore, media used in SCE assays should be stored in the dark, since certain media components produce reactive SCE-inducing intermediates on exposure to fluorescent light (Monticone and Schneider, 1979).

Coded and randomized slides should be read. All experiments should be repeated at least once (Perry *et al.*, 1984) with higher and lower concentrations of S9 mix if a negative response is achieved. Even for an apparently unambiguous positive response with a greater than twofold increase in SCEs over the background level at the highest dose, and with at least two consecutive dose levels with an increased SCE response, a repeat study is necessary to show a consistent response.

The quality of differential staining will determine the ease and accuracy of SCE scoring, and, to eliminate variation, results from different observers should occasionally be compared. Furthermore, to avoid observer bias, scorers should have slides from different treatment groups equally distributed among them, as with all cytogenetic studies.

HUMAN MONITORING

People exposed to environmental mutagens can be examined for chromosome damage in peripheral blood lymphocytes. Briefly, a sample of blood is taken per individual (about 10 ml) and chromosome preparations are made in the usual way (Evans and O'Riordan, 1975) from the lymphocytes, which have been stimulated into division by a mitogen such as PHA. This is because lymphocytes are normally in the resting or G_0 stage. A detailed questionnaire is also taken from the individual at the time of blood sampling relating to life-style habits. These could act as confounding factors in study interpretation when increases in chromosome damage are found. Such exogenous life-style factors include smoking, drinking alcohol and caffeine, therapeutic drug usage, X-ray examinations, recent viral infections, etc. Endogenous factors (age, gender, etc.) are also taken into account. Such human monitoring questionnaires and appropriate study designs have been described by ICPEMC Committee (Carrano and Natarajan, 1988), and many human monitoring studies have been described in a special issue of *Mutation Research* (Anderson, 1988).

HUMAN GENOME PROJECT

One of the most exciting recent developments in cytogenetics was the launching of the Human Genome Project in 1986 by the Department of the Environment in the USA. It is now supported by two federal departments, the Department of the Environment as well as the National Institutes of Health (US Department of Energy, 1990; US Human Genome Project, 1990).

The ultimate goal of the project is to analyse the structure of human DNA, to determine the location of all human genes on chromosomes.

An overall budget of 200 million dollars per year for approximately 15 years has been earmarked. Fiscal years 1988 to 1990 were a period for getting organized and getting research under way, and 5 year goals have been identified for the fiscal years 1991 to 1995 inclusive.

There are various scientific goals for these first 5 years.

Mapping and Sequencing the Human Genome

The human genome consists of up to 50 000–100 000 genes located on 23 pairs of chromosomes. One chromosome of each pair is derived from the father and the other from the mother. Each chromosome contains a long molecule of DNA, the basic chemical of the genes. The DNA is a double-stranded molecule in which each strand is composed of a linear array of bases

or nucleotides. There are four different bases (adenine, A, thymine, T, cytosine, C, and guanine, G). The bases on the DNA strand are precisely paired with the bases on the other strand (A opposite T and G opposite C). The order of the four bases on the DNA strand determines the information content of a particular gene or piece of DNA. The length of the genes varies, ranging from about 2000 to 2×10^6 base-pairs. Mapping is the process which determines the spacing and position of genes, or other genetic landmarks on chromosomes, relative to one another. There are two types of maps, *genetic* and *physical*, which differ in the methods used to construct them and in the measurements used to determine the distance between genes. Sequencing determines the order of the nucleotides or base-pairs in a DNA molecule.

To date, about 1700 (less than 2 per cent) of the human genes have been mapped. The first complete human genome to be sequenced will be a composite of sequences from many sources from long-established cell lines. The sequence will be a generic sequence representative of humans in general. It is presumed that functionally important DNA is conserved among humans. Also, DNA regions of particular interest, such as genes involved in genetic disease, will be sequenced.

Genetic Maps

Genetic maps can be used for the identification of genes associated with genetic disease and other biological properties, and are also used to guide in the construction of physical maps. Genetic maps are constructed by determining the frequency with which two marker genes are inherited together. Those that lie close together are inherited together more frequently than those genes that are further apart. Genetic studies of families determine how frequently two genes are inherited together. The distance between genes is measured in centimorgans. Two markers are 1 centimorgan apart when during transmission from parents to children they are separated 1 per cent of the time. The average distance for a centimorgan is about 10^6 base-pairs.

Useful genetic mapping tools are the DNA markers, known as restriction fragment length polymorphisms (RFLPs) and used to detect variation among individuals. Techniques such as denaturing-gradient gel electrophoresis have been adapted to detect variations in DNA sequences. For the first 5 years the Genome Project hopes to create a map of 2–5 centimorgans which would require up to 1500 such markers. Each marker should be identified by a sequence-tagged site (STS) (see below).

Physical Maps

The numbers of nucleotide pairs constitute the units of physical length of the distance between sites on physical maps. These can be constructed in different ways derived from recombinant DNA techniques. These allow the isolation and cloning of DNA fragments and the identification of specific sequence markers on DNA, and determine the distance between and order of such chromosome markers.

There are two general types of physical maps. One is the cytogenetic map, based on microscopic analysis; this records the location of genes and DNA markers relative to visible landmarks on the chromosomes. Precision in locating markers is rather low at about 10×10^6 base-pairs. The numbers of mapped markers on the human genome is now about 4500; another example of this type of physical map is the long-range restriction map, which records the order of and distance between specific sequences, known as restriction sites on chromosomes. Map resolution of this type is about 100 000 to 2×10^6 base-pairs. The other type of physical map consists of a collection of cloned pieces of DNA comprising a complete chromosomal segment or chromosome and the order of cloned pieces. The technology for constructing overlapping clone sets, known as 'contigs', is constantly improving. A collection of ordered clones provides the starting material for sequencing.

Improvements in several techniques have made the initial stages in the construction of physical maps of large genomes easier, such as pulsed-field gel electrophoresis, yeast artificial chromosome cloning, the polymerase chain reaction (PCR), fluorescence *in situ* hybridization and radiation hybrid analysis.

Of the 24 (23 pairs and X + Y) different human chromosomes, numbers 3, 4, 5, 11, 16, 17, 18, 19, 21, 22 and X are currently under investigation. There are still several barriers to the inexpensive, rapid and routine construction of physical maps, mainly due to the short length of DNA over which an uninterrupted set of overlapping clones can be established. Contigs exist of between 2 and 6 cosmid clones. A cosmid can carry a maximum of 40 000 base-pairs and is a type of vector. The length of DNA over which the physical map shows continuity should be longer, at up to 2×10^6 base-pairs.

It is also difficult to compare one mapping method with another and to combine maps constructed by different methods into a single map. Olson *et al.* (1989) proposed a system whereby data from any variety of physical mapping techniques can be reported in a common language. Here each mapped element, an individual clone, contig or sequenced region, is defined by a unique sequence-tagged site (STS) which is a short DNA sequence shown to be unique. A map can be constructed showing the order and spacing of STSs. The STS system can be represented electronically and stored in a database. This can be publicly available and should enable the recovery by any scientist of any mapped chromosomal region which can readily be checked by other laboratories.

DNA Sequencing

To date, the only organisms for which a complete DNA sequence has been determined are viruses (e.g. the Epstein–Barr virus of 170 000 base-pairs). Bacteria are 4.5×10^6 base-pairs long and attempts are being made to sequence bacterial DNA. The human genome, at 3×10^9 base-pairs of DNA, is nearly 1000 times longer than a bacterial genome, so an increase in the speed and a reduction in the cost of sequencing technology will be required. The cost will have to be reduced from the current cost of up to $5 per base-pair to below 50 cents a base-pair before large-scale sequencing will be cost-effective. Machines are now available that automatically identify the order of base-pairs in appropriately prepared DNA samples. One approach to lowering costs is further automation, but new methods should continue to be sought.

Model Organisms

Information derived from studies of the biology of model organisms is useful in the interpretation of data obtained in studies of humans and in understanding human biology. Those identified as useful for comparative purposes are the bacterium *Escherichia coli*, the yeast *Saccharomyces cerevisiae*, the fruit fly *Drosophila melanogaster*, the worm *Caenorhabditis elegans* and the laboratory mouse.

Other Goals and UK Contribution

Other interrelated goals of the Program are the development of capabilities for collecting, storing, distributing and analysing the data produced; the development of programmes addressed to understanding the ethical, legal and social implications of the human genome project, which includes stimulating public discussion of issues; and the development of policy options to assure that the information is used for the benefit of the individual and society. Appropriate technologies need to be created to achieve all these objectives.

In 1989 the UK Secretary of State for Education and Science awarded £11 M (US$21 million) to the Medical Research Council (MRC) for the initiation of a National Human Genome Mapping Project (HMGP) to co-ordinate and expand UK activities in human genome mapping and to provide a link with genome projects in other countries. The new funds were distributed over a 3-year period from April 1989 to March 1991 after which £4.5 M was to be incorporated into the MRC annual funding baseline. The UK Project will have a few areas identified for strategic development. One example is that instead of attempting large-scale sequencing or mapping, the UK programme will concentrate on identifying and isolating as many genes as possible and characterising them in biological terms. The assumption is that sequencing a few hundred bases of cDNA would determine what kind of protein the gene codes for and how interesting the gene would be to investigators. This approach will indicate which genes have already been sequenced and avoid duplication of effort (Human Genome News, 1982).

REFERENCES

Adams, J. M., Gerondakis, S., Webb, E., Corcoran, L. M. and Cory, S. (1983). Cellular *myc* gene is altered by chromosome translocation to an immunoglobulin locus in murine plasmacytomas and is rearranged similarly in human Burkitt lymphomas. *Proc. Natl Acad. Sci. USA*, **80**, 1982–1986

Adler, I.-D. (1984). Cytogenetic tests in mammals. In Venitt, S. and Parry, J. M. (Eds), *Mutagenicity Testing, a Practical Approach*. IRL Press, Oxford, pp. 275–306

Advisory Committee on Dangerous Pathogens (1984). *Categorisation of Pathogens According to Hazard and Categories of Containment*. HMSO, London

Albanese, R. (1987). Mammalian male germ cell cytogenetics. *Mutagenesis*, **2**, 79–85

Albanese, R. and Middleton, B. J. (1987). The assessment of micronucleated polychromatic erythrocytes in rat bone marrow. Technical and statistical considerations. *Mutation Res.*, **182**, 323–333

Albanese, R., Mirkova, E., Gatehouse, D. and Ashby, J. (1988). Species-specific response to the rodent carcinogens 1,2-dimethylhydrazine and 1,2-dibromochloropropane in rodent bone marrow micronucleus assays. *Mutagenesis*, **3**, 35–38

Ames, B. N., McCann, J. and Yamasaki, E. (1975). Methods for detecting carcinogens and mutagens with the *Salmonella*/mammalian microsome mutagenicity test. *Mutation Res.*, **31**, 347–64

Anderson, D. (1988). Human Monitoring. Special issue. *Mutation Res.*, **204**, 353–551

Anderson, D. (1990). Male mediated F_1 abnormalities. Special issue. *Mutation Res.*, **229**, 103–246

Anderson, D. and Richardson, C. R. (1981). Issues relevant to the assessment of chromosome damage *in vivo*. *Mutation Res.*, **90**, 261–272

Anderson, D., Jenkinson, P. C., Dewdney, R. S., Francis, A. T., Godbert, P. and Butterworth, K. R. (1989). Chromosome aberrations, mitogen induced blastogenesis and proliferative rate index in peripheral lymphocytes from 106 control individuals in the UK population. *Mutation Res.*, **204** (3), 407–420

Ashby, J. (1985). Is there a continuing role for the i.p. injection route of exposure in short term rodent genotoxicity assays. *Mutation Res.*, **156**, 239–243

Ashby, J. and Mirkova, E. (1987). A re-evaluation of the need for multiple sampling times in the mouse bone marrow micronucleus assay. Results for dimethylbenzanthracene. *Environ. Mutagen.*, **10**, 297–305

Barbacid, M. (1987). *Ras* genes. *Ann. Rev. Biochem.*, **56**, 779–828

Bender, M. A., Griggs, H. G. and Bedford, J. S. (1974). Mechanisms of chromosomal aberration production. III. Chemicals and ionising radiation. *Mutation Res.*, **23**, 197–212

Bowden, G. T., Hsu, I. C. and Harris, C. C. (1979). The effect of caffeine on cytotoxicity, mutagenesis and sister chromatid exchanges in Chinese hamster cells treated with dihydrodiol epoxide derivatives of benzo(a)pyrene. *Mutation Res.*, **63**, 361–370

Boyum, A. (1968). Separation of lymphocytes and erythrocytes by centrifugation. *Scand. J. Clin. Invest.*, **21**, 77–85

Bradley, M. O., Hsu, I. C. and Harris, C. C. (1979). Relationships between sister chromatid exchange and mutagenicity, toxicity and DNA damage. *Nature*, **282**, 318–320

Braithwaite, I. and Ashby, J. (1988). A non-invasive micronucleus assay in rat liver. *Mutation Res.*, **203**, 23–32

Brook, J. D. (1982). The effect of 4CMB on germ cells of the mouse. *Mutation Res.*, **100**, 305–308

Brook, J. D. and Chandley, A. C. (1985). Testing of 3 chemical compounds for aneuploidy induction in the female mouse. *Mutation Res.*, **157**, 215–220

Brook, J. D. and Chandley, A. C. (1986). Testing for the chemical induction of aneuploidy in the male mouse. *Mutation Res.*, **164**, 117–125

Brusick, D. (1987). Genotoxicity produced in cultured mammalian cell assays by treatment conditions. Special issue. *Mutation Res.*, **189**, 1–80

Carrano, A. V. and Natarajan, A. J. (1988). Considerations for population monitoring using cytogenetic techniques. ICPEMC Publication No, 14, *Mutation Res.*, **204**, 379–406

Cattanach, B. M. (1982). The heritable translocation test in mice. In Hsu, T. S. (Ed.), *Cytogenetic Assays of Environmental Mutagens*. Allanheld, Osmun and Co., Totowa, New Jersey, pp. 289–323

Cawood, A. D. and Breckon, G. (1983). Synaptonemal complexes as indicators of induced structural change in chromosomes after irradiation of spermatogonia. *Mutation Res.*, **122**, 149–154

Chandley, A. C. (1981). The origin of chromosomal aberrations in man and their potential for survival and reproduction in the adult human population. *Ann. Genet.*, **24**, 5–11

Cifone, M. A., Myhr, B., Eiche, A. and Bolisfoldi, G. (1987). Effect of pH shifts on the mutant frequency at the thymidine kinase locus in mouse lymphoma L5178Y TK+/− cells. *Mutation Res.*, **189**, 39–46

Cole, R. J., Taylor, N., Cole, J. and Arlett, C. F. (1981). Short term tests for transplacentally active carcinogens. I. Micronucleus formation in foetal and maternal mouse erythroblasts. *Mutation Res.*, **80**, 141–157

The Collaborative Study Group for the Micronucleus Test (1986). Sex Differences in the micronucleus test. *Mutation Res.*, **172**, 151–163

The Collaborative Study Group for the Micronucleus Test (1988). Strain differences in the micronucleus test. *Mutation Res.*, **204**, 307–316

Connell, J. R. (1979). The relationship between sister chromatid exchange, chromosome aberration and gene mutation induction by several reactive polycyclic hydrocarbon metabolites in cultured mammalian cells. *Int. J. Cancer.*, **24**, 485–489

Connell, J. R. and Medcalf, A. S. (1982). The induction of SCE and chromosomal aberrations with relation to specific base methylation of DNA in Chinese hamster cells by *N*-methyl-*n*-nitrosourea and dimethyl sulphate. *Carcinogenesis*, **3**, 385–390

Croce, C. (1987). Role of chromosome translocations in human neoplasia. *Cell*, **49**, 155–156

Dean, B. J. and Danford, N. (1984). Assays for the detection of chemically-induced chromosome damage in cultured mammalian cells. In Venitt, S. and Parry, J. M. (Eds), *Mutagenicity Testing. A Practical Approach*. IRL Press, Oxford, pp. 187–232

Department of Health (1989). *Report on Health and Social Subjects. 35 Guidelines for the Testing of Chemicals for Mutagenicity*. Committee on Mutagenicity of Chemicals in Food, Consumer Products and the Environment. HMSO, London

Edwards, A. J., Moon, E. Y., Anderson, D. and McGregor, D. B. (1993). The effect of simultaneous exposure to bromodeoxyuridine and methyl methansulphonate on sister chromatid exchange frequency in cultured human lymphocytes and its mutation research (in press) *Mutation Res.*

Ehrenburg, L. and Wachtmeister, C. A. (1977). Safety precautions in work with mutagenic and carcinogenic chemicals. In Kilbey, B. J., Legator, M., Nichols, W. and Ramel, C. (Eds), *Handbook of Mutagenicity Test Procedures*. Elsevier, Amsterdam, pp. 401–410

European Communities (1984). *Official Journal of the European Community*, L251, **27**, 132

Evans E. P., Breckon, G. and Ford, C. E. (1964). An air-drying method for meiotic preparations from mammalian testes. *Cytogenet. Cell Genet.*, **3**, 289–294

Evans, H. J., and O'Riordan, M. L. (1975). Human peripheral blood lymphocytes for the analysis of chromosome aberrations in mutagen tests. *Mutation Res.*, **31**, 135–148

Friend, S. H., Bernards, R., Rogely, S., Weinburg, R. A., Rapaport, J. M., Albert, D. M. and Dryja, T. P. (1986). A human DNA segment with properties of the gene that predisposes to retinoblastoma and osteosarcoma. *Nature*, **323**, 643–646

Galloway, S. M. and Wolff, S. (1979). The relation between chemically induced SCEs and chromatid breakage. *Mutation Res.*, **61**, 297–307

Gilbert, F. (1983). Chromosomes, genes and cancer: A classification of chromosome abnormalities in cancer. *J. Natl Cancer Inst.*, **71**, 1107–1114

Hansmann, I. (1973). Induced chromosomal aberrations in pronuclei, 2-cell stages and morulae of mice. *Mutation Res.*, **20**, 353–367

Hansmann, I. and El-Nahass, E. (1979). Incidence of non-disjunction in mouse oocytes. *Cytogenet. Cell Genet.*, **24**, 115–121

Hayashi, M., Sofuni, T. and Ishidate, M. (1983). An application of acridine orange fluorescent staining to the micronucleus test. *Mutation Res.*, **120**., 241–247

Hayashi, M., Sutou, S., Shimada, H., Sato, S., Sasaki, Y. K. and Wakata, A. (1989). Difference between intraperitoneal and oral gavage application in the micronucleus test. The 3rd collaborative study by CSGMT/JEMS.MMS. *Mutation Res.*, **223**, 329–344

Heddle, J. A. and Bodycote, D. J. (1970). On the formation of chromosomal aberrations. *Mutation Res.*, **9**, 117–126

Henderson, L. (1986). Transplacental genotoxic agents: cytogenetic methods for their detection. In de Serres, F. J. (Ed.), *Chemical Mutagens. Principles and Methods for Their Detection*, Vol. 10. Plenum Press, New York, pp. 327–355

Henry, M., Lupo, S. and Szabo, K. T. (1980). Sex difference in sensitivity to the cytogenetic effects of ethyl methane sulphonate in mice demonstrated by the micronucleus test. *Mutation Res.*, **69**, 385–387

Holden, H. E. (1982). Comparison of somatic and germ cell models for cytogenetic screening. *J. Appl. Toxicol.*, **2**, 196–200

Human Genome News, National Centre for Human Genome Research, Vol. 2, No. 6, March 1992, p. 1

IARC (1979). *Handling Chemical Carcinogens in the Laboratory; Problems of Safety*, Scientific Publications, No. 33. International Agency for Research on Cancer, Lyons

ISCN (1985). *An International System for Human Cytogenetic Nomenclature*. Report of the Standing Committee on Human Cytogenetic Nomenclature. Harnden, D. G. and Klinger, H. P. (Eds), Karger, Basel, Switzerland

Ishidate, M. Jr (1988a). *Data Book of Chromosomal Aberration Tests in vitro*. Elsevier, Amsterdam

Ishidate, M. Jr (1988b). A proposed battery of tests for the initial evaluation of the mutagenic potential of medicinal and industrial chemicals. *Mutation Res.*, **205**, 397–407

Ishidate, M. Jr and Harnois, M. C. (1987). The clastogenicity of chemicals in mammalian cells. Letter to the Editor. *Mutagenesis*, **2**, 240–243

Ishidate, M. Jr, Harnois, M. C. and Sofuni, T. (1988). A comparative analysis of data on the clastogenicity of 951 chemical substances tested in mammalian cell cultures. *Mutation Res.*, **195**, 151–213

Ishidate, M. Jr, Sofuni, T., Yoshikawa, K., Hayashi, M., Nohmi, T., Sawada, M. and Matsooka, A. (1984). Primary mutagenicity screening of food additives currently used in Japan. *Fd Chem. Toxicol.*, **22**, 623–636

JMHW (1984). *Guidelines for Testing of Drugs for Toxicity*. Pharmaceutical Affairs Bureau, Notice No. 118. Ministry of Health and Welfare, Japan

Joint Directives of the Japanese Environmental Protection Agency, Japanese Ministry of Health and Welfare and Japanese Ministry of International Trade and Industry, 31 March 1987

Kato, H. (1973). Induction of sister chromatid exchanges by UV light and its inhibition by caffeine. *Exptl Cell Res.*, **82**, 383–390

Kato, H. (1974). Induction of sister chromatid exchanges by chemical mutagens and its possible relevance to DNA repair. *Exptl Cell Res.*, **85**, 239–247

Kirkland, D. J. and Garner, R. C. (1987). Testing for genotoxicity-chromosomal aberrations *in vitro* — CHO cells or human lymphocytes? *Mutation Res.*, **189**, 186–187

Kirkland, D. J., Marshall, R. R., McEnaney, S., Bidgwood, J., Rutter, A. and Mullineux, S. (1989). Aro-

clor-1254 induced rat liver S-9 causes chromosome aberrations in CHO cells but not in human lymphocytes: A role for active oxygen? *Mutation Res.*, **214**, 115–122

Klein, G. and Klein, E. (1985). Evolution of tumours and the impact of molecular oncology. *Nature*, **315**, 190–195

Korenberg, J. R. and Freedlender, E. F. (1974). Giesma technique for the detection of sister chromatid exchanges. *Chromosoma*, **48**, 355–360

Koufos, A., Hansen, M. F., Copeland, N. G., Jenkins, N. A., Lampkin, B. C. and Cavanee, W. K. (1985). Loss of heterozygosity in three embryonal tumours suggest a common pathogenetic mechanism. *Nature*, **316**, 330–334

Lambert, B., Lindblad, A., Holmberg, K. and Francesconi, D. (1982). The use of sister chromatid exchange to monitor human populations for exposure to toxicologically harmful agents. In Wolff, S. (Ed.), *Sister Chromatid Exchange*. Wiley, New York, pp. 149–182

Latt, S. A. (1973). Microfluorometric detection of deoxyribonucleic acid replication in human metaphase chromosomes. *Proc. Natl Acad. Sci. USA*, **70**, 3395–3399

Latt, S. A., Allen, J. W., Bloom, S. E., Carrano, A., Falke, E., Kram, D., Schneider, E., Schreck, R., Tice, R., Whitfield, B. and Wolff, S. (1981). Sister chromatid exchanges: a report of the gene-tox program. *Mutation Res.*, **87**, 17–62

Latt, S. A., Allen, J. W., Rogers, W. E. and Juergens, L. A. (1977). *In vitro* and *in vivo* analysis of sister chromatid exchange formation. In Kilbey, B. J. *et al.* (Eds), *Handbook of Mutagenicity Test Procedures*. Elsevier, Amsterdam, pp. 275–291

Latt, S. A. and Loveday, K. S. (1978). Characterisation of sister chromatid exchange induction by 8-methoxypsoralen plus near UV light. *Cytogenet. Cell Genet.*, **21**, 184–200

Latt, S. A., Schreck, R. R., Loveday, K. S., Dougherty, C. P. and Shuler, C. F. (1980). Sister chromatid exchanges. *Adv. Human Genet.*, **10**, 267–331

Leonard, A. (1975). Tests for heritable translocation in male mammals. *Mutation Res.*, **31**, 291–298

Leonard, A. (1973). Observations on meiotic chromosomes of the male mouse as a test of the potential mutagenicity of chemicals. In Hollender, A. (Ed.), *Chemical Mutagens. Principles and Methods for Their Detection*, Vol. 3. Plenum Press, New York, pp. 21–56

Lovell, D. P., Anderson, D., Albanese, R., Amphlett, G. E., Clare, G., Ferguson, R., Richold, M., Papworth, D. G. and Savage, J. R. K. (1989). Statistical analysis of *in vivo* cytogenetics assays. In Kirkland, D. J. (Ed.), *UKEMS Sub-committee on Guidelines for Mutagenicity Testing. Report. Part III. Statistical Evaluation of Mutagenicity Test Data*. Cambridge University Press, Cambridge, pp. 184–232

MacGregor, J. J., Weir, C. M. and Gould, D. H.

(1980). Clastogen-induced micronuclei in peripheral blood erythrocytes: The basis of an improved micronucleus test. *Environ. Mutagen.*, **2**, 509–514

MacGregor, J. T., Heddle, J. A., Hite, M., Margolin, B., Ramel, C., Salamone, M. R., Tice, R. R. and Wild, D. (1987). Guidelines for the conduct of micronucleus assays in mammalian bone marrow erythrocytes. *Mutation Res.*, **189**, 103–112

MacGregor, J. T., Wehr, C. M. and Langlas, R. G. (1983). A simple fluorescent staining procedure for micronuclei and RNA in erythrocytes using Hoechst 33258 and pyronin Y. *Mutation Res.*, **120**, 269–275

Madle, S. and Obe, G. (1980). Methods for analysis of the mutagenicity of indirect mutagens/carcinogens in eukaryotic cells. *Human Genet.*, **56**, 7–20

Maron, D. M. and Ames, B. N. (1983). Revised methods for the *Salmonella* mutagenicity test. *Mutation Res.*, **113**, 173–215

Minden, M. D. (1987). Oncogenes. In Tannock, I. F. and Hill, R. P. (Eds), *The Basic Science of Oncology*. Pergamon Press, New York, pp. 72–88

Mirkova, E. and Ashby, J. (1987). Relative distribution of mature erythrocytes, polychromatic erythrocytes (PE) and micronucleated PE in mouse bone marrow smears: Control observations. *Mutation Res.*, **182**, 203–211

Monticone, R. E. and Schneider, E. L. (1979). Induction of SCEs in human cells by fluorescent light. *Mutation Res.*, **59**, 215–221

Morimoto, K., Sato, M. and Koizumi, A. (1983). Proliferative kinetics of human lymphocytes in culture measured by autoradiography and sister chromatid differential staining. *Exptl Cell Res.*, **145**, 249–356

MRC (1981). *Guidelines for Work with Chemical Carcinogens in Medical Research Council Establishments*. Medical Research Council, London

Natarajan, A. T., Tates, A. D., van Buul, P. P. W., Meijers, M. and de Vogel, N. (1976). Cytogenetic effects of mutagens/carcinogens after activation in a microsomal system *in vitro*. *Mutation Res.*, **37**, 83–90

Newton, M. F. and Lilly, L. J. (1986). Tissue specific clastogenic effects of chromium and selenium salts *in vivo*. *Mutation Res.*, **169**, 61–69

OECD (1983). *OECD Guidelines for the Testing of Chemicals*. No. 475. Genetic toxicology: *in vivo* mammalian bone marrow cytogenetic test—chromosomal analysis. Adopted 4 April 1984

Olson, M., Hood, L., Cantor, C. and Botstein, D. (1989). A common language for physical mapping of the human genome. *Science*, **245**, 1434–1435

Painter, R. B. (1980). A replication model of sister-chromatid exchange. *Mutation Res.*, **70**, 337–341

Pascoe, S. and Gatehouse, D. (1986). The use of a simple haematoxylin and eosin staining procedure to demonstrate micronuclei within rodent bone marrow. *Mutation Res.*, **164**, 237–243

Perry, P. E. and Evans, H. J. (1975). Cytotological detection of mutagen/carcinogen exposure by sister chromatid exchange. *Nature*, **258**, 121–125

Perry, P., Henderson, L. and Kirkland, D. (1984). Sister chromatid exchange in cultured cells. In *UKEMS Sub-committee on Guidelines for Mutagenicity Testing. Report. Part IIA*, pp. 89–121

Perry, P. E. and Thomson, E. J. (1984). Sister chromatid exchange methodology. In Kilbey, B. J. *et al.* (Eds), *Handbook of Mutagenicity Test Procedures*, 2nd edn. Elsevier, Amsterdam, pp. 495–529

Perry, P. E. and Wolff, S. (1974). New Giemsa method for the differential staining of sister chromatids. *Nature*, **251**, 156–158

Phillips, R. A. (1987). The genetic basis of cancer. In Tannock, T. F. and Hill R. P. (Eds), *The Basic Science of Oncology*. Pergamon Press, New York, pp. 24–51

Preston, R. J., Au, W., Bender, M. A., Brewen, J. G., Carrano, A. C., Heddle, J. A., McFee, A. F., Wolff, S. and Wassom, J. S. (1981). Mammalian *in vivo* and *in vitro* cytogenetic assays. *Mutation Res.*, **87**, 143–188

Preston, R. J., San Sebastian, J. R. and McFee, A. F. (1987). The *in vitro* human lymphocyte assay for assessing the clastogenicity of chemical agents. *Mutation Res.*, **189**, 175–183

Revell, S. H. (1974). The breakage-and-reunion theory and the exchange theory for chromosome aberrations induced by ionising radiations: A short history. In Lett J. T., and Zelle, M. (Eds), *Advances in Radiation Biology*, Vol. 4. Academic Press, New York, pp. 367–415

Richardson, C., Williams, D. A., Allen, J. A., Amphlett, G., Chanter, D. O. and Phillips, B. (1989). Analysis of data from *in vitro* cytogenetic assays. In Kirkland, D. J. (Ed.), *UKEMS Sub-committee on Guidelines for Mutagenicity Testing. Report. Part III. Statistical Evaluation of Mutagenicity Test Data*. Cambridge University Press, Cambridge, pp. 141–154

Richold, M., Chandley, A., Ashby, J., Gatehouse, D. G., Bootman, J. and Henderson, L. (1990). *In vivo* cytogenetics assays. In Kirkland, D. J. (Ed.), *UKEMS Sub-committee on Guidelines for Mutagenicity Testing. Report. Part I. Revised Basic Mutagenicity Tests. UKEMS Recommended Procedures*. Cambridge University Press, Cambridge, pp. 115–141

Romagna, F. and Staniforth, C. D. (1989). The automated bone marrow micronucleus test. *Mutation Res.*, **213**, 91–104

Salamone, M. F. and Heddle, J. (1983). The bone marrow micronucleus assay: rationale for a revised protocol. In de Serres, F. J. (Ed.), *Chemical Mutagens. Principles and Methods for Their Detection*. Plenum Press, New York, pp. 111–149

Schmid, W. (1976). The micronucleus test for cytogenetic analysis. In Hollaender, A. (Ed.), *Chemical Mutagens. Principles and Methods for Their Detection*, Vol. 4. Plenum Press, New York, pp. 31–53

Scott, D., Danford, N., Dean, B., Kirkland, D. and

Richardson, C. (1983). *In vitro* chromosome aberration assays. In Dean, B. J. (Ed.), *UKEMS Subcommittee on Guidelines for Mutagenicity Testing. Report. Part I. Basic Test Battery*. UKEMS, Swansea, pp. 41–64

Scott, D., Dean, B. J., Danford, N. D. and Kirkland, D. J. (1990). Metaphase chromosome aberration assays *in vitro*. In Kirkland, D. J. (Ed.), *UKEMS Sub-committee on Guidelines for Mutagenicity Testing. Report. Part I. Revised Basic Mutagenicity Tests. UKEMS Recommended Procedures*. Cambridge University Press, Cambridge, pp. 63–86

Shelby, M. D. (1986). A case for the continued use of the intraperitoneal route of exposure. *Mutation Res.*, **170**, 169–171

Shtivelman, E., Lifshitz, B., Gale, R. P. and Canaani, E. (1985). Fused transcript of *abl* and *bcr* genes in chronic myelogenous leukaemia. *Nature*, **315**, 550–554

Tates, A. D., Neuteboom, I., Hofker, M. and den Engelese, L. (1980). A micronucleus technique for detecting clastogenic effects of mutagens/carcinogens (DEN, DMN) in hepatocytes of rat liver *in vivo*. *Mutation Res.*, **74**, 11–20

Taylor, J. H. (1958). Sister chromatid exchanges in tritium labelled chromosomes. *Genetics*, **43**, 515–529

Thompson, E. D. (1986). Comparison of *in vivo* and *in vitro* cytogenetic assay results. *Environ. Mutagen.*, **8**, 753–767

Thust, R., Mendel, J., Schwarz, H. and Warzok, R. (1980). Nitrosated urea pesticide metabolites and other nitrosamides. Activity in clastogenicity and SCE assays, and aberration kinetics in Chinese hamster V79-E cells. *Mutation Res.*, **79**, 239–248

Topham, J., Albanese, R., Bootman, J., Scott, D. and Tweats, D. (1983). *In vivo* cytogenetic assays. In Dean, B. (Ed.), *Report of UKEMS Sub-committee on Guidelines for Mutagenicity Testing*. Part I, pp. 119–141

Tsuchimoto, T. and Matter, B. E. (1979). *In vivo* cytogenetic screening methods for mutagens with special reference to the micronucleus test. *Archs Toxicol.*, **42**, 239–248

US Department of Energy (1990). *The Human Genome (1989–1990)*. Program Report. Office of Energy Research, Office of Health and Environmental Research

US Human Genome Project (1990). *Understanding Our Genetic Inheritance. The First Five Years FY 1991–1995*. US Department of Health and Human Services, US Department of Energy. National Technical Information Service. US Department of Commerce, Springfield, Virginia

Waters, D. B. (Ed.) (1980). Safe handling of carcinogens, mutagens, teratogens and highly toxic substances. Ann Arbor, Science Publishers Inc., U.S.A.

Wolff, S. (1977). Lesions that lead to SCEs are different from those that lead to chromosome aberrations. *Mutation Res.*, **46**, 164

Wolff, S., Bodycote, J. and Painter, R. B. (1974). Sister chromatid exchanges produced in Chinese hamster cells by UV-irradiation to different stages of the cell cycle: The necessity for cells to pass through S. *Mutation Res.*, **25**, 73–81

Wolff, S. and Perry, P. (1974). Differential staining of sister chromatids and the study of sister chromatid exchange without autoradiography. *Chromosoma*, **48**, 341–353

Yunis, J. J. (1983). The chromosomal basis of human neoplasia. *Science*, **221**, 227–236

FURTHER READING

Garewal, H. S., Ramsey, L., Kaugars, G. and Boyle, J. (1993). Clinical experience with the micronucleus assay. *Journal of Cellular Biochemistry*, **17**, 206–212

Kirsch, I. R. (1993). *The Causes and Consequences of Chromosomal Aberrations*. CRC Press, Boca Raton, Florida

Tucker, J. D., Auletta, A., Cimino, M. C. Dearfield, K. L., Jacobson-Kram, D., Tice, R. R. and Carrano, A. V. (1993). Sister chromatid exchanged: second report of the Gene-Tox program. *Mutation Research*, **297**, 101–180

37 Carcinogenicity and Genotoxic Carcinogens

Douglas McGregor

INTRODUCTION

Carcinogenesis is a multistep process which occurs through a variety of incompletely understood mechanisms. The information upon which evaluations of carcinogenic potential are made comes from epidemiology and animal experiments. Frequently, the animal experiments conducted with high-volume production chemicals, or chemicals which are important for some other reason, give the first indications that special care may be necessary in handling the chemical because it is carcinogenic. On other occasions, the primary information may come from observations upon human disease patterns. This chapter is a description of some of the problems associated with carcinogenicity experiments and a discussion of what the results might mean, particularly for those substances which are so-called genotoxic carcinogens. Non-genotoxic carcinogens are discussed in Chapter 38.

GENETIC FACTORS IN CARCINOGENESIS

An association of abnormal mitotic metaphase chromosomes with cancer cells has been known for more than a century, but chromosomal aberrations seemed to exhibit no specific pattern with particular neoplastic diseases and it was far from clear whether the aberrations were causative or secondary events arising during tumour development. The first documentation of a non-random chromosomal aberration with a neoplastic disease was the reciprocal translocation between chromosomes 9 and 22 (t(9,22)), giving the Philadelphia chromosome, seen in chronic myeloid leukaemia (Nowell and Hungerford, 1960). Since then, it has been shown that specific reciprocal translocations are prevalent in leukaemias and lymphomas and that they also occur in 3 per cent of all neoplasms (reported by Solomon et al., 1991). More than 100 recurrent translocations have been described (Mitelman et al., 1990). In addition,

progression towards increased malignancy appears to be characterized by increased genetic instability, manifest as translocations, deletions, chromosomal breaks, ploidy changes and nondisjunctions.

The genetic instability of tumour cells is well documented, but the mechanisms involved are not yet defined. They may involve mutations in DNA repair and synthesis genes, but evidence for this mechanism in man is restricted to instability genes in association with inherited chromosomal fragility syndromes, such as xeroderma pigmentosum and ataxia telangiectasia. Comparison of point mutation rates in tumorigenic and non-tumorigenic cells does not reveal any marked difference, whereas the rate of gene amplification is clearly higher in tumorigenic cells. Thus, amplification of base sequences encoding the CAD protein (a multifunctional enzyme: carbamoyl phosphate synthase, aspartate transcarbamylase and dihydroorotase) cannot be demonstrated in cells from man, hamster or rat ($<10^{-9}$), whereas amplification occurs in tumorigenic cells from each of these species at about 10^{-4} (Tisty et al., 1989; Tisty, 1990).

Dominant Oncogenes

The finding that the avian retroviral src gene had evolved from a captured cellular gene (Stehelin et al., 1976) was to guide much future research and the development of the concept of oncogenes. These are dominantly acting mutant forms of normal cellular genes (proto-oncogenes) which play a physiological growth-regulating role (reviewed by Bishop, 1987), many of them having protein kinase activity, particularly for the phosphorylation of tyrosine residues.

When mouse NIH 3T3 fibroblasts are transfected with DNA from human tumours, the result is malignant transformation of the fibroblasts. Oncogenes were isolated from these cells (Shih et al., 1981) and were found to be homologues of retroviral transforming genes (Der et al., 1982). About 100 oncogenes have been discovered since the early 1980s by use of these transfection assays. However, only a few of the oncogenes have a demonstrated involvement in human carcinogenesis, although, in an altered form, they function as oncogenes in experimental systems. Apart from a few viruses, such as human papilloma virus (HPV) and hepatitis B virus (HBV), which may introduce foreign DNA, genetic alterations in human neoplasia entirely result from changes in structure and/or function of the cell's own genome. The proto-oncogenes are known or suspected to code for proteins acting as growth factors, growth factor receptors, secondary messengers that transduce signals through the cytoplasm and transcription factors that regulate gene expression within the nucleus (Table 1). In addition, the *bcl*-2 gene product appears to be localized on mitochondrial membranes and functions, not by stimulating growth, but in apoptosis, by preventing the programmed cell death of B lymphocytes.

The c-*myc* family and c-*ras* of proto-oncogenes are clearly important in human carcinogenicity, whereas, at present, no major role in human cancer has been found for *fos, myb, src* and *jun*, which are central to normal mammalian cell growth and differentiation (Nowell, 1991). Nevertheless, oncogenes have been reported in 10–30 per cent of human cancers (Slamon *et al.*, 1984) and some less prominent oncogenes could

act in collaboration with the more manifest ones. Exposure to some tumour promoters may cause transient increases in *fos, jun, sis* and *myc* expression; and in the case of c-*fos* this transient expression in NIH 3T3 cells gives a protein that activates or induces the synthesis of functions that accelerate mutation frequency (van den Berg *et al.*, 1991). Oncogenes are capable of cell immortalization and transformation *in vitro* and normally control a wide variety of cellular functions, such as proliferation, differentiation, morphology, intercellular communication and motility (Barbacid, 1987; Bishop, 1987). Their functions are affected by the cytogenetic processes mentioned earlier. For example, the t(9,22) translocation of chronic myeloid leukaemia results in the activation of the c-*abl* proto-oncogene, while t(8,14), t(2,8) and t(8,22) translocations in Burkitt's lymphoma all result in deregulated c-*myc* expression. There are many examples of proto-oncogenes located close to chromosomal breakage points in leukaemias and other neoplasms.

The prevalence of oncogenes in particular human tumours has its counterpart in chemically induced animal tumours. Some of these animal oncogenes show specific genetic changes involving growth factor receptors (*neu*), signal transducing systems (*ras*) or nuclear DNA-binding pro-

Table 1   Some proto-oncogenes involved in growth regulation. Modified from Hunter (1991) and Stoler (1991)

	Proto-oncogenes	Function
Growth factor	*sis*	PDGF
	hst	FGF family
	int-2	FGF family
	fgf-5	FGF family
Receptor	*erb-b*	EGF receptor ⎱ protein tyrosine
	fms	CSF 1 receptor ⎰ kinases
Transduction	*ras*	Membrane-associated GTP-binding/GTPase
	abl,src	PTKs
	mil/raf	Ser/Thr kinases
2nd messengers		
Transcription/other nuclear functions	*erb-a*	Dominant negative mutant thyroxine (T_3) receptor
	fos	Combines with c-*jun* product to form AP-1
	ets	Binds PEA-3 sites
	jun	AP-1
	myc	DNA binding sites unresolved

teins (*myc*). The *ras* proto-oncogene mutations are particularly important and result in gene activation or amplification. The mutations are often consistently carcinogen-specific (e.g. G:C→A:T transitions at the second base of codon 12 in H-*ras*, induced by methylating agents such as NMU and MNNG; A:T→T:A transversions at the second base of codon 61 in H-*ras*, induced by DMBA), but several polycyclic aromatic hydrocarbons other than DMBA do not induce consistent changes in the *ras* oncogene expressed in the induced tumours (Balmain and Brown, 1988).

Mutations in *ras* are, in some cases, very early events in carcinogenesis, but proto-oncogene activation may also occur late. In a transgenic mouse carrying *pim*-1, a single dose of ENU induced lymphomas, most of which expressed c-*myc* and some also expressed K-*ras* or N-*ras*. However, the data suggested that at least some of the *ras* mutations were late events and therefore not induced by the NMU treatment (Breuer *et al.*, 1991). Both NMU and ENU also induce gliomas and schwannomas in which *neu* is activated by specific T:A→A:T transversions within the transmembranal domain. However, adducts formed by NMU or ENU which might lead to this type of transversion have not been identified, so either the adduct is very minor but biologically important or the activation of *neu* occurs late in tumour development (Balmain and Brown, 1988). Currently, this type of observation is sparse, but they could be important for the interpretation of data in which oncogene expression is found in advanced neoplasms.

Tumour Suppressor Genes

Malignant transformation cannot be described simply in terms of proto-oncogene activation. Familial studies have shown that mutations associated with loss of function are important in neoplasia and these are strongly supported by experimental work. Fusion of mouse fibroblasts with carcinoma cells, or fusion of two varieties of sarcoma, resulted in cells which were initially non-tumorigenic (Harris *et al.*, 1969). As the hybrid clones were cultured *in vitro*, there was reversion to the malignant phenotype, which was always associated with loss of specific chromosomes. In mouse, the re-emergence of malignancy was strongly associated with the loss of chromosome 4 (Evans *et al.*, 1982). In human/

rodent cell hybrids, the reappearance of malignancy was also associated with the loss of certain human chromosomes, particularly chromosome 11 (Klinger and Shows, 1983). Powerful evidence for the insufficiency of oncogene activity for the malignant phenotype is the finding that the hybrid of normal fibroblasts fused with EJ bladder carcinoma cells, which contain an activated H-*ras* gene, are non-tumorigenic, even though H-*ras* gene expression continued at high levels (Noda *et al.*, 1983). Similarly, the tumorigenicity of K-*ras*-transformed mouse cells is suppressed when they are fused with non-tumorigenic mouse cells, although the K-*ras* gene continues to be expressed at high levels (Craig and Sager, 1985). It also emerged from this kind of experiment that fusion of a transformed bladder epithelium cell line with differentiated normal bladder epithelial cells resulted in suppression of tumorigenicity, whereas fusion with undifferentiated fibroblasts did not (Summerhayes and Franks, 1979; Cowell, 1980; Cowell and Franks, 1984). Thus, factors were present in normal, differentiated cells which suppressed malignancy. The concept arose that these factors were coded for in antioncogenes, or tumour suppressor genes. A number of these genes have been reported for a variety of human tumours (Table 2). Tumour suppressor genes may ultimately be more interesting than oncogenes, since loss of genetic material occurs far more frequently than does activation of a gene function.

The p53 suppressor gene may be the most frequently involved gene in human carcinogenesis, but shows complex behaviour. The majority of p53 mutations in human tumours occurs in the evolutionarily highly conserved domains in exons 5–8. The mis-sense mutations are predominantly GC → TA transitions and >95 per cent code amino acids that are entirely conserved in mouse, rat, monkey and man (Hollstein *et al.*, 1991). In squamous cell carcinoma of the skin, however, UV-specific CC → TT double-base and dipyrimidine C → T substitutions are also found which apparently do not occur in p53 of internal organs (Brash *et al.*, 1991). All mutations of this gene so far examined have lost the ability to suppress transformation. Some of these may be dominant negative mutations that inhibit the function of normal p53 by complex formation, while others not only have lost suppressor activity, but also can act, with the p21 product of *ras*, as dominant, co-operating oncogenes. There is even evidence

Table 2   Representative tumour suppressor genes incriminated in human tumours. Modified from Bishop (1991)

Neoplasm	Chromosomal locus	Tumour suppressor gene
Astrocytoma; carcinoma of the breast, colon, liver, oesophagus and lung; osteosarcoma	17q12–13.3	*p53*
Retinoblastoma; osteosarcoma; carcinomas of the breast, bladder and lung	13q14	*RB1*
Wilms' tumour	11p13 (p15)	*WT1*
Carcinomas of the lung and kidney	3p21	*PTPase* γ
Carcinoma of the colon	18q21-ter	*DCC*
Neurofibromatosis type 1	17q11.2	*NF1*
Carcinoma of the colon	5q21–22	*MCC*
Familial adenomatous polyposis of colon	5q15–22	*FAP*
Tumours of the parathyroid, pancreas, pituitary and adrenal cortex	11q13	*MEN-1*
Carcinoma of the liver	16q22.1–23.2	?
Carcinoma of the lung	3p21	?
Carcinoma of the kidney	3p12–14	?
Neuroblastoma	1p36.1	?

? = no currently adopted nomenclature.

that, in some cases, p53 truly behaves as a recessive oncogene (Marshall, 1991). Interaction between the products of an oncogene and a tumour suppressor gene has been described for the retinoblastoma gene product, p105[RB], which may play a role in transcriptional regulation (Mitchell, 1991) and is one of the targets of the transforming gene E1A of adenovirus-12 (Whyte *et al.*, 1988; Whyte *et al.*, 1989), of SV40 large T (Decaprio *et al.*, 1988) and of HPV-16 E7 protein (Dyson *et al.*, 1989). These DNA tumour virus oncoproteins may, therefore, mediate transformation by inactivating the RB gene by forming a complex with p105[RB].

These processes are believed to form part of the genetic basis for multistep carcinogenicity. While the viral introduction of specific genes to cells very rarely occurs in human carcinogenesis, it appears that there are a very large number of growth regulatory genes, both stimulatory and inhibitory, that do contribute significantly to the development of human cancer. The complexities of the actions and interactions of these genes have yet to be detailed, and it is probable that many important genes are currently unknown. While it is to be expected that most of this research should be directed towards understanding human cancer, there is a place for similar work on induced tumours in rats and mice, which play such an important part in carcinogen identification.

GENOTOXIC CARCINOGENS

Chemicals which increase carcinogenic risks have been categorized as 'genotoxic' and 'non-genotoxic', a process which can have effects upon the manner in which the chemicals are handled in the regulatory arena. Butterworth (1990) has defined a genotoxic agent as one for which a *primary biological activity* of the chemical or a metabolite is alteration of the information encoded in the DNA. Chemicals exhibiting such activity can usually be identified by assays that measure reactivity with DNA, induction of mutations, induction of DNA repair or cytogenetic effects (see Chapters 35 and 36). Many of these assays have been considered to be predictive of carcinogenicity.

Non-genotoxic chemicals are those that lack genotoxicity as a primary biological activity. While these agents may yield genotoxic events as a secondary result of other induced toxicity, such as forced cellular growth, their primary action does not involve reactivity with the DNA (see Chapter 35).

Two assumptions are made in formulating this distinction: that genotoxic carcinogens are biologically active at all doses and that non-genotoxic carcinogens have biologically significant effects only above a particular threshold dose. This division arises because genotoxic chemicals interact directly with nuclear DNA, of which there is basically a single copy within each cell (although there may be multiple copies of particular genes), while non-genotoxic chemicals react with non-DNA molecules, of which there are many copies. Thus, damage to non-DNA molecules will have biologically important consequences only when a sufficiently large proportion is inactivated so that first-order kinetics of their reactions are no longer followed. The validity of this division is questionable from two points of view.

First, a chemical which interacts with DNA will also react with other nucleophiles, and these latter reactions are quantitatively dominant and could be as important in the carcinogenic process as the reactions with DNA. *For no chemical is its mode of carcinogenic action known.* Consequently, it is less presumptive to define genotoxic chemical carcinogens as chemical carcinogens which are known to interact with DNA, rather than as chemicals which are carcinogens *because* they interact with DNA. The carcinogenic response might directly involve DNA damage, but this is seldom – if ever – sufficient to explain the response. Genotoxicity in general terms does not, by itself, prove that the carcinogen is acting through a genotoxic mechanism. It does not even provide evidence for this mechanism, although it does strongly suggest its plausibility. Genotoxicity is at least evidence that a chemical interacts with biological molecules to induce an adverse response. The demonstration of genotoxicity indicates that the responsible chemical could initiate (although it might not be sufficient for) the neoplastic process, that the substance is bioavailable and that it has the potential to interfere with biological processes, the disruption of which may play multiple roles in neoplasia. Biological elements in this process could include, for example, some cell population death with subsequent proliferation of a fraction of the survivors, or loss of communication and homoeostatic control between cells within a tissue.

Second, some non-genotoxic carcinogens may be involved in reactions which generate radicals and other charged species. The metabolism of xenobiotics usually involves the cytochrome *P*-450 system, in which electron transfer to the xenobiotic substrate occurs with varying efficiency. Active oxygen species are inevitable products of this inefficiency, so, while neither the xenobiotic nor any of its metabolites might be involved in reactions with DNA, the potential for DNA damage always exists.

By far the best-studied short-term predictive test for carcinogenicity is the *Salmonella* mutation test of Ames. But in recent years there has been forceful questioning of what short-term test results mean, particularly following the publication of the US National Toxicology Program (NTP) results with 114 chemicals (Tennant *et al.*, 1987; Zeiger *et al.*, 1990). This represents about one-third of the National Cancer Institute (NCI)/ NTP chemicals tested for carcinogenicity in rats and mice. The short-term genotoxicity tests evaluated were the *Salmonella* mutation assay, the mouse lymphoma L5178Y tk$^{+/-}$ mutation assay, the Chinese hamster ovary (CHO) cell assay for chromosomal aberrations and the CHO cell assay for sister chromatid exchanges (SCE). The conclusions drawn from these studies are:

(1) The tests did not perform as well as expected in predicting rodent carcinogens.
(2) No test complements any other.
(3) No battery predicts rodent carcinogens any better than any other.
(4) No test predicts rodent carcinogens any better than any other.
(5) No potency correlations emerged (i.e. strong rodent carcinogens were not predicted better than weak ones and strong genotoxic agents were no more likely to be rodent carcinogens than weak ones).

It appeared that none of the three mammalian cell *in vitro* assays used in this programme gave any improvement over the predictions possible with the use of *Salmonella* alone. Later, the use was advocated of the *Salmonella* assay in conjunction with chemical reactive group 'structural alerts' (Ashby, 1978; Ashby and Tennant, 1988; Ashby *et al.*, 1989).

Structure–Activity Relationships (SAR)

Chemical structural features associated with carcinogenesis have been analysed by Ashby and colleagues (Purchase *et al.*, 1978; Ashby and Tennant, 1991). The derived structural alerts were identified empirically from comparison of chemically related rodent carcinogens and 'non-carcinogens'. There was, therefore, some judgement as to which chemical moieties were responsible for the biological responses. Such judgements were based upon the analyses of Arcos *et al.* (1968) and Arcos and Argus (1974) and the electrophilicity theory of chemical carcinogenesis developed by Miller and Miller (1977). Owing to the method of their derivation, structural alerts identify molecules which react with nucleophilic groups on cellular macromolecules and give overall predictions which are not significantly different from those obtained from bacterial mutation assays. Therefore, structural alerts aid in the identification of chemicals which are both carcinogenic and mutagenic. These alerts have been summarized as a non-existent macromolecule (Tennant and Ashby, 1991; Figure 1).

In this same period, the use of computers facilitated the search for structural fragments and physicochemical properties that can be correlated with toxicological observations. A basic approach is that of Free and Wilson (1964). It requires a wide range of chemical structures to avoid repetition of the data considered and treats a wide range of substituents additively. A peculiarity of this system is that structural features may be identified as correlating with the biological response when they have no clear biological or chemical role in the activity under consideration. Two important SAR systems have been developed from this basis: those of Enslein and Klopman.

The more useful molecular descriptors in the Free–Wilson system, as developed by Enslein *et*

al. (1987), are substructural keys and molecular connectivities. The latter form a system devised by Kier and Hall (1976) for the quantitative evaluation of molecular structure through quantum mechanics. Substructural fragments describe atom–bond combinations considered to be representative of functional groups, such as rings, polycyclic ring systems and aliphatic moieties.

A variant of the Free–Wilson procedure is the computer-automated structure evaluation (CASE) system of Klopman (1984), in which key substructures have an indicator role, but not necessarily a functional one. The computer selects its own descriptors automatically from a learning set composed of active and inactive molecules. The descriptors are single, continuous fragments that are embedded within the complete molecule. The descriptors also consist of either activating or inactivating fragments. Entry of a chemical unknown to the computer results in the generation of all possible fragments ranging from 3 to 10 non-hydrogen atoms accompanied by their hydrogens. These fragments are then compared with the previously identified activating and inactivating descriptors.

All three of these better-known SAR approaches to carcinogen identification perform

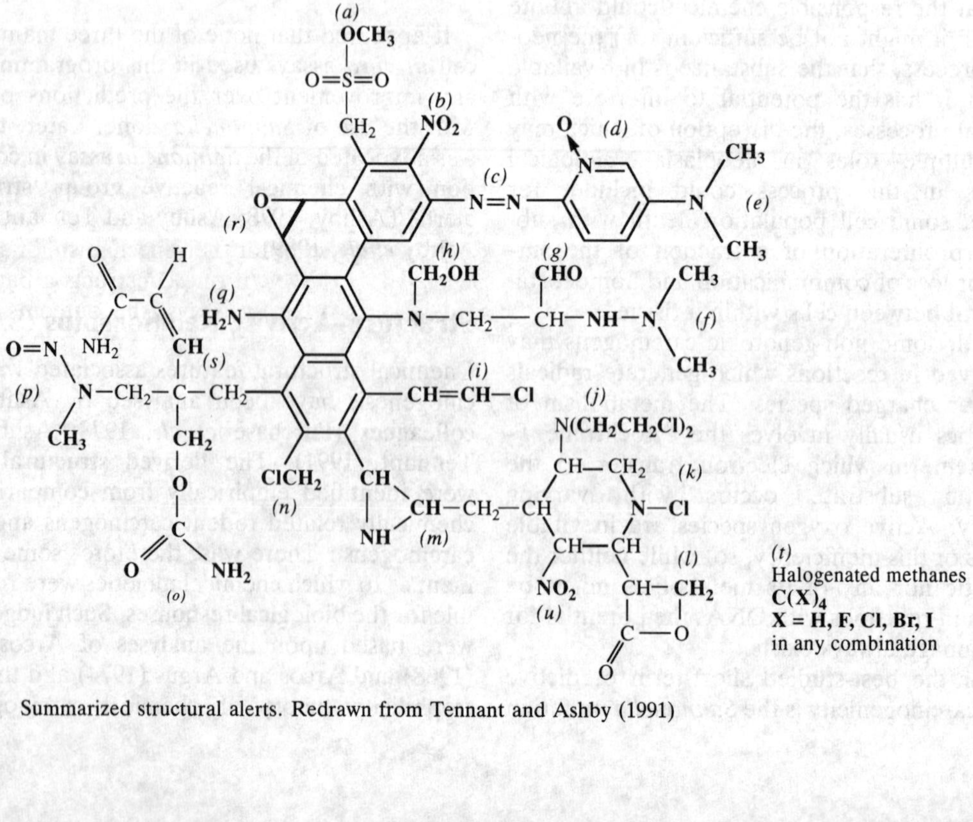

Figure 1   Summarized structural alerts. Redrawn from Tennant and Ashby (1991)

well in that role, but it is far from clear how mechanistic information can be derived from them. The exercise of structural alerts would appear to come closest to this objective, since they do correlate so very well with bacterial mutagenicity data. A key feature of SAR systems is the recognition that predictions are, strictly, in reference only to a particular, well-defined, end-point. The more complex the end-point (e.g. carcinogenesis), the lower the probability of successful recognition of a mechanism.

The use of structural alerts in conjunction with *Salmonella* mutation data appeared to introduce a very high level of redundancy, since there were no significant differences between the predictions of either the structural alert analysis or the *Salmonella* test alone (McGregor, 1989, 1990).

The reason is probably that *Salmonella* responds to chemicals readily recognized as electrophilic substances, while the structural alerts were accumulated largely on the basis of carcinogenicity results (Ashby, 1978) available at a time when the data were more clearly skewed towards potent carcinogens than is currently the case. Thus, it is highly probable that *Salmonella* testing is an experimental method and structural alert analysis is a theoretical method of demonstrating the electrophilicity of a chemical. This is a good basis for prediction of carcinogens that are also genotoxic, but its weakness is that it only permits the recognition of chemical groups which may interact with DNA; it leaves unconsidered those groups which may not themselves interact with DNA, but which generate species that are genotoxic (e.g. active oxygen). Its strength is that it forces special consideration of non-genotoxic mechanisms (see Chapter 38).

Genotoxic Characteristics of Carcinogens

One approach to the identification of carcinogens with genotoxic activity is to examine the characteristics of those carcinogens which are active in a very-high-specificity genotoxicity-based predictive assay. There is always a trade-off between specificity and sensitivity, but one example of a reasonable candidate assay is the *in vitro* hepatocyte unscheduled DNA synthesis (UDS) assay (i.e. *not* in cell lines). Published UDS data on 249 compounds for which carcinogenicity data were available contained 103 chemicals which induced

UDS (and 10 others giving inconclusive results). The sensitivity of the assay was 52 per cent (96/184), while its specificity was 100 per cent (22/22), unless chemicals giving inconclusive results in carcinogenicity tests were considered to be non-carcinogens, in which case the specificity was reduced to 85 per cent (48/55) (McGregor, unpublished).

An alternative basis for the recognition of a genotoxic carcinogen has been a carcinogen which is active in the widely used *Salmonella*/microsome mutation test (Ashby and Tennant, 1988, 1991; Tennant and Ashby, 1991). Among 301 chemicals tested in two rodent species by the US National Toxicology Program, there were 162 carcinogens and 100 chemicals giving no evidence of carcinogenicity (for 39 chemicals the data were equivocal). The *Salmonella* assay gave positive responses for 56 per cent of the carcinogens and 25 per cent of the so-called non-carcinogens. The correlations can also be studied after separation of the chemicals into different classes (Table 3). For aromatic amines, nitro-aromatics and alkylating agents, the proportion of mutagenic chemicals was high, irrespective of whether they had been shown to be carcinogenic or not. There was, however, a weakly increased likelihood of being carcinogenic, especially in more than one species, if the chemicals were active in the *Salmonella* mutation assay. There was no warning, given by the *Salmonella* test, of carcinogenic potential among those compounds not containing structural alerts. The problem with the use of single assays such as the UDS and *Salmonella* assays is that they leave us with many carcinogens which may yet be genotoxic (in other assays) and this activity may be important for their mechanism of carcinogenicity. However, if one constructs a battery of several genotoxicity assays, the outcome is that almost all chemicals demonstrate some type of activity.

Chemicals evaluated within the programme of the International Agency for Research on Cancer (IARC) are grouped according to the available evidence as: Group 1 (the agent is carcinogenic to humans); Group 2A (the agent is probably carcinogenic to humans); Group 2B (the agent is possibly carcinogenic to humans); Group 3 (the agent is not classifiable as to its carcinogenicity to humans); and Group 4 (the agent is probably not carcinogenic to humans). Chemicals assigned to the first four groups and for which carcinogenic

Table 3 Activity in the *Salmonella*/microsome mutation assay of different groups of chemicals which have been tested for carcinogenicity in the US National Toxicology Program standard bioassay. Adapted from Ashby and Tennant (1991)

Groups	Aromatic amino/nitro		Alkylating agents		Non-reactive halogenated[a]		Non-reactive no halogen[a]		Minimally reactive[a]	
	No. in group	% *Salm.* pos.	No. in group	% *Salm.* pos.	No. in group	% *Salm.* pos.	No. in group	% *Salm.* pos.	No. in group	% *Salm.* pos.
All carcinogens	59	93	30	83	26	0	15	0	16	13(2)
Two-species carcinogens	33	100	17	88	10	0	5	0	7	14(1)
One-species carcinogens	26	85	13	75	16	0	10	0	9	11(1)
Equivocal evidence	8	63(5)	5	60	8	13(1)	10	0	5	0
No evidence	17	71	11	55	16	6(1)	36	3(1)	15	7(1)

[a] Non-reactive = non-alerting structure (see Figure 1); minimally reactive = non-alerting structure, but may be considered to have some potential reactivity with DNA.
( ) Number of *Salm.* pos. (*Salmonella*-positive) chemicals, where the total number of chemicals in a group is small.

potency data were available were analysed in an attempt to identify characteristics of their behaviour in experimental carcinogenicity and genotoxicity studies which correlate with these groupings (McGregor, 1992). This represents an extension and development of an earlier analysis (Bartsch and Malaveille, 1989) based upon the extent of testing, rather than assay sensitivity. Carcinogenic potency information was derived from the Carcinogenic Potency Database (CPDB) (Gold *et al.*, 1984, 1986, 1987, 1989b) and expressed as TD_{50} values—i.e. the chronic dose rate, in mg per kg body weight per day, which would give half of the animals tumours within some standard experiment time, the 'standard life-span', for the species (Peto *et al.*, 1984).

The information relating to genotoxicity was very heterogeneous, so it was categorized as briefly described in Figure 2 (full details in McGregor, 1992). The genotoxicity categories D → A represent groups of assays for which there is a perceived increase in specificity for the prediction of what are currently operationally defined as carcinogens; assay sensitivity decreases in the same direction.

Most of these chemicals fall into the genotoxicity groups A and B—i.e. they are active in those assays which are less sensitive for mutagenicity, UDS induction and/or clastogenicity. All of the Group 1 rodent carcinogens considered were in these genotoxicity groups and, where data existed, 85 per cent of Group 2A, 74 per cent of Group 2B and 59 per cent of Group 3 chemicals. This trend, however, was insufficient to permit these *particular* genotoxicity groupings to form a sound basis for any simple evaluation for man of

rodent carcinogenicity data. Furthermore, there did not appear to be any powerful linkage between carcinogenic potency in rodents and genotoxicity: the most potent carcinogen in both rat and mouse (TCDD) was apparently non-genotoxic, while the least potent rat carcinogen (phenacetin) was mutagenic in the *Salmonella* assay. Nevertheless, it was notable that all rat carcinogens in Groups 1 and 2A and all mouse carcinogens in Group 1 were genotoxic in *Salmonella* and/or clastogenicity assays *in vivo*. Those few Group 2B carcinogens with TD_{50} values of about 1 mg kg^{-1} day^{-1} also were genotoxic agents in categories A and B (apart from TCDD). Agents placed in genotoxicity categories C and D tended to be carcinogens with TD_{50} values higher than approximately 2 mg kg^{-1} day^{-1}.

Transgenic Animals in Carcinogenicity Testing

Advances in molecular biology in recent years have opened up the possibility of approaches to carcinogenicity testing different from the more traditional approaches. It is now possible to transfer new or altered genes to the germ-line of mammals. These transgenic animals can then be used in short-term *in vivo* tests for carcinogenicity and may be useful for research into the characterization of critical, genotoxic events in carcinogenesis. Transgenes used so far are hepatitis B viral fragments, *pim*-1, viral-H-*ras*, c-H-*ras*, c-*myc* and c-*neu* (Table 4). Animals carrying genes commonly involved in human tumours (e.g. *ras*, *myc*, p53) may prove to be particularly valuable in carcinogen research, but it is too early to make

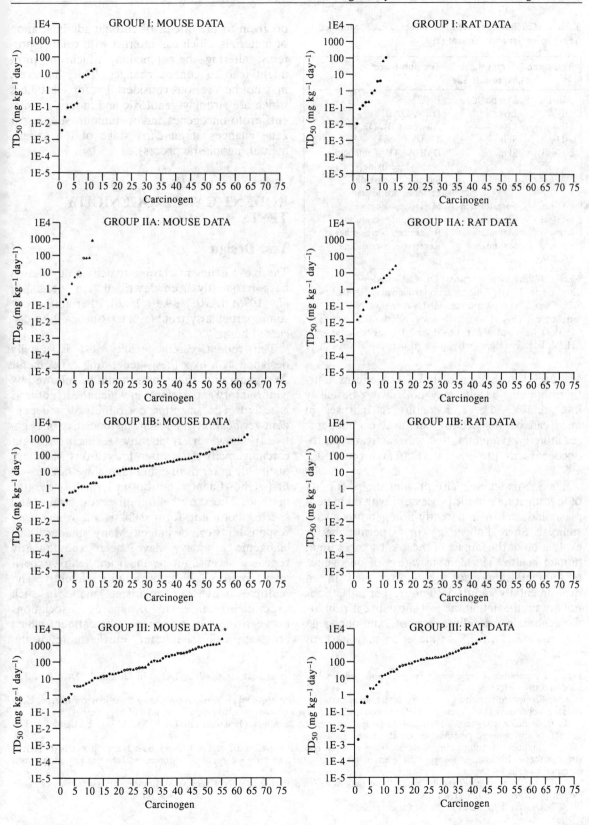

Table 4 Carcinogens tested in transgenic mice. Modified from Griesemer and Tennant (1992)

Transgene	Target tissue expression site	Test substance[a]
pim-1	Lymphoid	ENU
HBV[b]	Liver	DEN, DAB
HBV[c]	Liver	Aflatoxin B$_1$, DEN
v-H-*ras*	Skin	TPA
c-H-*ras*	Skin	DMBA, TPA, teleocidin, benzoyl peroxide, butanone peroxide, acetone, acetic acid
c-H-*ras*	Forestomach	MNU
v-H-*ras*	Mammary	Reserpine, *p*-cresidine
c-myc	Mammary	Reserpine, *p*-cresidine
c-neu	Mammary	Reserpine, *p*-cresidine
H2-K-*fos*	Skin	

[a] ENU, *N*-ethyl-*N*-nitrosourea; DEN, *N*-ethyl-*N*-nitrosamine; DAB, dimethylaminoazobenzene; DMBA, 7,12-dimethylbenzanthracene; MNU, *N*-methyl-*N*-nitrosourea; TPA, 12-*o*-tetradecanoyl-phorbol-13-acetate.
[b] HBV, a fragment of hepatitis B virus lacking the core gene.
[c] HBV, large envelope polypeptide of hepatitis B virus.

any useful evaluation of these procedures. Furthermore, the results may not always be easily interpretable—e.g. endogenous retroviruses in mice can be induced by chemical carcinogens, resulting in viraemia that can activate proto-oncogenes by proviral insertion (Warren *et al.*, 1987).

Transgenic animals also present the possibility of investigating genetic processes involved in neoplasia induced by apparently non-genotoxic substances. Such knowledge may permit better evaluation of the impact of these substances upon human health. The demonstration of oncogenes or tumour suppressor genes expressed in an experimentally induced tumour, perhaps, does not always mean that the test substance is primarily genotoxic (see discussion of late oncogene expression, p. 895). Consideration may have to be given to the effects of chronic administration of materials which can interact with cellular proteins, altering their function, which, in turn, might lead to genetic changes. This, however, may not be a serious consideration for substances which are strongly genotoxic and induce consistent proto-oncogene and/or tumour suppressor gene changes at an early stage of the experimental, neoplastic process.

RODENT CARCINOGENICITY TESTS

Test Design

The basic issues in chronic toxicity study design have frequently been described (e.g. Sontag *et al.*, 1976; IARC, 1980, 1986); therefore, only some particularly troublesome issues will be discussed here.

The rodent carcinogenicity test is usually designed as a hypothesis-generating experiment. As a generality, these tests should be followed by confirmatory experiments in which the hypothesis is tested. The scientific desirability of independent verification of a result, be it positive or negative, is, however, frequently lacking from these carcinogenicity data, often for reasons which are justifiable in terms of either animal welfare or—at first sight—finance, but not in terms of scientific method. The use of different sexes, strains and species does not form a basis on which data responsibility can be judged. Many 'standard' carcinogenicity assays have been subsequently repeated because the results from the first experiment could not be interpreted confidently. The multiple pairwise comparisons made in such experiments can result in apparent associations between tumour incidence and treatment which are statistically significant. Furthermore, if the

Figure 2 (opposite) Carcinogenic potency and genotoxicity of chemicals classified by IARC in Groups 1, 2A, 2B and 3. Modified from McGregor (1992).

●, A. Significant responses in: *in vivo* mammalian assays for chromosomal aberrations (including bone marrow micronucleus tests); unscheduled DNA synthesis (UDS) assays, either *in vivo* or *in vitro* with primary cultures of hepatocytes.

▲, B. Significant responses in: mutation assays using either *Salmonella typhimurium* TA1535, TA1537, TA1538, TA98 or TA100, or any cultured mammalian cell at the *hprt* locus.

○, C. Significant responses in: mutation assays using *S. typhimurium* TA102 or TA104, or mouse lymphoma cells (*tk* locus); sister chromatid exchange assays with mammalian cells either *in vitro* or *in vivo*; chromosomal aberration assays with mammalian cells *in vitro*.

△, D. No significant responses. Since there may have been testing in only a very small number of assays, this category cannot be clearly distinguished from the next one.

▽, N.D.—no data found in the two sources used.

investigators choose to analyse only the increases in tumour incidence, then any random nature of such associations is masked and it becomes more difficult to override them with other considerations.

Moderate control tumour incidences (e.g. 15–25 per cent) can allow the statistically significant demonstration of both increases and decreases in tumour incidence. Partly because of prejudice, the presence of a decrease in tumour incidence (which occurs in many experiments) has often been viewed as an interpretative problem, whereas an increase can be more readily attributed to the action of the chemical under test.

If, however, in control group animals site- or tissue-specific tumour incidences are low, then only increases in tumour incidence are likely to reach statistical significance, while if they are very high, then only significant decreases can be expected. In the latter case the animal strain would probably be considered as inappropriate for this kind of experiment.

The currently accepted design for carcinogenicity testing is for rats and mice to be exposed for at least 2 years. Rarely is any other species used. For each species, 50 M + 50 F per group are dosed with a vehicle or the test agent in that vehicle. Daily observations are made, and if animals become moribund during the experiment, then they are killed so that their tissues are not lost through autolysis. All animals are subjected to autopsy and almost 40 different tissues are taken from each animal for histological examination. All observations are recorded, summarized and analysed.

The objective is to expose a statistically acceptable number of animals to the highest dose that they will tolerate without reducing their life-span for reasons other than tumour development. A series of preliminary toxicity tests is conducted, beginning with either an LD_{50} determination or, preferably, a rising dose tolerance study. This initial study is followed by a 2 week and then a longer (4 or 13 week) toxicity study, the purpose of which is to identify a minimally toxic dose, as manifested by reduced body weight gain, reduced food intake, altered appearance or altered behaviour patterns, and non-neoplastic histology observed at the end of the experiment. This is the so-called maximum tolerated dose (MTD) determination.

Maximum Tolerated Dose

There seems to be general agreement that this measurement is necessary, but there are differences over its definition or what should be done with it. Twenty-seven different guidelines were described by the International Life Sciences Institute for the selection of doses in chronic toxicity/carcinogenicity studies (ILSI, 1984). Among these, the most commonly used definition is that adopted by the US National Cancer Institute (Sontag *et al.*, 1976) and the US National Toxicology Program. This states: 'The MTD is defined as the highest dose that can be predicted not to alter the animals' normal longevity from effects other than carcinogenicity.' In practical terms, the MTD is the dose which, in the three-month study, 'causes no more than a 10% weight decrement, as compared to the appropriate control groups, and does not produce mortality, clinical signs of toxicity, or pathological lesions (other than those that may be related to a neoplastic response) that would be predicted to shorten an animal's natural life span'. Ideally, this is precisely what should happen in the carcinogenicity test, but in reality the prediction of the MTD made on the evidence of sequential toxicity studies may be incorrect. In the carcinogenicity test, animals may die too early, thereby invalidating the study, or the predicted toxicity may not be realized, which invites the criticism that higher dose levels could have been used.

Other considerations in establishing the MTD value are metabolism and pharmacokinetics. Disproportionate changes in these parameters with increasing dose may signal saturation of metabolic pathways that are dominant at lower—and, therefore, more probably encountered—human dose levels.

It has been proposed, however, that metabolic and pharmacokinetic considerations should not be used to establish the MTD, but only to determine a lower dose level (IARC, 1980, 1986). The use of inappropriate metabolism for reducing the importance of a carcinogenic response has been criticized (Haseman, 1985) on the grounds that it is up to the protagonists of this opinion to demonstrate '. . . explicitly how this overload produced carcinogenic effects'. It is indeed necessary to have a sound basis for introducing the argument of inappropriate metabolism and it would be preferable for this inappropriateness to be demonstrated in advance of the carcinogenic experiment; but the mechanism leading to a carcinogenic response is not known for any chemical at any dose level. It would seem to be sufficient to demonstrate a plausible metabolic overload mechanism supported by a reasonable amount of data.

Discussion of the MTD is important because it is clearly needed for the demonstration of a carcinogenic response in many instances. In the US National Toxicology Program (NTP) feeding studies (1979–1983), 62 per cent (8/13) chemicals were judged to be carcinogenic on the basis of effects observed only at the MTD; at $0.5 \times$ MTD no carcinogenic effects occurred (Haseman, 1985). The basic problem is that the rodent carcinogenicity bioassay as currently conducted is insensitive: in relation to human populations, the numbers of rodents exposed are exceedingly low. Hence, it is readily conceded that some means must be used to compensate for the low statistical power inherent in the assay and that the use of high dose levels may be one device with which to achieve this end. At the same time, however, the use of such high dose levels does raise legitimate concerns regarding the mechanisms and relevance of carcinogenesis in these experiments.

It appears that the MTD is not required to demonstrate the carcinogenicity in rodent studies of those compounds known to be human carcinogens. Apostolou (1990) listed the appropriate rodent carcinogenicity data and doses for 13 human carcinogens to demonstrate that the lowest observed effective doses ranged from $0.005 \times$ MTD to $0.5 \times$ MTD. Since, in many cases, the MTD was not known but was assumed to be the highest tested dose, the real MTD fractions may be even lower than these estimated fractions in some cases. A conclusion one may reach from these data is that a carcinogen of potency sufficient to allow its detection at $<0.5 \times$ MTD in rodent tests is required before the relatively insensitive epidemiological methods permit detection in human populations. It would be wrong to conclude, however, that a substance showing a carcinogenic effect only at the MTD in the standard bioassay is not a human carcinogen. All that can be said of these compounds is that they may not be recognizable human carcinogens, and this question must remain open unless we can demonstrate that the mechanism of tumour induction is dependent upon the minimally toxic effect.

Pathology

The primary information for carcinogenicity evaluation is generated by pathologists. These professionals, like any other group of professionals, vary in their training and experience, and these are characteristics which may influence the evaluation in a number of ways. Some of these are listed below.

(1) Differences in terminology may be important when considering controversial lesions.

(2) Lack of consistency throughout a study is likely when a pathologist has only recently become involved with rodent carcinogenicity tests. Training is usually in a clinical situation, where each animal is unique and there is not the same need for consistency as there is in a rodent carcinogenicity study consisting of 500 animals.

(3) Unfamiliarity with the observed lesion in that particular species may cause problems in interpretation.

There is often, among non-pathologists, a suspicion that pathology is highly subjective and that pathologists are uncertain of their own discipline, as shown, for example, by a great reluctance on their part to evaluate tissues without prior knowledge of the treatment. Such criticism is unfair and, indeed, demonstrates a lack of understanding of biology in general and pathology in particular. Certainly, there is the possibility that treated animals might be examined more thoroughly than the controls and that knowledge of treatment of the animal might influence the terminology used to diagnose a lesion. But randomized, 'blind' slide reading is not the solution in the initial, routine evaluation of histological slides. If slide reading were 'blind', then there would be a loss of information about the controls, particularly in long-term studies, where many lesions in senile animals will be found. The other, sometimes stated, objection to 'blind' slide reading—that autopsy data are also important in diagnosis—is correct, but can be overcome through suitable coding of the information.

Possible bias introduced by knowledge of the treatment can be corrected in several ways, but the use of a two-stage process would seem to be most efficient:

(1) An initial evaluation is performed with full knowledge of the animal's history, including treatment.

(2) A second evaluation of specific lesions is then carried out. This should be done blind, either by the same pathologist or, preferably, by the same and a second pathologist.

Differences in evaluation between pathologists should always be discussed by them to resolve these differences; they may be due to subtle differences in diagnosis and do not indicate incompetence in one of the pathologists. It is quite unacceptable for a study sponsor to shop around until he finds a pathologist who gives—for whatever reason—the result he is looking for without giving an opportunity for interaction with all of the other evaluators. Sometimes these diagnoses are given years apart, during which time understanding of the pathogenesis of lesions may change, and even the first pathologist may not arrive at the same conclusion as he did some years ago.

Evaluation of the data is not purely a statistical exercise. A number of important factors should be considered, as follows: (1) dose–effect relationship; (2) a shift towards more anaplastic tumours in organs where tumours are common; (3) earlier appearance of tumours; (4) presence of preneoplastic lesions.

The language used to describe the carcinogenic response has masked its complexity and presents a stumbling block to its understanding among non-histopathologists. Benign or malignant neoplasms do not arise without some precursor change within normal tissue. An important concept in carcinogenicity evaluation is that of neoplastic progression, which was derived from studies on skin tumours (Berenblum and Shubik, 1947) and expanded to a number of other tissues (Foulds, 1969, 1975). There is, on many occasions, a far from clear distinction between normal and hyperplastic tissue, between hyperplastic and 'benign' neoplasia and between benign and malignant neoplasia.

Hyperplasia and benign and malignant neoplasia are convenient medical terms with prognostic significance. Hyperplasia can occur either as a regenerative response to injury, with no neoplastic connotations, or as a sustained response to a carcinogenic agent. It is an increase in the number of normal cells retaining normal intercellular relationships within a tissue. This normality may break down, resulting in altered growth patterns and altered cellular differentiation—a condition which may be described as atypical hyperplasia

or presumptively as preneoplastic lesions. There are four sequelae of hyperplasia: (1) persistence without qualitative change in either structure or behaviour; (2) permanent regression; (3) regression, with later reappearance; (4) progression to develop new characteristics indicating increased probability of malignancy. The last of these is the least likely to occur in experimental multistage models, such as in mouse skin or rat liver, where large numbers of hyperplastic lesions may occur, but notably fewer carcinomas develop from them.

Benign neoplasms in most rodent tissues apparently arise in hyperplastic foci—e.g. squamous cell papillomas of the skin and forestomach. Furthermore, these papillomas seldom demonstrate autonomous growth and even fewer progress to squamous cell carcinoma (Burns *et al.*, 1976; Colburn, 1980). This decisive progression to carcinoma, when it occurs, provides powerful evidence for the multistage theory of carcinogenesis: the new, malignant cells arising as a focus within the papilloma or even in an area of hyperplasia, since the papilloma is not a necessary intermediate stage. In other organs benign neoplasia is usually characterized by well-differentiated cell morphology, a fairly uniform growth pattern, clear demarcation from surrounding tissues and no evidence of invasion. The progression towards malignancy involves anaplasia (loss of differentiation) and pleomorphism (variety of phenotypic characteristics within the neoplasm). These changes may be focal in an otherwise benign neoplasm and may vary in degree and extent. Evidence of invasion of the surrounding tissues or of metastasis are not essential characteristics of malignancy, although their presence strengthens the diagnosis.

Grouping of Tumours for Analysis

The grouping together of certain tumour types can be an asset to statistical analysis, but it must be done carefully, with full appreciation of the biology and whatever is known of the pathogenesis of the lesions. Grouping for analysis of all animals showing neoplasia, irrespective of the tumour type, is inappropriate because the incidence in most treatment control groups can be very high and, in US National Toxicology Program studies, approaches 100 per cent in rats and 50–70 per cent in mice (Table 5).

Table 5 Tumour-bearing animals in control groups from rodent studies. Haseman, unpublished summary of US NTP data

Control animals for 2 year NTP bioassay	No. of animals	% with tumours		
		Malignant	Benign	Total
B6C3F1 mice				
male	1692	42	35	64
female	1689	45	33	64
F344 rats				
male	1596	55	95	98
female	1643	38	76	88
Osborne–Mendel rats				
male	50	26	68	78
female	50	12	80	88
Sprague–Dawley rats				
male	56	9	36	39
female	56	30	68	79

There may be similar high incidences of tumours in ageing people, but the real prevalence of tumours in human populations is uncertain. In the USA, where autopsies are uncommon, over one-third reveal previously undiagnosed cancers when they are conducted (Silverberg, 1984). A single type of neoplasm, renal adenoma, is present in 15–20 per cent of all adult kidneys (Holm-Nielsen and Olsen, 1988), although it is unclear whether these 2–6 mm foci of proliferating tubular and papillary epithelium represent small carcinomas or benign precursors of renal cell carcinomas. Irrespective of the significance of these lesions in human pathology, the presence of similar foci in a rodent carcinogenicity experiment would trigger the recording of renal tumour-bearing animals and, hence, their consideration in the statistical and pathological evaluation processes.

The independent analysis of every different diagnosis in rodent studies would also mask significant effects in many cases, while enhancing them in others. Benign and malignant neoplasms of a particular histogenesis are often grouped because the one is seen as a progression from the other. However, this grouping may result in a non-significant difference from the controls because there has been an acceleration of progression towards malignancy, the incidence of benign neoplasms decreasing while the malignant neoplasms increase. Guidelines are available for 'lumping' or 'splitting' tumour types (McConnell et al., 1988), but in using them the basis for the classification of neoplastic lesions should be clarified, especially when data generated over several or many years are being coupled, since diagnostic

criteria and ideas regarding tumour histogenesis may have changed. Reliance on tabulated results alone can lead to serious misinterpretation by those not closely connected with a particular study. For this very important reason, the pathology and toxicology narrative should be full and clear. If it is not, then there will always be doubts about future interpretations, even if these doubts are not, in reality, justified.

Historical Controls

The use of historical control data, to either support or refute an apparent treatment-related response, assumes that there is a greater stability in the accumulated data variation than in the much smaller concurrent control group and that the experiments performed over a period (perhaps several years) were done under identical conditions with animal stocks which did not vary. If these conditions were to be met, then the larger historical control group would provide a basis for increasing the power of the assay. When a higher incidence of a tumour that is rarely seen in untreated controls (e.g. brain tumours in rats) is found in treated animals, or when an unusually low incidence of a tumour type that normally has a variable and often high incidence is found in controls with respect to treated animals (e.g. mammary tumours in rats), a comparison with historical control data may provide a clearer insight into the possible biological significance of the finding.

Various factors can influence the incidence of spontaneous tumours in rodents (van Zwieten *et al.*, 1988), but it is clear that flaws in the randomization process are not commonly considered. An unexpected incidence of tumours in a control group might suggest some bias in the distribution of the animals to their groups at the beginning of the experiment. If such bias had been properly eliminated, then the unexpected incidence should also have occurred in the treated groups. The absence from the treated group of an anomalous low incidence indicates a treatment effect. Thus, a high tumour incidence in a treatment group claimed to be within the historical control range and therefore not attributable to treatment only indicates that, in the absence of randomization bias, if the control group tumour incidence had been in the expected range, then the treatment group incidence would have been even higher. However, it is probable that, in most situations, it cannot be assumed that conditions have remained constant over years and it cannot be assumed that animal stocks have not changed with time.

Outbred strains, such as Sprague–Dawley (SD) and Wistar rats, are genetically variable. The strain characteristics vary both with time and with the colony from which they are derived. MacKenzie and Garner (1973) showed how SD rats from different suppliers differed substantially in their incidence of spontaneous neoplasms. It has also been shown that Wistar rats from four colonies exhibit substantial genetic differences (Yamada *et al.*, 1979) and there appears to be considerable overlap in the genetic characteristics of SD and Wistar rat strains, which cannot be reliably distinguished from each other. A further important characteristic of Wistar rats is that the degree of heterozygosity (a measure of inbreeding) varied in the Yamada *et al.* (1979) investigation from 0 per cent (i.e. this supply of 'outbred' Wistars was fully inbred) to 38 per cent. Thus, at most, the outbred strain had only one-third of the heterozygosity that was expected of a fully outbred population and the variability in this value would, in most cases, be unknown because it is not normally checked.

The arguments for the use of outbred as opposed to inbred stocks for certain types of study are twofold (Gill, 1980): (1) they serve as better models for human populations, which are heterogeneous; (2) heterogeneity is particularly useful for first-level screening.

Both proffered reasons, however, are similar and refutable by the same argument. An experiment, with outbred animals, that would truly mimic a human population, would require very large numbers. Because only a portion of the exposed animal population might be responsive, the sensitivity of the assay performed could be low unless this factor was incorporated into the design. However, since the heterozygosity of so-called outbred strains is both low and variable, the modelling objective is confounded from the start. While it is not the only outcome, one important result from the use of outbred animals is that a biological unknown factor is introduced which can lead to difficulties in reproducing an effect with the 'same' outbred strain, adding to confusion in the literature, and the total unreliability of carefully accumulated historical control data to which reference can be made with well-recognized statistical methods.

Many of these problems should be overcome, theoretically, by the use of isogenic strains. Where these are used and—an important caveat—the environmental conditions have been constant and well-controlled, historical control data may be useful, particularly in the assessment of rare events, such as the occurrence of uncommon neoplasms. Isogenic strains are the result of brother × sister mating for >20 generations and F_1 hybrids between such strains. No strain can become fully inbred, but for all practical purposes they can be considered as a stock of genetically identical individuals which can be characterized and, within similar environmental conditions, they can be expected to exhibit the same phenotype over time and in different laboratories (Festing, 1990). However, in spite of the expected lower variance in isogenic strains, when tumour incidence is considered the results are disappointing; there are substantial differences in the experiences of laboratories using F344 rats (Tarone *et al.*, 1981; Table 6).

The reliability of the historical data is increased when variables are minimized by considering experiments in the same laboratory, with the same strain of animals from the same source and kept under the same husbandry conditions, and where the pathology is evaluated by the same pathologist. Peer review can aid pathology evaluation when different pathologists have been involved in the studies. Also, reliability increases when the data are derived from studies temporally close (e.g. 3–5 years) to the study in question. Even when historical control tumour data

Table 6 Variability in tumour incidence in F344 rats in 6 laboratories. From Tarone *et al.* (1981)

Tumour type or site	Sex	% of tumours in rats at different laboratories						All laboratories
		1 (*n*=8)	2 (*n*=7)	3 (*n*=8)	4 (*n*=22)	5 (*n*=11)	6 (*n*=16)	
Pituitary	M	18*	17*	30	31	13*	7	20*
		7–34	0–29	22–40	10–65	0–33	0–21	
Adrenal phaeochromocytoma	M	14	16	5	11	9	8	11*
		6–26	13–21	0–12	0–30	0–21	0–20	
Mammary fibroadenoma	F	22	24	9	17	6	11	15*
		12–32	8–38	4–20	5–30	0–15	0–20	
Endometrial stromal polyp	F	15*	25	18	12*	10*	10*	15*
		4–31	10–33	8–38	0–30	0–30	0–30	

* Significant heterogeneity. $P < 0.05$.

are peer-reviewed and re-examined with uniform and currently acceptable criteria applied, differences in the incidences of certain tumours do occur with time (van Zwieten *et al.*, 1988). These authors also point out that the incidence of non-neoplastic changes in shorter studies (e.g. 13 weeks) also varies. In general, the best controls are those concurrent with treatment; resorting to historical controls should be done with great caution and only to support an apparent effect, not to refute one.

Evaluation of High-dose Effects

Given at a sufficiently high dose level, any chemical will induce biological damage. This is an understanding in toxicology that is beyond dispute. This position has been tentatively advanced a step further by several people in recent years as a result of the examination of carcinogenicity data from tests conducted at the MTD. It has given rise to the notion that carcinogens might be recognizable by their systemic toxicity, although there is not necessarily a causal connection. The possibly tautologous nature of the correlation has been discussed in the literature (Bernstein *et al.*, 1985; Crouch *et al.*, 1987) and the experimental evidence for the hypothesis is restricted to a small number of chemicals. Thus, among 99 chemicals tested for carcinogenicity and site-specific toxicity in long-term rodent studies by the NTP, only 7 of he 53 which were shown to be carcinogenic exhibited target organ toxicity that could have

been causal to the observed neoplasms (Hoel *et al.*, 1988). Nevertheless, correlations as high as 0.79 have been calculated for mouse LD_{50} and TD_{50} values† among the NCI/NTP carcinogens (Zeise *et al.*, 1986), although the correlation was reduced to 0.73 when non-NCI/NTP data were included in the analysis (Metzger *et al.*, 1989).

The effects upon the physiology of rodents of life-long exposure to doses in the neighbourhood of the MTD may be expected to be so severe that some perturbation of the ageing process incidence is inevitable (Salzburg, 1989). In the case of a pharmaceutical substance given at a dose which inhibits almost all of some particular aspect of biological activity, the animal is driven into an altered equilibrium as a consequence of the changed biochemical milieu. The toxicity engendered by such treatment may be a response to the desired, but exaggerated, pharmacology; but drugs seldom—perhaps never—have a single action and there may be substantial biological effects which were not designed into the drug. These effects will be of an unspecified nature characteristic of any chemical, and so concern regarding effects on ageing could be extended to any substance submitted to a life-span, high-dose animal experiment. Since the development of most neoplasms is age-related, tumour incidence would be one of the factors affected, the response being manifest as either an increase or a decrease in tumour yield. Among 170 NCI studies pub-

† See p. 900 for definition.

lished as of 1980, 97 per cent showed statistically significant dose-related modifications in at least one species or sex and 70 per cent of them showed statistically significant dose-related modifications of tumour patterns that involved one type of tumour increasing with dose, while another type of tumour was decreasing with dose (Salzburg, 1983). The same situation prevails with the more recent NTP data, at least up to 1986 (Salzburg, 1988). Theoretically, high-dose effects on tumour incidence need not be primarily on the organ or tissue in which the change is found, particularly if hormonal control mechanisms are involved.

In an attempt to accommodate these conflicting responses within experiments, Salzburg (1989) used principal component analysis to describe a tumour profile, which is a weighted combination of site-specific tumours; non-parametric techniques are then used to compare these tumour profile scores across groups. However, this combination technique has been criticized by Haseman (1990) for having no biological significance and for being misapplied to experiments in which the resulting differences in tumour profiles were due to survival differences and data coding errors. Nevertheless, the problem of increases and decreases in the incidence of different tumour types is one which must be faced and not simply brushed aside.

Identification of Non-carcinogens

Since the proof of a negative statement is philosophically impossible, then the identification of chemicals which can be said to have no carcinogenic potential also is impossible. The most that can be said regarding carcinogenic inactivity is that activity has not been demonstrated within the operational definition that has been selected. This operational definition includes a testing programme restricted to rodents and a statistical power which varies from experiment to experiment according to the numbers of animals at risk in control and treatment groups from particular tumour types. While rejection of the null hypothesis is always presented in reports, the power of the experiment to demonstrate its rejection is seldom, if ever, presented when no significant treatment effect has been shown. This is not identical with asserting that all chemicals are carcinogens, although this also may be correct, provided that the circumstances in which carcinogen-

icity becomes recognizable can be defined. This kind of reasoning may lead one to conclude that there is no strict dividing line separating carcinogens from non-carcinogens and that epidemiological or laboratory studies of a particular power may fail to demonstrate an effect, whereas a higher-power study may do so.

There is a very high prevalence of carcinogens described in the open literature today, in contrast with the situation to be found 20 years ago. Gold *et al.* (1989a) reported a prevalence of 51 per cent among 955 chemicals tested and entered to the Carcinogen Potency Database (CPDB). This included the NCI/NTP data, where the prevalence was 48 per cent among 251 chemicals (currently the prevalence is 54 per cent among 301 chemicals). Yet, in 1969, Innes *et al.* reported their results with 120 chemicals, largely pesticides and industrial chemicals, in which the prevalence of carcinogens was only 9 per cent. It is plausible that the 9 per cent prevalence of carcinogens in the Innes *et al.* (1969) study is partially due to low statistical power, low doses and short observation time.

CARCINOGENIC RISK ASSESSMENT

Assessment of carcinogenic risk involves a number of steps: (1) hazard identification; (2) mechanism elucidation; (3) quantification of risk based upon the mechanism.

If, as has been suggested, all substances are hazardous, then the methods used for what we refer to as 'hazard identification' are, in fact, telling us something about the potency of the chemical. With all its difficulties, the 'hazard identification' process remains the easiest part of the process leading to quantitative risk assessment. Mechanism of action is the next, extremely important undertaking, and must involve a broad range of disciplines, including pathologists, toxicologists, metabolic chemists, pharmacokinetic specialists and molecular biologists. Mechanistic studies have always been interesting, but they have now achieved a very high level of importance in the evaluation of the toxicology of a compound. Today it would be difficult to overestimate their importance. There are few general principles which can be applied to understanding mechanisms of action, each carcinogenic entity being studied on a case-by-case basis, although genetic toxicity has been a high-profile consideration in most mechanistic studies. Nevertheless, each chemical structure is unique and it is a serious error to attempt to group chemicals—without experimental evidence—on the basis of either their structural similarities, or similarities in their effects. Chemicals sharing particular active groups can have very different effects and particular effects may be achieved by different mechanisms.

Quantification of risk is the ultimate step, although investigators in this field do not pretend that a solution to the problem is at hand. The best that they can offer at the moment are mathematical models which fit the observed data and may have a foundation in biology.

ACKNOWLEDGEMENTS

I am indebted to Drs J. R. P. Cabral, H. Vainio and H. Yamasaki, of the International Agency for Research on Cancer, for their helpful and constructive comments on this manuscript.

REFERENCES

Apostolou, A. (1990). Relevance of maximum tolerated dose to human carcinogenic risk. *Regulatory Toxicol. Pharmacol.*, **11**, 68–80

Arcos, J. C. and Argus, M. F. (1974). *Chemical Induction of Cancer*, Vols IIA and IIB. Academic Press, New York

Arcos, J. C., Argus, M. F. and Wolf, G. (1968). *Chemical Induction of Cancer*, Vol. I. Academic Press, New York

Ashby, J. (1978). Structural analysis as a means of predicting carcinogenic potential. *Br. J. Cancer* **37**, 904–923.

Ashby, J. and Tennant, R. W. (1988). Chemical structure, *Salmonella* mutagenicity and extent of carcinogenicity as indicators of genotoxic carcinogenesis among 222 chemicals tested in rodents by the U. S. NTP. *Mutation Res.*, **204**, 17–115

Ashby, J. and Tennant, R. W. (1991). Definitive relationships among chemical structure, carcinogenicity and mutagenicity for 301 chemicals tested by the U.S. NTP. *Mutation Res*, **257**, 229–308

Ashby, J. Tennant, R. W. Zeiger, E. and Stasiewicz, S. (1989). Classification according to chemical structure, mutagenicity to *Salmonella* and level of carcinogenicity of a further 42 chemicals tested for carcinogenicity by the U.S. National Toxicology Program. *Mutation Res.*, **223**, 73–103

Balmain, A. and Brown, K. (1988). Oncogene activation in chemical carcinogenesis. *Adv. Cancer Res.*, **51**, 147–182

Barbacid, M. (1987). *Ras* genes. *Ann. Rev. Biochem.*, **56**, 779–827

Bartsch, H. and Malaveille, C. (1989). Prevalance of genotoxic chemicals among animal and human carcinogens evaluated in the IARC Monograph Series. *Cell Biol. Toxicol.*, **5**, 115–127

Berenblum, I. and Shubik, P. (1947). The role of croton oil applications associated with a single painting of a carcinogen, in tumour induction in the mouse's skin. *Br. J. Cancer*, **1**, 379–383

van den Berg, S., Kaina, B., Rahmsdorf, H. J., Ponta, H. and Herrlich, P. (1991). Involvement of *fos* in spontaneous and ultraviolet light-induced genetic changes. *Mol. Carcinogen.*, **4**, 460–466

Bernstein, L., Gold, L. S., Ames, B. N., Pike M. C. and Hoel, D. G. (1985). Some tautologous aspects of the comparison of carcinogenic potency in rats and mice. *Fund. Appl. Toxicol.*, **5** 79–86

Bishop, J. M. (1987) The molecular genetics of cancer. *Science*, **235**, 305–311

Bishop, J. M. (1991). Molecular themes in oncogenesis. *Cell*, **64**, 235–248

Brash, D. E., Rudolph, J. A., Simon, J. A., Lin, A., McKenna, G. J., Baden, H. P., Halpern, A. J. and Pontén, J. (1991). A role for sunlight in skin cancer: UV-induced p53 mutations in squamous cell carcinoma. *Proc. Natl Acad. Sci. USA*, **88**, 10124–10128

Breuer, M., Wientjens, E., Verbeek, S., Slebos, R. and Berns, A. (1991). Carcinogen-induced lymphomagenesis in *pim*–1 transgenic mice: Dose dependence and involvement of *myc* and *ras*. *Cancer Res.*, **51**, 958–963

Burns, F. J., Vanderlaan, M., Snyder, E. and Albert, R. E. (1976). Induction and progression kinetics of mouse skin papillomas. In Slaga, T. J., Sivak, A. and Boutwell, R. K. (Eds), *Carcinogenesis*, Vol. 2, *Modifiers of Chemical Carcinogenesis*. Raven Press, New York, pp. 91–96

Butterworth, B. E. (1990). Consideration of both genotoxic and nongenotoxic mechanisms in predicting carcinogenic potential. *Mutation Res.*, **239**, 117–132

Colburn, N. H. (1980). Tumor promotion and preneoplastic progression. In Slaga, T. J., Sivak, A. and Boutwell, R. K. (Eds), *Carcinogenesis*, Vol. 5, *Modifiers of Chemical Carcinogenesis*. Raven Press, New York, pp. 33–56

Cowell, J. K. (1980). Consistent chromosome abnormalities associated with mouse bladder epithelial cell lines transformed *in vitro*. *J. Natl Cancer Inst.*, **65**, 955–961

Cowell, J. K. and Franks, L. M. (1984). The ability of normal mouse cells to reduce the malignant potential of transformed mouse bladder epithelial cells depends upon their somatic origin. *Int. J. Cancer*, **33**, 657–667

Craig, R. W. and Sager, R. (1985). Suppression of

tumorigenicity in hybrids of normal and oncogene-transformed CHEF cells. *Proc. Natl Acad. Sci. USA*, **82**, 2062–2066

Crouch, E., Wison, R. and Zeise, L. (1987). Tautology or not tautology? *J. Toxicol. Environ. Hlth*, **20**, 1–10

DeCaprio, J. A., Ludlow, J. W., Figge, J. Shew, J.-Y., Huang, C.-M., Lee, W.-H., Marsilio, E., Paucha, E. and Livingston, D. M. (1988). SV40 large tumor antigen forms a specific complex with the product of the retinoblastoma susceptibility gene. *Cell*, **54**, 275–283

Der, C. J., Krontiris, T. G. and Cooper, G. M. (1982). Transforming genes of the human bladder and lung carcinoma cell lines are homologous to the *ras* genes of Harvey and Kirsten sarcoma viruses. *Proc. Natl Acad. Sci. USA*, **79**, 3637–3640

Dyson, N., Howley, P. M., Munger, K. and Harlow, E. (1989). The human papilloma virus–16 E7 oncoprotein is able to bind to the retinoblastoma gene product. *Science*, **243**, 934–936

Enslein, K., Borgstedt, H. H., Tomb, M. E., Blake, B. W. and Hart, J. B. (1987). A structure-activity prediction model of carcinogenicity based on NCI/NTP assays and food additives. *Toxicol. Industr. Hlth*, **3**, 267–287

Evans, E. P., Burstenshaw, M. D., Brown, B. B., Hennion, R. and Harris, H. (1982). The analysis of malignancy by cell fusion. IX. Re-examination and clarification of the cytogenetic problem. *J. Cell Sci.*, **56**, 113–130

Festing, M. F. W. (1990). Use of genetically heterogeneous rats and mice in toxicological research: A personal perspective. *Toxicol. Appl. Pharmacol.*, **102**, 197–204

Foulds, L. (1969). *Neoplastic Development*, Vol. 1. Academic Press, New York

Foulds, L. (1975). *Neoplastic Development*, Vol. 2. Academic Press, New York

Free, S. M. and Wilson, J. W. (1964). A mathematical contribution to structure-activity studies. *J. Med. Chem.*, **7**, 395–399

Gill, T. J. III (1980). The use of randomly bred and genetically defined animals in biomedical research. *Am. J. Pathol.*, **101**, S22-S32

Gold, L. S., Bernstein, L., Magaw, R. and Slone, T. H. (1989a). Interspecies extrapolation in carcinogenesis: Prediction between rats and mice. *Environ. Hlth Perspect.*, **81**, 211–219

Gold, L. S., Sawyer, C. B., Magaw, R., Backman, G. M., de Veciana, M., Levinson, R., Hooper, N. K., Havender, W. R., Bernstein, L., Peto, R., Pike, M. C. and Ames, B. N. (1984) A carcinogenic potency data-base of the standardized results of animal bioassays. *Environ. Hlth Perspect.*, **58**, 9–319

Gold, L. S., Slone, T. H., Backman, G. M., Eisenberg, S., Da Costa, M., Wong, M., Manley, N. B., Rohrbach, L. and Ames, B. N. (1989b). Third chronological supplement to the carcinogenic potency database: Standardized results of animal bioassays published through December 1986 and by the National Toxicology Program through June 1987. *Environ. Hlth Perspect.*, **84**, 215–285

Gold, L. S. Slone, T. H., Backman, G. M. Magaw, R., Da Costa, M., Lopipero, P., Blumenthal, M. and Ames, B. N. (1987). Second chronological supplement to the carcinogenic potency database: Standardized results of animal bioassays published through December 1984 and by the National Toxicology Program through May 1986. *Environ. Hlth Perspect.*, **74**, 237–329

Gold, L. S., de Veciana, M., Backman, G. M., Magaw, R. Lopipero, P., Smith, M., Blumenthal, M., Levinson, R., Bernstein, L. and Ames, B. N. (1986). Chronological supplement to the carcinogen potency database standardized results of animal bioassays published through December 1982. *Environ. Hlth Perspect.*, **67**, 161–200

Griesemer, R. and Tennant, R. (1992). Transgenic mice in carcinogenicity testing. In Vainio, H., Magee, P., McGregor, D. and McMichael, A. (Eds), *Mechanisms of Carcinogenesis in Risk Identification*. IARC Scientific Publications No. 116. IARC, Lyon, pp. 429–436

Harris, H., Miller, O. J., Klein, G., Worst, P. and Tachibana, T. (1969). Suppression of malignancy by cell fusion. *Nature* **223**, 363–368

Haseman, J. F. (1985). Issues in carcinogenicity testing: Dose selection. *Fund. Appl. Toxicol.*, **5**, 66–78

Haseman, J. K. (1990). Use of statistical decision rules for evaluating laboratory animal carcinogenicity studies. *Fund. Appl. Toxicol.*, **14**, 637–648

Hoel, D. G., Haseman, J. K., Hogan, M. D., Huff, J. and McConnell, E. E. (1988). The impact of toxicity on carcinogenicity studies: implications for risk assessment. *Carcinogenesis*, **9**, 2045–2052

Hollstein, M., Sidransky, D., Vogelstein, B. and Harris, C. C. (1991). p53 Mutations in human cancers. *Science*, **253**, 49–53

Holm-Nielsen, P. and Olsen, T. S. (1988). Ultrastructure of renal adenoma. *Ultrastruct. Pathol.*, **12**, 27–39

Hunter, T. (1991). Cooperation between oncogenes. *Cell*, **64**, 249–270

Innes, J. R. M., Ulland, B. M., Valerio, M. G., Petrucelli, L., Fishbein, L., Hart, E. R., Pallota, A..J., Bates, R. R., Falk, H. L., Gart, J. J., Mlein, M., Mitchell, I. and Peters, J. (1969). Bioassay of pesticides and industrial chemicals for tumorigenicity in mice: A preliminary note. *J. Natl Cancer Inst*, **42**, 1101–1114

International Agency for Research on Cancer (IARC) (1980). Long-term and short-term screening assays for carcinogens: A critical appraisal. *IARC Monogr. Eval. Carcinogen. Risk Chem. Man Suppl.*, **2**, 21–83

International Agency for Research on Cancer (IARC) (1986). *Long-term and short-term assays for carcinogens: A critical appraisal.* IARC Scientific Publications No.83, pp. 15–83

International Life Sciences Institute (ILSI) (1984). The

selection of doses in chronic toxicity/carcinogenicity studies. In Grice, H. C. (Ed.), *Current Issues in Toxicology*. Springer-Verlag, New York, pp. 9–49

Kier, L. B. and Hall, L. H. (1976). Molecular connectivity in chemistry and drug research. *Medical Chemistry*, Vol. 14, Academic Press, New York, pp. 1–257

Klinger, H. P. and Shows, T. B. (1983). Suppression of tumorigenicity in somatic cell hybrids. II. Human chromosomes implicated as suppressors of tumorigenicity in hybrids with Chinese hamster ovary cells. *J. Natl Cancer Inst.*, **71**, 559–569

Klopman, G. (1984). Artificial intelligence approach to structure-activity studies. Computer-automated structure evaluation of biological activity of organic molecules. *J. Am. Chem. Soc.*, **106**, 7315–7321

McConnell, E. E., Solleeld, H. A., Swenberg, J. A. and Boorman, G. A. (1988). Guidelines for combining neoplasms for evaluation of rodent carcinogenesis studies. In Grice, H. C. and Ciminera, J. L. (Eds), *Carcinogenicity*. Springer-Verlag, New York, pp. 183–196

McGregor, D. (1989). Comments on the proposed use of *Salmonella* and structural alerts for the prediction of rodent carcinogens. *Mutation Res.*, **222**, 300–306

McGregor, D. (1990). *In vitro* mammalian cell genotoxicity assays: their use and interpretation. In Mendelsohn, M. L. and Albertini, R. J. (Eds), Mutation and the Environment, Part B. Wiley-Liss, New York, pp. 159–169

McGregor, D. (1992). Chemicals classified by I.A.R.C.: their potency in rodent carcinogenicity tests and their genotoxicity and acute toxicity. In Vainio, H., Magee, P., McGregor, D. and McMichael, A. (Eds). *Mechanisms of Carcinogenesis in Risk Identification*. IARC Scientific Publications No. 116. IARC, Lyon pp. 323–352

MacKenzie, W. F. and Garner, F. M. (1973). Comparison of neoplasms in six sources of rats. *J. Natl Cancer Inst.*, **50**, 1243–1257

Marshall, C. J. (1991). Tumor suppressor genes. *Cell*, **64**, 313–326

Metzger, B., Crouch, E. and Wilson, R. (1989). On the relationship between carcinogenicity and acute toxicity. *Risk Anal.*, **9**, 169–177

Miller, J. A. and Miller, E. C. (1977). Ultimate chemical carcinogens as reactive mutagenic electrophiles. In Hiatt, H. H., Watson, J. D. and Winsten, J. A. (Eds), *Origins of Human Cancer*, Cold Spring Harbor Laboratory, pp. 605–628

Mitchell, C. D. (1991). Recessive oncogenes, antioncogenes and tumor suppression. *Br. Med. Bull.*, **47**, 136–156

Mitelman, F., Kaneko, Y. and Trent, J. M. (1990). Report of the committee on chromosome changes in neoplasia. *Cytogenet. Cell Genet.*, **55**, 358–386

Noda, M., Selinger, Z. Scolnick, E. M. and Bassin, R. H. (1983). Flat revertants isolated from Kirsten sarcoma virus-transformed cells are resistant to the action of specific oncogenes. *Proc. Natl Acad. Sci. USA*, **80**, 5602–5606

Nowell, P. C. (1991). How many human cancer genes? *J. Natl Cancer Inst.*, **83**, 1061–1064

Nowell, P. C. and Hungerford, D. A. (1960). A minute chromosome in human granulocytic leukemia. *Science*, **132**, 1497

Peto, R., Pike, M. C., Bernstein, L., Gold, L. S. and Ames, B. N. (1984). The TD$_{50}$: A proposed general convention for the numerical description of the carcinogenic potency of chemicals in chronic-exposure animal experiments. *Environ. Hlth Perspect.*, **58**, 1–8

Purchase, I. F. H., Longstaff, E., Ashby, J., Styles, J. A., Anderson, D., Lefevre, P. A. and Westwood, R. F. (1978). An evaluation of 6 short-term tests for detecting organic chemical carcinogens. *Br. J. Cancer*, **37**, 873–959

Salzburg, D. (1983). The lifetime feeding study in mice and rats—an examination of its validity as a bioassay for human carcinogens. *Fund. Appl. Toxical.*, **3**, 63–67

Salzburg, D. (1988). The aggregation of incidence data in carcinogenicity assays. In Grice, H. C. and Ciminera, J. L. (Eds), *Carcinogenicity*. Springer-Verlag, New York, pp. 197–205

Salzburg, D. (1989). Does everything 'cause' cancer: An alternative interpretation of the 'carcinogenesis' bioassay. *Fund. Appl. Toxicol.*, **13**, 351–358

Shih, C., Padhy, L. C., Murray, M. and Weinberg, R. A. (1981). Transforming genes of carcinomas and neuroblastomas introduced into mouse fibroblasts. *Nature*, **290**, 261–264

Silverberg, S. G. (1984). The autopsy and cancer. *Arch. Pathol. Lab. Med.*, **108**, 476–478

Slamon, D.-J., De Kernion, J. B., Verma, I. M. and Cline, M. J. (1984). Expression of oncogenes in human malignancies. *Science*, **224**, 256–262

Solomon, E., Borrow, J. and Goddard, A. D. (1991). Chromosome aberrations and cancer. *Science*, **254**, 1153–1160

Sontag, J. M., Page, N. P. and Saffiotti, U. (1976). *Guidelines for Carcinogen Bioassay in Small Rodents*. DHHS Publication (NIH) 76–801, National Cancer Institute, Bethesda, Md

Stehelin, D., Varmus, H. E., Bishop, J. M. and Vogt, P. K. (1976). DNA related to the transforming gene(s) of avian sarcoma viruses is present in normal avian DNA. *Nature*, **260**, 170–173

Stoler, A. B. (1991). Genes and cancer. *Br. Med. Bull.*, **47**, 64–75

Summerhayes, I. C. and Franks, L. M. (1979). Effects of donor age on neoplastic transformation of adult mouse bladder epithelium *in vitro*. *J. Natl Cancer Inst.*, **62**, 1017–1023

Tarone, R. E., Chu, K. C. and Ward, J. M. (1981). Variability in the rates of some common naturally occurring tumors in Fischer 344 rats and (C57BL/6N × C3H/HeN)F$_1$ (B6C3F$_1$) mice. *J. Natl Cancer Inst.*, **66**, 1175–1181

Tennant, R. W. and Ashby, J. (1991). Classification according to chemical structure, mutagenicity to *Salmonella* and level of carcinogenicity by the U.S. National Toxicology Program. *Mutation Res.*, **257**, 209–227

Tennant, R. W., Margolin, B. H., Shelby, M. D., Zeiger, E. Haseman, J. K., Spalding, J., Caspary, W. J., Resnick, M., Stasiewicz, S., Anderson, B. and Minor, B. (1987). Prediction of chemical carcinogenicity in rodents from *in vitro* genetic toxicity assays. *Science*, **236**, 933–941

Tisty, T. D. (1990). Normal diploid human and rodent cells lack a detectable frequency of gene amplification. *Proc. Natl Acad. Sci. USA*, **87**, 3132–3136

Tisty, T. D., Margolin, B. H. and Lum, K. (1989). Differences in the rates of gene amplification in non-tumorigenic and tumorigenic cell lines as measured by Luria-Delbrück fluctuation analysis. *Proc. Natl Acad. Sci. USA*, **86**, 9441–9445

Warren, W., Lawley, P. D., Gardner, E., Harris, G., Ball, J. K. and Cooper, C. S. (1987). Induction of thymomas by *N*-methyl-*N*-nitrosourea in AKR mice: interaction between the chemical carcinogen and endogenous murine leukaemia viruses. *Carcinogenesis (Lond.)*, **8**, 163–172

Whyte, P., Buchkoich, K., Horowitz, J. M., Friend, S. H., Raybuck, M., Weinberg, R. A. and Harlow, E. (1988). Association between an oncogene and an anti-oncogene: the adenovirus E1A proteins bind to the retinoblastoma gene product. *Nature*, **334**, 124–129

Whyte, P., Williamson, N. M. and Harlow, E. (1989). Cellular targets for transformation by the adenovirus E1A proteins. *Cell*, **56**, 67–75

Yamada, J., Nikaido, H. and Matsumoto, S. (1979). Genetic variability within and between outbred Wistar strains of rats. *Exptl Anim.*, **28**, 259–269

Zeiger, E., Haseman, J. K., Shelby, M. D., Margolin, B. H. and Tennant, R. W. (1990). Evaluation of four *in vitro* toxicity tests for predicting rodent carcinogenicity: confirmation of earlier results with 41 additional chemicals. *Environ. Mol. Mutagen.*, **16** (suppl.18), 1–14

Zeise, L., Crouch, E. A. C. and Wilson, R. (1986). A possible relationship between toxicity and carcinogenicity. *J. Am. Coll. Toxicol.*, **5**, 137–151

van Zweiten, M. J., Majka, J. A., Peter, C. P. and Burek, J. D. (1988). The value of historical control data. In Grice, H. C. and Ciminera, J. L. (Eds), *Carcinogenicity*. Springer-Verlag, New York, pp. 39–51

FURTHER READING

Boutwell, R. K. and Riegel, I. L. (1990). *The Cellular and Molecular Biology of Human Carcinogenesis*. Academic Press, San Diego

Dragan, Y. P., Sargent, L., Xu, Y-D, Xu, Y-H and Pitot, H. (1993). The initiation promotion-progression model of rat hepato-carcinogenesis. *Proceedings of the National Academy of Sciences* USA, **80**, 95–99

Pitot, H. C. (1993). The molecular biology of carcinogenesis. *Cancer*, **72**, 962–970

Rowland, I. R. (1991). *Nutrition, Toxicity, and Cancer*. CRC Press, Boca Raton, Florida

38 Epigenetic Carcinogenesis

C. L. Berry

INTRODUCTION

For many tumours and probably for the majority occurring in man, a heritable change in the genetic material—more generally a number of such changes—provides the fundamental alteration in cellular biology which results in the production of a neoplasm. However, it is clear that other mechanisms may produce tumours, acting either alone or in concert with genetically determined events. This process, of *epigenetic carcinogenesis*, is best considered in terms of specific examples, for generalizations are difficult in this field despite the frequency with which they are employed. Nevertheless, it is reasonable to say that in many examples of epigenetic carcinogenesis affected tissues show a sequence of changes including hypertrophy, hyperplasia, a loss of uniform response with focal hyperplasia, adenoma and adenocarcinoma. As the latter term implies, this is a sequence often but not exclusively documented in glandular tissues.

GENERAL FEATURES OF NON-GENOTOXIC CARCINOGENS

Certain general statements can be made about many non-genotoxic carcinogens. However, with what can be described as a 'mixed bag' end-point reached by many routes, there are a wide range of exceptions, some of which we shall discuss as a way of exploring the data. The general points include:

- The carcinogens are non-mutagenic—a matter of definition.
- They show no evidence of other chemical reactivity with DNA.
- There are no common factors in the structure of compounds acting in this way.
- Threshold effects in dosage are clearly evident.
- The effects of a particular compound are usually limited to one organ and/or species.

THYROID CARCINOGENESIS

Hormonal feedback loops, changes in thyroid hormone synthesis, cellular receptor activity, variation in rates of hormone release and metabolism, and direct interference with cell function may all operate to produce the sequence of growth leading to neoplasia described above in the thyroid gland. Thyroid neoplasia may develop following any stimulus which results in prolonged and excessive thyroid stimulating hormone (TSH) secretion.

Bielschowsky (1953) first reported thyroid tumours in the rat due to iodine deficency, and Axelrod and Leblond (1955) used a low-iodine diet to induce thyroid neoplasia in this animal, with the occurrence of pituitary tumours in the test animals suggesting overstimulation of that gland. Subsequent experiments produced tumours following TSH administration (Sinha *et al.*, 1965). In man excessive production of TSH occurs in chronic iodine deficiency and following subtotal thyroidectomy, and may be accompanied by neoplasia. The sequence is most clearly evident in dyshormogenetic goitres, where failure of the production of thyroxine leads to pronounced pituitary drive. Increased production of TSH due to inadequate levels of thyroid hormone production may be induced by any of the following failures of the mechanisms of normal thyroid metabolism in dyshormogenesis:

- Failure of iodine trapping.
- Peroxidase deficiency, resulting in the failure of intrathyroidal iodine binding.
- Failure of iodotyrosine coupling.
- Dehalogenase deficiency leading to failure of deiodination of iodotyrosine residues.
- Production of abnormal iodoproteins due to defects in thyroglobulin synthesis.

In this type of thyroid disease the gland may become very large and weights of several hundred grams are not uncommon. Nodules are almost invariably present, and microscopically hyperplasia, often with many cells with pleomorphic nuclei, is inevitable. It is important to note that, rather like some experimental lesions, the progression of these changes to truly malignant behaviour with metastasis is rare (Crooks *et al.*, 1963).

In animals experimental work has shown that the pattern of stimulation of the gland by TSH is also critical; both duration and continuity are important. In general, a period during which the TSH level is allowed to return to normal has a protective effect with regard to tumour production. As Williams and his group in Cardiff have shown, alterations in the normal pattern of thyroid growth occur in three phases (see Stringer *et al.*, 1985). There is initially a rapid growth phase (4–8 weeks), followed by a period in which growth is limited but where the important change of loss of normal response of thyroid follicular cells to normal growth mechanisms occurs (see below). This is followed by the appearance of multiple follicular cell proliferations (tumours).

In the initial rapid growth phase, responses begin at concentrations within the normal physiological range of TSH levels but response continues to well above this. In the plateau phase, a growth response can still be obtained to non-TSH stimuli (wounding) but the proliferative response to TSH is lost, although the functional response is preserved. These results were obtained in dissociated cells and were thus not attributable to locally acting factors dependent on tissue organization. In later work this group found that the proliferative response could be restored by the addition of insulin to the culture, which suggests that direct metabolic effects may have been acting as limiting factors—EGF (epidermal growth factor) was not effective as a growth stimulant (Smith *et al.*, 1986). However, growth desensitization in these experiments certainly appears to be associated with an altered dependence on certain growth factors.

Naturally occurring goitrogens are found in cabbage leaves, Brussels sprouts, turnips and mustard. Goitrin, the active goitrogen in turnips (L-5-vinyl-2-thiooxazoidone) is about as active as propylthiouracil (Haynes and Murad, 1985), and although TSH production may be increased after exposure to naturally occurring goitrogens, a role in thyroid carcinogenesis in man seems unlikely.

The Effects of Drugs

Nominally, it is simple to identify the steps in thyroid hormone synthesis and release and to identify the drugs likely to affect the processes involved. However, there is a need for caution, since extrinsic factors may affect target cell sensitivity and the pattern of exposure will affect the outcome dramatically. When the effects of the various factors acting on the demand for, and degradation of, thyroid hormone are added (see Figure 1), a more complex picture generally emerges *in vivo*. It is important to note, however, that the simultaneous administration of goitrogenic drugs (thiouracil—Bielschowsky, 1955; thiourea—Rosin and Ungar, 1957) and thyroid hormone has been shown to prevent the development of follicular cell neoplasia.

Some highly specific effects have been characterized. Aminoglutethimide was widely used as an anticonvulsant until reports of the development of goitre in children on the drug appeared. The drug acts directly on the thyroid cells by reducing the production of thyroxine and diiodotyrosine by inhibiting ^{125}I organification in a concentration-dependent manner, with no effect on I^- uptake by the cells. The related compounds glutethimide, nitroglutethimide and acetylaminoglutethimide had no effect, which suggests that the effect depended on a free amino group in the phenyl ring of the molecule (Brown *et al.*, 1986). The increase in thyroid gland size is thus triggered by a very clear metabolic block. With an antihistamine (SK&F 93479—see Atterwill and Brown, 1988) similar changes can be produced by a primary effect on T4 clearance, although the mechanisms of this effect—hepatocellular binding, uptake, increase in conjugation by hepatic uridine diphosphate glucuronyltransferase—are probably variable between compounds. They also differ for other thyroid active drugs which act by this general mechanism—for example, phenobarbitone (phenobarbital) (Cavalieri and Pitt-Rivers, 1981).

Of course blockage of effective thyroid function may be produced by more than one mechanism. Bromide inhibits the uptake of iodine by the thyroid gland, inhibits the oxidation of iodide to iodine and thus the incorporation of iodine into tyrosine residues, inhibits the coupling of tyrosine residues to thyronine and causes an increase of

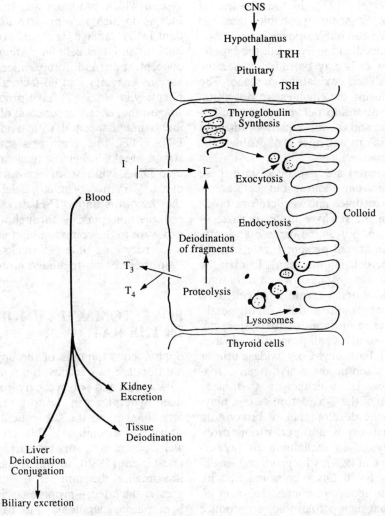

CNS

Hypothalamus

TRH

Pituitary

TSH

Thyroglobulin Synthesis

Exocytosis

I⁻ → I⁻

Blood

Colloid

Endocytosis

Deiodination of fragments

T_3

T_4

Proteolysis

Lysosomes

Thyroid cells

Kidney Excretion

Tissue Deiodination

Liver Deiodination Conjugation

Biliary excretion

Figure 1 Interactions of extracellular and cellular compartments in the synthesis, production and degradation of thyroid hormone. After Atterwill and Brown (1988) and others

NADH cytochrome *c* reductase activity (van Leeuwen *et al.*, 1988).

There is considerable public anxiety about the effects of pesticides in the food chain, and some of these compounds such as the dithiocarbamates (ethylenebisdithiocarbamates) and triazoles are goitrogeneic and carcinogenic in animals, under appropriate conditions of high and continuous dosage (O'Neil and Marshall, 1984). The food colouring erythrosine is also a thyroid carcinogen in this mode of dosing. The clear evidence of threshold effects and the large safety margin allow confident reassurance about theoretical risk in this well-understood example of carcinogenesis.

PEROXISOME PROLIFERATION AND NEOPLASIA

Peroxisomes are single-membrane-bound structures which increase in numbers dramatically in the rodent liver during exposure to certain lipid-lowering drugs and phthalate-ester plasticizers (Reddy and Lalwani, 1983). The increase in liver size accompanying this change can be directly related to increased synthesis of membranes and smooth endoplasmic reticulum, although mitochondrial volume density is not significantly altered (Reddy *et al.*, 1982). Total DNA in the liver increases in animals exposed to peroxisome proliferators over a period of days and will persist for weeks (Moody *et al.*, 1977) in the absence of hepatic necrosis. It seems probable that the increase in cell division is in response to the metabolic demands placed on the liver, but the rapidly proliferating liver cells may be more vulnerable to specifically induced (oxidative) damage. The compounds producing the changes are not mutagenic and the relationship between the proliferation of organelles and the subsequent production of liver tumours in rats and mice is of problematic significance for man.

Around 40 enzymes are associated with these organelles in different tissues, but catalase is found in all peroxisomes and is therefore taken as a 'marker'. In the rat liver urate oxidase, D-amino acid oxidase, polyamine oxidase and fatty acyl-CoA oxidase are all present (urate oxidase is not found in peroxisomes in man). In man the fatty acid ß-oxidation system of which fatty acyl-CoA oxidase is the first enzyme has been most studied in the syndrome of sudden infant death, where deficiencies in enzymes of the system are apparently involved in a small proportion of cases (see Berry, 1989). Fatty acyl-CoA oxidase utilizes molecular oxygen and produces hydrogen peroxide. There are clear data which appear to indicate that the induction of the ß-oxidation system plays a major role in the development of tumours in the liver in animals exposed to peroxisome proliferating compounds. In explaining the observations of Fahl *et al.* (1984), who produced single-strand breaks in SV40 DNA coincubated with peroxisomes from induced animals, Elliot *et al.* (1986) showed that such peroxisomes do produce higher levels of hydroxyl radical than untreated animals, under specific conditions. The induction of hydrogen peroxide-generating peroxisomal enzymes and the failure of epoxide metabolizing enzymes (cytosolic epoxide hydrolase, gluta-thione-*S*-transferase, microsomal epoxide hydrolase) to increase *pari passu*, results in an increased exposure to these damaging radicals. Compounds causing peroxisome proliferation do not increase the activities of peroxisome-associated enzymes uniformly—in general, catalase activity is around doubled when ß-oxidation enzyme activity is increased by a factor of 25 (Reddy *et al.*, 1982). This effect appears to be regulated at the transcriptional level (Reddy *et al.*, 1986).

However, there are some problems with this explanation, as Bentley *et al.* (1988) have pointed out. The differential response of parts of the system which produces and metabolizes peroxides, and which prevents activated oxygen-dependent DNA damage, is capable of definitive study only in 'an intact cellular system with the correct concentration and compartmentalization of the various enzymes and co-factors', and this group (Bentley *et al.*, 1987) have produced data which suggest that excess production of hydrogen peroxide is not associated with oxidative damage to DNA when this damage is sought directly (no strand breaks in hepatic nuclear DNA, unscheduled DNA synthesis in hepatocytes or induction of the formation of micronuclei in the liver). As the thyroid is under TSH drive, the stimulus to cell division persists throughout the period of exposure to the compound but remains reversible for a very long time (95 weeks—Greaves *et al.*, 1986) before non-regulated growth supervenes.

FORESTOMACH TUMOURS IN THE RAT

Spontaneous tumours of the upper gastrointestinal tract are rare in rats, but a number of nitroso compounds and polycyclic hydrocarbons will produce hyperplasia in the forestomach with papillary change and the subsequent development of squamous carcinoma. This sequence has been well documented for fatty acids by Mori (1953) and Griem (1986), in which class of compounds the smaller the number of carbon atoms the greater the effect—propionic acid (3C) producing hyperplasia, papilloma and carcinoma; butyric acid and valeric acid (4 and 5C) hyperplasia and papillomas only; and lauric acid (12C) no significant change. The shorter-chain acids which produce epithelial change may be carcinogenic after appropriate duration of administration; this was not always adequately explored. The antioxidant butylated hydroxyanisole (BHA), widely used as a food additive, produces this sequence in rats, mice and hamsters.

Although some of the compounds producing this effect produce epithelial necrosis in the forestomach, this change is not necessary for the later development of hyperplasia (Toledo, 1965). The oesophagus is not affected.

To illustrate the difference between the effects of genotoxic and non-genotoxic compounds in the same system, aristolochic acid, a phenanthrene carboxylic acid obtained from the medicinal plant

Aristolochia clematis L. which is genotoxic, produces the sequence of hyperplasia, papillomatosis and squamous carcinoma in the rat (Mengs, 1983) and the mouse (Mengs, 1988), but with this compound adenocarcinoma of the forestomach also develops, together with tumours in other tissues and organs. It is possible in the mouse to achieve 100 per cent tumour incidence.

Comparison of the effects of this type of compound in animals with and without a forestomach have been made: the changes observed with BHA in rodents are not seen in dogs (Tobe *et al.*, 1986) or monkeys (Iverson *et al.*, 1986).

LIVER TUMOURS IN THE RAT

The clear indication of the significance of a continuous stimulus to cell growth as a major factor in epigenetic carcinogenesis is clearly illustrated by the lesions found in the rodent liver as a result of the adaptive growth induced by xenobiotic compounds. The compounds vary widely in type (phenobarbitone, steroid hormones such as norethisterone, organochlorine pesticides such as DDT, hexachlorocyclohexane—HCH—and Ponceau MX are examples) but, in general, in the early stages of treatment they all produce liver enlargement by a combination of hypertrophy and hyperplasia of cells, with increases of total DNA content, parenchymal DNA synthesis and mitotic activity. There is no evidence of toxic injury to liver cells on conventional morphological examination, and Schulte-Hermann (1979) has suggested that liver tumour formation may be the result of promotion of tumours from pre-existent tumorigenic lesions as a result of prolonged and excessive stimulation of growth.

However, in many instances the use of histochemical and other methods indicates that an apparent similarity of growth response conceals differences in cellular response. In some cases (for example, with phenobarbitone and butylated hydroxytoluene) microsomal induction and an increase in smooth endoplasmic reticulum accompany the increase in liver size; changes not seen with coumarin or xylidine, which produced similar changes in liver size (see Grasso, 1979). These changes are themselves of major significance if they alter the metabolic handling of other xenobiotics. Examination of the activities of cells from liver nodules has shown them to be altered in both nuclear activating reactions and microsomal systems for drug metabolism (Pacifici *et al.*, 1988).

The suggestion that the cells of the altered foci in the liver which form after exposure to many xenobiotics represent an 'initiated' population (Schulte-Hermann, 1987) is at present speculative, and the basis for the assumption that their reduced susceptibility to toxins allows a prolonged proliferative response on exposure remains unclear. There are a number of changes in these cells which have been extensively characterized and are clearly variable after differing exposures.

OESTROGENS

In a review of the lesions occurring in the rat pituitary gland, Attia (1985) found that the majority of ageing rats displayed hyperplasia of prolactin producing (PRL) cells with the morphological criteria of high secretory activity. Somatotrophin producing (STH) cells showed evidence of similar functional hyperactivity and there was an increased relative proportion and apparent secretory activity of adrenocorticotrophin producing (ACTH) cells. Around half of the animals in this study had pituitary adenomas which were assigned to cell types on morphological criteria alone; the tumours were not characterized immunocytochemically or electron microscopically. Studies which include the use of current pathological methodology show that many of these tumours are likely to be prolactinomas, probably induced as a result of the changes in oestrogen production which occur with ageing rats (Lu *et al.*, 1979). Prolactin has a pronounced proliferative effect on rat mammary epithelial cells *in vivo* and *in vitro* (Nandi *et al.*, 1984), and this change probably underlies the increased incidence of mammary tumours in ageing rats—it has been known for many years that the administration of prolactin to normal rodents produces an increase in RNA synthesis in the mammary glands, followed by increased DNA synthesis and cellular proliferation (Pelc, 1968; Simpson and Schmidt, 1971).

BLADDER CARCINOGENESIS IN THE RAT

In rats a number of compounds act to produce bladder neoplasia, with a marked difference in incidence in the two sexes—the lesions are almost exclusively seen in males. The silicates which occur in many rat diets are precipitated in the urine under certain conditions and irritate the mucosa—a change apparently more common in males, owing to the large amounts of macromolecules excreted in their urine. Thus, there is a background of proliferative change against which other factors may act—urothelial transitional cell hyperplasia occurs and may be defined as an area (focal or diffuse) at least 3–4 cells thick in an inflated bladder, where normal bladders have a cell thickness of one or two flattened cells.

An example of a compound which operates in this way is 2-phenylphenol (OPP) and its sodium salt (SOPP). There is an additional point that two different mechanisms appear to act at different doses. Metabolic studies have shown that these compounds are converted into the sulphate and glucuronide conjugates at doses up to around 50 mg kg^{-1}; the conjugates are then excreted in the urine (Ernst, 1965; Nakao et al., 1983; Reitz et al., 1983). At doses above 200 mg kg^{-1} hydroxylation occurs with conversion into the 2,5-dihydroxybiphenyl form which is subsequently conjugated. Studies at very high dose (600 mg kg^{-1} OPP: Reitz et al., 1983) show that quinone compounds were formed via active intermediaries (semiquinones) in the rat. There are large sex differences in handling these compounds—in males eight times as much 2,5-dihydroxybiphenyl was formed as in females. The pathway via semiquinones has not been identified in dogs, cats or following dermal application in man, but the doses used may well not have revealed it (Savides and Oehme, 1980; Harke and Klein, 1981).

The tumours of the urinary tract which have occurred after exposure to OPP and SOPP have been observed predominantly in male rats. There appears to be a NEL of 250 mg kg^{-1} day^{-1} but a clear dose-related increase in incidence is seen above this level (see Hiraga and Fujii, 1981, 1984), which declines above 500 mg kg^{-1} day^{-1} for OPP and less markedly above 1000 mg kg^{-1} day^{-1} for SOPP. Data on the binding of metabolites to macromolecules in the urinary tract (Reitz et al., 1984) provide evidence for the

suggestion that the 2,5-dihydroxybiphenyl cannot be the oncogenic agent, an argument supported by noting that considerable amounts of the 2,5 compound are formed below doses of 200 mg kg^{-1} and transformed to conjugates—none of these metabolites are thus likely to be the carcinogen. However, injection of 0.05 per cent or 0.1 per cent 2-phenyl-1,4-benzoquinone resulted in evident hyperplasia of the bladder epithelium within 5 days. It has been suggested that saturation of the detoxification mechanism resulting in the production of free 2,5-dihydroxybiphenyl and its oxidation product, 2-phenyl-1,4-benzoquinone, allows the excretion of a bladder irritant in significant amounts at high doses in feeding studies.

However, there is also evidence of the influence of other factors. Both OPP and SOPP are irritant, and this may be an adequate explanation of bladder mucosal hyperplasia; in addition, there is clearly an effect attributable to changes in pH.

In the study of Fukushima et al. (1986) male F344 rats were given OPP or SOPP at 2 per cent in feed for a period of 24 weeks. Groups of treated animals also received ascorbic acid (AS), sodium ascorbate (SA), acid saccharin (SAC), sodium saccharin (SSAC), hippuric acid (HI) or sodium hippurate (SHI) at 5 per cent in the feed. Urinary sodium concentration was increased in all animals receiving sodium salts in the diet and in SOPP-treated animals. The pH value of the urine increased after SOPP, SA and SSAC, and urine osmolarity was decreased by SOPP, SA and SHI. OPP decreased osmolarity but did not affect urinary sodium concentrations. Histopathologically, the bladders showed epithelial thickening (4–8 cell epithelial thickness) at 8, 16 and 24 weeks after SOPP, and papillary and nodular changes at 16 and 24 weeks. Treatment with other sodium salts provoked some hyperplasia at 8 and 16 weeks but no papillary or nodular changes; these changes had regressed by 24 weeks. The authors concluded that a combination of raised urinary pH and sodium acted as promoting agents for SOPP; SHI raised urinary sodium but not pH and was without effect.

Fujii et al. (1987) did an essentially similar study in male F344 rats using NaHCO$_3$ to raise the urinary pH and NH$_4$Cl to lower it. Both OPP and SOPP were examined (at 1.25 per cent and 2 per cent in the diet, respectively). Changes were seen in all groups and can be summarized as follows: hyperplasia of the bladder epithelium occurred with OPP, OPP and bicarbonate and SOPP. SOPP with NH$_4$Cl had no significant effect. Tumours were significantly increased after OPP (12/31), SOPP (22/31) and OPP plus NaHCO$_3$ (20/31). Only 3 tumours were seen in 31 rats after SOPP and NH$_4$Cl. The oncogenic effects of OPP were promoted in alkaline urine; those of SOPP were inhibited in acid urine. The authors' view was that findings that suggested that SOPP was more carcinogenic than OPP related to the greater alkalinity of the former.

These studies have been considered in detail, since they shadow the well-known story of sodium saccharin and bladder neoplasia (see Cohen and Ellwein, 1990, for comment). This common route of development seen for a number of compounds with a clear dose-, sex- and species- specific effect typifies epigenetic carcinogenesis.

GLUTATHIONE AND CARCINOGENESIS

Reduced glutathione plays a major role in protecting cells from toxic chemicals and their metabolites. It produces conjugates subsequently excreted in the urine, protects the sulphydryl groups of certain enzymes (for example, oxidative enzymes) and helps maintain membrane integrity. Glutathione also protects specific sites from electrophilic attacks by alkylating metabolites. Induced deficiencies of glutathione thus allow the operation of metabolic routes which may well be damaging.

CONCLUSIONS

What is the importance of this form of carcinogenesis? Epigenetic neoplasia has a great significance in that the resolution of the mechanisms involved in the instances described above, and in others not considered here, has provided data of considerable significance in our understanding of cell growth and proliferation. In practical terms the stimulus to resolve some of the issues has come from regulatory toxicology; it is certain that the identification of a mechanism for an adverse effect greatly facilitates risk/benefit analyses and often permits much lower safety factors to be

set—some neoplastic end-points may simply not occur in man. Understanding of neoplasia in this framework makes both a practical and a theoretical contribution.

REFERENCES

Atterwill, C. K. and Brown, C. G. (1988). Mechanistic studies on the thyroid toxicity produced by certain drugs. *Arch. Toxicol.*, Suppl. 12, 71–79

Attia, M. A. (1985). Neoplastic and non-neoplastic lesions in ageing female rats with special reference to the functional morphology of the hyperplastic and neoplastic changes in the pituitary gland. *Arch. Toxicol.*, **57**, 77–83

Axelrod, A. A. and Leblond, C. P. (1955). Induction of thyroid tumours in rats by a low iodine diet. *Cancer*, **8**, 339–367

Bentley, P., Bieri, F., Muakkassah-Kelly, S., Staubli, W. and Waechter, F. (1988). Mechanisms of tumour induction by peroxisome proliferators. *Arch. Toxicol.*, Suppl. 12, 240–247

Bentley, P., Waechter, F. Bieri, F. and Staubli, W. (1987). Risks and benefits of agents which induce hepatic peroxisome proliferation. In Fahimi, H. D. and Sies, H. (Eds), *Peroxisomes in Biology and Medicine*. Springer, Berlin, Heidelberg, New York, pp. 309–314

Berry, C. L. (1989). Causes of sudden natural death in infancy and childhood. In Mason, J. K. (Ed.), *Paediatric Forensic Medicine and Pathology*. Chapman and Hall, London, pp. 165–177

Bielschowsky, F. (1953). Chronic iodine deficiency as a cause of neoplasia in thyroid and pituitary of aged rats. *Br. J. Cancer*, **7**, 203–213

Bielschowsky, F. (1955). Neoplasia and internal environment. *Br. J. Cancer*, **9**, 80–116

Brown, C. G., Fowler, K. and Atterwill, C. K. (1986). Assessments of thyroid toxicity using *in vitro* cell culture systems. *Fd Chem. Toxicol.*, **24**, 557–586

Cavalieri, R. R. and Pitt-Rivers, R. (1981). The effect of drugs on the distribution and metabolism of thyroid hormones. *Pharmacol. Rev.*, **33**, 55–80

Cohen, S. A. M. and Ellwein, L. B. (1990). Cell proliferation in carcinogenesis. *Science*, **249**, 1007–1011

Crooks, J., Greig, W. R. and Branwood, A. W. (1963). Dyshormogenesis and carcinoma of the thyroid gland. *Scott. Med. J.*, **8**, 303–307

Ernst, W. (1965). Umwandlung and Ausscheidlung von 2-Hydroxydiphenyl bei der Rat. *Arzneim. Forsch.*, **15**, 632

Elliot, B. M., Dodd, N. J. F. and Elcombe, C. R. (1986). Increased hydroxyl radical production in liver peroxisomal fractions from rats treated with peroxisome proliferators. *Carcinogenesis*, **7**, 795–799

Fahl, W. E., Lalwani, N. D., Watanabe, T., Goel, S. K. and Reddy, J. K. (1984). DNA damage related to increased hydrogen peroxide generation by hypolipidaemic drug-induced liver peroxisomes. *Proc Natl Acad. Sci. USA*, **81**, 7827–7830

Fujii, T., Nakamura, K. and Hiraga, K. (1987). Effects of pH on the carcinogenicity of o-phenylphenate in the rat urinary bladder. *Fd Chem. Toxicol.*, **25**, 359–362

Fukushima, S., Shibata, M.-A., Kurata, Y., Tamano, S. and Masui, T. (1986). Changes in the urine and scanning electron microscopically observed appearance of the rat bladder following treatment with tumour promotors. *Japan J. Cancer Res.*, **77**, 1074–1082

Grasso, P. (1979). Liver growth and tumourigenesis in rats. *Arch. Toxicol.*, Suppl. 2, 171–180

Greaves, P., Isarri, E. and Monoro, A. M. (1986). Hepatic foci of cellular and enzymatic alteration and nodules in rats treated with clofibrate or diethylnitrosamine followed by phenobarbital: Their rate of onset and their reversibility. *J. Natl Cancer Inst.*, **76**, 475–484

Griem, W. von (1986). Tumorigene Wirkung von Propionsäure an der Vormagenschleimhaut von Ratten im Futterungsversuch. *Bundesgesundheitsblatt.*, **28**, 322–327

Harke, H. P. and Klein, H. (1981). Zur Frage der Resorption von 2-phenylphenol aus Waschenden Handedisinfectionsmitteln. *Zbl. Bakt. Hyg. I Abt Orig B*, **174**, 274

Haynes, R. C. and Murad, F. (1985). Thyroid and antithyroid drugs. In Gilman, A. G., Goodman, L. S., Rall, T. W. and Murad, F. (Eds), *The Pharmacological Basis of Therapeutics*, 7th edn. Macmillan, New York, pp. 1389–1411

Hiraga, K. and Fujii, T. (1981). Induction of tumours of the urinary system in F344 rats by dietary administration of sodium o-phenylphenate. *Fd Cosmet Toxicol.*, **19**, 303

Hiraga, K. and Fujii, T. (1984). Induction of tumours in the urinary tract of F344 rats by the dietary administration of o-phenylphenol. *Fd Chem. Toxicol.*, **22**, 865

Iverson, F., Truelove, E., Nera, E., Lok, E., Clayson, D. B. and Wong, J. (1986). *Fd Chem. Toxicol.*, **24**, 1197–1200

Lu, K. H., Hopper, B. R., Vargo, T. M. and Yen, S. S. C. (1979). Chronological changes in sex steroid, gonadotrophin and prolactin secretion in ageing female rats displaying different reproductive status. *Biol. Reprod.*, **21**, 193–203

Mengs, U. (1983). On the histopathogenesis of rat forestomach carcinoma caused by aristolochic acid. *Arch. Toxicol.*, **52**, 209–220

Mengs, U. (1988). Tumour induction in mice following exposure to aristolochic acid. *Arch. Toxicol.*, **61**, 504–505

Moody, D. E., Rao, M. S. and Reddy, J. K. (1977). Mitogenic effect in mouse liver induced by a hypolipidemic drug, nafenopin *Virchows Arch. B*, **23**, 291–296

Mori, K. (1953). Production of gastric lesions in the rat by the diet containing fatty acids. *Gann*, **44**, 421–426

Nakao, T., Ushiyama, K., Kabashima, J., Nagai, F., Nakagawa, A., Ohno, T., Ichikawa, H., Kobayashi, H. and Hiraga, K. (1983). The metabolic profile of sodium o-phenylphenate after subchronic oral administration to rats. *Fd Chem. Toxicol.*, **21**, 325

Nandi, S., Imagawa, W., Tomooka, Y., McGrath, M. F. and Edery, M. (1984). Collagen gel culture system and analysis of estrogen effects on mammary carcinogenesis. *Arch. Toxicol.*, **55**, 91–96

O'Neil, W. M. and Marshall, W. D. (1984). Goitrogenic effects of ethylenethiourea on rat thyroid. *Pestic. Biochem. Physiol.*, **21**, 92–101

Pacifici, G. M., Eriksson, L. C., Glaumann, H. and Rane, A. (1988). Profile of drug metabolising enzymes in the nuclear and microsomal fractions from rat liver nodules and normal liver. *Arch. Toxicol.*, **62**, 336–340

Pelc, S. R. (1968). Turnover of DNA and function. *Nature*, **219**, 162–163

Reddy, J. K., Goel, S. K., Nemali, M. R., Carrino, J. J., Laffler, T. G., Reddy, M. K., Sperbeck, S. J., Osumi, T., Hashimoto, T., Lalwani, N. D. and Rao, M. S. (1986). Transcriptional regulation of peroxisomal fatty acyl-CoA oxidase and enoyl-CoA hydratase/3-hydroxyacyl-CoA dehydrogenase in rat liver by peroxisome proliferators. *Proc. Natl Acad. Sci. USA*, **83**, 1747–1751

Reddy, J. K. and Lalwani, N. D. (1983). Carcinogenesis by hepatic peroxisome proliferators:evaluation of the risk of hypolipidaemic drugs and industrial plasticisers to humans. *CRC Crit. Rev. Toxicol.*, **12**, 1–58

Reddy, J. K., Warren, J. R., Reddy, M. K. and Lalwani, N. D. (1982). Hepatic and renal effects of peroxisome proliferators: biological implications. *Ann. NY Acad. Sci.*, **386**, 81–110

Reitz, R. H., Fox, T. R., Quast, J. F., Hermann, E. A. and Watanabe, P. G. (1983). Molecular mechanisms involved in the toxicity of orthophenylphenol and its sodium salt. *Chem.–Biol. Interact.*, **43**, 99.

Reitz, R. H., Fox, T. R. Quast, J. F., Hermann, E. A. and Watanabe, P. G. (1984). Biochemical factors involved in the effects of orthophenylphenol (OPP) and sodium orthophenylphenol (SOPP) on the urinary tract of male F344 rats. *Toxicol. Appl. Pharmacol.*, **73**, 345

Rosin, A. and Ungar, H. (1957). Malignant tumours in the eyelids and the auricular region of thiourea treated rats. *Cancer Res.*, **17**, 302–305

Savides, N. C. and Oehme, F. W. (1980). Urinary metabolism of orally administered *ortho*-phenylphenol in dogs and cats. *Toxicology*, **17**, 355

Schulte-Hermann, R. (1979). Adaptive liver growth induced by xenobiotic compounds: its nature and mechanism. *Arch. Toxicol.*, Suppl. 2, 113–124

Schulte-Hermann, R. (1987) Initiation and promotion in carcinogenesis. *Arch. Toxicol.*, **60**, 179–181

Simpson, A. A. and Schmidt, G. H. (1971). Effect of prolactin on nucleic acid metabolism during lactogenesis in the rabbit. *J. Endocrinol.*, **51**, 265–270

Sinha, D., Pascal, R. and Furth, J. (1965). Transplantable thyroid carcinoma induced by thyrotropin. *Arch. Pathol.*, **79**, 192–198

Smith, P., Wynford-Thomas, D., Stringer, B. M. J. and Williams, E. D. (1986). Growth factor control of rat thyroid follicular cell proliferation. *Endocrinology*, **119**, 1439–1445

Stringer, B. M. J., Wynford-Thomas, D. and Williams, E. D. (1985). *In vítro* evidence for an intracellular mechanism limiting the thyroid follicular cell growth response to thyrotropin. *Endocrinology*, **116**, 611–615

Tobe, M., Furuya, T., Kawasaki, Y., Naito, K., Sekita, K., Matsumoto, K., Ochiai, Usui, A.,

Kobubo, T., Kanno, J. and Hayashi, Y. (1986). Six month toxicity study of butylated hydroxyanisole in beagle dogs. *Fd. Chem. Toxicol.*, **24**, 1223–1228

Toledo, J. D. (1965). Die Cytogenese des Vormagencarcinoms der Ratte durch *N*-Methyl-*N*-Nitrosurethan. *Beitr. Pathol. Anat.*, **131**, 63–120

Van Leeuwen, F. X. R., Hanemaaijer, R. and Loeber, J. G. (1988). The effect of sodium bromide on thyroid function. *Arch. Toxicol.*, Suppl. 12, 93–97

FURTHER READING

Butterworth, B. E. and Slaga, T. J. (1987). Nongenotoxic mechanisms in carcinogensis. *Cold Spring Harbor Laboratory*, Cold Spring Harbor, New York

39 Reproductive Toxicity

J. M. Ratcliffe, P. R. McElhatton and Frank M. Sullivan

INTRODUCTION

Reproductive toxicity can be defined as any adverse effect on any aspect of male or female sexual structure or function, or on the conceptus or on lactation, which would interfere with the production or development of a normal offspring which could be reared to sexual maturity, capable in turn of reproducing the species. This is a very wide definition and includes various types of toxicity which are often considered separately. For example, *teratogenicity* is the ability to cause gross structural malformations in the developing fetus; *behavioural teratogenicity* is a term which has been used to describe the ability to affect the developing fetus in such a way as to result in abnormal mental development to impair either the intellectual development or the behaviour of the offspring after birth. Since a good deal of central nervous system functional and biochemical development occurs not only *in utero* but also in the early postnatal period, it is possible that chemicals which affect lactation or which are transferred to the infant via the milk may also affect the normal development of the offspring in such a way as to produce permanent effects. The term *development toxicity* is often used now to include both of these different aspects of reproductive toxicity which can result in abnormal structural *or* functional development of the offspring following exposure of pregnant or lactating females, and is dealt with in Chapters 40 and 41. This chapter will concentrate on the other aspects of reproductive toxicity, viz. effects on the male and on the non-pregnant female and on the tests which are currently used to detect and investigate the mechanism of action of chemicals with reproductive toxic potential.

SCREENING TESTS IN ANIMALS FOR REPRODUCTIVE TOXICITY

These will be discussed in four sections dealing with (1) drugs, (2) pesticides, (3) food additives and (4) industrial chemicals.

Drug Testing

One important consequence of the thalidomide disaster was that virtually every country in the world introduced legal requirements for the testing of potential new drugs before these could be released for use by the general public. A major aim was to prevent a repetition of the teratogenic effects of thalidomide, so, not unnaturally, detailed reproductive tests were included as part of the testing battery. In 1966, under the direction of Dr Lehmann, the United States Food and Drug Administration (US FDA) published guidelines for a three-segment study for drug testing for adverse effects on fertility and pregnancy. This proved to be a classic design which is still used to this day with only minor modifications throughout the world (Sullivan, 1988).

Three-segment Reproduction and Teratogenicity Study

Normally three dose levels plus controls are used in each segment. Segment 1 of the study is the 'fertility and general reproductive performance' segment and is normally carried out on rats. In this, young male rats are treated for 60–80 days to cover the whole period of spermatogenesis. Female rats are treated for 14 days to cover three oestrous cycles and are then mated with the treated males, treatment of the males and females continuing during the mating period. Treatment of the females continues throughout the whole of pregnancy. Half of the females are killed at midterm for examination for dead and resorbing fetuses, and the remaining females are continued on treatment through parturition and lactation until weaning of the young, which is usually at 21 days postpartum. The young are reared till sexual maturity and tested for fertility. Modifications to this protocol in Europe are that half the females are killed just before term instead of midterm, so that full fetal examinations may be carried out. In addition, treatment is stopped at parturition, and the pups delivered naturally are tested for various behaviours during the rearing period. In general, however, European regulatory authorities will accept studies carried out to the USA design. In Japan there is a major difference in protocol design, in that treatment of the mated females is stopped on day 7 of gestation; otherwise the design is similar. With all of these designs, if an adverse effect is observed on fertility or pregnancy, then separate mating of treated males with untreated females and vice versa may be necessary to demonstrate whether the effect is on one sex only, and other studies may be necessary to investigate the exact nature of the effects observed.

Segment 2 of the study is the 'teratogenicity' or embryotoxicity segment and is normally carried out in two species, usually rats and rabbits. Mated animals are treated during the period of organogenesis (days 6–15 rats, 6–18 rabbits) and the pups are delivered by caesarean section on the day before expected parturition for examination. This is necessary in order to prevent loss of deformed fetuses by cannibalism, which happens in these species. The pups are examined for gross, soft tissue and skeletal defects by the use of appropriate dissection and staining techniques. In the USA and EEC, 20 pregnant rats are normally used per group. In Japan 30 pregnant rats are used per dose group and one-third of them are allowed to deliver their pups naturally. These are reared to weaning, and some behavioural and developmental tests are carried out before termination at weaning. This gives more information than the original design, especially on whether there is catch-up when developmental retardation is observed in the fetuses, as is often the case. This design is acceptable to most other regulatory authorities.

Segment 3 of the study is the 'peri-postnatal' segment. This is normally carried out on pregnant rats, which are treated during the last part of gestation, not covered by treatment in the segment 2 study, through parturition until weaning. This is to examine whether the drug has any adverse effects on parturition or lactation which have not been detected in the segment 1 study. Higher doses may be used in this segment than in the segment 1 study. Problems are commonly seen in the segment 3 study when non-steroidal anti-inflammatory agents which inhibit prostaglandin synthesis are tested, and when progestagens are tested, since both types of drugs can markedly prolong gestation in rodents and so lead

to parturition difficulties and resultant neonatal deaths. However, such effects do not preclude the use of these drugs in humans.

When positive results are observed in any of the segments in the reproduction studies, this will normally lead to further studies being carried out to investigate the mechanism of action. The effects observed may be extensions of their pharmacological actions which might be expected at the high doses used in the toxicity tests, but would not be expected at the lower doses used clinically. Sometimes the actions may be exerted on rodent-specific aspects of reproductive physiology and would not be a problem in humans. Differences in results between rats and rabbits may be due to metabolites which are produced in one species but not another. It is then important to know which metabolites are produced in humans and to be sure that these are adequately tested in the animal studies. It may sometimes be necessary to synthesize adequate quantities of human-specific metabolites and for animal tests to be repeated using these.

Pesticide Testing

The safety evaluation of pesticides for reproductive toxicity has to take into consideration several factors which are not relevant for drug testing. By their nature, pesticides are toxic compounds, since their use is to kill target species which may be plants, insects, fungi, etc., though they may have very low toxicity for mammals. First, consideration has to be given to the safety of workers handling these chemicals. Depending on their use, the exposure of operators may be considerable, and this has to be taken into account in the final risk assessment of safety in use and the need for protective clothing to be worn. For chemicals used on food crops there has to be residue data, so that exposure of the general public consuming the food can be calculated. For chemicals used on amenity lands such as parks, gardens and playing fields, consideration has to be given to exposure of the public using these facilities. The environmental ecological impact must also be examined, so that studies may have to be carried out to look for effects on beneficial species such as earthworms and bees, as well as on fishes, birds, predators, and so on. Reproduction tests on these latter species are outside the scope of this chapter but are of great environmental interest.

For tests related to operator exposure it is common to carry out the segment 1 and segment 2 tests described above for drugs. This covers possible effects on male and female fertility and teratogenicity. For pesticides leaving significant residues on food, it is usual to carry out a multigeneration study to test for long-term genetic or cumulative effects or effects on young developing animals. In such tests animals are treated continuously with the chemical, usually at three dose levels administered in the diet, through several generations.

Several different designs of multigeneration study have been used for pesticide testing. The original design proposed by the US FDA for testing food additives (Fitzhugh, 1968), which is a three-generation two-litter test, has been widely used. This involves treating young male and female rats with three dose levels of the test substance plus a control group and allowing them to produce two litters, F_{1a} and F_{1b}. Selected pups from the second (F_{1b}) litters are reared to maturity, still under treatment, and in turn are allowed to produce two litters (F_{2a} and F_{2b}). Again, selected pups from the second (F_{2b}) litters are reared to maturity, still under treatment, and allowed to produce two litters (F_{3a} and F_{3b}). The second (F_{3b}) litter are then subjected to full pathological and histopathological examination for any effects of long-term exposure. An immense amount of information is obtained in such studies, not only on the different aspects of fertility and pregnancy, but also on possible effects on growth and development of the young animals. In Europe, in an attempt to reduce the numbers of animals involved without significant loss of information, it is becoming common to perform this test using only two generations with two litters in each. In the USA a modified test using two generations with one litter in each is acceptable for pesticide testing. Recently designs have been used where a third litter is produced in one or two of the generations with the dams killed just before delivery for examination of the fetuses, so that the test includes a teratology element as well.

Food Additive Testing

The reproductive toxicity test requirements for the testing of food additives are less well defined in Europe than for the other classes of chemicals considered above (EEC, 1989; DHSS, 1982). In the USA, however, the US FDA have published an extensive account of the types of test which may be required, depending on the use, amount, frequency, and duration of exposure expected (US FDA, 1982). In general, fertility and teratogenicity are tested using the segments 1 and 2 of the drug testing scheme above, but sometimes modified so that the period of chemical exposure, especially in the teratology test, is extended to include most of gestation. Consideration has to be given also to whether the metabolism of the chemicals may alter on chronic administration, so that more than one dosing regimen may have to be used. For food chemicals where there is likely to be prolonged or extensive exposure, multigeneration studies are normally performed using one of the designs discussed above, usually a two-generation, two-litter test.

Industrial Chemicals Testing

In most industrialized countries there are now testing requirements for industrial chemicals when these are produced in significant amounts. In Europe, for example, under the requirements of the laws generally known as the 'Seventh Amendment', there is a stepwise system which permits regulatory authorities to require sequential testing for fertility, teratogenicity and multigeneration effects as the tonnage of chemical produced per year, or *in toto*, reaches certain critical values. The methods used are essentially the same as described above for drugs. There has, however, been good international co-operation under the auspices of the Organization for Economic Cooperation and Development (OECD) to establish mutually acceptable guidelines which have acceptance worldwide. As these are regularly updated, interested readers should obtain the most recent versions from the OECD.

MECHANISM OF ACTION OF CHEMICALS AFFECTING REPRODUCTION

When any adverse effects are detected in any of the above screening tests, then extrapolation to humans involves analysis of the mechanisms and sites of action of the chemicals causing the effects.

Some of the factors which have to be taken into account in analysing effects in males and females are considered in detail below, together with detailed descriptions of the types of toxic effects which can be produced in males and females.

Effects on the Male Reproductive System

Introduction

Exposure to a toxic agent may affect the male reproductive system at various stages of life: during fetal development of the gonads due to exposure of the pregnant mother; during the quiescent pre-pubertal period before active spermatogenesis begins; and post-pubertally during the long period of activity of spermatogenesis, which, although a gradual decline in testicular function occurs after middle age, continues into old age in man (Lipshultz and Howards, 1983). The two critical end-points of concern in male reproductive toxicology are (1) the production of sufficient sperm which are capable of fertilizing an egg and (2) the production of sperm with normal chromosome number and structure and genetic material. A toxic agent may produce alterations in spermatogenesis via an effect on the hypothalamo-pituitary-testicular axis, or affect accessory sex gland function or sexual function (libido, potency, ejaculation), with the result that fertilization fails to occur. However, a toxin may cause genetic or chromosomal damage to the germ cell, so that if a sperm carrying damaged genetic material fertilizes an egg, fetal death or a structural or functional abnormality in the newborn occurs (which may not become apparent until later life or even the subsequent generation).

In Western countries, about 15 per cent of couples are clinically infertile (i.e. have not conceived after one year of unprotected intercourse), although estimates vary widely in different countries (Belsey, 1984). An estimated 30 per cent of clinical infertility in couples has been attributed to the male, with a further 20 per cent due to a combination of male and female factors (Lipshultz and Howards, 1983). A considerable proportion of infertility (perhaps 30 per cent) is idiopathic, i.e. cannot be explained by diagnosed genetic, anatomical or organic conditions in either partner. Some 15–20 per cent of recognized pregnancies end in spontaneous abortion and a further unknown number of conceptions are aborted before pregnancy is diagnosed; approximately 50 per cent of recognized first-trimester abortions and about one-third of all recognized abortions up to 28 weeks are chromosomally abnormal, according to Warburton *et al.*, (1980); the frequency in early abortions is thought to be considerably higher. Approximately 6 per cent of perinatal deaths and 0.6 per cent of live births are chromosomally abnormal; further, an estimated 1 per cent of infants carry a gene for an autosomal dominant disease, of which possibly 20 per cent are new mutations (Wyrobek, 1989). It is not known, however, what proportion of these abnormalities are contributed by the male or could be attributable to toxic exposures. Nevertheless, a number of agents have been identified experimentally as affecting one or more aspects of male reproduction and mechanisms of toxicity elucidated by which they exert their effect; a number of agents have also been studied in humans. Below we shall first briefly describe the physiology of male reproduction, then outline the main methods by which reproductive toxicity can be studied in animals and man, and finally describe mechanisms and sites of action of toxic agents, using examples from experimental, clinical and epidemiological literature.

Physiology of the Male Reproductive System

The Hypothalamo–Pituitary–Testicular Axis

In the hypothalamus neuroendocrine neurons secrete gonadotrophic hormone releasing hormone (GnRH) into the hypophyseal portal system, where it is carried in the blood to the adenohypophysis or anterior pituitary. Here it stimulates the release of the gonadotrophic hormones, luteinizing hormone (LH) and follicle stimulating hormone (FSH). Prolactin is also released from the anterior pituitary under the control of dopamine released from neuron terminals in the median eminence. In contrast to the action of GnRH which stimulates LH and FSH release, the presence of dopamine inhibits the release of prolactin. In turn, the hypothalamic neuroendocrine neurons contain receptors for monamines (noradrenaline, dopamine, serotonin) and are thus affected by these CNS transmitters (and agents which affect these transmitters). The target of action of both LH and FSH is the testis; although the primary actions of each hormone are on different testicular cells (see below), there is increasing evidence that their functions may be more complex and overlapping than previously thought. The function of prolactin in males is less clear; it appears that prolactin may potentiate the effect of LH in the testis (for general reviews, see, e.g., Hansson *et al.*, 1981; Overstreet and Blazak, 1983; Lobl and Hafez, 1985; Cooke and Sharpe, 1988; Johnson and Everitt, 1988).

The Testis

The mammalian testis consists of two major compartments: the seminiferous tubules, in which spermatogenesis takes place, and the interstitial compartment. The intestitial space contains Leydig cells which produce testosterone and other androgens under the influence of LH. These cells are closely associated with blood vessels and lymphatics which facilitate transport into the seminiferous tubules. Most of the circulating testosterone produced by the testis is bound to plasma proteins. Androgens are responsible for controlling spermatogenesis, the growth and secretory activity of accessory sex glands, somatic masculinization, male behaviour and various metabolic functions. *In utero*, androgen secretion by the developing fetal testis, and critically in gestational weeks 4–6 in humans, is essential for sexual differentiation of the gonads; androgens control both the regression of the Müllerian ducts (which form female internal genitalia), the development of Wolffian ducts into the epididymis, vas deferens, seminal vesicle and ejaculatory duct, and the development of the urethra, penis, scrotum and prostate.

There are two major cell types in the seminiferous tubules; the spermatogonial cells, and the Sertoli cells. Sertoli cells have numerous functions, principally (a) the nutrition of developing sperm cells; (b) synthesis of androgen binding proteins, which permit the binding of testosterone within the tubular fluid of the adluminal compartment (note that the Sertoli cells themselves also have androgen receptors on them), (c) synthesis of inhibin, which is probably involved in feedback regulation of both LH and FSH in the pituitary; (d) secretion of fluid into the lumen of the tubule; and (e) maintenance of the blood–testis barrier (BTB). The BTB, first demonstrated by Setchell *et al.* (1969), consists principally of specialized Sertoli-cell/Sertoli-cell junctions within the seminiferous epithelium. The layers of myoid cells surrounding the seminiferous tubule epithelium also appear to retard the passage of molecules. Permeability to compounds appears to be determined primarily by molecular size (Dixon, 1983, 1985). Molecules smaller than about 0.36 nm or about 150 M.W. (e.g. water, urea) are transported easily. The rate-limiting factor for transport across the BTB is lipid solubility (Dixon, 1983). The permeability characteristics appear to be similar to those of the blood–brain barrier, membranes in the gastrointestinal tract, mammary gland and aqueous humour.

For general reviews of testicular function, see, e.g., Burger and de Kretser, 1981; d'Agata *et al.*, 1983; Schulze, 1984.

Spermatogenesis

Spermatogonia undergo several mitotic divisions in the basal compartment of the seminiferous tubule (separated from the adluminal compartment by the Sertoli cells). One population of dividing spermatogonia become stem cells which will go on to become spermatozoa, while the rest form a replacement population of spermatogonia. The last mitotic division of spermatogonia (after a characteristic number of divisions in different species) results in primary spermatocytes which push past the tight Sertoli cell junctions and enter the adluminal compartment, where they continue to divide meiotically into secondary spermatocytes and finally round spermatids. Thus, meiotically dividing spermatocytes and subsequent stages of spermatozoal development are protected by the blood–testis barrier provided by the Sertoli cells, whereas the spermatogonia are not. Cohorts of spermatogonia in a given region of the tubule divide and differentiate synchronously; because cohorts are differentiating at varying times, there is a net continuous release of mature spermatids from the tubule. One cycle of the seminiferous epithelium (the time between successive entries into spermatogenesis of any given Type A spermatogonia) is remarkably constant in different species (e.g. 12 days in rats, 16 days in man), as is the total time for spermatogenesis (the spermatogenic cycle), which is about four times the length of the seminiferous cycle. The *rate* of spermatogenesis does not appear to be affected by the action of exogenous agents. This regularity allows the identification of the precise stage of spermatogenesis affected by, e.g., experimental administration of a toxin. Agents can selectively cause degeneration of a given population of germ cells and thus eliminate subsequent stages of cells.

Spermiogenesis is the 'packaging' process by which round haploid spermatids become spermatozoa, and this occurs in close association with Sertoli cells. Immature spermatozoa (incapable of movement and fertilization) undergo maturation in the epididymis under androgen stimulation. It usually take about 20 days from late spermatid stage to ejaculation in man. During passage through the epididymis, the sperm chromosomes are condensed and packed into the sperm head complete with a cap, the acrosome, containing the enzymes required to penetrate the ovum. A mid-piece containing mitochondria and a tail are developed. In some species, e.g. the mouse, sperm morphology is highly characteristic of the species, but in man, depending on the classification system used, up to 40 per cent of sperm may be 'abnormal', without the oval head and usual tail shape (Belsey *et al.*, 1980). In most mammalian species there is a high degree of redundancy in sperm production, i.e. some 10^4–10^8 sperm are ejaculated. According to early work by Cohen (1975, 1977), at least part of this redundancy may be due to errors in crossing over of chromosome material during meiosis which render the sperm unsatisfactory for fertilization, since he found a correlation between chiasma frequency in different species and sperm numbers in the ejaculate. Clearly, there is also considerable wastage due to structural or functional deficiency in many sperm which reduces their viability, motility and ability to reach and penetrate the ovum. Sperm have to penetrate the cervical mucus of the female and combat the possible effect of sperm antibodies in the female tract before proceeding to the ovum. They must also reside for some period of time (usually several hours, depending on species) in the female tract to become 'capacitated' or capable of fertilization (Yanagimachi, 1981).

The seminal fluid consists of epididymal fluid and secretions of the accessory sex glands, principally from the prostate (30 per cent in man) and seminal vesicles (60 per cent in man), but also from the bulbourethral (Cowper's) glands and ampulla. The biochemical composition of the seminal fluid and its volume may affect the viability and motility of the spermatozoa after ejaculation, but in complex ways that are not clearly understood.

For general reviews, see, e.g., Burger and de Kretser, 1981; Mann and Lutwak-Mann, 1981; Burger *et al.*, 1989.

Libido, Potency and Ejaculatory Function

In man psychological factors are of critical importance in determining libido, but neurological integrity of the nervous system is also important, as centrally acting agents can affect libido in man and mating behaviour in mammals (see below). Potency in man is under parasympathetic nervous control; endocrine factors are less involved. The sympathetic nervous system controls ejaculation. In both cases psychological factors may be involved in disturbances of these functions (for review, see, e.g., Benson and McConnell, 1983).

Methods for Assessing the Effect of Toxic Agents on the Male Reproductive System

Studies of toxic agents and their mechanisms of effect on male reproduction can be divided into (a) experimental (usually using the rat, mouse or rabbit), (b) clinical (usually infertility clinic patients or patients undergoing specific drug treatments) and (c) epidemiological (studies of groups of men exposed occupationally or environmentally to some agent of concern). Clearly, a greater number of reproductive end-points and mechanisms can be studied in the laboratory than in the clinic or field setting. Examples of the techniques used in the laboratory include gross pathology and histology of the testis and accessory sex glands. Sperm analysis may be carried out to measure sperm viability, motility, swimming speed and morphology.

Studies in the mouse indicate that sperm shaping is under genetic control in this species, and that exposure to known mutagens increases the frequency of abnormal sperm shapes (Wyrobek, *et al.*, 1983a). There is also a correlation between induction of sperm abnormalities and an increase in germ cell mutations as tested by the dominant lethal, specific locus and heritable translocation tests (see below), which suggests that, in the mouse at least, abnormal morphology may predict for germ cell mutagenicity (Wyrobek *et al.*, 1983a). However, recent reviewers have argued that sperm shape does not necessarily predict for chromosomal or DNA damage within the sperm, particularly as damage to Sertoli cells may result in secondary morphological abnormalities

(Russell and Shelby, 1985; Working, 1989). Recently, chromosomal analyses of male germ cells have been developed which have been shown to detect germ cell mutagens (Working, 1989). Dixon and colleagues have used a method of measuring unscheduled DNA synthesis in sperm (which would not normally occur after the first replications of DNA before mitotic divisions in the spermatogonia), using incorporation of radiolabelled thymidine into sperm DNA following experimental mutagen treatment (Lee and Dixon, 1978). It has been shown to occur in spermatogonia and leptotene, zygotene, pachytene and diplotene stages in spermatocytes and round spermatids but not in elongated spermatids and spermatozoa, which indicates that DNA mutation induced in these stages cannot be repaired (Working, 1989). The swimming ability, capacitation and fertilizing capacity of mammalian sperm have also been studied *in vitro* (Katz *et al.*, 1989). Assays of seminal fluid to assess accessory sex gland function (e.g. of fructose and zinc) and assays of gonadotrophic hormones in blood and urine may also be conducted.

To determine the effect of a toxic agent on reproductive performance, mating behaviour (e.g. frequency of copulation) may be measured, usually in rodents. To determine the effect of treatment on the various stages of spermatogenesis, serial mating of treated males with untreated females is conducted and the number of implantations, fetal deaths or litter sizes determined: the effect of agents affecting the epididymal spermatozoa will be seen in the first mating and effects on stem cell spermatogonia in the last matings (Dixon, 1983). One of the most common tests of chromosomal damage in the germ cell in mammals is the dominant lethal mutation test (Bateman and Epstein, 1971; Ehling *et al.*, 1986). A dominant lethal mutation is one which results in the death of the early conceptus, and may be due to chromosome breakage, or non-disjunction, or irreparable fatal breaks in DNA strands in meiotic or post-meiotic cells. The mutation occurs prior to fertilization and, theoretically, could kill the zygote at any time during its development. However, in mice, for example, death is rarely seen after 10 days (half the gestational age) (Bateman and Epstein, 1971). It is not clear what the period of vulnerability is in humans, although recent studies of karyotyped human abortuses suggest that most lethal mutations are expelled in

the first trimester of pregnancy (Warburton *et al.*, 1980), often, as in the case of all monosomies except XO, too early to be detected. To determine the heritability of non-lethal chromosomal and genetic defects, heritable translocation and specific locus mutation tests and multigeneration tests in, e.g., mice may be conducted (Flamm and Dunkel, 1989). Behavioural and developmental tests of late effects of toxic exposure of the male on viable offspring have also been utilized.

In the clinical setting, investigations of infertility or the reproductive toxicity of drugs in humans may include a battery of tests on semen quality, including sperm count, viability, motility, velocity and morphology, and seminal fluid analyses (Belsey *et al.*, 1980; Amann, 1981; Dixon, 1983; Eliasson, 1983; Lipshultz and Howards, 1983; Assennato *et al.*, 1986); FSH, LH and testosterone levels in serum (Swerdloff and de Kretser, 1983); sperm–cervical mucus interaction assays (Kremer and Jager, 1976); *in vitro* fertilization assays using zona pellucida-free hamster eggs (Rogers, 1989); physical examination and testicular biopsy; psychological evaluation; and measurement of time to conceive in the individual couple (see, e.g., Lipshultz and Howards, 1983).

The epidemiological study of reproductive toxins presents considerable methodological difficulties, principally those of obtaining an adequate sample size, of being able to measure or estimate exposures or effects accurately and of being able to take into account other exposures or risk factors (e.g. age) which could explain an apparent association between exposure to a toxic agent and an effect on reproductive function (see, e.g. Bloom, 1981; Vouk and Sheehan, 1983; Lockey *et al.*, 1984). Further, a number of the tests which have been used in the clinical setting to diagnose the infertility of individuals are not suitable for epidemiological studies, for reasons of expense, practicality and/or unknown predictive value of the tests for infertility in populations (e.g. *in vitro* fertilization, sperm–cervical mucus interaction). Relatively few studies of reproductive outcomes (e.g. spontaneous abortions, birth defects) in partners of exposed men have been conducted, partly owing to the large sample sizes required and the difficulty of taking into account maternal factors and exposures. For example, approximately 170 pregnancies in each of an exposed and non-exposed group, representing about 2000 person-years of exposure are needed to detect a twofold increase in fetal deaths due to an exposure. The use of live birth rates to detect changes in fertility in exposed groups of men has been attempted, but is an insensitive measure of subfertility and presents problems of determining a standardized expected live birth rate (adjusted for, e.g., parity, race) particularly if existing vital statistics have to be used.

Recently, Wilcox and co-workers have developed a more sensitive measure of time to conception (Baird *et al.*, 1986), which requires about 55 pregnancies in each of an exposed and non-exposed group to detect a 50 per cent decrease in the probability of conceiving in any one non-contracepting menstrual cycle. This may still mean that more than 700 person-years of exposure per group must be studied (depending on the pregnancy rate) to obtain the required number of pregnancies. Reliance has thus been placed on studies of semen quality in exposed men. For example, recently developed techniques of semen analysis using mobile laboratory equipment have allowed the study of semen characteristics requiring fresh samples (e.g. sperm motility) to be evaluated in the occupational setting (Schrader *et al.*, 1987). The principal problems in the epidemiological study of male reproductive toxicology remain (a) determining the predictive value of experimental data in laboratory animals for humans; (b) determining the biological significance of alterations in semen quality in humans to male fertility and subsequent pregnancy outcomes; and (c) improving the methodologies for studying exposure to toxins on semen parameters and reproductive outcomes.

Mechanisms and Sites of Action of Male Reproductive Toxins

Several types of toxic agents will be considered here, which may be usefully classed into one of the following groups: physical agents (e.g. ionizing radiation); pharmaceutical (therapeutic) agents; recreational and illicit drugs; industrial or environmental chemicals, including agricultural chemicals; and biological, naturally occurring toxins. Although the modes of action of some chemicals or classes of agents have been discovered, it must be emphasized that the mechanisms of action of many agents known to affect one or more aspects of male reproduction have not been elucidated, and may involve multiple sites of action and complex activity.

Some general mechanisms of toxicity may be discussed first. A toxic substance may act in one or more of the following ways:

(1) An alteration in chromosome number or structure (e.g. translocations, deletions, or insertions of parts of chromosomes) or a gene mutation in the germ cell may occur. Although assessment of chromosomal abnormalities and genetic mutations in human sperm has not been possible until very recently, some data suggest that perhaps 2 per cent of human sperm are aneuploid (i.e. have numerical abnormalities) and 6 per cent have structural chomosomal abnormalities (Martin, 1985). It is possible that sperm with abnormal chromosomes are somehow selected out in the female tract before arrival at the ovum or they cannot fertilize the egg. If fertilization does take place, most chromosomal abnormalities would be expected to result in early, or occasionally late, fetal death through a dominant lethal effect—for example, virtually all monosomies and most trisomies are fatal. If the fetus survives, it may have a congenital abnormality or a genetic disorder which may be expressed at birth, later in life or in the next generation. Certain chromosomal abnormalities are entirely due to a paternal contribution (e.g. XYY), whereas in others the contribution is less—for example, 30 per cent of Down's syndrome (trisomy 21) and about 50 per cent of mutations of small segments of DNA (minisatellite mutations) are thought to be due to the male. The role of toxic exposures in the induction of genetic abnormalities is unknown.

(2) Spermatogenesis and normal sperm viability, motility and morphology may be affected by either direct cytotoxic action on spermatogonial cells or later sperm cells (including agents which interfere with normal meiosis, e.g. spindle poisons such as benomyl), an effect on Leydig cells or Sertoli cells, or an effect on the hormonal release and feedback of the hypothalamo–pituitary–testicular axis. Effects on accessory sex gland function secretions may also affect normal sperm function after ejaculation and seminal fluid volume. The net result may be impairment of fertility, due to low sperm numbers, failure of sperm to survive in the female tract or to swim up to the ovum, or their failure to fertilize due to a morphological abnormality or a functional deficit such as failure to capacitate.

(3) An effect on sexual behaviour (reduced

mating frequency or loss of libido, impotence or ejaculatory function) may occur, mediated by an effect on CNS or autonomic nervous system function.

Reproductive toxins may act directly because of structural similarity to an endogenous compound (e.g. agonists or antagonists of endogenous hormones), or because of general chemical reactivity (e.g. alkylating agents); these toxins usually have several sites of action (Mattison and Thomford, 1989). Other toxins may require metabolic activation before exerting their effects (e.g. cyclophosphamide, DBCP, polyaromatic hydrocarbons). Finally, some toxins act indirectly by inducing or inhibiting enzymes involved in steroid synthesis or clearance or by interfering with neuronal control of hormone levels or sexual function (Mattison and Thomford, 1989).

It is clear that in order to exert a toxic effect at a given site of action, the toxin or its metabolite must reach the site of action in sufficient concentration to overcome the detoxification and repair mechanisms in the cells of the tissue (Lee and Dixon, 1978). Apart from general aspects of the pharmacokinetics of absorption, distribution, metabolism and excretion of a toxic agent, several specific aspects of the male reproductive system's response to insult affect toxicity. These include (a) the resistance offered by the blood–testis barrier to testicular toxins; (b) local and systemic biotransformations (activation, detoxification) of chemicals; and (c) the capacity of spermatogenic cells to repair cell damage and damage to DNA (Lee and Dixon, 1978; Dixon, 1983).

The testis as well as the liver contains mixed-function oxidase systems which can metabolize (activate or detoxify) chemicals and also enzymes which are capable of conjugating toxic chemicals for elimination (Lee and Dixon, 1978). Mixed-function oxidase activity appears to be found principally in the interstitial tissue of the testis, whereas conjugating enzymes, such as epoxide hydrase and glutathione-*S*-transferase, are found mainly in the tubules. In general, the levels of these enzymes are considerably less than in the liver, but may be important in the local biotransformation of xenobiotics that penetrate the BTB. Certain compounds such as direct-acting alkylating agents can affect cells without activation, but several testicular toxins, such as dibromochloropropane, polycyclic hydrocarbons,

hydrazines and cytoxan, require metabolic activation first (Lee and Dixon, 1978). There may also be differences in the capacity of the testis to metabolize a given toxin at different stages of spermatogenesis, which may be one explanation for differences in sensitivity of different spermatogenic stages (Bateman and Epstein, 1971).

The timing of exposure is also of critical importance in determining toxicity. If exposure occurs *in utero*, normal sexual differentiation may be interrupted, resulting in anatomical abnormalities in the male gonads. Unlike in the female, however, where the complement of ova is developed *in utero*, the male gonad does not start to develop mature germ cells from the seminiferous epithelium until puberty, when spermatogenesis begins, so that pre-pubertal exposures would be expected to be of significance only if the testicular seminiferous cords or Leydig cells were irreparably damaged. Exposures to exogenous hormones such as sex steroids, if they delayed the onset of puberty and normal spermatogenesis, would be of importance if administered peri-pubertally. Once spermatogenesis has begun, the timing of exposure may alter the effect observed, depending on the stage(s) of spermatogenesis exposed and the agent involved. For example, in rodents early spermatids appear to be 2–3 times more sensitive to the effects of ionizing radiation on mutation induction than epididymal sperm (Bateman and Epstein, 1971), but late spermatids and epididymal sperm are more sensitive to the effects of alkylating agents.

Examples of Toxins and Their Mechanisms and Sites of Action

Toxins Which May Affect Germ Cell Chromosomes, Genes and DNA or RNA Synthesis

Toxins which can interfere with normal meiosis and the accompanying numerical and structural rearrangement of chromosomes, or which subsequently cause chromosomal or genetic damage, or which interfere with DNA synthesis or replication, are likely to be especially toxic to rapidly proliferating cells such as germ cells (Wudl and Sherman, 1983). Some oligopeptide antibiotics such as Netropsin and distamycin A form stable complexes with DNA and inhibit DNA and RNA synthesis (Kornberg, 1980). Similarly, certain planar polycyclic compounds such as acridine and actinomycin D intercalate with the DNA molecule and disrupt its structure and function. Alkylating agents, among other actions, covalently bind to DNA base molecules or DNA-binding proteins—for example, ethylnitrosourea is a potent mutagen, as shown by the specific locus test in the mouse, and induces reversible sterility in this species (Russell *et al.*, 1979). Other agents shown to be mutagenic in the mouse specific locus test include cyclophosphamide, methyl, ethyl and propyl methanesulphonate, procarbazine and triethylenemelamine (Russell *et al.*, 1981). A number of cancer chemotherapy drugs, such as niridazole, appear to suppress the meiotic division of spermatocytes (Mann and Lutwak-Mann, 1981).

Certain heavy metallic ions, such as mercury, lead and cadmium, can bind to phosphate, sulphydryl and imidazole groups in proteins and disrupt the activity of a number of enzymes, such as DNA polymerase. These metals are generally cytotoxic, as they also interfere with the action of mixed-function oxidases and phophorylases, and may affect the transport of ions across cell and mitochondrial membranes.

There are a large number of chemicals which have been tested for dominant lethal mutations in rodents. According to a review of the literature by Green (1985), 65 chemicals could be considered positive in this test. Joffe and Soyka (1981) have also reported data showing that certain compounds, such as morphine, methadone, alcohol and lead, increase the frequency of postnatal mortality in rodents; the mechanism of this effect has not been elucidated. Owing to the methodological difficulties discussed above, there are no cytogenetic data on the induction of chromosomal or genetic mutations by these agents in human sperm. Several have been shown to affect sperm quality (see below). Only a few agents have been studied in relation to spontaneous abortions, heritable birth defects or later effects in man, mainly owing to methodological difficulties such as the large sample sizes required, as discussed above.

Although some effects have been reported in man, none of the studies have provided conclusive evidence of a paternally mediated chromosomal or genetic effect on the fetus or offspring. Infante *et al.* (1976) reported an increase in spontaneous abortions among wives of men exposed to vinyl chloride. A number of early studies of lead-exposed men suggest an increased rate of abortion among their wives (see Rom, 1976). Anaesthetic gas exposure has also been linked to abortion in wives (Tomlin, 1979), although not in all studies (Knill-Jones *et al.*, 1975). There have been very few studies of paternal exposures and birth defects: a number of investigations using malformation registry data have not shown consistent associations (see Barlow and Sullivan, 1982). Specific exposures studied include exposure to 2,3,7,8-tetrachlorodibenzodioxin (TCDD) in 'Agent Orange', used in Vietnam, reported by Erickson *et al.* (1984), who found no association with malformations; and waste anaesthetic gas exposure among anaesthetists by Knill-Jones *et al.* (1975), who reported a significant increase in minor malformations, but this has not been confirmed in other studies. Recently Gardner *et al.* (1989) reported a significant increase in childhood leukaemia associated with occupational radiation exposure of the fathers; this is the first case where a link between a paternal exposure to radiation and childhood cancer has been demonstrated.

Toxins Which Affect Spermatogenesis and Sperm Quality

There have been a large number of studies of effects of drugs, narcotics and chemicals on sperm parameters, including sperm count, viability, motility, velocity, morphology and *in vitro* fertilizing capacity (see reviews by Wyrobek *et al.*, 1983a,b). It is often not easy to distinguish, however, even in experimental studies, whether observed effects on spermatogenesis are caused by direct effects on germ cells, damage to Leydig or Sertoli cells or effects on endocrine function, or by combinations of these effects. According to Bernstein (1984) there are a number of classes of organic compounds for which structure–activity relationships have been shown to predict for spermatotoxicity, and which have in fact been shown to affect sperm quality in animals (see Wyrobek *et al.*, 1983a). These include (a) straight-chain di- and tri-carbon compounds containing halogen atoms (e.g. ethylene dibromide, dibromochloropropane, halothane); (b) organochlorine compounds with a symmetrical chlorinated carbon bridge [e.g. dichlorodiphenyltrichloroethane (DDT), methoxychlor, heptachlor, chlordane and hexachlorophene pesticides]; (c) nitrobenzenes (e.g. 4-nitrobenzamide, dinoseb); (d) certain organophosphates (e.g. the pesticides dichlorvos, trichorfon); (e) aminobenzenes containing sulphonic, carboxylic or hydroxyl solubilizing groups (e.g. the drug sulphasalazine, used to treat ulcerative colitis); and (f) the glycol ether family of solvents, especially the methyl and ethyl forms. In addition, heavy metals and some of their compounds (see, e.g., Barlow and Sullivan, 1982; Davies, 1983), alkylating agents, antibiotics and antimetabolites used as cancer chemotherapeutic agents, such as cyclophosphamide, chlorambucil, adriamycin, cytosine arabinoside, vinblastine (Davies, 1983; Kinsella, 1989), other halogenated polycyclic hydrocarbons (e.g. polychlorinated and polybrominated biphenyls), as well as a number of other miscellaneous chemicals, and biologically occurring toxins (e.g. gossypol) are spermatotoxic (Davies, 1983).

A number of these agents have also been reported to affect semen quality in man, including the range of cancer chemotherapeutic drugs and the drugs prednisone and sulphasalazine (see Wyrobek *et al.*, 1983b); the recreational drugs alcohol, marijuana and, more equivocally, tobacco (Wyrobek *et al.*, 1983b); the industrial chemicals carbon disulphide (Lancranjan, 1972), lead (e.g. Lancranjan *et al.*, 1975; Assennato *et al.*, 1986); dibromochloropropane (e.g. Whorton *et al.*, 1977); ethylene dibromide (Ratcliffe *et al.*, 1985, 1987); chlordecone (Kepone) (Cannon *et al.*, 1978); chloroprene (Santoskii, 1976); and the glycol ether 2-ethoxyethanol (marginally) (Ratcliffe *et al.*, 1989). Physical agents shown to affect spermatogenesis in man include ionizing radiation (see Kinsella, 1989). With radiation exposure, spermatogonial cells are the most sensitive, showing morphological and quantitative changes at doses as low as 10 cGy. Spermatocytes are functionally damaged at 200–3000 cGy, when they cannot complete maturation division, and spermatids at approximately 600 cGy; recovery of testicular function is directly related to the dose received, taking up to 5 years at doses of approximately 600 cGy in some cases (Kinsella, 1989). Heating of the testis has also been shown to reversibly affect sperm count in man and other species; epididymal sperm seem to be most susceptible to short periods of increases in temperature of even 2–3°C, such as may occur with repeated hot tub use. Prolonged heating of the scrotum may affect earlier stages of spermatogenesis (Procope, 1965). Loss of sperm may be partly mediated by a decrease in androgen binding protein synthesis (Rich and de Kretser, 1977).

Toxins Which Affect Sexual Behaviour
The assessment of libido and potency presents difficulties in humans, particularly when studied epidemiologically, since reliance must be placed largely on self-reported symptoms and there is no good animal model (other than, e.g., mating frequency or ejaculatory capacity) for this complex area of sexual function. In humans a number of drugs which act on the CNS or the autonomic nervous system have been reported to affect libido, erectile potency or ejaculatory function (Woods, 1975). The two largest categories of drugs are antihypertensives and psychoactive drugs (Editorial, 1979). Antihypertensives may affect both erectile potency and ejaculation. Antidepressants may cause impotence via an anticholinergic action (tricyclics) or peripheral ganglionic blockade (monoamine oxidase inhibitors). Certain sedatives and tranquillizers, such as benzodiazepines and the phenothiazines, notably thioridazine, may act at several sites, by both decreasing libido at a central level and inhibiting autonomic nerve transmission at a peripheral level to impair ejaculation. It is possible that hypothalamic and pituitary function is also disturbed by phenothiazines, according to Woods (1975). Centrally acting drugs of abuse, including heroin, marijuana, alcohol, LSD and amphetamines, have all been reported to affect libido and potency in men, particularly after prolonged use. The use of anabolic steroids was reported to decrease libido and potency (together with other spermatotoxic effects in male athletes in one study) (Frasier, 1973). Some industrial chemicals have been reported to affect libido and/or potency, notably carbon disulphide, boric acid, lead and the pesticide Kepone (chlordecone) (Barlow and Sullivan, 1982), but findings are not consistent.

Toxins Which Affect Endocrine Function
Disruption of endocrine secretion, binding, feedback control or target activity can be affected by action at several sites. Often it is not clear, when an alteration in hormone activity is observed, whether this is the result of a primary effect on hormone secretion or a response to testicular damage or some other mechanism. Cimetidine, used in the treatment of peptic ulcer, appears to act by competing with dihydrotestosterone for

androgen receptors in the testis and accessory sex glands (Winters *et al.*, 1979), resulting in decreased sperm count, gynaecomastia, increased prolactin secretion and decreased prostate and seminal vesicle weight. LH receptors in Leydig cells have been shown to be depleted in rats exposed to ionizing radiation *in utero* (Rich and de Kretser, 1979). Men working on the production of oral contraceptives were found to have gynaecomastia (Harrington *et al.*, 1978); these exogenous steroids are thought to act by suppressing gonadotrophic hormone secretion. Some of the polycyclic chlorinated hydrocarbons [e.g. DDT, polychlorinated biphenyls (PCBs), hexachlorophene] may act either by oestrogen agonism or by inducing mixed function oxidases which increase the clearance of endogenous steroids (see Mattison, 1981); this may explain their observed effects on spermatogenesis.

There is one striking example of the effect of exogenous oestrogenic hormone exposure occurring *in utero* and affecting fetal gonadal development. Diethylstilboestrol (DES), a synthetic oestrogenic drug widely prescribed to pregnant women in the 1940s and 1950s to prevent miscarriage, premature delivery and toxaemia, exerted a dramatic effect on male fetal gonadal development by antagonizing the activity of fetal testosterone. The key aspect of the toxicity of DES is its lack of binding to maternal steroid binding protein or conjugation in fetal liver, processes which protect the developing male genital tract from damage by maternal oestrogens from the placenta and ovaries (Gill, 1989), Numerous structural and functional abnormalities of the reproductive system have been observed in the male offspring, including epididymal (spermatocoele) cysts, testicular hypoplasia, cryptorchidism, hypospadias, abnormal semen parameters and primary infertility (see, e.g., Gill *et al.*, 1979; Stenchever *et al.*, 1981; Whitehead and Leiter, 1981; and review by Gill, 1989). There are conflicting reports of testicular cancer in exposed males, perhaps due to methodological limitations (Gill, 1989).

Toxins Which Affect Accessory Sex Gland Function

There are relatively few examples of toxins which directly affect accessory sex glands. Alpha-chlorohydrin and 6-chloro-6-deoxy sugars affect glucose metabolism of epididymal spermatozoa,

and at high doses alpha-chlorohydrin damages the epithelium of the cauda epididymis, causing spermatocoeles (Zanefeld and Waller, 1989). Sulphasalazine, probably acting via an active metabolite, affects the fertilizing capability of sperm in rodents and man, apparently by inhibiting the acrosome reaction, either by an effect on epididymal function so that sperm maturation is impaired, or by a direct effect on the sperm (Zanefeld and Waller, 1989). Hexachlorophene has been found to impair ejaculation in rats by causing fibrosis of the prostate (Gellert *et al.*, 1978). Toxins which can impair motility of spermatozoa *in vitro* could, if found in the secretions of the seminal vesicles or prostate, affect motility of sperm after ejaculation. Imidazoles, such as the oral antifungal agent ketoconazole, have been shown to be transported into seminal fluid and to immobilize sperm (Zanefeld and Waller, 1989).

Effects on the Female Reproductive System

Introduction

Reproduction in the female mammal involves a complex series of interrelated steps under hormonal control via the hypothalamo–pituitary–ovarian axis. These steps involve follicular development, ovulation, ova transfer, fertilization, transport of the conceptus, and its subsequent implantation and development culminating in parturition. All of these processes are important and are the summation of many systemic, local, cellular and molecular interactions, which still remain poorly understood.

Because of the complexity of the reproductive system and the species differences involved, a description based on the human female will be used, with additional information given on other species where appropriate. Basically, female reproduction will be described under the following headings: general physiology of the female reproductive tract; the hypothalamo–pituitary–ovarian axis; the ovary, including ovarian cycles; and the various ways in which these systems can be adversely affected.

General Physiology of the Female Reproductive System

The female reproductive tract consists basically of paired gonads, or ovaries, and a system of hollow ducts, the oviducts, for transport of eggs to the exterior. The oviduct is modified in several ways according to the species and its characteristic mode of reproduction. In humans the oviducts consist of paired uterine tubes (Fallopian tubes) connected to a single midline uterus terminating in a vagina. All of these components are interrelated and are sensitive to hormonal changes which are controlled by the hypothalamo–pituitary–ovarian axis. This hormonal controlling system, is also responsible for the development of secondary sexual characteristics—for example, mammary gland development, fat disposition and, especially in humans, hair distribution and voice changes (Catt and Pierce, 1978; Page *et al.*, 1981; Takizawa and Mattison, 1983; Johnson and Everitt, 1988)

The Hypothalamo–Pituitary–Ovarian Axis

The hypothalamus is a complex structure involved in control of body temperature, integration of autonomic activity and the release of gonadotrophin releasing hormones (GnRH). The GnRH are carried in the blood via the hypothalamo–hypophyseal portal system to the anterior pituitary gland. The anterior lobe of the pituitary contains a variety of cells which release gonadotrophic hormones, follicle stimulating hormone (FSH), luteinizing hormone (LH), prolactin and other hormones. Prolactin release is under control of dopamine released from neurons in the median eminence (Leblanc *et al.*, 1976). Whereas GnRH stimulate the release of FSH and LH, dopamine inhibits the release of prolactin. The target organ for FSH and LH is the ovary. The role of prolactin is less clearly defined and its actions are more species-specific. In some rodents, for instance, it has the ability to maintain the corpus luteum (CL) and there is some evidence in humans that it may be involved in luteolysis and in lactation.

The release of GnRH from the hypothalamus is controlled by a number of feedback loops, principally from the hormones produced by the ovary (Yen and Lein, 1976). Although the exact mechanisms and site of action are not fully understood, it is generally thought that tonic release of FSH is involved in follicle growth. As the follicle grows, it secretes increasing amounts of sex steroids, predominantly oestrogen, which has a negative feedback effect on the hypothalamic pathways resulting in a decreased release of FSH from

the pituitary (Sadow *et al.*, 1980; Feder, 1981a; McCann, 1981).

In some mammals other factors such as temperature and light intensity also affect hormone secretion, presumably via other CNS mechanisms (Elliot and Goldman, 1981; Komisaruk *et al.*, 1981).

The Ovary

The ovary plays a central role in that it controls the production of gametes and sex steroids, which are regulated via the hypothalamic–pituitary pathways. The principal site of action of these ovarian hormones is the uterus, which responds by undergoing cyclical changes which enable conception and fetal development to occur.

The ovary develops from the germinal ridge and descends into the pelvis in the early part of fetal life. The germ cells, or oocytes, are formed before birth and develop to the primary oocyte stage, having undergone the first phase of meiosis (Ross and Schreiber, 1978; Feder, 1981c).

They remain in this resting oocyte–follicle complex until they are stimulated by gonadotrophin release at the onset of puberty (Moor and Warnes, 1979) to produce the characteristic mammalian graafian follicle. Thus, any agents that damage the oocytes will accelerate the depletion of this resting pool and may lead to a reduction in fertility. At maturity the ovary undergoes cyclical activity of a biphasic nature during which follicles undergo growth, maturation and regression.

In humans it is estimated that in excess of half a million follicles are present at birth; many of these die (atresia) and those that survive are continously reduced in number. It is estimated that fewer than 500 will be ovulated and fewer still will be fertilized to produce offspring (Sadow *et al.*, 1980; Page *et al.*, 1981).

These ovarian cycles are species-specific; some of the similarities and differences are described in the next section.

Ovarian Cycles

Ovarian cycles (i.e. oestrous cycles) and menstrual cycles in the higher primates and humans vary in their length and frequency of occurrence. Their duration may be a few days as in, for example, the mouse, or several weeks, as in humans and the horse. The term 'oestrus' refers to the period when the female is most receptive to the male (ie 'in heat'), which usually coincides with high levels of circulating oestrogen and subsequent stimulation of sexual excitement and behaviour patterns (Feder, 1981b). The human female does not exhibit oestrus behaviour as such, even though changes do occur in the reproductive organs, but there is no clear correlation between the secretion of oestrogens and sexual drive and libido.

Mammals having a succession of oestrous cycles (e.g. rodents) are called polyoestrous. In others, such as the goat, the cycles are limited to a particular season of the year (i.e. the breeding season). The interval between cycles is of relative quiescence and is termed 'anoestrus'. Other mammals, such as cats, dogs and ferrets, are monoestrus. They have one long sustained oestrus during the spring and occasionally another in late summer (Perry, 1971; Elliot and Goldman, 1981). In humans and the higher primates, such as the Old World monkey and apes, these cycles occur at approximately monthly intervals and are termed 'menstrual cycles' (*mensis*: Latin for month). These cycles differ from those of most other mammals in that there is external loss of blood (i.e. menstruation) at the end of each cycle.

In most mammals ovulation occurs spontaneously under hormonal control via the hypothalamo–pituitary–ovarian pathways, either during or just after oestrus. However, in some monoestrous animals such as the dog, the additional stimulus of mating is required to trigger ovulation (i.e. induced ovulation).

This complex series of events involved in the hormonal control of follicle maturation, ovulation, luteinization and luteolysis will be illustrated by reference to the human menstrual cycle. Significant species differences will be discussed where appropriate (Sadow *et al.*, 1980; Feder, 1981a,b; Page *et al.*, 1981; Takizawa and Mattison, 1983).

Menstrual Cycle

The complex process by which a single dominant follicle is selected for ovulation is not well understood (Bahr *et al.*, 1977; Takizawa and Mattison, 1983). However, it is generally accepted that tonic release of FSH from the pituitary stimulates follicular growth. As the follicle grows, it secretes sex steroids, predominantly oestrogen at this stage. As oestrogen levels increase, they eventually trigger off a reflex discharge of FSH and LH from the anterior pituitary which results in the release of a preovulatory LH surge. Oestrogen also has a negative feedback on the hypothalamic–pituitary pathways to decrease the amount of FSH released. Following the LH surge there is an increase in LH concentration in the follicular fluid which is associated with oocyte maturation, preovulatory progesterone secretion by the granulosa cells and the stimulation of prostaglandin (PG) synthesis. Ultimately this results in the rupture of the dominant follicle and the release of the oocyte—i.e. ovulation occurs (Chaslow and Pharriss, 1972; Delforge *et al.*, 1972; McNatty *et al.*, 1975). In some mammals there is a slight bloodstained discharge associated with ovulation which is quite different from menstruation.

Following ovulation the remaining follicles become atretic. The dominant follicle collapses and the granulosa cells begin to proliferate to form the corpus luteum. In humans the main hormone secreted by the corpus luteum for about 8–10 days is progesterone. If fertilization occurs, the conceptus, even prior to implantation, is thought to secrete substances which are recognized by the mother and prevent the breakdown (luteolysis) of the corpus luteum (Heap *et al.*, 1979). In the cow PG synthesis is suppressed by embryonically derived pregnancy-specific proteins (Goding, 1974). Similarly, in the pig, the blastocyst produces oestrogens which lead to maternal recognition of the conceptus and also inhibit PG synthesis. However, in primates such as monkeys, apes and man the conceptus secretes human chorionic gonadotrophin (HCG), which supports the corpus luteum and maintains a suitable endometrium.

If fertilization does not occur the corpus luteum undergoes luteolysis and its endocrine function ceases. Luteolytic mechanisms tend to be species-specific. In rodents, rabbits, cattle, sheep and pigs, PG via the utero-ovarian circulation play a major role. PG-induced vasoconstriction may also be a contributory factor (Karim, 1972; Cole and Cupps, 1977). In contrast, the primates do not seem to control luteolysis in this way. Although the mechanisms are poorly understood, it seems that alterations in the concentrations and interrelationship of various hormones, sex steroids, gonadotrophins, prolactin and PG initiate a feedback loop to the hypothalamus and trigger off the release of gonadotrophins—e.g. FSH and LH—to initiate the next cycle (Feder, 1981b; Takizawa and Mattison, 1983; Richardson, 1986; Johnson and Everitt, 1988).

Oviducts/Fallopian Tubes

The anatomy of the tubes is species-specific and is related to the way in which ovulation and fertilization occur. The tubes are the site of fertilization and their rich autonomic nerve innervation assists egg retention. The lumen of each tube is bathed with fluid whose composition and direction of flow are under control of sex steroids and the autonomic nervous system, and varies at different stages of the cycle. In general, egg transport from the ovary to the uterus seems to be a cumulative effect of co-ordinated cilial motility, muscle contractions and subsequent fluid flow. Tubular mobility is controlled by the synergistic effects of oestrogen and progesterone, and in humans during the luteal phase it is towards the uterus (Sadow *et al.*, 1980; Page *et al.*, 1981; Takizawa and Mattison, 1983).

The Uterus

The anatomy and physiology of the uterus are also species-specific. In many species the uterus acts simply for the transfer of sperm, while in others, such as rodents, cows and pigs, it acts as a sperm reservoir.

In humans the uterus undergoes hormonally dependent alterations in the endometrium during the cycle, to prepare the uterus for implantation and subsequent development of the conceptus. During the preovulatory phase the follicular-derived oestrogen increases uterine blood flow and stimulates endometrial development. After ovulation the synergistic actions of oestrogen and progesterone complete this process. The effects of progesterone on the oestrogen-primed endometrium are pleotropic, causing an increase in protein synthesis and formation of microvilli. There is increased vascularity, permeability and discharge of secretory products into the endometrial lumen of the glands which enables the conceptus to implant (Johnson and Everitt, 1988).

The time taken for the conceptus to implant varies with the species and is generally not known. However, it is known that receptivity for implantation has a limited time-span in rodents at 5–6 days and in humans at about 7 days (Psychoyos, 1962; Edwards, 1982). The myometrium, on the other hand, remains quiescent for most of pregnancy. However, towards the end of pregnancy it develops a co-ordinated pattern of contractions which assist in the expulsion of the fetus at parturition. There are many and varied theories as to the mechanisms controlling this, but on the whole it is accepted that PG synthesis and degradation is one of the key control factors (Porter and Finn, 1977; Yen, 1978; Challis and Lye, 1986; Johnson and Everitt, 1988).

Mechanisms of Action of Reproductive Toxins

As successful reproduction in the female relies on a complex system of hormonally controlled interrelated events, toxic insults at any one stage of this process can have profound detrimental effects on both the mother and the fetus. Agents may act directly on germ cells so that conception does not occur, or they may cause severe anomalies resulting in early abortions. Some of the abortuses have been shown to have chromosomal damage. Alterations in sex ratios may occur, but interpretation of existing data is difficult. Outcomes involving the prenatal period may involve low birth weights, stillbirths, neonatal deaths, chromosomal damage or gross structural malformations.

Just as there are species-specific differences in the physiology and hormonal control of the reproductive processes, there are also differences in the response to toxins. This may in part be explained by the interspecies differences in the pharmacokinetic responses—i.e. absorption, distribution, metabolism, excretion of a particular toxin. Other factors, such as gender differences and duration of exposure to the toxin, are also involved.

The principal action of toxins is to alter in some way the normal functioning of cells, organs or organisms. Toxins may inhibit ovulation, ovum transport, fertilization and implantation by altering the environment within the oviduct. In order for toxins to exert such effects, they must have adequate distribution to the target organ. Alternatively, they may have a much wider range of effects which may be non-specific and may act at many sites within the organism (Dixon, 1980; Mattison, 1981, 1983).

Mechanisms of Toxicity

Toxins may act directly or indirectly. Toxins may have a direct action because they bear structural similarities to an endogenous substance (e.g. hormones) or because of their chemical reactivity (e.g. alkylating agents). Others may act indirectly by requiring various processes prior to exerting their toxic effect or by metabolism to an active metabolite which may then exert its effect by direct mechanisms. In addition, some indirectly acting toxins exert their effects by altering the controlling mechanisms (e.g. inhibition of gonadotrophin release or enzyme induction–inhibition).

Toxins may exert their effects by more than one mechanism of action. The halogenated polycyclic hydrocarbons [e.g. PCB or polybrominated biphenyls (PBB)] behave in such a way, in that they may act indirectly by induction of microsomal monooxygenases or transferases or directly because of their steroid hormone agonist properties (Doull 1980; Neal, 1980).

Directly Acting Toxins Toxins which have structural similarities to biologically active molecules are generally agonists or antagonists of endogenous hormones. Oral contraceptives belong to this group, in that they act predominantly by suppression of gonadotrophin release. Workers who manufacture oral contraceptives experience a risk from this type of reproductive–endocrine toxicity (Harrington *et al.*, 1978). Exposure to other occupational and environmental substances which have oestrogenic or progestogenic activity may inhibit gonadotrophin release or ovarian function via the hypothalamus and pituitary pathways. Other chemically reactive compounds may be non-specific in their site of action. This category includes the alkylating agents, the toxic effects of which have been discussed above.

Indirectly Acting Toxins Indirectly acting toxins are substances that may require metabolic activation, and the metabolite thus formed may itself be chemically reactive or may mimic an endogenous molecule. Oxidation by microsomal monooxygenases is one of the mechanisms involved in removing hydrophobic xenobiotics from the body (Fleischer and Packer, 1978). It has been shown that the ovary has microsomal monooxygenases, epoxide hydrases and transferases capable of metabolizing many xenobiotics (Heinrichs and Juchau, 1980). The polar metabolites thus formed may undergo conjugation or be excreted directly. However, some of these metabolites are chemically reactive and are capable of interacting with cellular macromolecules in the same way as exogenously administered substances. Cyclophosphamide (Koyama *et al.*, 1977; Lentz *et al.*, 1977), DES (Metzler and McLachlan, 1978), ethanol (Ouellette *et al.*, 1977; Sullivan and McElhatton, 1986) and the polycyclic aromatic hydrocarbons (Felton *et al.*, 1978; Nebert, 1981) are examples.

Other indirectly acting toxins may affect enzymes—i.e. induce or inhibit enzyme systems, which in turn may stimulate or inhibit steroid production or excretion. As the reproductive system is controlled by hormonal feedback loops, substances which alter the steroid balance in any way may have a profound effect on the entire reproductive process. Rodent studies have shown that some of the polyhalogenated hydrocarbons (e.g. DDT, PCB, PBB) behave in this way. Some toxins may actually enhance rather than impair fertility. Oral contraceptives, for instance, exert fertility regulation via feedback inhibition of gonadotrophin secretion, and xenobiotics that stimulate clearance of the oestrogenic and/or progestogenic component in the oral contraceptive will cause a decrease in circulating levels and consequently may increase the probability of ovulation (reviewed by Mattison, 1983).

Interference with Detoxification Detoxification mechanisms are the methods by which biological organisms respond to toxic insults. Some of these mechanisms have been shown to be present in the ovary. They tend to have a relatively broad-based specificity, and may involve conjugation hydrolysis by epoxide hydratase in order to decrease the concentration of the toxin, or metabolism to a less toxic or more easily excreted metabolite and thus limit the activity of the toxin in the body. Impaired detoxification due to the nature of the substrate or enzyme deficiencies within the organism will enhance the toxic effects.

Repair Despite the presence of detoxification pathways within the cell, cellular or organ damage can still occur. In such a situation attempts are made to repair the damage by various mechanisms. The repair may simply involve alterations in protein synthesis to replace non-functioning proteins destroyed by the toxic insult, or more sophisticated repairs may be required if the DNA itself has been damaged, involving excision and subsequent replacement of the damaged DNA region. There is some evidence to suggest that mature oocytes are able to repair damage within the oocyte DNA prior to and after fertilization. However, it is not known whether the oocyte has other types of repair mechanism (Lehmann and Bridges, 1977; Dixon, 1980; Mattison, 1983).

A more detailed account of some of the reproductive toxins and their proposed modes of action is described below.

Sites and Mechanisms of Action of Some Reproductive Toxins

The Hypothalamo–Pituitary–Ovarian Axis
Chemicals can act at several levels, on the hypothalamus and pituitary, on the endocrine and ovulatory function of the ovary or on the tissues in the reproductive tract, and frequently may act at several sites.

The mode of action of the chemical may give some indication as to whether the toxic effects it produces are reversible or not. Drugs and other chemicals that alter gonadal function directly may well produce infertility via genetic effects which are irreversible, whereas those producing alterations in the nerve pathways in the hypothalamus, for instance, may cause disruption of fertility which is reversible.

Certain CNS drugs such as tranquillizers, barbiturates, narcotics and 'social' drugs such as marijuana have an inhibitory effect on hypothalamic–pituitary function by inhibiting gonadotrophin secretion. In animal studies effects such as suppression of ovulation, oestrus and fertility have been reported. Thus, the primary endocrine effect of inhibition of gonadotrophins induces a secondary effect on ovarian steroid synthesis, resulting in adverse effects on growth, development and function of the accessory organs.

As the nerve pathways to the hypothalamus are adrenergic and dopaminergic, drugs which alter catecholamine levels, either by inhibiting CNS activity (e.g. anaesthetics, sedatives, tranquillizers and analgesics) or by stimulating the CNS (e.g. psychotropic drugs, antidepressants and hallucinogens) can also affect the hypothalamic–pituitary control of gonadotrophin release. Such actions may result in alterations in the secretion of FSH, LH and prolactin which are important for follicle growth, oocyte maturation, ovulation and maintenance of the corpus luteum. However, the CNS and autonomic effects of such drugs are often difficult to distinguish. Drugs of abuse such as cocaine (Crack), Ecstasy, cannabis, mescaline and alcohol may also have adverse effects on reproduction, such as decreased fertility, an increase in spontaneous abortions, intrauterine growth retardation (IUGR) and postnatal behavioural problems in the offspring, but these effects are less well documented and their exact mechanisms of action are not known. The study of social drug use, and of drugs of abuse in pregnancy, is a complex one because, for example, it has been shown that heavy smokers are often also heavy drinkers and caffeine consumers. Similarly, smoking and alcohol consumption are common in addicts, which, combined with their general lifestyle and poor nutrition, makes identification of the individual contributions of each substance to any one adverse effect difficult.

Some of the drugs which have been studied more extensively are discussed below and have been reviewed by Rosen and Johnson (1982) Abel (1983); Gibson *et al.* (1983); Smith (1983); Armstrong (1986); Boobis and Sullivan (1986); and Johnson and Everitt (1988).

Major Drugs of Addiction Adverse reproductive effects such as a decreased sexual desire, menstrual irregularities, infertility and increased fetal loss have been reported (Wallach *et al.*, 1969; Weiland and Yunger, 1970; Finnegan, 1981). The adverse effects on early fetal and postnatal development following intrauterine exposure have been well documented (Ostrea and Chavez, 1979; Sullivan and McElhatton, 1986; Fulroth *et al.*, 1989). This has been partly attributed to altered function of the hypothalamo–pituitary axis and partly to altered ovarian function. Some of the narcotics are reported to cause a significant decrease in LH levels which may disrupt oocyte maturation and ovulation and interfere with the FSH–LH feedback loops to the hypothalamus.

Marijuana Marijuana is a complex group of drugs derived from the plant *Cannabis sativa*. Recent animal tests and human studies have indicated that chronic, sustained exposure is associated with reproductive dysfunction (Peterson, 1980; Abel, 1983; Hollister, 1986; Ellenhorn and Barceloux, 1988). A study of marijuana users has reported that these women had shorter menstrual cycles and that a higher proportion of these cycles was anovulatory or had shorter luteal phases

(Kolodny *et al.*, 1979). The psychoactive component is delta-9-tetrahydrocannabinol (THC) and it is thought that it inhibits the secretion of FSH and LH via a hypothalamic route, with secondary effects on the ovary. However, the Kolodny study did not confirm these effects as regards gonadotrophins or progesterone, but found a significant decrease in serum prolactin. Experimental studies have shown that the duration of gonadotrophin depression is dose-related and persists for up to 24 h after peak levels of the drug have occurred in the circulation. Furthermore, these effects can be reversed by giving LHRH. THC has also been shown to depress oestrogen production and the LH surge and thus inhibit ovulation in rhesus monkeys. Rodent studies have also indicated that there is a decrease in serum prolactin, possibly caused by THC inhibiting its release from the pituitary. Other studies indicate decrease or absence of oestrogen and gonadotrophins, but a marked rise in progesterone (Smith *et al.*, 1980). It would seem that the data within a species are variable and that there are species-specific differences.

Alcohol   The effects of alcohol on female reproduction have been studied in terms of its possible teratogenic effects on the offspring, producing the fetal alcohol syndrome (Jones and Smith, 1975), and also a wide range of other adverse effects such as increased spontaneous abortions (Harlap and Shiono, 1980), IUGR (intra-uterine growth retardation; Little, 1977), overall failure to thrive postnatally and some mental retardation (Streissguth *et al.*, 1978). As alcohol has significant pharmacological effects via the central nervous system in adults, it is probable that the hypothalamic–pituitary pathways and thus reproductive hormone control may also be adversely affected. Whether adverse effects on hormones occur in the developing fetal brain is not known (Root *et al.*, 1975). Chronic use of alcohol has been associated with various obstetric and gynaecological problems, such as menstrual disorders, recurrent miscarriages and infertility. However, there is no clearly defined evidence to assess whether alcohol consumption is the cause of such problems or vice versa (Abel, 1983; Boobis and Sullivan, 1986).

Studies in which female rats consumed alcohol showed atrophy of the ovaries, fallopian tubes and uteri, and the ovaries from these rats had fewer well-developed follicles, corpora lutea and secretory granules (Van Thiel *et al.*, 1978). It has been shown that infusions of alcohol in female rats cause inhibition of spontaneous LH release, but no inhibition of LH released by LHRH, so that ovulation may be affected by inhibition of LH release (Kieffer and Ketchel, 1970; Blake, 1974).

Gonadal Dysfunction Resulting from Cancer Chemotherapy

Alkylating agents (e.g. cyclophosphamide, chlorambucil, busulphan, nitrogen mustard), the vinca alkaloids (e.g. vincristine, vinblastine, vindesine) and radiation produce varying degrees of gonadal dysfunction which are not only dose-related, but also associated with the age at which the exposure occurs. In women irreversible sterility resulting in premature menopause and sexual dysfunction occurs at higher doses than in males. Lesser degrees of gonadal injury are associated with subfertility but normal sexual function. Age at the time of exposure is an important factor, in that children apparently sustain less gonadal damage for a given dose than do adults.

The ovaries of prepubertal girls are more resistant than those of adults to toxicity induced by cytotoxic chemotherapy, in that the majority who survive the illness go on to have normal menstrual cycles and serum gonadotrophin levels. Furthermore, post-mortem examination of some of the girls whose illness proved fatal showed that their ovaries were normal (Arniel, 1972; Pennisi *et al.*, 1975; Lentz *et al.*, 1977). In a study of prepubertal leukaemic children who died, cytotoxic therapy (usually prednisone, vincristine and occasionally methotrexate, 6-mercaptopurine, cytosine arabinoside and L-asparaginase) was shown to inhibit follicle development in the ovaries, as opposed to destruction of ova, which is sometimes seen in adults receiving similar therapy (Himelstein-Braw *et al.*, 1978).

In mature women treatment with cytotoxic drugs has variable effects on gonadal function and fertility. Age-dependent factors as well as dose and duration of treatment often determine the degree of toxicity observed. However, insufficient data are available to determine critical dose levels for a given age group (Warne *et al.*, 1973). Teenagers, for instance, may sustain impaired fertility, while serum hormone levels and menstrual cycles remain normal, whereas women in their 20s may develop clinical ovarian dysfunction, the reversibility of which is often dependent on the particular drug regimen. Abnormal ovarian function may manifest itself in terms of irregular or anovulatory cycles, alteration in serum gonadotrophins and oestradiol levels sometimes resulting in premature menopause (hot flushes, insomnia, irritability, depressed libido) and menopausal levels of oestradiol and gonadotrophins. The intensity of such symptoms is often age-related, in that they tend to be worse in younger women (Chapman, 1983). Although the critical age at which most women undergoing such treatment are likely to develop ovarian failure is not known, multiple drug exposure does seem to increase the risk factor. For instance, more than 80 per cent of women over the age of 25 years developed complete and irreversible ovarian failure after six cycles with MOPP or MVPP (Chapman *et al.*, 1979b; Schilsky *et al.*, 1981).

Cyclophosphamide alone may produce a reversible form of ovarian dysfunction or complete ovarian failure in which amenorrhoea, abnormal hormone levels or destruction of ova may occur (Kumar *et al.*, 1972; Uldall *et al.*, 1972; Rose and Davis, 1977). Cyclophosphamide seems to have an affinity for attacking the resting or small oocytes. As these are present throughout the life of the female in the same metabolic state, it cannot account for the age-dependent differences in sensitivity. However, there is evidence that the pathways for detoxification of the reactive metabolites do change with age, and this may be a key factor (reviewed by Mattison, 1981).

Busulphan use has also been associated with permanent amenorrhoea, a side-effect which also seems to be age-related (Belohorsky *et al.*, 1960; Schulz *et al.*, 1979). Autopsy data from a small number of women treated with busulphan have shown signs of ovarian atrophy (Belohorsky *et al.*, 1960; Heller and Jones, 1964).

Neither the vinca alkaloids nor nitrogen mustard alone seem to be associated with ovarian dysfunction. However, there have been occasional case reports of women who developed either reversible or permanent amenorrhoea after vinblastine therapy (Sobrinho *et al.*, 1971).

There are many secondary effects which follow on from ovarian toxicity, leading to early menopause, such as a greater risk of developing osteoporosis, cardiovascular disease and uterine cancer. To some extent these effects can be ameliorated by giving sequential hormone therapy or replacement therapy with oestrogen and progesterone (Gambrell, 1978; Chapman *et al.*, 1979a,b; Nordin *et al.*, 1980; Paganini-Hill *et al.*, 1981; Whitehead *et al.*, 1981).

6-Mercaptopurine, the active metabolite of azathioprine, has been shown in experimental rodent studies to reduce the fertility of female offspring exposed *in utero* (Gross *et al.*, 1977; Reimers *et al.*, 1980). It seems to act by causing premature ovarian failure, but whether the mechanism is oocyte destruction *per se* or inhibition of oogenesis is not known. The reproductive toxicity of this group of drugs is reviewed by Schardein (1985).

Ovotoxicity

Polycyclic aromatic hydrocarbons (PAH) are ubiquitous environmental pollutants. This group includes substances produced by combustion of fossil fuels contained in car exhaust fumes, smokestack emissions and cigarette smoke. The PAH group have been implicated as carcinogens, neurotoxins, hepatotoxins and reproductive toxins. They produce their reproductive toxicity by a variety of mechanisms, including induction of microsomal monooxygenases which alters hormone production and clearance, as well as metabolism to active intermediates and hormone agonist activity (Mattison *et al.*, 1983).

PAHs require conversion to reactive intermediates via microsomal cytochrome *P*-450 dependent monooxygenase and epoxide hydrase before they can exert their toxic effects within any biological system. Such converting enzymes are widely distributed throughout the body and are found in high levels in the liver and gonads. It has been demonstrated that in order to cause oocyte destruction PAH need to be distributed to the ovary and converted into one or more active intermediate(s) that cause oocyte destruction either by a direct action on the oocyte or by an indirect route via toxicity to the granulosa cells that support the oocyte within the follicle (Mattison and Ross, 1983). It is thought that differences in ovarian metabolism may account for strain and species differences in sensitivity to PAH-induced oocyte destruction. Treatment during pregnancy is capable of destroying the oocytes of a female fetus while *in utero* (Felton *et al.*, 1978).

The susceptibility of non-human primates or humans to oocyte destruction by PAH is not known. It has been shown, however, that women who smoke one or more packs of cigarettes per day have a menopause about 2 years earlier than non-smokers (Jick *et al.*, 1977). The mechanism suggested is that the PAH in cigarette smoke destroy the oocytes at an earlier age.

Oestrogenic Chemicals Many other halogenated hydrocarbons, including the pesticides–fungicides such as DDT, aldrin, 2,4,5-T, PCB, PBB, 2,4-D (2,4-dichlorophenoxyacetic acid), heptachlor, chlordane and hexachlorophene, can interfere with mammalian reproduction in two main ways: oestrogen agonist activity and induction of microsomal monooxygenase activity responsible for production and clearance of steroid hormones (Mattison, 1981; Barlow and Sullivan, 1982; Bulger and Kupfer, 1983; Safe, 1984; Schardein, 1985).

Treatment of neonatal rats with DDT has led to a dose-dependent premature vaginal opening culminating in an anovulatory syndrome with similarities to the human polycystic ovary disease. These effects, including the inhibition in the rise of gonadotrophins following ovariectomy, are attributed to the oestrogen agonist activity of DDT. The sites of action are thought to be the vagina and the hypothalamus; the neonatal treatment is believed to alter the patterning of the hypothalamus (Welch *et al.*, 1969; Bitman and Cecil, 1970; Gorski, 1971). Similar results have been reported for PCB (Gellert *et al.*, 1978).

By induction of the monooxygenase system both DDT and PCB can increase the length of oestrous cycles and decrease the frequency of implantation in the sexually mature mouse. Similar reproductive toxicity has been observed in other species (Ringer *et al.*, 1972; Linder *et al.*, 1974; Hansen *et al.*, 1975; Kihlstrom *et al.*, 1975; Spencer, 1982). A direct relationship between enzyme activity and inhibition of uterine weight response to oestrone has also been shown (Welch *et al.*, 1971). There is indirect evidence in primates also that the halogenated polycyclics can induce monooxygenase activity and thus impair fertility by similar mechanisms (Kolmodin *et al.*, 1969; Allen and Lambrecht, 1978).

Methoxychlor (bis-*p*-methoxy DDT) is much less oestrogenic, less toxic and less persistent, and has a shorter half-life than DDT in mammals. The reduced toxicity seems to be related to its rapid metabolism to more polar derivatives (Bulger and Kupfer, 1983; Schardein, 1985).

Chlordecone, a polychlorinated polycyclic compound, also has oestrogenic action on the murine uterus (Huber, 1965) and quail oviduct (Eroschenko and Wilson, 1975). There are conflicting data concerning its potential for reproductive toxicity in mice and rats in terms of teratogenicity (Ware and Good, 1967; Chernoff and Rogers, 1976; Khera *et al.*, 1976), and postnatal survival and development (Gaines and Kimbrough, 1970; Chu *et al.*, 1981). There have been no reports of effects in human pregnancy. However, it has been reported to cause loss of libido and sperm damage among manufacturing workers.

Genetic Abnormalities and the Effects of Irradiation

During the preimplantation stage the embryo is susceptible to toxic insults which may cause mutations. If the damage is not repaired or compensated for, it may result in early embryonic death. Radiation and chemical toxins have a wide range of effects on the preimplantation embryo (e.g. alterations in membrane permeability, disruption of the mitotic spindle and enzyme activity leading to cell disruption and possible death). These mutations can be inherited via the germ cells or they can occur in somatic cells during embryogenesis. The nature of these abnormalities varies from specific point mutation in the genome to chromosome derangement altering both numbers and structural arrangements. The majority of chromosome abnormalities occur during meiosis and gametogenesis, although some do occur during preimplantation development (Dean, 1983).

It has been known for many years that germ cell loss may be due to exposure to either radiation or chemicals. Sensitivity is often species-specific and may be dependent on the stage of germ cell maturation (Oakberg and Clark, 1964) as well as the age of the animal. There seems to be no general rule to determine radiosensitivity across the species. Oocytes from juvenile mice have the highest sensitivity known for any mammalian cell. There is less information available on the effects of chemical exposures, when compared with radiation; however, the increasing use of chemotherapy in humans is adding to our knowledge of such effects, as discussed above.

Ionizing Radiation High radiosensitivity in the

ovarian germ cells has been demonstrated in the mouse, prenatal squirrel monkey and prenatal pig (Dobson *et al.*, 1978; Erickson, 1978). Although, in the adult pig, germ cells are not particularly sensitive, exposure to continuous gamma radiation at 1 rad day^{-1} throughout gestation results in severe oocyte deficiency in the newborn (Erickson, 1978). Similar studies in dogs (Andersen *et al.*, 1961) and cows (Erickson and Reynolds, 1978) have shown that in these species also there are no serious effects on the germ cells of adults. The effects in squirrel monkeys have been reviewed by Dobson and Felton (1983). Prenatal exposures of 0.7 rad day^{-1} can completely kill off the germ cells, but in the adult the same exposure causes a less dramatic germ cell loss. In other primates, such as the rhesus monkey and Bonnet monkey, the results of experimental studies have been variable, but on the whole high sensitivity seems lacking (Baker and Beaumont, 1967; Andersen *et al.*, 1977). Very little data are available in the human female. However, it would seem that exposures of approximately 400 rad are associated with induction of sterility, with larger doses being required in younger women (Baker 1971; Baker and Neal, 1977). There have been reports of ovarian failure following abdominal radiotherapy, including treatment for childhood cancer (Shalet *et al.*, 1976; Stillman *et al.*, 1981) but this has not precluded the occurrence of pregnancies (Gans *et al.*, 1963; Vuksanovic, 1966).

There is significant concern about the extrapolation of the animal data, which are species- and strain-specific, to humans. Some studies have shown that the mechanism of action may be different (e.g. the extreme sensitivity of murine oocytes may be due to the vulnerability of the plasma membrane, not adverse effects on DNA)—i.e. it is a non-genetic type of effect. Thus, the genetic risks of radiation in humans, especially when it involves exposure of the primordial oocytes, may be overestimated by referring to mouse data unless this is taken into account (reviewed by Dean, 1983; Dobson and Felton, 1983).

Psychosexual Function

While it is widely accepted that drugs and other chemicals can affect male libido or cause impotence, the possibility that such effects can occur in women has been largely overlooked. In most mammals and subhuman primates sexual activity is closely linked to ovulation, and thus it is difficult to find an animal model for sexual dysfunction occurring in women. Drug-induced changes in female libido have been associated with the use of oral contraceptives, tranquillizers, monoamine oxidase inhibitors, heroin, methadone, cannabis, cytotoxic drugs and alcohol (Heinrichs and Gadallah, 1983; Griffin, 1986).

Studies by Chapman and her colleagues (Chapman *et al.*, 1979a,b) have reported the occurrence of ovarian failure in women treated with cytotoxic drugs, including MVPP for Hodgkin's disease. Ninety-two per cent (34) of these women reported a decrease in libido; 82 per cent had menstrual irregularities or amenorrhoea and a constellation of other menopausal-type symptoms.

Oral contraceptives have also been associated with decreased libido; however, the mechanism is not established, although some studies associate it with pill-induced depression. It has been shown that oral contraceptives abolish the hormone controlled mid-cycle peak in female-initiated sexual activity (Adams *et al.*, 1978). Cyproterone acetate, which is an antiandrogen used to treat severe acne and hirsutism in women, is also used in some cases as a contraceptive, and this too is associated with loss of libido in women.

Danazol, a drug which is used in the treatment of endometriosis and other menstrual disorders, inhibits pituitary gonadotrophin secretion and is frequently reported to cause loss of libido in women (Westerholm, 1977). The antiobesity drug fenfluramine, when used in high doses of around 240 mg day^{-1}, produces loss of libido as its main side-effect. It is reported that at this dosage 85 per cent of women treated may suffer loss of libido (Connell, 1977).

Miscellaneous Drug and Chemical Effects

Oral Contraceptives

The use of oral contraceptives has proved to be one of the most effective forms of reversible fertility control in use today, their efficacy being in the range of 97–99 per cent. The composition and actions of these 'pills' have been reviewed by Murad and Haynes (1985). Currently there are basically two main types: the classical combined type containing an oestrogen and a progestogen, and a progestogen-only type. In order to eliminate some of the side-effects associated with the high oestrogen content of the classical combined preparations, phased formulations containing a progestogen and variable amounts of oestrogen ('calendar packs') have been introduced. In addition, there is a postcoital pill, containing levonorgestrel and ethinyloestradiol (UK formulation), which is used in such a way that high dosages of each of the hormones are attained within a 12 h period.

The classical combined oral contraceptive preparation is considered to be the most effective for inhibiting ovulation. The effects of ovarian hormones on gonadotrophin release via the hypothalamic–pituitary axis have already been discussed. The predominant effect of oestrogen is to inhibit the release of FSH, while the continued action of progesterone inhibits the release of LH. Thus, ovulation may be inhibited by either inhibiting the ovulatory stimulus or preventing follicle growth; both of these actions have been observed in experimental studies. However, the orally active progestogens used in the pill cannot be directly equated with progesterone *per se*, because some are inherently oestrogenic, or androgenic, and some purely progestational, and consequently they may inhibit ovulation in different ways. Measurements of circulating FSH and LH have shown that the oestrogen and progestogen combination inhibits both hormones, which results in stable plasma FSH and LH and absence of early follicular FSH and mid-cycle FSH–LH peaks. The combined preparations may also have a direct effect on the genital tract, in that they alter the stage of development of the endometrium, thus making it unsuitable for implantation (Briggs, 1976). There are also changes in the viscosity of cervical secretions. At the time of ovulation these secretions are usually copious and watery and provide a good environment for sperm. Under the influence of progesterone these secretions become thick and mucoid in nature and provide a hostile environment. Although little is known about the co-ordinated movement of the fallopian tubes, uterus and cervix in the transport of eggs and sperm, it is generally accepted that the correct hormonal environment is essential for fertilization and implantation to occur.

Progestogen-only preparations have lower efficacy than the combined type and have been associated with a higher incidence of menstrual irregularities. However, they do provide a suitable alternative for those women in whom high oestrogen levels are to be avoided.

Low doses of progestogens may cause structural changes in the endometrium and alter the consistency of the cervical mucus without causing menstrual disruption. There are varying degrees of inhibition of FSH and LH and ovulation, and this may be associated with the reduced efficacy seen with this type of pill. When a daily administration regimen is used, menstruation does occur but the length of the cycle and the duration of the bleeding period vary considerably. Long-acting progestogens (e.g. medroxyprogesterone acetate) are often given at 3 monthly intervals and after an initial period of irregular bleeding give way to amenorrhoea and an atrophic endometrium.

Although there may be some initial impairment of fertility for some months after oral contraception has stopped, this is of a transitory nature in the majority of women (Vessey *et al.*, 1978). However, in a small number of women there is a more permanent infertility (Fletcher, 1986).

Diethylstilboestrol (DES)

DES is of interest in that it is a reproductive toxin with two possible mechanisms of action. It is an oestrogen agonist which causes changes on both the male and female reproductive tract in rodents (McLachlan and Dixon, 1977; Boylan, 1978; Vorherr *et al.*, 1979), and in humans has been reported to cause an increased risk of adenocarcinoma of the vagina in females exposed prenatally (Herbst *et al.*, 1971, 1975; O'Brien *et al.*, 1979). Some of the women exposed to DES *in utero* have vaginal abnormalities and there is evidence that they have irregular menstrual cycles and dysmenorrhoea and may be less fertile (Barnes *et al.*, 1980; Herbst *et al.*, 1980). Abnormal development of the uterus with a small hypoplastic T-shaped endometrial cavity has been seen in some of these women (Kaufman *et al.*, 1977; Haney, 1987).

Industrial Chemicals

The potential of industrial chemicals to cause reproductive toxicity has been reviewed by Barlow and Sullivan (1982), John *et al.*, (1984), Schardein (1985) and the American Medical Association Council in Scientific Affairs (1985). The major effects reported in female workers are as follows.

Menstrual irregularities and other gynaecological disorders have been associated with exposure to aniline, benzene, chloroprene, formaldehyde, inorganic mercury, PCB and toluene, but in many instances the lack of data precludes a critical risk evaluation being made (Zielhuis *et al.*, 1984; Commission of European Communities, 1986; Rosenberg *et al.*, 1987).

Other substances have been associated with infertility or spontaneous abortions. These include anaesthetic gases in both males and females, ethylene oxide, arsenic and lead, as well as some of the substances mentioned above—i.e. aniline, formaldehyde and benzene (Figá-Talamanca, 1984; Lemasters *et al.*, 1985; Sullivan and Barlow, 1985; Kline, 1986; Winder, 1987; Friedman, 1988; Van der Gulden and Zielhuis, 1989).

Factors such as decreased fetal growth, low birth weights and poor postnatal survival have been associated with exposures to carbon monoxide, PCB, vinyl chloride, toluene and formaldehyde (Fletcher *et al.*, 1986; Tabacova, 1986; Lemasters *et al.*, 1989).

Teratogenic effects and transplacental carcinogenesis have been omitted from this section, as they are discussed in Chapters 40 and 41.

Effects of Exercise

Although there have been reports associating strenuous exercise with adverse effects on the reproductive system, such as delayed menarche, menstrual irregularities or amenorrhoea, a cause–effect relationship is difficult to establish (Terjung, 1979; Cumming and Rebar, 1983). There seems to be a complex interplay of physical, hormonal, nutritional, environmental and psychological factors. One of the underlying concerns is whether or not so-called exercise-induced reproductive dysfunction is truly reversible once vigorous exercise has stopped.

The amenorrhoea associated with exercise is generally thought to be hypothalamic in origin (Speroff, 1981), but data are accumulating to suggest that other circulating hormones may also be involved (Shangold *et al.*, 1981). In a review by Cumming and Rebar (1983) it is postulated that exercise-induced amenorrhoea is caused by alterations originating in the periphery as well as from CNS abnormalities. Furthermore, they suggest that the amenorrhoea produced is reversible.

Adverse effects of strenuous exercise once pregnancy has been established have also been reported. These seem to be related to the complex physiological adjustments required in terms of metabolic, endocrine, respiratory and circulatory responses in both the mother and the foetus (Lotgering *et al.*, 1985).

REFERENCES

Abel, E. L. (1983). *Marihuana, Tobacco, Alcohol, Reproduction*. CRC Press, Boca Raton, Florida

Adams, D. B., Gold, A. R. and Burt, A. D. (1978). Rise in female-initiated sexual activity at ovulation and its suppression by oral contraceptives. *New Engl. J. Med.*, **299**, 1145–1150

Allen, J. R. and Lambrecht, L. (1978). Responses of rhesus monkeys to polybrominated biphenyls. *Toxicol. Appl. Pharmacol.*, **45**, 340

Amann, R. P. (1981). A critical review of methods for evaluation of spermatogenesis from seminal characteristics. *J. Androl.*, **2**, 37–58

American Medical Association Council in Scientific Affairs (1985). *Effects of Toxic Chemicals on the Reproductive System*. American Medical Association, Chicago

Andersen, A. C., Hendrickx, A. G. and Momeni, M. H. (1977). Fractional x-radiation damage to developing ovaries in the bonnett monkey (Macaca radiata). *Radiation Res.*, **71**, 398–405

Andersen, A. C., Schultz, F. T. and Hague, T. J. (1961). The effect of total body x-radiation on reproduction of the female beagle to 4 years of age. *Radiation Res.*, **15**, 745–753

Armstrong, D. T. (1986). Environmental stress and ovarian function. *Biol. Reprod.*, **34**, 29–39

Arniel, C. C. (1972). Cyclophosphamide and prepubertal testes. *Lancet*, **2**, 1259–1260

Assennato, G., Paci, C., Baser, M. E., Molinini, R., Candela, R. G., Altamura, B. M. and Giorgino, R. (1986). Sperm count suppression without endocrine dysfunction in lead-exposed men. *Arch. Environ. Hlth*, **41**, 387–390

Bahr, J. M., Ross, G. T. and Nalbandov, A. V. (1977). Hormonal regulation of the development, maturation and ovulation of the ovarian follicle. In Greep, R. O. and Koblinsky, M. A. (Eds), *Frontiers in Reproduction and Fertility Control*, Part 2. MIT Press, Cambridge, Mass., pp. 40–43

Baird, D. D., Wilcox, A. J. and Weinberg, C. R. (1986). Use of time to pregnancy to study environmental exposures. *Am. J. Epidemiol.*, **124**, 470–480

Baker, T. G. (1971). Radiosensitivity of mammalian oocytes with particular reference to the human female. *Am. J. Obstet. Gynecol.*, **110**, 746–761

Baker, T. G. and Beaumont, H. M. (1967). Radiosensitivity of oogonia and oocytes in the foetal and neonatal monkey. *Nature*, **214**, 981–983

Baker, T. G. and Neal, P. (1977). In Zuckerman, P. L.

and Weir, B. J. (Eds), *The Ovary*, Vol. 3. Academic Press, New York, pp. 1–58

Barlow, S. M. and Sullivan, F. M. (1982). *Reproductive Hazards of Industrial Chemicals*. Academic Press, London

Barnes, A. B., Colton, T., Gundersen, J., Noller, K. L., Tilley, B. C., Strama, T., Townsend, D. E., Hatab, P. and O'Brien, P. C. (1980). Fertility and outcome of pregnancy in women exposed *in utero* to diethystilbestrol. *New Engl J. Med.*, **302**, 609–613

Bateman, A. J. and Epstein, S. (1971). In Hollaender, A. (Ed.), *Chemical Mutagens*, Vol. 2. Plenum Press, New York, pp. 541–568

Belohorsky, B., Siracky, J., Sandor, L. and Klauber, E. (1960). Comments on the development of amenorrhea caused by myleran in cases of chronic myelosis. *Neoplasm*, **4**, 397–402

Belsey, M. A. (1984). Infertility: prevalence, etiology, and natural history. In Bracken, M. B. (Ed.), *Perinatal Epidemiology*, Oxford University Press, London, pp. 255–282

Belsey, M. A., Eliasson, R., Gallegos, A. J., Moghissi, K. S., Pauben, C. A. and Prasad, M. R. N. (1980). *Laboratory Manual for the Examination of Human Semen and Semen-Cervical Mucus Interaction*. Press Concern, Singapore

Benson, G. and McConnell, J. (1983). Erection, emission and ejaculation: physiological mechanisms. In Lipshultz, L. and Howards, S. S. (Eds), *Infertility in the Male*. Churchill Livingstone, New York, pp. 165–186

Bernstein, M. E. (1984). Agents affecting the male reproductive system: effects of structure and activity. *Drug Metab. Rev.*, **15**, 941–996

Bitman, J. and Cecil, H. C. (1970). Estrogenic activity of DDT analogs and polychlorinated biphenyls. *J. Agric. Fd Chem.*, **18**, 1108–1112

Blake, C. A. (1974). Localisation of the inhibitory actions of ovulation-blocking drugs on release of luteinizing hormone in ovariectomized rats. *Endocrinology*, **95**, 999

Bloom, A. (Ed.) (1981). *Guidelines for Studies of Human Populations Exposed to Mutagenic and Reproductive Hazards*. March of Dimes Birth Defects Foundation, White Plains, N.Y.

Boobis, S. and Sullivan, F. M. (1986). Effects of life-style on reproduction. In Fabro, S. E. and Scialli, A. R. (Eds), *Principles of Drug and Chemical Action in Pregnancy*. Marcel Dekker, New York, pp. 373–425

Boylan, E. S. (1978). Morphological and functional consequences of prenatal exposure to diethylstilbestrol in the rat. *Biol. Reprod.*, **19**, 854–863

Briggs, M. (1976). Biochemical effects of oral contraceptives. *Adv. Steroid Biochem. Pharmacol.*, **5**, 66–160

Bulger, W. H. and Kupfer, D. (1983). Estrogenic action of DDT analogs. *Am. J. Industr. Med.*, **4**, 163–173

Burger, H. and de Kretser, D. (1981). *The Testis*. Raven Press, New York

Burger, E. J. Jr, Tardiff, R. G., Scialli, A. R. and Zenick, H. (Eds) (1989). *Sperm Measures and Reproductive Success*. Progress in Clinical and Biological Research, Vol. 302. Alan R. Liss, New York

Cannon, S. B., Veazey, J. M. Jr, Jackson, R. S., Burse, V. W., Hayes, C., Straub, W. E., Landrigan, P. J. and Liddle, J. A. (1978). Epidemic Kepone poisoning in chemical workers. *Am. J. Epidemiol.*, **107**, 529–537

Catt, K. J. and Pierce, J. G. (1978). Gonadotropic hormones of the Adenohypophysis (FSH, LH, and prolactin) In Yen, S. S. C. and Jaffe, R. B. (Eds), *Reproductive Endocrinology*. W. B. Saunders, Philadelphia, London, Toronto, pp. 34–62

Challis, J. R. G. and Lye, S. J. (1986). In *Oxford Reviews of Reproductive Biology*, Vol. 8. Oxford University Press, Oxford, pp. 61–129

Chapman, R. M. (1983). Gonadal injury resulting from chemotherapy. *Am. J. Industr. Med.*, **4**, 149–161

Chapman, R. M., Sutcliffe, S. B. and Malpas, J. S. (1979a). Cytotoxic-induced ovarian failure in women with Hodgkin's Disease. I. Hormone function. *J. Am. Med. Assoc.*, **242**, 1877–1881

Chapman, R. M., Sutcliffe, S. B. and Malpas, J. S. (1979b). Cytotoxic-induced ovarian failure in women with Hodgkin's Disease. II. Effects on sexual function. *J. Am. Med. Assoc.*, **242**, 1882–1884

Chaslow, F. I. and Pharriss, B. B. (1972). Luteinizing hormone stimulation of ovarian prostaglandin biosynthesis. *Prostaglandins*, **1**, 107–117

Chernoff, N. and Rogers, E. H. (1976). Fetal toxicity of kepone in rats and mice. *Toxicol. Appl. Pharmacol.*, **31**, 302–308

Chu, I., Villeneuve, D. C., Secours, V. E., Valli, V. E. and Becking, G. C. (1981). Photomirex. Effects on reproduction in the rat. *Toxicologist*, **1**, 103

Cohen, J. (1975). Gametic diversity within an ejaculate. In Afzeluis, B. A. (Ed.), *The Functional Anatomy of the Spermatozoon*. Pergamon Press, Oxford, pp. 329–339

Cohen, J. (1977). *Reproduction*, Butterworths, London

Cooke, B. A. and Sharpe, M. (Eds) (1988). *The Molecular and Cellular Endocrinology of the Testis*. Serono Symposium Publications, Vol. 50. Raven Press, New York

Cole, H. H. and Cupps, P. T. (1977). *Reproduction in Domestic Animals*, 3rd edn. Academic Press, London and New York

Commission of European Communities (1986). *Organochlorine Solvents Health Risks to Workers*. No. Eur 10531 EN. Brussels–Luxembourg

Connell, P. H. (1977). In Dukes, N. M. G. (Ed.), *Side Effects of Drugs Annual*, Vol. 1. Excerpta Medica, Amsterdam, p. 4

Cumming, D. C. and Rebar, R. W. (1983). Exercise and reproductive function in women. *Am. J. Industr. Med.*, **4**, 113–125 d'Agata, R., Lipsett, M. B., Polosa, P. and van der Molen, H. J. (Eds) (1983). *Recent Advances in Male Reproduction: Molecular Basis and Clinical Implications*. Raven Press, New York

Davies, A. C. (1983). *Effects of Hormones, Drugs and Chemicals on Testicular Function*. Annual Research Reviews, Vol. 2. Eden Press, Montreal

Dean, J. (1983). Preimplantation development: Biology, genetics and mutagenesis. *Am. J. Industr. Med.*, **4**, 31–49

Delforge, J. P., Thomas, K., Roux, F., Carniero de Siqueira, J. and Ferin, J. (1972). Time relationships between granulosa cells and luteinization and plasma luteinization hormone discharge in humans. I. A morphometric analysis. *Fertil. Steril.*, **23**, 1–11

DHSS (1982). *Guidelines for the Testing of Chemicals for Toxicity*. Report on Health and Social Subjects 27. HMSO, London

Dixon, R. L. (1980). Toxic responses of the reproductive system. In Doull, J., Klassen, C. D. and Amdur, M. O. (Eds), *Casarett and Doull's Toxicology*, 2nd edn. Macmillan, New York, pp. 332–354

Dixon, R. L. (1983). Laboratory aspects of reproductive toxicology. In Vouk, V. B. and Sheehan, P. J. (Eds), *Methods for Assessing the Effects of Chemicals on Reproductive Functions*. Wiley, New York, pp. 149–162

Dixon, R. L. (1985). Aspects of male reproductive toxicology. In Hemminki, K., Sorsa, M. and Vainio, H. (Eds), *Occupational Hazards and Reproduction*. Hemisphere Publishing Corporation, Washington, D.C., pp. 57–71

Dobson, R. L. and Felton, J. S. (1983). Female germ cell loss from radiation and chemical exposure. *Am. J. Industr. Med.*, **4**, 175–190

Dobson, R. L., Koehler, C. G., Felton, J. S., Kwan, T. C., Wuebbles, B. J. and Jones, D. C. L. (1978). In Mahlum, D. D., Sikov, M. R., Hackett, P. L. and Andrew, F. D. (Eds), *Developmental Toxicology of Energy-related Pollutants*. US Department of Energy, Washington, D.C., pp. 1–14

Doull, J. (1980). Factors influencing toxicology. In Doull, J., Klassen, C. D. and Amdur, M. O. *Casarett and Doull's Toxicology*, 2nd edn. Macmillan, New York, pp. 70–83

Editorial (1979). Drugs and male sexual function. *Br. Med. J.*, **2**, 883–884

Edwards, R. G. (1982). *Conception in the Human Female*. Academic Press, London

EEC (1989). *Presentation of an Application for Assessment of a Food Additive Prior to its Authorisation*. Commission of the European Communities. Office for Official Publications of the European Commission, Luxembourg

Ehling, U. H., Chu, E. H. Y., de Carli, L., Evans, H. J., Hayashi, M., Lambert, B., Neubert, D., Thilly, W. G. and Vainio, H. (1986). In Montesano, R., Bartsch, H., Vainio, H., Wilbourn, J. and Yamasaki, H. (Eds), *Long-term and Short-term Assays for Carcinogenicity*. IARC Scientific Publications No. 86, Lyon

Eliasson, R. (1983). Morphological and chemical methods of semen analysis for quantitating damage to male reproductive function in man. In Vouk, V. B. and Sheehan, P. J. (Eds), *Methods for Assessing the Effects of Chemicals on Reproductive Functions*. Wiley, New York, pp. 263–270

Ellenhorn, M. J. and Barceloux, D. G. (1988). *Medical Toxicology*. Elsevier, New York, pp. 673–685

Elliot, J. A. and Goldman, B. D. (1981). In Adler, N. T. (Ed.), *Neuroendocrinology of Reproduction*. Plenum Press, New York, pp. 387–388

Erickson, B. H. (1978). Interspecific comparisons of the effects of continuous ionizing radiation on the primitive mammalian stem germ cell. In Mahlum, D. D., Sikov, M. R., Hackett, P. L. and Andrew, F. D. (Eds), *Developmental Toxicology of Energy-related Pollutants*. US Department of Energy, Washington, D.C., pp. 57–67

Erickson, B. H. and Reynolds, R. A. (1978). Oogenesis, follicular development and reproductive performance in the pre-natally irradiated bovine. In *Late Biological Effects of Ionizing Radiation*, Vol. II. International Atomic Energy Authority, Vienna, pp. 199–205

Erickson, J. D., Mulinare, J., McClain, P. W., Fitch, T. G., James, L. M., McClearn, A. B. and Adams, M. J. (1984). Vietnam veterans' risks from fathering babies with birth defects. *J. Am. Med. Assoc.*, **252**, 903–912

Eroschenko, V. P. and Wilson, W. O. (1975). Cellular changes in the gonads, liver and adrenal glands of Japanese quail as affected by the insecticide kepone. *Toxicol. Appl. Pharmacol.*, **31**, 491–504

Feder, H. H. (1981a). Experimental analysis of hormone actions on the hypothalamus, anterior pituitary, and ovary. In Adler, N. T. (Ed.), *Neuroendocrinology of Reproduction, Physiology and Behaviour*. Plenum Press, New York, pp. 243–278

Feder, H. H. (1981b). Estrous cyclicity in mammals. In Adler, N. T. (Ed.), *Neuroendocrinology of Reproduction, Physiology and Behaviour*, Plenum Press, New York, pp. 279–348

Feder, H. H. (1981c). Hormonal actions on the sexual differentiation of the genitalia and the gonadotrophin–regulating systems. In Adler, N. T. (Ed.). *Neuroendocrinology of Reproduction, Physiology and Behaviour*. Plenum Press, New York, pp. 89–126

Felton, J. S., Kwan, T. C., Wuebbles, B. J. and Dobson, R. L. (1978). Genetic differences in polycyclic–aromatic–hydrocarbon metabolism and their effects on oocyte killing in developing mice. In Mahlum, D. D., Sikov, M. R., Hackett, P. L. and Andrew, F. D. (Eds), *Developmental Toxicology of Energy-related Pollutants*. US Department of Energy, Washington, D.C., pp. 15–26

Figá-Talamanca, I. (1984). Spontaneous abortions

among female industrial workers. *Int. Arch. Occup. Environ. Hlth*, **54**, 163–171

Finnegan, L. P. (1981). The effects of narcotics and alcohol on pregnancy and the new born. *Ann. N.Y. Acad. Sci.*, **362**, 136–137

Fitzhugh, O. G. (1968). Reproduction tests. In Boyland, E. and Goulding, R. (Eds), *Modern Trends in Toxicology*. Butterworth, London, pp. 75–85

Flamm, W. G. and Dunkel, V. C. (1989). FDA procedures and policies to estimate risks of injury to the male reproductive system. In Burger, E. J., Tardiff, R. G., Scialli, A. R. and Zenick, H. (Eds), *Sperm Measures and Reproductive Success*. Progress in Clinical and Biological Research, Vol. 302. Alan R. Liss, New York, pp. 21–29

Fleischer, S. and Packer, L. (1978). *Biomembranes. Part C. Biological Oxidations, Microsomal, Cytochrome P-450 and Other Hemoprotein Systems*. Methods of Enzymology, Vol. 52, Academic Press, New York

Fletcher, A. P. (1986). Drug induced endocrine dysfunction. In D'Arcy, P. F. and Griffin, J. P. (Eds), *Iatrogenic Diseases*, 3rd edn. Oxford University Press, Oxford, pp. 358–381

Frasier, S. D. (1973). Androgens and athletes. *Am. J. Dis. Child.*, **125**, 479–480

Friedman, J. M. (1988). Teratogen update: Anaesthetic agents. *Teratology*, **37**, 69–77

Fulroth, R., Phillips, B. and Durand, D. J. (1989). Perinatal outcome of infants exposed to cocaine and/or heroin in utero. *Am. J. Dis. Child.*, **143**, 905–910

Gaines, T. B. and Kimbrough, R. D. (1970). Oral toxicity of Mirex in adult and suckling rats. With notes on ultrastructure and liver changes. *Arch. Environ. Hlth*, **21**, 7–14

Gambrell, R. D. (1978). The prevention of endometrial cancer in post-menopausal women with progestogens. *Maturitas*, **1**, 107–112

Gans, B., Bahry, C. and Levie, B. (1963). Ovarian regeneration and pregnancy following massive radiotherapy for dysgerminoma. *Obstet. Gynecol.*, **22**, 596–600

Gardner, M. J., Snee, M. P., Hall, A. J., Powell, C. A., Downes, S. and Terrell, D. (1989). Results of case-control study of leukaemia and lymphoma among young people near Sellafield nuclear plant in West Cumbria. *Br. Med. J.*, **300**, 423–434

Gellert, R. J., Wallace, C. A., Weismeier, E. M. and Shuman, R. M. (1978). Topical exposure of neonates to hexachlorophene: long-standing effects on mating behaviour and prostatic development in rats. *Toxicol. Appl. Pharmacol.*, **43**, 339–349

Gibson, G. T., Baghurst, P. A. and Colley, D. P. (1983). Maternal alcohol, tobacco and cannabis consumption and outcome of pregnancy. *Aust. N.Z. J. Obstet. Gynaecol.*, **23**, 15–19

Gill, W. B. (1989). Effects on human males of in utero exposure to exogenous sex hormones. In Mori, T. and Nagasawa, H. (Eds), *Toxicity of Hormones in Perinatal Life*, CRC Press, Boca Raton, Florida, pp. 162–177

Gill, W. B., Schumacher, G. F. B., Bibbo, M., Straus, F. H.II and Schoenberg, H. W. (1979). Association of diethylstilbestrol exposure in utero with cryptorchidism, testicular hypoplasia and semen abnormalities. *J. Urol.*, **122**, 36–39

Goding, J. R. (1974). The demonstration that $PGF_{2\alpha}$ is the uterine luteolysin in the ewe. *J. Reprod. Fertil.*, **38**, 261–271

Gorski, R. A. (1971). Gonadalt hormones and the perinatal development of neuroendocrine functions. In Martini, C. and Ganong, W. F. (Eds), *Frontiers in Neuroendocrinology*. Oxford University Press, New York, London, Toronto, pp. 237–290

Green, S. (1985). Current status of bioassays in genetic toxicology—the dominant lethal assay. *Mutation Res.*, **154**, 49–67

Griffin, J. P. (1986). Drug-induced sexual dysfunction. In D'Arcy, P. F. and Griffin, J. P. (Eds), *Iatrogenic Diseases*, 3rd edn. Oxford University Press, Oxford, pp. 513–524

Gross, A., Fein, A., Serr, D. M. and Nebel, L. (1977). The effects of imuran on implantation and early embryonic development in rats. *Obstet. Gynecol.*, **50**, 713

Haney, A. F. (1987). Structural and functional consequences of prenatal exposure to diethylstipbestrol in women. In McLachan, J. A., Pratt, R. M. and Market, C. L. (Eds), *Developmental Toxicology: Mechanisms and Risks*. Banbury Report No 26. Cold Spring Harbor Laboratory, Cold Spring Harbor, N.Y., pp. 271–285

Hansen, L. G., Byerly, C. S., Metcalf, R. L. and Bevill, R. F. (1975). Effect of a polychlorinated biphenyl mixture on swine reproduction and tissue residues. *Am. J. Vet. Res.*, **36**, 23

Hansson, V., Aakvaag, A. and Purvis, K. (Eds) (1981). *First European Workshop on Molecular and Cellular Endocrinology of the Testis*. Scriptor, Copenhagen

Harlap, S. and Shiono, P. H. (1980). Alcohol, smoking and incidence of spontaneous abortions in the first and second trimester. *Lancet*, **2**, 173–176

Harrington, J. M., Stein, G. F., Rivera, R. V. and de Morales, A. V. (1978). The occupational hazards of formulating oral contraceptives—a survey of plant employees. *Arch. Environ. Hlth*, **33**, 12–15

Heap, R. B., Flint, A. P. and Gadsby, J. E. (1979). Role of embryonic signals in the establishment of pregnancy. *Br. Med. Bull.*, **35**, 129–135

Heinrichs, W. L. and Gadallah, M. (1983). Adverse effects of environmental agents on mammalian female reproduction. In Vouk, V. B. and Sheehan, P. J. (Eds), *Methods for Assessing the Effects of Chemicals on Reproductive Function*. John Wiley & Son, SCOPE, **20**, 125–133

Heinrichs, W. L. and Juchau, M. R. (1980). Extrahepatic drug metabolism: the gonads. In Gram, T. E.

(Ed.), *Extrahepatic Metabolism of Drugs and Other Foreign Compounds*. S.P. Medical and Scientific Books, New York, pp. 319–332

Heller, R. H. and Jones, H. W. (1964). Production of ovarian dysgenesis in the rat and human by busulphan. *Am. J. Obstet. Gynec.*, **25**, 85–90

Herbst, A. L., Hubby, N. M., Blough, R. R. and Azizi, F. (1980). A comparison of pregnancy experience in DES-exposed and DES-unexposed daughters. *J. Reprod. Med.*, **24**, 62

Herbst, A. L., Poskanser, D. C., Robboy, S. J., Friedlander, L. and Scully, R. E. (1975). Prenatal exposure to Stilbestrol: A prospective comparison of exposed female offspring with unexposed controls. *New Engl J. Med.*, **292**, 334–339

Herbst, A. L., Ulfelder, H. and Poskanser, D. C. (1971). Adenocarcinoma of the vagina. Association of maternal stilbestrol therapy with tumour appearance in young women. *New Engl J. Med.*, **284**, 878

Himelstein-Braw, R., Peters, H. and Faber, M. (1978). Morphological appearance of the ovaries of leukemic children. *Br. J. Cancer*, **38**, 82–87

Hollister, L. E. (1986). Health aspects of cannabis. *Pharmacol. Rev.*, **38** (1), 1–20

Huber, J. J. (1965). Some physiological effects of the insecticide kepone in the laboratory mouse. *Toxicol. Appl. Pharmacol.*, **7**, 516–524

Infante, P. F., Wagoner, J. K., McMichael, A. J., Waxweiler, R. J. and Falk, H. (1976). Genetic risks of vinyl chloride. *Lancet*, **1**, 734–735

Jick, H., Porter, J. and Morrison, A. S. (1977). Relation between smoking and age of natural menopause. *Lancet*, **1**, 1354–1355

Joffe, J. M. and Soyka, L. F. (1981). Effects of drug exposure on male reproductive processes and progeny. *Period. Biol.*, **83**, 351–362

John, J. A., Wroblewski, D. J. and Schwetz, B. A. (1984). Teratogenicity of experimental and occupational exposure to industrial chemicals. In Kalter, H. (Ed.), *Issues and Reviews in Teratology*, Vol. 2. Plenum Press, London, New York, pp. 267–324

Johnson, M. and Everitt, B. (1988). *Essential Reproduction*, 3rd edn. Blackwell, London

Jones, K. L. and Smith, D. W. (1975). The fetal alcohol syndrome. *Teratology*, **12**, 1–10

Karim, S. M. M. (1972). Physiological role of prostaglandins in the control of parturition and menstruation. *J. Reprod. Fertil. Suppl.*, **16**, 105

Katz, D. F., Andrew, J. B. and Overstreet, J. W. (1989). Biological basis of *in vitro* tests of sperm function. In Burger, E. J., Tardiff, R. G., Scialli, A. R. and Zenick, H. (Eds), *Sperm Measures and Reproductive Success*. Progress in Clinical and Biological Research, Vol. 302. Alan R. Liss, New York, pp. 95–103

Kaufman, R. H., Binder, G. L., Gray, P. M. and Adam, E. (1977). Upper genital tract changes associated with exposure *in utero* to diethylstilbestrol. *Am. J. Obstet. Gynecol.*, **128**, 51

Khera, K. S., Villeneuve, D. C., Terry, G., Panopopio, L., Nash, L. and Trivett, G. (1976). Mirex—a teratogenicity, dominant lethal and tissue distribution study in rats. *Fd Cosmet. Toxicol.*, **14**, 25–29

Kieffer, J. D. and Ketchel, M. (1970). Blockade of ovulation in the rat by ethanol. *Acta Endocrinol.*, **65**, 117

Kihlstrom, J. E., Lundberg, C., Orberg, J., Danielsson, P. O. and Sydhoff, J. (1975). Sexual functions of mice neonatally exposed to DDT or PCB. *Environ. Physiol. Biochem.*, **5**, 54

Kinsella, T. J. (1989). Effects of radiation therapy and chemotherapy on testicular function. In Burger, E. J., Tardiff, R. G., Scialli, A. R. and Zenick, H. (Eds), *Sperm Measures and Reproductive Success*. Progress in Clinical and Biological Research, Vol. 302. Alan R. Liss, New York, pp. 157–171

Kline, J. K. (1986). Maternal occupation: Effects on spontaneous abortions and malformations. *Occ. Med: State of the Art Rev.*, **1**, 381–403

Knill-Jones, R. R., Newman, B. J. and Spence, A. A. (1975). Anaesthetic practice and pregnancy. *Lancet*, **ii**, 807–809

Kolmodin, B., Azarnof, B. and Sjoqvist, F. (1969). Effect of environmental factors on drug metabolism decreased plasma half-life of antipyrine in workers exposed to chlorinated hydrocarbon insecticides. *Clin. Pharmacol. Therap.*, **10**, 638

Kolodny, R. C., Webster, S. K., Tullman, G. D. and Donrbush, R. I. (1979). Chronic marihuana use by women: menstrual cycle and endocrine findings. Paper presented by the New York Postgraduate Medical School, 2nd Annual Conference. *Marihuana*, 28–29 June 1979

Komisaruk, B. R., Terasawa, E. and Rodriguez-Sierra, J. F. (1981). How the brain mediates ovarian responses to environmental stimuli. In Adler, N. T. (Ed.), *Neuroendocrinology of Reproduction, Physiology and Behaviour*. Plenum Press, New York, London, pp. 349–376

Kornberg, A. (1980). *DNA Replication*. W. H. Freeman, San Francisco

Koyama, H., Wada, T., Nishizawa, Y., Iwanaga, T., Aoki, Y., Terasawa, T., Kosaki, G., Yamamoto, T. and Wasa, T. (1977). Cyclophosphamide induced ovarian failure and its therapeutic significance in patients with breast cancer. *Cancer*, **39**, 1403–1409

Kremer, J. and Jager, S. (1976). The sperm-cervical mucus test: a preliminary report. *Fertil. Steril.*, **27**, 335–337

Kumar, R., Biggart, J. D. and McEvoy, J. (1972). Cyclophosphamide and reproductive function. *Lancet*, **1**, 1212–1214

Lancranjan, I. (1972). Alteration of spermatic liquid in patients chronically poisoned by carbon disulphide. *Med. Lav.*, **63**, 29–33

Lancranjan, I., Popescu, H. I., Gavanescu, O., Klepsch, I. and Serbanescu, M. (1975). Reproductive ability of workmen occupationally exposed to lead. *Arch. Environ. Hlth*, **30**, 396–401

Leblanc, H. G., Lachlebin, C. L., Abu-Fadil, S. and Yen, S. S. C. (1976). Effects of dopamine infusion on pituitary hormone secretion in humans. *J. Clin. Endocrinol. Metab.*, **43**, 668

Lee, I. P. and Dixon, R. L. (1978). Factors influencing reproduction and genetic toxic effects on male gonads. *Environ. Hlth Perspect.*, **24**, 117–127

Lehmann, A. R. and Bridges, B. A. (1977). D.N.A. repair. *Essays Biochem.*, **13**, 71–119

Lemasters, G. K., Hagen, A. and Samuels, S. J. (1985). Reproductive outcomes in women exposed to solvents in 36 reinforced plastic companies. I. Menstrual dysfunction. *J. Occup. Med.*, **27**, 490–494

Lemasters, G. K., Samuels, S. J., Morrison, J. A. and Brooks, S. M. (1989). Reproductive outcomes of pregnant workers employed at 36 reinforced plastics companies. II. Lowered birthweight. *J. Occup. Med.*, **31** (2), 115–120

Lentz, R. D., Bergstein, J., Steffes, M. W., Brown, D. R., Prem, K., Michael, A. F. and Vernier, R. L. (1977). Postpubertal evaluation of gonadal function following cyclophosphamide therapy before and during puberty. *J. Pediatr.*, **91**, 385–394

Linder, R. E., Gaines, T. B. and Kimbrough, R. D. (1974). The effect of polychlorinated biphenyls in rat reproduction. *Fd Cosmet. Toxicol.*, **12**, 63

Lipshultz, L. I. and Howards, S. S. (1983). Evaluation of the subfertile man. In Lipshultz, L. I. and Howards, S. S. (Eds), *Infertility in the Male*. Churchill Livingstone, New York, pp. 187–206

Little, R. E. (1977). Moderate alcohol use during pregnancy and decreased infant birth weight. *Am. J. Publ. Hlth*, **67**, 1154–1156

Lobl, T. J. and Hafez, E. S. E. (1985). *Male Fertility and Its Regulation*. MTP, Lancaster, Boston

Lockey, J. E., Lemasters, G. and Keye, W. R. (1984). *Reproduction: The New Frontier in Occupational and Environmental Health Research*. Alan R. Liss, New York

Lotgering, F., Gilbert, R. D. and Longo, L. D. (1985). Maternal and fetal responses to exercise during pregnancy. *Physiol. Rev.*, **65** (1), 1–36

McCann, S. (1981). CNS control of the pituitary: neurochemistry of hypothalamic releasing and inhibitory hormones. In Adler, N. T. (Ed.), *Neuroendocrinology of Reproduction, Physiology and Behaviour*. Plenum Press, New York, pp. 427–450

McLachlan, J. A. and Dixon, R. L. (1977). Teratologic comparisons of experimental and clinical exposures to diethylstilboestrol. *Teratogen. Carcinogen. Mutagen.*, **7**, 377–389

McNatty, K. P., Hunter, W. M., McNeilly, A. S. and Sawers, R. S. (1975). Changes in the concentrations of pituitary and steroid hormones in the follicular fluid of human graaffian follicles throughout the menstrual cycle. *J. Endocrinol.*, **64**, 555–571

Mann, T. and Lutwak-Mann, C. (1981). *Male Reproductive Function and Semen*. Springer-Verlag, Berlin

Martin, R. H. (1985) Chromosomal abnormalities in human sperm. In Dellero, V. L., Voytek, P. E. and Hollaender, A. (Eds), *Aneuploidy, Etiology and Mechanisms*, Part 2: *Etiological Aspects of Human Aneuploidy*. Plenum Press, New York, pp. 91–102

Mattison, D. (1981). Effects of biologically foreign compounds on reproduction. In Abdul-Karim, R. W. (Ed.), *Drugs During Pregnancy: Clinical Prespectives*. G. F. Stickley, Philadelphia, pp. 101–125

Mattison, D. R. (1983). *Reproductive Toxicology*. Pregnancy Research Branch, National Institute of Child Health and Human Development, National Institutes of Health, Bethesda, Maryland

Mattison, D. R. and Ross, G. T. (1983). Laboratory methods for evaluating and predicting specific reproductive dysfunctions: oogenesis and ovulation. In Vouk, V. B. and Sheehan, P. J. (Eds), *Methods of Assessing the Effects of Chemicals on Reproductive Functions*. Scope 20, Wiley, Chichester, pp. 217–246

Mattison, D. R., Shiromizu, K. and Nightingale, M. S. (1983). Oocyte destruction by polycystic aromatic hydrocarbons. *Am. J. Industr. Med.*, **4**, 191–202

Mattison, D. R. and Thomford, P. J. (1989). Mechanisms of action of reproductive toxicants. In Working, P. K. (Ed.), *Toxicology of the Male and Female Reproductive Systems*, Hemisphere Publishing Corporation, New York, pp. 101–129

Metzler, M. and McLachan, J. A. (1978). Peroxidase-mediated oxidation, a possible pathway for metabolic activation of diethylstilbestrol. *Biochem. Biophys. Res. Commun.*, **85**, 874–884

Moor, R. M. and Warnes, G. M. (1979). Regulation of meiosis in mammalian oocytes. *Br. Med. Bull.*, **35**, 99–103

Murad, F. and Haynes, R. C. Jr (1985). Adenohypophyseal hormones and related substances. In Gilman, G. A., Goodman, L. S., Rall, T. W. and Murad, F. (Eds), *The Pharmacological Basis of Therapeutics*, 7th edn, Macmillan, London, New York, Toronto, pp. 1362–1388

Neal, R. A. (1980). Metabolism of toxic substances. In Doull, J., Klaassen, C. D. and Amdur, M. O. (Eds), *Casarett and Doull's Toxicology*, 2nd edn. Macmillan, New York, pp. 56–69

Nebert, D. W. (1981). Birth defects and the potential role of genetic differences in drug metabolism. In Bloom, A. D. and James, L. S. (Eds), *Birth Defects, Original Article Series*, vol. 17, Alan R. Liss, New York, pp. 51–70

Nordin, B. E. C., Horsman, F. L., Crilly, R. G., Marshall, D. H. and Simpson, M. (1980). Treatment of spinal osteoporosis in postmenopausal women. *Br. J. Med.*, **280**, 451–454

Oakberg, E. F. and Clark, E. (1964). Species comparisons of radiation response of the gonads. In Carlson, W. D. and Gassner, F. X. (Eds), *Effects of Ionizing*

Radiation on the Reproductive System. Pergamon Press, Oxford, pp. 11–24

O'Brien, P. C., Noller, K. L., Robboy, S. J., Barnes, A. B., Kaufman, R. H., Tilley, B. C. and Townesend, D. E. (1979). Vaginal epithelial changes in young women enrolled in the National co-operative Diethylstilboestrol Adenosis (DESAD) Project. *Obstet. Gynecol.*, **53**, 300–308

Ostrea, E. M. Jr and Chavez, C. J. (1979). Prenatal problems (excluding neonatal withdrawal) in maternal drug addiction: A study of 830 cases. *J. Pediatr.*, **94**, 292–295

Oullette, E. M., Rosett, H. L., Rosman, N. P. and Weiner, L. (1977). Adverse effects on offspring of material alcohol abuse during pregnancy. *New Engl. J. Med.*, **297**, 528–530

Overstreet, J. W. and Blazak, W. F. (1983). The biology of reproduction: an overview. *Am. J. Industr. Med.*, **4**, 5–15

Paganini-Hill, A., Ross, R. K., Gerkins, V. R., Henderson, B. E., Arthur, M. and Mack, T. M. (1981). Menopausal estrogen therapy and hip fractures. *Ann. Int. Med.*, **95**, 28–31

Page, E. W., Villee, C. A. and Villee, D. B. (Eds) (1981). *Human-Reproduction. Essentials of Reproductive and Perinatal Medicine*, 3rd edn. W. B. Saunders, Philiadelphia, London and Toronto

Pennisi, A. J., Gruskin, C. M. and Lieberman, E. (1975). Gonadal function in children with nephrosis treated with cyclophosphamide. *Am. J. Dis. Child.*, **129**, 315–318

Perry, J. S. (1971). *The Ovarian Cycles of Mammals.* University Reviews in Biology. Oliver and Boyd, Edinburgh

Peterson, R. C. (1980). *Maryvana Research Findings 1980.* National Institute on Drug Abuse Research Monograph Series, Dept, Health and Human Services Publication No (ADM) 80–1001. US Government Printing Office, Washington, D.C.

Porter, D. G. and Finn, C. A. (1977). The biology of the uterus. In Greep, R. O. and Koblinsky, M. A. (Eds), *Frontiers in Reproduction and Fertility Control*, Part 2. MIT Press, Cambridge, Mass., pp. 146–156

Procope, B. J. (1965). Effect of repeated increase of body temperature on human sperm cells. *Int. J. Fertil.*, **10**, 333–340

Psychoyos, A. (1962). A study on the hormonal requirements for the ovum implantation in the rat by means of delayed nidation-inducing substances (chlorpromazine, trifluoperazine). *J. Endocrinol.*, **27**, 337–343

Ratcliffe, J. M., Clapp, D. E., Schrader, S. M., Halperin, W. E., Turner, T. and Hornung, R. (1989). Semen quality in workers exposed to 2-ethoxyethanol. *Br. J. Industr. Med.*, **46**, 399–406

Ratcliffe, J. M., Schrader, S. M., Meinhardt, T. J., Steenland, K., Clapp, D. E. and Turner, T. (1985). *Semen Evaluation of Timber Fumigators Exposed to Ethylene Dibromide.* NIOSH Report TA 83–244; NIOSH, Cincinnati, Ohio

Ratcliffe, J. M., Schrader, S. M., Steenland, K., Clapp, D. E., Turner, T. and Hornung, R. (1987). Semen quality in papaya workers with long term exposure to ethylene dibromide. *Br. J. Industr. Med.*, **44**, 317–326

Reimers, T. J., Sluss, P. M., Goodwin, J. and Seidel, G. E. (1980). Bi-generational effects of 6-mercaptopurine on reproduction in mice. *Biol. Reprod.*, **22**, 367

Rich, K. A. and de Krester, D. M. (1977). Changes in FSH and LH in serum and ABP in the testis and epididymis of the rat following exposure of the testis to local heating. *Proc. Endocrine Soc. Aust.*, **20**, 43–47

Rich, K. A. and de Krester, D. M. (1979). Effect of fetal irradiation on testicular receptors and testosterone response to gonadotrophin stimulation in the rat. *Int. J. Androl.*, **2**, 343–352

Richardson, M. C. (1986). Hormonal control of ovarian luteal cells. *Oxf. Rev. Reprod. Biol.*, **8**, 321–378

Ringer, R. K., Averlich, R. J. and Zabik, M. (1972). Effects on dietary polychlorinated biphenyls on growth and reproduction in mink. *164th Natl Am. Chem. Soc. Meet.*, **12**, 149

Rogers, B. J. (1989). Examination of data from programs of *in vitro* fertilisation in relation to sperm integrity and reproductive success. In Burger, E. J., Tardiff, G., Scialli, A. and Zenick, H. (Eds), *Sperm Measures and Reproductive Success*. Progress in Clinical and Biological Research, Vol. 302. Alan R. Liss, New York, pp. 69–89

Rom, W. M. (1976). Effects of lead on the female and reproduction: a review. *Mt. Sinai J. Med.*, **43**, 542–552

Root, A. W., Reiter, E. O., Andriola, M. and Duckett, G. (1975). Hypothalamic pituitary function in the fetal alcohol syndrome. *J. Pediatr.*, **87**, 585–588

Rose, D. P. and Davis, R. E. (1977). Ovarian function in patients receiving adjuvant chemotherapy for breast cancer. *Lancet*, **1**, 1174–1176

Rosen, T. S. and Johnson, H. L. (1982). Children of methadone-maintained mothers. Follow up to 18 months of age. *J. Pediatr.*, **101**, 192–196

Rosenberg, M. J., Feldblum, P. J. and Marshall, E. G. (1987). Occupational influences on reproduction. A review of recent literature. *J. Occup. Med.*, **29** (7), 584–591

Ross, G. T. and Schreiber, J. R. (1978). The ovary. In Yen, S. S. C. and Jaffe, R. B. (Eds), *Reproductive Endocrinology*. W. B. Saunders, Philadelphia, London, Toronto, pp. 63–79

Russell, L. B., Selby, P. B., von Halle, E., Sheridan, W. and Valvolic, L. (1981). The mouse specific-locus test with agents other than radiations. Interpretation of data and recommendations for future research. *Mutation Res.*, **86**, 329–354

Russell, L. B. and Shelby, M. D. (1985). Tests for

heritable genetic damage and evidence of gonadal exposure in mammals. *Mutation Res.*, **154**, 69–84

Russell, W. L., Kelly, E. M., Hunsicker, P. R., Bangham, J. W., Maddux, S. C. and Phipps, E. L. (1979). Specific locus test shows ethyl nitrosurea to be most potent mutagen in the mouse. *Proc. Natl Acad. Sci. USA*, **76**, 5818–5819

Sadow, J. I. D., Gulamhusein, A. P., Morgan, M. J., Napralin, N. J. and Petersen, S. A. (1980). *Human Reproduction, an Integrated View*. Croom Helm, London

Safe, S. (1984). Polychlorinated biphenyls (PCBs) and polybrominated biphenyls (PBBs): Biochemistry, toxicology and mechanism of action. *CRC Crit. Rev. Toxicol.*, **13**, 319–395

Sanotskii, I. (1976). Aspects of the toxicology of chloroprene: immediate and long term effects. *Environ. Hlth Perspect.*, **17**, 85–93

Schardein, J. L. (1985). *Chemically Induced Birth Defects*. Marcel Dekker, New York, Basel

Schilsky, R. L., Sherins, R. J., Hubbard, S. M., Wesley, M. N., Young, R. C. and De Vita, V. T. (1981). Long term follow up of ovarian function in women treated with MOPP chemotherapy for Hodgkins Disease. *Am. J. Med.*, **71**, 552–556

Schrader, S. M., Ratcliffe, J. M., Turner, T. and Hornung, R. (1987). The use of new methods of semen analysis in the study of occupational hazards to reproduction: the example of ethylene dibromide. *J. Occup. Med.*, **29**, 963–966

Schulz, K. D., Schmidt-Rhode, P., Weymar, P., Kunzig, H.-J. and Geiger, W. (1979). The effect of combination chemotherapy on ovarian, hypothalamic and pituitary function in patients with breast cancer. *Arch. Gynecol.*, **227**, 293–301

Schulze, C. (1984). *Sertoli Cells and Leydig Cells in Man*. Advances in Embryology and Cell Biology No. 88. Springer-Verlag, Berlin

Setchell, B. P., Voglmayr, J. K. and Waites, G. M. H. (1969). A blood−testis barrier restricting passage from blood lymph into rete testis fluid but not into lymph. *J. Physiol.*, **200**, 73–85

Shalet, S. M., Beardwell, C. G., Jones, P. H. M. and Pearson, D. (1976). Ovarian failure following abdominal irradiation in childhood. *Br. J. Cancer*, **33**, 655–658

Shangold, M. M., Gatz, M. L. and Thysen, B. (1981). Acute effects of exercise on plasma concentrations of prolactin and testosterone in recreational women runners. *Fertil. Steril.*, **35**, 699–702

Smith, C. G. (1983). Reproductive toxicity: Hypothalamic-pituitary mechanisms. *Am. J. Industr. Med.*, **4**, 107–112

Smith, C. G., Besch, N. F. and Asch, R. H. (1980). Effects of marihuana on the reproductive system. In Thomas, J. A. and Singhal, R. (Eds), *Advances in Sex Hormone Research*, vol. 7. Schwarzenberg, Baltimore, Munich, pp. 273–294

Sobrinho, L. G., Levine, R. A. and DeConti, R. C. (1971). Amenorrhea in patients with Hodgkin's disease treated with anti-neoplastic agents. *Am. J. Obstet. Gynecol.*, **109**, 135–139

Spencer, F. (1982). An assessment of the reproductive toxic potential of Aroclor 1254 in female Sprague-Dawley rats. *Bull. Environ. Contam. Toxicol.*, **28**, 290

Speroff, L. (1981). Getting high on running. *Fertil. Steril.*, **36**, 149–151

Stenchever, M. A., Williamson, R. A., Leonard, J., Karp, L. E., Shy, K. and Smith, D. (1981). Possible relationship between in utero exposure to diethylstilbestrol exposure and male fertility. *Am. J. Obstet. Gynecol.*, **140**, 186–193

Stillman, R. J., Schinfeld, J. S., Schiff, I., Gelber, R. D., Greenberger, J., Larson, M., Jaffe, N. and Li, F. P. (1981). Ovarian failure in long-term survivors of childhood malignancy. *Am. J. Obstet. Gynecol.*, **139**, 62–66

Streissguth, A. P., Herman, C. S. and Smith, D. W. (1978). Intelligence, behaviour and dysmorphogenesis in the fetal alcohol syndrome: a report on 20 patients. *J. Pediatr.*, **92**, 363–367

Sullivan, F. M. (1988). Reproductive toxicity tests: retrospect and prospect. *Human Toxicol.*, **17**, 423–427

Sullivan, F. M. and Barlow, S. M. (1985). The relevance for man of animal data on reproductive toxicity of industrial chemicals. In *Prevention of Physical and Mental Congenital Defects*, Part B. *Epidemiology, Early Detection and Environmental Factors*. Progress in Clinical and Biological Research. Alan R. Liss, New York, pp. 301–305

Sullivan, F. M. and McElhatton, P. R. (1986). The teratogenic and other toxic effects of drugs on reproduction. In D'Arcy, P. F. and Griffin, J. P. (Eds), *Iatrogenic Diseases*, 3rd edn. Oxford University Press, pp. 400–479

Swerdloff, R. S. and de Kretser, D. M. (1983). Endocrine evaluation of the infertile male. In Lipshultz, L. and Howards, S. S. (Eds), *Infertility in the Male*. Churchill Livingstone, New York, pp. 207–216

Tabacova, S. (1986). Maternal exposure to environmental chemicals. *Neurotoxicology*, **7** (2), 421–440

Takizawa, K. and Mattison, D. R. (1983). Female reproduction. In Mattison, D. R. (Ed.), *Reproductive Toxicology*. Alan R. Liss, New York, pp. 17–30

Terjung, R. (1979). Endocrine response to exercise. *Exerc. Sport Sci. Rev.*, **7**, 153–180

Tomlin, P. J. (1979). Health problems of anaesthetists and their families in the West Midlands. *Br. Med. J.*, **1**, 1280–1281

Uldall, P. R., Kerr, D. N. S. and Tacchi, D. (1972). Sterility and cyclophosphamide. *Lancet*, **1**, 693–694

US FDA (1982). *Toxicological Principles for the Safety Assessment of Direct Food Additives and Color Additives Used in Food*. US Food and Drug Administration, Bureau of Foods USA

Van der Gulden, J. W. J. and Zielhuis, G. A. (1989). Reproductive hazards related to perchlorethylene. A Review. *Int. Arch. Occup. Environ. Hlth*, **61**, 235–242

Van Thiel, D. H., Gavaler, J. S. and Lester, R. (1978). Alcohol induced ovarian failure in the rat. *J. Clin. Invest.*, **61**, 624

Vessey, M. P., Wright, N. H., McPherson, K. and Wiggins, P. (1978). Fertility after stopping different methods of contraception. *Br. Med. J.*, **1**, 265

Vorherr, H., Messer, R. H., Vorherr, U. F., Jordan, S. W. and Kornfeld, M. (1979). Teratogenesis and carcinogenesis in rat offspring after transplacental and transmammary exposure to diethylstilbestrol. *Biochem. Pharmacol.*, **28**, 1865

Vouk, V. B. and Sheehan, P. J. (Eds) (1983). *Methods for Assessing the Effects of Chemicals on Reproductive Functions*. John Wiley, New York

Vuksanovic, M. M. (1966). Pregnancy following ovarian irradiation. *Am. J. Roentgenol. Radium Ther. Nucl. Med.*, **97**, 951–956

Wallach, R. C., Jerez, E. and Blinick, G. (1969). Pregnancy and menstrual function in narcotic addicts treated with methadone. The methadone maintenances treatment. *Am. J. Obstet. Gynecol.*, **105**, 1226–1229

Warburton, D., Stein, Z., Kline, J. and Susser, M. (1980). Chromosome abnormalities in spontaneous abortion; data from the New York study. In Porter, I. H. and Hook, E. B. (Eds), *Human Embryonic and Fetal Death*. Academic Press, New York, pp. 261–287

Ware, G. W. and Good, E. E. (1967). Effects of insecticides on reproduction in the laboratory mouse. II. Mirex, Telodrin and DDT. *Toxicol. Appl. Pharmacol.*, **10**, 54–61

Warne, G. L., Fairley, K. F., Hobbs, J. B. and Martin, F. I. R. (1973). Cyclophosphamide-induced ovarian failure. *New Engl J. Med.*, **289**, 1159–1162

Welch, R. M., Levin, W. and Conney, A. H. (1969). Estrogenic action of DDT and its analog. *Toxicol. Appl. Pharmacol.*, **14**, 358–367

Welch, R. M., Levin, W., Kuntzman, W., Jacobson, M. and Conney, A. H. (1971). Effect of halogenated hydrocarbon insecticides on the metabolism and uterotropic action of estrogens in rats and mice. *Toxicol. Appl. Pharmacol.*, **19**, 234–246

Westerholm, B. (1977). Sex hormones, anabolic agents and related drugs. In Dukes, N. M. G. (Ed.), *Side Effects of Drugs Annual*, Vol. 1. Excerpta Medica, Amsterdam, pp. 292–311

Whitehead, E. D. and Leiter, E. (1981). Genital abnormalities and abnormal semen analyses in males exposed to diethylstilbestrol (DES) in utero. *J. Urol.*, **125**, 47–51

Whitehead, M. T., Townsend, P. T., Pryse-Davies, J., Ryder, T. A. and King, R. J. B. (1981). Effects of estrogens and progestins on the biochemistry and morphology of the postmenopausal endometrium. *New Engl J. Med.*, **305**, 1599–1605

Whorton, D., Krauss, R. M., Marshall, S. and Milby, T. H. (1977). Infertility in male pesticide workers. *Lancet*, **ii**, 1259–1261

Wieland, W. E. and Yunger, M. (1970). Sexual effects and side effects of heroin and methadone. In *Proceedings, Third National Conference on Methadone Treatment*. Government Printing Office, Washington, D.C.

Winder, C. (1987). Reproductive effects of occupational exposures to lead: Policy consideration. *Neurotoxicology*, **8** (3), 411–420

Winters, S. J., Banks, J. L. and Loriaux, D. L. (1979). Cimetidine is an antiandrogen in the rat. *Gastroenterology*, **76**, 504–509

Woods, J. S. (1975). Drug effects on human sexual behaviour. In Woods, N. F. and Woods, J. S. (Eds), *Human Sexuality in Health and Illness*. Mosby, Chicago, pp. 175–191

Working, P. K. (1989). Germ cell genotoxicity: methods for assessment of DNA damage and mutagenesis. In Working, P. K. (Ed.), *Toxicology of the Male and Female Reproductive Systems*. Hemisphere Publishing Corporation, New York, pp. 231–255

Wudl, L. R. and Sherman, M. I. (1983). Effects of chemicals on reproductive functions of mammals: mechanisms of cell injury and adaptive responses. In Vouk, V. B. and Sheehan, P. J. (Eds), *Methods for Assessing the Effects of Chemicals on Reproductive Functions*. Wiley, New York, pp. 171–198

Wyrobek, A. (1989). Markers for measuring germinal genetic toxicity and heritable mutations in people. In *Biological Markers in Reproductive Toxicology*. National Research Council, National Academy Press, Washington, D.C., pp. 119–140

Wyrobek, A. J., Gordon, L. A., Burkhart, J. G., Francis, M. W., Kapp, R. W., Letz, G., Malling, H. V., Topham, J. C. and Whorton, M. D. (1983a). An evaluation of the mouse sperm morphology test and other sperm tests in nonhuman mammals. *Mutation Res.*, **115**, 1–72

Wyrobek, A. J., Gordon, L. A., Burkhart, J. G., Francis, M. W., Kapp, R. W., Letz, G., Malling, H. V., Topham, J. C. and Whorton, M. D. (1983b). An evaluation of human sperm as indicators of chemically induced alterations of spermatogenic function. *Mutation Res.*, **115**, 73–148

Yanagimachi, R. (1981). Mechanisms of fertilization in mammals. In Mastroianni, L. Jr and Biggers, J. D. (Eds), *Fertilization and Embryonic Development in Vitro*. Plenum Press, New York, pp. 81–182

Yen, S. S. C. (1978). Physiology of human prolactin. In Yen, S. S. C. and Jaffe, R. B. (Eds), *Reproductive Endocrinology*. W. B. Saunders, Philadelphia, pp. 152–170

Yen, S. S. C. and Lein, A. (1976). The apparent paradox of the negative and positive feedback control system on gonadotrophin secretion. *Am. J. Obstet. Gynecol.*, **126**, 942

Zanefeld, L. J. D. and Waller, P. (1989). Non hormonal mediation of male reproductive tract damage: data from contraceptive drug research. In Burger, E. J., Tardiff, R. G., Scialli, A. R. and Zenick, H. (Eds), *Sperm Measures and Reproductive Success*. Progress in Clinical and Biological Research, Vol. 302. Alan R. Liss, New York, pp. 129–149

Zielhuis, R. L., Stijkel, A., Verberk, M. M. and Van de Poel-Bot, M. (1984). *Health Risks to Female Workers in Occupational Exposure to Chemical Agents*. Springer-Verlag, Berlin

FURTHER READING

Barlow, S. M. and Sullivan, F. M. (1982). *Reproductive Hazards of Industrial Chemicals*. Academic Press, London

Olshan, A. F. and Faustman, E. M. (1993). Male-mediated developmental toxicity. *Reproductive Toxicology*, **7**, 191–202

Richardson, M. (1993). *Reproductive Toxicology*. VCH, Verlagsgese Hschaft, Weinheim

Scialli, A. R. and Zinaman, M. (1993). *Reproductive Toxicology and Infertility*. McGraw Hill, New York

Thomas, J. A. and Ballantyne, B. (1990). Occupational reproductive risks: sources, surveillance and testing. *Journal of Occupational Medicine*, **32**, 547–554

40 Developmental Toxicology

Rochelle W. Tyl

INTRODUCTION

Human concern with birth defects is as ancient as human awareness. Throughout the nineteenth century, the prevailing view was that 'maternal impressions', maternal experience during the pregnancy, directly affected the newborn. Teratology, the study of monsters ('terata'), was essentially an observational 'art' with perceived supernatural implications. The widespread acceptance of the basic concepts of genetics early in the twentieth century provided a scientific basis for causation of congenital defects. The role of environmental insult in the production of birth defects in mammals inexorably followed, e.g. ionizing radiation (Hipple and Pagenstrecher, 1907; Warkany and Schraffenberger, 1947), sex hormones (Lillie, 1917; Greene, 1939, 1940), dietary deficiencies (Hale, 1933, 1935), and chemicals (Gilman *et al.*, 1948). The supposed inviolate safety of the human conceptus was refuted by German measles (rubella) epidemics in Australia in 1941 (Gregg, 1941) and in the USA in 1964 (Warkany, 1971) which resulted in thousands of children born with cataracts, deafness, and congenital heart disease. The thalidomide 'epidemic' in the late 1950s and early 1960s (Lenz, 1961, 1962; McBride, 1961), involving at least 8000 malformed children in 28 countries, confirmed the vulnerability of the human conceptus to environmental insult, especially in the first trimester of pregnancy, and precipitated worldwide concern for the safety of the unborn and the role of governmental intervention to ensure appropriate testing of drugs and other xenobiotics in pregnant mammals (Goldenthal, 1966; Wilson, 1979; Kelsey, 1982).

The early term for the study of birth defects, teratology, has been supplanted by a more general term, developmental toxicology, to enable inclusion of a more diverse spectrum of adverse developmental outcomes (which may be separate and distinct in aetiology or the result of a continuum of response) and to make overt the recognition that specific results of insult in one species

may not be the same in other species, including humans.

Developmental toxicity may be currently defined as any structural or functional alteration, reversible or irreversible, caused by environmental insult, which interferes with homeostasis, normal growth, differentiation, development, and/or behaviour. The targets for such insult(s) include the fertilized egg or zygote prior to implantation, or prior to the establishment of the three primary germ layers, the embryo during the period of major organ formation (i.e. organogenesis), the foetus in the post-embryonic period of histogenesis and the neonate or postnatal offspring, occurring or expressed through the postnatal period until sexual maturity (Tyl, 1987). The expressions of developmental toxicity encompass death, frank structural malformations, functional deficits and/or developmental delays (Wilson, 1973; Johnson and Christian, 1984). The vulnerability of the conceptus is viewed as due to qualitative or quantitative characteristics of both structure and functions. (1) It is composed of a small number of rapidly dividing undifferentiated cells, with absent or limited metabolic capabilities to alter or detoxify xenobiotics, repair lesions, etc. (2) There is the necessity for precise temporal and spatial sequencing of specific cell numbers and types, as well as specific cell products, for normal differentiation, including programmed cell death. (3) Sensitivities of certain cell types to certain insults may be unique to specific periods of cell movement, induction or differentiation (i.e. transient vulnerability during the period of formation of tissues or organs). (4) The immuno-surveillance system (to provide recognition of 'self' and detection of xenobiotics or lesions) is absent or immature in the prenatal or perinatal individual (Wolkowski-Tyl, 1981; Tyl, 1987).

Governmental regulation of the evaluation of test agents for developmental toxicity by formal testing guidelines and rules began soon after the worldwide thalidomide disaster by a letter from the Chief of the Drug Review Branch, US Food and Drug Administration (FDA), sent on

1 March 1966 to all corporate medical directors (Goldenthal, 1966), establishing Guidelines for Reproductive Studies for Safety Evaluation of Drugs for Human Use. These guidelines were promulgated 'as a routine screen for the appraisal of safety of new drugs for use during pregnancy and in women of childbearing potential.' Three phases or segments were proposed: Segment I, Study of Fertility and General Reproductive Performance, to provide information on breeding, fertility, nidation, parturition, neonatal effects and lactation (see Chapters 39 and 41); Segment II, Teratological Study, to provide information on embryotoxicity and teratogenicity; and Segment III, Perinatal and Postnatal Study, to provide information on late foetal development, labour and delivery, neonatal viability, and growth and lactation (US FDA, 1966). See Chapter 41.

Segment II testing guidelines are currently followed by FDA (since 1966), US Environmental Protection Agency (US EPA), Toxic Substances Control Act (TSCA) (US EPA, 1985b, 1987, 1989), Federal Insecticide, Fungicide and Rodenticide Act (FIFRA) (US EPA, 1982, 1984a, 1989), and US EPA Guidelines for the Health Assessment of Suspect Developmental Toxicants (1984b, 1986, 1989). International regulations also followed suit: Organization for Economic Cooperation and Development (OECD, 1981), United Kingdom, (1974) and Japan (1984).

In brief, the Segment II study consists of exposure of a pregnant rodent species (rats or mice) and a non-rodent species (usually rabbits) to the test agent during organogenesis, sacrifice of the maternal animals 1–2 days prior to the date of expected parturition, caesarean delivery of the gravid uterus, and thorough evaluation of the foetuses by examination of external, visceral (including craniofacial) and skeletal structures.

STANDARD SEGMENT II TESTING PROTOCOL

All current testing guidelines call for the use of a rodent and a non-rodent species. The rodent of choice is usually the rat: the CD (Sprague–Dawley) outbred albino, the Fischer 344 inbred albino, the Wistar outbred albino and the Long-Evans white and black hooded, and, less often,

the mouse: the CD-1 (Swiss) outbred albino, the non-Swiss outbred albino, the Swiss–Webster outbred albino or, rarely, the B_6C_3F black hybrid (any results in this hybrid are compounded by the segregating F_2 genotypes and phenotypes of the offspring). Both species satisfy the need for a small mammalian species with known, and relatively straightforward, husbandry requirements, short pregnancy, high fertility, large numbers of offspring, a low background incidence of spontaneous malformations and a reasonably well-known embryology. The mouse is the rodent of choice only when there is a good reason not to use the rat (i.e. metabolic differences which make the mouse a more appropriate surrogate for humans for a particular test agent). The rabbit of choice is the New Zealand White albino or Dutch Belted black and white. The rabbit is not a rodent; mice and rats belong to the order Rodentia, rabbits to the order Lagomorpha. The requirement for its use is predicated on the awareness that it was the only common test mammal in use in the 1960s which responded to thalidomide and, hopefully, would have indicated the prenatal risk to humans, and on the need to distinguish between agents with specific or unique species specificity (i.e. a rodent-specific teratogen) and those with more universal effects, presumably then also a greater potential risk to human development.

The animals are purchased from a reputable supplier, housed appropriately (light cycle, temperature, relative humidity, illumination, ventilation, noise levels, sanitation) with suitable caging, bedding (if used), certified food, and analysed potable water; they are free of intercurrent disease and of appropriate age and weight (see NIH Guide, 1985, for specific animal care and use requirements). The animals should be held for an acclimatization or quarantine period to adjust to husbandry procedures and to allow for evaluation of health status; i.e. viral serology, physical examination, check for intestinal parasites, histopathology of selected organs.

Rats and mice may be purchased timed-mated or mated in-house using breeding colony males of the same test strain. Rats are usually mated 1:1 (one male:one female); mice are mated 1:1 or 1:2. A 1:1 mating is preferred with the male used only once per study so that he contributes to the parentage of only one litter; if he is used more than once, he should not be represented more than once per dose group, in case he is responsible for the production of congenital malformations. Female mice become acyclic and anovulatory in the absence of a male (ovulation and oestrus cyclicity are triggered by a male pheromone present in urine) and may be primed prior to mating by close proximity to male mice (Whitten, 1956). Rabbits may be purchased timed-mated or mated in-house by natural mating or by artificial insemination (both usually after hormonal priming), with semen for artificial insemination collected from male breeders using an artificial vagina and a teaser female (Bredderman *et al.*, 1964) or electro-ejaculation, the latter being less humane. Logistical restrictions on the size of the male rabbit breeding colony may necessitate a given male siring more than one litter per study, or per dose group; in this case, he should be represented in all groups and no more than twice per group. Obviously, records of the identity of parentage must be scrupulously kept.

Rodents are usually housed overnight and females examined in the morning for evidence of a copulatory event. Mice are inspected for the presence of a retained vaginal copulatory plug, which is the product of the male copulatory gland and seminal vesicles or vesiculating glands at copulation. The copulatory plug in rats usually dries, shrinks, and falls out of the vaginal cavity within 6–10 h after copulation, so rats are examined by vaginal lavage or smear for the presence of vaginal sperm, or for a dropped plug if rats are housed in wire-bottom cages with a pan underneath; a retained copulatory plug may also occasionally be observed (Hafez, 1970). The day of observed copulation is usually designated gestational day (gd) 0, or less often, gd 1.

The current guidelines call for at least 20 rodent litters and at least 12 rabbit litters per group and at least four treatment groups, with three agent-exposed groups and a concurrent vehicle control group. The performing laboratory must know the in-house pregnancy rate of inseminated rabbits and sperm- or plug-positive rodents to determine the number of mated animals to put in the study to obtain at least the minimum numbers of litters required per group. Multiple breeding days are usually required to obtain the requisite number of inseminated rodents and rabbits and to allow a manageable number of animals on each necropsy day; this latter consideration is based on the type of evaluations to be done and the number of

technical staff. On each gd 0, inseminated animals are placed on study and assigned to groups; all groups should be represented each day, if possible, with approximately equal numbers per group per day. The animals may be randomly assigned or assigned by a stratified randomization procedure, with stratification by gd 0 body weight. Maternal gd 0 body weights should be equivalent across all groups in terms of group means, measures of variance such as standard deviation or standard error, and range.

The period of exposure of the maternal organism to the test agent is usually during the period of major organogenesis. This corresponds to gd 6–15 for rodents and gd 6–18 (US EPA, TSCA) or gd 7–19 (US EPA, FIFRA) for rabbits. This period of dosing, commencing after implantation and formation of the three primary germ layers (ectoderm, endoderm and mesoderm), continuing during formation of the major organ systems, and ending at the closure of the secondary palate, corresponds to approximately gd 8–60 in the human. It was specifically chosen to preclude effects on implantation so there would be conceptuses to evaluate and to maximize the chances of inducing and detecting structural changes in the conceptuses. The possible effects of the test agent on the reproductive and developmental processes prior to organogenesis are evaluated in Segment I or multigeneration studies discussed elsewhere in this book. This dosing period also precludes induction of maternal metabolizing enzymes prior to the presence of implanted conceptuses and allows for a postexposure recovery period prior to scheduled sacrifice close to term. Variations in the exposure period include exposure from implantation to scheduled sacrifice with no recovery period; exposure during the entire gestational period, gd 0 to term sacrifice; or exposure beginning prior to gd 0. These latter extended exposure periods may be useful and appropriate if the test agent, or route of administration, results in slow and/or limited systemic absorption and therefore delayed attainment of steady state or maximal blood levels in the maternal organism. Under these circumstances, the usual dosing period could result in the conceptuses being exposed to less than maximum levels during some or most of organogenesis and the misleading conclusion of little or no developmental toxicity (cf. Tyl *et al.*, 1993). Extended exposure periods may also be called for if bioaccumulation of or cumulative toxicity from parent compound or metabolites is an important aspect of known or potential human risk.

The guidelines specify the preferred route of administration as gavage (orogastric intubation) to deliver the largest possible bolus dose to maximize the potential of the test agent to cause maternal and developmental toxicity, i.e. 'worst case scenario'. Important considerations for gavage dosing include choice of vehicle (it should be innocuous and capable of maintaining the test agent in a stable homogeneous suspension or solution), use of dosing needle or catheter, dosing volume, and timing of dose to prefasted animals or animals allowed *ad libitum* feed and water. Use of other routes to simulate possible human exposure situations is becoming increasingly popular and is acceptable if scientifically defensible. These alternative routes include dosed feed, with considerations such as *ad libitum* or restricted availability, palatability, use of a solvent or vehicle, administration of microencapsulated material or capsules for larger animals; dosed in water with considerations of selected duration of availability and palatability; inhalation by whole body or nose-only exposure, the latter to preclude grooming and inadvertent ingestion or possible percutaneous absorption, and duration of daily exposures; cutaneous application with considerations of location and size of application site, occlusion or non-occlusion of application site, collaring, implications of localized skin irritation and slow systemic absorption (Francis and Kimmel, 1989; Kimmel and Francis, 1990; Tyl *et al.*, 1993); injection by intravenous, subcutaneous, intraperitoneal, intramuscular routes, or subcutaneous insertion (for implants or for minipumps for continuous infusion).

The extent of data collected in the in-life phase of the study on the responses of the maternal organism currently ranges from relatively minimal to very thorough. The rationale for minimal data collection usually is that other studies, for example those employing 14- to 28-day repeated dosing, have already provided information on adult toxicity including in-life parameters such as mortality, body weights, weight gain, clinical signs of toxicity, food and/or water consumption, etc. However, these other studies may not have employed females and never, intentionally, use pregnant animals. Pregnancy *per se* causes many physiological changes, which may alter over the duration of the pregnancy (Warshaw, 1977; Folb and Dukes, 1990). These changes include alterations in gastrointestinal function which may affect absorption rates of chemicals in the stomach and/or intestine, and ventilatory changes which may modify pulmonary uptake, absorption and/or elimination of chemicals with a 20–30 per cent increase in maternal oxygen consumption and greater oxygen debt after physical activity. Changes also occur in the cardiovascular system that alter haemodynamics (there is a 30–40 per cent increase in blood volume and a 33 per cent decrease in erythrocytes) and alter body water compartments which may influence distribution and elimination of chemicals. Plasma components also change, e.g. considerable alterations in plasma proteins, free fatty acids and other endogenous substances with roles in chemical binding, transport and disposition, decreases in plasma albumin in the first half of the pregnancy. If the chemical binds to albumin, the fall in albumin concentration capacity of a given plasma volume increases the concentration of the unbound or free form of the chemical and raises the apparent volume of distribution of the chemical. There are also decreases in plasma protein binding of chemicals especially in the last third of the pregnancy, with increases in the unbound chemical fraction (e.g. for diazepam, valproic acid, phenytoin, propanolol, etc.). Renal elimination is also normally enhanced and hepatic elimination may be modified, affecting xenobiotic elimination (Warshaw, 1977, Folb and Dukes, 1990).

Maternal data to be collected from Segment II studies are presented in Table 1. This list is modified from EPA guidelines (US EPA, 1984b, 1986, 1989) and also represents a consensus of a minimal list developed at a US EPA-sponsored workshop on Evaluation of Maternal and Developmental Toxicity held in 1986 (Kimmel *et al.*, 1987a and b; Schwetz and Tyl, 1987). Improvement on the presented list would include more frequent body weights during the dosing period, and weight change calculations, preferably daily, to detect early, possibly transient treatment-related effects; more frequent body weights, and weight changes, during the postexposure period to detect effects continued from the dosing period (e.g. body weights 24 h after last dose, and at least midway during the postdose period) and possible rebound and recovery. Food and/or water consumption frequency as described above

Table 1 Maternal endpoints of toxicity in Segment II developmental toxicity studies[a]

Mortality[b]
No. aborted (rabbits)
No. delivered early

No. (%) pregnant at sacrifice (includes all dams with implants)
No. (%) with live litters[c]
No. with totally non-live litters[d]

Body weights (minimal list)
   Gestational day (gd) 0
   First day of dosing
   24 h after last dosing
   Sacrifice day
   Corrected (or absolute) body weight (body weight at sacrifice minus gravid uterine weight)

Body weight changes
   Throughout gestation (gd 0 or exposure onset to sacrifice)
   Pre-exposure period (gd 0 to exposure onset)
   Exposure period
   Postexposure period (end of exposure to sacrifice)
   Corrected (or absolute) maternal weight (body weight change throughout gestation minus gravid uterine weight)

Food and water consumption (g/dam/day and/or g/kg/day)[e]

Clinical observations (from gd 0 to sacrifice)
   Incidence of clinical signs by dam, by gestational day and by dose group
   Recorded at and after dosing
   Findings at scheduled sacrifice (gross lesions)

Gravid uterine weight at sacrifice (includes all with implants)
   Apparent nongravid uteri stained for detection of early resorption sites[f]

Organ weights at sacrifice (e.g. liver, kidneys, spleen, etc.)
   Absolute
   Relative to corrected body weight and/or to brain weight.

[a] Source: table modified from EPA draft document (US EPA, 1984b) and from Schwetz and Tyl (1987).
[b] No. pregnant females dead/no. pregnant females on study; data from non-pregnant females should not be included in data analyses.
[c] Number of dams with one or more live foetuses at scheduled sacrifice.
[d] Litters with all implantations present as resorptions (early, middle and/or late) and/or dead foetuses at scheduled sacrifice.
[e] If the administration of test chemical is by dosed feed or dosed water, then the amount of chemical consumed may be determined, in mg/kg/day.
[f] Salewski (1964) and Dey (1989).

for body weights would enhance sensitivity for detection of toxicity, and aid in the interpretation of weight loss or reduced weight gain. Additional evaluations of physiological and/or biochemical status should be performed on study animals during and after the treatment period, such as more detailed behavioural evaluation, e.g. functional observational battery (FOB) (Irwin, 1968; Moser *et al.*, 1988), and specific non-invasive behavioural tests (e.g. motor activity). Clinical pathology may be appropriate in satellite or study females during the exposure period as well as at termination, such as haematology and clinical chemistry (RBC, WBC differential count, blood gases, enzyme assays for liver function, acetylcholinesterase if appropriate), and urinalysis. These tests may duplicate those performed in other studies, but pregnant animals may respond quantitatively or qualitatively differently (*vide supra*), and these data will be critical in interpretation of any observed developmental toxicity.

The concern for and emphasis on thorough evaluation of the maternal organism is based on the need to determine, when study results are interpreted, whether the maternal toxicity *per se* is responsible for the observed embryo/foetal results (Kavlock *et al.*, 1985; Chernoff *et al.*, 1989). Khera (1984, 1985) has identified a number of foetal malformations in rodents and rabbits which are observed in the presence of maternal toxicity, regardless of the agent, route or dose, with the clear implication that the maternal toxicity is the cause of the developmental toxicity, not the test agent. Mechanistic studies have also implicated the compromised status of the maternal organism as the cause for the adverse embryo/foetal outcome for drugs. For example, elevation of endogenous corticosteroids in mice, as a result of maternal stress irrespective of the source, results in cleft palate in offspring from susceptible strains (Barlow *et al.*, 1975, 1980; Hemm *et al.*, 1977); hypercapnia (elevated blood CO_2) in mice has been proposed as the cause of forelimb ectrodactyly in mice exposed to acetazolamide (Weaver and Scott, 1984a, b; Holmes *et al.*, 1988) and bradycardia (slowed heart rate) in mice from phenytoin administration has been suggested as the cause of cleft lip/palate in offspring (Millicovsky and Johnston, 1981; Watkinson and Millicovsky, 1983). In addition, maternal anaemia from diflunisal administration in rabbits has been shown to be the cause of skeletal defects in offspring (Clark *et al.*, 1984), maternal inanition (reduced food and water intake) in rabbits exposed to norfloxacin is the cause of the deaths and reduced body weights in the offspring (Clark *et al.*, 1986), and maternal uterine ischaemia (obstruction of uterine arterial blood flow) from hydroxyurea administration in rabbits has been shown to be the cause of embryo/foetal haemorrhages (Millicovsky and DeSesso, 1980a, b; Millicovsky *et al.*, 1981). For rats, hypokalaemia (reduced blood potassium) from indacrinone exposure has been shown to cause the observed foetal skeletal defects (Robertson *et al.*, 1981) and renal toxicity in rats from mercuric chloride exposure may be the cause of hydrocephalus in the offspring (da Costa e Silva *et al.*, 1984; Holt and Webb, 1988) If maternal toxicity *per se*, including even 'stress' from restraint, for example, is the cause of the developmental toxicity, then the classification of the test agent as a teratogen may be erroneous (Khera, 1984, 1985).

In addition, maternal toxicokinetics and metabolism of the test agent is essential to characterize the conditions under which the toxicity to dam or conceptuses is observed; these conditions include evidence of systemic exposure, blood levels of parent compound and/or metabolite(s), identification of metabolites, bioavailability, half-life,

evidence for or against bioaccumulation, etc. This last evaluation is specifically emphasized in testing guidelines suggested by a US EPA-sponsored work group concerned with studies utilizing the cutaneous route of exposure, mainly because of the anticipated slow (or no) absorption of test material across the intact skin and therefore the need to assess whether the route is indeed appropriate (Francis and Kimmel, 1989; Kimmel and Francis, 1990). The reality is that this information is necessary for studies by any route to extrapolate results from one species to another and for human risk assessment, i.e. the handling of the test agent by the test species must be characterized so that one can say that, for a specific test agent, maternal and/or developmental toxicity occurs in the presence of the parent compound or identified metabolite(s) at specific blood levels for a specified duration, with the expectation that another species that produces the same metabolite(s) at comparable levels for comparable duration will exhibit the same or similar toxicities. In the absence of metabolic information, one cannot assess whether the test animal is an appropriate surrogate for humans for specific test agents. At necropsy of maternal animals, the same additional endpoints should be assessed, to characterize the status of the test animals after the recovery period. Histopathology of target organ(s) and organ function tests may also be appropriate.

Reproductive and embryo/foetal data to be collected from Segment II studies are presented in Table 2. Again, this list is modified from the EPA draft document (US EPA, 1984b) and thoroughly assesses two of the four embryo/foetal endpoints: death and structural malformations, and also assesses developmental delays, but only in terms of delays in growth such as reduced body weight, reduced crown–rump length, and delays in structural development, such as reduced ossification relative to concurrent and historical control foetuses (usually designated as variations), especially in those skeletal districts that ossify late in prenatal development (Aliverti *et al.*, 1979). Double-staining of foetuses with alizarin red S for ossified bone and alcian blue for cartilaginous bone (Marr *et al.*, 1988, 1989) provides information on the status of bone not yet ossified, which may impact on the interpretation of the finding as a skeletal malformation or permanent skeletal variation (when there is no cartilage in a short bone or

Table 2 Reproductive and embryo/foetal endpoints of toxicity in Segment II developmental toxicity studies[a]

(1) All litters

    No. ovarian corpora lutea (CL)/dam
    No. uterine implantation sites/dam
    % Preimplantation loss: $\dfrac{(CL - Implantations)}{CL} \times 100$

    No. (%) resorptions/litter (early, mid and late, separated and pooled)
    No. (%) litters with resorptions
    No. (%) foetal deaths/litter
    No. (%) nonlive (foetal deaths plus resorptions) implants/litter
    No. (%) litters with nonlive implants
    % Postimplantation loss: $\dfrac{(Implantations - Live\ foetuses)}{Implantations} \times 100$

    No. (%) affected (nonlive plus malformed[b]) implants/litter
    No. (%) litters with affected implants

(2) Litters with live foetuses

    No. litters with live foetuses
    No. live foetuses/litter
    No. males/litter
    No. females/litter
    Sex ratio (% males)
    Foetal body weight/litter (all foetuses, male, females)
    Foetal crown–rump length/litter (all foetuses, males, females)
    Externally malformed and variant foetuses/litter
    Viscerally malformed and variant foetuses/litter (including craniofacial malformations)
    Skeletally malformed and variant foetuses/litter
    No. (%) malformed and variant foetuses/litter[b]
    No. (%) litters with malformed and variant foetuses[b]
    No. (%) malformed and variant males/litter[b]
    No. (%) malformed and variant females/litter[b]
    Incidence of individual malformations[c] (by foetuses, by litters and by dose)
    Incidence of individual variations[c] (by foetuses, by litters and by dose)
    Individual foetuses and their malformations and variations

[a] Source: table modified from EPA draft document (US EPA, 1984b).
[b] Malformed or variant includes foetuses with one or more malformations or variations (external, visceral and/or skeletal).
[c] A foetus may be represented more than once if it exhibited more than one category of malformations and/or variations.

for a missing bone, so no subsequent growth, ossification, or correction would be anticipated) versus a variation or transient delay in ossification (where there is cartilage with anticipated subsequent growth, ossification and possible correction).

There is apparent potential for extensive remodelling of the skeletal system in the postnatal period; extra ribs become vertebral arches (Wickramarantne, 1988; Chernoff, 1990), fused ribs and other skeletal malformations disappear prior to sexual maturity (Marr *et al.*, 1990, 1992). This plasticity of the skeletal system, if confirmed, will require a change in current perception of a malformation, or a wholesale revision of the current classification of morphological findings in term foetuses. The current definition of a malformation specifies a permanent morphological change which is incompatible with or detrimental to postnatal survival, normal growth and development. Short ribs, extra ribs, fused ribs, alterations in sternebrae (which fuse to form the sternum), alterations in vertebral centra and arches are currently designated malformations or variations depending on the laboratory; if these changes do not persist, their designation could change. The reverse situation is also true; i.e. findings commonly designated as variations, usually delays, in term foetuses may, in fact, sometimes develop into findings designated as malformations in postnatal life. For example, a dilated renal pelvis (reduced renal papilla) may or may not be the precursor of hydronephrosis, and dilated lateral ventricles of the foetal cerebral hemispheres may be the precursor to hydrocephaly in the postnatal organism. With strictly limited evaluations of term foetuses, 'frozen in time', there is no way to project the postnatal consequences of the initial findings. In addition, the term evaluation is based on structure; if the lungs, or kidneys, etc., are in the right location, the right size, shape and colour under a dissecting microscope, they are designated as normal; there is no assessment of microscopic integrity or of function. Additional evaluations of term foetuses should perhaps include biochemical assessment of organ function (Kavlock *et al.*, 1982), histological examination of structure, as well as postnatal assessment of the reversibility of detected structural lesions and of the structural and functional sequelae of the prenatal insult. The implications of this additional work, in terms of cost, time, etc., to evaluate even one chemical formulation in one species for developmental toxicity are enormous!

RANGE-FINDING STUDIES

Current regulatory requirements mandate observable maternal toxicity at the top dose but with constraints on the severity of the observed toxicity, e.g. no more than 10 per cent mortality, and with obvious constraints on the severity of the developmental toxicity. Thus, if there is extensive embryofoetal death, there will be no foetuses to evaluate for the other endpoints such as deficits, delays or malformations. Therefore, dose-setting is a critical component of the study design. Information from other types of studies, such as acute LD_{50} studies, involving only one dose to each animal, 14-day repeated dosing studies, or more lengthy studies, may be useful, but they do not involve females in some cases and never involve pregnant females. The state of pregnancy, *per se*, may affect the response to environmental insult, ameliorating or exacerbating the observed toxicity. There is no way, *a priori*, of anticipating the direction or extent of the change. Range-finding studies with pregnant animals should be employed to establish appropriate dose levels for the definitive developmental toxicity study.

Range-finding studies typically involve fewer animals per group (usually from five to ten) and more groups (at least four agent-exposed and up to eight or nine if necessary) than in a definitive study. Mating, assignment to the study on gd 0, dosing route, duration, and maternal in-life parameters (body weights, clinical observations, food and/or water consumption, etc.) are the same as in the definitive study. The maternal information obtained will enable selection of appropriate doses with and without maternal toxicity, for the definitive study. The termination of the in-life phase differs among practicing developmental toxicologists and laboratories: some studies terminate immediately after the last exposure so there is no maternal recovery period, and although a thorough maternal examination is performed at necropsy, only gravid uterine weight is taken and no information is collected on number or status of conceptuses. Some studies concluding at term, as in the definitive study, have maternal examination but with varying evaluations on the conceptuses ranging from (1) gravid uterine weight only; (2) gravid uterine weight plus status of conceptuses only (live, dead, resorptions); (3) gravid uterine weight, status of conceptuses and foetal body weights only, but no sex determination or examination of foetuses; (4) gravid uterine weight, status of conceptuses, foetal weights, sex and external examination (including examination for cleft palate) only; or (5) a complete evaluation of the products of conception, including external, visceral and skeletal evaluation of foetuses.

Because the objective of a range-finding study is to set doses based on maternal and usually some aspect of developmental toxicity, the most common study design is in-life procedures as described above until term and evaluation of conceptuses through external examination of foetuses. The liability of a thorough evaluation of foetuses is that with a small number of maternal animals per group, fully resorbed litters, malformations, small-for-age low body weight, so-called 'runt', foetuses, may occur spontaneously and markedly skew the results, especially if they occur in the vehicle control group (the basis for comparison) or in the high dose group, when the findings may not be, in fact, treatment- or dose-related. The liability of too cursory an evaluation of conceptuses is the risk of missing reductions in foetal body weight, a very sensitive indicator of developmental toxicity or other embryo/foetal effects, and therefore setting the lowest dose too high for the definitive study and not achieving a 'no observable adverse effect level' (NOAEL) for developmental toxicity.

STATISTICAL ANALYSES OF MATERNAL AND DEVELOPMENTAL TOXICITY DATA

As part of protocol development, the choice of statistical analyses should be made *a priori* although specific additional analyses may be appropriate once the data are collected. The unit of comparison is the pregnant female or the litter and *not* individual foetuses as only the dams are independently and randomly assorted into dose groups (Weil, 1970). The foetus is not an independent unit and cannot be randomly distributed to groups. Intralitter interactions are common for a number of parameters, e.g. foetal weight or malformation incidence. Two types of data are collected: ordinal/discrete data which are essentially present or absent (yes or no) such as incidence of maternal deaths, abortions, early deliveries, clinical signs, and incidence of foetal malformations or variations; and continuous data such as maternal body weights, weight changes, food and/or water consumption, organ weights (absolute or relative to body or brain weight) and foetal body weights per litter. For both kinds of data, three types of statistical analyses are performed. Tests for trends are available and appropriate to identify treatment-related changes in the direction of the data (increases or decreases), overall tests are performed for detecting significance among groups, and specific pairwise comparison tests (when the overall test is significant) to the concurrent vehicle control group values are the critical endpoint to identify statistically significant effects relative to the concurrent vehicle control group.

For ordinal data, the tests most commonly used are the Test for Linear Trend on Proportions, the chi-square (χ^2) Test for Independence (the overall test among all groups), and Fisher's exact test (if χ^2 is significant) for pairwise comparisons (Sokal and Rohlf, 1969). For continuous data, two sets of tests are commonly employed, depending on the number of units (dams) per group and whether the data are parametric or nonpara-

metric. Parametric data distribute on a bell-shaped curve (a Poisson distribution); non-parametric data do not, i.e. the distribution is skewed. One of two tests can be employed to determine if the data are parametric: Bartlett's test for homogeneity of variance [α level = 0.0001 (Winer, 1962)] or Levene's test for equal variances (Levene, 1960). Parametric tests have greater power and sensitivity than non-parametric tests so there are methods to 'massage' initially non-parametric data into a more parametric-like distribution, e.g. arcsine-square root transformation performed on litter-derived percentage data (Snedecor and Cochran, 1967), such as percentage pre- or postimplantation loss (percentage resorptions, dead foetuses/litter), percentage malformed or variant foetuses per litter. ANOVA and pairwise tests can then be run on the transformed data.

For groups with small numbers of dams, as in range-finding studies (or with non-parametric distribution of data), Jonckheere's test for trend (Jonckheere, 1954) is employed for trend analysis, Kruskal–Wallis analysis of variance by ranks (Siegel, 1956; Sokal and Rohlf, 1969) is used for overall significance determinations, and the Mann–Whitney U-test (if Kruskal–Wallis is significant) is used for pairwise comparisons (Siegel, 1956; Sokal and Rohlf, 1969).

For groups with a larger number of dams, as in definitive studies, or with parametric distribution of data, the GLM (general linear model) test for linear trend is used to identify trends (SAS Institute Inc., 1989a, b; 1990a, b, c). Analysis of variance (ANOVA) is run for overall comparisons and Dunnett's (Dunnett, 1955; 1964), or Williams' multiple comparison test (Williams, 1971; 1972) is used for pairwise comparisons (if ANOVA is significant). An alternative to Williams' or Dunnett's test for pairwise comparisons is the use of the pooled variance t-test with or without Bonferroni probabilities if ANOVA is significant and Levene's test indicates homogeneous variances; or the separate variance t-test is used with (or without) Bonferroni probabilities for pairwise comparisons, if Levene's test indicates heterogeneous variances and the ANOVA for unequal variances (Brown and Forsythe, 1974) is significant.

INTERPRETATION OF STUDY DATA

The interpretation of study results depends on the study design, the results obtained, and the background and experience of the person interpreting the study. The study protocol should have been designed to answer the scientific and/or regulatory question, or questions, the investigator posed. Therefore, the number of subject animals, the doses, route, and duration, as well as the evaluation parameters selected, should all have been chosen to bear directly on the goal(s) of the study.

Once the data are summarized and statistically analysed, the results are examined to determine if the question(s) asked have been answered. One hopefully obvious caveat is that given the usual level of significance chosen of $p < 0.05$, and the large number of parameters evaluated in a typical study, one out of 20 times (i.e. 0.05) a value will exhibit statistical significance by chance. Statistical analysis is a means to an end, study interpretation, and not an end in itself. The study director, or whoever interprets the data, should be able to evaluate the data in the context of the following six major aspects.

Statistical Significance Versus Biological Significance

A given parameter may exhibit one type of significance without the other. The presence of statistical significance is dependent on the number of animals per group, the intrinsic variation of the parameter, any additional treatment-induced variability, and the types of statistical tests employed (see above). For example, foetal body weight per litter is a sensitive indicator because it is a continuous variable within a narrow range; a mean value (95 per cent of the control value, i.e. 5 per cent reduction) is commonly statistically significantly different.

Dose–Response Pattern Based on Trends Analysis and Pairwise Comparisons to the Concurrent Vehicle Control Group

The response curve in developmental toxicity studies commonly assumes the shape of a hockey stick, with the flat 'blade' part in the region of low dose(s) where change in dose results in no observable effect, and with the 'handle' part in the range of high(er) dose(s) where a change in dose results in a large response, i.e. a steep slope.

However, there may be a change in incidence and/or severity with dose. For example, if higher doses result in deaths of conceptuses so that the litter size is smaller, then the foetal body weight per litter may be greater at these doses and obscure a possibly 'real' reduction in foetal weight from toxicity. Conversely, a mean litter size larger in one dose group may result in a lower foetal weight, by virtue of litter size, not toxicity. Male foetuses are heavier than female foetuses (Tyl, 1987), so a skew in sex ratio in a particular group may be reflected in a shift in foetal body weight per litter, unrelated to treatment. In addition, there may be an apparent increase in malformations at the mid-dose(s) but not at the top dose(s). However, treatment-related embryo-foetal deaths are increased at the high dose(s). Then there is the possibility that the more profoundly malformed conceptuses died at the top dose(s), so the dose–response curve for malformations is obscured. There may also be a change in the type of malformations, not just or necessarily only incidence, observed across doses as the severity shifts along a continuum of response. For example, dilated renal pelvis and/or dilated ureters may grade into hydronephrosis and/or hydroureter; dilated lateral ventricles may grade into hydrocephaly; reduced ossification may grade into short digits or limbs, which may in turn grade into missing digits or limbs, etc. The use of 'umbrella' terms such as nonlive (for resorptions plus dead foetuses), affected (nonlive plus malformed), or defects (for malformations and/or variations), and pooling all external, all visceral, all skeletal and also all malformations or variations for statistical analyses may detect an effect of treatment not obvious when the component parameters are evaluated separately. Conversely, statistically examining one specific type of malformation, (e.g. cardiovascular, urogenital or craniofacial, etc.) may detect an effect not obvious when all visceral malformations are pooled for statistical evaluation.

Consistency of Results

Within the study, are the effects observed consistent with the time of exposure to the conceptus? Are the effects observed consistent from dose to dose, with apparent exceptions discussed above? Are the effects on the maternal animal consistent with the effects of the chemical, if known? Between studies, how do the results from this study compare with results from other studies in terms of adult response (what types of results at which doses)? Are any differences observed from study to study based on design differences, such as the use of females, use of pregnant females, age of the animals, differences in route, duration of dosing, dose levels, differences in endpoints evaluated, etc.?

Transient Versus Permanent Effects

The observed effects on the maternal organism may be transient, limited to the first few days of exposure or to the treatment period (e.g. changes in body weight, weight gain, food consumption, clinical signs of toxicity) or to the first few hours after each dose (e.g. clinical signs of toxicity) with complete recovery prior to the next dose or after the dosing period is over. Conversely, the effects may persist until scheduled sacrifice. The effects on the conceptus may also be transient, but the nature of the standard developmental toxicity protocol precludes that assessment (see postnatal evaluations). The literature can provide guidance as to whether reduced foetal body weights, reduced ossification in skeletal districts, even skeletal malformations at term are transient or permanent effects of the treatment, i.e. would/could they resolve in the postnatal period?

Direct Versus Indirect Developmental Toxicity

If the study was designed to satisfy governmental regulatory requirements and testing guidelines, and the doses were appropriately selected, then the results should indicate demonstrable maternal toxicity at the top dose, and perhaps the mid dose as well, and possibly demonstrable developmental toxicity. If the developmental toxicity is observed at a dose (D), which is also maternally toxic (A) so the A/D ratio = 1.0, or maternal and developmental toxicity are both observed at the top dose and only maternal toxicity is observed at the mid dose (so the A/D ratio is <1.0), then one important aspect of interpretation is whether it is possible to ascertain if the developmental toxicity is due to the test agent or to the compromised status of the maternal organism. If the observed developmental toxicity occurs in the absence of demonstrable maternal toxicity (A/D ratio >1.0), then the conceptus may be uniquely or preferentially susceptible to the test agent (Fabro et al., 1982) and the agent may be, in fact, a primary developmental toxicant.

Alternatively the maternal parameters evaluated might not have been fully appropriate, sensitive or complete enough relative to the developmental parameters evaluated.

Comparison to Concurrent and Historical Controls

There may be an instance when the apparent effects observed in the treatment groups are not due to effects of the test agent but to the value(s) of the parameter(s) in the concurrent vehicle control group, e.g. maternal weight or weight gain heavier or lighter than usual, pregnancy rate higher (or lower), litter size smaller (and weight therefore heavier) or the converse (larger litters and therefore lighter weights than usual), incidence of foetal malformations and/or variations lower (or higher) than usual. The only way to detect the 'response' of the concurrent control group is to compare the data from this group with the historical control database for the laboratory. The current study data can then be put in the context of the historical control data. One cautionary note is that test animal strains change over time (e.g. development of a viral antibody free colony, genetic drift, founder effect for new rooms, from the supplier, etc.) so that the historical control database may not reflect the current background. One solution is to update the databases at least yearly and drop out older studies (e.g. greater than 3–5 years old) as new studies are added.

REGULATORY HEALTH ASSESSMENT

The US government's approach to health assessment of agents involves four major components: hazard identification, dose–response assessment, exposure assessment, and risk characterization (National Research Council, 1983). The US EPA has published guidelines for the health assessment of suspect developmental toxicants (US EPA, 1984b, 1986, 1989) which cogently present guidance on how the government uses, and is proposing to use, developmental toxicity data as part of their 'weight of evidence' approach to both the hazard identification and dose–response assessment components of risk assessment. This section relies heavily on the EPA guidelines (US EPA, 1984b, 1986, 1989).

Standard developmental toxicity studies are performed, under the appropriate governmental toxicity guidelines, for a drug early in the drug discovery period (as required by FDA, 1988), for a pesticide prior to registration (as required by US EPA, FIFRA) or for an industrial chemical (performed on a case-by-case basis under US EPA, TSCA). These studies provide information on the intrinsic capacity of the test agent to cause developmental toxicity, under conditions to maximize the opportunity, i.e. hazard identification, and the dosage or dosages at which the developmental toxicity (death, malformation, delays and/or deficits) is observed; i.e. dose–response assessment. Of the three or more dosage levels employed, the highest dose should result in overt maternal toxicity, including significantly reduced body weight, weight gain, and specific organ toxicity, with maternal mortality up to 10 per cent viewed as acceptable (US EPA, 1989). This dose level should characterize embryo/foetal outcome in a compromised dam/doe and should represent a 'worst case scenario' for hazard identification. However, the presence of maternal toxicity *per se* confounds the interpretation of observed developmental toxicity as these effects may reflect the status of the dam and not the test agent *per se* (see previous discussion under maternal toxicity data).

The low dose should be a 'no observable adverse effect level' (NOAEL) for both dams and conceptuses. The NOAEL is defined as the highest dose (or exposure concentration) at which no statistically significant and/or biologically relevant adverse effects are observed in 'any adequate developmental toxicity study' (US EPA, 1985b). The middle dose may or may not result in maternal and/or developmental toxicity and should be a 'lowest observable adverse effect level' (LOAEL). The LOAEL is defined as the lowest dose or exposure concentration at which a statistically significant and/or biologically relevant adverse effect is observed in 'any adequate developmental toxicity study' (US EPA, 1985b). The characteristics of the NOAEL (or the LOAEL) are that: (1) it is obviously experimentally derived and therefore dependent on the statistical power of the study, which is in turn, dependent on the number of animals employed, (2) it is dependent on the number and sensitivity of the parameters examined, and (3) its presence implies a 'threshold', i.e. a dose below which adverse effects

would not be observed, again with the same experimental caveats. The attainment of a NOAEL, or LOAEL, is critical for subsequent risk assessment processes as it is used to ultimately extrapolate to human exposure limits. But the NOAEL is *not* a characteristic of the population (all rats, all mice, etc.) but only of the group under test and, in a real sense, specific to the species, strain, laboratory, staff, specific time of performance, source and purity of test material, identity of any vehicle, parameters evaluated, etc. The NOAEL also does *not* provide information on the slope of the dose–response curve (steep or shallow), although it is obviously at the low end of the dose–response continuum. These characteristics are very important as regulators are usually extrapolating from relatively high dose levels in animal studies to relatively low exposure levels for humans, and the presence and location of the threshold is crucial to risk assessment.

Once a NOAEL or LOAEL is provided by the experimental data, the proposed next step is to define a reference dose for developmental toxicity (RfD$_{DT}$) according to the following equation (US EPA, 1989):

$$RfD_{DT} = \frac{NOAEL/LOAEL}{UF}$$

where 'UF' is an uncertainty factor. The RfD$_{DT}$ is defined as an estimate of the daily human exposure that is likely to be without appreciable risk of adverse developmental effect (US EPA, 1989) and is characterized by the use of NOAEL, or LOAEL if NOAEL unavailable, of most sensitive indicators for most appropriate (if known) and/or most sensitive mammalian species. If the NOAEL is used,

$$RfD_{DT} = \frac{NOAEL \text{ of most sensitive indicator}}{\underset{\substack{\text{variability} \\ \text{(UF)}}}{inter\text{species}} \times \underset{\substack{\text{variability} \\ \text{(UF)}}}{intra\text{species}}}$$

where the *inter-* and *intra*species variability factors are each assigned a value of 10. If the LOAEL is used,

$$RfD_{DT} = \frac{LOAEL \text{ of most sensitive indicators}}{\underset{\substack{\text{variability} \\ \text{(UF)}}}{inter\text{species}} \times \underset{\substack{\text{variability} \\ \text{(UF)}}}{intra\text{species}} \times \underset{\substack{\text{to NOAEL} \\ \text{(UF)}}}{LOAEL} \times \underset{\substack{\text{factor} \\ \text{(MF)}}}{modifying}}$$

where the *inter-* and *intra*species variability and the extrapolation from LOAEL to NOAEL are each assigned a value of 10 and the MF can be in the range of 1–10 to reflect the sensitivity of the endpoint(s) used, the adequacy of the doses tested, the confidence in the LOAEL, as well as the slope of the dose–response curve. The RfD_{DT} is based on a short duration of exposure to the adult with no uncertainty factor included for duration of exposures as extrapolations are made from test animal data to human exposure risk (US EPA, 1989). The RfD_{DT} is assumed to be below the threshold for an increase in adverse developmental effects in humans and is used for risk characterization along with human exposure assessments (US EPA, 1989).

A second use for NOAELs, or LOAELs, is in the calculation of a proposed margin of exposure (MOE) for developmental toxicity to be used in risk characterization. The MOE is defined as the ratio of the NOAEL from the most sensitive or appropriate species to the estimated human exposure level from all potential sources. If a NOAEL is not available, the LOAEL is used and the NOAEL is estimated from the LOAEL by dividing by a UF (usually 10). The MOE would then also be used for risk characterization (US EPA, 1989). If the MOE is very high relative to the estimated human exposure level, then risk would be considered low, as would concern for the human population.

The proposed weight of evidence (WOE) scheme for suspect developmental toxicants (US EPA, 1989) defines three levels of confidence for data used to identify developmental hazards and to assess the risk of human developmental toxicity:

- Definitive evidence for human developmental toxicity or for no apparent human developmental toxicity.
- Adequate evidence for potential human developmental toxicity or no apparent potential human developmental toxicity.
- Inadequate evidence for determining potential human developmental toxicity. The scheme may require scientific judgement based on experience to weigh the implications of study design, statistical analyses, and biological significance of the data (US EPA, 1989).

POSTNATAL EVALUATIONS

There is growing concern about postnatal sequelae to *in utero* structural and/or functional insult as well as a recognition that exposure to a developing system may result in qualitatively or quantitatively different effects than an exposure to an adult system. The nervous system, with its long developmental phase, involving proliferation, migration, and differentiation of cells and regions at different gestational and perinatal ages, and its complexity, is one for which there is especial concern (Rodier *et al.*, 1979). In response, the US EPA has developed a 'stand-alone' standardized developmental neurotoxicity screen (US EPA, 1988 for the TSCA version: US EPA, 1991 for the FIFRA version) to assess 'potential functional and morphological hazards to the nervous system which may arise in the offspring from exposure of the mother during pregnancy and lactation' (US EPA, 1988, p. 488). When this study design would be employed, i.e. the 'triggers' for its requirement, is still not fully established and will probably be decided on a case-by-case basis. Kimmel of US EPA (Kimmel, 1988) has suggested that the following classes of agents should be candidates for developmental neurotoxicity or behavioural teratology testing: agents that cause CNS malformations, drugs or chemicals that are psychoactive, agents that are adult neurotoxicants, agents that are hormonally active, and agents that are peptides or amino acids. The last agents might be antagonists or agonists of endogenous CNS chemical signallers and could easily cross the blood–brain barrier. She also suggests (Kimmel, 1988) that such testing protocols should assess sensory and motor function, neuromotor development, learning and memory, reactivity and/or habituation, reproductive behaviour and other functions such as social or aggressive behaviour.

The study design for the developmental neurotoxicity screen as currently mandated by both TSCA and FIFRA testing guidelines is very similar. The design will be described with differences noted. The design involves performance in Sprague–Dawley rats, at least three agent-exposed groups and one vehicle control group, and at least 20 usable litters in each group. The route of administration should be 'orally by intubation' (US EPA, 1988, p. 489). The FIFRA guidelines indicate that 'other routes of administration may be acceptable, on a case-by-case basis, with ample justification/reasoning for this selection' (US EPA, 1991, p. 34). If the agent has been previously shown to be developmentally toxic, 'the highest dose for this study shall be the highest dose which will not result in perinatal deaths or malformations sufficient to preclude a meaningful evaluation of neurotoxicity' (US EPA, 1988, p. 489; US EPA, 1991, p. 33). If there are no developmental toxicity study data, 'the highest dose shall result in overt maternal toxicity, with weight gain depression not to exceed 20 per cent during gestation and lactation'. The lowest dose should not result in either overt maternal or developmental neurotoxicity, while the intermediate dose(s) must be equally spaced between the highest and lowest doses. With gd 0 designated as the day of copulation, the dosing period extends from gd 6 to weaning (postnatal day 21) according to TSCA (US EPA, 1988, p. 489) and gd 6 to postnatal day 10 according to FIFRA (US EPA, 1991, p. 3). FIFRA states that dosing should not occur on the day of parturition for those dams who have not completed delivery (US EPA, 1991, pp. 33–34). Live pups should be counted and weighed at birth and on postnatal days 4, 7, 13, 17 and 21, and bi-weekly thereafter according to TSCA (FIFRA specifies at birth and on postnatal days 4, 11, 17 and 21 and at least once every 2 weeks thereafter). On postnatal day 4, litters are culled to yield eight pups with a 4:4 or 5:3 sex ratio; litters that cannot satisfy the number of sex ratio criteria are removed and retained pups are uniquely identified at this time. Additionally, FIFRA allows the use of litters with seven pups and a 4:3 sex ratio; TSCA does not. Developmental landmarks assessed on all appropriate pups include age of vaginal opening and testes descent (TSCA, 1989, p. 490) or preputial separation (FIFRA, 1989, p. 35). On postnatal day 4 after culling, pups are selected for specific behavioural assessments. Motor activity is monitored in an automated system with one pup/sex/litter on postnatal days 13, 17, 21, 45 ± 2 and 60 ± 2 (TSCA, p. 490; FIFRA deletes day 45, p. 35). The period of evaluation for motor activity will include the exploratory phase and the habituation phase. Auditory startle test, including magnitude and habituation of response, will be performed on one pup/sex/litter on postnatal days 22 and 60 (TSCA, p. 490); FIFRA allows day 60 ± 2 (p. 36). Active avoidance testing to evaluate

learning and memory on one pup/sex/litter begins on day 60 or 61 and continues for five consecutive daily sessions (TSCA, p. 490). FIFRA specifies tests for learning and memory to be performed around the time of weaning, postnatal days 21–24 and at adulthood, postnatal days 60 ± 2, with 'some flexibility' in the choice of test (FIFRA, p. 36). Necropsy and histopathology requirements probably differ the most widely between the two testing guidelines. TSCA calls for necropsy of one pup/sex/litter at weaning (on postnatal day 21) and necropsy of the remaining offspring after the last behavioural tests. At both necropsy times, at least six offspring per group, balanced between sexes and across litters, will be perfused with fixative *in situ*. Specified central and peripheral nervous system tissue will be removed and immersion fixed, embedded, sectioned, stained and examined histologically. Routine staining with hematoxylin and eosin is specified, with special stains required if further evaluation is necessary. In addition, at least ten animals per necropsy time, not used for histopathology, will be decapitated and the brains removed, chilled, weighed intact and regional brain weights obtained: the cerebellum, the medulla oblongata/pons (from the rhombencephalon), the diencephalon/midbrain, and the telencephalon (cerebrum). For FIFRA, one pup/sex/litter will be killed on postnatal day 11; six per sex will have their brains removed, weighed, immersion fixed and examined histologically with 'qualitative, semi-quantitative and simple morphometric analysis'; the remaining selected pups will have their brains removed and weighed. At the end of the study, one male or one female/litter will be killed, and the brains removed and weighed. In addition, six sex/dose groups (one male or one female per litter) will be killed for neuropathological evaluation, including 'qualitative, semi-quantitative and simple morphometric analysis'. For both agencies, the high dose and control tissues will be examined, with examination of mid and low dose specimens performed only if treatment-related effects are observed in the high dose tissues.

These tests are perceived as useful in the risk estimation process, to identify specific agents, or classes of agents, for which acceptable exposures in the adult may not be acceptable to the developing organism (US EPA, 1988), to elucidate long-term consequences of pre- and perinatal findings, to determine the relationship of lowest effective (or highest no-effect) dose for behavioural effects versus the dose for overt or general toxicity effects and to identify, for human exposures, those effects that may be important to monitor (Kimmel, 1988).

Although the developing nervous system has received the most attention from researchers and governmental regulators, there are many other systems with continuing proliferation and differentiation in the postnatal period. Evaluation of the postnatal sequelae of prenatal exposure has been done for three of these other systems. One group, employing known or suspect renal teratogens, administered the agents *in utero* and a series of kidney function tests were performed on the postnatal animals, *in vivo* and *in vitro*, until postnatal day 30. The objective was to identify any transient or permanent renal effects (structural and/or functional) expressed in the postnatal period (Daston *et al.*, 1988a, b). Another group (Christian and Johnson, 1979; Christian, 1983) evaluated the postnatal physiological development of the gastrointestinal tract after *in utero* exposure to agents. The immunosurveillance system has also been shown to exhibit effects in the young adult (Chapman and Roberts, 1984) or the older animal (Spyker and Fernandes, 1973) after *in utero* exposure to agents. Transplacental carcinogenesis, expressed in the adult from late gestational *in utero* exposure, is also well documented (Rice, 1976).

MALE-MEDIATED DEVELOPMENTAL TOXICITY

All of the previously described approaches focus on the maternal–placental–foetal unit as the subject of testing and the object of concern. However, increasing evidence has implicated the male as the cause of any of the classic four endpoints of developmental toxicity. Human male exposure, as operating room personnel, to waste anaesthetic gases, results in increased incidences of spontaneous abortions, stillbirths and congenital defects (Ad Hoc Committee, 1974). Male production worker exposure to Oryzalin has been implicated in congenital heart defects in their children (Rawls, 1980). The pesticide DBCP (1,2-dibromo-3-chloropropane) is a human male sterilant (Whorton *et al.*, 1977, 1979). Elevated caf-

feine consumption in men has been reported to result in spontaneous abortions, stillbirths, and premature births (Weathersbee and Lodge, 1977). In animal studies, exposure of the male to methadone (Soyka *et al.*, 1978), thalidomide (Lutwak-Mann, 1964), lead, narcotics, alcohol or caffeine (Anonymous, 1978) results in malformations in the offspring. Possible mechanisms of male-mediated developmental toxicity include genetic or epigenetic damage to the sperm, presence of the agent of its metabolite(s) in the semen which may affect the conceptus directly, or act on the gravid uterus (Lutwak-Mann *et al.*, 1967), or indirect or more systemic actions on the male affecting the hormonal milieu and perhaps libido (Joffe, 1979; Soyka and Joffe, 1980).

DEVELOPMENTAL TOXICITY SCREENING PROTOCOLS

Over 70 000 chemicals are listed in the TSCA Registry, with 1500–2000 new chemicals added each year; 20 000 chemicals are commonly found in the workplace (NIOSH list) with only <1 per cent tested for reproductive and developmental hazard potential. It is therefore necessary and appropriate to develop a fast, inexpensive, sensitive and accurate method or methods to prescreen the plethora of chemicals and concentrate resources on those identified by the screening test(s) as potential human health hazards. The development of the so-called Ames assay designed to detect mutations in *Salmonella* bacteria as a screen for human carcinogens, based on the assumption that DNA is DNA and the early view that all carcinogens were mutagens, provided additional impetus for the search for a screen in developmental toxicology. However, the mechanisms of action of developmental toxicants appear numerous and frustratingly difficult to identify (see section on Mechanisms).

A number of approaches have been taken to develop screening protocols (see, for example, Wilson, 1978; Kimmel *et al.*, 1982), herein arbitrarily classified into *in vivo, in vivo/in vitro* and *in vitro* categories. *In vivo* screens include developmental toxicity range-finding studies previously discussed, which also can be used to identify or prioritize agents that produce developmental toxicity for more rigorous testing, and the so-called Chernoff–Kavlock assay (Chernoff *et al.*, 1979;

Chernoff and Kavlock, 1980). In the Chernoff–Kavlock assay there are two phases. Phase 1 is a range-finding study and employs five dose groups plus a vehicle control group, with ten non-pregnant females per group; dosing is for 5 consecutive days. Data collected to determine the minimally toxic dose (the MTD) include mortality, body weights, body weight gains and treatment-related clinical signs of toxicity. Phase 2 is the definitive study and employs a block design of one dose (MTD) per chemical for one to four chemicals and a concurrent control group, with 24–50 timed-pregnant animals, usually mice, per group. Dosing is on gd 8–12, the date of a vaginal plug being designated gd 1. The earliest version of this study design (Chernoff and Kavlock, 1980) collected maternal weights at the beginning and end of the treatment period, and also weight change, with dams allowed to litter. Litters were counted, sexed, weighed and examined externally on postnatal days (pnd) 1 (date of birth) and 3, and then discarded. Derived data include number (per cent) pregnant; maternal weight gain; treatment period; number (per cent) with one or more live pups at birth (pnd 1); gestational length in days; number total, live and dead pups on pnd 1 and 3; sex ratio of pups on pnd 1 and 3; pup body weights (per sex per litter) on pnd 1 and 3; pup weight gain (per sex per litter) from pnd 1 to 3; survival index (= no. live pups pnd 3 + no. live pups pnd 1); prenatal loss (= no. uterine implants minus no. live pups at birth + no. uterine implants); and postnatal loss (= no. live pups at birth minus no. live pups on pnd 3 + no. live pups at birth). This protocol does not require extensive or intensive technical training in pup visceral or skeletal examinations and assumes that the pups will be their own assay system, i.e. if the pups survive and thrive, then they do not exhibit significant toxicity at a dose that is minimally toxic to the dam (the MTD) and they do not bear malformations or variations that preclude or affect normal early postnatal growth and development. If the pups exhibit toxicity (mortality pre- or postnatally, reduced weights and/or weight gain, obvious external malformations) at the MTD, then the test agent is a candidate for further classic developmental toxicity testing. Chernoff and Kavlock (1980) set up three levels of concern: if there is a pre- or postnatal mortality and/or malformations of the offspring, then the test agent has the 'highest priority' for further

testing; if the pups exhibit reduced weight gain, then the agent has a 'lower' priority for further testing; if there is no evidence of developmental toxicity, pre- or postnatally, then the agent has the 'lowest priority' for further testing. The block design described above provides comparisons among the test agents in the block, all at the MTD, for relative potency with regard to developmental toxicity.

Modifications to the initial protocol (US EPA, 1985a; Francis and Farland, 1987) include multiple dose levels of a given test agent, dosing during the entire period of major organogenesis, gd 6 to 15, and more thorough evaluation of pups on pnd 3 (including visceral and skeletal examinations) or a longer postnatal observation period (Gray and Kavlock, 1984); so that this protocol resembles more closely the classic Segment II protocol but with a postnatal component to assess viability and growth.

One *in vivo/in vitro* screening protocol (Beaudoin and Fisher, 1981) involves administration of the test agent to pregnant rodents, removal on gd 10 after one or more daily doses to the dam, explantation and culture of embryos for 24–48 h and evaluation of toxicity and teratogenicity. This protocol allows for the full mammalian complement of metabolizing enzymes in the dam to act on the conceptuses *in utero* and for the full range of early expression of developmental toxicity to be detected in the explanted embryos *in vitro*. The next step is one (New, 1976; Klein *et al.*, 1979; Chatot *et al.*, 1980) whereby explanted rat headfold embryos are cultured for 48 h in human, monkey or rodent serum after the serum donor had been exposed to the test agent. This protocol utilizes serum containing whatever metabolites, etc., are produced by and transported in the blood of the donor mammal, a condition duplicating embryonic exposure *in utero* (Rashbass and Ellington, 1988). In a fascinating offshoot of this work, serum from women who are chronic aborters has been used in the culture system to identify missing nutrients and the women were supplemented prior to and during subsequent pregnancies with some early apparent success (Ferrari *et al.*, 1991).

There are a number of fully *in vitro* screens employing mammalian, lower vertebrate and invertebrate species (Wilson, 1978; Daston and D'Amato, 1989). Explanted rat or mouse embryos are cultured in rodent serum to which is added the test agent or known metabolites for 24–48 h and the embryos are scored for viability, growth and development (Sadler, 1979). Portions of rodents, as intact organs or as dissociated cells (e.g. Wilk *et al.*, 1980), are also explanted and cultured in medium containing test agents and/or metabolites, and are scored for growth and differentiation. For example, dissociated limb bud cells or intact anlagen from older rodent or chick embryos are cultured in the presence of test agents for 6 days. They are scored for cartilage, by alcian blue staining, and/or ossified bone formation by alizarin red S staining (Wiger *et al.*, 1988, 1989). Dissociated midbrain cells from rodent embryos are cultured in micromass culture conditions and scored for neuronal outgrowth and characteristic neuronal cell differentiation (Flint and Orton, 1984). Murine embryonic salivary glands have also been cultured *in vitro* and exposed to test agents as a possible screen (Lyng, 1989). Embryonal palatal mesenchymal cells removed from rodents just prior to fusion of the palatal shelves are also cultured in the presence of test agents and assayed for interference with differentiation, including shelf fusion, programmed cell death, and cell transformation (Yoneda and Pratt, 1981; Abbot and Pratt, 1987). When explanted embryos, or parts thereof, are exposed to the test agent in culture, they are exposed only to the added test agent because metabolic capability is minimal or absent, so this study paradigm may expose embryos to situations they would not encounter *in utero* and therefore result in false positive or, worse, false negative study results. Cloned totipotent stem cell lines from murine embryonal teratocarcinoma (Martin, 1980) or pluripotent lines from neuroblastoma (Mummery *et al.*, 1984) are cultured, exposed to test agents, including those that are 'proteratogens' requiring metabolic activation, and the cultures scored for effects on differentiation. Both tumour lines are capable of extensive differentiation in culture; restriction of this capability is presumed to be indicative of potential developmental toxicity *in vivo*. In a novel approach to examine a fundamental property of differentiating cells, cell-to-cell communication by formation of gap junctions at cell membranes, Chinese hamster V79 lung cells in co-culture are exposed to the test agent and evaluated for disruption of cell-to-cell communication using 6-thioguanine sensitive and resistant cells or,

perhaps more pertinently, normal embryonal palatal mesenchyme cells in culture are exposed to the test agent and evaluated for inhibition of intercellular communication as assayed by transfer of H^3-uridine (Welsch, 1990).

Cell attachment is another presumed universal cell function during development and therefore a basis for a screen. Ascites or dissociated solid tumour cells are grown in culture in the presence of the test agent and scored for attachment, or inhibition of attachment, to surfaces coated with lectins, such as concanavalin A, as a measure of potential developmental toxicity (Braun *et al.*, 1979, 1982).

Explanted chick embryos at presomite or multiple somite stages (Wolkowski, 1970) or chick embryonic parts are cultured on egg-agar with the test agent incorporated into the medium and evaluated for growth (crown–rump length, protein, RNA and DNA content) and differentiation.

Amphibians have also been proposed for use in screening protocols. The FETAX system (Frog Embryo Teratogenesis Assay: *Xenopus*) involves exposure of early *Xenopus laevis* (African clawed frog) embryos at the notochord stage and/or as late premetamorphic larvae to test agents in the water. The embryos are evaluated for toxicity and teratogenicity, to the developing central nervous system, in the early embryo and to the developing skeletal system, in the metamorphosing tadpole. A teratogenic index (TI) is proposed to compare relative potencies of test agents and to identify any agents that affect development at doses below which general toxicity is observed; the TI is defined as LC_{50}/ED_{50} (the concentration lethal to 50 per cent of the animals divided by the concentration producing effects in 50 per cent of the animals) (Sabourin *et al.*, 1985; Dumont *et al.*, 1983).

Drosophila melanogaster (the fruit fly) is used in two ways: larvae are grown on feed containing the test agent, are allowed to pupate and emerging adults are scored for viability (toxicity) and malformations from alterations in imaginal discs present in the larvae and used to form adult structures (Schuler *et al.*, 1982, 1985; Ranganathan *et al.*, 1987), or early primary embryonic cell cultures are grown in medium containing the test agent and are scored for differentiation of embryonic cell types (Bournias-Vardiabasis *et al.*, 1983).

Synchronous cultures of *Artemia* spp. (brine shrimp) in sea water or rodent or human serum have also been suggested as a screen, with scoring for survival, growth and morphological and molecular differentiation after exposure directly to agents or to serum from agent-exposed individuals (Sleet, 1992).

Hydra attenuata (a coelenterate) is the source of the 'artificial embryo' assay (Johnson, 1980). The adult *Hydra*, a three-layered organism with a stalk and circumoral tentacles, can be dissociated and the cells pelleted by centrifugation. The cells of the pellet will sort and reaggregate by cell type and redifferentiate into an adult *Hydra*. The assay consists of pellets ('artificial embryos') and adult *Hydra* exposed to the test agent to determine the lowest effect concentration (or the highest no-effect concentration) of the developing 'embryo' as measured by inhibition of redifferentiation or abnormal differentiation, and of the adult as measured by mortality or overt damage to adult structures. An A/D ratio is calculated (Johnson *et al.*, 1987): i.e. the ratio of the adult toxicity lowest effect (or highest no-effect) concentration to the developmental toxicity lowest effect (or highest no-effect) concentration. The developers and users of this assay suggest that an A/D ratio of ≥3 indicates a unique or greater susceptibility of the developing organism relative to that of the adult and therefore a potential for mammalian development toxicity. They also claim that the A/D ratio is fairly consistent across widely divergent species and therefore predictive of relative risk (Johnson and Gabel, 1983; Johnson, 1984; Johnson *et al.*, 1988). However, a recent paper (Daston *et al.*, 1991) compared A/D ratios for 14 chemicals in four species, the mouse, *Xenopus*, the fathead minnow and *Drosophila*, and reported that there was no correlation of A/D ratios between species, that A/D ratios are not constant across the representative species and that 'there is no basis for using A/D for hazard assessment' (Daston *et al.*, 1991, p. 696). A subsequent paper (Setzer and Rogers, 1991) employed data simulations of developmental toxicity studies and concluded that no single index can quantify 'developmental hazard' as defined by an A/D ratio and if the concept is to be useful for hazard assessment it must be refined.

The consensus on screening assays appears to be that the *in vivo* protocols such as range-finding

designs and the Chernoff–Kavlock assay are appropriate and useful to prioritize chemicals for subsequent testing, to decide early in the chemical/drug development phase whether to pursue a particular formulation, to evaluate what effect changes in chemical structure have on toxicity, and to 'fill in the blanks' on a chemical series, all relative to the potential for developmental toxicity, including teratogenicity. The *in vivo/in vitro* assay requires the same number of maternal animals as do fully *in vivo* studies, requires sophisticated technical procedures for culturing embryos and provides for only a limited number of embryological endpoints due to the limitations on the length of time embryos can be maintained in culture. There does not appear to be an advantage in using this system as a screen.

The *in vitro* assays with mammalian embryos or tissues have two critical limitations. (1) The metabolic capabilities of the embryo are very limited and only the embryo is cultured. Any metabolic changes to the parent compound by the maternal organism and therefore the metabolites to which the embryo would be exposed *in vivo* are totally missing in the explant system. Therefore, the assay may result in findings irrelevant to the *in vivo* condition and therefore false positives or false negatives. Currently, attempts are being made to provide metabolic capability by co-culturing embryos with adult hepatocytes which are capable of and are the major source of metabolism of xenobiotics to obviate the first limitation. The presence of hepatocytes *per se* appears to be toxic to the explanted embryo so a further refinement is the addition of metabolizing enzymes such as the S9 fraction (9000 *g* supernatant from mammalian liver homogenate; Wiger *et al.*, 1989) or the *P*-450 complex to the culture medium to provide enzymatic manipulation of the parent compound. (2) The duration of sustained normal growth and development of embyros appears very limited, 24–48 h, to that the numbers of structures differentiating and the extent of differentiation are similarly limited. For example, during the culture period of early chick or mammalian embryos, the CNS is the dominant system developing; for slightly older embryos it is CNS, heart and the pharyngeal gill arches, with none of the systems completing growth and differentiation during the culture period. If the test agent does not affect the structures developing, or the stage(s) of the structures/systems developing during the culture period, then the agent may be classified as inactive, when in fact it may affect other later structures/systems or other later stages in the development of structures which are not present during the limited culture period. In addition, repair processes occurring *in vivo* will not be seen in the brief *in vitro* cultures (Fantel, 1981). A two-system approach, e.g. midbrain plus limb bud micromass culture assay (Flint and Orton, 1984), is an attempt to increase the number of systems evaluated, but it is still very limited relative to the tremendous range of developing systems which may be vulnerable. The *in vitro* assays are very useful in answering research-oriented questions, as the age of the embryos (as judged by somite number or other specific morphological signposts) can be precisely controlled, identity and concentration of the test agent are precisely controlled, and early responses can be observed and characterized. They can be used to identify the proximate teratogen by exposing the explanted embryos to specific metabolites which they cannot further transform, and to elucidate mechanisms of action of known teratogens at the organ, tissue, cellular, subcellular or molecular levels early in the toxic response, prior to cell death or demise of the embryo. The utility of non-mammalian (non-vertebrate) assays as predictors of potential mammalian developmental toxicity appears unclear at this time, although the concept of phylogenetically-conserved universal processes in embryonic development is attractive and compeling.

MECHANISMS

There is no mechanism fully understood for any developmental toxicant causing foetal malformations. Although in many cases the proximate teratogen is known and maternal and/or developmental toxicity is well characterized, what is not known is how the observed effects result in the malformation(s). The site(s) of action may be intranuclear, intracellular, at the cell membrane, extracellular, outside the conceptus, in the placenta or in the maternal organism. The mode(s) of action may be general or specific, biochemical, physiological or microstructural. It is also likely that the mechanism(s) will vary from agent to agent. The two extremes in mechanisms, from very specific to very general, may be exemplified

by those proposed for 2,3,7,8-tetrachlorodibenzo-*p*-dioxin (TCDD) and for valproic acid. TCDD produces cleft palate, and hydronephrosis at higher doses, in susceptible mouse strains. The putative mechanism for the induced cleft palate is that TCDD binds to certain epidermal growth factor (EGF) receptors and prevents the normal reduction in expression of certain EGFs in the medial epithelial cells of the palatal shelves just prior to fusion. Therefore, with TCDD, abnormally high levels of certain EGFs apparently continue to stimulate proliferation and differentiation of the cells normally destined to die, and the shelves do not fuse (Abbott and Birnbaum, 1990). Valproic acid causes neural tube defects, including exencephaly, in mice and spina bifida in humans. Nau and Scott (1986) have proposed that valproic acid and other weak acid teratogens (interestingly of which there are many) reach the mammalian embryo and lower the intracellular pH of the embryonic cells. It is noteworthy that the embryonic intracellular pH is more basic than the maternal intracellular pH, especially early in development, and changes over time. The specificity of the effect probably lies in the sensitivity of the target neural tube. The suggested mechanism for TCDD may explain the cleft palate but does not explain the hydronephrosis. The suggested mechanism for valproic acid (and other teratogens that are weak acids) does not explain the specificity and susceptibility of the targets as other weak acid teratogens do not affect the neural tube and lots of weak acids are not teratogens. Perhaps the most important barrier to understanding the mechanism(s) of abnormal development is that we do not know enough about the mechanism(s) of normal development.

Studies, performed initially on *Drosophila* embryos, indicated that sequential activation of a hierarchy of regulatory genes occurs during development of multicellular organisms. These genes regulate the transcription and translation of genetic information into structures and functions by orchestrating a precise temporal and spatial expression of structural genes, which in turn control differentiation, i.e. establishment of cell types and organ formation (Schöler, 1991). Numerous genes which control development have been isolated from *Drosophila* by genetic means. This is currently not possible in vertebrates due to the dearth of developmental mutants and the difficulty in their generation. Instead, a variety of genes have been identified in the mouse based on the similarity of their base sequence to the *Drosophila* regulatory genes. Many of these, such as *Hox* and *Pax* genes, appear to play a role in pattern formation during or after gastrulation in vertebrates (Blumberg *et al.*, 1991; Schöler, 1991). The mechanisms of these regulatory genes include genetic and epigenetic control. Genetic mechanisms include the role of genes in establishing the basic embryonic axes (cephalo–caudal, dorso–ventral), specifying specific embryonic regions, controlling the transition of cells from presumptive to determined, in the establishment of the fate of diverse cell types and ultimately, by transcription of DNA into messenger RNAs and the translation of messenger RNAs into proteins, specifying directly the differentiated patterns of gene expression, including inter- and intracellular molecules, structures, and functions. Epigenetic mechanisms include the interactions between cells, between cell types and between cells and the products of other cells. These interactions are mediated by signalling molecules such as diffusible growth factors, membrane-bound ligands, hormones, and components of the extracellular matrix and their appropriate receptors. The genetic and epigenetic roles are linked and integrated by so-called second messengers which translate molecular signals by individual cells into commands to produce specific effects on cell growth and patterns of gene activity (Angerer and Angerer, 1991).

Recent work has concentrated on classes of genes which encode regulatory transcription factors, such as the POU family containing genes designated *Oct-1* to *Oct-10* (Schöler, 1991); the *Hox* (homeobox-containing) genes (Holland and Hogan, 1988a, b; Boncinelli *et al.*, 1991) which organize segmentation and differentiation; the gene *int-1* (Wilkinson *et al.*, 1987) with demonstrated expression localized in different portions of the mammalian central nervous system; the genes which produce so-called heat shock proteins (hsp) in massive quantities in the embryo in response to stress (Walsh *et al.*, 1987), and, from the POU family specifically, the *Oct-3* genes which are expresssed in totipotent and pluripotent cells before gastrulation (undifferentiated cells) and in the germ cell lineage (Rosner *et al.*, 1991).

Abnormal expression of mutated genes from this regulatory class results in abnormalities in development which produce information on normal development as well as suggest mechanisms of action of xenobiotics. Examples of such genetic or epigenetic manipulations follow. *Undulated*, a mouse mutation involving a single base pair change in a putative transcription factor, results in abnormal vertebrae along the entire spinal column (Balling *et al.*, 1988). Dominant ectopic expression (expression in the wrong somites) of *Hox 1.1* transgenes results in specific malformations in cervical vertebrae in mice (Kessel *et al.*, 1990). Alterations of the *int-1* proto-oncogene in transgenic mice results in losses of large areas of the midbrain and cerebellum (McMahon and Bradley, 1990; Thomas and Capecchi, 1990). Specific degradation of Oct-3 messenger RNA (by injection of antisense Oct-3 oligonucleotides) in one-cell mouse embryos arrests development at the one-cell stage (Rosner *et al.*, 1991); injection of the antisense nucleotides into one-celled embryos just before mitosis (the first cleavage division of the embryo) does not block the first division but arrests development at the two-cell stage. Oct-3 may act as a transcription factor (but it is currently assumed that embryonic transcription begins at the two-cell stage) or it may regulate DNA replication in one-cell embryos (Rosner *et al.*, 1991). Oct-3 expression is observed in cells with undifferentiated phenotypes, with expression detected in all cells through the morula stage of development, in cells of the inner cell mass (ICM), which will form the embryo proper), in cells of the primitive ectoderm (but not in cells of the primitive endoderm which differentiate into extraembryonic tissues) after implantation during gastrulation, in the primordial germ cells as they migrate from the allantois into the genital ridge and in cells in the ovaries, specifically the mature oocytes, and testis. In the testis the specific cell types have not yet been identified but neither the Sertoli cells nor mature spermatozoa have detectable Oct-3 (Rosner *et al.*, 1991). It is clear that cell division, cell migration and differentiation are directed by regulatory gene classes which control which genes are expressed in which tissues at which times in development. The molecular approach to identifying these fundamental controlling factors of mammalian development may be the most fruitful in the long run in elucidating mechanisms of normal and abnormal development and providing mechanisms of action of developmental toxicants.

ACKNOWLEDGEMENTS

The author thanks Nathelle J. Gross for her diligent efforts 'above and beyond the call . . .' in preparing this manuscript.

REFERENCES

Abbott, B. D. and Pratt, R. M. (1987). Retinoids and EGF alter embryonic mouse palatal epithelial and mesenchymal cell differentiation in organ culture. *J. Craniofac. Genet. Dev. Biol.*, **7**, 219–240

Abbott, B. D. and Birnbaum, L. S. (1990). TCDD-induced altered expression of growth factors may have a role in producing cleft palate and enhancing the incidence of clefts after coadministration of retinoid and TCDD. *Toxicol. Appl. Pharmacol.*, **106**, 418–432

Ad Hoc Committee on the Effect of Trace Anesthetics on the Health of Operating Room Personnel (1974). Occupational disease among operating room personnel: a National Study. *Anesthesiology*, **41**, 321–340

Aliverti, V., Bonanomi, E., Giavini, E., Leone, V. G. and Mariani, L. (1979). The extent of foetal ossification as an index of delayed development in teratogenic studies on the rat. *Teratology*, **20**, 237–242

Angerer, L. M. and Angerer, R. C. (1991). Technology review. *In situ* hybridization—a guided tour. *Toxicol. Methods*, **1**, 2–29

Anonymous (1978). *Science*, **202**, 733

Balling, R., Deutsch, U. and Gruss, P. (1988). *Undulated*, a mutation affecting the development of the mouse skeleton, has a point mutation in the paired box of Pax 1. *Cell*, **55**, 531–535

Barlow, S. M., McElhatton, P. R. and Sullivan, F. M. (1975). The relation between maternal restraint and food deprivation, plasma corticosterone and cleft palate in the offspring of mice. *Teratology*, **12**, 97–104

Barlow, S. M., Knight, A. F. and Sullivan, F. M. (1980). Diazepam-induced cleft palate in the mouse: the role of endogenous maternal corticosterone. *Teratology*, **21**, 149–155

Beaudoin, A. R. and Fisher, D. L. (1981). An *in vivo/in vitro* evaluation of teratogenic action. *Teratology*, **23**, 57–61

Blumberg, B., Wright, C. V. E., De Robertis, E. M. and Cho, K. W. Y. (1991). Organizer-specific homeobox genes in *Xenopus laevis* embryos. *Science*, **253**, 194–196

Boncinelli, E., Simeone, A., Acampora, D. and Mavilio, F. (1991). Review: *HOX* gene activation by retinoic acid. *Trends in Genetics*, **7**, 329–334

Bournias-Vardiabasis, N., Teplitz, R. L., Chernoff, G. F. and Seecof, R. L. (1983). Detection of teratogens in the *Drosophila* embryonic cell culture test: assay of 100 chemicals. *Teratology*, **28**, 109–122

Braun, A. G., Emerson, D. J. and Nichinson, B. B. (1979). Teratogenic drugs inhibit tumour cell attachment to lectin-coated surfaces. *Nature*, **282**, 507–509

Braun, A. G., Buckner, C. A., Emerson, D. J. and Nichinson, B. B. (1982). Qualitative correspondence between *in vivo* and *in vitro* activity of teratogenic agents. *Proc. Natl Acad. Sci. USA.*, **79**, 2056–2060

Bredderman, P. J., Foote, R. H. and Yassen, A. M. (1964). An improved artificial vagina for collecting rabbit semen. *J. Reprod. Fertil.*, **7**, 401–403

Brown, M. B. and Forsythe, A. B. (1974). The small sample behaviour of some statistics which test the equality of several means. *Technometrics*, **16**, 129–132

Chapman, R. R. and Roberts, D. W. (1984). Humoral immune dysfunction as a result of parental exposure to diphenylhydantoin: correlation with the occurrence of physical defects. *Teratology*, **30**, 107–117

Chatot, C. L., Klein, N. W., Piatek, J. and Pierro, L. J. (1980). Successful culture of rat embryos on human serum: use in the detection of teratogens. *Science*, **207**, 1471–1473

Chernoff, N. (1990). Studies on maternal toxicity, formation of supernumerary ribs, and evidence for embryonic repair of xenobiotic-induced cellular injury. *Teratology*, **42**, 18A

Chernoff, N., Kavlock, R. J., Rogers, E. H., Carver, B. D. and Murray, S. (1979). Perinatal toxicity of maneb, ethylene thiourea, and ethylenebisisothiocyanate sulfide in rodents. *J. Toxicol. Environ. Health*, **5**, 821–834

Chernoff, N. and Kavlock, R. J. (1980). An *in vivo* teratology screen using pregnant mice. *J. Toxicol. Environ. Health*, **10**, 541–550

Chernoff, N., Rogers, J. M. and Kavlock, R. J. (1989). Review paper. An overview of maternal toxicity and prenatal development: considerations for developmental toxicity hazard assessments. *Toxicology*, **59**, 111–125

Christian, M. S. (1983). Postnatal alterations of gastrointestinal physiology, haematology and clinical chemistry. In Johnson, E. M. and Kochhar, D. (Eds), *Handbook of Experimental Pharmacology: Teratogenesis and Reproductive Toxicology*. Springer, Berlin, pp. 263–286

Christian, M. S. and Johnson, E. M. (1979). Postnatal alteration of non-CNS physiology evaluated in rats treated with teratogens during the foetal period. *Teratology*, **19**, 23A

Clark, R. L., Robertson, R. T., Minsker, D. H. *et al.* (1984). Diflunisal-induced maternal anemia as a cause of teratogenicity in rabbits. *Teratology*, **30**, 319–332

Clark, R. L., Robertson, R. T., Chennakatu, P. P. *et al.* (1986). Association between adverse maternal and embryo-foetal effects in Norfloxacin-treated and food-deprived rabbits. *Fund. Appl. Toxicol.*, **7**, 272–286

da Costa e Silva, A., Ribiero, R. C. J., Albuquerque,

R. H., Beraldo, P. S. S., Neves, F. A. R. and Marti- nelli, J. G. (1984). Effect of experimentally induced renal failure upon the fertility in rats. Fertility in uremic rats. *Nephron*, **36**, 252

Daston, G. P. and D'Amato, R. A. (1989). *In vitro* techniques in teratology. *Toxicol. Ind. Health*, **5**, 555–585

Daston, G. P., Rehnberg, B. F., Carver, B., Rogers, E. H. and Kavlock, R. J. (1988a). Functional terato- gens of the rat kidney. I. Colchicine, dinoseb and methyl salicylate. *Fundam. Appl. Toxicol.*, **11**, 381–400

Daston, G. P., Rehnberg, B. F., Carver, B. and Kav- lock, R. J. (1988b). Functional teratogens of the rat kidney. II. Nitrofen and ethylenethiourea. *Fundam. Appl. Toxicol.*, **11**, 401–415

Daston, G. P., Rogers, J. M., Versteeg, D. J., Sabou- rin, T. D., Baines, D. and Marsh, S. S. (1991). Interspecies comparisons of A/D ratios: A/D ratios are not constant across species. *Fundam. Appl. Toxi- col.*, **17**, 696–722

Dey, S. K. (1989). Embryo development and uterine interaction in the preimplantation period. *Society of Toxicology Symposium on Early Embryo Loss as a Factor in Reproductive Failure*. 28th Annual Meeting of SOT

Dumont, J. N., Schultz, T. W., Buchanan, M. and Kao, G. (1983). Frog embryo teratogenesis assay: Xenopus (FETAX)—a short-term assay applicable to complex mixtures. In Waters, M. D., Sandhu, S. S., Lewtas, J., Claxton, L. and Newnow, S. (Eds), *Symposium on the Application of Short-Term Bioas- says in the Analysis of Complex Environmental Mix- tures*. Plenum, New York, pp. 393–405

Dunnett, C. W. (1955). A multiple comparison pro- cedure for comparing several treatments with a con- trol. *J. Am. Stat. Assoc.*, **50**, 1096–1121

Dunnett, C. W. (1964). New tables for multiple com- parisons with a control. *Biometrics*, **20**, 482–491

Fabro, S., Schull, G. and Brown, N. A. (1982). The relative teratogenic index and teratogenic potency: proposed components of developmental toxicity risk assessment. *Teratog. Carcinog. Mutagen.*, **2**, 61–76

Fantel, A. G. (1981). Is there a future for embryo culture in teratogen screening? *Teratology*, **23**, 33A–34A

FDA (1988) (Food and Drug Administration). Good Laboratory Practice Regulations for Nonclinical Laboratory Studies. *Code of Federal Regulation (CFR)*, pp. 229–243, 1 April, 1988

Ferrari, D. A., Gilles, P. A. and Klein, N. W. (1991). Sera teratogenicity to cultured rat embryos in women with histories of spontaneous abortion. *Teratology*, **43**, 460 (P141)

FIFRA (1989) (Federal Insecticide, Fungicide, and Rodenticide Act). Environmental Protection Agency; Good Laboratory Practice Standards; Final Rule. *Federal Register*, **54**, 34051–34074, 17 August, 1989 (40-CFR-792)

Flint, O. P. and Orton, T. C. (1984). An *in vitro* assay for teratogens with cultures of rat embryo midbrain and limb bud cells. *Toxicol. Appl. Pharmacol.*, **76**, 383–395

Folb, P. I. and Dukes, M. N. G. (Eds) (1990). *Drug Safety in Pregnancy*. Elsevier Scientific Publishing Co., New York

Francis, E. Z. and Farland, W. H. (1987). Application of the preliminary developmental toxicity screen for chemical hazard identification under the Toxic Sub- stances Control Act. *Teratogen. Carcinogen. Mutagen.*, **7**, 107–117

Francis, E. Z. and Kimmel, C. A. (1989). Proceedings of the workshop on the acceptability and interpre- tation of dermal developmental toxicity studies. *Teratology*, **39**, 453

Gilman, J., Gilbert, C. and Gilman, G. C. (1948). Preliminary report on hydrocephalus, spina bifida and other congenital anomalies in rats produced by trypan blue. *S. Afr. J. Med. Sci.*, **13**, 47–90

Goldenthal, E. I. (Chief, Drug Review Branch—Div- ision of Toxicological Evaluation, Bureau of Scien- tific Standards and Evaluation), *Guidelines for Reproduction Studies for Safety Evaluation of Drugs for Human Use*, letter dated 1 March, 1966

Gray, L. E. and Kavlock, R. J. (1984). An extended evaluation of an *in vivo* teratology screen utilizing postnatal growth and viability in the mouse. *Terato- gen. Carcinogen. Mutagen.*, **4**, 403–426

Greene, R. R., Burrill, M. W. and Ivy, A. C. (1939). Experimental intersexuality: the effect of antenatal androgens on sexual development of female rats. *Am. J. Anat.*, **65**, 415–469

Greene, R. R., Burrill, M. W. and Ivy, A. C. (1940). Experimental intersexuality: the effects of estrogens on the antenatal sexual development of the rat. *Am. J. Anat.*, **67**, 305–345

Gregg, N. M. (1941). Congenital cataract following German measles in the mother. *Tr. Ophth. Soc. Australia*, **3**, 35–46

Hafez, E. S. E. (Ed.) (1970). *Reproduction and Breed- ing Techniques for Laboratory Animals*. Lea and Febiger, Philadelphia, PA

Hale, F. (1933). Pigs born without eyeballs. *J. Hered.*, **24**, 105–106

Hale, F. (1935). The relation of vitamin A to ano- phthalmos in pigs. *Am. J. Ophth.*, **18**, 1087–1093

Hemm, R. D., Arslanoglou, L. and Pollock, J. J. (1977). Cleft palate prenatal food restriction in mice: association with elevated maternal corticosteroids. *Teratology*, **15**, 243–248

Hipple, V. and Pagenstrecher, H. (1907). Über den Einfluss des Cholins und der Röntgenstrahlen auf den Ablauf der Gravidität. *Münch. Med. Wochen- schr.*, **54**, 452–456

Holland, P. W. H. and Hogan, B. L. M. (1988a). Spatially restricted patterns of expression of the homeobox-containing gene *Hox 2.1* during mouse embryogenesis. *Development*, **102**, 159–174

Holland, P. W. H. and Hogan, B. L. M. (1988b). Expression of homeo box genes during mouse development: a review. *Genes Dev.*, **2**, 773–782

Holmes, L. B., Kawanishi, H. and Munoz, A. (1988). Acetozolamide: maternal toxicity, pattern of malformations, and litter effect. *Teratology*, **37**, 335–342

Holt, D. and Webb, M. (1988). The toxicity and teratogenicity of mercuric mercury in the pregnant rat. *Arch. Toxicol.*, **58**, 243

Irwin, S. (1968). Comprehensive observational assessment: Ia. A systematic, quantitative procedure for assessing the behavioural and physiologic state of the mouse. *Psychopharmacologic (BERL)*, **13**, 222–257

Japan (1984). *Japanese Guidelines of Toxicity Studies*. Notification No. 118 of the Pharmaceutical Affairs Bureau, Ministry of Health and Welfare. 2. Studies of the effects of drugs on reproduction. Yakagyo Jiho Co., Tokyo, Japan

Joffe, J. M. (1979). Influence of drug exposure of the father on perinatal outcome. *Clinics Perinatol.*, **6**, 21–36

Johnson, E. M. (1980). A subvertebrate system for rapid determination of potential teratogenic hazards. *J. Environ. Pathol. Toxicol.*, **4**, 153–156

Johnson, E. M. (1984). A prioritization and biological decision tree for developmental toxicity safety evaluations. *J. Am. Coll. Toxicol.*, **3**, 141–147

Johnson, E. M. and Gabel, B. E. G. (1983). An artificial 'embryo' for detection of abnormal developmental biology. *Fundam. Appl. Toxicol.*, **3**, 243–249

Johnson, E. M. and Christian, M. S. (1984). When is a teratology study not an evaluation of teratogenicity? *J. Am. Coll. Toxicol.*, **3**, 431–434

Johnson, E. M., Christian, M. S., Dansky, L. and Gabel, B. E. G. (1987). Use of the adult developmental relationship in prescreening for developmental hazards. *Teratog. Carcinog. Mutagen.*, **7**, 273–285

Johnson, E. M., Newman, L. M., Gabel, B. E. G., Boerner, T. F. and Dansky, L. A. (1988). An analysis of the Hydra assay's applicability and reliability as a developmental toxicity prescreen. *J. Am. Coll. Toxicol.*, **7**, 111–126

Jonckheere, A. R. (1954). A distribution-free k-sample test against ordered alternatives. *Biometrika*, **41**, 133–145

Kavlock, R. J., Chernoff, N., Rogers, E., Whitehouse, D., Carver, B., Gray, J. and Robinson, K. (1982). An analysis of fetotoxicity using biochemical end points of organ differentiation. *Teratology*, **26**, 183–194

Kavlock, R. J., Chernoff, N. and Rogers, E. H. (1985). The effect of acute maternal toxicity on foetal development in the mouse. *Teratogen. Carcinogen. Mutagen.*, **5**, 3–13

Kelsey, F. O. (1982). Regulatory aspects of teratology: role of the Food and Drug Administration. *Teratology*, **25 (2)**, 193–199

Kessel, M., Balling, R. and Gruss, P. (1990). Vari-

ations of cervical vertebrae after expression of a *Hox 1.1* transgene in mice. *Cell*, **61**, 301–308

Khera, K. S. (1984). Maternal toxicity—a possible factor in foetal malformations in mice. *Teratology*, **29**, 411–416

Khera, K. S. (1985). A possible etiological factor in embryo-foetal deaths and foetal malformations of rodent–rabbit species. *Teratology*, **31**, 129–153

Kimmel, C. A. (1988). Current status of behavioural teratology: science and regulation. *CRC Crit. Rev. Toxicol.*, **19**, 1–10

Kimmel, C. A. and Francis, E. Z. (1990). Proceedings of the workshop on the acceptability and interpretation of dermal developmental toxicity studies. *Fundam. Appl. Toxicol.*, **14**, 386–398

Kimmel, G. L., Smith, K., Kochhar, D. M. and Pratt, R. M. (1982). Proceedings of the Concensus Workshop on *In Vitro* teratogenesis Testing. *Teratogen. Carcinogen. Mutagen.*, **2**, 221–374

Kimmel, G. L., Kimmel, C. A. and Francis, E. Z. (Eds) (1987a). Special issue: evaluation of maternal and developmental toxicity. *Teratogen. Carcinogen. Mutagen.*, **7**, 203–338

Kimmel, G. L., Kimmel, C. A. and Francis, E. Z. (1987b). Implications of the consensus workshop on the evaluation of maternal and developmental toxicity. *Teratogen. Carcinogen. Mutagen.*, **7**, 329–338

Klein, N. W., Volger, M. A., Chatot, C. L. and Pierro, L. J. (1979). The use of cultured rat embryos to evaluate the teratogenic activity of serum: cadmium and cyclophosphamide. *Teratology*, **19**, 35A

Lenz, W. (1961). Kindliche Missbildungen nach Medikament-Einnahme wahrend der Gravidität? *Deutsch. Med. Wochenschr*, **86**, 2555–2556

Lenz, W. (1962). Thalidomide and congenital abnormalities. *Lancet*, **i**, 45

Levene, H. (1960). Robust tests for equality of variance. In Olkin *et al.* (Eds), *Contributions to Probability and Statistics*. Stanford University Press, Stanford, CA, pp. 273–292

Lillie, F. R. (1917). The free-martin: a study of the action of sex hormones in the foetal life of cattle. *J. Exp. Zool.*, **23**, 371–452

Lutwak-Mann, C. (1964). Observations on progeny of thalidomide-treated male rabbits. *Br. Med. J.*, **1**, 1090–1091

Lutwak-Mann, C., Schmid, K. and Keberle, H. (1967). Thalidomide in rabbit semen. *Nature*, **214 (5902)**, 1018–1020

Lyng, R. D. (1989). Test of six chemicals for embryotoxicity using foetal mouse salivary glands in culture. *Teratology*, **39**, 591–599

McBride, W. G. (1961). Thalidomide and congenital abnormalities. *Lancet*, **ii**, 1358

McMahon, A. P. and Bradley, A. (1990). The *Wnt-1 (int-1)* protooncogene is required for development of a large region of the mouse brain. *Cell*, **62**, 1073–1085

Marr, M. C., Myers, C. B., George, J. D. and Price,

C. J. (1988). Comparison of single and double staining for evaluation of skeletal development: the effects of ethylene glycol (EG) in CD® rats. *Teratology*, **37**, 476

Marr, M. C., Myers, C. B., Price, C. J., Morrissey, R. E. and Schwetz, B. A. (1989). Developmental stages of the CD® rat skeleton. *Teratology*, **39**, 468

Marr, M. C., Price, C. J., Myers, C. B., Morrissey, R. E. and Shwetz, B. A. (1990). Developmental stages of the CD® rat skeleton after maternal exposure to ethylene glycol (EG). *Teratology*, **41**, 576 (P40)

Marr, M. C., Price, C. J., Myers, C. B. and Morrissey, R. E. (1992). Developmental stages of the CD® (Sprague–Dawley) rat skeleton after maternal exposure to ethylene glycol. *Teratology*, **46 (2)**, 169–181

Martin, G. (1980). Teratocarcinomas and mammalian embryogenesis. *Science*, **209**, 768–775

Millicovsky, G. and De Sesso, J. M. (1980a). Cardiovascular alterations in rabbit embryos *in situ* after a teratogenic dose of hydroxyurea: an *in vivo* microscopic study. *Teratology*, **22**, 115–124

Millicovsky, G. and De Sesso, J. M. (1980b). Differential embryonic cardiovascular responses to acute maternal uterine ischaemia: an *in vivo* microscopic study of rabbit embryos with either intact or clamped umbilical cords. *Teratology*, **22**, 335–343

Millicovsky, G. and Johnston, M. C. (1981). Maternal hyperoxia greatly reduces the incidence of phenytoin-induced cleft lip and palate in A/J mice. *Science*, **212**, 671

Millicovsky, G., De Sesso, J. M., Kleinman, L. I. and Clark, K. E. (1981). Effects of hydroxyurea on haemodynamics of pregnant rabbits: a maternally mediated mechanism of embryotoxicity. *Am. J. Obstet. Gynecol.*, **140**, 747

Moser, V. C., McCormick, J. P., Creason, J. P. and MacPhail, R. C. (1988). Comparison of chlordomeform and carbaryl using a functional observational battery. *Fundam. Appl. Toxicol.*, **11**, 189–206

Mummery, C. L., van den Brink, C. E., van der Saag, P. T. and de Laat, S. W. (1984). A short-term screening test for teratogens using differentiating neuroblastoma cells *in vitro*. *Teratology*, **29**, 271–279

National Research Council (NRC), Committee on the Institutional Means for the Assessment of Risks to Public Health (1983). *Risk assessment in the Federal government: Managing the process*. Commission on Life Sciences, NRC, Washington, DC, National Academy Press, pp. 17–83

Nau, H. and Scott, W. J. Jr (1986). Weak acids may act as teratogens because they accumulate in the basic milieu of the early mammalian embryo. *Nature*, **323**, 276–278

New, D. A. T. (1976). Comparison of growth *in vitro* and *in vivo* of postimplantation of rat embryos. *J. Embryol. Exp. Morphol.*, **36**, 133–144

NIH Guide for the Care and Use of Laboratory Animals, PHS, NIH Publication No. 86–23, revised 1985

OECD (1981) (Organization for Economic Cooperation and Development). *Guideline for Testing of Chemicals: Teratogenicity*. Director of Information, Paris, France

Ranganathan, S., Davis, D. G. and Hood, R. D. (1987). Developmental toxicity of ethanol in *Drosophila melanogaster*. *Teratology*, **36**, 45–50

Rashbass, P. and Ellington, S. K. L. (1988). Development of rat embryos cultured in serum prepared from rats with streptozotocin-induced diabetes. *Teratology*, **37**, 51–62

Rawls, R. C. (1980). Reproductive hazards in the work place. *Chem. Eng. News*, **58**, 28–31

Rice, J. M. (1976). Carcinogenesis: a late effect of irreversible toxic damage during development. *Environ. Health Persp.*, **18**, 133–139

Robertson, R. T., Minsker, D. H., Bokelman, D. L., Durand, G. and Conquet, P. (1981). Potassium loss as a causative factor for skeletal malformations in rats produced by indacrinone: a new investigational loop diuretic. *Toxicol. Appl. Pharmacol.*, **60**, 142

Rodier, P. M., Reynoles, S. S. and Roberts, W. N. (1979). Behavioral consequences of interference with CNS development in the early foetal period. *Teratology*, **19**, 327–336

Rosner, M. H., Vigano, M. A., Rigby, P. W. J., Arnheiter, H. and Staudt, L. M. (1991). Perspective. Oct-3 and the beginning of mammalian development. *Science*, **253**, 144–145

Sabourin, T. D., Faulk, R. T. and Goss, L. B. (1985). The efficacy of three non-mammalian test systems in the identification of chemical teratogens. *J. Appl. Toxicol.*, **5**, 227–233

Sadler, T. W. (1979). Culture of early somite mouse embryos during organogenesis. *J. Embryol. Exp. Morph.*, **49**, 17–25

Salewski, E. (1964). Färbemethode zum makroskopischen Nachweis von Implantationsstellen am Uterus der Ratte. *Naunyn-Schmiedebergs Arch. Exp. Pathol. Pharmakol.*, **247**, 367

SAS Institute Inc. (1989a). *SAS® Language and Procedures: Usage*, Version 6, First Edition, SAS Institute Inc., Cary, NC

SAS Institute Inc. (1989b). *SAS/STAT® Users' Guide*, Version 6, Fourth Edition, Volumes 1 and 2, SAS Institute Inc., Cary, NC

SAS Institute Inc. (1990a). *SAS® Language: Reference*, Version 6, First Edition, SAS Institute Inc., Cary, NC

SAS Institute Inc. (1990b). *SAS® Language: Procedures Guide*, Version 6, Third Edition, SAS Institute Inc., Cary, NC

SAS Institute Inc. (1990c). *SAS® Companion for the VMS™ Environment*, Version 6, First Edition, SAS Institute Inc., Cary, NC

Schöler, H. R. (1991). Review: Octamania: the POU

factors in murine development. *Trends Genetics*, **7**, 323–329

Schuler, R. L., Hardin, B. D. and Niemeier, R. W. (1982). *Drosophila* as a tool for the rapid assessment of chemicals for teratogenicity. *Teratog. Carcinog. Mutagen.*, **2**, 293–301

Schuler, R. L., Radike, M. A., Hardin, B. D. and Niemeier, R. W. (1985). Pattern of response of intact *Drosophila* to known teratogens. *J. Am. Coll. Toxicol.*, **4**, 291–303

Schwetz, B. A. and Tyl, R. W. (1987). Consensus workshop on the Evaluation of Maternal and Developmental Toxicity Group III Report: Low Dose Extrapolation and Other Considerations for Risk Assessment—Models and Applications. *Teratogen. Carcinogen. Mutagen.*, **7**, 321–327

Setzer, R. W. and Rogers, J. M. (1991). Assessing developmental hazard: the reliability of the A/D ratio. *Teratology*, **44**, 653–665

Siegel, S. (1956). *Nonparametric Statistics for the Behavioral Sciences*, McGraw-Hill, New York

Sleet, R. B. (1992). Brine shrimp (*Artemia*): fish food with potential application as a prescreen to predict chemical hazard to human development. *Lab. Animal.*, **21**, 26–36

Snedecor, G. W. and Cochran, W. G. (1967). *Statistical Methods*, sixth edn. Iowa State University Press, Ames, IO

Sokal, R. R. and Rohlf, F. J. (1969). *Biometry*, W. H. Freeman, San Francisco, pp. 369–371, 299–340, 370–372, 589–595

Soyka, L. F. and Joffe, J. M. (1980). Male mediated drug effects on offspring. In Schwarz, R. H. and Yaffe, S. J. (Eds), *Progress in Clinical and Biological Research: Drugs and Chemical Risk to the Fetus and Newborn*. Alan R. Liss, New York, pp. 49–66

Soyka, L. F., Peterson, J. M. and Joffe, J. M. (1978). Lethal and sublethal effects on the progeny of male rats treated with methadone. *Toxicol. Appl. Pharmacol.*, **45**, 797–807

Spyker, J. M. and Fernandes, G. (1973). Impaired immune function in offspring of methylmercury treated mice. *Teratology*, **7**, 28A

Thomas, K. R. and Capecchi, M. R. (1990). Targeted disruption of the murine *int-1* proto-oncogene resulting in severe abnormalities in midbrain and cerebellar development. *Nature (Lond)*, **346**, 847–850

TSCA (1989) (Toxic Substances Control Act). Environmental Protection Agency: Good Laboratory Practice Standards; Final Rule. *Federal Register*, **54**, 34033–34050

Tyl, R. W. (1987). Developmental toxicity in toxicologic research and testing. In Ballantyne, B. (Ed.), *Perspectives in Basic and Applied Toxicology*. John Wright, Bristol, pp. 203–238

Tyl, R. W., York, R. G. and Schardein, J. L. (1993). Reproductive and developmental toxicity studies by cutaneous administration. In Wang, R. G., Knaak, J. B. and Maibach, H. I. (Eds), *Health Risk Assess-*

ment: Dermal and Inhalation Exposure and Absorption of Toxicants. CRC Press, Boca Raton, FL, pp. 229–261

US EPA (1982). Environmental Protection Agency: *Teratogenicity Study. Pesticide Assessment Guidelines. Subdivision F.* Hazard Evaluation: Human and Domestic Animals. EPA-540 9-82-025, pp. 126–130

US EPA (1984a). Environmental Protection Agency: *Pesticides Assessment Guidelines, Subdivision F.* Hazard Evaluation: Human and Domestic Animals (Final Rule). Available from NTIS (PB86–108958), Springfield, VA

US EPA (1984b). Environmental Protection Agency: Proposed Guidelines for the Health Assessment of Suspect Developmental Toxicants and Requests for Comments. *Federal Register*, **49** (227), 46324–46331, 23 November, 1984

US EPA (1985a). Environmental Protection Agency: Preliminary Developmental Toxicity Screen. *Federal Register*, **50** (Sept. 27), 39428

US EPA (1985b). Environmental Protection Agency: Developmental Toxicity Study. Toxic Substances Control Act Test Guidelines; Final Rules. *Federal Register*, **50** (Sept. 27), 39433

US EPA (1986). Environmental Protection Agency: Guidelines for the health assessment of suspect developmental toxicants. *Federal Register*, **51**, 34028–34040

US EPA (1987). Environmental Protection Agency: Toxic substances control act test guidelines: Final rule. *Federal Register*, **50**, 39412

US EPA (1988). Environmental Protection Agency: Paragraph 795.250. Developmental Neurotoxicity Screen. 40 CFR Ch. 1 (7–1–88 Edition), pp. 488–493; *Federal Register*, **53**, 5957, February 26, 1988

US EPA (1989). Environmental Protection Agency: Proposed amendments to the guidelines for the health assessment of suspect developmental toxicants; requests for comments; notice. *Federal Register*, **54** (2), 9386–9403, March 6, 1989

US EPA (1991). Environmental Protection Agency: *Pesticide Assessment Guidelines—Subdivision F.* Hazard Evaluation: Human and Domestic Animals Addendum 10—Neurotoxicity Series 81, 82 and 83. Developmental Neurotoxicity Study, pp. 32–48, March 1991

US FDA (1966). Food and Drug Administration: *Guidelines for Reproduction Studies for Safety Evaluation of Drugs for Human Use*, Washington DC

United Kingdom (1974). Committee on Safety of Medicines: *Notes for Guidance on Reproduction Studies*. Department of Health and Social Security, London UK

Walsh, D. A., Kelin, N. W., Hightower, L. E. and Edwards, M. J. (1987). Heat, shock and thermotolerance during early rat embryo development. *Teratology*, **36**, 181–191

Warkany, J. (1971). *Congenital Malformations—Notes*

and Comments. Year Book Medical Publications, Chicago, IL

Warkany, J. and Schraffenberger, E. (1947). Congenital malformations induced in rats by roentgen rays. *Am. J. Roentgenol. Radium Ther.*, **57**, 455–463

Warshaw, C. J. (1977). *Guidelines on Pregnancy and Work*. NIOSH Research Report (The American College of Obstetricians and Gynecologists), US Department, HEW, Rockville, MD (Contract No. 210-76-0159)

Watkinson, W. P. and Millicovsky, G. (1983). Effects of phenytoin on maternal heart rate in A/J mice: possible role in teratogenesis. *Teratology*, **28**, 1–8

Weathersbee, P. S. and Lodge, J. R. (1977). Caffeine: its direct and indirect influence on reproduction. *J. Reprod. Med.*, **19**, 55–63

Weaver, T. E. and Scott, W. J. Jr (1984a). Acetazolamide teratogenesis: association of maternal respiratory acidosis and ectrodactyly in C57BL/6J mice. *Teratology*, **30**, 187–193

Weaver, T. E. and Scott, W. J. Jr. (1984b). Acetazolamide teratogenesis: interactions of maternal metabolic and respiratory acidosis in the induction of ectrodactyly in C57BL/6J mice. *Teratology*, **30**, 195–202

Weil, C. S. (1970). Selection of the valid number of sampling units and a consideration of their combination in toxicological studies involving reproduction, teratogenesis or carcinogenesis. *Fd. Cosmet. Toxicol.*, **8**, 177–182

Welsch, F. (1990). Teratogens and cell-to-cell communication. In De Mello, W. C. (Ed.), *Cell Intercommunication*. CRC Press, Boca Raton, FL, pp. 133–160

Whitten, W. K. (1956). Modification of the ooestrus cycle of the mouse by external stimuli associated with the male. *J. Endocrinol.*, **13**, 399–404

Whorton, D., Krauss, R. M., Marshall, S. and Milby, T. H. (1977). Infertility in male pesticide workers. *Lancet*, **ii**, 1259–1261

Whorton, D., Milby, T. H., Krauss, R. M. and Stubbs, H. A. (1979). Testicular function in DBCP exposed pesticide workers. *J. Occup. Medicine*, **21**, 161–166

Wiger, R., Støttum, A. and Brunborg, G. (1988). Estimating chemical developmental hazard in a chicken embryo limb bud micromass system. *Pharmacol. Toxicol.*, **62**, 32–37

Wickramarantne, G. A. de S. (1988). The post-natal fate of supernumerary ribs in rat teratogenicity studies. *J. Appl. Toxicol.*, **8**, 91–94

Wiger, R., Trygg, B. and Holme, J. A. (1989). Toxic effects of cyclophosphamide in differentiating chick limb and culture using rat liver 9,000g supernatant or rat liver cells as an activating system: an *in vitro*

short-term test for proteratogens. *Teratologicy*, **40(6)**, 603–613

Wilk, A. C., Greenberg, J. M., Horician, W. A., Pratt, R. M. and Martin, G. (1980). Detection of teratogenic compounds using differentiating embryonic cells in culture. *In Vitro*, **16**, 269–276

Wilkinson, D. G., Bailes, A. and McMahon, A. P. (1987). Expression of the proto-oncogene *int-l* is restricted to specific neuronal cells in the developing mouse embryo. *Cell*, **50**, 79–88

Williams, D. A. (1971). A test for differences between treatment means when several dose levels are compared with a zero dose control. *Biometrics*, **27**, 103–117

Williams, D. A. (1972). The comparison of several dose levels with a zero dose control. *Biometrics*, **28**, 519–531

Wilson, J. G. (1973). *Environment and Birth Defects*. Academic Press, New York (Environmental Sciences: An Interdisciplinary Monograph Series)

Wilson, J. G. (1978). Review of *in vitro* systems with potential for use in teratogenicity screening. *J. Environ. Pathol. and Toxicol.*, **2**, 149–167

Wilson, J. G. (1979). The evolution of teratological testing. *Teratology*, **20**, 205–212

Winer, B. J. (1962). *Statistical Principles in Experimental Design*. McGraw-Hill Book Co., NY

Wolkowski, R. M. (1970). Effect of actinomycin D on early axial development in chick embryos. *Teratology*, **3**, 389–398

Wolkowski-Tyl, R. M. (1981). Reproductive and teratogenic effects: no more thalidomides? *ACS Symposium Series: The Pesticide Chemist and Modern Toxicology*, **160**, 115–155

Yoneda, T. and Pratt, R. M. (1981). Interaction between glucocorticoids and epidermal growth factor *in vitro* in the growth of palatal mesenchymal cells from the human embryo. *Differentiation*, **19**, 194–198

FURTHER READING

Kimmel, C. A. and Buelke-Sam, J. (1994). *Developmental Toxicity*. 2nd edn. Raven Press, New York

Kimmel, C. A., Generoso, W. M., Thomas, R. D. and Bakshi, K. S. (1993). A new frontier in understanding the mechanisms of developmental abnormalities. *Toxicology and Applied Pharmacology*, **119**, 159–165

Schardein, J. L. (1993). *Chemically Induced Birth Defects*. Marcel Dekker, Inc., New York

Villeneuve, D. C. and Koeter, H. B. W. M. (1993). Proceedings of the international workshop on *In Vitro* methods in reproductive toxicology. *Reproductive Toxicology*, **7**, Supplement No. 1

41 Neonatal Toxicology

Sam Kacew

INTRODUCTION

In the strictest sense neonatal toxicology involves an abnormal responsiveness of newborns directly to therapeutic agents, recreational chemicals, drugs of abuse, or inadvertent exposure to environmental chemicals. Included in the definition of environmental exposure is the contact of an individual with chemicals in the workplace, termed occupational exposure. Environmental exposure can also arise through atmospheric, water, food or ground contamination, be it related to direct spraying of crops by farmers or an industrial accident, such as in Bhopal, or leaching at a hazardous waste site as occurred at Love Canal. In addition to direct contact of the newborn to chemicals, *in utero* exposure to drugs or environmental chemicals can also be manifested in altered newborn growth and functional development. Of necessity one must also consider the fact that newborn development can be modified by direct exposure to pharmacological and environmental chemicals through the mother's milk. Thus, to be able adequately to evaluate the effects of pharmacological and toxicological agents on the newborn, some consideration must be given to the role of drugs and environmental contaminants during pregnancy as well as after birth as reviewed by Schardein and Keller (1989). It should be noted that exposure to a chemical during pregnancy may take years before the toxicity becomes overt in the offspring; a notorious example being the use of diethylstilboestrol to prevent miscarriage which was found 20 years later to result in vaginal cancer in the female offspring.

In consideration of the use of therapeutic agents for management of disease in the mother and neonatal consequences, a dilemma can occur. Therapeutic drugs are, in specific circumstances, administered maternally to treat ailments, yet in the newborn can serve as a source of toxicity. Therapeutic agents are administered directly for the management of newborn disease, yet can in high doses produce adverse toxic reactions. A potentially dangerous, but not particularly emphasized problem is the abuse of the 'over-the-counter' (OTC) or self-administered drugs as a source of neonatal toxicity (Lock and Kacew, 1988). On the other hand, recreational or socially-used agents including alcohol and tobacco have been recognized as developmental toxicants in the foetus and newborn for many years. In addition to the socially used agents, one should be aware of the high levels of morbidity and mortality amongst newborn infants passively addicted to drugs of abuse, e.g. opioids as a result of maternal drug dependence.

Therapeutic agents form only a small fraction of the total number of chemicals in current use. At present it has been estimated that there are more than 60 000 chemicals in the commercial market; however, less than 20 per cent of these have been evaluated for their toxicological potential in adults. Because it was falsely perceived that an infant was merely a small adult, toxicological data were not obtained for neonates. Hence, substantially less toxicity data are available for newborns exposed to chemicals. With the realization that the newborn responds uniquely to drugs and chemicals, the aim of this chapter is to provide a general background on the developing infant from foetus to neonate and the consequences of toxicant exposure.

CHEMICAL EXPOSURE DURING PREGNANCY

During the pregnant state, inadvertent exposure to chemicals will affect two distinct individuals, the mother and foetus. Similarly, the obstetrician in the treatment of disease must consider not only the mother but also the developing foetus. However, little information is available on the influence of chemicals on maternal responses, with consequently even less known about foetal physiology. In reality the effects of chemicals on foetal status can be measured only through indirect techniques in the human. As outlined by Newton

(1989) the methodology used to assess foetal health status includes the following. (1) The measurement of various metabolic parameters in maternal serum. In particular the measurement of maternal serum α-fetoprotein at 15–20 weeks gestation is an index for a neural tube defect. (2) The aspiration of amniotic fluid (amniocentesis) at midtrimester is used to measure the concentrations of compounds which will predict neonatal distress syndrome with the most common index being the lecithin/sphingomyelin ratio. There is also cordocentesis, the aspiration of umbilical cord blood, for the determination of haemolytic disease. (3) The use of ultrasound especially in a high-risk population, such as a patient with hypertension, is very effective in predicting abnormal birth weight. (4) Foetal status is assessed by the electronic monitoring of foetal heart rate which is indicative of the balance between parasympathetic and sympathetic influences on the heart. A depression in the foetal heart rate can result in hypoxia. Although these different modes of foetal surveillance are available to the physician for screening infants in the high-risk group, the underlying causative factors involved in foetal injury and toxicity cannot be pinpointed with certainty. Finally it should be emphasized that any diagnostic test can by itself have dire consequences including maternal morbidity from tocolysis or neonatal morbidity from iatrogenic preterm delivery (Newton, 1989).

During the course of pregnancy a mother is likely to take a number of drugs for medicinal purposes. In the management of preterm labour to prevent preterm birth and neonatal morbidity in suitable patients, various agents such as alcohol, β-sympathomimetics, magnesium sulphate and calcium channel blockers may be utilized. Although these drugs stop labour, the incidence of preterm birth is not decreased (Newton, 1989). With the use of ritodrine, the only approved tocolytic agent, the high frequency of cardiovascular complications is indicative of the extreme caution and close supervision which is necessary. With many more women in the workforce there is an increased potential for interactions between therapeutic agents and a variety of chemicals present in the occupational environment. Furthermore, a large number of women indulge in a variety of recreational chemicals. Alcohol, as an example, is well known to influence drug action. The consequences attributed to the exposure to

a pharmaceutical product should be advantageous to the mother; however, in many instances the effects can be deleterious to the foetus. Thus it may be stated that the foetus is at some jeopardy as a result of exposure to foreign chemicals.

A subject that has received little attention but is now recognized as an important factor for foetal growth is the maternal diet and nutritional status. This has been recently reviewed by Basu (1988). In normal circumstances nutrients essential for foetal growth and development require an active transport system for them to be moved from the maternal circulation to the foetal circulation against a concentration gradient. However, as Basu (1988) points out, nutritional deficiency related to chemical or drug ingestion is not uncommon during pregnancy. As an example, chemical-induced vitamin B deficiency in the mother has resulted in stillbirth and low birth weight infants. A drug-induced deficiency in vitamin A has produced hydrocephalus and ocular defects; in vitamin D, has caused skeletal abnormalities; in vitamin K, has resulted in brain haemorrhage; and in vitamin E has caused anencephaly and cleft palate. Nutritional status also affects the process of drug absorption. Normally drugs cross the placenta by simple diffusion. A drug-induced destruction of maternal intestinal flora or the induction of vomiting may result in a nutritional imbalance. Consequently, maternal drug levels will rise with higher amounts transported to the foetus. The importance of chemical-induced nutritional deficiency in foetal development is difficult to delineate and more often than not overlooked.

There are a number of physicochemical factors that will influence the transfer of drugs from the maternal circulation to the foetus and thus will have a bearing on any subsequent foetal manifestations. The amount of a chemical that is transferred to the foetus is dependent on physicochemical properties such as lipid solubility, the degree of ionization and the molecular weight. Lipophilic drugs tend to diffuse across the placenta readily, while highly ionized compounds penetrate the placental membrane slowly. The molecular weight of an agent affects placental transfer with larger molecules crossing the placental barrier less readily. Foetal outcome is dependent on a pharmacodynamic system between mother and infant. The degree of protein binding of drug or chemical and/or its metabolic derivative in the mother ultimately determines the concentration of agent available for transfer to the foetus. The duration of exposure plays an important role in placental transfer and therefore subsequent foetal outcome. Furthermore, maternal metabolism is a determining factor for the amount of drug to be transferred to the foetus. In extensive reviews Juchau (1981, 1990) and Parke (1984) demonstrated that placental and/or foetal metabolism affects neonatal development and toxicity. The concentration of chemical in the foetal blood supply and elimination processes must also be considered in determination of foetal manifestations.

The physiological condition of the mother will affect placental transfer and foetal effects. In maternal diabetes the normal process of foetal lung maturation is delayed and manifested as infant respiratory distress syndrome (Bourbon and Farrell, 1985). The risk factor for foetal cerebral palsy is significantly increased in maternal thyroid disease or seizure patients (Newton, 1989). In the foetus itself genetic predisposition will affect neonatal development. The inability to metabolize phospholipid with subsequent accumulation results in Niemann–Pick and Tay–Sach's disease (Matsuzawa *et al.*, 1977). Inborn errors of metabolism associated with enzymic deficiency are a source of foetal toxicity (reviewed by Stanbury *et al.*, 1966).

It has been estimated that as of 1984 complete toxicological data are only available on approximately 18 per cent of the 53 500 chemicals used in commerce (Vorhees, 1986). The lack of information on single chemical exposure is self-evident but even less is known about the interaction between two drugs or a drug and an environmental agent on foetal outcome. Certain neonates can be subjected to at least four different drug preparations in the course of therapy (Aranda *et al.*, 1983). The manner in which drug–chemical interaction affects the foetus is a matter that requires intensive investigation. The adverse effects on the foetus of a mother who works in a smelting plant and smokes or an asthmatic mother who works in a plastics manufacturing firm remain to be established. In attempting to describe environmental or occupational pollutant interaction the consideration is primarily outdoors; however, indoor air pollution and foetal consequences must also be considered with respect to drug–chemical interactions.

A summary of the factors that influence the transfer of chemicals from the maternal circulation to the foetus and thus have a bearing on any subsequent foetal manifestations are presented in Table 1. An integral component which is frequently overlooked is the effect of paternal chemical exposure on foetal outcome. Exposure of males to lead, morphine, ethanol or caffeine has been shown to be associated with decreased birth weight and neonatal survival (Soyka and Joffe, 1980; Hill and Kleinberg, 1984a). It was suggested that the observed foetal manifestations arising from paternal chemical exposure may result from direct damage to spermatozoa or an alteration in the intrauterine environment such that normal development cannot occur. Exposure of females to formaldehyde, benzene, toluene, pesticides, etc. has been reported to produce menstrual disorders, increased rates of abortion, decreased foetal growth and low birth weight infants (Schrag and Dixon, 1985). Although the precise mechanisms are not known, female reproductive functions including oogenesis, steroidogenesis and ovulation can be affected by chemicals with subsequent foetal manifestations. It should be noted that damage to primary oocytes frequently results in cell death (Sonawane and Jaffe, 1988). However, genetically damaged oocytes can survive and become fertilized with the embryo dying at the stage of implantation. Basler *et al.* (1976) indicated that a small fraction of oocytes, with chemically induced damage, reach the embryonic stage but subsequently develop malformations and congenital childhood disorders.

The stage of foetal development at the time of chemical exposure will have a bearing on foetal outcome. During the first week of development after fertilization, the embryo undergoes the process of cleavage and gastrulation. Exposure to drugs such as antimetabolites, ergot alkaloids or diethylstilboestrol, at this stage can result in termination of pregnancy (Roberts, 1986). Organogenesis is the next developmental stage covering weeks 2–8 of gestation. Exposure to drugs including thalidomide, alcohol, lithium, phenytoin and isotretinoin during this phase can result in serious structural abnormalities (Arena and Drew, 1986; Manson, 1986; Roberts, 1986). Chemicals such as cigarette smoke, heavy metals or carbon monoxide may affect development during the remaining gestational period ranging from 9 weeks to 9 months. Predominant effects are alteration in the

Table 1 Factors affecting placental transfer and foetal drug effects

Physicochemical properties	The ability of drugs to reach the foetus are dependent on water solubility, lipid solubility and molecular weight
Pharmacokinetics	Foetus effects observed are dependent on drug concentration in maternal circulation, in foetal blood supply, placental and foetal drug metabolism, and elimination
Nutrition	Nutritional deficiency in the mother can influence placental transfer of essential nutrients to foetus
Physiological status	The absence of maternal hormones can alter the ability of foetus to cope with chemicals
Duration of exposure	A single administration of a high dose of a drug can produce damage to the same extent as chronic, low dose treatment
Genetic	Inborn errors of metabolism can predispose a foetus to enhanced toxicity
Drug interactions	The presence of more than one drug and/or chemical can increase susceptibility of the foetus
Environment	Various factors in outdoor or indoor environment can modify drug kinetics and thereby affect placental transfer
Developmental stage	Teratogenic agents act selectively on developing cells

Source: adapted from Lock and Kacew (1988) and Kacew and Lock (1990).

differentiation of the reproductive and central nervous systems (Roberts, 1986). Consequently, altered brain function and growth retardation are some of the principle adverse effects due to exposure at this stage. The relationship between stage of development and type of effect is illustrated in Table 2. As outlined by Schardein and Keller (1989) there are four established classes of developmental toxicity in animals which can be directly compared with humans. Intrauterine growth retardation, which is manifested as a decrease in foetal body weight in animals or as a low birth weight in humans, constitutes the first class of developmental toxicity. Newton *et al.* (1987) demonstrated a higher perinatal death rate associated with intrauterine growth retardation. Similarly, in growth-retarded infants there is an increased incidence of congenital anomalies, neurological deficits and learning disabilities (Christianson *et al.*, 1981; Miller, 1981). The estimated frequency in humans of intrauterine growth retardation is 7 per cent (Schardein and Keller, 1989). It is of interest that the risk of intrauterine growth retardation is increased in a chronic hypertensive mother (Newton, 1989). It is well established that in chronic hypertension the mother would normally be receiving medication. However, the influence of this medication on the manifestation (intrauterine growth retardation or perinatal mortality) is not known.

The second type of developmental toxicity is termed embryolethality and is manifested as resorption in animals or as spontaneous abortion with expulsion of product prior to the 20th week in humans, with an estimated frequency of 11–25 per cent (Hook 1981). It is believed that the predominant effect of toxicant exposure on development is spontaneous abortion (Stellman, 1979). In addition, spontaneous abortion is closely linked with the presence of congenital malformations. The abortive process may thus be considered as a mechanism to terminate an abnormal conception (Haas and Schottenfeld, 1979). Death in the developing foetus beyond 20 weeks of gestation results in stillbirth or foetal death. When calculated per 1000 live births the frequency of stillbirth is 7–9. Finally, death occurring within the first 28 days of life is termed neonatal death with an estimated frequency of 6–8 per 1000 live births (Newton, 1989). Neonatal death can result from infection, an accident or sudden infant death syndrome. However, Buehler *et al.* (1985) proposed that an increased percentage of neonatal death was merely a result of a postponement of lethal processes which were prevented from proceeding because of technological support systems. The role of chemicals in this latter phenomenon has yet to be established but it should be noted that the responsiveness to toxicants in numerous cases is cumulative and delayed.

The third class of developmental toxicity is congenital malformation and in general is manifested

Table 2 Relationship between developmental stage and foetal outcome

Developmental stage	Target system	Observed effect
Spermatozoa	Whole body	Decreased birth weight
		Neonatal mortality
Oocyte	Whole organism	Cell death
		Congenital anomalies
Placenta	Cardiovascular	Interference with active transport
		Alterations in maternal–foetal circulation
	Metabolism	Biosynthesis of nutrients
		Biotransformation of xenobiotics
Embryo	Whole organism	Intrauterine growth retardation
		Congenital anomalies
Foetus	Whole body	Growth retardation
	Reproductive and kidney	Genitourinary abnormalities
	Bone	Skeletal anomalies
Neonate	CNS	Neurobehavioural abnormalities
		Withdrawal symptoms
		Altered mental ability
	Reproductive	Altered fertility
	Respiratory	Respiratory depression
	Musculature	Hypotonia
	Whole organism	Neonatal death

Source: adapted from Lock and Kacew (1988), Hill and Kleinberg (1984a,b) and Kacew and Lock (1990).

as structural deformities. The congential malformations are distinctly different from the behavioural or functional abnormalities. Congenital malformations are associated with intrauterine growth retardation but are also considered a major cause of perinatal mortality (Newton, 1989). Approximately 14–18 per cent of infant death recorded was attributed to congenital malformations (Warkany, 1957; Newton *et al.*, 1987).

The fourth class of developmental toxicity is termed functional disorder and excludes those abnormalities considered as outright terata (Schardein and Keller, 1989). In this category are included behavioural functions such as learning ability and neuromotor ability as well as sensorimotor, reproductive and respiratory functions. In the broadest sense impairment or deficits in any biological system would fall into this category. Functional disorders are one of the major causes of perinatal mortality (Newton, 1989) and are

associated with congenital abnormalities (Smith and Bostian, 1964).

A perspective of the potential seriousness of the problems associated with drug use during pregnancy and the consequence to the foetus is gained from examination of Table 3. In addition, this table illustrates the effects of maternal occupational and/or environmental chemical exposure on foetal outcome. Although this table is extensive, it is by no means all-encompassing when one considers that there are currently over 60 000 chemicals available on the commercial market. Furthermore, there are two additional categories of agents to be described later, the over-the-counter (OTC) preparations and drugs of abuse, which deserve special attention. There are several important points to note with respect to Table 3. First, some of the effects shown to occur in humans by one group of investigators could not necessarily be confirmed by other scientists in this same species. Second, the route of

Table 3   Maternal exposure to industrial chemicals, environmental agents or drugs with foetal consequences

Toxicant	Foetal consequences
Acetazolamide	Electrolyte imbalance, haematological changes, forelimb defects[a]
Amantidine	Single ventricle, pulmonary atresia, skeletal anomalies[a]
Aminophylline	Tachycardia, gagging, vomiting, nervousness, opisthotonos, digit defects
Aminopterin	Multiple gross anomalies, foetal death, prenatal and postnatal growth retardation, renal anomalies, craniofacial abnormalities
Androgens	Masculinization of female foetus
Arsenic	Reduction in litter size, growth retardation[a], congenital anomalies[a]
Atropine	Tachycardia, dilated non-reactive pupils, skeletal anomalies[a], cytolytic effect on brain[a]
Azathioprine	Abnormal lymphocyte chromosomes at birth
β-Adrenergic agonists	Increase in foetal heart rate, foetal cardiac arrhythmias, foetal hyperglycaemia, hypotension
Benzene	Spontaneous abortion[a], stillbirth[a], congenital anomalies[a]
Bromides	Postnatal growth retardation, neurobehavioural abnormalities, acneform rash
Bupivacaine	Hyperirritability, incessant crying, meconium staining, metabolic acidosis, hypotonia, apnea, methaemoglobinaemia
Busulfan	Intrauterine, and postnatal growth retardation
Cadmium	Congenital anomalies[a], growth retardation[a]
Carbimazole	Goitre, hypothyroidism
Carbon disulphide	Spontaneous abortion, premature birth
Carbon monoxide	Stillbirth, functional neurological deficits, mental retardation
Chlorambucil	Renal agenesis, various foetal abnormalities[a]
Chloramphenicol	Increased risk of 'gray-baby' syndrome, cleft lip, cleft palate
Chlordiazepoxide	Newborn withdrawal
Chloroquine	Ototoxicity
Chlorpromazine	Extrapyramidal dysfunction, neonatal CNS depression, congenital malformations (?), gastrointestinal dysfunction, curled toe[a], intrauterine growth retardation[a]
Chlorpropamide	Hypoglycaemia
Cimetidine	Sexual dysfunction[a]
Clomiphene	Meningomyelocele, decreased birth weight, multiple births
Corticosteroids	Malpositioned kidney, decreased birth weight, increased antenatal death rate, electrolyte imbalance, increased lung maturity, increased risk of infection, cleft palate[a], skeletal abnormalities[a]
Cyclizine	Cleft palate[a], micrognathia[a], microstomia[a]
Cyclophosphamide	Digital defects, flattened nasal bridge, ectrodactyly, palatal anomalies, single coronary artery, bone marrow suppression
Cytarabine	Congenital malformations[a], cleft palate[a], club foot[a]
Dextropropoxyphene	Withdrawal symptoms
Diazepam	'Floppy' infant syndrome, newborn behaviour abnormalities, cleft lip and palate (?)
Diazoxide	Hyperglycaemia, hypertrichosis, languginosa, alopecia
Diethylstilboestrol	Vaginal adenocarcinoma, vaginal adenosis, penile abnormalities, epididymal cysts, hypotrophic testes, hypoplastic uterus, cervical gross defects

continued

Table 3 (continued)

Toxicant	Foetal consequences
Dimethylformamide	Foetal mortality
Dioxin (2,3,7,8,-TCDD)	Foetal death, low birth weight
Ergot	Spontaneous abortion, CNS symptoms, Poland syndrome
Ethchlorvynol	Lethargy, hypotonia, neurobehavioural
Ethylene oxide	Spontaneous abortion, reduced foetal weight[a], congenital malformations[a]
Ethinyl oestradiol	VACTEL anomalies, congenital heart defects, feminization of male foetus, trunco–conal great vessel malformation
5-Fluorouracil	Abortion, craniofacial abnormalities
Formaldehyde	Spontaneous abortion, low birth weight
Frusemide (furosemide)	Delay in renal maturation[a]
Glutethimide	Withdrawal manifestations, increased resorption rate[a]
Griseofulvin	Skeletal anomalies[a], eye defects[a], CNS dysfunction[a]
Haloperidol	Extrapyramidal dysfunction, neonatal CNS depression, congenital malformations (?), gastrointestinal dysfunction, curled toe[a], intrauterine growth retardation[a]
Halothane	Neonatal inability to habituate to auditory stimuli
Heparin	Perinatal and neonatal mortality incidence higher than with warfarin
Hexachlorobenzene	Stillbirths, neonatal mortality
Hydrochlorothiazide	Thrombocytopenia, hypoglycaemia, electrolyte imbalance
Hydroxyurea	Microphthalmia[a], hydrocephaly[a], decreased postnatal learning[a], palate and skeletal defects[a]
Hydroxyzine	Hypotonia, nervousness, myoclonic jerks, inability to read
Idoxuridine	Exophthalmos[a], club foot[a]
Imipramine	Respiratory difficulties, irritability, feeding difficulty, urinary retention, limb anomalies, encephaly, profuse sweating, skeletal anomalies[a]
Indomethacin	Neonatal pulmonary hypertension, disturbed cardiopulmonary adaptation, cleft lip and palate, infant death
Insulin	Growth retardation[a], skeletal anomalies[a], hypoglycaemia
Iodide	Goitre, abnormal neonatal thyroid function
Iodine (radioactive)	Hypothyroid, mental retardation, exophthalmos, goitre
Lead	Neurological deficits, spontaneous abortion, stillbirth, neonatal mortality
Lignocaine (lidocaine)	Seizures
Lithium	Congenital heart disease, goitre, hypotonia, hypothermia, neonatal cyanosis, poor sucking
Manganese	Foetal death[a]
Meclizine	Omphalocele, ectromelia, foetal death, cleft palate[a], incomplete skeletal ossification[a], macrostomia[a]
Mepivacaine	Foetal bradycardia
Meprobamate	Congenital heart disease, withdrawal symptoms, malformed diaphragm, behavioural abnormalities[a]
6-Mercaptopurine	Abortion, craniofacial abnormalities
Mercury	Growth retardation, spontaneous abortion, CNS dysfunction, cerebral palsy, foetal mortality
Methaqualone	Vertebral and rib defects[a]

continued overleaf

Table 3 (continued)

Toxicant	Foetal consequences
Methotrexate	Agenesis of frontal bones, cranial synostosis, abortion, unusual facies, postnatal growth retardation
Methoxyflurane	CNS depression, skeletal anomalies[a]
Methyltestosterone	Pseudohermaphroditism of female foetus
Methylthiouracil	Hypothyroidism, goitre
Mitomycin C	Defects of palate, skeleton and brain[a]
Molybdenum	Neurological defects[a], demyelination[a], symmetrical degeneration of white matter[a], foetal death[a]
Nitrofurantoin	Hemorrhage, anaemia
Nitrogen mustard	Small malpositioned kidney, bone marrow suppression
Novobiocin	Interference with bilirubin conjugation
Oral contraceptives	Congenital heart defects, limb reduction anomalies, VACTEL anomalies
Oxytocin	Hyperbilirubinaemia, delayed adaptation to extrauterine life, convulsions
Paraldehyde	Decreased adaptation to extrauterine life
Penicillamine	Abnormal connective tissue
Phenobarbitone (phenobarbital)	Acute: decreased hearing capacity, CNS depression, decreased incidence of neonatal hyperbilirubinaemia, haemorrhage, anaemia
	Chronic: infant withdrawal symptoms include tremulousness, excess crying, hyperphagia, hyperacusia, foetal addiction
Phenytoin	Foetal hydantoin syndrome: craniofacial abnormalities, limb abnormalities, mental and growth deficiency, congenital heart disease and hernias, coagulation defects, neonatal haemorrhage
Phthalate plasticizers	Intrauterine growth retardation[a], foetal mortality[a]
Polychlorinated biphenyls	Low birth weight, hypotonia, subcutaneous oedema, skin pigmentation, hyporeflexia
Procarbazine	Small, malpositioned kidney[a], anencephaly[a], congenital anomalies[a], CNS defects[a]
Progestins	Masculinization of female foetus, clitoral enlargement, lumbosacral fusion, VACTEL anomalies
Propranolol	Hypoglycaemia, bradycardia, apnea, prolonged labour, hypocalcaemia, intrauterine growth retardation, intrapartum asphyxia
Propylene oxide	Resorption[a], reduced foetal weight[a]
Propylthiouracil	Goitre, foetal death, hypothyroidism
Quinacrine	Increased foetal death rate[a]
Quinine	Mental retardation, ototoxicity, congenital glaucoma, genitourinary abnormalities, foetal death, anaemia
Reserpine	Nasal congestion and discharge, lethargy, hypothermia, bradycardia
Scopolamine	Lethargy, tachycardia, fever, respiratory depression
Styrene	Congenital anomalies
Styrene oxide	Reduced foetal weight[a], congenital malformations[a]
Sulphonamides	Methaemoglobinaemia, haemorrhage, anaemia, jaundice
Tetracyclines	Tooth discoloration, enamel hypoplasia, retardation in bone growth

continued

Table 3 *(continued)*

Toxicant	Foetal consequences
Thalidomide	Limb anomalies
Thallium	Reduced birth weight, alopecia, neonatal death
Tolbutamide	Foetal death, failure to thrive, apnoeic spells
Toluene	Intrauterine growth retardation, congenital anomalies, CNS dysfunction
Trimeprazine	Extrapyramidal dysfunction, neonatal CNS depression, congenital malformations (?), gastrointestinal dysfunction, curled toe[a], intrauterine growth retardation[a]
Trimethadione	Characteristic facies (V-shaped eyebrows and low ears), cardiac anomalies, ophthalmic anomalies, developmental delay, mental deficiency, growth retardation, conductive hearing loss
Valproic acid	Spina bifida
Vincristine	Small, positioned kidney[a], eye defects[a], cranial abnormalities[a], skeletal anomalies[a]
Warfarin	Embryopathy includes nasal hypoplasia and stippling of bone, ophthalmic abnormalities such as optic atrophy, cataracts and microphthalmia, developmental retardation, seizures, foetal mortality
Xylene	Congenital malformations[a], stillbirth[a], sacral agenesis[a]
Zinc	Hydrocephalus, hydroencephaly

[a] Non-human studies.

Sources: Hill and Stern (1979), Hill and Kleinberg (1984a,b), Kimmel *et al.* (1984), Lane and Hathaway (1985), Weber (1985), Arena and Drew (1986) Hill and Tennyson (1985), Kavlock *et al.* (1986), Roberts (1986), Hays and Pagliaro (1987), Lock and Kacew (1988), Kacew and Lock (1990).

exposure, particularly in the occupational workplace, has created difficulties in verification of chemical-induced effects. Exposure to benzene via inhalation produces developmental toxicity in the human while subcutaneous administration did not appear to induce malformations in rabbits or guinea pigs (Schardein and Keller, 1989). Third, the wide variation at the time and duration of exposure has resulted in conflicting evidence on chemical-induced effects. Fourth, the specificity of the response must be considered. In the case of styrene, where maternal occupational exposure induced developmental toxicity, an equivalent effect was not seen in four animal species (Murray *et al.*, 1978; Schardein and Keller, 1989). Fifth, the causative factor or chemical has also been a subject of controversy. In the case of developmental toxicity arising from 2,4,5-T (2,4,5-trichlorophenoxyacetic acid), a chlorophenoxy herbicidal component of Agent Orange, there are conflicting reports as to whether dioxin or 2,4,5-T is the culprit. Furthermore, if both chemicals are responsible, the contribution of each component towards the foetal outcome, which is spontaneous abortion, is still being debated (Hay,

1982). In the occupational field, discovery of the causative factor is compounded as individuals are subjected to a number of solvents at one time. For example, several solvents are used in the manufacture of pesticides, pharmaceutical products, paints, detergents, perfumes, fuels, dyes, etc. The finding that one solvent by itself in animal studies does not produce developmental toxicity is thus not surprising when compared with human data where exposure is usually to a number of solvents (Schardein and Keller, 1989). Finally, the differences in susceptibility between various animal species has been a subject of concern to scientists. Does the appearance of chemical-induced developmental toxicity in only one species establish that this agent is a teratogen? In spite of these uncertainties any reports of potential adverse effects of a chemical or drug on the unborn child should be taken into consideration by a physician. In the case of drugs there should be clear indication that the benefits derived by the mother from a specific drug greatly outweigh the risk to the foetus. By being overly cautious, the risks of chemical-induced foetal manifestations will be decreased.

In industrialized society, the overuse of self-administered or over-the-counter preparations during pregnancy is a growing problem. An increased knowledge combined with excessive advertisements has created the misconception that over-the-counter agents are necessary and safe even during pregnancy. It has been estimated that even when 200 active ingredients were used in over-the-counter preparations, the total number of products available was much higher, in the range of 100 000 to 500 000 (Moxley *et al.*, 1973). The potential foetal consequences attributed to maternal usage of over-the-counter preparations is shown in Table 4. Ingestion of a proper diet is sufficient to provide the necessary requirement for vitamins and iron. However, the erroneous belief that vitamin supplements provide extra energy and create a feeling of 'well-being' has resulted in the ingestion of quantities of vitamins vastly in excess of the recommended dietary allowance. This widespread nutritional self-medication promoted through effective, massive advertising can have dire consequences on the foetus and reiterates the fact that essential nutrients, in excess, are not safe. The use of over-the-counter mixtures of vitamins and minerals is not effective in abolishing iron deficiency anaemia and this practice should be discouraged. Although there is an increased demand for iron in pregnancy, the prophylactic use of iron to correct the deficiency should be carried out with caution. The misconception that frequent bowel movements are essential has resulted in the misuse of cathartics among some women. It is generally acknowledged that morning sickness is self-limiting and that antihistamines should be avoided. However, as can be seen in Table 4, maternal ingestion of antihistamines for this condition has occurred with consequent foetal effects. The antihistamines, along with antitussive agents, also constitute many cold remedies. Non-discriminant use of cold remedies during pregnancy thus serves as a source of drug exposure to the foetus. The utilization of antacids for conditions such as heartburn or reflux oesophagitis, when merely tilting the head to an upright position is sufficient to alleviate this condition, is an example of self-medication that is not necessary but does put the foetus at risk. The use of aspirin and paracetamol (acetaminophen) as well as other non-steroidal anti-inflammatory drugs such as ibuprofen or naproxen is not warranted during pregnancy (Table 4). It is even more disturbing in that aspirin is an ingredient in over 200 products (Leist and Banwell, 1974). In general the consumer would thus utilize a product without the realization that aspirin was being ingested. The controversy over the foetal consequences arising from coffee or tea drinking is still ongoing. However, it is generally accepted that a greater consumption would inevitably result in higher caffeine or theophylline levels in mother and foetus. As a consequence the potential for birth defects, irritability and tachycardia in infants of these beverage-consuming mothers is increased (Hill and Kleinberg, 1984a). An issue that still remains to be considered is the interaction between two over-the-counter preparations or between a required medication and an over-the-counter preparation. In a situation where a mother is being treated for a peptic ulcer with cimetidine, it is conceivable that there is simultaneous consumption of large quantities of tea (theophylline). Cimetidine, by preventing the metabolism of theophylline, results in increased theophylline concentrations and potentially a high risk of toxicity. Another example is the ingestion of iron to correct iron deficiency anaemia. If the mother is ingesting iron plus a multi-vitamin preparation, the latter preparation interferes with iron absorption. Consequently, less iron is available and the haematological response is impaired. The presence of over-the-counter preparations and concerted advertising may be a fact of life; however, increased awareness of the dangers associated with the use of self-medication must be stressed.

Drugs of abuse constitute those chemicals that are generally self-administered but are utilized for non-medicinal purposes and are not socially acceptable in a given culture. Included in this category of agents are tobacco (nicotine) and excess alcohol which are becoming increasingly unsociable and subject to greater restriction (Table 5). The campaigns for smoke-free environments in public places as well as against 'drinking and driving' are designed to point out the socially unacceptable attributes of these chemicals. It should be noted that passive smoking, which is exposure of a non-smoker to air contaminated by tobacco products, has been associated with adverse effects on foetal growth and development (Bottoms *et al.*, 1982). The epidemic associated with narcotic dependence in women and neonatal addiction was reviewed by Finnegan (1988). It is

Table 4 Foetal consequences attributed to active ingredients in over-the-counter preparations

Drug	Indication or source	Foetal effect
Aloe	Laxative	Increased intestinal peristalsis, release of meconium *in utero*, kidney damage
Aluminum compounds	Antacids	Reduced body weight[a], neurobehavioural dysfunction[a]
Betadine (Povidone-iodine)	Antiseptic	Goitre, hypothyroidism
Caffeine	Coffee	Neonatal irritability, reduced birth weight, limb reduction abnormalities[a], decreased ossification[a], tachycardia
Casathranol	Laxative	Congenital anomalies
Codeine	Antitussive	Cleft palate and lip[a], withdrawal symptoms[a], delayed ossification[a]
Dextromethorphan	Antitussive	Respiratory depression, withdrawal symptoms
Ferrous sulphate	Iron deficiency anaemia	Congenital malformations, gastrointestinal upset
Hexachlorophene	Soaps	Congenital malformation
Hexylresorcinol	Antiseptic	Liver toxicity, bone marrow depression, convulsions
Magnesium sulphate	Laxative	Hypotonia, hyporeflexia, CNS and respiratory depression, decreased adaptation to extrauterine life, convulsions
Magnesium trisilicate	Antacid	Kidney damage
Paracetamol (acetaminophen)	Analgesic, antipyretic	Foetal renal damage, renal failure, congenital cataracts, polyhydramnios
Phenylpropanolamine	Decongestant	CNS irritability, ear and eye defects[a], hypospadias[a]
Pseudoephedrine	Antitusive	Alkalosis
Pyridoxine	Nutrient	Convulsions
Salicylates	Analgesic, antipyretic	Gastrointestinal haemorrhage, neonatal petechiae, cephalohaematoma, bleeding tendency, low birth weight, increased perinatal mortality, neonatal pulmonary hypertension
Sodium bicarbonate	Antacid	Metabolic alkalosis, circulatory overload, oedema, congestive heart failure
Theophylline	Tea	Tachycardia, vomiting, teratogenic[a]
Vitamin A	Nutrient	Spontaneous abortion, hydrocephalus, cardiac abnormalities, teratogenesis[a], behavioural and learning disabilities[a], postnatal growth retardation[a]
Vitamin D	Nutrient	Supravalvular aortic stenosis, elfin facies, mental retardation, increased foetal death[a], skeletal anomalies[a]
Vitamin K (menadione)	Nutrient	Jaundice, haematological abnormalities

[a] Non-human studies.

Sources: see Table 3.

clearly established that maternal narcotic addiction is a significant health problem associated with a high incidence of prematurity, low birth weight infants and increased neonatal mortality. Although there are a number of complicating factors to be considered in narcotic-dependent mothers, which are not entirely attributable directly to the drug, it is evident that foetal morbidity and mortality are dire consequences. Despite the fact that data are not conclusive on the effects of hallucinogens such as marijuana, phencyclidine, mescaline or lysergic acid diethyl-

Table 5   Maternal ingestion of drugs of abuse with consequent foetal effects

Substance (classification)	Foetal consequence
Alcohol	Foetal alcohol syndrome, growth deficiency, abnormal facies, CNS disturbances
Amphetamines (stimulant)	Intrauterine growth retardation, cardiovascular anomalies, biliary tract atresia, prematurity, neonatal lethargy, withdrawal symptoms
Cannabis (marijuana)	Neurobehavioural abnormalities, teratogenesis[a], neural tube defects[a], foetal death[a], intrauterine growth retardation[a], abnormal neonatal behaviour[a]
Cocaine (stimulant)	Mental retardation, motor dysfunction, microcephaly
Heroin (narcotic)	Withdrawal symptoms in neonate, sudden infant death, respiratory CNS depression, thrombocytosis, intrauterine growth retardation, neonatal dependence
Lysergic acid diethylamide (hallucinogen)	Neurobehavioural abnormalities, foetal mortality[a], intrauterine growth retardation[a], congenital anomalies[a]
Meperidine (narcotic)	Withdrawal symptoms in neonate, sudden infant death, respiratory and CNS depression, thrombocytosis, intrauterine growth retardation, neonatal dependence
Mescaline (hallucinogen)	Increased resorption rate[a], CNS defects[a], intrauterine growth retardation[a]
Methadone (narcotic)	Withdrawal symptoms in neonate, sudden infant death, respiratory and CNS depression, thrombocytosis, intrauterine growth retardation, neonatal dependence
Morphine (narcotic)	Withdrawal symptoms in neonate, sudden infant death, respiratory and CNS depression, thrombocytosis, intrauterine growth retardation, neonatal dependence
Tobacco and nicotine (smoking)	Decreased foetal size[a], cleft palate[a], skeletal anomalies[a]
Phencyclidine (hallucinogen)	Abnormal facies, dislocated hip, cerebral palsy

[a] Non-human studies.

Sources: see Table 3.

amide, the scanty evidence available warrants avoidance of these chemicals during pregnancy. It should be noted that other drugs that are abused but appear in Table 3 include the barbiturates and the antidepressant tranquillizers such as diazepam and imipramine. In addition, the effects of volatile solvent abuse (glue sniffing) on foetal outcome are not established and thus included in this table. However, it has been estimated that there are over 1 million solvent abusers in the USA (Mikhael and Peel, 1984). In a recent study, inhalation of toluene by human pregnant mothers was reported by Hersh *et al.* (1985) to produce microcephaly, CNS dysfunction, craniofacial and limb anomalies, as well as impaired growth. Morbidity and mortality among newborn infants is a factor with therapeutically necessary drugs. However, the incidence of these complications is far greater in infants of maternal drug-of-abuse users. Despite this knowledge and awareness among the general population, the epidemic of drug abuse continues to increase.

CHEMICALS, DRUGS AND BREAST-FEEDING

The physiological process of breast-feeding plays a critical role in human infant development. As outlined by Lawrence (1989) breast-feeding provides not only essential nutrition but also protection against infection and other immunological disorders. It has been suggested that the incidence of gastrointestinal disease, respiratory ailments, otitis media and allergies occurs at a lower frequency in lactating infants (Chen *et al.*, 1988). Although the data are less conclusive, breast-feeding is believed to provide protection against obesity, arteriosclerosis, coeliac disease and other metabolic disorders (Lawrence, 1989). With respect to the mother, breast-feeding is known to create a special psychological bond between infant and mother which ultimately leads to a socially healthier child (Newton and Newton, 1967). In addition, lactation enhances maternal postpartum recovery and body weight returns to prepartum levels more rapidly. The distinct advantages of breast-feeding and breast milk are widely appreciated, and it is recommended that the barriers which keep women from initiation or continuation of this physiological process be decreased (Lawrence, 1989).

The nursing mother can serve as a source of neonatal exposure to drugs. No matter whether the agent is an over-the-counter medication or prescribed by a physician most drugs are detectable in breast milk. The presence of a drug in maternal milk may be construed as a potential hazard to the infant even though only 1–2 per cent of total intake is likely to be found there (Riordan, 1987). Hence the primary consideration in maternal drug therapy is the risk to the nursing infant rather than the mere presence of xenobiotic in the milk. Based on the numerous advantages of breast-feeding, the benefit of this physiological process in the majority of cases far exceeds the potential risk. Although it may be inadvertent, the lactating infant also derives environmental chemicals from the mother. These chemicals are excreted in breast milk and pose a serious potential hazard to the infant. Unlike drug therapy, which can be voluntarily terminated, environmental exposure may be chronic and consequently more toxic.

Several factors play a role in determining the quantity of a drug that will be transferred to breast milk. The amount of drug that is actually available for transfer to milk is dependent on certain maternal factors. As outlined in recent reviews (Nation and Hotham, 1987; Riordan, 1987), the dosage, frequency as well as route of drug administration are factors to consider in the mother. Following maternal intake the pharmacokinetic principles of absorption, distribution, metabolism and excretion of agent will play a role in determination of drug levels in the milk. The duration of exposure of the infant to lactational drugs can thus vary, dependent on maternal pharmacokinetics. If one considers the infant, the amount and frequency of feeding will affect the concentration of drug ingested. Furthermore, the flow and pH of blood to the breast, the composition and pH of milk, the rate of milk production as well as resorption of drug from milk into the maternal circulation are factors affecting the amount of drug reaching the infant. Finally, the most important factors influencing drug excretion into breast milk are the physicochemical features of the compound. The physicochemical characteristics, including degree of ionization, molecular weight, lipid solubility and protein-binding capacity, will affect the ability to traverse the mammary gland epithelium and thus be available to the suckling infant. The greater the degree of maternal plasma protein drug binding the less is the amount of agent available for diffusion through mammary alveolar membranes. This can be significant as drugs bind more readily to plasma proteins as opposed to milk proteins. For those drugs and chemicals that bind to milk proteins, one has to consider accumulation and the phenomenon of delayed responsiveness. Despite the lack of extensive data on the factors determining to what extent drug or chemical exposure may pose a toxic risk to the suckling infant, it is evident that in industrialized societies the lactational route of exposure must be considered as one of the initial sources of adverse effects.

As indicated by Roberts (1986) the critical factor to consider during breast-feeding is whether the drug utilized poses a documented risk to the infant. From the information available, it is generally believed that few drugs fall into the category of agents that initiate significant and predictable toxicity. Certain drugs should be totally avoided during lactation and mothers should be encouraged to restrict the intake of over-the-counter preparations as well as reduce social drug ingestion. The maternal use of routes of drug administration can be altered in certain conditions to minimize infant exposure, e.g. in asthma an inhaled bronchodilator being preferred to an oral medication. As the concentration of drug is a key factor in potential toxic outcome, it is self-evident that the minimal dose necessary for satisfactory treatment of a maternal disorder should be utilized, or the feeding schedule adjusted to minimize chemical levels in the milk. The fact that various drugs are present in breast milk (Riordan, 1987; Nation and Hotham, 1987) but do not appear to pose a risk to the infant, should not be deemed to indicate that it is safe to utilize the agent during lactation. A nursing mother should not be discouraged from utilizing drugs if maternal health is at stake. However, excessive use should be cautioned against or alternate, safer therapy should be sought.

In Western society with the advent of maternal leave, occupational exposure of nursing mothers to chemicals is diminished and consequently the lactational route does not appear to serve as a source for toxic agents. In contrast, environmental exposure or exposure via accidents and hazardous waste sites has resulted in chemical accumulation in breast milk. The human maternal ingestion of a fungicide, in the form of hexachlorobenzene-treated wheat, resulted in chemical accumulation in breast milk. Suckling infants subsequently developed symptoms of a disease, pembe yara, and porphyria cutanea tarda (Cam and Nigogosyan, 1963; Peters *et al.*, 1982). This accident occurred in Turkey but signficantly high concentrations of hexachlorobenzene have been

reported elsewhere, especially North America (Kitchin and Kacew, 1988). The manifestations are presented in Table 6. The Minamata Bay disaster in which nursing mothers ingested mercury-contaminated fish resulted in severe neurological disorders in human infants (Matsumoto *et al.*, 1965). Ingestion of polychlorinated biphenyl-contaminated rice oil by nursing mothers was thought to produce low birth weight human infants, growth retardation, abnormal skin pigmentation as well as bone and tooth defects

Table 6   Chemicals or drugs in breast milk and associated potential toxicity

Environmental chemical or drug	Adverse effects
Alcohol	Drowsiness, diaphoresis, growth retardation, Cushing's syndrome, decreased milk ejection reflex
Aloe	Increased bowel activity
Aluminum	Developmental retardation
Amantidine	Urinary retention, vomiting, skin rash
Amiodarone	Potential pulmonary toxicity
Amphetamines	Irritability, poor sleeping pattern
Androgens	Suppress lactation
Atropine	May suppress lactation, anticholinergic effects
Bendroflumethiazide	Suppresses lactation
Bromide	Rash, weakness, absence of cry
Bromocriptine	Suppresses lactation
Caffeine	Irritability, wakefulness
Cannabis	Drowsiness
Cathartics	Abdominal cramping, colic-like syndrome
Chloral hydrate	Sedation
Chloramphenicol	Possible bone marrow suppression, refusal to eat, vomiting
Chlorothiazide	May suppress lactation
Chlorpromazine	Drowsiness, lethargy, gynaecomastia in males, galactorrhea in females
Cimetidine	Suppresses gastric acidity in infant, inhibits drug metabolism, CNS stimulation
Clemastine	Drowsiness, irritability, refusal to feed, neck stiffness
Clomiphene	Suppresses lactation
Codeine	Bradycardia
Cyclophosphamide	Immune suppression
Diazepam	Sedation, accumulates in infant
Ergotamine	Vomiting, diarrhea, convulsions, suppresses lactation
Oestrogens	Feminization
Frusemide (furosemide)	Suppresses lactation
Glutethimide	May cause sedation

continued

Table 6 (continued)

Environmental chemical or drug	Adverse effects
Gold salts	Rash, inflammation of kidney and liver
Heroin	Neonatal narcotic dependence
Hexachlorobenzene	Severe skin disease, anaemia, porphyria, neonatal mortality
Indomethacin	Convulsions
I^{131}	Thyroid suppression
I^{125}	Risk of thyroid cancer
Isoniazid	Pyridoxine deficiency development, hepatotoxicity
Lead	Behavioural abnormalities
Levodopa	Suppresses lactation
Lithium	CNS disturbances, cardiovascular dysfunction
Mercury	Cerebral neuronal degeneration, mental retardation
Metergoline	Suppresses lactation
Methadone	Signs of opiate withdrawal if rapidly withdrawn
Methimazole	Decreased thyroid function
Methotrexate	Immune suppression
Metoclopramide	Increases milk production, galactorrhea
Metronidazole	Secreted into milk to same level as plasma; thus CNS and haematopoietic adverse effects too risky
Mirex	Cataracts
Morphine	Prolongs habituation
Nalidixic acid	Haemolytic anaemia
Nicotine (excess)	Shock, restlessness, decreased milk production, increased risk of infection
Nitrofurantoin	Haemolysis in glucose-6-phosphate dehydrogenase-deficient infant
Novobiocin	Hyperbilirubinaemia
Oral anticoagulants (ethyl biscoumacetate)	Cephalohaematoma, increased risk of bleeding problems
Oral contraceptives	Breast enlargement, decrease in milk production and protein content, feminization, decreased weight gain
Phenindione	Haemorrhage
Phenobarbitone (phenobarbital)	Sedation, decreased responsiveness, methaemoglobinaemia, poor suck reflexes
Phenytoin	Methaemoglobinaemia
Prednisone	Growth suppression, adrenal suppression
Prostaglandins	Suppress lactation
Salicylates	Metabolic acidosis, rash
Sulphonamides	Increased risk of kernicterus, allergic manifestations, neonatal jaundice
Tetracycline	Possible permanent staining of developing teeth
Theophylline	Irritability, fretful sleep
Tolbutamide	Jaundice, hypoglycaemia
Vitamin B_6 (pyridoxine)	Suppresses lactation

Source: adapted from Lock and Kacew (1988), Nation and Hotham (1987), Riordan (1987) and Kacew and Lock (1990).

(Yamaguchi *et al.*, 1971). In extensive studies in North Carolina, Rogan *et al.* (1986) measured the levels of polychlorinated biphenyls in human milk and found an associated hypotonicity and hyporeflexia in nursing infants. The symptoms associated with aluminum during lactation in mice include a reduced body weight and developmental retardation (Golub *et al.*, 1987). Exposure to pesticides such as mirex through gestation and lactation was found to result in a dose-related incidence of irreversible cataracts in rat pups (Chernoff *et al*, 1979). High concentrations of other organochlorine insecticides including DDT, dieldrin, lindane and chlordane have been found in human mother's milk (Virgo, 1984). Although the consequences of parent insecticides are not known in humans, Rogan *et al.* (1986) found that DDE, a metabolite of DDT, produced hyporeflexia in human infants. Fahim *et al.* (1970) demonstrated decreased growth and enhanced neonatal death among pups of dams given DDT during lactation. Early functional development characterized by a righting reflex, visual-evoked responsiveness and body temperature control is altered and delayed in pups of dams receiving lead during the lactational period (Kimmel, 1984). In the case of cigarette smoking there is a greater risk in human infants of respiratory infection and other infection from breathing smoke-filled air than from nicotine levels in breast milk (Riordan, 1987).

A somewhat more obscure but potentially no less serious situation is the use of certain consumer products which are used without warning or labels. Cosmetic preparations are known to contain oestrogens. Incidents include a 5-year-old boy using a hair cream who was found to develop gynaecomastia, and an 8-month-old girl treated for diaper rash developed enlarged breasts and pubic hair. Oestrogens are a component of oral contraceptives and accumulate in breast milk. It has been reported that use of oral contraceptives during lactation results in infant feminization and reduced weight gain (Riordan, 1987). The combination of a cosmetic and oral contraceptive would undoubtedly cause even higher milk oestrogen content and may result in feminization.

The physiological process of breast-feeding should be encouraged under most circumstances despite the presence of drugs. Most drugs are usually compatible with breast-feeding. The issue of environmental chemicals and breast-feeding needs to be addressed.

CHEMICALS, DRUGS AND NEONATAL TOXICITY

The pharmacokinetic principles applied in paediatric drug therapy are, in general, similar to those utilized for adults. However, data obtained in adult studies are not always applicable to rational therapy in infants or young children. The infant must be regarded as a distinct organism. Lack of appreciation of this fact could result in serious harm and potentially death. During infancy and childhood the body weight and composition is continuously changing such that the pharmacodynamic aspects of drug therapy are not predictable. Furthermore, in most cases the approval of drugs for adult therapy is not accompanied by adequate data to allow for use in children (Rane and Wilson, 1976). Despite the informational inadequacies the utilization of drugs in infants seems to be increasing. In their extensive studies, Aranda *et al.* (1982, 1983) reported that there were more than 30 different preparations that were administered at least once to the neonate. In addition, infants were subjected to polypharmacy as evidenced by at least four different drugs per baby in approximately 50 per cent of the patient population.

Drug utilization and consequent toxicity has also increased among the non-hospitalized paediatric population (Wiseman *et al.*, 1987a). Indeed, the prescribing habits of general practitioners was compared with the habits of hospital physicians for the condition of acute gastroenteritis in children. Over a 5-year period Choonara *et al.* (1987) found that general practitioners prescribed significantly more medicines than did hospital physicians. When one considers that gastroenteritis is self-limiting, this indicates that drug utilization is still too high in non-hospitalized children. Furthermore, Eskola and Poikolainen (1985) listed the number of drug poisonings in children aged 0–6 years and demonstrated a relationship to the season with recurring peaks over a 3-year period. Various investigators have also reported on a correlation between season and drug poisoning (Basavaraj and Forster, 1982; Paulozzi, 1983). In addition to inadvertent or accidental exposure, failure to comply with the proper use of drugs can either lead to toxicity as a result of excess amount or to ineffective therapy from underdosing. Compliance failure in children can occur when parents are inadequately instructed, or where patients refuse to take the drugs as directed. Failure to comply is not restricted solely to the home but can occur in a hospital (Becker *et al.*, 1972; Wilson, 1973). It is evident that the pharmacokinetic principles of drug utilization are dependent on proper paediatric compliance.

Unlike drugs, an infant is not normally administered a chemical that has no direct therapeutic potential. The potential for infants to be exposed to environmental agents is equivalent to adults in ambient air. Significant industrial pollution and photochemical smog in severe cases can produce respiratory irritation, oedema and hyperplasia. A concentration-dependent immunological response can occur as a consequence of exposure to certain chemicals. Because the lung cells of neonates are not fully developed, this population is more susceptible to the toxic actions of chemicals. As a general rule the potential risk of toxicity to chemicals or drugs is far higher in the neonate compared with the adult. In purulent otitis media, ear irrigations are carried out with aqueous merthiolate. However, in an 18-month-old infant, mercury toxicity, as manifested by metabolic acidosis, hypertension, renal failure and congestive heart failure, developed (Rohyans *et al.*, 1984). The use of this compound in adults did not appear to induce this severe reaction.

The pharmacokinetic principles to be discussed are applicable to chemicals or drugs. The route of exposure for environmental chemicals is primarily via inhalation; however, one should be aware of accidental poisoning from ingestion of household chemicals or toxic plants as well as topical application. A number of important characteristics exist that distinguish drug therapy in infants from adult medication protocols. For example, after intramuscular administration, drug absorption is partially dependent on blood in the muscle bed. Abnormal drug absorption following intramuscular injection can occur in premature infants where muscle mass is small and blood flow to the musculature is poor. Examples of adverse effects attributed to altered drug absorption are the reaction of infants to cardiac glycosides and anticonvulsants. The intramuscular route is not applicable to chemicals as a means of exposure.

In the infant, absorption from the gastrointesti-nal tract of an orally administered drug or chemical differs from that in adults. In both adults and infants the rate and extent of drug absorption is dependent on the degree of ionization which, in turn, is influenced by pH. Within the first 24 h of life gastric acidity increases rapidly and this is followed by an elevation in alkalinity over the next 4–6 weeks. These conditions result in drugs existing in the infant gastrointestinal tract in different states of ionization than might be observed in adults. Other factors that modify gastrointestinal drug or chemical absorption in the young infant as summarized by Roberts (1986) include an irregular neonatal peristalsis, a greater gastrointestinal tract surface to body ratio, and enhanced intestinal β-glucuronidase activity. The significance of the β-glucuronidase is that it releases drug bound glucuronide to the free form and thus increases drug bioavailability. The bioavailability of drug is also related to the diurnal pattern. In general the urinary pH is acidic during sleep. In infants where the tendency is to sleep for a greater portion of the day, acid drug excretion would decrease in the presence of a low pH; and hence the bioavailability of sulphonamides would be enhanced during the sleep period. In contrast, the bioavailability of basic drugs would be reduced during the sleep phase.

Differences exist in the organ distribution of drugs or chemicals between newborns and adults. In the newborn a higher percentage of body weight is represented by water, thus extracellular water space is proportionally larger (Friis-Hansen, 1961). To initiate a receptor response the distribution of drugs or chemicals must occur predominantly in the extracellular space, thus the concentration of drug or chemical reaching the receptor sites would be higher in neonates. Furthermore, the ability of newborns to bind drugs in plasma is significantly less than adults. (Rane and Wilson, 1976). This is supported by the findings of Gorodischer *et al.* (1976) who reported a twofold increase in myocardial digoxin levels in infants as compared with adults. Similarly, a fivefold higher myocardium/serum ratio was subsequently found in infants administered digoxin in comparison with adults (Park *et al.*, 1982). In addition to digoxin, significantly less plasma protein binding in the infant compared with the adult was noted for salicylates, diazoxide, phenytoin, propranolol, phenobarbitone, theophylline, penicillin and lignocaine (lidocaine). As a further complication, drug binding in neonates is also reduced by endogenous substrates including free fatty acids and bilirubin (Fredholm *et al.*, 1975). This again suggests that neonates could be expected to be more susceptible to the effects of free drug circulating in the plasma.

Enhanced susceptibility to adverse reactions in the neonate is a consideration for establishing dosing guidelines on the side of safety. In view of this fact theophylline was recommended at a dose sufficient to produce a blood level of 6–10 μg ml^{-1} for the treatment of apnoea of prematurity (Jones and Baillie, 1979). With more extensive study Gal and Gilman (1986) found that a neonate could tolerate a dose as high as that producing a level in serum of 20 μg ml^{-1} theophylline and apnoeas were eliminated. Based on this growing amount of information it was suggested that the dosing guidelines and therapeutic range should be re-evaluated. This is simply an example of the need to re-examine the current knowledge of paediatric responsiveness to drugs. Thus acquired data can be used subsequently to establish a more effective therapeutic regimen in the newborn.

Differences also exist with respect to drug metabolizing enzymes. It has been clearly demonstrated that the drug or chemical inactivation rate is generally slower in newborns (Parke, 1984; Juchau, 1990). However, one can not generalize about the drug metabolizing capacity in newborns as there is a marked variability among infants and this capacity is highly dependent on the drug being examined (Rane *et al.*, 1974). Furthermore, certain metabolic pathways exist uniquely in the neonate (Takkieddine *et al.*, 1981; Parke, 1984). Although drug metabolism is a means of chemical inactivation, it is also a process utilized to form an active component. In an effort to obtain a therapeutically effective regimen this factor must be considered in light of the fact that hepatic drug metabolizing enzyme capacity is age-related. The appreciation of the role of drug metabolism in therapeutics is suggestive that further study is necessary to maximize the ability of the physician to calculate a desired drug dosage.

The ability of the neonate to eliminate drugs or chemicals via the kidney, the major excretion pathway, is significantly limited by the state of development of these organs. It is well established that the half-life of several antibiotics is prolonged in the neonatal period owing to a decreased glomerular filtration rate (Axline *et al.*,

1967). However, the glomerular filtration rate reaches the level seen in adults by 5 months of age (West *et al.*, 1948). In addition, the renal tubular secretory capacity increases during the first few months to attain adult values at 7 months of age. Consequently, an agent eliminated via the secretory renal pathway would have a threefold longer half-life in the infant. Aranda and Stern (1983) found that the clearance of phenytoin and phenobarbitone (phenobarbital) was rapid in the first week or two of age yet theophylline and caffeine clearance remained low until the age of 6 weeks. In a recent study Leff *et al.* (1986) attributed the need for a greater dosage of phenytoin in infants compared with the adult as a result of increased metabolic clearance in the infant. The knowledge of clearance rates is essential in consideration of initial as well as subsequent drug dosage in the patient.

The morphological and metabolic responsiveness of the newborn to chemical or drug exposure can also result in less damage compared with the adult. Various investigators demonstrated that exposure of newborns to ozone or nitrogen dioxide produced less pulmonary damage than in mature animals (Freeman *et al.*, 1974; Ospital *et al.*, 1977) The phospholipidosis induced in pulmonary tissue by chlorphentermine was found to occur in adults at a much lower dose, suggesting that newborns are less sensitive (Kacew, 1984). Similarly, newborns were responsive to the nephrotoxic action of gentamicin but at much higher drug concentrations compared with adults (Kacew, 1985). The increased resistance of newborns to aminoglycoside nephrotoxicity was suggested to be associated with lower kidney antibiotic content (Kacew *et al.*, 1989). The basis for these differences in responsiveness between newborns and adults still warrants further study. It is evident that the predictability of neonatal toxicity is subject to a number of complex factors.

CHEMICALS, DRUGS AND OLDER CHILDREN

Within the context of this chapter, the final stage constitutes the older child where patterns of drug disposition are far less important than dose calculation based on normal growth. As the child grows, the pathways of drug or chemical biotransformation and metabolism are similar to those noted in the adult. In addition, the total body water distribution, albeit on a smaller scale, is similar in the child and adult. Despite these recognized similarities, barbiturates produce CNS stimulation in the child as compared with sedation in the adult (Camfield *et al.*, 1979). In a study of 1327 children attending outpatient clinics, the incidence of adverse drug reactions was 0.75 per cent (Sanz and Boada, 1987). The nature of these adverse reactions was slight, occurred predominantly in females and was associated with polypharmacy. As in the cases of the neonate, polypharmacy is believed to play an important role in initiation of adverse drug reactions.

There are other problems associated with therapy, the major component being compliance. At this stage of development the physician is still reliant on an adult, who at the best of times may not be consistent. Ultimately the onus is on the physician adequately to inform the responsible individual of the necessity for compliance and the consequences resulting from failure to adhere.

The developing organism is unique in its responsiveness to drugs or chemicals, and predictability of therapeutic effectiveness based on the adult can lead to grave consequences in the neonate and child. It should be emphasized that adverse drug or chemical reactions may take years to become overt whether the compound is administered to the mother or directly to the child, an example being diethystilboestrol-induced vaginal carcinoma in children 18 years later. Although the current trend is geared towards use of drugs, the role of the physician should be aimed towards caution rather than overuse. Concurrently, with the greater availability of over-the-counter drugs, adequate education of the dangers of these compounds should be promoted. Wiseman *et al.* (1987b) recently demonstrated that prescription medications were more frequently involved in accidental poisoning in children compared with over-the-counter drugs. It is of interest that packaging of drugs is now an important consideration in accidental childhood poisoning.

The aim of this chapter was to describe in greater detail the effects of drugs currently and frequently prescribed by the paediatrician. Furthermore, it is hoped that an awareness was created of the potential toxicity to environmental agents despite the fact that direct exposure might only have taken place via the mother. Neonatal toxicity should be considered as complex as adult toxicity and not merely as an extension of effects seen in the mature population.

REFERENCES

Aranda, J. V. and Stern, L. (1983). Clinical aspects of developmental pharmacology and toxicology. *Pharmacol. Ther.*, **20**, 1–51

Aranda, J. V., Collinge, J. M. and Clarkson, S. (1982). Epidemiologic aspects of drug utilization in a newborn intensive care unit. *Semin. Perinatol.*, **6**, 148–154

Aranda, J. V., Clarkson, S. and Collinge, J. M. (1983). Changing pattern of drug utilization in a neonatal intensive care unit. *Am. J. Perinatol.*, **1**, 28–30

Arena, J. M. and Drew, R. H. (1986). Teratogenicity. In Arena, J. M. and Drew, R. H. (Eds), *Poisoning: Toxicology, Symptoms, Treatments*, 5th edn. Charles C. Thomas, Springfield, IL, 997–1007

Axline, S. G., Yaffe, S. J. and Simon, H. J. (1967). Clinical pharmacology of antimicrobials in premature infants. *Pediatrics*, **39**, 97–107

Basavaraj, D. S. and Forster, D. P. (1982). Accidental poisoning in young children. *J. Epidemiol. Community Health*, **36**, 31–34

Basler, A., Buselmaier, B. and Rohrborn, G. (1976). Elimination of spontaneous and chemically induced aberrations in mice during early embryogenesis. *Hum. Genet.*, **33**, 121–130

Basu, T. K. (1988). Nutritional factors and dispositions of pharmacological chemicals in prenatal and neonatal life. In Kacew, S. and Lock, S. (Eds), *Toxicologic and Pharmacologic Principles in Pediatrics*. Hemisphere Publishing, Washington, DC, pp. 17–40

Becker, M. H., Drachman, R. H. and Kirscht, J. P. (1972). Predicting mothers' compliance with paediatric medical regimes. *J. Pediat.*, **81**, 843–854

Bottoms, S. F., Kuhnert, B. R., Kuhnert, P. M. and Reese, A. L. (1982). Maternal passive smoking and foetal serum thiocyanate levels. *Am. J. Obstet. Gynecol.*, **144**, 787–791

Bourbon, J. R. and Farrell, P. M. (1985). Fetal lung development in the diabetic pregnancy. *Pediat. Res.*, **19**, 253–267

Buehler, J. W., Hogue, C. J. R. and Zaro, S. M. (1985). Postponing or preventing death? Trends in infant survival, Georgia, 1974 through 1981. *J. Am. Med. Assoc.*, **253**, 3564–3567

Cam, C. and Nigogosyan, G. (1963). Acquired toxic porphyria cutanea tarda due to hexachlorobenzene. *J. Am. Med. Assoc.*, **183**, 88–91

Camfield, C. S., Chaplin, S., Doyle, A. B., Shapiro, S. H., Cummings, C. and Camfield, P. R. (1979). Side-effects of phenobarbital in toddlers; behavioural and cognitive aspects. *J. Pediat.*, **95**, 361–365

Chen, Y., Yu, S. and Li, W. X. (1988). Artificial

feeding and hospitalization in the first 18 months of life. *Pediatrics*, **81**, 58–62

Chernoff, N., Linder, R. E., Scotti, T. M., Rogers, E. H., Carver, B. D. and Kavlock, R. J. (1979). Fetotoxicity and cataractogenicity of mirex in rats and mice with notes on kepone. *Environ. Res.*, **18**, 257–269

Choonara, I. A., Shoo, E. E. and Owens, G. G. (1987). Prescribing habits for children with acute gastroenteritis: a comparison over 5 years. *Br. J. Clin. Pharmacol.*, **23**, 362–364

Christianson, R. E., van den Berg, B. J., Milkovich, L. and Oechsli, F. W. (1981). Incidence of congenital anomalies among white and black live births with long-term follow-up. *Am. J. Public Health*, **71**, 1333–1341

Eskola, J. and Poikolainen, K. (1985). Seasonal variation and recurring peaks of reported poisonings during a 3-year period. *Hum. Toxicol.*, **4**, 609–615

Fahim, M. S., Bennett, R. and Hall, D. G. (1970). Effect of DDT on the nursing neonate. *Nature*, **228**, 1222–1223

Finnegan, L. P. (1988). Influence of maternal drug dependence on the newborn. In Kacew, S. and Lock, S. (Eds), *Toxicologic and Pharmacologic Principles in Pediatrics*. Hemisphere Publishing, Washington, DC, pp. 183–198

Fredholm, B. B., Rane, A. and Persson, B. (1975). Diphenylhydantoin binding to proteins in plasma and its dependence on free fatty acid and bilirubin concentration in dogs and newborn infants. *Pediat. Res.*, **9**, 26–30

Freeman, G., Juhos, L. T., Furiosi, N. J., Mussenden, R. and Weiss, T. A. (1974). Delayed maturation of rat lung in an environment containing nitrogen dioxide. *Am. Rev. Resp. Dis.*, **110**, 754–759

Friis-Hansen, B. (1961). Body water compartments in children: changes during growth and related changes in body composition. *Pediatrics*, **28**, 169–181

Gal, P. and Gilman, J. T. (1986). Concerns about the food and drug administration guidelines for neonatal theophylline dosing. *Ther. Drug Monitor*, **8**, 1–3

Golub, M. S., Gershwin, M. E., Donald, J. M., Negri, S. and Keen, C. L. (1987). Maternal and developmental toxicity of chronic aluminium exposure in mice. *Fundam. Appl. Toxicol.*, **8**, 346–357

Gorodischer, R., Jusko, W. J. and Yaffe, S. J. (1976). Tissue and erythrocyte distribution of digoxin in children. *Clin. Pharmacol.*, **19**, 256–263

Haas, J. F. and Schottenfeld, D. (1979). Risks to the offspring from occupational exposure. *J. Occup. Med.*, **21**, 607–613

Hay, A. (1982). Vietnam and 2,4,5-T. In Hay, A. (Ed.), *The Chemical Scythe*. Plenum Press, New York, pp. 147–185

Hays, D. P. and Pagliaro, L. A. (1987). Human teratogens. In Pagliaro, L. A. and Pagliaro, A. M. (Eds), *Problems in Pediatric Drug Therapy*, 2nd edn. Drug Intelligence Publications, Hamilton, IL, pp. 51–191

Hersh, J. H., Podruch, P. E., Rogers, G. and Weisskopf, B. (1985). Toluene embryopathy. *J. Pediat.*, **106**, 922–927

Hill, L. M. and Kleinberg, F. (1984a). Effects of drugs and chemicals on the foetus and newborn. *Mayo Clin. Proc.*, **59**, 707–716

Hill, L. M. and Kleinberg, F. (1984b). Effects of drugs and chemicals on the foetus and newborn (second of two parts). *Mayo Clin. Proc.*, **59**, 755–765

Hill, R. M. and Stern, L. (1979). Drugs in pregnancy: effects on the foetus and newborn. *Drugs*, **17**, 182–197

Hill, R. M. and Tennyson, L. M. (1985). Maternal drug therapy: effect on foetal and neonatal growth and neurobehaviour. *Neurotoxicology*, **7**, 121–139

Hook, E. B. (1981). Human teratologic and mutagenic markers in monitoring about point sources of pollution. *Environ. Res.*, **25**, 178–203

Jones, R. A. K. and Baillie, E. (1979). Dosage schedule for intravenous aminophylline in apnea of prematurity based on pharmacokinetic studies. *Arch. Dis. Child*, **54**, 194–199

Juchau, M. R. (1981). Enzymatic bioactivation and inactivation of chemical teratogens. In Juchau, M. R. (Ed.), *The Biochemical Basis of Chemical Teratogenesis*. Elsevier North Holland, Amsterdam, pp. 63–94

Juchau, M. R. (1990). Fetal and neonatal drug biotransformation. In Kacew, S. (Ed.), *Drug Toxicity and Metabolism in Pediatrics*. CRC Press, Florida, pp. 15–34

Kacew, S. (1984). Role of age in amphiphilic drug-induced pulmonary morphological and metabolic responses. *Fed. Proc.*, **43**, 2592–2596

Kacew, S. (1985). Gentamicin or chlorphentermine induction of phospholipidosis in the developing organism: role of tissue and species in manifestation of toxicity. *J. Pharmacol. Exp. Ther.*, **232**, 239–243

Kacew, S. and Lock, S. (1990). Developmental aspects of paediatric pharmacology and toxicology. In Kacew, S. (Ed.), *Drug Toxicity and Metabolism in Pediatrics*. CRC Press, Florida, pp. 1–13

Kacew, S., Hewitt, W. R. and Hook, J. B. (1989). Gentamicin-induced renal metabolic alterations in newborn rat kidney: lack of potentiation by vancomycin. *Toxicol. Appl. Pharmacol.*, **99**, 61–71

Kavlock, R. J., Rehnberg, B. F. and Rogers, E. H. (1986). Chlorambucil induced congenital renal hypoplasia: effects on basal renal function in the developing rat. *Toxicology*, **40**, 247–258

Kimmel, C. A. (1984). Critical periods of exposure and developmental effects of lead. In Kacew, S. and Reasor, M. J. (Eds), *Toxicology and the Newborn*. Elsevier Science Publishers, Amsterdam, pp. 219–235

Kitchin, K. T. and Kacew, S. (1988). Some pharmacokinetic and metabolic factors affecting the neonatal toxicity of halogenated hydrocarbons found in the Great Lakes. In Kacew, S. and Lock, S. (Eds), *Toxi-*

cologic and Pharmacologic Principles in Pediatrics. Hemisphere Publishing, Washington DC, pp. 223–253

Lane, P. A. and Hathaway, W. E. (1985). Vitamin K in infancy. *J. Pediat.*, **106**, 351–359

Lawrence, R. A. (1989). Breastfeeding and medical disease. *Med. Clin. North Am.*, **73**, 583–603

Leff, R. D., Fischer, L. J. and Roberts, R. J. (1986). Phenytoin metabolism in infants following intravenous and oral administration. *Dev. Pharmacol. Ther.*, **9**, 217–223

Leist, E. R. and Banwell, J. G. (1974). Products containing aspirin. *N. Engl. J. Med.*, **291**, 710–712

Lock, S. and Kacew, S. (1988). General principles in paediatric pharmacology and toxicology. In Kacew, S. and Lock, S. (Eds), *Toxicologic and Pharmacologic Principles in Pediatrics*. Hemisphere Publishing, Washington, DC, pp. 1–15

Manson, J. M. (1986). Teratogens. In Klaassen, C. D., Amdur, M. O. and Doull, J. (Eds), *Casarett and Doull's Toxicology: The Basic Science of Poisons*, 3rd edn. Macmillan Publishing, New York, pp. 195–220

Matsumoto, M., Koya, G. and Takeuchi, T. (1965). Fetal Minamata disease. *J. Neuropathol. Exp. Neurol.*, **24**, 563–574

Matsuzawa, Y., Yamamoto, A., Adachi, S. and Nishikawa, M. (1977). Studies on drug-induced lipidosis. *J. Biochem.*, **82**, 1369–1377

Mikhael, N. Z. and Peel, H. W. (1984). Maternal drug abuse and subsequent effects on the newborn. In Kacew, S. and Reasor, M. J. (Eds), *Toxicology and the Newborn*. Elsevier Science Publishers, Amsterdam, pp. 101–120

Miller, H. C. (1981). Intrauterine growth retardation. An unmet challenge. *Am. J. Dis. Child.*, **135**, 944–948

Moxley, J. H., Yingling, G. L. and Edwards, C. C. (1973). The Food and Drug Administration's over-the-counter drug review: why review OTC drugs? *Fed. Proc.*, **32**, 1435–1437

Murray, F. J., John, J. A., Balmer, M. F. and Schwetz, B. A. (1978). Teratologic evaluation of styrene given to rats and rabbits by inhalation or by gavage. *Toxicology*, **11**, 335–343

Nation, R. L. and Hotham, N. (1987). Drugs and breast feeding. *Med. J. Australia*, **146**, 308–313

Newton, E. R. (1989). The foetus as a patient. *Med. Clin. North Am.*, **73**, 517–540

Newton, N. and Newton, M. (1967). Psychologic aspects of lactation. *N. Engl. J. Med.*, **277**, 1179–1188

Newton, E. R., Kennedy, J. L. and Louis, F. (1987). Obstetric diagnosis and perinatal mortality. *Am. J. Perinatol.*, **4**, 300–304

Ospital, J. J., Hacker, A. D., Elysayed, N., Mustafa, M. G. and Lee, S. D. (1977). Influence of age on the effect of ozone exposure in rat lungs. *Am. Rev. Resp. Dis.*, **115**, S235

Park, M. K., Ludden, T., Arom, K. V., Rogers, J. and Oswalt, J. D. (1982). Myocardial versus serum digoxin concentrations in infants and adults. *Am. J. Dis. Child.*, **136**, 418–420

Parke, D. V. (1984). Development of detoxication mechanisms in the neonate. In Kacew, S. and Reasor, M. J. (Eds), *Toxicology and the Newborn*. Elsevier Science Publishers, Amsterdam, pp. 3–31

Paulozzi, L. J. (1983). Seasonality of reported poison exposures. *Pediatrics*, **71**, 891–893

Peters, H. A., Gocmen, A., Cripps, D. J., Bryan, G. T. and Dogramaci, I. (1982). Epidemiology of hexachlorobenzene-induced porphyria in Turkey. *Arch. Neurol.*, **39**, 744–749

Rane, A. and Wilson, J. T. (1976). Clinical pharmacokinetics in infants and children. *Clin. Pharmacokinet.*, **1**, 2–24

Rane, A., Garle, M., Borga, O. and Sjoqvist, F. (1974). Plasma disappearance of transplacentally transferred phenytoin in the newborn studied in mass fragmentography. *Clin. Pharmacol. Ther.*, **15**, 39–45

Riordan, J. (1987). Drugs excreted in human breast milk. In Pagliaro, L. A. and Pagliaro, A. M. (Eds), *Problems in Pediatric Drug Therapy*, 2nd edn. Drug Intelligence Publications, Hamilton, IL, pp. 195–258

Roberts, R. J. (1986). Developmental aspects of clinical pharmacology. In Spector, R. (Ed.), *The Scientific Basis of Clinical Pharmacology*. Little, Brown and Company, Boston, pp. 153–170

Rogan, W. J., Gladen, B. C., McKinney, J. D., Carreras, N., Hardy, P., Thullen, J., Tinglestad, J. and Tully, M. (1986). Neonatal effects of transplacental exposure to PCBs and DDE. *J. Pediat.*, **109**, 335–341

Rohyans, J., Walson, P. D., Wood, G. A. and MacDonald, W. A. (1984). Mercury toxicity following merthiolate ear irrigations. *J. Pediat.*, **104**, 311–313

Sanz, E. and Boada, J. (1987). Adverse drug reactions in paediatric outpatients. *Int. J. Clin. Pharm. Res.*, **7**, 169–172

Schardein, J. L. and Keller, K. A. (1989). Potential human developmental toxicants and the role of animal testing in their identification and characterization. *CRC Crit. Rev. Toxicol.*, **19**, 251–339

Schrag, S. D. and Dixon, R. L. (1985). Reproductive effects of chemical agents. In Dixon, R. L. (Ed.), *Reproductive Toxicology*. Raven Press, New York, pp. 301–319

Smith, D. W. and Bostian, K. E. (1964). Congenital anomalies associated with idiopathic mental retardation. *J. Pediat.*, **65**, 189–196

Sonawane, B. R. and Yaffe, S. J. (1988). Drug exposure *in utero*: reproductive function in offspring. In Kacew, S. and Lock, S. (Eds), *Toxicologic and Pharmacologic Principles in Pediatrics*. Hemisphere Publshing, Washington, DC, pp. 41–65

Soyka, L. F. and Joffe, J. M. (1980). Male-mediated drug effects on offspring. *Prog. Clin. Biol. Res.*, **36**, 49–66

Stanbury, J. B., Wyngaarden, J. B. and Frederickson, D. S. (1966). Inherited variation and metabolic abnormality. In Stanbury, J. B., Wyngaarden, J. B. and Frederickson, D. S. (Eds), *The Metabolic Basis of Inherited Disease*. McGraw-Hill, New York, pp. 3–20

Stellman, J. M. (1979). The effect of toxic agents on reproduction. *Occupat. Health Safety*, **48**, 36–40

Takkieddine, F. N., Tserng, K. Y., King, K. C. and Kalhan, S. C. (1981). Postnatal development of theophylline metabolism in preterm infants. *Semin. Perinatol.*, **5**, 351–358

Virgo, B. B. (1984). Pesticides and the neonate. In Kacew, S. and Reasor, M. J. (Eds), *Toxicology and the Newborn*. Elsevier Science Publishers, Amsterdam, pp. 253–267

Vorhees, C. V. (1986). Principles of behavioural teratology. In Riley, E. P. and Vorhees, C. V. (Eds), *Handbook of Behavioral Teratology*. Plenum Press, New York, chap. 2

Warkany, J. (1957). Congenital malformations and paediatrics. *Pediatrics*, **19**, 725–733

Weber, L. W. D. (1985). Benzodiazepines in pregnancy—academical debate or teratogenic risk. *Biol. Res. Pregnan.*, **6**, 151–167

West, J. R., Smith, H. W. and Chasis, H. (1948). Glomerular filtration rate, effective renal blood flow, and maximal tubular excretory capacity in infancy. *J. Pediat.*, **32**, 10–18

Wilson, J. T. (1973). Compliance with instructions in the evaluation of therapeutic efficacy: a common but frequently unrecognized major variable. *Clin. Pediat.*, **12**, 333–340

Wiseman, H. M., Guest, K., Murray, V. S. G. and Volans, G. N. (1987a). Accidental poisoning in childhood: a multicentre study. 1. General epidemiology. *Hum. Toxicol.*, **6**, 293–301

Wiseman, H. M., Guest, K., Murray, V. S. G. and Volans, G. N. (1987b). Accidental poisoning in childhood: a multicentre study. 2. The role of packaging in accidents involving medications. *Hum. Toxicol.*, **6**, 303–314

Yamaguchi, A., Yoshimura, T. and Kuratsune, M. (1971). A survey of pregnant women having consumed rice oil contaminated with chlorobiphenyls and their babies. *Fukuoka Acta Med.*, **62**, 117–122

FURTHER READING

Kacew, S. and Reasor, M. J. (1984). *Toxicology of the Newborn*. Elsevier, Amsterdam

PART SIX: REGULATORY TOXICOLOGY

42   Overview of Regulatory Agencies

G. E. Diggle

The opinions expressed in this overview are the author's own and are not necessarily those of the regulatory agencies mentioned here. Advice concerning the regulatory position of specific products should be obtained directly, in writing, from the appropriate agencies. The author's views do not in any way commit the UK Department of Health, London.

INTRODUCTION

Regulatory agencies in many countries have responsibilities ranging from the control of nuclear power installations to the licensing of domestic pets. This overview deals with the agencies which are concerned specifically with chemical substances. The major strategic objective of regulation in this context is to ensure that the benefits of the substances controlled are not outweighed by their adverse effects. In controlling chemical products, agencies must take account of many kinds of adverse effects, including, for example, those arising from explosive or flammable characteristics, as well as from their toxicological properties. However, it is the latter which are considered here.

Chemical products are conventionally divided into broad categories, such as agrochemicals, pharmaceuticals, industrial chemicals, and so on. However, more precise classifications are required for many regulatory purposes. For example, the term 'agrochemicals' is sometimes used in a narrow sense to refer to agricultural pesticides, but it is also used to denote a much wider group which includes fertilizers, agricultural pesticides and growth regulators. Non-agricultural pesticides such as wood preservatives are not, of course, included in this group. It sometimes happens that a particular substance is regulated as an agricultural pesticide when used for plant protection but as a veterinary medicine when used, for example, for the elimination of ectoparasites from farm animals.

Pharmaceutical products include medicines for human and veterinary use, and many (but not all) countries possess a medicines statute under which both groups are regulated. Human medicines comprise a very wide variety of product types. These include substances of biological origin, ranging from blood products, such as factor VIII for the treatment of haemophilia-A, to antibiotics. In addition to preparations of fine chemicals and other 'orthodox' pharmaceuticals for use in humans, many classes of unorthodox 'alternative' or traditional formulations are also covered by the controls exercised by many regulatory agencies: such formulations include homoeopathic, herbal and anthroposophic remedies. Certain medical devices and surgical products may also be regulated by agencies responsible for the control of medicines for human use.

Veterinary medicines include a wide range of products. Many of these are used for purposes similar to those for which most human medicines are employed, such as the treatment, prevention and diagnosis of disease. However, there is also a number of pharmacologically active agents which are administered to animals for other purposes, such as promoting growth, increasing lactation and modifying the timing of oestrus.

Additives and contaminants comprise major categories of food chemicals. Additives consist of colourants, flavourings, preservatives, antioxidants, emulsifiers and similar substances. In some countries the inclusion of additives in food products is regulated under legislation which requires the establishment of a need for the substances concerned, as well as their safety. Food contaminants include adventitious substances which migrate from packaging materials and naturally occurring compounds (Diggle, 1992), as well as residues from pesticides, veterinary drugs and industrial chemicals. Foods may also be contaminated with unwanted substances present in environmental air, soil and water. The control of food contaminants is a particularly difficult area of regulatory toxicology. Novel foods constitute a related category which includes, for example, substances produced by recombinant DNA technology and other biological means.

'*Industrial chemicals*' is generally understood to refer to substances which are used, often in very large quantities, in manufacturing industries. In many countries, therefore, industrial chemicals are controlled by regulations which are primarily concerned with occupational exposures. Occupational exposure to toxic chemicals can, of course, also occur in small-scale usage—for example, in the administration of parenteral antineoplastic products to patients—and the same 'industrial' safety legislation can be expected to apply in such circumstances, in most countries.

Cosmetics comprise a relatively circumscribed category, and it is usually clear whether a particular product falls within the category or not. However, with this category, as with others, there are some exceptions to this generalization. Two examples of product types which may or may not fall under the cosmetics legislation of any individual country illustrate the point. The first example is the so-called 'eye-brightener' (i.e. eye drops which cause vasoconstriction in the conjunctival vasculature). The second example consists of those orally administered products which are used to change the colour of the skin.

It is clear that the chemical products controlled by regulatory agencies cover an extremely wide range extending from crude technical-grade mixtures produced in bulk to the carefully formulated preparations of fine chemicals which constitute many medicines. In addition to products, agencies are also concerned with chemical contaminants, such as those which occur in the environment and in food. There are no fixed boundaries between the broad categories of chemicals mentioned above. In the case of an injectable cytotoxic drug, for example, questions of safety arise for the nurse administering it and the workers manufacturing it, as well as for the patient receiving it: both pharmaceutical and occupational safety legislation will, therefore, apply.

MANAGEMENT OF TOXICOLOGICAL RISK

For each category of chemical product, the primary concern of regulatory agencies is human safety. Other aspects, such as the need for and the effectiveness of products, must also be taken into account, but considerations of safety take precedence. 'Risk' and 'hazard' are used in a variety of senses and often inconsistently in everyday English, but also by those who should know better.

In the present context, 'hazard' refers to the intrinsic toxicological properties of a chemical: its hepatotoxicity, its cutaneous irritancy, its carcinogenicity, and so on. 'Risk' on the other hand, is used here to refer to the likelihood (probability) that an adverse event will occur when a product containing a hazardous chemical is used in permitted ways. Mutagenic risk, for example, might be defined as: 'The probability that a disease or other health detriment will occur in the offspring of a member of the exposed population, as the result of an adverse mutation induced by the chemical'.

'Safety' denotes the extent to which risks have been eliminated, and the unattainable ideal of complete safety implies the absence of any risks. In theory, satisfactory balances of risk and benefit are sought, in which the risks associated with products are outweighed by their advantages. In practice, such assessments are often difficult to make and are frequently based upon incomplete information. Often benefits are merely expressed in the form of unsubstantiated claims and, even when they are quantified, the basis may be unsound. Similarly, toxicological risks are usually extremely difficult to quantify, because of inadequacies in data and in mechanistic understanding. Even when risks can be expressed in a toxicologically meaningful way, the estimates obtained are usually associated with very wide margins of uncertainty and can serve as little more than 'upper bounds' for use in the more conservative approaches.

Regulatory agencies are particularly concerned with 'risk management', which includes such approaches as controlling the ways in which a chemical is used and the uses for which products containing it may be marketed. The objective, which is rarely stated in formal terms, is in all cases to ensure that products are only used for purposes and under conditions in which the risks to the exposed populations are considered to be acceptable in the circumstances.

One of the major tasks of the toxicologist in the area of risk management is the establishment of regulatory standards. Examples in the area of food chemical toxicology include the maximum residue limits (MRLs) for pesticides and for veterinary drugs, and the acceptable daily intakes (ADIs) for these residues and other substances present in food, such as additives. The ADI is the upper limit of lifetime exposure to the chemical which is acceptable on public health grounds and, in the UK, ADIs are determined by the Department of Health. In the case of food contaminants, this figure may be referred to as the tolerable daily intake, or TDI, to emphasize the principle that food contamination is undesirable.

When it is known that the toxicological phenomena associated with a compound only appear above a certain daily dosage level, the procedure followed is straightforward and makes use of the concept of the 'no observed adverse effect level' (NOAEL), which is determined in the most sensitive species by means of the most discriminating test. In such cases, it is the NOAEL which is normally used to derive the standard, usually after a safety factor has been applied.

The principles are well illustrated by the standard approach to risk management applied to food chemicals possessing NOAELs, such as additives. Here the ADI is obtained by dividing the NOAEL by the chosen safety factor. There are several ways in which this approach can be used. In the case of a new additive, the regulatory agency decides the safety factor, usually in the light of independent expert advice. The NOAEL is then divided by this factor to give the ADI. Food consumption data are submitted, and used to estimate the maximum likely daily intake which would occur if the chemical was present in the types of food and at the concentrations proposed in the application submitted to the agency. A comparison between the maximum total intake expected and the ADI provides the measure of safety which constitutes the basis for regulatory decisions about the foods and the concentrations in which the additive may be used. Alternatively, a comparison may be made between the known dietary intake of an existing additive and the ADI: if the difference is not judged to be adequate, then regulatory action is taken. This was the procedure undertaken, for example, in the UK in the case of saccharin, recently.

In the case of veterinary drugs, the regulatory standard is the MRL. The veterinary drug MRL is based on the NOAEL divided by a safety factor (i.e. on the ADI), together with data on food consumption. In a typical example the MRL might refer to the maximum limit for the residue of an antibacterial in pig carcass muscle. The time–concentration, or depletion, curve in the living pig is then used to determine the withdrawal period between administration and slaughter which must be enforced in order to ensure that the MRL is not exceeded.

For pesticides it is the MRL, again, which is the regulatory standard, although in this case it is determined by field trials using good agricultural practice. However, it is essential that the pesticide MRL should also satisfy the criterion of consumer safety. Consumer exposure is calculated (on the basis of MRL and food intake data) and compared with the ADI, which is again derived by applying a safety factor to the NOAEL. Regulatory agencies are responsible for establishing and enforcing conditions of pesticide use which ensure that exposures do not exceed ADIs.

The ADI approach can be applied to any unwanted effect, provided that a NOAEL can be established, but it must be stressed that this approach does not provide any means for the calculation of risk when the ADI is exceeded by any particular amount. In other words, the probability that the relevant toxicological effect (whether it be carcinogenesis or some other endpoint) will occur cannot be calculated from the amount by which actual intake exceeds ADI. There should, of course, be no excess risk at all if the ADI is not exceeded. Moreover, the safety factor used in setting an ADI should ensure that there is unlikely to be any appreciable added risk if the ADI is exceeded by only small amounts, or for only short periods.

The ADI method is appropriate for the great majority of food chemicals, but for those which produce cancer in laboratory animals there are problems with this approach. Although a NOAEL may appear in a carcinogenicity study, the possibility that this same dose would produce a carcinogenic effect detectable in a much larger group of animals can rarely be excluded. In such a case it is inappropriate to attempt to set an ADI. Instead a 'weight of evidence' approach is employed, by most regulatory agencies, in which all the toxicological evidence, and not only that from the animal carcinogenicity study, is taken into account in assessing whether there is any possibility at all that the test substance could exert carcinogenic effects in man. If, for example, the chemical cannot be absorbed from the human gastrointestinal tract, if it is shown unequivocally to be innocuous to DNA, or if it is broken down completely and rapidly by a metabolizing enzyme present in man but not in the test species, then this might possibly provide some degree of reassurance.

If, however, this approach suggests that there is any possibility that the carcinogenic effect seen in test animals could occur in consumers, then the chemical is considered to be unacceptable as a food additive; contaminants are regulated in accordance with the 'as low as possible' principle. The policy of the UK Department of Health on food chemical safety can therefore be briefly summarized as follows. For substances possessing NOAELs (the great majority), the ADI approach is appropriate for regulatory purposes. Animal carcinogens which have not been shown unequivocally to possess NOAELs are assessed by means of the 'weight of evidence' approach, and if this fails to provide adequate reassurance, then the 'as low as possible' criterion is appropriate in regulatory control.

The difficulties, discussed above, in applying the ADI approach to animal carcinogens have led to particular problems in the United States, following the famous 1959 'Delaney' amendment of the Food, Drug and Cosmetic Act 1938. This originated as an attempt to improve consumer protection by preventing the addition to human food of any substance which had been shown to cause cancer in animals. It was hoped that this measure would provide a way out of interminable legal and scientific debates about whether particular animal carcinogens possessed true no-effect levels and whether their carcinogenicity could be expressed in humans. Saccharin causes cancer in rodents and, in accordance with the 'no threshold, no safe dose' philosophy implicit in the Delaney clause, had to be banned. But the carcinogenic effects of saccharin only occur at high dosage, in only one strain of rat, in only male animals and only in one organ—the bladder!

Toxicological common sense prevailed in the case of saccharin, although it required an Act of Congress to restore it to the market. The Delaney amendment remains in force to this day, although intense legal wrangles over many years have produced various 'solutions' to this unnecessary,

man-made problem. The most interesting of these has been the development of the virtually safe dose (VSD) concept. The VSD is the dose corresponding to an acceptable level of risk (ALR). Risk, in this context, means the probability, or likelihood, that fatal cancer will be caused by the chemical concerned in the consumer population (it may be expressed as lifetime or annual risk). Risk, according to the argument, will not exceed the ALR, provided that the exposure does not rise above the VSD. To apply this in practice requires two things: first, the courageous political decision to set the ALR, and, second, some technique for determining the probability that the chemical concerned will cause human cancer in the low-dose range. (At one point, the US courts attempted to facilitate the process of setting the ALR by reaffirming the *de minimis* principle, which avers that the law is not concerned with trifles.)

The second of these requirements has proved to be quite intractable. Attempts have been made to develop mathematical methods for interpolating from the relatively enormous doses used in animal carcinogenicity studies (because of limitations in the numbers of animals which can be used) to the very low doses relevant to consumer exposure. This procedure is known as quantitative risk analysis (QRA) and is, as many US regulators readily acknowledge, controversial and fraught with difficulties. The major difficulties arise from the fact that the commonly used models have no biological basis and have never been validated.

Mathematically, each model produces an equation which gives, as a function of dose, the probability that the dose will give rise to a carcinogenic response. By selecting appropriate parameters in the equations and making other adjustments, the graph of the equation is fitted optimally to the animal test data, while the precise shape near the origin, far from the data, crucially determines the probability estimate provided by the model. There is very wide variation between the results produced by different models (and often within the same model) when parameters are altered to reflect assumptions about the unknown shape of the dose–response curve in the region of the origin. These assumptions must always, of course, be made clear to the risk manager, as must the goodness of fit achieved and the confidence levels of the risk estimates.

These mathematical models fall into several distinct categories, including 'tolerance distribution', 'mechanistic', 'time to tumour' and 'two-stage growth' models. An equation which is sublinear (downwardly convex) in the low-dose region produces a more 'optimistic' result than one which is linear (Figure 1A,B). For a given dose, the estimated carcinogenic response is smaller when the curve is sublinear than when it is linear. As the true shape of the curve in the low-dose region is unknown, it is usually considered prudent to be 'conservative' (i.e. to err on the side of safety) and employ an equation which is linear in this region. This approach intentionally produces pessimistic estimates, which are of interest to regulators considering worst-case interpretations.

The risk estimate figures produced by these computer-based models should always be accompanied by the all-important confidence limits, together with details of the assumptions which have been made. Without this essential accompanying information, such estimates are scientifically meaningless and there is always a danger that they will be taken at face value and unduly influence, or even exert a thrall over, those who do not appreciate the uncertainties involved. Unfortunately, however, estimates do tend to become separated from their proper context, and to be used in isolation, often leading to a good deal of unnecessary public alarm. These models are little used in regulatory work outside the USA. It is particularly important that these difficulties should not be allowed to affect new regulatory systems which are currently under development (Diggle, 1992).

REGULATORY APPROACHES

There is great variation in the approaches and the procedures adopted by regulatory agencies throughout the world for the control of chemicals of different categories. In the case of pharmaceuticals, for example, controls are negligible in some developing countries, while in Norway the marketing of a product is not authorized unless safety, need, effectiveness, cost and quality are considered to be satisfactory. There may also be considerable differences in the regulatory approach to a compound within a particular country, when it is used as an active ingredient in different categories of product (e.g. pesticide and veterinary medicine).

Regulatory agencies sometimes place special emphasis on particular aspects of their work reflecting earlier toxicological incidents in the countries concerned. In Japan, for example, particular attention is paid to the environmental effects of industrial chemicals, which must satisfy the requirements of two separate statutes. One of these emphasizes testing for bioaccumulation and biodegradability, and it may be seen as a response to recent concerns about environmental contaminants such as polychlorinated biphenyls and earlier instances of heavy metal contamination. In one of these, cadmium-containing effluents entered rice fields and thus passed into the diet, causing itai-itai ('ouch-ouch') disease, characterized by osteomalacia, fractures, protein-

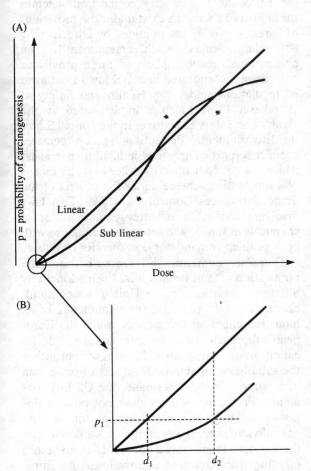

Figure 1   (A) The asterisks represent the results of an animal carcinogenicity study. (B) The 'acceptable' risk, p_1, is attained at a dose of either d_1 or d_2, according to which model is used.

uria and glycosuria. In another, episodes of mercury poisoning occurred at Minimata and Niigata, following the accumulation of methyl mercury in fish from heavily polluted water nearby.

Similar comments apply to the evolution of the Pharmaceutical Affairs Law in Japan following the establishment of the association between subacute myelo-optic neuropathy (SMON) and the use of clioquinol. In the UK the present Health and Safety at Work Act 1974 was enacted following the Aberfan tragedy, and the (now superseded) voluntary scheme for ensuring the safe use of pesticides was set up following the deaths of workers exposed to dinitro compounds.

The regulations administered by agencies are also greatly influenced by the legislative backgrounds of the countries concerned, and this accounts for many national differences. In France, for example, studies of drug pharmacokinetics in normal human volunteers were not permitted until the end of 1988, when new legislation came into effect. Before this, such studies were proscribed under the erstwhile legal framework, which derived from the Code Napolèon. In the UK, on the other hand, volunteer studies have always been allowed and, unlike clinical trials in patients, are not regulated by the Medicines Act 1968, although there are strict guidelines which are almost invariably observed. One result of these differences has been the relatively rapid development of Phase 1 studies of new drugs in the UK.

Despite variations in national regulatory approaches resulting from differences in historical, cultural and legislative backgrounds, many broad similarities exist. For example, there is a general tendency to control industrial chemicals by means of so-called 'notification' schemes, while pharmaceuticals are frequently regulated by means of 'licensing' systems. Procedures are known by such names as 'notification', 'licensing,' 'certification', 'approval', 'registration', 'clearance', etc. Actual usage is often loose and misunderstandings are common. The subtleties of language implied in the proper use of these terms frequently perish on passing through the administrative machinery of the EC, and some terms may not be recognizable when they emerge. 'Food supplements', for example, have become 'dietary integrators'.

Notification Schemes

The emphasis of a notification scheme, such as those often used for new industrial chemicals, is different from that of a licensing system. The primary purpose of a notification scheme is not to enable regulatory agencies to decide whether or not marketing authorizations should be granted. On the contrary, it is to ensure that when products are marketed, the agency is aware of their existence and that they will be used as safely as possible. This is generally achieved by means of appropriate testing, classification and labelling, by setting exposure limits in the workplace, and by ensuring adequate methods for storage, handling, disposal and the treatment of accidental spillages and of injuries caused by the chemical. For example, in the member states of the European Community notification schemes for industrial chemicals exist under the provisions of Directive 67/548, as amended by Directive 79/831 (the so-called 'sixth amendment'). The occupational health aspects of these provisions have been incorporated into UK law in the form of regulations under the Health and Safety at Work Act 1974, which is implemented by the Health and Safety Executive. In the United States the Environmental Protection Agency regulates chemicals (particularly new industrial chemicals) which are not controlled by other laws, by means of a notification scheme under the powers of the Toxic Substances Control Act 1976. Two laws involving notification schemes regulate industrial chemicals in Japan, and separate compliance with both of them is mandatory, as mentioned above.

There are numerous differences between the notification schemes which have been adopted by different countries. In the United States notification must take place before manufacture of an industrial chemical commences, while the European approach specifies premarketing notification. In the European and Japanese approaches the submission of standardized sets of basic data is required. On the other hand, the US Environmental Protection Agency does not possess this power, although it can request specific data on an individual-case basis if it is considered that there is need to evaluate a potential hazard before granting manufacturing approval. In the European schemes notification that production has reached specified annual tonnages is required, and this may trigger further data requirements.

An important distinction is to be made between voluntary and statutory notification schemes. In the former notification is invited by the regulatory agency, while in the latter it is mandatory. In the United Kingdom voluntary schemes have in the past been applied to pharmaceuticals and to pesticides. Under the pharmaceuticals scheme, set up in 1963, some 600 companies sought the advice of the Committee on Safety of Drugs (the 'Dunlop Committee') on their products up to September 1971, when licensing under the Medicines Act 1968 was implemented. It was then found that some 3600 companies had pharmaceutical products subject to licensing. In the case of pesticides the voluntary Pesticide Safety Precautions Scheme operated in the UK from 1957 until the introduction of the Control of Pesticides Regulations, under the Food and Environmental Protection Act 1985. Under the voluntary scheme trade associations agreed that their member companies would submit data to, and obtain clearance from, the regulatory authorities before marketing new products. Novel foods and food processes are currently the subject of a voluntary notification scheme in the UK.

Licensing Systems

A licence, in this context, is a formal written permission granted for a specified period by a regulatory agency, which authorizes the marketing of a chemical product. The essence of a licensing system (as opposed to a notification scheme) is that the agency receives an application for marketing authorization which it may or may not grant. Licences, unlike 'approvals' and 'clearances', are usually granted for a limited period, and require renewal. Distinct elements (including application, registration, assessment, representations and decision) comprise a typical licensing system.

The application is usually required to be in a prescribed format, giving details of the proposed product and its intended uses. In general, the formal application must be accompanied by scientific data, the nature and amount of which are usually indicated by the agency's guidelines. When an application is submitted, the agency must first decide whether it is adequate for assessment. If, for example, the data are obviously grossly deficient, if the documentation is not clear or is of poor quality, or if it is not in an approved language, then the agency may reject the application at this stage. If the application is deemed to be adequate for further consideration, it is then 'registered' (see below) for formal assessment. Assessment is typically carried out by the professional staff of the agency, but in most systems there is also provision for independent expert advice. If the results of assessment are favourable, a licence is granted. If not, it is usually possible for the applicant to make representations, involving the submission of arguments and, often, further data. It is only when all rights to make representations have been exhausted, without success, that an application is finally refused. Once granted, a marketing authorization may be revoked or suspended—for example, when evidence of a previously unrecognized hazard comes to light.

The existing regulatory arrangements for pharmaceutical products afford many examples of licensing systems. In the European Community, Council Directive 65/65 provides the basis for the control of medicines in the member states. The Medicines Act 1968 (as amended to comply with Community law) provides for the licensing of medicines in the United Kingdom; this statute was enacted following the thalidomide tragedy, which became known in 1961. In the United States the controls provided by the Food and Drugs Act 1906 were greatly strengthened 32 years later (following the 'sulfanilamide elixir' tragedy) when the Food, Drug and Cosmetic Act 1938 was enacted. This statute has been amended on a number of occasions and remains in force today. In Japan control is exercised through the Pharmaceutical Affairs Law.

Clearance

'Clearance' is a rather loose term, which can be used to refer to statutory processes for marketing authorizations, but which is more usually employed in the context of voluntary schemes. Before pesticides were controlled in the UK under the Food and Environmental Protection Act 1985, 'clearances' were given under the Pesticides Safety Precautions Scheme.

Approval

'Approval' is used widely and in a variety of senses, but usually to denote a statutory process.

Under present arrangements in the UK, pesticides may receive provisional or full approval under the Control of Pesticides Regulations, which were made under Part 3 of the Food and Environmental Protection Act 1985. In the case of agricultural pesticides in the UK, approvals are issued by the Ministry of Agriculture, Fisheries and Food. Non-agricultural products such as wood preservatives, masonry washes and anti-fouling paints are subject to approval by the Health and Safety Executive. Approvals, unlike licences, are usually issued for an unlimited period.

Certification

Certification is the issue of a document which attests to a particular fact—for example, the fact that the clinical trial of a pharmaceutical has been authorized. In the UK applications can be made for clinical trial certificates: however, a system has been devised which, with the subtle logic so favoured in the UK (Shah, 1988), makes it easier, faster and more economical to apply for exemptions from the requirement for certificates. In some countries the procedures involved in applications for clinical trial authorization resemble those used to obtain marketing authorization, with provisions for making representations when applications are not immediately successful. In other countries notification schemes operate.

In the case of agricultural pesticides in the UK, an 'experimental permit' rather than a certificate is issued to enable trials to take place.

Registration

'Registration' is a loose term. To state that a product is 'registered' may mean that it has been notified, or that it is licensed, or merely that it has been accepted for assessment. This confusing term has caused problems in international regulatory affairs on several occasions. In one instance the regulatory agency of a developing country was asked to grant marketing authorization for a product which was said to be 'already registered' in another state, and a licence number was cited. Subsequent investigation established that the product had in fact never received marketing authorization in that country, although it had (as is normal practice) been allocated a 'licence number', solely for reference purposes, while

assessment and representation procedures were under way.

DATA REQUIREMENTS

Many agencies publish data requirements, i.e. lists of tests whose results are required for regulatory purposes. In addition, agencies may also issue test guidelines or protocols indicating, in varying amounts of detail, how the individual tests should be conducted. Many guidelines for the testing of chemicals have been published by the Organization for Economic Cooperation and Development, and these have been adopted by most countries having significant data requirements (OECD, 1981). Nevertheless, in practice, there still exist some differences between national test guidelines, and these differences give rise to the unnecessary repetition of studies. Such duplication without scientific justification results in excessive costs and an unnecessary expenditure of toxicological resources, including laboratory animals.

A detailed comparison, for pesticides and industrial chemicals, has been made between the protocols published by the OECD and by the regulatory agencies in the European Community, the United States and Japan (ECETOC, 1985). The authors considered that the OECD guidelines were the most widely recognized internationally, and therefore used these as yardsticks. Various recommendations were made for ensuring common approaches without loss of flexibility, involving, in some cases, proposals for updating the OECD guidelines by adopting some of the better features from others. Indeed the OECD emphasises the need regularly to update its existing guidelines, and the 'Updating Panel' has established a timetable for the review of all the existing guidelines on toxicity testing.

The data requirements of many regulatory agencies concerned with pharmaceutical products have been summarized and compared by Alder and Zbinden (1988). As the authors pointed out, national drug safety guidelines differ in many respects. As well as differences in data requirements, there is also a good deal of variation in the degree of detail in which the guidelines express themselves. In a telling section of the book, 'A Look Behind Drug Regulatory Guidelines', Professor Zbinden considered the quality of guidelines for drug safety testing and discussed their practical application in regulatory toxicology.

Regular, informal contacts between agencies enable regulatory approaches to specific problems to be discussed and a good deal of cross-fertilization occurs in this way. The close liaison which occurs between the agencies of the Nordic Community constitutes an excellent example. Denmark, as a member of the EC as well as the Nordic Community, plays a unique role. In recent years the consistency of the guidelines issued by the different member states of the EC has improved considerably for all the categories of regulated chemicals, as a result of the ongoing programme of European legislation. Government scientists and doctors from the UK, the US and Canada meet informally every year to discuss a wide range of health issues, including regulatory problems. This annual meeting, known as the Tripartite Conference, was established in the late 1960s by the Chief Medical Officer in the UK and his counterparts in the US and Canada. It provides a valuable opportunity for a free exchange of views between specialists, and is held in turn in the UK, the US and Canada.

REGULATORY SYSTEMS AND ORGANIZATIONS

The nature of chemical safety regulation is best illustrated by outlining some of the most developed regulatory systems and organizations. The following descriptions give the clearest examples of controls for the major categories of chemical products, the work of agencies, some of their major problems and differences between national approaches.

The European Communities (EC)

Three separate communities were merged in 1967 to form the EC. These were:

- The European Coal and Steel Community (ECSC), which was established in 1952 with the purpose of putting the means of war under a common system of supranational control, using the economic approach devised by Schuman and Monnet.
- The European Atomic Energy Community

(EURATOM), which was established in 1957.
- The European Economic Community (EEC), which was also established in 1957, by means of the Treaty of Rome.

The objectives of the EEC are economic, and the Treaty of Rome contains no provisions concerned with chemical safety. However, it became apparent at an early stage that a good deal of 'harmonization' would be required to ensure that national differences in the regulatory control of products were not to restrict the free movement of these goods. The ongoing programme of EC legislation which originally stemmed from this requirement has resulted in the creation of a large body of European law concerning, among many other things, chemical safety. This is of great importance in regulatory toxicology, as European law takes precedence over domestic statutes in the member states (Germany, France, Italy, Belgium, the Netherlands, Luxembourg, the United Kingdom, Ireland, Denmark, Greece, Portugal and Spain). Article 36 of the Treaty of Rome allows for restriction of imports 'to protect the health of humans, animals or plants' provided this does not act as a 'disguised restriction on trade'.

The Treaty of Rome provides for the introduction of laws and other instruments through which the aims of the EEC are pursued. In descending order of power, these instruments are: Regulations, Directives, Recommendations and Opinions. Member states must obey Regulations as they stand, while Directives set out general principles which are incorporated by member states into new 'domestic' legislation. Recommendations and opinions are, as their names imply, not binding on member states. Council Directives must be agreed by the Council of Ministers, while Commission Directives are issued by the officials of the EC, the European Commission. The procedures for the regulation of chemicals are provided by Council Directives. For example, the framework for the regulation of pharmaceuticals is set out in Council Directive 65/65, while a daughter instrument (Council Directive 75/319) provides for advisory machinery and multistate applications. Commission Directives do not require Council approval, and deal with more detailed matters such as methods of analysis and technical advances: for example,

Commission Directives are used to promulgate revisions of the lists of substances annexed to the Council Directive on cosmetics, 76/768.

Industrial chemicals are subject to a number of important Council Directives, which ensure a considerable degree of harmonization throughout the EC. The Dangerous Substances Directive 67/548 is fundamental to the system. The sixth amendment of this directive sets out a 'notification' (registration) scheme, which covers all new chemicals (i.e. those not already included in the EC inventory), other than categories which are covered by other legislation, including drugs, pesticides, cosmetics and food additives. The purpose of the scheme is to ensure that member states are aware of new chemicals entering the market at a rate greater than 1 tonne per year. The scheme does not provide for the grant of any form of marketing authorization, however. Notifications are made to the 'competent' authority of the member state in which the chemical is first marketed. A 'base-set' of physicochemical, toxicity and ecotoxicity data must accompany the notification. The authority must be informed when the marketing rate reaches 10, 100 and 1000 tonnes per year, and there are further data requirements at these stages. The requirements for the base-set include data on acute toxicity, eye and skin irritancy, skin sensitization, 28 day repeated dose toxicity and mutagenicity studies. The notification must be submitted at least 45 days before marketing. This is a 'harmonized' procedure, and notification in one member state results in notification throughout the Community.

The EC approach differs from that adopted in the US, where the Environmental Protection Agency (EPA) regulates industrial chemicals under the provisions of the Toxic Substances Control Act 1976 (TOSCA). In the US manufacturers must submit to EPA a 'premanufacture notice' at least 90 days before commencing production of chemicals, whereas in the EC manufacture (but not marketing) can take place before notification. Under TOSCA, EPA cannot demand a basic set of data on each chemical, although it can specify studies which must be performed on a case-by-case basis before granting manufacturing authorization.

Both the EC and US systems differ from the Japanese approach, which is based upon two quite separate statutes. These are the Chemical Substances Control Law ('Law 44') of 1986, which is implemented jointly by the Ministry of International Trade and Industry (MITI) and the Ministry of Health and Welfare (MHW), and the Industrial Safety and Health Law 1972, which is administered by the Ministry of Labour (MOL). Separate compliance with both statutes is required before a new industrial chemical may be marketed. The emphasis of Law 44 is on the prevention of adverse human effects occurring indirectly via the environment, whereas the EC and US approaches focus on direct effects, both on humans and on the environment. Under Law 44, new compounds must be tested for biodegradation. No further testing is required for substances which biodegrade readily to produce safe degradation products, but compounds which do not must be tested for bioaccumulation potential and must undergo a battery of mutagenicity tests and 28 day repeat-dose toxicity studies. A preliminary estimate of bioaccumulation potential may be made from the compound's octanol–water partition coefficient; if this is not satisfactory, *in vivo* studies are required, using fish (carp). As with the US (but not EC) system, premanufacture notification is required. The requirements of the Industrial Safety and Health Law also include premarket notification and the submission of mutagenicity test results.

Returning now to the EC and the Dangerous Substances Directive, further provisions have been introduced which regulate classification and labelling. Two directives cover this area, one dealing with '*substances*' (defined as 'chemical elements and their compounds, as they occur in the natural state or produced by industry'), and the other with '*preparations*' ('mixtures or solutions composed of two or more substances'). For substances and preparations the labelling requirements, and the classification system upon which they are based, are fully harmonized throughout the EC. The system provides criteria for nine categories of hazard: harmful, toxic, very toxic, irritant, corrosive, flammable, very flammable, oxidizing, and explosive. Labelling phrases and symbols are specified for each category. Although the classification of substances and preparations has the same basis, allowance is made for the dilution of hazardous substances in preparations by means of concentration cut-off limits. Preparations which are covered by other provisions (e.g. pharmaceuticals) are of course excluded from the scheme.

The Community has attempted to create a system of multistate approval for pesticides. It has been able to agree on a prohibition Directive for pesticides (79/117) and this is currently in force. It is used for banning the use of unacceptably hazardous substances for use as pesticides throughout the Community. The genotoxic carcinogen ethylene oxide, for example, is prohibited under this Directive. Where special needs exist, individual member states may apply for 'derogations' under the Directive, which in effect allows the implementation of bans to be delayed. An acceptance Directive (91/414) was adopted in 1991, which will eventually lead to a list of accepted active ingredients. Approvals will continue to be granted, at the level of the individual states, of products containing active ingredients on the accepted list (EC, 1991). Non-agricultural pesticides will be dealt with in further Directives. Such pesticides include wood preservatives and marine antifouling paints.

Pharmaceutical products, including veterinary drugs as well as medicines for human use, are still controlled separately in each member state by the appropriate national regulatory agency. Two approaches for increasing the freedom of movement of these products have been considered intensively for some years: 'mutual recognition', under which each member state accepts the marketing authorizations of every other one; second, the establishment of a centralized EC agency which issues authorizations valid for all member states. It is highly unlikely that agreement to mutual recognition could be achieved in the foreseeable future, if only because of the considerable differences in the practice of medicine which exist between the 12 nations of the Community. For example, such diagnoses as '*spasmophilia*' and '*crise de foie*' are familiar to French physicians but do not appear to exist in British medicine. Similar comments apply to a condition known as 'vegetative dystonia' in German medical practice. It has been pointed out (Payer, 1989) that there are no fewer than 85 medicinal products on the German market for the treatment of a condition, *niedriger Blutdruck*, or 'low blood pressure', which would actually result in lowered premiums for life insurance in other countries!

A degree of co-ordination of national regulation for pharmaceuticals has already been achieved through the 'multistate' procedure which enables marketing authorization to be obtained in more than one member state at the same time. This now applies to veterinary drugs (Directive 81/851), as well as human medicines (75/319). Under the procedure a company which has already obtained marketing authorization for its product in one member state may apply for authorization in two or more of the remaining states. If any member state raises 'reasoned objections', the matter is referred to the Committee for Proprietary Medicinal Products (CPMP) in the case of a human medicine, or to the Committee for Veterinary Medicinal Products (CVMP) in the case of a pharmaceutical for animal use. The Committee provides an opinion, which, however, is not binding. The applicant receives copies of all reasoned objections, and the member state which issued the original marketing authorization is responsible for presenting the applicant's responses to the Committee. The procedure incorporates time limits to prevent unnecessary delays: objections must be raised within 120 days and each regulatory agency has 60 days after receipt of the Committee's opinion to take its own decision. So far, nearly all applications using this multistate procedure have resulted in objections from at least one member state. In the case of new medicines produced by means of recombinant DNA technology, a member state receiving an application must co-ordinate the assessments of other member states, together with the applicant's responses, and seek a non-binding opinion from the CPMP (or CVMP). The procedure, based upon the provisions of Directive 87/22, may also be used for other innovatory products, such as those using novel delivery systems and manufacturing processes and those which represent significant therapeutic innovations.

The regulation of cosmetics is an area of complete harmonization throughout the EC. The Cosmetics Directive (76/768, as amended) controls all cosmetic products by means of lists of permitted substances which may be used in them. These are lists of preservatives, colouring agents and UV filters, and there is a list of substances which cannot be used. Some permitted substances are only allowed to be used on a provisional basis, until further toxicological data are provided, and these must be submitted within a specified timespan. The lists, which appear as annexes to the Directive, are brought up to date by means of new Commission Directives which adapt the Cosmetics Directive 76/768 to technical progress. An expert committee, the Scientific Committee on Cosmetology (SCC), provides advice on the content of the lists (i.e. on substances), although individual products and formulations are not considered by the SCC. Manufacturers are, of course, under a general requirement to ensure the safety of their products, and this principle is incorporated into Article 2 of the Directive.

The foundations of the single market in foodstuffs are now in place. The Community's food law harmonization programme has helped to set higher standards of food safety and improved food labelling. The main framework directives on labelling, additives, flavourings, contact materials, special dietary foods and food inspection have already been adopted, as have other important directives, for example on nutrient labelling, lot marking, and extraction solvents.

Expert advice is provided by the Scientific Committee for Food (SCF), which consists of experts from the member states and advises on food safety, including the safety of additives. When an additive is considered to be acceptable, an acceptable daily intake (ADI) is specified by the committee. If the anticipated exposure is likely to approach the ADI, a list of foods to which it must be restricted is also provided. The advice of the SCF is submitted to a working group of national representatives which decides (by a system of voting) whether the additive will be added to the appropriate list. It is likely that the procedures adopted will allow individual member states to grant provisional authorizations for up to 3 years, although the additive must in these cases also be submitted for inclusion in the appropriate daughter Directive, after consideration by the SCF. Similarly, a member state may suspend an authorization temporarily, if information becomes available which suggests that the substance may endanger human health, but other member states must be informed and reasons provided.

The United States Food and Drugs Administration (FDA)

The FDA has, over many decades, acquired a distinctive regulatory style. Nevertheless, the responsibilities and activities of this important and influential organization are similar in many ways to those encountered elsewhere. The following outline of some of the FDA's developmental milestones and current tasks illustrates features of regulatory agencies throughout the world.

The Food and Drugs Act 1906 was the first US statute to regulate these categories of products, although the powers provided by the Act were very limited. The marketing of quack medicines for the treatment of major disease and the sale of dangerous preparations for minor ailments had always been an extremely serious problem in the US. Radium salts, for example, were promoted for conditions ranging from venereal disease to hypertension (Diggle, 1987a, 1988a). The Act concentrated on products containing harmful adulterants and those which did not contain the claimed ingredients. No premarketing approval was required, and the onus of proof rested firmly on the Department of Agriculture. Moreover, there were no requirements for safety testing by manufacturers.

The enactment of the 1906 statute was the direct result of intense pressure by the United States Department of Agriculture (USDA), which had submitted more than 100 Bills to Congress proposing regulatory controls. These efforts were further rewarded in 1927 by the creation of the Food, Drug and Insecticide Administration, the precursor of the present FDA. The long-standing concerns of the USDA, arising from the large numbers of dangerous and quack products on the market, were seen to be fully justified in 1937, when some 107 people died as a result of taking a medicine labelled 'Elixir of Sulphanilamide'. The account of the investigation, and of the behaviour of those involved, is compelling reading (Secretary of Agriculture, 1937). It emerged that diethylene glycol had been used as the solvent in the formulation, sulphanilamide being insoluble in aqueous solvents. The product had not undergone safety testing, but had merely been examined for colour, flavour and smell. The only legal basis for action by the FDA under the 1906 Act was that the product did not contain a claimed ingredient (the word 'elixir' traditionally implied the presence of ethanol, whereas diethylene glycol had been included instead). In a press statement the manufacturer denied responsibility (Secretary of Agriculture, 1937), claiming that the deaths must have been caused by sulphanilamide, and could not possibly have been foreseen.

A most important result of this tragedy was the

enactment of the Food, Drug and Cosmetic Act 1938. This law contained major new provisions, including the requirement for safety testing, although there was still no requirement for the submission of the test data to the FDA before marketing could be authorized. Other improvements included requirements for manufacturer 'registration' and factory inspection. There were also new provisions to permit the seizure of products which did not meet the new requirements, by means of court injunctions. The 1938 Act was amended in 1951 to include controls for 'prescription drugs' (the Durham–Humphrey amendment).

It was in 1962 that the Act was further modified (the Kefauver–Harris amendment) to include requirements for the submission of data on safety and efficacy, before marketing authorization could be granted. This major advance was an immediate result of the thalidomide tragedy, in which thousands of neonates throughout Western Europe were found to be affected by the normally rare deformity phocomelia, as a result of the use in pregnancy of this tranquillizer during a specific stage of organogenesis. It is to the great credit of the FDA's medical staff that the incidence of thalidomide-induced phocomelia in the US was relatively very small. Marketing authorization had never been granted by the FDA, and women who could be pregnant were excluded from the permitted clinical trials; the only cases which did occur involved patients whose doctors did not supervise this criterion adequately.

The FDA commenced a large-scale review of 'over the counter' pharmaceuticals in 1966. In 1976 the Medical Device amendments were introduced; this improvement was made as a result of long-standing concerns about the availability of fraudulent and unsafe products of this kind (Drew, 1986; Diggle, 1987b, 1988b).

The present procedure for the marketing authorization of pharmaceuticals in the US implements the Kefauver–Harris amendment. A new drug application (NDA) is approved only when the FDA is satisfied that the criteria of safety, effectiveness and quality have been met adequately. Neither relative effectiveness in comparison with other drugs nor price can be taken into account by the review team, which generally consists of doctor, pharmacologist, toxicologist, chemist, statistician and pharmacist. In theory the NDA should be processed within 180 days,

although in practice this period is frequently exceeded (Diggle and Griffin, 1982). Independent advice may be obtained from expert advisory committees, but their advice is not binding on the FDA. If the FDA is satisfied with the application, an 'approval letter' is issued and the product may then be marketed. Alternatively, the FDA may issue an 'approvable' letter indicating that marketing authorization would be granted if specified additional data were submitted or conditions met. However, if the FDA does not consider that the NDA can be granted, a 'not approvable' letter is issued. Information submitted to the FDA is confidential, with the exception of data which can be released under the US Freedom of Information Act. FDA staff prepare and publish a 'summary basis for approval' for each new chemical entity. The FDA procedures for regulating pharmaceuticals differ in some respects from those used by EC countries such as the UK. In the UK it is not unusual for pharmaceutical companies to attend hearings to defend their applications (Griffin and Diggle, 1981), but this is less common in the US. The FDA requires original patient documentation, duly signed by the investigating physicians. Exceptionally, detailed information on manufacturing plant is also required, but there is no equivalent to a requirement which exists in the EC system for an 'expert report'.

The history of the FDA's role in ensuring the safety of the American food supply has proceeded along analogous lines of development. There has always been particular emphasis on the involvement of consumers in decision-making and regulatory processes.

Today, the parent organization of the FDA is the Department of Health and Human Services, rather than the USDA, and the administration is organized in the form of six centres:

Center for Drug Evaluation and Research
Center for Devices and Radiological Health
Center for Veterinary Medicine
Center for Biologics Evaluation and Research
National Center for Toxicological Research
Center for Food Safety and Applied Nutrition

The work of the FDA in relation to food may be illustrated by the activities of the Center for Food Safety in the area of food additives. The legal basis is the 1958 Food Additive amendment of the 1938 Act, and statutory responsibility is vested in regulatory agencies of some individual states, as well as the FDA (42 states have adopted the provisions of the 1958 amendment into their own legislation). New food additives are subject to a system of premarketing approval, under which the substance must be shown to be 'safe'. In this context 'safe' means not injurious to the health of humans or animals and, in particular, not carcinogenic. Some 2700 substances are approved for use under this procedure. Some substances added to food do not fall within the legal definition of 'food additives'. These exceptions include substances 'generally recognized as safe' (GRAS), pesticides on or in raw foods, and substances which were in use before 6 September 1958 and are also presumed to be safe.

The so-called 'Delaney Clause' is a provision of section 409 of the Act, which applies to food additives, but not to other categories of regulated chemicals, as is popularly believed! This provision, introduced in 1958, states that an additive will not be considered to be safe if it has been found to 'induce cancer' in man or animal species. There is no reference to dosage or to whether genotoxic mechanisms have been excluded or to whether 'cancer' refers to benign as well as malignant tumours. This has led to two kinds of regulatory difficulties.

First, substances such as saccharin, which induces tumours only at extremely high doses, and which are not genotoxic, were nevertheless deemed to be 'unsafe'. As a result an Act of Congress was needed to reverse the initial ban on saccharin!

Second, it has been held that genotoxic carcinogens are unsafe, even at the smallest levels detectable. With modern analytical methods, quantities can be detected which are so low that the risk to consumers must be extremely small in relation to other everyday risks. In 1982 the FDA adopted a new policy under which a carcinogenic impurity in an additive might be permitted, provided that it posed a 'negligible' risk. 'Negligible risk' was defined as a probability of less than 0.000001 that an induced tumour would occur in the lifetime of a consumer. Thus, aniline is acceptable as an impurity in tartrazine at levels up to 0.5 ppm. Recent proposals advocate that the figure for negligible risk should be revised upwards.

Chemical contaminants in food, as distinct from additives, demand a good deal of FDA attention. The major health concerns associated with contaminants in fresh fruits and vegetables arise from pesticide residues. The FDA is responsible for ensuring compliance with maximum residue levels (MRLs) under the 1938 Act (Pesticide Chemical amendment 1954). However, the Insecticide, Fungicide and Rodenticide Act charges the Environmental Protection Agency with responsibility for setting MRLs on the basis of toxicological data. The FDA carries out random testing of some 15 000 shipments of raw food commodities, including fruit and vegetables, each year. When illegal residue levels are detected, the FDA is able to seize the commodity, impose an injunction and prosecute the seller. Commodities can also be turned away at ports of entry; Congress has recently asked the FDA to increase surveillance at borders. There are two special circumstances in which pesticides are regarded, for the FDA's purposes, as food additives. These are: first, when the concentration of the residue becomes greater in the food itself than in the raw commodity, as during the formation of raisins; second, when the pesticide is applied to the food (rather than the crop) after harvesting. In these circumstances, the risk criterion of 0.000001 is applied, in the case of a tumorigenic substance.

Unlike pesticide MRLs, which are determined by the Environmental Protection Agency, tolerance levels for veterinary drug residues in meat and poultry are set by the FDA. However, monitoring and testing are carried out under the animal drug residues programme of the Food Safety Inspection Service (US Department of Agriculture). When drug levels in excess of tolerances are detected, it is the FDA which takes enforcement action. Some 8000 inspectors of the Inspection Service are stationed in slaughtering and processing plants throughout the US. The legal basis for their work is provided by two statutes, the Meat Inspection Act and the Poultry Products Inspection Act. Approximately 7200 slaughtering and processing plants are involved in the programme and much of the work is, of course, concerned with the visual inspection of carcasses for signs of microbiological, rather than chemical, contamination. The development of improved methods for 'traceback' and the recall of carcasses and meat products containing excessive chemical residues, together with more comprehensive systems for testing, are currently receiving much attention.

The Nordic Council

The Nordic Council is a vehicle for co-operation between the governments of the Nordic countries. It was created in 1952 by Denmark, Iceland, Norway and Sweden, and Finland joined in 1955. Greenland has been represented since 1984. Recommendations are made to the Nordic Council of Ministers (founded in 1971), which ensures that appropriate action is taken by governments (each government appoints a minister for Nordic co-operation). Some 60 joint institutions and committees deal with specific subjects, including food safety and the testing of drugs. Denmark has been a member of the EC since 1972 and the other Nordic countries have also entered into various agreements with the Community. Finland has signed an agreement with the Council for Mutual Economic Assistance (CMEA), the Eastern European organization for co-operation.

These links are helping to maintain common approaches to shared areas of concern, such as food safety. There is extensive trade in food between the EC and the Nordic countries, and the EC's work in the field of food safety regulation has been allowed to exert an influence on the inter-Nordic programme of food safety co-operation (Nordisk Ministerrad, 1988). The Nordic Working Group on Food Toxicology (NMT) is responsible for co-ordinating methods for assessing the health risks arising from contaminants, including residues of pesticides, veterinary and radioactive materials.

Despite the considerable degree of co-operation which exists between Nordic regulatory agencies, their approaches are by no means identical in every respect, and some of the existing systems possess a great deal of individuality. The Norwegian approach to the regulation of medicines is noteworthy in this respect. In Norway marketing authorizations for pharmaceuticals have been required since 1928. The statute enacted in that year established that the criteria for authorization were to be: safety, medical need, therapeutic efficacy, cost and pharmaceutical quality. This act also provided for the control of advertising. In 1958 the wholesale supply of medicines was nationalized, with the establishment of Norsk Medisinaldepot, the state company. The legislation was revised and consolidated by means of the Poison and Drug Act 1964, and a reorganization of the regulatory agency,

the Norwegian Medicines Control Authority, was undertaken in 1974.

Although the cost of a product is a criterion for final marketing authorization, it is only considered after the other criteria have been assessed and found to be satisfactory. The Authority is assisted in its work by a number of expert advisory committees, including the Specialities Committee, which approves new products. The members are specialists in medicine and pharmacy, and are appointed by the Minister of Social Affairs; the committee is chaired by the Director General of Public Health.

The Norwegian legislation is unusual in that it contains a 'need' clause. This states that marketing authorization will '. . . only be granted for preparations which are medically justified and which are considered to be needed . . .'. The 'need' clause enables the relative effectiveness of different products to be taken into account when they are assessed for marketing authorization. This is not possible under the legislation of many other countries.

Another practical effect of the need clause is to limit the number of products on the market containing any particular active ingredient, the number of products in each case depending on the size of the patient population requiring the drug. The marketing of 'me too' and 'combination' products is particularly limited. The intention of this approach is to promote rational therapy and to reduce confusion among prescribers, patients and distributors. A physician can always obtain a special licence which enables him to prescribe an unauthorized product for a particular use in a named patient. In such cases the prescription, which must state the indication and provide full information about the product, is forwarded to the Medicines Control Agency. The product is then obtained from the Norsk Medisinaldepot. Halse and Lunde report that only a minor portion of these special prescriptions relate to important drugs, urgently needed in hospital practice. The majority represent products which '. . . the patients persuaded their doctors to prescribe. An example is pills of procaine in combination with 23 different minerals and vitamins in very small quantities. This preparation is advertised as being effective for various geriatric purposes' (Halse and Lunde, 1978).

Despite the individuality of the Norwegian regulatory system for pharmaceuticals, the

Nordic guidelines on the evaluation of drugs (Nordic Council on Medicines, 1986) ensure uniformity of the data requirements throughout the region. Moreover, a medical prescription issued in one Nordic country is recognized in all others.

INTERNATIONAL ORGANIZATIONS

Although they are not regulatory agencies, some of the organizations within the framework of the United Nations and its associated bodies are of particular relevance in the context of this chapter. These are the International Programme on Chemical Safety, the International Agency for Research on Cancer, the International Register of Potentially Toxic Chemicals, the International Environmental Information System, and the Codex Alimentarius Commission. Other relevant bodies include the Organization for Economic Co-operation and Development, the International Courts and the Council of Europe.

The International Programme of Chemical Safety (IPCS)

The IPCS is based in Geneva and was sponsored jointly by three specialized agencies of the United Nations—the World Health Organization, the International Labour Organization, and the UN Environment Programme. Its major aim is to assess the effects of chemicals on health and on the environment, and to publish these assessments. In support of this aim, the IPCS is also developing risk-assessment, laboratory and epidemiological methods which are intended to give internationally comparable results. Other activities include the development of toxicological expertise in these areas, in the follow-up of chemical accidents and in mechanistic aspects of toxicology. The IPCS produces numerous publications in its 'Environmental Health Criteria' and 'Health and Safety Guide' series, and it has recently started to publish a companion series of International Chemical Safety Cards (ICSC). The IPCS also collaborates with the Commission of the European Communities (CEC) in the evaluation of antidotes used in the management of poisoning, and the results of these evaluations are published jointly.

The International Agency for Research on Cancer (IARC)

The IARC is an international research organization based in Lyon, concerned with the identification of environmental causes of human cancer. It carries out laboratory work as well as epidemiological studies in various parts of the world where different environmental conditions apply. The research programme is particularly concerned with aetiological factors in carcinoma of the stomach, oesophagus and other important sites, and with exploring the possible role of pesticides and viruses in human cancer.

The IARC was the first international biomedical body and was the outcome of a French proposal. The founding countries were France, the United Kingdom, the United States, the Federal Republic of Germany and Italy. The IARC was established in 1965 (during the 18th World Health Assembly) as an autonomous body within the World Health Organization. In addition to the founding countries, the following countries participate today: Australia, Belgium, Canada, Finland, Japan, the Netherlands, Norway, Sweden and the Russian Federation. The IARC monographs provide authoritative, up-to-date assessments of the carcinogenic risk for humans associated with a wide range of compounds.

International Register of Potentially Toxic Chemicals (IRPTC)

IRPTC was founded in 1976 and is based in Geneva. Its objective is to reduce the risks associated with chemical contamination of the environment, and it constitutes a valuable source of information about regulations and standards. IRPTC exists within the framework of the United Nations Environment Programme and it is particularly concerned with the needs of developing countries. It provides a query-response service and maintains a register on some 500 chemicals, as well as general information files on more than 40 000 chemicals. The IRPTC *Bulletin* is published twice a year, and there is a unique series of monographs (published in conjunction with the Russian Federation) on the hazards of pesticides and other chemicals. In addition, in conjunction with the IPCS, IRPTC is developing a Computerized Registry of Chemicals Being Tested for Toxic Effects (CCTTE).

International Environmental Information System (INFOTERRA)

INFOTERRA is an environmental information network, involving 123 countries, founded in 1977 as part of the United Nations Environment Programme. Its major centres are in Geneva and Nairobi. It possesses a register of information sources, and its major function is to refer enquiries to the appropriate sources, rather than providing substantive information as such. The International Directory contains descriptions of some 6000 sources, and there is a network of national focal points in the participating countries. Relevant references are Hofsten and Ekstrom (1986) and Ekstrom and Kidd (1989).

The Codex Alimentarius Commission

The term 'Codex Alimentarius' translates roughly from the Latin as 'food code'. Although the Codex Alimentarius Commission is not itself a regulatory agency, it is responsible for a system of standards, guidelines and codes of practice which many agencies throughout the world utilize, to differing extents, in formulating their regulations. The Codex system is concerned with two major aspects of food: the facilitation of trade in foodstuffs and food safety. The Commission is a subsidiary body of the Food and Agriculture Organization of the United Nations (FAO) and the World Health Organization (WHO). A major aspect of the Commission's work is making proposals to governments for new standards, guidelines and codes.

In carrying out its work, the Commission is assisted by a network of committees. One group of committees deals with specific commodities, such as the Codex Committee on Fats and Oils, which is hosted by the UK, first met in 1964 has been revitalized following a long period of inactivity. A second group of Codex committees deals with general subjects, such as food labelling. Three of these 'general subject' committees are of special importance in the present context. These are: the Codex Committee on Food Additives and Contaminants (CCFAC), the Codex Committee on Pesticide Residues (CCPR) and the Codex Committee on Residues of Veterinary Drugs in Foods (CCRVDF). The CCFAC is hosted by the government of the Netherlands and the first session took place in 1964. The CCPR is also hosted by the government of the Netherlands and the initial meeting occurred in 1966. The terms of reference of CCPR (q.v.) also include 'environmental and industrial contaminants showing chemical or other similarity to pesticides'. The CCRVDF first met in 1986 in the United States and it is hosted by the government of that country. Expert advice on scientific aspects, including toxicology, is required in conjunction with the work of these three committees, which are made up of government and trade delegations. In the case of the CCFAC and the CCRVDF, independent specialist advice is provided by the Joint (FAO/WHO) Expert Committee on Food Additives (JECFA). The Joint Meeting on Pesticide Residues (JMPR) plays a similar part in relation to the work of the CCPR. The advice of these expert committees is addressed to the Directors-General of FAO and WHO. Finally, the Joint Expert Committee on Food Irradiation (JECFI), which is a subsidiary body of the FAO and the International Atomic Energy Agency (IAEA), also provides advice in conjunction with the work of the CCFAC.

New Codex standards are 'elaborated' by the appropriate committee (together with the relevant expert group) and, following a series of consultative steps, are sent by the Commission to governments for acceptance. The work of elaborating a new standard may follow a decision either of the Commission or of the committee concerned. Such standards include, for example, maximum residue levels (MRLs) for pesticide residues in specific food commodities and tolerances for veterinary drug residues in the carcasses of food-producing animals.

Individual governments may or may not accept Codex standards and MRLs. Countries which decide upon full acceptance may implement Codex standards by incorporating them into their own national legislation. Joint decisions on acceptance may be taken by intergovernmental groups, such as the European Communities. In some countries, where food controls are based upon general commodities, governments may nevertheless use Codex standards for non-statutory purposes, such as allowing free distribution of imported foodstuffs which conform.

If the present (Uruguay) round of talks under the General Agreement on Tariffs and Trade (GATT) succeed, there may be an obligation upon member states to accept Codex MRLs for pesticides and veterinary drug concentrations in imports.

The Organization for Economic Co-operation and Development (OECD)

Twenty-four countries, including the US, Japan and the EC member states, take part in the work of the OECD. The organization is based in Paris and was established in 1960. The OECD chemicals programme constitutes an important part of the OECD's work, and in 1984 a co-operative agreement with the three United Nations agencies which sponsor the IPCS (see above) was signed.

An important aspect of the OECD chemicals programme relates to the harmonization of test methods for assessing health effects, environmental effects (ecotoxicity and accumulation/degradation) and physicochemical properties. To this end the OECD has published guidelines on the testing of chemicals for toxicity, and these are updated as necessary. Guidance on the principles of good laboratory practice (GLP) and monitoring for compliance have also been published. The Mutual Acceptance of Data agreement has done much to reduce the duplication of studies and unnecessary testing. This agreement requires OECD member countries to accept data provided that they conform with the relevant OECD test guidelines and are generated in compliance with the OECD principles of GLP (OECD, 1981).

Member countries receive assistance in examining and refining their risk management policies. This work includes case studies of risk management approaches to specific chemicals and chemical groups. The exchange of information on banned and severely restricted chemicals is continuing to be encouraged by the OECD.

The Organization's EXICHEM database is used to assist member countries to identify opportunities for co-operation in the investigation of specific existing chemicals, and to facilitate negotiations about the conduct of such work. EXICHEM is available on computer diskette and can be run on compatible personal computers. The secretariat examines the database twice yearly and makes suggestions on potential candidate chemicals for co-operative work. Such work is undertaken as part of the OECD 'clearinghouse' programme.

In 1989 the OECD compiled a list of chemicals which are produced in large quantities and which

have been examined for data availability. Additional data required for hazard assessment will be identified and accorded priorities.

The International Courts

Although there are major differences between the three international courts, they all become involved with the regulation of chemicals from time to time.

The European Court of Justice, based at Luxembourg, was set up under the terms of the Treaty of Rome and is the judicial body of the EC. Its judgements overrule those of the national courts, and it ensures that member states incorporate into national laws the intentions of the Directives, including those concerned with chemical safety. The Court also ensures that new domestic legislation of this kind, as well as the Regulations of the EC itself, are enforced.

The International Court of Justice, or 'World Court', based at The Hague, is the principal judicial body of the United Nations. Its work includes the provision of legal advice to United Nations bodies, including the World Health Organization and its agencies.

The European Court of Human Rights, based at Strasbourg, has been the guardian of the European Convention on Human Rights since its creation in 1953. It became involved in a prominent toxicological issue when it upheld the right of a British newspaper to publish information about the thalidomide tragedy.

The Council of Europe (COE)

The COE was founded in 1949, is based in Strasbourg and has a membership of 21 European governments. It co-operates closely with other international organizations, including the UN, the EC and the OECD. One of the Council's objectives is the introduction of uniform health regulations, and 12 of the member countries co-operate particularly closely to encourage protection against food contamination and to support harmonization of legislation in this field. Aspects of this work cover flavourings, packaging materials, and pesticide and veterinary drug residues. Other work has been carried out on toxic substances in cosmetics, and on adverse effects of medicines and detergents. Seventeen of the COE's member countries co-operate in producing the *European Pharmacopoeia*.

THE FOUNDATIONS OF EFFECTIVE REGULATION

If it is to enjoy a reputation for soundness, a regulatory agency must possess recognizable expertise in two related areas: toxicological judgement and administrative skill. The most elaborate scientific evaluation is wasted if appropriate regulatory action is not put into effect as a result: and this requires administrative skill. Similarly, deft implementation of regulations could be seen as capriciousness or high-handedness if it were not based on sound science. The meeting-point of the two skills is, above all, the area in which decisions are made about which risks necessitate regulatory action, and about which approaches (e.g. informal persuasion or formal proceedings?) are likely to secure the desired result most efficiently.

Regulatory toxicologists must frequently seek independent toxicological judgements outside their agencies. This ensures that there is access to the best expert advice available and it provides demonstrable assurance that the actions of agencies are well-founded and objective. In the UK the standards of independent advice available to

agencies are extremely high. Statutory committees, whose members are appointed by ministers, provide advice on some categories of chemical products. In the case of pesticides advice is provided by the Advisory Committee on Pesticides, to assist officials who regulate these products in accordance with the Food and Environmental Protection Act 1985. Pharmaceuticals are controlled by means of the Medicines Act 1968, which provides for the establishment of the Medicines Commission; section 4 of the Act provides for the creation of advisory committees whose members are appointed by ministers, with advice from the Commission. These committees are: the Committee on Safety of Medicines (Figure 2), the Committee on the Review of Medicines, the Committee on Dental and Surgical Materials and the Veterinary Products Committee. In the case of industrial chemicals, the Advisory Committee on Toxic Substances (ACTS) advises the Health and Safety Executive, which is responsible for implementing the Health and Safety at Work Act 1974. The members of ACTS are appointed by the Health and Safety Commission, which is in turn appointed by Ministers. Three non-statutory committees have also been established to provide

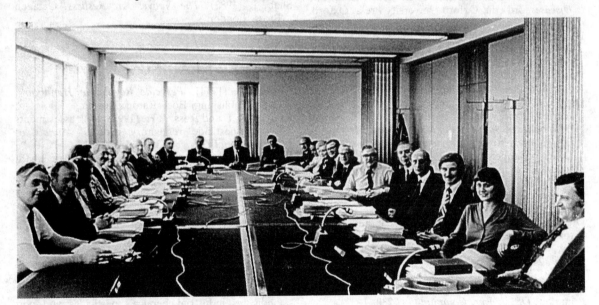

Figure 2   Committee on Safety of Medicines Meeting on 26 June 1980

Members and Secretariat, from left to right: Dr G. Diggle (DHSS), Dr R. Corcoran (DHSS), Dr L. Hill (DHSS), Professor M. Rawlins, Dr F. Fish, Dr M. Richards, Professor A. Read, Professor A. Goldberg, Professor D. G. Grahame-Smith, Dr J. Griffin (DHSS), Dr Gerald Jones (DHSS—Medical Assessor), Professor Sir Eric Scowen (Chairman), Mr P. Allen (DHSS—Secretary), Mr N. Williams (DHSS), Professor W. J. Cranston, Professor F. A. Jenner, Professor B. M. Hibbard, Dr J. M. Holt, Professor J. H. Girdwood, Professor J. W. Dundee, Mr R. Butcher (DHSS), Mr M. Parke (DHSS), Dr J. Calderwood (DHSS), Dr N. Taylor (DHSS), Dr G. Venning (DHSS)

foci of specialized expertise in toxicology. These are the Committees on Toxicity, Carcinogenicity and Mutagenicity of Chemicals in Food, Consumer Products and the Environment. Members are appointed by the Chief Medical Officer, and these sister committees are consulted by statutory committees, regulatory agencies and government departments.

ACKNOWLEDGMENTS

I acknowledge with gratitude the advice of numerous colleagues in regulatory toxicology during the preparation of this chapter, and particularly that of Dr R. Scheuplein (Washington), Dr Ola Westbye (Oslo) and Dr R. Fielder (London).

REFERENCES

Alder, S. and Zbinden, G. (1988). *National and International Drug Safety Guidelines*. MTC Verlag Zollikon

Diggle, G. E. (1987a). Iatrogenic neoplasia. In D'Arcy, P. F. and Griffin, J. P. (Eds), *Iatrogenic Diseases*, 3rd edn. Oxford University Press, Oxford, 811–856

Diggle, G. E. (1987b). Adverse effects of biomedical devices—Parts I and II. *Adv. Drug Reaction Bull.*, Nos. 124, 125

Diggle, G. E. (1988a). Carcinogenic drugs. *Adv. Drug Reactions Acute Poisoning Rev.*, **3**, 147–152

Diggle, G. E. (1988b). Safety aspects of implantable surgical devices. In *Proceedings First International Conference on Interfaces in Medicine and Mechanics*. Biomaterials Research Group, University of Wales College of Medicine

Diggle, G. E and Griffin, J. P. (1982). Licensing times in granting marketing authorisations for medicines: A comparison between the UK and USA. *Pharm. Int.*, **3**(7), 230–236

Diggle, G. E. (1992). Risk assessment and natural toxins. *Natural Toxins*, **1**, 71–72

Drew, G. (1986). Medical devices. *FDA Consumer*, May, 24–27

EC (1991). Council directive of 15th July 1991 concerning the placing of plant protection products on the market. *Off. J. Eur. Communities*, **230**, 1–31

ECETOC (1985). *Recommendation for the Harmonisation of International Guidelines for Toxicity Studies*. European Chemical Industry Ecology and Toxicology Centre, Monograph No. 7

Ekstrom, G. and Kidd, H. (Eds) (1989). *World Directory of Pesticide Control Organisations*. Royal Society of Chemistry, London

Griffin, J. P. and Diggle, G. E. (1981). A survey of medicinal products licensed in the UK 1971–1981. *Br. J. Clin. Pharmacol.*, **12**, 453–463

Halse, M. and Lund, P. (1978). Norway. In Wardell, W. M. (Ed.) *Control and Use of Therapeutic Drugs—An International Comparison*. American Enterprise Institute for Public Research, Washington, D.C.

Hofsten, B. and Ekstrom, G. (1986). *Control of Pesticide Applications and Residues in Food*. Swedish Science Press, Stockholm

Nordic Council on Medicines (1986). *Evaluation Reports on Proprietary Medicinal Products*. NLL Publication 17, Box 607, S–751 25 Uppsala, Sweden

Nordisk Ministerrad (1988). *The Nordic Programme of Cooperation in the Field of Foodstuffs*. Copenhagen

OECD (1981). Decision of the OECD Council Concerning the Mutual Acceptance of Data in the Assessment of Chemicals (C–81–30-final)

Peyer, J. (1989). *Medicine Culture—Notions of Health and Sickness in Britain, the US, France and West Germany*. Victor Gollancz, London

Richardson, M. (1986). *Toxic Hazard Assessment of Chemicals*. Royal Society of Chemistry, London

Secretary of Agriculture (1937). Report of the Secretary of Agriculture submitted in response to resolutions in the House of Representatives and Senate. *J. Am. Med. Assoc.*, **109**, 1985 ff

Shah, I. (1988). *The Natives Are Restless*. Octagon Press, London

FURTHER READING

Greene, J. (1994). *Pesticide Regulation Handbook*. Lewis Publishing, Boca Raton, Florida

Kreiger, R. I. and Ross, J. H. (1993). Risk assessments in the pesticide regulatory process. *Annals of Occupational Hygiene*, **37**, 565–578

Marr, A. P. and Scales, M. D. C. (1993). A review of documentation requirements for preclinical sections, for marketing submissions in the European Community, Japan and the USA. *Adverse Drug Reactions and Toxicology Reviews*, **12**, 253–262

Weisburger, J. H. (1994). Does the Delaney clause in the U.S. Food and Drug News prevent human cancers? *Fundamental and Applied Toxicology*, **22**, 483–493

Specific areas (drugs, veterinary products, veterinary medicines, industrial chemicals, pesticides, and food additives) are considered in Chapters 47–52 in Ballantyne, B., Marrs, T. C. and Turner, P. (Eds), *General and Applied Toxicology, Vol. 2*. Stockton Press, New York, pp. 1091–1156

PART SEVEN: TOXICOLOGY IN SPECIAL SITUATIONS

43 Pharmaceutical Toxicology

P. F. D'Arcy

INTRODUCTION

The development of potent and effective drugs continues to be associated with a concern regarding their safety. The administration of biologically active compounds to man must always be accompanied by some element of risk that cannot be avoided even by the most careful and exhaustive scientific and clinical study of the drug before it is introduced. Safety, efficacy and quality are the three statutory requirements in the UK guiding the evaluation and approval for subsequent use of any pharmaceutical product. Regulation in the pharmaceutical industry arose out of the concept of protecting the population—indeed, safeguarding the public health is the first objective stated in Directive 65/65 of the European Community.

It is salutary to look back in recent time and realize that the Committee on Safety of Drugs (the Dunlop Committee), which was established on a voluntary basis in the UK in 1963, was not directly concerned with drug efficacy. The voluntary arrangements were dominated by safety; the Committee's remit did not impose upon it any responsibility to consider the efficacy of drugs except insofar as their safety was concerned. It is only since 1971 that an integrated regulatory system concerned with all the three requirements—safety, efficacy and quality of medicinal products—was introduced into the UK through the implementation of the Medicines Act of 1968.

This enactment placed special emphasis on considerations of safety in relation to the issue of both Product Licences (Section 19.1) and Clinical Trials Certificates (Section 36.2). In contrast with its provisions in respect of efficacy, the Medicines Act allowed the Licensing Authority to take account of comparative safety (Section 19.2) in deciding applications. Moreover, the Act took a broad view of safety by including not only potential dangers to patients themselves, but also hazards to the community and to those administering the drugs; it also covered interference with diagnosis, treatment or prevention of disease (Section 132.2). Comparable requirements within the European Community are contained in the relevant EEC Directives (Commission of the European Communities, 1984). Matters which have potential financial implications, such as clinical need and comparative efficacy, are specifically excluded from both the Medicines Act in the UK and the EEC Directives.

In attempting to ensure the safety of drugs the Licensing Authority and the Committee on Safety of Medicines in the UK rely on three strategies—the control of quality, rigorous pre-marketing safety studies and post-marketing surveillance. Quality is controlled in relation to both manufacture and wholesale selling and, as a consequence, toxicity due to product defects is now exceptional (Rawlings, 1989).

There are no priorities within safety, quality and efficacy, for all three requirements are equally weighted. Default in any one will jeopardize marketing approval or continuation of clinical use. Stephens (1988) summed up the situation thus: '. . . in future it will no longer be sufficient for pharmaceutical companies to plan their clinical trial programme for a new drug on the basis of showing that it is efficacious and that secondarily no adverse drug reactions (ADRs) were noted. The cost half of the cost/benefit ratio now demands that equal effort must be put into active research for adverse reactions as in the proof for efficacy.' Thus, the evaluation of the toxic potential of a new molecule must be an active search, not merely a passive observation of what toxicity emerges during preliminary studies and subsequent clinical use.

RESPONSIBILITY

The discovery of the ADR profile of a new drug prior to marketing lies entirely within the sphere of the pharmaceutical company and, therefore, the company has the responsibility for providing adequate information. After a drug is marketed, the responsibility for extending the knowledge base of its adverse reactions spreads also to all the prescribers of that drug, as well as to specific organizations set up for that purpose.

The predominant objective of all national and international drug regulations is to ensure the safety of marketed medicinal products during normal conditions of use. It could be defined as protecting the public health and safeguarding the public purse, for such procedures also ensure that the patient gets value for money spent on the medication.

DRUG DISASTERS (Pre- and Post-thalidomide)

Modern drug regulation in the UK was conceived in the aftermath of the thalidomide disaster. There is evidence that earlier disasters were equally troublesome, although perhaps not so well publicized as thalidomide. There have also been other disasters before and since thalidomide (see Table 1).

For example, jaundice and hepatic necrosis ('yellow atrophy of the liver') reached epidemic levels following the use of organo-arsenicals such as salvarsan to treat syphilis in soldiers returning from World War I.

Amidopyrine was commonly used as an anti-pyretic and analgesic and it took almost half a century of common use to recognize that it caused agranulocytosis.

The ill-fated Elixir of Sulfanilamide produced by the old established Massengil Company in the United States not only heralded the new era of the sulphonamide drugs, but also during September and October 1937 directly caused at least 76 deaths due to the renal toxicity of its 72 per cent content of the solvent diethylene glycol; many of the victims were children. The sulphanilamide disaster shocked the country and was instrumental in Congress reacting by passing the Food, Drug and Cosmetic Act in 1938, which required all new drugs to be demonstrated to be safe.

Stalinon, a preparation designed to treat boils, led to a two-year prison sentence for its French inventor; it contained diiodoethyl tin and isolinoleic acid esters and was associated with raised intracranial pressure. The product was alleged to have killed 102 people and permanently affected 100 more, some survivors having residual paraplegia.

Table 1 Notable drug disasters or discovery of important adverse effects

1920s	Organo-arsenicals (jaundice and hepatic necrosis)
1933	Amidopyrine (agranulocytosis)
1937	Elixir of Sulfanilamide—Massengil (diethylene glycol toxicity)
1957	Stalinon (raised intracranial pressure)
1960s	Phenacetin (renal damage)
1960s	Thalidomide (teratogenicity)
1960s	Clioquinol (subacute myelo-opticoneuropathy)
1967	Phenytoin (rickets, osteomalacia)
1970s	Practolol (oculomucocutaneous syndrome)
1970s	Metamizol (novaminsulfon) (blood dyscrasias)
1979, 1991	Triazolam (Halcion) (excitation reactions and acute psychic derangement)
1982	Benoxaprofen (Opren) (photosensitivity, oncholysis, fatal hepatic reactions in the elderly)
1983	Osmosin (indomethacin dumping) (ulceration and intestinal perforation)
1983	Zimeldine (Zelmid) (neurotoxicity)
1983	Zomepirac (Zomax) (serious allergic and anaphylactic reactions)
1984	Alphaxalone (anaphylaxis)
1984	Fenclofenac (Flenac) (skin rashes, gastrointestinal disorders and suspected carcinogenicity)
1984	Feprazone (Methrazone) (skin rashes, gastrointestinal disorders, thrombocytopenia and haemolytic anaemia)
1986	Domperidone injection (cardiotoxicity)
1986	Nomifensine (Merital) (immune haemolytic anaemia)
1990	Propess, controlled-release PGE2 (dinoprostone) (uterine hypertonus and foetal distress syndrome)
1991	Terolidine (Micturin) (cardiac arrythmias)
1992	Propofol (Diprivan) (fatal neurologic, cardiac and renal toxicity, and hyperlipidaemia in children)
1992	Medicinal products containing extracts from the plant germander (*Teucrium* spp.) (hepatitis)
1992	MMR vaccines (Pluserix-MMR; Immravax) (meningitis caused by mumps vaccine component in children)

Phenacetin was first used in 1887 and is an effective analgesic and antipyretic; unfortunately, however, it also has a long and somewhat controversial association with chronic renal disease, especially in the Swedish town of Huskvana, where local custom among the munition workers involved the frank abuse of Hjorton's Powders, which contained caffeine, phenacetin and phenazone.

The thalidomide tragedy is well known, as also is the SMON (subacute myelo-opticoneuropathy) epidemic in Japan due to the use of clioquinol for enteric disorders; both have received much publicity and were directly responsible for a greater awareness of the public of adverse drug reactions and a demand through their legislators for stricter controls over medicines.

Practolol, a very useful member and forerunner of the beta-blockers, gave rise to oculomucocutaneous syndrome and was withdrawn from general use.

Metamizol (novaminsulfon), a non-steroidal anti-inflammatory agent, was associated with blood dyscrasias.

The hypnotic agent triazolam, a benzodiazepine derivative, was associated with excitation reactions and acute psychic derangement: reactions that were complicated in 1979 by media-induced suggestion and excitement in the Netherlands—the 'so-called' Halcion story. The Licensing Authority withdrew this medicine from the UK market in October 1991; an appeal is in progress.

Osmosin is worthy of particular mention because it was the formulation and not its indomethacin content that was the problem. This sustained-action (release) formulation 'dumped' its contents into the gut, causing ulceration and fatal intestinal perforation.

The non-steroidal anti-inflammatory agents (NSAIDs) have been singularly unfortunate in their marketing history. Benoxaprofen caused fatal hepatic reactions in the elderly patient and photosensitivity and onycholysis on a massive scale. It had a very short market life and it well illustrated the suddenness with which a true epidemic of adverse events can occur. Zomepirac, another NSAID, was withdrawn because of the large numbers of incidents of serious anaphylaxis and allergic reactions that were associated with its use, while fenclofenac was withdrawn from the UK market in 1984, owing to a cluster of ADRs, including skin rashes, gastrointestinal disorders and suspected carcinogenicity. In the same year feprazone was withdrawn because of associated skin rashes, gastrointestinal disorders, thrombocytopenia, and haemolytic anaemia. Other problems with marketed drug products have followed in succeeding years.

The thalidomide tragedy looms so ponderously over the history of adverse drug reactions that it causes other events that have since occurred to pale into insignificance and even suggests that since 1961 the worst of the problems have been solved. This is just not so! The number of patients gravely injured or killed in epidemics of drug-induced disease since then is a vast multiple of the number of thalidomide victims. Although much information has been gained about the circumstances leading to these individual disasters, there is little in these collections of data that will serve to prevent other drug disasters occurring that are qualitatively different from those that have gone before. The range of injuries produced is so wide that no single solution to the detection of future drug-induced disasters before they occur seems likely to emerge.

REGULATIONS CONCERNED WITH SAFETY

Pharmaceutical toxicology is quite a different field from industrial or pesticide toxicity evaluations. The techniques employed and the methodology used are similar but the orientation is different. Since there is no way of providing the complete safety of a new drug before it comes into widespread use, it becomes a question of at what stage of development the risks should be defined. The easy answer is: as soon as possible, so that as few patients as possible are exposed to unnecessary risks. The regulatory authority must therefore weigh the advantages of the efficacy of a new drug, compared with the normal prognosis of the disease with known therapy, against the risks involved in marketing the new drug without full knowledge of its adverse reaction burden. At the same time the regulatory authority has to decide whether to leave the detection of the more rare side-effects to be discovered by the present testing systems or whether they should institute a major surveillance programme so that these risks may be known earlier.

The regulation of medicines by society has been expressed by Lasagna (1989) as being time-bound, country-bound and person-bound. It is time-bound both because of what are thought to be socially necessary changes over the years and because the sciences of medicine and pharmacology are constantly evolving. It is country-bound because each nation, in setting up its own regulatory system, will be guided by the particular needs of its citizens for medicines, its economy, its political philosophy and the quality and extent of its scientific establishment and its health care delivery system. It is person-bound because no matter what the letter of the law may be for regulating medicines, or the nature of the published regulations, there is always the opportunity for value judgements to be made by those implementing the laws and regulations.

In considering the role of regulation, it is useful to be realistic about what can and what cannot be achieved by regulations, even when based on scientific rules of evidence and on accepted approaches to decision making. Traditionally, the most ancient and in a sense the least controversial function of regulation has been to ensure that a medicine is accurately labelled as to its contents, and the nature of the ingredients and their amounts (Lasagna, 1989). It is more difficult, however, to delineate the safety and efficacy of the medicine proposed for registration. Since the ability to explore the full dose–response curve for a drug's toxicity is not ethically possible in humans, it is necessary to rely to a great extent on animal studies to achieve insights into this relationship.

THE USE OF ANIMALS IN SAFETY TESTING

There are powerful scientific, ethical and regulatory reasons for exploring the effect of potential therapeutic candidates in animals before they are administered to man. There are also strong and public emotive reasons why they should not be used. However, the low proportion of significant toxic reactions in humans with new medicines, compared with the number tested and introduced, supports the contention that toxicity studies in laboratory animals are, in the main, predictive for man. There are also many positive occurrences between the findings in animal toxicity tests and adverse reactions in humans, particularly for dose- and time-related toxic effects (Table 2). On the contrary, there have been well-publicized accounts of failures of experimental toxicology and false alarms resulting from apparently irrelevant toxicological observations in animals. The overall success of the current preclinical safety evaluation process is difficult to assess. Although useful information could be obtained

Table 2   Some toxic reactions that occur in both animals and man. Source: Morton (1990)

Acrylamide	Peripheral neuropathy
Aniline	Methaemoglobinaemia
Asbestos	Mesothelioma
Atropine	Anticholinergic effects
Benzene	Leukaemia
Bleomycin	Pulmonary fibrosis
Carbon disulphide	Nervous system toxicity
Carbon tetrachloride	Hepatic necrosis
Cis-platinum	Nephropathy
Cobalt sulphate	Cardiomyopathy
Cyclophosphamide	Haemorrhagic cystitis
Cyclosporin A	Nephropathy
D&C Yellow	Eczema
Diethylene glycol	Nephropathy
Diethylaminoethoxyhexoestrol	Phospholipidosis of liver
Doxorubicin	Cardiomyopathy
Emetine	ECG abnormalities
Ethylene glycol	Obstructive nephropathy
Frusemide (furosemide)	Hypokalaemia
Gentamicin	Nephropathy and ototoxicity
Hexacarbons	Peripheral neuropathy
Hexachlorophene	Spongiform encephalopathy
Isoniazid	Peripheral neuropathy
Isoprenaline (isoproterenol)	Stenocardia
Isothiocyanates	Goitre
Isotretinoin (prenatal)	Multiple malformations
Kanamycin	Cochlear toxicity
Methanol	Blindness (monkey)
Methoxyflurane	Nephropathy (Fischer rat)
8-Methoxypsoralen	Phototoxicity
Methyl mercury	Encephalopathy
Morphine	Physical and psychological dependence
MPTP	Parkinsonism
Musk ambrette	Photosensitivity
2-Naphthylamine	Bladder cancer (dog)
Neuroleptic drugs	Galactorrhoea
Nitrofurantoin	Testicular damage

continued

Table 2 (continued)

Paracetamol (Acetaminophen)	Hepatic necrosis
Paraquat	Lung damage and fibrosis
Phenformin	Lactic acidosis
Phenothiazine NP 207	Retinopathy (pigmented animals)
Penicillamine	Loss of taste
Pyridoxine	Sensory neuropathy
Scopolamine	Behavioural disturbances
Slow-release potassium	Intestinal ulceration
Thalidomide (prenatal)	Phocomelia (monkey, rabbit)
Triparanol	Cataract
Vinyl chloride	Angiosarcoma of the liver
Vitamin A	Osteopathy
Vitamin D	Nephrocalcinosis

by retrospective analysis of data obtained for compounds that have been used extensively in the clinic, to date this has received only limited systematic study (Lumley and Walker, 1990).

In 1989, the Sixth Centre for Medicines Research (CMR), held in the Ciba Foundation in London, provided the opportunity for an international group of experts from the pharmaceutical industry, academia and the regulatory authorities to review critically and discuss past methodologies which have been employed to assess the efficacy of animal toxicity testing procedures in predicting qualitative toxicity in man. Conventional animal toxicological studies have three purposes: they attempt to define a compound's general toxicological profile; they are expected to reveal those target organs/systems demanding special study during clinical trials; and, it is hoped, they will provide a basis for predicting human safety (Rawlings, 1989). A most important aspect of the correlation of toxic effects between man and animals is the selection of animal species in which the drug is absorbed, distributed, metabolized and excreted in a similar manner to man.

The value of multispecies toxicity studies and parallel metabolic studies has been well established (Morton, 1990). Yet despite wide experience with animal studies, their validity remains uncertain (Zbinden, 1981). Only a few investi-

gators (Fletcher, 1978; Griffin, 1983; Laurence *et al.*, 1984) have attempted to correlate findings during human use with those observed during preclinical toxicity studies, and even these have been limited in scale and scope (Rawlings, 1989). Routine animal toxicity tests are most useful when there are no important qualitative differences between species and where one can make up for the difficulty in demonstrating certain adverse effects with clinically relevant doses in animals by administering the drug at very high doses, on the assumption that more sensitive individuals will respond in similar fashion when given smaller doses of the drug (Lasagna, 1989).

CARCINOGENICITY AND MUTAGENICITY TESTING

Unfortunately, there is current reliance on carcinogenicity and mutagenicity tests whose power and reliability are in question. Morton (1990) has summarized problems with the evaluation of animal mutagenicity and carcinogenicity tests and their prediction of potential carcinogenicity in humans.

For many years potential new drugs have been tested at high doses in long-term carcinogenicity studies in rodents prior to regulatory approval and broad clinical use. These studies have been costly in test chemicals, animals, laboratory facilities and staff, and research time. Although the overall database on animal bioassays has been greatly expanded by the United States National Cancer Institute and the National Toxicology Program, the prediction of human carcinogenicity is still problematic. In many studies the results have varied between species, strains and sexes of the animals tested. The incidence of tumours observed has not always been dose-related and the relevance of these studies to human carcinogenesis is still not clear.

Short-term mutagenicity tests are expected to detect genotoxic carcinogens, and a strong rationale has been developed for the use of these tests early in the process of drug development. Although neither a positive nor a negative result in short-term tests can be considered fully definitive, the International Agency for Research on Cancer has noted that the majority of chemicals that have given sufficient evidence of inducing human tumours are genotoxic (International Agency for Research on Cancer, 1987).

During recent years, however, it has become evident that the early estimates of the predictability of the mutagenicity tests for the carcinogenic properties of most chemicals were too optimistic (Shelby and Stasiewicz, 1984; Tennant *et al.*, 1987). A careful validation of *in vitro* tests against the results of long-term rodent carcinogenicity tests by Tennant *et al.* (1987) found that none of the short-term tests were necessarily predictive. In fact, it was suggested that no combination of the available *in vitro* mutagenicity tests (e.g. Ames bacterial mutation; L5178Y mammalian mutation; rat hepatocyte DNA repair; CHO cell cytogenetics) was significantly better than a single test. Furthermore, Clayson (1987) has suggested that short-term tests cannot be expected to detect all types of carcinogens, since mutations may only be related to the initiation phase of the complex process of carcinogenesis. Further evidence has been given by Morton (1990), who has described and quoted mutagenicity testing in the laboratories of Eli Lilly and Company; in these validation studies most of the known human or animal carcinogens were detected in the broadly used and well-accepted battery of *in vitro* and *in vivo* mutagenicity tests. However, when research compounds were tested in this tier, the number of positive findings was relatively small and in no case did a compound produce a positive response in more than one test.

TRANSLATION OF RESULTS FROM ANIMALS TO MAN

When one moves from animals to humans, a conservative approach is usually taken, starting with doses in healthy volunteers at only a fraction of those which produce significant toxicity in the most sensitive animal species. It is generally agreed that in these earliest human studies, and in the subsequent clinical trials in Phases I and II, one can gain considerable insight into those adverse reactions that occur with some frequency. However, it is usually not possible to detect in the studies the truly rare serious side-effect, to say nothing of the side-effect that is long delayed in its onset, or occurs as a result of an interaction with basic disease processes, or with other drugs.

All that will eventually be known about the drug's effects, both good and bad, will never be known at the time of initial marketing of a compound. The lesson is obvious: efficient and skilful postregistration observations must be relied upon to identify and prove cause–effect relationships between the taking of a drug and the occurrence of an untoward event.

Prospective studies designed to assess the relevance and predictive value of animal toxicity studies for man are rarely possible for ethical reasons (Brimblecombe, 1990). Substances showing marked toxicity in animals can only rarely, for ethical reasons, be administered to man. Prospective studies are, therefore, only possible with substances showing an acceptable toxicological profile in animals. In general, there is a paucity of data in this area. However, although retrospective collection and analysis of data are less satisfactory, they are none the less important alternatives. Such data are available, for example, within pharmaceutical companies, but analysis of larger databases such as those in regulatory authorities or those collected from a number of companies (for example, by the Centre for Medicines Research) has the potential for yielding more valuable information. Brimblecombe (1990) has suggested that retrospective studies can take a number of forms:

(1) Re-evaluation of data from animal studies when unwanted effects occur subsequently and unexpectedly in man.
(2) Design of specific animal studies to elucidate mechanisms of unwanted effects which have been observed in man.
(3) Pooling of data from a number of sources to increase the size of the database and to enable more meaningful 'epidemiological-type' analyses to be performed.
(4) Reviews of the history of individual compounds which have been, or are in, development.

Bass (1990), in summarizing the toxicologist's viewpoint on what could be learned by examining the data in the files of regulatory authorities, stated that data in those files highlighted the problem areas that exist in extrapolating the results of animal studies to man. Since animal toxicity studies should be performed for the sake of man, this implies differences for each developmental product; thus, it is no longer appropriate to work to generalized and rigid guidelines. Flexibility in itself seems insufficient if the pharmaceutical manufacturer does not know how the regulatory authorities will react to the test programmes envisaged, and if revision through interaction with the clinical level is not included. Bass concluded that the question to be answered is not whether studies available retrospectively have been of relevance to man and to what extent or percentage, but how to make such studies useful and relevant in the future. Thus, early interaction between the pharmaceutical manufacturer and the regulatory authority may be needed case by case. This, he believes, should reduce the overall number of toxicological studies, rendering those remaining as requirements more relevant.

Fletcher (1990), expressing the clinician's viewpoint, commented on the number of guidelines that have been introduced since 1977 which were similar but not identical: the toxicology guidelines of the Committee for Proprietary Medicinal Products (CPMP); the OECD toxicity testing guidelines; the Annexes of the Sixth Amendment Directive of the EEC, which were also toxicological guidelines; and the Guidelines for Good Laboratory Practice. The problem with these is that they have codified and ritualized toxicity testing, so that there is very little flexibility. In his view this was not ideal, for what was needed was a possibility of matching toxicological requirements to particular compounds.

There is a great deal of potential in examining the files of regulatory authorities, as these have a unique value in that they cover a whole range of compounds and therapeutic classes, providing the full range of toxicological and clinical testing. However, access to data held by regulatory authorities is strictly limited, since any one company has access only to information on its own compounds and the only place in which the totality exists is with the regulatory authorities. Fletcher (1990) has suggested how the situation could be improved. First, the inclusion of toxicokinetics in current safety evaluation studies would provide the opportunity to compare pharmacokinetics and metabolism in animals with man and could prevent inappropriate conclusions being drawn with regard to animal and human conditions. Second, there is an urgent need for closer co-operation between toxicologists and clinicians in the industry. Finally, detailed analyses of toxi-

cological and clinical data available from regulatory authorities should be carried out.

Fletcher (1990) has suggested that this could be approached by tabulating and analysing all the anatomical, physiological and toxicological findings for particular groups of chemically or therapeutically similar compounds. This would give insight into whether they were consistent or inconsistent and what could and could not be relied upon. He also suggested an analysis of time relationships to identify situations that have proved to be consistently unreliable, inappropriate or irrelevant. This should provide evidence as to whether long-term tests—for example, in dogs—were irrelevant.

Lumley (1990) has provided interesting information on the termination of development by companies as a result of clinical toxicity. Eighteen pharmaceutical companies in the UK, Switzerland and the USA gave information on 29 compounds for which they terminated development between 1975 and 1986. These data are summarized in Table 3. Almost one-half of the clinical effects causing termination (14) were effects that are difficult to identify in animal tests, including CNS disturbances and blood dyscrasias or skin reactions/allergies, and only two of these (both blood dyscrasias) were detected in animal tests. Lumley concluded, from these data, that it was not possible to draw any conclusions as to why some adverse reactions were predicted and others were not. More information would be needed—for example, on number of animals, species used, duration of exposure to drug in animals and man, comparative metabolism and pharmacokinetic data, and dose levels in animals and man. Without these data the predictive value of animal studies for man was doubtful.

Heywood (1990) has commented that many adverse reactions in man—in particular, immunotoxicity, allergy, hypersensitivity and effects on bone marrow—are unpredictable in animal models. The correlation between target system toxicity in the rat and a non-rodent species is around 30 per cent and the best guess for the correlation of adverse reactions in man and animal toxicity data is somewhere between 5 and 25 per cent. Table 4 shows major adverse reactions reported since 1975 and whether they can be predicted in animal studies; only 14 per cent showed adverse reactions that could have been predicted. Table 5 shows compounds withdrawn

Table 3 Compounds: development terminated due to clinical toxicity. Source: Lumley (1990)

Therapeutic class	Phase of testing	Approx. No./vol. patients tested	Clinical toxicity	Predicted (Y/N) or confirmed (C) in animal tests
1. GI	Clinical trial	2000	Raised liver enzymes	C
2. CVS	n/a	n/a	Abnormal liver function tests	n/a
3. CVS	Post-market		Hepatic necrosis	N
4. CVS	Phase I/II		Increased transaminases	Y
5. Respiratory	n/a	n/a	Abnormal liver function tests	n/a
6. NSAID	Phase III	2000	Raised liver enzymes	N
7.	Clinical trial	n/a	Raised liver enzymes	N
8. Antiallergy	Clinical trial	100s	Hepatoxicity	C
9. Antisecretory	Volunteers		Liver abnormalities	Y
10. CVS	Volunteers	3	Rashes	N
11. Skin	Phase II	150	Skin reactions	N
12. Prostaglandin inhibitor	n/a	n/a	Topical reaction	n/a
13. Spermicide	Volunteers	<10	Local irritability	N
14. Antiinfective	Volunteers		Pain on injection	N
15. Endocrine	Phase II	35	Allergy	N[a]
16. CNS	Phase II	14	Allergy	N
17. n/a	Volunteers		Anaphylactic reaction	N
18. GI	Volunteers	10s	Tachycardia	N
19.	Phase II	60	Postural hypotension	Y[b]
20. Antiallergy	Volunteers	10s	Flushing	N
21. GI	Clinical trial	100s	Granulocytopenia	C
22. Thrombolytic	Volunteers	10s	Haemorrhage	Y
23. n/a	Phase II	200–300	Blood dyscrasias	N
24. CNS	Volunteers	40	White cell count decreased	N
25. GI	Volunteers		CNS disturbances	N
26. CNS	Phase II	40	CNS effects	N
27. Steroid	Volunteers	10	Adrenal suppression	C
28. Leukotriene-D4 antagonist	n/a	n/a	GI effects (high dose)	n/a
29. Antiinfective	n/a	n/a	n/a	n/a

[a] Partially expected from chemical structure.
[b] Nausea/vomiting which would have limited clinical use was also observed.
n/a = Not available.

from the UK clinical market since 1980; anti-inflammatories and analgesic agents represent nearly 50 per cent of compounds that have been withdrawn, the second most important group being centrally active compounds, which includes anaesthetics and antiemetics.

HARMONIZATION OF REGULATIONS—REDUCED NUMBER OF ANIMALS NEEDED

The International Conference on Harmonization of Technical Requirements for Registration of Pharmaceuticals for Human Use, held in Brussels from 5 to 7 November 1991, has had important implications for animal safety testing. This tripar-

tite conference, representing mainly the Commission of the European Communities, the US Food and Drug Administration and the Japanese Ministry of Health and Welfare, together with the pharmaceutical industry as represented by the International Federation of Pharmaceutical Manufacturers Associations, the European Federation of Pharmaceutical Industry Associations, the US Pharmaceutical Manufacturers Association and the Japanese Pharmaceutical Manufacturers Association, discussed harmonization of regulatory requirements between the three regions the USA, the European Community and Japan. The Conference was preceded by 2 years of preparatory technical discussions aimed at ensuring that good-quality, safe and effective medicines are developed and registered in the

Table 4 Major adverse reactions in man since 1960: predictability in animal tests. Source: Heywood (1990)

Drug	ADR	Predictable in animals
Anti-inflammatory drugs	Gastrointestinal	Yes
	Haematological	Yes
	Skin rashes	No
Alphaxalone	Anaphylaxis	No
Benoxaprofen	Fatalities, skin rashes, photosensitivity	No
Chloramphenicol	Aplastic anaemia	No
Clioquinol	Neurotoxicity	Yes
Domperidone	Cardiotoxicity	No
Halothane	Jaundice	Yes
Lincomycin, clindamycin	Pseudomembranous colitis	No
Methysergide	Retroperitoneal fibrosis	No
Nomifensine	(Immune haemolytic anaemia)	No
Oral contraceptives	Thromboembolism	No
Phenacetin	Nephropathy	No
Phenformin	Lactic acidosis	No
Phenothiazines	Dyskinesia	Questionable
Phenylbutazone	Aplastic anaemia	No
Practolol	Oculomucocutaneous syndrome	No
Propanidid	Allergy	No
Stilboestrol	Vaginal cancer in female offspring	No (mice)
Sulphamethoxypyridazine	Haematological, dermatology	Questionable
Sympathomimetic aerosols	Asthmatic death	No
Triazolam	Amnesia	No
Zimeldine	Neurotoxicity	No

most efficient and cost-effective manner. Within this objective there was an intent to minimize the use of animal testing without compromising the regulatory obligations of safety and effectiveness. These recommendations should be adopted within a short period, with considerable savings in resources and the numbers of animals used.

In the Workshop on Safety, agreement was reached on all aspects of single-dose studies—in particular, on dropping LD_{50} determination. The tests which will replace the determination of LD_{50} will have a testing protocol which uses the fewest number of animals possible for the approximation of the highest non-lethal or the lowest lethal dose. In the area of repeated-dose safety studies, agreement was reached on the questions of delayed toxicity and appropriate dosing levels as well as on the reduction from 12 to 6 months duration for long-term studies. In specific circumstances, in non-rodents, 12 month studies may be requested.

In the area of reproductive toxicity, the existing guidelines were regarded as equivalent and, in addition, a tripartite guideline will be recommended in 1992.

For safety studies in biotechnology it emerged from the scientific discussions that requirements are equivalent and the major points of convergence were underlined.

Discussions on timing of toxicity studies versus clinical trials, and appropriate exposures for carcinogenicity studies, were productive, and harmonized regulations will be made within 2 years.

THE NUMBERS GAME

With all the reports on ADRs that appear in the literature each year from official drug regulatory bodies and from investigating clinicians, it may be difficult to understand why toxic reactions to drugs are so often undetected initially. Some individual reasons for this can be pinpointed: for example, in most clinical trials on new drugs patients are usually selected by criteria which may differ from those of patients treated in later clinical practice. Drugs which are to be mainly used in the very old are commonly tested on much younger populations (e.g. benoxaprofen) and drugs considered safe or effective in younger adults may be neither in the very old.

The 'numbers game' probably exerts influence as well. If an ADR is likely to occur in x per cent

Table 5 Compounds withdrawn from the UK market for clinical adverse reactions. Source: Heywood (1990)

Year	Compounds withdrawn	Clinical adverse reactions
1980	Phenacetin	Nephrotoxicity and carcinogenicity
1981	Clioquinol	Neurotoxicity
1982	Benoxaprofen (Opren)	Skin rashes Photosensitivity Onycholysis, GI tract Fatalities in elderly
	Phenformin	Metabolic
1983	Indomethacin (Osmosin)	Small intestine perforation
	Indoprofen (Flosint)	GI tract and carcinogenicity
	Propanidid	Allergy
	Zimeldine (Zelmid)	Neurotoxicity
	Zomepirac (Zomax)	Allergy
1984	Alphaxalone	Anaphylactic shock
	Fenclofenac (Flenac)	Rashes, GI tract Carcinogenicity
	Feprazone (Methrazone)	Rashes, GI tract Thrombocytopenia Haemolytic anaemia
	Oxyphenbutazone	Haematology, GI tract
1986	Domperidone injectable (Benzamide)	Cardiotoxicity
	Guanethidine eyedrops	Ophthalmological
	Nomifensine (Merital)	Haemolytic anaemia (immune)
	Sulphamethoxypyridazine	Haematological Dermatological
	Suprofen (Suprol)	Reversible renal insufficiency

of patients, then there is no guarantee that this probability will be uniformly distributed among the finite and relatively small population that is involved in the typical clinical trial. It is only when a larger population of patients are involved that the true extent of the *x* percentage is revealed. It may take a period of relatively extensive clinical use before the true extent of the ADR is revealed; this was so for benoxaprofen, chloramphenicol, ticrynafen (tienilic acid), halothane, practolol and the sulphonamides, and, in a different context, the same is true of the hazards of cigarette smoking.

DO MEDICINES REGULATIONS PROTECT THE PUBLIC BUT HINDER RESEARCH?

Griffin (1989) holds that medicines regulations have safeguarded the public. There is no doubt that the pharmaceutical industry has improved its standards of toxicological screening, clinical pharmacology, pharmacokinetic studies and clinical trial evaluation as a result of the guidelines that have been laid down by the UK regulatory authorities and the Committee for Proprietary Medicinal Products, which was set up in 1975 (Directive 75/319/EEC) and plays an important role in the application of harmonized regulations regarding medicinal products within the EEC. It is Griffin's personal view that the safety and efficacy of medicinal products have been improved more by the pharmaceutical industry striving to adhere to the standards laid down by the test procedures than as a result of any regulatory scrutiny of the data derived therefrom. He qualifies his view, however, by adding that the fact that data are scrutinized must encourage the adherence to the standards set. He also holds that collection of adverse reaction data is of no value if they are not analysed and interpreted adequately and are then communicated in such a form that they can modify the behaviour of the prescribing doctor.

There has, however, been a price to pay, and it is evident, for example, from a review of licensing applications in the UK during the 1970s that regulation did hinder research. Deregulation, in the form of the Clinical Trial Exemption scheme, has provided a stimulus to innovation without presenting a hazard to the population. Not only is regulation a deterrent to innovation, but also regulatory delay erodes effective patent term and reduces financial returns. Research initiatives are also reduced by high licensing fees. Futhermore, the existence in Europe of 12 regulatory authorities consumes scarce technical and scientific resources that could be better employed (Griffin, 1991).

HOW SAFE HAVE NEW DRUGS BEEN?

Perhaps the final question to be asked in this review is: How safe have drugs been? In this respect, it is worth remembering the words of Inman: 'No worthwhile drug is entirely without risk, but few have been responsible for large-scale disasters' (Inman, 1980). Of the more than 350 new chemical entities introduced in the United States from 1960 to 1982, only eight were removed from the market for safety reasons. That 22 year record argues that the balance between relative risk and providing new therapies is an excellent one (Spilker and Cuatrecasas, 1990). The predominant objective of all national and international drug regulations is to ensure freedom from undue toxicity (i.e. to ensure the safety) of marketed medicinal products during normal conditions of use. Total safety is probably an untenable goal since the use of any therapeutic agent is inevitably attended by a small risk that the patient may react adversely to it. Absolute safety in drug treatment is probably not achievable, although much can be done, and is being done, to reduce hazard.

REFERENCES

Bass, R. (1990). What can be learnt by examining the data in the files of regulatory authorities?—the toxicologist's viewpoint. In Lumley, C. E. and Walker S. R. (Eds), *Animal Toxicity Studies: Their Relevance for Man*. CMR Workshop Series. Quay Publishing, Lancaster, pp. 33–39

Brimblecombe, R. (1990). The importance of retrospective comparisons. In Lumley, C. E. and Walker, S. R. (Eds), *Animal Toxicity Studies: Their Relevance for Man*. CMR Workshop Series, Quay Publishing, Lancaster, pp. 15–19

Clayson, D. B. (1987). The need for biological risk assessment in reaching decisions about carcinogens. *Mutation Res.* **185**, 243–269

Commission of the European Communities (1984). *The Rules Governing Medicaments in the European Communities*. Office for Official Publications of the European Communities, Luxembourg

Fletcher, A. P. (1978). Drug safety testing and subsequent clinical experience. *J. Roy. Soc. Med.*, **71**, 693–696

Fletcher, P. (1990). What can be learnt by examining the data in the files of regulatory authorities? The clinician's viewpoint. In Lumley, C. E. and Walker, S. R. (Eds), *Animal Toxicity Studies: Their Relevance for Man*. CMR Workshop Series. Quay Publishing. Lancaster, pp. 41–46

Griffin, J. P. (1983) Repeat-dose long-term toxicity studies. In Balls, M., Riddell, R. J. and Worden, A. N. (Eds), *Animals and Alternatives in Toxicity Testing*. Academic Press, London, pp. 98–103

Griffin, J. P. (Ed.) (1989). Medicines control within the United Kingdom. In D'Arcy, P. F. and Harron, D. W. G. (Exec. Eds), *Medicines: Regulation, Research and Risk*. The Queen's University of Belfast, pp. 1–25

Griffin, J. P. (1991). Are regulations a stimulus to innovation? In Walker, S. R. (Ed.), *Creating the Right Environment for Drug Discovery*. CMR Workshop Series. Quay Publishing, Lancaster, p. 93

Heywood, R. (1990). Clinical toxicity—could it have been predicted? Post-marketing experience. In Lumley, C. E. and Walker S. R. (Eds), *Animal Toxicity Studies: Their Relevance for Man*. CMR Workshop Series. Quay Publishing, Lancaster, pp. 57–67

Inman, W. H. W. (Ed.) (1980). The United Kingdom. In *Monitoring for Drug Safety*. MTP, Lancaster, p. 9

International Agency for Research on Cancer (1987). *IARC Monographs on the Evaluation of Carcinogenic Risks to Humans*. Suppl. 7. *Overall Evaluations of Carcinogenicity: An Updating of IARC Monographs*, Vols 1–42. Lyon

Lasagna, L. (1989). Setting the scene—the role of regulation. In Walker, S. R. and Griffin, J. P. (Eds) *International Medicines Regulations: A Forward Look to 1992*, Kluwer, Dordrecht, Boston, London, pp. 19–26

Laurence, D. R., Maclean, A. and Weatherall, M. (1984). *Safety Testing of New Drugs*. Academic Press, London

Lumley, C. E. (1990). Clinical toxicity: could it have been predicted? Pre-marketing experience. In Lumley, C. E. and Walker, S. R. (Eds), *Animal Toxicity Studies: Their Relevance for Man*. CMR Workshop Series, Quay Publishing, Lancaster, pp. 49–56

Lumley, C. E. and Walker, S. R. (Eds) (1990). *Animal Toxicity Studies: The Relevance for Man*. CMR Workshop Series, Quay Publishing, Lancaster, p. vii

Morton, D. (1990). Expectations from animal studies. In Lumley, C. E. and Walker, S. R. (Eds), *Animal Toxicity Studies: Their Relevance for Man*. CMR Workshop Series, Quay Publishing, Lancaster, pp. 3–13

Rawlings, M. D. (1989). Objectives and achievements of medicines regulation in the UK. In Walker S. R. and Griffin, J. P. (Eds), *International Medicines Regulations: A Forward Look to 1992*. Kluwer, Dordrecht, Boston, London, pp. 93–100

Shelby, M. D. and Stasiewicz, S. (1984). Chemicals showing no evidence of carcinogenicity in long-term two species rodent studies; the need for short-term test data. *Environ. Mutagen.*, **6**, 871–876

Spilker, B. and Cuatrecasas, P. (1990). *Inside the Drug Industry*. Prous Science, Barcelona, p. 53

Stephens, M. D. B. (1988). *The Detection of New Adverse Drug Reactions*, 2nd edn. Stockton Press, New York, p. 1

Tennant, R. W., Margolin, B. H., Shelby, M. D.,

Zeiger, E., Haseman, J. K., Spalding, J., Caspary, W., Resnick, M., Stasiewicz, S., Anderson, B. and Minor, R. (1987). Prediction of chemical carcinogenicity in rodents from *in vitro* genetic toxicity assays. *Science*, **236**, 933–941

Zbinden, G. (1981). Scope and limitation of animal models for the prediction of human toxicity. In Brown, S. S. and Davies, D. S. (Eds), *Organ-Directed Toxicity*. Pergamon Press, Oxford, pp. 3–7

FURTHER READING

Herman, R. L. (1991). Symposium on the management of adverse exposure information: phase 1 through epidemiology. *Drug Information Journal*, **25**, No. 2

Heykants, J. and Meuldermans, W. (1994). Nonclinical kinetics and metabolism studies in support of the safety assessment of drugs. *Drug Information Journal*, **28**, 163–172

Mann, R. D., Rawlins, M. D. and Auty, R. M. (1993). *A Textbook of Pharmaceutical Medicine Current Practice*. Darthenon Publishing Group

Monro, A. (1993). How useful are chronic (life-span) toxicology studies in rodents in identifying pharmaceuticals that pose a carcinogenic risk to humans. *Adverse Drug Reactions and Toxicology Reviews*, **12**, 5–34

Scales, M. D. C. and Mahoney, A. (1991). Animal toxicology studies on new medicines and their relationship to clinical exposure: a review of international recommendations. *Adverse Drug Reactions and Toxicology Reviews*, **10**, 155–168

Sjoeberg, P. (1994). Toxicokinetics in preclinical safety assessment: views of the Swedish Medical Products Agency. *Drug Information Journal*, **28**, 151–157

Wolff, R. K. and Dorato, M. A. (1993). Toxicologic testing of inhaled pharmaceutical aerosols. *Critical Reviews in Toxicology*, **23**, 343–369

44 Toxicology of Medical Devices

Paul N. Adams

INTRODUCTION

Medical devices have been known since pre-history. Archaeological discoveries, such as trephined skulls and cuneiform writings, show that whatever doubts we may hold about their diagnoses, early humans had the ability to use tools to alter anatomy and physiology without killing at least some of the patients.

DEFINITIONS

The term 'medical device' covers many different types of instrument, apparatus, appliance, material or other article, whether used alone or in combination. It is intended by the manufacturer for use in human beings for the following purposes:

- Diagnosis, prevention, monitoring, treatment or alleviation of disease, injury or disability.
- Investigation, replacement or modification of the anatomy or of a physiological process.
- Control of conception.

As defined here it does not achieve its principal intended action in or on the human body by pharmacological, chemical, immunological or metabolic means, but it may be assisted in function by such means.

CLASSIFICATION OF DEVICES

There are many different ways of classifying devices. For the purpose of toxicological assessment, a functional classification is now suggested.

In practice, devices may be used: (1) *outside the body*, e.g. beds, wheelchairs, *in vitro* diagnostics; (2) *on the body* by an expert, e.g. instruments, X-ray equipment, anaesthetic machines, defibrillators; and (3) *in intimate contact with the body*, e.g. heart valves, pacemakers, wound dressings, sutures, contact lenses, implants.

Those devices in intimate contact with the body may be subdivided into:

- Onplants which have contact with intact skin, e.g. ostomy appliances, splints, adhesive dressings.
- Onplants that have contact with damaged tissue, e.g. burn, granulation and ulcer dressings.
- Implants which have contact with intact natural channels, e.g. urinary catheters, nasogastric tubes, contact lenses.
- Implants which have contact with bone.
- Implants which have contact with soft tissue.
- Implants which have contact with blood.
- Devices used for circulating blood.

All these may be subdivided into devices used at operation (a few hours), short-term (less than a month) and long-term (either continuously or intermittently).

This chapter focuses on devices which have prolonged intimate body contact, although the principles will apply to all devices. In such devices, toxicity may be a serious clinical problem and a toxicological appraisal is needed for at least four different reasons.

- The patient will want to be confident in the use of the product.
- The professional user, hospital or clinic will want to be sure that the product is safe for the sake of good practice and liability.
- The manufacturer will want to produce a safe product which will not induce additional disease in the patient or liability in law.
- In many countries, the rules governing the sale of devices may demand an assessment of safety.

DIFFERENCES BETWEEN DRUGS AND DEVICES

The differences between drugs and devices may appear obvious but there is a surprising overlap of characteristics. It is valuable to explore this borderline in order to build a rationale for a special approach to toxicity testing of devices.

Implanted and onplanted medical devices have the same general purposes of diagnosis, prevention and treatment as drugs but appear to differ in that efficacy seems to be determined by physical rather than chemical mechanisms. However, the transfer of drug substances across cell membranes and the interaction of molecules at receptor sites are as physicochemical at the microcellular level as cardiac stimulation by the pulsing of a pacemaker. The divide between drug and device cannot therefore be made by purpose, or ultimately by effector mechanism.

The distinction is essentially morphological. A drug is a substance that can have many forms and is effective irrespective of its form (providing that the optimal amount of drug reaches the target organs), whereas a device depends on the physical attributes of its form to achieve its effect.

The combination of drug and device poses interesting problems. It is sometimes necessary for regulatory purposes to determine whether it is the drug or device which achieves the principal or intended function. A capsule may appear to be a device but it exists only as the vehicle for the drug and is considered to be a pharmaceutical form. An object such as a transdermal patch appears to be a device but it exists solely for the purpose of containing and releasing the integral nitroglycerine as does a more conventional sustained release pharmaceutical preparation; both are considered pharmaceutical forms of the drug. An insulin pump is a device acting as a delivery mechanism for the drug but is independent of it in the same way as an infusion set, and is not a part of the pharmaceutical form. Steroids are clearly drugs, but when coated onto the tip of a pacing wire to overcome the problem of exit block due to endocardial fibrosis, the drug does not have an independent function or change the nature of the wire but rather acts adjunctively to assist its function.

The practical purpose of these distinctions is to identify which regulations apply to any product. Safety evaluation of combination devices will often require separate testing of the drug and device and also of the device as a whole.

SCOPE OF DEVICE SAFETY TESTING

The distinction between toxicity testing and other safety testing is less clear for devices than for drugs. While the majority of drugs are transitory within the body, most implanted material is retained for longer periods of time.

No non-living substance is likely to be totally inert in the immunocompetent human body. Indeed, some materials rely on biodegradation (e.g. absorbable sutures) or biotransformation (e.g. hydroxyapatite frameworks) to achieve their effect. Thus biocompatibility is a greater priority than inertness. Biocompatibility is defined (in ISO/TR 9966) as, 'a state of desirable reaction of living tissues to non-viable materials'.

Toxicology classically looks for a chemical substance which can be characterized and put through a variety of dose-ranging biological tests to detect target organ toxicity, teratogenicity, mutagenicity, carcinogenicity, or hypersensitivity.

Free chemicals are released from many devices as leachables of the product *per se* and also as residues of raw ingredients, processing agents, finishing agents, sterilizing agents and packaging. Adventitious contamination may occur in manufacture or as the result of chemical breakdown on sterilization or storage. So, in common with pharmaceuticals, tests of integrity and chemical purity are necessary to identify changes to the product in manufacture and storage; and standard tests for toxicity, mutagenicity, carcinogenicity, etc. can be performed on extracts.

The physical nature and effects of devices, despite whatever solution or leaching may occur, will produce special challenges in safety evaluation. The manifestations of toxicity—alteration of cell structure, changes in cell metabolism, cell death, loss of cell membrane integrity, reduced cell adhesion, altered rates of cell proliferation and biosynthetic activity—may all be produced directly by physical stimuli in the absence of noxious chemicals.

Electrical energy is useful for cautery, diathermy and defibrillation, but causes burns if incorrectly applied. Heat is necessary for moulding medical thermoplastics but the retained energy may burn skin or tissue. Cryoprobes are intended to cause cell damage but are used selectively in therapy.

Thus cellular disruption may be the result of heat, extreme cold, electricity or radiation causing burns; ultraviolet radiation may result in melanoma or basal cell carcinoma; aggressive adhesives on non-conformable dressings may produce physical separation within the skin layers.

Unlike drugs that are widely distributed in the body and are responsible for systemic or target organ effects, a device is most likely to induce toxicity locally, although the effect may be distant: a good example is the intravascular catheter. Damage may result either from a physical effect of the device (such as erosion of a vessel wall by a catheter), or the effect of plasticizer leaching, (inducing brittleness and fracture of a catheter tip which may embolize). Fracture may also occur as an expression of the mechanical properties of the material after repeated flexion. Interaction with local tissue or particular body fluids may constitute unique hazards which might not have been foreseen on the basis of dose-ranging toxicity of leachables alone; for example, the fibrin sheathing of a vascular catheter may be stripped on removal and then embolize. Another example is the accumulation of silicone lubricant in the kidney.

The presence of artificial valves cause rheological changes such as turbulence and high fluid shear stresses which cause changes in platelet and clotting function, and haemolysis of red cells. The same is true for blood pumps and dialysis machines.

The effect of soft contact lenses on the cornea has been shown to increase the incidence of *Pseudomonas* keratitis. Contributing factors include the deposition of fats and proteins on the lenses, the variability of patient compliance in disinfection regimes and changes to tear film proteins, but the underlying cause is inadequate oxygen transmission through the lens, especially on extended wear. Hydrogel lenses demonstrate other toxicity mechanisms; they will absorb and adsorb topical ocular drugs and cleansing agents, and with time may concentrate them in the lens to exceed the threshold of toxicity for the cornea.

We have seen that a medical device may be unsafe if it causes new pathology, but it is also unsafe if it fails to perform its intended function. The fatigue fracture of a heart valve's wire outflow strut caused dozens of fatalities, and reoperation of other patients would be accompanied by the usual morbidity. This principle is seen with devices as diverse as drip flow monitors, insulin pumps, anaesthetic machines, synthetic vascular grafts, orthopaedic cements, and CSF shunts.

TOXICITY ASSESSMENT OF DEVICES

It is against this background that the toxicologist is asked to make an assessment of the safety of the device to ensure that the material is compatible with the biological systems with which it comes into contact and that it will perform its intended function in that environment. The safety assessment of devices must therefore weigh the possibility of risk against the benefit of its intended use, assuming that the device will be handled according to the instructions in those conditions and subpopulations for which it is suitable.

The majority of medical devices carry some degree of risk, however small, which is composed of the intrinsic risk of the device and the extrinsic risk from placement or manipulation by professional or patient.

As there are so many variables to be considered, there is no single test that can provide a toxicological profile; thus each device with its fingerprint of leachables, contaminants and surface characteristics will demand a customized programme of testing the substances, materials and the device itself. Neither is it possible to extrapolate from the data on related materials, particularly plastics, as small differences in formulation and processing can produce polymers with greatly dissimilar toxicity.

Toxicity testing will recognize the possible presence of chemical leachables and contaminants but also looks for specific device effects. All tests should be performed in accordance with Good Laboratory Practice and should include negative, and where appropriate positive, controls. Tests should be used so that their results give a comparative profile against other products and materials with known clinical correlation.

The advice of an experienced toxicologist is essential if the selection of tests and their evaluation is to give a view of the likelihood of safe use in humans. Even then, the preclinical tests are only indicative and require clinical exposure to confirm suitability and safety.

DIFFERENT TYPES OF TOXICITY TEST

The purpose of the different tests is to identify possible noxious effects of the material or device in humans by challenging model biological systems. These systems may be live animals or cell culture. It is now generally accepted that the LD_{50} is an outmoded and wasteful test of acute toxicity and *in vitro* methods are preferred.

Acute toxicity can be tested *in vitro* by cell culture cytotoxicity and haemocompatibility tests. In animals, systemic toxicity, and local toxicity (skin irritation, subdermal irritation, mucous membrane irritation, sensitization and implantation tests) can be evaluated, as well as biocompatibility with specialized tissues.

In vitro mutagenicity tests of leachables can give a rapid profile of tumorigenic potential and there are cell culture models to detect the propensity of solid material, apart from leachables, to produce tumours. Many materials implanted in the rat have shown a tendency to induce tumours. There has been a steady trickle of published reports of associations of tumours with devices in humans and although there has been no validation of tumorigenicity of a particular device, it is important to eliminate tumorigens and to develop suitable tests to pinpoint causal relationships that may exist.

TOXICITY TESTING OF EXTRACTS

Materials are initially chosen for devices because of their physical properties. A programme of toxicity testing and significance evaluation should be completed before the device or material is tested in humans.

Most devices, when subjected to extraction procedures, will yield leachables. It is necessary to know the toxic potential of these substances, both systemically and locally. Toxicity is usually dose-related and therefore the rate of leaching to the body should be estimated. It may be that the rate of leaching is so small and the systemic sink so large that most toxic substances undergo massive dilution and no toxicity is seen. However, some compounds are toxic even at high dilution, and allergens may provoke cell-mediated hypersensitivity reactions on minimal dose challenge.

Local effects are more likely than generalized toxicity and some tissues (e.g. the cornea, inner ear or nervous tissue) are specially sensitive. Not all toxicity is deleterious: for example, povidone iodine is toxic to epidermal cells and fibroblasts, but the first priority for wound healing is a reduction in bacteria after which wound healing may progress, albeit at a slower rate, despite the presence of the antiseptic. This is important in the evaluation of impregnated wound dressings which may show high toxicity with cell culture methods.

A typical programme will start by *in vitro* screening to assess acute toxicity, mutagenicity, haemocompatibility and teratogenicity (if appropriate) of the leachables/contaminants, either directly or by reference to previous validated research. Confirmation of the *in vitro* toxicity assessment can be gained by intracutaneous injection of extracts into the rabbit.

It must also be remembered that the materials may release other potentially toxic substances after sterilization or storage. If unusual or uncharacterized molecules are found it may be better to invest in cleaning the process rather than justifying their presence. Toxic products may also be found after prolonged implantation as the result of biodegradation. Indeed, biodegradation may be integral to the function of some devices, such as absorbable sutures and dressings, and toxic breakdown products should be excluded.

IMPLANT TOXICITY

The difficulties surrounding the toxicological evaluation of leachables testing are partly overcome by implantation into a mammalian model.

At varying intervals, the biological reactions to the implanted material can be seen and compared with positive and negative controls. As a screening method this is expensive and wasteful but unless the *in vitro* test is completely negative, implantation tests are necessary to confirm a presumption of negative or minimal toxicity. Much experimental work has used the rat or rabbit implantation models and a host of standard practices have been agreed, as detailed later in this chapter.

Apart from the effects of leachables and some of the gross physical effects of implants, the solid material/device should also be tested for its capacity to induce inflammatory responses, hypersensitivity, thrombosis and tumours.

The typical response to a biomaterial implanted for some time is acute inflammation followed by resolution with or without scarring, chronic inflammation and giant cell formation, calcification, local necrosis followed either by chronic inflammation or scarring, and enclosure of the device in a fibrous sac or sheath. Some of these reactions are in response to the surgical intervention rather than to the implant, so it is important to have adequate controls.

Assessment of the implant depends on the correlation of the tissue into which it is implanted and the tissue types that it will meet in the human. Thus compatibility may need to be tested with bone, cartilage, blood, teeth, corneal or neural tissue.

The rat is an economical laboratory animal and is often used for implantation studies up to two years; for longer studies the rabbit is used. Good comparative data are available for interpretation of results. Implantation may be subcutaneous, intramuscular, or into specialized tissues. The material to be tested can either be placed in contact with the tissue or put in a cage or chamber so that only tissue fluids come into contact with the sample.

Irritation studies of mucous membrane are probably best modelled in the hamster cheek pouch. Irritation is commonly tested in the rabbit or guinea pig, but mouse, dog, pig and monkey are also used.

One of the most fascinating effects of implants (especially into rats) is their ability to induce tumours. The tendency of small animals to produce tumours in association with solid implants seems to be related to a non-porous, smooth surface with critical minimum dimensions. It may be that the critical size of the surface, if multiplied in the ratio of the rat/human body weight, would be so large that implantation of such dimensions in the human would be unlikely. Thus the animal pathology may give a distorted view of the likely response in humans.

CELL CULTURE

Apart from bacterial and mammalian mutagenicity tests, *in vitro* experiments assess acute toxic effects. Cell culture experiments use a variety of techniques based on either a fresh isolate from fragments of tissue or cell suspension (primary cell culture) which grow to confluence and then age and die, or single cell clones (continuous cell culture) which have an indefinite capacity to grow and replicate. The continuous cell lines have the advantage of being consistent, reliable and reproducible. They act as a standard with a documented history, they have fewer biological variables and may be tuned to particular toxicity concerns by using a variety of tissues and species with a range of doses and exposure periods. As a result these methods can be very efficient in screening and are often more sensitive than acute toxicity tests in animals. Early cell culture methods merely estimated the numbers of living or dead cells but now morphological analysis by electron microscopy reveals a spectrum of microcellular changes; and cell function tests measure biochemical parameters indicating the nature of cell stress.

Although many modifications have been made, cell culture tests are of four main types: gel diffusion, direct contact, extract dilution and cell function tests.

Gel diffusion uses agar or agarose to cover a cell monolayer. A sample of the material or extract is placed on top of the gel providing a concentration gradient of diffusibles. Agarose allows a faster diffusion of uncharged molecules and is as sensitive as the rabbit intramuscular implantation test.

Direct contact of the test material on to a culture layer is more sensitive than the rabbit intramuscular implantation test but care must be taken to avoid physical damage to the cells by pressure or movement of the sample.

Extracts may be serially diluted in the nutrient media and provide a quantitative comparison with reference extracts. Inevitably the correlation with animal tests will depend on the nature of the eluants.

Cell function tests are a very precise way of registering cellular response to any insult. In particular, inhibition of cell growth can be measured with considerable sensitivity.

With increasing complexity of test methodology, the results may be less reproducible; and increasing sensitivity may not assist the prediction of risk to humans as the impact of a material on the body systems may be much less intense than in the culture plate.

These *in vitro* culture methods are measures of acute toxicity only but correlate well with more wasteful animal tests. However, evidence of lack of chronic toxicity requires animal implantation.

Haemocompatibility is vital for many devices. Potential for thrombosis, toxicity including loss of integrity of cellular elements, and changes to rheological parameters can all be tested *in vitro* but correlation is variable so care in interpretation is essential.

STANDARDS

Because of the need to compare test results of different materials against clinical information, it is highly desirable that testing should be done according to fixed and agreed protocols. Each standard test (practice) has been developed by a consensus of scientists based on an appraisal of original research, and represents a generic approach to testing. Specific tests or modifications of the generic tests may still be needed for novel devices.

Toxicology of devices is a relatively young science. Although Dixon and Rickert published their implant irritancy test for dental materials in 1933, it was not until the late 1950s and early 1960s that more refined implantation tests were

collected by the Pharmaceutical Manufacturers' Association and the Society for Plastic Industries in the USA, and thereafter became incorporated into the United States Pharmacopeia in 1965. Since then standards organizations on both sides of the Atlantic have continued to search for predictive safety tests.

Currently, the International Standards Organisation (ISO), and the British Standards Institution (BSI) set benchmarks that are accepted in the UK. In the USA the American National Standards Institute (ANSI) acts as the coordinating and consensus body for national organizations such as the American Dental Association (ADA) and the American Society for Testing Materials (ASTM). The United States Pharmacopeia also states test methods. Other standards bodies which have published on device toxicology are AFNOR (France), Canadian Standards Association (CSA), and DIN (Germany).

In Europe the European Committee for Standardization (CEN) have decided not to create separate standards for biocompatibility but to adopt future ISO standards as a basis for conformity assessment of products under the European Medical Device Directives. These ISO standards will be constructed using and refining existing national standards.

Table 1   Range of tests required for devices in different applications

Type of device, material or application	Test												
	CYT	SI	IM	BC	H	CA	LTI	MMI	SAT	SDI	S	M	P
External devices:													
Intact surfaces		X								X			
Breached surfaces	X	X							X	X	X		
Externally communicating devices with:													
Intact natural channels								X		X			
Body tissues/fluids													
Intraoperative	X								X	X			X
Short-term	X		X						X	X			X
Long-term	X		X						X	X	X		X
Blood pathology	X		X	X	X				X	X	X		X
Implanted devices contacting:													
Bone	X					X	X		X		X	X	X
Tissue/tissue fluid	X		X			X	X		X	X	X	X	X
Blood	X		X	X	X	X	X		X	X	X	X	X

CYT = cell culture cytotoxicity; SI = skin irritation test; IM = intramuscular implantation; BC = blood compatibility; H = haemolysis test; CA = carcinogenicity; LTI = long-term implant; MMI = mucous membrane irritation; SAT = systemic acute toxicity; SDI = subdermal irritation; S = sensitization; M = mutagenicity; P = pyrogenicity

SELECTING APPROPRIATE METHODS FOR TOXICITY TESTING

Published standards (BS/5736 Pt1 and ASTM F 748–87) underline the need for a customized approach and to select tests on the basis of what is already known of the chemistry and biological effects of the materials. However, unexpected results should be carefully followed up.

For each material or device, testing will depend on the likely duration of tissue contact, the type of tissue and the 'intensity' of exposure (surface area of contact or quantity of leachables).

Initial screening for cytotoxicity is best done using cell cultures. In this closely controlled environment, cellular changes in different tissue types can be measured after exposure to test substances. This versatile method can detect toxic leachables in extracts or by direct contact with the material or device.

Table 1, based on the ASTM standard practice F748–87, indicates the range of tests required for devices in different applications.

BIBLIOGRAPHY

Anderson, D. (1990). *In vitro* models. *Drug Safety*, **5** (Suppl. 1), 27–39

Benjamin, W. J. (1991). Assessing the risks of extended wear. *Optometry Clin.*, **1**, 13–31

Brandl, H., Gross, R. A., Lenz, R. W. and Fuller, R. C. (1990). Plastics from bacteria and for bacteria: poly (beta-hydroxy) alkanoates as natural, biocompatible and biogradable polyesters. *Adv. Biochem. Eng. Biotechnol.*, **41**, 77–93

Cooper, M. L., Laxer, J. A. and Hansbrough, J. F. (1991). The cytotoxic effects of commonly used topical antimicrobial agents of human fibroblasts and keratinocytes. *J. Trauma*, **31**, 775–782, 782–784

Duffy, D. M. (1990). Silicone: a critical review. *Adv. Derm.*, **5**, 93–107, 108–109

Duntley, P., Siever, J., Korwes, M. L., Harpel, K. and Heffner, J. E. (1992). Vascular erosion by central venous catheters. Clinical features and outcome. *Chest*, **101**, 1633–1638

Ellender, G., Feik, S. A. and Gaviria, C. (1990). The biocompatibility testing of some dental amalgams *in vivo. Aust. Dent. J.*, **35**, 497–504

Galanti, J. O., Lemons, J., Spector, M., Wilson, P. D. Jr and Wright, T. M. (1991). The biological effects of implant materials. *J. Orthop. Res.*, **9**, 760–775

Goering, P. L. and Galloway, W. D. (1989). Toxicology of medical device material. *Fundam. Appl. Toxicol.*, **13**, 193–195

Goldring, S. R., Flannery, M. S., Petrison, K. K.,

Evins, A. E. and Jasty, M. J. (1990) Evaluation of connective tissue cell responses to orthopaedic implant materials. *Connect. Tissue Res.*, **24**, 77–81

Grunkemeier, G. L. and Rahimtoula, S. H. (1990). Artificial heart valves. *Ann. Rev. Med.*, **41**, 251–263

Irwin, J. C. (1989). Legal aspects of urologic prosthetic devices. *Urol. Clin. North Am.*, **16**, 165–174

Jansen, J. A., van der Waerden, J. P. and de Groot, K. (1989). Epithelial reactions to percutaneous implant materials: *in vitro* and *in vivo* experiments. *J. Invest. Surg.*, **2**, 29–49

Jansen, J. A., van der Waerden, J. P. and de Groot, K. (1991). Fibroblast and epithelial cell interactions with surface treated implant materials. *Biomaterials*, **12**, 25–31

McKeehan, W., Barnes, D., Reid, L., Stanbridge, E., Murakami, H. and Sato, G. H. (1990). Frontiers in mammalian cell culture. *In Vivo Cell. Devel. Biol.*, **26**, 23

Metz, S. A., Chegini, N. and Masterson, B. J. (1990). *In vivo* and *in vitro* degradation of nonfilament absorbable sutures, PDS and Maxon. *Biomaterials*, **11**, 41–45

Mond, H. G. and Stokes, K. B. (1992). The electrode–tissue interface: the revolutionary role of steroid elution. *PACE. Pacing Clin. Electrophysiol*, **15**, 95–107

Monrad Aas, I. H. (1991). Malpractice. *Qual. Assur. Health Care*, **3**, 21–39

Northup, S. J. (1989). Current problems associated with toxicity evaluation of medical device materials and future research needs. *Fundam. Appl. Toxicol.*, **13**, 196–204

Phillips, J. C., Gibson, W. B., Yam, J., Alden, C. L. and Hard, G. C. (1990). Survey of the QSAR and *in vitro* approaches for developing non-animal methods to supersede the *in vivo* LD_{50} test. *Food Chem. Toxicol.*, **28**, 375–394

Price, J. M. (1987). The liabilities and consequences of medical device development. *J. Biomed. Mater. Res.*, **21** (A1 Suppl.), 35–38

Propp, D. A., Clive, D. and Hennesfent, B. R. (1988). Catheter embolism. *J. Emerg. Med.*, **6**, 17–21

Santavirta, S., Gristina, A. and Konttinen, Y. T. (1992). Cemented versus cementless hip orthoplastry. A review of prosthetic biocompatibility. *Acta Orth. Scand.*, **63**, 225–232

Schoen, F. J. (1987). Cardiac valve prostheses: pathological and bioengineering considerations. *J. Card. Surg.*, **2**, 65–108

Silbert, J. A. (1991). Complications of extended wear. *Optometry Clin.*, **1**, 95–122

Staewen, W. S. (1990). Biomedical standards: what do they offer clinical engineering? *Biomed. Instrum. Technol.*, **24**, 51–53

Sunderman, F. W. Jr (1989). Carcinogenicity of metal alloys in orthopedic prostheses: clinical and experimental studies. *J. Fund. Appl. Toxicol.*, **13**, 205–216

Vince, D. G., Hunt, J. A., Wiliams, D. F. (1991).

Quantitative assessment of the tissue response to implanted biomaterials. *Biomaterials*, **12**, 731–736

Ward, J. J., Thornbury, D. D., Lemons, J. E. and Dunham, W. K. (1990). Metal-induced sarcoma. A case report and literature review. *Clin. Orthop. Rel. Res.*, **252**, 299–306

Williams, D. C. and Frolik, C. A. (1991). Physiological and pharmacological regulation of biological calcification. *Int. Rev. Cytol.*, **126**, 195–292

Zbinden, G. (1988). Reduction and replacement of laboratory animals in toxicological testing and research. Interim report 1984–1987. *Biomed. Environ. Sci.*, **1**, 90–100

FURTHER READING

Conine, D. L., Naumann, B. D. and Hecker, L. H. (1992). Setting health-based residue limits for contaminants in pharmaceuticals and medical devices. *Quality Assurance: Good Practice, Regulation, and Law*, **1**, 171–180

45 Toxicological Evaluation of Recombinant DNA-derived Proteins

John A. Thomas

INTRODUCTION TO BIOTECHNOLOGY

Genetic engineering represents a technology for producing a large number of biologically active polypeptides and proteins. These large-sized molecules can more readily be biosynthesized by cellular systems using prokaryotic and eukaryotic cells than by conventional synthetic organic chemistry. Through biotechnology or recombinant DNA-derived proteins, there is the potential to biosynthesize therapeutically useful molecules both for human and veterinary medicine. The definition of biotechnology is somewhat vague or generic, depending on the bioscientific discipline. However, the NIH Recombinant DNA Advisory Committee (RAC) has defined r-DNA as 'either molecules which are constructed outside living cells by joining natural or synthetic DNA segments to DNA molecules that can replicate in a living cell or DNA molecules that result from their replication'. Actually, both mammalian and plant cells can be genetically manipulated leading to products that can potentially be very beneficial to society. Such genetically engineered molecules must not only be proven useful or efficacious, but more importantly must be free from overt or serious toxicity.

Biotechnology is not a recent innovation, but it has increased in its degree of biochemical sophistication. There are numerous milestones in biotechnology and genetically engineered products (Table 1).

The art (or science) of brewing dates back to 7000 BC and is represented by a simple biological system (i.e. yeast) that can convert sugar to ethyl alcohol. In a contemporary sense, present day genetic engineering could not have been possible without the discovery of the double helical nature of DNA by Watson and Crick. The field was further enhanced by the 1973 discovery of prokaryotic restriction enzymes. Restriction enzymes are rather specific chemical scissors which can be used to cut segments of the DNA molecules. Such

Table 1 Selected milestones in biotechnology

Date	Discovery or invention
7000 BC	Brewing
1882	Tubercular bacillus; blood antibodies
ca. 1900	Term 'gene' used
ca. 1914	Production of glycerin by fermentation
ca. 1914	Production of acetone by fermentation
1928	Discovery of penicillin
1952	Discovery of double helix of DNA
1969	Immobilization of enzymes
1973	Discovery of restriction enzymes
1975	Hybridoma – monoclonal antibodies
ca. 1980	Production of interferon
1982	Clinical use of rDNA insulin
1985	Clinical trials: rDNA tPA; rDNA, IL-2
1987	FDA approves tPA
1988	Clinical trials: EGF, EPO, HGH, factor VIII
1989	Clinical trials: GM-CSF
1990	FDA approves use of G-CSF
1991	Clinical trials and/or FDA approval of EPO, *alpha*-interferon, *beta*-interferon, TNF, Hepatitis B vaccine

segments can subsequently be re-spliced into plasmids that are capable of replicating new or foreign proteins. The discovery of hybridoma technologies led to the production of monoclonal antibodies which then allowed for a method of detection of genetically engineered molecules.

Recombinant DNA human insulin was the first biopharmaceutical to be approved by the US Food and Drug Administration (FDA) for the treatment of diabetes mellitus. From a toxicological standpoint, this first genetically engineered agent (i.e. hormone) did not pose significant safety issues. In general, its efficacy and safety (i.e. toxicological testing) was reasonably established despite potential species differences. Another early addition to a genetically engineered hormone was human growth hormone (HGH). While the introduction of genetically engineered drugs was heralded by hormones, subsequent chimeric proteins have begun to involve therapies that extend beyond simple hormone replacements.

Despite a decade of advances in biotechnology, only 12 drugs have been approved for therapeutic use. Nevertheless, more than 100 genetically engineered drugs or vaccines are either in clinical trials or under regulatory review. All of these agents have been subjected to efficacy testing, but more importantly safety or toxicological batteries of preclinical assessments. Such assessments involve both immunological and non-immunological assessment.

REGULATORY CONSIDERATIONS

In the USA, the Food and Drug Administration (FDA) has the regulatory responsibility for approving genetically engineered products, particularly those that are to be used as either diagnostic or therapeutic agents. Approximately 300 monoclonal antibody-based diagnostic kits, about 15 rDNA probes for infectious diseases and 12 therapeutic drugs have been approved by the FDA. The US Department of Agriculture (USDA) and the US Environmental Protection Agency (EPA) are other regulatory agencies that become involved if the product is contained in a foodstuff or otherwise might pose an environmental concern. The Bureau of Biologicals of the FDA is generally responsible for approval of genetically engineered products. By definition, a biological product is 'any virus, therapeutic serum, toxin, antitoxin vaccine, blood, blood component or derivative, allergenic product, or analogous product . . . applicable to the prevention, treatment or cure of diseases or injuries of man'. The FDA applies the same regulations and standards for a IND (Investigational New Drug) for a biological as it does for a drug. Likewise good manufacturing practices (GMPs) apply to both biologicals and drugs (Miller and Young 1988).

The approval of rDNA-derived products sometimes represents some unique criteria. It is possible that the recombinant's product may differ in molecular structure from that of the natural substance. Thus, certain human recombinant growth hormones contain an extra N-terminal amino acid (e.g. methionine). Conversely, bacterial-produced recombinant products may have the same amino acid sequence as the natural product, but the molecular stoichiometry might differ. It is not uncommon for large protein-like molecules to fold or otherwise assume non-physiological

conformational orientations. It is also possible for genetic variants of recombinant proteins to occur during fermentation processes leading to mutations in the gene's coding sequences. Similarly, fermentation processes may produce partial products or peptides that can potentially evoke toxicological responses. Documentation of biosynthetic agents through rDNA technology should fulfil requirements for documentation for new drugs produced by more conventional methodologies (Sjodin, 1988). The identity, purity and reproducible quality of the recombinant product must be established and documented. Toxicological or safety testing must be appropriately applied to batches of product.

Toxicity testing on recombinant products includes the customary clinical chemistry and histopathology. A sensitive and quantitative analysis of circulating antibodies is required. In fact, a highly specific monoclonal antibody (Mab) must be developed very early in order to monitor the biodistribution of the recombinant product, both for pharmacokinetic and toxicokinetic information. Test for immunotoxicity is important for FDA submissions for recombinant products. Whether the intended therapeutic use of the recombinant protein product involves a single administration or a multiple administration can affect the agent's potential for immunogenicity.

The phases of drug development for a new drug and for a biological product do not differ to any great extent (Esber, 1988) (Figure 1). These phases consist of the preclinical phase, a clinical investigational or IND phase, the marketing application and the postmarketing phase. The marketing application specified by US Federal Food, Drug and Cosmetic Act is the New Drug Application (NDA). For the biological product or recombinant, the licence application includes

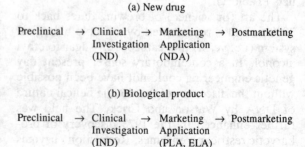

(a) New drug

Preclinical → Clinical → Marketing → Postmarketing
             Investigation Application
             (IND)   (NDA)

(b) Biological product

Preclinical → Clinical → Marketing → Postmarketing
             Investigation Application
             (IND)   (PLA, ELA)

Figure 1 Phases in drug development

both the US Product License Application (PLA) and the Establishment License Application (ELA). Whether a drug or a biological, the issues remain safety, purity, potency and efficacy. There is a pharmacological basis for the safety assessment of recombinant human proteins (Cossum, 1989).

GENERAL PHARMACOLOGICAL PRINCIPLES

As the majority of recombinant substances are relatively large protein molecules (Table 2), there are a number of physicochemical characteristics that must be considered in their pharmacological and toxicological evaluation (Table 3). Generally, large molecular weight substances are very poorly absorbed by the oral route of administration. For example, either recombinant human insulin or recombinant human growth hormone (HGH) must be administered by a parenteral route of administration thus bypassing the proteolytic environment of the stomach. Because these recombinant products are usually proteins, glycoproteins or peptides, they are often antigenic and hence can provoke immune responses. Finally, blood aminopeptidases and other proteolytic enzymes often result in recombinant proteins having a rather brief biological half-life.

An early consideration in planning for the toxicological assessment of a prospective recombinant substance is the therapeutic use of the product (Table 4). Diagnostic recombinant products (e.g. monoclonal antibody kits) are non-invasive and require less rigorous toxicological evaluation. Replacement products (i.e. hormones), such as insulin or HGH, represent physiological supplements and hence reduce the likelihood of suprapharmacological levels causing side-effects. Also, the replacement of otherwise physiologically active substances minimizes provocation of the immune system. Substances that require multiple injections to achieve a desired therapeutic effect (e.g. immunomodulators), particularly if they do not mimic a physiological mediator, are prone to alter the immune system.

Pretest considerations for assessing the toxicology of recombinant substances include factors ranging from physicochemical properties to selecting the most suitable animal model (Table 5). During the early discovery or advent of recombinant technologies, it was often difficult to secure sufficient amounts of the potential product and hence it was necessary to resort to *in vitro* test

Table 3 General pharmacological and toxicological characteristics of large molecular weight substances

Poor oral absorption
Usually protein or protein-like
Often antigenic
Brief biological half-life
Provocation of immune response, causing reduced therapeutic effectiveness (i.e. resistance)

Table 4 rDNA-derived protein: therapeutic use/purpose

Short-term/acute regimen Single injection (e.g. Hepatitis B vaccine)
Intermediate regimen Multi-injections (e.g. tPA)
Prolonged administration Years (5–10) (e.g. hGH)
Lifetime replacement Hormonal and/or genetic (e.g. insulin, factor VIII)

Table 2 Selected rDNA-derived therapeutic products

Agent	Molecular weight (approx.)	Chemical composition
tPA(s)	25 000 – 100 000	Glycoprotein
Insulin	5100	Protein
Erythropoietin	36 000	Glycoprotein
Interferon	17 000 – 25 000	Glycoproteins
HGH	21 500	Protein
Hepatitis B vaccine	Various subunits	Glycoprotein
Factor VIII	>1 000 000 (200 000 – >300 000 subunits)	Glycoprotein

Table 5 Pretest considerations for rDNA-derived proteins

Solubility	Acute versus chronic administration
Choice of vehicle	Species (small versus large animal)
Stability in solution	Dose ranging/standards
Route of administration	Comparison to prototype

systems or small animals. Increasingly, gene amplification systems have been incorporated into the replication clones so that reasonably sufficient amounts of end-product are now available. With newer recombinant products, it has also not always been possible to identify a comparable prototype.

Some recombinant products have vastly different pharmacological profiles (Table 6). While they may all be represented as protein substances, they have different onsets of action. The biological response may be very rapid (e.g. tPA) or it may require years (e.g. HGH) before its pharmacological efficacy is established. Some endpoints used for either pharmacological or toxicological endpoints may be very objective (e.g. blood clotting), while still others may be less objective or even subjective (e.g. immunomodulators). Immunopharmacological agents or agents affecting the immune system may involve many complex biochemical interactions with lymphokines, cytokines, complement, kinins, autacoids and even neuropeptides (Pope, 1989).

TOXICOLOGICAL TESTING: CLONED PROTEINS

Proteins that are coincidentally used as drugs (or more appropriately hormones) have been used for many years. Animal-derived proteins (e.g. insulin-ovine, bovine and porcine) have been used therapeutically for several decades in the medical management of diabetes mellitus. Usually, patients receiving animal insulin possess titres of antibody, but these are seldom either of immunological significance or associated with refractiveness to the hormone. Human proteins as drugs represent somewhat of a dilemma, in that these same substances become foreign proteins in the experimental animal. Thus species selection takes on an even greater significance in an effort to extrapolate to humans (Marafino *et al.*, 1988). The toxicological testing protocol of a recombinant product should contain both an immunological evaluation, i.e. safety, and a non-immunological evaluation, i.e. safety and efficacy (Table 7). Immunogenicity testing may involve both *in vitro* and *in vivo* systems. The non-immunological evaluation is product-specific and the animal testing strategy is focused on the therapeutic use of the substance. When the studies begin to examine the protein's biodistribution, it is usually necessary to have some means of measurement or identification. The development of a radioimmunoassay or a specific monoclonal antibody is often the only means for the product's detection.

Table 7 Toxicological testing of rDNA-derived proteins

(1) Immunological evaluation (safety)
    Immunogenicity testing
        In vivo (single versus multiple injection)
        In vitro

(2) Non-immunological evaluation (safety and efficacy)
    Product specific
    Pharmacological/toxicological profile
        In vitro tests
        In vivo tests (acute versus chronic)

Table 6 Selected pharmacological properties of rDNA-derived agents

Agent	Pharmacology		
	Action	Onset	Endpoint
tPA	Clot dissolution	Rapid	Rapid (minute)
Insulin	Hypoglycaemic	Rapid/intermediate	Intermediate (minutes/hours)
Erythropoietin	Anti-anaemic	Rapid/intermediate	Intermediate (days)
Interferon	Immunomodulator	Rapid/intermediate	Long (month/years)
HGH	Protein anabolic	Intermediate	Long (years)

Alternatively, large protein molecules can be iodinated and hence some insight into their biodistribution can be obtained, but usually not into their metabolic fate. Target organ accumulation (or lack of) can be ascertained with iodinated protein, but may lack some degree of specificity.

Many new drug candidates, both recombinant and others, are being developed for the sole therapeutic purpose of affecting the immune system (Norbury, 1985). There is little uniform consensus of what constitutes a general battery of immunotoxicological procedures. The multiplicity of cell types that comprise the immune system precludes the use of a single test that evaluates all of the possible immunological changes. All immunological assays should be supplemented with routine clinical chemistries, haematology and histopathology. Potential allergenicity, including both immediate and delayed type hypersensitivity, should be included in the toxicological evaluation. A basic immunotoxicological profile should include lymphoproliferation, popliteal lymph node enlargement, antibody response and natural killer cells.

All of these assays represent a reasonable immunotoxicological profile. The National Toxicology Program (NTP) (Luster *et al.*, 1986) has proposed a two-tiered approach to determine immunotoxicity. Tier I, or screen, includes immunopathology, humoral-mediated immunity (IgM antibody plaques), cell-mediated immunity (T cell response to mitogens) and non-specific immunity (natural killer cell activity). Tier II is more comprehensive and includes immunopathology (B and T cell response), humoral-mediated immunity (IgG antibody response), cell-mediated immunity (cytotoxic T cell lysis of tumour cells), non-specific immunity (macrophage function) and host resistance challenge modes (tumour cell, bacterial and viral systems).

SAFETY EVALUATION OF SPECIFIC RECOMBINANT PRODUCTS

Insulin

Insulin was the first recombinant product to be approved by the FDA and is used for the treatment of diabetes mellitus (Galloway and Chance, 1983). Because mammalian insulins are simple proteins, prokaryotic cell systems could be employed. Insulin has been cloned from *E. coli* either by constructing a gene that produces proinsulin or by constructing a gene for the A-chain and a gene for the B-chain of the insulin molecule. In the latter cloning strategy, the A-chain and the B-chain are assembled chemically.

Insulin represented a relatively easy recombinant product to produce, in that the amino acid sequence had already been established and safety and efficacy did not have to be subject to overly rigorous pharmacological or toxicological evaluation. Nevertheless, recombinant insulin underwent a rather extensive battery of physicochemical and toxicological tests (Table 8). This battery of physicochemical tests assured molecular integrity and purity. As prokaryotic systems are used, and because this necessitates harvesting the insulin from the *E. coli* by bursting its plasma membrane, testing for endotoxins and/or pyrogens is required. In addition to this battery of tests (Table 8), metabolic clearance rates of recombinant insulin labelled with radioactive iodine (^{125}I) were compared with ^{125}I-labelled porcine insulins. Thus, preclinical toxicological evaluation of recombinant insulin proceeded rapidly to clinical trials and eventual approval by the FDA.

Human Growth Hormone (HGH) and Somatotropin

Unlike insulin, which was never in short supply for the treatment of diabetes, human growth hormone had to be obtained from the limited cadaver sources of pituitary glands prior to the advent of recombinant HGH. Similar to insulin, the physiological actions of HGHs were known and hence

Table 8 Evaluative tests for human insulin (rDNA)

USP rabbit hypoglycaemia assay
Insulin radioreceptor assay
In vitro bioassays
Insulin radioimmunoassay
Amino acid composition and sequence
HPLC fragment analysis
Polyacrylamide gel electrophoresis
HPLC: identity and purity
Absorption and circular dichroic spectra
Zinc insulin crystalization
X-ray diffraction analysis
Limulus test for endotoxin
USP rabbit pyrogen test
E. coli polypeptide radioimmunoassay

it was perhaps not subjected to overly rigorous toxicological testing. Another factor that accelerated the cloning of both insulin and HGH was that the amino acid sequences had already been established for each hormone. Such information facilitated molecular confirmation and purity testing. However, HGH is a more complex molecule (Chawia *et al.*, 1983) than insulin and has a considerably larger molecular weight.

Initial efforts to clone rHGH resulted in an additional terminal amino acid, methionine. Subsequent safety and efficacy testing comparing methionine HGH with HGH failed to reveal any significant biological difference despite the presence of an additional amino acid.

Despite the established safety of human cadaver GH, several safety and efficacy tests were required for regulatory agency approval of rHGH (Table 9). The human pituitary dwarf responds only to monkey or human growth hormone. However, several animal species of GH will promote growth in the hypophysectomized rat. Hence, this rat model has been used extensively in rHGH assessment.

Recombinant bovine somatotropin (rbSt) has been evaluated with respect to its safety and efficacy in lactating dairy cows (Marcek *et al.*, 1989). The advent of rbSt makes it possible for increased milk production. Toxicological assessments revealed this recombinant hormone not to be a teratogen nor to have any side-effects on the neonate. It is not antigenic, and has little effect on blood chemistry and haematology.

Tissue Plasminogen Activator (tPA) and Clotting Factors

tPA is an endogenous trypsin-like serine protease that is used clinically to lyse blood clots. There are both natural and recombinant 'clot busters'. The pharmacology and therapeutic use of this thrombolytic agent has been extensively reviewed (Collen *et al.*, 1989). rtPA is similar to, or identical with, the physiological plasminogen activators in blood. rtPA does not induce an antibody response and it is more fibrin-specific than most or all other known thrombolytic agents (Collen *et al.*, 1989).

Several safety and efficacy tests were recommended for rtPA (Table 10). Both rodent and non-rodent species are recommended and at dose projections of one, three and ten times that anticipated for clinical trials. Considerable efforts were devoted to establishing reliable and reproducible quantitative clot dissolution models in rabbits and in dogs. The use of ^{125}I-labelled fibrinogen as a means of monitoring clot dissolution aided in establishing the thrombolytic properties of rtPA (Cossum, 1989).

Advances in other recombinant products that affect blood clotting have also been approved for clinical use. Blood clotting factor VIII has been cloned, tested for its safety and efficacy, and approved for clinical use. Likewise, factor VIII:C (antihaemophilic factor) has been cloned and expressed. These complex glycoproteins are subjected to the same rigorous purity and stability assurances as other recombinant products. They do, however, necessitate special animal models to determine blood clotting efficacy. Special inbred colonies of dogs that exhibit genetically defective blood clotting disorders can be used to study the effectiveness of recombinant factor VIII and factor VIII:C. In both instances it is necessary to develop a specific monoclonal antibody (Mab) to measure these factors.

Table 9 Summary for FDA basis for approving rHGH

Provide lyophilized product
Stability and purity (e.g. SDS, PAGE, NPLC)
Absence of contaminants (*E. coli* proteins/peptides)
Efficacy data (e.g. weight gain in rats)
Comparison of natural versus rHGH
Acute and subacute toxicity data (rats and monkey)
Immunotoxicology (e.g. autoantibodies)
Clinical trials (4-year period)

Table 10 Some recommended toxicity testing for tPA

Acute toxicity (1, 3 and 10 × clinical dose) (4 species)
Subchronic toxicity (rat, dog or monkey)
Guinea pig maximization test
Cardiopulmonary function in dogs (3 × clinical dose)
Ames test
Cytogenetic tests in rats (1, 3 and 10 × clinical dose)
Peripheral vein – clot dissolution model (rabbit)
Coronary artery – clot dissolution model (dog)
Pharmacokinetics studies in rabbit (iodinated tPA)

Erythropoietin (EPO)

EPO is a hormone synthesized primarily by the kidney. It regulates the production of red blood cells by the erythroid marrow. Recombinant human erythropoietin (r-HuEPO) has been cloned and expressed in Chinese hamster ovary. r-HuEPO (Epogen) has now been used clinically for 1–2 years and appears to enhance the quality of life of anaemic patients (Winearls, 1989; Evans *et al.*, 1990). Perhaps the most significant milepost in the eventual development of r-HuEPO was establishing a specific radioimmunoassay (RIA) for its detection. This RIA for EPO led to its isolation, fractionation and amino acid sequencing. Both a bioassay and eventually a Mab assay were required for it to be properly evaluated for safety and efficacy (Table 11). Early bioassays for EPO often involved using the stimuli of anoxia in experimental animals (e.g. mice) for quantifying subsequent increase in red blood cells. Mab assays rendered such bioassays obsolete.

Interferons (INF)

The interferons have been examined for their anticancer and anti-infective properties. Animal models (e.g. rhesus monkey) used to evaluate antimalarial and antiviral properties of human interferon gamma (HuINFg) and human interferon alpha no. 2 (HuINFa2) have proved quite useful in toxicological testing (Cossum, 1989). The chimpanzee is a better subhuman primate model than either the rhesus or the cynomolgus, but cost and limited availability precludes their widespread use for safety evaluation of rHuINFs. At least two INFs (e.g. Roferon-A and Interon-A) have been approved for clinical use.

The preclinical testing and development of INFa2a (Roferon-A) involves a thorough and progressive battery of immunological and non-immunological evaluations (Trown *et al.*, 1986). Both acute and subchronic toxicity tests were completed in several species including subhuman primates (Table 12). Preclinical tests not only examined different species but various routes of administration were studied; local tolerance tests, dose ranging, reproductive assessment, and reversibility of INF-induced changes were recorded. Of four animal models examined, and after 2–13 weeks of INF administration, antibody titres were detected in the cynomolgus monkey, the guinea pig and the rabbit. Other safety and efficacy evaluations for INF included antitumour activity, *in vitro* antiproliferation studies, inhibition of human tumour colony formation, nude mouse studies and pharmacokinetics in African green monkeys using ELISA.

Unlike evaluating recombinant hormones (e.g. insulin, HgH), some information obtained from the preclinical testing of INF was less meaningful.

Table 11 Some suggested toxicological tests for EPO

Purity (contaminants, pyrogenicity)
Bioassay and Mab assay
Acute toxicity (2 species)
Subchronic toxicity (2 species)
Antigenicity (guinea pig)

Genotoxicity
  Ames test
  Cytogeneticity testing

Pharmacokinetics

Table 12 INF toxicity testing: acute and subchronic

Studies/species	Routes of administration	Weeks of treatment
Acute parenteral toxicity studies		
Single dose studies		
Mouse	Intramuscular	
	Intravenous	
	Subcutaneous	
Rat	Intramuscular	
	Intravenous	
	Subcutaneous	
Rabbit	Intramuscular	
	Intravenous	
Ferret	Intramuscular	
	Subcutaneous	
LD$_{50}$		
Mouse	Intravenous	
Local tolerance studies		
Rat	Venous irritation	
Mouse	Venous irritation	
Rabbit	Muscle irritation	
Subchronic toxicity studies		
Squirrel monkey	Intramuscular	2
Rhesus monkey	Intramuscular	4
Mouse	Intramuscular	5
Cynomolgus monkey	Intramuscular	13

Source: modified from Trown *et al.* (1986).

Table 13   Selected list of biologically active lymphokines

Lymphokine	Major biological activity
IL-1	Enhanced IL-2 receptor expression on T-cells
IL-2	Enhanced T cell proliferation
IL-3	Proliferation/differentiation of granulocytes, macrophages, etc.
IL-4	Stimulation of class II MHC antigen
IL-5	Differentiation of antigen-primed B-cells and cytotoxic cells
IL-6	Terminal differentiation of antigen-primed B-cells
IL-7	Growth and maturation of precursor B-cells
TNF	T-cell proliferation and lymphatic secretion
IFNg	Antiviral and antineoplastic activity

Source: modified from Pope (1989).

Certain human proteins are species-restricted but the fact that INFa2a is a protein that is antigenic in experimental animals may have compromised toxicological endpoints. Thus the development of neutralizing antibodies to INFa2a in laboratory animals may not only affect its antiviral and anti-tumor properties, but they might also mask adverse effects produced by the recombinant product.

Lymphokines

There are a large number of lymphokines (Table 13) (Pope, 1989). Many of these natural products have been studied; others, such as interleukin-2 (IL-2), have been cloned. Human IL-2 has undergone preclinical and clinical testing as an anti-cancer agent (Winkelhake and Gauny et al., 1990). Initial testing of recombinant lymphokines involves various *in vitro* tests using both normal and neoplastic cell systems. Testing for antineoplastic activity involved both *in vitro* and *in vivo* tumour models. Recently, at least two recombinant cytokines (G-CSF and GM-CSF) have been undergoing regulatory review for possible approval by the FDA for the treatment of bone marrow suppression associated with cancer therapy (Dozier, 1991). These haematopoietic colony-stimulating factors, granulocyte colony stimulating factor (G-CSF) and granulocyte–macrophage colony stimulating factor (GM-CSF), act as chemical messengers between cells to stimulate the proliferation of blood cell precursors in bone marrow. These recombinant products promote full maturing and functionality of circulating blood cells. GM-CSF (e.g. leukine, prokine) is manufactured using yeast cells to express the GM-CSF gene. The Chinese hamster ovary cell and *E. coli* have also been used to express rGM-CSF.

Growth Factors

There may be as many as 30 or more cellular growth factors (van Brunt and Klausner, 1988). Their nomenclature is often confusing, but they are perhaps best known by their initials, EGF (epidermal growth factor), FGF (fibroblast growth factor), PDGF (platelet derived growth factor), TGF (alpha and beta transforming growth factors) and IGF (insulin growth factor). A principal therapeutic interest lies in their wound healing properties. Some may stimulate endothelial cell growth (e.g. capillary growth), and growth of bone and connective tissue. Recombinant EGF has undergone clinical trials for healing corneal transplants and non-healing corneal defects. All of these growth factors represent challenges to the toxicologist to insure the safety and efficacy of the recombinant products.

ACKNOWLEDGEMENTS

The author expresses his sincere appreciation to Mrs Betty L. Patton and Ms Kaye Nolan for their excellent editorial assistance in the preparation of this chapter.

REFERENCES

Chawia, R. K., Parks, J. S. and Rudman, D. (1983). Structural variants of human growth hormone: biochemical, genetic, and clinical aspects. *Ann. Rev. Med.*, **34**, 519–547

Collen, D., Lijnen, H. R., Todd, P. A. and Goa, K. L. (1989). Tissue-type plasminogen activator. *Drugs*, **38**, 346–388

Cossum, P. A. (1989). Pharmacologic basis for the safety assessment of recombinant human proteins. *J. Am. Coll. Toxicol.*, **8**, 1133–1138

Dozier, N. (1991). Hematopoietic growth factors: focus on GM-CSF. *US Pharmacist*, **16**: H1-H8

Esber, E. C. (1988). Regulatory concerns for biologics: United States perspectives. In Marshak, D. R. and Liu, D. J. (Eds), *Banbury Report 29: Therapeutic Peptides and Proteins: Assessing the New Technologies*. Cold Spring Harbor Laboratory, New York, pp. 265–273

Evans, R. W., Rader, B., Manninen, D. L. and the Cooperative Multicenter EPO Clinical Trial Group (1990). The quality of life of hemodialysis recipients treated with recombinant human erythropoietin. *JAMA*, **263**, 825–830

Galloway, J. A. and Chance, R. E. (1983). Human insulin rDNA: from rDNA through the FDA. In Lemberger, L. and Reidenberg, M. M. (Eds), *Proceedings of the Second World Conference on Clinical Pharmacology and Therapeutics*. Washington, American Society for Pharmacology and Experimental Therapeutics, pp. 503–520

Luster, M. I., Dean, J. H. and Moore, J. A. (1986). In Hayes, A. W. (Ed.), *Principles and Methods of Toxicology*. Raven Press, New York, pp. 561–586

Marafino, B. J., Young, J. D., Greenfield, I. L. and Kopplin, J. R. (1988). The appropriate toxicological testing of recombinant human proteins. In Marshak, D. R. and Darrell, T. L. (Eds), *Therapeutic Peptides and Proteins: Assessing the New Technologies*. Cold Spring Harbor Laboratory, New York, pp. 175–187

Marcek, J. M., Seaman, W. J. and Nappier, J. L. (1989). Effects of repeated high dose administration of recombinant bovine somatotropin in lactating dairy cows. *Vet. Hum. Toxicol.*, **31**, 455–460

Miller, H. I. and Young, F. E. (1988). FDA and biotechnology: Update 1989. *Biotechnol.*, **6**, 1385–1392

Norbury, K. C. (1985). Immunotoxicological evaluation: an overview. *J. Am. Coll. Toxicol.*, **4**, 279–290

Pope, B. L. (1989). Immunopharmacology: a new frontier. *Can. J. Physiol. Pharmacol.*, **67**, 537–545

Sjodin, L. (1988). Regulatory aspects of drugs produced by recombinant DNA technology. In Marshak, D. R. and Liu, D. J. (Eds), *Banbury Report 29: Therapeutic Peptides and Proteins: Assessing the New Technologies*. Cold Spring Harbor Laboratory, New York, pp. 293–297

Trown, P. W., Wills, R. J. and Kamm, J. J. (1986). The preclinical development of Roferon[R]-A. *Cancer*, **57**, 1648

Van Brunt, J. and Klausner, A. (1988). Growth factors speed wound healing. *Biotechnol.*, **6**, 25–30

Winearls, C. G. (1989). Treatment of the anaemia of chronic renal failure with recombinant human erythropoietin. *Drugs*, **38**, 342–345

Winkelhake, J. L. and Gauny, S. S. (1990). Human recombinant interleukin-2 as an experimental therapeutic. *Pharmacol. Rev.*, **42**, 1–25

FURTHER READING

Ducatman, A. M. and Liberman, D. (1991). The biotechnology industry. *Occupational Medicine*, **6**, No. 2, 157–322

Thomas, J. A. and Myers, L. A. (1993). *Biotechnology and Safety Assessment*. Lewis Publishers, Boca Raton, Florida

46 Epidemiology in Relation to Toxicology

John A. Tomenson and Lisa P. Brown

INTRODUCTION

Epidemiology is sometimes simply defined as the study of patterns of health in groups of people (Paddle, 1988). Behind this deceptively simple definition lies a surprisingly diverse science, rich in concepts and methodology. For instance, the group of people might consist of only two people. Goudie *et al.* (1985) described a father suffering from rheumatoid arthritis and his daughter with vertigo. In both father and daughter the pattern of affected areas was remarkably similar, which might suggest that the distribution of joint lesions in rheumatoid arthritis is genetically determined. At the opposite extreme, studies of the geographic distribution of diseases using national mortality and cancer incidence rates have provided clues about the aetiology of several diseases such as cardiovascular disease and stomach cancer. The patterns of health studied are also wide-ranging, and may include the distribution, course and spread of disease. The term 'disease' also has a loose definition in the context of epidemiology, and might include ill-defined conditions such as Organic Solvent and Sick Building Syndromes or consist of an indirect measure of impairment such as biochemical and haematological parameters or lung function measurements.

McMahon and Pugh (1970) observe that epidemiology has evolved from the study of striking outbreaks of disease or epidemics, and note that modern epidemiology can still be regarded as the study of epidemics if a broad view is taken as to what constitutes an epidemic. Clearly epidemiology has a very wide scope, but the aim of this chapter is to describe the relationship between epidemiology and toxicology. For this reason, discussion will be mainly limited to the role epidemiology plays alongside toxicology in the assessment of the hazards of chemical and physical agents and the recommendation of safe conditions under which we may come into contact with them.

Both toxicology and epidemiology are considered by many to be relatively new scientific disciplines. Toxicology, however, has a longer tradition and in the twentieth century it has come to be regarded as a science in its own right and not simply a branch of pharmacology. In order to survive, our prehistoric ancestors had to be aware which foods were harmful, and they were naturally led to experiment in order to cure natural ailments or develop antidotes to poisons. There is evidence that poisons were used for hunting and fishing and that prehistoric man was aware of the therapeutic benefits of certain natural substances. There are many early examples of toxicological writings such as the Papyrus Ebers of the ancient Egyptians, written about 1500 BC, and the Sanskrit medical writings in the Ayur Veda, which date back to around 900 BC. Decker (1987) provides a good description of the early history of the science of poisons and the rapid development of analytical toxicology during the nineteenth and twentieth centuries. In contrast, epidemiologists can quote Hippocrates to demonstrate that the ancient Greeks were aware that health may be connected with a person's environment.

However, there the similarity with toxicology ends, for it was not until the seventeenth century that the beginnings of quantitative epidemiology started to appear. John Graunt, who in 1662 published his *Natural and Political Observations . . . on the Bills of Mortality*, is often credited as being the pioneer of quantitative epidemiology, although McMahon and Pugh (1970) note that, since the techniques of Graunt saw no further epidemiological application for almost 200 years, it is more appropriate to regard Graunt as a forerunner than a founder of epidemiology. Although the nineteenth century saw important work by people such as William Farr and John Snow, most of the theory and quantitative methods of epidemiology have really only come into being during the past four decades.

Epidemiology and toxicology differ in many other ways but principally in that epidemiology is essentially an observational science, in contrast to the experimental nature of toxicology. The opportunistic approach of epidemiology has been commented upon by several authors (e.g. Paddle, 1988; Utidjian, 1987). The epidemiologist often has to make do with historical data which have been collected for reasons which have nothing to do with epidemiology. Nevertheless, the availability of personnel records such as lists of new starters and leavers, payrolls and work rosters and exposure monitoring data collected for compliance purposes has enabled many epidemiological studies to be conducted in the occupational setting. Thus, the epidemiologist has no control over who is exposed to an agent, the levels at which they are exposed to the agent of interest, or the other agents to which they may be exposed. The epidemiologist has great difficulty in ascertaining what exposure has taken place and certainly has no control over life-style variables such as diet and smoking.

Despite the lack of precise data, the epidemiologist has one major advantage over the toxicologist: an epidemiology study documents the actual health experiences of human beings subjected to real-life exposures in an occupational or environmental setting. Indeed Smith (1988) has recently expressed the view that uncertainty in epidemiology studies resulting from exposure estimation may be equal to or less than the uncertainty associated with extrapolation from animals to man. Regulatory bodies such as the US Environmental Protection Agency (EPA) are starting to change their attitudes towards epidemiology and recognize that it has a role to play in the process of risk assessment. However, there is also a complementary need for epidemiologists to introduce more rigour into the conduct of their studies and to introduce standards akin to the Good Laboratory Practice standards under which animal experiments are performed.

HISTORY OF EPIDEMIOLOGY

As noted in the introduction, awareness of certain epidemiological principles can be traced back to the days of Hippocrates, but it was a further 2000 years before epidemiology truly began to emerge. The analysis by John Graunt of the weekly Bills of Mortality and christenings recorded in the parish registers of London is generally regarded to be the first example of an epidemiological study. He reported higher death rates and birth rates for males than for females, and examined the influence of various factors on the spread of the plague. However, the greatest achievement of Graunt was to recognize the importance of studying biological phenomena in groups of people. Edmund Halley, the English Astronomer Royal, was another seventeenth century scientist who was interested in population mortality rates. Halley made a study of the records of births and deaths kept in the Silesian city of Breslau (now Wrocław in Poland) since 1584 and drew up a life-table which was published in 1693. Casina Stabe, a seventeenth century Italian physician, has received comparatively little recognition. However, the following extract from *De Morbis Artificum* (*Diseases of Workers*) written by Ramazzini in 1713 (Ramazzini, 1964), demonstrates clearly that Stabe understood the basic principles of epidemiology:

A few years ago a violent dispute arose between a citizen of Finale, a town in the dominion of Modena, and a certain business man, a Modenese, who owned a huge laboratory at Finale where he manufactured sublimate. The citizen of Finale brought a lawsuit against this manufacturer and demanded that he should move his workshop outside the town or to some other place, on the ground that he poisoned the whole neighbourhood whenever his workmen roasted vitriol in the furnace to make sublimate. To prove the truth of his accusation he produced the sworn testimony of the doctor of Finale and also the parish register of deaths, from which it appeared that many more persons died annually in that quarter and in the immediate neighbourhood of the laboratory than in other localities. Moreover, the doctor gave evidence that the residents of that neighbourhood usually died of wasting disease and disease of the chest; this he ascribed to the fumes given off by the vitriol, which so tainted the air near by that it was rendered unhealthy and dangerous for the lungs. Dr Bernardino Corradi, the commissioner of ordnance in the Duchy of Este, defended the manufacturer, while Dr Casina Stabe, then the town physician, spoke for the plaintiff. Various cleverly worded documents were published by both sides, and this dispute which was literally 'about the shadow of smoke', as the saying is, was hotly argued. In the end the jury sustained the manufacturer, and vitriol was found not guilty. Whether in this case the legal expert gave a correct verdict, I leave to the decision of those who are experts in natural science.

During the nineteenth century modern epidemiological theory began to take shape. In 1836 the registration of births, marriages and deaths became compulsory in England, and William Farr, appointed Registrar General for England and Wales in 1839, established a pattern for the reporting of mortality data which has continued to this day. Farr looked at mortality in a variety of occupational settings and established a procedure for linking mortality data to occupational groupings derived from census data. A Parisian physician who taught Farr, Pierre-Charles Alexandre Louis, is given much credit for introducing numerical techniques to occupational epidemiology (Lilienfeld and Lilienfeld, 1977). Louis also taught another eminent Victorian epidemiologist, William Guy (see Weed, 1986, for a discussion of some of Guy's work). Another Victorian pioneer in epidemiology was John Snow, who was famous for demonstrating the relationship between the incidence of cholera in certain London boroughs and faecal contamination of the water supply. McMahon and Pugh (1970) give a more detailed description of the work of Farr and Snow. The work of Farr and Snow is extremely well known but there were also many other excellent epidemiological studies conducted during the nineteenth century. Florence Nightingale, well known as the Lady of the Lamp, was also a reformer who knew how medical statistics could benefit her causes. She was a firm friend of William Farr, and one example of her work was a mortality table for hospital nurses and attendants showing a greatly increased prevalence of communicable diseases (Newell, 1984).

This progress continued into the twentieth century, and Utidjian (1987) points out that during the early years of the twentieth century there were a number of important occupational morbidity studies. In addition, there was much work done by actuaries in the insurance business which is often overlooked and predates the conventional landmarks of classical epidemiology. After the pioneering work of Graunt and Halley it was a further generation before James Dodson laid the foundations of actuarial science. Dodson calculated a scale of premiums based on the Bills of Mortality for London in the years 1728–1750. The life insurance business then developed steadily over the next 150 years. From the beginning of the twentieth century, the insurance companies of the USA and Canada have conducted many large-scale investigations of the mortality associated with various impairments. The first large-scale mortality study by the insurance companies, reported in 1903, *The Specialised Mortality Investigation*, was notable in that the results were reported as mortality ratios.

Having given due recognition to the nineteenth century fathers of epidemiology such as Farr and Snow, it is still fair to say that epidemiology has only begun to develop as a science in the last 40 years. Greenland (1987), writing about the evolution of epidemiological ideas, stated that the period from World War II up to the early 1980s encompasses the two 'golden eras' of epidemiological development. In Greenland's view, a foundation for epidemiological research was created during the years 1946–1966 and this coincided with the conduct of the first major studies of chronic disease. The second golden era, stretching from the mid-1960s to the early 1980s, saw the development of a theoretical framework for epidemiology, clarification of concepts such as confounding and interaction and the emergence of case–control methodology. A brief description of the different types of epidemiology study is given in a later section.

There is no doubt that the post-World War II period has seen a tremendous upsurge in epidemiological activity and a parallel rise in concern over environmental and occupational health matters. The work of Doll and Hill (1950, 1954) was of great importance in demonstrating that cigarette smoking causes lung cancer, but it also established the methodology of case–control and cohort studies. However, the British doctors' cohort study reported by Doll and Hill (1954) was prospective and credit must also be given to the bladder cancer study by Case *et al.* (1954), which played a major role in establishing the credibility of the historical cohort study. Not only does the work of Case stand up to scrutiny more than 30 years later, but also this study and the work of Cornfield (1951) on case–control studies have legitimized the use of retrospectively collected data and led to the historical cohort and case–control studies becoming the major techniques in modern cancer and mortality epidemiology.

The Framingham Heart Study initiated in 1949 to study risk factors for cardiovascular diseases was another major landmark in the development of epidemiology as a science. In addition to making a significant contribution to our understanding of the aetiology of cardiovascular disease, the Framingham study spurred the development of a large body of epidemiological methodology (e.g. Cornfield, 1962). However, despite the undoubted progress during the last 40 years, the science of epidemiology is still in its infancy. Rothman (1986) points to disagreements and confusion about the most basic concepts or measures leading to profound differences in the interpretation of data, and Feinstein (1988) notes that, despite peer review approval, current epidemiological methods need substantial improvement to produce trustworthy scientific evidence.

EPIDEMIOLOGICAL END-POINTS

The end-points studied by epidemiologists and toxicologists serve to illustrate some of the major differences between the two sciences. An excellent review of epidemiological end-points and their measurement is provided in a WHO publication on guidelines on studies in environmental epidemiology (World Health Organization, 1983). The end-points studied by epidemiologists and toxicologists are broadly similar—namely organ malfunction, death, carcinogenesis, birth defects and mutagenesis. However, only in the case of cancer is the epidemiologist likely to obtain the same quality of information about the end-point as is the toxicologist. An epidemiologist conducting a study of workers exposed to a hepatotoxin will be reliant on haematology and clinical chemistry laboratory test results. The toxicologist will of course also make use of the same indicators of liver malfunction but will also have access to other measures of subacute or chronic toxicity such as the organ weight at necropsy and histopathology. Even in the case of a discrete end-point such as death, the epidemiologist is reliant on death certificates for information. Many studies of the accuracy of death certificates have shown that the individual causes listed on the certificate are often identified incorrectly. The quality and limitations of death registration data

are discussed in the decennial occupational mortality supplement of the Office of Population Censuses and Surveys (OPCS) (1986), in England and Wales. It is noted there that the errors are generally greater for deaths of the elderly and for deaths from certain conditions, notably cerebrovascular disease. As an illustration, Doll and Peto (1981) argue that in recent years the old have received increasingly careful medical attention, which must affect artefactually the trends in cancer death certification rates. Consequently they restricted a study of trends in cancer incidence to people under the age of 65.

The epidemiologist is not at a total disadvantage, for there are certain health responses that the toxicologist would find difficult to measure in experimental studies of animals. The neurobehavioural tests for studies of Organic Solvent Syndrome are one such example (World Health Organization, 1985). Results in human studies cannot usually be replicated or explored in animal models, because we do not know how animals 'think' or 'feel'. However, the study of reproductive disorders typifies the difficulties that epidemiologists sometimes face in obtaining health response data. The toxicological approach to the study of reproductive effects is described in Chapter 43 and is a well-established feature of regulatory submissions for agrochemicals and pharmaceutical products. The epidemiologist has considerable difficulty in measuring the reproductive efficiency of couples. Male functional performance has been measured in some industry studies using semen collected from workforce volunteers (e.g. Dobbins, 1987), but such an approach would be unacceptable in occupational and environmental studies in many countries. Decreased libido and functional disorders may be revealed by questionnaires but the value of such an approach has yet to be proven. Questionnaires have also been used to estimate the occurrence of menstrual disorders in women and to measure the reproductive efficiency of couples (Levine *et al.*, 1980). Kallen (1988) comprehensively reviews the end-points studied in reproductive epidemiology and the methods for collecting and interpreting data on spontaneous abortion and malformations. However, fetal loss rates are extremely difficult to quantify and the event may not even be noticed by the woman herself in the first trimester.

Questionnaires have been described in the discussion of reproductive epidemiology and represent another major difference between toxicology and epidemiology. The use of symptom questionnaires is widespread in epidemiology and makes it possible to compare symptom prevalence in groups of individuals exposed to different agents. In the case of respiratory and cardiovascular epidemiology, standardized questionnaires are an extremely important research tool and considerable efforts have been made to ensure their validity and reproducibility (e.g. Medical Research Council, 1976; Rose *et al.*, 1982). Questionnaires are also used to quantify a number of ill-defined conditions such as stress (Goldberg, 1972), Sick Building Syndrome (Finnegan *et al.*, 1984) and allergy to laboratory animals (Botham *et al.*, 1987). They also form an important component of the range of neurological examination methods and the techniques used in epidemiological studies for assessing neurotoxic effects.

MEASUREMENT OF EXPOSURE

Wegman and Eisen (1988) make the valid point that epidemiologists have placed much greater emphasis on the measure of response than on the measure of exposure. They claim that this is because most epidemiologists have been trained as physicians and are consequently more oriented towards measuring health outcomes. It is certainly true that a modern textbook of epidemiology such as Rothman (1986) says very little about what the epidemiologist should do with exposure assessments. However, this is probably as much a reflection of the historical paucity of quantitative exposure information as a reflection on the background of epidemiologists. Nevertheless, it is surprising how many epidemiological studies do not contain even a basic qualitative assessment of exposure. Table 1 shows the quality of exposure data in 52 mortality studies of pesticide applicators reviewed by Brown (1990). Almost half, 24, do not even specify the pesticides to which applicators were potentially exposed. The contrast between epidemiology and toxicology is never more marked than in the area of estimation of dose response. Not only can the toxicologist carefully control the conditions of the exposure to the agent of interest, but also he can be sure that his animals have not come into contact with any other toxic agents. The industrial

Table 1 Quality of exposure data in 52 mortality studies of pesticide applicators (Brown, 1990)

Information on exposure	Number
Do not specify compounds or give exposure assessments	24
Compounds named (no exposure assessment)	10
Exposure assessment by questionnaire (personal or next of kin)	14
Exposure assessment by hygiene measurements	3
Biological monitoring data	1

epidemiologist conducting the study of workers exposed to a hepatotoxin described in the previous section will certainly have to control for alcohol intake and possibly for exposure to other hepatotoxins in the work and home environment. Nevertheless, it can be argued that epidemiology studies more accurately measure the effect on human health of 'real-life' exposures.

In occupational studies it is often necessary to assess exposure retrospectively. Few companies have either recorded or kept quantitative exposure data over even the working lifetimes of their current employees.

Most manufacturing processes change considerably over time, as do the exposures experienced by the workforce. In addition, the ingredients and chemical reactions may not be well documented and can greatly complicate the characterization of exposure. Often the epidemiologist has to rely on anecdotal evidence and careful detective work by an industrial hygienist to construct a matrix of exposures by job title and time-period. Occasionally attempts are made to estimate past exposures by reconstructing redundant industrial processes. Ayer *et al.* (1973) describe the reconstruction of an old granite shed to estimate dust levels. Even if quantitative exposure data are available, obtained by either static monitor or personal sampler, it will almost certainly have been collected to determine compliance with internal or external regulations. More emphasis is placed on recording the higher levels which occur after spillages and plant malfunction, and this may render the exposure data inappropriate for use to define normal exposures encountered in the jobs. It is to be hoped that, in future, epidemiologists and hygienists can develop sampling strategies that generate exposure data suitable for both compliance and epidemiological purposes.

If an exposure matrix has been constructed with quantitative estimates of the exposure in each job and time-period, then it is a simple matter to estimate cumulative exposure. It is a more difficult process when, as commonly, only a qualitative measure of exposure is available— e.g. high, medium and low. Even when exposure measurements are available, it may not be sensible to make an assumption that an exposure which occurred 20 years ago is equivalent to the same exposure yesterday. The use of average exposures may also be questionable, and peak exposures may be more relevant in the case of outcomes such as asthma and chronic bronchitis. Noise is a good example of an exposure which must be carefully characterized and where the simple calculation of a cumulative exposure may be misleading. There is now evidence that hearing loss due to noise is dependent on the amount of hearing already lost because of ageing (Robinson, 1987). It is also important to distinguish between continuous, intermittent and impulse noise when investigating noise-induced hearing loss. A further factor which is often not considered is the use of personal protective equipment. For instance, in the studies of noise-induced hearing loss it is rare to see an attempt made to correct for the protection afforded by ear-plugs, hearing-muffs, etc.

EPIDEMIOLOGICAL STUDY DESIGNS

This section provides a brief introduction to the most important types of studies conducted by epidemiologists. It is an attempt to briefly describe the principles of the major types of epidemiological studies in order to assist the toxicologist to understand the reporting of epidemiological studies and the assumptions made by epidemiologists. The next section of this chapter will discuss the similarities and differences between the methodologies of toxicology and epidemiology.

Cohort Studies

Historical Cohort Study

When the need arises to study the health status of a group of workers, there is often a large body of historical data which can be utilized. If sufficient information exists on individuals exposed in the past to a potential workplace hazard, then it may be possible to undertake a retrospective cohort study. The historical data will have been collected for reasons which have nothing to do with epidemiology. Nevertheless, the availability of personnel records such as starters' and leavers' registers, payrolls, work rosters and individuals' career records has enabled many epidemiological studies to be conducted—in particular, mortality studies.

The principles of a historical cohort study can also be applied to follow a cohort of workers prospectively. This approach will be discussed further in the next subsection, although it should be emphasized that many historical data studies have a prospective element in so far as they are updated after a further period of follow-up. The discussion of historical cohort studies in this section will concentrate on mortality and cancer incidence studies. However, there is no reason why hearing loss, lung function or almost any measure of the health status of an individual should not be studied retrospectively if sufficient information is available.

Mortality and cancer incidence studies are unique among retrospective cohort studies in that they can be conducted using national cancer and mortality registers even if there has been no medical surveillance of the workforce. A historical cohort study also has the advantages of being cheaper and providing estimates of the potential hazard much earlier than a prospective study. However, historical cohort studies are beset by a variety of problems. Principal among these is the problem of determining which workers have been exposed and, if so, to what degree. In addition, it may be difficult to decide what is an appropriate comparison group. It should also be borne in mind that in epidemiology, unlike animal experimentation, random allocation is not possible and there is no control over the factors which may distort the effects of the exposure of interest, such as smoking and standard of living.

The principles of historical cohort studies as

they apply within a large chemical company in the UK are described in the following subsections.

Cohort Definition and Follow-up Period

A variety of sources of information are used to identify workers exposed to a particular workplace hazard, to construct an occupational history and complete the collection of information necessary for tracing (see below). It is essential that the cohort be well defined and that criteria for eligibility be strictly followed. This requires that a clear statement be made about membership of the cohort so that it is easy to decide whether an employee is a member or not. It is also important that the follow-up period be carefully defined. For instance, it is readily apparent that the follow-up period should not start before exposure has occurred. Furthermore, it is uncommon for the health effect of interest to manifest itself immediately after exposure, and allowance for an appropriate biological induction (or latency) period may need to be made when interpreting the data.

Tracing

In the UK the vital status (alive, dead, emigrated or untraced) and the causes of death of members of a cohort study are ascertained by use of the National Health Service Central Register (NHSCR) of the UK. In the authors' Company it is also possible to ascertain the vital status of a large proportion of cohort members by use of company mortality registers and personnel records. NHSCR provides assistance to a wide variety of medical research projects in the UK. In addition to ascertaining the status of an individual on a given date, NHSCR will also flag live individuals and notify the study manager when they die. Consequently, it is a relatively simple matter to update a mortality study after a further period of follow-up.

Comparison Subjects

The usual comparison group for many studies is the national population. However, it is known that there are marked regional differences in the mortality rates for many causes of death. Regional mortality rates exist in the UK (e.g. Gardner *et al.*, 1984) but have to be used with caution because they are based on small numbers of deaths and estimated population sizes. In some situations the local rates for certain causes may be highly influenced by the mortality of the work-

force being studied. Furthermore, it is not always easy to decide what the most appropriate regional rate for comparison purposes is, as many employees may reside in a different region from that in which the plant is situated.

An alternative or additional approach is to establish a cohort of unexposed workers for comparison purposes. However, workers with very low exposures to the workplace hazard will often provide similar information. A good discussion of the issues is found in the proceedings of a conference entirely devoted to the subject (Medical Research Council Environmental Epidemiology Unit, 1984).

Analysis and Interpretation

In a cohort study the first stage in the analysis consists of calculating the number of deaths expected during the follow-up period. In order to calculate the expected deaths for the cohort, the survival experience of the cohort is broken down into individual years of survival known as 'person-years'. Each person-year is characterized by the age of the cohort member and the time-period when survival occurred and the sex of the cohort member. The person-years are then multiplied by age, sex and time-period specific mortality rates to obtain the expected number of deaths. The ratio between observed and expected deaths is expressed as a standardized mortality ratio (SMR) as follows:

$$\text{SMR} = 100 \times \frac{\text{observed deaths}}{\text{expected deaths}}$$

Thus, an SMR of 125 represents an excess mortality of 25 per cent. An SMR can be calculated for different causes of death and for subdivision of the person-years by factors such as level of exposure and time since first exposure.

Interpretation of cohort studies is not always straightforward, and there are a number of selection effects and biases that must be considered (Rothman, 1986). Cohort studies routinely report that the mortality of active workers is less than that of the population as a whole. It is not an unexpected finding, since workers usually have to undergo some sort of selection process to become or remain workers. Nevertheless, this selection effect, known as the 'healthy worker' effect, can lead to considerable arguments over the interpretation of study results, particularly if the cancer mortality is as expected, but the all-cause mortality is much lower than expected. Weed (1986) gives an interesting historical account of attempts to understand the process of occupational selection. However, even an experimental science such as toxicology is not without a similar problem of interpretation, viz. the problem of distinguishing between the effects of age and treatment on tumour incidence (Peto *et al.*, 1980).

Proportional Mortality Study

There are often situations where one has no accurate data on the composition of a cohort but does possess a set of death records (or cancer registrations). Under these circumstances a proportional mortality study may sometimes be substituted for a cohort study. In such a mortality study the proportions of deaths from a specific cause among the study deaths is compared with the proportion of deaths from that cause in a comparison population. The results of a proportional mortality study are expressed in an analogous way to those of the cohort study with follow-up. Corresponding to the observed deaths from a particular cause, it is possible to calculate an expected number of deaths based on mortality rates for that cause and all causes of death in a comparison group and the total number of deaths in the study. The ratio between observed and expected deaths from a certain cause is expressed as a proportional mortality ratio (PMR) as follows:

$$PMR = 100 \times \frac{\text{observed deaths}}{\text{expected deaths}}$$

Thus, a PMR of 125 for a particular cause of death represents a 25 per cent increase in the proportion of deaths due to that cause. A proportional mortality study has the advantage of avoiding the expensive and time-consuming establishment and tracing of a cohort, but the disadvantage of little or no exposure information.

Prospective Cohort Study

Prospective cohort studies are no different in principle from historical cohort studies in terms of scientific logic, the major differences being timing and methodology. The study starts with a group of apparently healthy individuals whose health

and exposure is studied over a period of time. As it is possible to define in advance the information that is to be collected, prospective studies are theoretically more reliable than retrospective studies. However, long periods of observation may be required to obtain results.

Prospective cohort studies or longitudinal studies of continually changing health parameters such as lung function, hearing loss, blood biochemistry and haematological measurements pose different problems from those encountered in mortality and cancer incidence studies. The relationships between changes in the parameters of interest and exposure measurements have to be estimated and, if necessary, a comparison made of changes in the parameters between groups. These relationships may be extremely complicated, compounded by factors such as ageing, and difficult to estimate, as there may be relatively few measurement points. Furthermore, large errors of measurement in the variables may be present because of factors such as within-laboratory variation and temporal variation within individuals. Missing observations and withdrawals may also cause problems, particularly if they are dependent on the level and change of the parameter of interest. These problems may make it difficult to interpret and judge the validity of analytical conclusions. Nevertheless, prospective cohort studies provide the best means of measuring changes in health parameters and relating them to exposure.

Case–Control Study

In a case–control study (also known as a case–referent study) two groups of individuals are selected for study, of which one has the disease whose causation is to be studied (the cases) and the other does not (the controls). In the context of the chemical industry, the aim of a case–control study is to evaluate the relevance of past exposure to the development of a disease. This is done by obtaining an indirect estimate of the rate of occurrence of the disease in an exposed and unexposed group by comparing the frequency of exposure among cases and controls.

Principal Features

Case–control and cohort studies complement each other as types of epidemiological study. In a case–control study the groups are defined on the basis of the presence or absence of a given disease and, hence, only one disease can be studied at a time. The case–control study compensates for this by providing information on a wide range of exposures which may play a role in the development of the disease. In contrast, a cohort study generally focuses on a single exposure but can be analysed for multiple disease outcomes. A case–control study is a better way of studying rare diseases because a very large cohort would be required to demonstrate an excess of a rare disease. In contrast, a case–control study is an inefficient way of assessing the effect of an uncommon exposure, when it might be possible to conduct a cohort study of all those exposed.

The complementary strengths and weaknesses of case–control and cohort studies can be used to advantage. Increasingly, mortality studies are being reported which utilize 'nested' case–control studies to investigate the association between the exposures of interest and a cause of death for which an excess has been discovered. However, case–control studies have traditionally been held in low regard, largely because they are often badly conducted and interpreted. There is also a tendency to overinterpret the data and misuse statistical procedures. In addition, there is still considerable debate among leading epidemiologists themselves as to how controls should be selected—e.g. Poole, (1986) and Schlesselman and Stadel (1987).

Analysis and Interpretation

In a case–control study it is possible to compare the frequencies of exposures in the cases and controls. However, what one is really interested in is a comparison of the frequencies of disease in the exposed and the unexposed. The latter comparison is usually expressed as a Relative Risk (RR), which is defined as

$$RR = \frac{\text{rate of disease in exposed group}}{\text{rate of disease in unexposed group}}$$

It is clearly not possible to calculate the RR directly in a case–control study, since exposed and unexposed groups have not been followed in order to determine the rates of occurrence of the disease in the two groups. Nevertheless, it is possible to calculate another statistic, the Odds Ratio (OR), which, if certain assumptions hold,

is a good estimate of the RR. For cases and controls the exposure odds are simply the odds of being exposed, and the OR is defined as

$$OR = \frac{\text{cases with exposure}}{\text{controls with exposure}} \bigg/ \frac{\text{cases without exposure}}{\text{controls without exposure}}$$

An OR of 1 indicates that the rate of disease is unaffected by exposure. An OR greater than 1 indicates an increase in the rate of disease in exposed workers.

Matching

Matching is the selection of a comparison group that is, within stated limits, identical with the study group with respect to one or more factors such as age, years of service, smoking history, etc., which may distort the effect of the exposure of interest. The matching may be done on an individual or group basis. Although matching may be used in all types of study, including follow-up and cross-sectional studies, it is more widely used in case–control studies. It is common to see case–control studies in which each case is matched to as many as three or four controls.

Nested Case–Control Study

In a cohort study the assessment of exposure for all cohort members may be extremely time-consuming and demanding of resources. If an excess of death or incidence has been discovered for a small number of conditions, it may be much more efficient to conduct a case–control study to investigate the effect of exposure. Thus, instead of all members being studied, only the cases and a sample of non-cases would be compared with regard to exposure history. Thus, there is no need to investigate the exposure histories of all those who are neither cases nor controls. However, the nesting is only effective if there are a reasonable number of cases and sufficient variation in the exposure of the cohort members.

Other Study Designs

Descriptive Studies

There are large numbers of records in existence which document the health of various groups of people. Mortality statistics are available for many countries and even for certain companies (e.g. Pell *et al.*, 1978; Paddle, 1981). Similarly, there is a wide range of routine morbidity statistics—in particular, those based on cancer registrations (Waterhouse *et al.*, 1982). These health statistics can be used to study differences between geographic regions (e.g. maps of cancer mortality and incidence presented at a recent Symposium, Boyle *et al.*, 1989), occupational groups and time-periods. Investigations based on existing records of the distribution of disease and of possible causes are known as descriptive studies. It is sometimes possible to identify hazards associated with the development of rare conditions from observation of clustering in occupational or geographical areas. The report by Creech and Johnson (1974) on 3 cases of haemangiosarcoma in vinyl chloride workers at the B. F. Goodrich Chemical Company is a good example. At that time only 25 cases a year of haemangiosarcoma were reported for the whole of the United States. However, much more detailed information on the population at risk (age, sex, size, etc.) and valid comparison rates are usually required to allow sensible interpretation of mortality and morbidity statistics.

Cross-sectional Study

Cross-sectional studies measure the cause (exposure) and the effect (disease) at the same point in time. They compare the rates of diseases or symptoms of an exposed group with an unexposed group. Strictly speaking, the exposure information is ascertained simultaneously with the disease information. In practice, such studies are usually more meaningful from an aetiological or causal point of view if the exposure assessment reflects past exposures. Current information is often all that is available but may still be meaningful, because of the correlation between current exposure and relevant past exposure.

Cross-sectional studies are widely used to study the health of groups of workers who are exposed to possible hazards but do not undergo regular surveillance. They are particularly suited to the study of subclinical parameters such as blood biochemistry and haematological values. Cross-sectional studies are also relatively straightforward to conduct in comparison with prospective cohort studies and are generally simpler to interpret.

Intervention Study

Not all epidemiology is observational, and experimental studies have a role to play in evaluating the efficiency of an intervention programme to prevent disease—e.g. fluoridation of water. An intervention study at one extreme may closely resemble a clinical trial with individuals randomly selected to receive some form of intervention—e.g. advice on reducing cholesterol levels. However, in some instances it may be a whole community that is selected to form the intervention group. The selection may or may not be random. The toxicologist might argue that even if selection was random, such a study of two communities, each consisting of many individuals, was in a sense a study of only two subjects. However, he should ask himself first whether the 'three rats to a cage' design of many subacute toxicity studies really generates three independent responses per cage.

THE EPIDEMIOLOGY–TOXICOLOGY INTERFACE

Beginning in the early 1990s the protection of human health from chemicals in the workplace, market place and environment has become a universally recognized goal. The approach towards this goal has developed over time and can be roughly characterized by three processes (Friess, 1987): (1) the development of some form of human dose–response relationship for an adverse health effect; (2) the assessment of risk for that effect under specific exposure conditions; and (3) the setting of permissible exposure limits for the chemical in various exposure scenarios. At the beginning of the twentieth century the US government passed the first Food and Drug Act, aimed at regulating the widespread adulteration of food with chemical additives. To identify some chemicals and to emphasize the problems, Dr Harvey Wiley conducted the first toxicology studies for regulatory purposes on behalf of the Bureau of Chemistry (which subsequently became the Food and Drug Administration) by setting up feeding experiments with 12 healthy, male volunteers (Glocklin, 1987). It soon became apparent that there were insidious, even life-threatening, toxicities lurking in foodstuffs and patent medicines which went far beyond the transient gastrointestinal upsets or general malaise that Dr Wiley's so-called 'poison squad' would have been willing to accept. The ethical concerns with human studies quickly led to the use of animals in safety testing. By developing strains of laboratory animals and maintaining them in good health and in a controlled environment, it was possible to carry out reproducible experiments, and the science of experimental toxicology came into existence (Zapp, 1981). However, ever since toxicologists came to rely on surrogate models for man, arguments about trans-species prediction in assessing human health hazards have been a major issue (Brown and Paddle, 1988).

Methodological Differences

The interface between epidemiology and toxicology is sometimes fraught. The toxicologist argues that the tighter specification of animal studies, and the absence of the social and environmental factors which confuse the issue in human studies, should lead one to regard the animal studies as more informative. However, the epidemiologist would counter that the greater relevance of the species, and the greater relevance of the dose in that species, make the epidemiological data more informative.

The toxicologist will have noticed certain similarities between the prospective cohort study and the carcinogenesis bioassay and other approaches to chronic toxicity testing. The use of national mortality statistics for comparison purposes may seem odd to the toxicologist but is analogous to the use of historical information in toxicology studies. The most obvious difference, however, is the inability of the epidemiologist randomly to assign workers to the different exposure groups. Randomization does play a part in epidemiology, as can be seen in the description of intervention studies. The cross-sectional study will also be recognized by the toxicologist as being the analogue of a subacute toxicity study. Although many of the study end-points are similar (e.g. haematology and clinical chemistry test results), the epidemiologist will also study a much larger range of health effects such as respiratory function (lung function testing and X-ray changes) and blood pressure. However, unlike the toxicologist, the epidemiologist is unable to look for histopathological changes in the tissues of subjects. The studies that will seem most alien to the toxicologist are the retrospective studies. They clearly have no counterpart in toxicology or any other experimental science, although it is interesting to note that Schlesselman (1982) claims that

the case–control approach was formalized within the field of sociology during the 1920s.

The major differences between the methodologies of laboratory and epidemiological studies are summarized in Table 2. The differences become most apparent when one considers carcinogens. It is both unethical and impractical to expose humans to compounds and wait and see (typically 15–30 years) whether cancers result. Animal studies are not so constrained by either ethics or time. A rodent bioassay can be completed within 3 years (animal life-span = 2 years; pathological and quantitative analyses up to 1 year) and therefore toxicology may be described as a prospective study, while epidemiology is largely retrospective. Chapters 9–14 of this book will also testify to the more sophisticated techniques that are afforded to animal toxicology for individual organ analyses, be they ongoing, interim or final evaluations. The poorer quality of some epidemiological end-points, particularly those based on death certification, has already been discussed. The epidemiologist has little control over the health of subjects on entry but, as noted previously, the health of an employee at recruitment is likely to be better than average. However, the health of a subject at recruitment will be one factor that influences the response of the subject to exposure to the agent under study. In addition, there may be many other confounding factors such as age, smoking habits, alcohol consumption, diet and exposure to other hazards at work and at home. By comparison, the toxicologist can be confident of minimal confounding effects and pure compound exposure, and has the reassurance provided by his trial control data of detecting genuine compound-related effects.

A further difference between the two types of study is in the pattern and level of exposure. Both animal and human studies may be investigating the same chemical but the means to the end is quite different. Suppose that the compound of interest is a pesticide used in spraying corn maize. Then two potential human groups to study would be: (1) applicators, having exposure seasonally to significant amounts, then periods of no exposure at all (i.e. pulse doses), and possibly concurrent exposure to other chemicals; and (2) the general population, who may consume the product on average twice a week in only very small amounts as a food contaminant. Not only is the pattern and level of exposure different for the two groups

Table 2 Differences between animal and human studies

Parameter	Animal study	Human study
Ethics	Provided that governmental animal cruelty/rights acts are not contravened, then it is perfectly acceptable to knowingly expose the animal to carcinogens, mutagens, teratogens, etc.	It is unethical to knowingly and deliberately expose humans to carcinogens, mutagens, teratogens, etc.
Conduct	Good laboratory practice (strict adherence to GLP)	Protocol for study (protocol may change during study)
Subject observation	Monitored case histories (record of animal health throughout study)	Exhaustive follow-up (sometimes subjects are untraceable/disappear)
Dose	Regulated exposure (defined dose at defined intervals)	Defined exposed group (it may only be known whether there was a potential for exposure but not at what level)
Length of exposure	Depending on the suspected effect of the chemical (generally lifetime for carcinogens, throughout organogenesis for teratogens, generations for reprotoxins)	Various (depending on whether chemical is an occupational, market place or environmental hazard)
Pattern of exposure	Single chemicals at around the maximum tolerated dose, dose levels constant	Mixed exposure at varied levels (usually 'pulse' exposure)
Comparison groups	Randomized uniformity (control group known to have no exposure, otherwise identical with exposed group)	Valid unexposed group (it can only be assumed that the only different variable is exposure)
Genetic homogeneity	Generally 'inbred' strain used; hence, high degree of genetic homogeneity	High degree of heterogeneity
Death	Standardized necropsy (every animal subject to pathological examination)	High degree of heterogeneity
Relevance	Extremely relevant to the species in which data were generated (trans-species relevance unknown)	Extremely relevant to man

of humans potentially at risk, but also the routes of exposure are dissimilar. The applicators are exposed by skin absorption, inhalation and oral routes to more than one pesticide, while the general population is exposed by the oral route. The toxicology study, however, would be conducted as a 7 days a week, lifetime feeding study with the only control variable being the single pesticide of interest. Dose levels would be defined around the maximum tolerance dose (MTD), and some subfraction thereof.

These three different exposure scenarios—(1) human, 'pulse dose' to more than one chemical; (2) human, intermittent very low doses and (3) animal, constant high levels—exemplify how exposure patterns, levels and routes can vary not only within a species, but also between species. Epidemiologists of necessity study populations of great genetic heterogeneity and of wide age distribution (at least within 16–65 years for industrial working age range and lifetime years for environmental agents). They are populations exposed intermittently to largely unknown concentrations of the toxicant of interest, by an ill-defined combination of routes, almost never in isolation, for outcomes or effects which are rarely determinable or even definable in the precise terms which are demanded of animal studies (Utidjian, 1987).

Species Differences

There are a number of biological factors which may enhance the susceptibility of an individual to experience adverse health effects from exposure to toxic substances. These include age, sex, genetic composition, nutritional status and pre-existing disease conditions (Calabrese, 1986). The extent or magnitude to which predisposing factors enhance susceptibility to toxic substances is known only to a limited extent. The conversion of estimated risks from animal studies conducted at high doses to estimated risks for humans at lower doses involves several considerations: (1) scaling for differences in size, life-span, metabolic rate (*quantitative differences*); (2) adjustment for differences in route of exposure or absorption (*qualitative differences*); (3) adjustment for bio-chemical and pharmacokinetic differences (*qualitative and quantitative differences*); (4) consideration of interspecies differences in inherent susceptibility (*qualitative differences*). These four considerations can be grossly divided between quantitative and qualitative differences. Considerations (2), (3) and (4) are considered to be qualitative, as generally the pharmacokinetics, pharmacodynamics and mechanism of action for individual toxins in a variety of species by different routes have many data gaps.

In terms of dose comparisons between animal studies and man, the quantitative differences assume greater importance over the qualitative differences because the database is more complete. The preferred scaling factor involves relating the dose to the species surface area, since this allometric relationship is a reflection of basal metabolic rate (Zeuthen, 1953; Freireich *et al.*, 1966; Funaki, 1974). Trans-species comparisons of toxicity have shown that surface area scaling provides the best correlation (Crump *et al.*, 1977; Crump, 1981; Davidson *et al.*, 1986), and consequently this approach has been adopted by the EPA (US EPA, 1980).

The allometric relationship between toxicity and species surface area may indeed provide an adequate, if not refined, method for cross-species predictivity. However, the literature is scattered with examples that reveal either marked underestimation or overestimation of the risks for man. Formaldehyde is an example where risk assessments based on animal data have overestimated the risks for man. The dose levels at which animal tumours were observed (Kerns *et al.*, 1983) resulted in overestimation of the risks for man (US EPA, 1987), which directly conflict with several epidemiology studies (Acheson *et al.*, 1984; Blair *et al.*, 1986). On the other hand, there are examples where epidemiology has revealed toxic effects in man at far lower levels than the animal models would predict—e.g. vinyl chloride

(Purchase, 1985) and benzene (Wong, 1987). Indeed there are several reviews which address the relative species sensitivity to specific carcinogens (Anderson and Campbell, 1985; Williams *et al.*, 1985; Dybing, 1986; Gregory, 1988), and it would appear that these conflicts (Purchase, 1980a, 1985; Brown and Paddle, 1988) are due not to quantitative differences but to metabolic or mechanistic qualitative species differences. It might then be appropriate to suggest that more metabolic and biochemically orientated investigations in species differences could result in a greater understanding of the frequent anomalies between toxicology and epidemiology study results.

Site Concordance and Predictability

Sir Richard Doll has noted that most recognized occupational cancers have been discovered as a result of clinical intuition or epidemiological observation. However, most could have been avoided if modern toxicological techniques had been employed to test the substances used before humans were exposed to them in the industrial environment (Doll, 1984). Virtually all of the chemicals that have been demonstrated to be causative agents of cancer in humans also produce cancer in a variety of animal models (Henschler, 1987). On the basis of this substantial background of evidence that human carcinogens can be revealed in animal models, it has been widely assumed that chemicals that are carcinogenic in animal models are likely to be potential cancer hazards to man. This assumption has been reinforced by instances in which chemicals have been demonstrated to be carcinogenic in animals before subsequent identification of cancer causation in humans; examples of this are vinyl chloride (Maltoni, 1977) and bis(chloromethyl) ether (Van Duuren *et al.*, 1972).

Doll (1981) commented on the agreement between carcinogenicity testing results in rats and mice for 250 chemicals reported by Purchase (1980b). The agreement between rats and mice for 83 per cent of compounds is substantially higher than would be expected by chance (50 per cent). Henschler (1987) concluded that 96 per cent of the 56 occupational carcinogens in the 1984 German MAK list were predictable by animal experiments. The only two compounds that were given as possible errors in predictability were arsenicals and benzene. It would be very comforting indeed to feel that toxicology provides such an adequate safety testing system/network to avoid epidemiologically discovered errors. However, one cannot judge a screening test in terms of its sensitivity alone. The International Agency for Research on Cancer (IARC, 1987) classified 50 chemicals and industrial processes as human carcinogens, and of these there was sufficient evidence to classify 21 as carcinogenic to both humans and experimental animals. Table 3 shows that at least 16 of these 21 agents could be considered to exhibit site concordance of tumours in test animals and humans. However, many of these agents produce tumours at several

Table 3   Site concordance between man and rat and/or mice for 21 compounds with sufficient evidence of carcinogenicity in humans and experimental animals (IARC, 1987)

Agree	Disagree	Debatable
Aflatoxins	Benzene	2-Naphthylamine[b]
4-Aminobiphenyl	Benzidine	Nickel and nickel compounds[c]
Asbestos	Melphalan[a]	
Bis(chloromethyl)ether and chloromethyl methyl ether (technical grade)		
Chlorambucil		
Chromium compounds, hexavalent		
Coal-tar pitches		
Coal-tars		
Cyclophosphamide		
Diethylstilboestrol		
Erionite		
Methoxsalen + UV-A		
Mineral oil, untreated and mildly treated		
Shale oils		
Tobacco smoke		
Vinyl chloride		

[a] Acute non-lymphocytic leukaemia in man and lymphosarcomas in rats and mice.
[b] Bladder cancer reported in one rat study.
[c] Nickel carbonyl and nickel acetate produced lung tumours in rats and mice, respectively.

sites and there is agreement in respect of only one site. Nevertheless, compounds for which tumours are induced in the animals but at sites not in accordance with the human data can generally be reasoned by virtue of differential metabolism— e.g. benzidine and 2-naphthylamine. It is apparent that human carcinogens are generally characterized by overt genetic toxicity (Shelby, 1988) and that tumour induction for genotoxins is ubiquitous trans-species.

Although it may be possible to examine the sensitivity of experimental testing in animals as an indicator of carcinogenicity in humans, it is extremely difficult to examine its specificity. IARC (1987) classify only one chemical, caprolactam, as probably not carcinogenic. Other agents are classified as having evidence suggesting lack of carcinogenicity in experimental animals, but no agent (including caprolactam) is classified as such in terms of human carcinogenicity. Thus, we cannot estimate how many times animal testing wrongly predicts carcinogenicity in humans.

SUMMARY

Utidjian (1987) provides for several compounds a comprehensive review of the ways in which epidemiology has historically interacted with animal toxicity studies. Utidjian concludes that epidemiology has started to lose its historic role as the initiating or hypothesis-generating discipline and has become a secondary tool to confirm, refute or quantify human carcinogenic effects, the animal carcinogenesis bioassay being responsible for this change in role. This is undoubtedly true to some degree, and Utidjian cites acrylonitrile, formaldehyde, ethylene oxide and acrylamide as examples where the results of animal carcinogenesis bioassays have triggered a flurry of epidemiology studies. However, cancer is not the only health effect of interest to medical investigators and regulators. For instance, Axelson *et al.* (1976) first described the syndrome now known as Organic Solvent Syndrome or 'Danish painters' disease' and a tentative association between the syndrome and chronic exposure to solvents. The report not only led to much epidemiological work, but also stimulated toxicologists to take a greater interest in neurobehavioural effects. Even in the case of carcinogenesis, the increasing interest taken by IARC in occupations and mixtures is likely to strengthen the hand of epidemiology. It is clear in the case of nickel and chromium that epidemiological evidence first indicated that certain nickel and chromium compounds must be carcinogens. However, the early studies led to much speculation as to what the specific carcinogenic agent or agents might be. Animal studies were conducted in an attempt to elucidate the situation, and the combination of evidence from the two disciplines has led to the identification of certain chromium compounds as human carcinogens, although the nickel debate continues. Epidemiology will undoubtedly continue to point the first finger of suspicion at occupations or processes that involve a mixture of compounds. The case–control study has an important role to play as a hypothesis generator and is a particularly potent research tool in the Scandinavian countries, where there exist computerized record systems linking census information and health data.

There can be little doubt that the relationship between epidemiology and toxicology should be an interaction. Although the two disciplines are methodologically very different and sometimes generate conflicting results, they should be seen as complementary. In this chapter we have tried to describe the strengths and weaknesses of each discipline and to indicate the need for co-operation between epidemiologists and toxicologists. Both share a common goal—human health protection. Toxicology in essence is animal epidemiology, and epidemiology can be viewed as an opportunistic analysis of the inadvertent exposure of humans to toxicants. Kamrin (1988) goes further when describing the different types of toxicity testing, and includes epidemiology as the fourth major study design alongside acute toxicity testing, subacute toxicity testing and chronic toxicity testing in animal experiments. The toxicologist must be prepared to recognize the greater relevance of epidemiology to assessing risks to humans, but the epidemiologist must also be prepared to acknowledge the high degree of site concordance (for overt genotoxins) and the additional number of non-concordants (but with carcinogenic activity) of the 50 known human carcinogens. Sir Richard Doll (1981), in an article on the relevance of epidemiology to policies for the prevention of cancer, concluded that '. . . no rational person would want to learn by counting dead bodies if he could possibly learn by other means how their particular causes of death could have been avoided' and 'Epidemiology may not be the method of choice for the discovery of preventative measures, as it requires some people to have been affected before it can be employed; but at present its use is essential . . .'. These remarks clearly indicate the need for both toxicologists and epidemiologists to be aware of the contributions their respective disciplines can make in assessing human health hazards.

REFERENCES

Acheson, E. D., Barnes, H. R., Gardner, M. J., Osmond, C., Pannett, B. and Taylor, C. D. (1984). Formaldehyde in the British chemical industry. *Lancet*, **1**, 611–616

Anderson, R. L. and Campbell, R. (1985). A review of the environmental and mammalian toxicology of nitrilotriacetic acid. *CRC Crit. Rev. Toxicol.*, **15**, 1–102

Axelson, O., Haue, M. and Hogstedt, C. (1976). A case-referent study on neuropsychiatric disorders among workers exposed to solvents. *Scand. J. Work Environ. Hlth*, **2**, 14–20

Ayer, H. E., Dement, J. M., Busch, K. A., Ashe, H. B., Levadie, B. T. H., Burgess, W. A. and Diberardins, L. (1973). A monumental study: reconstruction of a 1920 granite shed. *Am. Industr. Hyg. Assoc. J.*, **34**, 206–216

Blair, A., Stewart, P., O'Berg, M., Gaffey, W., Walrath, J., Ward, J., Bales, R., Kaplan, S. and Cubitt, D. (1986). Formaldehyde. *J. Natl Cancer Inst.*, **76**, 1071–1084

Botham, P. A., Davies, G. E. and Teasdale, E. L. (1987). Allergy to laboratory animals: a prospective study of its incidence and of the influence of atopy on its development. *Br. J. Industr. Med.*, **44**, 627–632

Boyle, P., Muir, C. S. and Grundmann, E. (1989). *Cancer Mapping*. Springer-Verlag, Berlin

Brown, L. P. (1990). *A Review of the Mortality and Morbidity of Pesticide Manufacturers and Applicators*. Internal report of the British Agrochemicals Association

Brown L. P. and Paddle, G. M. (1988). Risk assessment: animal or human model? *Pharm. Med.*, **3**, 361–374

Calabrese, E. J. (1986). Animal extrapolation and the challenge of human heterogeneity. *J. Pharm. Sci.*, **75**, 1041–1046

Case, R. A. M., Hosker, M. E., McDonald, D. B. and Pearson, J. T. (1954). Tumours of the urinary bladder in workmen engaged in the manufacture and use of certain dyestuff intermediates in the British chemical industry. Part 1. The role of aniline, benzidine, alpha-naphthylamine and beta-naphthylamine. *Br. J. Industr. Med.*, **11**, 75–104

Cornfield, J. (1951). A method of estimating comparative rates from clinical data. Applications to cancer
of the lung, breast and cervix. *J. Natl Cancer Inst.*,
11, 1269–1275

Cornfield, J. (1962). Joint dependence of risk of coronary heart disease on serum cholesterol and systolic
pressure: a discriminant function analysis. *Fed.
Proc.*, **2**, 58–61

Creech, J. L. and Johnson, M. N. (1974). Angiosarcoma of the liver in the manufacture of vinyl chloride. *J. Occup. Med.*, **16**, 150–151

Crump, K. S. (1981). An improved procedure for low-
dose carcinogenic risk assessment from animal data.
J. Environ. Pathol. Toxicol., **5**, 675–684

Crump, K. S., Guess, H. A. and Deal, L. L. (1977).
Confidence intervals and test of hypothesis concerning dose-response relations inferred from animal carcinogenicity data. *Biometrics*, **33**, 437–451

Davidson, I. W. F., Parker, J. C. and Beliles, R. P.
(1986). Biological basis for extrapolation across
mammalian species. *Regulatory Toxicol. Pharmacol.*, **6**, 211–237

Decker, W. J. (1987). Introduction and history. In
Haley, T. J. and Berndt, W. O. (Eds), *Toxicology*.
Hemisphere Publishing Corporation, Washington,
D.C., pp. 1–19

Dobbins, J. G. (1987). Regulation and the use of negative results from human reproductive studies: the
case of ethylene dibromide. *Am. J. Industr. Med.*,
12, 33–45

Doll. R. (1981). Relevance of epidemiology to policies
for the prevention of cancer. *J. Occup. Med.*, **23**,
601–609

Doll, R. (1984). Epidemiological discovery of occupational cancers. *Scand. J. Work Environ. Hlth*, **10**,
121–138

Doll, R. and Hill, A. B. (1950). Smoking and carcinoma of the lung. Preliminary report. *Br. Med. J.*,
iii, 739–748

Doll, R. and Hill, A. B. (1954). The mortality of doctors in relation to their smoking habits. A preliminary report. *Br. Med. J.*, **ii**, 1451–1455

Doll, R. and Peto, R. (1981). The causes of cancer:
quantitative estimates of avoidable risks of cancer in
the United States today. *J. Natl Cancer Inst.*, **66**,
1191–1308

Dybing, E. (1986). Predictability of human carcinogenicity from animal studies. *Regulatory Toxicol. Pharmacol.*, **6**, 399–415

Feinstein, A. R. (1988). Scientific standards in epidemiologic studies of the menace of daily life. *Science*,
242, 1257–1263

Finnegan, M. J., Pickering, C. A. C. and Burge, P.
S. (1984). The sick building syndrome: prevalence
studies. *Br. Med. J.*, **289**, 1573–1575

Freireich, E. J., Gehan, E. A., Rall, D. P., Schmidt,
L. H. and Skipper, H. E. (1966). Quantitative comparison of toxicity of anticancer agents in the mouse,

rat, hamster, dog, monkey and man. *Cancer Chemother. Rep.*, **50**, 219–244

Friess, S. L. (1987). History of risk assessment. In
Rohlich, G. (Ed.) *Pharmokinetics in Risk Assess-
ment. Drinking Water and Health*, Vol. 8. National
Academy of Science, Washington, D.C., pp. 3–7

Funaki, H. (1974). Drug toxicity (LD50) and dosis
medicamentosa for children in terms of body surface
area and body weight (preliminary report). *J. Kyoto
Pref. Univ. Med.*, **83**, 467–477

Gardner, M. J., Winter, P. D. and Barker, D. J. P.
(1984). *Atlas of Mortality from Selected Diseases in
England and Wales 1968–78.* Wiley, Chichester

Glocklin, V. C. (1987). Current FDA perspective on
animal selection and extrapolation. In Roloff, M. V.
(Ed.), *Human Risk Assessment: The Role of Animal
Selection and Extrapolation*. Taylor and Francis,
London, pp. 15–22

Goldberg, D. (1972). *The Detection of Psychiatric Illness by Questionnaire*. Maudsley Monograph,
London

Goudie, R. B., Jack, A. S. and Goudie, B. M. (1985).
Genetic and developmental aspects of pathological
pigmentation patterns. *Curr. Top. Pathol.*, **74**,
132–138

Greenland, S. (Ed.) (1987). *Evolution of Epidemiologic Ideas: Annotated Readings on Concepts and
Methods*. Epidemiology Resources Inc., Chapel Hill

Gregory, A. R. (1988). Species comparisons in evaluating carcinogenicity in humans. *Regulatory Toxicol.
Pharmacol.*, **8**, 160–190

Henschler, D. (1987). Risk assessment and evaluation
of chemical carcinogens—present and future
strategies. *J. Cancer Res. Clin. Oncol.*, **113**, 1–7

IARC (1987). *Evaluation of Carcinogenic Risks to
Humans. Overall Evaluations of Carcinogenicity: An
Updating of IARC Monographs Vols 1–42.* IARC,
Lyon (IARC Monographs, Supplement 7)

Kallen, B. (1988). *Epidemiology of Human Reproduction*, CRC Press, Boca Raton, Florida

Kamrin, M. A. (1988). *Toxicology*, Lewis Publishers,
Chelsea, Michigan

Kerns, W. D., Pavkov, K. L., Donofrio, D. J., Gralla,
E. J. and Swenberg, J. A. (1983). Carcinogenicity
of formaldehyde in rats and mice after long term
inhalation exposure. *Cancer Res.*, **43**, 4382–4392

Levine, R. J., Symons, M. J., Baloch, S. A., Arndt,
D. M., Kaswandik, N. T. and Gentile, J. W. (1980).
A method for monitoring the fertility of workers. *J.
Occup. Med.*, **32**, 781–791

Lilienfeld, A. M. and Lilienfeld, D. E. (1977). What
else is new? An historical excursion. *Am. J. Epidemiol.*, **105**, 169–179

McMahon, B. and Pugh, T. F. (1970). *Epidemiology,
Principles and Methods*. Little, Brown, Boston

Maltoni, C. (1977). Vinyl chloride carcinogenicity: an
experimental model for carcinogenesis studies. In
Hiatt, H. H., Watson, J. D. and Winsten, J. A.

(Eds), *Origins of Human Cancer*. Cold Spring Harbor Laboratory, New York, pp. 119–146

Medical Research Council (1976). *Questionnaire on Respiratory Symptoms and Instructions for Its Use*. MRC, London

Medical Research Council Environmental Epidemiology Unit (1984). *Expected Numbers in Cohort Studies*. MRC, Southampton (Scientific Report No. 6)

Newell, D. J. (1984). Present position and potential developments: some personal views. Medical statistics. *J. R. Statist. Soc. A*, **147**, 186–197

OPCS (1986). *Occupational Mortality 1979–80, 82–83*. HMSO, London

Paddle, G. M. (1981). A strategy for the identification of carcinogens in a large, complex chemical company. In Peto, R. and Schneiderman, M. (Eds), *Quantification of Occupational Cancer: Banbury Report 9*. Cold Spring Harbor Laboratory, New York, pp. 177–186

Paddle, G. M. (1988). Epidemiology. In Anderson, D. and Conning, D. M. (Eds), *Experimental Toxicology: The Basic Principles*. Royal Society of Chemistry, London, pp. 436–456

Pell, S., O'Berg, M. and Karrh, B. (1978). Cancer epidemiologic surveillance in the Du Pont company. *J. Occup. Med.*, **20**, 725–740

Peto, R., Pike, M. C., Day, N. E., Gray, R. G., Lee, P. N., Parish, S., Peto, J., Richards, S. and Wahrendorf, J. (1980). Guidelines for simple, sensitive significance tests for carcinogenic effects in long-term animal experiments. *IARC Monogr. Eval. Carcinog. Risk Chem. Man*, Suppl. 2, 311–426. International Association for Research on Cancer, Lyon

Poole, C. (1986). Exposure opportunity in case-control studies. *Am. J. Epidemiol.*, **123**, 352–358

Purchase, I. F. H. (1980a). Range of experimental evidence in assessing potential human carcinogenicity. *Arch. Toxicol.*, Suppl. 3, 283–293

Purchase, I. F. H. (1980b). Validation of tests for carcinogenicity. *IARC Sci. Publ.*, **27**, 343–349

Purchase, I. F. H. (1985). Carcinogenic risk assessment: a toxicologist's view. In Hoel, D. G. (Ed.), *Risk Quantitation and Regulatory Policy: Banbury Report 19*. Cold Spring Harbor Laboratory, New York, pp. 175–186

Ramazzini, B. (1964). *De Morbis Artificum Diatriba (Diseases of Workers)*. Translated from the Latin text of 1713 by Wright, W. C. Hafner, New York

Robinson, D. W. (1987). *Noise Exposure and Hearing: A New Look at the Experimental Data*. Health and Safety Executive, London (HSE Contract Research Report 1/1987)

Rose, G. A., Blackburn, H., Gillum, R. A. and Pricas, R. J. (1982). *Cardiovascular Survey Methods*, 2nd edn. WHO, Geneva (Monograph Series No. 56)

Rothman, K. J. (1986). *Modern Epidemiology*. Little, Brown, Boston

Schlesselman, J. J. (1982). *Case-Control Studies: Design, Conduct, Analysis*. Oxford University Press, New York

Schlesselman, J. J. and Stadel, B. V. (1987). Exposure opportunity in epidemiologic studies. *Am. J. Epidemiol.*, **125**, 174–178

Shelby, M. D. (1988). The genetic toxicity of human carcinogens and its implications. *Mutat. Res.*, **204**, 3–15

Smith, A. H. (1988). Epidemiologic input to environmental risk assessment. *Arch. Environ. Hlth*, **43**, 124–127

US Environmental Protection Agency (1980). Guidelines and methodology used in the preparation of health effects assessment chapters of the consent decree water quality criteria. *Federal Register*, **45**, 79347–79357

US Environmental Protection Agency (1987). *Environmental Protection Agency Assessment of Health Risks to Garment Workers and Certain Home Residents from Exposure to Formaldehyde*. Office of Pesticides and Toxic Substances, Washington, D.C.

Utidjian, H. M. D. (1987). The interaction between epidemiology and animal studies in industrial toxicology. In Ballantyne, B. (Ed.), *Perspectives in Basic and Applied Toxicology*. John Wright, Bristol, pp. 309–329

Van Duuren, B. L., Katz, C., Goldschmidt, B. M., Frenkel, K. and Sivak, A. (1972). Carcinogenicity of halo-ethers. II. Structure-activity relationships of analogs of bis(chloromethyl) ether. *J. Natl Cancer Inst.*, **48**, 1431–1439

Waterhouse, J. A. H., Muir, C. J., Shanmugaratnam, K. and Powell, J. (Eds) (1982). *Cancer Incidence in Five Continents*, Vol. IV. International Agency for Research on Cancer, Lyon (IARC Scientific Publication No. 42)

Weed, D. L. (1986). Historical roots of the healthy worker effect. *J. Occup. Med.*, **28**, 343–347

Wegman, D. H. and Eisen, E. A. (1988). Epidemiology. In Levy, B. S. and Wegman, D. H. (Eds), *Occupational Health. Recognizing and Preventing Work-related Disease*. Little Brown, Boston, pp. 55–73

Williams, G. M., Reiss, B. and Weisburger, J. H. (1985). A comparison of the animal and human carcinogenicity of environmental, occupational and therapeutic chemicals. In Flamm, W. G. and Lorentzen, R. J. (Eds), *Mechanisms and Toxicity of Chemical Carcinogens and Mutagens*. Princeton Scientific Publishing, Princeton, N.J., pp. 207–248

Wong, O. (1987). An industry wide study of chemical workers occupationally exposed to benzene. II. Dose response analyses. *Br. J. Industr. Med.*, **44**, 348–395

World Health Organization (1983). *Guidelines on Studies in Environmental Epidemiology*. WHO, Geneva (Environmental Health Criteria Series No. 27)

World Health Organization (1985). *Neurobehavioural Methods in Occupational and Environmental Health*. WHO, Copenhagen

Zapp, J. A. (1981). Industrial toxicology, retrospective and prospect. In Clayton, G. D. and Clayton, F. E. (Eds), *Patty's Industrial Hygiene and Toxicology*, Vol. 2A, 3rd edn. Wiley, Chichester, pp. 1197–1219

Zeuthen, E. (1953). Oxygen uptake as related to body size in organisms. *Q. Rev. Biol.*, **28**, 1–11

FURTHER READING

Checkoway, H., Pearce, N. E. and Crawford-Brown, D. J. (1989). *Research Methods in Occupational Epidemiology*. Oxford University Press

Monson, R. R. (1990). *Occupational Epidemiology*. 2nd edn. CRC Press, Boca Raton, Florida

Sackett, D. L., Haynes, R. B., Guyatt, G. H. and Tugwell, P. (1991). *Clinical Epidemiology*. Little, Brown and Company, Boston

World Health Organization (1986). Epidemiology of occupational health. *WHO Regional Publications, Euoropean Series No. 20*. World Health Organization, Geneva

47 Forensic Toxicology: A Broad Overview of General Principles

Ronald C. Backer

Toxicology is the study of poisons and how they impact on biological systems. As a science, toxicology is concerned with the physical and chemical properties of toxic substances, their physiological and clinical effects, and their qualitative and quantitative methods of analysis in biological and nonbiological materials (Poklis, 1980). Methods of treatment for poisoning, including the development of specific antidotes, are also an important aspect of toxicology. The American Board of Forensic Toxicology defines forensic toxicology as the application of toxicology for the purposes of the law. When forensic is used as an adjective it means 'pertaining to the courts of justice' or 'to the administration of justice'. Therefore, forensic toxicology literally means the study of the effects of poisons for the administration of justice.

THE TOXICOLOGY PROCESS

Toxicology plays an important part in the medicolegal investigation of death. It answers the question of whether alcohol, other drugs and or chemical poisons were the cause or a contributory cause of the death. The laboratory can analyse biological specimens including blood, urine, vitreous, bile, tissues (liver, brain, kidney, spleen) and non-biologicals such as pills, air samples and clothing for many toxicants.

Once the laboratory has determined the absence or presence of a drug or chemical toxicant, the toxicologist will give an opinion as to whether the findings are significant and how they may have been related to the death. As drug effects may differ from individual to individual and depend on many factors [health status of an individual, age, sex, combinations of drugs detected, quantity of drug taken, manner of dosing (oral, inhalation, injection) and rate of consumption], interpretation is a difficult and complex task based on knowledge and experience.

FOUNDATIONS OF TOXICOLOGY

Knowledge about poisons existed as long ago as the ancient writings of the Egyptians which made reference to poisons from plants. A passage from an ancient papyrus has been translated as 'Speak not of the name of Yao under penalty of the peach', indicating knowledge of a poison (hydrocyanic acid) in parts of the peach tree or fruit (Gettler, 1956). The papyrus Ebers from 1500 BC also mentions antimony, copper, hyoscyamus, lead and opium as poisons. Writings from India during the period 600 to 100 BC mention poisons including gold, copper, iron, lead, silver and tin. Socrates was executed in 339 BC with an extract of hemlock. A book entitled *The History of Plants* published in 300 BC by Theophrastus refers to medicinal and poisonous plants.

Numerous poisonings have been recorded in the history of the first 1800 years after Christ. Nine of the successors of Charlemagne (Holy Roman Empire) died before the 1400s of poisonings. Famous poisonings included five popes, many cardinals, and several kings. It became commonplace for kings to have 'tasters' of their food. In 1552 Nux Vomica (strychnine) was described.

Many poisonings occurred in England, France and Italy during the 16th and 17th Centuries. Spara in the 1650s was the leader of a secret poisoning society in Rome. In the 1700s Madame Toffana of Naples poisoned over 600 victims with white arsenic. The poisons most frequently used in this period were hemlock, aconite, opium, arsenic and corrosive sublimate (mercury).

Up until the late 1700s convictions of perpetrators of homicidal poisonings were based on circumstantial evidence. In 1781, Joseph Plenic stated that the detection and identification of the poison in the organs of the deceased was the only true sign of poisoning.

Mathiew J. B. Orfila (1787–1853) was a Spanish chemist who became a professor of legal medicine at the University of Paris. He published the first complete work of international importance on the subject of poisons and legal medicine in 1813. The publication was entitled: *Traité des Poisons Tirés des Règnes Mineral Vegetal et Animal, ou Toxicologie Générale*. Orfila is considered the 'Father of Toxicology'. He identified several different disciplines of toxicology including pharmaceutical, clinical, industrial and environmental. He established many of the guiding principles of toxicology including the need for adequate proof of identity and quality assurances. These principles still hold true today. They are:

(1) Experience is paramount for credibility and reliability.

(2) All facts surrounding the case must be given to the analysts.

(3) All the evidence must be submitted properly identified and labelled and sealed.

(4) All tests should be run and properly recorded.

(5) Reagents must be pure, blank tests must be run.

(6) All tests should be repeated and compared to spiked knowns.

Devising analytical methods for the determination of poisons in human organs was one of Orfila's most important accomplishments. In 1839, Orfila extracted arsenic from human tissues using a procedure for identification developed several years before by James Marsh. This evidence was used in court (1840) to convict Marie Lafarge of a homicidal poisoning. This was the first time toxicological data had been used as evidence in a trial. He was also the instructor of Robert Christison (1779–1882), a British physician who returned to Great Britain after his education. Christison became a professor of legal medicine at the University of Edinburgh and is considered the first British toxicologist. In 1829, he wrote the text *Treatise on Poisons* which was introduced into the USA in 1845.

Some of the major events that led to the development of chemical toxicology (Gettler, 1956), were:

- In 1836, the development of a test for arsenic by James M. Marsh.
- In 1839, Orfila successfully applied the Marsh test to identify arsenic extracted from liver, kidneys, spleen, muscle and heart.

- In 1844, Freenius and von Babo developed a procedure for the systematic search for all mineral poisons. The procedure used wet ashing with chlorine.
- In 1850, Stas developed a procedure for the extraction of nicotine from human tissues. The method was modified in 1856 by Otto to give purer extracts of alkaloids. This modified procedure is commonly called the Stas–Otto Method.
- In 1874, Salami proved that decomposition can create artefacts and that extreme caution must be used in identification of poisons after death.

During the period from the 1830s to the early 1900s, analysis of tissue from human organs for toxicants still remained extremely rare. Most analyses were performed on gastric contents. Likewise, most tests were only performed in a qualitative manner. However, as more procedures were developed using 'wet ashing' and the Stas–Otto technique some quantitative procedures also began to appear. Quantitative methods for alcohol were introduced in 1852 by Cotte based on the reduction of chromic acid. Electrolytic deposition techniques for metals were first used in 1862. In 1879, a method for the quantitation of arsenic was devised by Gutzeit. A quantitative procedure for carbon monoxide using palladium chloride reduction was introduced in 1880 by Fodor. Quantitative methods for alkaloids were introduced in 1890.

In 1918, New York replaced its coroners' system with the Medical Examiner's Office after members of the New York Academy of Medicine demonstrated that the medicolegal investigations carried out by politically-appointed coroners were not adequate to protect the public's interest. A toxicology laboratory was established immediately. The chief forensic toxicologist of this laboratory was Alexander O. Gettler, the 'Father of American Toxicology'. During the first 30 years of the laboratory, the only analytical instruments were a Duboscq colorimeter, an analytical balance, a pH meter, a filter photometer, and a van Slyke manometric gas analysis apparatus. Despite the lack of the existence of more sophisticated analytical equipment, the laboratory was able to analyse biologicals for alcohol, cyanide, fluoride, carbon monoxide poisonings, thallium, and the micro-isolation of volatile toxic substances from tissue.

In 1935, Dr Gettler instituted a graduate course in toxicology at New York University (NYU) Graduate School. He trained many renowned toxicologists over the years including H. C. Freimuth, C. J. Umberger, I. Ellerbrook, A. Stolman, F. Rieders, J. O. Baine, S. Kaye, I. Sunshine, L. Goldbaum, A. Freireich, M. Feldstein and H. Schwartz.

PROFESSIONAL ORGANIZATIONS, CERTIFICATION, AND INSTRUMENTATION

In 1949 the American Academy of Forensic Sciences was formed to promote the practice of the forensic sciences, including forensic toxicology. Since that time several other organizations have been formed which have only forensic toxicologists as members. Two such organizations are the International Association of Forensic Toxicologists (1963) and the Society of Forensic Toxicologists (1970).

The three decades from 1960 to 1990 has seen an astronomical growth in technology applied to the science of forensic toxicology. Sophisticated instrumentation including thin-layer chromatography, spectophotometry, gas chromatography, immunoassays, mass spectrometry and high-pressure liquid chromatography have all been applied successfully to analyses in the area of forensic toxicology. These analytical techniques will be discussed below (pp. 1085–1090).

Until the early 1980s forensic toxicology was primarily concerned with medical examiners' cases and blood alcohol concentrations (BACs) in driving under the influence (DUI) cases. However, with the advent of testing for drugs in the armed services and the workplace, the birth of a new area of forensic toxicology occurred, Forensic Urine Drug Testing (FUDT). The demand for 'certified' forensic toxicologists to direct 'certified forensic urine drug testing laboratories' has caused a shortage of 'Board Certified Forensic Toxicologists' in the US. Toxicology certification is available from several sources including the American Board of Forensic Toxicology and the American Association of Clinical Chemists. In other countries similar qualifications are available, e.g. the Diploma in Forensic Pathology of the Royal College of Pathologists in the UK. Another new frontier in the 1980s for forensic toxicologists has been the testing for driving under the influence of drugs other than alcohol (DUID). This chapter will focus on traditional post-mortem forensic toxicology.

THE FORENSIC LABORATORY

The forensic toxicology laboratory is responsible for demonstrating the absence or presence of chemical substances in biological and non-biological specimens in connection with medicolegal investigations. The laboratory must be capable of analysing a wide variety of toxic substances. Alcohol, antidepressants, barbiturates, benzodiazepines (minor tranquillizers), carbon monoxide, chlorinated hydrocarbons, cocaine, heavy metals (arsenic, antimony, bismuth and mercury), insecticides, lead, opium alkaloids, non-barbiturate sedative hypnotics, phenothiazines, and stimulants are among the most frequently encountered substances in the forensic laboratory.

The toxicology laboratory is responsible for the handling of evidence and must maintain a proper chain of evidence with receipts or records for the transfer and storage of materials to be analysed. The specimens should be properly refrigerated until transported to the laboratory. Specimens must be delivered to the laboratory with proper identification of the specimen affixed to each container. The information on the container label should include the name of the deceased, the case number, date of sampling and the type of sample (Figure 1). When the specimens are delivered to the laboratory, they must be accompanied by a proper transmittal form that shows the name,

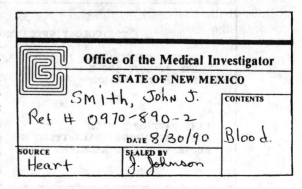

Figure 1 Label for specimen container

case number, date and types of specimens being transmitted (Figure 2). Any discrepancies in the form and the samples should be noted on the transmittal form and signed and dated by the receiving person in the laboratory and the person making the delivery. Additional documentation includes: a laboratory work sheet (Figure 3) and a report form (Figure 4).

Specimen Storage

Ideally, storage capacity should be adequate to store all specimens indefinitely. This idea is impractical because storage space is usually limited. A written policy must be established concerning disposal of samples. The policy should include the effective date of the policy, the length of time specimens will be held and a mechanism by which a request can be made for an extension of storage. Figure 5 is an example of a form to request extended specimen storage. A reasonable length of storage is 2 years; this will allow for adjudication of most court proceedings, both criminal and civil.

Specimens are usually kept refrigerated (4 °C) during the time they are being analysed (short-term storage) and then in a freezer (−10 °C) until disposed of (long-term storage). It has been calculated that approximately 0.85 cubic metres of freezer space is required to store the specimens from 500 cases (Backer, 1981).

THE FORENSIC TOXICOLOGIST

The role of the forensic toxicologist in the forensic investigations is to determine whether various toxicants were present or absent in the specimens submitted to the laboratory. He must be a first-rate analytical chemist and be knowledgeable about the effects of poisons. He must know the 'older' techniques in addition to the newly evolving ones.

The major responsibilities of the forensic toxicologist include: on-the-scene investigation, preservation of chains of evidence (external and internal), oral and written reports, consultation (pathologist, police, attorneys), expert testimony, research and development, education (self and others) and above all the ability to interpret the meaning of the concentration of the toxicant. The absence of a particular toxicant may be as important to a particular case as the detection of the substance in lethal concentrations. For example, finding subtherapeutic concentrations of anti-epileptic drugs is important in convulsion-related deaths. The presence of low concentrations of carboxyhaemoglobin in a suspected fire death always raises questions about the actual cause of death.

The forensic toxicologist is responsible for all the results that are reported by the laboratory. He must be familiar with all the procedures used by the laboratory and capable of developing new methods when they are needed. He must recognize that all laboratories have analytical limitations and be knowledgeable of when and where outside sources should be utilized.

The forensic toxicologist must have the proper educational background and professional experience necessary to interpret the laboratory's results. He must be knowledgeable of the specificity and sensitivity of the equipment and procedures utilized in the analyses. The forensic toxicologist must be capable of defending the results in judicial proceedings to a reasonable degree of

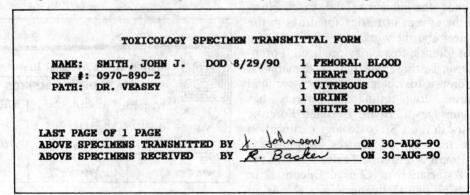

Figure 2   Form for specimen transmittal

```
                    TOXICOLOGY WORK SHEET


   NAME - SMITH, JOHN J.          DATE OF DEATH- 8/29/90

   MEDICAL EXAMINER - S. PEASEY, M.D.    DATE OF REQUEST-8/30/90

   REF# - 0970-890-2              DECOMPOSED -NO

   BRIEF HISTORY - FOUND WITH WHITE POWDER, RAZOR BLADE, AND
                   STRAW AT SCENE; SUSPECT COCAINE OVERDOSE


   SPECIMENS                 TEST

   BLOOD (HEART  ) - 1       ALCOHOL -_X_
   BLOOD (FEMORAL) - 1       UR DRUG -_X_
   BLOOD (      ) -          BL DRUG -_X_
   URINE          - 1        OTHER (specify)
   BILE           -          ANALYZE UNKNOWN WHITE POWDER
   VITREOUS       - 1
   KIDNEY         -
   BRAIN          -
   OTHER (      ) -



   RESULTS:

   ANALYSTS    DATE              TEST
   J. Robb     8/3/90    Ht Bld Alc 43.42 mmol/L
   R. Backer   9-1-90    fem bld Alc 41.25 mmol/L
   R. Backer   9-1-90    White Powder Coc-pos GC/ms
   R. Backer   9-2-90    Ht Bld Coc - 19.80 μMol/L GC/ms
   R. Backer   9-2-90    fem Bld Coc  14.85 μMol/L GC/ms
   R. Backer   9-2-90    DAS urine coc present - all others-
                         None detected
```

Figure 3 Laboratory work sheet

medical and scientific certainty. His reputation will be reinforced by his work record, evidence of professional growth through peer reviewed publications, presentations at professional meetings, membership of professional societies, and 'Board Certifications' in the USA, and equivalent in other countries.

One must always remember that the most important criteria in the interpretation of results are the circumstances surrounding the death. In the case of a low carboxyhaemoglobin in the above mentioned example, it would be important to know if the fire victim had been given oxygen or had been doused with petrol (gasoline). In either of these circumstances the carboxyhaemoglobin might be less than 10 per cent of total hae-

moglobin. Another example in which the toxicology results help to complete the circumstances is as follows: a person was last seen alive 6 hours prior to his body being found with a gunshot wound to the back of his head. When last seen he was sharing a marijuana joint with his friend. Analysis of the blood of the deceased revealed a concentration of 60 ng ml^{-1} of delta-9-THC and 100 ng ml^{-1} of THC-acid. This result would indicate that the person had died less than 1–2 hours after smoking the marijuana cigarette. This type of information aids in the investigation and helps to narrow the time of death estimation.

Even in cases where circumstances make the cause of death obvious the laboratory may be able to solve some questions such as was the

0970-890-2

Smith, John J.
2224 Saxton Court
Albuquerque, New Mexico

Age 49   Sex M   Race Anglo

TOXICOLOGY REPORT
OFFICE OF THE MEDICAL INVESTIGATOR
STATE OF NEW MEXICO
University of New Mexico, School of Medicine
Albuquerque, New Mexico 87131

Toxicology Bureau   8/30/90
Received by_____   Date_____

SPECIMEN:

1 Femoral Blood   1 Heart Blood
1 Vitreous   1 Urine
1 White Powder

EXAMINATION REQUESTED:

x Alcohol   x Drugs of Abuse   x Identify White Powder

RESULTS:

Alcohol, Heart Blood, GLC
Ethanol 43.42 mmol/L

Alcohol, Femoral Blood, GLC
Ethanol 41.25 mmol/L

Drugs of Abuse, Urine, EIA
Cocaine: Present (parent and metabolites)
No other drugs detected

Basic Drug Screen, Heart Blood, GC/MS
Cocaine 19.8 umol/L; Benzoylecgonine – present
No other drugs detected

Basic Drug Screen, Femoral Blood, GC/MS
Cocaine 14.85 umol/L; Benzoylecgonine – present
No other drugs detected

X Final Report	Amended Report	Laboratory No. 0970-890-2
REQUESTED BY S. Peasey, M.D.	REVIEWED 9/9/90 RCB	SIGNATURE OF TOXICOLOGIST *Ronald C. Backer, Ph.D.* DATE 9/11/90

UNM · OMI · 010   Distribution: White · Case File; Canary · District Medical Investigator;

Figure 4   Toxicology report sheet

Office of the Medical Investigator
STATE OF NEW MEXICO

University of New Mexico
School of Medicine
Albuquerque, New Mexico 87131
(505) 277-3053

REQUEST FOR EXTENDED SPECIMEN STORAGE

DATE _____

NAME OF REQUESTOR _____

AGENCY AND MAILING ADDRESS _____

NAME OF DECEASED _____ COUNTY OF DEATH ____

DATE OF DEATH _____ OMI CASE # _____

REASON FOR REQUEST _____

I am aware that if a written confirmation of this request is
not received within two weeks that it is my responsibility to
call the Office of the Chief Forensic Toxicologist and
confirm that the request has been received.

_____
Name of Requestor

Mail to: Chief Forensic Toxicologist
Office of the Medical Investigator
University of New Mexico
School of Medicine
Albuquerque, NM 87120

Figure 5 Request form for extended storage

homicide drug-related; was the deceased sexually molested (acid phosphatase); did the person jump out the window because he was 'high' on some type of drug (PCP, LSD, etc.).

SPECIMENS

As the autopsy usually occurs before the investigation into circumstances surrounding the case is final, it is important to obtain adequate types and volumes of specimens at the time of the autopsy (Table 1). The specimens collected in a specific medical examiner's case may differ depending on the circumstances. However, in all medicolegal investigation cases a blood specimen should be obtained when blood is available. The analysis of a post-mortem specimen is only as reliable as the

Table 1 Typical samples for toxicological analysis

Type	Quantity	Analysis
Blood (heart, femoral)*	20 ml	Volatiles, drugs
Urine	20 ml	Drugs, heavy metals
Bile	20 ml	Narcotics, other drugs
Kidney	entire	In absence of urine
Liver	20 g	Many drugs
Gastric contents	Total	Drugs taken orally
Vitreous humor	Both eyes	Alcohol, glucose, drugs and electrolytes

* Should contain preservative—sodium fluoride 10 mg ml^{-1}

conditions surrounding its collection (Plueckhahn, 1968). Proper collection of specimens often requires the addition of preservatives and/or enzyme poisons to protect the specimen from post-mortem changes, such as bacterial production of ethanol or other alcohols or their loss. A commonly employed agent for this purpose is sodium fluoride at a concentration of at least 10 mg ml^{-1} of specimen.

Traditionally heart blood has been collected at autopsy. However, recent studies have shown with drugs like propoxyphene, tricyclic antidepressants (amitriptyline, imipramine, doxepin, etc.) and many others that heart blood concentrations can increase post-mortem (Andrenyak and Backer, 1988; Bandt, 1981; Jones, 1986; Prouty and Anderson, 1984, 1990). Some reports show a relationship between post-mortem interval (time from death to autopsy) and concentration increase (Bandt, 1981; Jones, 1986; Prouty and Anderson, 1984, 1990). This concentration difference in heart blood and other peripheral sites is referred to as 'anatomical site concentration differences' or 'post-mortem redistribution'. A list of some of the drugs in which anatomical site concentration differences have been shown can be found in Table 2. Peripheral blood concentrations have been shown to be more reliable with these drugs when compared with peri-mortem concentrations (Andrenyak and Backer, 1988; Apple and Bandt, 1988; Prouty and Anderson, 1984, 1990). Therefore, in all suspected drug overdoses or in cases of unknown causes of death a femoral blood specimen should be collected and analysed.

It is also of interest that some drugs even within the same specimen do not show an increase while others do. Table 3 shows the analytical data from

Table 2 Drugs shown to have significant anatomical site concentration differences

Alprazolam	Maprotiline
Amantadine	Methamphetamine
Amitriptyline	Metoprodol
Amoxapine	Nordoxepin
Amphetamine	Norfluoxetine
Brompheniramine	Norpethidine
Caffeine	Norpropoxyphene
Chlordiazepoxide	Nortriptyline
Chlorpheniramine	Pethidine
Cocaine	Phencyclidine
Desipramine	Propoxyphene
Diphenhydramine	Propranolol
Doxepin	Thioridazine
Doxylamine	Trimipramine
Fluoxetine	Verapamil
Imipramine	

Table 3 Case data showing heart and femoral concentrations in a multiple drug overdose

Specimen	Carisoprodol	Propoxyphene
Heart blood	31.1 µmol l^{-1}	11.22 µmol l^{-1}
Femoral blood	30.3 µmol l^{-1}	5.54 µmol l^{-1}

an actual post-mortem case study with multiple drugs, carisoprodol and propoxyphene. The carisoprodol heart/femoral concentration ratio (H/F) was 1.02 and the propoxyphene H/F was 2.03. Other authors have proposed that drug concentrations in liver specimens are a better indicator of toxicity (Apple and Bandt, 1988; Prouty and Anderson, 1990; Roetlger, 1990).

Some studies have reported that heart blood alcohol concentrations also change during the post-mortem interval (Bowden and McCallum, 1949; Turkle and Gifford, 1957; Briglia et al., 1986). The authors of these studies recommend that femoral blood specimens be used for alcohol determinations in post-mortem cases. In several other studies it has been shown that heart blood concentrations of alcohol did not change post mortem in intact bodies and that concentration differences of ethanol in heart and femoral blood are minor and more likely represent the expected differences seen in the absorptive phases of alcohol consumption (Plueckhahn, 1968; Backer et al., 1980; Prouty and Anderson, 1984). However, in cases where bacterial infiltration of the body is likely a femoral specimen is recommended.

PROCEDURAL APPROACH

The particular approach that a laboratory takes for testing biological specimens is dictated by the type of services it provides. Therefore, a laboratory serving a hospital emergency room will be interested in rapid turnaround times for the common drugs of abuse. Laboratories testing for chemical substances to determine the cause of death typically utilize a large variety of different types of tests including screening tests, chromatographic methods (spectrophotometric, thin-layer, gas, mass spectrometry, high-pressure liquid chromatography) and immunoassays. The post-mortem forensic laboratory must be prepared to analyse for a number of commonly encountered analytes. Table 4 gives a list of frequently

Table 4 Frequently encountered substances in post-mortem cases

A. Gases and volatiles
    Alcohols, chlorinated hydrocarbons, aromatic
    hydrocarbons, carbon monoxide, cyanide

B. Acids
    Barbiturates, salicylates, paracetamol
    (acetaminophen)

C. Neutrals
    Glutethimide, ethchlorvynol, meprobamate,
    carisoprodol

D. Bases
    Cocaine, propoxyphene, opium alkaloids,
    antidepressants, benzodiazepines

E. Metals   Arsenic, mercury

encountered substances which a post-mortem toxicology laboratory should be capable of screening and quantitating. The following section describes some of the commonly employed types of tests and their general applications.

TYPES OF TESTING

Colorimetric Screening Test

Screening tests are usually performed directly on biological specimens with little or no sample preparation (Widdop, 1986). Some of the most common substances tested for include phenothiazines, imipramine, desipramine, trimipramine, halogenated compounds, salicylates, paracetamol (acetaminophen), ethchlorvynol (Finkle and Bath, 1971) and heavy metals (Gettler and Kaye, 1950). These tests are rapid and informative but only presumptive. As many of them only identify a class of compounds, they usually require further identification of the specific toxicant and confirmation.

Steam Distillation

Volatile substances can be separated from blood, urine or tissue homogenates by steam distillation. The specimen is made either acidic with hydrochloric acid or basic with solid magnesium oxide. Steam is passed into the solution and the aqueous distillate collected by condensation. Analytes distillable from acidic solutions include ethanol, methanol, phenols, halogenated hydrocarbons,

cyanide and ethchlorvynol. Distillates from basic solutions will contain volatile basic drugs such as amphetamines, meperidine, methadone and nicotine. The distillates can then be analysed by various techniques including colorimetric tests, immunoassays, spectroscopy and various chromatographic methods including thin-layer, gas and liquid chromatography.

Microdiffusion

Microdiffusion is a convenient, rapid separation technique that allows for the analyte to be either detected as it is isolated (alcohols, carbon monoxide) or to be captured in an appropriate medium and tested by various techniques (cyanide, methanol, phenols, chlorinated hydrocarbons, sulphides). The technique of isolation utilizes a Conway microdiffusion dish (Figure 6). A comprehensive review of microdiffusion applications has been described in the literature (Feldstein and Klendshoj, 1957). A microdiffusion method for ethchlorvynol has also been described (Peel and Freimuth, 1972).

Spectroscopy

Spectroscopy is based on the principle that substances either gain or lose energy when subjected to electromagnetic radiation. Identification of the substance may be possible by noting the wavelengths at which the energy change takes place. The energy changes are proportional to the quantity of the analyte present and therefore the method can also be used for quantitation. The common types of spectroscopy utilized in the forensic laboratory include visible, ultraviolet, fluorometry, atomic absorption and infrared.

Chromatography

Chromatography is a separation technique utilizing a partitioning process. Mixtures of drugs and their metabolites are commonly separated by chromatography. Chromatography requires a stationary or fixed phase, which may be a liquid or solid absorbed on an inert support having a large surface area, and a moving or mobile phase of a liquid or gas. In a chromatographic method, analytes within a mixture are moved by the mobile phase while the different interactions of the individual analytes with the stationary phase

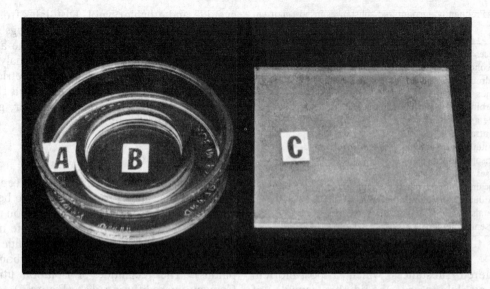

Figure 6 Conway microdiffusion dish. The separation dish, on the left, contains an outer (A) and an inner (B) chamber separated by an annular wall. Sample and reacting agents are placed in the outer compartment, and solution to absorb released vapour placed in the central compartment. A ground glass plate (C) is placed over the dish to seal it. Since the height of the annular wall is less than that of the outer wall, there is a space between the annular wall and the sealing plate which allows diffusion of vapour, released during the reaction, to pass into the absorption compartment.

cause separation from other components. After separation the components are identified by various means including colorimetric, electrolytic, and/or spectrophotometric.

Most chromatographic techniques require an extraction of the specimen before analysis. The extent of the 'clean-up' prior to chromatography depends on many variables including the nature of the matrix, the concentration of the analyte of interest and the type of chromatography. Liquid–liquid extraction is one of the most common separation techniques. Other types of extraction techniques commonly employed include liquid–solid such as charcoal, and solid phase extractions.

Thin-Layer Chromatography (TLC)

This is a rather simple separation technique which does not require a lot of expensive equipment. An extract of a biological specimen is applied as a concentrated spot at the origin of a TLC plate. The plate is placed in a developing tank with just enough solvent to submerge the bottom 1–1.5 cm. As the solvent (mobile phase) moves up the plate by capillary action, drugs and their metabolites are separated depending on the polarity of the solvent system and the solubility characteristics of the compounds in the extract. Visualization is accomplished with colour reagents and long- and

short-wave ultraviolet light. The distance the compound travelled from the origin divided by the distance the solvent travelled from the origin is called the R_f or migration value. The R_f value along with the colour reactions are used for qualitative and semi-quantitative results.

In general, TLC is a fairly sensitive technique. The specificity of TLC can be increased by using multiple chromatogenic sprays. Most spray reagents are non-destructive and the analytes can be removed and tested by other analytical techniques. The major disadvantages of TLC include the need for extraction prior to analysis and that the experience of the chromatographer will affect the quality of the results. Some excellent reviews of different TLC separation and visualization techniques can be found in the literature (Davidow *et al.*, 1968; Bussey and Backer, 1974; Moffat, 1986).

With some drugs a confirmation test can be performed directly on the TLC plate or the spot after removal without further extraction. A procedure for pethidine confirmation by fluorometry directly on TLC spots without extraction is described below. The spot corresponding to pethidine is removed with a spatula and placed in a 10 ml beaker and then processed as follows. To the TLC scrapings add 5 drops of Marquis

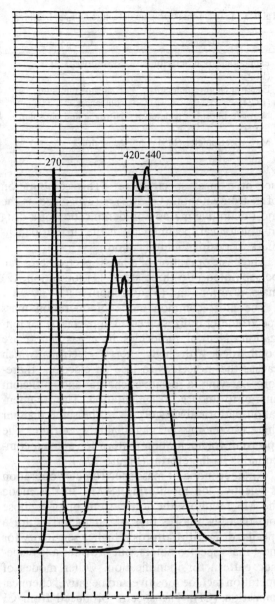

Figure 7 Spectrofluorometry of pethidine

reagent (8–10 drops of 40 per cent formaldehyde in 10 ml concentrated sulphuric acid) and heat in an oven at 110°C for 10 min. Then add 1 ml distilled water and observe under long-wave ultraviolet light. A blue fluorescence indicates that pethidine may be present. To confirm its presence (Dal Cortivo, 1970), add 2 ml of water and scan in a spectrofluorometer, excitation 270 μm, emission 420 and 440 μm (Figure 7).

TLC drug identification systems can be purchased from commercial sources. One system,

Toxi-LAB, available from Analytical Systems, Irvine, California, utilizes silica-gel impregnated paper and dips rather than sprays for visualization. Its chromatogram is subjected to four visualization steps (stages), the colours and R_f values are noted for each stage. A compendium of photograms showing the R_fs and colours in each stage for hundreds of drugs are supplied by the manufacturer. The advantage of this type of system is that it makes everything available including extraction tubes, visualization reagents, the photo compendium, confirmation systems, drug standards, continual updates on new drugs, and technical assistance. The disadvantage is the cost, but much of that is offset by technician time savings in not having to prepare visualization reagents, extraction tubes, and less technical training necessary to be proficient at identification. The identification process is also available on computer disk.

Gas Liquid Chromatography (GLC)

Like TLC, GLC is a separation technique. It is one of the most widely used techniques for drug analysis, for both screening and confirmation procedures. It uses an inert gas, such as nitrogen or helium as the mobile phase. An extract of the biological specimen is dissolved in a small amount of organic solvent (usually 25–100 μl) and then injected into a heated injector. The sample is vaporized and swept on to the column by the carrier gas (mobile phase). The identification of compounds in GLC is by retention time.

The column is in an oven with a temperature controller. The vaporized sample is carried through the column by a controlled flow rate of the mobile phase. The stationary phase interacts with the sample causing the analytes within the mixture to separate. The retention time is a measure of the elapsed time from the injection of the extract into the gas chromatograph until the apex of the detector response.

A column's capability to separate analytes can be modified by using different types and amounts of liquid phases (stationary phases) absorbed on an inert solid phase. Types of columns used include packed and capillary columns. Packed columns are usually glass, 1–2 metres in length and 3–6 mm in diameter. Figure 8 shows a typical separation of a mixture of volatiles (alcohols and acetone) using a 2 m packed column (0.2 per cent Carbowax 1500 on Carbopack C, Supelco,

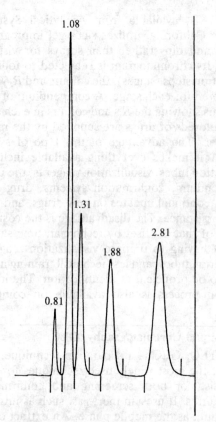

Figure 8 Separation of a volatile mixture on a packed column. Methanol (0.81), acetone (1.08), ethanol (1.31), 2-propanol (1.88), *n*-propanol (2.81)

Table 5 Gas chromatographic detectors and applications

Detector	Compounds
Flame ionization detector (FID)	Most drugs
Electron capture detector (ECD)	Halogen-containing substances
Nitrogen phosphorus detector (NPD)	Nitrogen and phosphorus
Mass spectrometer (MS)	Most drugs

Bellefonte, Pennsylvania). Capillary columns usually offer better separation than packed columns. They are commonly made of fused silica, 10–100 metres in length and have a diameter of between 0.25 and 0.60 mm. The stationary phase is a thin film (usually 0.25–1.0 μm). With most drugs non-polar stationary phases such as polydimethylsiloxane or polydiphenyldimethylsiloxane are commonly employed. Figure 9 shows a chromatogram of the separation of 'basic drugs' with a 30 metre capillary column (polydiphenyldimethylsiloxane).

There are several common types of detectors used in the toxicology laboratory. Table 5 lists commonly utilized detectors and their applications.

Gas Chromatography/Mass Spectrometry (GC/MS)

GC/MS combines the separating powers of the gas chromatograph with the discriminating abilities of a mass spectrometer. This combination of instrumentation (GC/MS) is recognized as the most definitive method of identification of a drug in a biological specimen and is the current benchmark of positive identification.

The basic operation of a mass spectrometer can be separated into three steps: (1) ionization, (2) mass filtration, and (3) detection.

The most common mode of operation mass spectrometer utilizes electron impact (EI) for ionization. Neutral molecules in a gas phase are bombarded with high energy electrons which causes the molecules to lose an electron, therefore carrying a positive charge and sufficient energy to undergo fragmentation. The fragmentation pattern always occurs in the same manner thereby creating an identifiable spectrum. The spectrum fragmentation pattern for a given compound is its fingerprint (Figure 10A).

Another mode of mass spectrometer operation is selective ion monitoring (SIM). In this mode the MS monitors the ion current of only those ions of a few masses that are characteristic for a specific drug. SIM affords a higher sensitivity for most mass spectrometers, but provides a less specific pattern for identification. Other modes of operation include 'positive and negative' chemical ionization (CI). The spectra produced from CI are typically less complex and more sensitive than EI spectra (Figure 10B).

Liquid Chromatography (LC)

LC is one of the oldest analytical separation techniques. The technique was a slow separation process when first developed because the mobile phase flowed through a column by gravity only. Modern techniques referred to as high-performance liquid chromatography (HPLC) utilize pumps to pass the mobile phases through columns at pressures exceeding 1000 psi. The major components of a basic high-performance liquid chro-

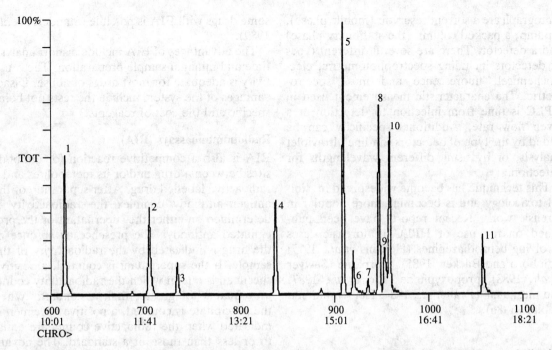

Figure 9 Separation of a 'basic drug' mixture. Pethidine (1), ketamine (2), phencyclidine (3), methadone metabolite (4), methadone (5), methaqualone (6), propoxyphene (7), cocaine (8), nortriptyline (9), imipramine (10), codeine (11)

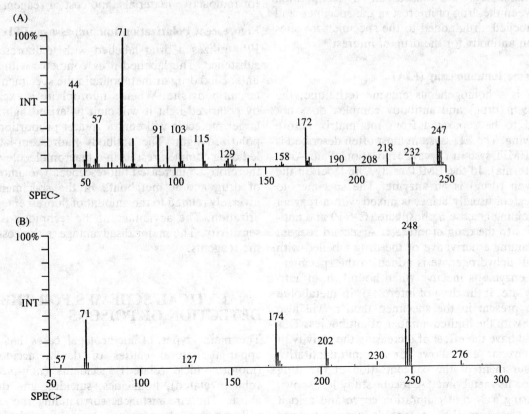

Figure 10 (A) EI spectrum and (B) positive CI spectrum of pethidine

matograph are a solvent reservoir (mobile phase), a pump, a packed column (the stationary phase) and a detector. There are several different types of detectors including spectrophotometric, electrochemical, fluorescence and mass spectrometric. The characteristic measurement used in HPLC is time from injection to detection at a given flow rate. Additional specificity can be added by the type of detectors, on-line ultraviolet analysis, or by using different wavelengths for detection.

This technique has become widespread in clinical toxicology and is becoming more popular in forensic work. Recent reports have been published on the use of HPLC in forensic cases involving benzodiazepines (Hoskins *et al.*, 1977; Edinboro and Backer, 1985), morphine (Sawyer *et al.*, 1988), propoxyphene (Rio *et al.*, 1987) and marijuana (Peat *et al.*, 1984; Isenschmid and Caplan, 1986).

Immunoassays

Immunoassays are based on a competition between the drug of interest in the specimen and a 'labelled' drug added to the specimen for sites on an antibody for the drug of interest.

Enzyme Immunoassay (EIA)

EIA is a homogeneous enzyme technique, the antigen (drug) and antibody complex does not need to be separated from the matrix before assaying. The EIA system most often described is the EMIT system (Syva Corporation, Palo Alto, California). In the EMIT assay, the label on the antigen (drug) is an enzyme. The specimen to be tested, usually urine, is mixed with a reagent containing glucose 6-phosphate (G-6-P) and antibodies to the drug of interest. A second reagent containing a derivative of the drug labelled with G-6-P dehydrogenase is added to the specimen. The enzyme is inactive when bound to an antibody site. If the drug of interest or its metabolite were present in the specimen then it will also react with the limited number of antibodies. This would have the effect of increasing the activity of the enzyme and allows for a semi-quantitative measurement of the concentration of the drug and/or its metabolite. A recent study has shown by using a 5-point calibration curve and a logit data transform that reasonable quantitation of

some drugs with EIA is possible (Standefer *et al.*, 1989).

The advantages of EIA include a short analysis time and minimal sample preparation. The sensitivity is adequate for most drugs of abuse. Disadvantages of the system include the tests not being specific and the cost of reagents.

Radioimmunoassays (RIA)

RIA is also a competitive reaction for antibody sites between a drug and/or its metabolites and a radioactive labelled drug. After separation of the antigen–antibody complex the radioactivity is determined on either the supernatant or the precipitated antibody. The presence or absence of the drug is indicated by the radioactivity of the sample. If the supernatant is counted, a positive specimen is one in which the radioactivity counts are equal to or greater than a standard. When the precipitate is counted, a positive specimen is indicated when the radioactive counts are equal to or less than those of a standard. The advantages of RIA are its sensitivity and small sample size. The disadvantages are incubation time, need for radioactive materials, and cost of reagents.

Fluorescent Polarization Immunoassays (FPI)

FPI utilizes a drug labelled with a fluorescent substance. The labelled drug competes with the unlabelled drug or metabolite in the specimen for an antibody site. When a fluorophore is excited by polarized light it will emit polarized light. A larger molecule will emit a greater proportion of polarized light. The antibody–fluorescent-labelled drug complex results in a macromolecule and therefore an increased fluorescence. The amount of drug and/or metabolite in the specimen is inversely related to the amount of fluorescent polarization. The advantage of the technique is its sensitivity. The major disadvantage is the cost of the reagents.

ANALYTICAL SCHEMES FOR THE DETECTION OF POISONS

The major types of medicolegal cases include apparent natural causes of death, accidents (motor vehicle related), accidents (non-motor vehicle related), homicides, suicides, and drug abuse. The circumstances surrounding the case will usually determine the types of toxicology tests that are required. In almost all cases a volatile screen (VS) will be required. Other types of protocols include a Drugs of Abuse Screen (DAS), a General Drug Screen (GDS), an Acidic/Neutral Screen (ANS), and a Basic Drug Screen (BDS). Figure 11 outlines the flow of specimens through the laboratory using the protocols described below.

The most frequently requested test in a forensic toxicology laboratory is a volatile screen (VS) for ethanol. There are many different types of techniques available for ethanol analysis such as oxidative, enzymatic or gas chromatographic. The most popular method in forensic applications for determining ethanol is GLC. GLC has the ability to separate commonly encountered volatiles including ethanol, methanol, acetone, and isopropanol providing the required specificity and sensitivity to measure ethanol as low as 2.2 mmol l^{-1} (10 mg dl^{-1}). A typical GLC procedure, using flame ionization detection (FID) for ethanol would employ an internal standard such as n-propanol or t-butyl alcohol. The peak height or area responses of ethanol to the internal standard would be compared with a series of aqueous standards with the same amount of internal standard for quantitation. Direct injection analysis procedures for alcohols have been described (Jain, 1971; Winek and Carfagna, 1987) as well as headspace procedures using both packed columns (Dubowski, 1977) and capillary columns (Penton, 1987). Figure 8 is a GLC chromatogram of a volatile analysis of alcohols and acetone from a head-space injection using n-propanol as an internal standard.

There are instances when a suitable blood specimen is not available for analysis (such as traumatic injuries) or when the body is decomposing. Endogenous (post-mortem neoformation) production of alcohol is a well-known occurrence (Blackmore, 1968). In cases where a suitable blood specimen is not available it may be possible to analyse various other biological specimens and at least make an estimate of the blood concentration (Backer *et al.*, 1980). Vitreous humor has been shown to be a fluid useful in the determi-

DRUG ANALYSIS FLOW CHART

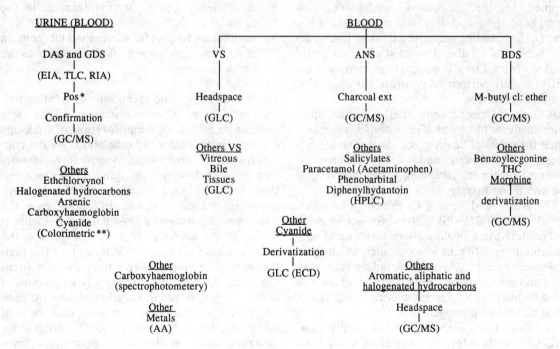

* If a drug is detected then the appropriate blood screen is initiated.
** If a colorimetric test is positive an appropriate confirmation is performed.

Figure 11 Flow diagram of laboratory protocols

nation of alcohol in the absence of blood and in decomposing bodies (Coe, 1972; Zumwalt *et al.*, 1982). The finding of ethanol in the vitreous humor and/or urine of a cadaver is consistent with an exogenous (ingested before death) source of alcohol. In Zumwalt's study of 130 decomposing bodies the highest concentration of endogenous ethanol was 47.8 mmol l^{-1} (220 mg dl^{-1}).

Another problem in ethanol determinations arises in embalmed cases. Embalming fluid can contain ethanol (Winek, 1984) and the embalming process has been reported to reduce the ethanol concentration by 52 per cent when it is free of ethanol (Bronstein and Park, 1984; Backer, 1989). Ethanol concentrations in vitreous humor have been shown to be useful in embalmed cases. In a series of cases where pre-embalmed and post-embalmed vitreous alcohol concentrations were determined (Coe, 1976; Scott *et al.*, 1974), 78 per cent of the time the post-embalmed concentration was within 6.5 mmol l^{-1} (30 mg dl^{-1}) of the usually higher pre-embalmed specimen's ethanol concentration.

A Drugs of Abuse Screen (DAS) commonly tests for amphetamines, barbiturates, benzodiazepines, cocaine, marijuana, methadone, propoxyphene, phencyclidine and opiate alkaloids. The DAS should be requested in most homicides and accidental deaths. The most common methodology for a DAS is an enzyme immunoassay (EIA) usually performed on urine but applicable to other specimens.

A General Drug Screen (GDS) is a broad spectrum analysis for many drugs and is necessary when the cause of death is not clear. The GDS is usually a TLC method and is applicable to many different specimens including urine, blood, gastric and tissue homogenates.

The Acidic and Neutral Drug Screen (ANS) is usually a GC (GC/MS) method for acidic drugs and neutral drugs including barbiturates and non-barbiturate sedative hyponotics such as glutethimide and muscle relaxants including meprobamate and carisoprodol. The ANS method is applicable to many types of specimens including blood, urine and tissue homogenates.

The Basic Drug Screen (BDS) is usually a GC (GC/MS) method for the analysis of many basic drugs such as propoxyphene, cocaine, antidepressants, opiates (codeine, oxycodone, hydromorphone, meperidine), calcium channel blockers, and many others.

Miscellaneous protocols that are also needed for other commonly encountered analytes include cyanide, carboxyhaemoglobin, arsenic and other metals, pesticides, aromatic, aliphatic and chlorinated hydrocarbons, and vitreous chemistries such as sodium, chloride and glucose. There are many different published texts that can be referred to for protocols to analyse these and other analytes (Sunshine, 1971; Moffat *et al.*, 1986; Baselt and Cravey, 1989).

INTERPRETATION OF RESULTS

After the analyses of specimens for a particular case are complete, the forensic toxicologist must interpret the findings as to the physiological effects of the analytes in retrospect to their concentrations. The specific questions that must be answered are whether the concentrations of any analyte or combinations of analytes were:

- sufficient to cause the death?
- sufficient to have affected the actions of the decedent so as to have caused the death?
- insufficient to have any involvement in the cause of death?
- insufficient to protect the individual from an underlying mechanism of death such as an epileptic seizure?

Many factors must be taken into account including the route of administration. The most common methods of administration of toxicants are oral, intravenous and inhalation. As the concentrations of drugs administered intravenously that result in fatalities are quite often much less than found in oral overdoses it can be very important to know the route. In forensic cases the route may not always be known unless evidence is found at the scene such as a syringe and the decedent has very recent injection sites. The toxicology finding may answer some questions about the route, for example, finding a large amount of drug or even intact medication in the stomach contents is a good indication of an oral route of administration. However, some drugs are absorbed very rapidly, such as tricyclic antidepressants, and even when massive overdoses are ingested only traces may be found in the gastric contents. It is important to point out that with most analytes the presence of the drug in the gastric contents is not sufficient proof that it was the agent or one of a combination of toxicants that caused the death. It must be documented that sufficient absorption of the substance occurred to result in a toxic concentration of the analyte in blood and/or liver. Other findings such as extremely high lung concentrations of a drug or chemical are very suggestive of an inhalation route.

It has always been assumed that the concentration of most analytes in heart blood paralleled the physiological consequences. This premise has been shown to be untrue in recent years (Prouty and Anderson, 1984, 1990; Jones and Pounder, 1987; Andrenyak and Backer, 1988). It is now known that the concentration of many analytes increases in both heart and peripheral blood specimens during the post-mortem interval. These anatomical site concentration differences have shown that in most cases femoral blood is more likely to be a better indicator of the peri-mortem (at death) concentration of the analyte (Table 2). Reference to common tabulations of toxic concentrations of analytes (Winek, 1976; Baselt *et al.*, 1975; Baselt and Cravey, 1977; Stead and Moffat, 1983) must be used with extreme caution because most are based on heart blood findings. The liver concentration and/or brain concentration of an analyte may be extremely important in the determination of the involvement of an analyte in the cause of death. The toxic concentrations of many analytes in liver can be found in tabular form (McBay, 1973; Baselt and Cravey, 1977). The concentration ratios of the analyte in blood to liver are often very helpful in interpretation of the involvement of the analyte (Stajic *et al.*, 1979). With some drugs like methadone the therapeutic (or maintenance concentration) overlaps the concentrations found in overdoses. However, it has been postulated that the concentration ratio of 1,5-dimethyl-3,3-diphenyl-2-ethylidenepyrrolidine, a major metabolite of methadone, in liver to kidney is always less than or equal to 1 in an overdose of methadone (Thompson, 1976). The ratio of blood propoxyphene concentrations to its major metabolite, norpropoxyphene, has also been investigated in predicting toxicity (Caplan *et al.*, 1977; Hartman *et al.*, 1988).

Drugs taken in combination can be more toxic than if considered separately. Knowledge of the interaction of toxicants will be paramount to proper interpretation of the toxicity of any analyte. Most analytes are more toxic in the presence of alcohol. The toxicity of barbiturates and alcohol has been studied (Cimbura *et al.*, 1972). Unfortunately, information about most combinations of analytes is not well known and the toxicologist must quite often deal with them on an individual basis. Experience with similar cases or published reports will be the only information the forensic toxicologist can rely on in predicting the toxicity of many analyte combinations.

Other factors that must be considered in the interpretative process by the forensic toxicologist are the age, sex, body weight, genetic factors, tolerance, environmental exposures and general health status of the individual. All of these factors can influence the response to a given concentration of an analyte or combinations of analytes. Liver disease may prevent the metabolism of an analyte allowing multiple dosing to result in accumulation of the drug to toxic concentrations, or an underlying condition such as atherosclerotic cardiovascular disease will make the presence of an analyte at a given concentration more toxic. Environmental exposure as well as abusive uses of halogenated hydrocarbons can result in sensitization of myocardial tissues, making an individual more susceptible to a cardiac arrhythmia (Reinhardt *et al.*, 1971).

CONCLUSION

Post-mortem forensic toxicology has changed dramatically in the past 20 years. Some of the major changes have been related to analytical techniques such as immunoassays, high-performance liquid chromatography and the role of gas chromatography/mass spectrometry in positive identification of toxicants. The knowledge that the concentrations of many drugs are not stable post mortem has also caused considerable debate and change in the toxicologist's ability to interpret his analytical findings.

The next 20 years promise to see the introduction of many additional analytical techniques and the increasing role of the forensic toxicologist in new areas of employment such as drugs in the work place and driving under the influence of drugs other than alcohol programmes. Perhaps, however, the most demanding change on the horizon for the forensic toxicology profession is the certification of laboratories by outside governmental agencies.

REFERENCES

Andrenyak, D. M. and Backer, R. C. (1988). Postmortem concentrations of propoxyphene and norproproxyphene in blood obtained from different anatomical locations. Presented at the *40th Annual Meeting of the American Academy of Forensic Sciences*, Philadelphia, Pennsylvania

Apple, F. S. and Bandt, C. M. (1988). Liver and blood postmortem tricyclic antidepressant concentrations. *Am. J. Clin. Pathol.*, **89**, 794–796

Backer, R. C. (1981). The forensic laboratory. In Cravey, R. H. and Baselt, R. C. (Eds), *Introduction to Forensic Toxicology*. Biomedical Publications, Davis, California, pp. 142–150

Backer, R. C. (1989). Determination of alcohol-postmortem consideration in embalmed and decomposed cases. Presented at the *41st Annual Meeting of the American Academy of Forensic Sciences*, Las Vegas, Nevada

Backer, R. C., Pisano, R. V. and Sopher, I. M. (1980). The comparison of alcohol concentrations in postmortem fluids and tissues. *J. Forensic Sci.*, **25**, 327–331

Bandt, C. W. (1981). Postmortem changes in serum levels of tricyclic antidepressants. Presented at the *33rd Annual Meeting of the American Academy of Forensic Sciences*, Los Angeles, California

Baselt, R. C. and Cravey, R. H. (1977). A compendium of therapeutic and toxic concentrations of toxicologically significant drugs in human biofluids. *J. Anal. Toxicol.*, **1**, 81–101

Baselt, R. C. and Cravey, R. H. (Eds) (1989). *Disposition of Toxic Drugs and Chemicals in Man*, 3rd edition, Year Book Medical Publishers, Chicago, Illinois

Baselt, R. C., Wright, J. A. and Cravey, R. H. (1975). Therapeutic and toxic concentrations of more than 100 toxicologically significant drugs in blood, plasma, or serum: a tabulation. *Clin. Chem.*, **21**, 44–62

Blackmore, D. J. (1968). The bacterial production of ethyl alcohol. *J. Forensic Sci. Soc.*, **8**, 73–78

Bowden, K. M. and McCallum, N. E. W. (1949). Blood alcohol content: some aspects of its postmortem uses. *Med. J. Aust.*, **2**, 76–81

Briglia, E. J., Hauser, C., Giaquinta, P. and Dal Cortivo, L. A. (1986). Distribution of ethanol in post-mortem specimens. Presented at the *International Symposium on Driving Under the Influence of Alcohol and/or Drugs*, Quantico, Virgina

Bronstein, A. and Park, M. (1984). Comparison of ethanol in pre and post embalmed blood specimens. *Society of Forensic Toxicologists' Newsletter, ToxTalk*, **8**, No. 2, 3

Bussy, R. and Backer, R. C. (1974). Thin-layer chrom-

atographic differentiation of amphetamine from other primary-amine drugs in urine. *Clin. Chem.*, **20**, 302–304

Caplan, Y. H., Thompson, B. C. and Fisher, R. S. (1977). Propoxyphene fatalities: blood and tissue concentrations of propoxyphene and norpropoxyphene and a study of 115 medical examiner cases. *J. Anal. Toxicol.*, **1**, 27–35

Cimbura, G., McGarry, E. and Daigle, J. (1972). Toxicological data for fatalities due to carbon monoxide and barbiturates in Ontario. *J. Forensic Sci.*, **17**, 640–644

Coe, J. I. (1972). Use of chemical determinations on vitreous humor in forensic pathology. *J. Forensic Sci.*, **17**, 541–546

Coe, J. I. (1976). Comparative postmortem chemistries of vitreous humor before and after embalming. *J. Forensic Sci.*, **21**, 583–586

Dal Cortivo, L. (1970). Fluorometric determination of microgram amounts of meperidine. *Anal. Chem.*, **42**, 941–942

Davidow, B., Li-Petri, N. and Quane, B. (1968). A thin-layer chromatographic screening procedure for detecting drug abuse. *Am. J. Clin. Pathol.*, **38**, 714–719

Dubowski, K. M. (1977). *Manual for the Analysis of Ethanol in Biological Liquids*. U.S. Department of Transportation, No. DOT-TSC-NHTSA–76–4, Washington, DC

Edinboro, L. E. and Backer, R. C. (1985). Preliminary report on the application of a high pressure liquid chromatographic method for alprazolam in postmortem blood specimens. *J. Anal. Toxicol.*, **9**, 207–208

Feldstein, M. and Klendshoj, N. C. (1957). The determination of volatile substances by microdiffusion analysis. *J. Forensic Sci.*, **2**, 39–58

Finkle, B. S. and Bath, R. J. (1971). Ethychlorvynol, type A procedure. In Sunshine, I. (Ed.), *Manual of Analytical Toxicology*. The Chemical Rubber Co., Cleveland, Ohio, pp. 150–151

Gettler, A. O. (1956). History of forensic toxicology. *J. Forensic Sci.*, **1**, 3–25

Gettler, A. O. and Kaye, S. (1950). A simple and rapid analytical method for Hg, Bi, Sb and As in biological materials. *J. Lab. Clin. Med.*, **35**, 146–151

Hartman, B., Miyada, D., Pirkle, H., Sedgwick, P., Cravey, R., Tennant, F. and Wolen, R. (1988). Serum propoxyphene concentrations in a cohort of opiate addicts on long-term propoxyphene maintenance therapy. *J. Anal. Toxicol.*, **12**, 25–29

Hoskins, W. M., Richardson, A. and Sanger, D. G. (1977). The use of high pressure liquid chromatography in forensic toxicology. *J. Forensic Sci. Soc.*, **17**, 185–188

Isenschmid, D. S. and Caplan, Y. H. (1986). A method for the determination of 11-nor-delta-9-tetrahydrocannabinol-9-carboxylic acid in urine using high performance liquid chromatography with electrochemical detection. *J. Anal. Toxicol.*, **10**, 170–174

Jain, N. C. (1971). Direct blood-injection method for gas chromatographic determination of alcohols and other volatile compounds. *Clin. Chem.*, **17**, 82–85

Jones, G. R. (1986). Postmortem redistribution of drugs. Further evidence of major changes. *38th meeting, American Academy of Forensic Sciences*, Abstract K1. New Orleans, Louisiana.

Jones, G. R. and Pounder, D. J. (1987). Site dependence of drug concentrations in postmortem blood—a case study. *J. Anal. Toxicol.*, **11**, 184–190

McBay, A. J. (1973). Toxicological findings in fatal poisonings. *Clin. Chem.*, **19**, 361–365

Moffat, A. C. (1986). Thin-layer chromatography. In Moffat, A. C., Jackson, J. V., Moss, M. S. and Widdop, B. (Eds), *Clarke's Isolation and Identification of Drugs*, 2nd edition, The Pharmaceutical Press, London, pp. 160–177

Moffat, A. C., Jackson, J. V., Moss, M. S. and Widdop, B. (Eds) (1986). *Clarke's Isolation and Identification of Drugs*, 2nd edn. The Pharmaceutical Press, London

Peat, M., Deyman, M. E. and Johnson, J. R. (1984). High performance liquid chromatography-immunoassay of delta-9-tetrahydrocannabinol and its metabolites in urine. *J. Forensic Sci.*, **31**, 110–119

Peel, H. W. and Freimuth, H. C. (1972). Methods for the determination of ethchlorvynol in biological tissue. *J. Forensic Sci.*, **17**, 688–692

Penton, Z. (1987). Gas-chromatographic determination of ethanol in blood with 0.53 mm fused silica open tubular columns. *Clin. Chem.*, **33**, 2094–2095

Plueckhahn, V. D. (1968). The evaluation of autopsy blood alcohol levels. *Med. Sci. Law*, **8**, 168–176

Poklis, A. (1980). Toxicology. In Eckert, W. G. (Ed.), *Introduction to Forensic Sciences*. C. V. Mosby Company, St. Louis, Missouri, pp. 79–101

Prouty, R. W. and Anderson, W. H. (1984). Documented hazards in the interpretation of postmortem blood concentrations of tricyclic antidepressants. Presented at the *36th Annual Meeting of the American Academy of Forensic Sciences*, Anaheim, California

Prouty, R. W. and Anderson, W. H. (1990). The forensic implications of site and temporal influences on postmortem blood-drug concentrations. *J. Forensic Sci.*, **35**, 243–270

Reinhardt, C. F., Azar, A., Maxifield, M. E., Smith, P. E. and Mullins, L. S. (1971). Cardiac arrhythmias and aerosol 'sniffing'. *Arch. Environ. Hlth*, **22**, 265–279

Rio, J., Hodnett, N. and Bidanset, J. H. (1987). The determination of propoxyphene, norpropoxyphene, and methadone in post-mortem blood and tissue by high-performance liquid chromatography. *J. Anal. Toxicol.*, **11**, 222–224

Roetlger, J. R. (1990). The importance of blood collection site for the determination of basic drugs: a case with fluoxetine and diphenhydramine overdose. *J. Anal. Toxicol.*, **14**, 191–192

Sawyer, W. R., Waterhouse, G. A., Doedens, D. J. and Forney, B. (1988). Heroin, morphine, and hydromorphone determination by high performance liquid chromatography. *J. Forensic Sci.*, **33**, 1146–1155

Scott, W., Root, I. and Sanborn, B. (1974). The use of vitreous humor for determination of ethyl alcohol in previously embalmed bodies. *J. Forensic Sci.*, **19**, 913–916

Stajic, M., Caplan, Y. H. and Backer, R. C. (1979). Detection of drugs using XAD–2 Resin. II: analysis of liver in medical examiner's cases. *J. Forensic Sci.*, **24**, 732–744

Standefer, J., Backer, R. C. and Archuletta, M. S. (1989). Comparison of quantitative results: EMIT assay vs TDX for drugs of abuse. Presented at the *41st Annual Meeting of the American Academy of Forensic Sciences*, Las Vegas, Nevada

Stead, A. H. and Moffat, A. C. (1983). A collection of therapeutic, toxic and fatal blood drug concentrations in man. *Hum. Toxicol.*, **3**, 437–464

Sunshine, I. (Ed.) (1971). *Manual of Analytical Toxicology*. The Chemical Rubber Co., Cleveland, Ohio

Thompson, B. C. (1976). Chemical diagnosis of methadone related death. Doctoral Thesis, University of Maryland, Baltimore, Maryland

Turkel, H. W. and Gifford, H. (1957). Erroneous blood alcohol findings at autopsy; avoidance by proper sampling technique. *J. Am. Med. Assoc.*, **164**, 1077–1079

Widdop, B. (1986). Hospital toxicology and drug abuse screening. In Moffat, A. C., Jackson, J. V., Moss, M. S. and Widdop, B. (Eds), *Clarke's Isolation and Identification of Drugs*, 2nd edn. The Pharmaceutical Press, London, pp. 3–34

Winek, C. L. (1976). Tabulation of therapeutic and lethal drugs and chemicals in blood. *Clin. Chem.*, **22**, 832–836

Winek, C. L. (1984). Reply to research query. *Society of Forensic Toxicologists' Newsletter, Toxtalk*, No. 4, 4

Winek, C. L. and Carfagna, M. (1987). Comparison of plasma, serum, and whole blood ethanol concentrations. *J. Anal. Toxicol.*, **11**, 267–268

Zumwalt, R. E., Bost, R. O. and Sunshine, I. (1982). Evaluation of ethanol concentrations in decomposed bodies. *J. Forensic Sci.*, **27**, 549–554

FURTHER READING

Ballantyne, B. and Marrs, T. C. (1987). Post-mortem features and criteria for the diagnosis of acute lethal cyanide poisoning. In Ballantyne, B. and Marrs, T. C. (Eds), *Clinical and Experimental Toxicology of Cyanides*. Wright, Bristol, pp. 217–247

Curry, A. S. (1988). *Poison Detection in Human Organs*. 4th edn. Charles C. Thomas, Springfield, Illinois

Knight, B. (1991). *Forensic Pathology*. Oxford University Press

48   Air Pollution

Robert L. Maynard and Robert E. Waller

EPIDEMIOLOGICAL ASPECTS

Introduction

Insofar as the general public is exposed to a complex mixture of air pollutants that cannot readily be reproduced in the laboratory, much of the information on adverse effects must ultimately come from field studies. Controlled human exposures in the laboratory to individual pollutants or to relatively simple mixtures have a complementary role to play, helping to define exposure–effect relationships, at least for short-term readily-reversible effects. There are, however, fundamental problems in conducting and interpreting epidemiological studies. The mixture of pollutants is liable to vary from time to time and place to place and it can be characterized only by observations on a few index substances. Hence great care is required in extrapolating from findings in one set of circumstances to others. Adverse effects observed may result from, or be compounded by, other environmental or life-style factors, and it is particularly difficult to separate out effects of air pollution in respect of long-term effects. The most obvious and dramatic effects have in fact been seen in relation to episodes of high pollution, such as in the major London 'smog' of December 1952, when there was an immediate impact on morbidity and mortality, clearly related to the exceptionally high concentrations of pollutants from domestic coal fires (Ministry of Health, 1954).

Common Air Pollutants

While there is a wide range of pollutants from specific industrial sources that can have adverse effects on people occupationally exposed, and sometimes on others living in the vicinity, the emphasis for the present purpose is on a range of pollutants that are ubiquitous in the general environment and that come mainly from the combustion of fossil fuels (coal, oil products or gas), for heating, power generation or transport. As indicated above, the resultant mixture is of complex composition, but two broad types are now recognized, characterized in each case by observations on the principal constituents.

The traditional air pollution problem in much of the UK and in other parts of the world where coal has been used for industrial, or more particularly domestic purposes, has as its main constituents smoke, or other particulate matter, and sulphur dioxide (SO_2), the latter imparting a reducing quality in the chemical sense. The burning of heavier grades of oil in power stations, industrial or commercial premises also contributes to the SO_2 content. This mixture, when present in high concentration, is sometimes referred to as the 'London smog' complex, or just 'winter smog'.

The more recent development of the past few decades has been the emergence of the 'Los Angeles smog' or 'summer smog' complex that has oxidizing properties, with ozone as a principal constituent. It arises from photochemical reactions taking place in the air, sometimes at a considerable distance from the source of the primary pollutants, between volatile organic compounds and oxides of nitrogen. Motor vehicle emissions are important contributors to the sources, and the highest and most persistent concentrations of photochemical pollutants have been experienced in Los Angeles, with its exceptionally high vehicle density coupled with high sunlight intensity for much of the year and an unusual combination of topographic and climatological features leading to poor natural ventilation over the whole of the Los Angeles basin.

The two types of pollution complex can coexist, but more generally they exhibit their seasonal patterns, with photochemical pollution being of little or no consequence in the winter months in temperate climates. Some components, such as oxides of nitrogen, are however common to both types of pollution, being emitted from all fuel combustion processes, whether stationary or vehicular.

The main pollutants of concern in relation to

health, as components of traditional or photochemical pollution, are outlined below, further information on properties, methods of measurement and distribution being available in other publications (WHO, 1987).

Smoke and Other Suspended Particulate Matter

Suspended particulate matter is a generic term for finely divided solid or liquid particles that are small enough to remain in suspension for periods of hours or days, being capable of travelling long distances during that time. Such particles commonly have effective diameters less than 1 μm, but they may extend up to 5 or 10 μm. Close to sources, or in strong winds, somewhat larger particles can be present, and some samplers used for monitoring purposes have a (50 per cent) cut-off at about 10 μm to limit the range of collected particles to those small enough to penetrate to the thoracic region of the respiratory tract, the material then being referred to as 'PM$_{10}$'.

Black smoke is one component of suspended particulates, produced in the incomplete combustion of coal or oil. Its assessment is based on its soiling properties, generally by collecting small samples on filter paper and measuring the reflectance of the stain produced (International Standards Organization, 1991a). Results are expressed in terms of concentrations of equivalent 'standard smoke', and while the units used are μg m^{-3} it is important to recognize that this is a separate type of measurement from direct gravimetric observations, and there is no uniform relationship between the two.

Other components of suspended particulates include inorganic ash, largely from coal-burning, fine dusts from some industrial processes, acid sulphates or nitrates formed as secondary pollutants by atmospheric reactions and residues of lead compounds from leaded petrol (where used).

Sulphur Dioxide

The irritant acidic gas sulphur dioxide (SO$_2$) often accompanies smoke and other suspended particulates, produced from sulphur impurities in coal and oil. Routine monitoring methods have in the past been based on the measurement of 'net acid gas' by titration, linked with simultaneous assessment of black smoke (British Standards Institution, 1969), but currently continuous instruments using the ultraviolet fluorescence principle are widely used (International Standards Organ-

ization, 1991b). Such instruments not only produce data averaged over periods of 24 h that may be required for regulatory purposes, but they display shorter-period peaks that can be of concern in relation to acute effects on health.

As indicated above, some of the SO$_2$, once emitted into the air, may undergo conversion to particulate sulphates (notably ammonium sulphate) or sulphuric acid. Such material is often associated with other particulate matter, and 'acid particles' were a common feature of former London smogs (Waller, 1963). The routine determination of particulate acid is a difficult task, but with increasing concern about the role of such components in either winter or summer 'smog' in relation to effects on health, some methods suitable for research purposes have been developed (Koutrakis *et al.*, 1989).

Oxides of Nitrogen

The mixture of oxides of nitrogen emitted to air from combustion processes, mainly through the fixation of atmospheric nitrogen, is often referred to as NO$_x$, comprising nitric oxide (NO) and nitrogen dioxide (NO$_2$). Concentrations are measured with continuously recording instruments based on the chemiluminescence principle (International Standards Organization, 1985) and the highest values in outdoor air are generally found close to traffic in busy streets.

Volatile Organic Compounds

The importance of this group of compounds is not so much in relation to direct effects on health as to their role as precursors, with oxides of nitrogen, in the photochemical production of oxidant (summer smog) pollution. Motor vehicle emissions of unburnt or partially burnt fuel provide the main source, and while gas chromatographic techniques are required to identify and measure individual components, there is some routine monitoring of total hydrocarbons, results being expressed in terms of equivalent amounts of methane (CH$_4$). One component of interest in relation to possible direct effects on health is benzene (C$_6$H$_6$), present at a level of a few per cent in petrol and emitted to air as an exhaust product or through evaporative losses.

Ozone

The photochemical reactions between volatile organic compounds and oxides of nitrogen yield a complex mixture of oxidants of which ozone is the main component (PORG, 1987). It is the ozone that is routinely monitored, using continuous instruments on chemiluminescence or ultraviolet absorption principles. The distribution of this pollutant differs from most others in that concentrations may be relatively uniform over large regions and are not necessarily highest in city centres. This is due to the finite time required for the photochemical reactions to take place as precursor pollutants drift away from their sources and to primary nitric oxide, from traffic, scavenging some of the ozone in busy streets.

Carbon Monoxide

Outdoor concentrations of this pollutant are dominated by traffic sources, principally from petrol-engined vehicles, although emissions can be greatly reduced by the use of catalytic convertors in exhaust systems. The highest values are found very close to traffic falling away sharply at increasing distances from busy roads. Continuous measurements can be made with infrared absorption or electrochemical instruments. Much carbon monoxide is also emitted from stationary combustion sources but dispersion and dilution factors are such that they have little effect on concentrations at ground level. Indoors, unflued heating or cooking appliances can contribute to carbon monoxide concentrations, and with faulty operation or blockages in flued appliances, lethal concentrations can be reached. For people who smoke, intake of carbon monoxide is in general dominated by their own smoking.

Lead

The organo-lead compounds that have been widely used to improve the octane rating of petrol are largely burnt in the engine and emitted as fine particles of inorganic lead compounds. Such sources provide the main contribution to lead-in-air concentrations, although locally some smelters or other industrial sources can be important. The phasing-out of leaded petrol that has occurred, or is occurring, in many countries has substantially reduced air lead concentrations in recent years. Monitoring is generally carried out by collecting samples over extended periods on filters and analysing by atomic absorption spectrophotometry or X-ray fluorescence.

Polycyclic Aromatic Hydrocarbons

The incomplete combustion of fossil fuels, wood or organic material in general leads to the production of a wide range of polycyclic aromatic hydrocarbons (PAHs), some of which are of possible concern in relation to health because of their carcinogenic properties. The five-ringed member, benzo[a]pyrene (BaP), is often used as an index substance in this respect, although other components have potential adverse effects. The PAHs are largely adsorbed on smoke particles, and can be collected with them on filter papers, although some have appreciable vapour pressures at ambient temperatures and for completeness, additional vapour phase collection may be incorporated. The analytical methods now favoured are glass capillary gas chromatography with mass-spectrometric detection or high-performance liquid chromatography (Bjorseth, 1983; Hansen *et al.*, 1990).

Patterns of Exposure to Air Pollutants

The most difficult step in associating air pollution with effects on health is the assessment of exposure. Most monitoring of pollutant concentrations is carried out at fixed sites, albeit chosen to be as representative as practicable of the exposure of the population living or working in the area, but that can provide no more than a rough guide. There is a basic problem in that there can be large differences in concentrations between indoor and outdoor air, but beyond that there are several different types of situation in respect of sources, each needing a different approach.

The simplest type to deal with is the 'area' source where a multiplicity of similar sources are distributed throughout a heavily populated area, in which case concentrations may not vary too severely from one location to another. This was the situation in many large urban areas of the UK, up to the 1950s, when domestic coal fires were the main sources of air pollution (by smoke and sulphur dioxide), and the majority of households had at least one such fire. A limited number of strategically placed samplers could then provide a reasonable index of exposure of large population groups. Even if the absolute exposures differed across a town, the pattern of day-to-day variation was consistent, depending primarily on the general weather picture.

Point sources, such as individual or a few scattered industrial chimneys, present more difficult problems as the plumes are liable to be blown around in different directions by the wind, leading to large differences in concentrations in respect of both place and time. In such circumstances average concentrations at any one location may be below a level anticipated to have adverse effects but there could still be occasional transient peaks that could be of relevance to acute effects on health.

A third situation arises in respect of traffic, because of the very low level of the emissions, within the breathing zone. Exposures then depend critically on how close people are to traffic in a busy street, a few metres making an important difference. Fixed site monitors can be used to identify 'hot spots' and to indicate the pattern of distribution but they are of limited value in assessing exposures of individuals or population groups.

Finally, ozone and related photochemical pollutants fall into a category of their own for, as mentioned above, their mode of formation leads to relatively uniform concentrations over large regions, with a tendency for concentrations in rural less-populated areas to be as high as, or higher than, those in city centres. A reasonable picture of exposures can then be obtained with a modest number of monitors, although there are problems in the vicinity of busy streets, where the concentrations of primary pollutants from traffic may be high but ozone values are liable to be reduced.

Some of the above problems can be overcome to a limited extent through the use of personal samplers, sometimes simple passive ones that do not require any power supply, or miniaturized battery-operated instruments that can be worn by individuals in specific epidemiological studies. Such approaches are particularly valuable when assessing 'total' exposures, indoors and out in the course of the day, but it can be costly to provide and maintain such equipment for more than a modest number of people. Biological uptake measures can be useful for a limited range of pollutants, the prime example being for carbon monoxide. Because this gas has a strong affinity for haemoglobin, exposures can be assessed directly on small blood samples or indirectly by measurements of carbon monoxide in exhaled air. Tobacco smoking provides a relatively potent

source of carbon monoxide however, and the role of environmental sources can only be assessed this way in non-smokers. Similarly, uptake of lead can be determined directly on blood, but dietary sources also contribute, and exposure from lead in the air cannot readily be separated out.

Studies Related to Sulphur Dioxide/ Particulates Complex, 'Winter Smog'

Acute Effects

Mortality
Historically the most widely studied and most clearly demonstrated adverse effects of air pollution on health have been short-term changes in morbidity and mortality associated with sharp increases in concentrations of smoke and sulphur dioxide, notably where coal has been widely used for domestic heating and industrial purposes. The most notorious event was the London fog of December 1952, which lasted for 5 days with concentrations of sulphur dioxide averaging 1.34 ppm ($3830 \ \mu g \ m^{-3}$) in central areas over the peak days. Smoke concentrations were such as to grossly overload the samplers, a conservative estimate of the maximum being $4460 \ \mu g \ m^{-3}$. For each pollutant, such concentrations are of the order of 100 times typical urban values today. A sudden and unprecedented increase in daily deaths occurred, and it was estimated that during and just after the fog the total number of deaths in Greater London was some 4000 more than would otherwise have been recorded (Ministry of Health, 1954). The impact was largely among the elderly and chronic sick, the interpretation being that their deaths were precipitated by the highly irritant pollution, some weeks, months or years sooner than they would otherwise have occurred. Comprehensive records of morbidity were not available but reports from hospitals and general practitioners indicated a steep rise in respiratory ailments.

Subsequent studies (Martin and Bradley, 1960) showed that smaller increases in daily deaths in Greater London were associated with more modest episodes of high pollution (smoke and sulphur dioxide) and through the 1960s daily deaths were monitored continuously along with records of emergency admissions to hospital. The way in which each of these indices responded in a further major episode, in December 1962, is illustrated in Figure 1. Whether such effects could be ascribed more particularly to the smoke, sulphur dioxide or associated pollutants was not clear. The judgement of a WHO group (WHO, 1979) considering these and related findings was that increases in daily deaths became discernible with 24 h average concentrations of black smoke and sulphur dioxide, each exceeding about 500 $\mu g\,m^{-3}$, although no actual threshold was implied.

Subsequent re-analyses of the data using multiple regression techniques (Mazumdar *et al.*, 1982; Ostro, 1984; Schwartz and Marcus, 1990) have attempted to resolve this but the outcome depends very much on the models and assumptions introduced, and the best that can be said is that these effects related very specifically to the kind of complex, including coal smoke, sulphur dioxide and probably reaction products such as sulphuric acid, present in the former London 'winter smogs', and that any extrapolation to conditions today needs to be undertaken with caution.

There are, however, reported effects of pol-

lution complexes elsewhere, including sulphur dioxide and particulates of various kinds, on daily mortality. In the Ruhr area of Germany increases in deaths have been seen in episodes of high pollution (Wichmann *et al.*, 1989), effects being detected at levels of sulphur dioxide and particulates consistent with London findings. There has also been concern in recent years about high levels of air pollution in Athens, and while the particulates there come mainly from motor vehicles rather than coal burning, small increases in daily mortality have been related to smoke and sulphur dioxide concentrations (Hatzakis *et al.*, 1986). An association between daily mortality and levels of pollutants, including particulates at relatively low concentrations, has also been reported from the intensive study of air pollution and health in Steubenville, in the USA (Schwartz and Dockery, 1992). The statistical approach used, treating daily deaths in terms of a Poisson distribution, has also been applied to data from Detroit (Schwartz, 1991), linking them with concentrations of total suspended particulates (TSP), which were predicted on a daily basis from less frequent (one in six days) observations, with a knowledge of meteorological conditions. An association with TSP was reported, within a relatively modest range of particulate concentrations.

In France investigations have been carried out in two large cities, Lyons and Marseilles, demonstrating an apparent delayed effect of pollution, with an association between sulphur dioxide concentration and mortality up to 10 days later (Derriennic *et al.*, 1989). Similar associations were not demonstrated with concentrations of particulates, although as in other studies there were inter-relationships with temperature. An earlier study in Paris (Loewenstein *et al.*, 1983) had also shown links between sulphur dioxide concentrations and respiratory deaths.

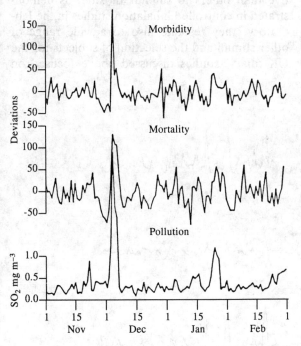

Figure 1 Day to day variations in deaths and emergency admissions to hospital in Greater London, winter 1962–63, each plotted as deviations from 15-day moving averages. Corresponding daily average concentrations of sulphur dioxide are shown, as an index of the sulphur dioxide/particulates complex. Source: Waller (1991)

Morbidity

In addition to increases in emergency admissions to hospital, as mentioned above, there is much general information on increased illness, particularly for respiratory conditions, as seen in general practitioner consultations, hospital out-patient attendances or sickness-absence records when pollution by sulphur dioxide/particulates has been high. People with existing respiratory impairment are particularly susceptible to such effects, those with established chronic bronchitis often reporting that their condition is worse in the kind of weather associated with high pollution. This feature was exploited in a series of studies in London and elsewhere in the UK in the 1950s and 1960s, in which large groups of bronchitic patients recruited at chest clinics maintained daily records of changes in their condition, using small pocket diaries. Numerical scores were assigned to the simple 'better', 'same', 'worse' entries enabling a mean illness score to be calculated for the group, relating that in turn to average smoke and sulphur dioxide concentrations (see Figure 2) and also to weather variables. Up to the mid-1960s, a remarkably close association was seen between peaks in the illness score and those in either smoke or sulphur dioxide concentrations (Lawther *et al.*, 1970) but as the implementation of the Clean Air Act 1956 gained momentum, such peaks, both in illness and in pollutant concentrations, largely disappeared by the late 1960s (Waller, 1971). This is illustrated in Figure 3, showing results for a repeat study 10 years after the earlier one. While it was not implied that there was any threshold for such effects, the overall conclusion from these studies was that significant consistent increases in the illness score were seen when concentrations of sulphur dioxide exceeded about 500 μg m^{-3} together with black smoke exceeding about 250 μg m^{-3}, each as the

mean of 24 h averages at representative outdoor sites in the study area. Important riders were that no conclusion could be reached about one of these pollutants without the other, nor about the role of other associated pollutants, and that effects might have been related more to short-period peak values during the day rather than to the mean values that were monitored.

One of the other studies of this type considered originally by the WHO group related to a relatively small panel of asthmatics living around an old coal-fired power station in the USA that was liable to produce local peaks of sulphur dioxide and particulates (Cohen *et al.*, 1972). The authors reported increases in asthma attacks when the 24 h mean concentration of sulphur dioxide exceeded 200 μg m^{-3} or total suspended particulates (determined gravimetrically) exceeded 150 μg m^{-3}. In these circumstances however, exposure would have been to sharp transient peaks, very much higher than the daily means, as the wind blew the plume around in various directions. While asthmatics are often more sensitive than others to sulphur dioxide, as demonstrated in controlled inhalation studies in the laboratory, they respond also to a wide range of other stimuli and the selection of subjects for the UK 'diary' studies discussed above focused on

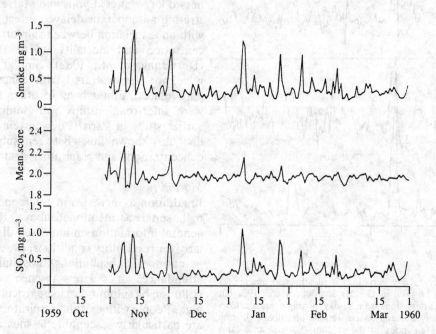

Figure 2   Daily changes in the condition of bronchitic patients in relation to air pollution, winter 1959–60

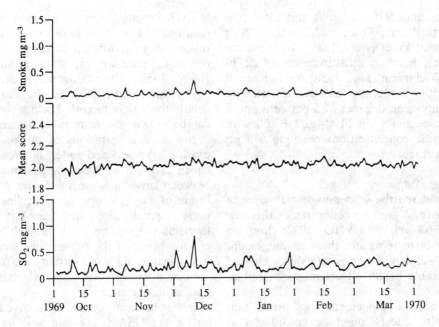

Figure 3 Daily changes in the condition of bronchitic patients in relation to air pollution, winter 1969–70

people with chronic bronchitis rather than asthma.

Functional Changes
To examine possible effects of the more moderate levels of pollution by sulphur dioxide/particulates experienced in the UK and elsewhere in western Europe or the USA over the past two decades, sensitive objective measurements have been included in most studies. These generally include indices of ventilatory capacity such as $FEV_{0.75}$, FEV_1 or FVC. To make such measurements daily on selected groups in anticipation of possible peaks in pollution is a difficult task, but in a study among schoolchildren in the USA (Dockery *et al.*, 1982) $FEV_{0.75}$ and FVC were measured before and after days with relatively high pollution, and regression equations were developed for each child, relating these measurements to concentrations of sulphur dioxide and total suspended particulates. While individually there were some increases and some decreases in lung function as pollution increased, the balance for the group as a whole was towards a negative slope, representing a median reduction of the order of 1 per cent in FVC and $FEV_{0.75}$ over the range of pollution observed (the highest values for each pollutant being about 275 μg m^{-3}). The authors later noted that if attention were directed to the 25 per cent

of children having the more extreme negative slopes, the average reduction was about 4 per cent, and the minimum level of such effects was judged to be 180 μg m^{-3} total suspended particulates, 24 h average, in the presence of sulphur dioxide (at a numerically similar concentration). The justification for such an interpretation is, however, dubious on statistical grounds (Brunekreef *et al.*, 1987) and all the changes were within the range of normal variation and too small to have subjective effects.

An opportunity for a somewhat similar type of study arose in The Netherlands in an episode of relatively high pollution that affected central and western Europe in 1985 (Dassen *et al.*, 1986). A small temporary decline in FVC, FEV_1 and other expiratory flow measures was observed among a group of schoolchildren when concentrations of sulphur dioxide and suspended particulates (either total, or fine fraction), as 24 h averages were each in a range of 200–250 μg m^{-3}. The decline in lung function was not larger than about 5 per cent on a group mean basis and follow-up measurements suggested that values had returned to baseline about 3 weeks after the episode. In a further episode in Europe in 1987, small transient declines in ventilatory function were again observed among schoolchildren in The Netherlands, with sulphur dioxide reaching 300 μg m^{-3}, black smoke about 100 μg m^{-3} and total suspended particulates 300 μg m^{-3}, each as 24 h averages (Brunekreef *et al.*, 1989). In the same episode, lung function measurements made in Germany (Wichmann *et al.*, 1988) on a group of patients with moderate airway obstruction showed group mean declines of 5 per cent and 7 per cent, respectively, in FEV$_1$ and FVC, with sulphur dioxide concentrations reaching 540 μg m^{-3}, 24 h average.

Acute Effects: Summary

Having considered the epidemiological evidence outlined above, a group meeting under the auspices of WHO in 1990 (WHO, 1992) drew up data (Table 1) to represent the best judgement of levels of sulphur dioxide/particulates beyond which detectable health effects might be anticipated.

On this basis a judgement was made that adverse health effects might be considered as 'severe' with 24 h average concentrations of sulphur dioxide and black smoke each (simultaneously) above about 400 μg m^{-3}. As stressed above, such effects must be considered to be related to the whole ('winter smog') pollution complex and they might more properly be linked to the (often much higher) peak values experienced during the episodes that had been studied.

Chronic Effects

Mortality

The high death rates from respiratory diseases in urban as compared with rural areas and the high national rates in some countries where there has been much air pollution have long been taken as indicators of a role of such pollution in the development of chronic respiratory disease. In the UK investigations of the wide differences in death rates from bronchitis and some other conditions between different towns have been carried out using data for the years around the 1951 (Daly, 1959), 1961 (Gardner *et al.*, 1969) and 1971 (Chinn *et al.*, 1981) censuses, to define more clearly the 'urban factor'. The net conclusion that can be drawn now from these descriptive studies is that as concentrations of smoke and sulphur dioxide have declined under the provisions of the Clean Air Act 1956, apparent associations between bronchitis mortality and contemporary levels of air pollution have declined, although there are indications that exposure to the high levels that existed earlier in life still have residual effects. Much of the present-day local variations in respiratory disease mortality is associated with socioeconomic factors, within which smoking may play an important part.

Somewhat analogous studies have been carried out in the USA (Lave and Seskin, 1977) using data on total suspended particulates or total sulphate concentrations as indices of pollution exposure. Statistical associations have been demonstrated, but again it is unclear to what extent confounding with socioeconomic factors is involved, and whether the pollution indices are appropriate. In a review of these studies (Evans *et al.*, 1984) it was concluded that while there was evidence of a causal relationship between mortality and air pollution of the particulates/sulphur dioxide type, the nature of any specific pollutant could not be identified in this way and the strength of the association could have been either under- or overestimated.

Table 1 Levels of 24h average concentrations of air pollutant mixtures containing sulphur dioxide and particulate matter above which specific acute effects on human health are expected on the basis of observations made in epidemiological studies

| SO$_2$ (μg m^{-3}) | Particles (μg m^{-3}) | | Health effects | Overall classification of effects |
	Black smoke	Gravimetric		
200		200	Small, transient decrements in lung function (FVC, FEV$_1$) in children and adults which may last for 2–4 weeks. Magnitude of the effect is in the order of 2–4% of group mean.	*Moderate*
250	250		Increase in respiratory morbidity among susceptible adults (chronic bronchitics) and possibly children	*Moderate*
500	500		Increase in mortality among elderly, chronically ill people	*Severe*

Note: effects on human health are thought to become severe at levels of 400 μg m^{-3} for each of SO$_2$ and particles.

Morbidity

In view of the difficulty of allowing adequately for possible confounding factors in studies based purely on death certification, as above, further investigations of the role of air pollution in the gradual development of respiratory disease have been undertaken through epidemiological surveys. For this purpose, the standardized questionnaires on respiratory symptoms (MRC, 1976) developed originally in the 1950s for studies on occupational factors, have proved invaluable. These include questions on cough, phlegm, breathlessness, wheezing and history of acute respiratory illness, together with detailed enquiries into smoking habits and opportunities to include occupational and residential histories, linking with possible air pollution exposure. This latter aspect has, however, remained a weak feature as quantitative assessment of exposures, particularly in relation to past conditions, has generally been difficult. What has emerged by now is that smoking is the dominant factor in the development of chronic respiratory symptoms but exposure to urban air pollution, from birth onwards, can play a contributory role (Waller, 1989).

Some early studies (Holland *et al.*, 1965) examining effects of pollution in urban and rural areas within and between the UK and the USA were carried out on a specific group (telephone workers) to minimize effects of occupational or socioeconomic factors. Differences in symptom prevalence were shown that were not attributable to smoking habits, but the pollution measurements were not comparable enough between the UK and the USA for quantitative interpretation. Another study carried out in the UK while pollution levels were still high (Lambert and Reid, 1970) was based on a general population sample, demonstrating a continuous relationship with both smoking and levels of air pollution (smoke and sulphur dioxide). Further extensive surveys of respiratory symptoms were carried out in the USA, notably in Berlin, New Hampshire (Ferris *et al.*, 1973; 1976) where a papermill had led to relatively high concentrations of sulphur dioxide, and in the heavily polluted city of Cracow in Poland. Collectively, the findings from the available studies were considered by a WHO group (WHO, 1979) to indicate an increased prevalence of respiratory symptoms among adults when mean annual concentrations of smoke and of sulphur dioxide each exceeded about 100 μg m^{-3}.

A somewhat separate approach to examining medium- to long-term effects of exposure to air pollution has been to concentrate on children, avoiding to a large extent problems related to occupational exposures or to smoking. Two early studies in the UK (Douglas and Waller, 1966; Lunn *et al.*, 1967, 1970) each demonstrated an increasing incidence of respiratory infections among children with increasing levels of pollution. The same WHO group (WHO, 1979) considered that such effects became apparent with levels of smoke and sulphur dioxide consistent with those noted in respect of adults, namely, beyond about 100 μg m^{-3} annual average for each of these pollutants. In retrospect, however, one cannot be sure that confounding variables linked with socioeconomic conditions were adequately accounted for, in particular the role of environmental tobacco smoke indoors in enhancing respiratory symptoms in young children (Colley, 1974).

Functional Changes

Some of the earlier studies on the prevalence of respiratory symptoms described above also included measurements of lung function, usually spirometric observations of $FEV_{0.75}$, FEV_1, FVC or peak expiratory flow readings. To obtain sensitive assessments of possible air pollution effects in recent years, with the generally lower exposures experienced, such measurements have become a more important part of epidemiological surveys.

In one particular long-running series (Van der Lende *et al.*, 1986) respiratory symptoms and lung function have been examined in an industrial and a rural area, each repeated at 3-year intervals. While FEV_1 values have remained lower in the industrial than in the rural area, possibly attributable to exposures to relatively high levels of sulphur dioxide and other pollutants in earlier years, before the surveys began, findings overall have not been clear-cut.

The overall conclusion in respect of chronic effects of air pollution is that adverse effects of prolonged exposures to the very high levels of pollution by sulphur dioxide/particulates, notably from domestic coal-burning sources, have been detectable in the past in terms of enhanced morbidity and mortality from respiratory diseases, and that situation still persists in a number of countries around the world. Elsewhere, while there could still be residual effects, they are difficult to detect in the face of other important factors, especially smoking.

Studies Related to the Photochemical Complex, 'Summer Smog'

Acute Effects

Mortality

The photochemical complex, with ozone as a principal component, has never been associated with any substantial increases in daily mortality such as have occurred with 'winter smog'. However, there have been a number of investigations of possible associations in the Los Angeles area, where there is a large population yielding a substantial number of deaths per day, and where levels of photochemical pollutants are particularly high. The most recent study of this type (Kinney and Ozkaynak, 1991) considered daily deaths from all causes combined (excluding accidents and violence) and cardiovascular and respiratory causes individually in relation to temperature, concentrations of primary motor vehicle related pollutants (carbon monoxide, nitrogen dioxide and a particular measure of aerosols) as well as photochemical oxidants (ozone). The principal result was an association between total mortality and ozone levels on the previous day, but temperature and nitrogen dioxide levels were also linked with mortality. The changes in daily deaths attributable to ozone (or to inter-related components of the photochemical complex) were small, and it was shown that a combined variable of temperature, ozone lagged one day, and nitrogen dioxide concentration could account for 4 per cent of the variance in daily mortality.

Morbidity and Functional Changes

There are reports of acute respiratory symptoms including chest discomfort (Schwartz and Zeger, 1990) and cough, shortness of breath or pain on deep inspiration (Lippmann, 1989b) associated with relatively high concentrations of ozone and associated photochemical pollutants, but most investigations have been based primarily on objective measurements of lung function. The majority of the studies reported to date have been carried out in North America and have involved ventilatory capacity measurements, such as FEV_1 or peak flow repeated daily on groups of children

attending summer camps. Such a design offers advantages not only in terms of easy access to compliant subjects, but also in terms of exposure, as ozone levels reach their maxima in sunny summer weather, and concentrations of this secondary pollutant can be as high, or higher, in rural areas away from the sources of the primary (motor-vehicle related) pollutants than close to them. The associated outdoor activities also contribute to enhancement of effects because, as seen in the toxicological section, exercising in moderate concentrations of ozone increases the likelihood of observing (transient) changes in lung function. The magnitude of the changes associated with ambient concentrations is small in relation to either intra- or inter-subject variations, and the statistical analyses have generally involved within-subject regressions of the lung function measures on ozone concentrations, as averaged over 1–8 h periods. While the regression coefficients vary widely between subjects, some being positive and some negative, the average for each group is negative, indicating a loss of about 3 per cent of the predicted FEV_1 with ozone concentrations in the region of 100 ppb (200 $\mu g \ m^{-3}$) (Department of Health, 1991). Such concentrations are common in Southern California and are reached or exceeded in occasional 'summer smog' episodes in the UK. While the changes are in general too small to notice subjectively, and are transient, some recent work (Berry *et al.*, 1991) has indicated that intense exposures in episodes can lead to decrements in peak flow persisting for several days.

A summary of expected acute effects of exposure to photochemical smog, characterized in terms of ozone concentrations, as assessed by a WHO group, is reproduced as Table 2.

Chronic Effects

The approach to considering possible long-term effects of exposure to photochemical pollutants has been similar to that concerning the sulphur dioxide/particulates complex, but it suffers from the same risks of confounding by smoking or various socioeconomic factors and little definitive information has emerged regarding chronic effects in terms of mortality. Most of the reported studies have been done in Southern California or some other areas of the USA with a long history of pollution of this type. Comparisons have been made (Detels *et al.*, 1987; Knudson *et al.*, 1983)

Table 2 Expected acute effects of photochemical smog on days characterized by maximum 1h average ozone concentrations as indicated for children and non-smoking young adults on the basis of observations made in toxicological, clinical and epidemiological studies (chronic effects are not considered)

Ozone level ($\mu g\,m^{-3}$)	Eye, nose and irritation (in all people)	Average FEV_1 decrement (in active people outdoors)		Imposed avoidance of time and activity outdoors	Respiratory, inflammatory and clearance response, hyper-reactivity (active people outdoors)	Respiratory symptoms (primarily in adults)	Overall classification of effect
		Population	Most sensitive 10% of population				
<100	No effect	None	None	None	None	None	–
200	In few sensitive subjects	5%	10%	None	Mild	Some chest tightness, cough	*Mild*
300	<30% of people	15%	30%	Some individuals	Moderate	Increased symptoms	*Moderate*
400	>50% of people	25%	50%	Many individuals	Severe	Further increase of symptoms	*Severe*

between average annual rates of change in lung function values in areas differing in levels of photochemical pollutants, and while a reasonably consistent picture has emerged, indicating a possible dose–response relationship between ozone concentrations and the rate of decline in lung function, uncertainty remains (Lippmann, 1989a) about how effectively actual exposures have been ascertained and whether confounding factors have been accounted for adequately.

TOXICOLOGICAL ASPECTS OF AIR POLLUTANTS

Photochemical Air Pollution

Photochemical air pollution is the term given to the mixture of compounds produced as a result of the action of sunlight on primary pollutants produced in large part by the burning of fossil fuels. Petrol engines and to a lesser extent diesel engines emit nitric oxide which is rapidly oxidized to nitrogen dioxide. Ozone, a strong oxidizing agent, combines readily with nitric oxide and this accounts for the low levels of ozone recorded in busy city streets. The nitric oxide is said to form an ozone sink.

Nitrogen dioxide absorbs solar radiation and the following series of reactions occurs:

$$NO_2 + h\nu \rightarrow NO + O^{\cdot}$$
$$O^{\cdot} + O_2 \rightarrow O_3$$
$$NO + O_3 \rightarrow NO_2 + O_2$$

It will be appreciated that this 'ozone cycle' will not lead to the net production of ozone. However, the first reaction may be driven strongly to the right by the presence of catalysts, including volatile organic compounds, thus increasing the rate of ozone production relative to its breakdown. Also peroxyradicals can play a part in oxidizing nitric oxide to nitrogen dioxide and thus less ozone is lost in the third reaction of the cycle. In hot sunny weather a build up of ozone is produced.

Other compounds produced during photolysis of primary pollutants include peroxyacyl nitrates, hydrogen peroxide, secondary aldehydes, nitric acid, fine particulates and short-lived radicals (WHO, 1987). Of these only peroxyacetyl nitrate will be considered.

Ozone

Occurrence and Production
Ozone is the component of photochemical pollution on which most attention has been focused. The notorious photochemical smog of Los Angeles was demonstrated in the 1950s to contain high concentrations of ozone, and ozone is often assumed to be a component of the air pollution

found in other cities. This is not always true: the ozone sink described above often leads to rather low levels of ozone in close proximity to heavy traffic.

High levels of ozone are found in the stratosphere. Tropospheric infolding produces peak ozone levels as high as 120 μg m^{-3} in areas remote from industrial or vehicular generation of the primary pollutants which take part in the photochemical pollution of ozone. Formation of ozone takes place in air masses which drift away from urban and industrialized areas and thus in many parts of the world mean ozone levels are highest in rural areas. In Los Angeles special topographic conditions, remarkable vehicle density and strong sunlight have led, in the past, to ozone levels of 1500 μg m^{-3}. Levels in Los Angeles are today lower than this and seldom exceed 600 μg m^{-3}. Levels in the UK reached a peak in 1976 when for a 2-week period peak hourly averages in parts of southern England exceeded 400 μg m^{-3}. The combination of pollutant drift from Europe and exceptional sunny weather accounted for this.

As expected, ozone levels are highest in the afternoon when formative processes have had time to work on the primary pollutants. Ozone levels tend to fall at night but during ozone episodes concentrations may be maintained leading to a day to day escalation in peak levels.

Ozone is a very reactive compound and levels indoors are lower than those outside as a result of ozone reacting with furnishings and fittings.

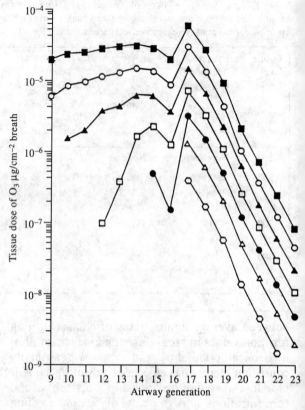

Figure 4 Predicted tissue deposition of ozone for various regions of the human lung. Model analysis used a tidal volume of 500 ml and a respiratory frequency of 15 breaths per min. Source: Miller *et al.* (1978). Tracheal ozone concentration (μg m^{-3}): ■, 4000; ○, 2000; ▲, 1000; □, 500; ●, 250; △, 125; ○, 62.5

Toxicokinetics of Ozone

Much of what is known of the kinetics of ozone uptake derives from the work of Miller *et al.* (1978). This work suggests that the peak local ozone dose in terms of mass per unit surface area (μg cm^{-2}) occurs at the terminal bronchiole in both man and laboratory animals (Figure 4).

Gerrity and Wiester (1987) reported total percentage respiratory uptake of ozone to be 96 per cent of the inspired mass in man and 44 per cent in rats. Despite this difference the authors concluded that the mass dose per unit surface airway area was similar in man and rats. Increased minute volume has been calculated to have a significant effect in increasing local ozone dose at the terminal airways.

Effects of Ozone on Health

Three particularly important reviews of aspects of the toxicology of ozone have been published in recent years (Menzel, 1984; Lippmann, 1989a; Mustafa, 1990). The present authors have both contributed to a recent review of the acute effects of ozone episodes in the UK (Department of Health, 1991) which deals at length with the topic. The following comments are based in part on that review.

Biochemical and Histopathological Effects of Ozone

Ozone is a strong oxidizing agent and reacts with a range of cellular components. Lipids in the cell membrane are susceptible to oxidation and the production of free radicals may lead to chain reactions and further membrane damage. Aldehyde formation leads to destabilization of cell membranes and impairment of functioning of normal permeability control processes. Elevation of cytosolic Ca^{2+} has been suggested (Orrenius, 1987) to play a role in cell damage and activation of phospholipases can lead to the initiation of inflammatory cascades with production of arachidonic acid derivatives.

Protective systems which defend cells against oxidant attack include the superoxide dismutase (SOD)/catalase system and glutathione peroxidase which catalyses the conversion of glutathione to oxidized glutathione with toxic peroxides being converted to non-toxic lipid alcohols (Department of Health, 1991). Glutathione has been shown to be present in high concentrations in the lining fluid of the respiratory tract (Cantin *et al.*, 1987) and this may represent the first line of defence against ozone.

Type I alveolar cells located in alveolar ducts and respiratory bronchioles appear to be the most sensitive of lung cells to ozone attack. Plopper *et al.* (1979) have demonstrated cell damage at ozone concentrations of 400 μg m^{-3}. The importance of Clara cells, their susceptibility to damage by ozone, and their role in repair of the epithelium of the terminal airways has been stressed by Richards (Department of Health, 1991). Many animal studies have involved exposure to high concentrations of ozone for long periods; Moffat *et al.* (1987) exposed bonnet monkeys to 800 or 1280 μg m^{-3} ozone, for 8 h per day for 90 days and demonstrated significant changes in respiratory bronchioles. These included peribronchiolar inflammation and hypertrophy and hyperplasia of non-ciliated bronchiolar cells. As is the case with many studies of the effects of air pollutants in animals, these studies are of more value in clarifying the site and mode of action of ozone than in predicting likely effects produced by ambient exposures in humans.

Tolerance has been demonstrated to be developed by animals to the effects of ozone (Mustafa and Tierney, 1978). It may be that the mechanism underlying the enhanced resistance of mice to the effects of high doses of ozone is related to the decrease in response to ozone demonstrated in humans after a primary exposure (see below).

Ozone has been demonstrated to impair the capacity of the lung to resist bacterial infection (US Environmental Protection Agency, 1986). The exact mechanism involved has not been iden-

tified but damage to epithelial surfaces, impairment of macrophage functioning, and impaired mucociliary clearance have been suggested.

Effects of Ozone on Humans

Numerous experimental studies of the effects of ozone on humans have been reported. These were reviewed by Tattersfield (Department of Health, 1991). The paper by Hazucha (1987) provides a useful compilation of data from human studies. McDonnell *et al.* (1983) report studies involving a range of concentrations of ozone and Hazucha *et al.* (1989) have commented on the mechanisms involved.

From these reviews and reports of studies the following conclusions are drawn:

(1) Exposure to ozone at concentrations in excess of 160 μg m^{-3}, particularly while subjects undertake moderate to vigorous exercise, will lead to reproducible, statistically significant changes in indices of lung function including FEV_1, specific airways resistance, vital capacity, and total lung capacity in sensitive individuals.

(2) A curvilinear dose–response relationship between ozone concentration and change in indices of lung function exists. This relationship is shown in Figure 5 (from Hazucha, 1987).

(3) No threshold of effect has been demonstrated (Menzel and Wolpert, 1989).

(4) As a group, asthmatics do not appear more sensitive to low concentrations of ozone than the normal population, although Kreit *et al.* (1989) demonstrated that exposure to 800 μg m^{-3} ozone for 2 h led to a greater fall in FEV_1 in asthmatic subjects than in controls. Other indices of lung function showed a similar change in both groups. Koenig *et al.* (1987) failed to demonstrate a difference in sensitivity between asthmatics and normal subjects. However, among normal individuals a considerable range of sensitivity to ozone has been demonstrated. Some 10 per cent of the population may well be unusually sensitive to ozone: identification of this group prior to exposure to ozone is not currently possible.

The exact mechanisms by which ozone produces changes in lung function are not understood. A decrease in FEV_1 and an increase in airway resistance indicate a bronchoconstrictive element as does a fall in vital capacity.

In addition to the controlled studies referred

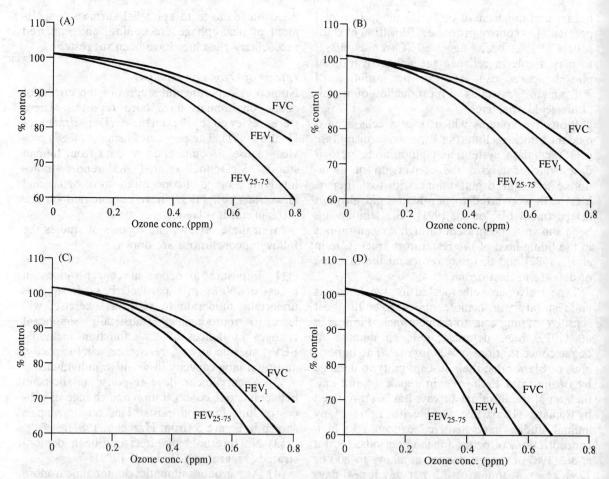

Figure 5 Ozone concentration–response regression curves of forced vital capacity (FVC), forced expiratory volume at 1 s (FEV$_1$) and mean forced expiratory flow between 25 and 75 per cent of FVC (FEV$_{25-75}$) grouped by exercise load. (A) Light exercise, (B) moderate exercise, (C) heavy exercise, and (D) very heavy exercise. Source: Hazucha (1987)

to above, extensive field studies of the effects of ozone on lung function have been conducted. Kinney *et al.* (1988) have provided a useful summary of the results of a number of these studies. Classic studies include those of Lippmann and his associates (Lippmann *et al.*, 1983; Lioy *et al.*, 1985; Spektor *et al.*, 1988). Anderson (Department of Health, 1991) reviewed these studies and concluded that they confirmed the effects predicted by chamber studies; indeed the response to ozone tended to be greater, exposure for exposure, in the field studies. The role of other pollutants in the response recorded in the field studies is difficult to quantify. Interestingly, the field studies which have examined the effects of ozone on indices of lung function in children have shown little association between ozone levels and

symptoms. In adult studies cough and pain on inspiration have been recorded. Schelegle and Adams (1986) have shown that performance in athletic events may be impaired by elevated ambient ozone concentrations.

As noted above in the section on animal studies, tolerance or adaptation has been demonstrated to be developed in humans after exposure to ozone (Horvath *et al.*, 1981). The mechanism of effect is again unknown, but on repetitive exposure for 5 days peak responses were seen on day 2 and minimal responses on day 5. Adaptation to ozone seems to last from 7 to 20 days.

Peroxyacetyl Nitrate (PAN)

Early observation of the effects of Los Angeles photochemical smog demonstrated eye, nose and throat irritation when ozone concentrations exceeded 200 μg m^{-3}. Controlled studies of the effects of pure ozone have not consistently demonstrated eye irritation at such concentrations and it may be that other compounds of the photochemical mix were responsible for the effect. PAN is an eye irritant and is found in photochemical smog. At the levels usually encountered PAN is accepted as being unlikely to pose a serious threat to health. In addition to PAN a number of aldehydes and acrolein have been identified in photochemical smog. It is possible that these play a role in the production of eye, nose and throat irritation.

Nitrogen Dioxide

Nitrogen dioxide is generated in large quantities as a result of burning fossil fuels for heating, power generation and as petrol and diesel oil in motor vehicles. In many developed countries nitrogen dioxide forms a significant proportion of the air pollutant mixture outdoors during both summer and winter. Nitrogen dioxide is formed largely from nitric oxide which makes up the majority of the nitrogen oxides emitted by combustion processes. Conversion of nitric oxide to nitrogen dioxide is rapid, particularly in the presence of ozone (see above).

Interestingly, nitrogen dioxide levels may be higher indoors than out as unvented heating appliances and gas stoves unequipped with extraction hoods are an important source. Tobacco smoke also contributes to indoor nitrogen dioxide levels.

Toxicokinetics of Nitrogen Dioxide

Like ozone, nitrogen dioxide is poorly absorbed by the upper respiratory tract and peak tissue doses occur at the junction of the conducting airways and the gas exchange zone of the lung (Miller *et al.*, 1982). As is the case for most inhaled compounds, exercise leading to increased ventilation and an increased oral inspiratory flow, raises the proportion of the inspired gas which reaches the lower airways.

Biochemical and Histopathological Effects

A particularly detailed account of the cellular effects of nitrogen dioxide has been provided by Guidotti (1978). Mustafa and Tierney (1978) have also dealt with the biochemical changes in detail. As in the case of ozone, oxidant attack on components of cell membranes appears to be a major cause of injury. It has been suggested that nitrogen dioxide may combine with water to form nitric acid (Goldstein *et al.*, 1980; Overton and Miller, 1988) although Samet and Utell (1990) have pointed out that uncertainty remains over the role of nitric acid in the damage-producing process.

An effect was reported by Guidotti (1978): the capacity of nitrogen dioxide (0.33 per cent) to raise the surface tension of films of egg lecithin (phosphatidylcholine) and phospholipid extract of *Escherichia coli*, was not confirmed when films of dipalmitoyl lecithin were studied. An increase in the surface tension exerted by lung washings was, however, reported by Arner and Rhoades (1973) from studies of rats exposed to 0.3 ppm nitrogen dioxide for 9 months. The relevance of these studies to the understanding of the effects of nitrogen dioxide on the fluid flux across alveolar capillaries is considerable.

At high concentrations, nitrogen dioxide produces severe effects on the lungs including damage to cilia, stripping of bronchiolar epithelium, impairment of macrophage function, delayed pulmonary oedema, emphysema and interstitial fibrosis. These changes are associated with exposure to levels well in excess of those present in ambient air but are relevant in cases of 'silo-fillers' disease' where individuals are exposed to very high concentrations of nitrogen dioxide. Welders working in box section steel work are also at risk (see Chapter 22). Recently attention has focused on the capacity of nitrogen dioxide to impair the defence mechanisms of the lung against bacteria and viruses. This work has been linked with the suggestion that exposure to nitrogen dioxide increases the likelihood of respiratory infections in humans (see below). In some of these studies exposure regimens have involved exposure of experimental animals to levels of nitrogen dioxide in excess of 1 ppm for long periods and few studies have attempted to replicate conditions of common ambient exposure. Ehrlich and Henry (1968) demonstrated that chronic exposure to 0.5 ppm of nitrogen dioxide increased mortality and reduced clearance of *Klebsiella pneumoniae* from the lungs of mice. Studies by Richters *et al.* (1987) and Richters and Damji (1988) showed that long-term (7–12 week) exposures to 0.25 or 0.35 ppm of nitrogen dioxide affected splenic T lymphocyte populations. These latter studies show results at concentrations low enough to be of relevance to those exposed to fumes from gas cookers.

Effects of Ambient Concentrations of Nitrogen Dioxide on Humans

The effects of low concentrations of nitrogen dioxide on humans remain ill-understood. Here two kinds of data will be considered: those relating to the effects of low concentrations of nitrogen dioxide on indices of lung function, and those relating to epidemiological studies designed to investigate the effects of long-term exposure to nitrogen dioxide on susceptibility to infections.

Effects of Nitrogen Dioxide on Indices of Lung Function As with other irritant gases, asthmatics might be expected to be sensitive to lower concentrations of nitrogen dioxide than normal individuals. Clear changes in indices of lung function have been recorded in individuals exposed to more than 2.5 ppm of nitrogen dioxide either at rest or during exercise, for periods of up to 2 h (Beil and Ulmer, 1976). At a concentration of 1 ppm and less no consistent changes have been recorded in normal individuals (WHO, 1987). Effects have been recorded in asthmatic subjects at concentrations below 1 ppm; the report of Orehek *et al.* (1976) that exposure to 0.1 ppm nitrogen dioxide potentiated the response to carbachol challenge records the lowest concentration at which effects have been demonstrated. The results of this study have not been confirmed by other workers (Hazucha *et al.*, 1983) although Kleinman *et al.* (1983) demonstrated increased sensitivity in asthmatics at 0.2 ppm. Bauer *et al.* (1986) demonstrated potentiation of exercise-induced bronchospasm and airway hyper-reactivity after cold air provocation as a result of exposing asthmatics to 0.3 ppm of nitrogen dioxide. Rubinstein *et al.* (1990) failed to demonstrate an increased sensitivity to sulphur dioxide after exposing asthmatics to 0.3 ppm of nitrogen dioxide. Bauer *et al.* (1984) demonstrated small changes in indices of lung function in exercising asthmatics exposed to 0.3 ppm of nitrogen dioxide. The changes recorded were of the order of a 10 per cent decrement in FEV_1 and were not considered as 'necessarily adverse' by the panel of experts contributing to the WHO Guidelines on Air Quality (WHO, 1987). Considerable inter-subject variability of response was demonstrated

in these studies but it seems likely that exercising asthmatics might show reproducible changes in indices of lung function as nitrogen dioxide concentrations approach 0.5 ppm.

The significance of small changes in indices of lung function is discussed below.

Epidemiological Studies of the Effects of Nitrogen Dioxide on Respiratory Infections The association between indoor concentrations of nitrogen dioxide and the use of gas for cooking has led to a number of studies of respiratory disease amongst children living in gas-using homes as compared with those from homes not using gas. Speizer *et al.* (1980) demonstrated that children from homes using gas for cooking were significantly more likely to suffer from respiratory illness before the age of 2 years. In later studies the association between gas use and respiratory illness was found to be weaker and statistically not significant (Ware *et al.*, 1984). Other studies including those of Florey *et al.* (1979), Melia *et al.* (1983), Ogsten *et al.* (1985) and Koo *et al.* (1990) failed to show a clear effect. In 1989 Goings *et al.* reported a 3-year study of adults exposed for short periods to either fresh air or levels of nitrogen dioxide ranging from 0.1 ppm to 0.3 ppm and then exposed to intranasally administered influenza virus (live, attenuated cold-adapted influenza A/Korea/82 reassortant virus). Although exposure to nitrogen dioxide produced a small increase in the likelihood of infection the results were not statistically significant.

In conclusion, the assertion that indoor pollution by nitrogen dioxide leads to an increase in respiratory disease has not been proven. In passing it may be noted that the association between childhood respiratory infections and maternal smoking is much more firmly established.

Sulphur Dioxide, Particulates and Acid Aerosols

Sulphur Dioxide

Toxicokinetics of Sulphur Dioxide
Sulphur dioxide is soluble in water and considerable absorption occurs in the upper airways including the nose and mouth. Absorption is concentration dependent with more than 90 per cent of inspired sulphur dioxide being absorbed at high

concentrations. However, at low concentrations, Strandberg (1964) demonstrated that only 5 per cent of inspired sulphur dioxide was taken up in the upper respiratory tract of rabbits. The significance of this finding to estimating likely upper airway exposure in humans, given the interspecies differences in nasal structure, may be questioned.

Effects of Sulphur Dioxide on Humans

Sulphur dioxide produces bronchoconstriction when inhaled in high concentration by both humans and common laboratory animals. In humans bronchoconstriction, monitored by measurement of airway resistance, is regularly seen on exposure to concentrations of sulphur dioxide in excess of 5.0 ppm. In normal individuals effects are only occasionally seen at, or below, 1.00 ppm (Frank *et al.*, 1962). Other features include increased response with deep breathing and a decline rather than further increase in airway resistance with prolonged exposures (Lawther *et al.*, 1975). Asthmatics have been shown to be more sensitive to sulphur dioxide than normal individuals. Studies by Sheppard *et al.* (1980, 1981a,b), Jaeger *et al.* (1979) and Linn *et al.* (1980, 1982) have shown that small changes in indices of lung function might be expected on inhalation of sulphur dioxide at concentrations as low as 0.5 ppm. The WHO Expert Panel (WHO, 1987) accepted that effects of concern to health were demonstrable in exercising asthmatics at concentrations down to about 1000 μg m^{-3}.

It is accepted that sulphur dioxide exerts its bronchoconstrictor effects by stimulating receptors in the airways. These receptors are vagally innervated and the response is mediated by the efferent vagal innervation of the airways (Widdicombe, 1954). Afferent fibres running in sympathetic nerves are also thought to be involved in the reflex.

Acid Aerosols

Folinsbee (1989) has pointed out the difficulties in studying the effects of acid aerosols on the respiratory tract. These difficulties apply equally to attempts to estimate the likely effects of an often inadequately characterized aerosol. Table 3 compares the factors of importance in studies of ozone and acid aerosols (Folinsbee, 1989).

Amdur (1986) considered the toxicology of acid aerosols under three headings. This is helpful and the following account follows Amdur's approach.

Sulphuric Acid Aerosols

There is no doubt that high levels of sulphuric acid aerosols can be dangerous to health. Kitagawa (1984) showed that so-called 'Yokkaichi asthma' was caused by the release of sulphuric acid from a titanium dioxide plant in Japan. The effects of exposure to lower levels of sulphuric acid are, however, not easy to define. Lippmann in 1985 reviewed the effects of airborne acidity on health and stated that it was not possible to be certain about whether ambient levels of airborne acidity were having an effect on health in North America. Studies by Bates and Sizto (1989) and Schenker *et al.* (1983) have suggested that morbidity from respiratory disease is related to air pollution and have argued, on the basis of strengths of association, that acid aerosols play a significant part in the effect.

Studies by Amdur (1958) and Amdur *et al.* (1978) using guinea pigs have shown that sulphuric acid is more potent than sulphur dioxide as a bronchoconstrictor and that the response to sulphuric acid depends both on concentration and the size of the aerosol particles inhaled. Interestingly, peak responses were recorded when very small particles were inhaled <1.0 μm mass median diameter (MMD).

The effects of sulphuric acid aerosols on mucociliary clearance in the airways has been studied in both humans and animals (Schlesinger *et al.*, 1978). Clearance is slowed by exposure to sulphuric acid and in this, as well as other effects, sulphuric acid is markedly more active than sulphur dioxide.

Though asthmatics might be expected to be more sensitive to acid aerosols than normal subjects, experimental studies have yielded conflicting results. In asthmatic adolescents effects have been demonstrated at a concentration of 100 μg m^{-3} (Ericsson and Camner, 1983), and in adult asthmatics at 350 μg m^{-3} (Utell and Morrow, 1986). In both these studies subjects undertook exercise during exposure to the acid aerosol.

Particulate Sulphates

The role of particulate sulphates is difficult to determine. Unfortunately, airborne acid sulphate is often reported in terms of 'total sulphate' and,

Table 3   Comparison of factors important in exposure to ozone and sulphuric acid

Factor	Ozone	Acid aerosol
Factors affecting dose		
Exposure duration	Yes	Yes
Ventilation	Yes	Yes
Oral/nasal partitioning	Minimal effect	Important
Concentration	Yes	Yes
Particle size (MMAD)	No	Yes
Particle distribution (σ_g)	No	Yes
Humidity	Minimal effect	Yes
Temperature	Minimal effect	Yes
Surface properties	No	Yes
Deposition/loss in upper airways	Fairly consistent	Highly variable
Air-phase neutralization	No	Yes
Reactions on airway surface	Forms byproducts	Mucus buffering
		Forms byproducts
Ease of measurement of		
sensitive physiological end point	Yes (spirometry)	No (clearance)
Ease of generation and control		
of artificial environment	Simple	Complex

without further analysis to identify the species present, it is not possible to predict the effects.

Sulphates present in air include: ammonium sulphate, ammonium bisulphate, ammonium metabisulphite, ammonium sulphite and ammonium bisulphite. These are produced by reactions of ammonia with sulphuric and sulphurous acid. Neutralization of inhaled acid by oral ammonia is a complicating factor in volunteer studies designed to investigate the effects of inhaled acid. There is also the further complication that sulphate particles and droplets undergo hygroscopic growth and neutralization as they pass along the airways. In many countries haze is produced by ammonium sulphate aerosols. Amdur (1961) studied the relative potency of a range of sulphates and ranked them as shown in Table 4. It is interesting to note that ammonium sulphate is markedly more active than sodium sulphate. It is also interesting that ammonium sulphate is more active than the more acidic salt ammonium bisulphate. Clear explanations for the differing effects are not available, and it cannot be assumed that the same pattern would occur in humans.

Effects of Particulates on the Response to Sulphur Dioxide

Amdur showed that the effects of sulphur dioxide may be potentiated by inert aerosols of small size. Humidity was found to play an important part in

Table 4   Relative irritant potency of sulphates

Sulphuric acid	100
Zinc ammonium sulphate*	33
Ferric sulphate†	26
Zinc sulphate*	19
Ammonium sulphate	10
Ammonium bisulphate	3
Cupric sulphate	2
Ferrous sulphate	0.7
Sodium sulphate‡	0.7
Manganous sulphate†	−0.9§

* Data of Amdur and Corn, 1963.
† Data of Amdur and Underhill, 1968.
‡ Particle size: 0.1 µm.
§ Resistance decreased; change not significant.

the effect, a more marked effect being seen at higher humidity values. More marked potentiation was demonstrated by the same author with particulates capable of converting sulphur dioxide to sulphuric acid in the particle surface water film. Manganese, vanadium, and ferrous iron were effective in this way (Amdur and Underhill, 1968).

The Problem of Predicting Effects on Human Populations from Measurements of Particulate Concentrations

In addition to the particulates mentioned above a range of other particulates occur in ambient air. Carbonaceous particles, particles of silicates, metals and other salts are also present. Measurement of particulates by means of reflectance methods or gravimetric determinations allow statements about particle concentrations to be made. From the above description it will be realized at once that the response likely to be produced on inhalation of particulate aerosols is likely to be critically dependent not only on the distribution of particle size but also on particle composition. As far as acidic effects are concerned the active component is likely to be hydrogen ion (H^+). Lippmann (1989a) arranges a series of measurements in increasing order of value as significant predictors of the effects on health of the sulphate–particulate mix; total suspended particulates, inhalable particles, fine particles and sulphates. Of course sulphuric acid would be better yet.

Carbon Monoxide

Toxicokinetics

Carbon monoxide is readily absorbed across the respiratory tract and binds avidly to haemoglobin. The affinity of haemoglobin for carbon monoxide is some 250 times greater than its affinity for oxygen. In addition to reducing the capacity of the blood to transport oxygen, carbon monoxide causes the oxyhaemoglobin dissociation curve to shift to the left, reducing the amount of oxygen unloaded at the tissues. A reduction in unloading of oxygen is particularly serious in tissues such as myocardium where 60–70 per cent of the oxygen in arterial blood is usually extracted in comparison with 25 per cent in many other tissues. The reduction in the oxygen carrying capacity of the blood and the shift of the oxyhaemoglobin dissociation curve explain the majority of the toxicological effects of carbon monoxide. Other mechanisms may play a smaller role including the binding of carbon monoxide to intracellular components such as myoglobin in muscle cells and cytochrome oxidase (Coburn, 1979). It has been suggested that the formation of carboxymyoglobin in the subendocardium could explain the electrocardiographic changes and decrements in work capacity seen, particularly in patients with a compromised coronary circulation, at comparatively low levels of blood carboxyhaemoglobin.

Exposure to low concentrations of carbon monoxide does not lead to immediate complete equilibration of the blood with the gas. Comroe (1974), using a ratio of 210 for the affinity of haemoglobin for carbon monoxide compared with oxygen, illustrated this as follows:

(1) Given that air contains 21 per cent oxygen, and that the affinity ratio is 210, then at full equilibration breathing air containing 0.1 per cent carbon monoxide (i.e. an $O_2 : CO$ ratio of 210 : 1) will lead to 50 per cent of the haemoglobin being HbCO and 50 per cent HbO_2.

(2) Assuming a blood volume of 6 l and that at 50 per cent equilibrium each litre of blood contains 100 ml CO (at a normal haemoglobin concentration 200 ml of oxygen are transported in each litre of blood) 6 l of blood will contain 600 ml CO.

(3) Assuming a minute volume of 6 l, and assuming that all inspired air becomes alveolar air, then when breathing 0.1 per cent CO the volume of CO reaching the alveoli per minute is 6 ml.

(4) Assuming all of this diffuses into the blood and combines with haemoglobin then 100 min will be required for 600 ml of CO to cross into the blood and bring the carboxyhaemoglobin level to 50 per cent.

It will be obvious that the rate of equilibration of the blood with carbon monoxide will depend on the minute volume, the diffusing capacity for

Table 5 Predicted carboxyhaemoglobin levels for subjects engaged in different types of work

Carbon monoxide concentration		Exposure time	Predicted COHb level for those engaged in work		
ppm	mg m^{-3}		Sedentary	Light	Heavy
100	115	15 min	1.2	2.0	2.8
50	57	30 min	1.1	1.9	2.6
25	29	1 h	1.1	1.7	2.2
10	11.5	8 h	1.5	1.7	1.7

carbon monoxide, pulmonary blood flow, and the carbon monoxide concentration of the inspired gas.

Coburn *et al.* (1965) has modelled the uptake of carbon monoxide and Table 5 is derived from his equations.

Effects of Carbon Monoxide on Humans

In compiling the WHO Air Quality Guidelines for Europe (WHO, 1987) reference to EPA reports (US Environmental Protection Agency, 1979 and 1984) was made. These reports identified four types of health effects likely to be associated with exposure to carbon monoxide: (1) cardiovascular, (2) neurobehavioural, (3) fibrinolysis, and (4) perinatal. Of these, most stress was laid on the cardiovascular and neurobehavioural effects. Table 6 shows the likely health effects of exposure to carbon monoxide resulting in different percentage concentrations of carboxyhaemoglobin.

From the discussion of the mode of action of carbon monoxide certain groups of individuals are likely to be particularly affected by exposure to the compound. These are:

- Patients with angina pectoris or presymptomatic coronary insufficiency.
- Pregnant women and young infants.
- Those suffering from chronic obstructive pulmonary disease.
- Patients suffering from anaemia.
- Individuals with abnormal haemoglobin and a reduced oxygen carrying capacity.
- People living at high altitude.

Table 6 Human health effects associated with carbon monoxide exposure: lowest-observed effect levels

Carboxyhaemoglobin concentration (%)	Effects
2.3–4.3	Statistically significant decrease (3–7%) in the relation between work time and exhaustion in exercising young healthy men
2.9–4.5	Statistically significant decrease in exercise capacity (i.e. shortened duration of exercise before onset of pain) in patients with angina pectoris and increase in duration of angina attacks
5–5.5	Statistically significant decrease in maximal oxygen consumption and exercise time in young healthy men during strenuous exercise
<5	No statistically significant vigilance decrements after exposure to carbon monoxide
5–7.6	Statistically significant impairment of vigilance tasks in healthy experimental subjects
5–17	Statistically significant diminution of visual perception, manual dexterity, ability to learn or performance in complex sensorimotor tasks (e.g. driving)
7–20	Statistically significant decrease in maximal oxygen consumption during strenuous exercise in young healthy men

DEFINITION OF ADVERSE HEALTH EFFECTS

In many developed countries, levels of air pollution have declined over the past few decades and it has become more difficult to detect clear effects of air pollution on health. In the 1950s and 1960s in England the winter coal smoke and sulphur dioxide smogs were shown to increase mortality among those suffering from cardiovascular and respiratory diseases. It has also been demonstrated that raised levels of sulphur dioxide correlated with patients' self-reported exacerbations of their bronchitis. Epidemiological studies continue to reveal that exposure to pollutants may affect people, though with decreasing levels of pollution more sensitive indicators may be required to indicate an effect. Also, as pollutant levels have fallen more emphasis has been placed on individuals who may be more sensitive to given pollutants than other individuals. This is particularly the case as regards the effects of sulphur dioxide on asthmatics. Interestingly, those supposed to be likely to be sensitive to ozone, asthmatics, have not been shown to be as a group more sensitive than normal individuals.

It has also recently been realized that for many pollutants the dose–response curve may not show a threshold and thus it will be impossible to define

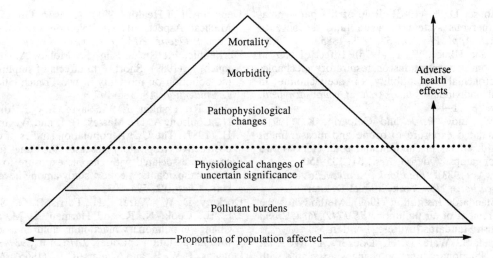

Figure 6 Spectrum of biological response to pollutant exposure. Source: American Thoracic Society (1985)

a no-effect level. It is accepted by some workers that this is the case for ozone.

These observations place a responsibility on the toxicologist to define what he considers to be a significant effect when commenting on the effects of low concentrations of pollutants on humans. This problem was considered by the American Thoracic Society in 1985 (American Thoracic Society, 1985) when the now well-known pyramid of effects was defined. This is shown in Figure 6.

It will be seen from Figure 6 that physiological changes of uncertain significance are not included as adverse health effects. The definition of how large a change in an index of physiological functioning need be recorded before it is classed as an adverse effect has not been resolved. Some authorities regard changes in indices of lung function of less than the recorded day to day variation in the index as defined in a group of individuals as insignificant. Others regard all statistically significant, reproducible changes as of medical significance. It is clear that only properly organized, long-term cohort studies will allow the accurate determination of the importance of small changes in indices of physiological functioning.

REFERENCES

Amdur, M. O. (1958). The respiratory response of guinea pigs to sulfuric acid mist. *AMA Arch. Ind. Health*, **18**, 407–414

Amdur, M. O. (1961). The effect of aerosols on the response to irritant gases. In Davies, C. N. (Ed.), *Inhaled Particles and Vapours*. Pergamon Press, Oxford, pp. 281–292

Amdur, M. O. (1986). Air pollutants. In Klaasen, C. D., Amdur, M. O. and Doull, J. (Eds), *Casarett and Doull's Toxicology: The Basic Science of Poisons*. Macmillan Publishing Company, New York, pp. 801–824

Amdur, M. O. and Underhill, D. W. (1968). The effects of various aerosols on the response of guinea pigs to sulfur dioxide. *Arch. Environ. Health*, **16**, 460–468

Amdur, M. O., Dubriel, M. and Creasia, D. A. (1978). Respiratory response of guinea pigs to low levels of sulfuric acid. *Environ. Res.*, **15**, 418–423

American Thoracic Society (1985). Guidelines on what constitutes an adverse respiratory health effect, with special reference to epidemiologic studies of air pollution. *Am. Rev. Respir. Dis.*, **131**, 666–668

Arner, E. C. and Rhoades, R. A. (1973). Long-term nitrogen dioxide exposure: effects on lung lipids and mechanical properties. *Arch. Environ. Health*, **25**, 156–160

Bates, D. V. and Sizto, R. (1989). The Ontario air pollution study: identification of the causative agent. *Environ. Health Perspect.*, **79**, 69–72

Bauer, M. A., Utell, M. J., Morrow, P. E., Speers, D. M. and Gibb, F. R. (1984). 0.3 ppm nitrogen dioxide inhalation potentiates exercise induced bronchospasm in asthmatics. *Am. Rev. Respir. Dis.*, **129**, A151 (abstract)

Bauer, M. A., Utell, M. J., Morrow, P. E., Speers, D. M. and Gibb, F. R. (1986). Inhalation of 0.3 ppm nitrogen dioxide potentiates exercise induced bronchospasm in asthmatics. *Am. Rev. Respir. Dis.*, **134**, 1203–1208

Beckett, W. S., McDonnell, W. F., Horstmann, D. H.

and House, D. E. (1985). Role of the parasympathetic nervous system in acute lung response to ozone. *J. Appl. Physiol.*, **59**, 1879–1885

Beil, M. and Ulmer, W. T. (1976). Effect of NO_2 in workroom concentrations on respiratory mechanics and bronchial susceptibility to acetylcholine in normal individuals. *Int. Arch. Occup. Environ. Health*, **38**, 31–44

Berry, M., Lioy, P. J. and Gelperin, K. (1991). Accumulated exposure to ozone and measurement of health effects in children and counselors at two summer camps. *Environ. Res.*, **54**, 135–150

Bjørseth, A. (1983). *Handbook of Polycyclic Aromatic Hydrocarbons*. New York, Marcel Dekker

British Standards Institution (1969). Methods for the measurement of air pollution. *BS 1747, Parts 2 and 3*. British Standards Institute, London

Brunekreef, B., Ware, D. H., Dockery, D. W. *et al.* (1987). Pulmonary function changes associated with air pollution episodes: a re-analysis of the Steubenville and Ijmond alert studies. Paper 87–33.7 presented at the *80th Annual Meeting of APCA*, New York

Brunekreef, B., Lumens, M., Hoek, G., Hofschreuder, P., Fischer, P. and Biersteker, K. (1989). Pulmonary function changes associated with an air pollution episode in January 1987. *JAPCA*, **39**, 1444–1447

Cantin, A. M., North, S. L., Hubbard, R. C. and Crystal, R. G. (1987). Normal alveolar epithelial lining fluid contains high levels of glutathione. *J. Appl. Physiol.*, **63**, 152–157

Chinn, S., Florey, C. V., Baldwin, I. G. and Gorgol, M. (1981). The relation of mortality in England and Wales 1969–73 to measurements of air pollution. *J. Epidemiol. Commun. Health*, **35**, 174–179

Coburn, R. F. (1979). Mechanisms of carbon monoxide toxicity. *Prev. Med.*, **8**, 310–322

Coburn, R. F., Forster, R. E. and Kane, P. B. (1965). Considerations of the physiological variables that determine the blood carboxyhaemoglobin concentration in man. *J. Clin. Invest.*, **44**, 1899–1910

Cohen, A. A., Bromberg, S., Buechley, R. W., Heiderscheit, L. T. and Shy, C. M. (1972). Asthma and air pollution from a coal-fuelled plant. *Am. J. Public Health*, **62**, 1181–1188

Colley, J. R. T. (1974). Respiratory symptoms in children and parental smoking and phlegm production. *Br. Med. J.*, **2**, 201–204

Comroe, J. H. (1974). *Physiology of Respiration*, 2nd edn. Year Book Medical Publishers, Chicago, pp. 192–193

Daly, C. (1959). Air pollution and causes of death. *Br. J. Prev. Soc. Med.*, **13**, 14–27

Dassen, W., Brunekreef, B., Hoek, G., Hoschreuder, P., Staatsen, B., Schouten, E. and Biersteker, K. (1986). Decline in children's pulmonary function during an air pollution episode. *JAPCA* **36**, 1223–1227

Department of Health (1991). Advisory Group on the Medical Aspects of Air Pollution Episodes. *First Report: Ozone*. HMSO, London

Derriennic, F., Richardson, S., Mollie, A. and Lellouch, J. (1989). Short-term effects of sulphur dioxide pollution on mortality in two French cities. *Int. J. Epidemiol.*, **18**, 186–197

Detels, R., Tashkin, J. W., Sayre, J. W., Rokaw, S. N., Coulson, A. H., Massey, F. J. and Wegman, D. H. (1987). The UCLA population studies of chronic obstructive respiratory disease. 9. Lung function changes associated with chronic exposure to photochemical oxidants: a cohort study among never-smokers. *Chest*, **92**, 594–603

Dockery, D. W., Ware, J. H., Ferris, B. G., Speizer, F. E., Cook, N. R. and Herman, S. M. (1982). Change in pulmonary function in children associated with air pollution episodes. *JAPCA* **32**, 937–942

Douglas, J. W. B. and Waller, R. E. (1966). Air pollution and respiratory infection in children. *Br. J. Prev. Soc. Med.*, **20**, 1–8

Ehrlich, R. and Henry, M. C. (1968). Chronic toxicity of nitrogen dioxide. I. Effect on resistance to bacterial pneumonia. *Arch. Environ. Health*, **17**, 860–865

Ericsson, G. and Camner, R. (1983). Health effects of sulfur oxides and particulate matter in ambient air. *Scand. J. Work Environ. Health*, **9** (Suppl. 3) 1–52

Evans, J. S., Tosteson, T. and Kinney, P. L. (1984). Cross-sectional mortality studies and air pollution risk assessment. *Environ. Int.*, **10**, 55–83

Ferris, B. G., Higgins, I. T. T., Higgins, M. W. and Peters, J. M. (1973). Chronic nonspecific respiratory disease in Berlin, New Hampshire 1961–67. A follow-up study. *Am. Rev. Respir. Dis.*, **107**, 110–122

Ferris, B. G., Chen, H., Puleo, S. and Murphy, R. L. (1976). Chronic nonspecific respiratory disease in Berlin, New Hampshire, 1967–1973. A further follow-up study. *Am. Rev. Respir. Dis.*, **113**, 475–485

Florey, C. V., Melia, R. J. W., Chinn, S., Goldstein, B. D., Brooks, A. G. F., John, H. H., Craighead, I. B. and Webster, X. (1979). The relationship between respiratory illness in primary school children and the use of gas for cooking: III. Nitrogen dioxide, respiratory illness and lung function. *Int. J. Epidemiol.*, **8**, 347–353

Folinsbee, L. J. (1989). Human health effects of exposure to airborne acid. *Environ. Health Perspect.*, **79**, 195–199

Frank N. R., Amdur, M. O. and Worcester, J. L. (1962). Effects of controlled exposure to SO_2 on respiratory mechanics in healthy male adults. *J. Appl. Physiol.*, **17**, 252–258

Gardner, M. J., Crawford, M. D. and Morris, J. N. (1969). Patterns of mortality in middle and early old age in the County Boroughs of England and Wales. *Br. J. Prev. Soc. Med.*, **23**, 133–140

Gerrity, T. R. and Wiester, M. J. (1987). Experimental measurement of the uptake of ozone in rats and human subjects. *APCA 80th Annual Meeting*, New York

Goings, S. A., Kulle, T. J., Bascom, R., Sauder, L. R., Green, D. J., Hebel, J. R. and Clements, M. L. (1989). Effect of nitrogen dioxide exposure on susceptibility to influenza virus infection in healthy adults. *Am. Rev. Respir. Dis.*, **139**, 1075–1081

Goldstein, E., Goldstein, F., Peek, N. F. and Parks, N. J. (1980). Absorption and transport of nitrogen oxides. In Lee, S. D. (Ed.) *Nitrogen Oxides and their Effects on Health*. Ann Arbor Science, Ann Arbor, Michigan, pp. 143–160

Guidotti, T. L. (1978). The higher oxides of nitrogen: inhalation toxicology. *Environ. Res.*, **15**, 443–472

Hansen, A. M., Olsen, I. L. B., Holst, E. and Poulsen, O. M. (1990). Validation of a high performance liquid chromatography/fluorescence detection method for the simultaneous quantification of fifteen polycyclic aromatic hydrocarbons. *Ann. Occup. Med.*, **35**, 603–612

Hatzakis, A., Katsouyanni, K., Kalandidi, A., Day, N. and Trichopoulos, D. (1986). Short-term effects of air pollution on mortality in Athens. *Int. J. Epidemiol.*, **15**, 73–81

Hazucha, M. J. (1987). Relationship between ozone exposure and pulmonary function changes. *J. Appl. Physiol.*, **62**, 1671–1680

Hazucha, M. J., Ginsberg, J. F., McDonnell, W. F., Haak, E. D., Pimmel, R. L., Salaam, S. A., House, D. E. and Bromberg, P. A. (1983). Effects of 0.1 ppm nitrogen dioxide on airways of normal and asthmatic subjects. *J. Appl. Physiol.*, **53**, 730–739

Hazucha, M. J., Bates, D. V. and Bromberg, P. A. (1989). Mechanism of action of ozone on the human lung. *J. Appl. Physiol.* **67**, 1535–1541

Holland, W. W., Reid, D. D., Seltzer, R. and Stone, R. W. (1965). Respiratory disease in England and the United States. *Arch. Environ. Health*, **10**, 338–343

Horstmann, D., McDonnell, W., Abdul-Salaam, S., Folinsbee, L. and Ives, P. (1989). Changes in pulmonary function and airway reactivity due to prolonged exposure to typical ambient ozone levels. In Schneider, T., Lee, S. D., Walters, G. J. R. and Grant, L. D. (Eds), *Atmospheric Ozone Research and its Policy Implications*. Elsevier, Amsterdam, The Netherlands, pp. 755–762

Horvath, S. M., Gliner, J. A. and Folinsbee, L. J. (1981). Adaptation to ozone: duration of effect. *Am. Rev. Respir. Dis.*, **123**, 496–499

International Standards Organization (1985). Ambient air—determination of the mass concentration of nitrogen oxides—chemiluminescence method. *ISO/7996*. Paris, ISO

International Standards Organization (1991a). Ambient air—determination of a black smoke index. *ISO/DIS 9835*. Paris, ISO

International Standards Organization (1991b). Ambient air—determination of sulphur dioxide, ultra-violet fluorescence method. *ISO/DIS 10498*. ISO, Paris

Jaeger, M. J., Tribble, D. and Wittig, H. J. (1979). Effect of 0.5 ppm sulphur dioxide on the respiratory function of normal and asthmatic subjects. *Lung*, **156**, 119–127

Kinney, P. L. and Ozkaynak, H. (1991). Associations of daily mortality and air pollution in Los Angeles County. *Environ. Res.*, **54**, 99–120

Kinney, P. L., Ware, J. H. and Spengler, J. D. (1988). A critical evaluation of acute ozone epidemiology results. *Arch. Environ. Health*, **43**, 168–173

Kitagawa, T. (1984). Cause analysis of the Yokkaichi asthma episode in Japan. *JAPCA* **34**, 743–746

Kleinman, M. T., Bailey, R. M., Linn, W. S., Anderson, K. R., Whynot, J. D., Shamoo, D. A. and Hackney, J. D. (1983). Effect of 0.2 ppm nitrogen dioxide on pulmonary function and response to bronchoprovocation in asthmatics. *J. Toxicol. Environ. Health*, **12**, 815–826

Knudson, R. J., Lebowitz, M. D., Holberg, C. J. and Burrows, B. (1983). Changes in the normal maximal expiratory flow-volume curve with growth and ageing. *Am. Rev. Respir. Dis.*, **127**, 725–734

Koenig, J. Q., Covert, D. S., Marshall, S. G., van Belle, G. and Poerson, W. E. (1987). The effects of ozone and nitrogen dioxide on pulmonary function in healthy and asthmatic adolescents. *Am. Rev. Respir. Dis.*, **136**, 1152–1157

Koo, L. C., Ho, J. H-C., Ho, C-Y., Matsuki, H., Shimizu, H., Mori, T. and Tominaga, S. (1990). Personal exposure to nitrogen dioxide and its association with respiratory illness in Hong Kong. *Am. Rev. Respir. Dis.*, **141**, 1119–1126

Koutrakis, P., Fasano, A. M., Slater, J. L., Spengler, J. D., McMarthy, J. F. and Leaderer, B. P. (1989). Design of a personal annular denuder sampler to measure atmospheric aerosols and gases. *Atmos. Environ.*, **23**, 2767–2774

Kreit, J. W., Gross, K. B., Moore, T. B., Lorenzen, T. J., D'Arcy, J. and Eschenbacher, J. W. L. (1989). Ozone-induced changes in pulmonary function and bronchial responsiveness in asthmatics. *J. Appl. Physiol.*, **66**, 217–222

Lambert, P. M. and Reid, D. D. (1970). Smoking, air pollution and bronchitis in Britain. *Lancet*, **i**, 853–857

Lave, L. B. and Seskin, E. P. (1977). *Air Pollution and Human Health*. Johns Hopkins University Press, Baltimore

Lawther, P. J., Waller, R. E. and Henderson, M. (1970). Air pollution and exacerbations of bronchitis. *Thorax*, **25**, 525–539

Lawther, P. J., MacFarlane, A. J., Waller, R. E. and Brooks, A. G. F. (1975). Pulmonary function and sulphur dioxide, some preliminary findings. *Environ. Res.*, **10**, 355–367

Linn, W. S., Bailey, R. M., Shamoo, D. A., Venet, T. G., Wightman, L. H. and Hackney, J. D. (1982).

Respiratory responses of young adult asthmatics to sulfur dioxide exposure under simulated ambient conditions. *Environ. Res.*, **29**, 220–232

Linn, W. S., Jones, M. P., Bailey, R. W., Kleinman, M. T., Spier, C. E., Fischer, D. A. and Hackney, J. D. (1980). Respiratory effects of mixed oxides of nitrogen and sulfur dioxide in human volunteers under simulated ambient exposure. *Environ. Res.*, **22**, 431–438

Lioy, P. J., Vollmuth, T. A. and Lippmann, M. (1985). Persistence of peak flow decrement in children following ozone exposures exceeding the National Ambient Air Quality Standard. *JAPCA*, **35**, 1068–1071

Lippmann, M. (1985). Airborne acidity: estimates of exposure and human health effects. *Environ. Health Perspect.*, **63**, 63–70

Lippmann, M. (1989a). Background and health effects of acid aerosols. *Environ. Health Perspect.*, **79**, 3–6

Lippmann, M. (1989b). Health effects of ozone: a critical review. *JAPCA*, **39**, 672–675

Lippmann, M., Lioy, P. J., Leikauf, G., Green, K. B., Baxter, D., Morandi, M., Pasternack, B., Fife, D. and Speizer, F. E. (1983). Effects of ozone on the pulmonary function of children. *Adv. Mod. Environ. Toxicol.*, **5**, 423–426

Loewenstein, J. C., Bourdel, M. C. and Bertin, M. (1983). Influence de la pollution atmosphérique (SO₂-poussières) et des conditions météorologiques sur la mortalité à Paris entre 1969 et 1976. *Rev. Epidemiol. Santé Publique*, **31**, 143–161

Lunn, J. E., Knowelden, J. and Handyside, A. J. (1967). Patterns of respiratory illness in Sheffield infant school-children. *Br. J. Prev. Soc. Med.*, **21**, 7–16

Lunn, J. E., Knowelden, J. and Roe, J. W. (1970). Patterns of respiratory illness in Sheffield junior school-children. *Br. J. Prev. Soc. Med.*, **24**, 223–228

McDonnell, W. F., Horstman, D. H., Hazucha, M. J., Seal, E., Haak, E. D., Salam, S. A. and House, D. E. (1983). Pulmonary effects of ozone exposure during exercise: dose response characteristics. *J. Appl. Physiol.*, **54**, 1345–1352

Martin, A. E. and Bradley, W. (1960). Mortality fog and atmospheric pollution. An investigation during the winter of 1958–59. *Mon. Bull. Minist. Health Pub. Health Lab. Serv.*, **19**, 56–72

Mazumdar, S., Schimmel, H. and Higgins, I. T. T. (1982). Relation of daily mortality to air pollution: an analysis of 14 London winters, 1958–1971/72. *Arch. Environ. Health*, **37**, 213–220

Medical Research Council (1976). *Questionnaire on Respiratory Symptoms*. Medical Research Council, London

Melia, R. J. W., Florey, C. V., Sittampalam, Y. and Watkins, C. (1983). The relation between respiratory illness in infants and gas cookers in the UK: a preliminary report. In *Air Quality VIth World Congress*. Proceedings of the International Union of Air Pollution Prevention Associations, Paris France. Paris, France, SEPIC(APPA), pp. 263–269

Menzel, D. B. (1984). Ozone: an overview of its toxicity in man and animals. *J. Toxicol. Environ. Health*, **13**, 183–204

Menzel, D. B. and Wolpert, R. L. (1989). Is there a threshold for human health risk from ozone? In Schneider, T., Lee, S. D., Wolters, G. J. R. and Grant, L. D. (Eds), *Atmospheric Ozone Research and its Policy Implications*. Elsevier Science Publishers, Amsterdam

Miller, F. J., Menzel, D. B. and Coffin, D. L. (1978). Similarity between man and laboratory animals in regional pulmonary deposition of ozone. *Environ. Res.*, **17**, 84–101

Miller, F. J., Overton, J. H., Meyers, E. T. and Graham, J. A. (1982). Pulmonary dosimetry of nitrogen dioxide in animals and man. In Schneider, T. and Grant, L. (Eds), *Air Pollution by Nitrogen Oxides*. Elsevier, Amsterdam, pp. 377–386

Ministry of Health (1954). *Mortality and Morbidity during the London Fog of December*. HMSO, London

Moffat, R. K., Hyde, D. M., Plopper, C. G., Tyler, W. S. and Putney, L. F. (1987). Ozone-induced adaptive and reactive cellular changes in respiratory bronchioles of bonnet monkeys. **12**, 57–74

Mustafa, M. G. (1990). Biochemical basis of ozone toxicity. *Free Radic. Biol. Med.*, **9**, 245–265

Mustafa, M. G. and Tierney, D. F. (1978). Biochemical and metabolic changes in the lung with oxygen, ozone and nitrogen dioxide toxicity. *Am. Rev. Respir. Dis.*, **118**, 1061–1090

Ogsten, S. A., Florey, C. V. and Walker, C. H. M. (1985). The Tayside infant morbidity and mortality study: effect on health of using gas for cooking. *Br. Med. J.*, **290**, 957–960

Orehek, J., Massari, J. P., Gayrard, P., Grimaud, C. and Charpin, J. (1976). Effect of short-term, low level nitrogen dioxide exposure on bronchial sensitivity of asthmatic patients. *J. Clin. Invest.*, **57**, 301–307

Orrenius, N. P. (1987). Perturbation of thiol and calcium homeostasis in cell injury. In Fowler, B. A. (Ed.), *Mechanisms of Cell Injury; Implications for Human Health*. John Wiley, Chichester and New York, pp. 115–125

Ostro, B. (1984). A search for a threshold in the relationship of air pollution to mortality: a re-analysis of data on London winters. *Environ. Health Perspect.*, **58**, 397–399

Overton, J. H. and Miller, F. J. (1988). Dosimetry modelling of inhaled toxic reactive gases. In Watson, A. Y., Bates, R. R. and Kennedy, D. (Eds), *Air Pollution, the Automobile and Public Health*. National Academy Press, Washington DC, pp. 367–385

PORG (1987). Photochemical Oxidants Review

Group. *Ozone in the United Kingdom*. Department of the Environment, London

Plopper, C. G., Dungworth, D. L., Tyler, W. S. and Chow, C. K. (1979). Pulmonary alterations in rats exposed to 0.2 and 0.1 ppm ozone: a correlated morphological and biochemical study. *Arch. Environ. Health.*, **34**, 390–395

Richters, A. and Damji, K. S. (1988). Changes in T lymphocyte subpopulations and natural killer cells following exposure to ambient levels of nitrogen dioxide. *J. Toxicol. Environ. Health*, **25**, 247–256

Richters, A., Damji, K. S. and Richters, V. (1987). Immunotoxicity of nitrogen dioxide. *J. Leukocyte Biol.*, **42**, 413–414

Rubinstein, I., Bigby, B. G., Reiss, T. F. and Boushey, H. A. (1990). Short-term exposure to 0.3 ppm nitrogen dioxide does not potentiate airway responsiveness to sulphur dioxide in asthmatic subjects. *Am. Rev. Respir. Dis.*, **141**, 381–385

Samet, J. M. and Utell, M. J. (1990). The risk of nitrogen dioxide: what have we learned from epidemiological and clinical studies? *Toxicol. Ind. Health*, **6**, 247–262

Schelegle, E. S. and Adams, W. C. (1986). Reduced exercise time in competitive simulations consequent to low level ozone exposure. *Med. J. Sci. Sports Exerc.*, **18**, 408–414

Schenker, M. B., Speizer, F. E., Samet, J. M., Gruhl, J. and Batterman, S. (1983). Health effects of air pollution due to coal combustion in the Chestnut Ridge region of Pennsylvania: results of cross sectional analysis in adults. *Arch. Environ. Health*, **38**, 325–330

Schlesinger, R. B., Lippmann, M. and Albert, R. E. (1978). Effects of short-term exposure to sulfuric acid and ammonium sulfate aerosols upon bronchial airway function in the donkey. *Am. Ind. Hyg. Assoc. J.*, **39**, 275–286

Schwartz, J. (1991). Particulate air pollution and daily mortality in Detroit. *Environ. Res.*, **56**, 204–213

Schwartz, J. and Marcus, A. (1990). Mortality and air pollution in London: a time series analysis. *Am. J. Epidemiol.*, **131**, 185–194

Schwartz, J. and Zeger, S. (1990). Passive smoking, air pollution and acute respiratory symptoms in a diary study of student nurses. *Am. Rev. Respir. Dis.*, **141**, 62–67

Schwartz, J. and Dockery, D. W. (1992). Particulate air pollution and daily mortality in Steubenville, Ohio. *Am. J. Epidemiol.*, **135**, 12–19

Sheppard, D., Wong, W. W., Uehara, C. F., Nadel, J. A. and Boushey, H. A. (1980). Lower threshold and greater responsiveness of asthmatic subjects to sulfur dioxide. *Am. Rev. Respir. Dis.*, **122**, 873–878

Sheppard, D., Saisho, A., Nadel, J. A. and Boushey, H. A. (1981a). Exercise increases sulfur dioxide-induced broncho-constriction in asthmatic subjects. *Am. Rev. Respir. Dis.*, **123**, 486–491

Sheppard, D., Nadel, J. A. and Boushey, H. A.

(1981b). Inhibition of sulfur dioxide-induced bronchoconstriction by disodium cromoglycate in asthmatic subjects. *Am. Rev. Respir. Dis.*, **124**, 257–259

Speizer, F. E., Ferris, B., Bishop, Y. M. M. and Spengler, J. (1980). Respiratory disease rates and pulmonary function in children associated with NO_2 exposure. *Am. Rev. Respir. Dis.*, **121**, 3–10

Spektor, D. M., Lippmann, M., Lioy, P. J., Thurston, G. D., Citak, K., James, D. J., Bock, N., Speizer, F. E. and Hayes, C. (1988). Effects of ambient ozone on respiratory function in active normal children. *Am. Rev. Respir. Dis.*, **137**, 313–320

Strandberg, L. G. (1964). SO_2 absorption in the respiratory tract. Studies on the absorption in rabbits, its dependence on concentration and breathing pace. *Arch. Environ. Health*, **9**, 160–166

US Environmental Protection Agency (1979 and 1984). *Air Quality Criteria for Carbon Monoxide* (Report No EPA-600/8-79-022) and *Revised Evaluation of Health Effects Associated with Carbon Monoxide Exposure*: Addendum to the 1979 Air Quality Criteria Document for Carbon Monoxide (Report No. EPA-600/8-83-033F), Washington DC

US Environmental Protection Agency (1986). *Air Quality Criteria for Ozone and Other Photochemical Oxidants*. 4 volumes, (Report No. EPA-600/8-84-020F) Washington DC

Utell, M. J. and Morrow, P. E. (1986). Effects of inhaled acid aerosols on human lung function: studies in normal and asthmatic subjects. In Lee, S. D., Schneider, T., Grant, L. D. and Verkerk, P. J. (Eds), *Aerosols: Research, Risk Assessment and Control Strategies*. Lewis Publishers, Chelsea, Michigan, pp. 671–698

Van der Lende, R., Schouter, J. P., Rijcken, B. and van der Muelen, A. (1986). Longitudinal epidemiological studies on effects of air pollution in the Netherlands. In Lee, S. D., Schneider, T., Grant, L. D. and Verkerk, P. J. (Eds), *Aerosols: Research, Risk Assessment and Control Strategies*. Lewis Publishers, Chelsea, Michigan, pp. 731–742

Waller, R. E. (1963). Acid droplets in town air. *Int. J. Air Water Pollut.*, **7**, 773–778

Waller, R. E. (1971). Air pollution and community health. *J. R. Coll. Physicians Lond.*, **5**, 362–368

Waller, R. E. (1989). Atmospheric pollution. *Chest*, **96**, 363S–368S

Waller, R. E. (1991). Field investigation of air. In Holland, W. W., Detels, R. and Knox, G. (Eds), *Oxford Textbook of Public Health*. Oxford University Press, Oxford. 2nd edn, **2**, pp. 435–450

Ware, J. H., Dockery, D., Spiro, A., Speizer, F. E. and Ferris, B. G. (1984). Passive smoking, gas cooking and respiratory health of children living in six cities. *Am. Rev. Respir. Dis.*, **129**, 366–374

Wichmann, H. E., Sugiri, D., Seraluj-Islam, M., Haake, D. and Roscovanu, A. (1988). Pulmonary function and carboxyhaemoglobin during the smog episode of January 1987. *Zentralbl. Bakteriol. Mikrobiol. Hyg. Ser. B*, **187**, 31–43

Wichmann, H. E., Müller, W., Allhoff, P., Beckmann, M., Bocker, N., Csicsaky, M. J., Jung, M., Molik, B. and Schoeneberg, G. (1989). Health effects during a smog episode in West Germany in 1985. *Environ. Health Perspect.*, **79**, 89–99

Widdicombe, J. G. (1954). Respiratory reflexes from the trachea and bronchi of the cat. *J. Physiol.*, **123**, 55–70

World Health Organization (1979). *Sulfur Oxides and Suspended Particulate Matter*. Environmenal Health Criteria No. 8, World Health Organization, Geneva

World Health Organization (1987). *Air Quality Guidelines for Europe*. WHO Regional Publications, European Series No. 23, World Health Organization, Copenhagen

World Health Organization (1992). *Acute Health Consequences of Winter-type and Summer-type Smog Exposures*. World Health Organization, Copenhagen

FURTHER READING

Callabrese, E. J. and Kenyon, E. M. (1991). *Air Toxics and Risk Assessment*. Lewis Publishers, Chelsea, Michigan

Gammage, R. B . and Kaye, S. V. (1987). *Indoor Air and Human Health*. Lewis Publishers, Inc., Chelsea, Michigan

Griffin, R. D. (1994). *Principles of Air Quality Management*. Lewis Publishers, Boca Raton, Florida

Lippman, M. (1992). *Environmental Toxicants*. Van Nostrand Reinhold, New York

Pitts, J. N. (1993). Atmospheric formation and fates of ambient air pollutants. *Occupational Medicine*, **8**, 631–662

Witorsch, P. (1994). *Air Pollution and Lung Disease in Adults*. Lewis Publishers, Boca Raton, Florida

49   Toxicology of Chemical Warfare Agents

Robert L. Maynard

HISTORICAL INTRODUCTION

Throughout history humans have sought more effective means of killing and disabling their fellow men. Stones, clubs, spears, bows and arrows, gunpowder, muskets, rifles, high-explosives, machine-guns, tanks, warplanes, rockets and nuclear weapons comprise an apparently unending catalogue of increasing military sophistication designed for the destruction of one's enemies while exposing one's forces to decreasing risk. Accompanying this development of military hardware, the effects of which are based on the physical disruption of men or materials, has been a very much less marked development of chemical means of attack. Some chemicals have been used as a means of killing and others as a means of incapacitating. Recently, attempts have been made to stem the development of chemical weapons but it is a sad reflection on the world that in 1993 more countries than ever have acquired, or are in the process of acquiring, the means to wage a chemical war.

Chemical weapons probably began with smoke and flame, and the hurling of various concoctions of pitch and sulphur (Greek Fire) dates from classical times. Irritant smokes were described by Plutarch, hypnotic substances by the Scottish historian Buchanan, compounds allegedly capable of producing incessant diarrhoea by classical Greek authors (SIPRI, 1971) and preparations containing the saliva of rabid dogs by Leonardo da Vinci (1452–1519) (Reprint Society, 1938).

At the time these authors were writing, chemistry and chemical technology were in their infancy and the chemical weapons developed had probably only a marginal effect on the outcome of battles or wars. However, during the medieval period the widespread use of poisons acquired, rightly, an evil reputation and the use of such compounds came to be despised by military men. The use of poisons was seen as running counter to the tenets of chivalrous conduct and this view has persisted and lies close to the root of the objections raised during the twentieth century to the use of chemical weapons (Haldane, 1925).

At the end of the nineteenth century the first international convention to address, among other topics, chemical warfare was held. This, the First Hague Convention (1899), led to a wide-ranging prohibition of the use of chemicals in war: 'The contracting powers agree to abstain from the use of all projectiles the sole object of which is the diffusion of asphyxiating or deleterious gases.' (Prentiss, 1937).

Despite this prohibition, chemical warfare was used on a large scale during World War I, some 113 000 tons of chemical weapons being used in all (Prentiss, 1937). Lefebure (1921) reported that on 9 March 1918 German forces fired some 200 000 mustard gas shells. This resulted in many casualties but compared with the total casualties produced during World War I the number of casualties from chemical warfare was low. This is shown in Table 1 (Prentiss, 1937).

From the figures given in this table a number of deductions can be made: (1) The proportion of deaths attributable to chemical warfare during World War I was low. (2) The ratio of dead to injured among those affected by chemical warfare was very low. (3) Ill-prepared forces, e.g. Russian troops on the Eastern Front, suffered badly. These observations have been examined in detail elsewhere (Maynard, 1988) and have been adduced by some as evidence of the efficacy of chemical warfare and by others as evidence of its inefficacy. Space here does not permit an examination of these interpretations.

After World War I a widespread campaign to ban chemical warfare was mounted and The Geneva Protocol, promulgated in 1925, encapsulated widely held opinion. However, during the Italian campaign in Ethiopia (1935–36) Italian troops used mustard gas on a large scale against unprotected native forces (SIPRI, 1971). Many casualties were produced. During the late 1930s fear that fascist countries might use chemical warfare on a substantial scale during a future war led to the incorporation of anti-gas drills into Air

Table 1   Chemical warfare and other casualties during World War I

Country	Battle casualties due to gas			Total battle deaths	Total wounds including battle deaths
	Non-fatal	Death	Total		
Russia	419 340	56 000	475 340	1 416 700	6 366 700
France	182 000	8 000	190 000	1 131 500	5 397 500
British Empire	180 597	8 109	188 706	585 533	2 590 509
Italy	55 373	4 627	60 000	541 500	1 488 500
USA	71 345	1 462	72 807	52 842	272 138
Germany	191 000	9 000	200 000	1 478 000	5 694 058
Austria/Hungary	97 000	3 000	100 000	1 000 000	4 620 000
Other	9 000	1 000	10 000	684 436	1 580 318
Total	1 205 655	91 198	1 296 853	6 890 511	28 009 723

Wounded due to chemical warfare as percentage of all wounded (including fatalities): 4.63%.
Deaths due to chemical warfare as percentage of total chemical warfare injured: 7.03%.
Deaths due to chemical warfare as percentage of all deaths: 1.32%.
UK forces deaths due to chemical warfare as percentage of total UK forces deaths: 4.3%.
Source: After Prentiss (1937).

Raid Precautions (ARP) in the UK and the issue of gas masks to all troops and civilians. These fears were not demonstrated to have been justified during World War II despite the production of large quantities of chemical warfare munitions by both sides. Germany's reluctance to use chemical weapons has never been satisfactorily explained, particularly as she had what many might have been considered a great advantage in having synthesized the very toxic nerve agents which were unknown to the Allied Powers. The discovery of large stocks of these compounds, the acquisition of the means of production by the USSR and the worsening state of international relations, led to the expansion of research into chemical warfare in both the UK and the USA during the years following World War II.

The UK's programme of research, designed to produce chemical weapons, sometimes described as 'offensive research' (in contrast to work on antidotes and means of protection: 'defensive research'), was halted permanently in 1956 with the decommissioning of the nerve agent production plant at the Chemical Defence Establishment out-station at Nancekuke in Cornwall. Production of nerve agents continued in the USA until 1969 and began again in 1981 in order to produce the components of the so called 'binary weapon system' (Meselson and Perry Robinson,

1980). Production in the USSR probably continued in parallel with that in the USA.

Accusations and reports of the use of chemical weapons have been common since World War II. Those of their use by Egyptian forces in The Yemen (1963–67) seem better supported than many others. US forces used defoliants and irritants on a large scale during the war in Vietnam. That this represented a use of chemical warfare has been strenuously denied by US sources and the view that the use of CS (2-chlorobenzylidene malononitrile) tear-gas, which had been sanctioned for use in the USA against rioting civilians, could not be regarded as an exercise in chemical warfare has been voiced.

Iraq, during the Iran–Iraq war in the early and mid-1980s used chemical weapons on a large scale. Mustard gas and probably the nerve agent tabun were used (UN, 1987). Many casualties resulted, and in one particularly distressing incident, at Halabja, some 5000 civilians were killed. Death from chemical warfare on this scale had not been known since the gas cloud attacks of 1915 and attracted international condemnation.

Among less well-known accusations are the use of 'Yellow Rain' in South East Asia (Seagrave, 1981) and the use of 'knock down agents' and 'black body agents' by USSR forces in Afghanistan. During 1988 reports that Libya had constructed a chemical warfare production plant appeared in the press. This report fuelled fears that terrorists might acquire access to chemical weapons.

In 1988 major steps were taken by both the USA and the USSR towards a verifiable ban on chemical weapons. Expansion of the capacity to wage chemical warfare has, however, continued in a number of other countries.

CONCEPTS OF USE OF CHEMICAL WEAPONS

It is often assumed that chemical weapons would be used during a war to kill as many of the opposing forces as possible. This is fallacious and misrepresents the professed purpose of modern warfare. Modern warfare is, it is generally agreed, waged to compel governments to amend their actions and not to annihilate populations (Fotion and Elfstrom, 1986). It is a fact of military experience that the weapon systems which produce many casualties are likely to be more effective than systems which produce fatalities. Casualties require evacuation, nursing care and may sap morale. Because of this chemical weapons would more likely be used to incapacitate than to kill. Some established chemical weapons such as mustard gas are rather ineffective as regards killing (death rate in mustard casualties during World War I was about 2 per cent) although particularly effective as incapacitants (Haldane, 1925).

Chemical weapons can be effectively defended against by the use of protective clothing including a respirator, gloves, boots and special over-garments. Prophylactic drugs play a much less important part in providing protection. Physical protection inevitably carries the penalty of impaired performance and commanders might be loath to institute such measures. Indeed aggressors might consider their use, or expression of willingness to use, chemical warfare as successful if they forced their opponents into protective clothing. Because of this, a policy of intelligent avoidance of contaminated areas would be likely to be observed. This has led to the development of the concept of use of chemical warfare agents as agents of 'Ground Denial' rather than as deliberate producers of casualties. Such an effect could well be exploited by an aggressor by attacks on centres of strategic and tactical importance, some

'behind the lines'. Such a use would inevitably lead to the exposure of civilians, probably less well-trained and protected than members of the Armed Forces, and the production of many civilian casualties. Lethal chemical warfare compounds could be used in high concentrations to permit the rapid breakthrough by well-protected troops through strongly defended points.

These concepts of use permit a number of categories of chemical warfare agent to be defined (see Figure 1). Only a few well-known chemical warfare agents have been included in Figure 1. Other compounds such as lewisite could well appear in more than one category. CS has been included as a non-persistent agent on the grounds of its rapid hydrolysis in contact with water.

It should be remembered that military concepts of use could well vary from area to area and reports of the use of specific chemical warfare agents may prove very difficult to understand unless details of the operational scenario are available.

STANDARD CLASSIFICATION OF CHEMICAL WARFARE AGENTS

A number of different classifications of chemical warfare agents have been devised. Two broad systems, 'medical' and 'service', are in general

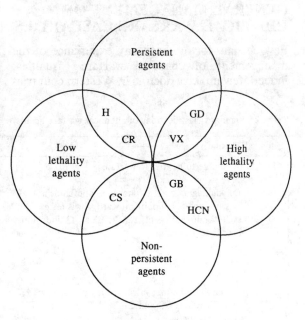

Figure 1 Categories of chemical warfare agents

use and are compared in Table 2 (HMSO, 1972). Both of these systems would be regarded today as outmoded by many experts. Several of the compounds listed in the Table, e.g. LSD (lysergic and diethylamide) and DM (10-chloro-5,10-dihydrophenarsazine), are no longer seen as likely to be used in war and chlorine and arsine are very unlikely to be used.

The possible means of production of chemical weapons have also changed in recent years as genetic engineering and the production of chemicals on a large scale by cultures of bacteria and yeasts have been developed. Today, chemical weapons and biological weapons are considered to form a spectrum ranging from the classical chemical weapons, such as nerve agents and mustard gas, to the classical biological agents, such as the anthrax bacillus or the smallpox virus. Between the two extremes are compounds originally discovered as natural products, e.g. bacterial toxins, and which were classified as biological weapons, but which are in fact chemicals. The chemical–biological warfare spectrum is shown in Figure 2 (Pearson, 1988). Useful though this classification is it is likely that the simple military classification will remain in widespread use as it lends itself to use in training and defining standard means of dealing with casualties.

GENERAL MANAGEMENT OF CHEMICAL WARFARE CASUALTIES

Few civilian doctors have any experience of the management of chemical warfare casualties; indeed, few military doctors in Western countries have ever seen a chemical warfare casualty. If casualties are to be well cared for and the carers not to be placed at risk a number of key points must be borne in mind.

(1) Early treatment of casualties is essential.

(2) Attendants must be adequately protected from contamination.

(3) Decontamination of casualties is the priority once life-saving measures, including the establishment of adequate ventilation and the administration of antidotes, have been undertaken. Fullers' earth is an excellent decontaminant for liquid agents. Any source of water will suffice as a means of removing liquid agents from the eyes.

(4) Casualties should be moved as soon as possible after decontamination into a clean environment where clinicians may work under conditions with which they are familiar. Defence of this environment must be absolute.

(5) Casualties will range from the mildly affected to the moribund and the rules of triage must be rigorously applied if optimal use is to be made of clinical resources.

(6) Early identification of the agent responsible for the poisoning will be of great value to the clinician and every effort should be made to use such detectors and monitors as are available.

(7) Some casualties will require intensive nursing and should be moved along evacuation routes as quickly as possible.

Table 2 Standard classifications of chemical warfare agents

Medical classification	Service classification
(1) Agents liable to be met in warfare	
Nerve agents (G and V)	Lethal agents (nerve)
Lung-damaging agents (phosgene and chlorine)	Lethal agents (choking)
Vesicant agents (sulphur mustard, lewisite, etc.).	Damaging agents (blister)
Psychotomimetic agents (LSD, BZ: 3-Quinuclidinyl benzilate)	Incapacitating agents (mental)
Miscellaneous agents	
Cyanide	Lethal agents (blood)
Arsine	
Herbicides	–
(2) Agents liable to be met in riot control/or war	
Sensory irritants CS and CR	Riot control agents
Vomiting agents, e.g. DM	Incapacitating agents (physical)

CHEMICAL–BIOLOGICAL WARFARE SPECTRUM

Mustard	Toxic industrial, pharmaceutical and agricultural chemicals	Peptides	Saxitoxin	Modified/tailored bacteria and viruses	Bacteria
Nerve agents			Mycotoxins		Viruses
Cyanide			Ricin		Rickettsia
				← Agents of biological origin →	
← Agents not found in nature →		← Designer drug modification →			
Classification CW	Emerging CW	Bioregulators	Toxins	Genetically manipulated BW	Traditional BW

CW = chemical warfare; BW = biological warfare. Source: after Pearson (1988).

Figure 2 Chemical–biological warfare spectrum

VESICANT COMPOUNDS

Vesicant compounds were introduced as chemical warfare agents on 12 July 1917 when German forces used sulphur mustard at Ypres (Prentiss, 1937). Mustard gas became the most effective chemical warfare agent used during World War I, 14 000 British casualties being produced during the first 3 months of its use and 120 000 by the end of the war (HMSO, 1923). This efficacy earned for mustard gas the sobriquet 'King of the Battle Gases' but, despite this, it carried only a low lethality. This low lethality, of the order of 2 per cent, was one of the points which convinced J. B. S. Haldane (1925) of the desirability of chemical warfare as compared with conventional warfare.

Physicochemical Properties of Mustard Gas

'Mustard gas' is an unfortunate misnomer as the compound which at room temperature gives off vapour and smells of mustard, garlic or leeks, is a liquid with a boiling point of 217°C. Sulphur mustard is often referred to as HS [Hun Stoff] or more commonly as H. The nitrogen mustards are referred to as HN1, HN2 and HN3. The formulae and some of the characteristics of the mustards are shown in Table 3.

Sulphur mustard is poorly miscible with water but on mixing hydrolysis takes place leading to the production of thiodiglycol and hydrochloric acid (Figure 3). The low miscibility and solubility of sulphur mustard in water leads to lengthy persistence of the compound in the field, particularly if protected from wind and rain. Sulphur mustard

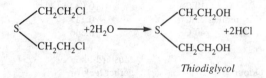

Thiodiglycol

Figure 3 Hydrolysis of sulphur mustard

vapour passes quickly through clothing, although properly designed, modern military protective clothing provides good protection. Sulphur mustard in the liquid state passes quickly through ordinary surgical rubber gloves and heavy gloves made of butyl rubber should be worn when decontaminating casualties. The standard issue UK (Mark 6) respirator provides excellent protection against mustard gas vapour (HMSO, 1972).

Absorption of Sulphur Mustard

Sulphur mustard, as a liquid or vapour, is lipid soluble and is absorbed across the skin. Renshaw (1946) demonstrated that 80 per cent of a sample of sulphur mustard placed on the uncovered skin evaporated. Cameron *et al.* (1946) demonstrated, in rabbits, that some 80 per cent of inhaled vapour was absorbed in the nose. Clinical experience suggests that the majority of inhaled sulphur mustard is absorbed in the upper airways.

Toxicity of Sulphur Mustard

The toxicity of sulphur mustard as an incapacitating agent is militarily of much greater importance than its capacity to kill in terms of LD_{50}, and compared with the nerve agents, sulphur mustard

Table 3   Physicochemical characteristics of mustard vesicants

Characteristic		H		HN₁	HN₂	HN₃
Formula		$S\begin{cases}CH_2CH_2Cl\\CH_2CH_2Cl\end{cases}$	$C_2H_5N\begin{cases}CH_2CH_2Cl\\CH_2CH_2Cl\end{cases}$		$CH_3N\begin{cases}CH_2CH_2Cl\\CH_2CH_2Cl\end{cases}$	$N\begin{cases}-CH_2CH_2Cl\\-CH_2CH_2Cl\\CH_2CH_2Cl\end{cases}$
Appearance		Yellowish, oily liquid	◄——————— Colourless or yellowish ———————► oily liquids			
M.P. °C		14	−34		−60	−4
B.P. °C		217	85		75	138
S.G.		1.27	1.09		1.15	1.24
V.P. mmHg	10°C	0.032	0.0773		0.130	0.00272
	25°C	0.112	0.2500		0.427	0.01090
	40°C	0.346	0.7220		1.250	0.03820
Odour		Mustard-like, garlic, leek or horseradish-like	Soapy or fishy			

is a comparatively non-toxic compound. Intravenous LD_{50} figures include the following: rat, 3.3 mg kg⁻¹; mice, 8.6 mg kg⁻¹ (Anslow *et al.*, 1948). Much more important are the effects of exposures to differing concentration/time products (Ct products). These are listed in Table 4.

Figure 4 shows the interdependence of concentration and time in defining the effects of mustard gas vapour.

Table 4   Effects of sulphur mustard vapour on humans

Exposure dose mg min m⁻³	Effects
20–50	Onset of eye effects
70	Mild reddening of the eyes—tearing
100	Partial incapacitation from eye effects
100–400	Erythema of skin
200	Total incapacitation from eye effects
200–1000	Skin burns produced
750–10 000	Severe incapacitation from skin effects

[a] The effects of sulphur mustard vapour on the skin are very dependent on ambient temperature and the range shown for skin burns encompasses the effects of decreasing ambient temperature from 80 to 50°F.

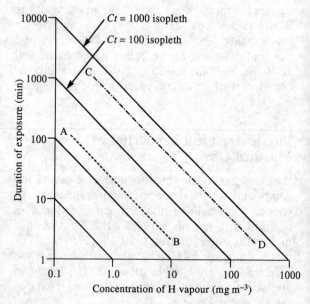

Figure 4   Effects of sulphur mustard vapour on humans. Lines AB and CD are offered as guides to early eye effects (AB: Ct = 20 mg min m⁻³) and skin burns of significance (CD: Ct = 500 mg min m⁻³). Because of uncertainty regarding the Ct = a constant, relationship, extrapolation to extremes of time and concentration will be inaccurate

Mechanism of Action of Sulphur Mustard

Sulphur mustard is an alkylating agent and a detailed account of the mode of action of such compounds will be found in Chapter 35 and in the works of Goodman and Gilman (1980) and Fox and Scott (1980). Both sulphur mustard and the various nitrogen mustards are bifunctional alkylating agents possessing two side chains capable of undergoing cyclization. Crosslinking of guanine in nucleic acids results from this property. Crosslinked guanine molecules are shown in Figure 5.

Binding of the ethylenesulphonium ion (sulphur mustard) or the ethylimmonium ion (nitrogen mustard) to DNA produces a range of effects including:

- Alkylated guanine residues tend to form base pairs with thymine rather than with cytosine, leading to coding errors and hence inaccurate protein synthesis.
- Damaged guanine residues may be excised from the DNA molecule.
- A pair of guanine residues may become crosslinked as shown below. This is considered by some as the most serious effect of alkylating agents on DNA.

Repair to DNA may take place as long as damage is not too widespread. Jaurez-Salinas *et al.* (1979) reported the polymerization of NAD under the influence of poly(ADP ribose)polymerase enzyme as part of the DNA repair process. Papirmeister *et al.* (1984a,b) suggested that the reduction in the cellular levels of NAD following DNA repair could lead to cell death.

Early work by Dixon (1946) suggested a correlation between skin injury and inhibition of glycolysis. Although the effects of alkyating agents such as mustard on nucleic acids are usually

stressed it should be recalled that they also alkylate a wide range of other cellular components and enzymes. Membrane proteins at both the plasmalemma and the surfaces of intracellular organelles are liable to alkylation.

Despite this apparent understanding of how the alkylating agents act no clear explanation of how mustard produces blisters is yet available. Miskin and Reich (1980) proposed increased protease synthesis and release after mustard-induced damage to cells. Release of such enzymes would be expected to set up an inflammatory response and would explain some of the effects of sulphur mustard. Acute inflammation does not, however, usually lead to blistering.

The cholinomimetic effects of nitrogen mustard may be explained by cyclization leading to the formation of a quaternary ammonium compound (Figure 6).

Histopathology of the Skin Effects of Sulphur Mustard

Extensive experimental work was undertaken during World War I to discover the effects of sulphur mustard on human skin. This work has been reported in detail by Ireland (1926).

Volunteer studies were undertaken involving exposure of personnel to various concentrations of sulphur mustard; in some instances biopsies of damaged skin were taken. In one study small quantities (0.0004 ml drops) of sulphur mustard were placed on the skin. Small blisters were produced. The evolution of the lesions was followed by a timed series of biopsies.

Early vacuolation of the deeper layers of the epidermis was reported as were nuclear changes in the stratum granulosum. Capillary dilatation and leukocyte diapedesis were also noted. These changes were established some 30 min after exposure. Later separation at the dermo–epidermal junction occurred with liquefaction of the epidermis near the centre of the lesion. Epithelial cells of hair follicles and sweat glands were also affected. These changes were maximally

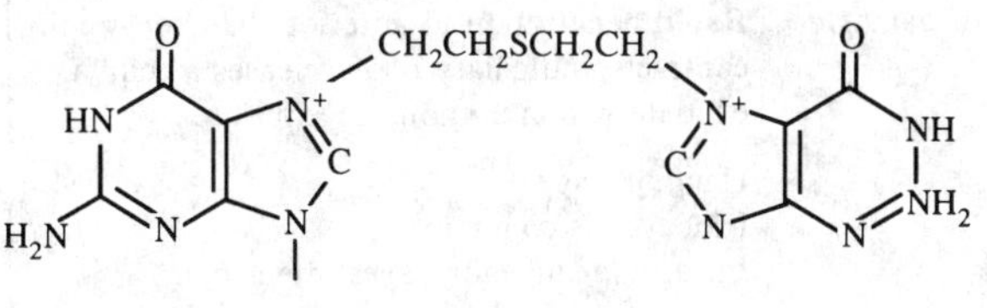

Figure 5 Crosslinking of guanine residues by sulphur mustard

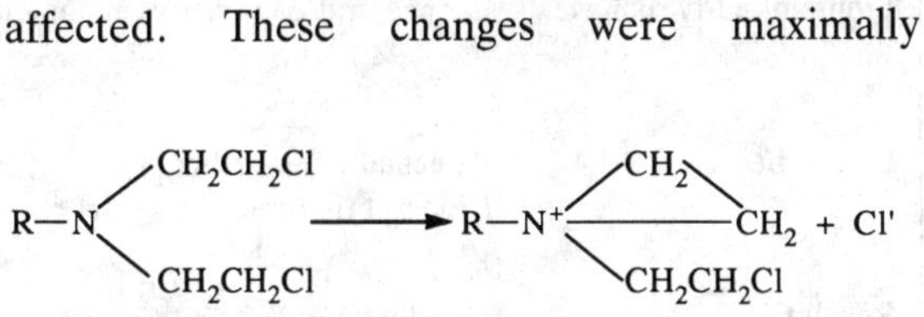

Figure 6 Formation of a quaternary ammonium compound

developed by 18 h after exposure. Necrosis was followed by formation of an eschar by 72 h, sloughing by 4–6 days, a pigmented scar being present by 19 days.

Histochemical studies by Vogt *et al.* (1984) have confirmed the above and, furthermore, have demonstrated two phases of increased capillary permeability. Papirmeister (1984a,b) has undertaken detailed studies using athymic human-skin-xenografted mice and has extended the above descriptions to the ultrastructural level. His papers should be consulted for details.

Histopathology of the Effects of Sulphur and Nitrogen Mustard on the Eyes

These effects were investigated in detail by Mann (1948) who divided the compounds into two groups. These are described in Table 5. Note that the division does not correspond with the usual classification: sulphur mustard/nitrogen mustard.

Histopathology of the Effects of Mustard Gas on the Respiratory Tract

Several reports are available (Warthin and Weller, 1919; HMSO, 1923; Vedder, 1925; Ireland, 1926). These effects are largely confined to the conducting airways, with damage being particularly marked in the larger airways. The pseudostratified ciliated columnar epithelium becomes necrotic and sloughs; haemorrhages and inflammatory changes occur in the lamina propria and a false, diphtheritic membrane of sloughed cells, blood and exudate is formed. In severe cases damage to the submucossa and other layers of the airway wall may occur. Surface repair is by squamous metaplasia and complete restoration of a normal ciliated epithelium is suspected to be slow.

In the deeper lung, damage is usually less marked although severe exposure can produce haemorrhagic pulmonary oedema. During World War I this was clearly recorded at post mortem and found to be most marked in the alveoli adjacent to conducting airways. Repair of damage at the alveolar level involves initial organization of the exudate and its subsequent removal by macrophages. Extensive fibrotic changes following exposure to mustard gas have not been demonstrated.

Histopathology of the Effects of Mustard Gas on Bone Marrow

Alkylating agents in general have profound effects on rapidly dividing tissues and damage to the cells of the bone marrow produces an aplastic anaemia (Smith, 1986). The granulocyte series is first affected followed by the megakaryocytes and finally the erythropoietic series. In mustard gas casualties the peripheral white cell count has been observed to begin to fall on about the fourth day post-exposure after an initial post-exposure rise.

Symptoms and Signs of Exposure to Mustard Gas

The following is based on the accounts of Vedder (1925) and Warthin and Weller (1919) and the author's observations of Iranian casualties during 1985 and 1986. The comprehensive review of Willems (1989) should be consulted for further

Table 5   Mann's classification of mustards by effects on the eye

Group	'Mustard gas group'	'Nitrogen mustard group'
Compounds	Sulphur mustard and HN_3	HN_1 and HN_2
Latent period	Present, may be some hours	Absent
Limits of early damage	Cornea and conjunctiva main site of damage	Rapid penetration to anterior chamber, pupil contracts and ciliary body releases a cellular exudate within an hour of exposure
Later effects	Petechial haemorrhages Iridocyclitis rare	Haemorrhage Iridocyclitis common Intraocular haemorrhages often seen
Resolution	Usually complete	Permanent damage likely

Source: Modified from Mann (1948).

details. The symptoms and signs are listed in Table 6.

Clinical Investigations

Blood should be taken for estimation of thiodiglycol. Regular chest X-rays and standard haematological investigations are clearly indicated. Pulmonary function testing should be undertaken in all whose respiratory problems appear to be resolving particularly slowly.

Management of Mustard Gas Casualties

As already stated casualty management divides into two parts.

First Aid

Casualties should be moved quickly from the source of contamination by adequately protected attendants and decontaminated thoroughly with fullers' earth. Washing of the skin with kerosene to remove liquid contamination was strongly advocated by Vedder (1925) but if undertaken should be continued for 30 min.

Medical Management

There is no specific therapy for mustard gas lesions and no antidote has been demonstrated to be clinically effective in removing mustard from the body. Despite this, considerable amelioration of the effects may be achieved and secondary infection prevented.

Management of Skin Lesions

Large blisters should be aspirated aseptically as they are likely to be broken accidentally. Blister fluid is not harmful despite the oft repeated assertion that it contains free mustard and may cause damage to attendants. That blister fluid is harmless was conclusively demonstrated in volunteer studies by Sulzberger (1943). After aspiration blisters should be covered with sterile dry dressings. Treatment by exposure seems to be as effective as by wet dressings and demands less nursing care. A variety of ointments have been used in cases of mustard gas burns although none has been shown to enhance their rate of healing. Silver sulphadiazine cream (Flamazine) has been widely used and is useful in preventing secondary infection.

Table 6 Symptoms and signs of exposure to mustard gas

Time post-exposure	Symptoms and signs
20–60 min	Nausea, retching and eye smarting have all been reported. More commonly a latent period of up to an hour occurs and was clearly recorded at first hand by Adolph Hitler from experience in 1918 (Hitler, 1925)
2–6 h	Inflammation of the eyes occurs with intense and burning eye pain. Lachrymation, blepharospasm, photophobia and rhinorrhoea appear; the face becomes reddened and the voice hoarse
6–24 h	Blisters develop on skin exposed to vapour or liquid. The blisters are delicate and are often rubbed off by the patient turning in bed. Blisters are not *per se* painful although if they occur over flexure lines at joints, pain may be produced on moving. The warm areas of the body are particularly liable to blistering with the axillae, inguinal folds, perineum and genitalia being badly affected. In contrast the palms and soles appear to invariably escape blistering
24–48 h	Blistering becomes more marked and fresh crops of blisters appear. Coughing develops and sloughed tissue is expectorated. Intense itching of the skin may occur and frequently prevents sleep. Darkening of the skin, due to an increase of melanin in the basal layer of the epidermis, occurs and areas of dark brown or black hyperpigmentation are produced. Eye effects are maximal at this time and patients may be temporarily blinded
48 h–6 weeks	Blisters heal slowly and healing areas of skin are sensitive and secondary blistering may be produced by friction. Peeling of areas of hyperpigmentation to leave areas of hypopigmentation occurs and a striking piebald appearance may be produced. The eye problems resolve slowly and persistent roughening of the cornea may be observed
6 weeks–6 months	Many patients will have recovered by 6 weeks although in some the process takes much longer. A state of functional neurosis was described during World War I with depression and continuous eye problems. Persistent lachrymation and photophobia represent a particularly difficult problem

Severe itching and pain from damaged skin has been reported and in some cases narcotic analgesics have been used. This is probably unnecessary in the majority of cases and a milder analgesic combined with a sedative would be more appropriate therapy.

Most mustard gas burns are superficial or partial thickness burns. Deeper burns are occasionally seen and for these skin grafting should be considered as this may increase the rate of healing. Recent work by Rice (1993, personal communication) has shown that in animal models light abrasion of mustard-damaged skin enhances the rate of healing.

Management of Eye Lesions
Early decontamination of liquid splashes in the eye is essential as a delay of more than a few minutes may make later decontamination ineffective and allow serious damage to occur (HMSO, 1972). For damaged eyes the following are recommended:

- Daily saline irrigations.
- The use of petroleum jelly on the follicular margins to prevent sticking.
- Chloramphenicol eye drops to prevent infection.
- Mydriatics, e.g. hyoscine drops, to prevent iridolenticular adhesions and to reduce pain caused by spasm of the ciliary muscle.
- It has been suggested that if eye pain is particularly severe local anaesthetic drops should be used, amethocaine hydrochloride being recommended. Ophthalmological opinion should be sought before local anaesthetic or corticosteroid drops are used.
- Potassium ascorbate (10 per cent) and sodium citrate (10 per cent) drops 'alternately, each once an hour, i.e. half hourly drops, for 14 h or the waking day', are also recommended.
- Dark glasses to alleviate photophobia.
- Perhaps most important of all: constant reassurance that blindness will not be produced and that recovery *will* occur, albeit slowly.

Management of Lesions of the Respiratory Tract
Antibiotic cover is recommended if the respiratory effects are more than very mild. Codeine linctus is of value in preventing coughing at night. Mucolytics including acetylcysteine have been used in some cases although evidence of their efficacy is lacking. In cases of very severe respiratory damage a chemical pneumonitis may be produced and may demand intensive care. Respiratory physicians and anaesthetists should be consulted if evidence of deteriorating respiratory function appears.

Management of Depression of the Bone Marrow
Until recently no treatment has been available to restore the damaged bone marrow. However, the recent introduction of granulocyte colony stimulating factor (GCSF) has led to the hope that this might be useful in such cases.

Prognosis of Mustard Gas Casualties

Most mustard gas casualties recover fully. In a small proportion of cases late-onset corneal problems producing blindness occur (Mann, 1948). Sulphur mustard is a recognized carcinogen and a study in Japanese mustard gas-factory workers demonstrated an increase in the incidence of cancer (Yamada, 1963). The risk of cancer occurring as a result of a single exposure to sulphur mustard is exceedingly low.

LEWISITE

Lewisite, developed as a chemical warfare agent in 1918 by Lee Lewis, has never been proven to have been used in war. Despite this it has acquired a reputation as an agent of likely great effectiveness and lethality. In fact this is unlikely to be true. In the early 1920s Lewisite was considered as a compound likely to produce more severe effects than mustard gas and was nicknamed 'The Dew of Death'. It has retained its place in the standard lists of chemical warfare agents although often as a mixture with sulphur mustard, the Lewisite lowering the freezing point of the mustard and making it more effective under cold conditions. Fears that Lewisite might be used during World War II prompted the work of Peters, Thompson and Stocken (Peters *et al.*, 1945; Peters 1948, 1953) and led to the development of the chelating agent dimercaprol or British Anti-Lewisite (BAL). The view that Lewisite is rather unlikely to be used in war has limited interest in the compound and only a short account of its effects and the recommended management of those effects will be provided.

Physicochemical Properties of Lewisite

These are shown in Table 7. Unlike sulphur mustard, Lewisite decomposes rapidly on contact with water or even in a 'damp atmosphere' (Sartori, 1939). The reaction taking place is shown in Figure 7.

Absorption of Lewisite

Lewisite is absorbed rapidly through the skin and mucous membranes. Its distribution in the body follows that of other arsenical compounds.

Toxicity of Lewisite

Lewisite has a much higher systemic toxicity than sulphur mustard and 0.5 ml allowed to remain on the skin would be expected to produce severe poisoning; 2.0 ml allowed to remain in contact with the skin has been said to represent a lethal dose in humans (Vedder, 1925). Because of its systemic toxicity few volunteers have been

exposed to Lewisite and data available regarding the effects of vapour on the skin are scanty. It is the author's impression that Lewisite vapour is more toxic to the skin and eyes than mustard gas vapour and the effects could be expected at lower concentrations.

Mechanism of Action of Lewisite

Peters *et al.* (1945) demonstrated that Lewisite attacked the pyruvate dehydrogenase system by combining with the co-enzyme lipoic acid to form a cyclic compound (Figure 8). The essential and ubiquitous nature of lipoic acid accounts for the widespread effects of Lewisite on the body. Interestingly, as in the case of sulphur mustard, the exact link between the primary biochemical effect of Lewisite and the production of blisters remains unknown. It should be recalled that other arsenical compounds such as sodium arsenite are not vesicants.

Effects of Lewisite on Humans

Both in terms of histopathology and general patterns of symptoms and signs it is believed that Lewisite would produce effects similar to those described above for mustard gas. However, certain important differences exist and instead of repeating much of the above only these will be considered:

- Exposure of the eyes to Lewisite vapour is immediately painful and the damage produced is likely to be more severe than that produced by mustard gas vapour. Liquid contamination of the eyes is particularly painful, dangerous and demands immediate treatment.
- Skin blisters produced by Lewisite appear more quickly post-exposure than those pro-

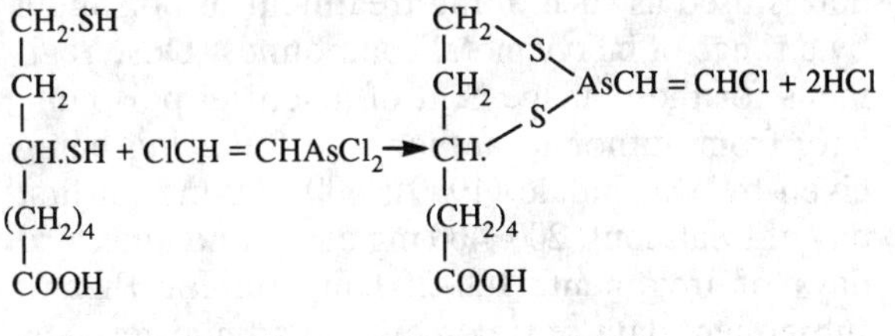

Table 7 Physicochemical characteristics of Lewisite

Formula	$ClCH = CH\,As\,Cl_2$
M.W.	207.32
M.P. °C	−13
B.P. °C	190
V.P. mmHg	0°C : 0.087
	10°C : 0.196
	20°C : 0.394
	40°C : 1.467
S.G.	0°C : 1.9200
	10°C : 1.9027
	30°C : 1.8682
Appearance	A colourless oily liquid. Impure samples may be blue-black in colour and smell, faintly, of geraniums

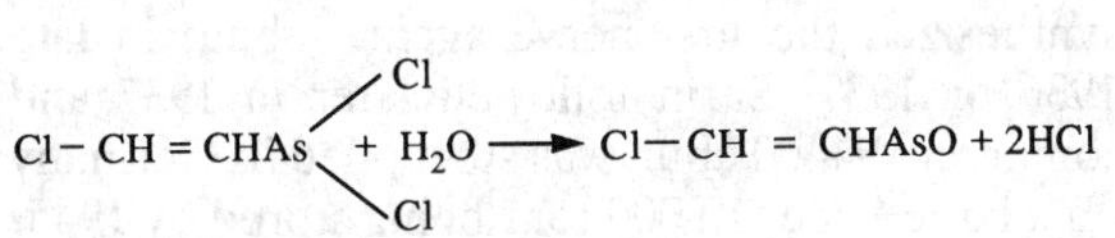

$$Cl-CH = CHAs\diagdown^{Cl}_{Cl} + H_2O \longrightarrow Cl-CH = CHAsO + 2HCl$$

Figure 7 Hydrolysis of Lewisite

$$
\begin{array}{l}
CH_2.SH \\
\quad| \\
CH_2 \\
\quad| \\
CH.SH \\
\quad| \\
(CH_2)_4 \\
\quad| \\
COOH
\end{array}
+ ClCH = CHAsCl_2 \longrightarrow
\begin{array}{l}
CH_2\diagdown_S \\
\quad|\quad\quad\diagdown AsCH = CHCl + 2HCl \\
CH_2\diagup_S \\
CH.\diagup \\
\quad| \\
(CH_2)_4 \\
\quad| \\
COOH
\end{array}
$$

Figure 8 Reaction between Lewisite and lipoic acid

duced by mustard gas (Friedenwald and Hughes, 1948).

- The inflammatory response associated with Lewisite lesions is likely to be more severe than that associated with mustard lesions.
- Healing of Lewisite induced skin lesions is likely to be more rapid than of those occurring as a result of exposure to sulphur mustard. Hunter (1978) described a case of blistering following exposure of another vesicant arsenical compound, phenyl dichlorarsine, and reported that the skin lesions healed by the tenth day.
- The collapse of the bone marrow seen in severe cases of mustard gas poisoning would not be expected after exposure to Lewisite. Goyer, however, has pointed out that large doses of arsenical compounds can lead to leukopenia (1986).

Clinical Investigations

Blood and urine should be analysed for arsenic. Under military conditions analysis should certainly be undertaken as information regarding the identity of chemical weapons used on the battle field might be of tactical importance.

Management of Lewisite Casualties

First Aid

This is as described for mustard gas.

Medical Treatment

Perhaps the most cheering difference between Lewisite and sulphur mustard is that specific therapy is available for the former but not for the latter.

Dimercaprol (BAL) binds the arsenical groups of Lewisite and produces a harmless complex. BAL competes avidly with binding sites in the body for arsenic and removes arsenic from them. BAL is available in a form suitable for injection and is used as such in the treatment of poisoning by a range of heavy metal compounds. Dose regimens for the management of arsenical poisoning vary from author to author, the following being given by Martindale (1989): 400–800 mg on first day of treatment, 200–400 mg on second and third days of treatment, 100–200 mg on fourth and subsequent days of treatment, all administered as divided doses.

For an alternative regimen the HMSO publication *Medical Manual of Defence Against Chemical Agents* (HMSO, 1972) should be consulted. It is unlikely that one would need to continue treatment for more than about 14 days.

Marked reactions may be produced by the injection of BAL including tachycardia, nausea, vomiting, headache and sweating. Individual doses should not exceed 3 mg kg^{-1} and an interval of at least 4 h should separate these doses.

BAL may also be prepared as an ointment or as eye drops. Both preparations contain 5–10 per cent dimercaprol. BAL ointment should not be used in conjunction with silver sulphadiazine (Flamazine) as chelation of silver will occur.

Recently, newer chelating agents have been proposed as replacements for BAL in the management of poisoning. The work of Granziano *et al.* (1978), Lenz *et al.* (1981) and Aposhian *et al.* (1982, 1984) should be consulted for details. Despite the apparent advantages of some of the newer compounds in the treatment of systemic arsenic poisoning in experimental animals it should be remembered that the high lipid-solubility of BAL will probably lead to the ointment retaining its place in the management of Lewisite burns.

Prognosis of Lewisite Casualties

Given that adequate, early decontamination followed by the administration of BAL is undertaken the prognosis should be good.

In war, eye splashes with liquid lewisite would, fortunately, be expected to be rare but if such did occur the difficulties of immediate decontamination under battle field conditions could well lead to serious eye damage.

NERVE AGENTS

Nerve agents, produced first in Germany during the late 1930s, are often described as second generation chemical weapons to distinguish them from those used during World War I. Schrader synthesized the first nerve agent, tabun, in late 1936 or 1937. Sarin followed later in 1937 and soman in 1944. Tabun was stockpiled in Germany on a large scale, 12 000 tons being stored by 1945. Sarin was produced on a smaller scale with some 600 tons being available by 1945. Tabun, sarin and soman are usually referred to by the abbreviations GA, GB and GD, respectively. Other G agents exist including GE and GF but these are less well known. During the 1950s another group of nerve agents was developed and stockpiled in large quantities. These were the rather more toxic V agents including VE, VM and VX (Tammelin, 1957). Of these only VX has become well known. The history of the development of the nerve agents has been presented in some detail by Holmstedt (1963). In this section only GA, GB, GD and VX will be considered and will be referred to by these abbreviations.

Physicochemical Properties of Nerve Agents

These are shown in Table 8.

Military Use of Nerve Agents

Nerve agents may be disseminated on the battlefield by a variety of means and may be encountered as vapour, liquid or artificially thickened liquid in the case of GD. GB is a comparatively volatile compound and presents a severe vapour hazard when encountered in the liquid state. VX on the other hand is a compound of very low volatility and presents little vapour hazard. The standard UK military respirator provides excellent protection against the effects of nerve agent vapour.

Toxicity of Nerve Agents

Nerve agents are probably the most toxic compounds yet produced on a large scale. Many studies of their toxicity have been undertaken using animal models and a very wide range of LD_{50} values are known. A small selection of these values are shown in the Table 9. Fortunately, the number of accidental exposures of people to nerve agents has been small and, in consequence, information on the lethal doses of the compounds in humans is scarce. Many volunteers have, however, been exposed to low concentrations of nerve agents and the effects of such exposures are well understood. A recent account (Maynard

Table 8 Physicochemical properties of nerve agents[a]

Characteristic		Tabun GA	Sarin GB	Soman GD	GF	VX
Formula		(structural formula)	(structural formula)	(structural formula)	(structural formula)	(structural formula)
M.W.		162.3	140.1	182.18	180.14	267.36
S.G. (20°C)		1.073	1.0887	1.022	1.133	1.0083
M.P. °C		−49	−56	−80	−12	−20
B.P. °C		246	147	167	–	300
	°C					
	0	0.004	0.52	0.044	0.006	
V.P.	10	0.013	1.07	0.11	0.017	
mmHg	20	0.036	2.10	0.27	0.044	0.00044
	30	0.094	3.93	0.61	0.104	
	40	0.23	7.1	–	0.234	
	50	0.56	12.3	2.60	0.501	

Source: From Maynard and Beswick (1992)
[a] GA = ethyl *N*-dimethylphosphoramidocyanidate;
  GB = isopropyl methylphosphonofluoridate;
  GD = 1,2,2-trimethylpropyl methylphosphonofluoridate;
  GF = cyclohexyl methylphosphonofluoridate;
  VX = *O*-ethyl *S*-[2-(diisopropylamino)ethyl]methylphosphonothioate.

Table 9 Toxicity of nerve agents

Species	Route	Term	Units	GA	GB	GD	VX
Rat	Inhalation	$L(Ct)_{50}$	mg m^{-3} 10 min	304[1]	150[2]	–	–
	Intravenous	LD_{50}	µg kg^{-1}	66[1]	39[3]	44.5[4]	–
	Subcutaneous	LD_{50}	µg kg^{-1}	193[5]	103[6]	75[7]	12[5]
Mouse	Inhalation	$L(Ct)_{50}$	mg m^{-3} 30 min	15[1]	5[8]	1[8]	–
	Intravenous	LD_{50}	µg kg^{-1}	150[1]	113[9]	35[10]	–
	Subcutaneous	LD_{50}	µg kg^{-1}	250[11]	60[8]	40[8]	22[11]
Guinea pig	Inhalation	$L(Ct)_{50}$	mg m^{-3} 2 min	393[1]	128[12]	–	–
	Subcutaneous	LD_{50}	µg kg^{-1}	–	30[13]	24[14]	8.4[15]

Source: 1 Gates and Renshaw (1946); 2 Rengstorff (1985); 3 Fleisher (1963); 4 Pazdernik *et al*. (1983); 5 Jovanovic (1983); 6 Brimblecombe *et al*. (1970); 7 Boskovic *et al*. (1984); 8 Lohs (1960); 9 Schoene and Oldiges (1973); 10 Brezenoff *et al*. (1984); 11 Maksimovic *et al*. (1980); 12 Bright *et al*. (1991); 13 Coleman *et al*. (1968); 14 Gordon and Leadbeater (1977); 15 Leblic *et al*. (1984).

and Beswick, 1992) should be consulted for details. Table 10 gives some indication of the approximate lethal toxicity figures for nerve agents in humans.

Absorption of Nerve Agents

Nerve agents in the liquid form are absorbed rapidly across the unbroken skin and mucous membranes. Vapour is not absorbed across the skin in significant amounts, although it is absorbed across the cornea in sufficient quantities to produce miosis as a local effect. Absorption of vapour by the lung is rapid and more than 80 per cent of inhaled agent is absorbed. This important point should be borne in mind whenever the $L(Ct)_{50}$ figure for a volatile nerve agent is quoted. During exercise, respiratory minute volume is increased but the absorption of the high percentage of the inhaled vapour is maintained. The $L(Ct)_{50}$ of the compound is therefore ventilation-dependent. For example the $L(Ct)_{50}$ for GB in resting humans is approximately 100 mg min m^{-3}. On exercise, producing a fivefold increase in minute volume, this value could fall to 20 mg min m^{-3}.

Mechanism of Action of Nerve Agents

Nerve agents are organophosphorus anticholinesterases (anti AChEs) and exert their toxic effects by long lasting inhibition of acetylcholinesterase (AChE) at sites of activity of acetylcholine (ACh) in the body. The action of anticholinesterase compounds has been discussed at length in chapter 62 and by Koelle (1963), Taylor (1980) and Murphy (1986) and will not be considered here. One point should, however, be borne in mind: many organophosphorus compounds undergo a reaction generally known as 'ageing' after they have combined with AChE (Fleisher and Harris, 1965). The rate at which this reaction occurs varies with the anti-AChE and is particularly rapid in the case of GD. Ligtenstein (1984) has compiled data illustrating this point (see Table 11).

The values given in Table 11 should not, of course, be taken as representative of the half-lives of ageing of the nerve agents at human synaptic or neuromuscular junctions and are shown only for the purposes of comparing the rates of ageing of different agent–enzyme complexes. Differences in rates of ageing are important as regards the treatment of nerve agent poisoning with oximes (see below).

Table 10 Estimated values for toxicity of nerve agents in humans

Species	Route	Term	Units	GA	GB	GD	VX
Human	Inhalation	$L(Ct)_{50}$	mg min m^{-3}	150	70–100	40–60	–
	Intravenous	LD_{50}	mg kg^{-1}	0.08	0.01	0.025	0.007
	Percutaneous	LD_{50}	mg kg^{-1}	–	–	–	0.142

Table 11 Ageing of organophosphorus–AChE complexes

Nerve agent	Enzyme[a]	Ageing half-life	Reference
GA	BEA	46 h	de-Jong and Wolring (1978)
GB	BEA	12 h	Benschop and Keijer (1966)
GD	BEA	4 min	de-Jong and Wolring (1980)
VX	BEA	>12 days	de-Jong (1983)

[a] BEA = bovine erythrocyte acetylcholinesterase.

Source: modified from Ligtenstein (1984).

Clinical Effects of Nerve Agents

The clinical effects of nerve agents may be deduced by recalling the sites of action of ACh in the body (Koelle, 1975). As well as acting at autonomic ganglia, peripheral parasympathetic terminals and the neuromuscular junction, it should be recalled that ACh also plays an important role in transmission within the CNS.

The symptoms and signs of antiAChE poisoning have been described in Chapter 52 and will not be described in detail here. Table 12 shows the symptoms and signs of nerve agent poisoning in terms of short-term exposure and AChE depression. The effects of systemic exposure leading to similar degrees of depression of AChE are also shown.

Information from volunteer studies on the effects of nerve agents relates only to comparatively short duration exposures and, in the main, to exposures to concentration–time profiles of less than 30 mg min m^{-3}. It will be noted that considerable variations in the expected degrees of depression of AChE have been indicated in Table 12. This is important and all workers have stressed the considerable variation in the effects observed in different individuals at identical levels of AChE depression. This point will be returned to in the next section.

Table 12 Signs and symptoms of nerve agent poisoning

Short-term Ct mg min m^{-3}	AChE inhibition % (±SD)	Symptoms and signs Vapour exposure	Systemic exposure (eyes protected)
2	?	Incipient miosis, ? slight headache	Nil
5	20 ± 10	Miosis, headache, rhinorrhoea, eye pain, injection of conjunctivae, tightness of chest	? Tightness of chest
5–15	20–50 ± 10	Eye signs maximal, bronchospasm in some	Symptoms in some, ? bronchospasm
15	50 ± 10	Effects as above but more severe	Wheezing, salivation, nausea, vomiting, miosis, local sweating, muscle fasciculation in cases of skin contamination
40	80 ± 10	As above but more severe with weakness, involuntary micturition and defaecation, paralysis and convulsions	
100	100	Respiratory failure Death	

Clinical Investigations

Measurement of whole blood, erythrocyte and plasma cholinesterase activities are often undertaken in cases of organophosphorus compound poisoning. Plasma contains butyrylcholinesterase and red cells contain acetylcholinesterase. It is often assumed that a measurement of the level of active, i.e. uninhibited, red cell cholinesterase will provide an accurate reflection of levels of AChE at synaptic and neuromuscular junctions and thus reflect the severity of the poisoning which the patient has sustained. This is not so. Willems (1989) studied the patterns of cholinesterase depression in 53 cases of poisoning by organophosphorus insecticides and showed there was a poor correlation between clinical severity of poisoning and the extent of enzyme depression. It is difficult to imagine that a better relationship would exist in cases of nerve agent poisoning.

Management of Nerve Agent Poisoning

First Aid

Casualties should be removed from risk of further contamination and decontaminated by adequately protected and trained attendants. Contaminated clothing should be removed as quickly as possible taking care not to transfer liquid from the casualty's clothing to his skin. If protective clothing has been worn then this should be decontaminated with fullers' earth before being removed. Under battlefield conditions clean areas occupied by staff not wearing respirators and protective clothing must be protected at all costs. Monitoring equipment should be used to confirm adequate decontamination before casualties are transferred into these clean areas. One of the most serious consequences of nerve agent poisoning is respiratory failure produced by inhibition of the medullary centres. If respiration can be maintained while the drugs discussed below are administered then the casualty's chances of recovery will be much enhanced. Under battlefield conditions the artificial ventilation of casualties presents formidable problems. 'Ambu' style bags (protected by suitable rubber coverings and equipped with adequate filters) and oro-pharyngeal airways can reduce these problems.

Medical Treatment

Drug therapy for nerve agent poisoning, as for poisoning by other antiAChE compounds, divides into three: (1) cholinolytics such as atropine, (2) reactivators of the inhibited AChE:oximes, and (3) anticonvulsants, e.g. diazepam or other benzodiazepines. To these should be added oxygen which may be needed in cases of respiratory failure. The use of oxygen will not be considered further here.

In addition to the above, research has been undertaken to try to provide drugs, which if taken in advance of exposure to nerve agents, would reduce the effects of the exposure and make the treatment of poisoning resulting from that exposure the more effective. This research has been most successfully prosecuted in the UK and all UK forces would be issued with pyridostigmine bromide tablets (30 mg three times daily) for use should the risk of exposure to nerve agents be deemed significant.

Cholinolytics

Atropine is the drug of choice and should be given intramuscularly or preferably intravenously, in aliquots of 2 mg, as soon as possible after poisoning. To enable servicemen to self-administer atropine and in some cases oxime, a wide variety of autoinjection devices have been developed commercially. Most contain 2 mg of atropine per injection and permit injection through clothing. Speed of administration as soon as the first signs of poisoning are detected is critical as the progress of symptoms and signs may be very rapid. It is essential therefore that servicemen should be well trained in the recognition of the early signs of poisoning and in the use of the autoinjection devices.

As in cases of poisoning by other organophosphorus compounds large total doses of atropine are often said to be likely to be needed. However, in casualties surviving to reach hospital it is unlikely that the heroic doses of atropine reported by some who were managing cases of organophosphorus pesticide poisoning would be required.

The dangers of atropine overdose should always be borne in mind:

- Drying of bronchial secretions making them tenacious and difficult to remove; the careful use of suction may be required.

- Large doses of atropine may induce arrhythmias particularly if the myocardium is hypoxic as a result of respiratory failure.
- Bladder dysfunction may necessitate catheterization.

Atropine drops are sometimes recommended for the relief of visual impairment and eye pain caused by contraction of the iris and spasm of the ciliary muscle. Atropine drops may be expected to relieve the eye pain to some extent but seem to do little to improve vision. The combination of mydriasis and impairment of accommodation seems to produce at least as severe an impairment of vision as the miosis produced by exposure to the nerve agent. The use of oxime, instead of atropine, eye drops has been suggested but not widely adopted.

Oximes
The oximes, developed in the early 1950s (Wilson and Ginsburg, 1955; Wegner-Juaregg, 1956) represented a major step forward in the treatment of nerve agent poisoning. Hydroxylamine was the first compound demonstrated to be capable of reactivating the AChE/nerve agent complex. More effective oximes followed and the work of Davies and Green (1956, 1959) and others led to the development of pralidoxime methanesulphonate (pralidoxime mesylate or P2S). This compound and other pralidoxime salts have maintained their place as the oximes of choice in the treatment of organophosphorus poisoning in many countries. P2S is included in the autoinjection device issued to the UK Armed Forces.

P2S is a monopyridinium oxime; its chemical structure is shown in Figure 9.

A number of bispyridinium oximes have been developed including obidoxime (Toxogonin) and those of the series of oximes referred to as the Hagedorn, or H, oximes (Oldiges and Schoene, 1970). The structures of some of the better known compounds are shown in Figure 10.

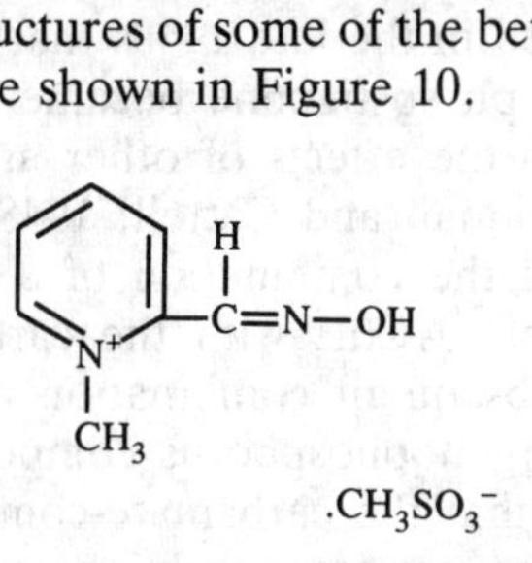

Figure 9 Pralidoxime methanesulphanate (P2S)

If P2S is used it should be given intramuscularly, as soon as possible after poisoning, or better by slow intravenous injection, at a dose of 30 mg kg^{-1}. The dose should be repeated at 15 min intervals to a total dose of 2 or possibly 4 g. It should be remembered that very little experience of management of nerve agent casualties has been accumulated. Oximes should be administered carefully and a close watch kept on the patient's condition. Side-effects include headache, disturbances of vision and muscular weakness and care should be taken to monitor the patient's condition before and after the administration of oxime to permit differentiation between the signs of deepening organophosphorus toxicity and the side-effects of therapy. If given too quickly, bronchospasm and laryngospasm may occur. The use of an intravenous infusion of 2 g of P2S in 250 ml of normal (0.9 per cent) saline delivered over 30 min has also been recommended. Ligtenstein (1984) has made a strong case for the continuation of the use of oximes beyond the often suggested limit of a day or two.

The choice of oxime, if more than one is available, may be difficult. The following points should be recalled:

- Pralidoxime (PAM) salts are probably still the most widely available oximes.
- PAM is likely to be markedly more effective in cases of GB and VX poisoning than in cases of GA and GD poisoning.
- Although obidoxime (Toxogonin) (3–6 mg kg^{-1} iv 4 hourly) is likely to be effective in cases of GA, GB and VX (but not GD) poisoning, cases of liver damage following its use have been reported.
- The Hagedorn oximes such as HI6 and HGG12 have been shown to be effective in GD poisoning in some animal models but are rather less effective than had been hoped in GA poisoning (Wolthuis and Kepner, 1978; Harris *et al.*, 1981; Clement, 1981, 1982a,b; Clement and Lockwood, 1982).
- The recently developed Hagedorn oxime HLö–7 (pyrimidoxime) is effective both in GA and GD poisoning in some animal models (Eyer *et al.*, 1989).
- In general the Hagedorn oximes are unstable in solution and demand more complex autoinjection devices than the conventional oximes (Eyer *et al.*, 1989).

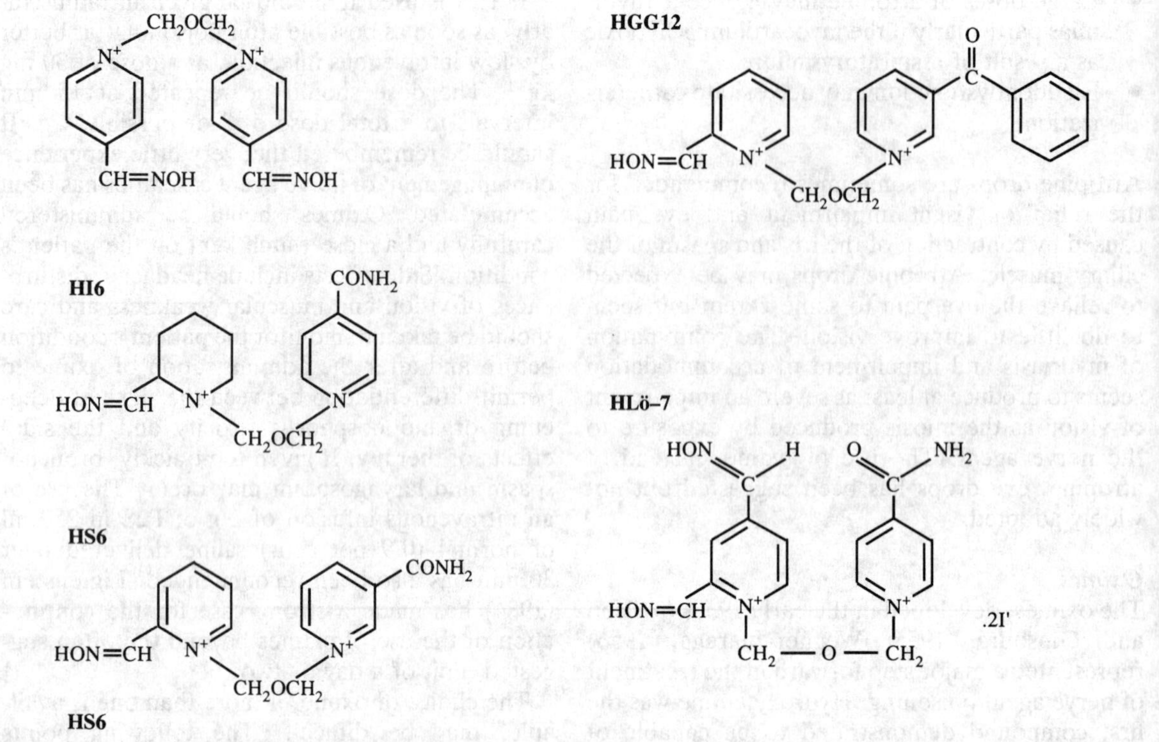

Figure 10 Structure of some of the better-known oximes

In addition to the above it should be recalled that atropine and oximes are synergistic in their effects and the administration of atropine and oxime has been shown to raise the LD_{50} of some nerve agents in animal models by a factor of more than 20 (Inns and Leadbeater, 1983). GD remains a major problem and the publications of Wolthuis and Kepner (1978), and Wolthuis *et al.* (1981) and Clement (1981, 1982a,b) should be consulted for details of the intractability of poisoning with GD and for arguments regarding the use of H oximes.

Anticonvulsants
Diazepam has come to be regarded as a valuable addition to the combination of atropine and oxime in the management of nerve agent poisoning. Nerve agent poisoning, and particularly poisoning with GD in monkeys, is often complicated by convulsions and the control of these convulsions with diazepam has been shown to enhance the likelihood of survival (Lipp, 1972, 1973). A number of theories have been put forward to explain this effect, including the suggestion that diazepam may prevent the rise in cyclic

GMP levels observed in the CNS of animals suffering GD-induced convulsions (Lundy and Magor, 1978). Recent work has however cast doubt on this theory (Liu *et al.*, 1988).

Diazepam should be given in a dose of 5 mg orally, intramuscularly or better intravenously. Diazepam is not suitable for combination in solution with atropine and P2S but a recently-developed lysine–diazepam conjugate is. This has been incorporated in the autoinjection devices issued to the UK Armed Forces.

Prophylaxis and Pretreatment Against Nerve Agent Poisoning
It was noted in the late 1940s that cats given the carbamate physostigmine became comparatively resistant to the effects of other antiAChE compounds (Gilman and Cattell, 1948). It was suggested that the combination of a proportion of the available AChE with the carbamate would prevent subsequent combination of the enzyme with the organophosphorus compound and, furthermore, that the carbamate-combined enzyme would, later, spontaneously reactivate and provide the body with a supply of normal uninhibited

enzyme. This hypothesis is now generally accepted. A great deal of work has been done in developing the carbamate pyridostigmine bromide for use in this way and Inns and Leadbeater (1983) summed up work on the efficacy of pretreatment, combined with the treatment detailed above, in cases of GD poisoning in guinea pigs. Table 13 shows some of the results obtained.

Pyridostigmine is a quaternary carbamate and as such does not readily penetrate the blood–brain barrier. Physostigmine, a tertiary carbamate, penetrates the blood–brain barrier to a greater extent and has been suggested as an alternative to pyridostigmine. The short biological half-life and side-effects of physostigmine may, however, render it unsuitable for general issue to servicemen.

Prognosis of nerve agent casualties

Animal studies have suggested that the combination of the pretreatment and treatment described above would probably be effective in cases of nerve agent poisoning. It is, however, difficult to extrapolate from such work to the case of the soldier poisoned on the battlefield at a considerable distance from medical attention. For those casualties who have self-administered one or perhaps more of their autoinjection devices but who are slipping deeper into the effects of the nerve agent the prognosis can hardly be other than poor. Those who sustain a dose of nerve agent sufficient to produce respiratory failure are unlikely to survive. It is believed that self-administration of therapy will delay the onset of symptoms and signs of nerve agent poisoning and make it more likely that the poisoned man will survive and reach medical attention.

Long-term Effects of Nerve Agent Poisoning

It is well known that organophosphorus compounds can produce permanent damage to the nervous system. These effects, thought to be dependent on the combination of the organophosphate with the enzyme known as neuropathy target esterase (NTE), have been studied in detail by Johnson and commented on in Chapter 52. Studies in animal models have demonstrated that the nerve agents are capable of producing these effects, but only when administered to animals protected by the prior administration of atropine and oxime, in doses many times in excess of their LD_{50}s. It is likely that a soldier who survives nerve agent poisoning on the battlefield will not have been exposed to a dose of nerve agent capable of inducing neuropathy.

PULMONARY OEDEMA-INDUCING COMPOUNDS

During World War I the chemical warfare compounds with the highest lethality were those which induced pulmonary oedema, and included chlorine and phosgene. Phosgene was first used by German forces on 19 December 1915 and soon acquired a reputation as a dangerous compound: 85 per cent of deaths resulting from exposure to chemical warfare compounds during World War I were caused by phosgene (HMSO, 1972). Despite this, well-protected troops using modern respirators should not be placed at serious risk as a result of exposure to these compounds, and little development of pulmonary oedema-producing compounds for use as chemical warfare agents has taken place since World War I. During World

Table 13 Effectiveness of oximes and bispyridinium compounds against Soman poisoning in guinea pigs receiving various supporting drug treatments. Pyridostigmine 0.32 μmol kg^{-1} im) was injected 30 min before challenge with soman(sc). One minute after poisoning P2S (130 μmol kg^{-1}) was injected im with atropine (50 μmol kg^{-1}). Diazepam (25 μmol kg^{-1}) was given as a separate im injection

Compound	Protective ratio (95% confidence limits)			
	Atropine	Atropine, diazepam	Pyridostigmine, atropine	Pyridostigmine, atropine, diazepam
–	1.5 (1.2–1.9)	2.2 (1.8–2.7)	5.2 (4.1–6.6)	8.7 (5.7–14)
P2S	1.7 (1.5–1.9)	2.5 (1.9–3.1)	6.8 (5.4–8.5)	14 (10–19)

Source: modified from Inns and Leadbeater (1983).

War I great efforts to develop other pulmonary-damaging compounds were made and a large number of compounds were used, albeit sometimes on a comparatively small scale. Accounts dating from the 1920s should be consulted for details of these compounds. Among accounts generally available, that of Prentiss (1937) is particularly detailed and reliable.

During World War I phosgene acquired a particularly evil reputation as it was soon realized that men who had inhaled a potentially lethal dose of the compound might show few symptoms and signs during the first few hours following exposure (Vedder, 1925). Early diagnosis was therefore difficult. It was further noted that men in the symptomless latent period could collapse with florid pulmonary oedema if exposed to physical stress (HMSO, 1923). It will be appreciated that the sensible clinical advice to rest all those thought to have been exposed, for 24–48 h, preferably in bed, was ill-received by commanders in the field.

While phosgene might not present a severe toxicological risk to modern troops it is not detected by the various detectors and monitors in general military use, and troops thought to be at risk would be forced to don respirators and accept the concomitant drop in their performance. As stated in the introduction to this chapter, inducing this drop in performance might well have been all for which the aggressor had hoped, and thus phosgene remains a significant chemical warfare agent.

Phosgene is produced in large quantities in peacetime by the chemical industry and cases of industrial accidents occur from time to time. The general effects of lung damaging compounds have been described in Chapters 20 and 22 and only those aspects of the toxicology of phosgene of chemical warfare importance are mentioned here.

Physicochemical Properties of Phosgene

These are given in Table 14.

Likely Mode of Exposure

Phosgene is rapidly dispersed by wind and is regarded as an agent of short persistence likely to be used only in surprise attacks. It may however linger in cellars, tunnels and hollows as it

Table 14 Physicochemical properties of phosgene

Formula	$COCl_2$
M.W.	99
M.P. °C	−118
B.P. °C	8.2
Vapour density	3.5
V.P. mmHg	−13.7°C : 335
	−10 °C : 365
	0 °C : 555
	8.2°C : 760
Odour	Stifling odour of new-mown hay

is heavier than air. Lefebure (1921) described experiments undertaken during World War I in an attempt to convert phosgene into a more persistent compound by impregnating porous powders with the gas. These experiments do not seem to have been successful.

Absorption of Phosgene

Phosgene is not absorbed to a significant extent through the skin; it is of course absorbed by the lung. Nash and Pattle (1971) studied the reaction of phosgene with water at moist surfaces and concluded that the rate of hydrolysis would render penetration by phosgene of more than 'a few tens of microns' unlikely.

Toxicity of Phosgene

The toxicity of phosgene has been widely studied, and Table 15 shows the range of toxicity encountered in different species.

As in the case of nerve agents $L(Ct)_{50}$ is dependent on the respiratory state and will fall with exertion.

Mechanism of Action of Phosgene

Despite its long history, the exact mechanism of action of phosgene remains obscure. The hypothesis that phosgene acts by combining with water and forming hydrochloric acid (Winternitz, 1920; Vedder, 1925), which then produces tissue damage, was challenged by the work of Nash and Pattle (1971). These authors showed that the 'maximum concentration of acid in a blood–air barrier of thickness 1 μm, in contact with 25 ppm

Table 15   Toxicity of phosgene

Species	Route	Term	Units	Value	Source
Rat	Inhalation	LC_{50}	mg m^{-3} per 30 min	1400	NTIS[a]
Mouse	Inhalation	LC_{50}	mg m^{-3} per 30 min	1800	NTIS
Dog	Inhalation	LC_{50}	mg m^{-3} per 20 min	4200	NTIS
Monkey	Inhalation	LC_{50}	mg m^{-3} per 1 min	600	NTIS
Rabbit	Inhalation	LC_{50}	mg m^{-3} per 30 min	1000	NTIS
Rat	Inhalation	LC_{LO}	ppm per 30 min	50	NIOSH[b]
Dog	Inhalation	LC_{LO}	ppm per 30 min	80	NIOSH
Rat	Inhalation	100% mortality	ppm per 20 min	37	

[a] NTIS = National Technical Information Service.
[b] NIOSH = National Institute for Occupational Safety and Health.

The values quoted in Table 15 are often described in toxicological data bases as LC_{50} values, e.g. the 'LC_{50} of phosgene for a 30 minute exposure in mice is 1800 mg m^{-3}'. Attempts to convert such values to $L(Ct)_{50}$ values by simple multiplication should be avoided as it is known that the $L(Ct)_{50}$ of phosgene is time-dependent.

It will be noted that as the duration of the exposure is increased the $L(Ct)_{50}$ value rises. This has also been noted by Ballantyne (1977) for hydrogen cyanide.

A widely quoted statement of the toxicity of phosgene to humans is . . . '50 ppm may be rapidly fatal' (for phosgene 1.0 mg m^{-3} = 4.419 ppm, at STP)

Table 16   Variations in lethal index of phosgene with duration of exposure (dogs). After Prentiss (1937)

Time of exposure (min)	Minimum lethal dose (mg l^{-1})	Lethal index
2	2.00	4000
5	1.10	5500
10	0.55	6500
15	0.46	6900
20	0.37	7400
25	0.30	7500
30	0.27	8100
45	0.20	9000
60	0.17	10200
75	0.16	12000

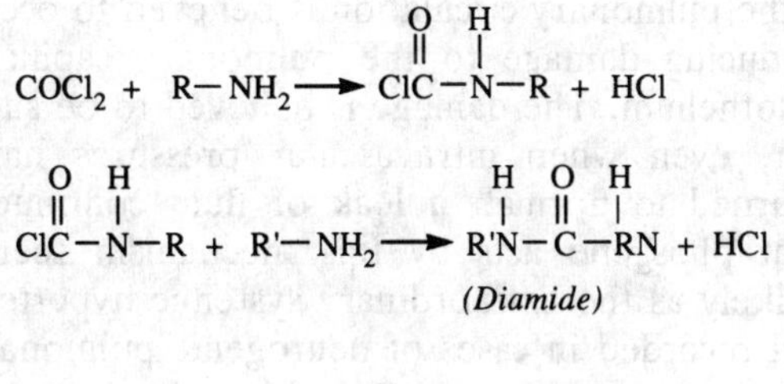

of phosgene is 7×10^{-10} M, which is negligible. Buffering by tissue constituents would prevent any significant change in pH'. At high concentrations it was accepted that the formation of hydrochloric acid might play a role.

Potts *et al.* (1949) proposed that phosgene combined with the amino groups of proteins to form diamides (Figure 11). Diller (1978) proposed a series of reactions to explain the combination of phosgene with a wider range of chemical groups (Figure 12). Frosolono and Pawlowski (1977) studied the biochemical changes produced by phosgene in various lung fractions prepared from rats exposed to close to an $L(Ct)_{50}$ of phosgene. A number of enzymes showed decreased activity

Figure 11   Formation of diamides

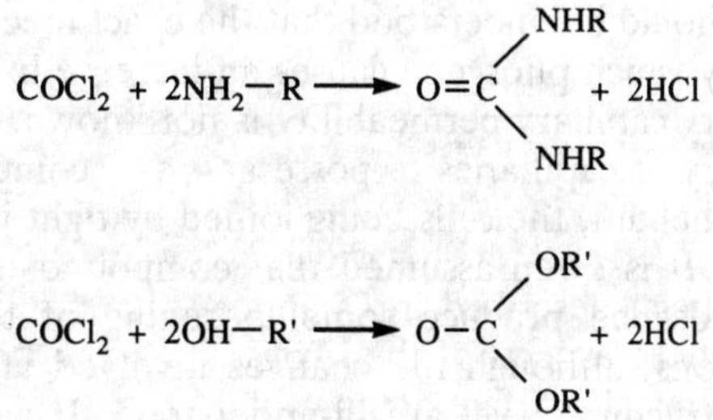

Figure 12   Reactions to explain the combination of phosgene with a wider range of chemical groups

but the data did not allow a distinction to be drawn between reduction in enzyme activity as a result of direct inhibition and that resulting from loss from damaged cells.

In addition to the above, efforts have been made to produce a pathophysiological hypothesis to explain the production of pulmonary oedema. Phosgene clearly damages the blood–air barrier in the lung and allows the leak of fluid from the pulmonary capillaries. At first this leak may be contained by increased flow in the pulmonary lymphatic system but later an increase in fluid in the connective tissue spaces occurs and finally fluid spills over into the alveoli. This sequence, the standard pattern of 'permeability' as compared with 'hydrostatic' pulmonary oedema, has been most competently reviewed by Staub (1974), Teplitz (1979) and Robin (1979) and is discussed at greater length in Chapter 22. Some authors, including Everett and Overholt (1968) and Ivanhoe and Meyers (1964), have suggested that phosgene could lead to massive reflex vasoconstriction and the production of oedema as in neurogenic pulmonary oedema (NPE). In this condition a sudden redistribution of blood from the systemic to the pulmonary circulation is believed to occur producing damage to the pulmonary capillary endothelium. The damage is believed to be such that, even when intravascular pressures have returned to normal, a leak of fluid continues. That phosgene acts by this mechanism seems unlikely as the extraordinary systemic hypertension recorded in cases of neurogenic pulmonary oedema has not been observed in animal models of phosgene poisoning.

It should be understood that the exact mechanism by which phosgene causes an increase in pulmonary capillary permeability is not known. Pulmonary capillaries possess a complete endothelium, the cells being joined by tight junctions. It is often assumed that compounds such as phosgene produce some loosening of these junctions, although the changes involved at the ultrastructural level are ill-understood. It would be particularly interesting to know whether phosgene produces any change in the pattern of strands of particles, revealed upon the p-face of the cell membrane by freeze–fracture techniques, which appear to be important in the structure of the tight junction.

Histopathology of Phosgene-induced Lung Damage

The light microscopic appearances of phosgene-damaged lungs were accurately described by Winternitz in 1920. Since then many studies have

been carried out, Pawlowski and Frosolono's work (1977) at the ultrastructural level being particularly valuable. The sequence of changes described by Pawlowski is as follows:

- The epithelium of the terminal bronchiole appeared to be first affected. Intracellular vesiculation of ciliated epithelial cells and Clara cells was observed. These effects appeared very soon after exposure.
- An increase in the amount of extracellular fluid visible in the interalveolar septae was noted.
- Frank oedema of cells of the interalveolar septae was observed.
- Swelling of type II alveolar cells was noted.
- Type I alveolar cells showed areas of focal disruption.
- Interalveolar septae became widely distended with fluid.
- Oedema fluid appeared in alveolar spaces.

Oedema fluid in phosgene-induced lung damage is protein-rich and, by light microscopy, classically eosinophilic. Damage to type II alveolar cells is interesting although a clear demonstration of a decline in surfactant production in phosgene-induced oedema appears to be lacking. It is, however, known that by lowering the surface tension of the lining film of the alveoli, surfactant may reduce the forces acting to move fluid out of pulmonary capillaries (Pattle, 1965). Damage to cells which produce surfactant would then be expected to enhance the likelihood of alveolar oedema.

Symptoms and Signs of Phosgene Exposure

Because of the extensive use of phosgene during World War I many detailed accounts of its effects on humans are available, Ireland (1926) and Vedder (1925) providing particularly valuable accounts. Accidental exposures occur and Diller (1978), Seidelim (1961), Fruhman (1974) and Bradley and Unger (1982) have also provided accounts.

Some authors describe eye irritation, coughing, lacrimation, choking and a feeling of tightness of the chest as early symptoms and signs of phosgene exposure. Doubtless these do occur in some patients, but it was clearly demonstrated during World War I that an absence of such effects did not preclude serious and sometimes lethal exposure.

The hallmark of phosgene poisoning has been recognized to be the occurrence of a latent period intervening between exposure and the onset of the symptoms and signs of pulmonary oedema. This period may range from 30 min to 24 h depending, in part, on the severity of the exposure. During this period it is notoriously difficult to distinguish the mildly exposed from the severely exposed.

During World War I emphasis was placed on the value of the so-called 'tobacco reaction' in identifying those exposed to phosgene, as it had been repeatedly observed that smokers who were exposed to phosgene complained of a metallic taste on next lighting a cigarette. Once the latent period is over dyspnoea, a painful cough and cyanosis appear rapidly. Increasing quantities of, initially whitish but later pink, fluid are expectorated, a marked efflux of fluid, the 'champignon d'écume', sometimes appearing just before death. The cause of death is usually cardiac failure and circulatory collapse caused by the hypoxia.

A World War I description of a chemist dying some hours after a brief exposure to a high concentration of phosgene during a laboratory accident gives the clinical picture:

His condition now rapidly deteriorated. Every fit of coughing brought up large quantities of clear, yellowish, frothy fluid of which about 80 ounces (2272 ml) were expectorated in one and a half hours. His face became of a grey, ashen colour, never purple, though the pulse remained fairly strong. He died at 6.50 pm without any great struggle for breath. The symptoms of irritation were very slight at the onset; there was then a delay of at least four hours and the final development of serious oedema up to death took little more than an hour though the patient was continually rested in bed.

(Vedder, 1925)

Management of Phosgene Poisoning

First Aid
Casualties should be removed from risk of further exposure by suitably-protected attendants. Because phosgene would not be encountered in the liquid state decontamination with fullers' earth is unnecessary.

Medical Treatment
The management of phosgene poisoning is the management of permeability pulmonary oedema. No antiphosgene drug of any proven value has been discovered although hexamethylenetetramine is discussed briefly below. Steroids, antibiotics, bronchodilators, respiratory stimulants and cardiac stimulants have all been suggested, although none has received universal support. Two measures are, however, generally agreed.

Rest
All persons thought to have been exposed to phosgene should be confined to bed. It was demonstrated repeatedly during World War I that exertion during the latent period following exposure to phosgene could precipitate acute and fatal pulmonary oedema.

Oxygen
Patients unable to maintain an adequate arterial oxygen tension when breathing air should be given supplementary oxygen. This was stressed during World War I by Barcroft (1920) and Haldane (1917) when experience in the management of phosgene poisoning was unrivalled.

Of measures not commanding universal support the following should be considered:

Corticosteroids
Arguments both for and against the use of steroids in pulmonary oedema have been plentiful for some years and have been considered by Everett and Overholt (1968), Diller (1978) and Bradley and Unger (1982). Everett reported the successful use of glucocorticoids, Diller also supported their use although Bradley found the evidence of their efficacy unconvincing. It is known that inflammatory changes are likely to occur in lung tissue damaged by phosgene and that these changes involve the release of mediators which are likely to increase capillary permeability and therefore worsen the oedema. That such release can be prevented by the prophylactic administration of corticosteroids seems likely; that such release can be reduced significantly once initiated, remains doubtful. Some clinicians, perhaps the majority, have felt that the lack of serious side-effects usually associated with the

short-term administration of large doses of corticosteroids and the seriousness of permeability pulmonary oedema, justifies the use of these drugs. Others have felt that the lack of clear evidence of efficacy should preclude their use.

Prichard and Lee (1987) recently considered the question of the use of steroids in high permeability pulmonary oedema in the *Oxford Textbook of Medicine* and concluded: 'Until a conclusive answer is produced, clinicians will continue to use steroids in large doses despite the absence of adequate supportive clinical data.' In some military manuals (HMSO, 1987) the use of a large single dose of corticosteroid as soon as possible after exposure has been advocated.

Antibiotics   The provision of antibiotic cover in phosgene poisoning has been supported by both Diller (1978) and Everett and Overholt (1968). During World War I the absence of antibiotics made pneumonia a feared complication of lung damage arising as a result of exposure to a variety of chemical warfare compounds. The choice of antibiotics is wide, penicillin G, amoxycillin and chloramphenicol all having been recommended.

Of measures not receiving wide support only one will be considered.

Hexamethylenetetramine ('Hexamine', 'Methanamine', HMT)
Hexamine is used prophylactically as an antimicrobial drug in cases of recurrent urinary tract infections. It has been demonstrated to be of value, in animal models, if given before exposure to phosgene. Stravrakis (1971) argued that hexamine was also of value if given post-exposure in cases of phosgene poisoning and recommended the administration of 20 ml of a 20 per cent solution, intravenously, as soon as possible after exposure. Diller (1978) reviewed the use of hexamine and concluded that there was no firm evidence to support the view that hexamine is of value if given *after* poisoning.

As in all cases of permeability pulmonary oedema the administration of intravenous fluids should be approached with great caution.

Long-term Effects of Phosgene Poisoning

Chronic bronchitis and emphysema have been reported as a consequence of exposure to phosgene (Cucinell, 1974).

HYDROGEN CYANIDE

Of the poisons known to the general public, cyanide, arsenic and strychnine are perhaps the best known and it is often assumed that cyanide would be a dangerous chemical warfare agent. Despite this, hydrogen cyanide has been but little used as a chemical warfare agent and its physicochemical and toxicological characteristics make it unsuitable for such use on any other than a fairly small scale. It has, however, been used as a means of judicial execution and was used for the large scale murder of prisoners in German concentration camps during World War II.

Only France used hydrogen cyanide as a chemical warfare agent during World War I, the first use of hydrogen cyanide shells being on the Somme on 1 July 1916 (Prentiss, 1937). German respirators offered poor protection against hydrogen cyanide although this was quickly remedied and hydrogen cyanide lost most of its advantages over the alternative lethal compound, phosgene. It will be recalled that phosgene has a density equal to 3.5 times that of air but that hydrogen cyanide is less dense than air. Rapid dispersion of hydrogen cyanide greatly reduced its value as a chemical warfare agent. Prentiss (1937) commented: 'Because of its extreme volatility and the fact that the vapors are lighter than air, it is almost impossible to establish a lethal concentration of hydrocyanic acid in the field and this is particularly true when the gas is put over in artillery shells.' Few authorities today believe that hydrogen cyanide would be used on a large scale as a chemical warfare agent although it has retained its place in military chemical warfare handbooks on the grounds that successful use, at high concentration, on selected targets could probably be achieved.

In view of the above, the discussion of hydrogen cyanide as a chemical warfare agent will be limited; a discussion of the antidotal management of cases of poisoning will be found in Chapter 12.

Physicochemical Characteristics of Hydrogen Cyanide

These are shown in Table 17. Below 26°C hydrogen cyanide occurs as a colourless to yellowish-brown liquid. In its usual slightly impure state it is unstable, although it is said to be stable when highly purified. On standing, polymerization

Table 17   Physicochemical properties of hydrogen cyanide

Formula	HCN
M.W.	27.02
Vapour density	: 0.93 × that of air
B.P. (760 mm Hy)	: 26°C
M.P.	: −14°C
V.P. mmHg	°C
165	−10
256	0
600	20
757	26

takes place and the compound may present an explosive hazard. The risk of explosion may be much reduced by the addition of a small quantity of an organic acid, e.g. phosphoric acid. Prentiss (1937) commented: 'Anhydrous hydrocyanic acid is extremely unstable and is quickly decomposed with the formation of a black resinous mass.' This tendency to decomposition led to difficulties with munitions and Sartori (1939) commented: 'Even in the anhydrous condition it cannot be kept long as it gradually decomposes, occasionally with explosive force. Filled in projectiles it soon becomes harmless.' Hydrogen cyanide smells of almonds although not all individuals are able to detect the odour. The capacity to detect hydrogen cyanide rapidly wanes on exposure owing to failure of cells of the olfactory mucosa.

Absorption of Hydrogen Cyanide

Hydrogen cyanide vapour is readily absorbed across the lung but only to an insignificant extent across the skin.

Toxicity of Hydrogen Cyanide

The $L(Ct)_{50}$ value for hydrogen cyanide in humans is not known with any accuracy. It is, however, known that the $L(Ct)_{50}$ value is likely to be very time-dependent. This is shown by the estimates of human toxicity given in Table 18. The variation in $L(Ct)_{50}$ with time is believed to relate to the detoxification of cyanide, by enzymatic conversion to thiocyanate. Ballantyne and Schwabe (1981) have shown the variation in graphical form (Figure 13).

Further guidance on the estimated toxicity of hydrogen cyanide may be gained from Table 19.

Table 18   Estimated toxicity of hydrogen cyanide in humans

Duration of exposure (time)	Concentration (C) mg m⁻³	$L(Ct)_{50}$ mg min m⁻³
15 s	2400	660
1 min	1000	1000
10 min	200	2000
15 min	133	4000

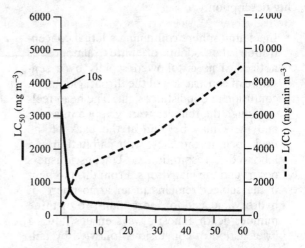

Figure 13   Acute lethal inhalation toxicity of hydrogen cyanide vapour.—LC_{50} of hydrogen cyanide (mg m⁻³). ---Corresponding $L(Ct)_{50}$ values (mg min m⁻³). From Ballantyne and Schwabe (1981). Reproduced with the permission of the authors

Table 19   Estimated toxicity of hydrogen cyanide in humans

Toxic effects	Concentration mg m⁻³
Mild symptoms on inhalation for many hours	24–48
Maximum tolerance limit for 1 h	50–60
Hazardous to life on inhalation for 30–60 min	112–150
Death in 5–10 min	240–360
Death in 5 min	420
Death after several breaths	1000

Symptoms and Signs of Hydrogen Cyanide Poisoning

It is often assumed that exposure to a given concentration of hydrogen cyanide either produces sudden death or very few ill-effects. In military circles this is often summed up by the observation that the use of hydrogen cyanide leaves 'the quick and the dead' but no incapacitated or partly incapacitated individuals. This is incorrect. Work in animal models (D'Mello, 1987) has shown that exposure to sublethal doses of hydrogen cyanide can produce incapacitation. Dizziness and nausea have been recorded in people exposed to sublethal quantities of hydrogen cyanide, the effects lasting for some hours.

At lethal concentrations, collapse and death are rapid. Vedder (1925) has provided the following description:

> In an atmosphere containing a lethal concentration the odour of bitter almonds is noticed. This is followed rapidly by a sensation of constriction of the throat, giddiness, confusion and indistinct sight. The head feels as though the temples were gripped in a vice and there may be pain at the back of the neck, pain in the chest with palpitation and laboured respiration. Unconsciousness occurs and the man drops. From this moment if the subject remains in an atmosphere of hydrocyanic acid for more than two or three minutes death almost always ensues, after a brief period of convulsions followed by failure of respiration.

Management of Hydrogen Cyanide Poisoning

Here only a few points of relevance to battlefield casualties will be made:

- The usual points regarding the rapid removal of casualties from the risk of further contamination should be noted.
- Decontamination of casualties is unnecessary unless the clothing is contaminated with liquid hydrogen cyanide. This is very unlikely.
- All forms of treatment currently available demand intravenous administration. This will probably be impossible on the battlefield and the author knows of no NATO country which intends to issue to non-medical personnel the equipment necessary for such treatment.
- Bearing the last point in mind it is likely that casualties who reach aid-posts will be incapacitated by sublethal doses of hydrogen cyanide. Given that adequately-trained medical orderlies, nursing staff or medical staff are available then antidotal therapy would be used. When deciding which therapy to recom-

mend it should be borne in mind that the exact diagnosis of the cause of collapse may, under battlefield conditions, be difficult and treatment known to produce severe side-effects if given to casualties who have, in fact, not been exposed to hydrogen cyanide should perhaps be avoided.

Prophylaxis in Hydrogen Cyanide Poisoning

It is generally accepted that treatment of casualties suffering from hydrogen cyanide poisoning, under battlefield conditions, will be difficult and often unsuccessful. Because of this, attempts to provide a measure of pharmacological protection against the effects of hydrogen cyanide have been made. The conversion of a fraction of haemoglobin to methaemoglobin, thus providing a ready-made binding site for the cyanide, has been a favoured line of research and in 1948 Gilman and Cattell reported studies undertaken during World War II in America. *p*-Aminopropiophenone was found to be the best compound tested for the production of methaemoglobinaemia and oral doses of 2.0 mg kg^{-1} were given to volunteers. This produced a methaemoglobinaemia of some 20–30 per cent. This was maintained by repeated dosing over 7 days without ill-effects although 'at the end of this period there were observed the beginnings of a haemolytic anaemia'. Methaemoglobin levels of up to 15 per cent were not found to interfere with exercise at light work loads. Animal work was reported to have shown that such levels of methaemoglobin (15 per cent) would have provided protection against ten lethal doses of hydrogen cyanide. On the battlefield, recalling the difficulty likely to be experienced in establishing a lethal concentration of cyanide, such a level of protection would be very valuable. Recent work by Bright (1987) in dogs has confirmed the above results although the issue of *p*-aminopropiophenone to troops for use in anticipation of an attack with hydrogen cyanide has, as far as is known, not been undertaken by any country.

LESSER CHEMICAL WARFARE AGENTS

In addition to the compounds described above many other substances have been considered, although in the main rejected, as possible chemical warfare agents. During World War I dozens, probably hundreds, of compounds were examined and during World War II several hundred mustard derivatives and variants were synthesized. The large number of compounds in this group which *could* be used in war makes any detailed consideration of individual compounds impossible. Instead a few comments will be made on some older compounds of interest and on the riot control agents which could be encountered during modern warfare.

Early Irritant Compounds

Smoke from fires, used since classical times to discommode forces defending strong positions, exerted its effects by producing choking and eye irritation. In the early twentieth century the Paris police force used grenades containing ethyl bromoacetate against rioters and it has been alleged that some of the police involved, later conscripted into the French Army, used the same grenades against German forces. The use of ethyl bromoacetate seems to have been taken up by the French and was also studied in London at Imperial College. (The military abbreviation for ethyl bromoacetate, SK, is said to stand for South Kensington, the location of Imperial College.) German workers also studied irritants and on 27 October 1914 at Neuve-Chapelle, HE shells containing lead balls embedded in the irritant *o*-dianisidine chlorosulphonate were deployed (SIPRI, 1971). This incident was followed by the use of other compounds including xylyl bromide, chloroacetone, benzyl bromide and iodide, ethyl and methyl chlorosulphonate, 2-chloroacetophenone and bromobenzyl cyanide. Prentiss (1937) held the latter to be the most powerful irritant introduced during the war. In addition to the lacrimators more toxic irritant smokes were developed. These included diphenylchlorarsine (DA), chlorodihydrophenarsazine (DM or Adamsite), and diphenyl cyanarsine (DC).

These compounds were described as vomiting agents and as well as producing nausea and vomiting produced acute pain in the nose, uncontrollable sneezing, coughing, eye pain and lacrimation (HMSO, 1972). The marked sneezing led to these compounds being termed sternutators (Latin *sternuto . . .* sneezing). Of these compounds only Adamsite has survived to modern use and has been used as a riot control agent, although not in the UK.

Other arsenical compounds developed during World War I included methyl-, ethyl- and phenyl-dichlorarsine, collectively known as 'The Dicks' (HMSO, 1972). These were vesicant compounds of considerable toxicity and were developed in an attempt to find a 'faster acting mustard gas' which would incapacitate casualties on contact. Attempts were also made to develop compounds combining irritancy with the lethality of hydrogen cyanide. Cyanogen bromide and chloride were produced, both effective irritants, capable of killing. Despite this, neither proved a very successful chemical warfare agent (Prentiss, 1937).

Modern Riot Control Compounds

The development of modern riot control compounds has been dominated by the perceived desirability of developing a compound with the following characteristics:

- Rapid incapacitating effect even when used against highly motivated individuals.
- Insignificant toxicity even to the very young or the very elderly bystander.
- Capacity for easy dissemination.
- Capacity for easy decontamination.
- Long shelf-life.
- Low cost.

It will be appreciated that these are difficult criteria to meet in full. At first glance the first two criteria listed might appear likely to be mutually exclusive and yet each is met remarkably well by compounds such as CS and CR [dibenz(b.f)-1,4-oxazepine] discussed below.

A detailed review of those compounds which might be considered for use today in riot control has been provided by Ballantyne (1977) and much of the present account has been based on his work. Information on the individual compounds is given in Table 20.

Table 20   Riot control agents

Com-pound	Formula	Toxicometrics				V.P.	Water solubility	Onset of effects	Recovery
		$L(Ct)_{50}$ Rat (pure compound) mg min m^{-3}	$L(Ct)_{50}$ Human (estimated) mg min m^{-3}	TC_{50} Human eyes μg m^{-3}	IC_{50} Human mg m^{-3}	20°C mmHg	20°C		
DM	(phenarsazine chloride: N, As, Cl)	3700–12 710	11 000–35 000	–	25–220	2×10^{-13}	Insoluble	Delayed for some hours	1–2 h
CN	C–CH$_2$Cl (‖ O)	3700–18 800	8 500–25 000	0.3	20–50	5.4×10^{-3}	4.4×10^{-3}	At once	20 min
CS	CH=C(CN)$_2$, Cl	88 480	25 000–150 000	4×10^{-3}	3.6	3.4×10^{-5}	2.0×10^{-4} (rapid hydrolysis)	At once	20 min Erythema for up to 24 h
CR	(dibenzoxazepine: O, N=CH)	>425 000	>100 000	4×10^{-3}	0.7	5.9×10^{-5}	3.5×10^{-4}	At once	20 min Erythema for up to 1 h

Dangers Associated with Exposure to Riot Control Compounds

Despite the low toxicity of these compounds exposure is not entirely without risk. The following points should be borne in mind.

- Exposure to levels much in excess of those anticipated, for example in a closed room, might produce significant toxic effects. DM in large doses may produce corneal necrosis and pulmonary damage. CN (2-chloroaceto-phenone) in large doses may produce corneal damage particularly if the compound enters the eye in the form of powder. Five deaths due to the pulmonary damage following exposure to high concentrations of CN in enclosed spaces have been reported (Gonzales *et al.*, 1954; Stein and Kirwan, 1964).
- Exposure to irritants may produce transient although significant elevations of blood pressure. These have generally been regarded as not likely to do harm in healthy individuals, although those suffering from hypertension, aneurysms or myocardial disease might be placed at some risk (Ballantyne *et al.*, 1976).
- Hysteria and panic may be produced by exposure to irritants particularly if the means of escape from exposure are blocked. Secondary injuries may be produced by stampeding crowds.
- Each of the compounds listed in the above table, with the exception of CR, can produce contact sensitization (Holland and White, 1972; Rothberg, 1970).

Management of Casualties Exposed to Riot Control Agents

As for all other compounds discussed in this chapter removal of casualties from the risk of further contamination by adequately protected attendants is of first priority. Contaminated clothing should be removed and placed in polythene bags: CS and CR are notorious for spreading during decontamination of casualties. Lacrimation, blepharospasm, blepharoconjunctivitis and eye pain disappear quickly after removal from an irritant cloud. The effects on the eyes may be initially so distressing that casualties may require a great deal of reassurance that permanent eye damage has not been produced. The eyes should be kept open and those who have been regularly exposed to CS advise standing with the eyes open 'facing the wind'. Irrigation of the conjunctival sacs with 0.9 per cent saline brings rapid, although in the author's personal experience, sometimes temporary, relief.

Skin should be decontaminated with soap and water. In the case of CS, hydrolysis occurs quickly and decontamination is rapidly accomplished. Showering is often advised but it should be remembered that CR and to a lesser extent CS may be washed out of the hair and produce secondary contamination of the eyes. Erythema generally subsides without treatment although primary contact dermatitis may require treatment with corticosteroid ointment.

ALLEGED CHEMICAL WARFARE AGENTS

One of the commonest misconceptions regarding chemical warfare is represented by the view that compounds of great toxicity must, *ipso facto*, be likely effective chemical warfare agents. This view is so commonly put that it may be worth noting that in assessing the potential of a compound as a putative chemical warfare agent a number of factors have to be considered of which acute toxicity is only one and probably not the most important. These criteria include:

- Ease of manufacture in large quantities. Chemical warfare waged on a small scale during a major war is unlikely to produce significant results. It is sometimes argued that assassinations have been carried out using small quantities of highly toxic compounds. This is true, but assassination should not be confused with chemical warfare.
- The conditions of storage of the compound should not be demanding and the compound should not deteriorate on storage.
- The compound should be easy to disperse using inexpensive munitions and should not be destroyed by the dispersal system.

- The compound should be active in the form in which it is likely to be encountered by the opposing forces: a compound only active by the intravenous route would be an unsatisfactory chemical warfare agent.
- On the whole, compounds producing severe and care-demanding incapacitation are more effective chemical warfare agents than those which are inevitably lethal.
- It should be possible to protect one's own forces against the effects of the chosen compound without excessive expense or loss of efficiency.
- The compound should offer advantages when compared with already available compounds which meet the above criteria.

A rigorous application of these criteria will serve to remove many substances from accounts which purport to list possible or probable chemical warfare agents. In assessing the *probability* that a compound would be used as a chemical warfare agent the question: *Why should this compound be chosen?* should always be asked rather than the question: *Could this compound be used as a chemical warfare agent?*

A considerable range of exotic compounds have been examined as potential chemical warfare agents: batrachotoxin, tetrodotoxin, saxitoxin, palytoxin, botulinus toxin, staphylococcal enterotoxin B, ricin and abrin have all been examined in detail.

Ricin was used to assassinate G. Markow in 1978. Figures are not available for the toxicity of staphylococcal enterotoxin B when absorbed by inhalation although it is felt the compound would be significantly more toxic when administered in this way than by ingestion.

During the early 1980s considerable attention was paid to toxins of fungal origin: mycotoxins. It was alleged that a group of mycotoxins known as trichothecenes had been used in South-East Asia. The compounds on which attention centred were: T2 toxin (*Merck Index*, 11th edn, ref no. 9711) and nivalenol (*Merck Index*, 11th edn, ref no. 6581).

T2 is a caustic skin irritant which may cause dizziness, nausea, vomiting, diarrhoea and haemorrhage. The LD_{50} of T2 toxin (oral, rat) is 4.0 mg kg^{-1}. Nivalenol, also known to be capable of producing similar effects, has an LD_{50} (ip, mice) of 40 μg kg^{-1}. Further discussion of the toxicity of these compounds may be found in the work of Tatsuno (1968), Wade (1981), Rosen and Rosen (1982) and Marasas *et al.* (1969). Irrefutable evidence that these compounds were deliberately used as chemical warfare agents, is, however, lacking. During the Soviet occupation of Afghanistan it was alleged that Soviet forces had used chemical warfare agents against rebel tribesmen. No clear identification of the compounds alleged to have been used has appeared and the effects reported—the induction of unconsciousness with recovery with few ill-effects an hour or so later and the production of blackened and very rapidly decaying bodies—have been hard to explain.

In examining reports of alleged uses of chemical warfare agents factors such as the likely naivity of observers, deliberate attempts to mislead and the more common causes of death in war should be borne in mind. Before dismissing such reports, however, it should also be remembered that small-scale use of chemicals on an *ad hoc* basis might occur during a war waged by poorly disciplined forces.

All the compounds considered thus far have been characterized as likely to have effects on humans. If the definition of chemical warfare is widened a little and the attack on food production resources or woodland, which provides hiding places for troops, is included then a number of herbicidal compounds could also be considered. Such compounds may be *per se* toxic to humans or, in the forms deployed, contain toxic contaminants. During the Vietnam War American forces used large quantities of herbicides, including the phenoxyacetates 2,4-D and 2,4,5-T, some preparations being contaminated with TCDD (tetrachlorodibenzodioxin). The mixture was often referred to as Agent Orange (Young *et al.*, 1978). Exposure to the mixture has been alleged to have produced long-term effects in both Vietnamese and American veterans. Details of the toxic effects of herbicides may be found in Chapter 52.

CONCLUSIONS

Chemical warfare has a long history although only in the twentieth century has it been developed as a means of waging war on a large scale. In the late 1980s moves to ban the production and stockpiling of chemical weapons have been made and may yet prove completely successful between

countries involved in these negotiations. It should, however, be recalled that treaties have been violated in the past and that a number of countries currently believed to have acquired or to be acquiring chemical weapons are not involved in treaty negotiations. It seems therefore that although the risk of chemical warfare has diminished during the past decade such a risk still exists.

BIBLIOGRAPHY

In addition to the sources identified in the text a particular series of books deserve mention: *The Problem of Chemical and Biological Warfare*, vols 1–6, published by the Stockholm International Peace Research Insitute (SIPRI) 1971–75. ISBN numbers: 91-85114-10-3, 16-2, 17-0, 11-1, 13-8, 18-9.
This invaluable work contains a wealth of information on all aspects of chemical warfare.

REFERENCES

Anslow, W. P., Karnofsky, D. A., val-Jager, B. and Smith, H. W. (1948). Intravenous, subcutaneous and cutaneous toxicity of bis(*b*-chloroethyl)sulphide (mustard gas) and various derivatives. *J. Pharmacol. Exp. Ther.*, **93**, 1–9

Aposhian, H. V., Mershon, M. M., Brinkley, F. B., Hsu, C. A. and Hackley, B. E. (1982). Anti-Lewisite activity and stability of meso-dimercaptosuccinic acid and 2,3-dimercapto-1-propanesulfonic acid. *Life Sci.*, **31**, 2149–2156

Aposhian, H. V., Carter, D. E., Hoover, T. D., Hsu, C. A., Maiorino, R. M. and Stine, E. (1984). DMSA, DMPS and DMPA as arsenic antidotes. *Fundam. Appl. Toxicol.*, **4**, S58–S70

Ballantyne, B. (1977). Riot control agents: biomedical and health aspects of the use of chemicals in civil disturbances. *The Medical Annual*, John Wright, Bristol, pp. 7–41

Ballantyne, B. and Schwabe, P. H. (1981). *Respiratory Protection: Principles and Applications*. Chapman and Hall, London, p. 113

Ballantyne, B., Gall, D. and Robson, D. C. (1976). Effects on man of drenching with dilute solutions of *o*-chlorobenzylidine malononitrile CS and dibenz(b,f)-1:4-oxazepine (CR). *Med. Sci. Law.*, **16**, 159–170

Barcroft, J. (1920). Discussion on the therapeutic uses of oxygen. *Proc. Roy. Soc. Med. London*, Section of therapeutics and pharmacology, **xiii**, 59

Benschop, A. P. and Keijer, J. H. (1966). The correlation between aging of phosphylated cholinesterases and unimolecular solvolysis of related reference compounds. *PML Report*, Prins Mauritz Laboratory TNO, Rijswick, Netherlands

Bosković, B., Kovacević, V. and Jovanović, D. (1984). 2-PAM chloride HI6 and HGG12 in soman and tabun poisoning. *Fundam. Appl. Toxicol.*, **4**, 106–115

Bradley, B. L. and Unger, K. M. (1982). Phosgene inhalation, a case report. *Tex. Med.*, **78**, 51–53

Brezenoff, H. E., McGee, J. and Knight, V. (1984). The hypertensive response to soman and its relation to brain acetylcholinesterase inhibition. *Acta Pharmacol. Toxicol.*, **55**, 270–277

Bright, J. E. (1987). A prophylaxis for cyanide poisoning. In Ballantyne, B. and Marrs, T. C. (Eds), *Clinical and Experimental Toxicology of Cyanides*. Wright, Bristol, pp. 359–382

Bright, F. E., Inns, R. H., Tuckwell, N. J., Griffiths, G. D. and Marrs, T. C. (1991). A histochemical study of changes observed in the mouse diaphragm after organophosphate poisoning. *Human and Experimental Toxicology*, **10**, 9–14

Brimblecombe, R. W., Green, D. M., Stratton, J. A. and Thompson, P. B. (1970). The protective actions of some anticholinergic drugs in sarin poisoning. *Br. J. Pharmacol.*, **39**, 822–830

British Medical Association and The Royal Pharmaceutical Society of Great Britain (1989). *British National Formulary*, No. 18, September. BMA and The Pharmaceutical Press, London

Cameron, G. R., Gaddum, J. H. and Short, R. H. D. (1946). The absorption of war gases by the nose. *J. Path.*, **LVIII**, 449–457

Clement, J. G. (1981). Toxicology and pharmacology of bispyridinium oximes. Insight into the mechanism of action vs soman poisoning *in vivo*. *Fundam. Appl. Toxicol.*, **1**, 193–202

Clement, J. G. (1982a). HI–6: reactivation of central and peripheral acetylcholinesterase following inhibition by soman, sarin and tabun *in vivo* in the rat. *Biochem. Pharmacol.*, **31**, 1283–1287

Clement, J. G. (1982b). Plasma aliesterase—a possible depot for soman (pinacolyl-methylphosphonofluoridate) in the mouse. *Biochem. Pharmacol.*, **31**, 4085–4088

Clement, J. G. and Lockwood, P. A. (1982). HI–6, an oxime which is an effective antidote in soman poisoning: a structure activity study. *Toxicol. Appl. Pharmacol.*, **64**, 140–146

Coleman, I. W., Patton, G. E. and Bannard, R. A. (1968). Cholinolytics in the treatment of anticholinesterase poisoning V. The effectiveness of Parpanit with oximes in the treatment of organophosphorus poisoning. *Can. J. Physiol. Pharmacol.*, **46**, 109–117

Cucinell, S. A. (1974). Review of the toxicity of long-term phosgene exposure. *Arch. Environ. Health*, **28**, 272–275

Davies, D. R. and Green, A. L. (1956). The kinetics of reactivation by oximes of cholinesterase inhibited

by organophosphorus compounds. *Biochem. J.*, **63**, 529–535

Davies, D. R. and Green, A. L. (1959). 2-Hydroxyiminoethyl-N-methylpyridine methanesulphonate and atropine in the treatment of severe organophosphorus poisoning. *Br. J. Pharmacol.*, **14**, 5–8

De-Jong, L. P. A. and Wolring, G. Z. (1978). Effect of 1-(AR)alkyl-2-hydroxyiminomethylpyridinium salts on reactivation and ageing of acetylcholinesterase inhibited by diethylphosphoramide-cyanidate (Tabun). *Biochem. Pharmacol.*, **27**, 2229–2235

De-Jong, L. P. A. and Wolring, G. Z. (1980). Reactivation of acetylcholinesterase inhibited by 1,2,2'-trimethylpropylmethyl-phosphonofluoridate (Soman) with HI6 and related oximes. *Biochem. Pharmacol.*, **29**, 2379–2387

De-Jong, L. P. A. (1983). Personal communication to Ligtenstein, D. (1984)

Diller, W. F. (1978). Medical phosgene problems and their possible solution. *J. Occup. Med.*, **20**, 189–193

Dixon, H. (1946). Biochemical research on CW agents. *Nature*, **158**, 432–438

D'Mello, G. D. (1987). Neuropathological and behavioural sequelae of acute cyanide toxicosis in animal species. In Ballantyne, B. and Marrs, T. C. (Eds), *Clinical and Experimental Toxicology of Cyanides*. Wright, Bristol, pp. 156–183

Everett, E. D. and Overholt, E. L. (1968). Phosgene poisoning. *JAMA*, **205**, 103–105

Eyer, P., Ladstetter, B., Schafer, W. and Sonnenbichler, J. (1989). Studies on the stability and decomposition of the Hagedorn oxime HLO–7 in aqueous solution. *Arch. Toxicol.*, **63**, 59–67

Fleisher, J. H. (1963). Effects of *p*-nitrophenyl phosphonate (EPN) on the toxicity of isopropyl methyl phosphonofluoridate (GB). *J. Pharmacol. Exp. Ther.*, **139**, 390

Fleisher, J. H. and Harris, L. W. (1965). Dealkylation as a mechanism for ageing of cholinesterase after poisoning with pinacolyl methylphosphonofluoridate. *Biochem. Pharmacol.*, **14**, 641–650

Fotion, H. and Elfstrom, G. (1986). *Military Ethics*. Routeledge and Kegan Paul, London

Fox, M. and Scott, D. (1980). The genetic toxicology of nitrogen and sulphur mustard. *Mutat. Res.*, **75**, 131–168

Friedenwald, J. S. and Hughes, W. F. (1948). The effects of toxic chemical agents on the eye and their treatment. In Andrus, E. C. *et al.* (Eds), *Advances in Military Medicine*, vol. II. Ch. XXXIX. Little Brown, Boston

Frosolono, M. F. and Pawlowski, R. (1977). Effect of phosgene on rat lungs after single high level exposure 1. Biochemical alterations. *Arch. Environ. Health*, **32**, 271–277

Fruhman, G. (1974). Vorkommen und Behandlung des Lungenödems nach Inhalation von Reizgas. *Med. Klin.*, **69**, 22–26

Gates, M. and Renshaw, B. C. (1946). Fluorophosphates and other phosphorus containing compounds. In *Summary Technical Report of Division 9*, vol. I, Parts I and II. Office of Scientific Research and Development. NTIS PB 158508, Washington DC, pp. 131–155

Gilman, A. and Cattell, M. (1948). Systemic agents: action and treatment. In Andrus, E. C. *et al.* (Eds), *Advances in Military Medicine*, vol. 2. Little Brown, Boston, 546–564

Gonzales, T. A., Vance, M., Helpern, M. and Umberger, C. J. (1954). *Legal Medicine*. Appleton-Century Crofts, New York

Goodman, L. S. and Gilman, A. (1980). *The Pharmacological Basis of Therapeutics*, 6th edn. Macmillan, London, Billière Tindall, New York

Gordan, J. J. and Leadbeater, L. (1977). The prophylactic use of 1-methyl, 2-hydroxyiminomethylpyridinium methanesulfonate (P2S) in the treatment of organophosphate poisoning. *Toxicol. Appl. Pharmacol.*, **40**, 109–114

Goyer, R. A. (1986). Toxic effects of metals. In Klaassen, C. D., Amdur, M. O. and Doull, J. (Eds), *Casarett and Doull's Toxicology: The Basic Science of Poisons*. 3rd edn, Macmillan, London, pp. 582–635

Graziano, J. H., Cuccia, D. and Friedheim, E. (1978). The pharmacology of 2,3-dimercaptosuccinic acid and its potential use in arsenic poisoning. *J. Pharmacol. Exp. Ther.*, **207**, 1051–1055

Haldane, J. B. S. (1925). *Callinicus: A Defence of Chemical Warfare*. Kegan Paul, French, Trubner, London

Haldane, J. S. (1917). The therapeutic administration of oxygen. *Br. Med. J.*, **1**, 181

Harris, L. W., Stitcher, D. L. and Heyl, W. C. (1981). Protection and induced reactivation of cholinesterase by HS-6 in rabbits exposed to soman. *Life Sci.*, **29**, 1747–1753

Hitler, A. (1925). *Mein Kampf*, vol. I

HMSO (1923), *History of the Great War: Medical Services [Diseases of the War]*, vol. II. HMSO, London

HMSO (1972, 1987). *Medical Manual of Defence Against Chemical Agents*. (JSP312). HMSO, London

Holland, P. and White, R. G. (1972). The cutaneous reactions produced by *o*-chlorobenzylidine malononitrile and ω-chloracetophenone when applied directly to the skin of human subjects. *Br. J. Dermatol.*, **86**, 150–154

Holmstedt, B. (1963). Structure activity relationships of the organophosphorus anticholinesterase agents. In Koelle, G. B. (Ed.), *Cholinesterases and Anticholinesterase Agents. Handbuch der Exp. Pharm., Erganzungsuk.* **15**, pp. 428–485

Hunter, D. (1978). *The Diseases of Occupations*, 6th edn. Hodder and Stoughton, London

Inns, R. H. and Leadbeater, L. (1983). The efficacy of bispyridinium derivatives in the treatment of organophosphate poisoning in the guinea pig. *J. Pharm. Pharmacol.*, **35**, 427–433

Ireland, M. M. (1926). *Medical Aspects of Gas Warfare*, vol. XIV of *The Medical Department of the United States in the World War*, Washington DC

Ivanhoe, F. and Meyers, F. H. (1964). Phosgene poisoning as an example of neuroparalytic acute pulmonary edema: the sympathetic vasomotor reflex involved. *Dis. Chest*, **46**, 211–218

Jovanović, D. (1983). The effect of bis-pyridinium oximes on neuromuscular blockade induced by highly toxic organophosphates in rat. *Arch. Int. Pharmacodyn. Ther.*, **262**, 231–241

Juarez-Salinas, H., Sims, J. L. and Jacobson, M. K. (1979). Poly(ADP-ribose) levels in carcinogen treated cells. *Nature*, **282**, 740–741

Kleinberger, G., Pichler, M. and Weiser, M. (1981). 2,3-Dimercaptosuccinic acid in human arsenic poisoning. *Arch Toxicol.*, **47**, 241–243

Koelle, G. B. (1963). Cholinesterases and anticholinesterase agents. In Koelle, G. B. (Ed.), *Cholinesterases and Anticholinesterase Agents. Handbuch der Exp. Pharm., Erganzungsuk.* **115**, 428–485

Koelle, G. B. (1975). Neurohumoral transmission and the autonomic nervous system. In Goodman, L. S. and Gilman, A. (Eds) *The Pharmacological Basis of Therapeutics*, 5th edn. Macmillan, London, 404–444

Leblic, C., Coq, H. M. and Le-Moan, G. (1984). Etude de la toxicité de l'eserine, VX et le paraoxon pour établir un modèle mathematique de l'extrapolation à être humain. *Arch. Belg.* **Suppl.** 226–242

Lefebure, V. (1921). *The Riddle of the Rhine*. Collins, London

Lenz, K., Hruby, K., Druml, W., Eder, A., Gaszner, A., Kleinberger, G., Picher, M. and Weiser, M. (1981). 2,3-Dimercaptosuccinic acid in human arsenic poisoning. *Arch. Toxicol.*, **47**, 241–243

Ligtenstein, D. A. (1984). On the synergism of the cholinesterase reactivating bispyridinium-aldoxime HI6 and atropine in the treatment of organophosphate intoxications in the rat. PhD Thesis, University of Amsterdam

Lipp, J. A. (1972). Effect of diazepam upon soman-induced seizure activity and convulsions. *Electroencephalogr. Clin. Neurophysiol.*, **32**, 557–560

Lipp, J. A. (1973). Effect of benzodiazepine derivatives on soman-induced seizure activity and convulsions in the monkey. *Arch. Int. Pharmacodyn.*, **202**, 244–251

Liu, D. D., Ueno, E., Hoi, K. and Hoskins, B. (1988). Evidence that changes in levels of cyclic nucleotides are not related to soman induced convulsions. *Neurotoxicology*, **9**, 23–28

Lohs, von K. (1960). Zur Toxicologie und Pharmakologie organischer Phosphorsäuster. *Dtsh. Gesundheitswesen*, **15**, 2179–2133

Lundy, P. M. and Magor, G. F. (1978). Cyclic GMP concentrations in cerebellum following organophosphate administration. *J. Pharm. Pharmacol.*, **30**, 251–252

Marasas, W. F. O., Bamburg, J. R., Smalley, E. B., Strong, F. M., Ragland, W. L. and Degurse, P. E. (1969). Toxic effects on trout, rats and mice of T-2 toxin produced by the fungus *Fusarium tricinctum*. *Toxicol. Appl. Pharmacol.*, **15**, 471–482

Maksimović, M., Bosković, B., Radović, L., Tadić, V., Deljac, V. and Binenfeld, Z. (1980). Antidotal effects of bis-pyridinium 2 mono oxime carbonyl derivatives in intoxication with highly toxic organophosphorous compounds. *Acta Pharm. Jugosl.*, **30**, 151–160

Mann, I. (1948). An experimental and clinical study of the reaction of the anterior segment of the eye to chemical injury, with special reference to chemical warfare agents. *Br. J. Ophthalmol.*, Monogr. Suppl. **XIII**

Martindale. (1989). *The Extra Pharmacopoeia*, 29th edn. The Pharmaceutical Press, London

Maynard, R. L. (1988). *The Ethics of Chemical Warfare: An Historical Perspective*. Royal College of Defence Studies, London

Maynard, R. L. and Beswick, F. W. (1992). Organophosphorus compounds as chemical warfare agents. In Ballantyne, B. and Marrs, T. C. (Eds), *Clinical and Experimental Toxicology of Organophosphates and Carbamates*. Butterworth Heinemann, Oxford, pp. 373–385

Meselson, M. and Perry Robinson, J. (1980). Chemical warfare and chemical disarmament. *Scientific American*, **242**, 34–43

Miskin, R. and Reich, E. (1980). Plasminogen activator: induction of synthesis by DNA damage. *Cell*, **19**, 217–224

Murphy, S. D. (1986). Toxic effects of pesticides. In Klaassen, C. D., Amdur, M. O. and Doull, J. (Eds), *Casarett and Doull's Toxicology: The Basic Science of Poisons*, 3rd edn. Macmillan, London, pp. 519–581

Nash, T. and Pattle, R. E. (1971). The absorption of phosgene by aqueous solution and its relation to toxicity. *Ann. Occup. Hyg.*, **14**, 227–233

Oldiges, H. and Schoene, K. (1970). Pyridinium und Imidazolinium—Salze als Antidote genüber Soman und Paraoxonvergiftungen bei Mäuse. *Arch. Toxicol.*, **26**, 293–305

Papirmeister, B., Gross, C. L., Patrali, J. P. and Hixson, C. J. (1984a). Pathology produced by sulfur mustard in human skin grafts on athymic nude mice: I. Gross and light microscopical changes. *J. Toxicol. Cutaneous Ocul. Toxicol.*, **3**, 371–392

Papirmeister, B., Gross, C. L., Petrali, J. P. amd Meier, H. L. (1984b). Pathology produced by sulfur mustard in human skin grafts on athymic nude mice: II. Ultrastructural changes. *J. Toxicol. Cutaneous Ocul. Toxicol.*, **3**, 393–408

Pazdernik, T. L., Cross, R., Nelson, S., Samson, F. and McDonough, J. (1983). Soman-induced depression of brain activity in TAB treated rats: 2-deoxyglucose study. *Neurotoxicity*, **4**, 27–34

Pattle, R. E. (1965). Surface lining of lung alveoli. *Physiol. Rev.*, **45**, 28–79

Pawlowski, R. and Frosolono, M. F. (1977). Effect of phosgene on rat lungs after single high level exposure II. Ultrastructural alterations. *Arch. Environ. Health*, **32**, 278–283

Pearson, G. S. (1988). Chemical Defence. *Chemistry in Britain* **24**, 657–658

Peters, R. (1948). Development and theoretical significance of British Anti Lewisite BAL. *Br. Med. Bull.*, **5**, 313–318

Peters, R. (1953). Significance of lesions in the pyruvate oxidase system. *Br. Med. Bull.*, **9**, 116–121

Peters, R., Stocken, L. A. and Thompson, R. H. S. (1945). British Anti Lewisite [BAL]. *Nature*, **156**, 616–619

Potts, A. M., Simon, F. P. and Gerard, R. W. (1949). The mechanism of action of phosgene. *Arch. Biochem.*, **24**, 329–337

Prentiss, A. M. (1937). *Chemicals in War*. McGraw-Hill Book Company, New York

Prichard, J. S. and Lee, G. deJ. (1987). *Pulmonary Oedema*. In Weatherall, D. J., Ledingham, J. G. G. and Warrell, D. A. II (Eds), *Oxford Textbook of Medicine*. Oxford University Press, Oxford

Rengstorff, R. H. (1985). Accidental exposure to sarin: vision effects. *Arch. Toxicol.*, **56**, 201–203

Renshaw, B. (1946). *Mechanisms in Production of Cutaneous Injuries by Sulfur and Nitrogen Mustards. Chemical Warfare Agents and Related Chemical Problems*, vol. I, chap. 23, US Office of Science Research and Development, National Defense Research Committee, Washington DC, pp. 79–518

Reprint Society (1938). *The Notebooks of Leonardo Da Vinci*. The Reprint Society, England

Robin, E. D. (1979). Permeability pulmonary edema. In Fishman, A. P. and Renkin, E. M. (Eds), *Pulmonary Edema*. American Physiological Society, Bethesda, Maryland

Rosen, R. T. and Rosen, J. D. (1982). Presence of four *Fusarium* mycotoxins and synthetic material in 'yellow rain'. Evidence for the use of chemical weapons in Laos. *Biomed. Mass Spectrom.*, **9**, 443–450

Rothberg, S. (1970). Skin sensitization potential of the riot control agents BBC, DM, CN and CS in guinea pigs. *Milit. Med.*, **135**, 552–556

Sartori, M. (1939). *The War Gases—Chemistry and Analysis*. J and A Churchill, London

Scaife, J. F. (1959). Oxime reactivation studies of inhibited true and pseudocholinesterase. *Can. J. Biochem. Physiol.*, **37**, 1301–1311

Schneeberger, E. E. (1979). Barrier function of intercellular junctions in adult and fetal lungs. In Fishman, A. P. and Renkin, E. M. (Eds), *Pulmonary Edema*. American Physiological Society, Bethesda, Maryland

Schoene, K. and Oldiges, H. (1973). Efficacy of pyridinium salts against tabun and sarin poisoning *in vivo* and *in vitro*. *Arch. Int. Pharmacodyn. Ther.*, **204**, 110–123

Seagrave, S. (1981). *Yellow Rain: A Journey Through the Terror of Chemical Warfare*. M. Evans, New York

Seidelim, R. (1961). The inhalation of phosgene in a fire extinguisher accident. *Thorax*, **16**, 91–93

SIPRI (1971). Stockholm International Peace Research Institute. *The Problem of Chemical and Biological Warfare*. vol. 1. *The Rise of Chemical Weapons*

Smith, R. P. (1986). Toxic responses of the blood. In Klaassen, C. D., Amdur, M. O. and Doull, J. (Eds), *Casarett and Doull's Toxicology: The Basic Science of Poisons*. Macmillan, London, pp. 223–244

Staub, N. C. (1974). Pathogenesis of pulmonary oedema. *Am. Rev. Respir. Dis.*, **109**, 356–372

Stavrakis, P. (1971). The use of hexamethylenetetramine (HMT) in the treatment of acute phosgene poisoning. *Ind. Med. Surg.*, **40**, 30–31

Stein, A. A. and Kirwan, W. E. (1964). Chloracetophenone (tear gas) poisoning: a clinicopathological report. *J. Forensic Sci.*, **9**, 374–382

Sulzberger, M. B. (1943). The absence of skin irritants in the contents of vesicles. *US Navy Med. Bull.*, **41**, 1258–1262

Tammelin, L. E. (1957). Dialkoxy-phosphorylcholines, alkoxy-methyl-phosphorylthiocholines and analogous choline esters. *Acta Chem. Scand.*, **11**, 1340–1349

Tatsuno, T. (1968). Toxicologic research on substances from Fusarium nivale. *Cancer Res.*, **28**, 2393–2396

Taylor, P. (1980). Anticholinesterase agents. In Goodman, L. S. and Gilman, A. (Eds), *The Pharmacological Basis of Therapeutics*. 6th edn, Pergamon Press, New York, chap. 6

Teplitz, C. (1979). Pulmonary cellular and interstitial edema. In Fishman, A. P. and Renkin, E. M. (Eds), *Pulmonary Edema*. American Physiological Society, Bethesda, 97–111

United Nations Reports: S/16433[1984], S/17911[1986], S/18852[1987]. United Nations Organization, New York

Vedder, E. B. (1925). *The Medical Aspects of Chemical Warfare*. Williams and Wilkins, Baltimore USA

Vogt, R. F., Dannenberg, A. M., Schofield, B. H., Haynes, N. A, and Papirmeister, B. (1984). Pathogenesis of skin lesions caused by sulphur mustard. *Fundam. Appl. Toxicol.*, **4**, S71–S83

Wade, N. (1981). Toxin warfare charges may be premature [Editorial]. *Science*, **214**, 34

Warthin, A. S. and Weller, C. V. (1919). *The Medical Aspects of Mustard Gas Poisoning*. Henry Kimpton, London

Wegner-Jauregg, T. (1956). Experimentelle Chemotherapie von durch phosphorhaltige Anti-Esterasen hervorgerufenen Vergiftungen. *Arzneim.-Forsch.*, **6**, 194–196

Willems, J. L. (1989). Clinical management of mustard gas casualties. *Ann. Med. Milit. Belg.*, **3**, S1–S61

Wilson, I. B. and Ginsburg, S. (1955). A powerful reactivator of alkyl phosphate inhibited acetylcholinesterase. *Biochim. Biophys. Acta*, **18**, 168–170

Winternitz, M. C. (1920). *Pathology of War Gas Poisoning*. Yale University Press, Newhaven

Wolthuis, O. L. and Kepner, L. A. (1978). Successful oxime therapy one hour after soman intoxication in the rat. *Eur. J. Pharmacol.*, **49**, 415–425

Wolthuis, O. L., Berends, F. and Meeter, E. (1981). Problems in the therapy of soman poisoning. *Fundam. Appl. Toxicol.*, **1**, 183–192

Yamada, A. (1963). On the late injuries following occupational inhalation of mustard gas with special reference to carcinoma of the respiratory tract. *Acta Path. Jap.*, **13**, 131–155

Young, A. L., Calcagni, J. A., Thalken, C. E., Tromblay, J. W. (1978). The toxicology, environmental fate and human risk of herbicide agent orange and its dioxin. *USAF OEHL Technical report 78–92*, National Technical Information Centre (AD-A062–143), US Department of Commerce, Springfield VA

FURTHER READING

Compton, J. A. F. (1987). *Military Chemical and Biological Agents*. Telford Press, Caldwell, New Jersey

Somani, S. M. (1992). *Chemical Warfare Agents*. Academic Press, San Diego

50 Veterinary Toxicology

Wilson K. Rumbeiha and Frederick W. Oehme

INTRODUCTION

Veterinary toxicology is a diverse discipline with many subspecialities dealing with the health and care of animals, the relevance of animals in studying human disease, and the concern for domestic and wild animals in the environment. As these themes cannot all be addressed adequately in the space of one chapter, the focus will be on the classic role of veterinary medicine in understanding and managing the chemically induced disorders of domestic animals. Domestic animals have basic anatomical, physiological and biochemical differences and it is, therefore, not surprising that each animal species may often react differently to the same toxicant. Those interspecies differences will be emphasized.

Approximately 10 per cent of veterinary clinical practice is devoted to the diagnosis and treatment of poisonings in animals. The range of animals varies from small domestic animals, i.e. cats and dogs, to food-producing animals, i.e. dairy and beef cattle and swine, to horses, pet birds, zoo animals and occasionally wild game, such as rabbits and fish. The small animals react to chemicals more or less in the same way as humans because the species are all monogastrics. The ruminants (i.e. cattle and sheep), however, react differently from the monogastrics. The ruminants have evolved a unique digestive tract structure and microbial flora which play a major role in the fermentation of the forage ingested. The ruminant's microflora are usually capable of metabolizing toxic chemicals. As an example, cattle are more susceptible to nitrate poisoning than the horse, while dogs and cats are very resistant. Cattle are very susceptible to nitrate poisoning because the microbes in their digestive tract will convert nitrates to the proximate toxic metabolite, nitrite. Dogs, because of their relatively small gastrointestinal microbial population, are resistant to nitrate poisoning. The horse may succumb to nitrate poisoning because of the microorganisms in the caecum in its posterior digestive tract. However, by the time nitrate reaches the caecum, more than 70 per cent will have been absorbed; little will be available for biotransformation into the toxic nitrite ion. The horse will therefore require three-fold higher nitrate concentrations to be poisoned than will cattle.

Physiological differences among species can markedly alter the susceptibility of animals to toxicants. Birds, including pet birds, are more sensitive to toxic vapours and gases than mammals. Canaries have been used in mines to test for the presence of poisonous gases because their elaborate respiratory system will make them succumb to lower concentrations of toxic gases than humans. Biochemical differences also contribute to differential susceptibility between and within species. Cats are more susceptible to paracetamol (acetaminophen) poisoning than other domestic animals (Welch et al., 1966). The cat's glucuronyl transferase activity for conjugating paracetamol (acetaminophen) is much lower than in other domestic species and feline haemoglobin is more susceptible to oxidation than that of other animals (Rumbeiha and Oehme, 1992a). Therefore, cats given what would be considered a therapeutic dose for humans will die of methaemoglobinaemia. Biochemical differences are also found within the same species; for example, the Boston terrier is much more susceptible to copper poisoning than other species of dogs. Most biochemical differences are of genetic origin.

Adequate comprehension of the variability in toxicity from chemicals in the domesticated species requires understanding the anatomy, physiology and biochemistry of the affected animals. The other general factors that affect the toxicity of chemicals must also be considered when dealing with clinical toxicities in domestic animals. These factors include the animal's age, sex, health, and nutritional status, concurrent exposure to other chemicals, and the environment in which it lives (Osweiler et al., 1985). The effects of these and other factors in modifying the outcome of poisoning can be of vital significance in determining its outcome and also indicates the appropriate management options. There is a vast literature in this area which interested readers can consult for detailed discussions (Osweiler *et al.*, 1985; Hayes, 1991).

COMMON TOXICOSES OF DOGS AND CATS

Dogs and cats are commonly poisoned by pesticides, herbicides, household products such as antifreeze, and drugs often used by humans such as paracetamol (acetaminophen). By far the most commonly reported toxicities in these small animals involve insecticides because of overzealous use of these products by owners in controlling fleas and ticks on their pets (Trammel *et al.*, 1989).

The insecticides most commonly involved in poisoning dogs and cats are organophosphates and carbamates, pyrethrins and pyrethroids, and chlorinated hydrocarbons. The organophosphate and carbamate insecticides have a common mode of action which is the inhibition of acetylcholinesterase (Fikes, 1990). Acetylcholinesterase is an enzyme which breaks down acetylcholine, a neurotransmitter in autonomic ganglia and at cholinergic nerve endings. The inhibition of acetylcholinesterase by organophosphate and carbamate compounds causes acetylcholine to accumulate and results in persistent firing of cholinergic nerve fibers. Affected animals are overexcited and show increased respiratory rates, muscle tremors, and excessive salivation. Treatment of animals poisoned by organophosphate compounds involves administration of atropine and prolidoxime. Cases involving carbamates can only be treated with atropine. The organophosphate and carbamate compounds have a relatively high acute toxicity compared with chlorinated hydrocarbons but have a lower residual activity. As such, organophosphate compounds have largely replaced the organochlorines for insecticide use because of environmental concerns.

The chlorinated hydrocarbons (CH) were among the first insecticide compounds to be used but have fallen into disfavour because of their persistence in the environment (Smith, 1991). Typical examples include DDT and lindane. The toxicity of these compounds in small animals is characterized by central nervous system (CNS) signs including ataxia and convulsions. Small animals are usually poisoned accidentally by being sprayed or by drinking concentrates of CH intended for spraying on crops. Although most of the organochlorines are burned or their use highly restricted in Western countries, they are still widely used in developing countries. Therefore, cases of chlorinated hydrocarbon insecticide poisoning are still present mainly in developing countries.

Another class of insecticides which is commonly involved in small animal poisoning involves plant products: pyrethrins and their synthetic congeners the pyrethroids. These products are currently enjoying a resurgence because of their selective insecticidal properties and absence of environmental persistence (Valentine, 1990). These compounds are metabolized in the body mainly in the liver by glucuronidation. The cat is the most sensitive domesticated animal to pyrethrin toxicity because of the low activity of the glucuronide conjugating system in this species. Young cats less then 6 weeks of age are the most sensitive. Pyrethroid compounds formulated with the insect repellant diethyltoluamide (DEET) were responsible for several deaths in cats and dogs in the early 1980s. Pyrethroids interfere with sodium channels in nerves causing them to fire repetitively (Casida *et al.*, 1983). Clinical signs of pyrethroid poisoning in small animals include muscle fasciculations and tremors, ataxia and excitement. There is no antidote for pyrethrin poisoning but treatment consists of symptomatic treatment such as decontamination procedures and sedation (Valentine, 1990).

Rodenticides

Rodenticide poisoning is commonly encountered in small animals. Rodenticides are widely used around farm houses to control rodents such as rats and mice which destroy property and farm produce. Several classes of rodenticides are currently in use. These include the anticoagulant rodenticides (warfarin and the second generation rodenticides such as brodifacoum), zinc phosphide, strychnine, compound 1080, and arsenic compounds. Small animals are poisoned either by consuming baits directly or through consumption of carrion of animals which have died of rodenticide poisoning. The clinical signs will vary with the compound involved and in the majority of cases occur in dogs because of their indiscriminate eating habits. Strychnine and anticoagulant rodenticides are the most frequently reported offenders. Strychnine poisoning in dogs is a rapidly developing syndrome characterized by tonic–clonic seizures. These signs are a result of strychnine competitively blocking the inhibitory neurones in the brain (Heisser *et al.*, 1992). The animals start showing signs within 20 min to 1 h of ingesting strychnine and if the animal has ingested a sufficient amount, death from anoxia occurs fairly acutely. Anoxia results from paralysis of respiratory muscles. Treatment of strychnine poisoning is symptomatic and involves general decontamination procedures, use of sedatives such as phenobarbitone (phenobarbital) and diazepam, maintenance of adequate urine output and respiratory support. The sedatives control the seizures and cause muscles to relax (Boyd and Spyker, 1983; Maron *et al.*, 1971).

The anticoagulant rodenticides have been in use for a fairly long time. Because of the long time required to take effect, some strains of rats became genetically resistant to the so-called first generation anticoagulant rodenticides, such as warfarin. This led to the introduction of second generation rodenticides, such as brodifacoum. Unlike the first generation rodenticides which took at least 24–48 h to take effect, the second generation rodenticides act fairly acutely; clinical signs can be evident within a few hours and have a long residual action. These anticoagulant rodenticides act by inhibiting vitamin K-dependant factors (VII, IX and X), decreasing prothrombin synthesis, and by directly damaging blood capillaries (Coon and Wallis, 1972). Clinically, animals poisoned by anticoagulant rodenticides are weak, have swollen joints because of bleeding into the joint cavities, may show bleeding from the nostrils and may pass blood-stained faeces. Treatment of anticoagulant rodenticide poisoning involves blood transfusions if the bleeding is severe or heparin and vitamin K_1 injections. Early intervention involves general decontamination procedures to limit further absorption of toxicants, especially in the case of exposure to second generation rodenticides, followed by vitamin K_1 therapy (Pelfrene, 1991).

The toxicity of zinc phosphide is due to phosphine gas which is produced by acid hydrolysis in the stomach. Animals with partially filled stomachs are more sensitive to zinc phosphide poisoning than those on empty stomachs because of higher acid secretion precipitated by the pres-

ence of food. Phosphine gas is then absorbed systemically and exerts its effects in the lungs. Poisoned animals exhibit respiratory difficulties because of the build up of fluid in the lungs. The cause of death is respiratory failure (Stephenson, 1967). Supportive therapy including respiratory support is recommended in cases of zinc phosphide poisoning but the prognosis is poor as no effective antidote is available.

Compound 1080 (sodium fluoroacetate) is a very lethal toxicant which acts by blocking the Embden–Meyerhof pathway thereby depriving cells of energy. *In vivo*, fluoroacetate is metabolized to fluorocitrate which inhibits mitochondrial aconitase. This blocks ATP production (Buffa and Peters, 1950). Affected animals are initially uneasy, become excitable and will run in one direction and finally fall down in seizures and die of anoxia. There is no antidote to Compound 1080 and, invariably, poisoned animals die.

Cholecalciferol (Quintox) is a newly introduced rodenticide which has recently been reported to be widely involved in the poisoning of dogs. The compound alters calcium homeostasis by promoting calcium absorption from the gut and also by mobilizing calcium from bones. Consequently, poisoned animals have increased blood calcium levels. The calcium is subsequently deposited in soft tissues, such as muscle, liver, heart, and kidneys. Mineralization of soft tissue interferes with normal function of these organs. Clinically the animals do not show signs until 24–48 h after ingestion of the bait. The affected animals are depressed, have reduced urine production and the urine is of low specific gravity. Severely poisoned animals have haematemesis, azotaemia and cardiac arrhythmias (Dorman, 1990). Animals with renal impairment are more susceptible to cholecalciferol poisoning than those with normal renal function. Cholecalciferol poisoning requires protracted treatment which may last as long as 3 weeks in severe intoxications (Livezey *et al.*, 1991). The treatment consists of fluid therapy to assist the kidneys excrete calcium, corticosteroids to depress inflammation, and calcitonin to enhance calcium resorption into bones.

Several other rodenticides can cause poisoning in small animals but less frequently because these rodenticides are used less often. Red squill and thallium have been used as rodenticides for a very long time. Red squill acts as a cardiotoxicant and causes death by cardiac arrest. Red squill also causes convulsions and paralysis. Thallium is a general systemic toxicant. It has high affinity for sulphydryl groups throughout the body. Thallium causes cracking at the corners of the lips and also hair loss. α-Naphthylthiourea (ANTU) causes death by inducing lung oedema, subsequently leading to anoxia. White phosphorus is a hepatorenal toxicant. Animals poisoned by white phosphorus have severe abdominal pain, hepatomegaly, and signs of hepatic insufficiency such as prolonged bleeding and hypoglycaemia. In general, cases of rodenticide poisoning in small animals should be regarded as emergencies. General decontamination procedures such as vomiting induced with either hydrogen peroxide or apomorphine, use of activated charcoal to bind the unabsorbed toxicants, or enterogastric lavage should be employed to minimize absorption of the toxicant.

Herbicides

Herbicides are not widely involved in small animal toxicity despite their frequent use around farms. However, toxicity in dogs arising from consumption of concentrates of herbicides during mixing is occasionally reported. The triazine herbicides act by inhibiting photosynthesis and are generally safe products. The LD_{50} of these compounds in the rat is at least 1900 mg kg^{-1} of body weight. Therefore, toxicity in dogs can only occur following ingestion of large doses of concentrates. In experimental situations, triazine-herbicide-poisoned dogs become either excited or depressed, have motor incoordination and may show clonic–tonic spasms. Some inorganic arsenic compounds are used as herbicides. Inorganic arsenicals are general protoplasmic poisons and are therefore hazardous to both plant and animal life. Affected dogs have severe abdominal pain, bloody diarrhoea, and vomiting and the vomitus may contain mucous shreds from erosion of the intesinal epthelium.

Paraquat, although restricted in use in Western countries, is a very toxic herbicide which is readily available in developing tropical countries. Following intake, paraquat is rapidly metabolized in the liver and lungs with secondary oxygen radical production. It is these secondary radicals which cause injury to tissues, especially the lungs. Poisoned animals die of respiratory failure acutely (see Chapter 22).

Unlike other animals the dog appears to be sensitive to chlorphenoxy herbicides such as 2,4-D. In the dog the oral LD_{50} is 100 mg kg^{-1} of body weight. Ventricular fibrillation is the cause of death in severely poisoned dogs. Ingestion of sublethal doses induces myotonia, stiff extremities, ataxia, paralysis, coma and subnormal temperatures (Stevens and Sumner, 1991).

Chlorates are herbicides which have been used on roadsides. Chlorates are rapidly metabolized in the liver to the chlorate ion which induces methaemoglobinaemia in both cats and dogs. Cats, however, because of the greater susceptibility of their haemoglobin molecule to oxidation, are more susceptible to chlorate poisoning than dogs. Organophosphate herbicides, e.g. glyphosate and merphos, are weak cholinesterase inhibitors and are of moderate toxicity in dogs and cats. Carbamate herbicides are not inhibitors of acetylcholinesterase and are moderately toxic in dogs. The LD_{50} of most of the carbamate herbicides is at least 5000 mg kg^{-1} of body weight.

Household Chemicals

Antifreeze is one of the household products most commonly involved in small animal poisoning. The active ingredient in antifreeze is ethylene glycol. The characteristic sweet taste of this compound makes it very attractive to small animals. Ethylene glycol is metabolized in the liver by the alcohol dehydrogenase pathway into glycollic acid and oxalate and the former contributes to acidosis which is characteristic of ethylene glycol poisoning. The oxalic acid binds calcium in the blood to produce calcium oxalate crystals which are filtered in the glomerulus into renal tubules where they cause blockage of the tubules (Grauer and Thrall, 1982). Consequently, affected animals have renal failure characterized by anuria and uraemia. The binding of blood calcium to oxalate causes hypocalcemia which, if severe, can lead to death. Ethylene glycol poisoning is treated by giving ethanol if the animal is presented within 4 h of suspected ingestion and by giving fluids containing sodium bicarbonate to facilitate flushing out the calcium oxalate crystals from the kidney and also to correct the acid–base imbalance. Alcohol dehydrogenase, an enzyme which breaks down ethanol to acetic acid and water, prefers ethanol to ethylene glycol and in the presence of both substrates will metabolize ethanol leaving ethylene glycol to be excreted unchanged in the urine. 4-Methylpyrazole is a new drug reported to have antidotal properties against ethylene glycol.

Household products such as sink cleaners, dish washing detergents, toilet cleaners, etc. are common causes of poisoning in small animals. The majority of the cleaning detergents are corrosive compounds which contain either strong alkali, acids or phenolic compounds (Coppock *et al.*, 1988). These compounds therefore act as contact poisons causing coagulative necrosis of the tissues which they contact. Following ingestion of these products the dog or cat will vomit, have severe abdominal pain, and may have diarrhoea. The vomitus and faeces may be bloody. Animals may also show other signs depending on the specific ingredients of the offending products. For example, products containing phenolic derivatives will cause acidosis and hepatotoxicty. In general, treatment following ingestion of household products is symptomatic and involves the administration of adsorbents such as activated charcoal, gastrointestinal protectants such as peptobismol and correction of systemic disturbances such as the acidosis which may accompany the poisoning. Animals should also be administered plenty of glucose and fed a high protein diet.

Garbage Poisoning

Garbage poisoning is a frequently encountered problem in small animals. This condition is also referred to as enterotoxicosis or endotoxaemia depending on whether poisoning is from bacterial infection or ingestion of bacterial endotoxins. Dogs that are not well fed and/or not closely supervised may eat garbage. Cats may also be affected but only rarely because they are discriminate eaters. The bacteria most commonly involved are coliforms, staphylococci, *Salmonella*, and occasionally *Clostridium botulinum*. In enterotoxaemia affected animals develop a bacteraemia after eating infected carrion, clinical signs normally appearing at least 24–48 h after ingestion of the infected carrion. The condition is characterized by severe abdominal pain, anorexia, fever, vomiting and a bloody diarrhoea. In endotoxaemia the poisoning results from the bacterial endotoxins which are normally present in bacterial cell walls. The clinical signs are generally indistinguishable from those of enterotoxaemia,

except that in the later there is no bacteraemia (which can be ruled out by culturing the blood). Although rare in occurrence, botulism is a rapidly developing fatal disease which can result from ingesting bones contaminated with *Clostridium botulinum*. In small animals the disease is characterized by an ascending paralysis. At first there is weakness and incoordination in the muscles of the hind limbs and as the paralysis progresses anteriorly there are dyspnoea and convulsions.

Garbage poisoning is rarely a severe condition in small animals because the animals invariably vomit and reduce the amount of toxicant ingested. However, in severe cases medical attention will be required. If the cat or dog is presented early after ingestion then general decontamination procedures should be instituted. Anti-inflammatory corticosteroids and antibiotics should be given, further treatment involving tender supportive therapy.

Heavy Metals

Lead and arsenic are the heavy metals most frequently involved in small animal poisoning. Lead poisoning is more commonly reported in the dog than the cat, but both are susceptible. The sources of lead poisoning in the dog include ingested leaded objects such as lead weights and paint chips in old houses that are being renovated. The clinical signs of lead poisoning in the dog primarily involve the CNS. The dogs are often presented having abdominal pains, diarrhoea and CNS involvement. Lead poisoning is a chronic disease in dogs but the overt central nervous signs may appear suddenly. Lead poisoning causes blood dyscrasia characterized by reticulocytosis and occasionally anaemia. Similar clinical signs are elicited in the cat. Treatment consists of giving chelating agents such as calcium versanate, dimercaprol (BAL), succimer (DMSA), or D-penicillamine.

Arsenic is the active ingredient in some insecticides, rodenticides and herbicides. Inorganic arsenic and the aliphatic organic arsenicals are rapidly absorbed from the gut, skin and lungs and are more toxic than cyclic organic arsenicals which are used as feed additives (Furr and Buck, 1986). Trivalent arsenic is the proximate toxicant of the pesticide arsenicals and it reacts with the sulphydryl groups of proteins throughout the body. It is therefore a general poison, inhibiting all sulphydryl-containing enzymes. The clinical signs of inorganic arsenic poisoning in dogs include severe abdominal pain, bloody diarrhoea, anorexia and hair loss, etc. as discussed earlier under herbicides. Treatment involves decontamination, chelation therapy with BAL and supportive therapy.

Plant and Mushroom Poisonings

Although one would not expect dogs and cats to eat plants (toxic or non-toxic), plant poisoning is surprisingly often reported in these species (Fowler, 1981). Because of their exploratory nature, puppies and kittens are most often involved. Boredom and change of environment are some of the predisposing factors to plant ingestion in dogs and cats. Poisonous ornamental plants, e.g. *Rhododendron*, and plants used around fences such as cassia and oak are mostly involved. The subject of poisonous plants is a vast one and because the clinical signs are similar in food-producing and small animals, this subject will be dealt with extensively under food-producing animals. In addition, interested readers may consult a good review of plant poisonings in small companion animals (Fowler, 1981).

Occasionally dogs or cats will eat or be fed poisonous mushrooms by uninformed owners. *Amanita muscaria* and *A. pantherima* are acutely toxic and induce signs within 15–30 min of ingestion. These two mushroom species cause nervous signs which include salivation, pupillary constriction, muscular spasms, drowsiness or excitement, and eventually coma and death, in severe intoxications. Ibotenic acid and muscimol are the active ingredients. However, *A. phaloides*, *A. virosa* and *A. verna* induce gastrointestinal signs which are evident 6–12 h after ingestion. The signs include violent vomiting, diarrhoea, dehydration, and muscle cramps and these mushrooms also cause hepatic insufficiency. Phalloidin and alpha- and beta-amanitine are the principal poisons in this group (Fowler, 1981).

COMMON TOXICOSES IN FOOD-PRODUCING ANIMALS

This section will address toxicoses commonly encountered in cattle, swine and small ruminants. Swine differ from all other animals in this cate-

gory in that they have a simple stomach (monogastrics) whereas the rest have a compound stomach. Most of the toxicants discussed under small animals also affect food-producing animals but there are some toxicants which are peculiar or predominantly seen only in food-producing animals. Toxicoses which are frequently encountered in ruminants include non-protein nitrogen toxicoses, copper, lead, arsenic, mycotoxicoses, nitrite poisoning, plant poisoning, and algae poisoning. In swine, salt poisoning, mycotoxicoses, organic arsenicals, plant poisoning and gases generated in swine-confinement operations are often involved.

Poisoning by Non-Protein Nitrogen Compounds

Non-protein nitrogenous sources in food-producing animals include urea, biuret, and ammoniated feeds. These compounds are cheap sources of nitrogen which is required by the animals for protein synthesis. Non-protein nitrogen poisoning is a common problem and is often seen in animals that are not gradually introduced to diets containing these compounds. It is an acute fatal condition which is characterized by bloating, intense abdominal pain, ammonia on the breath, frequent urination, and frenzy. Often several animals will be affected. In ruminant animals the rumen microflora normally convert urea to ammonia, and the ammonia is rapidly utilized by the liver for protein synthesis. However, in cases of excess ammonia production, the blood ammonia concentration builds up to toxic levels very quickly and induces CNS derangement (Lloyd, 1986). Therefore, in addition to gastrointestinal signs, the animals will show fulminating central nervous signs. Treatment of the condition involves giving a weak acid such as vinegar and plenty of cold water orally. The rationale behind giving cold water and acetic acid is to slow down the action of urease, the enzyme responsible for breaking down urea to ammonia, which requires high temperature and pH for optimal function. The cold water lowers the temperature and the acetic acid lowers the pH. Infusions of calcium and magnesium solutions should be given to alleviate tetany (Osweiler *et al.*, 1985; Lloyd, 1986).

Other sources of non-protein nitrogen (urea) poisoning in ruminants involve accidental ingestion of nitrogen-based fertilizers, such as ammonium phosphate (Gosselin *et al.*, 1976). Occasionally cattle break into drums or bags of fertilizers containing these nitrogen-based compounds. Prognosis is grave in most cases if several animals are affected. In cases where only a few valuable animals are affected, a rumenotomy can be performed. Although small ruminants have the same anatomical predisposition to suffer from non-protein nitrogen poisoning, they are rarely involved probably because they are not often fed rations containing these compounds.

Nitrate–Nitrite Poisoning

Excessive exposure of ruminants to nitrates causes nitrite toxicity, an acute rapidly fatal disease. The commonest source of nitrates in ruminants is through consumption of forage grown on heavily fertilized fields that have accumulated a lot of nitrates (Ridder and Oehme, 1974). All common animal feeds such as sorghum, alfalfa, milo, etc. can accumulate excessive amounts of nitrates (Clay *et al.*, 1976). Another common source of nitrates is contaminated drinking water. Nitrates are highly water soluble and underground water contamination can occur from heavily fertilized fields (Menzer, 1991). Run-off from fertilized fields is another source of contamination to surface pools and ponds. Nitrates are broken down to nitrites by rumen microflora, and under normal circumstances the nitrite ion is rapidly utilized for ammonia synthesis, but in cases of excessive acute intake of nitrate, the nitrite ion is absorbed into the blood stream. In blood the nitrite ion reacts with haemoglobin to form methaemoglobin. Methaemoglobin is incapable of oxygen transport and the animal compensates for the anoxia by increasing the respiratory rate. Therefore affected animals will be hyperventilating, have brownish mucous membranes and will be weak. Chronic intake of nitrates has been reported to cause reproductive problems, such as abortion, but experimental results are inconclusive (Osweiler *et al.*, 1985). Besides reacting with haemoglobin, the nitrite ion also replaces iodine in the thyroid gland thereby interfering with the function of the thyroid hormone. Treatment of nitrate/nitrite poisoning involves intravenous infusion of 1 per cent methylene blue at a dose of 1.5 mg kg^{-1} of body weight and withdrawal of the offending feed.

Copper–Molybdenum Poisoning

Sheep are more susceptible to copper poisoning than cattle but cattle are more sensitive to molybdenum poisoning than sheep. The *in vivo* relationship between copper and molybdenum is well understood, copper excess inducing molybdenum deficiency and *vice versa*. The most frequent cause of copper poisoning in sheep is feeding them, by uninformed farmers, feed meant for cattle. Copper is an essential element for cattle and is usually added to their feeds but molybdenum is not considered essential and is therefore not added. Cattle feeds therefore have high copper and no molybdenum and feeding this ration to sheep upsets the normal copper/molybdenum ratio *in vivo*. Copper toxicity in sheep is an acute condition which develops after a chronic copper intake. During the chronic phase copper is stored in the liver until a certain critical concentration is reached and, following stressful conditions such as transportation or insufficient feed or water intake, a massive hepatic release of copper may be triggered, producing a haemolytic crisis (Osweiler *et al.*, 1985). Affected sheep have haemoglobinuria, are weak and death occurs acutely. The massive release of haemoglobin can block the renal tubules inducing renal failure and the prognosis is poor for animals already showing clinical signs. Chelation therapy using D-penicillamine is recommended for exposed animals not showing clinical signs.

In cattle molybdenosis is characterized by a foamy diarrhoea which may be bloody; affected cattle also have depigmented hair. Molybdenosis is a subacute to chronic condition and occurs when the ratio of copper/molybdenum is 2:1 or less. The condition has a geographical distribution and occurs in areas deficient in copper or where there is an excess of molybdenum, in parts of the USA (California, Oregon, Nevada and Florida) (Buck, 1986). Treatment of this condition involves copper supplementation in the feed.

Lead Poisoning

Despite an awareness of the dangers of lead poisoning in humans and domestic species, it is surprisingly the most frequently encountered heavy metal toxicity in food-producing animals. Lead poisoning is more commonly seen in cattle than in other food-producing animals. Young animals are mostly affected because of their curiosity and indiscriminate feeding habits. There are several sources of lead for cattle and discarded batteries and leaded water pipes are the commonest sources. Quite often uninformed owners will discard or store old batteries in farm environments, and cattle will lick them. Discarded leaded pipes, especially those used around oil wells, are a common source of lead poisoning (Blood and Rodostits, 1989). Lead interferes with haem synthesis and causes renal and CNS lesions as in small animals. Affected animals are initially anorectic. They may become belligerent and blind at the terminal stages of the disease. Once the CNS signs have appeared the prognosis is poor but treatment with chelating agents, e.g. calcium disodium EDTA and DMPS, may be of value.

Arsenic

Arsenic poisoning is second to lead as the most frequently reported heavy metal toxicant in food-producing animals. Arsenic is present in the environment in two forms: inorganic and organic. Inorganic arsenic is often incorporated into pesticides, which are the most common sources of arsenic poisoning in cattle. Inorganic arsenicals are also used as herbicides and cattle are sometimes exposed by eating grass clippings from recently sprayed forage. Inorganic arsenic poisoning is a rapidly developing and fatal disease (Radeleff, 1970). Affected animals show severe gastrointestinal abnormalities with minor CNS involvement, and have severe abdominal pain, haemorrhagic diarrhoea, and are depressed. Usually these signs appear 24–36 h after exposure.

Phenylarsonic arsenicals are less toxic to mammals than the inorganic arsenicals. Phenylarsonic compounds are usually incorporated into swine and poultry feed for disease-control purposes and also to improve weight gain. Examples of these compounds include arsenilic acid, 3-nitroarsenilic acid and 4-nitroarsenilic acid. Organic arsenicals are also available as trivalent and pentavalent compounds, the trivalent forms being more toxic than the pentavalent compounds. These phenylarsonic compounds are peripheral nervous system (PNS) toxicants. They cause demyelination of the peripheral nerve fibres leading to ataxia and paralysis of the hind quarters. The condition occurs frequently in swine kept on feed containing 10 000 ppm arsenic for at least 10 days or 200 ppm arsenic for 30 days. Therefore, unlike inorganic arsenic poisoning which is an acute form of the disease, poisoning by phenylarsonic compounds has an insidious onset. In addition, organic arsenic is commonly involved in toxicities in swine because of its incorporation into swine feeds, whereas inorganic arsenic poisoning is commonly seen in cattle.

Treatment of inorganic poisoning is by decontamination procedures and the use of BAL antidote. Use of demulcent to coat the gastrointestinal tract and antibiotics are also recommended. Treatment of organic arsenic poisoning involves withdrawal of the feed involved. Affected pigs should be culled.

Selenium Poisoning

Selenium poisoning is a regional problem occurring in areas where the selenium content in soil is high. Selenium is absorbed and concentrated by selenium-accumulating plants such as *Astragalus*. Cattle, sheep, goats and swine are exposed by consuming these indicator plants and acute selenium poisoning occurs when animals consume plants containing more than 10 000 ppm. This is characterized by sudden death or the animal may have laboured breathing, abnormal movement and posture, frequent urination, diarrhoea and death. Because plants containing high selenium concentration are unpalatable they are rarely consumed by animals so that acute selenium poisoning is rare. However, chronic selenium poisoning is common. Chronic consumption of plants containing as low as 50 ppm of selenium can cause chronic poisoning. Affected animals are anorexic, have impaired vision, wander, salivate excessively, are emaciated, lame and lose hair. Removal of animals from pastures that have high selenium concentrations is the recommended cure (Muth and Binns, 1964).

Mycotoxins

Some of the mycotoxins of veterinary interest include aflatoxins, deoxynivalenol (DON), diacetoxyscirpenol (DAS), T-2, zearalenone, ochratoxins and fumonisin B_1 (Cheeke and Shull, 1985; Keller *et al.*, 1990). Mycotoxins are especially a common problem in warm climates where high temperatures and relative humidity support fungal growth and favour mycotoxin production. All food-producing animals are susceptible and clinical signs will depend on the mycotoxins involved. Rarely is only one mycotoxin involved because several species of fungi, e.g. *Fusarium*, *Penicillium* and *Aspergillus*, coexist and often produce more than one type of mycotoxin. The common sources of aflatoxins to food-producing animals include corn and oats. When aflatoxins are ingested in parts per million quantities acute death can occur with the affected animals showing severe gastrointestinal pain and haemorrhage. Aflatoxins are severe hepatotoxicants; therefore hepatomegaly and jaundice may be observed in severe subacute cases. Quite often, however, aflatoxin poisoning is insidious following a chronic intake of parts per billion concentrations of aflatoxin over a prolonged period of time. Clinical signs include poor weight gain, decreased milk production and poor reproductive performance, including abortions. Virtually every organ function is affected by aflatoxins. The immune system of affected animals is impaired and they succumb to infectious diseases (Pier, 1981).

Toxicity due to T-2 mycotoxins has been reported in North America and some other parts of the world, including Germany, Hungary, France and South Africa. It is less common than aflatoxin toxicity. T-2 acts by interfering with the blood clotting mechanism. Affected animals have gastrointestinal bleeding and will pass blood-stained faeces. The animals will perform poorly, i.e. have low weight gain, decreased milk production and decreased food intake. T-2 is also an immunosupressant. All food-producing animals are susceptible to T-2 mycotoxicosis. Treatment consists of withdrawal of the contaminated feed and supportive care.

Zearalenone is an oestrogenic mycotoxin which often causes toxicity in swine, prepubertal swine being mostly affected. Swine are affected by consuming contaminated corn. Affected females show swelling of the vulva and excessive straining which may cause vaginal prolapse. In male animals zearalenone will cause decreased libido. There is no effective treatment apart from withdrawing the contaminated feed.

Other mycotoxins, including DON, DAS and ochratoxin, are not of major economic importance although they can be toxic to food-producing animals. DAS causes necrosis and erosion of the oral mucous membranes. Consequently, affected animals may refuse to feed and have impaired growth. DON also induces vomiting and feed refusal in swine. Ochratoxins cause renal problems including hydronephrosis, especially in swine. Ergot poisoning is occasionally encountered in livestock fed grain screenings contaminated with *Claviceps purpurea*. The active ingredients are ergotoxin and ergotamine which are vasoactive compounds. These compounds cause vasoconstriction of the peripheral vessels, especially those of the extremities, causing necrosis and gangrene of hooves and tail. Abortions and agalactia have been reported in cattle fed contamined feed. Therapy consists of discontinuation of the source of the toxicant and antibiotics to prevent secondary bacterial infection in necrotic tissues (Cheeke and Shull, 1985). Fumonisin B_1 is produced by *Fusarium moniliforme*, a worldwide fungus which predominantly grows on corn. Fumonisin B_1 causes pulmonary edema and respiratory distress in swine. Several deaths have been reported in swine fed contamined corn screenings (Colvin and Harrison, 1992).

Blue-Green Algae

Blue-green algae poisoning occurs late in summer and early autumn when algae form a scum on pond water. Because of husbandry practices cattle are most frequently involved. Algae of the genus *Anabaena* are the ones most frequently involved. There are two distinct syndromes in blue-green algae poisoning: hepatotoxic and neurotoxic. The neurotoxic type is peracute and cattle that drink water containing the neurotoxic principle anatoxin A can die within a few minutes and are found close to the pond. On the other hand, the hepatotoxic type causes an acute poisoning characterized by lethargy and jaundice (Beasley *et al.*, 1989) and death may occur within 2–3 days after drinking contaminated water. Blue-green algae poisoning has been reported in North America and the UK. Treatment involves supportive therapy in animals affected with the liver syndrome. Because of the peracute nature of the blue-green-algae-induced neurological syndrome there is hardly time for treatment and the prognosis is poor.

Toxic Gases

Toxic gases are of primary concern in closed animal housing, especially swine operations. In intensive swine confinement operations, with buildings designed to save on energy, toxic gases can accumulate in swine houses causing serious health consequences in cases of ventilation failure. These toxic gases are generated from the decomposition of urine and faeces, respiratory excretion and operation of fuel-burning heaters. The most important gases are ammonia, carbon monoxide, methane and hydrogen sulphide. A number of vapours which cause odours of manure decomposition, such as organic acids, amines, amides, alcohols, carbonyls and sulphides, are also produced. Respirable particles may be loaded with endotoxins and are also a major health problem in swine housed in confinement operations (Osweiler *et al.*, 1985).

Ammonia is highly lipid soluble and will react with the mucous membranes of the eyes and respiratory passages. At 100 ppm or greater, ammonia toxicosis will show as excessive tearing, shallow breathing, and clear or purulent nasal discharge. The irritation of the respiratory tract epithelium leads to bronchoconstriction and shallow breathing. Hydrogen sulphide poisoning is responsible for more animal deaths than any other gas and at 250 ppm and above, hydrogen sulphide causes irritation of the eyes and respiratory tract and pulmonary oedema. Concentrations of hydrogen sulphide above 500 ppm cause marked nervous system stimulation and acute death (O'Donogue, 1961). To prevent hydrogen sulphide poisoning manure pits should be agitated when pigs are not in the premises and proper ventilation should always be in place.

Carbon monoxide is produced by incomplete combustion of hydrocarbon fuels. Poisoning by carbon monoxide is caused by operating improperly vented space heaters or furnaces in poorly ventilated buildings. Carbon monoxide binds to haemoglobin forming carboxyhaemoglobin, thereby reducing the oxygen-carrying capacity of the blood and subsequently causing hypoxia. Concentrations of carbon monoxide greater than 250 ppm cause hyperventilation, respiratory distress; stillbirths have been reported (Carson and Dominick, 1982).

Nitrogen dioxide is a very poisonous gas which is responsible for causing silo fillers' disease in humans and the gas is also very toxic to animals. Nitrogen dioxide is produced during the first 2 weeks after the silage has been cut and put in the silo. Highest concentrations of the gas are reached during the first 48 h after filling the silo. Nitrogen dioxide dissolves in water to form nitric acid which is very corrosive to the respiratory tract and the lungs. As low as 4–5 ppm nitrogen dioxide can cause respiratory system disturbances (Osweiler *et al.*, 1985).

Exposure to sulphur dioxide at 5 ppm or higher causes irritation and salivation in swine. The gas is soluble in water forming the more toxic sulphuric acid, which causes eye and nasal irritation, and in severe cases haemorrhage and emphysema of the lungs (Osweiler *et al.*, 1985).

The effects of these toxicants singly and in combination is a hypofunctional respiratory system, and affected animals are predisposed to respiratory tract infections. The end result is retarded performance of the affected animals. It is therefore important to ensure that animal housing is adequately ventilated to provide animals with a healthy environment.

Toxic Plants

Plant poisoning is very common in areas where open grazing is practiced, such as in Africa. Interestingly though, plant poisoning is also widely reported in North America during the spring and autumn. The subject of poisonous plants is a wide one which cannot be adequately summarized here. However, the toxicity of some selected poisonous plants is summarized in Tables 1–8. In these tables the plants are discussed on the basis of the organs most prominently affected. It is important to realize, however, that these plants rarely affect only one organ. This presentation is an attempt to summarize the vast amount of literature on the subject.

Interested readers should consult the relevant literature for detailed discussions (Kingsburry, 1964; Cheeke and Shull, 1985). It is important to remember that the toxicity of a given plant can vary widely depending on the prevailing natural conditions. It is therefore not surprising that a given toxic plant may be toxic under certain conditions, e.g. during stressful drought conditions, but safe during other times.

Table 1 Toxic plants affecting the gastrointestinal tract of food-producing animals

Scientific name	Common name	Species commonly affected	Toxic parts and principle(s)	Clinical signs
Ricinus communis	Castor oil plant	Cattle, pigs	Seeds, leaves Ricin	Abdominal pain, vomiting, convulsions, dullness
Robinia pseudocacia	Black locust	Cattle, sheep	Bark, foliage, seed Robin, robitin, phasin	Anorexia, lassitude, posterior paralysis, cold extremities, dilated pupils
Phoradendron spp.	Mistletoe	Cattle, sheep	Berries β-Phenylethylamine, choline, tyramine	Vomiting, diarrhoea, bradycardia, sudden death
Ranunculus spp.	Buttercup	Cattle, goats, swine	Fresh foliage Protoanemonin	Blisters on lips, salivation, diarrhoea, tucked abdomen
Phytolacca dodecandra	Pokeweed	Cattle, sheep, swine	Foliage, unripe berries Oxalic acid, phytolaccotoxin, phytolaccin	Diarrhoea, dyspnoea, spasms, reduced milk, convulsions, ataxia
Sesbania spp.	Rattlebox	All	Seeds, foliage Sesbanine	Haemorrhagic diarrhoea, severe abdominal pain, coma, death
Agrostemma githago	Corn cockle	Cattle, swine	Seeds Githagenin	Diarrhoea, arched back
Quercus spp.	Oak	Cattle, sheep, swine	Acorns, buds, young leaves, flowers, seeds, stem Tannic acid, gallic acid	Abdominal pain, constipation or bloody diarrhoea
Euphorbia spp.	Spurge	Cattle, sheep	Whole plant Euphoron, euphorbin, cyanide	Diarrhoea (haemorrhagic or not), blisters of skin and oral mucous membranes, salivation, abdominal pain
Xanthium spp.	Cocklebur	Pigs, cattle, sheep	Seeds, cotyledons Carboxyatractlyloside	Anorexia, vomiting, tucked abdomen, depression, severe hypoglycaemia, weakness, convulsions

Salt Poisoning

Salt poisoning is frequently encountered in swine operations but can also occur in feedlot cattle. The causes of this condition are twofold. Most commonly, the pigs will be on a ration containing the recommended concentration of sodium chloride but management failure can favour conditions that can cause salt poisoning to occur. These poor management conditions include the sudden absence of water e.g. by freezing in winter or breakdown of the water supply, and possibility of the accidental addition of excessive amounts of salt to the ration. Salt poisoning has also been reported in swine operations even when the management situation is satisfactory, the only change being that the animals were moved into a new housing facility, as occurs after weaning. Apparently, the animals were not used to the new watering facilities in the new buildings and they did not know how to obtain the water and went without water while feeding on a normal ration. Clini-

Table 2 Toxic plants primarily affecting the liver of food-producing animals

Scientific name	Common name	Species commonly affected	Toxic parts and principle(s)	Clinical signs
Senecio spp.	Groundsel	Cattle, sheep, goats	Foliage Several alkaloids, e.g. jacobine, jacodine	Dullness, aimless walking, weakness, increased pulse, rapid respiration
Crotolaria sagitallis and *C. spectabilis*	Rattlebox	Cattle and swine mainly, but all species affected	Foliage and seeds Monocrotaline	Loss of appetite, weakness, emaciation incoordination, excitability, nervousness
Amsinkia intermedia	Fiddleneck	Pigs mainly but also sheep and cattle	Seeds Intermidine, lycopsamine, sincamidine	Unthrifty, icteric, haemorrhages of the gastrointestinal tract and subcutaneous tissues
Echium plantagineum	Viper's bugloss	Sheep mainly but also cattle and pigs	All parts are toxic Echiumine, echimidine	As for *Amsinkia*; contact dermatitis
Heliotropium	Heliotrope	Sheep	All parts Heliotrine, lasiocarpine, heleurine	As for *Amsinkia*; secondary photosensitization
Trichodesma europeum	–	All	Foliage Unidentified pyrolizidine alkaloids	As for *Amsinkia*
Lantana camara	–	Cattle, sheep, goats	All parts but especially foliage and berries Lantadine A and B	Severe gastroenteritis, bloody watery faeces, jaundice, secondary photosensitization
Helenium spp.	Sneezeweeds	Sheep and goats mainly but also cattle	All parts but especially leaves and flowers Helenaline, helanine, dugaldine	Severe abdominal pain, bloating, CNS involvement, e.g. head pressing
Hymenoxys	Bitterweed	Sheep, cattle, goats	All parts Hymenoxon	Unthriftiness, inappetance, salivation
Kochia scoporia	Kochia	Cattle	Foliage Unidentified alkaloids, + oxalates, nitrates and a thiamine antagonist	Unthriftiness, CNS signs, bleeding disorders, photosensitization
Agave lechaguilla	Agave	Sheep, goats, but also cattle	Foliage Unidentified saponins	Listlessness, primary photosensitization
Trifolium hybridum	Alsike clover	Pigs, sheep, cattle	Foliage Unidentified saponins	Listlessness
Lotus corniculatus	Birdsfoot trefoil	Cattle	Foliage Unidentified principles	Listlessness, bloat

cally, salt poisoning is a neurological disorder and the syndrome is acute. Affected pigs will spin on their hind quarters and fall down in convulsions. The pigs will also show a characteristic rhythmic pattern of convulsions which occur every 3–5 min.

Several pigs will be affected at the same time. The condition is corrected by provision of adequate but restricted amounts of water (Dunn and Leman, 1975).

Table 3 Toxic plants primarily causing CNS effects in food-producing animals

Scientific name	Common name	Species commonly affected	Toxic parts and principle(s)	Clinical signs
Dicentra cucullaria	Dutchman's breeches	Cattle	All parts but especially leaves and bulbs Isoquinaline-type alkaloids, e.g. apomorphine	Initially abdominal pain and diarrhoea; ataxia, trembling, respiratory distress, convulsions
Cicuta spp.	Water hemlock	Cattle, sheep, goats, pigs less often	Roots, stem base Cicutoxin, cicutol	Muscular spasms and spasmodic convulsions
Corydalis spp.	Fitweed	Sheep mostly but also cattle	Foliage Unidentified alkaloids	Clonic seizures, twitching of facial muscles
Asclepsia spp.	Milk weed	All	Foliage Cardenolides	Severe depression, ataxia, dilated pupils, laboured respiration
Gelsemium spp.	Carolina jessamine	Cattle, sheep, goats	Foliage, flowers Gelsemine and other strychnine-related alkaloids	Depression, muscle weakness, respiratory failure, convulsive movements preceding death
Calycanthus spp.	Sweet shrub	Cattle	Seeds Calycanthine	Seizures, severe tetanic spasms, muscular fasciculations
Eupatropium rugosum	White snakeroot	Young cattle, sheep	Foliage, passes in milk Tremetol	Depression, listlessness, trembling, laboured breathing
Haplopappus heterophylus	Rayless goldenrod	Cattle, sheep, goats	Foliage Tremetol	Depression, trembling, rare limb weakness
Sophora spp.	Mescal beans	Sheep mostly but also cattle and goats	All parts but seeds especially Cytisine, sophorine and nicotinic alkaloids	Nervousness, exercise-induced violent tremors, stiff gait
Xanthium spp.	Cocklebur	Pigs mostly but also cattle and sheep	Seeds, cotyledons Carboxyatractyloside	Depression, prostration, haunched posture, severe hypoglycaemia, extreme hypersensitivity, convulsions when recumbent
Ranunculus spp.	Buttercup	Cattle mostly but also sheep, goats, pigs	Fresh foliage Protoanemonin	Irritation of oral tissues, salivation, nervousness, paralysis, depression or excitement and convulsions

COMMON TOXICOSES OF HORSES

In comparison with cats and dogs and food-producing animals, horses are less frequently poisoned. The most commonly encountered equine toxicoses involve pesticides, snake bites, arsenic, selenium, monensin, cantharidin and mycotoxins (Oehme, 1987a). Most plants discussed above with regard to food-producing animals are also toxic to horses, but less frequently. Horses are very sensitive to monensin and cantharidin poisoning.

The pesticides most frequently encountered in equine poisoning are the organophosphate, car-

Table 4   Toxic plants affecting the autonomic nervous system of food-producing animals

Scientific name	Common name	Species commonly affected	Toxic parts and principle(s)	Clinical signs
Datura stramonium	Jimsonweed, thorn apple	Pigs mostly; sheep goats, cattle	All parts but especially seeds Atropine, scopolamine, hyoscyamine	Anticholinergic signs, e.g. dilated pupils, dry mouth, muscle twitching, incoordination, paralysis
Hyoscyamus niger	Henbane	All	Seed Hyoscyamine	As for *D. stramonium*
Solanum spp.	Nightshades	Pigs mostly; sheep, goats	Foliage, berries Solanine, dihydrosolanine, chaconine	Apathy, depression, dilated pupils, trembling, incoordination, muscular weakness, paralysis, convulsions
Physalis spp.	Groundcherry	Sheep	Tops and unripe berries Solanine and atropine-like alkaloids	Diarrhoea, trembling, hyperthermia, weakness, paralysis
Gelsemium spp.	Carolina jessamine	Cattle, sheep, goats	(see 'plants causing CNS effects')	
Lycium spp.	Matrimony vine	Calves and sheep	Foliage Unidentified solanaceous alkaloids	Excitement, convulsion
Lobelia spp.	Wild tobacco	Sheep, cattle, goats	Foliage and green fruits Lobeline and lobelidine	Profuse salivation, dilated pupils, narcosis
Conium maculatum	Poison hemlock	Cattle, pigs	Seeds most toxic; fresh Nicotinic alkaloids, e.g. coniine	Muscle tremors, ataxia, muscle weakness, frequent urination and defecation, respiratory failure
Lupinus spp.	Lupine	Sheep	Pods (seeds) Nicotinic alkaloids, Lupinine, lupanine	Laboured breathing, depression, salivation, ataxia, seizures
Sophora spp.	Mescal beans	(see 'plants causing CNS effects')		

bamate, and chlorinated hydrocarbon insecticides. Both the organophosphates and the carbamates are acetylcholinesterase inhibitors and the clinical presentation is similar to that of food-producing animals. Affected animals salivate profusely, and show muscle incoordination and ataxia. The chlorinated hydrocarbons are central nervous system stimulants and affected horses become excited, alert and in extreme cases go into convulsions. In the majority of cases the mode of exposure to pesticides is topical (Oehme, 1987b).

Horses are highly susceptible to monensin poisoning in comparison with other domesticated animals. Monensin is an ionophore which is normally incorporated into poultry feed to enhance the absorption of calcium and sodium from the gut. Horses are easily poisoned by accidentally consuming poultry feed containing recommended amounts of monensin. Affected animals can die suddenly without any premonitory signs. Monensin affects the cardiac and skeletal muscles and heart failure is the cause of death (Amend *et al.*, 1980).

Cantharidin is the toxic agent found in blister beetles. Several species of blister beetles are known and only a few contain cantharidin. Blister beetles are abundant in August and September at

Table 5 Toxic plants affecting the reproductive system of food-producing animals[a]

Scientific name	Common name	Species commonly affected	Toxic parts and principle(s)	Clinical signs
Veratrum californicum	False hellebore	Sheep	Roots and rhizomes mainly, but all parts are toxic Jervin, veratrosin, cyclopamine	Cyclopian-type congenital malformation, anophthalmia, cleft palate
Festuca arundinacea	Tall fescue	Sheep, cattle	Foliage Endophyte alkaloids, e.g. perlolidine, perloline	Abortion, still births, agalactia
Pinus ponderosa	Ponderosa	Cattle, sheep	Pine needles Unidentified	Last trimester abortions, stillbirths, premature deliveries, retained placenta
Gutierrezia microcephala	Broomweed	All	Foliage Unidentified saponins	Abortions, premature delivery, swelling of vulva
Cupressus macrocarpa	Monterey cypress	Cattle	Foliage Unidentified	Last trimester abortions, weakness, ataxia, death
Iva augatifolia	Sumpweed	Cattle	Foliage Unidentified	Abortion in last half of gestation

[a] Other plants that cause abortion include those containing nicotinic alkaloids (such as poison hemlock and tobacco), nitrate accumulating plants (such as locoweed), cyanogenic plants (such as sorghum), and oestrogenic plants (such as clovers and wheat germ).

the time that hay is harvested in North America. Horses may be poisoned by eating hay containing swarms of blister beetles. Affected horses show severe colic and will kick at their belly and roll; they may die of shock. There is no effective therapy for affected horses but treatment involves the use of pain killers such as banamine hydrochloride (Schmitz and Reagor, 1987).

Lead poisoning in horses is characterized by neurological abnormalities. Affected horses may either be depressed or excited. Colic and diarrhoea are also observed. Horses poisoned by lead also have difficult respiration with roaring because of laryngeal nerve paralysis. Abortions are also common.

Arsenic poisoning in horses is caused by consumption of foliage which has recently been sprayed by arsenic herbicides and the condition is normally acute and characterized by intense colic and haemorrhagic diarrhoea. As in food-producing animals, inorganic arsenic poisoning does not involve the nervous system which helps differentiate this condition from organophosphate or carbamate poisoning.

Selenium is an essential element but is toxic when excessive quantities are ingested. Exposure is usually through consumption of seleniferous (indicator) plants, e.g. *Astragalus*. Exposure to high quantities of selenium over a short period of time causes diarrhoea, which may be foul smelling and contain air bubbles, and neurological, cardio-vascular and respiratory signs. Death in these animals is from respiratory failure. Chronic exposure to excessive selenium is characterized by hoof abnormalities at the coronary bands and discolouration and loss of hair. The hoof deformities and pain cause lameness (Hultine *et al.*, 1979).

The plant poisonings commonly encountered in horses are those that cause gastrointestinal problems, liver damage, primary or secondary nervous system involvement, and sudden death. Plants such as castor bean, oleander and bracken fern cause colic and diarrhoea, Oleander also causing heart failure. Prolonged ingestion of some plants for several weeks can lead to liver damage and hepatic cirrhosis. Examples of commonly involved hepatotoxic plants include *Amsinckia*, *Senecio* and *Crotolaria* (Rumbeiha

Table 6 Toxic plants affecting the cardiovascular system of food-producing animals[a]

Scientific name	Common name	Species commonly affected	Toxic parts and principle(s)	Clinical signs
Digitalis purpurea	Foxglove	All (see 'plants causing CNS effects')		
Nerium oleander	Common pink oleander	All	Foliage and flowers Several digitoxin-like glycosides	Cardiac arrhythmias, unconsciousness, hypotension, dyspnoea
Convalaria spp.	Lily-of-the-valley	All	All parts Convallarine, convallatoxin, convallamarin	Tachycardia, diarrhoea, anorexia
Apocynum spp.	Dogbane	Cattle, sheep	All parts Cardiac glycosides, e.g. apocynamarin	Cardiac arrhythmias, fever, gastrointestinal pain, fever, gastric upset
Taxus spp.	Yew	All, but swine most sensitive	Foliage, bark, seeds Taxine	Acute heart failure (bradycardia)
Zygadenus spp.	Death camas	Sheep, cattle	All parts Zygacine	Lowered blood pressure, salivation
Brassica spp.	Kale, rape	Cattle, sheep, goats	Foliage *S*-Methylcysteine sulphoxide	Haemolytic anaemia, weakness, fast respiration, haemoglobinuria, staggering, collapse
Onion	Onion	All	All parts *n*-Propyl disulphide	As for *Brassica* spp.

[a] Several nitrate-accumulating plants, e.g. *Astragalus*, sudan grass, sorghum, corn and pigweed, cause methemoglobinemia. Some other plants, including sudan grass and sorghum, affect the cardiovascular system by virtue of their cyanogenic properties (see text).

and Oehme, 1992b). Liver damage may compromise the ability of the horse to detoxify ammonia which accumulates *in vivo* leading to CNS involvement. Plants that commonly cause CNS stimulation include larkspur, locoweed, lupin, water hemlock and fitweed. Common plants that cause CNS depression include black locust, bracken fern, horsetail, milkweed and white snake root. Like ruminants, horses will avoid eating toxic plants because they are not palatable. Therefore, consumption of poisonous plants will occur during drought conditions when the animals lack suitable pasture. Sudden death in horses can be caused by consumption of cyanide-containing plants such as sorghum. The cyanide ion forms a complex with cytochrome oxidase, which prevents transportation of electrons and utilization of oxygen by tissues throughout the body. As a consequence, blood is well oxygenated and cherry red. Treatment for this condition is an emergency and in the USA involves giving both sodium thiosulphate and sodium nitrite (other antidotes are used in other countries).

Horses, like other monogastrics, are more resistant to nitrate/nitrite poisoning than ruminants. However, horses can reduce nitrates to nitrites in the caecum but it takes three times more nitrate to produce a similar effect in the horse as in the ruminants.

Mycotoxins

Contaminated grains are sources of mycotoxin exposure in horses. The effects of mycotoxins are similar in the horse as for food-producing animals, the most commonly involved mycotoxins being aflatoxins, T-2 and fumonisin B_1. Aflatoxins will cause non-specific signs such as poor thriving, haemorrhages, and abortions. T-2 is a trichothecene mycotoxin which causes prolonged bleeding time in affected animals. A specific mycotoxin affecting horses is fumonisin B_1 which is produced by *Fusarium moniliforme* and has been responsible for the condition called equine leucoencephalomalacia. Horses are affected by the consumption of mouldy corn, and become anorectic

Table 7 Toxic plants affecting renal function of food-producing animals

Scientific name	Common name	Species commonly affected	Toxic parts and principle(s)	Clinical signs
Beta vulgaris	Beet	Sheep and cattle	Sugar beet tops Oxalates	Muscle tetany, renal failure
Rheum rhaponticum	Rhubarb	All	Foliage Oxalic acid, oxalates	Irritation of oral cavity and digestive tract, renal failure, death in convulsions
Halogeton spp.	Halogeton	All	Foliage and seeds Oxalates	Renal failure, dullness, weakness, slobbering
Sarobatus vermiculatus	Black grease-wood	Sheep, cattle	Foliage Oxalates	As for *Halogeton*
Rumex spp.	Curlydock	Sheep, cattle	Foliage Oxalic acid	As for *Halogeton*
Chenopodium spp.	Lambsquarters	All	All parts Oxalic acid	As for *Halogeton*
Amaranthus spp.	Rough pigweed	Pigs, cattle, sheep	Foliage Unidentified	Non-specific but related to perirenal oedema and nephrosis
Quercus spp.	Oak	Cattle, sheep	Young leaves, acorn, flowers, stem Tannic acid, gallic acid	Abdominal pain, constipation, frequent urination, renal failure

Table 8 Toxic plants causing primary photosensitization of food-producing animals

Scientific name	Common name	Species commonly affected	Toxic parts and principle(s)	Clinical signs
Hypericum perforatum	St. John's wort	Cattle, sheep, goats	Foliage Hypericin	Acute: increased respiration and heart rate, mild dermatitis Chronic: photosensitization of unpigmented areas of the skin, photophobia
Agave lecheguilla	Agave	Sheep, goats, cattle	Foliage Unidentified	As for *H. perforatum*
Fagopyrum esculantum	Buckwheat	All	All parts and seeds Fagopyrin	As for *H. perforatum*
Cymopterus watsonii	Spring parsley	Sheep, cattle	Foliage Psolalens	As for *H. perforatum*
Trifolium hybrium[a]	Alsike clover	Pigs, sheep, cattle	Foliage and seeds Unidentified	As for *H. perforatum*

[a] May be a secondary photosensitizer.

and initially depressed, but as the condition progresses animals become blind, walk aimlessly and may show head pressing, have difficulties with swallowing, and eventually die (Wilson *et al.*, 1990).

COMMON TOXICOSES OF POULTRY

This section will mainly address toxicoses in chicken, ducks and turkeys. However, there is much interest in the toxicology of wild birds, especially those kept in zoos, as well as pet birds. This discussion will emphasize toxicoses encountered in poultry. Readers interested in the general subject of avian toxicology are referred to LaBonde (1991).

Chemotherapeutic Drugs

Sulphonamides have been used as coccidiostats in poultry for four decades. Although sulphonamides have inhibitory action against coccidia and other pathogenic agents, they can be toxic to the host. In poultry, sulphonamide toxicity is characterized by blood dyscrasia, and renal and liver dysfunctions, and feeding chicken a mash containing as low as 0.2 per cent sulphonamides for 2 weeks is toxic. Clinically affected birds have ruffled feathers, are depressed, pale, icteric, have poor weight gain and prolonged bleeding time. In laying birds, sulphonamides cause a marked decrease in egg production, thin rough shells, and depigmentation in brown eggs. The temperature of affected birds is often elevated. At post mortem, haemorrhages are found in the skin, muscles (especially those of thighs and breast) and in internal organs. Once these signs are noticed the concentration of sulphonamides in the ration should be checked and the feed involved withdrawn (Peckham, 1978).

Other chemotherapeutic agents sometimes involved in poisoning poultry include coccidiostats such as nicarbazine, zoalene (3,5-dinitro-*o*-toluamide) and nitrophenide and the ionophore monensin. As little as 0.006 per cent nicarbazine causes mottled yolks and at 0.02 per cent there is a depressed rate of growth and depressed feeding efficiency. Feeding 0.025 per cent nicarbazine to day-old chicks for 1 week results in dullness, listlessness, weakness and ataxia. Feeding zoalene at least twice the recommended level of 0.025 per cent will cause nervous signs and depressed growth and feeding efficiency. The nervous signs include stiff neck, staggering, and tumbling over when the birds are excited. Nitrophenide possesses marked electrostatic properties and therefore sticks to the walls of the feed mixer. The last part of feed in the feed mixer will normally contain a high concentration of nitrophenide and has caused disturbances in posture and locomotion, retarded growth and mortality in chickens. Postural disturbances include a tilted position of the head, tremor of the neck and difficulty in the righting reflex (Peckham, 1978).

In general poultry are more resistant to monensin toxicity than mammals. There have been reports of monensin toxicity in turkeys accidentally fed rations containing 250 ppm monensin. There is a big difference in species susceptibility among poultry to monensin poisoning. Chickens and turkeys less than 2 weeks old are more resistant than older birds but keets (young guinea fowl) seem to be more susceptible than adult guinea fowl and the young of other species. For example, monensin at 200 ppm was not toxic for poults whereas 100 ppm was toxic for keets.

Cresol

Cresol was a commonly used disinfectant in poultry houses but has been gradually withdrawn and replaced by safer disinfectants. Nevertheless, cresol is still used in some countries. In chickens cresol poisoning usually occurs at 3–6 weeks of age. Affected chicks are depressed and have a tendency to huddle. There are signs of respiratory problems such as rales, gasping and wheezing, and in the event of prolonged exposure some chicks will have edema of the abdomen.

Sodium Chloride

All poultry and pigeons are susceptible to salt poisoning, young birds being more susceptible than adults. Although both acute and chronic forms of salt poisoning can occur, the chronic form is more commonly encountered and results from prolonged ingestion of feed containing a high salt content. Levels of 0.5 per cent and above in drinking water or 5–10 per cent in feed cause death in baby chicks. Signs of salt poisoning in poultry include anorexia, thirst, dyspnoea, opisthotonos, convulsions and ataxia. Increased water consumption may be the most significant early indicator of salt poisoning in poultry (Peckham, 1978).

Insecticides

Chlorinated hydrocarbon insecticides and organophosphate compounds are sometimes used inappropriately around poultry houses to control external parasites (LaBonde, 1991). Commonly involved organochlorine insecticides include chlordane, dieldrin, DDT, heptachlor and lindane. Occasionally birds are exposed by gaining access to sprayed grounds, such as golf courses. Chlordane causes chicks to chirp nervously, rest on their hocks and lie on their sides. The birds then become hyperexcitable as the condition progresses. In adult birds there is reduced food consumption, decreased body weight and a fall in production. Consumption of seeds dressed with dieldrin has been a source of exposure in wild birds. Affected birds are listless, have coordination problems while alighting, and severely poisoned birds show nervous signs characterized by lateral movements of the head and tremors of the head and neck. Birds die of violent convulsions. DDT toxicity in chickens is characterized by hyperexcitability and fine tremors in severe cases. Moderate cases are characterized by loss in weight, moulting, and reduced egg production. Lindane dust is frequently used in chicken houses. Adult chickens poisoned by lindane become anorectic, manifest opisthotonos, flapping of the wings, clonic muscle spasms, and they die in coma (Peckham, 1978).

The organophosphate compounds commonly involved include diazinon, malathion and parathion. Diazinon is used for chicken premises but is very toxic to ducklings; when used at rates recommended for chicken, 100 per cent mortality occurred in 1–2-week-old ducklings. Experimental studies suggest that goslings are three times more sensitive than ducks, chickens and turkeys. Poisoned birds are unable to stand, salivate profusely and manifest tremors of the head and neck. Brain cholinesterase levels in birds that die of organophosphate poisoning are on the average 69 per cent less than controls. Other organophosphate compounds commonly used in chicken premises include dichlorvos, malathion, and parathion. Birds poisoned by these compounds manifest similar signs to diazinon. Other signs that may be encountered include birds being depressed, ataxic, reluctant to move, paralysis, lachrymation, gasping, diarrhoea, crop stasis, and dyspnoea (Mohan, 1990). In general, ducks are more sensitive to organophosphate poisoning than chickens and care should be exercised when using this product in premises holding ducks (Mohan, 1990).

The carbamate insecticide carbaryl is widely used as a poultry insecticide. This compound is relatively safe to use but deaths have been reported in turkey poults kept in premises where the product had been applied at ten times the recommended rate. The clinical signs are similar to those caused by organophosphate poisoning.

Heavy Metals

Lead poisoning is not as common in poultry as in wild birds. Lead poisoning is the most common toxicity reported in avian species (LaBonde, 1991). Lead shot has caused losses in waterfowl populations in North America. All birds are susceptible to lead poisoning but most losses are reported in waterfowl because their feeding habits predispose them to lead ingestion. Characteristic signs of lead poisoning are those related to CNS derangement, such as ataxia, depression, paralysis of wings, or convulsions. In some cases the birds present anaemic, emaciated, regurgitating and weak. Green diarrhoea has also been reported in some affected birds (LaBonde, 1991).

Yellow phosphorus is a highly toxic element used as a rodenticide. Poultry and wild birds can be intoxicated by consumption of bait intended for rodents. Fragments of fireworks also are a common source of poisoning in free range birds. Affected birds are depressed, anorectic, have increased water consumption, and manifest diarrhoea, ataxia, paralysis, coma and death (Peckham, 1978).

Rodenticides

The effects of yellow phosphorus have been discussed in the preceding section. All rodenticides are potentially toxic to poultry and other birds. The clinical signs caused by rodenticides are similar to those in small animals. Birds occasionally consume baits containing anticoagulant rodenticides. The more potent second generation rodenticide-containing baits such as brodifacoum are especially dangerous to birds. These coumarin anticoagulants act by interfering with vitamin K recycling causing bleeding because of depletion of vitamin K-dependent clotting factors. Poisoned birds bleed from nares and subcutaneously, and have oral petechial; quite often they are also weak and depressed.

Of special interest, however, is secondary intoxication from consumption by free range birds of carrion of animals that died of rodenticide poisoning. Strychnine and sodium monofluoroacetate are compounds commonly involved because they cause acute death in primary victims and are present in high concentrations in carrion. Strychnine-poisoned birds manifest clinical signs within 2 h of ingesting the product. The birds become apprehensive, nervous and show violent tetanic convulsions which cause the birds to become exhausted and die of hypoxia. Sodium monofluoroacetate causes overstimulation of the CNS and also myocardial depression. Cardiac failure is the cause of death and this occurs within 1 h of consuming the product or contaminated carcasses (Peckham, 1978).

Mycotoxins

Mycotoxicoses are a common problem in the poultry industry in developing countries in the tropics. Aflatoxins are the most commonly involved mycotoxins and poultry are normally exposed by consumption of contaminated feed, especially corn. Some developing countries lack the resources adequately to screen contaminated corn. In some cases poultry feed is made from poor quality corn which has been rejected for human consumption, and often this poor quality feed is contaminated. Aflatoxicosis in poultry can be either acute or chronic depending on the exposure dose. Ducklings are more susceptible to aflatoxin than turkeys, pheasants or chickens (Butler, 1974). In acute cases affected birds become lethargic, their wings droop, and they manifest nervous signs, such as opisthotonos, and die with legs rigidly extended backward. Chronic consumption of at least 2.5 ppm aflatoxin in the diet causes a significant drop in performance, such as weight gain and egg production. Perhaps more important is the increased susceptibility of the affected flock to infection because chronic consumption of aflatoxins lowers the immunity of the birds. Aflatoxicosis is therefore a disease of serious economic consequences to the poultry industry in developing countries such as Uganda, both through lowered productivity and the death of affected birds.

Ergot poisoning has been reported in Europe where rye is commonly used as a feed. In acute ergot poisoning the comb is cold, wilted and cyanotic. The birds are weak, thirsty and have diarrhea. In severe cases the birds go into convulsions, paralysis and death. Ochratoxins have been reported to cause renal toxicity in poultry.

SUMMARY

In this chapter we have attempted to summarize the broad discipline of veterinary toxicology. We have given brief accounts of some selected common toxicities among different animal species so as to draw the attention of the reader to similarities and differences in their reaction to toxicants. Because some animals are more sensitive than others given the same toxicant, the diagnosis of some toxicoses may require the help of specialists within the veterinary profession. This chapter was not intended to be a detailed source of reference for diagnosis and treatment of animal poisonings, nor was it meant to be all inclusive. Rather it was a summary of the commonly encountered toxicoses in the veterinary profession. We suggest that interested readers consult the relevant references given in order to gain in-depth knowledge on subjects of interest. From the general overview of the subject it should be clear that all animals are susceptible to some type of toxicants and that some toxicants are toxic to all animals (including humans). It is therefore important to be cautious when handling chemicals around animals and we also need to provide a clean environment to all animals. Animals should be fed well-balanced quality food from reputable sources and suspect feed should be either avoided or checked for suspected toxicants before feeding. It is also vitally important to remember that all chemicals are poisons if the exposure is high enough. Therefore even some of the useful compounds we use around animals, e.g. growth promoters, can be fatal if used excessively or if given to species for which they are not intended. The susceptibility of sheep to feed containing copper that was intended for cattle, or of monensin in horses fed poultry feeds, are cases in point.

REFERENCES

Amend, J. F., Mellon, F. M. and Wren, W. B. (1980). Equine monensin toxicosis: some experimental clinicopathologic observations. *Comp. Contin. Ed. Pract. Vet.*, **2**, S175–S183

Beasley, V. R., Dahlem, A. M., Cook, W. O., Valentine, W. M., Lovell, R. A., Hooser, S. B., Harada, K., Suzuki, M and Carmichael, W. W. (1989). Diagnositic and clinically important aspects of cyanobacterial (blue-green) algae toxicoses. *J. Vet. Diag. Invest.*, **1**, 359–365

Blood, D. C. and Rodostits, O. M. (1989). *Veterinary Medicine*. Baillière Tindall, London, pp. 1241–1249

Boyd, R. E., and Spyker, D. A. (1983). Strichnine poisoning: recovery from profound lactic acidosis, hyperthermia and rhabdomyolysis. *Am. J. Med.*, **74**, 507–512

Buck, W. B., (1986). Copper-molybdenum. In Howard, J. L. (Ed.), *Current Veterinary Therapy: Food Animal Practice* 2, W. B. Saunders Co., Philadelphia, pp. 437–439

Buffa, P. and Peters, R. A. (1950). The *in vivo* formation of citrate induced by fluoroacetate poisoning and its significance. *J. Physiol. (Lond.)*, **110**, 488–500

Butler, W. H. (1974). Aflatoxin. In Purchase I. F. H. (Ed.) *Mycotoxins*. Elsevier Scientific Publishing Co., Amsterdam, pp. 1–28

Carson, T. L. and Dominick, M. A. (1982). Diagnosis and experimental reproduction of carbon monoxide induced fetal death in swine. *Am. Assoc. Vet. Lab. Diag.*, **25**, 403–410

Casida, J. E., Gammon, D. W., Glickman, A. H. and Lawrence, L. J. (1983). Mechanisms of selective action of pyrethroid insecticides. *Ann. Rev. Pharmacol. Toxicol.*, **23**, 413–438

Cheeke, P. R. and Shull, L. R. (1985). Mycotoxins. In Cheeke P. R. and Shull L. R. (Eds), *Natural Toxicants in Feeds and Poisonous Plants*. AVI Publishing Co., Connecticut, pp. 393- 476

Clay, B. R., Edwards, W. C. and Peterson, D. R. (1976). Toxic nitrate accumulation on sorghums. *Bovine Pract.*, **11**, 28–32

Colvin, B. M. and Harrison, L. R. (1992). Fumonisin-induced pulmonary edema and hydrothorax in swine. *Mycopathologia*, **117**, 79–82

Coon, W. W. and Wallis, P. W. (1972). Some aspects of pharmacology of oral anticoagulants. *Clin. Pharmacol. Ther.*, **11**, 312–336

Coppock, R. W., Monstrom, M. S. and Lillie, L. E. (1988). The toxicology of detergents, bleaches, antiseptics and disinfectants in small animals. *Vet. Hum. Toxicol.*, **30**, 463–473

Dorman, D. C. (1990). Anticoagulant, cholecalciferol, and bromethalin-based rodenticides. In Beasley, V. R. (Ed.), *The Veterinary Clinics of North America. Small Animal Practitioner: Toxicology of Selected Pesticides, Drugs and Chemicals*, **20**, 339–352

Dunn, H. W. and Leman, A. D. (Eds) (1975). *Diseases of Swine*, 4th edn, Iowa State University Press, Ames, pp. 854–860

Fikes, J. D. (1990). Organophosphorus and carbamate insecticides. In Beasley, V. R. (Ed.), *The Veterinary Clinics of North America: Toxicology of Selected Pesticides, Drugs and Chemicals*, **20**, 353–367

Fowler, M. E. (1981). *Plant poisoning in small companion animals*, Ralston Purina, St Louis, MO, pp. 1–4

Furr, A. and Buck, B. W. (1986). Arsenic. In Haward, J. L. (Ed.), *Current Veterinary Therapy: Food Animal Practice* 2, W. B. Saunders Co., Philadelphia, pp. 435–437

Gosselin, R. E., Hodge, H. C., Smith, R. P. and Gleason, M. N. (1976) (Eds). Ammonia. In *Clinical Toxicology of Commercial Products*, 4th edn. Williams and Wilkins, Baltimore, pp. 20–24

Grauer, G. F. and Thrall, M. A. (1982). Ethylene glycol (antifreeze) poisoning in the dog and cat. *J. Am. Anim. Hosp. Assoc.* **18**, 492–497

Hayes, W. J. Jr. (1991). Dosage and other factors influencing toxicity. In Hayes, W. J. Jr. and Laws, E. R. Jr. (Eds), *Handbook of Pesticide Toxicology*. Academic Press, San Diego, pp. 39–105

Heisser, J. M., Doya, M. R., Magnussen, A. R., Norton, R. L., Spyker, D. A., Allen, D. W. and Krasselt, W. (1992). Massive strichnine intoxication: serial blood levels in a fatal case. *Clin. Toxicol.*, **30**, 269–283

Hultine, J. D., Mount, M. E., Easiley, K. J. and Oehme, F. W. (1979). Selenium toxicosis in the horse. *Equine Pract.*, **1**, 57

Keller, W. C., Beasley, V. R. and Robens, J. F. (1990). *Proceedings of the Symposium on Public Health Significance of Natural Toxicants in Animal Feeds*, Alexandria, Virginia, February 1989, pp. 1–111

Kingsburry, J. M. (1964). *Poisonous Plants of the United States and Canada*, Prentice-Hall, Englewood Cliffs

LaBonde, J. (1991). Avian toxicology. In *Vet. Clin, North Am. Small Anim. Pract.*, **21**, 1329–1342

Lloyd, W. E. (1986). Urea and other non-protein nitrogen sources. In Howard, J. L. (Ed.), *Current Veterinary Therapy: Food Animal Practice* 2, W. B. Saunders, Philadelphia, pp. 354–356

Livezey, K. L., Dorman, D. C., Hooser, S. B. and Buck, W. B. (1991). Hypercalcemia induced by vitamin D_3 toxicosis in two dogs. *Canine Practice*, **16**, 126–132

Maron, B. J., Krupp, J. R. and Tune, B. (1971). Strychnine poisoning successfully treated with diazepam. *J. Pediatr.*, **78**, 697–699

Menzer, R. E. (1991). Water and soil pollutants. In Amdur M. O., Doull, J. and Klassen C. D. (Eds), *Casarett and Doull's Toxicology, the Basic Science of Poisons*, 4th edn. Pergamon Press, New York, pp. 872–902

Mohan, R. (1990). Dursban toxicosis in a pet bird breeding operation. In *Proceedings of Association of Avian Veterinary Conference*, Phoenix, pp. 112–114

Muth, O. H. and Binns, W. (1964). Selenium toxicity in domestic animals. *Ann. N.Y. Acad. Sci.* **III**, 583–590

O'Donohue, J. G. (1961). Hydrogen sulfide poisoning in swine. *Can. J. Comp. Med. Vet. Sci.*, **25**, 217–219

Oehme, F. W. (1987a). Toxicosis commonly observed in horses. In Robinson, N. E. (Ed.), *Current Therapy in Equine Medicine* 2, W. B. Saunders, Philadelphia, pp. 649–653

Oehme, F. W. (1987b). Insecticides. In Robinson, N. E. (Ed.), *Current Therapy in Equine Medicine* 2. W. B. Saunders, Philadelphia, pp. 656–660

Osweiler, G. D., Carson, T. L., Buck, W. B. and Van Gelder, G. A. (Eds). (1985). *Clinical and Diagnostic Veterinary Toxicology*, 3rd edn. Kendal/Hunt Publishing Co., Dubuque, pp. 27–39, 160–166

Peckham, M. C. (1978). Poisons and toxins. In Hofstad, M. S., Calnek, B. W., Hemboldt, C. F., Reid, W. M. and Yonder, H. W. Jr (Eds), *Diseases of Poultry*. Iowa State University Press, Iowa, pp. 895–933

Pelfrene, A. F. (1991). Synthetic organic rodenticides. In Hayes, W. J. Jr. and Laws, E. R. Jr. (Eds), *Handbook of Pesticide Toxicology*. Academic Press, San Diego, pp. 1271–1316

Pier, A. C. (1981). Mycotoxins and animal health. *Adv. Vet. Sci. Comp. Med.*, **25**, 185–243

Radeleff, R. D. (1970). *Veterinary Toxicology*, Lea and Febiger, Philadelphia, pp. 158–161

Ridder, W.E. and Oehme, F. W. (1974). Nitrate as an environmental animal and human hazard. *Clin. Toxicol.*, **7**, 145

Rumbeiha, K. W. and Oehme, F. W. (1992a). Methylene blue can be used to treat methemoglobinemia in cats without inducing Heinz body hemolytic anemia. *Vet. Hum. Toxicol.*, **34**: 120–122

Rumbeiha, K. W. and Oehme, F. W. (1992b). Emergency procedures for equine toxicoses. *Equine Pract.*, **14**, 26–30

Schmitz, D. G. and Reagor, J. C. (1987). Cantharidine (blister beetle) toxicity. In Robinson, N. E. (Ed.), *Current Therapy in Equine Medicine* 2. W. B. Saunders, Philadelphia, pp. 120–122

Smith, A. G. (1991). Chlorinated hydrocarbon insecticides. In Hayes, W. J. Jr. and Laws, E. R. Jr. (Eds), *Handbook of Pesticide Toxicology*, Academic Press, San Diego, pp. 731–916

Stephenson, J. P. B. (1967). Zinc phosphide poisoning. *Arch. Environ. Health*, **15**, 83–88

Stevens, J. T. and Sumner, D. D. (1991). Herbicides. In Hayes, W. J. Jr. and Laws, E. R. Jr, (Eds), *Handbook of Pesticide Toxicology*. Academic Press, San Diego, pp. 1317–1408

Trammell, H. L., Dorman, D. C., and Beasley, V. R. (1989). *Ninth Annual Report of the Illinois Animal Poison Information Center*, Kendal/Hunt, Dubuque

Valentine, W. M. (1990). Pyrethrin and pyrethroid insecticides. In Beasley, V. R. (Ed.), *The Veterinary Clinics of North America: Toxicology of Selected Pesticides, Drugs and Chemicals*, **20**, 375–385

Welch, R. M., Conney, A. H. and Burns, J. J. (1966). The metabolism of acetophenetidin and N-acetyl-*p*-aminophenol in the cat. *Biochem. Pharmacol.*, **15**, 521–531

Wilson, T. M., Ross, P. F., Rice, L. G., Osweiler, G. D., Nelson, H. A., Owens, D. L., Platner, R. D., Reggiardo, C., Noon, T. H. and Pickrell, J. W. (1990). Fumonisin B_1 levels associated with an epizootic of equine leucoencephalomalacia. *J. Vet. Diagn. Invest.*, **2**, 231–216

FURTHER READING

Bartik, M. and Piskae, A. (1981). *Veterinary Toxicology*. Elsevier, Amsterdam

51 Combustion Toxicology

James C. Norris and Bryan Ballantyne

GENERAL CONSIDERATIONS

Combustion toxicology deals with the nature and potential adverse effects of products resulting from the heating or burning of materials; these effects include irritation, incapacitation, toxicity and lethality. Although the major effort has been devoted to products generated in accidental fires, adverse effects may also result from exposure to products resulting from heating or burning materials in occupational and domestic situations. Two typical examples of illnesses resulting from the inhalation exposure to products resulting from heating polymers are meat wrappers' 'allergy' and polyfume fever. The former affects some workers wrapping meat in polyvinyl chloride (PVC) film. The sources of exposure come from the hot wire cutting (approximately 105 °C) of the film from rolls, heat sealing of the folded film ends, and thermal fixing of an adhesive label to the wrapped product, with the heating element temperature at around 200 °C (Levy, 1988). The major products from hot wire cutting of PVC film include di-2-ethylhexyl phthalate and hydrogen chloride, and those from the thermal attachment of labels include dicyclohexyl phthalate, phthalic anhydride, cyclohexyl ether and cyclohexyl benzoate (Levy et al., 1978; Vandevort and Brooks, 1979). Affected meat wrappers complain of cough, wheezing, shortness of breath, chest tightness, and symptoms and signs from irritation of the eyes and throat. The spectrum of the illness should be interpreted as a complex response to emissions from all phases of the wrapping procedure (Andrasch et al., 1975). Currently it is considered that exposure to the products from heating PVC in meat wrapping environments produces effects compatible with irritation of the eyes and respiratory tract; in those with pre-existing asthma or chronic obstructional airways disease there may be an exacerbation of the condition. The effects produced accord with respiratory tract irritation and hyperreactivity; the role of an immunological process (i.e. an asthmatic reaction) is questionable (Brooks, 1983). It is possible that it is a reaction similar to that described as the reactive airways dysfunction syndrome by Brooks et al. (1985). Polyfume fever is an example of illness resulting from exposure to the pyrolysis products of polytetrafluoroethylene (PTFE) after contamination of cigarettes with the polymer in an occupational environment. Workers smoking cigarettes contaminated with PTFE subsequently develop an 'influenza-like syndrome', characterized by cough, tightness of the chest, a choking sensation, and chills. There is characteristically a delay of several hours between exposure and the development of symptoms; recovery is complete within 12–48 h (Gantz, 1988). No long-term sequelae have been described. Thermal decomposition products up to 500 °C are principally the TFE monomer, but also perfluoropropene and other perfluoro compounds containing four or five carbon atoms. In the range 500–800 °C the major pyrolysis product is carbonyl fluoride (Hathaway et al., 1991).

Currently in the USA there are approximately 6000 deaths each year from fire, with a much larger number of non-lethal injuries (Alexeff and Packham, 1984; Gad, 1990a). Casualties occur during, or as a consequence of, exposure to a fire for various reasons, of which the following are the more important.

(1) *Direct physical trauma*: resulting from structural collapse of buildings.

(2) *Flame and heat*: direct thermal injuries to skin and/or respiratory tract, or secondary complications from primary thermal injuries.

(3) *Oxygen depletion*: this may be a primary factor and/or enhance the toxicity of respirable chemicals in the fire atmosphere.

(4) *Factors hindering escape*: these may increase the likelihood of further exposure to flame, heat, oxygen depletion, and toxic materials in the atmosphere. Escape may be hindered by physical injury, obscuring smoke, prior use of alcohol or narcotic drugs, panic, the presence of peripheral sensory irritants, or depression of CNS function from specific materials in the atmos-

phere. For example, alcoholic intoxication has been a significant factor in some fires and may have impeded escape. Thus, in one series of fire deaths in the UK, mainly occurring in dwellings, ethanol was present in the blood of most victims, and 59 per cent of the adults had blood ethanol concentrations >80 mg dl^{-1} or urine concentrations in excess of 107 mg dl^{-1}; the average blood ethanol concentration was 276 mg dl^{-1} (Harland and Wooley, 1979). In a study of fire deaths in Maryland, blood ethanol concentrations in excess of 150 mg dl^{-1} were found in 35 per cent of victims (Radford *et al.*, 1976).

(5) *Toxic substances in the atmosphere*: such materials vary considerably in their chemical nature and concentrations, and are released by heating and/or burning of materials involved in the fire. These toxic substances may produce acute effects, latent effects and, with repeated exposure, as for example with firemen, cumulative and/or long-term toxicity.

Smoke is a complex mixture of airborne solid and liquid particulates and gases which are evolved when materials undergo vaporization or thermal decomposition. Thermal decomposition may be conveniently described under the following conditions:

(1) *Anaerobic pyrolysis*: thermal breakdown and chemical conversion of materials in a low oxygen environment.

(2) *Oxidative pyrolysis*: thermal breakdown and chemical conversion of materials in a normal oxygen environment but in the absence of flaming ('smouldering').

(3) *Flaming combustion*: thermal breakdown and chemical conversion of materials in a normal oxygen environment in the presence of flaming.

All these processes may be operating at the same time at different geographical regions in a fire, or one may predominate. Pyrolysis is usually defined as the thermal degradation of a material at a temperature below the autoignition temperature. Flaming is the highly efficient burning of a material above the autoignition temperature in the presence of sufficient oxygen. Thermolysis is a generic term covering flaming, pyrolysis and smouldering.

The atmosphere in a fire is usually of extremely complex composition and, because of the con-

stantly changing conditions during the progress of a fire, the chemical composition (both nature and concentration of materials) varies markedly at different stages of the fire. Also, the characteristics and hazards of one fire may be entirely different from those of another. The chemical composition of the atmosphere and the concentrations of the individual constituents depend on a large number of variable factors; the most important of these include:

- The nature of the materials available for heating or burning.
- Phase of the combustion process.
- The potential for chemical and/or physical interactions between materials present in the fire atmosphere.
- The potential for additive or synergistic toxic effects.
- Temperature.
- Air flow and oxygen availability.

A review of the European and North American literature suggests that some 50–75 per cent of deaths that occur within a few hours of being involved in a fire result from the toxic effects of chemicals in the fire atmosphere. After about 12 h, the contribution of toxic effects to mortalities is considerably less. Over the past few decades the contribution of toxic chemicals to mortalities and non-fatal casualties has increased—for example, in the UK during the period 1955–74 the total number of fire fatalities increased by 70 per cent; those from burns and scalds fluctuated around 400–600 annually, while those attributed to the effects of gas and smoke showed a steady increase (Ballantyne, 1981). The increasing hazard from toxic materials was also shown by consideration of the total incidence of smoke casualties (i.e. fatal and non-fatal): there was a 600 per cent increase over the 19-year period. In the USA there are approximately 6000 deaths annually from fire, with smoke inhalation being responsible for about 80 per cent of the fatalities (Alexeff and Packham, 1984; Kaplan, 1988; Gad, 1990a). Also, the probability of death is increased for the fire victim by smoke inhalation and burns (Zawacki *et al.*, 1977, 1979; Shirani *et al.*, 1986). There are reasonable grounds to believe that the marked increase in smoke and gas casualties is related to the introduction of man-made materials for construction and furnishing. Combustion processes involving polymers result in the generation of a variety of lower molecular weight materials which may have significant irritant effects and acute and/or long-term toxicity. The nature and relative amounts of toxic products from combustion of polymers vary with both the nature of the polymeric material and the conditions of burning. The range of toxicity possible is reflected in the following examples of typical products from polymer combustion: acetaldehyde, acrolein, phosgene, hydrogen cyanide, carbon monoxide, hydrogen chloride, and vinyl chloride. It is of practical importance to note that the combustion products of some phosphorus-based fire retardants may present toxicological problems (Purser, 1992).

Lethalities resulting from inhalation of chemicals in a fire atmosphere may be due to local chemical injury to the respiratory tract and/or systemic toxicity following absorption of inhaled materials; the latter may include disturbance of biochemical mechanisms or transport processes, or tissue injury. Non-lethal adverse effects may result from more restricted or less severe local respiratory tract injury or systemic toxicity. It should also be appreciated that inhaled smoke and fumes may contain products of incomplete combustion which continue to release heat following inhalation, resulting in thermal injury to the laryngeal and tracheobronchial mucosa and, with sufficient penetration, to the alveolar epithelium. These thermal injuries will complement any chemically induced respiratory tract injury (Zachria, 1972). Smoke inhalation may lead to pulmonary oedema, in which there is increased permeability of the pulmonary microvasculature (Neimann *et al.*, 1989). Studies of experimentally produced smoke inhalation injury in sheep showed that the primary, and dose-responsive, injury was acute cell membrane damage in the trachea and bronchi leading to oedema, progressive necrotic tracheobronchitis with pseudomembrane formation, and airways obstruction (Hubbard *et al.*, 1991). Morphological changes occurring in the alveolar epithelium included intracellular oedema (Type I cells), changes in membrane-bound vacuoles (Type II cells), and interstitial oedema.

Although great emphasis has been placed on the acute toxic effects of fire atmospheres, there is also a potential for long-term adverse effects, particularly by repeated exposures. This is considered later in this chapter under a consideration of hazards of firefighting (pp. 1191–1193).

NATURE AND TOXICITY OF FIRE ATMOSPHERES

Thermal decomposition of a material may produce a wide variety of lower molecular species of differing toxicity and irritancy. The number, nature and relative proportions of the products depend on the material burned and the conditions of the combustion process. This may be illustrated by considering the simple burning of wood in an enclosed space (Table 1). Carbon, hydrogen and sulphur are available as the common combustible elements. In the early phase of burning, sulphur dioxide, water and carbon dioxide are produced, together with some carbon monoxide. As oxygen becomes depleted and burning becomes slower, more carbon monoxide and sulphur dioxide are formed. With further decrease in oxygen availability incomplete combustion occurs and hydrogen, methane, carbon monoxide and free carbon are produced. In the smouldering phase, hydrogen, methane, sulphur dioxide, carbon dioxide, carbon monoxide, free carbon and smoke are all produced. This simple example indicates that as a fire progresses and temperature increases, available oxygen decreases (in enclosed spaces); toxic, irritant and flammable gases are produced and obscuring smoke is formed. Additionally, with combustion of wood, other irritant and toxic materials may be produced; for example, formaldehyde, methanol, acetic acid and other organic irritants (DeKorver, 1976). Even in the apparently simple example of wood, a multiplicity of differing chemicals may be produced; for example, combustion of Douglas fir produced more than 75 discrete chemicals in the smoke (Packham and Hartzell, 1981). Smoke is usually defined as a complex mixture of airborne solid and liquid particulates and gases produced when a material undergoes thermal decomposition (Kaplan, 1988). Smoke may be obscuring, contain smouldering particles that can produce thermal injury to the respiratory tract, and contain toxic and irritant materials in gas or vapour form or absorbed on the surface of particulates.

As noted earlier, the widespread introduction of man-made polymeric materials into buildings and furnishings has been associated with a wider

Table 1 Products of the burning of wood in an enclosed space, and the influence of the stage of burning

Factor	Burning stage[a]			
	Free	Slowed	Incomplete combustion	Smouldering
Oxygen (%)	20	17	15	<13
Temperature (°C)	40	205	370	550
Products	SO_2 +	SO_2 +	SO_2 ++	SO_2 ++
	H_2O ++	H_2O ++	H_2O ++	H_2O ++
	CO_2 ++	CO_2 ++	CO_2 +++	CO_2 +++
	CO ±	CO +	CO ++	CO +++
			H_2 ±	H_2 +
			CH_4 +	CH_4 +
			Free C +	Free C +++
			Smoke +	Smoke +++

[a] + designation = relative proportion of product.

spectrum of toxicity than that produced from natural polymers (Alarie, 1985; Gad, 1990a). Products from the combustion of synthetic polymers may have a significant role in morbidity and mortality in fires (Ballantyne, 1981). At low temperatures (up to 400 °C) polymers decompose to give a range of complex products; at medium temperatures (400–700 °C) the complexity of products increases and complex organic species may develop; at high temperatures (>700 °C) complex organic molecules are unstable and decompose (Ballantyne, 1989).

Examples of the differing highly toxic and irritant chemical species produced by the combustion of synthetic polymers are shown in Table 2. This table shows a few major toxic products, but it must be emphasized that, depending on the condition of combustion, the number of chemical species produced by combustion of a specific polymer may be high. For example, polyvinyl chloride yields hydrogen chloride as a principal combustion product but about 75 other organic compounds are generated (Wooley, 1971; Dyer and Esch, 1976). Combustion of polyethylene yielded 55 compounds and polypropylene yielded 56 compounds (Mitera and Michal, 1985). With polypropylene, the main thermal degradation products are formaldehyde, acetaldehyde, 2-methylacrolein, acetic acid and acetone (Frostling *et al.*, 1984). Nitrogen-containing polymers may yield hydrogen cyanide and various cyanogens (see later; pp. 1186–1187).

Table 2 Examples of toxic and irritant chemicals that may be generated by combustion of commonly occurring materials

Material	Combustion products[a]	Reference
Polyvinylchloride	Hydrogen chloride	Dyer and Esch (1976)
	Carbon monoxide	Michal (1976)
Polyethylene	Formaldehyde	Morikawa (1976)
	Acrolein	
Polyacrylonitrile	Hydrogen cyanide	Morikawa (1978)
Polyurethane foams	Toluene di-isocyanate	Wooley (1974)
	Hydrogen cyanide	Bowes (1974)
	Carbon monoxide	
Polytetrafluorethylene	Hydrogen fluoride	Young *et al.* (1976)
	Carbonyl fluoride	

[a] These are not necessarily the only products generated but are given to illustrate the more toxic materials. The relative amounts of materials generated depends on the conditions of heating.

Factors Influencing Combustion Products and Their Toxicological Effects

The specific chemical species, and their relative proportions, produced during the combustion processes are dependent on various environmental factors (Table 3). These factors may, additionally, quantitively modify the toxic response. The more important factors are summarized below.

Oxygen Availability

The availability of oxygen in the burning area may significantly affect the generation of combustion products. For example, at 500–600 °C polyethylene gives a high acrolein yield with low atmospheric oxygen, and a low acrolein yield when atmospheric oxygen is high (Morikawa, 1976). An example of the influence of oxygen availability on toxicity is illustrated in Figure 1,

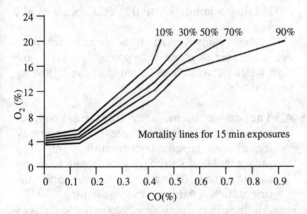

Figure 1 Mortality of male rats exposed for 15 min to atmospheres containing various proportions of oxygen and carbon monoxide. For any given carbon monoxide concentration, mortality increases with decreasing oxygen content. After Ballantyne (1981).

which shows that for any given atmospheric carbon monoxide content, lethal toxicity increases with decreasing oxygen content. Clearly this results, at least in part, from proportionately less oxygen being available to maintain vital process where oxygen transport is already compromised by carbon monoxide-induced hypoxia. This is also clearly relevant to practical fire situations, where carbon monoxide is ubiquitous and oxygen depletion common.

Temperature

The temperature in an area of burning or smouldering may significantly influence the products released into the atmosphere. Pyrolysis of polyurethane smoke at 300 °C yields polymeric smoke, but at 800 °C the smoke decomposes to *N*-containing materials, such as hydrogen cyanide, acetonitrile, acrylonitrile, pyridine and benzonitrile (Wooley, 1972).

Several studies have shown that environmental temperature may influence toxicity. Nomiyama *et al.* (1980) demonstrated an increase in acute toxicity for various organic solvents, heavy metals and agrochemicals at elevated environmental temperature. Sanders and Endecott (1991) showed, in laboratory rats, that incapacitation occurred earlier when exposure to carbon monoxide was combined with elevated temperature, compared with the effects of carbon monoxide or temperature alone.

INCAPACITATING FACTORS IN FIRES

Incapacitating effects are those that hinder escape from a fire by impairment of physical and/or

Table 3 Influence of various factors on the generation of thermolysis products from specific materials

Material	Variable	Observation	Reference
Polyurethane foam	Time	In the early stages both hydrogen cyanide and carbon monoxide produced; in the later stages only carbon monoxide	Bowes (1974)
Polyurethane foam	Temperature	Pyrolysis at 300 °C yields a polymeric smoke; at 800 °C smoke decomposes to N-containing materials, notably hydrogen cyanide, acetonitrile, acrylonitrile, pyridine and benzonitrile	Wooley (1972)
Polyethylene	Oxygen availability	Low oxygen atmosphere (500–600 °C) gives high acrolein yield; high oxygen atmosphere (500–600 °C) gives low acrolein yield.	Morikawa (1976)

mental functions. Clearly, obstacles, physical injury and dense smoke are physical factors which may impair mobility and escape. Hypoxia, discussed later, may impair mental functions by a wide range of effects ranging from impairment of judgement to loss of consciousness. Some substances encountered in fire atmospheres may be absorbed and affect CNS function and produce, for example, disturbance of consciousness, abnormalities of coordination, weakness, and decreased reaction and responsiveness times; volatile organic solvents, carbon monoxide and hydrogen cyanide are all examples of materials that produce such effects. These considerations on the effect of hypoxia and absorbed chemicals on behaviour and judgement clearly apply not only to impairment of escape but are also relevant to safe and effective performance by those occupationally involved in firefighting operations.

Many materials of widely varying chemical nature that are released in a fire are peripheral sensory irritants. They are thus capable of inducing excess tear production, eye discomfort, and blepharospasm. These ocular effects will clearly result in impairment of vision and thus influence the performance of coordinated tasks and escape from a critical situation.

HYPOXIA

Hypoxia is a condition in which there is a physiologically inadequate supply of oxygen to tissues or an impairment of the cellular utilization of oxygen. In the context of a fire, all of the following types of hypoxia may occur.

Hypoxic Hypoxia

This is present where there is a decrease in the arterial blood PO_2 resulting from inadequate availability of oxygen to blood in pulmonary alveolar capillaries. There is a reduction in the amount of oxygen in arterial blood, but no reduction in PaO_2. This may be a consequence of depletion of atmospheric oxygen in the inspired air, airways obstruction, lung injury sufficient to reduce diffusing capacity, low tidal volume, or increased dead space.

Anaemic Hypoxia

This is present when there is a decreased oxygen transporting capacity of the blood, as, for example, a reduced circulating erythrocyte mass. In a fire, anaemic hypoxia may occur from reduced haemoglobin oxygen binding sites which is frequently a result of carboxyhaemoglobin formation or the induction of methaemoglobinaemia.

Cytotoxic Hypoxia

This is a systemic effect where there is interference with the utilization of oxygen by cells. A classic example is that of inhibition of cellular cytochrome oxidase activity by cyanide.

Hypoxia is a broad term referring to inadequate tissue supply or utilization of oxygen for any reason; hypoxaemia refers only to decreased carriage of oxygen in arterial blood (as in hypoxic and anaemic hypoxia). Although tissue oxygen supply is decreased in hypoxaemia, significant damage does not occur until arterial oxygen saturation falls to about 50 per cent and PaO_2 falls to about 30 mmHg (Campbell *et al.*, 1984).

If of sufficient degree, hypoxia may result in death. Lesser degrees of hypoxia, however, are highly significant in fires because of the following possibilities:

- The development, sometimes insidious, of neurological abnormalities. These may include impaired coordination, impaired judgement, disturbance of consciousness ranging from drowsiness to coma and disorientation (Autian, 1976; Ganong, 1977). All these can clearly produce variable degrees of mental and/or physical incapacitation.
- Hypoxia may increase chemoreceptor activity, leading to an increase in the rate and depth of breathing. This could result in enhanced inhalation exposure to toxic materials in inspired air.
- As mentioned earlier, hypoxia may enhance the toxicity of some materials.

EXAMPLES OF COMMON MATERIALS IN FIRE ATMOSPHERES

Carbon Monoxide

Carbon monoxide is a major and ubiquitous component of fire atmospheres, often at potentially lethal concentrations (Jankovic *et al.*, 1991). Barnard (1979) measured carbon monoxide concentrations in 25 Los Angeles fires and found that in 12 per cent of fires the peak carbon monoxide was less than 100 ppm; in 40 per cent peak values were in the range 501–1000 ppm, 25 per cent in the range 500–1000 ppm, and 23 per cent more than 1000 ppm; the highest concentration measured was 3000 ppm. A major factor in the toxicity of carbon monoxide is generally considered to be related to its high affinity for haemoglobin, being about 250 times that of oxygen. A sufficient exposure to carbon monoxide causes an anaemic hypoxia. An additional factor influencing the toxicity of carbon monoxide is the fact that the presence of carboxyhaemoglobin (COHb) causes a shift-to-the-left of the oxygen–haemoglobin dissociation curve. As a consequence there is increased affinity of hemoglobin for oxygen, and thus at any given PO_2 the release of oxygen will be reduced compared with conditions where COHb is not present (Ayres *et al.*, 1973). Also, carbon monoxide inhibits cytochrome a_3; this will be a function of plasma carbon monoxide (Goldbaum *et al.*, 1976; Goldbaum, 1977).

Interpretation of COHb values, particularly at lower concentrations, needs to be undertaken carefully because of the influence of environment (rural or urban) factors, and cigarette smoking, on COHb concentrations (Ballantyne, 1981). Also, if dichloromethane is present, this may be endogenously converted to carbon monoxide (Hathaway *et al.*, 1991). Additionally, if analysis for COHb is not performed promptly in appropriately stored containers, analytical artefact losses may occur (Chance *et al.*, 1986; Levin *et al.*, 1990). The majority of individuals exposed to fire atmospheres will have elevated concentrations of COHb, the degree of which depends on the exposure time and exposure concentration. Low concentrations of COHb may indicate rapid death from trauma or extensive burning (Levin *et al.*, 1990; Mayes, 1991; Mayes *et al.*, 1992). When death is solely from carbon monoxide poisoning (for example coal gas poisoning) the COHb concentrations stated to be compatible with death from acute carbon monoxide poisoning are usually in the range 50–60 per cent. COHb concentrations [COHb] measured in fire victims may show a wide spectrum of values, some compatible with death from carbon monoxide poisoning, others significantly lower. For example, Harland

and Wooley (1979) in a sample of 90 fire deaths found [COHb] of more than 50 per cent in half the cases; those above 50 per cent had a mean value of 67 per cent and those below a mean of 18 per cent. In interpreting lower concentrations of COHb in fatal cases, it should be remembered that hypoxia may enhance the toxicity of carbon monoxide, and that carbon monoxide toxicity may be an interactive factor in the presence of other toxic substances and physical and thermal trauma. Patterns of [COHb] found in differing fires may reflect the circumstances of an individual specific fire. For example, in the MGM Grand Hotel fire 51.3 per cent of victims had [COHb] of more than 50 per cent; in this fire most of the victims were found in areas remote from the conflagration (Birky *et al.*, 1985). In contrast, in the DuPont Plaza Hotel fire in Puerto Rico, 80–85 per cent of the victims had [COHb] of less than 50 per cent; in this fire the majority of victims were burned and found in the area of the fire (Levin *et al.*, 1990).

Exposure to sublethal concentrations of carbon monoxide may result in various potentially adverse health effects. Of notable importance are neurological and behavioural effects, which could hinder the performances of skilled tasks or the recognition of, and escape from, a critical situation. These include headache, dizziness, disturbance of vision, confusion, difficulties in coordination, decreased reaction time, and drowsiness (Stewart, 1974; Zarem *et al.*, 1973). Additionally, acute exposure to carbon monoxide may produce cardiac arrythmias, myocardial damage, and circulatory failure (Stewart, 1974). Also, there may be aggravation of exercise-induced angina, decreased exercise tolerance, depression of the S–T segment in the ECG, and increased vulnerability to ventricular fibrillation (Anderson *et al.*, 1973; Aronow, 1976; DeBias *et al.*, 1976).

The human foetus is particularly sensitive to carbon monoxide because of several differences from the adult. Under steady-state conditions foetal [COHb] is around 10–15 per cent greater than the corresponding maternal blood [COHb]. Additionally, the partial pressure of oxygen in foetal blood is lower, at 20–30 mmHg, compared with the adult value of 100 mmHg (Longo, 1976, 1977; McDiarmid *et al.*, 1991). Furthermore, the fetal oxygen–haemoglobin dissociation curve lies to the left of the adult curve, resulting in greater tissue hypoxia at equivalent COHb concentrations. It is also considered that the foetal half-life of elimination of carbon monoxide is longer than in the mother (Margulies, 1986). Acute exposure to carbon monoxide concentrations that are non-lethal to the mother have been associated with foetal loss (Muller and Graham, 1955; Goldstein, 1965), or permanent neurological sequelae in the foetus (Cramer, 1982). These factors need to be considered in relation to pregnant women exposed to fire atmospheres, and the employment of women of childbearing age in the fire services.

Hydrogen Cyanide

Any material containing carbon and nitrogen will liberate hydrogen cyanide (HCN) under appropriate combustion conditions. In addition, various cyanogens may be produced such as acrylonitrile, acetonitrile, adiponitrile, benzonitrile and propionitrile (Stark, 1974; Wooley, 1982). Cyanogen has also been detected in the blood of fire victims (Anderson *et al.*, 1979; Symington *et al.*, 1978). Polymeric materials are a particularly notable source of HCN; for example, nylon (Purser and Wooley, 1983), polyacrylonitrile (Bertol *et al.*, 1983), polyurethanes (Jellinek and Takada, 1977), urea formaldehyde (Paabo *et al.*, 1979) and melamine (Moss *et al.*, 1951). Although some studies show that the evolution of HCN is proportional to the nitrogen content of polymeric materials (Morikawa, 1978), this is not a universal finding. Bertol *et al.* (1983) found that proportionately more HCN (1500 ppm) was evolved from polyacrylonitrile (19.0 per cent elemental nitrogen) than from wool (200 ppm; 14.3 per cent elemental nitrogen). Also, Urhas and Kullik (1977) found that with pyrolysis temperatures in the range of 625–925 °C, the yield of HCN was inversely related to the nitrogen content of three fibers. Both temperature and oxygen availability influence the yield of HCN from a nitrogen-containing material. The general effect of temperature on HCN yield from nitrogen-containing polymers is shown in Figure 2. Under anaerobic conditions, high temperatures result in the generation of HCN, the yield of which increases with increasing temperature. In oxidizing atmospheres, HCN is evolved at lower temperatures and as temperature increases so does HCN liberation, up to a maximum, and then decreases with further increase in temperature; a secondary rise

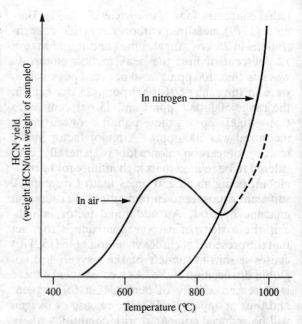

Figure 2 Graphical representation of HCN yields from nitrogen-containing polymers as a function of thermolysis temperature in oxidative and inert atmospheres. In air there is an initial increase in HCN yield followed by a decrease; a secondary increase in HCN yield may occur at higher temperatures. For anaerobic conditions the evolution of HCN begins at temperatures above those for oxidative conditions, and the yield increases with increasing temperature

in HCN may occur at even higher temperatures. Polyester and polyether flexible urethane foams decompose at relatively low temperature (200–300 °C) in inert atmospheres to produce a yellow smoke which is stable up to 800 °C; however, over the range of 800–1000 °C there is decomposition yielding HCN, acetonitrile, benzonitrile and pyridine as the major nitrogen-containing products (Wooley, 1972). These and many other studies indicate that the evolution of HCN varies with temperature, oxygen availability, the chemical nature of the nitrogen-containing material, and the burning time. Although these variables will differ at any given time, practical estimates for HCN generation have been made. For example, Morikawa (1978) calculated that if nylon is burned at 950 °C under restricted air conditions, then only 1.5 g is necessary to raise the HCN concentration to around 135 ppm in a 1 m³ space. Extrapolating data from combustion studies, Bertol *et al.* (1983) calculated that a toxic concentration of HCN could be developed in an average-sized room by the burning of 2 kg polyacrylonitrile.

Many independent studies using laboratory animals have shown that when animals are exposed to combustion products, principally from nitrogen-containing polymers, then HCN may be generated in amounts sufficient to produce physical incapacitation or lethality. Yamamoto (1975) studied the acute toxicity of combustion products from various fibres and found that in rats exposed for up to 30 min, signs of incapacitation developed most rapidly following exposure to polyacrylonitrile (less than 10 min). Blood removed after development of signs showed COHb concentrations were less than 10 per cent with polyacrylonitrile and wool, and in the range of 20–40 per cent for silk; blood cyanide concentrations ranged from 1.5 to 3.0 μg ml^{-1} for silk, 1.5–2.0 μg ml^{-1} for PAN, and less than 0.5 μg ml^{-1} for wool. Thus, under these conditions of combustion of silk and polyacrylonitrile, HCN was the major cause of incapacitation, and blood cyanide concentrations of potentially lethal significance developed. Purser *et al.* (1984) exposed primates to the combustion products from polyacrylonitrile, and a comparable group to HCN vapour. The pathophysiological effects were similar for the two groups: hyperventilation, loss of consciousness, bradycardia, and cardiac arrhythmias; following this, breathing was slowed and respiratory minute volume markedly decreased. For both groups there was a relationship between chamber HCN concentration and time to incapacitation. Blood cyanide concentrations in the polyacrylonitrile combustion group were similar to those in the HCN-alone group. Purser and Grimshaw (1984) exposed primates for 30 min to the products of pyrolysis of flexible polyurethane foam generated at 900 °C or oxidation thermal decomposition of rigid polyurethane foam at 600 °C. Signs included hyperventilation followed by loss of muscle tone and limb reflexes, and then loss of consciousness. Venous blood [COHb] at the end of the exposure period ranged from 17 to 28 per cent, and whole blood cyanide ranged from 1.9 to 2.3 μg ml^{-1}. They noted that the CNS effects could be extreme because of the cytotoxic hypoxia and circulatory failure, and that the hyperventilation might produce cerebral arterioconstriction owing to the induced hypocapnia. Thomas and O'Flaherty (1979) demonstrated that the products of pyrolysis of polyurethane foam

inhibited brain and heart cytochrome oxidase activity which was positively correlated with blood cyanide concentrations. These and many other studies involving exposure of animals to the products of combustion from various nitrogen-containing polymeric materials have shown that significant inhalation dosages of HCN may be received resulting in physical incapacitation, coma, or lethality.

As with animal studies, there is a wealth of information suggesting that humans exposed to combustion products have absorbed cyanide. The first detailed description of cyanide in the blood of fire victims was given by Wetherell (1966) who found cyanide in the blood of 39 of 53 individuals dying in fires; the average concentration was 0.65 μg ml^{-1} (range 0.17–2.20 μg ml^{-1}). Other representative studies are as follows. Hart *et al.* (1985) described five subjects with smoke inhalation who were comatose on admission to hospital; blood cyanide ranged from 0.35 to 3.9 μg ml^{-1} (average 1.62 μg ml^{-1}). The subject with the highest blood cyanide died 4 days after admission. In postcrash aeroplane fires, Mohler (1975) reported blood cyanide in victims in the range of 0.01–3.9 μg ml^{-1}. In some cases, increased cyanide concentrations clearly indicate death from acute cyanide poisoning; for example, Tscuhiya (1977) described two persons found dead after a fire involving a polyurethane mattress with blood cyanide concentrations of 7.2 and 23.0 μg ml^{-1}, respectively.

Exposure to HCN vapour released in a fire can lead to muscle weakness, difficulty in coordination, physical incapacitation, a confusional state, and partial or complete loss of consciousness. This clearly will impede escape from the area of a fire. The high concentration of cyanide measured in fire casualties has raised the question of the use of cyanide antidotes in cases of severe smoke inhalation (Daunderer, 1979; Hart *et al.*, 1985). HCN as a product of combustion, and its significance, has been reviewed by Ballantyne (1987).

TOXIC INTER-RELATIONSHIPS BETWEEN FIRE GAS COMPONENTS

As has been repeatedly stressed, the fire atmosphere is a continually varying complex of numerous chemicals of differing chemical structure and differing toxicity. The acute and long-term hazards of many, but not all, individual components are known to varying extents. The influence of interactive factors on known toxicity and the potential for additional interactive toxicity is, however, poorly understood. Nevertheless, studies have been conducted for a few binary chemical systems. Several illustrative examples are given below, which demonstrate that even with such simple binary systems the hazard may vary according to the relative proportions of the components.

Hydrogen Cyanide–Carbon Monoxide

As CO and HCN coexist in a fire, this is a highly practical consideration, and has been discussed in detail by Ballantyne (1987). The approaches have been variable and have included mortality studies, measurements of blood cyanide and COHb, and assessment of physiological functions. Moss *et al.* (1951) found that simultaneous exposure to CO (2000 ppm) and HCN (10–20 ppm), both at individually sublethal concentrations, caused death. Smith *et al.* (1976) found that the times to death for rats exposed to an atmosphere containing 450 ppm HCN and 13500 ppm CO (3.7 ± 0.4 min; mean $\pm$ SD) were slightly longer than for corresponding concentration of HCN alone (10.9 ± 2.0 min; mean $\pm$ SD) or CO alone (5.8 ± 1.2 min; mean $\pm$ SD). Norris *et al.* (1986) investigated the effect of a 3-min inhalation exposure of mice to CO (0.63–0.66 per cent) on the lethal toxicity of intraperitoneal KCN (4–9 mg kg^{-1}). A significantly lower LD$_{50}$ for KCN (6.51; 6.04–7.00 mg kg^{-1}; mean with 95% CL) was found in CO-pretreated animals than in air-alone controls (7.0; 7.36–8.45 mg kg^{-1}; mean with 95% CL). In further studies they found evidence for a synergism between CO and KCN. The authors suggested that this may have been the result of augmentation of the inhibition of cytochrome oxidase in the CNS. Pitt *et al.* (1979) investigated the effects of CO and HCN on cerebral circulation and metabolism in the dog. When given together, CO and HCN increased cerebral blood flow in an additive manner; however, a significant decrease in cerebral oxygen consumption occurred with combined exposure to CO and HCN, neither of which alone had an effect. Ballantyne (1984, 1987) investigated the effects of differing pro-

portions of HCN and CO in the atmosphere on lethal toxicity and on blood cyanide and COHb concentrations, and determined that the contribution of either substance to toxicity depends in their absolute and relative atmospheric concentrations. Thus, when there was a marked excess of CO, the presence of HCN lowered the lethal inhalation dosage for CO by a less than additive toxicity; i.e. HCN physiologically potentiated (by hyperventilation) the toxicity of CO. When there was excess CO with respect to HCN, but not sufficient to produce a clear biochemical evidence of death from CO, then the blood picture indicated death not primarily from either CO or HCN. In these circumstances, because of the less than additive toxicity, it is likely that both are acting at a common target site, probably cytochrome oxidase. When CO and HCN are present in equal mass proportions, biochemical evidence indicates that death results from acute cyanide poisoning.

Carbon Monoxide–Carbon Dioxide

Nelson *et al.* (1978) found the 30-min lethal concentration of CO to rats was 6000 ppm, which was decreased to 2560 ppm in the presence of 1.44 per cent CO$_2$. Redkey and Collison (1979) found more rapid times to death in rats exposed to 6000 ppm CO with 4.5 per cent CO$_2$ (16.8 ± 0.6 min) compared with 6000 ppm alone. Levin *et al.* (1989), in detailed studies, found that above a certain concentration of CO (4100 ppm) some rats will die, and adding CO$_2$ has no influence. Below 2500 ppm CO the addition of CO$_2$ (up to 17.7 per cent) is not sufficient to produce mortality. However, with a CO concentration range of 2500–4100 ppm (which produces few mortalities *per se*) CO$_2$ (more than 1.5 per cent) will produce a higher level of mortality. They noted that CO and CO$_2$ act together by (1) increasing the rate of COHb formation, (2) producing a severe acidosis which was greater than the metabolic acidosis from CO alone or respiratory acidosis from CO$_2$ alone, and (3) prolonging the recovery period from acidosis.

INVESTIGATION OF THE TOXICOLOGICAL HAZARDS OF FIRES

Investigation into, and assessment of, potential adverse health effects from the products of combustion are complex exercises because of the multiplicity of thermolysis products and the variability of factors affecting the qualitative and quantitative nature of the products and the biological responses to them. Therefore, in respect of most practical situations it is possible only to give an overview of the products likely to be present under given conditions of thermolysis, and a qualitative assessment of hazards. Although detailed studies have been carried out on some binary systems, allowing quantitative assessments for interactions to be made, the majority of studies have been conducted on overall combustion products. An outline of the various approaches to investigating toxicological hazards from fires is given below; details can be found in Gad (1990b) and Kaplan (1988).

Physicochemical Studies on Thermolysis Products

These laboratory studies are concerned with the analytical determination of the chemical nature and relative proportions of substances produced by thermolysis of materials under differing conditions. Ideally, the analyses should be conducted under the following conditions: simple heating, complete combustion, oxidative pyrolysis, and anaerobic pyrolysis. It is thus necessary to subject materials to a range of temperatures in atmospheres of differing oxygen content, with the resultant effluent being analyzed by appropriate instrumental procedures. In some instances, highly toxic materials may be generated over a narrow temperature range, and if a differential temperature study is not performed this may be missed. In addition to the influence of temperature and oxygen availability on the materials generated from combustion, it is important to study the nature of the materials generated as a function of time period in the combustion phase because the pattern may change appreciably. A few examples are given in Table 3 to illustrate the influence of variables on combustion products.

From a knowledge of the nature of the materials generated, under different conditions of combustion, it may be possible to give a hazard pattern for a given material providing that adequate information on toxicology is available. In some cases a major hazardous material may be identified from a large number of analytically detected substances produced by combustion of a specific material. With polyvinyl chloride (PVC) about 75 organic products have been detected on thermal decomposition, most being aliphatic or aromatic hydrocarbons (Wooley, 1971). However, a major product which begins to be liberated at 200–300 °C is hydrogen chloride, and it is estimated that 1 kg of PVC may yield about 400 g of hydrogen chloride on complete combustion. Hydrogen chloride causes sensory irritation of the eyes and respiratory tract, and in sufficient concentrations may cause inflammatory lesions in the respiratory tract. PVC combustion is recognized as a major hazard in fires involving modern buildings (Dyer and Esch, 1976).

The small-scale laboratory tests yield useful, though often preliminary, information on the nature of combustion products generated from specific materials under defined conditions and allow a qualitative assessment of the hazards that may be encountered for a specific material in a fire. The majority of fires, however, involve the burning of a multiplicity of materials including structural and furnishing components. In an attempt to obtain more reliable information it may be desirable to undertake large-scale experimental fires with appropriate instrumentation. Such tests are likely to be expensive and require careful planning, specifically with regard to sampling and analysis of the atmosphere. Guidance on the design of large-scale tests will clearly be obtained from preliminary small-scale laboratory combustion product studies.

Animal Exposure Studies

In the strictly physicochemical analytical approach to defining the nature and relative proportions of combustion products generated from specific materials, the likely hazard of the effluent smoke is determined by attempting to predict the probable combined toxicity of the constituents in the smoke from a knowledge of their individual toxicities. Such an approach may produce misleading predictions because there is the possibility of chemical and toxicological interactions, including synergism. Attempts have therefore been made to determine the toxicity of smokes from specific material by exposing animals to the products of thermolysis and monitoring for adverse effects by standard and special procedures. Such tests readily lend themselves to observations on irritancy and acute toxicity. Irritancy will give an index of potentially harassing and incapacitating properties of effluent smoke from the material, and the acute toxicity an indication of lethal potential or obvious non-lethal adverse effects such as lung damage, or neurobehavioural abnormalities. Such tests are frequently carried out with the smoke being generated under differing conditions of atmospheric oxygen content and thermolysis temperature. For comparative purposes the findings are frequently referred to tests from the burning of a standard material, usually wood. Although such tests give useful information in themselves, they are particularly valuable when viewed in the light of studies on the analysis of combustion products generated under similar conditions. Thus, when interpreting laboratory data in an attempt to define possible hazards from combustion products of materials it is highly desirable to have information on both the nature and relative proportions of combustion products and on their effects on experimental animals exposed to combustion products generated under similar conditions. Where appropriate facilities and expertise exist it is possible to combine analytical studies with animal exposure tests. Also, animal exposures have been performed in large-scale fire tests.

Problems may be encountered in defining the presence of novel or highly toxic materials for several reasons; first, because of the multiplicity of materials generated there may be limitations in analytical capability and second, the toxicology of some materials generated may be unknown. However, animal studies may draw attention to the presence of highly toxic, or unsuspected, materials in a test atmosphere. This may be illustrated by investigations on a fire-retarded polyurethane foam. The products from non-flaming combustion of a trimethylol-propane-based rigid urethane foam fire retarded with an organophosphate, *O,O*-diethyl-*N,N*-bis(2-hydroxyethyl)-aminomethyl phosphonate, were found to produce grand mal seizures in rats; similar effects were not observed when the foam was not fire retarded (Petajan *et al.*, 1974). Subsequent chemical analysis revealed the presence of 4-ethyl-1-phospha-2,6,7-trioxabicyclo[2,2,2]octane-1-oxide in the smoke (Voorhees *et al.*, 1975). This is a material of high acute toxicity (Kimmerle, 1976). Further work demonstrated no unusual toxicity when the flame-retarded polyurethane foam was either gradually or rapidly pyrolyzed to 800 °C in the absence of air; however, convulsions were observed when the material was flash pyrolyzed in the presence of air flow (Hilado and Schneider, 1977). See Purser (1992) for a discussion of caged bicyclophosphorus esters in combustion processes.

Combustion Toxicity Apparatus

Several apparatuses are currently available: the DIN 53-436 (a German standard), the radiant furnace (an ASTM draft standard), and the University of Pittsburgh furnace (an ASTM draft standard and legislated in the State of New York). The selection of the apparatus will depend on the combustion conditions that are to be simulated. Some possible combustion conditions are smouldering, flaming, preflashover and postflashover. These apparatuses have different capabilities for simulating these combustion conditions.

The DIN 53-438

The combustion device is a moving annular furnace encircling a quartz tube containing the test specimen. The intent of this design is to generate a consistent combustion environment for the time course of the experiment even though the animal exposure is dynamic. The furnace temperature is a fixed value during the experiment but that value can range between 100 and 900 °C. The animals are rats, and the exposure is head only. After the exposure, the animals are retained for a 2-week postexposure period. Selection of the temperature can determine the combustion conditions of the test specimen for non-flaming or flaming mode.

The Radiant Furnace

The combustion device is a set of four quartz lamps designed to subject the test specimen to a heat flux density ranging from 2 to 7 kW m^{-2}. The animal exposure to the combustion products is static. The animals are rats, and the exposure is head only. The rats are observed for 2 weeks after exposure. The combustion conditions can be selected by changing the heat flux density and implementing the use of a piloted ignition source. Thus, non-flaming and flaming conditions can be investigated. The LCt_{50} (median lethal concentration × time of exposure) value is expressed as (mg min l^{-1}). The methodology is currently an ASTM draft standard.

The University of Pittsburgh

The combustion device is basically a muffle furnace. The test specimen is subjected to a ramping temperature of 20 °C per min. The animal exposure to the combustion products is dynamic. The animals are mice, and the exposure is head only. After the test specimen has lost 1 per cent of its initial weight, the combustion products are presented to the animals. The exposure period is ended 30 min later. For 10 min after the exposure period the animals are observed. The combustion conditions are the same for all test specimens. However, the test specimen can react differently to those conditions, thereby combusting in a non-flaming or flaming mode. The critical variable appears to be the weight of the specimen. The smaller weight specimens will not necessarily spontaneously flame, while larger weight specimens may spontaneously flame. Thus, more than one LC_{50} value can be obtained for a test substance (Norris, 1990). The LC_{50} value is expressed as grams. This is the weight of the test specimen placed in the furnace which is calculated to kill 50 per cent of the animals. The State of New York legislated that certain building products be tested by this procedure and the results filed with the state before the products could be sold. New York City also uses this test for pass/fail criteria for some building materials. The methodology is currently an ASTM draft standard.

Studies on Exposed Human Populations

Valuable and unique information may be obtained about the adverse effects of exposure to fire atmospheres, and on the possible long-term hazards of recurrent exposures to fires, by appropriate studies on the victims of fires and on firefighters. Major sources of information have been derived from post-mortem examination of fire victims; clinical, radiological and clinical chemistry examination of non-lethal fire victims; and routine medical examination and special epidemiological studies of firefighters. In the context of

defining the requirement for respiratory and other protective equipment by firefighters based on the medical and epidemiological data, short-term repeated and chronic exposure situations as well as acute exposures all require consideration.

Toxic Hazard and Hazard Analysis

In 1986 the US National Institute of Building Sciences initiated a program to develop a performance toxicity test to characterize building products. This performance test was developed so that it incorporated additional fire parameters, such as the LC_{50} value, time to ignition, and mass loss rate. The concern was that regulation of products was to occur based solely on the LC_{50} values. As a hazard analysis was not available, this was viewed as an interim step until the complete hazard analysis could be established (Norris, 1988). The methodology is currently an ASTM draft standard.

The direction for the utilization of combustion toxicity data has been to include them in hazard analysis. These analyses include other fire performance parameters, such as time to ignition, flame spread, heat release rate, etc. The fire scenario is also a part of these analyses. The US National Institute of Standards and Technology has developed a hazard analysis called HAZARD 1 Fire Hazard Assessment Method (Bukowski *et al.*, 1989).

CHEMICAL HAZARDS TO FIREFIGHTERS

Firefighting is one of the most hazardous of professions, having an associated high level of morbidity and mortality, with the most important health concerns being as follows.

(1) *Trauma*: notably from falling objects, in rescue situations, and during close-in firefighting.
(2) *Thermal*: primary burns to the skin and respiratory tract, and heat stress. The latter is a function of environmental temperature, insulating properties of protective clothing, and endogenous heat production from severe physical exertion compounded by the additional weight of equipment such as self-contained breathing apparatus.

(3) *Ergonomic*: the high energy costs of fire-fighting may clearly be interrelated with, and compounded by, other health concerns.

(4) *Psychological*: these are multiple in nature and include the thought of personal security, victim rescue and loss, emotional scenes, and heavy social responsibility (Guidotti and Clough, 1992).

(5) *Toxic chemicals*: sequential exposures to smoke and chemicals, often at high concentrations, which are known or suspect of producing acute and/or long-term health problems. An outline of this aspect of health concern is presented below; details are available from Guidotti and Clough (1992).

Firefighters are recurrently exposed to a large variety of materials that may cause acute, cumulative, and/or chronic health problems; typical examples are carbon monoxide, hydrogen cyanide, sulphur dioxide, hydrogen chloride, phosgene, isocyanates, oxides of nitrogen, acrolein, acetaldehyde, asbestos, polycyclic aromatic hydrocarbons, and benzene. That such materials may be absorbed has been suggested by several studies; for example, that firefighters absorb HCN is indicated by increased serum thiocyanate concentrations (Levine and Radford, 1978). As expected, several studies have demonstrated that firefighters have increased blood COHb concentrations. Sammons and Coleman (1974) found a significant difference in COHb concentrations between non-smoking firemen (mean 5.0 per cent, range 2.5–13.9 per cent) and non-smoking controls (mean 2.3 per cent, range 1.0–11.7 per cent). Similarly, Radford and Levine (1976) found increased COHb concentrations in firemen after fighting a fire (4.53 per cent) compared with unexposed controls (2.17 per cent). Increased COHb concentrations were also found after fire-fighting by Loke *et al.* (1970) and Levy *et al.* (1976) (Figure 3).

Respiratory Disease

Several studies have shown that exposure to a fire atmosphere produces acute changes in pulmonary function and may be a factor in the development of chronic lung dysfunction. Musk *et al.* (1979) studied acute changes in firefighters during routine duties and found an average decrease of FEV_1 (forced expiratory volume in 1 s) of 0.05 l

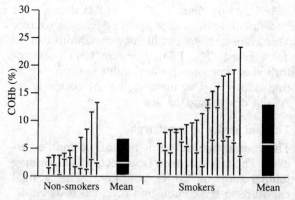

Figure 3 Increases in COHb concentration in firefighters following exposure to smoke. The lower bars represent COHb pre-exposure, and the upper bars the increase in COHb post-exposure. Drawn from data in Levy *et al.* (1976) and Loke *et al.* (1970) by permission

which was related to subjectively assessed smoke exposure; decreases in FEV_1 of 0.1 l or more were found in 30 per cent of cases. Brandt-Rauf *et al.* (1989) found that for firefighters not wearing respiratory protective equipment, there were statistically significant postfire decrements in FEV_1 and FVC (forced vital capacity). Pre- and postfire average FEV_1 values were respectively 3.80 l and 3.61 l, and FVC values 5.03 l and 4.81 l ($n = 14$).

For cumulative effects, Peabody (1977) reported a decrease in pulmonary function for San Diego firefighters which was significantly greater than that of the general population. Peters *et al.* (1974), over a 2-year period, found that the rate of decline in pulmonary function, measured by FVC and FEV_1, was twice the expected rate; these changes were significantly related to frequency of exposure. A raised risk for emphysema was found in a mortality study by Demers *et al.* (1992). The importance of respiratory protective equipment was shown in a study by Tepper *et al.* (1991) who reevaluated 632 Baltimore city firemen 6–10 years after baseline measurements, and found that in those who never wore a mask there was a 1.7 times greater decline than in mask wearers.

Cardiovascular Disease

Some epidemiological studies do not show an excess of cardiovascular disease among firemen (Beaumont *et al.*, 1991; Demers *et al.*, 1992). Summarizing the available evidence, Guidotti (1992) states that population-based mortality and disability surveillance studies suggest a relatively small but significant excess of disability, but not mortality, for non-malignant cardiovascular disease for firefighters. More targeted cohort and case-control studies do not support such an excess, but suggest a strong healthy worker effect. However, some studies suggest an excess of coronary artery disease (Musk *et al.*, 1978).

Reproductive Hazards

Many of the chemicals that are found in a fire atmosphere have been associated with potential adverse reproductive effects (McDiarmid *et al.*, 1991). In spite of this, little epidemiological evidence is available on the reproductive hazards of fire fighting. One study has indicated a possible excess of birth defects in children of firefighters (Olshan *et al.*, 1990). Also, it has been noted that peak carbon monoxide concentrations measured in fires could be immediately dangerous to an unprotected woman firefighter and her foetus (McDiarmid *et al.*, 1991). There is a clear need for further investigation into the reproductive hazards of firefighting.

Carcinogenic Hazards

Several known or suspect carcinogens are present, to variable extents, in fire atmospheres; for example, polycyclic aromatic hydrocarbons, acrylonitrile, vinyl chloride, asbestos, formaldehyde and PCBs. There are some inconsistencies between various studies on the possible excesses of cancers in firefighters. Biological monitoring for genotoxic effects, including sister chromatid exchanges and polycyclic aromatic hydrocarbon-DNA adducts in peripheral blood, suggests a potential for carcinogenic effects (Liou *et al.*, 1989). Particular sites for neoplasms, possibly occupationally related to firefighting, are buccal and pharyngeal (Mastromatteo, 1974), oesophageal (Beaumont *et al.*, 1991), colonorectal (Guidotti and Clough, 1992), brain (Howe and Burch, 1990; Demers *et al.*, 1992), lymphatic and leukaemic (Demers *et al.*, 1992). Documentation for an association between lung cancer and occupational exposures is inconsistent. A Danish study (Hansen, 1990) reported an SMR of 317 for older firefighters, but studies from San Francisco (Beaumont *et al.*, 1991) and Buffalo (Vena and Fielder, 1987) showed no excess. Cigarette smoking is a clear confounding factor (Liou *et al.*, 1989), although according to one study the incidence of smoking among firemen is not excessive compared with other occupations (Gerace, 1990). The excesses of certain cancers may be the result of interaction of several factors; for example, toxic substances, alcohol and smoking (Beaumont *et al.*, 1991). Ford *et al.* (1992) suggest that the immunological detection of serum β-transforming growth factor-related proteins may be a possible biomarker for monitoring firefighters for potential development of cancer.

REFERENCES

Alarie, Y. (1985). The toxicity of smoke from polymeric materials during thermal decomposition. *Ann. Rev. Pharmacol. Toxicol.*, **25**, 325–347

Alexeff, G. and Packham, S. C. (1984). Evaluation of smoke toxicity using concentration–time products. *J. Fire Sci.*, **2**, 362

Anderson, E. W., Andelman, R. J., Strauch, J. M. *et al.* (1973). Effect of low-level exposure on onset and duration of angina pectoris. *Ann. Intern. Med.*, **79**, 46–50

Anderson, R. A., Thomson, I. and Harland, W. A. (1979). The importance of cyanide and organic nitriles in fire fatalities. *Fire and Materials*, **3**, 91–99

Andrasch, R. H., Foster, F., Lawson, W. H. *et al.* (1975). Meat wrappers asthma: an appraisal of a new occupational syndrome. *J. Allergy Clin. Immunol.*, **55**, 130

Aronow, W. S. (1976). Effect of cigarette smoking and of carbon monoxide on coronary heart disease. *Chest*, **70**, 514–518

Autian, J. (1976). Medical aspects of toxicity resulting from fire exposures. In *Physiological and Toxicological Aspects of Combustion Products*. National Research Council, National Academy of Science, Washington, DC. pp. 47–56

Ayres, S. M., Giannelli, S. and Mueller, H. (1973). Carboxyhaemoglobin and the access to oxygen. *Arch. Environ. Health*, **216**, 8–15

Ballantyne, B. (1981). Inhalation hazards of fire. In Ballantyne, B. and Schwabe, P. H. (Eds), *Respiratory Protection: Principles and Applications*. Chapman and Hall, London. pp. 351–372

Ballantyne, B. (1984). Relative toxicity of carbon monoxide and hydrogen cyanide in combined atmospheres. *Toxicologist*, **4**, 69

Ballantyne, B. (1987). Hydrogen cyanide as a product of combustions and a factor in morbidity and mortality from fires. In Ballantyne, B. and Marrs, T. C. (Eds), *Clinical and Experimental Toxicology of Cyanides*, Wright, Bristol, pp. 248–291

Ballantyne, B. (1989). Toxicology. In *Encyclopedia of*

Polymer Science and Engineering, vol. 16. John Wiley, New York, pp. 879–930

Barnard, R. J. (1979). Coronary artery disease deaths in the Toronto Fire Department. *J. Occup. Med.*, **29**, 132–135

Beaumont, J. J., Chu, G. S. T., Jones, J. R., Schenker, M. B., Singleton, J. A., Piantanida, L. S. and Reiterman, M. (1991). An epidemiological study of cancer and other causes of mortality in San Francisco firefighters. *Am. J. Industr. Health*, **19**, 357–372

Bertol, E., Mari, F., Orzalies, G. and Volpato, I. (1983). Combustion products from various kinds of fibres: toxicologic hazards from smoke exposure. *Forensic Sci. Int.*, **22**, 111–116

Birky, M. M., Malek, D. and Paabo, M. (1985). Study of biological specimens obtained from victims of MGM Grand Hotel fire. *J. Anal. Toxicol.*, **7**, 265–271

Bowes, P. C. (1974). Smoke and toxicity hazards of plastics in fire. *Ann. Occup. Hyg.*, **17**, 143–157

Brandt-Rauf, P. W., Cosman, B., Fallon, L. F. Jr., (1989). Health hazards of firefighters: acute pulmonary effects after toxic exposure. *Br. J. Industr. Med.*, **46**, 209–211

Brooks, S. M. (1983). Bronchial asthma of occupational origin. In Rom, W. N. (Ed.), *Environmental and Occupational Medicine*. Little, Brown and Co., Boston, pp. 242–243

Brooks, S. M., Weiss, M. A. and Bernstein, I. L. (1985). Reactive airways dysfunction syndrome (RADS). *Chest*, **88**, 376–384

Bukowski, R. M., Peacock, R. D., Jones, W. W. and Forney, C. L. (1989). *HAZARD 1—Fire Hazard Assessment Method, NIST Handbook*, 146 (3 vols). National Institute of Standards and Technology, Washington, D.C.

Cade, J. F. (1984). Respiration. In Campbell, E. J. M., Dickinson, E. J., Slater, D. J. H., Edwards, C. R. W. and Sikora, E. K. (Eds), *Clinical Physiology*. Blackwell Scientific Publications, Oxford, pp. 96–153

Campbell, E. J. M., Dickinson, E. J., Slater, D. J. H., Edwards, C. R. W. and Sikora, E. K. (1984). *Clinical Physiology*. Blackwell Scientific Publications, Oxford, pp. 116–118

Chance, D. M., Goldbaum, L. R. and Lappas, N. T. (1986). Factors affecting the loss of carbon monoxide from stored blood samples. *J. Anal. Toxicol.*, **10**, 181–189

Cramer, D. R. (1982). Fetal death due to accidental maternal carbon monoxide poisoning. *J. Toxicol., Clin. Toxicol.*, **19**, 297–301

Daunderer, M. (1979). Fatal smoke inhalation of hydrogen cyanide from smouldering fires. *Fortsch. Med.*, **97**, 1401–1405

DeBias, D. A., Banerjee, C. M., Birkhead, N. C., Greene, C. H., Scott, S. D. and Harrer, W. V. (1976). Effect of carbon monoxide inhalation on ventricular fibrillation. *Arch. Environ. Health*, **31**, 42–46

DeKorver, L. (1976). Smoke problems in urban fire control. In *Physiological and Toxicological Aspects of Combustion Products*. National Research Council, National Academy of Sciences, Washington, DC, pp. 4–10

Demers, P. H., Heyes, N. J. and Rosenstock, L. (1992). Mortality among firefighters from three Northwestern United States Cities. *Br. J. Industr. Med.*, **49**, 664–670

Dyer, R. F. and Esch, V. H. (1976). Polyvinyl chloride toxicity in fires. *J. Am. Med. Assoc.*, **235**, 393–397

Ford, J., Smith, S., Luo, J.-C. (1992). Serum growth factors and oncoproteins in firefighters. *Occup. Med.*, **42**, 39–42

Frostling, H., Huff, A., Jacobsson, S., Pfaffli, P., Vainiotalo, S. and Zittino, A. (1984). Analytical, occupational and toxicologic aspects of the degradation products of polypropylene plastics. *Scand. J. Work Environ. Health*, **10**, 163–169

Gad, S. C. (1990a). In Gad, S. C. and Anderson, R. C. (Eds), *Combustion Toxicology*. CRC Press, Boca Raton, pp. 1–16

Gad, S. C. (1990b). Combustion toxicity testing. In Gad, S. C. and Anderson, R. C. (Eds), *Combustion Toxicology*. CRC Press, Boca Raton, pp. 81–128

Ganong, W. F. (1977). *Review of Medical Physiology*. Large Medical Publications, California, p. 511

Gantz, N. M. (1988). Infectious agents. In Levy, B. S. and Wegman, D. H. (Eds), *Occupational Health*, Little Brown and Co., Boston, pp. 281–295

Gerace, T. A. (1990). Road to a smoke-free service for Florida: policies and progress. *J. Public. Health Policy*, **11**, 206–217

Goldbaum, L. R. (1977). Is carboxyhemoglobin concentration the indicator of carbon monoxide toxicity? *Legal Med. Ann.*, **176**, 165–170

Goldbaum, L. R., Orellando, T. and Dergal, E. (1976). Mechanism of the toxic action of carbon monoxide. *Ann. Clin. Lab. Sci.*, **6**, 372–376

Goldstein, D. P. (1965). Carbon monoxide poisoning in pregnancy. *Am. J. Obstet. Gynecol.*, **9**, 526–528

Guidotti, T. L. (1992). Human factors in firefighting: ergonomic-, cardiopulmonary-, and psychogenic stress-related issues. *Int. Arch. Occup. Environ. Health*, **64**, 1–12

Guidotti, T. L. and Clough, V. M. (1992). Occupational health concerns of firefighting. *Ann. Rev. Public Health*, **13**, 151–171

Hansen, E. S. (1990). A cohort study on the mortality of firefighters. *Br. J. Industr. Med.*, **47**, 805–809

Harland, W. A. and Wooley, W. D. (1979). Fire fatality study—University of Glasgow. *Building Research Establishment Information Paper No. 18/79*. Fire Research Station, Borehamwood, Herts, UK

Hart, G. B., Strauss, M. B., Lennon, P. A. and Whitcraft, D. D. (1985). Treatment of smoke inhalation by hyperbaric oxygen. *J. Emerg. Med.*, **3**, 211–215

Hathaway, G. J., Proctor, W. H., Hughes, J. P. and Fishmann, M. C. (1991). *Chemical Hazards of the*

Workplace, 3rd edn. Van Nostrand Reinhold, New York, pp. 393–395; 485

Hilado, C. J. and Schneider, J. E. (1977). Toxicity studies of a polyurethane rigid foam. *J. Combust. Toxicol.*, **4**, 79–86

Howe, G. R. and Burch, J. D. (1990). Firefighting and risk of cancer: an assessment and overview of the epidemiologic evidence. *Am. J. Epidemiol.*, **132**, 1039–1050

Hubbard, G. B., Langinais, P. C., Shimazu, T. *et al.* (1991). The morphology of smoke inhalation injury in sheep. *J. Trauma*, **31**, 1477–1486

Jankovic, J., Jones, W., Burkhart, J. and Noonan, G. (1991). Environmental study of firefighters. *Ann. Occup. Hyg.*, **35**, 581–602

Jellinek, H. H. G. and Takada, K. (1977). Toxic gas evolution from polymers: evolutions of hydrogen cyanide from polyurethanes. *J. Polymer Sci.*, **15**, 2269–2288

Kaplan, H. L. (1988). Evaluating the combustion hazards of combustion products. In Gad, S. C. (Ed.), *Product Safety Evaluation Handbook*. Marcel Dekker, New York, pp. 409–470

Kimmerle, G. (1976). Toxicity of combustion products with particular reference to polyurethane. *Ann. Occup. Hyg.*, **19**, 269–273

Levin, B. C., Paato, M., Gurman, J. L. *et al.* (1989). Toxicologic interaction between carbon monoxide and carbon dioxide. *Toxicology*, **47**, 135–164

Levin, B. C., Rechani, P. R., Gurman, J. L. *et al.* (1990). Analysis of carboxyhemoglobin and cyanide in blood from victims of the Dupont Plaza Hotel fire in Puerto Rico. *J. Fire Sci.*, **35**, 151–168

Levine, S. and Radford, E. P. (1978). Occupational exposure to cyanide in Baltimore firefighters. *J. Occup. Med.*, **20**, 53–56

Levy, S. A. (1988). An overview of occupational pulmonary disorders. In Zeng, C. (Ed.), *Occupational Medicine*, 2nd edn. Year Book Medical Publishing, Chicago, pp. 201–225

Levy, A. L., Lum, G. and Abeles, F. J. (1976). Carbon monoxide in firemen before and after exposure to smoke. *Ann. Clin. Lab. Sci.*, **6**, 455–458

Levy, S. A., Storey, J. D. and Plashko, B. E. (1978). Meat worker's asthma. *J. Occup. Med.*, **15**, 116–117

Liou, S-H., Jacobson-Kram, D., Poirer, M. C., Nguyen, D., Strickland, P. T. and Tockman, M. S. (1989). Biological monitoring of firefighters: sister chromatid exchanges and polycyclic aromatic hydrocarbon–DNA adducts in peripheral blood cells. *Cancer Res.*, **49**, 4929–4935

Loke, J., Farmer, W. C., Mattham, R. A. (1970). Carboxyhemoglobin levels in firefighters. *Lung*, **154**, 35–39

Longo, L. D. (1976). Carbon monoxide effects on oxygenation of fetus in utero. *Science*, **194**, 523–525

Longo, L. D. (1977). The biological effects of carbon monoxide on pregnant women, fetuses, and newborn infants. *Am. J. Obstet. Gynecol.*, **129**, 69–103

McDiarmid, M. A., Lees, P. S. J., Agnew, J., Midzenski, M. and Duffy, R. (1991). Reproductive hazards of firefighting. 11 Chemical hazards. *Am. J. Industr. Med.*, **19**, 447–472

Margulies, S. L. (1986). Acute carbon monoxide poisoning during pregnancy. *Am. J. Emerg. Med.*, **4**, 516–519

Mastromatteo, E. (1974). Mortality in city firemen. *Arch. Industr. Health*, **20**, 1–7

Mayes, R. W. (1991). The toxicological examination of victims of the British Air Tours Boeing 727 Accident at Manchester 1988. *J. Forensic Sci.*, **36**, 179–184

Mayes, R., Levine, B., Smith, M. L. *et al.* (1992). Toxicologic findings in the USS Iowa Disaster. *J. Forensic Sci.*, **37**, 1352–1357

Michal, J. (1976). Toxicity of pyrolysis and combustion products of polyvinyl chloride. *Fire and Materials*, **1**, 57–62

Mitera, J. and Michal, J. (1985). The combustion products of polymeric materials. 11. GC-MS analysis of the combustion products of polyethylene, polypropylene, polystyrene and polyamide. *Fire and Materials*, **9**, 11–28

Mohler, S. R. (1975). Air crash survival: injuries and evacuation hazards. *Aviation, Space Environ. Med.*, **46**, 86–88

Morikawa, T. (1976). Acrolein, formaldehyde, and volatile fatty acids from smouldering combustion. *J. Combust. Toxicol.*, **3**, 135–150

Morikawa, T. (1978). Evaluation of hydrogen cyanide during combustion and pyrolysis. *J. Combust. Toxicol.*, **5**, 315–338

Moss, R. H., Jackson, C. F. and Saberlick, J. (1951). Toxicity of carbon monoxide and hydrogen cyanide gas mixtures. *Arch. Industr. Hyg. Occup. Med.*, **4**, 53–60

Muller, G. L. and Graham, S. (1955). Intrauterine death of the fetus due to accidental carbon monoxide poisoning. *N. Engl. J. Med.*, **252**, 1075–1078

Musk, A. W., Morison, B. R., Peters, J. M. and Peters, R. K. (1978). Mortality among Boston firefighters, 1915–1975. *Br. J. Industr. Med.*, **35**, 104–108

Musk, A. W., Smith, T. J., Peters, J. M. and McLaughlin, E. (1979). Pulmonary function in firefighters: acute changes in ventilatory capacity and their correlates. *Br. J. Industr. Med.*, **36**, 29–34

Nelson, G. L., Hixon, E. J. and Denine, E. P. (1978). Combustion product toxicity studies of burning plastics. *J. Combust. Toxicol.*, **5**, 222–238

Niemann, G.-F., Clark, W. R., Goyette, D. *et al.* (1989). Wood smoke inhalation increases pulmonary microvascular permeability. *Surgery*, **105**, 481–487

Nomiyama, K., Matsui, K. and Nomiyama, H. (1980). Environmental temperature, a factor modifying the acute toxicity of organic solvents, heavy metals, and agricultural chemicals. *Toxicol. Lett.*, **6**, 67–70

Norris, J. C. (1988). National Institute of Building

Sciences Toxicity Hazard Test. In *Proceedings of the Joint Meeting of the Fire Retardant Chemicals Association and the Society of Plastics Engineers*, Technomic Publishing, Lancaster, PA, pp. 146–155

Norris, J. C. (1990). Investigation of the Dual LC_{50} Values of Woods Using the University of Pittsburgh Combustion Toxicity Apparatus. *Standardization News STP*, **1082**, 57–71

Norris, J. C., Moore, S. J. and Hume, A. S. (1986). Synergistic lethality induced by the combustion of carbon monoxide and cyanide. *Toxicology*, **40**, 121–129

Olshan, A. F., Teschke, K. and Baird, P. A. (1990). Birth defect among offspring of firemen. *Am. J. Epidemiol.*, **131**, 312–321

Paabo, M., Birky, M. M. and Womble, S. E. (1979). Analysis of hydrogen cyanide in fire environments. *J. Combust. Toxicol.*, **6**, 99–108

Packham, S. C. and Hartzell, G. E. (1981). Fundamentals of combustion toxicology in fire hazard assessment. *J. Test Eval.*, **9**, 341

Peabody, M. D., (1977). Pulmonary function and the firefighter. *J. Combust. Toxicol.*, **4**, 8–15

Petajan, J. H., Voorhees, K. J., Packham, S. C., Baldwin, R. C., Einborn, I. N., Grunnet, M. L., Dinger, B. G. and Birky, M. M. (1974). Extreme toxicity from combustion products of a fire-retarded polyurethane foam. *Science*, **187**, 742–744

Peters, J. M., Therrault, G. P., Fine, L. J. and Wegman, D. H. (1974). Chronic effects of firefighting on pulmonary function. *N. Engl. J. Med.*, **291**, 1320–1322

Pitt, B. R., Radford, E. P., Qurtner, G. H. and Traystman, R. J. (1979). Interaction of carbon monoxide and cyanide on cerebral circulation and metabolism. *Arch. Environ. Health*, **34**, 354–359

Purser, D. A. (1992). Combustion toxicology of anticholinesterases. In Ballantyne, B. and Marrs, T. C. (Eds), *Clinical and Experimental Toxicology of Organophosphates and Carbamates*. Butterworth-Heinemann, Oxford, pp. 386–395

Purser, D. A. and Wooley, W. D. (1983). Biological studies of combustion atmospheres. *J. Fire Sci.*, **1**, 118–144

Purser, D. A. and Grimshaw, P. (1984). The incapacitative effects of exposure to the thermal decomposition products of polyurethane foams. *Fire and Materials*, **8**, 10–16

Purser, D. A., Grimshaw, P. and Berrill, K. R. (1984). Intoxication of cyanide in fires: a study in monkeys using acrylonitrile. *Arch. Environ. Health*, **39**, 394–400

Radford, E. P. and Levine, M. S. (1976). Occupational exposure to carbon monoxide in Baltimore firefighters. *J. Occup. Med.*, **18**, 628–632

Radford, E. P., Pitt, B., Halpin, B., Caplan, Y., Fisher, R. and Schwedia, P. (1976). Study in five deaths in Maryland, September 1971–January 1974. In *Physiological and Toxicological Aspects of Combustion Products*. National Research Council, National Academy of Science, Washington, DC, pp. 26–35

Redkey, F. L. and Collison, H. A. (1979). Effect of oxygen and carbon dioxide in carbon monoxide toxicity. *J. Combust. Toxicol.*, **6**, 208–212

Sammons, J. H. and Coleman, R. L. (1974). Firefighters occupational exposure to carbon monoxide. *J. Occup. Med.*, **16**, 543–546

Sanders, D. C. and Endecott, B. R. (1991). The effect of elevated temperature on carbon monoxide-induced incapacitation. *J. Fire Sci.*, **9**, 296–300

Shirani, K. Z., Puritt, B. A., McManus, W. F. and Mason, A. D. (1986). The influence of inhalation injury and pneumonia on burn mortality. *Proc. Am. Burns Assoc.*, **18**, 131

Smith, P. W., Crane, C. R., Sanders, D. C., Abbot, S. K. and Endecott, B. (1976). Effect of carbon monoxide exposure to carbon monoxide and hydrogen cyanide. In *Physiological and Toxicological Aspects of Combustion Products*. National Research Council, National Academy of Science, Washington, DC, pp. 75–88

Stark, G. W. V. (1974). Smoke and toxic gases from burning plastics. *Building Research Establishment Current Paper 5/74*. Building Research Establishment, Fire Research Station, Borehamwood, Herts., UK

Stewart, R. D. (1974). The effect of carbon monoxide on man. *J. Combust. Toxicol.*, **1**, 167–176

Symington, I. S., Anderson, R. A., Oliver, J. S., Thomson, I., Harland, W. A. and Kerr, W. J. (1978). Cyanide exposure in fires. *Lancet*, July 8, pp. 91–92

Tepper, A., Comstock, G. W. and Levine, M. (1991). A longitudinal study of pulmonary function in firefighters. *Am. J. Industr. Med.*, **20**, 307–316

Thomas, W. C. and O'Flaherty, E. J. (1979). Cytochrome a oxidase activity in tissues of rats exposed to polyurethane pyrolysis fumes. *Toxicol. Appl. Pharmacol.*, **49**, 463–472

Tscuhiya, Y. (1977). Significance of HCN generation in fire gases. *J. Combust. Toxicol.*, **3**, 363–370

Urhas, E. and Kullik, E. (1977). Pyrolysis gas chromatographic analysis of some toxic compounds from nitrogen-containing fibres. *J. Chromatog.*, **137**, 210–214

Vandevort, R. and Brooks, S. M. (1979). Polyvinyl chloride fibre decomposition products as an occupational illness. I. Environmental exposures and toxicology. *J. Occup. Med.*, **19**, 189–191

Vena, J. E. and Fielder, R. C. (1987). Mortality of a municipal-worker cohort. IV Firefighters. *Am. J. Industr. Med.*, **11**, 671–684

Voorhees, K. J., Einhorn, I. N., Hileman, F. D. and Wojcik, C. H. (1975). The identification of a highly toxic bicyclophosphate in the combustion products of a fire-related urethane foam. *Polymer Lett.*, **13**, 293–297

Wetherell, H. R. (1966). The occurrence of cyanide in blood in fire victims. *J. Forensic Sci.*, **11**, 167–172

Wooley, W. D. (1971). Decomposition products of PVC. *Br. Polymer. J.*, **3**, 186–193

Wooley, W. D. (1972). Nitrogen-containing products from the thermal decomposition of flexible polyurethane foam. *J. Combust. Toxicol.*, **1**, 259–267

Wooley, W. D. (1974). The production of free tolylene diisocyanate (TDI) from the thermal decomposition of flexible polyurethane foam. *J. Combust. Toxicol.*, **1**, 259–276

Wooley, W. D. (1982). Smoke and toxic gas productions from burning polymers. *J. Macromolec. Sci. Chem.*, **A17**, 1–33

Yamamoto, Y. (1975). Acute toxicity of the combustion products from various kinds of fibers. *Z. Rechtsmed.*, **77**, 11–26

Young, W., Hilando, C. J., Kourtides, D. A. and Parker, D. S. (1976). A study of the toxicity of pyrolysis gases from synthetic polymers. *J. Combust. Toxicol.*, **3**, 157–165

Zachria, B. A. (1972). Inhalation injuries in fires. In *Approach to Halogenated Fire Extinguishing Materials*. National Academy of Science, Washington, DC, pp. 42–52

Zarem, H. A., Rattenberg, C. L. and Harmer, M. A. (1973). Carbon monoxide toxicity in human fire victims. *Arch. Surg.*, **107**, 851–853

Zawacki, B. E., Jung, R. C., Joyce, J. and Rincon, E. (1977). Smoke, burns and the natural history of inhalation injury in fire victims. *Ann. Surg.*, **185**, 100–110

Zawacki, B. E., Azen, S. P., Imbus, S. H. and Chang, Y. (1979). Multifactorial probit analysis of mortality in burned patients. *Ann. Surg.*, **189**, 1–10

FURTHER READING

Gad, S. C. and Anderson, R. C. (1990). *Combustion Toxicology*. CRC Press, Boca Raton, Florida

McDiarmid, M. A., Lees, P. S. J., Agnew, J. Midzenski, M. and Duffy, R. (1991). Reproductive hazards of fire fighting. II. Chemical hazards. *American Journal of Industrial Medicine*, **19**, 447–472

Sarofim, A. F. and Suk, W. A. (1994). Health effects of combustion products. *Environmental Health Perspectives*, **102**, Supplement, 237–244

Shusterman, D. T. and Peterson, J. E. (1993). Section on smoke inhalation. *Occupational Medicine*, **8**, 415–504

52 Toxicology of Pesticides

Timothy C. Marrs

INTRODUCTION

Pesticides are an heterogeneous group of substances whose desired activity is the killing of unwanted living organisms, in a more or less specific manner. In order to review the toxicity of pesticides, some method of classification of them is needed. In this article, they are divided by class of action into insecticides, fungicides and herbicides, these groups being subdivided by chemical group. The fungicides are further subdivided into those used as wood preservatives and those used on crops. Some chemical groups have more than one type of pesticidal activity, and therefore appear in more than one category, for example, the carbamates and organophosphates.

The very definition of pesticides may vary, particularly in relation to regulatory affairs. Some veterinary products, for example organophosphorus (OP) sheep dips, are regulated in many countries under a different legislation from when the same active ingredients are used on arable commodities. Moreover, pesticide legislation often controls substances such as growth promoters and defoliants: some of these will be briefly discussed here.

There are a number of possible ways in which humans can be exposed to pesticides and thus the toxic effects of pesticides may have consequences for consumers of food as well as for production workers, formulators, farmers and other applicators. Moreover, pesticides used domestically in wood preservation or as household insecticides may be important sources of exposure of the general public. It should also be remembered that the more acutely toxic pesticides have been used for suicide and murder.

The effects of pesticide residues in food and water probably cause the greatest public concern. However, reports of clinical poisoning by residues seem to be extremely rare, certainly by comparison with occupational intoxication. The reasons for this are complex but may reflect a true rarity of poisoning or the fact that occupational poisonings are far more easily identified. Occupational intoxications would be expected to be more severe than food-borne poisonings, and the proximity of cause and effect in occupational poisoning certainly makes diagnosis easier. Food-borne pesticide intoxication, especially where clinical signs are non-specific or trivial, would probably pass unnoticed. This is particularly likely where the signs and symptoms could be ascribed to a microbiological cause. Acute poisoning, where pesticides had been used in accordance with regulations, seems likely to be a very uncommon occurrence, if it occurs at all, at least in developed countries. The problem of extreme consumers is taken into account when maximum residue limits (MRLs) are pronounced to be toxicologically acceptable by comparison with the acceptable daily intake (ADI). Bearing in mind that, as a minimum, a 100-fold safety factor is used in calculating ADIs from animal studies (WHO, 1990), residues of many multiples of the MRL would be necessary to produce acute poisoning. Thus it would seem highly unlikely that extreme consumption, by itself, could give rise to acute pesticide poisoning. In fact, analysis of reported consumer poisonings by pesticides shows that most reported instances occur from the following.

- Spillage of pesticides onto food during storage or transport.
- Eating grain or seed potatoes treated with pesticides, where the food article was not intended for human consumption.
- Improper application of pesticides or failure to observe harvest intervals.

The pesticides responsible have often been ones with low 50 per cent lethal doses (LD$_{50}$s), such as endrin, parathion or aldicarb or the rodenticides, such as thallium or sodium fluoride. Other pesticides that have produced morbidity by ingestion with food include organic mercury fungicides (Ferrer and Cabral, 1991).

Weighed against the disadvantages of pesticides that accrue from their toxic effects is the fact that insects and fungi are important sources of agricultural loss and give rise to much damage to buildings, particularly in those countries, such as the USA and Canada, where construction is often of wood. Furthermore, many insects carry diseases such as malaria and sleeping sickness, which in the absence of control measures may render land uninhabitable or agriculturally unusable; despite control measures these diseases continue to be major sources of morbidity and mortality. Also, fungal contamination of agricultural produce can give rise to conditions such as ergotism and aflatoxicosis.

In this chapter it is not possible to give more than an outline of the toxicology of the main groups of pesticides, pointing out the major problems which occur in the regulation of the use of pesticides and allowable residues in food and the treatment of poisoning arising from them.

INSECTICIDES

Many insecticides affect the nervous system of insects and, as many have some activity against the mammalian nervous system, in humans the neurotoxic effects of insecticides are often prominent. The main groups of insecticides are:

- Organochlorines
- Anticholinesterases
  A. Organophosphates
  B. Carbamates
- Pyrethroids
- Compounds of natural origin, including antibiotics, avermectins, derris (rotenone) and *Bacillus thuringiensis*.

Organochlorines

This group was formerly of great importance and includes DDT(*p,p'*-dichlorodiphenyltrichloroethane), HCH (1,2,3,4,5,6-hexachlorocyclohexane), the cyclodienes, dieldrin, endrin and heptachlor, and toxaphene. However, the use of organochlorines (OCs) has, in recent years, been severely restricted in most countries. This has been mainly as a result of the persistence of OCs in the environment, rather than their toxicity to mammals. Despite the fact that OCs are used much less than formerly, their toxicology is still important because they continue to be present in the environment and because, in the foodstuffs

imported into developed countries, their residues, sometimes above international MRLs, continue to be present (Working Party on Pesticide Residues, 1990) presumably due either to contamination from environmental sources or continued use in developing countries. OCs are excreted in breast milk (Siddiqui and Saxena, 1985) and their persistence is shown by the continuing presence of OCs in human milk, although usually at declining levels (Working Party on Pesticide Residues, 1992).

OCs produce changes in electrical activity in the CNS (Burchfiel *et al.*, 1976) and it is here that the most prominent effects of the OCs are seen. DDT produces tremor and incoordination in low doses and convulsions in high doses, whereas HCH and the cyclodienes may produce convulsions as the first sign of intoxication, together with fever by a central effect. As far as mechanisms are concerned, much of the work on OCs has been carried out on DDT, which appears to act by altering Na^+ and K^+ flux across nerve cell membranes (Hayes and Laws, 1991). Whilst the mechanism of toxicity of some OCs is ill-defined, it is noteworthy that the cyclodienes inhibit GABA-receptor-mediated Cl^- transport (Abalis *et al.*, 1986; Gant *et al.*, 1987). Furthermore they inhibit brain (and heart) calmodulin-regulated Ca^{2+} pump activity (Mehotra *et al.*, 1989). Chlorinated hydrocarbons produce microsomal enzyme induction and characteristic histopathological changes in the livers of experimental animals; tumours are seen in rodents. These tumours do not appear to be indicative of genotoxic carcinogenicity.

OC poisoning is treated symptomatically, and diazepam is usually used for the convulsions.

Anticholinesterases

Two groups of anticholinesterases, the organophosphates (OPs) and the carbamates, are widely used as agricultural insecticides. They are often more acutely toxic than the OCs. Their action is respectively to phosphorylate or carbamylate esterases, particularly the enzyme acetylcholinesterase, causing accumulation of the neurotransmitter, acetylcholine. A variety of cholinergic symptoms and clinical signs occurs in the parasympathetic system, such as bronchorrhoea, salivation, constriction of the pupil of the eye and abdominal colic. Sympathetic effects can also ensue, together with signs of CNS involvement, initially confusion and sometimes convulsions. Effects at the neuromuscular junction result in muscle fasciculation and later paralysis. The terminal event in fatal poisonings is respiratory paralysis, which may be of central or peripheral origin, or both. It is generally believed that, provided the patient survives, the symptoms and clinical signs of anticholinesterase poisoning are reversible. Moreover, histopathological changes from the anticholinesterase effects of OPs and carbamates are, *per se*, exiguous, being confined to the nervous system and muscles (including heart muscle). However, there is the recognition that survival after high doses of OPs (and possibly also lower doses) and after carbamate intoxication may result in long-term clinical and morphological changes in the CNS (see below).

It is often stated that the main difference between the OPs and the carbamates is that the former produce irreversible inhibition of acetylcholinesterase while the latter produce reversible inhibition: this is only true in a relative sense. With the exception of those substances that produce rapid ageing of the OP–acetylcholinesterase complex (the nerve agent soman), OP–acetylcholinesterase complexes have half lives for reactivation varying from a matter of hours to days. Nevertheless, the stability of the phosphorylated enzyme is generally greater than that of the carbamylated one, with the result that the symptoms and signs of intoxication persist longer.

The numerous cholinesterases in the body show different intensities of sensitivity to inhibitors. Although by no means always the case, plasma cholinesterase is usually the most sensitive cholinesterase to inhibition and reactivates slowly (Škrinjarić-Špoljar *et al.*, 1973), making the enzyme a useful marker of exposure. However, this sensitivity is usually combined with a poor correlation with cholinergic symptoms, so that plasma cholinesterase inhibition can usually be taken as a marker of exposure and no more. Erythrocyte acetylcholinesterase inhibition often correlates better with cholinergic symptomatology but reactivation can take place sufficiently fast to interfere with the validity of blood tests both in clinical and experimental situations unless care is taken (Mason *et al.*, 1992; FAO, 1993). The great sensitivity to inhibition and the poor correlation with the clinical cholinergic effects of inhibition of erythrocyte cholinesterase and, even

more so, plasma cholinesterase have resulted in the Joint Meeting on Pesticide Residues (JMPR) preferring to use the inhibition of brain cholinesterase when deriving acceptable daily intake levels (ADIs) for OPs (WHO, 1990). Presumably the JMPR did not consider the implications of peripherally-mediated intoxication (Ligtenstein, 1984).

Organophosphates

OP anticholinesterases are esters of phosphoric, phosphonic or phosphorothioic or related acids. They are akin to the chemical warfare nerve agents which, however, are often phosphonofluoridates. Many pesticidal OPs are phosphorothioates and those containing $P=S$ groups tend to be of lower mammalian toxicity than their corresponding phosphates and phosphonates. Thus paraoxon is much more toxic than parathion, as is malaoxon compared with malathion. The reason for this is that the $P=S$ phosphorothioates are inactive as anticholinesterases *in vitro* and only acquire toxicity after conversion of the $P=S$ moiety to a $P=O$ moiety, forming the oxon (WHO, 1986). Although OPs share their cholinergic symptomatology with the carbamates, the toxicology of OPs has certain features which, at the present time, do not appear to be shared with the carbamates. These features are organophosphate-induced delayed neuropathy (OPIDN) and the so-called intermediate syndrome. Because all the OP insecticides have the same anticholinesterase action, and this property is responsible for their acute lethal toxicity, quantitative differences in toxicity are partly the result of differences in absorption, distribution and metabolism. However, the rates of formation of the OP–acetylcholinesterase complex, the hydrolysis of this complex, and the ageing reaction (see above) must also be considered.

Inactivation of cholinesterases by OPs involves a reaction in which one substituent group, the leaving group, is lost, producing a dialkylphosphoryl enzyme. The vast majority of insecticides produce a dimethylphosphorylated enzyme or a diethylphosphorylated enzyme and the kinetics of reactivation are the same for each derivative regardless of the structure of the leaving group of the OP. Reactivation of the dimethylphosphorylated enzyme is considerably quicker than the diethyl equivalent and will occur within a few hours (WHO, 1986). Ageing, important with the nerve gas soman, is a reaction in which one alkyl group is lost to leave a monoalkylphosphoryl enzyme. Such derivatives are refractory to spontaneous or oxime-induced reactivation. The nerve agent soman (pinacolyl methylphosphonofluoridate) produces an unusual phosphorylated enzyme that ages with a half-time of a few minutes. No pesticidal OP gives rise to a complex that ages so fast, but therapeutic failure with oximes has been attributed to ageing with certain pesticides (Glickman *et al.*, 1984; Gyrd-Hansen and Kraul, 1984).

Senanayake and Karalliede (1987) reported a syndrome that followed therapy for and resolution of the cholinergic effects of OP intoxication. As the syndrome developed before the late effects of OPs, the authors called this syndrome the intermediate syndrome. Since 1987, other examples have been recorded, for instance that by Karademir *et al.* (1990). The syndrome comprises a proximal limb paralysis starting 1–4 days after poisoning. The progression is not altered by atropine or oximes and, as the sensorimotor muscles are affected, respiratory support is necessary until recovery occurs.

OPIDN is a symmetrical sensory–motor axonopathy, tending to be most severe in the long axons, occurring 7–14 days after exposure. The most disabling feature which may result is paralysis of the legs. Less severe cases exhibit a characteristic high stepping gait. Some recovery may occur, but there is no specific treatment (Barrett *et al.*, 1985). The initial event in the pathogenesis of the syndrome appears to be the inhibition of neuropathy target esterase (NTE). This is followed by an ageing reaction similar to that described above for soman with acetylcholinesterase (Johnson, 1975). However, the structural requirements for inhibition of acetylcholinesterase and NTE are different, as shown by tri-*o*-cresyl phosphate, a substance with little anticholinesterase activity but a powerfully neuropathic action, while many OPs with powerful anticholinesterase properties are devoid of the ability to produce OPIDN. It should be noted that the robustly anticholinesterase nerve agents have little propensity to cause OPIDN (Gordon *et al.*, 1983).

Many regulatory authorities demand the use of tests to detect the propensity for the development of OPIDN, with the result that those OPs in current use do not usually produce the syndrome.

The test is usually carried out in hens as these animals are very susceptible to the syndrome. However, mice and rats also develop OPIDN (Veronesi *et al.*, 1991) and the reported resistance of rodents to the development of OPIDN has been attributed to the use of young animals in those studies (Moretto *et al.*, 1992). It is possible that tests based on a rodent model may become available in the future. Several OPs not in current use as pesticides produce OPIDN, including mipafox and diisopropyl phosphorofluoridate (a common laboratory OP), while leptophos, also not currently used in most countries, has been reported several times to produce OPIDN. There is some limited experimental and clinical evidence that a few OPs currently used in some countries can produce OPIDN, for example EPN (*O*-ethyl *O*-*p*-nitrophenyl phenylphosphonate), cyanofenphos and trichloronat (El-Sabae *et al.*, 1981).

The behavioural toxicity of anticholinesterases, *inter alia* OPs, has been reviewed (D'Mello, 1993). As acute intoxication with OPs can cause major effects such as convulsions, respiratory failure and cardiac arrhythmias, all of which can result in anoxia, it is hardly surprising that major intoxication is sometimes associated with long-term CNS changes (Holmes and Gaon, 1956; Gershon and Shaw, 1961; Tabershaw and Cooper, 1966; Rodnitzky *et al.*, 1975; Korshak and Sato, 1977; Hirshberg and Lerman, 1984). Generalized or localized anoxia within the CNS from other causes, for example convulsions and carbon monoxide poisoning, is widely recognized as having long-term effects on brain function. More debatable is whether doses below those causing acute clinical intoxication can bring about changes in the CNS. A number of investigations into this problem have shown behavioural or psychological alterations, while others have failed to elicit any effects. Additionally, there are some studies where the details in the published paper make evaluation difficult (e.g. Durham *et al.*, 1965). Behavioural and fairly subtle electroencephalographic (EEG) changes were described by Duffy *et al.* (1979) after exposure to sarin. In addition, Burchfiel *et al.* (1976) described changes in the EEG of primates (rhesus monkey) after a single large dose or repeated small doses of sarin. Although these changes appear genuine, the numbers of animals in each dose group were small and it is extremely uncertain as to what extent the observations can be extrapolated to likely consumer or even operator exposure to OP pesticides.

More recently, an epidemiological study of the long-term effects of OP poisoning was undertaken by Savage *et al.* (1988). In this study 100 matched pairs of individuals with previous OP poisoning were compared with appropriate controls. Significant differences were not found in the EEG and blood chemistry, but such differences were found in psychometric testing and a test of motor reflexes. Among the exclusion criteria was poisoning within 3 months of the study, but very severe poisoning does not appear to have been excluded; the criteria for inclusion, *inter alia*, attendance at certain poisons units during a certain period. It is therefore possible that all the observed effects were caused by the severe poisonings, which would almost certainly have been included. Thus, there seems very little doubt, on theoretical, experimental and epidemiological grounds, that severe OP poisoning can cause long-term irreversible changes in brain function. In less intense poisoning the data are conflicting and few of the studies are above criticism. The most impressive studies relate to sarin, an OP nerve agent, and one might argue that nerve agents have properties not shared by OP pesticides, a possibility which some studies appear to support (e.g. Kadar *et al.*, 1992).

It should never be forgotten that OPs may have properties, some of which may be entirely independent of their anticholinesterase effects, including mutagenicity and carcinogenicity as well as organ-specific toxicity to the heart, liver, kidney and other organs (Singer *et al.*, 1987; Baskin and Whitmer, 1992; Pimentel and Carrington da Costa, 1992; Wedin, 1992; Yemano and Morita, 1992). A myopathy has been described post mortem in cases of human poisoning (de Rueck and Willems, 1975) and in experimental animals (Preusser, 1967; Wecker *et al.*, 1978).

The treatment of OP poisoning involves symptomatic treatment and the use of antidotes. Atropine, an anticholinergic compound, and an oxime enzyme reactivator such as pralidoxime chloride (2-PAM) or obidoxime is used, while convulsions and muscle fasciculation respond to diazepam. The antidotal treatment is only effective against acute poisoning and specific treatment is not available for OPIDN or other long-term effects.

Carbamates

In general the carbamates produce toxicity similar to that of organophosphates, but less severe. A major difference is that carbamate-inhibited cholinesterases reactivate more rapidly than enzyme inhibited by OPs, with the result that the effects do not last as long in carbamate poisoning. Indeed, reactivation of carbamylated enzyme may be fast enough to render detection of cholinesterase depression difficult in both experimental animals and clinical situations. However, an insecticidal carbamate, aldicarb, is one of the few pesticides that has given rise to poisoning in consumers of treated food. Residues have occurred in cucumbers, water-melons, squashes and similar products sufficient to cause illness, which in some cases was severe. Outbreaks have occurred in the USA and Canada (Hall and Rumack, 1992) and in the Irish Republic (Department of Agriculture and Food, 1992). The reason for these problems is that aldicarb, in other respects a satisfactory pesticide, has a high mammalian toxicity. Atropine is effective in carbamate poisoning but oximes are less so and there is some evidence that, with certain carbamates, oximes are harmful (Bismuth *et al.*, 1992).

Pyrethroids

Pyrethrins are natural insecticides produced from *inter alia* pyrethrum, a plant of the Compositae group, and are esters of pyrethric or chrysanthemic acids. The synthetic pyrethroids are structurally similar compounds rendered photostable by various substituent groups, such as chlorine, bromine or cyanide, on the basic structure. Some of the newer ones bear a more distant structural relationship to the pyrethrins. Because of their low mammalian toxicity, high insecticidal potency and lack of persistence in the environment, they have achieved widespread usage in agriculture, as household insecticides and in wood preservation. However, they are very toxic to aquatic organisms (Zitco *et al.*, 1979) and their lack of persistence can be a problem when the synthetic pyrethroids are used as wood preservatives. The advantageous properties of the synthetic pyrethroids result from the fact that they hydrolyze relatively easily, both in the mammalian body and in the environment. Consequently, bioaccumulation does not occur and they do not persist in soils. However, some pyrethroids are potent allergens and allergic rhinitis, asthma and extrinsic allergic alveolitis have been reported (Bismuth *et al.*, 1987).

The pyrethroids are neurotoxic by virtue of their action on voltage-dependent sodium channels (Vijverberg and van den Bercken, 1990), but pathological changes underlying the neurotoxic effects are scanty (Aldridge, 1990). Pyrethroids can be separated into two classes on the basis of the central neurotoxic syndrome that they produce by parenteral routes in animals. The CS syndrome consists of marked choreoathetosis, salivation, coarse tremor and convulsions and is a property of those pyrethroids with an α-cyano group (deltamethrin, cyfluthrin, cypermethrin, fenpropathrin, fenvalerate, flucythrinate and fluvalinate). The T syndrome is characterized by fine or coarse tremor, hypersensitivity to stimuli and aggressive sparring and is seen in those compounds without the cyano group (permethrin and resmethrin as well as the components of natural pyrethrum) (Aldridge, 1990). A few pyrethroids produce an intermediate TS-syndrome in experimental animals. As well as central effects, pyrethroids cause peripheral nerve damage with functional impairment (Rose and Dewar, 1983). Axonal degeneration has been described, but generally at near lethal doses and there is no evidence that pyrethroids can produce delayed neuropathy of the OP type (Aldridge, 1990).

Despite the findings in the central and peripheral nervous systems of animals, in humans the most prominent effect of the pyrethroids is to cause paraesthesia, mainly in the face, and little else, these effects being probably caused by repetitive firing of sensory nerve endings. Pruritis with blotch erythema, itching rhinorrhoea and lacrimation have also been described (Aldridge, 1990). Deltamethrin seems more potent and permethrin less so, in producing these effects. There is little evidence of any permanent effects in humans.

Specific treatment of the effects of synthetic pyrethroids is rarely necessary as systemic effects are very unusual in humans. Rapid hydrolysis by esterases means that any effects would be expected to be of short duration. Nevertheless, cases of severe poisoning with pyrethroids have been reported from some countries, for example China, and a few deaths have been recorded (He *et al.*, 1989).

Insecticides of Biological Origin Other Than Pyrethrum

Avermectins

Abamectin is the common name for a mixture of avermectin B1a and B1b, macrocyclic lactone disaccharide antibiotics from *Streptomyces avermitilis*. Abamectin is used as an insecticide and acaricide, while the dihydro derivative, ivermectin, is used to control nematodes and arthropods. Ivermectin is used additionally in the control of human onchocerciasis (Wright, 1986). The insecticidal activity is based on their action on GABAergic nerve transmission; because mammals only have GABAergic synapses in the CNS, the mammalian blood–brain barrier ensures a degree of specificity. A notable feature of this group of compounds is their low LD_{50}s, but these compounds are not usually of high toxicity by the dermal route on account of their large molecules and poor transdermal absorption.

Rotenone

The other insecticide of biological origin that is very well known is rotenone, under the name derris (actually the name of an Asiatic plant). Rotenone blocks mitochondrial electron transport and this is responsible for the toxic effects in mammals, including humans. It can also cause dermatitis.

Juvenile Hormone Analogues and Chitin Synthesis Inhibitors

The attraction of these two groups of insecticides is that they have no target organ or system in mammals.

The juvenile hormone analogues, which include hydroprene and methoprene, are of low acute toxicity (LD_{50} approximately 5 g kg^{-1}) and usually non-teratogenic and non-genotoxic (Hayes and Laws, 1991). Chitin synthesis inhibitors, such as diflubenzuron, are also generally of low toxicity.

FUNGICIDES

The fungicides are an heterogeneous group of chemicals that defy convenient chemical classification: their action is often on the cytoskeleton.

Fungicides Predominantly Used as Wood Preservers

Organometals

The organometals are in general fairly toxic compounds, many being neurotoxic. The organotins, such as tributyltin oxide, were, for a time, used extensively as wood preservatives but their use has been considerably restricted in the UK (Advisory Committee on Pesticides, 1990). Tributyltin oxide has immunotoxic properties (IPCS, 1990).

Phenols

One of the most widely used wood preservers has been pentachlorophenol, which is a potent fungicide. The main toxic action of pentachlorophenol and similar compounds in humans is to cause uncoupling of oxidative phosphorylation and hyperthermia.

Creosote

Coal-tar creosote, a widely used wood preserver in the UK, is a complex mixture which contains varying amounts of various carcinogens. The amount of benz[a]pyrene in some preparations has caused some concern. However, it is likely that irritancy reduces the potential of creosote for causing skin cancer and it probably presents little hazard to the public.

Fungicides Predominantly Used in Agriculture or Horticulture

Carbamate Fungicides and Thiabendazole

A number of carbamates, generally benzimidazole derivatives, possess fungicidal activity. They include benomyl and its hydrolysis product carbendazim as well as thiophanate and thiophanate-methyl. Thiabendazole, although not strictly a carbamate, shares many of the properties of the carbamate fungicides. The acute toxicity of the carbamate fungicides is usually low. Thus thiophanate has an oral LD_{50} of more than 5 g kg^{-1} in rodents (Hashimoto *et al.*, 1970).

Carbendazim and benomyl have detrimental effects on fertility of male rats (Carter and Laskey, 1982; Carter *et al.*, 1987) and under experimental conditions these two fungicides have been shown to be embryotoxic and teratogenic (Kavlock *et al.*, 1982: Janardhan *et al.*,

1984; Cummings *et al.*, 1990; Hoogenboom *et al.*, 1991). A major area of concern with benomyl and carbendazim has been the possibility of these two pesticides being spindle poisons. Furthermore, there is evidence that benomyl and carbendazim may be mutagenic (Kirkhart, 1980; Pandita, 1988; Albertini, 1989; Georgieva *et al.*, 1990). Some of these concerns are related to the effects of benomyl and carbendazim on microtubules and thus to their fungicidal effects, which are mediated through their binding to fungal tubulin and preventing polymerization.

Dithiocarbamates

The dithiocarbamates include two main groups of fungicides, the dimethyl dithiocarbamates thiram and ziram and the ethylenebis dithiocarbamates (EBDCs) maneb and zineb, the latter group being metabolized to ethylene thiourea. The dithiocarbamates are generally not highly toxic in acute exposure. A notable feature of them is that some are teratogenic. The ethylene thiourea metabolite of EBDCs causes reduced incorporation of iodine into thyroid hormones (T4 and T3); repeated administration produces thyroid hyperplasia that is initially reversible. Prolonged dosage produces follicular thyroid tumours (Hill *et al.* 1989). The data on the mutagenicity of dimethyl dithiocarbamates are generally sparse, but there is a suggestion that at least some of them are mutagenic (Tennant *et al.*, 1987; Hemavathy and Krishnamurthy, 1988; BG Chemie, 1992). A further feature of the dithiocarbamates is that they may produce alcohol intolerance.

Chloroalkyl Thio-Containing Fungicides

This group consists of captan, folpet and captofol. They are of low mammalian toxicity. However, because of the similarity of their molecules to thalidomide, there was considerable concern over their effect on reproductive and fetal development. The negative results of reproductive studies into the chloralkylthio fungicides suggest that another part of the thalidomide molecule is responsible for the teratogenicity of that drug (Hayes, 1982). There also have been concerns over the ability of some fungicides of this class to induce unusual gastrointestinal tumours in experimental animals (FAO, 1991).

Other Fungicides

There remains a heterogeneous group of fungicides that are used on crops, including phenols such as dinocap, diazines such as dazomet and the hydantoins. The hydantoins group include vinclozolin, which has recently been the cause of concern in the UK because of its reproductive toxicity (Advisory Committee on Pesticides, 1992). Other fungicides include the urea derivatives (linuron, monlinuron) and the OP pyrazophos. Although pyrazophos is used as a fungicide, it has anticholinesterase properties and, insofar as mammalian toxicity is concerned, has many features in common with OP insecticides (FAO, 1993).

HERBICIDES

Bipiridinium Herbicides

The most well known pesticide in this group is paraquat. This chemical is selectively toxic to the lungs, producing an acute alveolitis followed by fibrosis. Both type I and type II alveolar cells, as well as the Clara cells, are destroyed. Associated with this process, it has been noted that the lung tissue accumulates paraquat by a saturable uptake process (Rose *et al.*, 1974, 1976; Smith, 1982; Smith *et al.*, 1990). In experimental animals, the main result of paraquat toxicity seen histologically is a proliferative pneumonitis with fibroblasts, alveolar oedema, perivascular and peribronchial oedema and the accumulation of neutrophils and macrophages (Schoenberger *et al.*, 1984). The precise histological changes observed in rats depend on the dose of paraquat and time to death. In those dying early, haemorrhage and oedema are very prominent, while in those dying later there is greater evidence of fibrosis. These changes appear to occur largely independently of the route of administration of the paraquat, and it should be noted that in mice similar histopathological findings have been observed after exposure to paraquat aerosol (Popenoe, 1979).

Poisoning with paraquat in man initially produces damage to the gastrointestinal tract, including the mouth and pharynx, and to the liver and kidneys. Often partial recovery occurs and then from 10 days onwards clinical signs and symptoms referable to the respiratory tract develop (Higen-

bottam *et al.*, 1979; Schuster *et al.*, 1981). Death normally occurs from respiratory failure. There is no effective treatment for paraquat-induced lung damage and the only effective measures involve the prevention of absorption of the herbicide from the gastrointestinal tract.

Diquat differs from paraquat poisoning in that renal effects are more prominent and lung changes do not generally occur, presumably because diquat, unlike paraquat, is not concentrated in lung tissue (IPCS, 1984). An effect of diquat that has been extensively investigated is its ability to produce cataracts in experimental animals (Pirie and Rees, 1970). In human poisoning death is usually caused by renal failure (IPCS, 1984).

Phenoxy Herbicides

The phenoxy herbicides, which are widely used to destroy broad-leaved weeds, are chemical analogues of plant growth hormones. They include 2,4-D (2,4-dichlorophenoxyacetic acid), 2,4,5-T (2,4,5-trichlorophenoxyacetic acid), mecoprop and fenoprop. One herbicide of the group, namely 2,4,5-T, has caused concern because of its contamination with 2,3,7,8-tetrachlorodibenzo-*p*-dioxin (TCDD). The whole group has attracted some suspicion because of certain epidemiological studies linking non-Hodgkin's lymphoma and soft tissue sarcoma with the manufacture or application of herbicides. 2,4,5-T is rarely used nowadays, but 2,4-D is extensively used as a selective pesticide on lawns and on monocotyledonous crops. Because mutagenicity tests on 2,4-D have produced somewhat contradictory results, the International Association for Research on Cancer (IARC, 1982) concluded that the results on mutagenicity and carcinogenicity were inadequate for a proper evaluation to be made. However, it seems unlikely that pure 2,4-D is mutagenic.

2,4-D is a moderately toxic compound but, in humans, large doses are necessary to produce major toxic effects, which include alterations in consciousness, muscle fasciculation, vomiting and convulsions. Gross overdose produces stupor, muscle hypotonia and coma.

OP Herbicides

Two groups of organophosphates, both of which have a low or non-existent ability to produce cholinesterase inhibition, are used as herbicides. Glyphosate [*N*-(phosphonomethyl) glycine] is an inhibitor of amino acid synthesis in plants. In mammals it appears to be very non-toxic, with $LD_{50}s$ in the 5 g kg^{-1} range (Atkinson, 1985; FAO, 1987). In general this appears to be true in humans, where poisonings have usually shown that high doses are necessary to produce fatality. However, the lethal dose in humans seems to be somewhat variable, with some patients surviving doses that were fatal in others. Massive overdose of glyphosate produces gastric irritation, hypotension and pulmonary insufficiency, for which other constituents of the formulation may be to blame (Talbot *et al.*, 1991). *S,S,S*-Tributyl phosphorotrithioate (DEF) and *S,S,S*-tributyl phosphorotrithioite (merphos) are OPs that are used as defoliants because they produce leaf abscission. A notable feature of their toxicity is that in hens they produce OPIDN (Baron and Johnson, 1964).

Substituted Anilines

These are used as herbicides and include alachlor, propachlor and propanil. Some herbicides of this group have the general property of causing methaemoglobinaemia, as do many other aniline derivatives (Kiese, 1970). The probable mechanism of the methaemoglobinaemia is *N*-hydroxylation to the corresponding hydroxylamine, which then takes part in an intraerythrocytic cycle with the corresponding nitroso derivative at the same time generating methaemoglobin. If this were the mechanism, for propanil, the proximate methaemoglobin former would be *N*-hydroxy-3,4-dichloroaniline (McMillan *et al.*, 1990). In the case of propachlor, which is a tertiary amine, it would seem unlikely that the above mechanism would operate and data from the rat suggest that this is indeed the case (Panshina, 1973). However, it must be remembered that the rat is not a good experimental animal for demonstrating methaemoglobinaemia (Calabrese, 1983). As well as causing methaemoglobinaemia, propanil reduces red cell survival (McMillan *et al.*, 1991).

Alachlor is, like other substituted aniline herbicides, not a substance of high acute toxicity (Pesticide Manual, 1987). It is carcinogenic in rodents, producing posterior nasal and stomach tumours, possibly by a non-genotoxic mechanism (Berry, 1988).

TOXICITY OF COMBINATIONS OF PESTICIDES

There has been some concern as to the possible deleterious effects from multiple pesticide exposure, either as residues in food or at the workplace. Clinical effects from exposure to pesticide residues in food are exceedingly uncommon (see above) and therefore seem unlikely to be much of a problem. The workplace is more of a problem and raises the question of the safety of tank-mixing of pesticides and other sources of combined exposure. Frequently data on a particular combination are scanty and general principles are necessary for predictive purposes. The possible types of toxicological interaction between two pesticides are: (1) additive, (2) synergistic, and (3) antagonistic or they may act independently of one another. Often, compounds with the same toxic effects act additively, while in the case of pesticides with different toxic effects the combined effect is less than additive. If toxic effects were only determined by actions at receptors, this would probably always be the case. However, one has also to consider alteration by one pesticide of the pharmacokinetics or metabolism of the other and as a result interactions may be exceedingly complex. Thus, in combination the acute toxicity of OCs is usually additive, although potentiation and antagonism can occur. With pairs consisting of one OP and one OC, the same is true (Keplinger and Deichmann, 1967). It has been shown that some pairs of OPs exhibit greater than additive toxic effects when administered together (Dubois, 1961). Because of the predictive difficulty, experimental approaches have been proposed (GIFAP, 1988).

Note: These views are those of the author and do not necessarily reflect those of the Department of Health or the UK Government.

REFERENCES

Abalis, I. M., Eldefrawi, M. E. and Eldefrawi, A. T. (1986). Effects of insecticides on gaba-induced chloride influx into rat brain microsa. *J. Toxicol. Env. Hlth*, **18**, 13–23

Advisory Committee on Pesticides (1990). *Annual Report 1989*, HMSO, London, Edinburgh and Belfast

Advisory Committee on Pesticides (1992). *Annual*

Report 1991, HMSO, London, Edinburgh and Belfast

Albertini, S. (1989). Influence of different factors on the induction of chromosome malsegregation in *Saccharomyces cerevisiae* D61.M by Bavistan and assessment of its genotoxic property in the Ames test and in the *Saccharomyces cerevisiae* D7. *Mutat. Res.* **216**, 327–340

Aldridge, W. N. (1990). An assessment of the toxicological properties of pyrethroids and their neurotoxicity. *Crit. Rev. Toxicol.*, **21**, 89–103

Atkinson, D. (1985). Toxicological properties of glyphosate, a summary. In Grossbard, E. and Atkinson, D. (Eds), *The Herbicide Glyphosate*. Butterworths, London, pp. 127–133

Barrett, D. S., Oehme, F. W. and Kruckenberg, S. M. (1985). A review of organophosphorus ester-induced delayed neurotoxicity. *Vet. Hum. Toxicol.*, **27**, 22–37

Baron, R. L. and Johnson, C. H. (1964). Neurological disruption produced in hens by two organophosphorus esters. *Brit. J. Pharmac*, **23**, 295–304

Baskin, S. I. and Whitmer, M. P. (1992). Cardiac effects of anticholinesterases. In Ballantyne, B. and Marrs, T. C. (Eds), *Clinical and Experimental Toxicology of Organophosphates and Carbamates*. Butterworth-Heinemann, Oxford, pp. 135–144

Berry, C. L. (1988). The no-effect level and optimal use of toxicity data. *Reg. Toxicol. Pharmacol.*, **8**, 385–388

BG Chemie (1992). *Toxicological Evaluations 3. Potential Effects of Existing Chemicals*. Berufsgenossenschaft der chemischen Industrie. Springer, New York, Berlin, pp. 91–130

Bismuth, C., Baud, F. J., Conso, F., Frejaville, J. P. and Garnier, R. (1987). *Toxicologie Clinique*, 4th edn., Flammarion, Paris, p. 424

Bismuth, C., Inns, R. H. and Marrs, T. C. (1992). Efficacy, toxicology and clinical use of oximes. In Ballantyne, B. and Marrs, T. C. (Eds), *Clinical and Experimental Toxicology of Organophosphates and Carbamates*. Butterworth-Heinemann, Oxford, pp. 555–577

Burchfiel, J. L., Duffy, F. H. and Sim, van M. (1976). Persistent effects of sarin and dieldrin upon the primate electroencephalogram, *Toxicol. Appl. Pharmacol.*, **35**, 365–379

Calabrese, E. J. (1983). *The Principles of Animal Extrapolation*. John Wiley and Sons, New York, pp. 307–320

Carter, S. D. and Laskey, J. W. (1982). Effect of benomyl on reproduction in the male rat. *Toxicol. Lett.*, **11**, 87–94

Carter, S. D., Hess, R. A. and Laskey, J. W. (1987). The fungicide methyl 2-benzimidazole carbamate causes infertility in male Sprague-Dawley rats. *Biol. Reprod.*, **37**, 709–717

Cummings, A. M., Harris, S. T. and Rehnberg, G. L. (1990). Effects of methyl benzimidazole carbamate during early pregnancy in the rat. *Fund. Appl. Toxicol.*, **15**, 528–535

Department of Agriculture and Food (1992). *Press release 117/92*. Government Information Services, Dublin 2, Irish Republic

de Rueck, J. and Willems, J. (1975). Acute parathion poisoning: myopathic changes in the diaphragm. *J. Neurol.*, **208**, 309–314

D'Mello, G. D. (1993). Behavioural toxicity of anticholinesterases in humans and animals—a review. *Hum. Exp. Toxicol.*, **12**, 3–7

Dubois, K. P. (1961). Potentiation of the toxicity of organophosphorus compounds. In Metcalf, R. L. (Ed.), *Advances in Pest Control Research*, Vol 4. Interscience, New York, pp. 117–151

Duffy, F. H., Burchfiel, J. L. Bartels, P. H., Gaon, M. and Sim, van M. (1979). Long-term effects of an organophosphate upon the human electroencephalogram. *Toxicol. Appl. Pharmacol.*, **47**, 161–176

Durham, W. F., Wolfe, H. R. and Quinby, G. E. (1965). Organophosphorus insecticides and mental alertness. *Arch. Environ. Health*, **10**, 55–66

El-Sebae, A. H., Soliman, S. A., Ahmed, N. S. and Curley, A. (1981). Biochemical interaction of six OP delayed neurotoxicants with several neurotargets. *J. Environ. Sci. Health*, **816**, 465–474

FAO (1987). *Plant Production Paper No 78(2). Evaluation of Some Pesticide Residues in Food. Part 2—Toxicology*. Joint Meeting Proceedings: Food and Agricultural Organization of the United Nations, World Health Organization, Geneva

FAO (1991). *Pesticide Residues in Food. Toxicology Evaluations*. Joint Meeting Proceedings, Rome 17–26 September, 1990, Food and Agricultural Organization of the United Nations, World Health Organization, Geneva

FAO (1993). *Pesticide Residues in Food. Toxicology Evaluations*. Joint Meeting Proceedings, Rome, 20 September–1 October, 1992, Food and Agricultural Organization of the United Nations, World Health Organization, Geneva

Ferrer, A. and Cabral, R. (1991). Toxic epidemics caused by alimentary exposure to pesticides: a review. *Food Addit. Contam.*, **8**, 755–776

Gant, D. B., Eldefrawi, M. E. and Eldefrawi, A. I. (1987). Cyclodiene insecticides inhibit GABA-regulated chloride channels. *Toxicol. Appl. Pharmacol.*, **88**, 313–321

Georgieva, V., Vachkova, R., Tzoneva, R. and Kappas, A. (1990). Genotoxic activity of benomyl in different test systems. *Environ. Mol. Mut.*, **16**, 32–36

Gershon, S. and Shaw, F. H. (1961). Psychiatric sequelae of chronic exposure to organophosphorus insecticides. *Lancet*, **i**, 1371–1374

GIFAP (1988). *GIFAP Position Paper on Toxicology of Crop Protection Products in Combination*. Groupement International des Associations Nationales de Fabricants de Produits Agrochimiques, Brussels

Glickman, A. H., Wing, K. D. and Casida, J. E. (1984). Profenofos insecticide bioactivation in relation to antidote action and the stereospecificity of anticholinesterase inhibition, reactivation and aging. *Toxicol. Appl. Pharmacol.*, **73**, 16–22

Gordon, J. J., Inns, R. I., Johnson, M. K., Leadbeater, L., Maidment, M. P., Upshall, D. G., Cooper, G. H. and Rickard, R. L. (1983). The delayed neuropathic effects of nerve agents and some other organophosphorus compounds. *Arch. Toxicol.*, **52**, 71–82

Gyrd-Hansen, N. and Kraul, I. (1984). Obidoxime reactivation of organophosphate inhibited cholinesterase activity in pigs. *Acta Vet. Scand.*, **25**, 86–95

Hall, A. H. and Rumack, B. H. (1992). Incidence, presentation and therapeutic attitudes to anticholinesterase poisoning in the USA. In Ballantyne, B. and Marrs, T. C. (Eds), *Clinical and Experimental Toxicology of Organophosphates and Carbamates*. Butterworth-Heinemann, Oxford, pp. 471–493

Hashimoto, Y., Makita, T., Mori, T., Nishibe, T., Noguchi, T., Tsuboi, S. and Ohtu, G. (1970). Toxicological evaluations of thiophanate. (I) Acute and subacute toxicity of a new fungicide, thiophanate (active ingredient of NF–35), 1,2-bis-(ethoxycarbonyl-thioureido) benzene. *Pharmacometrics*, **4**, 5–21

Hayes, W. J. (1982). *Pesticides Studied in Man*. Williams and Wilkins, Baltimore

Hayes, W. J. and Laws, E. R. (1991). *Handbook of Pesticide Toxicology*. Academic Press, New York, pp. 612–613

He, F., Wang, S., Liu, L., Chen, S., Zhang, Z. and Sun, J. (1989). Clinical manifestations and diagnosis of acute pyrethroid poisoning. *Arch. Toxicol.*, **63**, 54–59

Higenbottam, T., Crome, P., Parkinson, C. and Nunn, J. (1979). Further clinical observations on the pulmonary effects of paraquat ingestion. *Thorax*, **34**, 161–165

Hemavathy, K. C. and Krishnamurthy, N. B. (1988). Cytogenetic effects of Cuman L, a dithiocarbamate fungicide. *Mutat. Res.*, **208**, 57–60

Hill, R. N., Erdreich, L. S., Paynter, R. O., Roberts, P. A., Rosenthal, S. L. and Wilkinson, C. F. (1989). Thyroid follicular cell carcinogenesis. *Fund. Appl. Toxicol.*, **12**, 629–697

Hirshberg, A. and Lerman, Y. (1984). Clinical problems in organophosphate poisoning: the use of a computerized information system. *Fund. Appl. Toxicol.*, **4**, S209–S124

Holmes, J. H. and Gaon, M. D. (1956). Observations on acute and multiple exposure to anticholinesterase agents. *Trans. Am. Clin. Chem. Assoc.*, **68**, 86–103

Hoogenboom, E. R., Ransdell, J. F., Ellis, W. G., Kavlock, R. J. and Zeman, F. J. (1991). Effects on the rat eye of maternal benomyl exposure and protein malnutrition. *Curr. Eye Res.*, **7**, 601–612

IARC (1982). *IARC Monographs* on the evaluation of carcinogenic risk of chemicals to man: some fumigants, the herbicides, 2,4-D and 2,4,5-T,chlorinated dibenzo-dioxins and miscellaneous industrial chemicals. Vol. 15, International Association for Research on Cancer, Lyon

IPCS (1984). International Programme on Chemical Safety. *Environmental Health Criteria 63. Paraquat and Diquat*. World Health Organization, Geneva

IPCS (1990). International Programme on Chemical Safety. *Environmenal Health Criteria 116. Tributyltin compounds*. World Health Organization, Geneva

Janardhan, A., Sattur, P. B. and Sisodia, P. (1984). Teratogenicity of methyl benzimidazole carbamate in rats and rabbits. *Bull. Environ. Contam. Toxicol.*, **33**, 257–263

Johnson, M. K. (1975). Organophosphorus esters causing delayed neurotoxic effects. *Arch. Toxicol.*, **34**, 259–288

Kadar, T., Cohen, G., Sahar, R., Alkalai, D. and Shapira, S. (1992). Long-term study of brain lesions following soman, in comparison with DFP and metrazol poisoning. *Hum. Exp. Toxicol.*, **11**, 517–523

Karademir, M., Ertürk, F. and Koçak, R. (1990). Two cases of organophosphate poisoning with development of intermediate syndrome. *Hum. Exp. Toxicol.*, **9**, 187–189

Kavlock, R. J., Chernoff, N., Gray, L. E., Gray, J. A. and Whitehouse, D. (1982). Teratogenic effects of benomyl in the Wistar rat and CD–1 mouse, with emphasis on the route of administration. *Toxicol. Appl. Pharmacol.*, **62**, 44–54

Keplinger, M. L. and Deichmann, W. B. (1967). Acute toxicity of combinations of pesticides. *Toxicol. Appl. Pharmacol.*, **10**, 586–595

Kiese, M. (1970). Drug-induced ferrihemoglobinemia. *Hum. Genetik.*, **9**, 220–223

Kirkhart, B. (1980). Micronucleus test on benomyl test substance was not benomyl but MBC. *US EPA report LSU 7553–19*, EPA, Washington D.C.

Korshak, R. J. and Sato, M. M. (1977). Effects of chronic organophosphate pesticide exposure on the central nervous system. *Clin. Toxicol.*, **11**, 83–95

Ligtenstein, D. A. (1984). On the synergism of the cholinesterase reactivating bispyridinium oxime HI-6 and atropine in the treatment of organophosphate intoxications in the rat. *MD Thesis*, Rijksuniversiteit te Leiden, Leyden, Netherlands

McMillan, D. C., McRae, T. A. and Hinson, J. A. (1990). Propanil-induced methemoglobinemia and hemoglobin binding in the rat. *Toxicol. Appl. Pharmacol.*, **105**, 530–537

McMillan, D. C., Bradshaw, T. P., Hinson, J. A. and Jollow, D. J. (1991). Role of metabolites in propanil-induced hemolytic anemia. *Toxicol. Appl. Pharmacol.*, **110**, 70–78

Mason, H., Waine, E. and McGregor, A. (1992). *In vitro* studies on human cholinesterase (ChE) and biological effect monitoring of organophosphorus pesticide exposure. *Hum. Exp. Toxicol.*, **11**, 557

Mehotra, B. D., Moorthy, K. S., Ravichandra Reddy, S.

and Desaiah, D. (1989). Effects of cyclodiene compounds on calcium pump activity in rat brain and heart. *Toxicology*, **54**, 17–29

Moretto, A., Capodicasa, E. and Lotti, M. (1992). Clinical expression of organophosphate-induced delayed neuropathy in rats. *Toxicol. Lett.*, **63**, 97–102

Pandita, T. K. (1988). Assessment of the mutagenic potential of a fungicide Bavistan using multiple assays. *Mutat. Res.*, **204**, 627–643

Panshina, T. N. (1973). Ramrod. In Medved, L. M. (Ed.) *Gigiena Primeninia Toksikologia Pesticidov Klinica Otravlenni*. Medizina, Leningrad (now St Petersburg), pp. 301–303

Pesticide Manual (1987). 8th edn. British Crop Protection Council, Thornton Heath

Pimentel, J. M. and Carrington da Costa, R. B. (1992). Effects of organophosphates on the heart. In Ballantyne, B. and Marrs, T. C. (Eds), *Clinical and Experimental Toxicology of Organophosphates and Carbamates*, Butterworth-Heinemann, Oxford, pp. 145–148

Pirie, A. and Rees, J. R. (1970). Diquat cataract in the eye. *Exptl Eye Res.*, **9**, 198–203

Popenoe, D. (1979). Effects of paraquat aerosol on mouse lung. *Arch. Pathol. Lab. Med.*, **103**, pp. 331–334

Preusser, H.-J. (1967). Die Ultrastructur der motorischen Endplatte im Zwerchfell der Ratte und Veränderungen nach Inhibierung der Acetylcholinesterase. *Z. Zellforsch.*, **80**, 436–457

Rodnitzky, R. L., Levin, H. S. and Mick, D. L. (1975). Occupational exposure to organophosphate pesticides, a neurobehavioral study. *Arch. Environ. Health*, **30**, 98

Rose, G. P. and Dewar, A. J. (1983). Intoxication with four synthetic pyrethroids fails to show any correlation between neuromuscular dysfunction and neurobiochemical abnormalities in rats. *Arch. Toxicol.*, **53**, 297

Rose, M. S., Smith, L. L. and Wyatt, I. (1974). Evidence for the energy dependent accumulation of paraquat into rat lung. *Nature*, **252**, 314–315

Rose, M. S., Lock, E. A., Smith, L. L. and Wyatt, I. (1976). Paraquat accumulation: tissue and species specificity. *Biochem. Pharmacol.*, **24**, 419–423

Savage, E. P., Keefe, T. J., Mounce, L. M., Heaton, R. K., Lewis, J. A. and Burcar, P. J. (1988). Chronic neurological sequelae of acute organophosphate pesticide poisoning. *Arch. Environ. Health*, **43**, 38–45

Schoenberger, C. I., Rennard, S. I., Bitterman, P. B., Fukuda, Y., Ferrans, V. J. and Crystal, R. G. (1984). Paraquat-induced pulmonary fibrosis. *Am. Rev. Resp. Dis.*, **129**, 168–173

Schuster, R., Erkelenz, I. and von Romatowski, H.-J. (1981). Frühbild der Lungenfibrose nach Zytostatika und Paraquatintoxikation. *Röntgenblatter*, **34**, 338–341

Senanayake, N. and Karalliede, I. (1987). Neurotoxic effect of organophosphorus insecticides: an intermediate syndrome. *N. Engl. J. Med.*, **316**, 761–763

Siddiqui, M. K. J. and Saxena, M. C. (1985). Placenta and milk as excretory routes of lipophilic pesticides in women. *Hum. Toxicol.*, **4**, 249–254

Singer, A. W., Jaax, N. K., Graham, J. S. and McLeod, C. G. (1987). Cardiomyopathy in soman and sarin intoxicated rats. *Toxicol. Lett.*, **36**, 243–249

Škrinjarić-Špoljar, M., Simeon, V. and Reiner, E. (1973). Spontaneous reactivation and aging of dimethylphosphorylated acetylcholinesterase and cholinesterase. *Biochim. Biophys. Acta*, **315**, 363–369

Smith, L. L. (1982). The identification of an accumulation system for diamines and polyamines into the lung and its relevance to paraquat toxicity. *Arch. Toxicol.*, **5** (Suppl.), 1–14

Smith, L. L., Lewis, C., Wyatt, I. and Cohen, G. M. (1990). The importance of epithelial uptake systems in lung toxicity. In Volans, G. N., Sims, J., Sullivan, F. M. and Turner, P. (Eds), *Basic Science in Toxicology*. Proceedings of the Vth International Congress of Toxicology, Brighton, England, 16–21 July, 1989. Taylor and Francis, London, pp. 233–241

Tabershaw, I. R. and Cooper, W. C. (1966). Sequelae of acute organic phosphate poisoning. *J. Occup. Med.*, **8**, 5–20

Talbot, A. R., Shiaw, M.-H., Huang, J.-S. *et al.* (1991). Acute poisoning with glyphosate-surfactant herbicide ('Roundup'): a review of 93 cases. *Hum. Exp. Toxicol.*, **10**, 1–8

Tennant, R. W., Margolin, B. H., Shelby, M. D. *et al.* (1987). Prediction of chemical carcinogenesis in rodents from *in vitro* genetic toxicity assays. *Science*, **236**, 933–941

Veronesi, B., Padilla, S., Blackmon, K. and Pope, C. (1991). Murine susceptibility to organophosphate-induced peripheral neuropathy (OPIDN). *Toxicol. Appl. Pharmacol.*, **107**, 311–324

Vijverberg, H. P. M. and van den Bercken, J. (1990). Neurotoxicological effects and the mode of action of pyrethroid insecticides. *Crit. Rev. Toxicol.*, **21**, 105–126

Wecker, L., Kiauta, T. and Dettbarn, W-D. (1978). Relationship between acetylcholinesterase inhibition and the development of a myopathy. *J. Pharm. Exp. Ther.*, **206**, 97–104

Wedin, G. P. (1992). Nephrotoxicity of anticholinesterases. In Ballantyne, B. and Marrs, T. C. (Eds), *Clinical and Experimental Toxicology of Organophosphates and Carbamates*. Butterworth-Heinemann, Oxford, pp. 195–202

WHO (1986). *Environmental Health Criteria 63. Organophosphorus Insecticides: a General Introduction*. World Health Organization, Geneva

WHO (1990). *Environmental Health Criteria 104. International Programme on Chemical Safety; Principles for the Toxicological Assessment of Pesticide Residues in Food*. World Health Organization, Geneva

Working Party on Pesticide Residues (1990). *Report 1988–1989*. HMSO, London, Edinburgh and Belfast

Working Party on Pesticide Residues (1992). *Report 1990–1991*. HMSO, London, Edinburgh and Belfast

Wright, D. J. (1986) Biological activity and mode of action of avermectins. In Ford, M. G., Lunt, G. C., Reay, R. C. and Usherwood, P. N. R. *Neuropharmacology of Pesticide Action*. Ellis Horwood, Chichester, England, pp. 174–202

Yemano, T. and Morita, S. (1992). Hepatotoxicity of trichlorfon and dichlorvos in isolated rat hepatocytes. *Toxicology*, **76**, 69–77

Zitko, V., McLeese, D. W., Metcalfe, C. D. and Carson, W. G. (1979). Toxicity of permethrin, decamethrin, and related pyrethroids to salmon and lobster. *Bull. Environ. Contam. Toxicol.*, **21**, 336–343

FURTHER READING

Ballantyne, B. and Marrs, T. C. (1992). *Clinical and Experimental Toxicology of Organophosphates and Carbamates*. Butterworth-Heinemann, Stoneham, Massachusetts

Hayes, W. J. and Laws, E. R. (1991). *Handbook of Pesticide Toxicology, Vols, 1, 2 and 3*. Academic Press, San Diego

Kaloyanova, F. P. and El Batawi, M. A. (1991). *Human Toxicology of Pesticides*. CRC Press, Boca Raton, Florida

53　Toxicology of Food and Food Additives

David M. Conning

INTRODUCTION

Since the 1850s when the illegal adulteration of foodstuffs caused a public scandal, there has been legislation to control the use of non-nutritious chemicals in food. During this century, concomitant with the growth of food technology, food legislation has expanded to cover virtually every aspect of food manufacture and packaging, and has extended to regulate the residues in foodstuffs of the considerable number of chemicals used in agricultural production.

Such legislation, together with that devoted to medicines, has to a considerable extent paralleled the development of the technology, if not the science, of toxicology. As the scope of toxicology has enlarged, so has the amount of food law. In addition, the regulation of food chemicals has been undertaken by almost all national governments and the whole framework is now truly global in character. Given the international nature of trade, considerable efforts are made to ensure that national requirements do not conflict, thereby constituting barriers to trade.

Nutrition science has also demonstrated remarkable growth during the twentieth century, but for much of that time has concentrated almost exclusively on the study of dietary deficiency that results in disease. This has resulted in major advances in the knowledge and understanding of the roles of individual nutrients, although much remains to be accomplished in elucidating the biochemical detail. During this time a few nutritionists have attempted to examine the influence of diet on health—that is the attainment of optimal health and disease resistance as opposed to the rectification of deficiency. Much of this work has been governed by an intuitive belief that the intensification of agricultural practice and the industrialization of food manufacture must diminish the nutritional value of foodstuffs.

The international comparisons of diet and heart disease, begun in 1947 (Keys, 1980), opened up a third line of development for nutrition science. This was the recognition that the excessive consumption of specified nutrients may be associated with certain conditions previously classified as age-related degenerative disease. By this time the concept of chronic toxicity had been identified by toxicology. Chronic toxicity is the induction of a disease process by the repeated administration of a small dose of a compound, over a long period of time. In most instances, but not all, the disease process itself is an age-related degenerative phenomenon, but the intensity is increased and the onset occurs earlier in the life-span when the toxic compound is present. Usually a dose can be identified which does not influence the natural disease process or provoke other toxic responses.

In many respects the notion that a given nutrient consumed repeatedly to excess over many years can induce or enhance a chronic disease process is a precise replication of the concept of chronic toxicity, and has led to the recognition of food toxicology or nutrition toxicology as a complementary science to both toxicology and nutrition. In that this concept embraces the genetic basis for age-related degenerative diseases, the analogy is quite close and could be a valuable adjunct in the study of disease mechanisms.

There are, however, other components of food which are toxic, the so-called natural toxicants. Until recent years these have been neglected as subjects of scientific study. With the present tendency towards a reduction in the use of agricultural chemicals, it is possible that natural toxicants, many of which constitute a plant's own defences against predators, will assume greater importance.

FOOD TOXICOLOGY

Nutrient Toxicity

Investigations of the relationship between diet and disease have concentrated in the main on two areas: (1) diet and vascular disease and (2) Diet and malignant disease.

Diet and Vascular Disease

Vascular disease accounts for approximately 40 per cent of deaths in the UK. Among males 31 per cent is due to coronary heart disease and 9 per cent to cerebrovascular disease. The figures among females are 23 per cent and 15 per cent, respectively. The median age of deaths is around 75 years, but a third of the deaths from ischaemic heart disease in males occur before the age of 65 years (DHSS, 1984).

Coronary Heart Disease

Coronary heart disease (CHD) consists of two elements—arterial degeneration (atherosclerosis) of the coronary arteries, which is part of a generalized degeneration of the arterial system, and coronary thrombosis resulting in myocardial ischaemic necrosis which may be fatal. Studies of patients with the condition have revealed a number of shared characteristics, now designated 'predisposing risk factors'. The most consistent include age, hypertension, raised blood cholesterol concentration, maleness, cigarette smoking and family history.

Other conditions that predispose to the disease are the hyperlipidaemias, diabetes, obesity and lack of physical exercise.

Many of these factors may be assumed to raise the concentration of blood lipids, increase the myocardial burden and decrease the potential blood supply should the main supply be compromised. Women are protected until the menopause (unless hyperlipidaemia is present), but thereafter develop the same susceptibility as the male.

Heavy cigarette smoking is associated with peripheral vascular disease, coronary heart disease and myocardial infarction, but the mechanism remains uncertain. It may be a combination of several factors such as vasoconstriction, increased platelet adhesiveness and blood coagulation.

Studies of the effects of diet have concentrated on the causes of the elevated blood cholesterol and the induction of thrombosis.

Blood Cholesterol

The seminal cross-population studies of Ancel Keys (1980) demonstrated that in males aged 40–59 years there was a direct association between the prevalence of CHD and serum cholesterol concentrations and a further association, though less striking, between blood cholesterol and the proportion of saturated fatty acids in the diet. This observation has been the basis of many national public health policies which attempt to achieve a reduced consumption of saturated fatty acids, mainly derived from animal fats, compensated by an increased consumption of polyunsaturated fatty acids, mainly derived from vegetable oils, to maintain the intake of adequate food energy.

Several large studies have attempted to decrease the incidence of CHD by reducing the blood concentrations of cholesterol through manipulations of the diet or the use of hypolipidaemic drugs. Such studies have not been strikingly successful. Although the prevalence of myocardial ischaemia has been slightly reduced in some instances, overall mortality has not been reduced. This may be because, in men over 65 years of age, there is an inverse relationship between mortality and blood cholesterol concentration (Kannel and Gordon, 1970).

The lipoprotein transport systems for serum cholesterol are known to be important in that low-density lipoprotein cholesterol (LDL) is strongly and directly associated with the risk of CHD, whereas high-density liproprotein cholesterol (HDL) is inversely related—that is, HDL cholesterol has a protective effect.

Serum concentrations of LDL cholesterol are governed by the availability of the LDL receptors on cell surfaces, especially of the liver, and this availability is genetically controlled. The LDL receptors govern the access of blood cholesterol to the hepatic cells, where it is metabolized and excreted in the bile. HDL represents an additional transport mechanism that reduces the deposition of cholesterol in the arterial wall (Goldstein *et al.*, 1983). Extreme reduction in the numbers of such receptors occurs in familial hypercholesterolaemia. The mechanism of action of saturated fatty acids in influencing LDL levels is not known, although it is now recognized that the most important fatty acids are C12 (lauric), C14 (myristic) and C16 (palmitic) acids. It is known also that monounsaturated fatty acids may be beneficial by causing an elevation of the circulating levels of HDL cholesterol.

Why LDL cholesterol exerts an adverse effect is not known but is thought to be related to an oxidative damage that occurs as the LDL particle passes through vascular endothelium. Such a change results in inactivation of macrophages after LDL particle ingestion, leading to the production of 'foamy' macrophages (that is, macrophages with accumulated fat), cellular disintegration and the possible release of growth factors which stimulate the proliferation of smooth muscle cells, another feature of the atheromatous lesion. Although highly speculative, this hypothesis has resulted in an analysis of the antioxidant protection known to be exercised in LDL particles by vitamin E and β-carotene, with the recognition that reduced dietary intake of vitamin E is an important additional 'risk factor' in CHD (Gey *et al.*, 1987).

The possible role of antioxidants in preventing the adverse effects of high circulating levels of LDL cholesterol is compatible with experimental animal studies which have suggested that atheromatous lesions are mainly due to oxidized cholesterol or oxidized cholesterol esters.

In terms of toxicology, therefore, the problem is the nature of the change in LDL particles which renders them toxic to vascular endothelium or intima, resulting in the degenerative change that characterizes atherosclerosis.

Thrombosis

Occlusion of a coronary artery by a thrombus is a common terminal event in CHD. It is likely that, before such a catastrophe, mural thrombi are formed on the damaged intima of diseased arteries and are incorporated into subendothelial plaques, thereby aggravating the condition. Considerations of the possible role of dietary components in this process have centred on the essential fatty acids (EFAs) linoleic and linolenic acids. These EFAs are known to be the precursors of the endoperoxides PGH2 and PGH3, which are converted, respectively, to prostaglandins and thromboxanes in vascular endothelium and platelets (Moncada and Vane, 1978) The hypothesis is that a dietary imbalance resulting in relative deficiency of synthesis of the linoleic pathway results in a relative excess of thromboxane A2 which promotes thrombosis. This hypothesis suggests that competition exists for the available cyclo-oxygenases, thereby influencing the final pathway.

It is known that a diet rich in marine products, with relatively high levels of eicosapentaenoic acid (EPA), causes a prolongation of the bleeding time and that even a modest increase in fish consumption reduces CHD mortality (Kromhout *et al.*, 1985). It has yet to be demonstrated that EPA and arachidonic acid compete for the available cyclo-oxygenase, or that the enzyme is limited in supply.

It is clear that atherosclerosis is a multifactorial disease and it is not possible at present to define the mechanism that explains the combined role of the known factors. The contemporary view (Figure 1) offers a scheme susceptible to experimental elucidation which may provide solutions in due course. In the meantime it must be correct that public health policies seek to remove the risk factors known to be influenced by diet and lifestyle.

Diet and Cancer

Energy and Fat in Experimental Carcinogenesis

The study of the carcinogenicity of chemicals has had a central place in the development of toxicology as a science, and it has been known since 1941 that diet plays a very important role in modulating tumour incidence and tumour induction times (Lavick and Baumann, 1941). Since the demonstration that restriction of energy consumption reduced the incidence of spontaneous tumours in experimental animals and the susceptibility of skin to chemical carcinogenesis, this finding has been extended subsequently to a wide variety of experimental animals and tumour models.

For example, the incidence of spontaneous mammary tumours in mice is greater in animals maintained on a high-fat diet than in those on a low-fat or a carbohydrate-rich diet, even when total energy consumption is identical. This observation, too, has been repeated in many studies, although the assumption that different diets have been isocaloric has depended on there being no significant changes in body weight or rate of weight gain rather than direct measurement. A confounding factor in many studies has been failure to recognize that the available energy from fat may be much greater in experimental animals than the accepted figure for man and that this value varies according to the length of the fatty acid chain. Thus, depending on the type of fat used in the preparation of the animal diets, the available energy may be greater than that computed. The use of body weight as a measure of energy consumption therefore requires much more precise measurement than has often been the case.

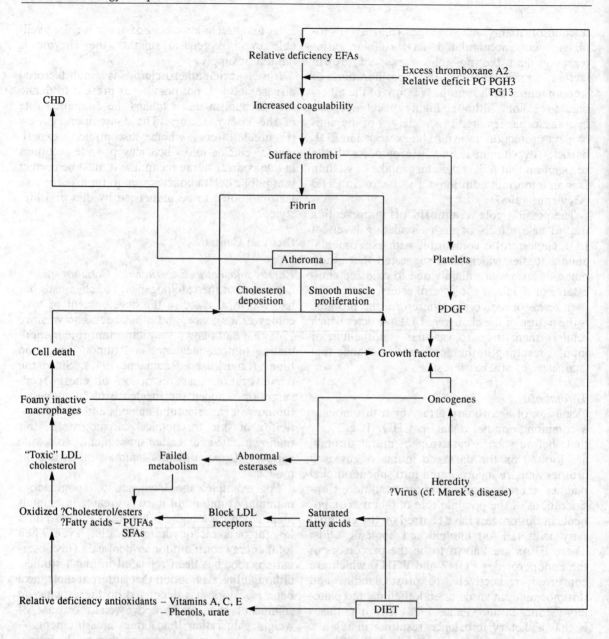

Figure 1 A scheme illustrating the possible interaction of a number of pathogenic factors in the development of atherosclerosis and coronary heart disease. CHD = coronary heart disease; PG = prostaglandin; PDGF = platelet derived growth factor; LDL = low-density lipoprotein; PUFAs = polyunsaturated fatty acids; SFAs = saturated fatty acids; EFAs = essential fatty acids

Further analysis of the roles of different types of fat has suggested that polyunsaturated fatty acids of the types found in vegetable oils (C16 to C20) are much more active in promoting carcinogenesis than saturated fatty acids, although the longer chain polyunsaturated acids found in fish oils also show much less activity (Carroll and Khor, 1975).

These confusing findings were resolved to some extent when it was shown, subsequently, that the essential fatty acids may be the critical moiety in experimental mammary carcinogenesis. Tumour yield increases as the EFA content of the diet is increased, a maximum response being obtained with a dietary content of about 4 per cent. Once this level is achieved, tumour yield may be further increased by the incorporation of greater percentages of fat but the type of fat is not important. This would suggest that EFAs have an important role in experimental carcinogenesis which is enhanced by energy consumption. The nature of the specific role is uncertain (Ip *et al.*, 1985). The position is further complicated by the finding that these properties of EFA may reside only with the linoleic series, which results in the synthesis of arachidonic acid, and that the linolenic series may actually be inhibitors of the carcinogenic process. It is known that eicosapentaenoic acids and decosahexaenoic acids inhibit arachidonic acid metabolism and it is possible that this is the important effect. Until more is known about the roles of prostaglandins, thromboxanes and leukotrienes, derivatives of arachidonic and eicosapentaenoic acids, in the carcinogenic process, no conclusions are possible.

Energy and Fat in Human Carcinogenesis

Epidemiological studies of human cancer in relation to dietary components are difficult on account of the virtual impossibility, in retrospective studies, of defining with any accuracy the precise consumption of nutrients for the many decades before the patient develops a tumour. Other confounding factors are insufficient dietary variance between cases and controls, failure to consider other factors such as smoking, the consumption of complex carbohydrates, dietary modification as a result of the presence of the disease itself, and family history. Prospective studies would be expected to avoid most of these factors.

Plotting age-adjusted death rates for breast cancer against the putative intake of fat or energy-from-fat demonstrates a direct relationship with a high coefficient of correlation, even though the quality of the dietary data from many countries is not good. A similar analysis reveals no relationship between death from breast cancer and the intake of polyunsaturated fatty acids.

The grossly obese demonstrate elevated mortality rates from cancer, mainly colorectal tumours in males and tumours of gall bladder, breast and uterus in females. The excess is not large.

Other studies have attempted to characterize the relationship between diet and the incidence of breast and colonic cancers by an analysis of religious sects or closed communities with strict dietary rules. In these studies the level of fat in the diet is assumed to equate with the amount of meat, since many communities control meat consumption, whereas none control fat consumption directly. Some studies have attempted to equate serum cholesterol measurements with the incidence of cancer, assuming the cholesterol to be dependent on fat consumption. All of these studies have given inconsistent results that do not allow a clear correlation between dietary fat and the incidence of cancer to be made (Kinlen, 1987).

Non-starch Polysaccharides

The possible protective role of non-starch polysaccharides (NSP) against the induction of colonic cancer was suggested by a comparison of African and Western diets (Burkitt and Trowell, 1975). This has stimulated considerable research but very little in the way of consolidated findings. Many studies have been confounded by the failure to recognize that NSPs as a class include compounds with very different biological effects, and the failure to compensate for the reduced energy content of diets high in NSP (BNF Task Force Report, 1990).

When properly controlled, there is no evidence at present that NSP has a consistent influence on experimental or human colonic carcinogenesis.

The Role of Antioxidants

Following the pioneering work of Miller and Miller (1966), the bioactivation of foreign compounds to yield electrophiles and radicals is now well established. If these reactive metabolites gain access to macromolecules such as enzyme proteins or nucleic acids, toxic damage may occur. In the case of DNA this could result, if unrepaired, in mutation which, in somatic cells, might produce cancer.

Since these ideas emerged in the 1960s, there have been a number of studies to examine the effect of dietary antioxidants on the incidence of human cancer. Most studies have concentrated on vitamin C, vitamin E and β-carotene, but more recently other carotenes have begun to be examined. The retrospective studies are hampered by the almost insurmountable difficulty of assessing nutrient intake and have depended on the habitual intake of fruit, vegetables and vegetable oils. Prospective studies also depend to a considerable extent on habitual food intake to achieve consistency. Better evaluation is obtained if serum levels can be measured, but the long-term preservation of antioxidants in serum samples may be unreliable.

Vitamin C Studies of vitamin C have given equivocal results. Case–control studies have suggested a reduced dietary intake in subjects with cancer of the cervix, mouth, larynx and stomach, but not in cancers of the colon, bladder, prostate and breast. None of the correlations are large (odds ratio <1.7). Animal studies in experimental carcinogenesis have shown variable results also, with different effects on tumours of different organs in the same study.

Analysis of a large number of studies involving assessment of either vitamin C intake or fruit intake has suggested a probable inhibition of cancer incidence.

Vitamin E The largest study to date involved over 21 000 men in Finland, and showed that higher serum levels of vitamin E were correlated with lower risk of subsequently developing cancer. This was particularly evident in male smokers. A 3 per cent reduction in serum levels was associated with a significant increase in incidence of, though not death from, cancer, at the time of publication. In this study, the serum samples were stored at −20 °C, which may not be adequate to preserve vitamin E concentrations.

Several animal studies have shown a strong inhibition of experimental carcinogenesis.

β-Carotene Early studies failed to distinguish between vitamin A and β-carotene intake, but since the review by Peto (Peto *et al.*, 1981) most have concentrated on β- and other carotenes. Most studies have shown an inverse relationship between dietary intake or serum levels and cancer incidence and mortality. This is particularly striking for lung cancer, even in long-term smokers. More recently it has been suggested that better inverse correlations may be obtained with lycopene or with 9-*cis*-β-carotene. Nevertheless, in animal studies β-carotene has been shown to suppress experimental carcinogenesis with a number of carcinogenic agents and at a variety of sites.

Selenium Several studies have suggested that selenium intake is inversely related to cancer incidence, particularly in respect of cancers of breast, colon and prostate. Animal studies have also demonstrated an inhibitory effect. The selenium content in the diet, however, depends on soil content and bioavailability and may not be consistent in all geographical locations.

Uric Acid Studies on the relationship of serum uric acid and total mortality have been negative. One study has examined the relationship with mortality from lung cancer, and found a significant inverse relationship which persisted after adjustment for age and smoking habits.

Overall, it may be concluded that a low dietary intake of antioxidant micronutrients is associated with an increased incidence of cancers and, in particular, lung cancer. Given the range of compounds studied, it is likely that the effect is related to the antioxidant property and that the compounds studied cannot be regarded only as markers for some other as yet unrecognized dietary component. Furthermore, the likely mechanism of action is based on a hypothesis for which there is considerable supporting evidence. Nevertheless, other dietary components, such as lycopene, may achieve much greater intake and tissue levels and have yet to be studied adequately.

Natural Toxicants

Plants produce a variety of toxic compounds as a defence against insect predators and fungal infections. The rate of production tends to be governed by the frequency of attack and, as a consequence of the widespread use of synthetic pesticides, most agricultural produce contains only small concentrations. With the trend towards reducing the use of synthetic compounds because of concern about environmental contamination, it is likely that the natural toxicants will assume greater importance as potential hazards for consumers. Attempts to increase the concentrations of natural toxins by plant breeding programmes have occasionally resulted in illness among consumers of the products. It must be recognized, however, that there are very few plant toxins that have caused human illness when consumed as part of a normal diet, although, if the criteria used to assess the safety of synthetic substances were used to judge natural toxins, many more would be included as potential hazards.

Substances that have caused human disease as a result of excessive consumption or inadequate processing usually occur in the diet when food is otherwise not available.

Proteins

Phytohaemagglutinins occur predominantly in beans and are normally removed by soaking in water for several hours prior to thorough cooking. They cause agglutination and lysis of erythrocytes and some are cytotoxic to the intestinal mucosa.

Lathyrogens

Lathyrogens are unusual amino acids (diaminobutyric or diaminopropionic acids) and aminonitriles that cause amyotrophic lateral sclerosis of the spinal cord resulting in spastic paralysis.

Glucosinolates

Glucosinolates are sulphur compounds metabolized to thiocyanates, isothiocyanate and cyclic thiocyanates, all of which inhibit thyroxine production, which results in goitre.

Cyanogens

A number of glycosides yield hydrocyanic acid on hydrolysis. The glycosides occur in a variety of nuts and fruits but the most important are linamarin and lotaustralin, which occur in cassava root and lima beans. Normal processing releases and removes the HCN before consumption.

Toxicity that may result from the consumption of usual dietary components in normal amounts is unusual, but occurs with two components with sufficient regularity to be noted.

Honey

Honey produced by bees that have foraged rhododendron or azalea contains the complex substances andromedol and desacetyl pieristoxin. These may cause cardiovascular collapse and acute peripheral neuropathies at very small dosage. Honey manufacturers take great care to ensure that their bees do not have access to such plants.

Potatoes

Potatoes produce the anticholinesterase glycoalkaloids α-solanine and α-chaconine. These compounds are heat resistant but occur at greatest concentrations in the green skins of immature potatoes. Poisoning is characterized by gastrointestinal symptoms and may be accompanied by central nervous depression (Whitaker *et al.*, 1973).

THE TOXICOLOGY OF FOOD ADDITIVES

A food additive is here defined as a substance used to facilitate some part of the processing or manufacture of a foodstuff, or deliberately added to a foodstuff to effect a particular characteristic. This definition excludes indirect additives derived from packaging, and contaminants, including the residues of agricultural chemicals.

Food additives may be classified according to their intended function. Although this does not necessarily coincide with their chemistry and therefore is not always directly pertinent to a study of toxicological properties, often such properties are related to the function rather than to the chemical structure and many additives are variants of a single structure, all having a similar function.

By far the most comprehensive surveys of the toxicology of food additives are those carried out by the Joint Expert Committee on Food Additives (JECFA) of the World Health Organization and the Food and Agriculture Organization of the United Nations. This committee has, over many years, reviewed toxicological data, both published and unpublished, on a large number of compounds, to determine the Acceptable Daily Intake (ADI). The ADI is the maximum amount of substance, in milligrams per kilogram body weight (mg kg^{-1}), that may be consumed daily for a lifetime without adverse effect. It is usually derived by determining the maximum dosage without detectable effect in an assay of long-term toxicological feeding studies in a number (at least 2) of animal species, divided by a safety factor of at least 100. This factor is said to encompass reduction by a factor of 10 to account for the difference in size between the human population and the test population of experimental animals, and by a factor of 10 to govern the variable sensitivity likely to be exhibited by man to the compound under test. It is clearly difficult to justify this derivation on scientific grounds and it has not been possible to test its efficacy in practice, but as a regulatory procedure it has served its purpose and is recognized as a convenient index by most authorities.

It may be noted in passing that the difficulty of assessing the efficacy of the ADI is due to the impossibility of determining the precise consumption of foods in which an additive is permitted, and the concentration of the additive that is actually used. Such assessments have been attempted for food colours and flavours, and some dietary analyses have been undertaken for selected additives.

Where a number of compounds are used for the same purpose, they may be allocated a 'Group ADI', which states the total permitted concentration of all the compounds in the group.

The Toxicology of Additives by Class (Table 1)

Acidity Regulators

Modification of acidity is an extremely important food manufacturing process having an influence on taste, texture and preservation. Many compounds are used for these purposes, most derived from simple organic acids, themselves natural body constituents, which exhibit little or no toxicity, except at overwhelming dosage.

A wide range of salts of phosphoric acid are accorded a group ADI of 70 mg kg^{-1} based on the dietary concentration that induces nephrocalcinosis in the rat. This effect, however, depends on the calcium–phosphate ratio in the diet, calcium deposition being more likely when the ratio falls below unity. Higher amounts of phosphate intake are permissible if the calcium intake is also high, and vice versa.

Fumaric acid and its sodium salt showed slightly increased mortality in the rat at a dietary concentration of 1.5 per cent but not at 1.2 per cent. Slight testicular atrophy was seen also.

Tartaric acid and its salts also showed no adverse effects at 1.2 per cent in the diet of rats. The ADI for tartrates (30 mg kg^{-1} day^{-1}) is greater than that of the fumarates (6 mg kg^{-1} day^{-1}), because only 20 per cent of ingested tartrate is absorbed.

Anticaking Agents

Phosphate compounds are again limited by the nephrocalcinosis that results from high dietary concentrations, but others, such as magnesium oxide or magnesium carbonate, various silicates and crystalline cellulose, show no toxicity by mouth.

Polydimethylsiloxane showed no toxicity at the highest dose administered (0.1 per cent) and was excreted unchanged in the faeces.

The ferrocyanides are said to cause renal enlargement at 0.5 per cent in the diet, with a minor degree of renal tubular damage.

Antifoaming Compounds

Propylene glycol alginate (also used as a thickener and an emulsifier) undergoes about 80 per cent hydrolysis in the small intestine, releasing propylene glycol, which is absorbed. Residual propylene glycoalginate and the released alginic acid and salts are excreted unchanged in the faeces. Long-term feeding studies in rats and mice have shown no adverse effects at levels up to 5 per cent in the diet.

Antioxidants

Antioxidants are an extremely important group of compounds used extensively to prevent the oxidation of fats and oils in foods, thereby preventing rancidity during distribution and storage. The oxidation process is catalysed by trace metals such as iron and copper. Antioxidants as a class, therefore, include compounds which themselves act as oxygen receptors and compounds which chelate trace metals.

Electron transfer, the major mechanism whereby living cells generate energy, itself produces oxygen free radicals which, if uncontained, would prove lethal. Living tissues are equipped with potent antioxidant mechanisms dependent on compounds that act as electron receptors or as metal chelators. These compounds are the so-called antioxidant vitamins ascorbic acid (vitamin C) and α-tocopherol (vitamin E), and various salts of citric, tartaric and phosphoric acid. The vitamins and their derivatives are regarded as nutrients and have not been subjected to extensive toxicological analysis. Where limits on intake have been suggested, the limit is often dependent on the maximum dose administered in a particular study rather than that which produced a response.

Table 1 Table of all JECFA ADIs by class

CLASS	Subclasses
Acidity regulator	Buffer, buffering agent, acid, base, alkali, pH adjusting agent
Anticaking agent	Anticaking agent, drying agent, dusting powder, antistick agent
Antifoaming agent	Antifoaming agent
Antioxidant	Antioxidant, antioxidant synergist, sequestrant
Bulking agent	Bulking agent
Carbonating agent	Carbonating agent
Clarifying agent	Clarifying agent
Colour	Colour, colour adjunct, colour fixative, colour retention agent, colour stabilizer
Emulsifier	Emulsifier, plasticizer, dispersing agent, surface-active agent, surfactant
Enzyme preparation	Enzyme preparation
Flavour enhancer	Flavour enhancer
Flavouring agent	Flavouring agent, seasoning agent
Flour treatment agent	Bleaching agent, dough conditioner, flour improver
Foaming agent	Whipping agent, aerating agent
Freezant	Freezant
Gelling agent	Gelling agent
Glazing agent	Coating, sealing agent, polish, dusting agent, release agent, lubricant
Humectant	
Preservative	
Propellant	
Raising agent	
Solvent, carrier	
Solvent, extraction	
Stabilizer	
Sweetener	
Thickener	

ADI = Acceptable daily intake (mg kg^{-1}).
NS = Not specified. An ADI is not necessary.
LGMP = Limited by good manufacturing practice and an ADI is not necessary.

CLASS	ADI
Acidity regulators	
Acetic acid, glacial	NS
Ammonium acetate	NS
Calcium acetate	NS
Potassium acetate	NS
Sodium acetate	NS
Ammonium hydrogen carbonate	NS
Magnesium hydrogen carbonate	NS
Potassium carbonate	NS
Potassium hydrogen carbonate	NS
Sodium carbonate	NS
Sodium hydrogen carbonate	NS
Sodium sesquicarbonate	NS
Citric acid	NS
Calcium citrate	NS
Potassium dihydrogen citrate	NS
Sodium dihydrogen citrate	NS
Triammonium citrate	NS
Tripotassium citrate	NS
Trisodium citrate	NS
Glucono delta lactone	NS
Calcium gluconate	NS
Hydrochloric acid	NS
Ammonium hydroxide	NS

continued overleaf

Table 1 (continued)

CLASS		ADI
Acidity regulators		
Calcium hydroxide		NS
Magnesium hydroxide		NS
Potassium hydroxide		NS
Sodium hydroxide		NS
Lactic acid		NS
Ammonium lactate		NS
Calcium lactate		NS
Magnesium lactate (DL-)		NS
Calcium malate (DL-)		NS
Potassium malate solution (DL-)		NS
Potassium hydrogen malate (DL-)		NS
Malic acid (DL-)		NS
Sodium hydrogen malate (DL-)		NS
Sodium malate (DL-)		NS
Calcium oxide		NS
Potassium sulphate		NS
Ammonium phosphate, dibasic	Group ADI	70
Ammonium phosphate, monobasic	Group ADI	70
Calcium phosphate, monobasic	Group ADI	70
Calcium phosphate, tribasic	Group ADI	70
Dicalcium pyrophosphate	Group ADI	70
Dipotassium hydrogen phosphate	Group ADI	70
Disodium pyrophosphate	Group ADI	70
Monopotassium monophosphate	Group ADI	70
Phosphoric acid	Group ADI	70
Potassium phosphate	Group ADI	70
Sodium phosphate, monobasic	Group ADI	70
Sodium phosphate, dibasic	Group ADI	70
Sodium phosphate, tribasic	Group ADI	70
Tetrapotassium pyrophosphate	Group ADI	70
Tetrasodium pyrophosphate	Group ADI	70
Magnesium gluconate	Group ADI	50
Potassium gluconate	Group ADI	50
Sodium gluconate	Group ADI	50
Tartaric acid (L(+)-)		30
Fumaric acid	Group ADI	6
Sodium fumarate	Group ADI	6
Adipic acid	Group ADI	5
Ammonium adipate	Group ADI	5
Potassium adipate	Group ADI	5
Sodium adipate	Group ADI	5
Anticaking agents		
Magnesium carbonate		NS
Magnesium hydrogen carbonate		NS
Cellulose, microcrystalline		NS
Cellulose, powdered		NS
Sodium, potassium and calcium salts of oleic acid		NS
Magnesium oxide		NS
Aluminium silicate		NS
Calcium aluminium silicate		NS
Calcium silicate		NS

continued

Table 1 (continued)

CLASS		ADI
Anticaking agents		
Magnesium silicate (synthetic)		NS
Silicon dioxide, amorphous		NS
Sodium aluminosilicate		NS
Talc		NS
Bone phosphate		70
Calcium phosphate, tribasic	Group ADI	70
Magnesium phosphate, tribasic		70
Tetrasodium pyrophosphate		70
Polydimethylsiloxane		1.5
Calcium ferrocyanide		0.025
Potassium ferrocyanide		0.025
Sodium ferrocyanide		0.025
Antifoaming agents		
Oxystearin		25
Propylene glycol alginate		25
Polydimethylsiloxane		1.5
Antioxidants		
Ascorbic acid		NS
Calcium ascorbate		NS
Potassium ascorbate		NS
Sodium ascorbate		NS
Citric acid		NS
Calcium citrate		NS
Potassium dihydrogen citrate		NS
Sodium dihydrogen citrate		NS
Tripotassium citrate		NS
Trisodium citrate		NS
Glucose oxidase from *Aspergillus niger*		NS
Lecithins		NS
Potassium lactate (solution)		NS
Sodium lactate (solution)		NS
Dipotassium hydrogen phosphate		70
Monopotassium monophosphate	Group ADI	30
Sodium phosphate, monobasic		70
Sodium phosphate, tribasic		70
Tartaric acid (L(+)-)		30
Potassium L(+)- tartrate	Group ADI	30
Potassium sodium L(+)- tartrate		30
Sodium L(+)- tartrate		30
Oxystearin		25
Isopropyl citrate mixture		14
Anoxomer		8
Isoascorbic acid	Group ADI	5
Sodium erythorbate		5
Thiodipropionic acid		3
Dilauryl thiodipropionate	Group ADI	3
Distearyl thiodipropionate		3
Calcium disodium ethylenediaminetetraacetate	Group ADI	2.5
Disodium ethylenediaminetetraacetate		2.5

continued overleaf

Table 1 (continued)

CLASS		ADI
Antioxidants		
Guaiac resin		2.5
Propyl gallate		2.5
Stannous chloride		2
Tocopherol, alpha- concentrate (D-)	Group ADI	2
Tocopherol, alpha- (DL-)	Group ADI	2
Tocopherol, alpha- concentrate mixed	Group ADI	2
Ascorbyl palmitate	Group ADI	1.25
Ascorbyl stearate	Group ADI	1.25
Sodium thiosulphate	Group ADI	0.7
Sulphur dioxide	Group ADI	0.7
Butylated hydroxyanisole		0.3
Tertiary butylhydroquinone		0.2
Butylated hydroxytoluene		0.125
Bulking agents		
Polydextroses A and N		NS
Carbonating agent		
Carbon dioxide		NS
Clarifying agents		
Tannic acid		NS
Polvinylpyrrolidone		50
Colours		
Beet red		NS
Caramel colour (I) (plain)		NS
Carbon, activated vegetable (food grade)		NS
Chlorophyll		NS
Insoluble polyvinylpyrrolidone		NS
Magnesium chloride		NS
Magnesium hydrogen carbonate		NS
Titanium dioxide		NS
Smoke flavourings		accept
Caramel colour III (ammonia process)		200
Caramel colour IV (ammonia–sulphate process)		200
Fast Green FCF		25
Grapeskin extract		25
Chlorophyll–copper complex		15
Chlorophyllin–copper complex, sodium and potassium salts		15
Brilliant Blue FCF		12.5
Quinoline Yellow		10
Tartrazine		7.5
Allura Red AC		7
Beta-apo-8′-carotenoic acid, methyl or ethyl ester	Group ADI	5
Beta-apo-8′-carotenal	Group ADI	5
Beta-carotene (synthetic)	Group ADI	5
Carmines		5
Indigotine		5

continued

Table 1 (continued)

CLASS		ADI
Colours		
Potassium nitrate	} Group ADI	5
Sodium nitrate		5
Azorubine		4
Ponceau 4R		4
Sunset Yellow FCF		2.5
Brown HT		1.5
Brilliant Black PN		1
Ferrous gluconate		0.8
Amaranth		0.5
Iron oxide		0.5
Riboflavin 5'-phosphate sodium	} Group ADI	0.5
Riboflavin		0.5
Turmeric oleoresin		0.3
Potassium nitrite	} Group ADI	0.2
Sodium nitrite		0.2
Curcumin		0.1
Red 2G		0.1
Annatto extracts		0.065
Canthaxanthin		0.05
Erythrosine		0.05
Emulsifiers		
Acetic and fatty acid esters of glycerol		NS
Citric and fatty acids of glycerol		NS
Lactic and fatty acid esters of glycerol		NS
Mixed tartaric, acetic and fatty acid esters of glycerol		NS
Mono- and diglycerides		NS
Lecithins		NS
Cellulose, microcrystalline		NS
Cellulose, powdered		NS
Gelatine, edible		NS
Hydroxypropyl starch		NS
Oxidized starch		NS
Sodium caseinate		NS
Sodium, potassium and calcium salts of oleic acid		NS
Trisodium citrate		NS
Bone phosphate		70
Calcium polyphosphates		70
Potassium phosphate		70
Potassium polyphosphates		70
Sodium phosphate, dibasic	Group ADI	70
Sodium phosphate, tribasic		70
Sodium polyphosphate, glassy		70
Tetrapotassium pyrophosphate		70
Tetrasodium pyrophosphate		70
Diacetyltartaric acid and fatty acid esters of glycerol		50
Stearyl citrate		50
Ammonium salts of phosphatidic acid		30
Calcium stearoyl lactate	} Group ADI	20
Sodium stearoyl lactate		20

continued overleaf

Table 1 (continued)

CLASS		ADI
Emulsifiers		
Ethyl hydroxyethyl cellulose		25
Hydroxypropyl cellulose		25
Hydroxypropyl methyl cellulose	Group ADI	25
Methylcellulose		25
Methyl ethyl cellulose		25
Polyglycerol esters of fatty acids		25
Polyoxyethylene (20) sorbitan monolaurate		25
Polyoxyethylene (20) sorbitan monooleate		25
Polyoxyethylene (20) sorbitan monopalmitate	Group ADI	25
Polyoxyethylene (20) sorbitan monostearate		25
Polyoxyethylene (20) sorbitan tristearate		25
Polyoxyethylene (8) stearate		25
Polyoxyethylene (40) stearate		25
Propylene glycol alginate		25
Propylene glycol esters of fatty acids		25
Sorbitan monolaurate		25
Sorbitan monooleate		25
Sorbitan monopalmitate	Group ADI	25
Sorbitan monostearate		25
Sorbitan tristearate		25
Sucroglycerides	Group ADI	10
Sucrose esters of fatty acids		10
Polyglycerol esters of interesterified ricinoleic acid		7.5
Cholic acid		1.25
Desoxycholic acid		1.25
Sodium aluminium phosphate, basic		0.6
Enzyme preparations		
Carbohydrase from *Bacillus licheniformis*		NS
Carbohydrase from *A. niger*		NS
Glucose isomerase from *Streptomyces violaceoniger*		NS
Glucose isomerase from *Actinoplanes missouriensis* (immob.)		NS
Glucose isomerase from *Bacillus coagulans* (immob.)		NS
Glucose isomerase from *Streptomyces olivaceous* (immob.)		NS
Glucose isomerase from *Streptomyces olivochromogenes* (immob.)		NS
Glucose isomerase from *Streptomyces rubiginosus* (immob.)		NS
Glucose isomerase from *A. niger*		NS
Lipase from *A. oryzae*		NS
Pepsin, avian		NS
Rennet from *Endothia parasitica*		NS
Rennet from *Mucor* spp.		NS
Bromelain		LGMP
Carbohydrases from malt		LGMP
Carbohydrase from *Rhizopus oryzae*		LGMP
Carbohydrase from *Saccharomyces* sp.		LGMP
Catalase from bovine liver		LGMP
Lipase, animal		LGMP
Mixed carbohydrase and protease from *Bacillus subtilis*		LGMP
Papain		LGMP
Pepsin (hog stomach)		LGMP
Rennet		LGMP
Rennet, bovine		LGMP
Rennet from *Bacillus cereus*		LGMP

continued

Table 1 (continued)

CLASS	ADI
Enzyme preparations	
Trypsin	LGMP
Amyloglucosidases from *A. niger*	1
Beta-glucanase from *A. niger*	1
Hemi-cellulase from *A. niger*	1
Pectinases from *A. niger*	1
Protease from *A. niger*	1
Beta-glucanase from *T. harzianum*	0.5
Cellulase from *T. reesei*	0.3
Flavour enhancers	
Glutamic acid (L(+)-)	NS
Calcium di-L-glutamate	NS
Magnesium di-L-glutamate	NS
Monoammonium L-glutamate	NS
Monopotassium L-glutamate	NS
Monosodium L-glutamate	NS
Guanylic acid	NS
Calcium 5'-guanylate	NS
Dipotassium 5'-guanylate	NS
Disodium 5'-guanylate	NS
Inosinic acid	NS
Calcium 5'-inosinate	NS
Disodium 5'-inosinate	NS
Potassium inosinate	NS
Calcium 5'-ribonucleotides	NS
Disodium 5'-ribonucleotides	NS
Lipase from *A. oryzae*	NS
Monoglyceride citrate	NS
Thaumatin	NS
Lipase, animal	LGMP
Maltol	1
Flavouring agents	
Acetic acid, glacial	NS
Citric acid	NS
Ethyl lactate	NS
Malic acid (DL-)	NS
Potassium malate solution (DL-)	NS
Sodium malate (DL-)	NS
Potassium chloride	NS
Paprika oleoresins	LGMP
Smoke flavourings	accept
Ethyl acetate	25
Ethyl butyrate	15
Ethyl vanillin	10
Vanillin	10
Fumaric acid ⎫ Group ADI	6
Sodium fumarate ⎬	6
Benzaldehyde ⎭	5

continued overleaf

Table 1 (continued)

CLASS		ADI	
Flavouring agents			
Benzyl acetate	} Group ADI	5	
Benzyl alcohol		5	
Amyl acetate		3	
Ethyl formate		3	
Isoamyl butyrate		3	
Ethyl heptanoate		2.5	
Ethyl nonanoate		2.5	
Eugenol		2.5	
Ethyl maltol		2	
Methyl anthranilate		1.5	
Gamma-nonalactone		1.25	
Gamma-undecalactone		1.25	
trans-Anethole		1.2	
Carvone (D-)	} Group ADI	1	
Carvone (L-)		1	
Ethyl laurate		1	
Maltol		1	
Cinnamaldehyde		0.7	
Citral		0.5	
Citronellol		0.5	
Geranyl acetate	Group ADI	0.5	
Linalol		0.5	
Linalyl acetate		0.5	
Ethyl methyl phenyl glycidate		0.5	
Methyl salicylate		0.5	
Piperonal		0.3	
Turmeric oleoresin		0.3	
Menthol (L- and DL-)		0.2	
Methyl *N*-methyl anthranilate		0.2	
Alpha-ionone	} Group ADI	0.1	
Beta-ionone		0.1	
Nonanal	} Group ADI	0.1	
Octanal		0.1	
Flour treatment agents			
Ammonium chloride		NS	
Ammonium lactate	} Group ADI	NS	
Calcium lactate		NS	
Magnesium lactate (DL-)		NS	
Calcium oxide		NS	
Calcium sulphate		NS	
Calcium phosphate, dibasic		70	
Protease from *A. niger*		1	

	Maximum treatment level (mg kg flour⁻¹)	Conditional level
Chlorine	2500	
Stearyl tartrate	500	
Potassium bromate	60	
Azodicarbonamide	45	
Benzoyl peroxide	40	75
Chlorine dioxide	30	75

continued

Table 1 *(continued)*

CLASS	ADI
Foaming agents	
Methyl ethyl cellulose	25
Oxystearin	25
Propylene glycol alginate	25
Quillaia extracts	5
Polydimethylsiloxane	1.5
Freezants	
Nitrogen	NS
Dichlorodifluoromethane	1.5
Gelling agents	
Carrageenan	NS
Furcellaran from *F. fastigiata*	NS
Gelatine, edible	NS
Pectin	NS
Potassium chloride	NS
Glazing agent	
Mineral oils	NS
Humectants	
Glycerol	NS
Triacetin	NS
Mannitol	NS
Polydextroses A and N	NS
Sodium hydrogen malate (DL-)	NS
Sodium lactate (solution)	NS
Sorbitol	NS
Sorbitol syrup	NS
Xylitol	NS
Ammonium polyphosphates	70
Bone phosphate	70
Calcium polyphosphates	70
Potassium polyphosphates	70
Sodium polyphosphate, glassy	70
Propylene glycol	25
Preservatives	
Acetic acid, glacial	NS
Calcium acetate	NS
Potassium acetate	NS
Sodium acetate	NS
Propionic acid	NS
Calcium propionate	NS
Potassium propionate	NS
Sodium propionate	NS
Sorbic acid	25
Calcium sorbate	25
Potassium sorbate	25
Sodium sorbate	25

Note: "Group ADI" brackets apply to Glycerol–Triacetin; Ammonium polyphosphates–Sodium polyphosphate, glassy; and Sorbic acid–Sodium sorbate.

continued overleaf

Table 1 (continued)

CLASS		ADI
Preservatives		
Sodium diacetate		15
Ethyl *p*-hydroxybenzoate	Group ADI	10
Methyl *p*-hydroxybenzoate	Group ADI	10
Propyl *p*-hydroxybenzoate	Group ADI	10
Benzoic acid	Group ADI	5
Calcium benzoate	Group ADI	5
Potassium benzoate	Group ADI	5
Sodium benzoate	Group ADI	5
Potassium nitrate	Group ADI	5
Sodium nitrate	Group ADI	5
Formic acid		5
Calcium disodium ethylenediaminetetraacetate	Group ADI	2.5
Disodium ethylenediaminetetraacetate	Group ADI	2.5
Nisin		
Calcium hydrogen sulphite	Group ADI	0.7
Potassium bisulphite	Group ADI	0.7
Potassium sulphite	Group ADI	0.7
Potassium metabisulphite	Group ADI	0.7
Sodium hydrogen sulphite	Group ADI	0.7
Sodium metabisulphite	Group ADI	0.7
Sodium sulphite	Group ADI	0.7
Sulphur dioxide	Group ADI	0.7
Pimaricin		0.3
o-Phenylphenol	Group ADI	0.2
Sodium *o*-phenylphenol	Group ADI	0.2
Potassium nitrate	Group ADI	0.2
Sodium nitrite	Group ADI	0.2
Hexamethylenetetramine		0.15
Diphenyl		0.05
Propellants		
Carbon dioxide		NS
Nitrogen		NS
Dichlorodifluoromethane		1.5
Raising agents		
Ammonium hydrogen carbonate		NS
Ammonium carbonate		NS
Potassium hydrogen carbonate		NS
Sodium hydrogen carbonate		NS
Glucono delta lactone		NS
Calcium phosphate, monobasic		70
Disodium pyrophosphate		70
Sodium aluminium phosphate, acidic		0.6
Solvents, carrier		
Glycerol		NS
Glycerol diacetate		NS
Glycerol monoacetate		NS
Triacetin		NS
Monoglyceride citrate		NS

continued

Table 1 (continued)

CLASS	ADI
Solvents, carrier	
Ethyl alcohol	LGMP
Ethyl acetate	25
Propylene glycol	25
Triethyl citrate	20
Polyethylene glycols	10
Butane-1,3-diol	4
Amyl acetate	3
Castor oil	0.7
Solvents, extraction	
Carbon dioxide	NS
Light petroleum	NS
Propane	NS
Toluene	NS
Acetone	LGMP
Dichloromethane	Lowest levels technologically attainable
Ethyl alcohol	LGMP
Heptane	LGMP
Hexane	LGMP
Methanol	LGMP
Nitropropane (2-)	Lowest levels technologically attainable
Trichloroethylene (1,1,2-)	Lowest levels technologically attainable
Stabilizers	
Acetylated distarch adipate	NS
Acetylated distarch phosphate	NS
Acid-treated starch	NS
Alkaline-treated starch	NS
Bleached starch	NS
Dextrins, roasted starch	NS
Distarch phosphate, A	NS
Distarch phosphate, B	NS
Hydroxypropyl distarch phosphate	NS
Monostarch phosphate	NS
Oxidized starch	NS
Phosphated distarch phosphate	NS
Starch acetate esterified with vinyl acetate	NS
Starch acetate esterified with acetic anhydride	NS
Starch sodium octenyl succinate	NS
Agar	NS
Carob bean gum	NS
Carrageenan	NS
Furcellaran from *F. fastigiata*	NS
Gelatine, edible	NS
Guar gum	NS
Gum arabic	NS
Pectin	NS
Tara gum	NS
Xanthan gum	NS
Cellulose, microcrystalline	NS
Polydextroses A and N	NS

continued overleaf

Table 1 (continued)

CLASS		ADI
Stabilizers		
Insoluble polyvinylpyrrolidone		NS
Mono- and diglycerides		NS
Sodium caseinate		NS
Calcium acetate		NS
Calcium chloride		NS
Calcium citrate		NS
Calcium gluconate		NS
Calcium hydroxide		NS
Calcium sulphate		NS
Magnesium chloride		NS
Tripotassium citrate		NS
Trisodium citrate		NS
Papain		LGMP
Ammonium polyphosphates	Group ADI	70
Calcium phosphate, monobasic	Group ADI	70
Disodium pyrophosphate	Group ADI	70
Potassium polyphosphates	Group ADI	70
Sodium phosphate, tribasic	Group ADI	70
Alginic acid	Group ADI	50
Ammonium alginate	Group ADI	50
Calcium alginate	Group ADI	50
Potassium alginate	Group ADI	50
Sodium alginate	Group ADI	50
Magnesium gluconate		50
Polvinylpyrrolidone		50
Potassium L(+)-tartrate	Group ADI	30
Potassium sodium L(+)-tartrate	Group ADI	30
Sodium L(+)-tartrate	Group ADI	30
Ethyl cellulose		25
Ethyl hydroxyethyl cellulose	Group ADI	25
Hydroxypropyl cellulose	Group ADI	25
Hydroxypropyl methylcellulose	Group ADI	25
Methylcellulose	Group ADI	25
Methyl ethyl cellulose	Group ADI	25
Sodium carboxymethyl cellulose	Group ADI	25
Calcium stearoyl lactate	Group ADI	20
Sodium stearoyl lactate	Group ADI	20
Calcium disodium ethylenediaminetetraacetate	Group ADI	2.5
Disodium ethylenediaminetetraacetate	Group ADI	2.5
Calcium hydrogen sulphite		0.7
Sweeteners		
Isomalt		NS
Lactitol		NS
Maltitol		NS
Maltitol syrup		NS
Mannitol		NS
Sorbitol		NS
Sorbitol syrup		NS
Thaumatin		NS
Xylitol		NS
Aspartame		40

continued

Table 1 (continued)

CLASS		ADI
Sweeteners		
Calcium cyclamates	} Group ADI	11
Sodium cyclamate		11
Acesulfame potassium		9
Trichlorogalactosucrose		3.5
Calcium saccharin		2.5
Potassium saccharin		2.5
Saccharin	} Group ADI	2.5
Saccharin (potassium and sodium salts)		2.5
Sodium saccharin		2.5
Thickeners		
Acetylated distarch adipate		NS
Acetylated distarch phosphate		NS
Acid-treated starch		NS
Alkaline-treated starch		NS
Amylose and amylopectin		NS
Bleached starch		NS
Dextrins, roasted starch		NS
Distarch phosphate, A		NS
Distarch phosphate, B		NS
Hydroxypropyl distarch phosphate		NS
Hydroxypropyl starch		NS
Monostarch phosphate		NS
Oxidized starch		NS
Phosphated distarch phosphate		NS
Starch acetate esterified with vinyl acetate		NS
Starch acetate esterified with acetic anhydride		NS
Starch sodium octenyl succinate		NS
Starches, enzyme-treated		NS
Cellulose, powdered		NS
Polydextroses A and N		NS
Agar		NS
Carob bean gum		NS
Carrageenan		NS
Furcellaran from *F. fastigiata*		NS
Guar gum		NS
Gum arabic		NS
Karaya gum		NS
Pectin		NS
Tara gum		NS
Tragacanth gum		NS
Xanthan gum		NS
Glycerol		NS
Sorbitol		NS
Sorbitol syrup		NS
Calcium polyphosphates		70
Pentapotassium triphosphate	} Group ADI	70
Pentasodium triphosphate		70
Alginic acid		50
Ammonium alginate		50
Calcium alginate	} Group ADI	50
Potassium alginate		50
Sodium alginate		50

continued overleaf

Table 1 (continued)

CLASS		ADI
Thickeners		
Propylene glycol alginate		25
Ethyl hydroxyethyl cellulose		25
Hydroxypropyl cellulose		25
Hydroxypropyl methyl cellulose	Group ADI	25
Methylcellulose		25
Methyl ethyl cellulose		25
Sodium carboxymethyl cellulose		25

Two groups of synthetic antioxidants, gallic acid esters and butylated hydroxytoluenes, warrant closer attention. Gallic acid esters (propyl, octyl and dodecyl) are used extensively. They can cause contact dermatitis. On ingestion, the gallates are hydrolysed, releasing the acid, which is absorbed. It is excreted unchanged in the urine or metabolized to 4-*O*-methylgallic acid and conjugated with glucuronic acid. In reproductive studies the gallates cause failure of the neonates to thrive at maternal dietary levels above 0.1 per cent. This effect is abolished if the pups are fostered and is thus due to a product in the maternal milk. The effect is not seen with propyl gallate.

The butylated phenols butylated hydroxytoluene (BHT) and butylated hydroxyanisole (BHA) are two synthetic antioxidants that are very widely used and not only in food products. The toxicology of these compounds has been studied in great detail over many years.

BHT is rapidly absorbed after ingestion, maximum tissue concentrations being achieved in 4 h in rats and mice. There is no evidence of tissue accumulation on repeated dosage but excretion is slow (half-life 7–10 days), probably owing to an enterohepatic circulation. In man absorption is rapid also but 50 per cent of the dose is excreted in the urine in 24 h. The remainder is excreted more slowly, and this could indicate that biliary excretion with an enterohepatic circulation also occurs in humans.

In the experimental animal the main metabolite is BHT acid, both free and conjugated, whereas in man this is a minor metabolite. The main metabolite is a benzofuran, excreted as a conjugate with glucuronic acid or mercapturic acid (Conning and Phillips, 1986).

Repeated exposure to BHT, by incorporation in the diet, results in liver enlargement and the induction of microsomal oxidases. The growth rate of animals is reduced and the life-span increased. No adverse effects occur in reproductive studies. In one study an increased incidence of hepatic tumours occurred in animals surviving beyond 111 weeks (the control animals survived much less well) at a dose equivalent, on a body weight basis, to 250 mg kg^{-1} day^{-1}, but not at lower doses (25 and 10 mg kg^{-1} day^{-1}). The ADI is currently set at a maximum of 0.125 mg kg^{-1}.

BHA is absorbed after oral administration and excreted in the urine conjugated directly with glucuronic acid or sulphate. The half-life in man is 2–5 days. At small dosage, BHA may be excreted unconjugated and at high dosage there may be metabolism to a hydroquinone. BHA shows no adverse effects on reproduction. It has, however, been shown at high dosage to induce malignant tumours of the forestomach in several animal species that possess a forestomach. This effect occurs at dietary concentrations of 1 per cent and 2 per cent but not at 0.5 per cent. The appearance of tumours is preceded by hyperplasia which is slowly reversible if treatment is stopped (Ito *et al.*, 1983).

These findings have resulted in further extensive studies of the roles of BHT and BHA as promoters of carcinogenesis, given that neither compound is genotoxic. Both have been shown, at high dosage, to promote tumours initiated by tissue-specific carcinogens and yet to inhibit carcinogenesis at low dosage. Similar studies with alpha-tocopherol, alone or with BHA and/or BHT, have consistently shown tumour inhibition.

It seems likely that at low dosage antioxidants reduce the likelihood of tumour formation, owing perhaps to a protective effect against free radical damage, but at high dosage, except for alpha-tocopherol, they may become oxygen donors and enhance the carcinogenic process.

Colours

Colouring materials are added to processed foodstuffs to restore or standardize colour. It is generally accepted that colour has an important role in making food attractive, but with advanced preservation techniques based on the rapid reduction of the temperature of cooked products, the need for added colour has become less. There is a general regulatory policy in the UK to reduce the use of colours except where the resultant product would be colourless, such as boiled sweets and other confectionery (Food Advisory Committee, 1987).

Colours used in food products may be classified in two groups—synthetic and natural. The synthetic colours can be produced to high specifications, whereas the natural colours are extracted and usually consist of mixtures. Some natural colours can be synthesized but this also usually results in mixtures that are nevertheless better characterized.

Synthetic Colours

Four main classes of compounds are used.

Azo dyes Compounds in which one or more azo groups ($-N=N-$) are present. They have been subjected to extensive toxicological study. They are, in general, poorly absorbed but the azo linkage is broken down by bacterial activity in the colon. The products are absorbed only to a minor extent and are usually excreted as glucuronide conjugates in the urine. The stimulus to bacterial metabolism of the large doses employed in toxicological studies commonly results in caecal hypertrophy. This may be associated, by mechanisms as yet unknown, with nephrocalcinosis in those experimental species susceptible to age-related nephrosclerosis such as the rat and mouse.

There have been a number of reports that azo dyes, and, in particular, tartrazine, are associated with food intolerance. Food intolerance is characterized by a reproducible, unpleasant reaction to a food or food ingredient. It may give rise to many symptoms, the commonest being migrainous headaches, gastrointestinal disturbance or manifestation of an allergic reaction. Although commonly called 'food allergies' the demonstration of an immunological basis is rarely achieved. The condition occurs most commonly in children under the age of 5 years and usually does not persist beyond the age of 7 or 8, although a minority of adults may exhibit adverse reactions to specific food components.

Claims have been made that attention deficit disorder, commonly called hyperactivity, is due to food intolerance. This rare condition occurs in early childhood and is characterized by short attention span, disruptive behaviour, volatile temperament and underachievement in school. Studies of dietary causes have given conflicting results, but it is likely that a small minority of cases are the result of intolerance to some dietary items, which may include some food additives. Regrettably, the doses used to elicit responses have been much larger than would be obtained from food and drink, and the possibility of pseudoallergic (anaphylactoid) reactions cannot be excluded. The syndrome itself is difficult to diagnose without considerable experience, and there can be little doubt that it has been considerably overdiagnosed (Lessof, 1987).

Triphenylmethane Dyes In general, triphenylmethane dyes are poorly absorbed and long-term toxicity studies have shown no adverse effects.

Fluorescein Dyes Based on fluoran, the main example is erythrosine, a molecule in which iodine is incorporated. This has given rise to some concern in relation to thyroid function, in that in the rat, at high dosage, there is evidence of hypertrophy and hyperplasia of the thyroid gland with an accompanying increase of the serum concentrations of thyroxine and protein-bound iodine, and a reduction in serum triiodothyronine (T_3). Such findings suggest that erythrosine stimulates the release of thyroid stimulating hormone, possibly by inhibiting the conversion of thyroxine to T_3, thereby reducing the feedback mechanism. The effect does not occur at the concentrations experienced in food usage, which are about 1000 times less than the minimal effect dosage.

Sulphonated Indigo Dyes Sulphonated indigo dyes are poorly absorbed and have demonstrated no adverse effects in several long-term toxicity studies.

Natural Colours

Natural colours are obtained from naturally occurring materials which may or may not be foods. Usually those derived from natural foods by physical means (pressing and filtration, or aqueous extracts) are accepted for use in foods. Usually they have not been subjected to rigorous toxicological study. Such studies will be required if their use increases substantially.

The main colours of this type are the ribo-flavins, cochineal carmine, the carotenes (with the exception of a carotenoid, canthoxanthin), the anthocyanins, chlorophyll and chlorophyllins, and beetroot red. Directly extracted annatto, but not the solvent extracted compound, is also included.

Of the naturally occurring compounds which are synthesized, caramel is by far the most important. It is very extensively used in cola drinks and beers. Caramels are formed when simple sugars are heated. The process involves dehydration and the formation of furans and fur-furaldehyde, which then degrade and polymerize to form brown-coloured compounds. The precise chemistry is unknown. Pyrolysis may occur but can be prevented in the presence of ammonium salts, acids, alkalis or sulphites.

Industrially, a wide range of caramels is pro-duced through the use of ammonia and ammonium sulphite. This has made the toxico-logical evaluation difficult. The position improved when the British Caramel Manufacturers Associ-ation specified six types of caramels (including starting materials) to which industrial use would be confined. This proposal was later modified by international industrial agreement and the modi-fied proposal has been accepted, provisionally, by the regulatory authorities.

Four main types of caramel have been speci-fied.

Alkali compounds, made with sodium or pot-assium hydroxide.
Ammonia compounds, made with ammonia or ammonium hydroxide, carbonate, bicar-bonate, phosphate or sulphate.
Sulphite compounds, made with sulphur dioxide, sulphurous acid, sodium or potas-sium sulphite, bisulphite or metabisulphite.
Ammonium sulphite compounds, made with ammonium sulphite or bisulphite, this group to be classified in two strengths.

In each case the process must be specified. Burnt sugar caramels, used essentially as flavouring agents, are additional to these groups.

Although many studies have been undertaken with many caramels, the main finding has been caecal enlargement in the rat, not considered to be of toxicological significance. Other adverse effects have been attributed to imidazole con-taminants at high dosage. With ammonia cara-mels, however, it was noted that rats developed lymphocytopenia, an effect enhanced by reduced dietary levels of vitamin B_6. It is thought that this effect is mainly due to the presence of a tetrahydroxybutyl imidazole (THI), although it cannot be excluded that other active compounds are present. It is not known whether this effect occurs in the other species, such as man, or whether it has any functional significance. Work proceeds and for the time being, the THI content of ammonia caramel is limited to 25 ppm.

As caramel colours represent 98 per cent usage of all colours in foodstuffs, they are of consider-able economic importance. More importantly, such widespread usage could have serious impli-cations for public health if adverse effects occur in man. At present there is no evidence that this is the case (Food Advisory Committee, 1987).

Emulsifiers

Food manufacture involves to a considerable extent, the mixing of ingredients, especially ingredients that are either fat- or water-soluble. Such mixing is greatly facilitated by the use of emulsifiers. These are usually chain-like mole-cules with a water-soluble group at one end and a fat-soluble group at the other. Additionally, the group includes some proteins and some simple salts of organic acids. Emulsifiers are almost invariably compounds and derivatives that occur naturally, the commonest being based on esters of fatty acids with glycerol or simple sugars. They have been extensively studied and generally are of low toxicity, the observed effects being associ-ated with the physical consequences of very large dosage, such as bladder stones and altered cal-cium–phosphate balance. Many studies con-ducted at lower dosage in man have shown no adverse effects.

Flavours

Modern food processes employ flavouring materials very extensively. This has resulted in the development of a wide range of flavouring materials. At present about six thousand flavour-ing agents have been identified of which about 3500 are in common use, many in complicated mixtures. It is a considerable technological challenge to develop for a particular foodstuff an identifiable and acceptable flavour from the large array of compounds that exist.

The vast majority of flavouring compounds occur naturally, having been identified through the laborious extraction of prepared foods. Having been characterized, the compounds are often synthesized. These are the so-called 'nature-identical' compounds. Their manufacture allows adherence to tighter specification than is possible with extracts of natural materials and, of course, improves their availability and reduces cost.

Flavour compounds are extremely potent, often eliciting a distinct flavour at molecular concentrations. As a consequence, although their use is widespread, the concentrations in food are very low indeed, and the amounts manufactured are small in comparison with foodstuffs themselves or industrial chemicals generally.

One result has been that very few of the compounds have been subjected to extensive toxicological testing, essentially because conventional toxicity studies are too insensitive to detect effects at the concentrations likely to be present in food, so that the resultant safety margins will be very large. An additional reason is that, for many flavouring substances, the amount of material required to mount a comprehensive toxicological analysis would be difficult to obtain (Food Additives and Contaminants Committee, 1976).

Flavouring substances are classified as follows. *Natural*—compounds that are extracted from foodstuffs and spices and used directly. They consist of complex mixtures and are generally regarded as offering no hazard where their usage does not greatly exceed that which occurs naturally.

Nature-identical—compounds that have been characterized as part of a natural flavour complex and synthesized. They are regarded, for regulatory purposes, as new chemicals requiring toxicological evaluation. Many have been subjected to such studies and the rest will be when priorities have been agreed.

Artificial—wholly new compounds with flavouring characteristics. In the UK, four such compounds comprise the bulk of consumption. These are: ethyl vanillin, ethylmaltol, ethylmethylphenylglycidate and butyl butyryl lactate.

All have given repeatedly negative responses in a variety of toxicological studies. The average individual consumption of these compounds in the UK does not exceed 16 μg kg^{-1} day^{-1} for each compound.

It is likely that in due course the use of flavouring substances will diminish as preservation techniques based on quick freezing are developed, but for the foreseeable future a substantial usage will remain, given the increasing popularity of processed foods and meals.

Flavour Enhancers

Flavour enhancers have the ability to intensify the flavour of cooked, processed foods without, at the concentrations used, adding flavour of their own. They have been in use for many centuries, although it is only in the last century or so that they have been chemically characterized. They are particularly popular with Japanese and Chinese cooks. The mode of action is not known but seems to involve both the taste buds and the tactile nerve endings in the buccal cavity, enhancing taste and imparting a satisfactory 'mouth feel'.

The compounds are salts of glutamic or guanylic acids, or of the nucleotides inosinic acid or ribonucleic acid. As naturally occurring compounds, they are not associated with adverse toxicity, except at very high dosage.

The commonest compound in use is monosodium glutamate (MSG). Adult diets normally contain approximately 20 g of MSG daily, of which not more than 0.7 g is 'added'. Quantities as high as 45 g day^{-1} (0.75 g kg^{-1} day^{-1}) have been consumed without adverse effect. One animal study showed that neonatal mice given 0.5 g kg^{-1} day^{-1} by mouth developed hypothalamic lesions, although these did not occur when MSG was given subcutaneously. Human breast milk contains 21.6 mg dl^{-1} of free L-glutamate.

Some people claim to experience a variety of symptoms such as tingling of the mouth and tongue, and weakness of the limbs, after the consumption of food reputedly containing MSG, the so-called 'Chinese restaurant syndrome'. This effect has not been confirmed by double-blind clinical trials but it remains a possibility that some individuals exhibit an idiosyncratic sensitivity. The mechanism remains obscure.

Preservatives

In many respects the history of mankind is characterized by his increasing ability to produce and preserve food. The origins of many preservation techniques, such as salting, pickling, acidification, smoking and dehydration, are lost in antiquity. Although many of these methods are still used today, food manufacture has latterly relied more on chemical expertise.

Chemical preservation depends on the ability of certain compounds to inhibit microbial growth, thereby preventing microbiological spoilage of foodstuffs. At the concentrations used, preservatives are not bactericidal.

Most chemical preservatives are simple acids or their salts, and exert their effect through a reduction of pH. The commonest are benzoic acid, acetic acid, propionic acid and sorbic acid. Sulphites, nitrites and nitrates are also in common use. Another major group is the ethyl and propyl esters of *para*-hydroxybenzoic acid, valuable because they exert an antimicrobial effect across a wide range of pH values.

Each compound is effective against a limited range of micro-organisms (bacteria, moulds, yeasts) in a particular type of foodstuff and tends to have been developed for that purpose, although there is a considerable overlap. Sorbic acid, for example, is used in chemically leavened baked goods; propionic and acetic acids in yeast-leavened baked goods; sulphites in wines and beers; benzoates or *para*-hydroxybenzoates in beverages, fruit juices, purées and pie fillings; nitrites and nitrates, almost exclusively, in meat products.

Benzoic Acid   Benzoic acid is conjugated in the liver and excreted in the urine as hippuric acid. This reaction was used for many years as a test of liver function in man. Absorption is rapid and excretion complete. The only adverse effects resulting from long-term administration at high dosage are gastric irritation and a possible disturbance of acid–base balance. Some individuals exhibit allergy to benzoates.

Para-hydroxybenzoic Acid Esters   Para-hydroxybenzoic acid esters are readily absorbed and metabolized in the liver. The main excretion product is *para*-hydroxybenzoic acid and its glucuronide conjugate. Hydroxyhippuric acid is also formed. Extensive studies in several species have shown only marginal effects on growth rate at high dosage. Some individuals may show allergic responses.

Sorbic Acid   Sorbic acid is readily absorbed and converted to the fully saturated caproic acid. It is then metabolized as any other fatty acid and is used as a source of energy. Extensive toxicity studies have revealed no adverse effects at 5 per cent in the diet.

The Sulphites   The sulphites are reactive chemicals and, in foods, tend to be bound to sugars and proteins. On absorption they are converted to sulphates. In *in vitro* studies, sulphite can bind to DNA, causing bacterial mutation. This effect has not been observed in mammalian systems. The only adverse effect seen in extensive toxicological studies has been slight reduction in litter size or litter weight in three-generation reproduction studies.

Between 4 per cent and 7 per cent of severely asthmatic patients exhibit sensitivity to sulphur dioxide, which may be released from sulphite in acid media or on ingestion. This seems particularly the case where sulphites are used, in spray form, to preserve salads. The prevalence in all asthmatics is 1–2 per cent. The mechanism is not known but is unlikely to be an immune effect. Hypersensitivity of bronchial receptors has been postulated.

The Nitrates and Nitrites   Nitrates are readily absorbed and excreted unchanged although a small percentage may be converted to nitrite. At high levels of intake this conversion may result in the formation of methaemoglobin. The ingestion of nitrite is, of course, much more likely to result in methaemoglobinaemia in neonates.

Nitrites can react with amines to produce volatile *N*-nitrosamines and, with ureas, amides, carbamates or guanidines, to form *N*-nitrosamides. These reactions occur endogenously as well as in response to exogenous nitrites. *N*-Nitrosamines and *N*-nitrosamides are potent animal carcinogens, although, in practice, the former are much more stable and therefore more important. The role of *N*-nitrosamines in human carcinogenesis is not known. The major source of nitrites to man is derived from nitrates in the diet, mainly from vegetables and from water. The use of nitrites in foods probably adds a negligible burden and, given its efficacy in controlling the growth of *Clostridium botulinum* and, hence, deadly botulism, its continued use is probably justified.

Nevertheless, this is a field of very active research aimed at the quantification of *N*-nitroso compounds in order to gauge the carcinogenic hazard.

Sweeteners

Sucrose is a unique food in that it confers not only sweetness but also textural characteristics that are indispensable to certain products such as baked confectionery. However, its energy content (3.75 kcal g^{-1}) has led to its association with being overweight. There is a general cultural perception that being overweight is undesirable and a consequent requirement to reduce energy consumption. This has resulted in a search for compounds that possess similar characteristics to sucrose but with less energy content. None has been found, but two groups of compounds have been developed which approximate certain technical functions.

Bulk Sweeteners

Bulk sweeteners are polyhydric alcohols (polyols and sugar alcohols) and most of those of use in foodstuffs occur naturally. They are five- or six-carbon molecules essentially similar to the equivalent sugar, except that the aldehyde group or linkage is replaced by an alcohol group. They are of equivalent sweetness to sucrose and, in cooking, show several of the technical characteristics, such as effects on viscosity, crystallization and stability. They tend to be hygroscopic, and this, associated with their reduced absorption after ingestion, results in the main toxicological hazard—the production of diarrhoea. Individuals vary in their susceptibility to this effect but, in general, ingestion of less than 20 g day^{-1} does not cause problems. In the experimental rat these compounds cause the caecal enlargement associated with bacterial fermentation, but no other effect. The reduced absorption confers a reduced energy contribution to the diet.

Intense Sweeteners

Intense sweeteners are chemical compounds that exhibit intense sweetness but contribute little or no energy to the diet. Their sweetness ranges from 30 to 2000 times the sweetness of sucrose, so that they are used in very small amounts. They have none of the technological characteristics of sugars or sugar alcohols.

Aspartame Aspartame is the methyl ester of phenylalanine and aspartic acid, and is approximately 180 times as sweet as sucrose. On ingestion, it is metabolized to the constituent amino acids and methanol. Very extensive toxicological studies in experimental animals and in man have not revealed adverse effects attributable to the compound. There is continuing discussion on the possible effects of intakes of phenylalanine but as yet no definite effects have been consistently observed. In the UK products containing aspartame must contain a statement warning phenylketonurics of the possible presence of phenylalanine.

The methyl ester undergoes hydrolysis in acid and aqueous products on storage, with the formation of a substituted piperazine. This, too, has been subjected to extensive study, with no adverse effects detected at acceptable dosage. The breakdown product is not sweet-tasting, so that extensive consumption is unlikely.

Cyclamic Acid—Sodium and Calcium Salts Cyclamic acid was used for many decades in combination with saccharin because it reduced the bitter aftertaste associated with the latter compound. Its regulatory approval was discontinued when it was claimed that a cyclamate–saccharin mixture caused bladder carcinoma in the rat, the putative agent being cyclohexylamine, a metabolite of cyclamate produced by bacterial fermentation in the gut. Subsequent study has demonstrated that neither cyclamate nor cyclohexylamine are carcinogenic or mutagenic but that the amine can cause testicular atrophy at high dosage in the rat. Humans vary in their ability to generate the amine and certainly cannot produce toxic amounts, given the likely concentrations of cyclamate in the diet. Nevertheless, the use of cyclamate remains severely restricted in the UK and is not permitted in the USA.

Saccharin—potassium, sodium and calcium salts Saccharin, discovered in 1879, has been used as an intense sweetener since the turn of the century. It is some 300 times sweeter than sucrose but is associated with a bitter aftertaste. For many years it was regarded as absolutely safe, being absorbed and excreted unchanged. A study of a cyclamate–saccharin mixture with added cyclohexylamine claimed to detect a carcinogenic effect which was initially attributed to cyclamate. Subsequent studies with cyclamate failed to confirm this conclusion. Since then attention turned to saccharin, and innumerable investigations have been undertaken with this compound and its salts.

These studies have examined whether saccharin is a complete carcinogen or is a promoter of carcinogenesis initiated by primary carcinogens. The main findings which have been confirmed in repeated studies are:

(1) Sodium saccharin induces bladder tumours in male (but not female) rats, when administered for the lifetime of the animals at dietary concentrations of 5 per cent and above, provided that the administration commences within 2 weeks of birth or is fed to the mother during pregnancy and is continued thereafter. It does not exhibit this effect in other species.

(2) Sodium saccharin is not mutagenic.

(3) Sodium saccharin at a dietary concentration of 5 per cent will promote bladder tumours initiated by a known bladder carcinogen, N-butyl-N-4-(hydroxybutyl)nitrosamine (BBN). This effect is shared with sodium ascorbate, sodium bicarbonate and sodium citrate. Several similar claims using other initiators or the implantation of pellets in the urinary bladder have not been confirmed by repeated experiments.

(4) Sodium saccharin, but not potassium and calcium saccharin or the free acid, at 5 per cent in the diet induces epithelial hyperplasia in the urinary bladder of the rat.

(5) Sodium saccharin results in increased pH of rat urine. Studies employing 5 per cent sodium cyclamate or sodium hippurate, which do not elevate urinary pH, have not resulted in the formation of bladder tumours.

The overall conclusion is that sodium saccharin is a bladder carcinogen for the male rat, provided that the compound is administered soon after birth and continued for a lifetime. The dose–response relationship is steep and suggests a threshold limit of 1 per cent in the diet, equivalent, on a body weight basis, to 500 mg kg^{-1} day^{-1}. Potassium and calcium saccharin, or the free acid, are not associated with these effects. The current ADI of 2.5 mg kg^{-1} incorporates a 200-fold safety factory and applies to all forms of saccharin. Such

an intake represents approximately 12 cans of a diet drink, sweetened with saccharin, per day (Munro, 1989).

REFERENCES

British Nutrition Foundation's Task Force (1990). *Report: Complex Carbohydrates in Foods*. Chapman and Hall, London

Burkitt, D. P. and Trowell, H. C. (1975). *Refined Carbohydrate Foods and Disease: Some Implications of Dietary Fibre*. Academic Press, London

Carroll, K. K. and Khor, H. T. (1975). Dietary fat in relation to tumorigenesis. *Prog. Biochem. Pharmacol.*, **10**, 308–353

Conning, D. M. and Phillips, J. C. (1986). Comparative metabolism of BHA, BHT and other phenolic antioxidants and its toxicological relevance. *Fd Chem. Toxicol.*, **24**, 1145–1148

DHSS (1984). Department of Health and Social Security Report on Health and Social Subjects 28: *Diet and Cardiovascular Disease*. HMSO, London

Food Additives and Contaminants Committee (1976). *Report on the Review of Flavourings in Food*. F.A.C./Rep./22, HMSO, London

Food Advisory Committee (1987). *Final Report on the Review of the Colouring Matter in Food Regulations 1973*. F.A.C./Rep./4, HMSO, London

Gey, K. F., Brubacher, G. B. and Stähelin, H. B. (1987). Plasma levels of antioxidant vitamins in relation to ischemic heart disease and cancer. *Am. J. Clin. Nutr.*, **45**, 1368–1377

Goldstein, J. L., Kita, T. and Brown, M. S. (1983). Lessons from an animal counterpart of familial hypercholesterolemia. *New Engl. J. Med.*, **309**, 288–296

Ip, C., Carter, C. A. and Ip, M. M. (1985). Requirement of essential fatty acid for mammary tumorigenesis in the rat. *Cancer Res.*, **45**, 1997–2001

Ito, N., Fukushima, S., Hagiwara, A., Shibata, M. and Ogiso, T. (1983). Carcinogenicity of butylated hydroxyanisole in F344 rats. *J. Natl Cancer Inst.*, **70**, 343–349

Kannel, W. B. and Gordon, T. (Eds) (1970). *Some Characteristics Related to the Incidence of Cardiovascular Disease and Death*. Framingham Study 16-year Follow-up. US Government Printing Office, Washington, D.C.

Keys, A. (1980). *Seven Countries. A Multivariate Analysis of Death and Coronary Disease*. Harvard University Press, Cambridge, Massachusetts and London

Kinlen, L. J. (1987). Diet and cancer. In Cottrell, R. (Ed.), *Food and Health*. Parthenon Publishing Group, Carnforth, UK, pp. 83–98

Kromhout, D., Bosschieter, E. B. and Cowlander, L. Cor. De. (1985). The inverse relationship between fish consumption and 20-year mortality from coronary heart disease. *New Engl. J. Med.*, **312**, 1205–1209

Lavik, P. S. and Baumann, C. A. (1941). Dietary fat and tumour formation. *Cancer Res.*, **1**, 181–187

Lessof, M. M. (1987). Allergies to food additives. *J. Roy. Coll. Physicians*, **21**, 237–240

Miller, E. C. and Miller, J. A. (1966). Mechanisms of chemical carcinogenesis: Nature of proximate carcinogens and interactions with macromolecules. *Pharmacol. Rev.*, **18**, 805–836

Moncada, S. and Vane, J. R. (1978). Pharmacology and endogenous roles of prostaglandin endoperoxides, thromboxane A2 and prostacyclin. *Pharmacol. Rev.*, **30**, 293–331

Munro, I. C. (1989). A case study: The safety evaluation of artificial sweeteners. In Taylor, S. L. and Scanlan, R. A. (Eds), *Food Toxicology: A Perspective on the Relative Risks*. Marcel Dekker, New York, pp. 151–168

Peto, R., Doll, R., Buckley, J. D. and Sporn, M. B. (1981). Can dietary β-carotene materially reduce human cancer rates? *Nature*, **290**, 201–208

Whitaker, J. R. and Feeney, R. E. (1973). Enzyme inhibitors in food. In *Toxicants Occurring Naturally in Foods*. National Academy of Sciences, Washington, D.C.

FURTHER READING

Morgenroth, V. (1993). Scientific calculation of the data-derived safety factors for the acceptable daily intake. Case study: diethyhexylphthalate. *Food Additives and Contamination*, **10**, 363–373

Nerin, C., Cacho, J. and Gancedo, P. (1993). Plasticizers from printing inks in a selection of food packagings and their migration to food. *Food Additives and Contamination*, **10**, 453–460

Ohta, T. (1993). Modification of genotoxicity by naturally occurring flavorings and their derivatives. *Critical Reviews in Toxicology*, **21**, 171–182

Quattrucci, E. (1992). Current issues with food preservation. Symposium. *Food Additives and Contaminants*, Vol. 9

Gregory P. Wedin

INTRODUCTION

Poisons of animal origin encompass a broad array of toxic agents that are possessed by thousands of animal species. The vast number of poisonous and venomous animals, as well as significant differences among these species, prohibits generalizations that would be necessary to review this topic extensively. The toxicity of these agents, therefore, will be reviewed by discussing representative animal species that are significant hazards to humans.

It is important first to distinguish between animals that are poisonous and those that are venomous. A venomous animal can produce venom in specialized glands or cells which can be administered in some way to its enemy or prey. Poisonous animals, on the other hand, possess a toxin(s) within their tissue that can have deleterious effects when ingested.

Considerable differences exist within the animal kingdom with respect to the venom apparatus, mode of envenomation and constituents of the venom. Venomous animals can either bite or sting their victims and some are capable of squirting or spitting venom. The venom of most species is a unique but complex proteinaceous mixture. The biochemical and pharmacological properties of most venoms are incompletely understood because of their complexity. Difficulties in obtaining sufficient venom and in extracting individual components further complicate this issue.

An animal may use its venom offensively or defensively. For example it may be used to subdue or kill its prey and to aid in digestion. Alternatively, it may be used to ward off predators. Many venoms are multipurpose and cannot be narrowly classified. The toxic manifestations from envenomation will be influenced by these functions and the corresponding venom constituents.

Most poisonous animals accumulate toxin through the marine food chain. Unicellular sea algae (dinoflagellates) are the most common initial source. A number of these dinoflagellates are responsible for the often publicized 'red tides' which are associated with poisonous shellfish.

Although people who live in regions inhabited by venomous or poisonous animals are at greatest risk for toxic exposure, such encounters can occur elsewhere. Venomous animals, for example, may be imported by hobbyists or shipped inadvertently in produce or other goods. Likewise, poisonous seafood may be shipped to distant markets. This may present a therapeutic dilemma to a practitioner unfamiliar with such exposures. Regional Poison Control Centers are staffed with specially trained professionals who can provide expert information and advice on the management of such cases. These centers also have access to the Antivenom Index which was developed to assist with locating the appropriate antivenin to exotic bites and stings. The Index is a joint effort of the American Association of Zoological Parks and Aquariums, the American Association of Poison Control Centers and the Arizona Poison and Drug Information Center and similar information sources are available in some other countries.

SNAKES

Snakes are probably the most well recognized of all venomous animals. Their notorious reputation is established in ancient history, myth, magic and religion. While some people adore and are fascinated by these creatures, others are inordinately fearful. As expected, snakes and snakebite have been extensively studied but because of the vast number and complexity of these species and their venoms, considerable work is still needed.

It is estimated that up to 1 million snakebites occur annually worldwide resulting in up to 40 000 deaths. Approximately 45 000 snakebites occur in the USA each year of which 8000 are inflicted by venomous species (Russell *et al.*, 1975). In the USA only about 9–14 deaths occur annually from venomous snakebite (Russell, 1980). In some countries, e.g. the UK, poisonous snakebites are uncommon but venomous snake-bite is a much more significant problem in other parts of the world. In India, for example, available data suggest that up to 200 000 snakebites occur annually with approximately 15 000 deaths (George *et al.*, 1987). Most bites are inflicted on the foot or leg. Accidental snakebites occur most often in children during daylight hours of warm summer months (Parrish, 1966; McNally and Reitz, 1987). Conversely, adult men are frequently victims of snakebites that could be easily avoided, bites which have been termed illegitimate (Curry *et al.*, 1989).

Over 3000 species of snakes are distributed throughout the world, primarily in temperate climates (Russell *et al.*, 1975). Approximately 300 of these snakes are significantly hazardous to humans. Snakes are members of the class Reptilia. There are five families of venomous snakes including the Colubridae, Crotalidae, Elapidae, Hydrophidae and Viperidae.

Only two snakes in the family Colubridae are significant hazards to humans, namely the boomslang (*Dispholidus typus*) and vine snake (*Thelotornis capensis*), which are found in southern Africa (Aitchison, 1990). Their venomous bite results primarily in a consumptive coagulopathy, delayed hemorrhage and related complications. Crotalidae species are distributed throughout the world and include the pit vipers such as rattlesnakes, copperheads and cottonmouths (Nelson, 1989; Kunkel *et al.*, 1983–84). These snakes most notably produce local tissue necrosis and coagulopathies. Elapids, which are found in Asia, Australia, Africa and the Americas, include such notorious creatures as cobras, mambas and coral snakes (Russell, 1983; Nelson, 1989). Predominantly neurotoxic effects result from the venomous bites of these snakes. The Viperidae family includes the true vipers, located in Africa, Europe and the Middle East (Nelson, 1989). The toxic effects of their bites are comparable to those of the Crotalidae. The Hydrophids include the sea snakes which are found in warm, shallow waters in the Indian and Pacific Oceans (Tu and Fulde, 1987). Although these snakes possess very potent neurotoxins, their short fangs and low venom output results in relatively few serious envenomations.

Toxic Manifestations

Snakes are often categorized by the primary toxic effects of their venom but this oversimplifies the problem. For example, several species of cobra, whose venoms are considered neurotoxic, may also produce significant local necrosis as well as potentially lethal cardiotoxic events (Blaylock, 1982; Kunkel *et al.*, 1983–84; Minton, 1990). Likewise, rattlesnakes generally produce local tissue damage and coagulopathies but minimal neurotoxicity. The bite of the Mojave rattlesnake (*Crotalus scutulatus*), however, produces less local swelling and pain but neurotoxicity can be a significant problem (Russell *et al.*, 1975; Kunkel *et al.*, 1983–84).

Snake venom is a complex mixture of proteins, enzymes, metals and other inorganic substances (Russell, 1983). The venom of some species, in fact, may contain up to 20 different components (Russell, 1983). However, relatively little is known about the composition of most venoms. The complex nature of snake venom as well as intra- and interspecies differences contribute to the variability and perplexity of snake venom poisoning.

The potential severity of envenomation is dependent on a number of factors, including the species of snake involved; its age and size; the location, number and depth of bites; and the total quantity of venom injected. Other important factors include the age and size of the victim and their general state of health. Not all strikes by snakes result in envenomation. So called 'dry bites' may occur in up to 30 per cent of crotalid bites, 50 per cent of elapid bites, and up to 75 per cent of sea snake bites (Kunkel *et al.*, 1983–84).

Local Toxic Effects

Envenomation by Crotalids and Viperids typically results in significant local toxic effects (Russell, 1980). Pain, swelling and oedema occur soon after the bite. In severe cases the oedema progresses rapidly. Within several hours the site may become ecchymotic and discoloured. Vesicles may also appear, which are usually filled with clear fluid but may become filled with blood in severe cases. Local tissue necrosis may also occur which is probably due to the direct action of the venom's enzymes. Pain and swelling are generally most severe following bites by eastern and western diamondback rattlesnakes and least severe following bites by copperheads and *Sistrurus* rattlesnake species (Russell *et al.*, 1975).

Coagulopathies

Snake envenomation may result in a variety of systemic manifestations. Probably the most significant but unpredictable are coagulopathies. Snakes within all families have been implicated with such disorders (Blaylock, 1982; Russell, 1983; Cable *et al.*, 1984). Both anticoagulant and procoagulant properties have been described but bleeding disorders occur most commonly.

Anticoagulation results from the constituents of snake venom that may (1) interfere with activation of clotting factors, (2) have fibrinolytic and fibrinogenolytic activity, (3) directly or indirectly activate plasminogen, or (4) directly act on phospholipids (Russell, 1983). Thrombocytopenia with or without other coagulopathies may result from intravascular clotting and consumption of platelets, sequestration of platelets at the site of envenomation or destruction of platelets by the venom (Riffer *et al.*, 1987). The degree of thrombocytopenia may directly correlate with the severity of envenomation (La Grange and Russell, 1970). Disseminated intravascular coagulation may complicate severe cases.

Snake venom constituents may interact at various points of the coagulation cascade to activate clotting factors or even prothrombin directly (Russell, 1983). Significant amounts of thrombin-like enzymes have also been identified in the venom of crotalids and viperids (Russell, 1983).

Cardiotoxicity

Cardiovascular shock is a common cause of death from crotalid envenomation and contributes to other systemic complications (Hardy, 1986). Shock results from ·increased capillary permeability which leads to third-spacing of fluids and intravascular volume depletion (Schaeffer *et al.*, 1979). Reduced cardiac output secondary to venom-induced cardiac changes, as well as the release of mediators such as bradykinins, histamine and serotonin, may also contribute to haemodynamic compromise (Curry and Kunkel, 1985; Christopher and Rodning, 1986).

Neurotoxicity

Neurotoxicity is primarily associated with envenomation by elapids and hydrophids. The venoms of these snakes are comparable but the venoms of sea snakes are more toxic (Tu and Fulde, 1987). The neurotoxin of sea snakes binds to postsynaptic acetylcholine receptors resulting in paralysis (Tu and Fulde, 1987). Respiratory paralysis is the primary cause of immediate death (Kitchens and van Mierop, 1987). The venom of elapids such as the banded krait contains presynaptic neurotoxins which inhibit the release of acetylcholine at the myoneural junction (Minton, 1990). Neurotoxic signs and symptoms include diplopia, slurred speech, deafness, paraesthesias, hyperaesthesia, muscle fasciculations, weakness, incoordination, trismus, pain, stiffness, drowsiness, apprehension, increased salivation, diaphoresis and convulsions (Russell, 1980; Blaylock, 1982; Tu and Fulde 1987; Kitchens and van Mierop, 1987; Nelson, 1989). Crotalid envenomation can also cause perioral paraesthesias, muscle fasciculations and weakness (Russell, 1980). The Mojave rattlesnake (*Crotalus scutulatus*) is a unique crotalid in that neurotoxic manifestations predominate.

Other Toxic Manifestations

Numerous other systemic toxic effects have been associated with snake bites. These may result from either direct actions of the venom or as complications of cardiovascular, neuromuscular or coagulation disorders. Renal failure may complicate crotalidae, hydrophidae and viperidae envenomation, which may result from disseminated intravascular coagulation, cardiovascular shock or hemolysis (George *et al.*, 1987; Nelson, 1989). A direct nephrotoxic effect of the venom is postulated as the primary cause of renal failure in *Vipera russelli* envenomation. Adult respiratory distress syndrome may develop in severe cases. The aetiology is unclear but shock, disseminated intravascular coagulation, multiple blood component transfusions and the venom itself are all postulated (Curry and Kunkel, 1985).

Management

A shroud of controversy veils the treatment of venomous snakebite. Rather than fully exploring all treatment issues and modalities, an overview of the generally accepted approach to management will be presented.

The most important first aid measures are to keep the victim calm, immobilize the bitten extremity and transport to the nearest appropriate healthcare facility. Incision and suction at the bite is generally impractical and potentially dangerous. It may be beneficial in a few select cases when it can be performed within a few minutes by a qualified individual using appropriate equipment. Likewise, the use of a lymphatic tourniquet to impede venom distribution is of questionable value and hazardous if done improperly. The use of a firm bandage wrapped around the affected extremity in conjunction with immobilization has been shown to delay elapid venom distribution (Sutherland *et al.*, 1979). Such an approach may have some utility in the management of elapid or hydrophid bites. The bandage is contraindicated following bites by snakes that cause tissue necrosis such as the crotalids and viperids. Cryotherapy is also contraindicated.

Correct indentification of the offending snake is important. Unfortunately, the victim often cannot give a detailed description of the snake and it is usually not available for examination. The use of immunological tests to identify snake venom in serum or other materials is currently used in some parts of the world. In Australia, for example, venom detection kits, which use the enzyme-linked immunosorbent assay (ELISA) technique, are an integral part of snakebite management (Minton, 1987).

Antivenin therapy is the cornerstone of snake-bite management worldwide. The choice of antivenin depends on the species of snake involved and available forms of antivenin. Antivenin may be monovalent (activity against only one species of snake) or polyvalent (activity against two or more species of snake). If available, monovalent antivenin is preferable when the offending species of snake is known with certainty. Polyvalent antivenins have been developed to treat many venomous species in a geographical area. In the USA, for example, Antivenin (Crotalidae) Polyvalent (Wyeth Laboratories, Philadelphia, PA) is active against all pit vipers in the western hemisphere and even some Asian species (Otten, 1983).

The clinical status of the patient and the species of snake involved guide antivenin therapy. It first must be determined if the patient was envenomated. The patient should be closely monitored for the development of local or systemic signs or symptoms as well as laboratory changes. Approximately 4–6 h of observation is generally necessary to rule out significant envenomation. There are, however, notable exceptions to these

fundamental guidelines. Bites by the eastern coral snake (*Micrurus fulvius*), for example, may produce minimal local toxic effects, but profound neurotoxicity may develop hours later. Likewise, the Mojave rattlesnake (*Crotalus scutulatus*) may produce minimal local effects, but neurotoxic manifestations can be delayed. Accordingly, prophylactic antivenin therapy is indicated for all definite bites by the eastern coral snake and other potentially neurotoxic envenomations (Otten, 1983).

The dose of antivenin is dependent on the species of the snake, the particular antivenin, and the severity of the envenomation. If indicated, antivenin should be administered as soon as possible following the bite. It is important to note that children should receive the same dose of antivenin as would an adult and possibly even more (Otten, 1983).

The initial dose of Antivenin (Crotalidae) Polyvalent for crotalid bites depends on the initial severity of the bite. Russell recommends grading the severity as minimal, moderate or severe (Russell, 1983). Minimal envenomations involve only local manifestations confined to the area of the bite and should be treated with three to five vials of antivenin. Moderate envenomations that involve progressive local effects, significant systemic manifestations and laboratory changes should be treated with six to ten vials. Severe envenomation, which should be treated initially with at least ten vials of antivenin, involves the entire extremity or part and there is serious systemic toxicity and laboratory changes. Additional doses of antivenin may needed if toxic effects persist following the initial dose (Russell, 1980). In severe cases 30 or more vials may be required.

All currently available snake antivenins are derived from hyperimmunized horse serum. As a result some patients will develop an immediate type I hypersensitivity reaction, which is IgE mediated (Otten and McKimm, 1983). To reduce the risk of unexpected hypersensitivity reactions all patients should be skin tested prior to administering any antivenin. In the event of an allergic response the potential risks and benefits from therapy must be weighed. Generally, if life or limb is at stake, antivenin therapy should be continued after taking appropriate precautions. Patients who are treated with antivenin also are likely to develop a delayed immune complex reaction commonly known as serum sickness. This is an IgG- and IgM-mediated process which results in the formation of antigen–antibody complexes and the subsequent activation of the complement system (Otten and McKimm, 1983). Acute IgE-mediated allergic reactions to antigens in the snake venom itself have also been reported (Hogan and Dire, 1990).

The allergenic nature of currently available antivenins is a significant limitation. It causes indecision as to whether to start therapy and restricts the dose of antivenin that can be safely administered. This is compounded by the fact that in some cases many vials of currently available antivenins are needed to adequately neutralize the venom. A promising approach to resolve this dilemma is the use of polyacrylamide gel affinity chromatography to produce purified antibodies (Russell *et al.*, 1985). The superior efficacy and safety of this product has been demonstrated in both *in vivo* and *in vitro* studies (Russell *et al.*, 1985). Purified Fab fragments of IgG may provide further pharmacokinetic, therapeutic and safety advantages (Sullivan, 1987). The application of monoclonal antibody technology may be useful for those species whose venom contains one main toxin, such as the elapids (Theakston, 1989). The use of monoclonal antibodies for crotalids or viperids, on the other hand, is impractical because of the complexity of their venoms (Sullivan, 1987; Theakston, 1989).

Local wound care should be provided as needed and tetanus immunization should be updated if necessary. The systemic manifestations of poisonous snakebite are managed with traditional supportive measures. As intravascular volume depletion is a primary cause of cardiovascular shock, adequate fluid replenishment is essential. Central venous pressure (CVP) and pulmonary artery wedge pressure (PAWP) should be used to guide therapy. Oxygen should be administered and appropriate respiratory support provided as needed. Whole blood or blood products may be needed to treat acute blood loss and coagulopathies. The use of anticholinesterase agents such as neostigmine bromide has been suggested as a means to treat the paralysis of elapid bites (Blaylock, 1982). Antivenin and appropriate supportive measures, however, should be sufficient.

GILA MONSTER

The Gila monster, *Heloderma suspectum*, is one of only a few known venomous lizards. There are five subspecies of Heloderma including: *Heloderma suspectum suspectum* and *H. s. cinctum* (banded Gila monster), which are found in southwestern USA; *H. horridum horridum* (beaded lizard), *H. h. exasperatum* and *H. h. alvarez*, which along with *H. s. suspectum* are found in Mexico (Russell and Bogert, 1981). *H. h. alvarez* and *H. h. horridum* are also located further south into Guatemala.

The Gila monster may be kept as an exotic pet; therefore, humans may be bitten and require treatment essentially anywhere. In fact, most bites by this venomous lizard result from careless handling rather than unsuspecting attacks in nature.

The Gila monster is a rather large, slow moving, nocturnal reptile. Adults may reach 55 cm in length (Russell and Bogert, 1981). They feed mostly on small animals and have few predators other than humans.

The Helodermatids have a much less sophisticated venom apparatus than snakes. It consists of two venom glands located in the lower jaw. A pair of venom ducts lead to venom-conducting grooved teeth. When the Gila monster bites, it passively injects venom as it is drawn up its teeth by capillary action.

The venom apparatus is used primarily in defence. When the Gila monster bites, it often holds on to crush its prey and to allow sufficient venom to be injected. The venom contains proteins and a number of enzymes. Serotonin, amine oxidase, phospholipase A, protease, lipase and hyaluronidase have all been identified (Russell and Bogert, 1981). The venom may also have bradykinin-releasing activity.

Toxic Manifestations

There have been sporadic reports of humans bitten by the Gila monster. The bite generally results in relatively minor local and systemic toxic effects. On the other hand, life-threatening reactions have been reported. Bites should be treated, therefore, as medical emergencies with appropriate evaluation and care.

The Gila monster has strong jaws which can inflict significant local pain from mechanical trauma. Several small puncture wounds may result. Occasionally teeth may become lodged in the tissue. Bluish discoloration around the bite may be noted but tissue necrosis is unlikely. Injected venom causes pain which can be intense and may radiate throughout the extremity.

Oedema generally develops more slowly and is less severe than that which occurs with snake bites but in some cases it can become quite marked and tense (Roller, 1976; Russell and Bogert, 1981). This may contribute to the pain of envenomation. Lymphadenopathy and lymphadenitis have also been reported (Russell and Bogert, 1981; Bou-Abboud and Kardassakis, 1988).

Other common manifestations include weakness, faintness or dizziness, diaphoresis, nausea, vomiting and hypotension. Profound hypotension has been reported in several cases (Heitschel, 1986; Piacentine *et al.*, 1986; Streiffer, 1986; Bou-Abboud and Kardassakis, 1988; Preston, 1989).

Other cardiovascular effects have been described including nonspecific electrocardiogram changes, ventricular arrhythmias, and myocardial infarction (Roller, 1976; Bou-Abboud and Kardassakis, 1988; Streiffer, 1986; Preston, 1989). Impaired renal function has also been reported which is probably a result of prolonged hypotension (Preston, 1989).

Laboratory abnormalities may include hypokalaemia and leucocytosis. Thrombocytopenia has been rarely reported (Russell and Bogert, 1981; Bou-Abboud and Kardassakis, 1988; Preston, 1989). Thrombocytopenia associated with reduced fibrinogen and increased prothrombin time, partial thromboplastin time and fibrin split products indicated a consumptive coagulopathy in two cases (Bou-Abboud and Kardassakis, 1988; Preston, 1989).

Management

Limited first aid can be provided. The first step often is to remove the lizard, which can be difficult. Several reasonable approaches include: (1) using a stick or similar device inserted in the back of the jaw to pry it off; (2) putting the affected extremity under water thereby causing the animal to release itself; or (3) lighting and holding a match under the Gila monster's jaw. Keep the patient warm, immobilize the extremity and transport to an appropriate healthcare facility.

The site of the bite should be thoroughly cleansed and examined for remaining teeth. An X-ray of the site may be helpful.

There is no commercially available Gila monster antivenin. Vital signs and laboratory indicies should be monitored closely. An electrocardiogram should also be obtained. Treatment is primarily symptomatic and supportive care.

HYMENOPTERA

Flying insects of the order hymenoptera are distributed worldwide. A few of the thousands of known species are significantly hazardous to humans. These include honeybees, bumblebees, wasps, hornets and yellow jackets. Honeybees and bumblebees belong to the family Apidae; the others belong to the family Vespidae.

The vespids are generally more aggressive and attack vigorously if disturbed. Honeybees account for most apidae stings and a person is most likely to be stung by honeybees when around flowering plants. Yellow jackets tend to nest on the ground or in decaying wood. They will scavenge for food and may be pests at picnics or around garbage cans. Hornets build nests in trees or shrubs; wasps often nest under eaves of buildings.

Their stinging apparatus consists of a modified ovipositor that is connected to a venom sac. They grasp the victim's skin with their claws and then jab their stinger into the skin. The stinger of honeybees is barbed so it and the venom sac remain attached to the victim's skin when the bee flies away, resulting in its demise. Vespids and the bumblebee are generally able to withdraw their stingers and are capable of stinging again. Some yellowjackets, however, may also lose their stinger.

Stings from these insects may result in manifestations ranging from minor local pain and swelling to life-threatening respiratory and cardiovascular compromise. These toxic effects may result from direct local and systemic effects of the venom as well as allergic reactions to venom proteins.

Toxic Manifestations

Up to 50 μl of venom may be injected with each sting. This dose is insufficient to produce systemic toxicity; however, venom constituents will produce local irritation and pain. If a person is stung many times at once then sufficient venom may be injected to produce toxicity. Systemic toxicity from bee stings resembles an allergic reaction. Toxicity from vespid stings may include an acute allergic-like response followed by delayed effects such as haemolysis, rhabdomyolysis and renal failure (Bousquet *et al.*, 1984).

The normal response to a hymenoptera sting consists of a small painful, urticarial lesion that lasts only a few hours. Approximately 10–17 per cent of people may develop a large local reaction that includes swelling and erythema greater than 5 cm in diameter which may last more than 24 h (Maguire and Geha, 1986; Reisman, 1989). This large local reaction may have an immunological origin.

The allergic reactions to hymenoptera stings deserve detailed discussion. The allergic response may range from exaggerated local effects to analphylaxis and death. It is estimated that hymenoptera stings account for at least 40–50 deaths annually in the USA, more deaths than result from all other venomous animals (Golden, 1989). The systemic allergic response to hymenoptera stings is IgE mediated. Recent evidence also suggests a role for indirect complement activation (Valentine *et al.*, 1990). There is considerable crossreactivity among the various vespids but crossreactivity between vespid and bee venoms is relatively uncommon (Wright and Lockey, 1990).

The incidence of systemic allergic reactions may be as low as 0.4–0.8 per cent in children but as high as 4.0 per cent in adults (Settipane *et al.*, 1972; Golden *et al.*, 1982). Up to 10–15 per cent of the population may be sensitized to hymenoptera venom but have not had an allergic response (Golden *et al.*, 1982).

Systemic allergic reactions may range from mild, primarily dermatological manifestations to life-threatening anaphylaxis. Mild systemic reactions consist of generalized urticaria, angiooedema, erythema and pruritus (Maguire and Geha, 1986). Gastrointestinal symptoms may also be present. Laryngeal oedema, bronchospasm and hypotension may be life-threatening in severe cases (Maguire and Geha, 1986).

There are limited data to characterize which patients may develop some, none, or all of these manifestations. Important factors include the age of the patient, history of prior stings, sensitization as documented by skin test or RAST (radioallergosorbent tests) and previous response to hymen-

optera stings. Approximately 75 per cent of the population is not sensitized to hymenoptera venom and will develop a normal local response, and less than 1 per cent will develop a systemic allergic reaction (Golden, 1989). Those who have previously had normal or large local reactions but have a positive skin test or RAST have a 10–20 per cent risk of developing a systemic reaction (Golden, 1989). Patients with a previous history of a systemic reaction who have a positive skin test or RAST have a 50 per cent chance of developing another systemic reaction (Golden, 1989).

It is commonly thought that patients develop more severe reactions with subsequent stings. While it is true that patients who are stung repeatedly within a relatively short time (weeks to months) are more likely to develop a systemic reaction, most patients develop more mild or similar reactions with subsequent stings (Golden, 1989; Valentine *et al.*, 1990). Insect sting allergy, in fact, is a self-limiting disease for most people (Reisman, 1989). In other words, the more time between stings the less likely a person is to have a serious systemic reaction.

The typical allergic response in children is much different from that in adults. Children are more likely to have cutaneous manifestations but less likely to develop hypotension (Golden, 1989). Also, children much less frequently develop recurrent systemic manifestations. In fact, children who have previously had non-life-threatening allergic reactions are unlikely subsequently to develop a life-threatening reaction (Schuberth *et al.*, 1983; Valentine *et al.*, 1990).

Management

First aid treatment for hymenoptera stings includes removing the stinger (if it remains) by scraping across the site with a blunt-edged object such as a credit card. Do not grab the stinger to pull it out as squeezing the venom sack will inject more venom. The area should be washed well with soap and water. Normal local reactions can be managed by applying ice to reduce swelling, oedema and pruritus. An antihistamine such as diphenhydramine may also help relieve pruritus. Large local reactions may be helped by elevating the extremity and administering an analgesic as well as a glucocorticoid such as prednisone. The combined use of H_1- and H_2-antagonists has been suggested as a means to decrease the severity of late phase cutaneous reactions (deShazo *et al.*, 1984).

Adrenaline is the drug of choice for systemic sting reactions. Subcutaneous administration is adequate in mild to moderate cases. In the event of hypotension, adrenaline (epinephrine) should be administered intravenously. Intravenous fluids and aggressive cardiopulmonary resuscitation should be provided if adrenaline (epinephrine) therapy alone is not adequate. Oral or intravenous antihistamines should only be used for cutaneous manifestations of hymenoptera allergy.

Patients who may develop systemic reactions should be prescribed an emergency kit that includes adrenaline (epinephrine) for subcutaneous injection. This includes those patients with a previous history of systemic allergic effects and those who have had large local reactions and have a positive skin test or RAST.

Venom immune therapy (VIT) may be useful in selected cases. It is presently indicated for those patients who previously have had life-threatening systemic reactions and have a positive skin test or RAST (Maguire and Geha, 1986). Adults are more likely candidates than children as they are at greater risk for developing a repeat systemic reaction. Immunotherapy, in fact, is unnecessary in most children (Valentine *et al.*, 1990). Other patients with less severe systemic reactions who have positive skin tests or RAST may benefit from VIT but the cost of therapy and other factors such as their age, medical history, occupation, outdoor activities or hobbies must be considered.

ANTS

Ants belong to the family Formicidae and comprise the third group of venomous hymenoptera. Thousands of ant species are distributed worldwide, some of which can inflict painful venomous stings. Local or systemic allergic reactions can also occur. Not all venomous ants sting. Some, such as the carpenter and weaver ants of the subfamiliy Formacinae, bite their prey and then spray venom into the wound. Formic acid, which is a potent cytotoxin, is the primary constituent of their venom (Rhoades *et al.*, 1977).

Fire ants (*Solenopsis spp*) are native to both North and South America. Fire ant envenom-

ation is a significant health hazard in the southern USA (Blum, 1984; Stafford *et al.*, 1989a). In fact, up to 60 per cent of the population in an infested area are stung each year (deShazo *et al.*, 1990). The red imported fire ant (*Solenopsis invicta*) has rapidly spread throughout the southern USA and has overtaken the less aggressive native species (*S. xyloni*), as well as the black imported fire ant (*S. richteri*). The imported fire ants of the USA are so named because they are thought to have been introduced via produce shipped from Brazil to Mobile, Alabama in 1939.

Ants sting to subdue their prey and as a means of defence. The fire ant grasps its victim with its mandibles, then using its head as a pivot it swings its abdominal stinger to inflict multiple stings (Diaz *et al.*, 1989). Unlike other hymenoptera, fire ants sting slowly and may inject venom for seconds to minutes (Stafford *et al.*, 1989b). With each sting the ant injects from 0.04 to 0.11 µl of venom (deShazo *et al.*, 1990).

The venom of most ants and other hymenoptera consists primarily of protein (Blum, 1984). Imported fire ant venom, on the other hand, is 90–95 per cent piperidine alkaloids and contains only 0.1 per cent protein (Hoffman *et al.*, 1988a). Four proteins have been identified, namely: *Sol i I, Sol i II, Sol i III* and *Sol i IV* (Hoffman *et al.*, 1988a). All these proteins are significant allergens.

Toxic Manifestations

Toxicity associated with fire ant envenomation is normally limited to the site of the sting. *In vitro* studies indicate that the venom has haemolytic, cytotoxic, bactericidal and insecticidal properties Adrouny *et al.*, 1959; Rhoades *et al.*, 1977). Multiple stings (approximately 10 000), however, have not resulted in systemic toxicity (Diaz *et al.*, 1989).

The local response to envenomation includes an initial weal and flare reaction. Superficial vesicals with clear fluid develop at the site of the sting within 4 h. This fluid is lost and replaced within 8–10 h by cloudy fluid which becomes purulent. A pustule develops within 24 h which may be surrounded by a red halo (Car *et al.*, 1957). This lesion is pathognomonic in the USA for fire ant stings (Lockey, 1990).

Large local reactions may also occur, which may be immunologically mediated (Diaz *et al.*,

1989). These reactions are characteristic of 'late-phase reactions' that occur secondary to ragweed (deShazo *et al.*, 1984). Systemic allergic reactions characteristic of those caused by other hymenoptera may also occur. The natural history of such responses has not been well studied but is probably comparable to that for other hymenoptera. Anaphylaxis may result in up to 1 per cent of stings (deShazo *et al.*, 1990).

The prevalence of asymptomatic sensitized people to fire ant venom is comparable to that which exists for other hymenoptera, approximately 16 per cent (Hoffmann *et al.*, 1988b). Crossreactivity may exist between bee or wasp venom and fire ant venom. *Sol i II* has been identified as the crossreactive protein (Hoffmann *et al.*, 1988b).

An important complication of fire ant stings is secondary infection (Parrin *et al.*, 1981). Neurological sequelae including seizures and mononeuropathy have also been reported (Fox *et al.*, 1982). The aetiology of such reactions is not known.

Management

First aid for fire ant envenomation is primarily thorough washing with soap and water. Although a number of therapeutic measures have been evaluated as a means to alter the development of pustules, neither topical nor parenteral therapies had any effect on developing lesions (Parrin *et al.*, 1981). A cold compress may help relieve some swelling and discomfort. The pustules should be bandaged to prevent excoriation. Large local reactions and systemic allergic reactions should be managed as previously described for other hymenoptera.

As with other hymenoptera the indications for immunotherapy are not clear. The relatively high risk for stings in sensitized people, however, causes many to undergo such therapy (Stafford *et al.*, 1989c). To confound the issue further, only whole body extracts are available for therapy, which contain variable quantities of venom. Some evidence of its effectiveness, however, has been presented (Hylander *et al.*, 1989).

SPIDERS

Spiders are arthropods of the order arachnidae. Most spiders are venomous; in fact, all but two families of spiders have venom glands. Thousands of venomous spiders are distributed worldwide; however, only a few are of significant medical importance. Most notable are spiders of the genus *Latrodectus* and *Loxosceles*.

Black Widow Spider

The true black widow spider (*Latrodectus mactans*) is found in temperate zones of North America including all of the USA except Alaska. Other *Latrodectus* species are distributed throughout the world (Rauber, 1983–84). The major differences between these species are in their body markings and habitats. *L. mactans* has a characteristic shiny black coloration with a red hourglass-shaped marking on its abdomen. Generally, these spiders are non-aggressive and bite defensively when threatened or disturbed. They are typically found in undisturbed, protected areas such as storage buildings, wood piles and garbage heaps. Female spiders make irregular funnel shaped webs in which to trap prey and suspend their egg sacs.

Only the females of this species are hazardous to humans. The male is too small to cause significant envenomation. The black widow has claw-like hollow fangs which are connected to two venom glands in its cephalothorax. The venom glands have striated musculature which controls the injection of venom. While there are some interspecies differences in venom constituents, the toxic fraction appears to be the same (Rauber, 1983–84).

The venom of the black widow, which is one of the most potent of all animal venoms, is primarily neurotoxic. The venom gland contains just less than 0.2 mg of venom (Binder, 1989). The mean lethal doses range from 0.005 to 1.0 mg kg^{-1} in various animal species (Edlich *et al.*, 1985). The venom acts at the neuromuscular synaptic junction causing the release of acetylcholine and noradrenaline (norepinephrin) from presynaptic vesicles (Rauber, 1983–84; Binder, 1989). This results in excessive neuromuscular stimulation and, as expected, other cholinergic and adrenergic signs and symptoms. The venom causes initial local muscle pain which then generalizes to involve primarily large muscle groups (Kobernick, 1984).

Toxic Manifestations

Most bites in humans occur above the waist on the forearm or torso (Moss and Binder, 1987). Bites are more prevalent during the late summer or early autumn, a time at which there are increased numbers of both young and mature spiders (Moss and Binder, 1987). Although the bite itself is often not initially painful and may go unnoticed, pain at the site is the most common early symptom of envenomation (Moss and Binder, 1987). Other common symptoms include abdominal pain and cramping as well as lower extremity pain and weakness. Hypertension, tachycardia, fever, leucocytosis, vomiting, restlessness, mental status changes, headache, rash, paraesthesiae, albuminuria, ptosis, and periorbital oedema have also been reported. In severe cases shock, coma, respiratory failure and pulmonary oedema may occur (Binder, 1989; La Grange, 1990). The mortality rate from black widow envenomation is probably less than 1 per cent (Binder, 1989).

Management

There are no specific first aid measures for black widow envenomation. The bite site should be thoroughly cleansed and tetanus immunization should be updated if necessary. Medical management is primarily directed at relieving muscle spasms and pain. Calcium gluconate, administered intravenously, has been shown to be both safe and effective (Binder, 1989). Centrally acting muscle relaxants such as methocarbamol and diazepam may also provide relief. Dantrolene sodium, a direct-acting muscle relaxant, has been used successfully and is reported to provide more pronounced and protracted relief (Ryan, 1983–84). Narcotic analgesics and sedatives may also be employed to help relieve pain and restlessness.

An equine-derived antivenin is available but is not used routinely in the USA because of the risks associated with horse serum-based products. In one study of a small number of patients there was no demonstratable difference between those who received antivenin and those who did not in terms of length of hospitalization, ancillary drug use for pain control, or clinical outcome (Moss and Binder, 1987). It is generally recommended

that antivenin be reserved for cases of severe envenomation in which standard measures are inadequate. It can also be used in life-threatening situations and in those at high risk for severe morbidity, such as the very young or old, and in those with underlying hypertension, cardiac or cerebrovascular disease. As with any equine-derived antivenin the risk for hypersensitivity reactions must be considered and appropriate skin testing and other precautions must be taken.

Necrotic Arachnidism

Bites of some spiders result in local tissue destruction and possibly systemic toxic effects. This condition has been referred to as necrotic arachnidism. The most notorious of these spiders are those of the genus *Loxosceles*. Spiders of this genus are distributed worldwide throughout North and South America, Africa, Australia, southern Russia, as well as the Mediterranean and Orient (Gendron, 1990). *Loxosceles* spiders are fawn to dark brown in colour with relatively long skinny legs and a characteristic violin-shaped marking on their dorsal carapace (Binder, 1989). The terms brown, violin, or fiddleback spider are used to describe these species. The brown recluse spider, *Loxosceles reclusa*, is the most significant species in the USA and this has been extensively studied and exemplifies the toxicity associated with these spiders.

The diagnosis of brown recluse envenomation and its actual incidence are difficult to establish because of other potential causes of necrotic wounds, including bites of other spiders and confusing medical conditions such as infections or toxic epidermal necrolysis (Russell and Gertsch, 1983). Diagnostic difficulties have also hampered attempts to study promising treatment modalities. For example, in one series of 95 cases of presumed brown recluse spider bite, only 17 cases could be confirmed and ultimately studied (Rees et al., 1987). A lymphocyte transformation test has been developed to aid in the diagnosis of *Loxosceles reclusa* envenomation but it is not routinely available (Berger et al., 1973a).

The brown recluse spider is distributed primarily in the south-central USA (Majeski and Durst, 1976). Most reported bites have occurred in Arkansas, Kansas, Missouri and Oklahoma. These spiders inhabit primarily warm, dry, secluded places and can be found both indoors and outdoors. The household cupboard (closet) is the most frequently reported site of discovery (Rees and Campbell, 1989). Other potential sites include wood piles, storage buildings, stored clothing, attics, basements and other quiet locations. The brown recluse is nocturnal and as a result most bites occur during the night (Rees and Campbell, 1989). These spiders are most active in summer months and hibernate during the winter.

Toxic Manifestations

The venom of the brown recluse is both cytotoxic and haemolytic. Studies of the venom have identified at least nine proteins, most notably a hyaluronidase which accounts for the spreading of injected venom, and sphingomyelinase D which likely contributes to its haemolytic and cytotoxic properties (Wasserman, 1988; Hobbs and Harrell, 1989; Rees and Campbell, 1989). The quantity of injected venom is relatively small and by itself is unlikely to cause significant injury. The destructive nature of the venom is apparently facilitated by complement activation and the subsequent inflammatory response (Rees *et al.*, 1983; Hobbs and Harrell, 1989). This results in endothelial cell damage, haemorrhage, infiltration of polymorphonuclear leucocytes and thrombosis of venules and arterioles causing necrosis (Berger *et al.*, 1973b).

The bite of a brown recluse spider results in little more than a stinging or prick sensation and may go unnoticed by the victim. The clinical manifestations following envenomation depend on the amount of venom injected, the site of envenomation, and the age, underlying health and immune status of the victim (Majeski and Durst, 1976; Wasserman and Anderson, 1983–84). Not all patients develop the characteristic necrotic lesion or potentially severe systemic effects. It may be that most often only minimal envenomation results and victims experience mild discomfort that resolves within a few days (Berger, 1973).

Most patients, even following significant envenomation, do not present for treatment until many hours after the bite, once the initial signs of a necrotic lesion become evident (Gendron, 1990). The most common presenting signs and symptoms include erythema, cellulitis, generalized rash, blister, pain, pruritus, malaise, chills and sweats (Rees *et al.*, 1987). The characteristic

lesion begins as a blister with surrounding ischaemic discolouration (Wasserman and Anderson, 1983–84; Hobbs and Harrell, 1989). An erythematous ring may surround this area giving a characteristic 'bulls eye' or 'halo' appearance (Wasserman and Anderson, 1983–84). The blister subsequently becomes a bluish macule, the centre of which generally sinks below surrounding tissue (Hobbs and Harrell, 1989). Over several days the necrotic lesion may progress resulting in an area of eschar which sloughs off after 7–14 days leaving an area of ulceration from 1 to 30 cm in diameter (Wasserman and Anderson, 1983–84; Hobbs and Harrell, 1989). Bites in fatty areas of the body tend to become more extensive (Wasserman and Anderson, 1983–84). It may take weeks to months for this area to heal by second intention. A small percentage of patients may develop persistent lesions which could subsequently progress to the development of pyoderma gangrenosum and pseudoepithelomatous hyperplasia (Rees *et al.*, 1987; Hoover *et al.*, 1990).

Systemic toxicity occurs less commonly and may not develop for 24–72 h after the bite. Systemic toxic effects may include fever, malaise, arthralgias, myalgias, rash, convulsions, haemolysis, thrombocytopenia, anaemia, and disseminated intravascular coagulation (Wasserman and Anderson, 1983–84). Nephrotoxicity may result as a complication of haemolysis and subsequent haemoglobinuria.

Management

The treatment of necrotic arachnidism, regardless of the spider involved, should consist of sound local wound management. This should include thorough cleansing, tetanus prophylaxis as necessary, immobilization, elevation and rest (Wasserman, 1988). Cool compresses may help relieve inflammation and pain (Gendron, 1990). Prophylactic antibiotics generally are not indicated and steroid therapy has not been found to be effective (Wasserman, 1988). Symptomatic relief can be provided with the use of antipruritic, analgesic and antianxiety agents.

In definite cases of brown recluse spider bite, in which there is progressive local involvement, dapsone therapy may help to limit the necrotic lesion and speed healing (Berger, 1984). It is postulated that dapsone may be effective by reducing polymorphonuclear leucocyte infiltration (King and Rees, 1983). Dapsone itself, however, may produce dose-dependent haemolytic anaemia, which is likely to be more severe in those with glucose-6-phosphate dehydrogenase deficiency. It should, therefore, be used cautiously and only when the diagnosis of *Loxosceles reclusa* envenomation is certain. Early excisional therapy should be avoided as it has been shown to be ineffective and potentially disfiguring or disabling (Wasserman and Anderson, 1983–84).

In cases of systemic involvement, therapy should be directed at specific complications. Systemic corticosteroids may help reduce venom-induced destruction of red blood cells. Platelets and packed red blood cells may be indicated in the presence of thrombocytopenia or anaemia, respectively. Good hydration should be maintained and renal function monitored. Alkalinization of the urine is indicated in the presence of haemoglobinuria or haematuria.

A brown recluse spider antivenin has been prepared and has been shown *in vitro* to abolish the dermonecrotic activity of brown recluse venom (Rees *et al.*, 1984). In a clinical trial involving 17 patients antivenin was comparably effective to dapsone therapy alone or dapsone in combination with antivenin (Rees *et al.*, 1987). Further evaluation of these therapeutic approaches is warranted. The development of a highly refined antivenin would be a tremendous therapeutic advance for brown recluse spider bites.

SCORPIONS

True scorpions are arachnids of the order scorpionida. There are approximately 650 species distributed worldwide, only a few of which are of significant medical importance (Curry *et al.*, 1983–84). All of these are in the Buthidae family. Scorpions primarily inhabit deserts and semi-arid regions. While scorpions are native to certain localities, it is important to recognize that they may be inadvertently transported in luggage or other goods to distant areas (Trestrail, 1981).

In the USA the most significant of all the scorpions is *Centruroides exilicauda* (bark scorpion) which is found primarily in Arizona, but also inhabits areas within New Mexico, California and Texas as well as Mexico (Likes *et al.*, 1984). A number of other scorpions which can produce significant envenomation may be found in South America, northern and southern Africa, India and the Middle East (Banner, 1989).

Scorpions are nocturnal and take shelter during the day under rocks, piles of debris, or may hide inside houses in clothing or shoes. The bark scorpion notoriously shelters under the loose bark of trees, and in crevices of dead trees or logs (Likes *et al.*, 1984). Scorpions feed primarily on insects, spiders and occasionally on other scorpions (Banner, 1989).

Scorpions have a hard exoskeleton and three primary body parts: the cephalothorax, to which are attached a pair of pincers; an abdomen, which has four pairs of legs; and a tail which is segmented and ends in a telson which contains the stinging apparatus. The telson contains two venom glands which lead via independent ducts to the stinger. The scorpion uses its pincers to grab its prey and then arches its tail over its body and head to inject venom. Likewise, the scorpion may grab the skin of humans and sting, sometimes repeatedly, in self-defence.

Toxic Manifestations

The venom of scorpions is primarily neurotoxic. This property appears to result from its effects on the activation and inactivation of sodium channels, which ultimately results in the release of catecholamines and acetylcholine (Wang and Strichartz, 1983; Banner, 1989). Other venom fractions exhibit enzymatic, anticholinesterase, coagulopathic, haemolytic, cardiotoxic and pancreatotoxic properties (Banner, 1989).

Most envenomations occur on the extremities. Adults are most commonly stung; however, children are more likely to develop serious toxicity (Curry *et al.*, 1983–84; Likes *et al.*, 1984). The sting of *Centruroides exilicauda* causes local pain, numbness, hyperaesthesia, salivation, agitation, wheezing, tachycardia, hypertension and muscle spasms (Likes *et al.*, 1984). In severe cases, cranial nerve and somatic motor abnormalities such as eye movement disorders, blurred vision, tongue fasciculations, impaired pharyngeal muscle control and jerking of the extremities may develop (Curry *et al.*, 1983–84). It is notable that the bark scorpion causes few if any local effects such as inflammation or swelling. In the presence of such findings other scorpion species are the likely culprit.

Centruroides and *Titus* scorpions are of importance in South America. Neurologic toxicity is the primary concern but it is important to note that with *Titus* species parasympathetic effects predominate (Banner, 1989). *Titus* scorpion envenomation may also produce significant local pain and erythema. This species has also been reported to produce pancreatitis (Bartholomew, 1970).

In South Africa, the most important genera of scorpions include *Parabuthus* and *Bothotus*. These scorpions most commonly sting their victims; however, certain species of *Parabuthus* are also capable of squirting venom for up to 1 meter (Newlands, 1978). If the venom enters the eye or open wound it can cause toxicity comparable to that of the spitting cobra. Local effects following envenomation by these South African scorpions include local burning and possibly swelling. Systemic toxicity may include muscle contractions, convulsions, perspiration, salivation, tachycardia, arrhythmias and irregular respirations (Newlands, 1978). Death may result from respiratory or cardiac failure.

Red scorpion (*Buthus tamulus*) envenomation in India can cause severe toxicity and death. Excessive release of catecholamines can result in myocardial damage, arrhythmias, cardiac failure and pulmonary oedema (Alagesan *et al.*, 1977; Rajarajeswari *et al.*, 1979; Bawaskar, 1982). Other reported manifestations in both fatal and non-fatal cases include profuse sweating, mydriasis, vomiting and priapism (Bawaskar, 1982).

The Middle East and northern Africa are inhabited with the yellow scorpion (*Leiurus quinquestriatus*) as well as *Androctonus* and *Buthus* species. The yellow scorpion also causes excessive release of catecholamines which can result in myocardial damage and congestive heart failure (Barzilay *et al.*, 1982). Arrhythmias and pulmonary oedema have also been reported (Alagesan *et al.*, 1977; Rahav and Weiss, 1990).

Management

First aid for scorpion envenomation consists of good local wound care including thorough cleansing and tetanus prophylaxis if necessary. Cold compresses can be applied to help relieve pain and inflammation if present. Systemic manifestations of envenomation can generally be managed conservatively with traditional supportive measures. Atropine sulphate may be indicated

to control excessive parasympathetic manifestations; however, this is often not necessary (Banner, 1989). Excessive adrenergic toxic effects can be controlled using adrenergic blocking agents such as the β-antagonist propranolol or possibly the shorter acting agent esmolol (Rachesky *et al.*, 1984; Banner, 1989). Severe hypertension, unresponsive to conservative measures, may respond to intravenous hydralazine or sublingual nifedipine (Sofer and Gueron, 1990). Recent evidence further suggests that vasodilator therapy can effectively control hypertension and the cardiac sequelae resulting from scorpion envenomation (Gueron and Sofer, 1990).

Antivenin therapy may have an important role in therapy for certain scorpion envenomations. Antivenin is available in India, Israel, South Africa, North Africa and Mexico (Banner, 1989). In the USA an antivenin for *C. exilicauda* has been derived from goat serum, but it is not approved by the Food and Drug Administration (Rachesky *et al.*, 1984). It has been used safely and successfully to relieve severe signs and symptoms of envenomation; however, experience to date is limited (Curry *et al.*, 1983–84). Experience with antivenin in other parts of the world is also limited and issues relative to safety, efficacy and specificity remain to be resolved (Banner, 1989).

JELLYFISH

The phylum Cnidaria (formerly Coelenterata) includes the subphylum Scyphoza, the true jellyfish. The Portuguese man-o'-war, although generally considered a jellyfish, is actually a Cnidarian of the subphylum Hydrozoa. Because of marked similarities, however, the Portuguese man-o'-war will be discussed here with the true jellyfish.

The most notable of these species are the box jellyfish (*Chironex fleckeri*), which inhabits the coastal waters of Australia and the Indo-Pacific region; the Portuguese man-o'-war (*Physalia physalis*), located in the more tropical waters of the Atlantic; the sea nettle (*Chrysaora quinquecirrha*), which is endemic to the Chesapeake Bay and the mid-Atlantic coastal waters of the USA; and the Pacific Portuguese man-o'-war (*Physalia utriculus*), which is often responsible for stings in Hawaiian waters. Other species of jellyfish can also be found in these and other waters throughout the world.

The hanging tentacles of jellyfish contain thousands of stinging organelles known as nematocysts. Within the nematocyst is a coiled thread-like structure coated with venom. In response to pressure or changes in osmolarity the nematocyst fires its thread which can penetrate the skin to cause envenomation.

The venom of jellyfish contains various polypeptides and enzymes. It is both toxic and allergenic. In animal studies the venom has been shown to produce dermonecrosis, vasopermeability, haemolysis, cardiotoxicity, neurotoxicity, musculotoxicity and cytotoxicity (Burnett *et al.*, 1987a). A kinin-like fraction has also been identified which is believed to account for pain (Burnett and Calton, 1987a).

Toxic Manifestations

The most common manifestations from Cnidaria envenomation are local toxic effects. Severe systemic and allergic reactions, as well as delayed or recurrent dermal effects, also may occur. The severity of envenomation is dependent on a number of factors including the species of jellyfish, the extent and duration of contact with tentacles and the resultant number of fired nematocysts, the amount of venom available in the nematocyst at the time of firing, the thickness of the skin, and the size, age and underlying health of the victim (Burnett *et al.*, 1987a; Lumley *et al.*, 1988).

Dermal contact with jellyfish tentacles typically results in linear, urticarial and painful eruptions which are the result of toxic effects of the venom (Burnett and Calton, 1987a). The sting of the Portuguese man-o'-war is generally considered more painful than that of the sea nettle, and the local pain from envenomation by the box jellyfish can be excruciating (Burnett *et al.*, 1987a). The resultant lesions may be vesicular, haemorrhagic, necrotizing or ulcerative (Burnett *et al.*, 1987a). Subacute or chronic reactions may include localized hyperhidrosis, desquamation, lymphadenopathy, angiooedema, urticaria, keloid formation, hyper- or hypopigmentation, local fat atrophy, contractions, vasospasm, gangrene and nerve damage (Burnett and Calton, 1987b; Burnett *et al.*, 1987a).

An allergic response may contribute to the local effects (Burnett *et al.*, 1983). In fact, a large local reaction comparable to that seen with hymenoptera stings has been described (Burnett and Calton, 1987a). Recurrent eruptions at the site of the initial sting and at distant sites have also been reported (Burnett *et al.*, 1983, 1987b). It has been postulated that an antigen depot must exist for this to occur. There is also evidence that individuals may crossreact with different animals of this phylum (Burnett *et al.*, 1987b). The potential for an anaphylactoid reaction must be considered.

Jellyfish envenomation may result in severe systemic toxic reactions and even death. The most common systemic toxic effects include headache, nausea, vomiting, malaise, weakness, perspiration and lachrymation (Burnett *et al.*, 1987a). More severe manifestations include hypotension, cardiac conduction disturbances, arrhythmias, respiratory depression, pulmonary oedema and cardiovascular collapse.

Death from jellyfish envenomation may result from either allergic or toxic mechanisms. The box jellyfish is the most toxic of all marine animals and has been implicated in most jellyfish related fatalities. It is not clear whether death results from cardiotoxicity or respiratory failure (Lumley *et al.*, 1988; Stein *et al.*, 1989). The precise aetiology, in fact, may be dose-dependent (Lumley *et al.*, 1988).

Management

Victims of jellyfish envenomation should be kept quiet and the affected limb should be immobilized because muscle activity may increase the firing of nematocysts. The exposed area should be rinsed with sea water. Fresh water is contraindicated as this too will increase nematocyst firing as a result of osmotic changes.

The next step is to inactivate the nematocysts which is a species-specific process. For most species this can be accomplished by flooding the area with household vinegar (5 per cent acetic acid). In the event of sea nettle or lion's mane jellyfish envenomation, a baking soda slurry is more appropriate (Burnett and Calton, 1987b). Nematocysts can then be removed from the skin by scraping with a blunt edged object such as a sea shell, credit card or by shaving with a razor. Application of a cold pack may help relieve mild to moderate pain (Exton *et al.*, 1989). Topical anesthetics or steroid creams as well as oral analgesics may benefit some patients. Hyperpigmentation can be treated with a bleaching agent such as topical hydroquinone (Kokelj and Burnett, 1990).

Systemic manifestations are managed with traditional supportive measures. The calcium channel antagonist verapamil hydrochloride has been shown to inhibit the action of box jellyfish cardiotoxin and prolong survival in mice (Burnett and Calton, 1983). This finding has been extended to other jellyfish species (Burnett *et al.*, 1985). It is, therefore, recommended that patients who manifest cardiac dysfunction should be treated with verapamil (Stein *et al.*, 1989). An antivenin is available for the box jellyfish from the Commonwealth Serum Laboratory in Melbourne, Australia.

Antihistamines may be useful if there is evidence of an allergic response to the venom. Anaphylactoid reactions should be managed accordingly. In the event of recurrent dermal eruptions a tapering dose of a corticosteroid may be employed.

In addition to the Portuguese man-o'-war another important Hydrozoan is fire coral. The fire coral, while not a true coral, is so named because of its marked resemblance to these species. Polyps which contain nematocysts protrude through pores of its calcareous skeleton. It typically produces only mild dermatitis and burning discomfort (Kizer, 1983–84). The subphylum anthosa includes the sea anemones which also contain modified nematocysts capable of inflicting stings and local effects as described for the cnidarians.

STINGRAYS

Another important coastal hazard is the stingray. Approximately 20 species have been described (Fenner *et al.*, 1989). These creatures are often found partially buried in the sand and are a significant hazard to beachcombers and to those who swim or play in shallow water. Although normally very docile, stingrays will lash their tails forward and sting with a spine located near the base of the tail if they are stepped on or otherwise abruptly disturbed. Some species of stingray contain more than one spine and are capable of inflicting multiple simultaneous stings (Grainger, 1987).

The stinging spine(s) of stingrays are covered by a venom-containing integumentary sheath. As the spine enters the victim this sheath may rupture resulting in the release of venom into the wound. The spines of stingrays vary by species and may range from 2.5 cm to 12 cm in length (Grainger, 1985). The spine is curved and serrated enabling it to inflict significant trauma in addition to envenomating the victim. A large stingray, in fact, is capable of inflicting fatal traumatic injury (Russell *et al.*, 1958).

Toxic Manifestations

Most stings are to the lower extremities (Russell *et al.*, 1958). The upper extremities, abdomen or thorax may be involved from careless handling or under extraordinary circumstances. The stingray's venom consists of a heat-labile protein that causes intense pain at the site of the sting which is out of proportion to the physical trauma. In the event that the wound is not characteristically painful and other toxic manifestations do not occur it is likely that the integumentary sheath had already been lost or it was not disrupted during the sting.

The venom can produce local tissue necrosis which complicates the healing process (Fenner *et al.*, 1989). It has also been shown in animal models to possess both cardiotoxic and neurotoxic properties (Russell *et al.*, 1958). Systemic manifestations from envenomation may include nausea; vomiting; diarrhoea; salivation; generalized oedema; headache; vertigo; syncope; respiratory depression and distress; cardiac conduction disturbances and arrhythmias; hypotension; muscle cramps, fasciculations, tremor and seizures; and death (Russell *et al.*, 1958; Grainger, 1985; Ikeda, 1989). Secondary infections are also possible.

Management

First aid for stingray envenomation consists of washing the wound with sea water and as soon as possible soaking the site in water that is as hot as the patient can tolerate for 30–90 min to denature the thermolabile venom (Russell *et al.*, 1958; Fenner *et al.*, 1989). The wound should then be surgically explored to remove any remaining fragments of the sheath or spine. Necrotic tissue should be debrided and an antiseptic should be used to cleanse the wound, which should be left open to heal by second intention. Tetanus immunization status should be updated if necessary and prophylactic antibiotics should be administered in serious cases (Fenner *et al.*, 1989). Narcotic analgesics may be necessary to control pain. No antivenin is available and systemic manifestations should be managed with traditional symptomatic and supportive care.

STINGING FISHES

Other venomous underwater creatures include fresh and salt water fishes. Common examples include the lionfish, scorpion fish, stone fish, catfish and weaver fish. All these fish sting with venomous spines associated with their fins. The sting of these fish is much less traumatic than that associated with the stingray but in other respects their stings are quite comparable.

Fish stings may be inflicted in those who swim or recreate in the oceans, seas or lakes; in those who fish for recreation or commercially; and in hobbyists who may keep a venomous species in their aquaria. The lionfish is popular with salt water aquarists and has been responsible for many stings to the hand and fingers (Kizer *et al.*, 1985; Trestrail and Al-Mahasneh, 1989).

Toxic Manifestations

Fish stings result in an initial sharp stabbing pain when the spine penetrates the skin. In some cases the spine may break free and remain lodged in the wound. Severe pain may ensue which can radiate to involve the entire extremity. The pain may be excruciating and incapacitating in some cases. Pronounced local swelling occurs commonly and vesicles may form at the puncture sites (Auerbach *et al.*, 1987). The vesicular fluid may itself be harmful, and prompt drainage of the fluid is recommended.

Systemic manifestations may occur with significant envenomation resulting from multiple stings or single stings from certain species such as the stone fish. These toxic effects may include nausea, vomiting, diaphoresis, bradycardia or tachycardia, conduction disturbances, hypotension, myocardial ischaemia, respiratory distress, muscle tremor, weakness, delirium, convulsions and death (Kizer *et al.*, 1985; Ell and Yates, 1989).

Management

As with the stingray the venom of these fish consists primarily of a heat labile protein. Accordingly, first aid treatment should include immersion of the affected site in water as hot as the patient can tolerate for 30–90 min. Afterwards the site should be thoroughly cleaned and in some cases the wound may need to be surgically explored to remove any remaining spine. Tetanus prophylaxis should be updated as necessary. Prophylactic antibiotics are not routinely necessary. It is important to recognize that failure to treat these inflictions promptly may result in permanent scaring and physical impairment (Kasdan *et al.*, 1987). Systemic manifestations should be managed with traditional supportive and symptomatic measures. An antivenin is available for the management of stone fish envenomation.

POISONOUS FISH AND SHELLFISH

In addition to those animals that can cause human poisoning by envenomation, several toxic syndromes may result from ingestion of various fish and shellfish. In some cases these animals excrete the toxin, but most concentrate toxins that are produced by dinoflagellates or bacteria. Fish can be categorized based on the tissue that contains the toxin (Halstead, 1964). Ichthyosarcotoxic fish, which cause most poisonings, have toxin in muscle, viscera, skin or mucus. Ichthyootoxic fish produce toxin concentrated in the gonads. Ichthyohaemotoxic fish, which rarely produce poisoning, have toxin in their blood. Toxic syndromes resulting from ingestion of poisonous aquatic life are unlike traditional food poisoning which is associated with ingestion of microbial contaminated foods.

Ciguatera Fish Poisoning

Ciguatera intoxication is the most common type of ichthyosarcotoxic fish poisoning. The primary responsible toxin, ciguatoxin, is produced by the dinoflagellate *Gambierdiscus toxicus* (Eastaugh and Shepherd, 1989). Although it has anticholinesterase activity, its primary mechanism of action is thought to be from competitive inhibition of calcium-regulated sodium channels (Eastaugh and Shepherd, 1989). Ciguatoxin is a heat-stable, lipid-soluble compound that is resistant to gastric acid (Estaugh and Shepherd, 1989). It can be excreted in breast milk which can cause toxicity in nursing infants (Blythe and deSylva, 1990). Maitotoxin, scaritoxin, lysophosphatidylcholine, ATPase inhibitor and possibly an indole-positive toxin may also contribute to toxicity (Sims, 1987). Toxins are concentrated up the food chain; as a result large fish are most likely to cause human poisoning. Hundreds of fish species have been reported to harbour ciguatoxin; common examples include the barracuda, grouper, snapper, amberjack and sea bass (Halstead, 1964).

Most outbreaks of ciguatera intoxication occur in the Caribbean and South Pacific. In the USA most cases have been reported in Hawaii and Florida (Hughes and Merson, 1976). Ciguatera poisoning, however, has also been associated with ingestion of fish caught from the southeastern USA coastal waters as far north as North Carolina (Morris *et al.*, 1990). The ability readily to transport fish great distances may result in ciguatera poisoning in virtually any geographic region. People of Chinese or Philippine descent are likely to be more severely affected but Hawaiians least affected (Sims, 1987). This ethnic variation is not well understood.

Toxic Manifestations

Ciguatera poisoning affects primarily the gastrointestinal and nervous systems. Signs and symptoms usually develop within 6 h; however, there is considerable variability. Common gastrointestinal effects include diarrhoea, vomiting and abdominal pain (Morris *et al.*, 1982). These symptoms generally occur early and resolve within 24 h. Other initial symptoms may include malaise, pain and weakness in the lower extremities, dysaesthesias including reversal of hot and cold sensation, and paraesthesias around the mouth and of the extremities (Hughes and Merson, 1976; Morris *et al.*, 1982). These effects may persist for weeks or months. Other common findings include rash, dry mouth, metallic taste, myalgias, arthralgia, visual disturbances, and a sensation of loose teeth. Bradycardia, hypotension and respiratory paralysis may occur in severe cases (Hughes and Merson, 1976).

Management

Gastrointestinal decontamination may be helpful if the toxic nature of the fish is recognized soon after ingestion. Treatment is primarily symptomatic and supportive care. Fluid and electrolyte balance should be monitored as well as the electrocardiogram. Atropine and intravenous fluids have been effective in the treatment of bradycardia and hypotension. Mannitol was found to improve neurological and gastrointestinal toxicity dramatically in a group of 24 patients (Palafox *et al.*, 1988). It is postulated that mannitol may have inactivated the toxin or competitively inhibited its action on the sodium channel.

Paralytic Shellfish Poisoning

Paralytic shellfish poisoning results from ingestion of contaminated bivalve molluscs such as clams and oysters. These molluscs concentrate neurotoxins known as saxitoxins, which are produced by a number of dinoflagellates including those of the *Gonyaulax* and *Pyridinium* species (Eastaugh and Shepherd, 1989; Rodrigue *et al.*, 1990). The toxin is a water soluble, heat and acid stable compound which cannot be destroyed by ordinary cooking (Auerbach and Halstead, 1989). The toxin acts by interfering with sodium conductance thereby inhibiting neuromuscular transmission.

Toxic Manifestations

As the name implies, paralytic shellfish poisoning primarily affects the nervous system. Prominent toxic effects include paraesthesias of the lips, face and extremities; headache; weakness; dizziness; vertigo; and difficulty walking (Hughes and Merson, 1976; Eastaugh and Shepherd, 1989). A sensation of floating has also been described (McCollum *et al.*, 1968). In severe cases muscle paralysis may occur. Death may result from respiratory arrest if adequate life-support cannot be provided. Some neurological symptoms such as headaches, memory loss and fatigue may persist for up to 2 weeks (Rodrigue *et al.*, 1990).

Management

Gastrointestinal decontamination should be performed if the toxic nature of the mollusc is recognized soon after consumption. The remainder of therapy is basically symptomatic and supportive care. Respiratory function should be monitored closely with ventilatory assistance provided as needed.

Neurotoxic Shellfish Poisoning

A milder intoxication, known as neurotoxic shell-fish poisoning, may result from ingestion of contaminated shellfish off the western Florida coast of the USA (Sakamoto *et al.*, 1987). The toxins, brevitoxins, from the dinoflagellate *Ptychodiscus brevis* stimulate postganglionic cholinergic nerve fibres (Grunfeld and Spiegelstein, 1974; Asai *et al.*, 1982). Toxic manifestations include nausea, vomiting, diarrhoea and paraesthesias. As with ciguatera poisoning, patients may experience the hot–cold reversal phenomenon (Hughes and Merson, 1976; Sims, 1987).

Domoic Acid Intoxication

A unique toxic syndrome was recently described that resulted from ingestion of contaminated mussels from Prince Edward Island in Canada (Perl *et al.*, 1990). Domoic acid was implicated as the responsible toxin, which was apparently produced by the marine algae *Nitzschia pungens*. Domoic acid is an excitatory neurotransmitter structurally similar to glutamic acid and kainic acid (Teitelbaum *et al.*, 1990).

The most common acute symptoms of intoxication included nausea, vomiting, abdominal cramps, diarrhoea, headache and memory loss (Perl *et al.*, 1990). In severe cases altered mental status, seizures, myoclonus and cardiovascular instability resulted. Death was reported in four cases. The initial widespread neurotoxicity and subsequent chronic residual memory impairment differentiates this syndrome from either paralytic or neurotoxic shellfish poisoning.

Tetrodotoxic Fish Poisoning

Tetrodotoxication is primarily associated with ingestion of the puffer fish and related fish of the order Tetraodontiformes. Other animals also may contain this neurotoxin, for example the Californian newt (*Taricha torosa*), Pacific goby (*Gobius criniger*), and Costa Rican frog (Tibballs, 1988).

Tetrodotoxin acts similar to saxitoxin in that it blocks neurotransmission by action on sodium channels (Narahashi, 1972). This results in motor, autonomic and sensory nerve impairment (Tibballs, 1988). It also has direct action on the medulla, stimulating the chemoreceptor trigger zone

and depressing the respiratory center (Eastaugh and Shepherd, 1989).

Toxic Manifestations

Prominent signs and symptoms of intoxication include persistent vomiting, paraesthesias, weakness, respiratory impairment, hypotension and bradycardia (Sims and Ostman, 1986; Tibballs, 1988). Other manifestations may include headache, dilated pupils, salivation, diaphoresis, myalgias, dysarthria, ataxia, muscle fasciculations and seizures (Sims and Ostman, 1986). Death may result in severe cases from respiratory failure or cardiovascular collapse.

Management

Treatment is primarily symptomatic and supportive care. Gastric lavage should be performed if it can be done soon after ingestion. Activated charcoal is also recommended. Ventilatory assistance may be required in severe cases. Hypotension and bradycardia should be managed with atropine and fluid therapy. Vasopressors, such as dopamine hydrochloride, may be required.

Scombroid Fish Poisoning

Scombroid fish poisoning is a toxic syndrome that resembles an acute allergic reaction. It results from ingestion of spoiled fish that is contaminated with histamine and possibly other toxins. Histamine is formed as a result of bacteria that cause enzymatic decarboxylation of histidine, which is normally present in the flesh of certain fish species (Lerke *et al.*, 1978). Fish most commonly involved are those of the suborder *scombroidei* such as the tuna, mackerel, bonito, skipjack and saury. Other marine fish such as the mahimahi have also been implicated in outbreaks of scombroid intoxication (Eastaugh and Shepherd, 1989).

The association between histamine and scombroid intoxication is unclear. Histamine has limited activity when administered orally because of rapid metabolism and elimination in the urine (Garrison, 1990). However, markedly elevated urinary histamine concentrations have been measured in symptomatic patients after ingestion of scombrotoxic fish (Morrow *et al.*, 1991). This evidence and the effectiveness of antihistamines to relieve symptoms of scombroid intoxication implicate histamine as the causative toxin. Other substances in spoiled fish such as cadaverine or putrescine might inhibit histamine-metabolizing enzymes, thereby allowing the absorption of histamine (Auerbach, 1990). This is an area that warrants further investigation.

Toxic Manifestations

Scombroid intoxication usually results in a relatively mild, self-limited syndrome, which usually begins within 1 h of ingestion and lasts for 8 h or less (Merson *et al.*, 1974; Hughes and Merson, 1976). Typical manifestations include nausea, diarrhoea, abdominal cramps, vomiting, throbbing headache, oral blistering or burning sensation, flushing, burning sensation of the skin, and urticaria. Tachycardia, palpitations, bronchospasm and respiratory distress may also occur (Merson *et al.*, 1974; Hughes and Merson, 1976; Blakesley, 1983).

Management

Treatment is primarily symptomatic and supportive care. If the fish is recognized as poisonous soon after ingestion the gastrointestinal tract should be decontaminated. Antihistamines such as diphenhydramine are the mainstay of therapy. The use of cimetidine in a few cases has been shown to dramatically relieve the signs and symptoms of scombroid intoxication (Blakesley, 1983; Auerbach, 1990). Bronchodilators may be needed in the event of bronchospasm.

It is important to differentiate between scombroid poisoning and fish allergy. An incorrect diagnosis of fish allergy will unnecessarily limit the diet of the patient. Considerations include the patient's prior response to ingestion of the implicated fish species and the response in others who consumed the same meal (Taylor *et al.*, 1989). The food can be analysed for the presence of histamine but at this time there are no diagnostic tests that can be performed on the patient (Lerke *et al.*, 1978; Taylor *et al.*, 1989).

ACKNOWLEDGEMENTS

The author acknowledges the careful and critical review of this chapter by David E. Seidler, MD, Kay A. Wallander, PharmD, and Lynn F. Durback, RN, BSN, CSPI and the expert technical assistance of Tina C. Means.

REFERENCES

Adrouny, G. A., Derbes, V. J. and Jung, R. C. (1959). Isolation of a hemolytic component of fire ant venom. *Science*, **130**, 449

Alagesan, R., Srinivasarnghavan, J., Balambal, R., Haranath, K., Subramanyam, N. and Thiruvengadam, K. V. (1977). Transient complete right bundle branch block following scorpion sting. *J. Indian Med. Assoc.*, **69**, 113–114

Aitchison, J. M. (1990). Boomslang bite – diagnosis and management: a report of 2 cases. *S. Afr. Med. J.*, **78**, 39–42

Asai, S., Krzanowski, J., Anderson, W. H., Martin, D. F., Polson, J. B., Lockey, R. F., Bukantz, S. C. and Szentivanyi, A. (1982). Effects of the toxin of red tide, *Ptychodiscus brevis*, on canine tracheal smooth muscle: a possible new asthma-triggering mechanism. *J. Allergy Clin. Immunol.*, **69**, 418–428

Auerbach, P. S. (1990). Persistent headache associated with scombroid poisoning: resolution with oral cimetidine. *J. Wild. Med.*, **1**, 279–283

Auerbach, P. S. and Halstead, B. W. (1989). Hazardous aquatic life. In Auerbach, P. S. and Geehr, E. C. (Eds), *Management of Wilderness and Environmental Emergencies*, 2nd edn. St Louis, C. V. Mosby Company, pp. 931–1028

Auerbach, P. S., McKinney, H. E., Rees, R. S. and Heggers, J. P. (1987). Analysis of vesicle fluid following the sting of the lionfish *Pterois Volintans*. *Toxicon.*, **25**, 1350–1353

Banner, W. (1989). Scorpion envenomation. In Auerbach, P. S. and Geehr, E. C. (Eds), *Management of Wilderness and Environmental Emergencies*, 2nd edn. St Louis, C. V. Mosby Company, pp. 603–616

Bartholomew, C. (1970). Acute scorpion pancreatitis in Trinidad. *Br. Med. J.*, **1**, 666–668

Barzilay, Z., Shaher, E., Motro, M., Shem-Tov, A. and Neufeld, H. N. (1982). Myocardial damage with life-threatening arrhythmia due to scorpion sting. *Eur. Heart J.*, **3**, 191–193

Bawaskar, H. S. (1982). Diagnostic cardiac premonitory signs and symptoms of red scorpion sting. *Lancet*, **1**, 552–554

Berger, R. S. (1973). The unremarkable brown recluse spider bite. *J.A.M.A.*, **225**, 1109–1111

Berger, R. S. (1984). Management of brown recluse spider bite. *J.A.M.A.*, **251**, 889

Berger, R. S., Millikan, L. E. and Conway, F. (1973a). An *in vitro* test for *Loxosceles reclusa* spider bites. *Toxicon.*, **11**, 465–470

Berger, R. S., Adelstein, E. H. and Anderson, P. C. (1973b). Intravascular coagulation: the cause of necrotic arachnidism. *J. Invest. Dermatol.*, **61**, 142–150

Binder, L. S. (1989). Acute arthropod envenomation. *Med. Toxicol. Adverse Drug. Exp.*, **4**, 163–173

Blakesley, M. L. (1983). Scombroid poisoning: prompt resolution of symptoms with cimetidine. *Ann. Emerg. Med.*, **12**, 104–106

Blaylock, R. S. M. (1982). The treatment of snakebite in Zimbabwe. *Cent. Afr. J. Med.*, **28**, 237–246

Blum, M. S. (1984). Poisonous ants and their venoms. In Tu, A. T. (Ed.), *Insect Poisons, Allergens and other Invertebrate Venoms*. New York, Marcel Dekker, pp. 225–242

Blythe, D. G. and deSylva, D. P. (1990). Mother's milk turns toxic following fish feast. *J.A.M.A.*, **264**, 2074

Bou-Abboud, C. F. and Kardassakis, D. G. (1988). Acute myocardial infarction following a Gila monster (*Heloderma Suspectum Cinctum*) bite. *West. J. Med.*, **148**, 577–579

Bousquet, J., Huchard, G. and Francois-Bernard, M. (1984). Toxic reactions induced by hymenoptera venom. *Ann. Allergy*, **52**, 371–374

Burnett, J. W. and Calton, G. J. (1983). Response of the box-jellyfish (*Chironex fleckeri*) cardiotoxin to intravenous administration of verapamil. *Med. J. Aust.*, **2**, 192–194

Burnett, J. W. and Calton, G. J. (1987a). Jellyfish envenomation syndromes updated. *Ann. Emerg. Med.*, **16**, 1000–1005

Burnett, J. W. and Calton, G. J. (1987b). Venomous pelagic coelenterates: chemistry toxicology, immunology and treatment of their stings. *Toxicon.*, **25**, 581–602

Burnett, J. W., Cobbs, C. S., Kelman, S. N. and Calton, G. J. (1983). Studies on the serologic response to jellyfish envenomation. *J. Am. Acad. Dermatol.*, **9**, 229–231

Burnett, J. W., Gean, C. J. and Calton, G. J. (1985). The effect of verapamil on the cardiotoxic activity of Portuguese man-o'-war (*Phisalia physalis*) and sea nettle (*Chrysaora quinquecirrha*) venoms. *Toxicon*, **23**, 681–689

Burnett, J. W., Calton, G. J., Burnett, H. W. and Mandojana, R. M. (1987a). Local and systemic reactions from jellyfish stings. *Clin. Dermatol.*, **5**, 14–28

Burnett, J. W., Hepper, K. P., Aurelian, L., Calton, G. J. and Gardepe, S. F. (1987b). Recurrent eruptions following unusual solitary coelenterate envenomations. *J. Am. Acad. Dermatol.*, **17**, 86–92

Cable, D., McGehee, W., Wingert, W. A. and Russell, F. E. (1984). Prolonged defibrination after a bite from a 'nonvenomous snake'. *J.A.M.A.*, **251**, 925–926

Car, M. R., Derbes, V. J. and Jung, R. (1957). Skin responses to the sting of the imported fire ant (Solenopsis Saevissima). *Arch. Dermatol.*, **75**, 475–488

Christopher, D. G. and Rodning, C. B. (1986). Crotalidae envenomation. *South. Med. J.*, **79**, 159–162

Curry, S. C. and Kunkel, D. B. (1985). Death from a rattlesnake bite. *Am. J. Emerg. Med.*, **3**, 227–235

Curry, S. C., Vance, M. V., Ryan, P. J., Kunkel, D. B. and Northey, W. T. (1983–84). Envenomation by the scorpion *Centruroides sculpturatus*. *J. Toxicol. Clin. Toxicol.*, **21**, 417–449

Curry, S. C., Horning, D., Brady, P., Requa, R.,

Kunkel, D. B. and Vance, M. V. (1989). The legitimacy of rattlesnake bites in central Arizona. *Ann. Emerg. Med.*, **18**, 658–663

DeShazo, R. D., Griffing, C., Kwan, T. H., Banks, W. A. and Dvorak, H. F. (1984). Dermal hypersensitivity reactions to imported fire ants. *J. Allergy Clin. Immunol.*, **74**, 841–847

DeShazo, R. D., Butcher, B. T. and Banks, W. A. (1990). Reactions to the stings of the imported fire ant. *N. Engl. J. Med.*, **323**, 462–466

Diaz, J. D., Lockey, R. F., Stablein, J. J. and Mines, H. K. (1989). Multiple stings by imported fire ants (*Solenopsis invicta*), without systemic effects. *South. Med. J.*, **82**, 775–777

Eastaugh, J. and Shepherd, S. (1989). Infectious and toxic syndromes from fish and shellfish consumption. *Arch. Intern. Med.*, **149**, 1735–1740

Edlich, R. F., Rodeheaver, G. T., Feldman, P. S. and Morgan, R. F. (1985). Management of venomous spider bites. *Curr. Concepts Trauma Care*, **7**, 17–20

Ell, S. R. and Yates, D. (1989). Marinefish stings. *Arch. Emerg. Med.*, **6**, 59–62

Exton, D. R., Fenner, P. J. and Williamson, J. A. (1989). Cold packs: effective topical analgesia in the treatment of painful stings by *Physalia* and other jellyfish. *Med. J. Aust.*, **151**, 625–626

Fenner, P. J., Williamson, J. A. and Skinner, R. A. (1989). Fatal and non-fatal stingray envenomation. *Med. J. Aust.*, **151**, 621–625

Fox, R. W., Lockey, R. F. and Bukantz, S. C. (1982). Neurologic sequelae following the imported fire ant sting. *J. Allergy Clin. Immunol.*, **70**, 120–124

Garrison, J. C. (1990). Histamine, bradykinin, 5-hydroxytryptamine, and their antagonists. In Gilman, A. G., Rall, T. W., Nies, A. S. and Taylor, P. (Eds), *Goodman and Gilman's The Pharmacologic Basis of Therapeutics*, 8th edn. New York, Pergamon Press, pp. 575–599

Gendron, B. P. (1990). *Loxosceles reclusa* envenomation. *Am. J. Emerg. Med.*, **8**, 51–54

George, A., Tharakan, V. T. and Solez, K. (1987). Viper bite poisoning in India: a review with special reference to renal complications. *Renal Failure*, **10**, 91–99

Golden, D. B. K. (1989). Epidemiology of allergy to insect venoms and stings. *Allergy Proc.*, **10**, 103–107

Golden, D. B. K., Valentine, M. D., Kagey-Sobotka, A. and Lichtenstein, L. M. (1982). Prevalence of hymenoptera venom allergy. *J. Allergy Clin. Immunol.*, **69**, 124

Grainger, C. R. (1985). Stingray injuries. *Trans. R. Soc. Trop. Med. Hyg.*, **79**, 443–444

Grainger, C. R. (1987). Multiple injuries due to stingrays. *J. R. Soc. Health*, **107**, 100

Grunfeld, Y. and Spiegelstein, M. Y. (1974). Effects of *Gymnodinium breve* toxin on the smooth muscle preparation of guinea pig ileum. *Br. J. Pharmacol.*, **51**, 67–72

Gueron, M. and Sofer, S. (1990). Vasodilators and

calcium blocking agents as treatment of cardiovascular manifestations of human scorpion envenomation. *Toxicon.*, **28**, 127–128

Halstead, B. W. (1964). Fish poisoning—their diagnosis, pharmacology and treatment. *Clin. Pharmacol. Ther.*, **5**, 615–627

Hardy, D. L. (1986). Fatal rattlesnake envenomation in Arizona: 1969–84. *J. Toxicol. Clin. Toxicol.*, **24**, 1–10

Heitschel, S. (1986). Near death from a Gila monster bite. *J. Emerg. Nurs.*, **12**, 259–262

Hobbs, G. D. and Harrell, R. E. (1989). Brown recluse spider bites: a common cause of necrotic arachnidism. *Am. J. Emerg. Med.*, **7**, 309–312

Hoffman, D. R., Dover, D. E. and Jacobson, R. S. (1988a). Allergens in hymenoptera venom. *J. Allergy Clin. Immunol.*, **82**, 818–827

Hoffman, D. R., Dover, D. E., Moffitt, J. E. and Stafford, C. T. (1988b). Allergens in hymenoptera venom. *J. Allergy Clin. Immunol.*, **82**, 828–834

Hogan, D. E. and Dire, D. J. (1990). Anaphylactic shock secondary to rattlesnake bite. *Ann. Emerg. Med.*, **19**, 814–816

Hoover, E. L., Williams, W., Koger, L., Murthy, R., Parsh, S. and Weaver, W. L. (1990). Pseudoepitheliomatous hyperplasia and pyoderma gangrenosum after a brown recluse spider bite. *South. Med. J.*, **83**, 243–246

Hughes, J. M. and Merson, M. H. (1976). Fish and shellfish poisoning. *N. Engl. J. Med.*, **295**, 1117–1120

Hylander, R. D., Ortiz, A. A., Freeman, T. M. and Martin, M. E. (1989). Imported fire ant immunotherapy: effectiveness of whole body extracts. *J. Allergy Clin. Immunol.*, **83**, 232

Ikeda, T. (1989). Supraventricular bigeminy following a stingray envenomation: a case report. *Hawaii Med. J.*, **48**, 162–163

Kasdan, M. L., Dasdan, A. S. and Hamilton, D. L. (1987). Lionfish envenomation. *Plast. Reconstr. Surg.*, **80**, 613–614

King, L. E. and Rees, R. S. (1983). Dapsone treatment of a brown recluse bite. *J.A.M.A.*, **250**, 648

Kitchens, C. S. and van Mierop, L. H. S. (1987). Envenomation by the eastern coral snake (*Micrurus fulvius fulvius*). A study of 39 victims. *J.A.M.A.*, **258**, 1615–1618

Kizer, K. W. (1983–84). Marine envenomations. *J. Toxicol. Clin. Toxicol.*, **21**, 527–555

Kizer, K. W., McKinney, H. E. and Auerbach, P. S. (1985). Scorpaenidae envenomation. A five-year poison center experience. *J.A.M.A.*, **253**, 807–810

Kobernick, M. (1984). Black widow spider bite. *Am. Fam. Physician*, **29**, 241–245

Kokelj, F. and Burnett, J. W. (1990). Treatment of a pigmented lesion induced by a *Pelagia noctiluca* sting. *Cutis*, **46**, 62–64

Kunkel, D. B., Curry, S. C., Vance, M. V. and Ryan, P. J. (1983–84). Reptile envenomations. *J. Toxicol. Clin. Toxicol.*, **21**, 503–526

La Grange, M. A. C. (1990). Pulmonary oedema from a widow spider bite. *S. Afr. Med. J.*, **77**, 110

La Grange, R. G. and Russell, F. E. (1970). Blood platelet studies in man and rabbits following *crotalus* envenomation. *Proc. West. Pharmacol. Soc.*, **13**, 99–105

Lerke, P. A., Werner, S. B., Taylor, S. L. and Guthertz, L. S. (1978). Scombroid poisoning: report of an outbreak. *West J. Med.*, **129**, 381–386

Likes, K., Banner, W. and Chavez, M. (1984). *Centruroides exilicauda* envenomation in Arizona. *West. J. Med.*, **141**, 634–637

Lockey, R. F. (1990). The imported fire ant: immunopathologic significance. *Hosp. Pract.*, **25**, 109–112, 115–124

Lumley, J., Williamson, J. A., Fenner, P. J., Burnett, J. W. and Colquhoun, D. M. (1988). Fatal envenomation by *Chironex fleckeri*, the north Australian box jellyfish: the continuing search for lethal mechanisms. *Med. J. Aust.*, **148**, 527–534

McCollum, J. P. K., Pearson, R. C. M., Ingham, H. R., Wood, P. C. and Dewar, H. A. (1968). An epidemic of mussel poisoning in north-east England. *Lancet*, **2**, 767–770

McNally, S. L. and Reitz, C. J. (1987). Victims of snakebite: a 5-year study at Shongwe Hospital, Kangwane, 1978–82. *S. Afr. Med. J.*, **72**, 855–860

Maguire, J. F. and Geha, R. S. (1986). Bee, wasp and hornet stings. *Pediat. Rev.*, **8**, 6–11

Majeski, J. A. and Durst, G. G. (1976). Necrotic arachnidism. *South. Med. J.*, **69**, 887–891

Merson, M. H., Baine, W. B., Gangarosa, E. J. and Swanson, R. C. (1974). Scombroid fish poisoning: outbreak traced to commercially canned tuna fish. *J.A.M.A.*, **228**, 1268–1269

Minton, S. A. (1987). Present tests for detection of snake venom: clinical applications. *Ann. Emerg. Med.*, **16**, 932–937

Minton, S. A. (1990). Neurotoxic snake envenoming. *Semin. Neurol.*, **10**, 52–61

Morris, J. G., Lewin, P., Hargrett, N. T., Smith, C. W., Blake, P. A. and Schneider, R. (1982). Clinical features of ciguatera fish poisoning: a study of the disease in the US Virgin Islands. *Arch. Intern. Med.*, **142**, 1090–1092

Morris, P. D., Campbell, D. S. and Freeman, J. I. (1990). Ciguatera fish poisoning: an outbreak associated with fish caught from North Carolina coastal waters. *South. Med. J.*, **83**, 379–382

Morrow, J. D., Margolies, G. R., Rowland, J. and Roberts, L. J. (1991). Evidence that histamine is the causative toxin of scombroid-fish poisoning. *N. Engl. J. Med.*, **324**, 716–720

Moss, H. S. and Binder, L. S. (1987). A retrospective review of black widow spider envenomation. *Ann. Emerg. Med.*, **16**, 188–192

Narahashi, T. (1972). Mechanism of action of tetrodotoxin and saxitoxin on excitable membranes. *Fed. Proc.*, **31**, 1124–1132

Nelson, B. K. (1989). Snake envenomation: incidence, clinical presentation and management. *Med. Toxicol. Adverse Drug. Exp.*, **4**, 17–31

Newlands, G. (1978). Review of Southern African scorpions and scorpionism. *S. Afr. Med. J.*, **54**, 613–615

Otten, E. J. (1983). Antivenin therapy in the emergency department. *Am. J. Emerg. Med.*, **1**, 83–93

Otten, E. J. and McKimm, D. (1983). Venomous snakebite in a patient allergic to horse serum. *Ann. Emerg. Med.*, **12**, 624–627

Palafox, N. A., Jain, L. G., Pinano, A. Z., Gulick, T. M., Williams, R. K. and Schatz, I. J. (1988). Successful treatment of ciguatera fish poisoning with intravenous mannitol. *J.A.M.A.*, **259**, 2740–2742

Parrin, J., Kandawalla, N. M. and Lockey, R. F. (1981). Treatment of local skin response to imported fire ant sting. *South. Med. J.*, **74**, 1361–1364

Parrish, H. M. (1966). Incidence of treated snakebites in the United States. *Public Health Rep.*, **81**, 269–276

Perl, T. M., Bedard, L., Kosatsky, T., Hockin, J. C., Todd, E. C. D. and Remis, R. S. (1990). An outbreak of toxic encephalopathy caused by eating mussels contaminated with domoic acid. *N. Engl. J. Med.*, **322**, 1775–1780

Piacentine, J., Curry, S. C. and Ryan, P. J. (1986). Life-threatening anaphylaxis following Gila monster bite. *Ann. Emerg. Med.*, **15**, 959–961

Preston, C. A. (1989). Hypotension, myocardial infarction, and coagulopathy following Gila monster bite. *J. Emerg. Med.*, **7**, 37–40

Rachesky, I. J., Banner, W., Dansky, J. and Tong, T. (1984). Treatments for *Centruroides exilicauda* envenomation. *Am. J. Dis. Child.*, **138**, 1136–1139

Rahav, G. and Weiss, A. T. (1990). Scorpion sting-induced pulmonary edema: scintigraphic evidence of cardiac dysfunction. *Chest*, **97**, 1478–1480

Rajarajeswari, G., Sivaprakasam, S. and Viswanathan, J. (1979). Morbidity and mortality pattern in scorpion stings. *J. Indian Med. Assoc.*, **73**, 123–126

Rauber, A. (1983–84). Black widow spider bites. *J. Toxicol. Clin. Toxicol.*, **21**, 473–485

Rees, R. S. and Campbell, D. S. (1989). Spider bites. In Auerbach, P. S., Geehr, E. C. (Eds), *Management of Wilderness and Environmental Emergencies*, 2nd edn. St Louis, C. V. Mosby Company, pp. 543–561

Rees, R. S., O'Leary, J. P. and King, L. L. (1983). The pathogenesis of systemic loxoscelism following brown recluse spider bites. *J. Surg. Research*, **35**, 1–10

Rees, R. S., Nanney, L. B., Yates, R. A. and King, L. E. (1984). Interaction of brown recluse spider venom on cell membranes: the inciting mechanism? *J. Invest. Dermatol.*, **83**, 270–275

Rees, R., Campbell, D., Rieger, E. and King, L. E. (1987). The diagnosis and treatment of brown recluse spider bites. *Ann. Emerg. Med.*, **16**, 945–949

Reisman, R. E. (1989). Studies of the natural history of insect sting allergy. *Allergy Proc.*, **10**, 97–101

Rhoades, R. B., Schafer, W. L., Newman, M., Lockey, R., Dozler, R. M., Wubbens, P. F., Townes, A. W., Schmid, W. H., Neder, G., Brill, T. and Wittig, H. J. (1977). Hypersensitivity to the imported fire ant in Florida. Report of 104 cases. *J. Fla. Med. Assoc.*, **64**, 247–254

Riffer, E., Curry, S. C. and Gerkin, R. (1987). Successful treatment with antivenin of marked thrombocytopenia without significant coagulopathy following rattlesnake bite. *Ann. Emerg. Med.*, **16**, 1297–1299

Rodrigue, D. C., Etzel, R. A., Hall, S., DePorras, E., Velasquez, O. H., Tauxe, R. V., Kilbourne, E. M. and Blake, P. A. (1990). Lethal paralytic shellfish poisoning in Guatemala. *Am. J. Trop. Med. Hyg.*, **42**, 267–271

Roller, J. A. (1976). Gila monster bite. *J.A.M.A.*, **235**, 249–250 (letter)

Russell, F. E. (1980). Snake venom poisoning in the United States. *Annu. Rev. Med.*, **31**, 247–259

Russell, F. E. (1983). *Snake Venom Poisoning*. Scholium International, Great Neck

Russell, F. E. and Bogert, C. M. (1981). Gila monster: its biology, venom and bite—a review. *Toxicon*, **19**, 341–359

Russell, F. E. and Gertsch, W. J. (1983). For those who treat spider or suspected spider bite. *Toxicon*, **21**, 337–339 (letter to the Editor)

Russell, F. E., Panos, T. C., Kang, L. W., Warner, A. M. and Colket, T. C. (1958). Studies on the mechanism of death from stingray venom—a report of two fatal cases. *Am. J. Med. Sci.*, **235**, 566–584

Russell, F. E., Carlson, R. W., Wainschel, J. and Osborne, A. H. (1975). Snake venom poisoning in the United States: experiences with 550 cases. *J.A.M.A.*, **233**, 341–344

Russell, F. E., Sullivan, J. B., Egen, N. B., Jeter, W. S., Markland, F. S., Wingert, W. A. and Bar-Or, D. (1985). Preparation of a new antivenin by affinity chromatography. *Am. J. Trop. Med. Hygiene*, **34**, 141–150

Ryan, P. J. (1983–84). Preliminary report: experience with the use of dantrolene sodium in the treatment of bites by the black widow spider *Latrodectus Hesperus*. *J. Toxicol. Clin. Toxicol.*, **21**, 487–498

Sakamoto, Y., Lockey, R. and Krzanowski, J. (1987). Shellfish and fish poisoning related to the ingestion of toxic dinoflagellates. *South. Med. J.*, **80**, 866–870

Schaeffer, R. C., Pattabhiraman, T. R., Carlson, R. W., Russell, F. E. and Weil, M. H. (1979). Cardiovascular failure produced by a peptide from the venom of the southern pacific rattlesnake *Crotalus viridis heller*. *Toxicon*, **17**, 447–453

Schuberth, K. C., Graft, D. F. and Kagey-Sobotka, A. (1983). Do all children with insect allergy need venom therapy? *J. Allergy Clin. Immunol.*, **71**, 140 (abstract)

Settipane, G. A., Newstead, G. J. and Boyd, G. R. (1972). Frequency of hymenoptera allergy in an atopic and normal population. *J. Allergy Clin. Immunol.*, **50**, 146–150

Sims, J. K. (1987). A theoretical discourse on the pharmacology of toxic marine ingestions. *Ann. Emerg. Med.*, **16**, 1006–1015

Sims, J. K. and Ostman, D. C. (1986). Pufferfish poisoning: emergency diagnosis and management of mild human tetrodotoxication. *Ann. Emerg. Med.*, **15**, 1094–1098

Sofer, S. and Gueron, M. (1990). Vasodilators and hypertensive encephalopathy following scorpion envenomation in children. *Chest*, **97**, 118–120

Stafford, C. T., Hutto, L. S., Rhodes, R. B., Thompson, W. O. and Impson, L. K. (1989a). Imported fire ant as a health hazard. *South. Med. J.*, **82**, 1515–1519

Stafford, C. T., Hoffman, D. R. and Rhoades, R. B. (1989b). Allergy to imported fire ants. *South. Med. J.*, **82**, 1520–1527

Stafford, C. T., Rhoades, R. B., Bunker-Soler, A. L., Thompson, W. O. and Impson, L. K. (1989c). Survey of whole body-extract immunotherapy for imported fire ant- and other hymenoptera-sting allergy. *J. Allergy Clin. Immunol.*, **83**, 1107–1111

Stein, M. R., Marraccini, J. V., Rothschild, N. E. and Burnett, J. W. (1989). Fatal Portuguese man-o'-war (*Physalia physalis*) envenomation. *Ann. Emerg. Med.*, **18**, 312–315

Streiffer, R. H. (1986). Bite of the venomous lizard, the Gila monster. *Postgrad. Med.*, **79**, 297–299, 302

Sullivan, J. B. (1987). Past, present, and future immunotherapy of snake venom poisoning. *Am. Emerg. Med.*, **16**, 938–942

Sutherland, S. K., Coulter, A. R. and Harris, R. D. (1979). Rationalization of first-aid measures for elapid snakebite. *Lancet*, **1**, 183–186

Taylor, S. L., Stratton, J. E. and Nordlee, J. A. (1989). Histamine poisoning (scombroid fish poisoning): an allergy-like intoxication. *J. Toxicol. Clin. Toxicol.*, **27**, 225–240

Teitelbaum, J. S., Zatorre, R. J., Carpenter, S., Gendron, D., Evans, A. C., Gjedde, A. and Cashman, N. R. (1990). Neurologic sequelae of domoic acid intoxication due to the ingestion of contaminated mussels. *N. Engl. J. Med.*, **322**, 1781–1787

Theakston, R. D. G. (1989). New techniques in antivenom production and active immunization against snake venoms. *Trans. R. Soc. Trop. Med. Hyg.*, **83**, 433–435

Tibballs, J. (1988). Severe tetrodotoxic fish poisoning. *Anaesth. Intensive Care*, **16**, 215–217

Trestrail, J. H. (1981). Scorpion envenomation in Michigan: three cases of toxic encounters with poisonous stow-aways. *Vet. Hum. Toxicol.*, **23**, 8–11

Trestrail, J. H. and Al-Mahasneh, Q. M. (1989). Lionfish sting experiences of an inland poison center: a retrospective study of 23 cases. *Vet. Hum. Toxicol.*, **31**, 173–175

Tu, A. T. and Fulde, G. (1987). Sea snake bites. *Clin. Dermatol.*, **5**, 118–126

Valentine, M. D., Schuberth, K. C., Kagey-Sobotka, A., Graft, D. F., Kwiterovich, K. A., Szklo, M., Lichtenstein, L. M. (1990). The value of immunotherapy with venom in children with allergy to insect stings. *N. Engl. J. Med.*, **323**, 1601–1603

Wang, G. K. and Strichartz, G. R. (1983). Purification and physiological characterization of neurotoxins from the venoms of scorpions *Centruroides sculpturatus* and *Leiurus quinquestriatus*. *Mol. Pharmacol.*, **23**, 519–533

Wasserman, G. S. (1988). Wound care of spider and snake envenomations. *Ann. Emerg. Med.*, **17**, 1331–1335

Wasserman, G. S. and Anderson, P. C. (1983–84). Loxoscelism and necrotic arachnidism. *J. Toxicol. Clin. Toxicol.*, **21**, 451–472

Wright, D. N. and Lockey, R. F. (1990). Local reactions to stinging insects (Hymenoptera). *Allergy Proc.*, **11**, 23–28

FURTHER READING

Harvey, A. L. (1991). *Snake Toxins*. Pergamon Press, New York

Jasperse, J. A. (1993). *Marine Toxins and New Zealand Shell Fish*. Miscellaneous Series, Royal Society of New Zealand, No. 24 (ISBN 0–9086544–44–8)

Meier, J. and Stocker, K. (1991). Effects of snake venoms on hemostasis. *Critical Reviews in Toxicology*, **21**, 171–187

Nhachi, C. F. B. and Kasilo, O. M. J. (1993). Poisoning due to insect and scorpion stings/bites. *Human and Experimental toxicology*, **12**, 123–125

Shier, W. T. and Mebs, D. (1994). *Handbook of Toxicology*. Marcel Dekker, Inc., New York

55 Radiation Toxicology

Gerald E. Adams and Angela Wilson

INTRODUCTION

The Nature of Radiation Action

Ionizing radiation causes many different types of damage in mammalian systems. These include effects in both proliferative and non-proliferative tissues, the induction of genetic abnormalities that in some circumstances can be passed on to offspring, and the induction of malignancy. The nature and severity of radiation-induced effects can vary with radiation type; the magnitude of the radiation dose and the period over which it is delivered; the age, sex and health status of the individual; and, particularly, the degree of post-irradiation care that may be available.

The energies of radiation emanating from X-ray sets, many radionuclides and particle accelerators are usually vastly in excess of the chemical bonds that are present in all biological molecules. Following interaction between radiation and any molecule, simple or complex, electron ejection, or ionization, is the primary event. The time-scale is governed by various factors, but a quantum of gamma-radiation or a high-energy particle will pass through a small molecule and impart energy to it in times of the order of 10^{-17} s. The subsequent physical, chemical and biological processes are complex and occur over very different time-scales. For example, the onset of malignancy does not occur in many instances until 20 or even 30 years after irradiation.

It is often convenient, though not necessarily rigorous, to classify radiation action into physical, chemical, cellular, and tissue effects.

The Physical and Chemical Stages

Radiation deposits energy in discrete packages in 'tracks' through the absorbing medium. The spatial distribution of energy deposition depends on the type of radiation, the composition of the medium and the energy of the radiation. The so-called densely ionizing radiations such as α-particles, neutrons and heavier particles, lose energy over much shorter distances than low

linear energy transfer (LET) radiations such as X- or γ-rays. LET is a measure of the rate at which energy is imparted to the absorbing medium per unit distance of track length. The biological effectiveness of the former type is generally greater in inducing most types of biological effect, including malignancy. Particulate radiations, with the exception of neutrons, are absorbed over short distances, except at extremely high energies. Following primary ionizations, the secondary electrons, which are still highly energetic, lose energy by various collisional and other interactions, thereby producing other ions, excited molecules and molecular fragments.

The chemical stage of radiation action is mainly concerned with the formation, diffusion and eventual reaction of the molecular fragments and other unstable entities. Because of the high energy of the radiations relative to the normal bond energies in molecules, radiation is absorbed fairly non-selectively. This is not necessarily true in all cases, particularly in materials abundant in heavy atoms, but it is certainly a sound approximation in biological material. The 'principle of equipartition of energy' implies that, in cellular material, about 80 per cent of the energy is initially deposited in the aqueous component. This is why so much attention has been given in the past to the study of the radiation chemistry of water—particularly, aqueous solutions or mixtures containing various biological molecules. There is now abundant evidence that damage to such molecules, particularly the nucleic acids, caused by free radicals, contributes to loss or change of intracellular function following irradiation. The continuing problem, however, is to distinguish those processes that are relevant to the observed cellular response to radiation from those that are not.

The Cellular Stage

Various morphological changes in the cell can often be observed shortly after irradiation. Local protrusions of the plasma membrane follow within minutes of exposure to relatively high doses of radiation. These are followed within hours by other membrane changes, including an increase in permeability and loss of essential enzymes. However, the more important effects concerning the loss of, or changes in, cellular function that occur at much lower doses can only be observed much later. For clonogenic cells *in vitro*, loss of reproductive capacity is evident only when the cells fail to divide. Subcellular effects, such as mutation and the induction of aberrant chromosomes, can only be observed when sufficient cell divisions have taken place to permit analysis. Mammalian cells are often at their most sensitive during mitosis and early in G phase. Resistance is usually greatest during early S phase, although this is very dependent on radiation quality, i.e. the type of radiation.

Repair processes occur in irradiated cells both *in vitro* and *in vivo*. When radiation is delivered at a low dose rate or in a series of multiple fractions separated by several hours, the overall effect on cell-kill is usually less than that for an acute dose of radiation. This phenomenon, more commonly seen with low LET radiation, is attributable to repair of sublethal injury. It is relevant to dose–response relationships for cell-kill and various sublethal effects such as mutation and cell transformation. Repair processes of various kinds occur both *in vitro* and *in vivo* and are responsible for the reduced severity of some radiation injuries when the exposure is protracted.

Radiation dose to tissue is expressed in terms of the quantity of absorbed energy per unit mass. The SI unit is the gray (Gy), which is defined as 1 joule of absorbed energy per kilogram. The older unit, the rad, which is still in common use, is equivalent to 100 erg g^{-1} and is equal to 0.01 Gy. A dose of 1 Gy of X-rays will cause about 2×10^5 separate ionizations within the mammalian cell. Of these, about 1 per cent occur in the genomic material and a major consequence of this is breakage of DNA strands. Of the many breaks that occur, almost all disappear within a few hours, probably by enzyme-mediated repair. Some breaks remain, however, probably as aligned double-strand breaks, and these are the major cause of loss of cell viability and also contribute to various types of sublethal injury. In many mammalian cells it is remarkable that, for this high dose of radiation, a substantial population of the cells retain a degree of reproductive capacity despite the large amount of chemical damage sustained by the cells. Much of the initial chemical damage caused by the radiation must therefore be of little consequence to the fate of the cell. It is likely that only a small part of the damage, caused perhaps by the rather rare local deposition of energy close to critical molecular sites, is important.

The Tissue Stage

The response time of mammalian tissues to radiation varies widely, as do their sensitivities. The general finding *in vitro* that mammalian cells are at their most radiation-sensitive during mitosis predicts that *in vivo* the mammalian fertilized egg cell (zygote) will be highly radiation-sensitive and that tissues with high rates of cell turnover will also be particularly sensitive. Both predictions are correct. Rapidly proliferating stem cells of the intestinal epithelium and the haematopoietic system are highly sensitive and respond more rapidly than do less sensitive cells, such as those in the lung and the basal layer of the skin, which have lower proliferation rates. Cells that do not divide, or do so only after an appropriate stimulus, e.g. parenchymal cells of the liver, are less sensitive still. Cells that divide only during embryogenesis are the least sensitive.

In this chapter the nature, origin and expression of radiation injury are classified according to the organ in which it occurs, and particularly with regard to the stochastic or non-stochastic nature of the pathological response. The International Commission on Radiological Protection (ICRP) made the distinction between stochastic and non-stochastic effects (ICRP, 1977). Stochastic effects are those for which the probability of an effect occurring, but not its severity, increases with radiation dose, without a threshold. In contrast, non-stochastic effects are those for which the severity of the effect depends on the magnitude of the dose, and for which a threshold dose exists, below which no detrimental effects are observable. The types of damage that result from injury to substantial populations of cells in tissues such as the eye, skin, lung, gonads, gastrointestinal tract and haematopoietic system are considered to be non-stochastic. On the other hand, stochastic effects can result from injury to a single cell or to a small number of cells, and include the induction of various hereditary defects and most types of cancer.

A further distinction is often made between the somatic and hereditary effects of radiation. Somatic effects refer to those which are manifest in the exposed individual, and include both non-stochastic and stochastic effects. The hereditary effects of radiation are of a stochastic nature and are transmitted via germ cell damage. The effects may be expressed in the immediate offspring or in later generations. Figure 1 (taken from ICRP, 1984) illustrates the essential features of stochastic and non-stochastic effects.

NON-STOCHASTIC EFFECTS

General

Non-stochastic radiation effects are due to radiation-induced cell killing with the accompanying disruption of functions for which the cells are responsible.

Cell death is most likely to occur when the irradiated cells attempt to resume dividing. This leads to a lack of replacement of mature cells which have been lost through natural senescence and death. For certain cell types, including lymphocytes and oocytes, radiation-induced cell death occurs during interphase. In general, the rate at which cells divide, differentiate, age and are lost from a given tissue will influence the rapidity with which that tissue exhibits radiation damage. Those tissues containing actively dividing cells will tend to exhibit greater radiosensitivity than do those composed of fully differentiated cells with little or no mitotic activity.

The life-span of the comparatively radioresistant mature cells represents a further factor influencing the interval between irradiation and the time when damage becomes evident in tissues with well-defined stem cell populations. In the case of fractionated or protracted exposures, stem cell division can partially compensate for cell killing and so reduce the effectiveness of the radiation.

Populations containing cells with a relatively short life-span, e.g. the gastrointestinal mucosa, will exhibit radiation damage much more quickly than populations where the cell life-span is

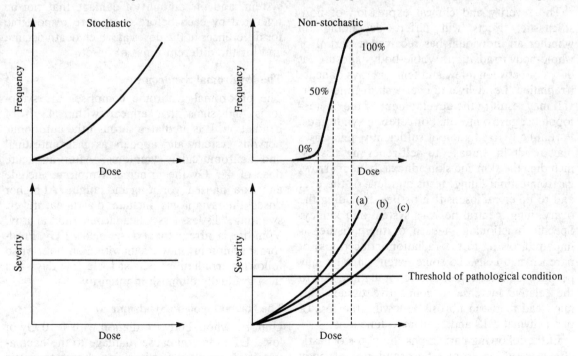

Figure 1 Dose–effect curves illustrating stochastic and non-stochastic effects. The upper and lower plots on the right of the figure show how the frequency and severity of a given radiation injury of a non-stochastic type increase with radiation dose in a population of mixed susceptibilities (a, b and c). The severity increases most rapidly with dose in the most sensitive group (curve a) and reaches a level of clinical detectability at a dose lower than those for the other two subgroups (curves b and c). The upper and lower plots on the left of Figure 1 illustrate that the frequency of a stochastic effect increases with radiation dose, but not the severity. Redrawn from ICRP (1984)

longer, e.g. blood cells of the circulatory system. On this basis it is possible to distinguish between early effects, which may appear within a few weeks, depending on the pattern of exposure, and later effects, which do not appear until months or years after irradiation.

In those tissues which lack a well-defined stem cell population and exhibit low cellular proliferations, radiation effects, although dose-dependent, may not appear for some time. These tissues, e.g. the liver, where the turnover of parenchymal cells is low, have much less protection from the effects of radiation in the absence of an ability to compensate for cell killing through stem cell proliferation.

Other factors, besides the proliferative ability of cells in a given tissue, which may contribute to a reduction in the effects of irradiation include tissue repopulation by surviving cells; the ability of differentiating, maturing and functioning cells to buffer stem cell damage; the ability of a tissue to undergo compensatory changes to maintain the supply of differentiated cells; and the tissue's functional reserve capacity.

The severity and clinical expression of non-stochastic effects will differ, depending on whether an individual has received a partial or whole-body irradiation. Whole-body exposures at doses of between a few and tens of grays of acute irradiation, i.e. delivered over a short time-interval, may result in the development of the haematopoietic, gastrointestinal or cerebral syndromes. Partial-body irradiation at sufficiently high doses may result in damage to self-renewing tissues, including the skin and skin adnexa, bone marrow, gastrointestinal lining, testis and lens of the eye, and to other radiosensitive tissues, including the ovary, lung, central nervous system and kidney. Specific functioning in each of these tissues is impaired, owing to the radiation-induced loss of parenchymal cells. To some extent damage may persist even after repair and repopulation, due to the relative increase in connective tissue. This may lead to tissue fibrosis following the loss of parenchymal cells and associated functions.

In the following paragraphs the non-stochastic effects resulting from whole and partial body irradiation are considered in detail. Subsequently the stochastic effects—namely radiation carcinogenesis and hereditary defects—are examined. The effects resulting from *in utero* irradiation are also discussed, although these are not easily classified as stochastic or non-stochastic.

Whole-body Irradiation

In man death may occur within a few weeks following acute radiation exposure. The survival time and mode of death is dose-dependent. A dose of 100 Gy can cause death from neurological damage within a few hours; 5–12 Gy can cause death from gastrointestinal injury within a few days; while 2.5–5 Gy may cause death from irreversible damage to the haematopoietic system in several weeks. The prodromal syndrome (see below) develops shortly after irradiation, and precedes the onset of neurological, gastrointestinal and haematopoietic syndromes. Although the exact cause of death in the neurological syndrome is uncertain, depletion of the stem cells in the critical self-renewing tissues of the gut epithelium and circulating blood cells causes death in the gastrointestinal and haematopoietic syndromes, respectively. Differences in the population kinetics of the gut epithelium and haematopoietic system, and the amount of damage that can be tolerated by each before death, are responsible for differences in the doses at which death occurs, and for the different times of onset.

The Prodromal Syndrome

The prodromal syndrome comprises the symptoms and signs that appear within 48 h of irradiation. It is mediated through the autonomic nervous system, and appears as gastrointestinal and neuromuscular symptoms. After an acute dose of 4–5 Gy the principal symptoms include anorexia, nausea, vomiting and fatigue. At higher doses the symptoms include diarrhoea, fever, sweating, listlessness, headache and apathy. Vomiting is infrequent at doses below 1 Gy. Prodromal symptoms may occur within an hour or so following irradiation, persist for a few days and then gradually diminish in intensity.

The Haematopoietic Syndrome

Uniform whole-body irradiation with 1–10 Gy of low-LET radiation causes damage to the haematopoietic system. Proliferating haematopoietic stem cells are highly radiosensitive and are sterilized by radiation, thereby reducing the body's supply of red and white cells and platelets. The full effect of the damage is not experienced until the number of circulating cells in the blood reaches a critical minimum value.

In human bone marrow the total number of nucleated cells is reduced at day 1 by 10–20 per cent after 1–2 Gy, by 25–30 per cent after 3–4 Gy, by 50–60 per cent after 5–7 Gy and by a maximum of 80–85 per cent after 8–10 Gy. Resistant cells such as macrophages, stromal cells, cells of the vascular epithelium and some mature granulocytes and eosinophils remain (IAEA, 1971).

The lymphocyte count is the most sensitive index of radiation injury in the blood: for a given dose, nadir levels are reached earlier than for other cell types. Lymphocytes undergo interphase death and their numbers decrease to about 50 per cent of normal by 48 h following a dose of 1–2 Gy.

Neutrophils show an initial increase over the first few days after irradiation, then a dose-related fall. Between 10 and 15 days after a dose of 2–5 Gy, there is a second abortive rise due to recovering haematopoiesis from precursor cell populations, followed by a second decline to about day 25. This is due to a lack of recovery in the stem cell population. With doses greater than 5 Gy the second abortive rise does not occur. The time-course for platelet loss is similar to that for granulocytes, but there is no second abortive rise. A decrease in platelet levels in the blood is associated with bleeding. Owing to the long life-span of radioresistant red blood cells (109–127 days in man), anaemia results only when there has been substantial bleeding.

Figure 2 shows data from accident cases, depicting the average time-courses for suppression and recovery of neutrophils, lymphocytes and platelets in man following irradiation.

Approximately 3 weeks after irradiation, symptoms including chills, fatigue, ulceration of the mouth and petechial haemorrhages of the skin develop as a result of the reduction in blood cell components. Infections and fever arise as a result of granulocyte depression and impairment of the immune system, while bleeding and possibly anaemia may develop from haemorrhage caused through platelet depression. Death, which is often caused by infection, will follow at this stage unless bone marrow regeneration has commenced. Where the radiation dose is less than 4–5 Gy, it is possible to treat the individual in response to specific symptoms—for example, by administering antibiotics for infection until the immune system has fully recovered.

Humans develop signs of haematological damage and recover from it much more slowly than do other mammals. Peak incidence of death occurs at about 30 days after irradiation, although deaths may continue for up to 60 days. The 50 per cent lethal dose or LD_{50} for man is therefore expressed as the $LD_{50/60}$ (i.e. the dose that causes 50 per cent mortality within 60 days), in contrast to the $LD_{50/30}$ for most animal species, where the peak incidence of death occurs between 10 and 15 days after irradiation.

The Gastrointestinal Syndrome

A whole-body dose of 10 Gy or more of low-LET radiation will produce the gastrointestinal syndrome in most mammals, resulting in death 3–10 days later. Signs and symptoms follow those of the prodromal phase, and include nausea, vomiting, increased lethargy, prolonged diarrhoea, loss of appetite, and loss of fluids and electrolytes. After a few days individuals show signs of dehydration; weight loss; gastric retention and decreased intestinal absorption; emaciation; and complete exhaustion. There is a marked reduction in the leukocyte count, and haemorrhages and bacteraemia may occur, aggravating the injury and contributing to death. The symptoms and subsequent death are due to the radiation-induced damage to the epithelium lining the gastrointestinal tract. A dose of about 10 Gy will sterilize a large proportion of the mitotic cells in the crypts of the intestinal mucosa. This arrests the continuous supply of new cells which normally move up the villi, differentiate to become functioning cells and eventually slough off. Sterilization of cells in the crypts prevents repopulation. After a few days, the villi begin to shrink and the intestinal lining is eventually denuded of villi.

The Neurological Syndrome

A radiation dose of more than about 100 Gy will cause death from cerebrovascular damage in most mammalian species within 2 days. The neurological syndrome is characterized by severe prodromal effects followed by transitory periods of depressed or enhanced motor activity. Severe nausea may occur within minutes, which is then followed by vomiting, disorientation, loss of co-ordination and muscular movement, respiratory

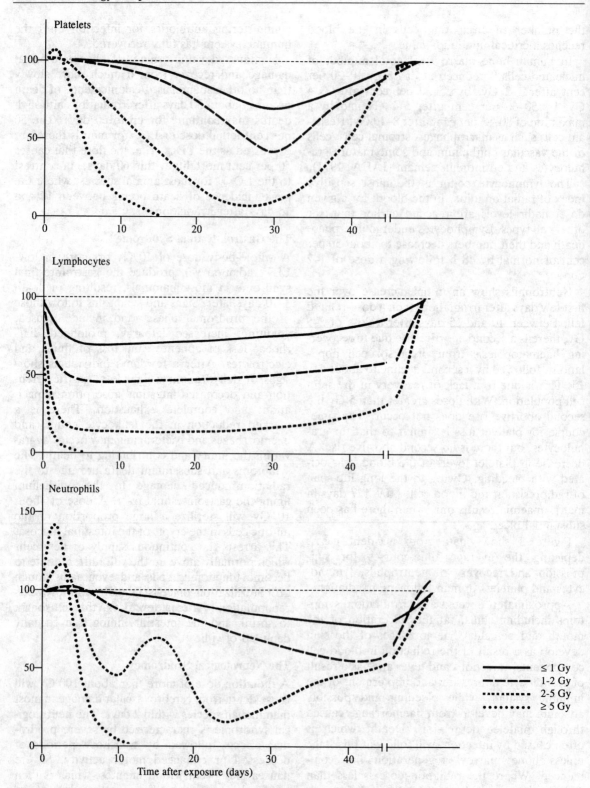

Figure 2 Schematic picture of average time-courses for various cells in the blood after various doses of radiation in man. Curves derived from accident case data. Redrawn from UNSCEAR (1988)

distress, diarrhoea, convulsive seizures, coma and eventually death.

The exact cause of death in the neurological syndrome is not fully understood. Although death is usually attributed to direct damage to the central nervous system, much higher doses are required to produce death if only the head is irradiated, which indicates that effects elsewhere in the body are also important. An increase in the fluid content of the brain due to leakage from small vessels creating a build-up of pressure inside the skull has been suggested as the cause of immediate death.

Effects from Partial Body Irradiation

Eye

The lens of the eye is one of the most radiosensitive tissues of the body. Exposure to ionizing radiation may cause a cataract, a term used to describe any detectable change in the normally transparent lens of the eye. This may range from tiny flecks in the lens to virtually complete opacification, causing blindness.

Radiation-induced cataracts arise through damage to the mitotic cells in the anterior epithelium of the lens. Under normal conditions these cells continue to proliferate throughout life and differentiate into lens fibres. Damage to the dividing cells results in abnormal lens fibres which are not translucent. These damaged cells and their breakdown products migrate posteriorly and accumulate beneath the capsule at the posterior pole of the lens, where they cause posterior displacement of the lens bow. If enough damaged cells accumulate, they become visible ophthalmologically as a dot, usually situated at the posterior pole.

During the early stages, radiation-induced cataracts are unique in that, unlike other radiation-induced effects, they can be distinguished in most cases from cataracts resulting from other causes. As the cataract enlarges, small granules and vacuoles appear around it, and by the time the opacity is a few millimetres in diameter, it may have developed a clear centre and have assumed a doughnut shape. The radiation dose received will determine whether the cataract remains stationary or continues to progress. If the cataract progresses, it becomes indistinguishable from other types of cataract.

In humans lens opacities may appear between 6 months and 35 years after irradiation. The latent period between irradiation and appearance of a cataract is dose-related. At high doses lens opacities develop within months, progress rapidly and produce vision-impairing cataracts. At lower doses the opacities develop more slowly, remain microscopic in size and cause no significant impairment of vision (Merriam *et al.*, 1972). A threshold dose of about 2 Gy X-irradiation in a single exposure is required for the induction of minimally detectable lens opacities; larger doses are required with fractionated or protracted exposures (Merriam *et al.*, 1972). Compared with the lens, other parts of the eye are less radiosensitive.

Skin

The effect of radiation on the skin is dependent on various factors, including dose, the depth and area of skin irradiated, and the anatomical location and its vascularity. It is also influenced by the age, hormonal status and genetic background of the irradiated individual. Within hours of irradiation, transitory erythema may occur, indicating capillary dilation brought about by the release of histamine-like substances from injured epithelial cells. Typically this persists for only a few hours. Two to four weeks later, one or more waves of deeper and more prolonged erythema usually appear. Thereafter, depending on the dose received, epilation, dry desquamation, moist desquamation and necrosis of the skin may occur.

The severity of the skin response is determined by the dose to the germinal cells in the basal layer of the epidermis. Since damage to these cells appears to be critical to the pathogenesis of erythema and desquamation, post-irradiation treatments using corticosteroids may decrease the severity of the desquamation reaction but will have no effect on erythema. In human skin the threshold dose of X- or gamma-rays required to produce erythema in a 10 cm^2 field range from 6–8 Gy for single, brief exposures to more than 30 Gy for highly fractionated or protracted exposures. Threshold doses for dry desquamation, moist desquamation and necrosis are higher, but also increase with fractionated or protracted exposures (Rubin and Casarett, 1968).

The effect of radiation-induced damage to the dermis appears later than does that to the epidermis or to the epidermal-associated hair follicles, principally because of the slower turnover of cell types in the dermis. The dermis contains connective tissue, sebaceous glands, muscle fibres, nerve plexuses and nerve fibres, sweat glands and blood vessels. The effects of high doses on blood vessels are visible as erythema and later as haemorrhages, which may appear as small (petechiae) or larger (purpura) lesions. The peak onset of purpura occurs 3–4 weeks after irradiation, and can be produced by doses of 4–6 Gy. Following high doses of radiation to the dermis, a second wave of erythema is produced as a result of damage to the deep dermal plexus of blood vessels.

Temporary epilation may result after a single brief exposure to 3–5 Gy of low-LET radiation and is most severe 2–3 weeks after irradiation. Permanent epilation may occur after a single exposure to more than 7 Gy, or to 50–60 Gy fractionated over a period of weeks. Hair on the scalp is more sensitive than the beard or body hair.

Skin on the anterior aspect of the neck, antecubital and popliteal areas is most sensitive to radiation, followed by that on the anterior surfaces of extremities, the chest and abdomen. Thereafter, skin on the face (not strongly pigmented), the back and posterior surfaces of extremities, the face (strongly pigmented), the nape of the neck and the scalp are of decreasing sensitivity. Skin on the palms and soles is least sensitive to radiation.

The long-term effects of radiation on the skin, which develop months or years after exposure, include changes in pigmentation; atrophy of the epidermis, sweat glands, sebaceous glands and hair follicles; fibrosis of the dermis; and increased susceptibility to trauma and chronic ulceration. These changes result in part from depletion of fibroblasts and in part from injury to blood vessels in the dermis. It is possible that the loss of epidermal cells may also contribute.

The Reproductive System

The germ cells of the ovary and testis are very radiosensitive and their irradiation impairs fertility in both sexes in a dose-dependent manner. In male mammals spermatozoa are continuously produced in the seminiferous tubules of the testes. Spermatogonial stem cells divide to produce primary spermatocytes, which, in turn, give rise to secondary spermatocytes, spermatids and mature spermatozoa. In humans the development of mature sperm from spermatogonial stem cells takes about 10 weeks.

Spermatogonial stem cells are more radiosensitive than are postspermatogonial cell stages. The second and third stages of spermatogenesis, from preleptotene spermatocytes through to the spermatids, are not affected by doses of less than 3 Gy. After such doses, postspermatogonial cells mature and a normal sperm count can be maintained for approximately 46 days, the time-period required for the development of spermatozoa from preleptotene spermatocytes. Thereafter, the sperm count will drop, approaching azoospermia by 10 weeks following a dose in excess of 1 Gy. Sterility will remain until the surviving 'stem' spermatogonia are able to repopulate the seminiferous tubules. In humans a dose of 2.5 Gy may cause temporary sterility for 1–2 years, while a dose of 6 Gy will often cause permanent sterility. The threshold dose for permanent sterility does not increase appreciably on fractionation of irradiation over days or even weeks.

The mature oocyte is the most radiosensitive germ cell stage in females. Exposure of both ovaries to an acute dose of more than 0.65–1.5 Gy can cause temporary sterility. With doses below 2–3 Gy, enough immature oocytes may survive to restore fertility. It has been estimated that the ovary can withstand 6–20 Gy of low-LET radiation in highly fractionated or protracted exposure regimes (Lushbaugh and Ricks, 1972; Lushbaugh and Casarett, 1976). The threshold dose for permanent sterility decreases with age, probably owing to the decrease in oocyte number with age.

An important consideration in germ cell irradiation is the potential increase in mutation incidence in the offspring. In general, irradiation of the female is less damaging than irradiation of the male in regard to the induction of mutations. This is due to the greater lethal radiosensitivity of mature oocytes, thereby decreasing the number of viable cells carrying mutations which could be passed to the offspring.

The genetic consequences of a given dose can be reduced if a time-interval is allowed between irradiation and conception. This is due to the variation of radiation sensitivity with stage of germ cell development. In males irradiation immediately prior to conception, so that mature sperm are irradiated, increases the sensitivity to mutation induction. This is a direct consequence of the greater resistance of mature sperm cells to the lethal effects of radiation. If the time-interval between irradiation and conception is longer, so that the sperm involved in fertilization are irradiated during an earlier developmental stage, then fewer mutations result.

The Digestive System

Radiation damage to the epithelial cells of the mucous membranes in the mouth and throat evokes inflammation and swelling, with ulceration and necrosis developing after high doses. Mucosal injury is greatest in the cheeks, soft palate and hypoglossal region, and less in the gums, hard palate, nose, posterior wall of the throat, tongue and larynx. Following doses of up to 10 Gy of low-LET radiation, the mucosal surfaces recover after 2–3 weeks. With doses of 10–20 Gy extensive mucosal necrosis occurs after 4–5 days and recovery is much slower (1.5–2 months).

The salivary glands are radiosensitive but may recover even after high doses, provided that the dose is given in a fractionated regimen. Following 50–70 Gy of conventionally fractionated X-rays, the salivary glands undergo necrosis, atrophy and fibrosis, which results in reduced salivary flow (Rubin and Casarett, 1968). In humans there may be a loss of taste after doses as low as 2.4–4.0 Gy (Congar, 1973).

The glandular mucosa of the stomach, small intestine and colon respond more rapidly and tolerate less radiation in a single exposure than do the squamous cell mucosa of the oral cavity, pharynx, oesophagus and anus. Radiation damage to the germinal epithelium in the mucosa interferes with cell renewal and may cause ulceration and, possibly, denudation of the affected mucosae. Exposure of a large part of the intestine to an acute dose in excess of 10 Gy may lead to the induction of the rapidly fatal gastrointestinal syndrome, as described earlier. With regard to long-term effects, fibrosis, stricture, intestinal perforation and fistula formation may develop months or years after exposure as complications arising from radiation injury to the gastrointestinal tract (Rubin and Casarett, 1968).

Of the parenchymatous organs of the digestive tract, the liver appears to have the lowest threshold for injury. Impaired liver function results from exposure of the whole organ to 30 Gy of conventionally fractionated therapeutic X-radiation. Changes which may include damage to centrilobular veins, with thrombosis and portal hypertension, may lead to hepatic failure, ascites and death (Kraut *et al.*, 1972; Wharton *et al.*, 1973). With partial irradiation of the liver, substantially larger doses can be tolerated.

The Respiratory System

The respiratory system can tolerate considerable localized radiation injury, as, for example, when a small part of a lung is heavily irradiated for therapeutic purposes. If, however, both lungs or a large proportion of lung tissue is irradiated with doses of greater than about 8 Gy, a fatal pneumonitis may develop after a latent period of 1–3 months. The earliest signs of radiation injury to the lungs are oedema and changes in blood circulation, which precede pneumonitis.

Individuals who survive the acute inflammatory phase of pneumonitis may later develop pulmonary fibrosis and cor pulmonale. With a whole-body dose of more than 8 Gy, bone marrow failure may occur before severe lung damage becomes evident. The target cell population responsible for pneumonitis after irradiation is unknown, but type-II alveolar cells are implicated and vascular injury may be contributory (Travis and Tucker, 1986; De Saint-Georges *et al.*, 1988).

In the case of the upper respiratory tract, including tissues of the nasopharynx, larynx, trachea and bronchi, doses in excess of 30 Gy in 2 Gy fractions are required to cause ulceration, atrophy and fibrosis (van den Brenk, 1971).

The Nervous System

Radiation-induced damage to the spinal cord, including demyelination and delayed necrosis of neurons in the white matter and damage to the fine vasculature, may develop between 6 months and 2 years after exposure (Rubin and Casarett, 1968). Typical neurological symptoms resulting from this damage include numbness, tingling, anaesthesia, paraesthesia, weakness and paralysis.

The brain is relatively resistant to radiation damage, with a dose of about 15 Gy required to produce deleterious effects. Necrosis of the brain, associated with demyelination and damage to cerebral vasculature, may occur within 1–3 years of receiving a dose of 55 Gy delivered over about 5½ weeks to the whole brain, or about 65 Gy delivered over 6½ weeks to a small part of the brain. This may lead to neurological symptoms and, in some cases, death. Many months after accidental or therapeutic irradiation in the range over 10 Gy, leukoencephalopathy, electroence-phalographic changes and functional disturbances have been reported in humans, especially children. In addition, detectable morphological and physiological changes in children have been reported following a dose of 1–6 Gy (Ron *et al.*, 1982). With regard to the peripheral nervous system, damage may occur at doses above 60 Gy delivered in conventional fractionated radio-therapy regimens (Rubin and Casarett, 1968).

The Cardiovascular System

The heart is not a particularly radiosensitive organ, but a dose of 40 Gy, in conventionally fractionated radiotherapy, may cause myocardial degeneration, while a dose of more than 60 Gy to the entire heart may lead to death from peri-cardial effusion or constrictive pericarditis. If only a part of the heart is irradiated, tolerance is greater, but degenerative changes and fibrosis in the exposed tissues may occur following a dose of 60 Gy.

A dose of 40–60 Gy will cause changes in the blood vessels in all organs (Rubin and Casarett, 1968). Vascular permeability and blood flow will increase in the early phases of the response. Endothelial cell degeneration, thickening of the basement membrane and progressive sclerosis will follow within a few months. Blood vessels may undergo late changes, including focal endo-thelial proliferation, thickening of the wall, nar-rowing of the lumen and decrease in blood flow. It has been suggested that vascular damage may play a major role in most forms of late radiation-induced tissue injury (Law, 1981).

The Endocrine System

Endocrine glands, including the thyroid, para-thyroid, adrenal and pituitary glands, have a low cell turnover rate in normal adults, and are there-fore relatively radioresistant, If, however, these glands are in a growing or proliferative state, they will be more radiosensitive.

In children irradiation of the thyroid gland by external gamma-radiation or internally deposited radioiodine can lead to hypothyroidism and growth retardation (Conard *et al.*, 1975). In adults thyroid damage with myxoedema has been reported to develop between 4 months and 3 years after fractionated X-ray therapy with doses of between 26 and 48 Gy for tumours in the neck (Markson and Flatman, 1965; Glatstein *et al.*, 1971).

The pituitary and adrenal glands are less radio-sensitive than the thyroid; in adults threshold doses of conventionally fractionated irradiation of about 45 and 60 Gy, respectively, are required to depress permanently the functioning of these glands (Rubin and Casarett, 1968). The threshold for severe functional damage following irradiation of the entire adult thyroid gland is approximately 25–30 Gy fractionated over 30 days; at lower doses subclinical damage may occur.

Although the female breast is relatively radio-resistant during adult life, normal breast develop-ment may be impaired if doses of more than 10 Gy of conventionally fractionated X-irradiation are administered before puberty (Rubin and Casarett, 1968).

The Urinary Tract

Of the organs of the urinary tract, the kidneys are most radiosensitive, followed by the bladder and the ureters. The threshold dose for a fatal nephritis-like reaction in the kidneys, which can develop 6–12 months after irradiation, is esti-mated to be about 23 Gy of X-rays delivered in fractions of about 1 Gy over a 5 week period (Maier, 1972).

Radiation-induced renal injury involves degenerative changes in the fine vasculature of the kidney and in the epithelium of the nephron itself (Rubin and Casarett, 1968; Law, 1981). His-tologically, degeneration and depopulation of the renal tubules can be detected in the kidney within 6–12 months after irradiation following doses of more than 10 Gy; with high doses depopulation may be permanent, with degenerative changes in the vasculature. If the individual survives for several years after irradiation, the kidneys shrink in size, the capsule thickens and adheres to the cortex, and there will be cortical thinning and disorganization.

The bladder is less radiosensitive than the kid-neys. With high doses complications, including cystitis, ulceration, fistula, fibrosis, contraction and urinary obstruction, may occur (Rubin and Casarett, 1968).

The Musculoskeletal System

Muscle, bone and cartilage are relatively resistant to the direct cytocidal actions of radiation. With doses exceeding 20 Gy administered during childhood in conventionally fractionated therapy, scoliosis, kyphosis, slipped upper femoral epiphysis and exostoses may be observed.

Early radiation damage in mature bone and cartilage is difficult to detect because of the paucity of cells, the abundance of matrix, the radioresistance of the matrix and the mature cells, and the normally slow turnover rate of most of the matrix. The principal factor in radiation damage to these tissues is the injury to the fine vasculature supplying these structures. The degeneration and loss of dependent cells is secondary to interference with the blood supply, with changes in the matrix secondary to either of these changes. In the event of a large degree of vascular and cellular damage where there is degeneration and loss of many of the bone or cartilage cells, this will eventually be reflected in changes in the matrix, with the development of 'radiation osteitis' or 'radiation chrondritis'. Whether or not the devitalized bone or cartilage results in structural disintegration depends on the degree at which occlusion of fine vasculature and loss of parenchymal cells occurs, and on the occurrence of complicating factors such as infection or trauma.

In a proliferative state, as, for example, in growing children, or during the healing of fractures, cartilage and bone may exhibit a greater response to radiation than when in the mature state. In children a dose of 1 Gy may cause some growth retardation, depending on the age at irradiation and the exposure conditions (Tefft, 1972; Blot, 1975). With doses exceeding 20 Gy, administered in conventionally fractionated radiotherapy in childhood, skeletal changes, including scoliosis, kyphosis, slipped upper femoral epiphysis and exostosis, may occur.

In adults, mature cartilage will tolerate 40 Gy fractionated over 4 weeks, or over 70 Gy fractionated over 10–12 weeks; mature bone will tolerate up to 65 Gy fractionated over 6–8 weeks (Parker, 1972). Although these doses may be tolerated by adult bone and cartilage without necrosis, these tissues may exhibit increased susceptibility to trauma in the long term (Rubin and Casarett, 1968).

Large radiation doses (500 Gy) are required to cause early necrosis of muscle which involves disruption of the fine vasculature and microcirculation, with increased capillary permeability, oedema and inflammation. At lower doses the acute oedematous and inflammatory response to vascular damage is more moderate and transient. However, the associated vascular damage and connective tissue reactions from acute interstitial oedema and inflammation may progress to cause delayed secondary degeneration, atrophy, or necrosis and fibrosis of irradiated muscles.

STOCHASTIC EFFECTS

The acute or early effects of radiation as described above result mainly from cell killing. By contrast, some late effects of irradiation result from damage to surviving cells which is transmitted to their progeny. Damage to germ cells may result in a genetic mutation that is expressed in a later generation; in the case of somatic cells, the result may be cancer induction in the exposed individual. Cancer and the induction of hereditary damage represent the stochastic effects of irradiation and are regarded as the principal risks to health from low doses of radiation.

Radiation Carcinogenesis

Radiation is effective both as a carcinogen and in the treatment of cancer. The use of radiation in cancer therapy is based on its cell-killing ability, when administered in sufficiently large doses to replicating malignant cells. For cancer induction sublethal doses of radiation are important.

Several general principles apply to the induction of tumours by radiation. As a carcinogen, radiation is unique in that it can cause cancer in almost every tissue of the body, and radiogenic cancers are indistinguishable from those cancers which arise naturally or as a result of other carcinogens. Leukaemia (except for chronic lymphatic leukaemia) is the most frequently induced cancer. Chronic lymphatic leukaemia, squamous cell carcinoma of the cervix and Hodgkin's lymphoma are not induced by radiation.

Prior to the appearance of an induced tumour there is a latency period, the length of which depends on the type of tumour, its growth rate and metastatic form. The latency period for leukaemia is 2–5 years, while for other tumours 10 or more years is usual. There is also a delay before the initially 'transformed' cell or cells begin to divide to form a tumour, and there may be a further delay before the tumour assumes the 'malignant' characteristics of growth and spread. Radiation carcinogenesis is thought to be a multistage process involving initiation, promotion and progression.

Various factors influence the probability that an individual exposed to radiation will develop cancer. Current information suggests that sex has little or no effect on radiation carcinogenesis, while increasing age is associated with a decrease in radiation-induced tumours. Irradiation conditions, including the dose delivered, the time-period over which the dose is received and the radiation quality, are also important. Genetic constitution may be influential. Other factors, such as the host's susceptibility, living habits and exposure to other toxic agents, may contribute to cancer development.

Populations exposed to moderate to high levels of radiation form the basis of radiation risk assessment and are fundamental to the development of models of radiation carcinogenesis in man. The most useful human data on the risk of radiation-induced cancer in terms of the length of time of follow-up and population size have been obtained from follow-up studies of the incidence of tumours in survivors of the Japanese atomic bombings at Hiroshima and Nagasaki during World War II, and from medically irradiated populations. Occupationally exposed individuals, e.g. certain groups of workers in the nuclear industry, also represent a potentially useful source of data, although as yet they have yielded little quantitative data on cancer risk estimates (Beral *et al.*, 1985, 1988; Smith and Douglas, 1986).

The Life Span Study of the Japanese atomic bomb survivors represents the largest single study population examined for age and sex trends with a wide range of doses, and currently has a follow-up period of over 45 years (Shimizu *et al.*, 1987, 1988). Of about 280 000 individuals who survived the bombings, 80 000 have been followed up, with about 24 000 deaths, 5000 of which were caused by cancer; some of these were in excess of the number expected and have therefore been attributed to radiation. For those survivors exposed as adults, almost the entire course of induced cancer is now known; however, for those exposed as children the picture is still incomplete.

Investigations of medically irradiated populations contributing useful information on the risk of radiation-induced cancer include the follow-up of over 14 000 ankylosing spondylitic patients given a single course of X-rays to ameliorate pain associated with the disease (Darby *et al.*, 1987), follow-up studies of patients irradiated as part of their treatment for cervical cancer (Boice *et al.*, 1988) or benign breast disease (Baral *et al.*, 1977) and follow-up of children irradiated for an enlarged thymus (Hempelmann *et al.*, 1975; Shore *et al.*, 1985) or for tinea capitus (scalp ringworm) (Ron *et al.*, 1988). In the ankylosing spondylitic patients, it has been shown that the relative risk for all neoplasms, other than leukaemia or colon cancer, more than 25 years after their first treatment, is lower than that in the earlier years (5–24.9 years after treatment) (Darby *et al.*, 1987). This is in contrast to the results of follow-up studies of the Japanese atomic bomb survivors (Darby *et al.*, 1985) and of patients irradiated as part of their treatment for cervical cancer (Boice *et al.*, 1985, 1988). In both instances the relative risk for all neoplasms (other than leukaemia and colon cancer) increased with time since exposure (Darby *et al.*, 1987).

As yet no study population has been followed up for a long enough period to yield the lifetime incidence of cancers following irradiation. The overall risk for an exposed population must therefore be extrapolated over time, using models based on limited data. Two such projection models are used: an additive risk model and a relative risk model. The additive or absolute model postulates that the annual excess risk arises after a period of latency and then remains constant. In this case the risk from radiation appears to be additional to the natural incidence. The relative or multiplicative risk model postulates that the distribution of excess risk follows the same pattern as the time distribution of natural cancers—i.e. the excess (after latency) is given by a constant factor applied to the age-dependent incidence of natural cancers in the population. Because the natural incidence of cancer increases with increasing age, this model predicts a large number of radiation-induced cancers in old age. While it is not possible to distinguish between the two models for most cancers, for leukaemia and bone cancer (which have shorter latency periods) it has been established that these fit the absolute risk model.

Most of the data relating to human radiation carcinogenesis are derived from exposures at high doses and dose rates from which it is impossible to deduce the shape of the dose–response relationship, especially at low doses. Frequently the data are fitted to linear and linear-quadratic relationships. The former assumes that the excess cancer incidence is proportional to dose; the latter implies that at low doses cancer incidence is proportional to dose but that at high doses it is proportional to dose squared. In extrapolating the risk of cancer from high to low doses, the linear model implies that the risk per rad is the same at high and at low doses; the linear-quadratic model implies a smaller risk per rad at low doses. Because risk estimates are associated with a large degree of uncertainty, and are dependent on the choice of model used to extrapolate from high to low doses, they should not be viewed as definitive, but as the best available estimates based on inadequate data. Despite the difficulties associated with estimating the risks of radiation-induced cancer, the number of fatal malignancies induced by sparsely ionizing radiation in the range of 1 Gy is reported to be of the order of 10^{-2} per sievert (UNSCEAR, 1988).

Dose–response relationships for radiation-induced cancers vary, depending on the tumour type and the radiation quality. For low-LET radiations, the incidence of many types of cancer increases with increasing dose, up to a maximum, which usually occurs in the dose region 3 and 10 Gy. Thereafter, the cancer incidence decreases with increasing dose. The shape of the dose–response curve is the result of two phenomena: a dose-related increase in the proportion of normal cells transformed into a malignant state, and a dose-related decrease in the probability that such cells may survive the radiation exposure. Both phenomena normally operate but to different degrees, depending on the dose and tumour type. The decreasing slope at high doses is attributed to the killing of the radiation-initiated cells from which tumours eventually arise.

For densely ionizing neutron irradiation, tumour induction in animals, in general, follows an almost linear curve at the lower end of the dose scale and exhibits little dose-rate dependence. For X- and gamma-rays the dose–response relationships tend to be curvilinear and concave at low doses. Tumour induction is dose-rate dependent, in that a reduction in the dose rate, or fractionation of the dose, reduces the tumour yield.

Hereditary Effects

General

Radiation-induced hereditary effects may be dominant or recessive, appearing in the first or later generations, respectively, and may involve changes to a single gene or to the gross structure of a chromosome. A gene mutation involves a change in the structure of DNA and may involve the base composition, the sequence, or both. Chromosomal changes can involve the loss or addition of a chromosome, chromosome breakage and translocation.

Radiation-induced mutations represent an increase in the frequency of the same mutations that already occur spontaneously or naturally within a species. Since radiation-induced mutations are indistinguishable from those which occur naturally, large sample sizes are necessary to detect any increase in their frequency caused by radiation. Human data relating to the genetic effects of radiation are scarce, with the exception of the follow-up of survivors of the atomic bombings of Hiroshima and Nagasaki (Neel *et al.*, 1989). Estimation of genetic risk from radiation in humans is therefore based predominantly on animal data. It should be noted, however, that the results of *in vitro* studies of human cells, in conjunction with the limited evidence from Hiroshima and Nagasaki, suggest that humans are not especially sensitive to the induction of chromosome aberrations and gene mutations by radiation (Neel *et al.*, 1989). Genetic risk is estimated on the basis that the doses received are genetically significant—i.e. that they are received by individuals before or during the reproductive period.

In using the data from animal studies to make quantitative estimates of genetic risks in man, three important assumptions are made unless there is evidence to the contrary:

(1) The amount of genetic damage induced by a given type of radiation under a given set of conditions is the same in human germ cells and in those of the test species used as the model.
(2) The biological factors (e.g. sex, germ cell stage and age) and physical factors (e.g. radiation quality and dose rate) affect the magnitude of the

damage in similar ways and to similar extents in humans and in the experimental species from which extrapolations are made.

(3) At low doses and at low dose rates of low-LET irradiation, there is a linear relationship between dose and the frequency of genetic effects.

The genetic risks from radiation can be estimated by either the direct method or the doubling dose method. The direct method estimates the incidence of genetic diseases resulting from mutations or chromosomal disorders as a function of dose, and ignores the natural rate of these diseases in a population. By contrast, the doubling dose method involves a comparison between the rate of radiation-induced genetic disorders and the spontaneous incidence of these diseases in the population, and is expressed in terms of the dose required to double the spontaneous incidence of gene or chromosomal disorders.

On the basis of animal experiments, which have shown an approximately linear increase in point-mutations with radiation doses of 1–100 mGy, it is assumed that the increased irradiation of humans will result in a proportional increase in mutation frequency (Searle, 1989). Point-mutation frequencies of between 1 and 10 per million cells per Gy for human lymphoblasts (Grossovsky and Little, 1985; Konig and Kiefer, 1988), and less than 20 mutations per million cells per Gy for erythroblasts in A-bomb survivors (Langlois *et al.*, 1987), have been reported.

Survivors of the A-bombs have been studied for four genetic indicators: (1) abnormal outcome of pregnancy (stillbirth, major congenital defects, or death during the first postnatal week); (2) childhood mortality; (3) sex chromosome abnormalities; (4) mutations resulting in electrophoretic variation in blood proteins (Schull *et al.*, 1981). For these four parameters, differences between the children of proximally and distally exposed survivors were in the direction expected if a genetic effect did result from irradiation. However, none of the findings was statistically significant.

On the basis of mouse data (Russell and Russell, 1956; Russell, 1965), the doubling dose for low-rate exposure in humans was estimated by the Biological Effects of Ionizing Radiation (BEIR) III Committee of the US National Academy of Sciences (National Research Council, 1980) to be in the range of 0.5–2.5 Sv. The corre-

sponding estimate in the 1986 UNSCEAR Report was 1 Gy (UNSCEAR, 1986).

Table 1 shows estimates of genetic damage, obtained according to the direct method. The estimates are expressed as the expected number per million of genetically abnormal children born in the first generation after irradiation, per 0.01 Gy of sparsely ionizing low dose rate irradiation (UNSCEAR, 1986, 1988).

The genetic effect of 0.01 Gy per generation of low-LET, low dose rate irradiation in a population of 10^6 liveborn estimated by the doubling dose method is given in Table 2. These values have been derived, assuming a doubling dose of 1 Gy.

Preconceptual Irradiation and Cancer Induction

There is considerable experimental evidence of the induction of genetic abnormalities by preconceptual irradiation of either parent. Searle (1989, and references therein) has estimated that the risk factors for a mutation at a specific locus in F_1 mice after paternal irradiation is about 0.001 per cent per Gy. From data such as these, UNSCEAR (1988) has estimated that the total genetic risk for all loci in F_1 and F_2 humans after parental irradiation is about 0.3 per cent. This is in line with risk estimates for general congenital malformations in the offspring of irradiated male mice (0.5 per cent per Gy) (Kirk and Lyon, 1984; Nomura, 1982).

Interest in the induction of cancer-proneness by preconceptual irradiation has been stimulated recently by the results of a reanalysis of the incidence of leukaemia in children living near the

Table 1 Risks of induction of genetic damage in man per 0.01 Gy at low dose rates of low-LET radiation, estimated using the direct method. From UNSCEAR (1986, 1988)

Risk associated with	Expected frequency per 10^6 of genetically abnormal children in the first generation after irradiation	
	Males	Females
Induced mutations having dominant effects	~10 to ~20	0 to ~9
Induced recessive mutations	0	0
Unbalanced products of induced reciprocal translocations	~1 to ~15	0 to ~5

Table 2 Effects of 0.01 Gy per generation of low-LET radiation at low dose rates on a population of 1 million liveborn, estimated using the doubling-dose method with an assumed doubling dose of 1 Gy. From UNSCEAR (1982, 1988)

Disorder	Current incidence per million offspring	Effect of 0.01 Gy per generation	
		First generation	Equilibrium
Autosomal dominant and X-linked diseases	10 000	15	100
Autosomal recessive diseases	2 500	Slight	Slow increase
Chromosomal diseases structural anomalies	400	2.4	4
numerical anomalies	3 000	Probably very small	Probably very small
Irregularly inherited	90 000	4.5	45
Total	105 900	~22	~150

nuclear installation at Sellafield in the UK. Gardner *et al.* (1990) reported that the raised incidence appeared to be associated with paternal employment at the plant and the recorded doses of radiation received by the fathers during the periods of their employment. It was suggested that these doses, although low, may have increased the risk of leukaemia in the offspring. The implication of the hypothesis is that if the association is truly causal, then it would follow that the risk of cancer arising from irradiation of pre- or postmeiotic germ cells must be very high.

The risk factors calculated from the data of Gardner *et al.* (1990) depend upon the period of preconceptual exposure assumed to be important. These would be in the range of about 2 per cent per Gy for a lifetime dose to about 20 per cent for a 6 month dose. The problem arises in that risk factors of these magnitudes are vastly in excess of those normally expected for mutation at defined loci, as determined in radiation genetic studies in the laboratory. There are some experimental data, however, that are supportive. Nomura *et al.* (1982, 1983, 1986) have reported the induction of lung tumours and leukaemia after paternal irradiation in three strains of mice. The risk factors were found to be dose-dependent and varied with mouse strain, the germ cell stage at the time of irradiation and the type of tumour induced. Some responses in the offspring were also noted for preconceptual irradiation of female mice. The risk factors of a few per cent per Gy found in some of the studies imply that, in these experimental systems, induced mutations leading to cancer induction occur at much higher frequencies than those normally found for other types of mutations arising from preconceptual irradiation.

Effects of Prenatal Irradiation

Developmental harm to an individual exposed to radiation *in utero* is not easily classified as a stochastic or a non-stochastic effect. Irradiation of the developing embryo and foetus may result in death, malformation or growth retardation. The observed effect is dependent on the radiation dose, the dose rate and the gestational stage at which irradiation occurs. Prenatal irradiation effects are due to the fact that foetal tissues are continuously differentiating and growing, and fetal development follows a predetermined pathway; irradiation of the developing organism with the subsequent killing of embryonic or foetal cells at critical developmental stages can cause disruption in the normal complex sequence of events.

Gestation may be divided into three major stages: preimplantation, which extends from fertilization until the embryo attaches to the uterine wall; organogenesis, which represents the period during which the major organs are developed; and the foetal stage, during which growth of the preformed structures occurs. The relative duration of each of these periods, the length of intrauterine life, and the state of differentiation or maturation of any one structure, with respect to the others, varies between different animal species. Table 3 shows the appropriate beginning and end of the major developmental

Table 3 Approximate time of beginning and end of the major developmental periods (in days post conception) in mammalian species. From UNSCEAR (1977)

Species	Preimplantation	Organogenesis	Foetal period
Hamster	0–5	6–12	13–16.5
Mouse	0–5	6–13	14–19.5
Rat	0–7	8–15	16–21.5
Rabbit	0–5	6–15	16–31.5
Guinea-pig	0–8	9–25	26–63
Dog	0–17	18–30	31–63
Man	0–8	9–60	61–270

periods in man and in some of the commonly used laboratory mammals.

The preimplantation period is most sensitive to the lethal effects of radiation. Irradiation at this stage does not result in growth retardation, and few if any abnormalities are produced. If the irradiated preimplantation embryo survives, it will continue to grow and develop normally. At the preimplantation stage the embryo consists of a small cluster of cells, so that, if a few cells are killed by radiation, one or two cell divisions will rectify the damage. If, however, a larger number of cells are killed, the embryo will die and become resorbed.

Irradiation during organogenesis can induce congenital defects. In the mouse a dose of 2 Gy during the period of maximum sensitivity can produce 100 per cent malformations in the offspring at birth (Russell and Russell, 1954), although in man radiation-induced malformations of structures other than the central nervous system are uncommon. This is probably related to the fact that the sensitive period for the induction of congenital malformations during organogenesis in humans represents a smaller fraction of the total period of gestation compared with that in small rodents. In humans, however, CNS development is occurring for much of the gestational period, which makes it a likely target for radiation-induced damage. Consequently, the principal effects of irradiation during the period of organogenesis in humans are microcephaly and mental retardation.

Embryos exposed to radiation in early organogenesis exhibit the most severe intrauterine growth retardation, from which there may be recovery later (i.e. temporary growth retardation). Irradiation in the foetal period leads to the greatest degree of permanent growth retardation.

Irradiation during the foetal period, which extends from about 14 days onward in the mouse, and 6 weeks onward in man, can result in damage to the haematopoietic system, liver, kidney and developing gonads, the latter affecting fertility. Higher radiation doses are required to cause lethality during the foetal stage than at earlier developmental stages. In man the most commonly reported effects of *in utero* irradiation are microcephaly, mental retardation and other central nervous system defects, and growth retardation. Other effects, including spina bifida, deformities, alopecia of the scalp, divergent squint and blindness at birth, are also recognized (Murphy and Goldstein, 1930). Table 4 summarizes the effects of radiation on the mammalian embryo and foetus.

Follow-up studies of individuals exposed *in utero* during the atomic bombings of Hiroshima and Nagasaki have shown that microcephaly can result from an air dose (Kerma) of 0.1–0.19 Gy. In addition, an increased incidence of severe mental retardation has been reported in the A-bomb survivors exposed *in utero* (Otake and Schull, 1984). A child was classified as severely mentally retarded when he/she was 'unable to perform simple calculations, to make simple conversation, to care for her/himself, or if he/she was completely unmanageable or has been institutionalized'. The probability of radiation-related severe mental retardation is essentially zero with exposure before 8 weeks after conception, is maximum with irradiation between 8 and 15 weeks, and decreases between 16 and 25 weeks. After 25 weeks and for doses below 1 Gy, no case of severe mental retardation has been reported. On the assumption that the induction of the effect is linear with dose, the probability of induction per unit dose was estimated at 0.4 and 0.1 per Gy at 8–15 and 16–25 weeks after

Table 4 Radiation effects on the mammalian embryo and foetus. From Hall (1988)

State of gestation	Growth retardation	Death	Congenital malformations	
			General	Microcephaly and mental retardation in humans
Preimplantation	None	Embryonic death and resorption	None	None
Organogenesis	Temporary	Neonatal death	High risk	Very high risk
Foetal period	Permanent	LD_{50} similar to that for adult	Less risk	High risk

conception, respectively (Otake and Schull, 1984). The period of highest risk of severe mental retardation coincides with the period of most rapid proliferation of neuronal elements, and with the migration of neuroblast cells from the proliferative zones to the cerebral cortex. It is thought that severe mental retardation results from radiation interfering with this normal sequence of events.

Prenatal irradiation with diagnostic X-rays has also been associated with the subsequent development of leukaemia and other childhood malignancies (MacMahon, 1962; MacMahon and Hutchison, 1964; Stewart and Kneale, 1970). In the Oxford Childhood Cancer study, irradiated children received between 1 and 5 films, with a dose of 0.2–0.46 rad per film. While these studies have been interpreted as indicating that relatively low doses of radiation result in an increased incidence of cancer during the first 10–15 years of life, by a factor of 1.5–2.0, they do not prove that *in utero* irradiation caused the malignancies. It has been suggested that the irradiated mothers represent a select group whose children are more prone to cancer and that the irradiation is coincidental. The strongest evidence in support of a causal relationship between irradiation and childhood cancer is that provided by Mole (1974) in an analysis of the Oxford data relating to twins. Twins who were X-rayed more frequently than singletons were found to have a higher incidence of childhood cancer.

REFERENCES

Baral, E., Larsson, L. E. and Mattsson, B. (1977). Breast cancer following irradiation of the breast. *Cancer*, **40**, 2905–2910

Beral, V., Fraser, P., Carpenter, L., Booth, M., Brown, A. and Rose, G. (1988). Mortality of employees of the Atomic Weapons Establishment 1951–82. *Br. Med. J.*, **297**, 757–770

Beral, V., Inskip, H., Fraser, P., Booth, M., Coleman, D. and Rose, G. (1985). Mortality of employees of the United Kingdom Atomic Energy Authority, 1946–1979. *Br. Med. J.*, **291**, 440–447

Blot, W. J. (1975). Growth and development following prenatal childhood exposure to atomic radiation. *J. Radiat. Res.*, **16** (Suppl.), 82–88

Boice, J. D., Day, N. E., Anderson, A. and 33 others. (1985). Second cancers following radiation treatment for cervical cancer. An international collaboration among cancer registries. *J. Natl Cancer Inst.*, **74**, 955

Boice, J. D., Engholm, G., Kleinerman, R. A., Blettner, M., Stovall, M., Lisco, H., Moloney, W. C., Austin, D. F., Bosch, A., Cookfair, D. L., Krementz, E. T., Latouret, H. B., Merrill, J. A., Peters, L. J., Schulz, M. D., Storm, H. H., Bjorkholm, E., Pettersson, F., Janine Bell, C. M., Coleman, M. P., Fraser, P., Neal, F. E., Prior, P., Won Choi, N., Gregory Hislop, T., Koch, M., Kreiger, N., Robb, D., Robson, D., Thomson, D. H., Lochumller, H., von Fournier, D., Frischkorn, R., Kjorstad, K. E., Rimpela, A., Pejovic, M.-H., Kirn, V. P., Stankusova, H., Berrino, F., Sigurdsson, K., Hutchison, G. B. and MacMahon, B. (1988). Radiation dose and second cancer risks in patients for cancer of the cervix. *Radiat. Res.*, **116**, 3–55

Conard, R. A., Knudson, K. D., Dobyns, B. M., Meyer, L. M. and 47 others. (1975). *A Twenty-year Review of Medical Findings in a Marshallese Population Accidentally Exposed to Radioactive Fallout*. Brookhaven National Laboratory, New York, BNL 50424

Congar, A. D. (1973). Loss and recovery of taste acuity in patients irradiated to the oral cavity. *Radiat. Res.*, **53**, 338–347

Darby, S. C., Doll, R., Gill, S. K. and Smith, P. G. (1987). Long term mortality after a single treatment course with X-rays in patients treated for ankylosing spondylitis. *Br. J. Cancer*, **55**, 179–190

Darby, S. C., Nakashima, E. and Kato, H. (1985). A parallel analysis of cancer mortality among atomic bomb survivors and patients with ankylosing spondylitis given X-ray therapy. *J. Natl Cancer Inst.*, **72**, 1

De Saint-Georges, L., Van Gorp, U. and Maisin, J. R. (1988). Response of mouse lung air-blood barrier to X-irradiation: ultrastructural and stereological analysis. *Scanning Microsc.*, **2/1**, 537–543

Gardner, M. J., Snee, M. P., Hall, A. J., Powell, C. A., Downes, S. and Terrell, J. D. (1990). Results of case–control study of leukaemia and lymphoma among young people near Sellafield nuclear plant in West Cumbria. *Br. Med. J.*, **300**, 423–429

Glatstein, E., McHardy-Young, S., Brast, N., Eltringham, J. G. and Kriss, J. P. (1971). Alterations in serum thyrotropin (TSH) and thyroid function following radiotherapy in patients with malignant lymphoma. *J. Clin. Endocr. Metab.*, **32**, 833–841

Grossovsky, A. J. and Little, J. B. (1985). Evidence for linear response for the induction of mutations in human cells by X-ray exposure below 10 rads. *Proc. Natl Acad. Sci. USA*, **82**, 2092–2095

Hall, E. J. (1988). *Radiobiology for the Radiologist*, 3rd edn. Lippincott, Philadelphia

Hempelmann, L. H., Hall, W. J., Phillips, M., Cooper, R. A. and Ames, W. R. (1975). Neoplasms in persons treated with x-rays in infancy: fourth survey in 20 years. *J. Natl Cancer Inst.*, **55**, 519–530

International Atomic Energy Agency (IAEA) (1971). *Manual on Radiation Haematology*. IAEA, Vienna

International Commission on Radiological Protection (ICRP) (1977). *Recommendations of the International Commission on Radiological Protection*. ICRP Publication No 26. Annals of the ICRP, Vol. 1, No. 3. Pergamon Press, Oxford

International Commission on Radiological Protection (ICRP) (1984). *Nonstochastic Effects of Ionizing Radiation*. ICRP Publication No 41. Annals of the ICRP, Vol. 14, No 3. Pergamon Press, Oxford

Kirk, K. M. and Lyon, M. F. (1984). Induction of congenital malformations in the offspring of male mice treated with x-rays at pre-meiotic and post-meiotic stages. *Mutation Res.*, **125**, 75–85

Konig, F. and Kiefer, J. (1988). Lack of dose rate effect for mutation induction by gamma-rays in human TK_6 cells. *Int. J. Radiat. Biol.*, **54**, 891–897

Kraut, J. E., Bagshaw, M. A. and Glatstein, E. (1972). Hepatic effects of irradiation. *Front. Radiat. Ther. Onc.*, **6**, 182–195

Langlois, R. G., Bigbee, W. L. and Kyoizumi, S. (1987). Evidence of increased somatic cell mutations at the glycophorin A locus in atomic bomb survivors. *Science*, **236**, 445–448

Law, M. F. (1981). Radiation-induced vascular injury and its relation to late effects in normal tissues. *Adv. Radiat. Biol.*, **9**, 37–73

Lushbaugh, C. C. and Casarett, G. W. (1976). The effects of gonadal irradiation in clinical radiation therapy: a review. *Cancer*, **37**, 1111–1120

Lushbaugh, C. C. and Ricks, R. C. (1972). Some cytokinetic and histopathologic considerations of irradiated male and female gonadal tissues, *Front. Radiat. Ther. Oncol.*, **6**, 228–248

MacMahon, B. (1962). Prenatal X-ray exposure and childhood cancer. *J. Natl Cancer Inst.*, **28**, 1173–1191

MacMahon, B. and Hutchison, G. B. (1964). Prenatal X-ray and childhood cancer: a review. *Acta Univ. Int. Contra Cancrum*, **20**, 1172–1174

Maier, J. G. (1972). Effects of radiations on kidney, bladder and prostate. *Front. Radiat. Ther. Oncol.*, **6**, 196–227

Markson, J. L. and Flatman, G. E. (1965). Myxoedema after deep X-ray therapy to the neck. *Br. Med. J.*, **1**, 1228–1230

Merriam, G. R., Szechter, A. and Focht, E. F. (1972). The effects of ionizing radiations on the eye. *Front. Radiat. Ther. Oncol.*, **6**, 346–385

Mole, R. H. (1974). Antenatal irradiation and childhood cancer causation or coincidence. *Br. J. Cancer.*, **30**, 199–208

Murphy, D. P. and Goldstein, L. (1930). Micromelia in a child irradiated *in utero. Surg. Gynecol. Obstet.*, **50**, 79–80

National Research Council (1980). Advisory Committee on the Biological Effects of Ionizing Radiation. BEIR III. National Academy of Sciences, Washington, D.C.

Neel, J. V., Schull, W. J., Awa, A. A., Satoh, C., Otake, M., Kato, H. and Yoshimoto, Y. (1989). The genetic effects of atomic bombs: problems in extrapolating from somatic cell findings to risk for children. In Baverstock, K. F. and Stather, J. W. (Eds), *Low Dose Radiation*. Taylor and Francis, London, pp. 42–53

Nomura, T. (1982). Parental exposure to x-rays and chemicals induces heritable tumours and anomalies in mice. *Nature*, **296**, 575–577

Nomura, T. (1983). X-ray-induced germ-line mutation leading to tumours. *Mutation Res.*, **121**, 59–65

Nomura, T. (1986). Further studies on x-ray and chemically induced germ line alterations causing tumors and malformations in mice. In Ramel, C., Lambert, B. and Magnusson, J. (Eds), *Genetic Toxicology of Environment Chemicals*. Part B: *Genetic Effects and Applied Mutagenesis*. Alan R. Liss, New York, pp. 13–20

Otake, M. and Schull, W. J. (1984). *In utero* exposure to A-bomb radiation and mental retardation: a reassessment. *Br. J. Radiol.*, **57**, 409–414

Parker, R. G. (1972). Tolerance of mature bone and

cartilage in clinical radiation therapy. In Vaeth, J. M. (Ed.), *Frontiers of Radiation Therapy and Oncology*, Vol. 6. Karger, Basel, and University Park Press, Baltimore, pp. 312–331

Ron, E., Modan, B. and Boice, J. D. Jr (1988). Mortality after radiotherapy for ringworm of the scalp. *Am. J. Epidemiol.*, **127**, 13–25

Ron, E., Modan, B., Floro, S., Harkedar, I. and Gurewitz, R. (1982). Mental function following scalp irradiation during childhood. *Am. J. Epidemiol.*, **116**, 149–160

Rubin, P. and Casarett, G. W. (1968). *Clinical Radiation Pathology*, Vols I and II. Saunders, Philadelphia

Russell, L. B. and Russell, W. L. (1954). An analysis of the changing radiation response of the developing mouse embryo. *J. Cell. Physiol.*, **43** (Suppl. 1), 103–149

Russell, L. B. and Russell, W. L. (1956). The sensitivity of different stages in oogenesis to the radiation induction of dominant lethals and other changes in the mouse. In Mitchell, J. S., Holmes, B. E. and Smith, C. L. (Eds), *Progress in Radiobiology*. Oliver and Boyd, Edinburgh, pp. 187–192

Russell, W. L. (1965). Studies in mammalian radiation genetics. *Nucleonics*, **23**, 53–56

Schull, W. L., Otake, M. and Neal, J. V. (1981). Genetic effects of the atomic bomb: a reappraisal. *Science*, **213**, 1220–1227

Searle, A. G. (1989). Evidence from mammalian studies on genetic effects of low level irradiation. In Baverstock, K. F. and Stather, J. W. (Eds), *Low Dose Radiation*. Taylor and Francis, London, pp. 123–138

Shimizu, Y., Kato, H. and Schull, W. J. (1988). Life Span Study Report 11, Part II: *Cancer Mortality in the Years 1950–1985 Based on the Recently Revised Doses (DS86)*. Hiroshima Radiation Effects Research Foundation RERF TR5–88

Shimizu, Y., Kato, H., Schull, W. J., Preston, D. L., Fujita, S. and Pierce, D. A. (1987). Life Span Study Report 11, Part I: *Comparison of Risk Coefficients for Site-specific Cancer Mortality Based on DS86 and T65DR Shielded Kerma and Organ Doses*. Hiroshima Radiation Research Foundation RERF TR12–87

Shore, R. E., Woodard, E., Hildreth, N., Dvoretsky, P., Hempelmann, L. and Pasternack, B. (1985). Thyroid tumors following thymus irradiation. *J. Natl Cancer Inst.*, **74**, 1177–1184

Smith, P. G. and Douglas, A. J. (1986). Mortality of workers at the Sellafield plant of British nuclear fuels. *Br. Med. J.*, **293**, 845–854

Stewart, A. and Kneale, G. W. (1970). Radiation dose effects in relation to obstetric X-rays and childhood cancers. *Lancet*, **1**, 1185–1188

Tefft, M. (1972). Radiation effect on growing bone and cartilage. *Front. Radiat. Ther. Oncol.*, **6**, 289–311

Travis, E. L. and Tucker, S. L. (1986). The relationship between functional assays of radiation response in the lung and target cell depletion. *Br. J. Cancer*, **53** (Suppl. VII), 304–319

United Nations Scientific Committee on the Effects of Atomic Radiation (UNSCEAR) (1977). *Sources and Effects of Ionizing Radiation*. Annex J: *Developmental Effects of Irradiation* in utero. United Nations, New York, pp. 655–710

United Nations Scientific Committee on the Effects of Atomic Radiation (UNSCEAR) (1982). *Sources and Biological Effects of Irradiation*. Annex I: *Genetic Effects of Irradiation*. United Nations, New York, pp. 425–569

United Nations Scientific Committee on the Effects of Atomic Radiation (UNSCEAR) (1986). *Genetic and Somatic Effects of Ionizing Radiation*. Annex B: *Dose-Response Relationships for Radiation-induced Cancer*. United Nations, New York, pp. 165–262

United Nations Scientific Committee on the Effects of Atomic Radiation (UNSCEAR) (1988). *Sources, Effects and Risks of Ionizing Radiation*. Annex E: *Genetic Hazards*, pp. 375–403. Annex F: *Radiation Carcinogenesis in Man*, pp. 405–543. Annex G: *Early Effects in Man of High Doses of Radiation*, pp. 545–612. United Nations, New York

van der Brenk, H. A. S. (1971). Radiation effects on the pulmonary system. In Berdjis, C. C. (Ed.), *Pathology of Irradiation*. Williams and Wilkins, Baltimore, pp. 569–591

Wharton, J. T., Declos, L., Gallagher, S. and Smith, J. P. (1973). Radiation nephritis induced by abdominal irradiation with the cobalt–60 moving strip technique. *Am. J. Roentgnol.*, **117**, 73–80

FURTHER READING

Baverstock, K. F. and Stather, J. W. (Eds) (1989). *Low Dose Radiation: Biological Bases of Risk Assessment*. Taylor and Francis, London

Hall, E. J. (1988). Radiobiology for the Radiologist, 3rd edition. J. B. Lippincott Company, Philadelphia

International Commission on Radiological Protection Publications. Pergamon Press, Oxford

International Symposium (1991). Radiation carcinogenesis in the whole body system. *Journal of Radiation Research*, **32**, No. 2 Supplements

Kollas, J. G. (1993). The health impact of major nuclear accidents. *Risk Analysis*, **13**, 503–508

Kramer, H. M. and Schnuer, K. (1992). Proceeding of seminar on dosimetry in diagnostic radology. *Radiation Protection and Dosimetry*, **43**, Nos. 1–4

Modan, B. (1993). Low dose radiation carcinogenesis – issues and interpretation. *Health Physics*, **65**, 473–480

National Council on Radiation Protection and Measurements Reports. 7910 Woodmont Avenue, Bethesda, MD 20814

National Research Council Advisory Committee on the

Biological Effects of Ionizing Radiation. BEIR Reports. National Academy Press, 2101 Constitution Avenue, N.W., Washington, D.C. 20418

Steel, G. G. (Ed.) (1989). *The Radiobiology of Human Cell and Tissues*. Taylor and Francis, London

United Nations Scientific Committee on the Effects of Atomic Radiation. Reports to the General Assembly, with Annexes. United Nations, New York

Valk, P. E. and Dillon, W. P. (1991). Radiation injury of the brain. *American Journal of Roentgenology*, **156**, 689–706

56 Toxicology and Disasters*

H. Paul A. Illing

INTRODUCTION

Disasters (great or sudden misfortunes: *Concise Oxford Dictionary*, 1990) occur from time to time. Because they are portrayed and analysed extensively in the news media and subjected to careful examination in subsequent public enquiries, they become entrenched in everyone's mind. Unfortunately, the ideas on how to handle or prevent potential disaster situations occurring have often been developed from the lessons learnt from analysing previous disasters. In many cases disasters can be avoided and the effects of accidents minimized by careful planning. In addition, by examining how to handle the consequences of an accident once it has occurred, it should be possible to mitigate the effects. It is these thoughts that have led to legislation aimed at considering the safety aspects of certain hazardous situations at an early stage in order to minimize the likelihood of their becoming disasters.

Some disasters are the consequence of a toxicant entering a biological system and creating a damaging pertubation to that system. These effects may be largely environmental (e.g. the consequences of an oil tanker spill in coastal waters) or they may affect human health, either directly (through ingestion of contaminated drinking water or inhalation of a toxicant as it is dispersed in air) or indirectly (e.g. via uptake, etc., into food species). Thus, a knowledge of the effects of toxicants can be important when examining disasters and potential disaster situations.

In this chapter concepts involved in planning to prevent disasters occurring are discussed first. This is followed by an evaluation of different types of disaster or serious incident involving toxicants. Although purely environmental effects should not be ignored, the examples chosen are all associated with human health effects. After-wards approaches to the planning associated with preventing disasters due to toxicants and mitigating their effects are discussed.

THEORETICAL CONSIDERATIONS

Many of the concepts used in analysing major hazards and minimizing their potential for causing disasters have their origin in engineering concepts associated with the design of military equipment, aircraft and nuclear plant. As a consequence, the definitions used need examining, especially as difficulties can ensue if toxicologists and chemical engineers employ different interpretations of the same words. Although 'hazard' and 'risk' are interchangeable terms to the general public, they have separate meanings in the context of risk assessment, so their definitions will be examined carefully.

Hazard

Hazard is an intrinsic property of a substance or situation. The Royal Society Study Group on Risk Assessment (1983) defined hazard as 'the intrinsic situation that in particular circumstances could lead to harm'. The Institution of Chemical Engineers Working Party Report (1985) used the words 'a physical situation with a potential for human injury, damage to property, damage to the environment or some combination of these' and went on to define a chemical hazard as 'a hazard involving chemicals or processes which may release its potential through agencies such as fire, explosion, toxic or corrosive effects'. Because the latter definition was intended for the process industries, it did not include potential radiation effects from nuclear plant failures. Such potential effects are also hazards (Health and Safety Executive, 1988a).

A toxicological definition of hazard called it

---

* The views expressed in this chapter are the author's personal opinions and should not be taken as an expression of the policy of the Health and Safety Executive.

'the qualitative nature of the adverse effect resulting from a particular toxic chemical, physical effect or inappropriate action' (Hodgson *et al.*, 1988). This toxicological definition uses carcinogenesis and asphyxiation as examples of toxic hazards. Thus, it is compatible with the engineering definitions.

A major industrial hazard is 'any man-made hazard which has the potential to cause large-scale injury and loss of life from a single brief event' (Health and Safety Executive, 1988a). Major industrial hazards include nuclear power stations as well as chemical process plant, and the definition of a major chemical hazard as 'an imprecise term for a large-scale chemical hazard' by the Institution of Chemical Engineers (1985) is entirely compatible. In circumstances where plant failure is not the cause of a disaster, the initiating event may be prolonged; thus, a major hazard can be any naturally occurring or man-made hazard that has the potential to cause large-scale injury and loss of life from a single event.

For chemicals or radiation to represent toxic hazards, they must be present in sufficient quantities to exert toxic effects on the individual. If they are to be major hazards, they must be present in quantities which, if released or dispersed, could result in effects being seen in many people.

Risk

Risk differs from hazard, as it involves a consideration of the probability or likelihood of a consequence occurring as well as what the consequence might be. The Royal Society study group (1983) defined risk as 'the probability that a particular adverse event occurs during a stated period of time or results from a particular challenge'. The Institution of Chemical Engineers (1985) extended the statement to 'the likelihood of a specific undesired effect occurring within a specified time or in specified circumstances'. They go on to say that 'it may be either a frequency (the number of events occurring in unit time) or a probability (the probability of a specified event following a prior event), depending on circumstances'. If risk is quantified, it is a statistically based parameter.

The Relationship Between Hazard and Risk

In engineering terms, for toxic risks the individual risk is obtained by identifying possible events resulting in hazardous releases, and by analysing potential failure mechanisms which would allow the release in order to determine their likely frequency and size (Health and Safety Executive, 1989a). The hazard is a quantitative statement of the potential consequences of a release. Central to this approach is the assumption that events occurring during ordinary use do not constitute a significant risk. Societal risk is expressed numerically as the frequency (F) that there will be a disaster harming more than a particular number (N) of people, and can be aggregated in the form of an F–N curve (Figure 1). Lees (1980), Marshall (1987) and Health and Safety Executive (1989a, b) give more detailed discussions of these ideas.

Toxicological risk has been called 'the probability that some adverse effect (e.g. cancer) will result from a given exposure to a chemical' (Hodgson *et al.*, 1988). When human data are available, they are the actual or estimated frequency of occurrence of an event in a population. However, the toxicological risk is often based on extrapol-

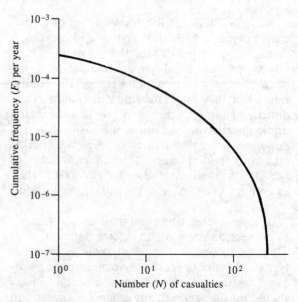

Figure 1   A *F*–*N* curve for societal risk. In assessing societal risk, a particular actuarial or estimated curve must be compared with a criterion curve. Actuarial curves (based on historic data) are usually only available for high-frequency–low-number events. Curves for low-frequency–high-number events are normally estimated

ation of information from animal studies. These studies indicate that the substance is hazardous to the animal and therefore that there is a (presumed substantial until otherwise proven) probability that the hazard may also occur in man.

For the purposes of analysing the potential health effects that could arise from a major hazard, the effects are considered as 'hazard to man' and the difficulties in extrapolating information to man are part of the uncertainty in defining the hazard.

Individual and Societal Risk

There are two principal types of risk which can arise from major hazards: individual risk and societal risk. The Health and Safety Executive (1988a) has called the individual risk associated with major industrial hazards 'the risk to any particular individual, either a worker or a member of the public'. A member of the public is considered to be 'either anybody living within a defined radius from the establishment or somebody following a particular pattern of life'. Societal risk was 'the risk to society as a whole, as measured, for example, of a large accident causing a defined number of deaths and injuries'. Although the individual risk remains the same for each person, the societal risk is governed also by the number of people likely to be affected. The individual risk of living 1 km from a major hazard (industrial or natural) remains the same irrespective of whether the hazard is located in an unpopulated area or in a city, but the societal risk is very different!

Risk Assessment and Risk Management

The concepts of hazard and risk are fundamental to analysing the causes of disasters and to preventing their recurrence. However, these concepts must be contained within a framework of analysis and management if they are to be applied usefully to a given situation. In practice there is a multistage process involved in handling any hazard (Figure 2), and most of the people analysing and managing hazards from industrial plants have engineering or chemistry backgrounds. Their specialisms cover plant design and failure rates, event and fault tree analyses, dispersion modelling for releases of clouds of substances and rates of combustion, etc., for explosions and burning gases (Lees, 1980; Withers, 1988). Geo-

logists are often the principal people interested in the causes of natural disasters involving toxicants. These are 'overt' disasters where a clear point source can be identified readily. Only when the substance released is a toxicant or is transformed into a toxicant will any toxicological input become important. This input will largely be in defining the hazard; it will be concerned with identifying whether the agents present are toxic and defining the combination of exposure size and duration likely to produce a given toxic effect. Clinical toxicologists are also able to advise on the treatment of victims following an incident, i.e. they can have a role in the event of an incident occurring.

'Disseminated' disasters are those which only become apparent because of evidence of effect. Identifying the cause when the effect is ill-health may require persistent, painstaking research. If the suspected cause is non-infective, the investigation team will need the assistance of toxicologists in identifying the agent responsible.

Often risk can be managed in more than one way. The aim of risk management is to reduce the risk, both in terms of the frequency of an event and in terms of the nature of the potential consequences to an acceptable or tolerable level (see Table 1 for definitions of acceptable and tolerable risk). This involves choices as to what chemical and physical agents are usable by society and in what circumstances. It involves selecting which processes to employ when manufacturing, using or disposing of these agents and their waste products. It also involves choices on where to site plants (in the case of man-made hazards) and methods of waste disposal, and whether to permit housing, etc., developments around major hazards. It is also concerned with examining how to handle the consequences of an untoward event at a particular site (emergency planning). What is an acceptable, or at least a tolerable, risk is a separate, but interlinked problem, which depends on a number of factors. Some of these factors are listed in Table 1. Ultimately, government decides whether a societally regulated risk is generally tolerable. Individuals or groups of individuals may attempt to vary the decision as it relates to their specific circumstances and perceptions. In the final analysis risk acceptability revolves around political and personal decisions, although it is to be hoped that such decisions are based on scientific data.

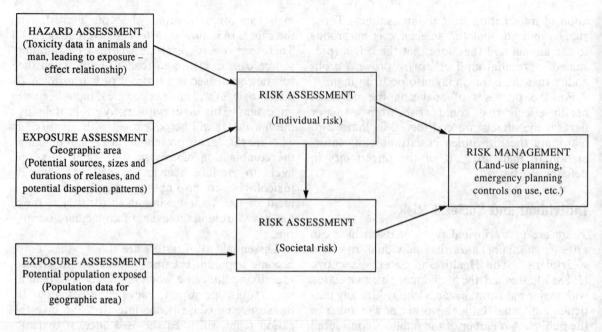

Figure 2 Block diagram illustrating the processes involved in risk assessment and risk management

DISASTERS AND SERIOUS INCIDENTS INVOLVING TOXICANTS

Many disasters are the results of major hazards fulfilling their potential for harm. They are part of a continuous spectrum of possible consequences which can arise from a point hazard. These consequences range from minor difficulties through serious incidents until, in the worst cases, they become disasters. Most of these disasters are not due to toxicants. Their primary effects are physical in nature, and include crush injuries and burns. Other disasters may be due to failure to meet adequate standards associated with ordinary exposures to potential toxicants. This failure may be because the appropriate knowledge was not available and the standard, in consequence, inadequate. Alternatively, it may be because of some accidental or intentional deviation from the standard. A classification of disasters is given in Table 2. This classification is based on the type of event which caused the disaster or serious incident.

Health effects due to toxicants may result from inhalation or from absorption through the skin or gastrointestinal tract. Inhaled toxicants may be gases, liquids (aerosol mists) or solids (dusts, fumes). Particle size is important when particu-

late material is inhaled, since, if inhaled, a particle may be deposited in the lung alveoli or, as a result of the 'tracheo-bronchial escalator', it may be swallowed. An inhaled toxicant may cause injury to the lung, it may restrict the transfer of oxygen (asphyxiation), or it may act systemically in a particular organ (including skin). Skin and eye effects are often phenomena of surface contamination.

Gastrointestinal absorption may contribute to the overall toxicity of inhaled material. However, it is the main route of entry for those toxicants which are transmitted to man in food or water supplies.

Examples of different types of disaster or serious incident with the potential for disaster now follow.

Natural Disasters

Disasters due to natural causes include phenomena caused by the movement of the earth's crust as well as the consequences of abnormal weather. In general, these types of disasters cause injuries due to physical effects or disease due to infective organisms. Toxicants are rarely involved, and then usually secondarily (e.g. due to water contamination), except in the cases of volcanoes and gas emission from lakes. Asphyxiation can be

Table 1 Various aspects of risk. Based on Royal Society Study Group (1983), Lovell (1986) and Health and Safety Executive (1988a,b)

Objective, actual or statistical risk	A statistically calculated risk evaluation.
Perceived risk	The combined evaluation that is made by an individual of the likelihood of an adverse event occurring in the future and its consequences.
Acceptable risk	An acceptable risk is one which, on objective criteria, should generally be regarded as not worth worrying about by those exposed to it.
Tolerable risk	A tolerable risk is one which society is prepared to live with in order to have certain benefits.
Accepted risk	People tend to accept the risks which they have experienced but are less prepared to accept new risks, even though, on 'objective' criteria, the risks are similarly acceptable. The new risk is regarded as worse.
Voluntary and involuntary risk	Certain risks are accepted willingly by choice (e.g. in sport) by individuals but are not accepted (even by the same individuals) if they are unable to choose to accept the risk.
Risk and benefit	Costs occur in reducing risks, either directly or indirectly. For example, many drugs used to treat cancers carry a significant risk that they will cause cancer in that patient at some future time; whooping cough vaccine may prevent severe illness and possible death in most recipients but can cause severe damage in a very few recipients. Risks to non-beneficiaries are regarded as worse than risks to beneficiaries.

Table 2 A classification of types of disasters involving toxic agents

Cause of disaster		Example
Natural	Volcanic	Vesuvius, AD 79; Mount St. Helens, 1980
	Non-volcanic	Lake Nyos, 1986
Man-made	Plant failures	Seveso, 1976; Bhopal, 1984; Chernobyl, 1986
	Fire	Manchester Airport, 1985; Kings Cross, 1987
	Food and drink adulteration	Ginger paralysis, 1930 Toxic oil, 1981
	Accidental contamination	North Cornwall, 1988 Epping jaundice, 1966
	Environmental contamination	Minamata and Niigata, 1951–1974
Interaction of man and nature	Mining, tunnelling Waste disposal	Love Canal, 1960s Minamata and Niigata 1951–1974

caused by emitted gases and irritant dusts, as well as respiratory dysfunction, bronchial obstruction and pulmonary oedema.

Volcanoes

Volcanic eruptions can be divided into two types—explosive and effusive. Each type may present different health hazards. In a volcanic eruption, magma (molten rock and associated dissolved gas below the earth's surface) is extruded to the surface. When it reaches the surface, it may appear as liquid (lava), fragments (pyroclastic debris) and exsolved gases. In effusive eruptions these flows are usually slow-moving, gas releases are steady and most of the limited amount of dust produced is non-respirable. Explosive eruptions tend to be more dangerous, the principal toxic hazards being hot ash release and gas emission. Volcanoes may change their nature from one type to the other.

The gas emitted by volcanoes is principally steam, but includes carbon dioxide, carbon monoxide, hydrogen sulphide, sulphur dioxide, hydrogen chloride and hydrogen. Plumes normally disperse by dilution in the atmosphere and are carried on the wind above human settlement. However, sulphur dioxide, hydrogen chloride or hydrogen fluoride may occasionally be present in sufficient quantities to contaminate air within settlements, water supplies and animal feedstuffs. Denser-than-air gases, principally carbon dioxide and hydrogen sulphide, can flow into valleys and low-lying basins and displace oxygen, giving rise to asphyxiation. A *nuée ardente* (a cinder cloud carrying trapped gases) can flow rapidly down slopes and may also endanger life.

Pyroclastic debris (tephra) and ash products vary in size. Blocks and bombs are large (over 64 mm), lapilli vary between 2 mm and 64 mm, and cinders and ashes are smaller particles. Lapilli and ash, when released to the atmosphere, rise in a hot convection cloud which may be transmitted widely (several hundred kilometres) downwind. Eventually they fall to earth and blanket large areas. Finer particles are deposited further away. The particles have the ability to cause darkness during daylight hours. Ash products include respirable particles containing significant levels of crystalline silica (quartz and cristobolite). Volcanic ash can affect the respiratory tract and eyes. Severe tracheal injury, pulmonary oedema and bronchial obstruction can occur, leading to death from pulmonary injury or suffocation. Ash may also act as a respiratory tract and eye irritant. Irritation and inflammation of the upper and lower respiratory tract may persist if low-level chronic exposure occurs.

Lava is molten rock, the liquid product from the volcano. It is derived from the molten magma, but differs from it because the dissolved gases in the magma escape with the reduction of pressure which occurs as the material approaches the surface.

Debris flows occur when loose rock mixes with surface water or groundwater and flows as a mass of rock, mud and water.

This description of volcanoes is inevitably very short and much simplified. More detailed information can be found in Sheets and Grayson (1979) and Newhall and Fruchter (1986).

Vesuvius, Italy, AD 79

Perhaps one of the best-known historic volcanic eruptions is that of Vesuvius in Italy in AD 79. A contemporary description of the eruption and its effects on one victim is provided by Pliny the Younger in two 'letters' to Tacitus (Radice, 1969). More detailed information on the eruption and its consequences has been obtained during archaeological investigation of the sites at Pompeii and Herculaneum, both of which were buried in the eruption (Jashemski, 1979; Sigurdsson *et al.*, 1985).

Vesuvius had been quiescent for many cen-

turies before the eruption of AD 79. The first sign of its reawakening was an earthquake in AD 62 which damaged almost all the buildings in Pompeii. Then came the eruption of AD 79. There were three phases to this eruption. The first stage was expulsion of the vent plug on 24 August. This was followed by expulsion of ashes. There were six surges and pyroclastic flows during the ash eruption.

Both Plinys were at Misenum when Vesuvius erupted, together with Pliny the Elder's sister (Pliny the Younger's mother). Pliny the Elder, who was in command of the Roman fleet at Misenum, gave instructions that a ship would be made ready so that he could investigate the phenomenon. However, by the time the ship got under way, with the elder Pliny, he changed the mission to one of attempting to rescue the people living along the shore of the bay at the foot of Vesuvius (see Figure 3). Pompeii and Herculaneum were probably being buried at this time, the former from deposition of lapilli and ashes and the latter from a mud and tephra flow. Pliny found his mission impossible because of the falling debris near the shore, and eventually made port at Stabiae, where he stayed the night. During the night the courtyard of the house in which he was staying filled with ashes and debris. On the morning of 25 August it was still dark at Stabiae after dawn. Pliny the Elder went to the shore to investigate the possibility of escape by sea, and died. Pliny the Younger described the death as because 'the dense fumes choked his breathing by blocking his windpipe which was constitutionally weak and narrow and often inflamed'. In modern terms this might be described as asphyxiation.

The crew of the ship later successfully got away, and the younger Pliny and his mother were evacuated from Misenum on 25 August as ashes started falling there. Both survived. Although the 'letters' only describe ash and lapilli, there was also a lava flow on the north side of the volcano. The results of excavations at Pompeii suggest that at least 2000 people died. Most deaths were probably due to asphyxiation caused by inhaling the hot ash material in the first surge of the ash eruption, but some might have been due to thermal shock (Sigurdsson *et al.*, 1985). Presumably many more deaths went unrecorded.

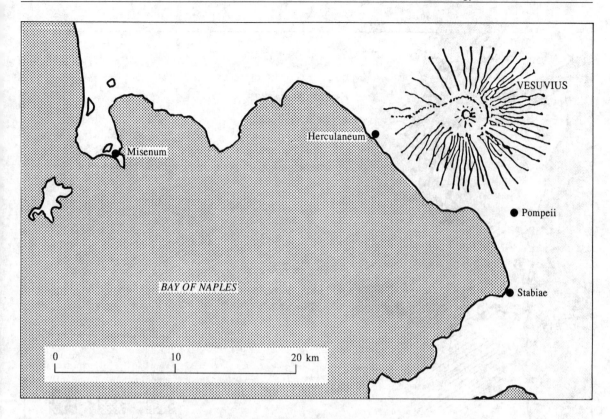

Figure 3 Sketch map of the Bay of Naples. Based on Jashemski (1979)

Mount St. Helens, USA, 1980

A much more recent volcanic eruption was that of Mount St. Helens, in the Cascade range in the west of North America. Premonitory earthquakes started on 20 March and, towards the end of April, a bulge developed in an area to the north of the summit (Buist and Bernstein, 1986). On 18 May a major earthquake occurred, the roof of the bulge slid downhill and an explosive blast took place. Large quantities of ash, superheated steam and gas were released. There were five additional explosions over the following 5 months and ash falls accompanied four of these eruptions. The dispersion pattern is shown in Figure 4; the main land areas covered by the vented material lay in a north-easterly direction from the volcano.

There were 35 known deaths and at least 23 people missing without trace following the eruption (Baxter *et al.*, 1981, 1983; Buist and Bernstein, 1986). Asphyxiation was the cause of death in 18 of the 23 victims autopsied. Ash probably acted as an irritant to the respiratory tract and eye, causing tracheal injury, pulmonary oedema and bronchial obstruction in those dying. The irritation of the respiratory tract continued as the result of chronic low-level exposure to ash, but there appeared to be few long-term sequelae. However, any potential pneumoconiotic effect from the single massive exposure to silica could not be detected within the short time-span since the eruption. Interview studies of patients with pre-existing chronic lung disease showed that the ashfall exacerbated the condition in these patients. There were dose-related increases in the prevalence of three psychiatric syndromes associated with disaster stress—namely generalized anxiety, major depression and post-traumatic stress. The duration of effect was related to the level of disaster stress suffered by the subject.

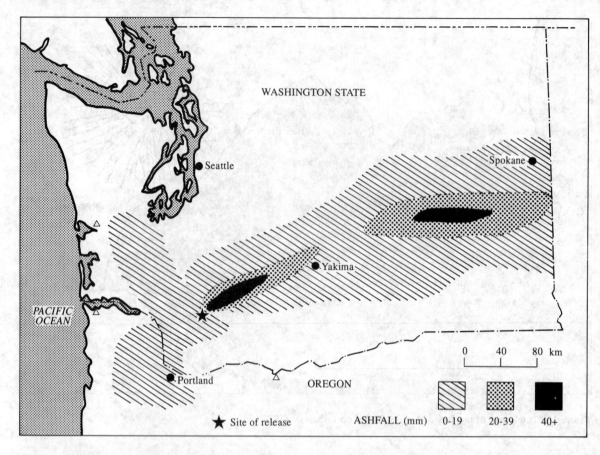

Figure 4 Sketch map of Washington State, showing deposition patterns of ash for the first three eruptions of Mount St. Helens in 1980. The star indicates the position of the volcano. Based on Baxter *et al.* (1981)

The toxic effects seen in the victims of the Mount St. Helens eruption were largely those due to the nature of the ash deposited. Fortunately, the toxic gases that were emitted were vented to the atmosphere and diluted to non-toxic levels through dispersion.

Other Natural Disasters

Lake Nyos, Cameroon, West Africa, 1986
Volcanoes are not the only natural phenomena which can cause major disasters due to toxic substances. On 21 August 1986 there was a catastrophic release of gas from Lake Nyos, Cameroon (Freeth and Kay, 1987; Kling *et al.*, 1987; Baxter *et al.*, 1989b). The cloud of gas was lethal at distances up to 10 km from the source. About 1700 people, 3000 cattle and many other animals died, mostly from asphyxiation. An earlier, smaller release from Lake Monoun, also

in Cameroon, had resulted in 37 deaths, presumably from similar causes.

The generally accepted cause of the disaster is that, because of the geochemical and geophysical characteristics of the Cameroon rocks and the geological conditions in the Lake Nyos area, waters rich in carbon dioxide develop. The gas accumulated in the lake to near-saturating conditions. Although the trigger mechanism for the release is unknown, a small disturbance would have been sufficient to cause degassing in the form of a large release of the carbon dioxide. The gas cloud produced was denser than air and dispersed through the river valleys. Simultaneously, a water surge resulted in the loss of about 200 000 t of water from the lake. The release was heard as a series of rumbling sounds lasting 15–20 s, and one observer reported seeing a white cloud rise from the lake.

Many people lost consciousness rapidly and

survivors woke 6–36 h after the event, weak and confused. Cutaneous erythema and bullae were present in about 19 per cent of survivors treated in hospital. Very limited pathological investigations on those dying suggested that carbon dioxide was the toxicant, as it appeared that the potential toxicants, carbon monoxide, cyanide or hydrogen sulphide, were not relevant to the cause of death. Reports of the odour of sulphur compounds were probably a result of the sensory hallucination due to exposure to high levels of carbon dioxide.

This disaster was a consequence of the special geology of the area. Therefore, although a rare event, it does illustrate that natural disasters involving toxicants are not confined to volcanic releases.

Man-made Disasters

Plant Failures

Plant failures are a well-known cause of major disasters. Those involving the release of toxic chemicals or radioactivity are relevant to toxicologists, and some examples are examined here. A much more comprehensive collection of case studies of the causes and consequences of chemical plant failure in major disasters, written from the chemical engineer/risk assessor's point of view, is given in Marshall (1987).

Seveso, Italy, 1976

An escape of toxic substances occurred at an industrial plant at Seveso, Italy, in 1976. The circumstances surrounding the escape and the potential health effects caused by the escape were investigated by a Parliamentary Commission of Enquiry (Orsini, 1977), and both the engineering and chemical aspects of the incident have been reviewed recently (Marshall, 1987; Skene *et al.*, 1989). The incident was important because of its influence on European Community legislation (the 'Seveso' Directive) concerned with major industrial chemical hazards.

The plant produced trichlorophenol by reacting tetrachlorobenzene with sodium hydroxide (Figure 5). Following the reaction, the solvent (ethylene glycol–xylene) was partially vacuum-distilled off by the end of shift, at which time the heating and agitation were switched off. Some 7.5 h later a safety plate on the reactor vessel burst and there was a consequent venting of the reaction mixture, including approximately 2–3 kg of the impurity dioxin (2,3,7,8-tetrachlorodibenzo-*p*-dioxin) to the atmosphere. Once in the atmosphere the dioxin was spread over a wide area downwind of the plant and settled on fields and houses. Three major zones were identified according to the levels of dioxins present in the vegetation and soil (Figure 6). The resident populations in the zones were 733, 4800 and 22 000 people, respectively, in the most contaminated, middle and least contaminated areas. A medical surveillance programme was undertaken on these people.

Apart from burns arising directly from contact with the caustic reaction products, the other major effect was chloracne. This was reported some 6 weeks after the accident, with a frequency correlating approximately to the levels of dioxins

Tetrachlorobenzene → NaOH → (Cl, Cl, Cl, ONa) → H⁺ → *Trichlorophenol* (Cl, Cl, Cl, OH)

2, 3, 7, 8-tetrachlorodibenzodioxin
(dioxin)

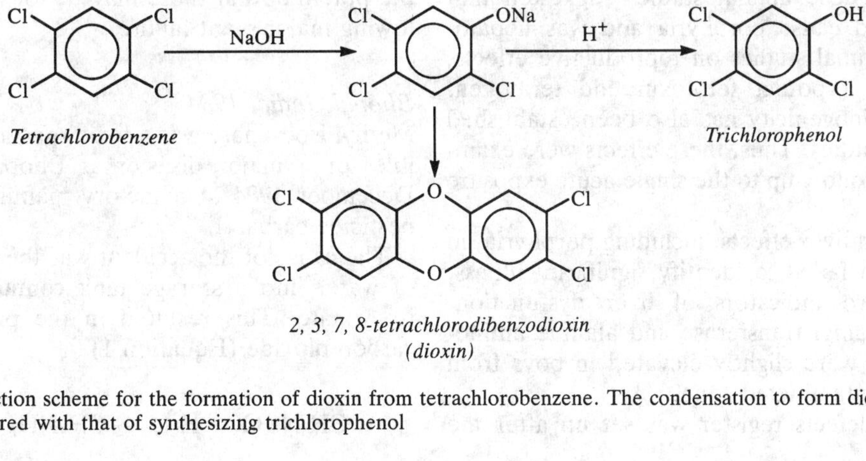

Figure 5 Reaction scheme for the formation of dioxin from tetrachlorobenzene. The condensation to form dioxin is a minor reaction compared with that of synthesizing trichlorophenol

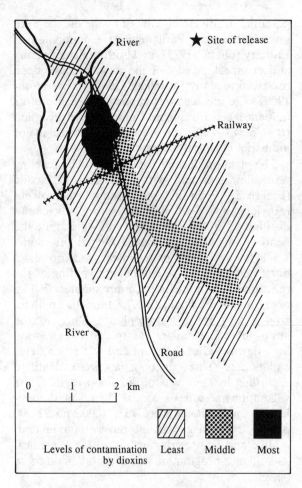

River

★ Site of release

Railway

River

Road

0   1   2 km

Levels of contamination   Least   Middle   Most
by dioxins

Figure 6 Sketch map of Seveso, showing areas of most, middle and least contamination by dioxin. Based on Marshall (1987)

in the soil. By the end of 1978 the chloracne had disappeared.

Repeated-dose animal studies suggested that dioxin could cause porphyria and was hepatotoxic. In animal studies on reproductive effects, dioxin was a potent fetotoxin and teratogen. Hepatocarcinogenicity has also been established in animal studies. Thus, these effects were examined in the follow-up to the single acute exposure at Seveso.

Studies on liver effects, including porphyria, in 700 children failed to identify significant illness, although two indicators of liver dysfunction, gamma-glutamyl transferase and alanine aminotransferase, were slightly elevated in boys from the most contaminated zone.

A birth defects register was set up after the

disaster. There were no birth defects that could be unequivocally linked to dioxin exposure among the limited number of births to residents of the high-exposure zone. In addition, although there were wide variations in the spontaneous abortion rate between zones, these could not be ascribed to dioxin. Examination of chromosomes in aborted tissue following artificially induced abortions suggested that there might have been a higher frequency of chromosomal aberrations in fetuses from mothers potentially exposed to dioxins, but it was not possible to establish whether these aberrations would have led to adverse reproductive outcomes.

Perhaps the greatest long-term worry from the Seveso incident was cancer. All those exposed have now been followed up for 10 years (Bertazzi *et al.*, 1989). There are no excesses of overall mortality or mortality due to all cancers. Risks of deaths from certain individual cancers and from cardiovascular disease were elevated, but they could not be related to exposure patterns. Although restricted by the short observation time and the small numbers of deaths from certain causes, the study seems to suggest that there have not been the feared large increases in the overall numbers of deaths from cancer.

The Seveso incident illustrates how an accidental release of a chemical may be perceived by the general public as a major disaster. So far, few, if any, human deaths have resulted from the single-dose exposure to dioxin. Those suffering chloracne or burns recovered. Fears of large numbers of people being affected by potential long-term effects have not been confirmed despite scientific study. Nevertheless, the Seveso incident is important, as it raised the general awareness of the potential that there may be for ill-health following major plant failure.

Bhopal, India, 1984
Methyl isocyanate was a toxic substance responsible for a major disaster at Bhopal, India, in December 1984 at a factory manufacturing the pesticide carbaryl.

The cause of the accident was the introduction of water into a storage tank containing methyl isocyanate. This resulted in the production of carbon dioxide (Equation 1)

$$CH_3NCO + H_2O \rightarrow CH_2NH_2 + CO_2 \quad (1)$$

The combination of rising temperature due to a runaway exothermic reaction coupled with gas evolution led to a build up of pressure which caused 30–35 t of methyl isocyanate to be vented to the atmosphere in a 2–3 h period (Marshall, 1987). The venting occurred during the night and the cloud dispersed over a densely populated area (Figure 7).

Estimates of the number of deaths which resulted from the release vary between 1700 and 5000, with up to 60 000 people being seriously injured (Bucher, 1987; Andersson, 1989). Survivors reported that the vapour cloud gave off considerable heat and had a pungent odour. Irritation, coughing and choking were early symptoms, and were followed by vomiting, defaecation and urination, and panic, depression, agitation, apathy and convulsions. Although severe eye effects, including temporary blindness, were seen in many survivors, they did not persist (Andersson *et al.*, 1988). Initial lung effects (oedema,

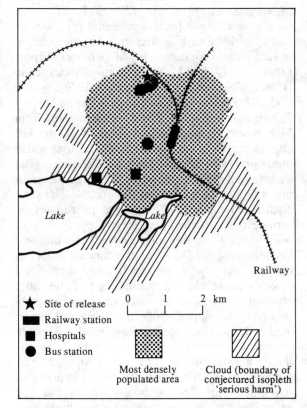

Figure 7 Sketch map of Bhopal, showing overlap between populated area and the approximate boundary for receiving serious harm from the vapour cloud. Based on Marshall (1987)

★ Site of release
■ Railway station
■ Hospitals
● Bus station

0   1   2 km

Most densely populated area   Cloud (boundary of conjectured isopleth 'serious harm')

Railway

Lake   Lake

focal atelectasis) were probable causes of death and led, in survivors, to more persistent changes in lung function, and possible fibrosis and inflammation. Serial studies showed that some survivors improved, that there was no change in some and that some worsened. Liver and kidney function appeared to be normal in survivors (Andersson *et al.*, 1988; Bucher, 1987).

The Bhopal incident illustrates many important points. First, although the reasons for the water entering the methyl isocyanate tank were never clearly identified, the consequences were made substantially worse than they need have been because several of the design safety features had been rendered unusable and because there were substantial numbers of shanty houses right up to the factory fence. Also, there was a paucity of toxicological data on methyl isocyanate prior to the incident, which has now been rectified by undertaking substantial studies in animals as well as following up the victims (Bucher, 1987). At the time of the incident there was only one substantial published report on the toxicity of methyl isocyanate, and that was restricted to an animal study on the acute effects following single exposure (Kimmerle and Eben, 1964).

Chernobyl, USSR, 1986
Chernobyl, 80 km north of Kiev, USSR (now Ukraine) was the site of probably the worst accident to have occurred at a nuclear plant.

In April 1986 a test was being conducted on a reactor during shut-down for routine maintenance (Chernobyl Report, 1986; Henderson, 1987; Bertazzi, 1989). However, the planning of the test was poor and safety devices were deliberately switched off to allow the test to proceed. By the time it was realized that something was wrong, uranium oxide fuel elements in the upper part of the core had probably started to disintegrate because of the high temperatures. Explosions followed which released considerable quantities of radioactivity to the atmosphere, much of which was dispersed over the Soviet Union and western and northern Europe.

By 1 year after the event only 31 people had died as a result of it. They died in the immediate aftermath of the accident, from acute radiation sickness. However, there could be a total of over 10 000 premature deaths due to cancers caused by the radioactivity, of which 35 might be in the UK, over the following 50 years (Henderson,

1987). This has to be set against the approximately 7 million anticipated deaths due to cancers in the UK over the same time.

The radioactivity from the accident was washed from the skies and entered food chains, notably in areas of high rainfall. In the UK this led to the banning of the sale for human consumption of sheep meat from badly affected areas for over a year. Subsequent to the accident, the people in the area around Chernobyl were evacuated. They have not been allowed to return and the area is being converted to a national park where human activity, including farming, is banned.

This disaster is one in which future illness and premature deaths are the primary effects on man. It is this fear of the future effects of radiation which has made the nuclear industry so heavily regulated in comparison with other industries.

Fire

Thermal injuries, heat stress and physical trauma from collapsing structures are obvious problems in major fires. However, fire statistics indicate that deaths consequent on being overcome by smoke are the most common type of death (Committee on Fire Toxicology, 1986). Such deaths and incapacitations are due to the evolution of toxic combustion products. As toxicants are likely to be funnelled upwards and diluted to non-toxic levels in unconfined fires, major fire disasters usually occur in confined spaces when it is not possible to escape from the effects of the toxic combustion products.

Smoke includes all airborne products from the pyrolysis and combustion of materials (Committee on Fire Toxicology, 1986). Full oxidation of substances present in fires would result in such products as carbon dioxide, water (steam), nitrogen dioxide, sulphur dioxide and chlorine. However, complete combustion rarely occurs and other products such as carbon monoxide, soot (particles), hydrogen cyanide, hydrogen chloride, hydrogen fluoride, acrolein and other organic materials are often present. The toxicity of fires therefore arises from the evolution of smoke (including gases, dust/fume and aerosol), containing irritants and asphyxiants and, potentially, carcinogens. Those most at risk will normally be the firefighters in close proximity to the fire, and thus near enough to inhale undispersed toxic smoke and gases.

Potentially, risks from acute health effects of dispersed combustion products may occur in warehouse fires such as that at Brightside, Sheffield (Health and Safety Executive, 1985). Onlookers who were in close proximity to the fire may have acquired sore throats and chest symptoms due to effects from the fire. However, potential combustion product toxicants were dispersed to levels thought too dilute to pose a risk to the general population within very short distances. Asbestos roofing materials were dispersed widely in this fire, but the longer-term health effects for people exposed to single doses of dispersed fire products were considered to be minimal.

Two examples of disasters in which the evolution of toxic combustion products from fires contributed significantly are given below. In both examples most of those who died were incapacitated by the effects of inhaling toxic smoke and gases in relatively confined spaces, and thus became unable to move to less polluted atmospheres.

Manchester Airport Crash, UK, 1985

One area where there is a potential for disasters due to toxic hazards is aircraft fires. An example of such a catastrophe was the Manchester Airport crash of 1985 (Air Accidents Investigation Branch, Department of Transport, 1989).

On 22 August 1985 a British Airtours Boeing 737 aircraft bound for Corfu was taking off from Manchester International Airport when the left engine suffered an uncontained failure which punctured a wing fuel tank access panel. The leaking fuel ignited and burnt as a large plume of fire trailing directly behind the engine. The crew abandoned take-off and cleared the runway by turning onto a taxiway as they stopped. A light wind carried the fire onto and around the rear fuselage (Figure 8). After the aircraft stopped, the hull was penetrated rapidly, and smoke and possibly flame entered through one of the cabin aft-doors which had just been opened. Fire subsequently developed inside the cabin and generated a dense black toxic/irritant smoke. Despite prompt attendance by the airport fire services, the aircraft was destroyed and 55 people (53 passengers, 2 crew) died, one after 6 days in hospital. All those who died on board the aircraft had general congestion and oedema of the lungs with carbon particles in the air passages, consistent with inhalation of smoke. The cause of death

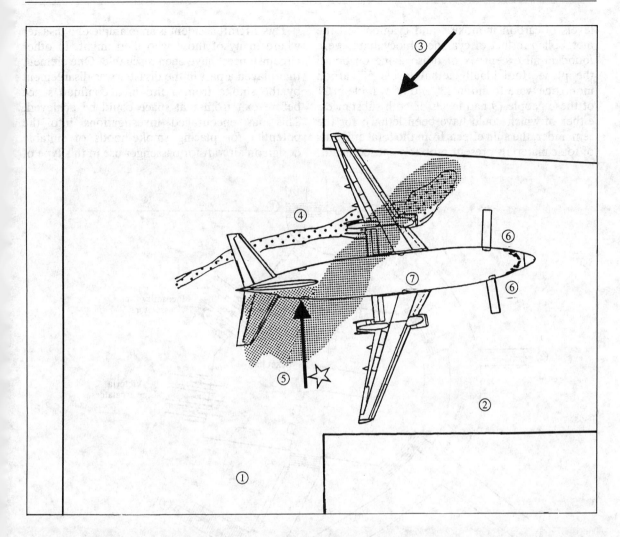

Figure 8 Sketch map to illustrate the position of the stopped plane in the Manchester Airport crash 1985. 1, Main runway; 2, taxiway; 3, wind direction (wind speed 6 knots); 4, pool of jet fuel from punctured tank; 5, plume of fire/smoke from ignited fuel; 6, forward emergency doors (used to escape). Star indicates rear emergency door through which flames/smoke may have penetrated cabin. Based on data in Air Accident Investigation Branch Report 8/88 (1989)

was inhalation of smoke for 48 people and direct thermal injury (burns) for only 6 passengers.

Of those engulfed by smoke, only 38 (47 per cent) survived. The survivors reported that a single breath of the cabin atmosphere was burning and painful, immediately causing choking. They experienced drowsiness and disorientation. Eight survivors actually collapsed, but recovered sufficiently to get out from the plane. Most of the deaths due to incapacitation might have been prevented if the people concerned had been protected from smoke or if external assistance had been more quickly available. All except one of

the survivors of the immediate accident made their exit within 7 min of the aircraft stopping. The only passenger recovered alive by firemen was taken out after 33 min; he died 6 days later from severe pulmonary damage and associated pneumonia.

The thermal decomposition products of cabin materials included toxic irritant gases, such as carbon monoxide, hydrogen chloride and hydrogen cyanide. Some fluorinated materials (used as decorative films) yielded hydrogen fluoride. It was probably the combined effects of toxic combustion products which caused death. Elevated levels of carbon monoxide and cyanide and the metabolic product of cyanide, thiocyanate, were found in all except six of those dying on board the plane. Individually lethal levels of carbon monoxide were found in 13, and of cyanide in 21 of these people (9 had levels of both substances, either of which could have been lethal); for the remainder, the sum effects from the total amounts of toxic materials present probably caused death.

This aircraft accident is an example of a disaster where many of those who died might, in other circumstances, have been rescuable. One element that played a part in the disaster was disablement by the smoke from a fire in a confined space before exit from that space could be achieved. This has encouraged investigations into the potential for placing smoke-hoods of suitable design on aircraft for passenger use in this type of

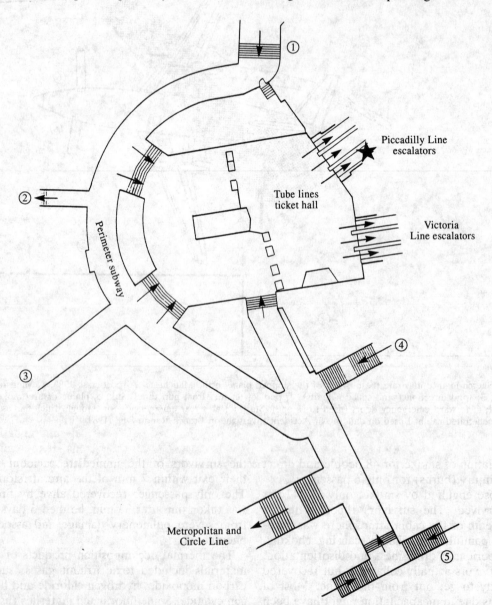

Figure 9   Sketch map of the layout of the subsurface ticket hall and subways at Kings Cross Underground station. 1, Entrance from Kings Cross main line station; 2, entrance from St. Pancras main line station; 3, entrance from Pancras Road; 4 and 5, entrances from Euston Road. Star indicates escalator in which fire started. Based on Fennel (1988)

emergency. Investigations into possible 'in-cabin' firefighting systems in order to slow down the development of toxic atmospheres were also undertaken as a consequence of this disaster.

Kings Cross (London) Underground Station, UK, 1987

Thirty-one people died and many more were injured in an escalator fire at Kings Cross Underground station. The fire took place in the evening at an extremely busy Underground station where four lines cross (Figures 9 and 10). Access to the three deep lines (Piccadilly, Victoria and Northern) is from the ticket hall below the main line station forecourt. The ticket hall is approached by subways from Kings Cross and St. Pancras main line stations and from street level. According to the Inquiry Report (Fennel, 1988), the fire started in the Piccadilly line escalator, among an accumulation of grease and detritus (dust, fibre and debris) on the running tracks, possibly as a result of a lighted match passing through the skirting board. This fire preheated the balustrades and decking, which were wooden. As a consequence of a 'trench' effect, the fire initially burnt cleanly and then produced dense, black smoke. 'Flashover' occurred as the fire erupted into the ticket hall. The deaths all

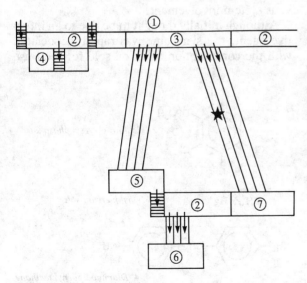

Figure 10 Sketch map of the levels of the components of Kings Cross Underground station. 1, Surface level (Kings Cross main line station forecourt); 2, subways; 3, ticket hall; 4, Metropolitan and Circle lines; 5, Victoria line; 6, Northern line; 7, Piccadilly line. Star indicates escalator on which fire started

occurred among people in the ticket hall at around the time 'flashover' occurred.

The inquiry did not pursue in detail the question of cause of death for the 31 people who died, but concluded that many deaths were due to the toxic effects of the smoke rather than to burns. In the report the Inspector says:

'After hearing expert evidence about the role of toxic gases in the fire and the findings of pathologists on post-mortem tests, I determined that the cause of death in individual cases could not be pursued any further in this Investigation. On the evidence available to me no reliable assessment could be made of the relative importance of various materials present in the station to the production of toxic fire fumes or to the sources of toxic materials found in the bodies. Although separate statutory Coroner's Inquests were held, the Coroner decided not to take the matter further.'

A major part of the inquiry focused on the procedures by which London Underground dealt with escalator fires. It was clear that the Underground lacked an adequate approach to safety in terms of their attitudes to safety matters, their attention to staff training in safety and their equipment and procedures to be used in emergencies. The lack of preparedness led to an emergency becoming a disaster.

Food and Drink

Mass poisonings due to contamination of food or drink may be considered disasters. Many episodes of this type of mass poisoning are the consequences of bacterial or fungal contamination of foods consumed by the victims. If the causative agent is pathogenic, then health can suffer. However, a portion of such poisonings is due to the introduction of a chemical toxicant into the consumed material, either directly or via a food chain.

Because of the indirect way in which the contamination affects man, it can be difficult to demonstrate cause and effect. Ill-health may occur indirectly, in a species (man) remote from that (e.g. wheat) to which the toxicant was administered, possibly after transmission through a food chain (fed to farm animals, etc.) or directly (in bread). It may be some time before the toxicant accumulates sufficiently for the victim to exhibit symptoms of ill-health, or for the ill-health to be manifest following ingestion. Consequently, considerable detective work may be needed in order to identify the cause of ill-health, and on occasion it may never be properly characterized.

A series of examples of incidents involving contamination of food or water follow. Further examples can be found in Aldridge (1987).

Adulteration of Food or Drink
Adulteration (debasing by adding other or inferior substances: *Concise Oxford Dictionary*, 1990) of foodstuffs and deliberate poisonings by admixture in food have gone on from time immemorial. Adulteration for commercial reasons was rife in the eighteenth and nineteenth centuries (see Smullen, 1989). Bread from bakers often contained chalk, lime, lead salts or even bone to make it look white. Leaves of hawthorn, sloe or ash were used to dilute tea. With hindsight several of these adulterants were toxic chemicals and may have had disastrous consequences for the recipients. Deliberate adulteration, when it occurs, is still capable of causing major disasters.

Ginger Paralysis, Mid-west and South-west USA, 1930   During Prohibition in the United States, the Prohibition Bureau ruled that the USP 'fluid extract of ginger' was a non-potable beverage and its sale was not restricted. This beverage was an alcoholic extract of material from the ginger plant and was freely drunk. An adulterated 'fluid extract of ginger' entered circulation through dealers (non-pharmacists), mainly in Ohio and Tennessee early in 1930. Cases of paralysis started occurring in mid-February. Adult men were the principal victims and those showing symptoms seemed to do so some 10 days to 3 weeks after drinking the suspect ginger extract (Smith and Elvove, 1930). Ultimately some 50 000 people were affected (Morgan, 1982).

The paralysis first appeared as soreness of the muscles of the arms and legs, with occasional numbness in the fingers and toes. Foot and wrist drop and weakness of the fingers developed. The symptoms were found in distal parts of the limbs and were more marked in the feet and legs. This neuropathy was a primary axonopathy caused by demyelination and dying back from the distal end of the long nerves. In some cases recovery was very limited (Aldridge, 1987).

In a very detailed piece of work, the causative agent was identified chemically as tri-*ortho*-cresyl phosphate (Figure 11; Smith and Elvove, 1930; Smith, 1930). Both the adulterated ginger extract and the presumed adulterant, tri-*ortho*-cresyl phosphate, were found to cause the symptoms of the neuropathy in calves, chickens and, to a much less marked degree, rabbits, but had little effect on monkeys or dogs following oral ingestion.

Toxic Oil Syndrome, Spain, 1981   Toxic oil syndrome was a previously unknown disease syndrome which appeared in Spain in May 1981, principally in Madrid and the north west provinces (World Health Organization, 1984; Aldridge, 1985, 1987). The epidemic was at its peak in mid-June and faded away thereafter. By March 1983, 340 deaths had occurred and over 20 000 cases had been recorded.

The disease developed in two phases. In the acute phase, a pleuropneumonia sufficient to cause respiratory distress and death in severe cases was present. This pleuropneumonia did not respond to antibiotic treatment and about 20 per cent of survivors did not recover completely. A chronic phase of the disease, a sensorimotor peripheral neuropathy of variable appearance, developed, together with sclerodermal-like skin changes. There was little evidence of central nervous system involvement.

Although initially thought to be due to an infective agent, the syndrome was rapidly associated with the consumption of an oil sold for food use

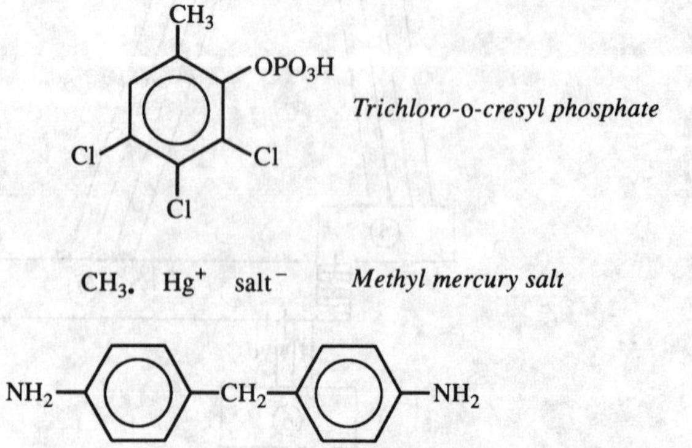

Trichloro-o-cresyl phosphate

$CH_3 \cdot Hg^+$ salt$^-$ *Methyl mercury salt*

NH_2—⬡—CH_2—⬡—NH_2

4, 4'-Diaminodiphenyl methane

$Al_2(SO_4)_3 \cdot 18H_2O$ *Alum (hydrated aluminium sulphate)*

Figure 11   Structures of chemicals implicated in disasters mediated through the food or water supplies

in 5 litre cans by itinerant salesmen. The oil was rapeseed oil, denatured with aniline, intended for industrial use. In most cases the oil had been re-refined, mixed with other seed oils, animal fats and poor-quality olive oil or chlorophyll, but in the cases of a small number of victims in the Seville area (well away from the main outbreak) the re-refined oil had not been further processed. The unsolved problem in toxic oil syndrome is the exact nature of the (presumed) chemical toxicant. Despite considerable effort aimed at its identification, the precise toxicant has not been identified.

Accidental Contamination

As opposed to deliberate addition of materials to foodstuffs or drinks, accidental addition of toxicants can also occur. If the toxicant is sufficiently effective and affects a large number of people, a major disaster could result.

Pollution of Drinking-water in North Cornwall, UK, 1988 Mass intoxications, in theory at least, could occur due to contamination of drinking-water supplies. That this is not such a remote possibility was demonstrated in 1988, when the South West Water Authority found that a truck load (20 t) of alum (aluminium sulphate; Figure 11) had accidentally been released into the drinking-water supply to Camelford, a small town in Cornwall, and the surrounding district (Lowermoor Incident Health Advisory Group, 1989). The material was delivered into the treated water reservoir at Lowermoor Treatment Works. The pH of the water dropped below 5 and aluminium levels were raised to over 10 mg l^{-1}, considerably above the 0.2 mg l^{-1} set on palatability grounds in the European Community Drinking Water Directive. Although initial advice from local sources suggested that little ill-health would occur, newspapers reported considerable acute health symptoms and speculated that there were potential long-term effects. The expert assessment was that the early symptoms of gastrointestinal disturbances, rashes and mouth ulcers were probably due to the incident, but short-lived. Later complaints of joint and muscle pain, memory loss, hypersensitivity and gastrointestinal disorders may have been induced because of 'sustained anxiety naturally felt by many people'. The expert committee concluded that there was no

adequate scientific foundation available for the speculation on potential long-term effects.

The incident is a sufficient reminder of the possibility of a disaster occurring as a result of contaminated water supplies. It also illustrates the difficulties which occur in allaying fears when the affected population receives initial advice which was, to quote the conclusions of the Advisory Group, 'contradictory, confusing and sometimes inappropriate'.

Contamination of Food During Storage—Epping Jaundice, UK, 1965 Epping Jaundice was an outbreak of jaundice which affected at least 84 people in the Epping area of London during February 1965 (Kopelman *et al.*, 1966a,b). It was traced to ingestion of wholemeal bread made from flour contaminated with 4,4'-diaminophenylmethane (structure in Figure 11). The chemical had spilled from a container on to the floor of a van which was carrying flour as well as chemicals.

In most of the cases jaundice and liver enlargement were preceded by severe, intermittent pains in the upper abdomen and lower chest areas of the body. Normally, these pains were of acute onset (50 patients), but sometimes onset was insidious (27 patients). Of the 57 patients further investigated, most had raised serum bilirubin, alkaline phosphate and aspartate aminotransferase levels. Needle biopsies were performed on 4 patients within 3 weeks of the onset of symptoms; all showed considerable evidence of portal inflammation and bile duct cholestasis and showed evidence of hepatocyte damage. The lesion was reproducible in mice given 4,4'-diaminophenylmethane (Schoental, 1968). The patients slowly recovered over succeeding weeks.

The jaundice was the result of an accidental, undetected (until too late) contamination of a foodstuff because it was stored during delivery adjacent to chemicals which were insufficiently securely contained within the packaging. The chemicals were absorbed by the flour through the sacking and, following baking, were present in the bread.

Poisoning Due to Consumption of Foodstuff Not Intended for Human Consumption—Methylmercury Poisoning in Iraq, 1971–1972
An outbreak of organomercurial poisoning due to the consumption of treated grain by farmers and their families occurred in Iraq in 1971–1972

(World Health Organization, 1976). There were 459 deaths and over 6000 further cases admitted to hospital.

Poisoning cases started to appear in hospitals in late December. Farming families only were affected, and the cause of the poisoning was identified as consumption of homemade bread, an important element of their diet, made from wheat treated with seed dressing. There was a latent period of up to 60 days from first consumption to the appearance of signs and symptoms of poisoning, and in many cases consumption of contaminated grain ceased before the symptoms occurred.

Symptoms included speech disturbances, abnormal behaviour, loss of auditory and visual acuity, and ataxia. The severity varied from minimal effects to severe disability and death. Most of those showing only mild or moderate symptoms were symptom-free 2 years later, although symptoms were still present in severe cases. Mercury levels in hair were found to be good indicators of the dose of mercury received.

Organomercurials, such as the methylmercury (Figure 11) involved in this episode, are fungicides, the methylmercury being used as a seed dressing to prevent wheat bunt and other crop diseases. Grain dressed with methylmercury was distributed to farmers between mid-September and early December, 1971. Although much of the wheat had been consumed before a cause–effect relationship had been established, surplus treated grain was withdrawn to storehouses once the cause of the outbreak was known. The problem arose because wheat intended as seed for next year's crop was eaten by the farmers and their families rather than used for its intended function.

Environmental Pollution — Minamata and Niigata, Japan, 1951–1974

The examples of major disasters arising from toxic substances so far discussed arise from contamination of the foodstuff. It is also possible for contamination to arise indirectly as a result of an environmental pollutant entering a food chain. Two examples of this occurred in Japan, at Minamata and Niigata (Tsubaki and Irukayama, 1977).

Over the period 1951–1974 there were over 700 recognized cases and 80 deaths due to 'Minamata disease', and over 2000 other people had applied for recognition as Minamata disease patients. The principal geographical areas affected were in two prefectures, Kumamoto and Kagoshima, which border Minamata Bay. The disease occurred mainly in fishermen and their families who consumed large quantities of locally caught fish containing high concentrations of mercury. The patients' nervous systems were affected, with symptoms of sensory, motor and visual involvement. Domestic cats (presumably also largely fed fish) exhibited similar clinical signs, and abnormal behaviour occurred among crows in the affected areas. Congenital effects also occurred.

The outbreak of poisoning at Niigata was first identified in 1965, with over 520 patients being identified by the end of 1974. The epidemic was also apparent in the domestic animal population.

In the Minamata outbreak the effects were due to organically bound mercury present in sludges from industrial plant. The mercury was used as a catalyst. Mercury from the sludge or from the waste-water outlet entered food chains and was bioconcentrated in both shellfish and fish. These were eventually consumed by man. At Niigata river fish from the lower reaches of the Agano river were the main foodstuff consumed which contained organic mercurial compounds. The source of the mercury was an industrial plant waste-water discharge containing low concentrations of mercury (Figure 11). Methylation took place in sediments and considerable bioconcentration occurred in the fish, as evidenced by the much higher levels of mercury in the fish when compared with the river water.

At both sites consumption of contaminated fish had gone on for a considerable time before the causes of the disease were identified. This points to the great difficulties involved in deriving a cause–effect relationship when the effect is remote from the source of the causative agent.

Although the particular examples chosen to illustrate this effect related to human health, other species may be the final consumer in a food chain. The story of the consequences of spraying persistent organochlorine insecticides, their bioconcentration in the food chain and their disastrous effects on raptor populations because the concentrations reached were sufficient to cause eggshell thinning and failure to reproduce effectively, summarized in Smith (1986), is well known.

Interactions of Man and Nature

Mining

In general, toxicants are unlikely to be a primary cause of a specific mining disaster, as the conditions causing ill-health are unlikely to develop suddenly. Historically, it is possible that disasters due to asphyxiation or the release of toxic gases occurred. Canaries were taken underground to act as fail-safe biological monitors for these effects. (When the singing ceased. . . .) Nowadays forced ventilation makes these events extremely rare.

People have died as a result of lung cancer due to exposure to radon in mines or of pneumoconiosis caused by exposure to coal dusts or silica, but the exposure to these agents was a consequence of inadequate working conditions rather than specific accidental exposures.

Waste Disposal

Inadequately thought-out disposal of wastes may cause major disasters.

Love Canal, USA

Love Canal was a waste disposal site which contained municipal and chemical waste disposed of over a period of 30 years up to 1953. Homes were built on the site during the 1960s. Leaching became a problem in the late 1960s, when chemical odours were detected in basements. These were followed by fears of potential ill-health which led to considerable psychological stress. Dibenzofurans and dioxins were identified in the organic phases of leachates and were presumably derived from the disposal of waste products of the manufacture of chlorinated hydrocarbons. Animal studies, conducted on the organic phase of the leachate, indicated that there could be risks of immunotoxic, carcinogenic and teratogenic effects (Silkworth *et al.*, 1984, 1986, 1989a,b). Low birthweights have been found in the offspring of residents of Love Canal (Vianna and Polan, 1984). Although follow-up was limited, no causal link has been established for exposure to chemicals and cancer in man (Janerich *et al.*, 1981). Nevertheless, serious social and psychological consequences have resulted from the use of the site for houses and the lack of understanding of the fears of residents initially apparent on the toxic properties of the chemicals dumped at the site (Holden, 1980).

Minamata and Niigata

The mercury poisoning at Minamata and Niigata, already described, were caused by the disposal of industrial wastes in such a manner that the toxicant was concentrated to dangerous levels in a food chain in the aqueous environment.

Conclusions

Toxicants, whether derived from nature or the chemical plant, can cause disasters. Identifying the cause is relatively easy when the toxicant is airborne and the ill-health occurs during or shortly after exposure. It is usually more difficult if the effect is mediated via the food or water supply and/or if the effect is not immediately apparent. The former have been called 'overt' disasters and the latter 'dilute' disasters (Bertazzi, 1989). As 'dilute' implies some diminution of effect, it might be better to refer to the latter type of disaster as a 'disseminated' disaster.

In overt disasters due to airborne toxicants there is usually a primary event such as volcanic eruption or a plant failure. This is followed by dispersal of the toxicant, which depends on the buoyancy in air of the material released and the meteorological conditions at the time of release. Any immediate dose received by man will depend on the level and duration of the exposure. Only very simple post-event preventative measures can be used to minimize the dose received. Although usually ill-health is immediate, long-term effects such as carcinogenicity could occur. However, they are difficult to link to a primary event and are chiefly known for releases of radioactivity. Toxic material can be deposited on to surfaces and containment, to prevent ill-health due to continuing lower-level exposures, may be difficult.

Most known airborne toxicants involved in major disasters affect the respiratory tract. Irritation, asphyxiation (chemically induced by binding of toxicant or physically induced by blockage of the respiratory tract) and pulmonary oedema are common (Schwartz, 1987). Cancers are frequent effects of radiation. Other toxic effects may occur in organs away from the respiratory system, although this appears to be rare. When airborne, the toxicant reaches the lung and respiratory system first; consequently they appear to be the most frequently affected organ systems.

By comparison, 'disseminated' disasters are more difficult to identify and are often identified by effect. Tracing the cause may take a considerable time, particularly if the ill-health effect took some time to develop. Consequently, it is more difficult to prevent exposures and it becomes more likely that a disaster will occur because of a voluntary oral intake of the food or water containing the toxic material. Organs other than the 'portal of entry' are more likely to be affected in such disasters, and withdrawal of the food, etc., causing the disaster may be too late to be an effective post-event preventative measure.

In the absence of sufficient authoritative and accurate information, popular speculation generally favours the worst possible outcomes, however improbable. This is likely to worsen psychiatric consequences of the event and to complicate the emergency response. The provision of timely, accurate advice in an understandable form is one need that must be considered when examining how to handle the consequences of a serious incident.

APPROACHES TO HANDLING MAJOR HAZARDS

One role of industry, individual governments and international organizations is to develop and implement procedures for preventing or minimizing the effects of potential or actual disasters. In most countries governments develop a series of legislative requirements in order to provide a framework of regulation within which to work. Rather than compare different national frameworks, this section will concentrate on conceptual approaches to handling the risks arising from major hazards.

Assessment of potential hazards and assessment and management of the likely consequences are the key elements in any process for dealing with major hazards. In the case of toxic hazards, one aspect of the hazard evaluation is an examination of the likely toxicity of the materials involved in the potential disastrous situation, including prediction of the amounts of toxic materials likely to cause these effects. Procedures can then be adopted for the assessment of the risks associated with the various uses. Interacting with, and dependent on the risk assessment will be the approaches available by which the risks can be managed. These procedures of risk management differ fundamentally according to the type ('overt' or 'disseminated') of potential disaster envisaged.

Criteria for Judging Risk

'Is it a risk?' is usually the first question asked when a potential hazard is being examined. Once the concept of risk has been explained, two questions will follow: 'what is the risk?' and 'is it acceptable/tolerable?' (see Table 1 for definitions). This involves trying to define in general what is an acceptable or tolerable risk. Once acceptability (tolerability) has been defined, a method is needed in order to compare the risk for the particular problem under study with acceptable risk. That method may be qualitative, of the form 'acceptable'/'non-acceptable', based on a judgement of the data available against broadly defined criteria. However, for many purposes, including much risk assessment, many quantitative, numerical approaches are adopted. These numerical approaches are called quantified risk analyses. These quantitative analyses render decision-making easier, especially when choosing between options, as they give a clearer indication of the magnitude of a risk or of the relative risks for different options.

Criteria for judging the acceptability of a human health risk depend on three factors: the risk level (the frequency with which the event will occur); the definition of the biological event (death, serious injury, etc.); and the status of the receiving individual (a 'normal' or a 'vulnerable' individual).

Criteria against which to judge environmental effects are more difficult as the importance of a loss has to be considered as well as the size of the effect. Descriptions of damage levels constituting a major disaster are therefore judgements. One set of such end-effect criteria is that published by the UK Dept. of Environment (1991).

Risk Comparisons

When comparing risks, it is necessary to ensure that the particular hazard for which the risk is being calculated is the same for all the risks being examined, both in terms of the biological event and for the type of recipient. For many risk comparisons, that event is 'death' (in reality, foreshortening of life, often such that death occurs during or shortly after the event) as a result of an event and the individual responding is a 'normal' person. Criteria for assessing this 'risk of death' have been obtained by comparisons with everyday risks associated with various activities (Royal Society Study Group, 1983; Health and Safety Executive, 1988a,b, 1989a). There are several levels of 'risk of death' that can be elaborated. At one level there is the 'trivial', 'negligible' or 'completely acceptable' risk. At the other extreme there is the 'intolerable' or 'unacceptable' risk. In between lies a range of risks which are tolerable under certain circumstances and/or provided they are minimized (Figure 12).

A risk of about 1 in 10^6 per year that the individual concerned will die from a given cause appears to be generally regarded in the United Kingdom as acceptable (Royal Society Study Group, 1983). This was justified by considering the death rates for different activities considered 'safe' (see Table 3 for some comparative risks of 'death'). The risk of death for workers in recognized dangerous occupations is of the order of 1 death per 10^3 per year; thus this is considered the highest bound of 'tolerable' risk for a lifetime risk. Any higher level is considered intolerable and unacceptable at all times. Because working in a 'risky' industry is, at least to some extent, voluntary, the individual risk just tolerable for a member of the general public living in the neighbourhood of a hazard is considered to be tenfold less (1 death per 10^4 per year) (Health and Safety

Executive, 1989a). This is approximately the risk from death in a road traffic accident and slightly less than the risk of developing any form of cancer. All of these risk criteria relate to individual risk and to average individuals.

A more conservative approach has been adopted in the Netherlands (Versteeg, 1988). It depends on the frequency of deaths from natural causes and is based on the idea that industrial activity should not increase the background mortality by more than 1 per cent. An upper bound of 10^6 deaths per year has been derived, with a lower bound of 10^8 per year being considered trivial.

In between the upper and lower bounds of acceptability lies a region where risks from known hazards should be reduced as far as reasonably practicable. This means that the cost of reducing the risk should not be disproportionate to the level of risk encountered. A small reduction in an already low risk may not be justified if it is very expensive.

'Overt' Disasters

Potential 'overt' disasters can be averted or minimized by a combination of land-use planning and emergency planning. Good land-use planning can minimize the potential risks of a disaster by restricting the size of any interaction of event and consequence. A hazardous process or a large store of hazardous material can be sited well away from large numbers of people. Potential developments involving significant numbers of members of the public can be sited away from natural or man-made major hazards.

There will remain a residue of risk after appropriate land-use planning has been achieved. Occasionally there will be the situation where inappropriate combinations of people and major hazards occurred prior to the time when the need for appropriate land-use planning became apparent. In addition, other considerations, such as a need for local employment, may mean that other factors were decisive when the plannning decision was made. The consequences, should the event occur, can still be substantially reduced, provided that appropriate emergency planning has been undertaken. This involves both enabling potential victims to survive better prior to treatment and making available appropriate treatment sufficiently rapidly.

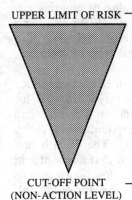

UPPER LIMIT OF RISK

INTOLERABLE/
UNACCEPTABLE RISK

TOLERABLE RISK (Only if risk reduction is impractical or cost grossly disproportionate)

MAY BE JUSTIFIABLE
Further control required to reduce risk 'so far as is reasonably practicable'

TOLERABLE RISK (If cost of risk reduction would exceed the improvement gained)

CUT-OFF POINT
(NON-ACTION LEVEL)

BROADLY
ACCEPTABLE RISK
(Detriment judged to be trivial/negligible)

Figure 12 Diagram to illustrate the approach to risk evaluation for major hazards. Based on Royal Society Study Group (1983) and Health and Safety Executive (1988a)

Table 3   Comparisons of risk of death from various causes

Cause of death	Risk (as annual experience) (per year)	Year of statistic
Cancer	2.8×10^{-3}	1985
Industrial accidents to deep-sea fishermen (UK registered vessels)	8.8×10^{-4}	1984
All violent deaths	4.0×10^{-4}	1985
Industrial accidents during quarrying	3.0×10^{-4}	1985
Industrial accidents during coal extraction and manufacture of solid fuel	1.1×10^{-4}	1986–7
Road accidents	1.0×10^{-4}	1985
Industrial accidents in construction	9.2×10^{-5}	1986–7
Industrial accidents in agriculture	8.7×10^{-5}	1986–7
Industrial accidents in offices, shops, warehouses, etc.	4.5×10^{-6}	1985
Gas incidents	1.8×10^{-6}	1981–5
Lightning	1.0×10^{-7}	Average over several years

Data on deaths due to industrial accidents are based on accidents to the employee; data on deaths due to other causes are averaged over the general population. Based on Health and Safety Executive (1988a)

Land-use Planning
Although the criterion of death can be employed in land-use planning, allowances need to be made for the uncertainties in developing this criterion for an individual within a population. Do we need the data for 5 per cent dying or 95 per cent dying? In addition, there may be serious, but sublethal, effects on health. These sublethal effects may be of great concern when handling toxic substances. In consequence, a broader concept, the 'dangerous dose', has also been employed. The dangerous dose is a description of the exposure conditions producing a level of toxicity (Health and Safety Executive, 1989a; Turner and Fairhurst, 1989):

(1) Severe distress will be caused to almost everyone.
(2) A substantial fraction will require medical attention.
(3) Some people are seriously injured and require prolonged treatment.
(4) Any highly susceptible people may be killed.

This type of criterion reflects that there is a range of individual ill-health effects and imprecision in the level of overall effect seen in the population.

The type of population being considered may also differ according to circumstances. Rather than examining the frequency of achieving a given biological effect in terms of the event occurring in an average individual in a 'normal' population, it may be that the consequence should be considered for an individual from a population containing a large number of particularly vulnerable (or susceptible) individuals.

If the biological effect being looked at changes and the type of individual being examined is different, then the numerical value of any risk criterion ought also to be altered. When quoting a risk criterion for it, it is therefore necessary also to mention the effect and the type of recipient. Otherwise confusion reigns.

Some arbitrary ratios have been enunciated for the relationship between the risk criteria for exposure conditions leading to 'death' and 'dangerous dose' in the same population (Health and Safety Executive, 1989a). The Health and Safety Executive has suggested that a risk of 1 in 10^{6} per year for a 'dangerous dose' corresponds to a risk of 3.3 in 10^{7} per year for risk of 'death'. Such a value will depend, in large measure, on the slope of the dose–response line; nevertheless, there is some evidence that might be considered to support the assumption. It can be calculated from a comparison of the relationship between classification on the basis of oral LD_{50} values (based on the criteria in Health and Safety Executive, 1988c) and on the basis of 'evident toxicity' following an oral dose to young, healthy rats (van den Heuval *et al.*, 1987) that the ratio between these events which yields the same classification is approximately 4:1. As 'evident toxicity' is a less severe effect than 'severe distress', a ratio of 3.3:1 is probably appropriate as a generalized, pragmatic assumption. Because risk is normally measured using logarithmic scales, this is a convenient value, as it represents a half-order of magnitude on such a scale.

A risk criterion of 3.3 in 10^7 per year for when there is a high proportion of 'highly susceptible' people receiving a 'dangerous dose' has also been proposed in place of the 1 in 10^6 per year for a individual from a population containing a normal balance of 'highly susceptible' individuals (Health and Safety Executive, 1989a). This is more arbitrary. The identity of the 'highly susceptible' people will depend on the effects seen, and this proportion will differ as effect differs. As homes for the elderly, caring institutions and long-stay hospitals are considered to contain a high proportion of 'highly susceptible' people, it would suggest that the occupants of such institutions are, in general, more susceptible to the effects of toxic chemicals. However, the choice of the ratio of 3.3:1 (again a half-order of magnitude) must be a pragmatic rather than a scientific decision.

Emergency Planning

Emergency planning is essentially concerned with handling the consequences after an event has occurred. It involves both immediate responses of emergency services and the medical management of the immediate and long-term health effects (Murray, 1990). Such planning is concerned with a much wider range of biological effects than death. These include 'severe health effect' (disability, requiring hospital treatment), and 'mild health effect' (discomfort or distress, detection or nuisance) (Baxter *et al.*, 1989a; Illing, 1989). ECETOC has defined three 'Emergency Exposure Indices', airborne concentrations for exposures lasting up to a specified time, below which direct toxic effects are unlikely to lead to one of death/permanent incapacity, disability or discomfort (ECETOC, 1991). Although hospital treatment may be essential for recovery from the severe health effects, it will usually have little

influence in the case of the milder effects (discomfort).

There is also a need to plan for an appropriately sized event. One proposal categorizes three types of release: small but likely accidents, severe but reasonably foreseeable events and large unlikely events (Baxter *et al.*, 1989a). If the severe, reasonably foreseeable event is chosen for planning purposes, then it should be possible to scale up or down the response for an individual event relatively readily.

'Disseminated' Disasters

Essentially, 'disseminated' disasters should only occur as a result of failure of a regulatory mechanism resulting in exposure to a toxicant. That failure may be because a new effect was uncovered by the disaster. Alternatively, a known effect might have occurred because of non-adherence to pre-existing regulatory requirements. The primary means of control has to be preventative, ensuring that, under normal conditions of exposure, the frequency of ill-health is acceptably low. A sufficiently rigorous enforcement system is also needed in order to ensure that failures in control which result in higher frequencies of ill-health do not occur. This type of approach is based on the conventional 'no effect' level and safety factors, leading to such concepts as maximum 'acceptable daily intake' and 'occupational exposure limits' (Royal Society Study Group, 1983). Where carcinogenic or other stochastic risks are concerned, the approach will be to minimize exposure as far as is reasonably practicable.

Determining Risk Levels

Determination of risk levels is required for overt hazards. There are essentially similar processes for determining risk levels for land-use planning and emergency planning (Health and Safety Executive, 1989a; ECETOC, 1991). The process can be divided into seven steps (Health and Safety Executive, 1989a):

(1) Identification of possible hazardous release events.

(2) Identification and analysis of the failure mechanisms which would allow a release to occur.

(3) Estimation of rates and durations of the release.

(4) Estimation of the frequencies of releases using the analysis of failure mechanisms.

(5) Estimation of the injury consequences of releases, taking account of mitigating factors.

(6) Combination of the frequencies and consequences to determine the overall risk levels.

(7) Judgement of the significance of the risk levels (by comparison with appropriate criteria).

Although this process was described for land-use planning in the vicinity of major industrial hazards in the UK, it can also be used more generally. Essentially, it can be described as three elements—a description of a source, a model for looking at the dispersion of the substance and a means of entering into the dispersion model parameters describing the conditions which will give a biological effect.

The source term for inputting into the dispersion model can be obtained by 'fault tree' analysis of the frequency of events (failure rates), by 'event tree analysis' leading to an estimate of failure rates or by engineering judgement based on historical event frequency. The actual method(s) chosen will depend on the type of release being studied and the available data. The sizes and durations of the postulated/actual releases are also examined (Health and Safety Executive, 1989a). For land-use planning there is a continuum of event frequency and size of release. Usually, sets of release sizes and durations are selected from the continuum and assigned appropriate frequencies. However, for emergency planning the process can be simplified by using the 'severe, but reasonably forseeable event' as the appropriate basis on which to plan (Baxter *et al.*, 1989a). This event was exemplified as a large hole in or fracture of a liquid chlorine pipe or of a road tanker delivery coupling at a chlorine installation. Scaling a response up or down should then be possible when an event actually occurs if the plan is sufficiently flexible.

The modelling then required is concerned with the dispersion of the toxic cloud. Several models have been described (examples include Fryer and Kaiser, 1979; Jagger, 1983; Baldini and Komosinsky, 1988; Kakko, 1989; review: McQuaid, 1989). In general, these models require a knowledge of the buoyant density of the cloud under different weather conditions. The dispersal conditions need to be combined with a function describing the combination of exposure concentration and time resulting in a defined effect. For example, one concentration–time combination may be described as the 'dangerous dose' for land-use planning, while a different combination could be used for the outer boundary for 'discomfort' for emergency planning. When combined with the information on the source, the model is then used to calculate 'isopleths'. These are boundaries of areas within which, at a point time, the concentration–time combination of exposure to the toxic substance would exceed those expected to give the identified biological effect. An overall isopleth envelope can then be calculated for a given set of release conditions by combining the individual isopleths for each time point post-event.

The information on the various isopleth envelopes for different types of release and meteorological conditions, when combined using a knowledge of the frequencies with which these conditions occur, gives a generalized 'contour' for all source terms and dispersal conditions. This contour is a risk statement for individual risk for a person within the specified boundary. An estimate of societal risk can then be obtained if data on the distribution of people within the geographic area are inputted.

In view of the complexity of these systems, computer programs have been developed to carry out the calculations associated with the models. The aim of the toxicologist is to find appropriate information on which to base a function describing the concentration and time relationship for a particular biological effect or combination of effects.

The Contribution of Toxicology to Hazard and Risk Assessment

The most likely direct hazards arising from a major accidental release of a toxic substance are the biological consequences of short-term exposure during dispersal of the toxicant. Longer-term or delayed effects should be considered as well as those more immediately apparent. Indirect consequences due to contamination of food or water supplies or to inhalation of dusts following settlement and subsequent disturbance are potentially important, but less immediate, problems, and should be amenable to post-event measures aimed at preventing significant exposure.

The Data Available

In theory, at least, the ideal assessment of toxicity of a potential major hazard substance or agent would be based on accurate observations of the appropriate effect in man. Reliable reports on severe effects in man are, fortunately, few, and mainly as a result of accidental exposure or exposure in wartime. Controversy often surrounds the exposure levels associated with such studies (Withers and Lees, 1987; Marshall, 1989). Results from studies on sublethal effects in man may be more plentiful. Nevertheless, the data on most substances are restricted to accidental exposures, often affecting only one or two people and rarely containing accurate exposure information. Except for radioactivity, human evidence concerning long-term effects of single exposures to most agents and substances is virtually non-existent. Further studies which require deliberate exposure of men (or women) to dangerous levels of a substance or agent are unethical.

As a consequence of the limited human data, heavy reliance has to be placed on animal and other experiments in attempting to predict the adverse effects in the human population. Often those animal data are confined to short-term effects (sometimes only lethality) following single exposures. Prior to Bhopal, the information available on the toxicity of methyl isocyanate was confined to a single published paper (Kimmerle and Eben, 1964) on short-term effects following acute exposure (Bucher, 1987). Also, many animal studies on the types of substances which might constitute major hazards were performed a long time ago and the data are, by modern standards, of poor quality.

In view of the very variable nature of the toxicity information, it is essential to evaluate this information critically and to understand the uncertainties introduced as a consequence of the nature and quality of the data (Illing, 1989; Marshall, 1989; Turner and Fairhurst, 1989; ECETOC, 1991). This means that assessments will normally be conducted using the original reports or published papers.

As the information may be required for quantitative risk analysis, where possible it will need to be described in numerical terms. Uncertainty has to be handled by sensitivity analysis. By inputting various potential values for particular effects into the risk assessments, it is possible to discover the differences that variation of the input parameter will have in terms of the outcome, the areas of the map covered by the contour envelope related to a particular risk value. This sensitivity analysis is an essential part of the overall risk assessment.

Usually there are few, if any, data on the immunological, carcinogenic or reproductive effects likely after single exposures to major hazard substances/agents. Indirect effects, mediated through food chain uptake and bioconcentration or disturbing settled material also need to be considered. If data are available, they should be evaluated. However, that evaluation will normally be descriptive as, except for the effects of radioactivity, there is currently no satisfactory way of obtaining the data in a form suitable for more quantitative approaches.

Problems of Extrapolation

The difficulties encountered in extrapolating from data in animals in evaluating the hazard to man, and, hence, the risk, are similar, whatever the nature of the hazard and risk being examined may be. The ways in which these extrapolations can be carried out have been described in great detail elsewhere (Tardiff and Rodricks, 1987). Three principal problems—interspecies variation, population heterogeneity (interindividual variation) and route-to-route extrapolation—are particularly relevant when data for major hazard substances are being examined.

Interspecies variation in biological effects is an important area of uncertainty in the evaluation. Toxicokinetic and toxicodynamic relationships between species, together with information on the relevant biochemical parameters in man, can lead to a better understanding of the relevance of results in a particular species for man. Physiologically based toxicokinetic models for extrapolation between species have been developed in other areas of toxicology (National Research Council, 1987) and are being used in the evaluation of the relevance of carcinogenic studies in animals for man. As many major hazard substances are lung toxicants, models based on the structure and function and on access of inspired area to the different parts of the lung (see, e.g., Davidson and Schroter, 1983; Miller *et al.*, 1985) may also be important. As substances are taken into blood and more slowly exhaled, owing to the development of tissue reservoirs of the material, but nevertheless mediate their effect at the lung surface, the models for lung may need incorporating into toxicokinetic models. This type of modelling has not yet been applied to major hazard toxicants, probably because of a lack of suitable data. Nevertheless, it would help considerably in reducing the uncertainty of interspecies extrapolation. The models and the data are likely to be developed over the next few years.

In the absence of appropriate toxicokinetic models, extrapolation between species is more judgemental. Allometric scaling is an obvious technique to use. As both lung surface area (for absorption) and body weight or body surface area (for effect) can both be scaled allometrically, they are, in general, less applicable to inhalation studies when compared with studies using other routes of administration. The only possible approach often is to take the exposure effect data based on the most sensitive relevant species and check it against any relevant human data.

In addition to interspecies variation, it is necessary to consider interindividual variation and the nature of the population being studied. Animal experiments, particularly those performed in recent years, have been conducted using animals specially bred to limit variations in response, and are usually young, healthy individuals. In many older studies much less closely defined animals were used. The general human population is more heterogeneous still, containing groups of individuals who must be considered 'highly susceptible' because of age, genetic constitution or disease state. These interindividual variations are a factor which adds to the uncertainty when extrapolating from animal studies to effects in man or when extrapolating from a small sample to a large population.

Occasionally, toxicity data may be used which were obtained for a different route of exposure from that for which they are being assessed (Pepelco and Withey, 1985; Pepelco, 1987). For example, in the absence of sufficient inhalation data it may be possible, in some circumstances, to make use of oral data and to relate them to equivalent inhalation exposures. However, comparisons cannot be made if there are substantial differences in the toxicokinetics for the two routes. Often, effects on the lung are critical. These can be considered local effects, in which case it is not appropriate to extrapolate from oral data. Great caution is required when extrapolating data from studies using different routes of exposure.

Modelling the Toxicity Information

The best way of relating exposure level, duration and effect for quantitative risk assessment is probably based on toxicokinetic and toxicodynamic modelling, similar to that used for workplace exposure to inhaled gases and vapours. However, appropriate data are not available for most, if not all, major hazard substances, so other, more pragmatic, approaches are adopted.

A generally available pragmatic approach is based on the need to obtain: (1) a concentration–time relationship, usually based on the mid-point (LC_{50} or EC_{50}) of the effect(s) being examined and (2) an appropriate set of exposure conditions that are taken to result in a particular level of effect in the population (Turner and Fairhurst, 1989; ECETOC, 1991).

As the concentration–time $(c.t)$ relationships often have to be based on LC_{50} or EC_{50} data for various times (they are frequently the only data available), they normally refer to mid-point concentration, that where the effect is seen in 50 per cent of the population. In general, the values have to be adjusted to yield the boundary between effects (disability with few immediate deaths for 'dangerous dose'; discomfort with few disabled in the case of defining zones where people needing hospital treatment are likely to be located). The dose response may also need to be adjusted to account for differences in the make-up of the populations being examined. It must be emphasized that any boundary will be approximate because of the nature of the data and the models being used.

In the early years of this century, studies on the acute inhalation toxicity for a limited number of gases yielded mortality data suggesting the following relationship:

$$c.t = \text{constant} \qquad (2)$$

(Haber, 1924). This is usually known as the Haber rule. More recent observations have suggested a more general relationship:

$$c^n.t = \text{constant} \qquad (3)$$

(ten Berge *et al.*, 1985; Klimisch *et al.*, 1987;

Marshall, 1989). An alternative form of this equation, which can be used to plot data, is

$$n \log c = - \log t + \text{constant} \qquad (4)$$

(this constant is the logarithmic value of the constant in Equation 3). Although a wide range of values for n have been cited, usually the value appears to be close to 1 or 2. Where it is possible, the relationship should be derived from experimental data, ideally from a single series of experiments in the same laboratory and using the same strain of animal. If data are combined from different laboratories and different strains or species, the relationship generated may represent interlaboratory or interspecies (or interstrain) vari-

ation rather than a genuine concentration–time relationship.

Frequently there are insufficient data to verify the relationship and the value of $n=1$ is used. It is probably adequate when extrapolating to longer times, where it usually overestimates the consequences. However, the Haber rule could seriously underestimate if data are not available for short periods and extrapolation of information from longer exposure periods is undertaken. Because of underlying assumptions about 'steady-state' toxicokinetics inherent in any of these relationships, they are all likely to be over-estimates at very short time intervals (say, less than 5 min) while equilibration to some form of pseudo steady state is taking place.

Usually it is also necessary to define the con-

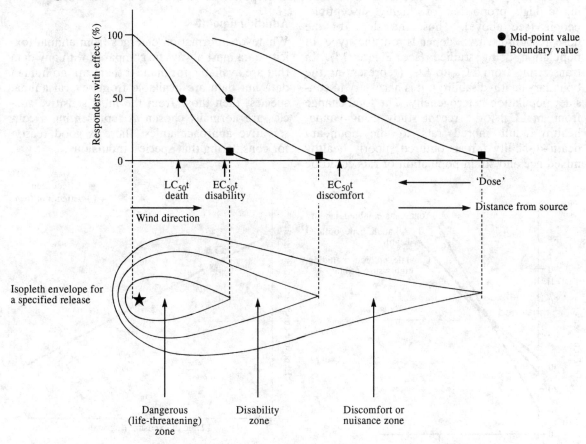

Figure 13 Diagram to illustrate the correlation between response and isopleth envelope. 'Dose' is the combined exposure concentration and duration function for the particular effect. The isopleth envelope described is that bounding the overall combination of concentrations and durations of exposure for a release, and can be built up from a series of isopleths describing the dispersion at different intervals after the start of the release. A combination of isopleth envelopes becomes a risk estimate when it incorporates the frequencies for different source and dispersion conditions

centration–time combination for a boundary condition rather than for the mid-point value for an effect (Figure 13). Ideally this should be obtained from experimental data. Often it has to be derived from the slope of the dose–response curve. If data on the slope are not available, it may be possible to use an arbitrary ratio gleaned from generalized information available in the literature. Based on the comparison of the slightly weaker criterion 'evident toxicity' and LD_{50} for the same classification for oral toxicity in young healthy adult rats (where the ratio was 4–5-fold; see above), the ratio for the relationship between 'dangerous dose' and LC_{50} could be about a three-fold reduction in concentration in the same population.

A further reduction in concentration of 3–4-fold has been suggested for transfer from a general healthy population to a population containing a high proportion of 'highly susceptible' people (see above). Thus, the slope of the dose–response curve depends on the type of population being studied (see Figure 14). In transferring from LC_{50} to LC_x (representing the boundary death–disability), it is necessary to consider population heterogeneity. The total change from an LC_{50} for a recent study using young, healthy adult inbred rats to the boundary death–disability for an outbred, poorly healthy mixed age and strain population of rats could be

an order of magnitude (tenfold) or more. A similar order of magnitude change has been proposed in moving from the criterion of death in a normal human population to 'dangerous dose' for a population containing a large number of 'highly susceptible' people (Health and Safety Executive, 1989a; see above).

As an alternative to the approach to concentration–time relationships outlined above, it is sometimes possible to describe mathematically a line for the boundary conditions of the concentration–time relationship using scatter diagrams, showing all concentrations and times at which the effect occurred (Figure 15) (ECETOC, 1991). This approach normally requires access to more detailed data, including, ideally, the results for individual animals. It also can suffer from problems relating to population heterogeneity and interspecies and interlaboratory variation.

Additional points

Whatever information emerges from animal toxicity data must always be compared with any data that are available for man. If there are no human data but data are available from several animal species, then those from the most sensitive species are normally chosen as representing a conservative approach unless there is good reason for considering that species anomalous.

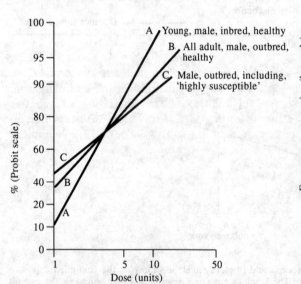

Figure 14   Diagram to illustrate hypothetical dose–response lines for different populations

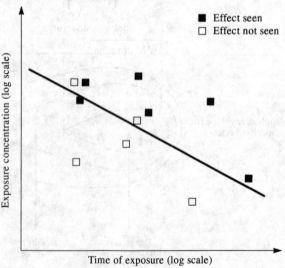

Figure 15   Idealized scatter diagram of hypothetical relationship for an exposure–time relationship for an effect. By plotting on logarithmic axes, the slope of the boundary line can be used to derive n. In the example shown the slope is $-n$ and $n = 2$.

The data are generally being used predictively in order to describe geographic areas where effects may occur or where the risk levels are associated with particular consequences. Best estimates are therefore usually considered preferable to more 'conservative' values based on the more severe confidence limit for the data. How closely defined the geographic areas affected by the risk analysis are when the toxicity data are limited in quality and quantity needs to be checked by uncertainty analysis in which the more extreme toxicity interpretations can be compared with the best estimate. Great accuracy is not required in view of the approximate nature of the overall evaluation.

Outcomes

The requirements from the overall assessment of the toxic risks are different for land-use planning and for emergency planning.

Land-use Planning

The outcome from a quantitative risk analysis is a risk statement based on a series of isopleth envelopes. This statement can be judged against predetermined criteria to decide whether a risk is acceptable in 'objective' terms. The risk assessor can recommend that no objection be raised to the proposed development or that the new development should not go ahead. Acceptance by the general population may depend on different, often subjective, criteria. There is a political process associated with land-use planning (in the United Kingdom, based on the local authority with access to a planning inquiry on behalf of central government) in order to allow expression of the objective and subjective opinions on the development. A decision then has to be taken by the local authority councillors or a government minister on behalf of society as a whole.

Emergency Planning

In emergency planning the aim is to delineate appropriate zones over which to provide public information on the types of hazard and the protective measures that can be taken to ameliorate the likely damage. It is also to help delineate ways of tackling the problems likely to emerge post-event; to guide general emergency planning, search and rescue, and planning for the medical needs of casualties, including setting permissible exposures for people involved. The type of medical planning required is discussed in greater detail elsewhere (Baxter *et al.*, 1989a; Murray, 1990)

CONCLUDING REMARKS

Disasters can be caused when large amounts of toxicants interact with a (human) population and cause deleterious effects on that population. They can occur in many forms; some result from natural causes and many from man's efforts. Describing the consequences of past disasters is the first stage to preventing or ameliorating the effects of future potential disasters.

There has been an 'explosion' of interest in major hazards. As yet this has not been followed through with the development of approaches to handling the toxicity data required when toxic hazards are being examined. Using toxicity data to predict the type and size of untoward biological effects for varying exposure conditions is still in its infancy. Both new techniques and new data are needed for many toxic major hazard substances.

In general, sites which contain toxicants causing them to be classified as major hazards are classified because of the quantity of toxicant present. There is no change in the toxicity of the substance. Unfortunately, the evidence concerning the toxicity of many of these toxicants is limited, as was clearly demonstrated in the case of methyl isocyanate pre-Bhopal. Often, further experimental work is needed to develop a proper database on which to take decisions.

Toxicologists can make a massive contribution to our ability to handle certain types of major hazard. We can contribute to new information, new techniques, better legislation and better public information. Preventing disasters due to toxic effects is an area ripe for development (pardon the pun!).

REFERENCES

Air Accidents Investigation Branch, Department of Transport (1989). *Report on the Accident to Boeing 737–236 Series 1, G-BGJL at Manchester International Airport on 22 August 1985*. Aircraft Accident Report 8/88. HMSO, London

Aldridge, W. N. (1985). Toxic oil syndrome. *Human Toxicol.*, **4**, 231–235

Aldridge, W. N. (1987). Toxic disasters with food contaminants. In Chambers, P. L. (Ed.), *Attitudes to Toxicology in the European Economic Community*. Wiley, Chichester

Andersson, N. (1989). Long-term effects of methyl isocyanate. *Lancet*, **i**, 1259

Andersson, N., Kerr Muir, M., Mehra, V. and Salmon, A. G. (1988). Exposure and response to methyl isocyanate: results of a community based survey in Bhopal. *Br. J. Industr. Med.*, **45**, 469–475

Baldini, R. and Komosinsky, P. (1988). Consequence analysis of toxic substance clouds. *J. Loss Prevention Process Industr.*, **1**, 147–155

Baxter, P. J., Davies, P. C. and Murray, V. (1989a). Medical planning for toxic releases into the community: the example of chlorine gas. *Br. J. Industr. Med.*, **46**, 277–285

Baxter, P. J., Ing, R., Falk, H. *et al.* (1981). Mount St. Helens eruptions, May 18 to June 12, 1980. An overview of the acute health impact. *J. Am. Med. Assoc.*, **246**, 2585–2589

Baxter, P. J., Ing, R., Falk, H. and Plikaytis, B. (1983). Mount St. Helens eruptions: The acute respiratory effects of volcanic ash in a North American community. *Arch. Environ. Hlth*, **38**, 138–143

Baxter, P. J., Kapila, M. and Mfonfu, D. (1989b). Lake Nyos disaster, Cameroon, 1986: the medical effects of large scale emission of carbon dioxide. *Br. Med. J.*, **298**, 1437–1441

Bertazzi, P. A. (1989). Industrial disasters and epidemiology. A review of recent experiences. *Scand. J. Work Environ. Hlth*, **15**, 85–100

Bertazzi, P. A., Zocchetti, C., Pesatori, A. C. *et al.* (1989). Ten year mortality study of the population involved in the Seveso incident in 1976. *Am J. Epidemiol.*, **129**, 1187–1200

Bucher, J. R. (1987). Methyl isocyanate: a review of health effects research since Bhopal. *Fund. Appl. Toxicol.*, **9**, 367–379

Buist, A. S. and Bernstein, R. S. (Eds) (1986). Health effects of volcanos: An approach to evaluating the health effects of an environmental hazard. *Am. J. Public Hlth*, **76**, Suppl.

Chernobyl Report (1986). *Nature*, **323**, 25

Committee on Fire Toxicology (1986). *Fire and Smoke: Understanding the Hazards*. National Academy Press, Washington D.C.

Davidson, M. R. and Schroter, R. C. (1983). A theoretical model for the absorption of gases by the bronchial wall. *J. Fluid Mech.*, **129**, 313–335

Department of the Environment (1991). Interpretation of major accident to the Environment for the purposes of the CIMAH Regulations. Dept of Environment (Toxic Substances Division), London

ECETOC (1991). Emergency exposure indices for industrial chemicals. *Technical Report No. 43*. European Chemical Industry Ecology and Toxicology Centre, Brussels

Fennel, D. (1988). *Investigation into the King's Cross Underground Fire*. HMSO, London

Freeth, S. J. and Kay, R. L. J. (1987). The Lake Nyos gas disaster. *Nature*, **325**, 104–105

Fryer, L. S. and Kaiser, G. D. (1979). *DENZ—A Computer Program for the Calculation of Dispersion of Dense Toxic or Explosive Gases in the Atmosphere*. Safety and Reliability Directorate Report 152. UK Atomic Energy Authority, Culcheth

Haber, F. (1924). *Fünf Vorträge aus den Jahren 1920–1923*. Springer Verlag, Berlin

Health and Safety Executive (1985). *The Brightside Lane Warehouse Fire*. HMSO, London

Health and Safety Executive (1988a). *The Tolerability of Risk From Nuclear Power Stations*. HMSO, London

Health and Safety Executive (1988b). *Comments Received on the Tolerability of Risk from Nuclear Power Stations*. HMSO, London

Health and Safety Executive (1988c). *Approved Code of Practice: Classification and Labelling of Substances Dangerous for Supply*. HMSO, London

Health and Safety Executive (1989a). *Risk Criteria for Land Use Planning in the Vicinity of Major Industrial Hazards*. HMSO, London

Health and Safety Executive (1989b). *Quantified Risk Assessment: Its Input to Decision Making*. HMSO, London

Henderson, M. (1987). *Living with Risk: The British Medical Association Guide*. Wiley, Chichester, pp. 115–118

Hodgson, E., Mailman, R. B. and Chambers, J. E. (1988). *Macmillan Dictionary of Toxicology*. Macmillan Reference Books, Basingstoke

Holden, C. (1980). Love Canal residents under stress. *Science*, **208**, 1242–1244

Illing, H. P. A. (1989). Assessment of toxicology for major hazards: Some concepts and problems. *Human Toxicol.*, **8**, 369–374

Institution of Chemical Engineers Working Party (1985). *Nomenclature for Hazard and Risk Assessments in the Process Industries*. Institution of Chemical Engineers, Rugby

Jagger, S. (1983). *Development of CRUNCH: A Dispersion Model for Continuous Release of a Denser than Air Vapour into the Atmosphere*. Safety and Reliability Directorate Report 229. UK Atomic Energy Authority, Culcheth

Janerich, D. T., Burnett, W. S., Feck, W. *et al.* (1981). Cancer incidence in the Love Canal area. *Science*, **212**, 1404–1407

Jashemski, W. P. (1979). Pompeii and Mount Vesuvius. In Sheets, P. D. and Grayson, D. K. (Eds), *Volcanic Activity and Human Ecology*. Academic Press, New York, pp. 587–622

Kakko, R. (1989). Vapor cloud modelling in the assessment of major toxic hazards. *J. Loss Prevention Process Industr.*, **2**, 102–107

Kimmerle, G. and Eben, A. (1964). Zur Toxizität von Methylisocyanat und desen quantitative Bestimmung in der Luft. *Arch. Toxicol.*, **20**, 235–241

Klimisch, H. J., Bretz, R., Doe, J. E. and Purser, D. A. (1987). Classification of dangerous substances in the European Economic Community: a proposed revision of criteria for inhalation toxicity. *Regulatory Toxicol. Pharmacol.*, **7**, 21–34

Kling, G. W., Clark, M. A., Compton, H. R. *et al*, (1987). The 1986 Lake Nyos gas disaster in Cameroon, West Africa. *Science*, **236**, 169–174

Kopelman, H., Robertson, M. H., Sanders, P. G. and Ash, I. (1966a). The Epping Jaundice. *Br. Med. J.*, **1**, 514–516

Kopelman, H., Scheuer, P. J. and Williams, R. (1966b). The liver lesion of the Epping Jaundice. *Quart. J. Med.*, **35**, 553–564

Lees, F. P. (1980). *Loss Prevention in the Process Industries*. Butterworths, London

Lovell, D. P. (1986). Risk assessment—General principles. In Richardson, M. L. (Ed.), *Toxic Hazard Assessment of Chemicals*. Royal Society of Chemistry, London, pp. 207–222

Lowermoor Incident Advisory Group (1989). *Water Pollution at Lowermoor, North Cornwall*. Cornwall and Isles of Scilly Health Authority, Truro

McQuaid, J. (1989). Dispersion of chemicals. In Bourdeau, P. and Green, G. (Eds), *Methods for Assessing and Reducing Injury from Chemical Accidents*. Wiley, Chichester, pp. 157–187

Marshall, V. (1989). Prediction of human mortality from chemical accidents with especial reference to the lethality of chlorine. *J. Hazard. Mat.*, **22**, 13–56

Marshall, V. C. (1987). *Major Chemical Hazards*. Ellis Horwood, Chichester

Miller, F. J., Overton, J. H., Jakot, R. H. and Menzel, D. B. (1985). A model of the regional uptake of gaseous pollutants in the lung. *Toxicol. Appl. Pharmacol.*, **79**, 11–27

Morgan, J. P. (1982). The Jamaica ginger paralysis. *J. Am. Med. Assoc.*, **248**, 1864–1867

Murray, V. (1990). *Major Chemical Disasters: medical aspects of management*. International Congress and Symposium Series Number 155. Royal Society of Medicine Services, London

National Research Council (1987). *Pharmacokinetics in Risk Assessment*. National Academy Press, Washington, D.C.

Newhall, C. G. and Fruchter, J. S. (1986). Volcanic activity: A review for health professionals. *Am. J. Public Hlth*, **76**, Suppl., 10–24

Orsini, B. (1977). *Parliamentary Commission of Enquiry on the Escape of Toxic Substances on 10 July 1976 at the ICMESA Establishment and the Consequent Potential Dangers to Health and the Environment Due to Industrial Activity. Final Report*. English translation. Health and Safety Executive, London

Pepelco, W. E. (1987). Feasability of route extrapolation in risk assessment. *Br. J. Industr. Med.*, **44**, 649–657

Pepelco, W. E. and Withey, J. R. (1985). Methods for route to route extrapolation. *Toxicol. Industr. Hlth*, **1**, 153–170

Radice, B. (translator) (1969). *Letters of the Younger Pliny*. Penguin Books, Harmondsworth

Royal Society Study Group (1983). *Risk Assessment*. Royal Society, London

Schoental, R. (1968). Carcinogenic and chronic effects of 4,4'-diaminodiphenylmethane. *Nature*, **219**, 1162–1163

Schwartz, D. A. (1987). Acute inhalation injury. In Rosenstock, L. (Ed.), *Occupational Medicine: State of the Art Reviews—Lung Disease*. Hanley and Belfus, Philadelphia, pp. 297–318

Sheets, P. D. and Grayson, D. K. (1979). *Volcanic Activity and Human Ecology*. Academic Press, New York

Sigurdsson, H., Carey, S., Cornell, W. and Pescatore, T. (1985). The eruption of Vesuvius in AD 79. *Nat. Geog. Res.*, **1**, 332–387

Silkworth, J. B., Cutler, D. S., Antrim, L. *et al.* (1989a). Teratology of 2,3,7,8-tetrachlorobenzo-*p*-dioxin in a complex environmental mixture from Love Canal. *Fund. Appl. Toxicol.*, **13**, 1–15

Silkworth, J. B., Cutler, D. S. and Sack, G. (1989b). Immunotoxicity of 2,3,7,8-tetrachlorodibenzo-*p*-dioxin in a complex environmental mixture from the Love Canal. *Fund. Appl. Toxicol.*, **12**, 302–312

Silkworth, J. B., McMartin, D. N., Rej, R. *et al.* (1984). Subchronic exposure of mice to Love Canal soil extracts. *Fund. Appl. Toxicol.*, **4**, 231–239

Silkworth, J. B., Tsumasonis, C., Briggs, R. G. *et al.* (1986). The effects of Love Canal soil extracts on maternal health and fetal development in rats. *Fund. Appl. Toxicol.*, **7**, 471–485

Skene, S. A., Dewhurst, I. C. and Greenberg, M. (1989). Polychlorinated dibenzo-*p*-dioxins and polychlorodibenzofurans: The risks to human health. A review. *Human Toxicol.*, **8**, 173–203

Smith, M. I. (1930). The pharmacological action of certain phenol esters, with special reference to the etiology of so-called ginger paralysis. *Public Hlth Reps*, **45**, 2509–2524

Smith, M. I. and Elvove, E. (1930). Pharmacological and chemical studies on the cause of so-called ginger paralysis. *Public Hlth Reps*, **45**, 1703–1716

Smith, S. (1986). Assessing the ecological and health effects of pollution. In Hester, R. E. (Ed.), *Understanding Our Environment*. Royal Society of Chemistry, London, pp. 226–290

Smullen, I. (1989). Bread and bones. *Country Life*, **183**, No. 12, 237

Tardiff, R. G. and Rodricks, J. V. (Eds) (1987). *Toxic Substances and Human Risk: Principles of Data Interpretation*. Plenum Press, New York

ten Berg, W. F., Zwart, A. and Appelman, L. M. (1985). Concentration mortality response relationship for irritant and systemically acting gases and vapours. *J. Hazard. Mat.*, **13**, 301–309

Tsubaki, T. and Irukayama, K. (1977). *Minamata Disease*. Kodansha/Elsevier, Tokyo

Turner, R. M. and Fairhurst, S. (1989). *Assessment of the Toxicity of Major Hazard Substances*. Specialised Inspector Report 21. Health and Safety Executive, London

van den Heuval, M. J., Dayan, A. D. and Shillaker, R. O. (1987). Evaluation of the BTS approach to the testing of substances and preparations for their acute toxicity. *Human Toxicol.*, **6**, 279–291

Versteeg, M. F. (1988). External safety policy in the Netherlands: an approach to risk management. *J. Hazard. Mat.*, **17**, 215–222

Vianna, N. J. and Polan, A. K. (1984). Incidence of low birth weight among Love Canal residents. *Science*, **226**, 1217–1219

Withers, J. (1988). *Major Industrial Hazards. Their Appraisal and Control*. Gower Technical Press, Aldershot

Withers, R. M. J. and Lees, F. P. (1987). The assessment of major hazards: the lethal toxicity of chlorine. Part 3. Cross checks. *J. Hazard. Mat.*, **15**, 301–342

World Health Organization (1976). Conference on intoxication due to alkyl-mercury treated seed. *Bull. World Hlth Org.*, **53**, Suppl.

World Health Organization (1984). *Toxic Oil Syndrome*. Report of a WHO Meeting, Madrid, 21–25 March 1983. World Health Organization, Copenhagen

FURTHER READING

Beck, B. D., Conolly, R. B., Doursun, M. L., Guth, D., Hattis, D., Kimmel, C. and Lewis, S. C. (1993). Improvements and quantitative noncancer risk assessment. *Fundamental and Applied Toxicology*, **20**, 1–14

Cote, R. P. and Wells, P. G. (1991). *Controlling Chemical Hazards*. Unwin Hyman, London

Bourdeau, P. and Green, G. (1989). Methods for assessing and reducing injury from chemical accidents. *IPCS Joint Symposia No. 11*. John Wiley and Sons, Chichester

Hallenbeck, W. H. and Cunningham, K. M. (1986). *Quantitative Risk Assessment for Environmental and Occupational Health*. Lewis Publishers, Inc., Chelsea, Michigan

Paustenbach, D. J. (1989). *The Risk Assessment of Environmental Hazards*. John Wiley and Sons, New York

57 Ethical, Moral and Professional Issues, Standards and Dilemmas in Toxicology

D. W. Vere

WHAT ARE OUR DUTIES?

These are easy to state in abstract, but very difficult to work through in application. There seems to be wide agreement that our duties are beneficence (doing good, to others as well as to self), non-maleficence (avoiding harm), respect for autonomy or an individual's self-determining choices, and justice, which means perhaps equity rather than just equality of treatment of others. In addition, people should respect agreed formulations of good conduct, or codes ('deontology'), pay active attention to the possible or foreseeable consequences of what they are doing, to see that these will be beneficial to others (utilitarianism, consequentialism), and be truthful. Lastly, it helps to have a hierarchy (or pecking order) of 'goods'; this was Mills's only answer to Bentham's problem of whether it was better to be a contented pig or a discontented Socrates (Gillon, 1985). This seems as fine as 'liberty, fraternity, equality', until one tries to apply it all to toxicology.

THE TOXICOLOGICAL ENVIRONMENT OF ETHICAL DECISIONS

Why is there difficulty? Perhaps it is easiest to show the reasons if one compares toxicology with medicine, where ethics has been applied and debated for a very long time, and that not without difficulty. General awareness of ethics in toxicology seems to have been a more recent development. This seems odd, considering the extensive role of poisoners in former times; perhaps it reflects the fact that it is somewhat easier to kill someone by misapplied medicine than by deliberate poisoning. In medicine, decisions are largely atomized to individual problems. A doctor, or a small group of medical people, discuss with one patient what may be their best treatment. Autonomy is well ventilated; beneficence for *that patient*

is the aim. Issues of consequence do arise, but justice is considered little except where the provision of services to groups of patients are concerned, and there only very partially. But toxicology concerns groups, often very large groups, whether of people or of animals. The aim is risk avoidance or containment in general, not just for an individual. The difference between medical and toxicological ethics is seen in clearest relief with clinical trials, where risks to one and to all can be in conflict (Cancer Research Campaign Working Party, 1983). Are the pathological tests made in early phase I and II trials 'safeguards', or 'monitoring' the action of a new drug, or are they 'human toxicology' or tests on 'human guinea-pigs'? They are, of course, in some senses, both, but the name one uses for them sets the minds of hearers towards sympathy or hostility, much as the same set of actions can be called those of a 'freedom fighter' or of a 'terrorist', depending on one's presuppositions.

This problem is seen very clearly when a chemical process benefits most while harming a few. Dry cleaning benefits everyone, but can cause liver damage to a tiny minority. The inverse is just as true. Signal benefits for some can cost all overmuch: cars and spray cans for the wealthy nations may have damaged the climate of the world. The geographical context of the toxicological problems can be much broader than those of medicine.

A similar dilemma exists over the time-course of human actions: for most of medicine the time-course of effects does not transcend one life; in toxicology it may be short-lived, but can cover many generations or even reach permanence. This is well seen in the era of remanent organohalogen insecticides and their effects, a story which seems likely to recur with dioxins and polyhalogenated biphenyls.

Perhaps the most obvious difference between the ethics of medicine and of toxicology resides in the part played by autonomy. In medicine the patient, or the experimental subject, is a person who can and should know about his or her own situation and express 'informed consent'. In toxicology the subjects of experiments, or of disaster, are animals; or if they are humans, those people may well be ignorant of the dangers about them, or are already the unwitting victims of them. So the whole atmosphere of ethical decision-making is different for these subjects from that in medicine. There is far more paternalism; for example decisions are often made on behalf of the subjects, and often this is by those who already 'have an interest' in the outcome of the tests or procedures in question. There neither is, nor can be, 'informed consent' to chemical exposure, unless it be refusal to purchase, having read package warnings.

Last, the purview of toxicology is vastly wider than that of medicine. Medicine is about human illness, its remedies and prevention. Toxicology is about this in many ways, but it is also about natural pollutants, animal experiments, drugs in man's environment, weapons, microbiological toxins and hazards (when the toxin is chemical), pesticides and agrochemicals, sewerage and water treatment, biotechnology, radiation hazards and manufacturing pollutants.

Any of these aspects of toxicology can interact with others, so that it can be very hard even for experts to foresee the potential repercussions of a process, and to take responsible action about them. Because the public is often unaware of potential problems, unless they glare threateningly from media reports, there is great suspicion and vivid imagination, factors which may themselves impede helpful and satisfactory efforts to offset the feared ill-effects. So futile media debates about suspected toxicological hazards are almost daily events.

Since toxicological problems are so complex, they have an added dimension beyond the problems of many other subjects in that they can seldom be thought through once and for all; as time moves on, new aspects appear, and a second or third ethical assessment must be made. For example, it may be impossible at first to foresee how a toxin or metabolite may accumulate in animal tissues, or to collect sufficient instances of adverse effects to discover how often late manifestations of poisoning occur (such as carcinogenesis or teratogenesis). The usage of a product may change, and with it the toxicity profile; an example is the fact that chilled foods have probably always contained *Listeria* organisms, but it is only their newer methods of use which encourage *Listeria* to multiply and so to intoxicate. Every new productive process, be it a manufactured chemical, a drug or a food that is made, needs to be monitored at inception, during restricted trials, and after marketing.

WHAT ARE THE DIFFICULTIES OF BEING DUTIFUL?

No one can reach decisions about something which they cannot define or measure. The toxicologist faces daunting problems already, for several reasons.

First, there is biostatistical uncertainty. The practical problems here are that experience with small numbers can rarely lead to conviction, whereas to obtain large numbers may require immense outlays of resource or time. Toxicological tests are often judged by their alpha probabilities; can a positive outcome of a test be claimed? But with smaller number tests the beta probability matters as much or more, if the result is to be 'we saw no evidence of the suspected effect'.

The next technical problem concerns the interpretation of tests: everyone naturally values expert opinions on histology, or the metabolic profile of a drug, or the likely risks of intoxication with stated plasma levels of a toxin. But how many experts does one need? Their disagreements are often wide once their number exceeds unity, yet many 'expert' committees are advised by a single pathologist, for example.

Then there is the vexed issue of when and how to warn if one thinks one has a signal. Thalidomide was a case in point: the first six cases of phocomelia were denied reporting space on evidential grounds, correctly in scientific terms, but wrongly in terms of the known eventual outcome. Even when a rigorous effort is made to achieve a significant noise-to-signal ratio, the data are often skewed by selection bias.

The next difficulty concerns the fact that many intoxicants merely amplify a natural but rare event. An example is failure of neural development in tadpoles, a rare spontaneous event whose frequency is amplified enormously, and in a dose-related manner, by calcium antagonist drugs. Hence, in such a human situation, no one can point to one case and conclude that the drug did it; yet that is exactly what a court decided in the Mekdeci case in 1979, a decision reversed in 1981 (Smithells and Sheppard, 1978; *Current Problems*, 1981). Equally, one cannot look at an insignificant signal and conclude therefrom that the drug did not do it.

Last, there is the problem that a metabolite or a decomposition product may prove intensely toxic, perhaps only in certain situations. The net effect of these scientific and technical aspects of measure and detection is to obscure resolution of problems, so that ethical argument sways readily in either direction. Just as for smoking and lung cancer, it has proved immensely difficult to show an association between even expected toxicities and known toxins, a point demonstrated elegantly by a recent review of the human risks of dioxins and related compounds (Skene *et al.*, 1989).

As if science did not involve problems enough, ethics itself imports more into toxicological debate. Ethical decisions have to take account of the cost/harm versus gain/benefit ratios of any set of proposals. Who is to decide the hierarchy of values for any proposal? The problems are that interested parties differ inevitably in their value judgements; this is well seen in the question as to whether or not laboratory animals should suffer to test cosmetics. No doubt, cosmetic users want protection for themselves, and animal rights protesters for the animals. And may not the outcome depend as much on adjunctive issues as upon the main ones: Are alternative tests possible? Have they been sought? How much suffering is inflicted? These issues are compounded by the fact that some tests (e.g. the LD_{50} test) have been enjoined by regulators in situations where many others involved wanted to be rid of them. Sometimes things which could well be changed seem to roll on by sheer momentum (Walker and Dayan, 1986).

Animal testing is an especially thorny issue, well exposed in a recent book by Rollin (1989), where the assumptions about animal pain made by many scientists in past years are questioned on common-sense logical grounds: if animals do not *perceive* pain, why do we use them to test analgesics? To argue that this is simply because their responses model well for analgesic effects in humans begs the whole question; it is simply a reductionist argument. We often use Occam's razor, and the simplest explanation has

undoubted appeal; but how often is the simplest explanation shown to be the correct one in biology? The Occam postulate is a good test, but one which should always be tested, if only because it is so often wrong, and also because it has no necessary logical force in any single case. It is a useful initial postulate—no more.

The second ethical problem about animals is the question as to whether or not they differ from man, and if so, how? The infliction of suffering on animals, if we assume that they do suffer, in order to avoid human ills is justifiable only if we take them to be of a lower order, of less significance than, ourselves. ('You are of more value than many sparrows' [Matthew: 10, 26–31]). But even this is not to assert that animals are of *no* value; there still has to be a value judgement about *how much* suffering it is justifiable to inflict—hence our laws which regulate animal experimentation.

Similar ethical issues arise about resource allocation: How much is it right to pay volunteers for experiments? When is it necessary to halt development of an 'orphan' drug on grounds of market size? If a safe product has been found, how long should an older product remain on the market because major capital investment has gone into its production plant?

What Can be Done?

First, a set of clear objectives ('goods') needs to be defined, without attempting to arrange them in any hierarchy. It must be good, other things being equal, to gain new knowledge, to create wealth, to prevent hazard, to conserve natural resources and to keep to codes which have been generally agreed, such as the Helsinki declaration on human experiment, and the various guidelines for 'good clinical practice', 'good laboratory practice' and 'good animal husbandry'. But even in their statement, it is at once clear that these 'goods' will at times conflict: it is obviously easy to create wealth while causing hazard, to gain knowledge by exploiting natural resources. It is possible to warn publicly to gain recognition, even when the evidence is inadequate, and to fail to warn when a warning is needed for fear of spreading needless alarm. So, some general conclusions emerge:

(1) It is essential to discover facts about all

the envisageable aspects of a problem, and to consider their interactions and their likely repercussions on people, on animals and on the environment.

(2) This assessment must contain a hierarchy of value judgements, based upon the best knowledge available. This is the 'state of the art' justification for ethical judgements.

(3) The balance points must be found by considerations of 'natural justice'—not those of self or sectarian interest.

(4) It must never be assumed that a bit of good justifies a lot of evil: ends do not justify means.

(5) Given all goodwill, there will inevitably be mistakes, hurts and losses if there are to be any new things at all, as every mother knows.

So what? What can be done in practice? Obviously, where the public has interests, the public needs to be interested; but so often this is difficult because industry operates competitively (even within the same company!), and free sharing of information is impossible in this imperfect world. Regulatory authorities exist, and guarantee industrial confidence as essential to their very operation. They do seek to operate on a base of sound science, with members declaring personal interests, in strict confidence towards industry yet aiming at public safeguard. But these very safeguards exist because there is secrecy; hence, debate inevitably polarizes, becomes adversarial and frequently comes to appeal. This is the very opposite of wise, ethical judgement, but perhaps it is the best that can be done in a realm where competition generates secrecy rather than openness. But everyone, every company, every scientific group has the opportunity to consider what they are doing first, so that a regulatory hand need not interfere with what they are doing. Whether as regulator or regulated, no one can do better than his or her present knowledge will allow: the 'state of the art' has to be the determinant of fame or blame.

When mistakes or adversities occur, they should be compensated; how? Most scientists and doctors want 'no fault' indemnity; the problems are that governments will not fund the higher potential claims, and lawyers (who tend to be determinist and free from biostatistical qualms of any kind) want 'strict liability'. 'Strict liability' seems to secure exactly what it destroys, natural justice, because it is proof-, not hurt-, dependent

(Laurence, 1989). It is also unscientific and irrational in the sense that its attributions of blame fall upon manufacturers in a biased way (Royal Commission on Civil Liability, 1974).

It is at this point that the discussion enters an unreal world, one might say a nightmare, in terms of something frighteningly unreal which nevertheless exists. This is the realm of public risk perception, the media presentation of matters toxicological and the impact of political decisions on such things. These issues cannot be presented here in detail; several points emerge in general. The most obvious is that distorted perceptions of risk, real or potential, will abound in the ethical environment of toxicological decisions. Whether deliberate or fear-driven, these distortions will not just go away. There is no point in being outraged rationally by them; they do not arise from evidenced grounds without bias, being reasoned from selected information. They are to do with people and their emotions. Often, they are linked to words or other fear cues. 'Nuclear' is an obvious example; it is interesting to reflect, while driving through a 'nuclear-free zone', how much radiation from natural and medical sources abounds within it. Many protesters at Chernobyl fallout must have enjoyed an equal burden sniffing the radon in a week's holiday in Cornwall. It was delightfully expressed in that misprint about 'the unclear threat'. But in the problem of public explanations and relations, suspicions and interpretations must always enter the ethical analysis.

The second point about public perceptions is that the amount of fear and noise evoked is greater when the perceived risk seems greater. Many scientists, engineers and policy-staters seem to expect public fears to retreat when a risk can be shown to be vanishingly small. This will not happen, since people are reacting to their perception of the risk size were the unthinkable to occur or were they the person affected. Three Mile Island is a case in point: the fact that the nuclear power plant was successfully shut down did not reassure those who envisaged what would have happened had it not been contained successfully.

A third generality is that public fears should not be countered by derision, however witty and factual these remarks may be. Destructive humour suggests insincerity and carelessness, and reaps its own reward.

Perhaps the greatest ethical burden concerns

the clash between establishments and value judgements. Animal tests, causing some apparent suffering, became established, whether as a part of regulatory requirements or in the shape of an expensive laboratory process or plant of which they form an integral part. Then value perceptions changed. Which force will win, the changed perception or the money and effort enshrined in the established process?

This problem is exacerbated because one of the opposing forces is external, and the other internal to the company or institution involved. There may be no natural forum for debate between the two groups of proponents. Often this sort of ethical tension becomes prolonged until a flashover occurs, either through the media or even as physical violence.

Where there has to be uncertainty, what methods are open to help people to do their best? Those which are available are (1) analysis of decisions by ingredient factors; (2) peer review; (3) scale containment; (4) ongoing review; (5) risk analysis, in those cases where this can be done.

(1) Breaking a proposal down to identify all its ingredient factors guards against overlooking the vulnerable. It helps to consider:

(a) The impact severity of a potential hazard— that is, the product of intensity and range. The neglect of one abandoned caesium source in Brazil caused intense damage to a small number of those who handled it; ozone from photochemical smog causes some damage to large numbers of city dwellers; the human 'cost' of both kinds of hazard could be considered to be comparable.

(b) Vulnerable subgroups.

Sometimes these can be anticipated, as when the chemical cousins of known toxins are released into an environment. But biological mechanisms are subtle enough to outwit most such anticipations. Occasionally they succeed, as when it was foreseen by chemists that the drug alclofenac could yield an epoxide metabolite in man (Mercia *et al.*, 1983) More often they are discovered as the result of release into human or animal populations, as with thalidomide. Even when an adverse effect can be anticipated quite strongly,

minor chemical differences often decide whether or not it appears, and what its impact may be. For example, it is well known that a wide variety of inhibitors of 5-hydroxytryptamine uptake into neurons cause disorders of immunity in man. But these disorders vary from drug to drug. These inhibitors have such potential value in psychiatry that firms continue to prepare new compounds for human testing. The only way to discover their potential for immunological damage is to test them in man.

(2) Whatever the degree of likelihood of harm may be, it is an incontrovertible ethical onus on any experimenter or supplier of new chemical agents to try to anticipate toxic hazards and to seek expert opinion about potential risks. This leads naturally to the question of peer review. For new human experiments in medicine, all projects are referred to a research ethics committee. The problems with animal experiments are dealt with in the UK by a government inspectorate under the Animal Procedures Act. But this is concerned with limiting animal suffering and cruelty, not with the wider ethical questions which might arise from animal experiments. Pesticides and agrochemicals are regulated through a somewhat, but necessarily, cumbrous process: the Food and Agriculture Organization of the United Nations at Rome, and the World Health Organization Expert Group on pesticide residues in food, meet and publish recommendations on maximum residue limits, acceptable daily intakes and pesticide use practice ('good agricultural practice'). Evidence is also collected on continued evaluation of human exposure, including the results of volunteer testing. Most of the recommendations are based on animal tests for toxicity, mutagenicity and growth to preformalized schedules. There are supervised trials of new agrochemicals and a review of toxicological databases. But all these digested facts issue as recommendations proposed for use by the member governments of the respective agencies. Important though they are, they cannot substitute effectively for local vigilance in manufacture, distribution and control in relation to the chemical environment, especially since not all governments are members of these agencies. Similarly, industrial safety is governed in the United Kingdom under the Factories Inspectorate, a system aimed to ensure conformity to safety regulations. None of these bodies

can influence greatly either the broader ethical issues of chemical exposure or local decisions about the release of industrial chemicals. This has become very apparent with regard to toxic waste disposal, whether from hospital chimneys (burning polyvinyl chloride) or nitrate fertilizer in soil and river pollution. However good the regulations, they will not work without the local will to implement them, costly though that can often be.

(3) Another way to maximize safety and reduce risk is by scale containment. Exposures can be increased in a graded fashion so that, should adverse effects appear, they will be on a small scale and they can be studied. The problem here is that small-scale exposures seldom yield sufficient data to demonstrate an adverse effect unambiguously. As already shown with dioxins, a known and much studied group of toxins, even quite wide human exposure in accidents has so far failed to reveal definite long-term hazards (Skene *et al.*, 1989). Planned exposures in critical experiments are not possible for ethical reasons; accidental exposures are usually too ill-defined and too riddled with litigation to yield clear scientific information.

(4) Ongoing review of successively wider releases of new chemical agents seems essential, but is almost impossible to achieve. For new drugs, successive stages of initial tests in healthy volunteers and clinical trials are reviewed by regulatory authorities, which may also require postmarketing surveillance (PMS) or 'monitored release' (MR) schemes. Unfortunately, PMS and MR often fail, although some have been successful in revealing new and unexpected toxicities. But such schemes cannot be mounted for industrial chemical exposures. In any case, it is often impossible to discriminate between natural disease and chemical toxicity; for example, a worker who becomes jaundiced after solvent exposure may have a problem which resists all efforts at firm diagnosis.

(5) Risk analyses can seldom be made. Risk ratios can be calculated only if all cells of a fourfold table can be denumerated; these are the numbers exposed and not exposed as columns, and the numbers with or without a defined adverse event as rows. These four totals are almost never all available. Partial analyses can be done using case controls and specialized statistical tests such as the Mantel–Haentzel procedure. But

the work involved is often substantial and the results debatable unless confirmed. All in all, risk analyses have contributed little to the detection and control of toxicological problems.

Again, the overriding problem in this difficult ethical area is the fact that most industrial development is competitive and so is secret until marketing occurs. The business of ethics is to act in prospect so as to maximize good and minimize harm, to one and to all. Its business is not detection and recrimination after some adverse event, although it is involved in securing justice for the victims. The law tends to be determinist, requiring proof of cause; justice for the victims of an accident of uncertain cause is therefore attained uncertainly, and involves costly hearings, enquiries or tribunals.

There are also four ethical paradoxes which bedevil any agreed policies. These are: (1) the value assessment of resources; (2) autonomous choice to accept risk—the 'self' or 'others' paradox; (3) differences between societies; (4) health versus survival.

Resource assessment   There is no easy way to decide the value of resources to any community or sector of a community. Natural resources are 'given', but are consumable. It may be our farmland against your climate when it comes to felling forests; this global example illustrates a problem which repeats endlessly upon lesser scales. The suggested solution is to live in balance with nature, to recycle, to return what has been taken. But this cannot be done with some toxic wastes; these can only be destroyed or stored, often at immense cost.

Choices, self and others   Chemical glues are necessary evils. I may resolve never to give them to children, but children may decide to take the risk of glue-sniffing. How paternalistic should a person, a company, a society be in seeking to protect those who accept the risk of self-harm? What is the balance of autonomy with deontology or consequentialism here. We accept risky sports: how much risk from intoxication should be accepted? Attitudes differ in bizarre ways towards various toxins: compare ethanol and nicotine with cannabis and amphetamine, counting deaths.

Differences between societies   There are enormous differences worldwide between societies about the amount of toxicological risk they will accept. Some of this relates obviously to the relative wealth of societies, some to the value set upon human life which their culture suggests or accepts. But the size of the differences between the protection afforded by various states to their citizens shows how impossible it is to state absolute values here. This is not to say that there is disagreement among peoples about what is or might be desirable, but there is enormous variation in the will and in the means to attain proper goals (Yudkin, 1978). Even within one society with decided health objectives in the United Kingdom, there are considerable regional differences in attainment of the agreed goals (DHSS, 1980). Griffin (1987) has reported remarkable variations in drug exposure and adverse reaction reporting rates between cultures.

Health versus survival Good health and survival are not synonymous. There have been, and still are, times and places where the acceptance of a heavy toxicological burden is the price of survival. In some degree this happened in the industrial revolution in Britain: chronic bronchitis was the price and became known as 'the English disease' in mainland Europe. But this burden was accepted unwittingly; in many third world countries toxic industries are accepted deliberately as the only way to expand a weak economy, and widespread pollution has occurred as a result, often as a legacy for later generations.

CONCLUSIONS

In conclusion, it can be said that whereas it seems desirable for the same ethical considerations that apply to medicine to be used for toxicological work, there are often immense difficulties in so doing. These relate chiefly to the broader scope of toxicological work: animals as well as people, populations as well as individuals, and resource use on major scales. It also relates to the biostatistical uncertainty of prospective assessment of toxic hazard, and the difficulty of knowing when to warn. Because these problems exist, agreement is often reached on policies which benefit some but risk many, or which benefit soon but risk later, simply because it is so difficult to weigh the various risk probabilities prospectively. These risks vary differently in time and even well-informed and careful people may disagree

strongly about the value judgements which should be made about each step of such complex processes. The central problem is that, if there is to be progress of any kind, there must be exploratory advance. These advances always carry risks, some foreseeable but some not. There will always be those whose vote is to try progress and take risk, and others who think it better to wait, and possibly not see. And biological systems are amazingly resilient in the face of threat; adaptive processes are remarkably strong. For this reason it is often the anticipated threats which prove to be unimportant and the unforeseeable which do most subtle damage. We can only seek to act responsibly, using the best current standards of due care, examining what has been done continuously for unforeseen hazards. Failure is to be seen chiefly in this last aspect, in the thorny but necessary process of public information and in the secrecy which is imposed upon innovation by the competitive nature of industry.

REFERENCES

Cancer Research Campaign Working Party in Breast Conservation (1983). Informed consent: ethical, legal and medical implications for doctors and patients who participate in randomised clinical trials. *Br. Med. J.*, **286**, 1117–1121

Current Problems (1981). Data Sheet changes—Debendox, *Current Problems*, **6**, July 1981. Also *Daily Mirror*, Monday July 1984, p. 1; *Hospital Doctor*, June 16, 1983, p. 24

Department of Health and Social Security (1980). *Inequalities in Health*. DHSS, London

Gillon, Raanan (1985). *Philosophical Medical Ethics*. Wiley, Chichester, pp. viii, 9–13

Griffin, J. P. (1987). Differences between Protestant and Catholic religious ethics impinges on medical issues. *Int. Pharm. J.*, **1**, 145–148

Laurence, D. R. (1989). Ethics and law in clinical pharmacology. *Br. J. Clin. Pharmacol.*, **27**, 718

Mercia, M., Ponselet, F., de Meester, C., McGregor, D. B., Willins, M. J., Leonard, A. and Fabry, L. (1983). *In vitro* and *in vivo* studies on the potential mutagenicity of alclofenac, dihydroxyalclofenac and alclofenac epoxide. *J. Appl. Toxicol.*, **3**, 230–236

Rollin, B. (1989). *The Unheeded Cry: Animal Consciousness, Animal Pain and Science*. Oxford University Press

Royal Commission on Civil Liability (1974). *The First Circular of the Royal Commission on Civil Liability and Compensation for Personal Injury*, Para. 6, p. 2

Skene, S. A., Dewhurst, I. C. and Greenberg, M. (1989). Poly chlorinated dibenzo-*p*-dioxins and polychlorinated dibenzyofurans: the risks to human health. A review. *Human Toxicol.*, **8**, 173–203

Smithells, R. W. and Sheppard, S. (1978). Teratogenicity testing in humans: a method demonstrating safety of Bendectin. *Teratology*, **17**, 31–35

Walker, S. R. and Dayan, A. D. (1986). *Long-term Animal Studies, Their Predictive Value for Man.* MTP, Lancaster

Yudkin, J. S. (1978). Provision of medicines in a developing country. *Lancet*, **1**, 810–812

FURTHER READING

Bulger, R. E., Heitman, E. and Reiser, S. J. (Eds) (1993). The use of animals in biological research. Part VII. In *The Ethical Dimensions of the Biological Sciences.* Cambridge University Press. pp. 173–198

Orlans, F. B. (1993). *In the Name of Science. Issues in Responsible Animal Experimenation.* Oxford University Press

Weitzner, M. I. (1993). *Developments and Ethical Considerations in Toxicology.* Royal Society of Chemistry, London

INDEX

Index